MVFOL

LEXI-COMP'S

Pediatric Dosage Handbook

Including
Neonatal Dosing, Drug Administration
& Extemporaneous Preparations

10th Edition

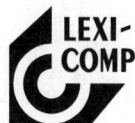

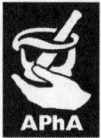

LEXI-COMP'S

Pediatric Dosage Handbook

Including
Neonatal Dosing, Drug Administration,
& Extemporaneous Preparations

10th Edition

LEXI-COMP'S

Pediatric Dosage Handbook

Including
**Neonatal Dosing, Drug Administration,
& Extemporaneous Preparations**

10th Edition

Carol K. Taketomo, PharmD
Pharmacy Manager
Children's Hospital of Los Angeles
Los Angeles, California

Jane Hurlburt Hodding, PharmD
Director, Pharmacy Services
Miller Children's Hospital
Long Beach, California

Donna M. Kraus, PharmD, FAPhA
Associate Professor of Pharmacy Practice
Departments of Pharmacy Practice and Pediatrics
Pediatric Clinical Pharmacist
University of Illinois at Chicago
Chicago, Illinois

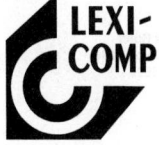

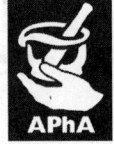

This data is intended to serve the user as a handy reference and not as a complete drug information resource. It does not include information on every therapeutic agent available. The publication covers 692 commonly used drugs and is specifically designed to present important aspects of drug data in a more concise format than is typically found in medical literature or product material supplied by manufacturers.

The nature of drug information is that it is constantly evolving because of ongoing research and clinical experience and is often subject to interpretation. While great care has been taken to ensure the accuracy of the information presented, the reader is advised that the authors, editors, reviewers, contributors, and publishers cannot be responsible for the continued currency of the information or for any errors, omissions, or the application of this information, or for any consequences arising therefrom. Therefore, the author(s) and/or the publisher shall have no liability to any person or entity with regard to claims, loss, or damage caused, or alleged to be caused, directly or indirectly, by the use of information contained herein. Because of the dynamic nature of drug information, readers are advised that decisions regarding drug therapy must be based on the independent judgment of the clinician, changing information about a drug (eg, as reflected in the literature and manufacturer's most current product information), and changing medical practices. Therefore, this data is designed to be used in conjunction with other necessary information and is not designed to be solely relied upon by any user. The user of this data hereby and forever releases the authors of this data for any and all liability of any kind that might arise out of the use of this data. The editors are not responsible for any inaccuracy of quotation or for any false or misleading implication that may arise due to the text or formulas as used or due to the quotation of revisions no longer official.

The authors, editors, and contributors have written this book in their private capacities. No official support or endorsement by any federal or state agency or pharmaceutical company is intended or inferred.

The publishers have made every effort to trace the copyright holders for borrowed material. If they have inadvertently overlooked any, they will be pleased to make the necessary arrangements at the first opportunity.

If you have any suggestions or questions regarding any information presented in this data, please contact our drug information pharmacist at (330) 650-6506.

This manual was produced using the FormuLex™ Program —
A complete publishing service of Lexi-Comp Inc.

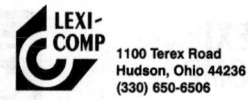
LEXI-COMP
1100 Terex Road
Hudson, Ohio 44236
(330) 650-6506

ISBN 1-59195-058-9 (Domestic Edition)

ISBN 1-59195-059-7 (International Edition)

TABLE OF CONTENTS

PREFACE

This tenth edition of the *Pediatric Dosage Handbook* is designed to be a practical and convenient guide to the dosing and usage of medications in children. The pediatric population is a dynamic group, with major changes in pharmacokinetics and pharmacodynamics taking place throughout infancy and childhood. Therefore, the need for the evaluation and establishment of medication dosing regimens in children of different ages is great.

Special considerations must be taken into account when dosing medications in pediatric patients. Unfortunately, due to a lack of appropriate studies, most medications commonly used in children do not have FDA approved labeling for use in pediatric patients. Only 30% of drugs used in children in a 1988 survey carried FDA approval in their labeling. Seventy-five percent of medications listed in the *1990 Physicians Desk Reference* carry some type of precaution or disclaimer statement for use in children.[1]

The FDA Modernization Act of 1997, the Children's Health Act of 2000, and the Best Pharmaceuticals for Children Act of 2002 will help to increase pediatric drug studies. The FDA Modernization Act of 1997 was signed into law on November 21, 1997 (Section 111, Public Law 105-115, 105th Congress). This bill **encourages** pharmaceutical companies to conduct pediatric drug studies by allowing 6 months of market exclusivity to certain designated drugs. A list of drugs, for which additional pediatric information may produce pediatric healthcare benefits, was required by this law to be developed by the U.S. Department of Health and Human Services (HHS), with input from the American Academy of Pediatrics, the Pediatric Pharmacology Research Unit Network,[2] and the U.S. Pharmacopoeia. To date, the FDA has received 324 proposals from pharmaceutical companies to conduct pediatric drug studies under this Act and has issued 264 written requests for studies. If these pediatric studies are completed as the FDA has specified, then these medications will qualify for the 6 month patent extension or additional market exclusivity. Seventy-three products have already had their marketing patents extended by this law and pediatric labeling changes have occurred for 49 of these products[3]. The FDA submitted a required report on the Pediatric Exclusivity Provision to Congress in January 2001[4]. This report described the effectiveness, short comings, and economic impact of the Pediatric Exclusivity Provision. It also gave suggestions for modifications and ways to address gaps in the statute.

The pediatric section of the FDA Modernization Act was renewed by Congress and signed into law January 4, 2002. This new law, called the Best Pharmaceuticals for Children Act, reauthorizes the use of the 6-month patent extension to **encourage** pharmaceutical companies to conduct pediatric drug research. This law, which remains in effect until October 2007, calls for the establishment of an Office of Pediatric Therapeutics within the FDA and establishes an FDA Pediatric Pharmacology Advisory Committee and a Pediatric Subcommittee of the Oncologic Drugs Advisory Committee. It also creates a research fund for pediatric studies of drugs that are off patent, grants a special "priority status" to pediatric labeling changes, requires the Department of Health and Human Services (along with the Institute of Medicine) to conduct a study to assess federally funded pediatric research and calls for the development of a Final Rule that will require drug labeling to include a toll-free number to report adverse events[5].

The 1998 Pediatric Final Rule was an FDA regulation, titled "Regulations Requiring Manufacturers to Assess the Safety and Effectiveness of New Drugs and Biological Products in Pediatric Patients; Final Rule"[6]. This important regulation **required** that manufacturers conduct pediatric studies for certain new and marketed drugs and biological products. This requirement was mandatory, and its scope included new drugs (ie, new chemical entities, new dosage forms, new indications, new routes of administration, and new dosing regimens) and certain marketed drugs (ie, where the drug product offered meaningful therapeutic benefit or had substantial use in pediatric patients, AND the absence of pediatric labeling posed a risk). This FDA regulation became effective April 1, 1999, but studies mandated under this rule were not required to be submitted to the FDA before December 2, 2000. The 1998 Pediatric Final Rule and the authority of the FDA to **require** manufacturers to conduct pediatric studies was challenged with a law

PREFACE *(Continued)*

suit. In March 2002, the FDA requested a 2-month stay on the lawsuit, so it could publish a notice and suspend the 1998 Pediatric Final Rule for 2 years. During the 2 year suspension of the Rule, the FDA planned to study whether the Best Pharmaceuticals for Children Act of 2002 made the 1998 Final Rule unnecessary. After multiple organizations lobbied Congress and the president, the Secretary of Health and Human Services announced in April 2002, that the FDA would continue to defend the Pediatric Final Rule of 1998 in court. Unfortunately, on October 17, 2002, the U.S. District Court for the District of Columbia barred the FDA from enforcing the Pediatric Final Rule. The court ruled that the FDA did not have the authority to issue the Rule. Currently, the government is working with Congress to enact legislation to **require** pharmaceutical manufacturers to conduct pediatric studies and to help reinstate the Pediatric Final Rule through appropriate legislation.

The Children's Health Act of 2000 was signed into law on October 17, 2000. This important law establishes a Pediatric Research Initiative (headed by the Director of the NIH) and provides funds to increase support for pediatric clinical research. These two important laws, plus other FDA regulations, such as the FDA labeling changes[7] that required expanded information in the Pediatric Use section of the package insert for all prescription drugs, will certainly help to increase and disseminate pediatric drug information.

Currently, however, most commonly used pharmacy references do not include information regarding pediatric dosing, drug administration, or special pediatric concerns. It is, therefore, not surprising that in order to obtain pediatric dosing information, oftentimes the pediatric clinician is faced with extensive literature searches to arrive at a logical dose. This handbook was developed with the intent to serve as a compilation of recommended pediatric doses found in the literature and to provide relevant clinical information regarding the use of drugs in children.

This new edition incorporates additions and revisions in a format which we hope the user will find beneficial. As with each edition, drug monographs have been updated and revised. Eighteen new medications have been added. Ten monographs have been deleted because the drugs are no longer available in the U.S.: Brompheniramine, clioquinol, droperidol and fentanyl, d-xylose, ethacrynic acid, mezlocillin, niclosamide, plicamycin, sulfamethoxazole, and tubocurarine. This brings the total number of drug monographs to 692. New monographs added to this edition include: Aprepitant, atomoxetine, caspofungin, colistimethate, danazol, esomeprazole, fexofenadine, irinotecan, lactic acid and ammonium hydroxide, laronidase, loratadine and pseudoephedrine, megestrol, mometasone, pantoprazole, pimecrolimus, rasburicase, voriconazole, and zonisamide. In addition, 6 new extemporaneous preparations have been added to this edition. This brings the total number of drug monographs with extemporaneous preparations to 74 and the total number of "recipes" to 103.

Three new appendix pieces have been added to this edition including The Catch-up [Immunization] Schedule for Children Age 4 Months Through 6 Years, Catch-up [Immunization] Schedule for Children Age 7 Through 18 Years, and a table listing Total Blood Volume by age. Appendix material has been updated to include the 2003 Childhood and Adolescent Immunization Schedule and the following tables were updated or revised: Antihypertensive Agents by Class, Asthma: Guidelines for the Diagnosis and Management of Asthma, Corticosteroids (Topical), Extravasation Treatment, OTC Cough and Cold Preparations (Pediatric), Multivitamin Products, and Dosage and Administration Guidelines for Vaccines Available in U.S.

We hope this edition continues to be a valuable and practical source of clinical drug information for the pediatric healthcare professional. We welcome comments to further improve future editions.

Footnotes

1.   Food and Drug Letter, Washington Business Information, Inc. November 23, 1990.

2.   "NIH Funds Network of Centers for Pediatric Drug Research," *Am J Hosp Pharm*, 1994, 51:2546.

3. Birenbaum D, "Fruits of the Pediatric Initiatives: A CDER Update," March 27, 2003, http://www.fda.gov/cder/pediatric/presentation/dlb2-DIA-Mar2003/index.htm.

4. Department of Health and Human Services, U.S. Food and Drug Administration, "The Pediatric Exclusivity Provision, January 2001: Status Report to Congress," http://www.fda.gov/cder/pediatric/reportcong01.pdf.

5. Birenbaum D, "Pediatric Initiatives: A Regulatory Perspective of the U.S. Experience," June 17, 2002, http://www.fda.gov/cder/pediatric/presentation/Ped Init 2002 DB/index.htm.

6. Department of Health and Human Services, Food and Drug Administration, 21CFR Parts 201, 312, 314, and 601, Regulations Requiring Manufacturers to Assess the Safety and Effectiveness of New Drugs and Biological Products in Pediatric Patients; Final Rule,' *Fed Regist* 1998, 63(231):66631-72.

7. "Pediatric Use Drug Labeling NDA Supplements Due by December 1996 - FDA Final Rule; Agency Establishing Pediatric Subcommittee to Track Implementation," *F-D-C Reports - The Pink Sheet*, Wallace Werble Jr, Publisher, December 19, 1994.

ACKNOWLEDGMENTS

The *Pediatric Dosage Handbook* exists in its present form as the result of the concerted efforts of the following individuals: Robert D. Kerscher, publisher and president of Lexi-Comp Inc; Lynn D. Coppinger, managing editor; Barbara F. Kerscher, production manager; Mark F Bonfiglio, BS, PharmD, RPh, director of pharmacotherapy resources; Joni L. Stahura, BS, PharmD, pharmacotherapy specialist; Matthew Fuller, PharmD, clinical pharmacy specialist, psychiatry (VA Medical Center, Brecksville, OH); Leonard L. Lance, RPh, BSPharm, pharmacist; David C. Marcus, director of information systems; Stacy S. Robinson, project manager; Alexandra Hart, composition specialist; and Julian I. Graubart, American Pharmacists Association (APhA), Director of Books and Electronic Products.

Special acknowledgment goes to all Lexi-Comp staff for their contributions to this handbook.

Special thanks goes to Chris Lomax, PharmD, director of pharmacy, Children's Hospital, Los Angeles, who played a significant role in bringing APhA and Lexi-Comp together.

Some of the material contained in the book was a result of pediatric pharmacy contributors throughout the United States and Canada. Lexi-Comp has assisted many pediatric medical institutions to develop hospital-specific formulary manuals that contain clinical drug information as well as dosing. Working with these pediatric clinical pharmacists, pediatric hospital pharmacy and therapeutics committees, and hospital drug information centers, Lexi-Comp has developed an evolutionary drug database that reflects the practice of pediatric pharmacy in these major pediatric institutions.

The authors wish to thank their families, friends, and colleagues who supported them in their efforts to complete this handbook.

In addition, Dr Taketomo would like to thank Robert Taketomo, PharmD, MBA and Chris Lomax, PharmD for their professional guidance and continued support, and the pharmacy staff at Childrens Hospital, Los Angeles for their assistance.

Dr Kraus would like to especially thank Keith A. Rodvold, PharmD, for his ongoing professional and personal support.

Dr Hodding would like to thank Glenn Hodding, PharmD, Carl Kildoo, PharmD, and the pediatric pharmacists at Miller Children's Hospital for their continued professional and personal support.

EDITORIAL ADVISORY PANEL

EDITORIAL ADVISORY PANEL *(Continued)*

EDITORIAL ADVISORY PANEL *(Continued)*

11

EDITORIAL ADVISORY PANEL *(Continued)*

ABOUT THE AUTHORS

Carol K. Taketomo, PharmD

Dr Taketomo received her doctorate from the University of Southern California School of Pharmacy. Subsequently, she completed a clinical pharmacy residency at the University of California Medical Center in San Diego. With over 26 years of clinical experience at one of the largest pediatric teaching hospitals in the nation, she is an acknowledged expert in the practical aspects of pediatric drug distribution and clinical pharmacy practice. She currently holds the appointment of Adjunct Assistant Professor of Pharmacy Practice at the University of Southern California School of Pharmacy.

In her current capacity as Pharmacy Manager at Children's Hospital of Los Angeles, Dr Taketomo plays an active role in the education and training of the medical, pharmacy, and nursing staff. She coordinates the Pharmacy Department's quality assurance and drug use evaluation programs; maintains the hospital's strict formulary program; and is the editor of the house staff manual. Her particular interests are strategies to influence physician prescribing patterns and methods to decrease medication errors in the pediatric setting. She has been the author of numerous publications, and is an active presenter at professional meetings.

Dr Taketomo is a member of the American Pharmacists Association (APhA), American Society of Health-System Pharmacists (ASHP), California Society of Hospital Pharmacists (CSHP), and Southern California Pediatric Pharmacy Group.

Jane Hurlburt Hodding, PharmD

Dr Hodding earned a doctorate and completed her pharmacy residency at the University of California School of Pharmacy in San Francisco. She has held teaching positions as Assistant Clinical Professor of Pharmacy at UCSF as well as Assistant Clinical Professor of Pharmacy Practice at the University of Southern California in Los Angeles. Currently, Dr Hodding is the Director, Pharmacy Services at Miller Children's Hospital in Long Beach, California.

Throughout her 26 years of pediatric pharmacy practice, Dr Hodding has actively pursued methods to improve neonatal intensive care, pediatric intensive care, pediatric hematology/oncology, and parenteral nutrition. She has published numerous articles covering neonatal medication administration and aminoglycoside and theophylline clearance in premature infants.

Dr Hodding is a member of the American Pharmacists Association (APhA), American Society of Health-System Pharmacists (ASHP), California Society of Hospital Pharmacists (CSHP), Children's Oncology Group, and Southern California Pediatric Pharmacy Group. She is frequently an invited speaker on the topics of Monitoring Drug Therapy in the NICU, Fluid and Electrolyte Therapy in Children, Drug Therapy Considerations in Children, and Parenteral Nutrition in the Premature Infant.

Donna M. Kraus, PharmD

Dr Kraus received her Bachelor of Science in Pharmacy from the University of Illinois at Chicago (UIC). She worked for several years as a hospital pediatric/obstetric satellite pharmacist before earning her doctorate degree at the UIC. Dr Kraus then completed a postdoctoral pediatric specialty residency at the University of Texas Health Science Center in San Antonio. She has served as a pediatric intensive care clinical pharmacist for 15 years and currently is an ambulatory care pediatric clinical pharmacist, specializing in pediatric HIV pharmacotherapy and patient/parent medication adherence. Dr Kraus has also served as a clinical pharmacist consultant to a pediatric long-term care facility for over 18 years. She currently holds the appointment of Associate Professor of Pharmacy Practice in both the Departments of Pharmacy Practice and Pediatrics at the University of Illinois in Chicago.

ABOUT THE AUTHORS *(Continued)*

In her 26 years of active pharmacy experience, Dr Kraus has dealt with pediatric pharmacy issues and pharmacotherapy problems. She is an active educator and has been a guest lecturer in China, Thailand, and Hong Kong. Dr Kraus has played a leading role in the advanced training of postgraduate pharmacists and has been the Director of the UIC (ASHP accredited) Pediatric Residency and Fellowship Program for 16 years. Dr Kraus' research areas include pediatric drug dosing and developmental pharmacokinetics and pharmacodynamics. She has published a number of articles on various issues of pediatric pharmacy and pharmacotherapy.

Dr Kraus has been an active member of numerous professional associations including the American Pharmacists Association (APhA), American Society of Health-System Pharmacists (ASHP), Illinois Pharmacists Association (IPhA), American College of Clinical Pharmacy (ACCP), Illinois College of Clinical Pharmacy (ICCP), and the Pediatric Pharmacy Advocacy Group (PPAG). She served as Chairperson of the ASHP Commission on Therapeutics, and was an APhA, Academy of Pharmaceutical Research and Science, Member-at-Large. Dr. Kraus also served as an Editorial Board member of the *American Journal of Health-System Pharmacy* and the *Journal of Pediatric Pharmacy Practice.* Currently, she serves as an Editorial Board member of *The Journal of Pediatric Pharmacology and Therapeutics.* Dr. Kraus was recently awarded Fellow status by the American Pharmaceutical Association and is the APhA designated author for this handbook.

DESCRIPTION OF SECTIONS AND FIELDS USED IN THIS HANDBOOK

The *Pediatric Dosage Handbook, 10th Edition* is organized into a drug information section, an appendix, and a therapeutic category & key word index.

Drug information is presented in a consistent format and provides the following:

Generic Name	U.S. adopted name. "Tall Man" lettering appears for look-alike generic drug names as recommended by the FDA. See "FDA Differentiation Project: The Use of "Tall Man" Letters" on page 25. The symbol [DSC] appears after the generic name of drugs that have been recently discontinued.
Pronunciation Guide	Phonetic listing of generic name
Related Information	Cross-reference to other pertinent drug information found in the Appendix
U.S. Brand Names	Common trade names used in the U.S. The symbol [DSC] appears after trade names that have been recently discontinued.
Canadian Brand Names	Common trade names used in Canada
Available Salts	Lists the various salt forms of the drug for selected monographs. For the majority of drugs, this information can be found in the dosage forms field.
Synonyms	Other names or accepted abbreviations for the generic drug
Therapeutic Category	Unique systematic classification of medications
Generic Available	Indicated by a "Yes" or "No" as to whether a generic form of the drug is available. Specific generic dosage forms (or exceptions) are listed in parentheses.
Use	Information pertaining to appropriate indications or use of the drug
Restrictions	Drug Enforcement Agency (DEA) classification for federally scheduled controlled substances
Pregnancy Risk Factor	Five categories established by the FDA to indicate the potential of a systemically absorbed drug for causing birth defects
Contraindications	Information pertaining to inappropriate use of the drug, or disease states and patient populations in which the drug should not be used
Warnings	Hazardous conditions related to use of the drug
Precautions	Disease states or patient populations in which the drug should be cautiously used
Adverse Reactions	Side effects are grouped by body system and include a listing of the more common and/or serious side effects. Due to space limitations, every reported side effect is not listed.
Drug Interactions	For select drugs that have demonstrated involvement with cytochrome P450 enzymes, the initial line of this field identifies the drug as a substrate, inducer, or inhibitor of specific isoenzymes (eg, CYP1A2). A summary of this information can also be found in a tabular format within the appendix. The remainder of the field presents a description of common or significant interactions between the drug listed in the monograph and other drugs or drug classes that are commonly used in pediatric patients. Due to space limitations, the reader is advised to read the drug interaction field of both drugs involved in the interaction.
Food Interactions	Possible interactions between the drug listed in the monograph and certain foods and/or nutritional substances
Stability	Storage, refrigeration, and compatibility information
Mechanism of Action	How the drug works in the body to elicit a response
Pharmacodynamics	Dose-response relationships including onset of action, time of peak action, and duration of action
Pharmacokinetics	Drug movement through the body over time. Pharmacokinetics deals with absorption, distribution, protein binding, metabolism, bioavailability, half-life, time to peak concentration, elimination, and clearance of drugs. Pharmacokinetic parameters help predict drug concentration and dosage requirements.

DESCRIPTION OF SECTIONS AND FIELDS USED IN THIS HANDBOOK (Continued)

Usual Dosage	The amount of the drug to be typically given or taken during therapy
	Please note that doses for neonates are often listed by postnatal age (PNA) (eg, PNA ≤7 days) and/or by body weight (eg, 1200-2000 g)
	When both milligram and milligram per kilogram doses are listed, the milligram per kilogram dosing method is preferred. If using a milligram dosing guideline according to age, special care and lower doses should be used in children who have a low weight for their age. When ranges of doses are listed, initiate therapy at the lower end of the range and titrate the dose accordingly. References are listed at the end of drug monographs to support doses listed when little dosing information exists.
	For select drugs, the dosing adjustment in renal impairment or dosing interval in renal impairment is given according to creatinine clearance (Cl_{cr}). Since most studies that recommend dosing guidelines in renal dysfunction are conducted in adult patients, Cl_{cr} is usually expressed in units of mL/minute. However, in order to extrapolate the adult information to the pediatric population, one must assume that the adults studied were of standard surface area (ie, 1.73 m^2). Therefore, although the value of Cl_{cr} listed for dosing adjustment in renal impairment or dosing interval in renal impairment may be expressed in mL/minute, it is assumed to be equal to the same value in mL/minute/1.73 m^2.
	To calculate the dose in a pediatric patient with renal dysfunction, first calculate the normal dose (ie, the dose for a patient without renal dysfunction), then use the guidelines to adjust the dose. For example, the normal piperacillin dose for a 20 kg child is 200-300 mg/kg/day divided every 4-6 hours. If one selected 300 mg/kg/day divided every 6 hours, the dose would be 1.5 g every 6 hours in normal renal function. If Cl_{cr} was 20-40 mL/minute/1.73 m^2, the dose would be 1.5 g every 8 hours and if Cl_{cr} was <20 mL/minute/1.73 m^2, the dose would be 1.5 g every 12 hours.
Administration	Information regarding the recommended final concentrations and rates for administration of parenteral drugs are listed when appropriate, along with pertinent oral, ophthalmic, and topical administration information.
Monitoring Parameters	Laboratory tests and patient physical parameters that should be monitored for safety and efficacy of drug therapy are listed when appropriate.
Reference Range	Therapeutic and toxic serum concentrations are listed when appropriate
Test Interactions	Listing of assay interferences when relevant; (S) = Serum; (U) = Urine
Patient Information	Advice, warnings, precautions, and other information of which the patient should be informed
Nursing Implications	Comments regarding nursing care of the patient are offered when appropriate
Additional Information	Other data and facts about the drug are offered when appropriate
Dosage Forms	Information with regard to form, strength, and availability of the drug. The symbol [DSC] appears after dosage forms that have been recently discontinued. U.S. brand names appear in this field when more than one brand name exists for a medication. For dosage forms that are available as generic products and multiple brand names, the generic dosage forms are listed first, followed by the U.S. brand names and dosage form descriptions. Important information about ingredients found in specific dosage forms appears in brackets at the end of the dosage form entry. The following items are listed if present: Alcohol content, benzoic acid, benzyl alcohol, metabisulfites, sodium benzoate, sulfites, tartrazine, phenylalanine, aspartame, and flavor. Other ingredients may be listed if information was readily available. Since commercial formulations may change, the reader should check a current package insert for all possible ingredients.

(continued)

Extemporaneous Preparations | Directions for preparing liquid formulations from solid drug products. May include stability information and references (listed when appropriate).

References | Bibliographic information referring to specific pediatric literature findings, especially doses

Appendix

The appendix offers a compilation of tables, guidelines, and conversion information which can often be helpful when considering patient care. This section is broken down into various sections for ease of use.

Therapeutic Category & Key Word Index

This index provides a useful listing by an easy-to-use therapeutic classification system. Also listed are controlled substances, preservative free, sugar free, and alcohol free medications.

DEFINITION OF AGE GROUP TERMINOLOGY

Information in this handbook is listed according to specific age or by age group. The following are definitions of age groups and age-related terminologies. These definitions should be used unless otherwise specified in the monograph.

Gestational age (GA)	The time from conception until birth. More specifically, gestational age is defined as the number of weeks from the first day of the mother's last menstrual period (LMP) until the birth of the baby. Gestational age at birth is assessed by the date of the LMP and by physical exam (Dubowitz score).
Postnatal age (PNA)	Chronological age since birth
Postconceptional age (PCA)	Age since conception. Postconceptional age is calculated as gestational age plus postnatal age (PCA = GA + PNA).
Neonate	A full-term newborn 0-4 weeks postnatal age. This term may also be applied to a premature neonate whose postconceptional age (PCA) is 42-46 weeks.
Premature neonate	Neonate born at <38 weeks gestational age
Full-term neonate	Neonate born at 38-42 weeks (average ~40 weeks) gestational age
Infant	1 month to 1 year of age
Child/Children	1-12 years of age
Adolescent	13-18 years of age
Adult	>18 years of age

FDA PREGNANCY CATEGORIES

Throughout this book there is a field labeled Pregnancy Risk Factor and the letter A, B, C, D, or X immediately following which signifies a category. The FDA has established these five categories to indicate the potential of a systemically absorbed drug for causing birth defects. The key differentiation among the categories rests upon the reliability of documentation and the risk:benefit ratio. Pregnancy Category X is particularly notable in that if any data exists that may implicate a drug as a teratogen and the risk:benefit ratio is clearly negative, the drug is contraindicated during pregnancy.

These categories are summarized as follows:

A   Controlled studies in pregnant women fail to demonstrate a risk to the fetus in the first trimester with no evidence of risk in later trimesters. The possibility of fetal harm appears remote.

B   Either animal-reproduction studies have not demonstrated a fetal risk but there are no controlled studies in pregnant women, or animal-reproduction studies have shown an adverse effect (other than a decrease in fertility) that was not confirmed in controlled studies in women in the first trimester and there is no evidence of a risk in later trimesters.

C   Either studies in animals have revealed adverse effects on the fetus (teratogenic or embryocidal effects or other) and there are no controlled studies in women, or studies in women and animals are not available. Drugs should be given only if the potential benefits justify the potential risk to the fetus.

D   There is positive evidence of human fetal risk, but the benefits from use in pregnant women may be acceptable despite the risk (eg, if the drug is needed in a life-threatening situation or for a serious disease for which safer drugs cannot be used or are ineffective).

X   Studies in animals or human beings have demonstrated fetal abnormalities or there is evidence of fetal risk based on human experience, or both, and the risk of the use of the drug in pregnant women clearly outweighs any possible benefit. The drug is contraindicated in women who are or may become pregnant.

SYMBOLS & ABBREVIATIONS USED IN THIS HANDBOOK*

°C	degrees Celsius (Centigrade)
<	less than
>	greater than
≤	less than or equal to
≥	greater than or equal to
µg	microgram
µmol	micromole
AAP	American Academy of Pediatrics
AAPC	antibiotic associated pseudomembranous colitis
ABG	arterial blood gas
ABMT	autologous bone marrow transplant
ACE	angiotensin-converting enzyme
ACLS	advanced cardiac life support
ADH	antidiuretic hormone
AED	antiepileptic drug
AHCPR	Agency for Health Care Policy and Research
AIDS	acquired immunodeficiency syndrome
ALL	acute lymphoblastic leukemia
ALT	alanine aminotransferase (formerly called SGPT)
AML	acute myeloblastic leukemia
ANA	antinuclear antibodies
ANC	absolute neutrophil count
ANLL	acute nonlymphoblastic leukemia
APTT	activated partial thromboplastin time
ARDS	adult respiratory distress syndrome
ASA (class I-IV)	American Society of Anesthesiology physical status classification of surgical patients according to their baseline health
	ASA I: Normal healthy patients
	ASA II: Patients having controlled disease states (eg, controlled hypertension)
	ASA III: Patients having a disease which compromises their organ function (eg, decompensated CHF, end stage renal failure)
	ASA IV: Patients who are extremely critically ill
AST	aspartate aminotransferase (formerly called SGOT)
ATP	adenosine triphosphate
AUC	area under the curve (area under the serum concentration-time curve)
A-V	atrial-ventricular
BMT	bone marrow transplant
BPD	bronchopulmonary disease
BSA	body surface area
BUN	blood urea nitrogen
CAD	coronary artery disease
CADD	computer ambulatory drug delivery
cAMP	cyclic adenosine monophosphate
CBC	complete blood count
CDC	Center for Disease Control and Prevention
CF	cystic fibrosis
CFC	chlorofluorocarbons
CHF	congestive heart failure
CI	cardiac index
Cl_{cr}	creatinine clearance
CLL	chronic lymphocytic leukemia
CML	chronic myelogenous leukemia
CMV	cytomegalovirus
CNS	central nervous system
COPD	chronic obstructive pulmonary disease

(continued)

CPK	creatine phosphokinase
CPR	cardiopulmonary resuscitation
CRF	chronic renal failure
CSF	cerebrospinal fluid
CT	computed tomography
CVA	cerebral vascular accident
CVP	central venous pressure
CYP	cytochrome
d	day
D_5/LR	dextrose 5% in lactated Ringer's
D_5/NS	dextrose 5% in sodium chloride 0.9%
D_5W	dextrose 5% in water
D_5/^{1}/$_4$ NS	dextrose 5% in sodium chloride 0.2%
D_5/^{1}/$_2$ NS	dextrose 5% in sodium chloride 0.45%
D_{10}W	dextrose 10% in water
DIC	disseminated intravascular coagulation
DL_{co}	pulmonary diffusion capacity for carbon monoxide
DNA	deoxyribonucleic acid
[DSC]	discontinued
DVT	deep vein thrombosis
ECHO	echocardiogram
ECMO	extracorporeal membrane oxygenation
EEG	electroencephalogram
EKG	electrocardiogram
ESR	erythrocyte sedimentation rate
ESRD	end stage renal disease
E.T.	endotracheal
FDA	Food and Drug Administration (United States)
FEV_1	forced expiratory volume exhaled after 1 second
FSH	follicle-stimulating hormone
FVC	forced vital capacity
g	gram
G-6-PD	glucose-6-phosphate dehydrogenase
GA	gestational age
GABA	gamma-aminobutyric acid
GE	gastroesophageal
GERD	gastroesophageal reflux disease
GFR	glomerular filtration rate
GI	gastrointestinal
GVHD	graft versus host disease
GU	genitourinary
h	hour
Hct	hematocrit
HDL-C	high density lipoprotein cholesterol
Hgb	hemoglobin
HFA	hydrofluoroalkane
HIV	human immunodeficiency virus
HMG-CoA	hydroxymethyl glutaryl coenzyme A
HPLC	high performance liquid chromatography
HSV	herpes simplex virus
ICP	intracranial pressure
IDDM	insulin-dependent diabetes mellitus
IgG	immune globulin G
I.M.	intramuscular
INR	international normalized ratio
ILCOR	International Liaison Committee on Resuscitation
I.O.	intraosseous
I & O	input and output
IOP	intraocular pressure

SYMBOLS & ABBREVIATIONS USED IN THIS HANDBOOK* *(Continued)*

IQ	intelligence quotient
I.T.	intrathecal
ITP	idiopathic thrombocytopenic purpura
I.V.	intravenous
IVH	intraventricular hemorrhage
IVP	intravenous push
JRA	juvenile rheumatoid arthritis
kg	kilogram
L	liter
LDH	lactate dehydrogenase
LDL-C	low density lipoprotein cholesterol
LE	lupus erythematosus
LH	luteinizing hormone
LP	lumbar puncture
LR	lactated Ringer's
M	molar
MAC	*Mycobacterium avium* complex
MAO	monoamine oxidase
MAP	mean arterial pressure
mcg	microgram
mg	milligram
MI	myocardial infarction
min	minute
mL	milliliter
mM	millimole
mo	month
MOPP	mustargen (mechlorethamine), Oncovin® (vincristine), procarbazine, and prednisone
mOsm	milliosmoles
MRI	magnetic resonance image
MRSA	methicillin-resistant *Staphylococcus aureus*
NAEPP	National Asthma Education and Prevention Program
NCI	National Cancer Institute
ND	nasoduodenal
ng	nanogram
NG	nasogastric
NIDDM	noninsulin-dependent diabetes mellitus
NMDA	n-methyl-d-aspartate
nmol	nanomole
NMS	neuroleptic malignant syndrome
NPO	nothing per os (nothing by mouth)
NS	normal saline (0.9% sodium chloride)
½NS	0.45% sodium chloride
NSAID	nonsteroidal anti-inflammatory drug
NYHA	New York Heart Association
O.R.	operating room
OTC	over-the-counter (nonprescription)
PABA	para-aminobenzoic acid
PALS	pediatric advanced life support
PCA	postconceptional age
PCP	*Pneumocystis carinii* pneumonia
PCWP	pulmonary capillary wedge pressure
PDA	patent ductus arteriosus
PE	pulmonary embolism
PICU	Pediatric Intensive Care Unit
PIP	peak inspiratory pressure

(continued)

PNA	postnatal age
prn	as needed
PSVT	paroxysmal supraventricular tachycardia
PT	prothrombin time
PTH	parathyroid hormone
PTT	partial thromboplastin time
PUD	peptic ulcer disease
PVC	premature ventricular contraction
PVR	peripheral vascular resistance
qsad	add an amount sufficient to equal
RAP	right arterial pressure
RDA	recommended daily allowance
RIA	radioimmunoassay
RNA	ribonucleic acid
RSV	respiratory syncytial virus
S-A	sino-atrial
S.C.	subcutaneous
S_{cr}	serum creatinine
SIADH	syndrome of inappropriate antidiuretic hormone
S.L.	sublingual
SLE	systemic lupus erythematosus
SSRI	selective serotonin reuptake inhibitor
STD	sexually-transmitted disease
SVR	systemic vascular resistance
SVT	supraventricular tachycardia
SWI	sterile water for injection
T_3	triiodothyronine
T_4	thyroxine
TCA	tricyclic antidepressant
TIA	transient ischemic attack
TIBC	total iron binding capacity
TNF	tissue necrosis factor
TPN	total parenteral nutrition
TSH	thyroid stimulating hormone
TT	thrombin time
UA	urine analysis
UTI	urinary tract infection
V_d	volume of distribution
V_{dss}	volume of distribution at steady-state
VF	ventricular fibrillation
VMA	vanillylmandelic acid
VT	ventricular tachycardia
VZV	varicella zoster virus
w/v	weight for volume
w/w	weight for weight
y	year

*Other than drug synonyms

SAFE WRITING

Health professionals and their support personnel frequently produce handwritten copies of information they see in print; therefore, such information is subjected to even greater possibilities for error or misinterpretation on the part of others. Thus, particular care must be given to how drug names and strengths are expressed when creating written health-care documents.

The following are a few examples of safe writing rules suggested by the Institute for Safe Medication Practices, Inc.*

1. There should be a space between a number and its units as it is easier to read. There should be no periods after the abbreviations mg or mL.

Correct	Incorrect
10 mg	10mg
100 mg	100mg

2. Never place a decimal and a zero after a whole number (2 mg is correct and 2.0 mg is **incorrect**). If the decimal point is not seen because it falls on a line or because individuals are working from copies where the decimal point is not seen, this causes a tenfold overdose.

3. Just the opposite is true for numbers less than one. Always place a zero before a naked decimal (0.5 mL is correct, .5 mL is **incorrect**).

4. Never abbreviate the word unit. The handwritten U or u, looks like a 0 (zero), and may cause a tenfold overdose error to be made.

5. IU is not a safe abbreviation for international units. The handwritten IU looks like IV. Write out international units or use int. units.

6. Q.D. is not a safe abbreviation for once daily, as when the Q is followed by a sloppy dot, it looks like QID which means four times daily.

7. O.D. is not a safe abbreviation for once daily, as it is properly interpreted as meaning "right eye" and has caused liquid medications such as saturated solution of potassium iodide and Lugol's solution to be administered incorrectly. There is no safe abbreviation for once daily. It must be written out in full.

8. Do not use chemical names such as 6-mercaptopurine or 6-thioguanine, as sixfold overdoses have been given when these were not recognized as chemical names. The proper names of these drugs are mercaptopurine or thioguanine.

9. Do not abbreviate drug names (5FC, 6MP, 5-ASA, MTX, HCTZ, CPZ, PBZ, etc) as they are misinterpreted and cause error.

10. Do not use the apothecary system or symbols.

11. Do not abbreviate microgram as µg; instead use mcg as there is less likelihood of misinterpretation.

12. When writing an outpatient prescription, write a complete prescription. A complete prescription can prevent the prescriber, the pharmacist, and/or the patient from making a mistake and can eliminate the need for further clarification. The legible prescriptions should contain:

    a. patient's full name

    b. for pediatric or geriatric patients: their age (or weight where applicable)

    c. drug name, dosage form and strength; if a drug is new or rarely prescribed, print this information

    d. number or amount to be dispensed

    e. complete instructions for the patient, including the purpose of the medication

    f. when there are recognized contraindications for a prescribed drug, indicate to the pharmacist that you are aware of this fact (ie, when prescribing a potassium salt for a patient receiving an ACE inhibitor, write "K serum leveling being monitored")

*From "Safe Writing" by Davis NM, PharmD and Cohen MR, MS, Lecturers and Consultants for Safe Medication Practices, 1143 Wright Drive, Huntington Valley, PA 19006. Phone: (215) 947-7566.

FDA NAME DIFFERENTIATION PROJECT: THE USE OF "TALL MAN" LETTERS

Confusion between similar drug names is a frequent cause of medication errors. For years, The Institute For Safe Medication Practices (ISMP), has urged generic manufacturers to use a combination of capital and lower case letters (eg, chlorproMAZINE and chlorproPAMIDE) to help distinguish drugs with look-alike names, especially when they share similar strengths. The FDA's Office of Generic Drugs has acted upon this suggestion and initiated the "Name Differentiation Project," to help decrease medication errors that result from look-alike drug names. From March to May 2001, the Office of Generic Drugs issued 142 letters encouraging manufacturers to revise product labeling and labels to visually differentiate the established drug name with the use of "Tall Man" letters.

The ISMP recommends that hospitals follow suit by making similar changes in their pharmacy-prepared labels, preprinted order forms, pharmacy and physician order entry systems, computer-generated medication administration records, drug storage location labels, and other print or electronic use of the drug name.

Lexi-Comp Medical Publishing will begin using these "Tall Man" letters for the drugs suggested by the FDA. The "Tall Man" lettering will appear in the generic name field of the monograph.

The following is a list of product names and recommended FDA revisions.

Drug Product	Recommended Revision
acetazolamide	aceta**ZOLAMIDE**
acetohexamide	aceto**HEXAMIDE**
bupropion	bu**PROP**ion
buspirone	bus**PIR**one
chlorpromazine	chlorpro**MAZINE**
chlorpropamide	chlorpro**PAMIDE**
clomiphene	clomi**PHENE**
clomipramine	clomi**PRAMINE**
cycloserine	cyclo**SERINE**
cyclosporine	cyclo**SPORINE**
daunorubicin	**DAUNO**rubicin
dimenhydrinate	dimenhy**DRINATE**
diphenhydramine	diphenhydr**AMINE**
dobutamine	**DOBUT**amine
dopamine	**DOP**amine
doxorubicin	**DOXO**rubicin
glipizide	glipi**ZIDE**
glyburide	gly**BURIDE**
hydralazine	hydr**ALAZINE**
hydroxyzine	hydr**OXY**zine
medroxyprogesterone	medroxy**PROGESTER**one
methylprednisolone	methyl**PREDNIS**olone
methyltestosterone	methyl**TESTOSTER**one
nicardipine	ni**CAR**dipine
nifedipine	**NIFE**dipine
prednisolone	predniso**LONE**
prednisone	predni**SONE**
sulfadiazine	sulfa**DIAZINE**

FDA NAME DIFFERENTIATION PROJECT: THE USE OF "TALL MAN" LETTERS *(Continued)*

Drug Product	Recommended Revision
sulfisoxazole	sulfi**SOXAZOLE**
tolazamide	**TOLAZ**amide
tolbutamide	**TOLBUT**amide
vinblastine	vin**BLAS**tine
vincristine	vin**CRIS**tine

References

FDA, "Name Differentiation Project." Available at http://www.fda.gov/cder/drug/MedErrors/nameDiff.htm.

Institute for Safe Medication Practices. "New Tall-Man Lettering Will Reduce Mix-Ups Due to Generic Drug Name Confusion," *ISMP Medication Safety Alert*, September 19, 2001. Available at: http://www.ismp.org.

Institute for Safe Medication Practices. "Prescription Mapping, Can Improve Efficiency While Minimizing Errors With Look-Alike Products," *ISMP Medication Safety Alert*, October 6, 1999. Available at: http://www.ismp.org.

U.S. Pharmacopeia, "USP Quality Review: Use Caution-Avoid Confusion," March 2001, No. 76. Available at: http://www.usp.org.

SELECTED REFERENCES

Dorr RT and Von Hoff DD, *Cancer Chemotherapy Handbook*, 2nd ed, Norwalk, CT: Appleton & Lange, 1994.

Drug Interaction Facts, St Louis, MO: J.B. Lippincott Co (Facts and Comparisons Division), 2003.

Facts and Comparisons, St Louis, MO: J.B. Lippincott Co (Facts and Comparisons Division), 2003.

Feigin RD and Cherry JD, *Textbook of Pediatric Infectious Diseases*, 4th ed, Philadelphia, PA: WB Saunders Company, 1998.

Hale T, *Medications and Mother's Milk*, 8th ed, Amarillo, TX: Pharmasoft Medical Publishing, 1999.

Handbook on Extemporaneous Formulations, Bethesda, MD: American Society of Health-System Pharmacists, 1987.

Handbook of Nonprescription Drugs, 13th ed, Washington, DC: American Pharmaceutical Association, 2002.

Jacobs DS, DeMott WR, Grady HJ, et al, *Laboratory Test Handbook with Key Word Index*, 5th ed, Hudson, OH: Lexi-Comp Inc, 2001.

Jenson HB and Baltimore RS, *Pediatric Infectious Diseases - Principles and Practice*, 2nd ed, Philadelphia, PA: Saunders, 2002.

Lacy CF, Armstrong LL, Goldman MP, et al, *Drug Information Handbook*, 11th ed, Hudson, OH: Lexi-Comp, Inc, 2003.

Mandell GL, Bennett JE, and Dolin R, *Principles and Practice of Infectious Diseases*, 5th ed, Philadelphia, PA: Churchill Livingstone, 2000.

McEvoy GK, *AHFS Drug Information*, 45th ed, Bethesda, MD: American Society of Health-System Pharmacists, 2003.

Nahata MC and Hipple TF, *Pediatric Drug Formulations*, 4th ed, Cincinnati, OH: Harvey Whitney Books Company, 2000.

Nelson JD and Bradley JS, *Nelson's Pocket Book of Pediatric Antimicrobial Therapy*, 15th ed, Philadelphia, PA: Lippincott Williams & Wilkins, 2002.

PDR® Generics™, 2nd ed, Montvale, New Jersey: Medical Economics Co, 1996.

Phelps SJ, *Teddy Bear Book: Pediatric Injectable Drugs*, 6th ed, Bethesda, MD: American Society of Health-System Pharmacists, 2002.

Physician's Desk Reference, 57th ed, Montvale, NJ: Medical Economics Co, 2003.

Pickering LK, ed, *2000 Red Book, Report of the Committee on Infectious Diseases*, 25th ed, Elk Grove Village, IL: American Academy of Pediatrics, 2000.

Piscitelli SC and Rodvold KA, eds, *Drug Interactions in Infectious Diseases*, Totowa, NJ: Humana Press Inc, 2001.

Pizzo PA and Poplack DG, *Principles and Practice of Pediatric Oncology*, 4th ed, Philadelphia, PA: Lippincott Raven Publishers, 2001.

Pronsky ZM, *Powers and Moore's Food Medication Interactions*, 11th ed, Pottstown, PA: Food Medication Interactions, 2000.

Radde IC and MacLead SM, *Pediatric Pharmacology and Therapeutics*, St. Louis, MO: Mosby, 1993.

Rogers MC and Helfaer MA, *Handbook of Pediatric Intensive Care*, 3rd ed, Baltimore, MD: Lippincott Williams & Wilkins, 1998.

Rogers MC and Nichols DG, *Textbook of Pediatric Intensive Care*, 3rd ed, Baltimore, MD: Williams & Wilkins, 1996.

Rudolph AM, *Rudolph's Pediatrics*, 21st ed, Norwalk, CT: Appleton & Lange, 2002.

Toro-Figueroa LO, Levin DL, and Morriss FC, *Essentials of Pediatric Intensive Care Manual*, St Louis, MO: Quality Medical Pub, Inc, 1992.

Trissel L, *Handbook of Injectable Drugs*, 12th ed, Bethesda, MD: American Society of Health-System Pharmacists, 2001.

Trissel LA, *Trissel's Stability of Compounded Formulations*, 2nd ed, Washington, DC: American Pharmaceutical Association, 2000.

United States Pharmacopeia Dispensing Information (USP DI), 23rd ed, Englewood, CO: Micromedex, Inc, 2003.

Yaffe SJ and Aranda JV, *Pediatric Pharmacology: Therapeutic Principles in Practice*, Philadelphia, PA: WB Saunders Company, 1992.

ALPHABETICAL LISTING OF DRUGS

♦ **A200® Lice [OTC]** see Permethrin on page 885

♦ **A-ase** see Asparaginase on page 132

Abacavir (uh BACK ah veer)

Related Information
Adult and Adolescent HIV on page 1327
Pediatric HIV on page 1323

U.S. Brand Names Ziagen®

Therapeutic Category Antiretroviral Agent; HIV Agents (Anti-HIV Agents); Nucleoside Reverse Transcriptase Inhibitor (NRTI)

Generic Available No

Use Treatment of HIV-1 infection in combination with other antiretroviral agents. (**Note:** HIV regimens consisting of **three** antiretroviral agents are strongly recommended)

Pregnancy Risk Factor C

Contraindications Hypersensitivity to abacavir or any component; **do not rechallenge** patients who have experienced hypersensitivity reactions to abacavir, potentially fatal hypersensitivity reactions may occur (see Warnings)

Warnings Fatal hypersensitivity reactions may occur; discontinue therapy immediately in patients who show signs or symptoms of hypersensitivity reaction such as fever, fatigue, skin rash, respiratory symptoms (cough, dyspnea, pharyngitis), and GI symptoms (nausea, vomiting, diarrhea, or abdominal pain). Carefully consider the diagnosis of hypersensitivity reaction in patients who present with acute onset respiratory symptoms, even if other diagnoses, such as bronchitis, flu-like illness, pharyngitis, or pneumonia, are possible. Skin rash may be maculopapular or urticarial, but can be variable in appearance; erythema multiforme has been reported; hypersensitivity reaction may occur without a rash. Other symptoms may include edema, lethargy, malaise, arthralgia, myolysis, myalgia, paresthesia, shortness of breath, mouth ulcerations, conjunctivitis, headache, lymphadenopathy, and abnormal findings on chest x-ray (ie, infiltrates that can be localized). Laboratory abnormalities include increases in liver function tests, elevated CPK or serum creatinine, and lymphopenia.

Do not restart abacavir after a hypersensitivity reaction occurs; more severe symptoms can recur within hours and may include: Anaphylaxis, renal failure, hepatic failure, respiratory failure, ARDS, life-threatening hypotension and death. Fatal hypersensitivity reactions have occurred following the reintroduction of abacavir in patients whose therapy was interrupted for other reasons. These patients had no identified history or had unrecognized symptoms of abacavir hypersensitivity. Reactions occurred within hours. In some cases, signs of a hypersensitivity reaction may have been previously present, but attributed to other medical conditions (acute onset respiratory diseases, gastroenteritis, reactions to other medications). If abacavir (or Trizivir®) is to be restarted following an interruption in therapy, the patient must first be evaluated for previously unsuspected symptoms of hypersensitivity. **Do not restart** abacavir (or Trizivir®) if hypersensitivity is suspected or cannot be ruled out. Hypersensitivity reactions occur in ~5% of adult and pediatric patients; most hypersensitivity reactions occur within the first 6 weeks of therapy, but can occur at any time; call the Abacavir Hypersensitivity Reaction Registry at 1-800-270-0425 to facilitate reporting and collection of information on patients experiencing abacavir hypersensitivity reactions (see Additional Information)

Cases of lactic acidosis, severe hepatomegaly with steatosis and death have been reported; prolonged nucleoside use, obesity, and prior liver disease may be risk factors; use with extreme caution in patients with other risk factors for liver disease; discontinue abacavir in patients who develop laboratory or clinical evidence of lactic acidosis or pronounced hepatotoxicity

Precautions Fat redistribution and accumulation [ie, central obesity, peripheral wasting, facial wasting, breast enlargement, dorsocervical fat enlargement (buffalo hump), and cushingoid appearance] have been observed in patients receiving antiretroviral agents (causal relationship not established). Always use abacavir in combination with other antiretroviral agents; do not add abacavir as a single agent to antiretroviral regimens that are failing; resistance to abacavir develops relatively slowly, but cross resistance between abacavir and other nucleoside reverse transcriptase inhibitors (NRTIs) may occur; limited response may be seen in patients with HIV isolates containing multiple mutations conferring resistance to NRTIs or in patients with a prolonged prior NRTI exposure (see Additional Information)

Systemic exposure of abacavir at 6-32 times the normal human exposure, increased the incidence of tumors (malignant and nonmalignant) in mice and rats; myocardial degeneration was seen in mice and rats receiving abacavir for 2 years at 7-24 times the expected human exposure; the clinical relevance of these 2 findings is currently unknown

Adverse Reactions

Central nervous system: Insomnia, fever, headache, malaise, fatigue

Dermatologic: Rash (see Warnings); erythema multiforme. **Note:** Suspected toxic epidermal necrolysis and Stevens-Johnson syndrome have been reported but patients also received medications known to be associated with these rashes; due to the similarities between these rashes and abacavir hypersensitivity reactions, abacavir should be discontinued and never restarted in such patients.

Endocrine & metabolic: Mild elevations of blood glucose, hypertriglyceridemia, lactic acidosis, fat redistribution and accumulation (see Precautions)

Gastrointestinal: Nausea, vomiting, diarrhea, anorexia; pancreatitis (rare)

Hepatic: Hepatomegaly with steatosis; elevated liver enzymes (rare)

Neuromuscular & skeletal: Asthenia

Respiratory: Cough

Miscellaneous: Hypersensitivity reaction (see Warnings)

Drug Interactions Use with ethanol increases abacavir AUC by 41% and prolongs half-life by 26%; abacavir may increase the clearance of methadone by 22% (a small number of patients may require an increase in methadone dosage)

Food Interactions Food does not significantly affect AUC

Stability Store tablets and oral solution at room temperature; oral solution may be refrigerated; do not freeze

Mechanism of Action A carbocyclic analogue that is converted within cells to the active metabolite carbovir triphosphate; carbovir triphosphate serves as an alternative substrate to deoxyguanosine-5'-triphosphate (dGTP), a natural substrate for cellular DNA polymerase and reverse transcriptase; carbovir triphosphate inhibits HIV viral reverse transcriptase by competing with natural dGTP and by becoming incorporated into viral DNA causing chain termination

Pharmacokinetics

Absorption: Rapid and extensive

Distribution: Apparent V_d: Adults: 0.86 ± 0.15 L/kg

CSF to plasma AUC ratio: 27% to 33%

Protein binding: 50%

Metabolism: In the liver by alcohol dehydrogenase and glucuronyl transferase to inactive carboxylate and glucuronide metabolites; not significantly metabolized by cytochrome P450 enzymes

Bioavailability: Tablet: 83%; solution and tablet provide comparable AUCs

Half-life:

Infants ≥3 months and Children ≤13 years: 1-1.5 hours

Adults: 1.54 ± 0.63 hours

Time to peak serum concentration: Infants ≥3 months and Children ≤13 years: Within 1.5 hours

Elimination: ~83% of dose excreted in the urine (1.2% as unchanged drug, 30% as 5'-carboxylic acid metabolite, 36% as the glucuronide, and 15% as other metabolites); 16% eliminated in feces

Clearance (apparent): Single dose 8 mg/kg:

Infants ≥3 months and Children ≤13 years: 17.84 mL/minute/kg

Adults: 10.14 mL/minute/kg

Usual Dosage Oral (use in combination with other antiretroviral agents):

Neonates: Not approved for use

Infants 1-3 months: Not approved for use; doses of 8 mg/kg twice daily are being studied

Infants ≥3 months, Children, and Adolescents: 8 mg/kg twice daily (maximum: 300 mg twice daily)

Adults: 300 mg twice daily

Administration Oral: May be administered without regard to food

Monitoring Parameters Signs and symptoms of hypersensitivity reaction; serum glucose and triglycerides, viral load, CD4 counts

Patient Information Abacavir is not a cure for HIV. Take abacavir everyday as prescribed; do not change dose or discontinue without physician's advice. If abacavir is stopped for any reason, notify physician before restarting therapy. If a dose is missed, take it as soon as possible, then return to normal dosing schedule; if a dose is skipped, do **not** double the next dose

Stop taking abacavir and notify physician immediately if skin rash or 2 or more of the following sets of symptoms occur: Fever, GI symptoms (nausea, vomiting, diarrhea or abdominal pain), flu-like symptoms (severe tiredness, achiness, or generally ill feeling), or respiratory symptoms (sore throat, shortness of breath, cough). If you experience an allergic (hypersensitivity) reaction to abacavir (or Ziagen® or Trizivir®), **never** take abacavir (or Ziagen® or Trizivir®) again.

(Continued)

Abacavir *(Continued)*

HIV medications may cause changes in body fat, including an increase in fat in the upper back and neck, breasts, and trunk; a loss of fat from the face, arms, and legs may also occur.

Nursing Implications Inform patients of the possibility of a fatal hypersensitivity reaction and the signs and symptoms (see Warnings)

Additional Information The patient Medication Guide, which includes written manufacturer information, should be dispensed to the patient with each new prescription and refill; the Warning Card describing the hypersensitivity reaction should be given to the patient to carry with them. A familial predisposition to the abacavir hypersensitivity reaction has been reported; use abacavir with great caution in children of parents who experience a hypersensitivity reaction to abacavir (see Peyriére, 2001). Recent stories have identified genetic markers which may help predict which patients are at risk for developing the abacavir hypersensitivity reaction; further studies are needed (see Hetherington, 2002 and Mallal, 2002). Oral solution contains methylparaben and propylparaben (preservatives) and propylene glycol

Reverse transcriptase mutations of K65R, L74V, Y115F, and M184V have been associated with abacavir resistance; at least 2-3 mutations are needed to decrease HIV susceptibility by 10-fold. A recent multicenter study, conducted in previously untreated HIV-infected children (median age: 5.3 years; range: 0.3-16.7 years), demonstrated that abacavir-containing antiretroviral regimens were more effective than regimens containing the NRTI combination of zidovudine and lamivudine; after adjusting for use of nelfinavir and controlling for baseline factors, the NRTI combination of abacavir and lamivudine showed the largest and most durable reduction in viral load, compared to the combination of zidovudine and lamivudine or zidovudine and abacavir; further studies are needed (see Penta, 2002).

Dosage Forms Available as abacavir sulfate; mg strength refers to abacavir
Solution, oral: 20 mg/mL (240 mL) [strawberry-banana flavor]
Tablet: 300 mg

References

Center for Disease Control and Prevention, "Guidelines for Using Antiretroviral Agents Among HIV-Infected Adults and Adolescents. Recommendations of the Panel on Clinical Practices for Treatment of HIV," *MMWR*, 2002, 51(RR-7):1-55.

Collura JM and Kraus DM, "New Pediatric Antiretroviral Agents," *J Pediatr Health Care*, 2000, 14(4):183-90.

Foster RH and Faulds D, "Abacavir," *Drugs*, 1998, 55(5):729-36.

Hetherington S, Hughes AR, Mosteller M, et al, "Genetic Variations in HLA-B Region and Hypersensitivity Reactions to Abacavir," *Lancet*, 2002, 359(9312):1121-2.

Hughes W, McDowell JA, Shenep J, et al, "Safety and Single-Dose Pharmacokinetics of Abacavir (1592U89) in Human Immunodeficiency Virus Type 1-Infected Children," *Antimicrob Agents Chemother*, 1999, 43(3):609-15.

Kline MW, Blanchard S, Fletcher CV, et al, "A Phase I Study of Abacavir (1592U89) Alone and in Combination With Other Antiretroviral Agents in Infants and Children With Human Immunodeficiency Virus Infection," *Pediatrics*, 1999, 103(4):e47; http://www.pediatrics.org/cgi/content/full/103/4/e47.

Mallal S, Nolan D, Witt C, et al, "Association Between Presence of HLA-B•5701, HLA-DR7, and HLA-DQ3 and Hypersensitivity to HIV-1 Reverse-Transcriptase Inhibitor Abacavir," *Lancet*, 2002, 359(9308):727-32.

Paediatric European Network for Treatment of AIDS (PENTA), "Comparison of Dual Nucleoside-Analogue Reverse-Transcriptase Inhibitor Regimens With and Without Nelfinavir in Children with HIV-1 Who Have Not Previously Been Treated: The PENTA 5 Randomised Trial," *Lancet*, 2002, 359(9308):733-40.

Panel on Clinical Practices for Treatment of HIV Infection, "Guidelines for the Use of Antiretroviral Agents in HIV-Infected Adults and Adolescents," February 4, 2002, http://www.aidsinfo.nih.gov.

Peyriére H, Nicolas J, Siffert M, et al, "Hypersensitivity Related to Abacavir in Two Members of a Family," *Ann Pharmacother*, 2001, 35(10):1291-2.

Working Group on Antiretroviral Therapy and Medical Management of HIV-Infected Children, "Guidelines for the Use of Antiretroviral Agents in Pediatric HIV Infection," December 14, 2001, http://www.aidsinfo.nih.gov.

Working Group on Antiretroviral Therapy and Medical Management of HIV-Infected Children, "Guidelines for the Use of Antiretroviral Agents in Pediatric HIV Infection. Hyperlink Supplement I: Pediatric Antiretroviral Drug Information," December 14, 2001, http://www.aidsinfo.nih.gov.

♦ **Abacavir, 3TC, and AZT** *see* Abacavir, Lamivudine, and Zidovudine *on page 32*
♦ **Abacavir, 3TC, and ZDV** *see* Abacavir, Lamivudine, and Zidovudine *on page 32*
♦ **Abacavir, Lamivudine, and Azidothymidine** *see* Abacavir, Lamivudine, and Zidovudine *on page 32*

Abacavir, Lamivudine, and Zidovudine

(uh BACK ah veer, la MI vyoo deen, & zye DOE vyoo deen)

U.S. Brand Names Trizivir®

Synonyms Abacavir, 3TC, and AZT; Abacavir, 3TC, and ZDV; Abacavir, Lamivudine, and Azidothymidine; Abacavir, Zidovudine, and Lamivudine; ABC, 3TC, and AZT; ABC, 3TC, and ZDV; Azidothymidine, Abacavir, and Lamivudine; Azidothymidine, Lamivudine and Abacavir; AZT, Abacavir, and 3TC; AZT, Abacavir, and Lamivudine; AZT, ABC, and 3TC; Compound S, Abacavir, and 3TC; Compound S, Abacavir, and

Lamivudine; Compound S, ABC, and 3TC; Lamivudine, Abacavir, and Zidovudine; Lamivudine, Zidovudine, and Abacavir; 3TC, Abacavir, and AZT; 3TC, Abacavir, and ZDV; 3TC, Abacavir, and Zidovudine; 3TC, ABC, and AZT; 3TC, ABC, and ZDV; ZDV, Abacavir, and 3TC; ZDV, Abacavir, and Lamivudine; ZDV, ABC, and 3TC; Zidovudine, Abacavir, and Lamivudine

Therapeutic Category Antiretroviral Agent; HIV Agents (Anti-HIV Agents); Nucleoside Analog Reverse Transcriptase Inhibitor (NRTI)

Generic Available No

Use Treatment of HIV-1 infection (either alone or in combination with other antiretroviral agents) (**Note:** HIV regimens consisting of **three** antiretroviral agents are strongly recommended; data on the use of this triple NRTI combination regimen in patients with baseline viral loads >100,000 copies/mL is limited)

Pregnancy Risk Factor C

Contraindications Hypersensitivity to abacavir, lamivudine, zidovudine, or any component. **Do not rechallenge** patients who have experienced hypersensitivity reactions to abacavir, potentially fatal hypersensitivity reactions may occur (see Warnings)

Warnings Fatal hypersensitivity reactions to abacavir may occur; discontinue therapy immediately in patients who show signs or symptoms of hypersensitivity reaction such as fever, fatigue, skin rash, respiratory symptoms (cough, dyspnea, pharyngitis) and GI symptoms (nausea, vomiting, diarrhea, or abdominal pain). Carefully consider the diagnosis of hypersensitivity reaction in patients who present with acute onset respiratory symptoms, even if other diagnoses, such as bronchitis, flu-like illness, pharyngitis, or pneumonia, are possible. Skin rash may be maculopapular or urticarial, but can be variable in appearance; erythema multiforme has been reported; hypersensitivity reaction may occur without a rash. Other symptoms may include edema, lethargy, malaise, arthralgia, myolysis, myalgia, paresthesia, shortness of breath, mouth ulcerations, conjunctivitis, headache, lymphadenopathy, and abnormal findings on chest x-ray (ie, infiltrates that can be localized). Laboratory abnormalities include increases in liver function tests, elevated CPK or serum creatinine, and lymphopenia.

Do not restart abacavir or Trizivir® after a hypersensitivity reaction occurs; more severe symptoms can recur within hours and may include: Anaphylaxis, renal failure, hepatic failure, respiratory failure, ARDS, life-threatening hypotension, and death. Fatal hypersensitivity reactions have occurred following the reintroduction of abacavir in patients whose therapy was interrupted for other reasons. These patients had no identified history or had unrecognized symptoms of abacavir hypersensitivity. Reactions occurred within hours. In some cases, signs of a hypersensitivity reaction may have been previously present, but attributed to other medical conditions (acute onset respiratory diseases, gastroenteritis, reactions to other medications). If abacavir or Trizivir® is to be restarted following an interruption in therapy, the patient must first be evaluated for previously unsuspected symptoms of hypersensitivity. **Do not restart** abacavir or Trizivir® if hypersensitivity is suspected or cannot be ruled out. Hypersensitivity reactions occur in ~5 % of adult and pediatric patients; most hypersensitivity reactions occur within the first 6 weeks of therapy, but can occur at any time; call the Abacavir Hypersensitivity Reaction Registry at 1-800-270-0425 to facilitate reporting and collection of information on patients experiencing abacavir hypersensitivity reactions (see Additional Information).

Cases of lactic acidosis, severe hepatomegaly with steatosis, and death have been reported in patients receiving nucleoside analogues; prolonged nucleoside use, obesity, and prior liver disease may be risk factors; use with extreme caution in patients with other risk factors for liver disease; discontinue Trizivir® in patients who develop laboratory or clinical evidence of lactic acidosis or pronounced hepatotoxicity.

The major clinical toxicity of lamivudine in pediatric patients is pancreatitis; discontinue therapy if clinical signs, symptoms, or laboratory abnormalities suggestive of pancreatitis occur. Zidovudine is associated with hematologic toxicity including granulocytopenia and severe anemia requiring transfusions; use with caution in patients with ANC <1000 cells/mm³ or hemoglobin <9.5 g/dL; discontinue treatment in children with an ANC <500 cells/mm³ until marrow recovery is observed; use of erythropoietin, or filgrastim may be necessary in some patients; prolonged use of zidovudine may cause myositis and myopathy; zidovudine has been shown to be carcinogenic in rats and mice.

Trizivir® contains abacavir, lamivudine, and zidovudine as a fixed-dose combination; do not use in patients weighing <40 kg, in patients with renal dysfunction (Cl$_{cr}$ ≤50 mL/minute) who require lamivudine and zidovudine dosage adjustment, or in patients with hepatic dysfunction (mild to moderate hepatic dysfunction or liver cirrhosis) who (Continued)

Abacavir, Lamivudine, and Zidovudine *(Continued)*

require zidovudine dosage adjustment. Concomitant use of Trizivir® with abacavir, lamivudine, or zidovudine is not recommended.

Precautions Fat redistribution and accumulation [ie, central obesity, peripheral wasting, facial wasting, breast enlargement, dorsocervical fat enlargement (buffalo hump), and cushingoid appearance] have been observed in patients receiving antiretroviral agents (causal relationship not established). Resistance to abacavir develops relatively slowly, but cross resistance between abacavir and other nucleoside reverse transcriptase inhibitors (NRTIs) may occur; limited response may be seen in patients with HIV isolates containing multiple mutations conferring resistance to NRTIs or in patients with a prolonged prior NRTI exposure. HIV-infected patients who are coinfected with hepatitis B may experience clinical symptoms or laboratory evidence of hepatitis when lamivudine is discontinued; most cases are self-limited, but fatalities have been reported; monitor patients closely for at least several months after discontinuation of abacavir, lamivudine, and zidovudine.

Systemic exposure of abacavir at 6-32 times the normal human exposure, increased the incidence of tumors (malignant and nonmalignant) in mice and rats; myocardial degeneration was seen in mice and rats receiving abacavir for 2 years at 7-24 times the expected human exposure; the clinical relevance of these 2 findings is currently unknown

Adverse Reactions See Abacavir *on page 30*, Lamivudine *on page 650*, and Zidovudine *on page 1163*

Drug Interactions See Abacavir *on page 30*, Lamivudine *on page 650*, and Zidovudine *on page 1163*

Food Interactions Food decreases the rate, but not the extent of absorption (see Yuen, 2001).

Stability Store at room temperature 25°C (77°F)

Mechanism of Action See Abacavir *on page 30*, Lamivudine *on page 650*, and Zidovudine *on page 1163*

Pharmacokinetics One Trizivir® tablet is bioequivalent, in the extent (AUC) and rate of absorption (peak concentration and time to peak concentration), to one abacavir 300 mg tablet, one lamivudine 150 mg tablet, plus one zidovudine 300 mg tablet; See Abacavir *on page 30*, Lamivudine *on page 650*, and Zidovudine *on page 1163*

Usual Dosage Oral:

Children: Not intended for pediatric use; product is a fixed-dose combination

Adolescents and Adults:

<40 kg: Not recommended; product is a fixed-dose combination

≥40 kg: 1 tablet twice daily

Dosage adjustment in hepatic impairment: Mild to moderate hepatic dysfunction or liver cirrhosis: Not recommended (use individual antiretroviral agents to reduce dosage)

Dosage adjustment in renal impairment: Cl_{cr} ≤50 mL/minute: Not recommended (use individual antiretroviral agents to reduce dosage)

Administration May be administered without regard to meals

Monitoring Parameters Signs and symptoms of abacavir hypersensitivity reaction, lactic acidosis, pronounced hepatotoxicity, anemia, bone marrow suppression, and pancreatitis; serum glucose and triglycerides, viral load, CD4 counts, CBC with differential, platelets, hemoglobin, MCV, reticulocyte count, liver enzymes, serum amylase, bilirubin, renal and hepatic function tests

Patient Information Trizivir® is not a cure for HIV. Take Trizivir® every day as prescribed; do not change dose or discontinue without physician's advice. If Trizivir® is stopped for any reason, notify physician before restarting therapy. If a dose is missed, take it as soon as possible, then return to normal dosing schedule; if a dose is skipped, do **not** double the next dose. Avoid alcohol. Notify physician if persistent severe abdominal pain, nausea, or vomiting occurs.

Trizivir® contains abacavir (also called Ziagen®). Abacavir may cause a potentially fatal allergic (hypersensitivity) reaction. Stop taking Trizivir® and notify physician immediately if skin rash or 2 more of the following sets of symptoms occur: Fever, GI symptoms (nausea, vomiting, diarrhea, or abdominal pain), flu-like symptoms (severe tiredness, achiness, or generally ill feeling), or respiratory symptoms (sore throat, shortness of breath, cough). If you experience an allergic (hypersensitivity) reaction to Trizivir® (or abacavir or Ziagen®), **never** take Trizivir®, abacavir or Ziagen® again.

HIV medications may cause changes in body fat, including an increase in fat in the upper back and neck, breasts, and trunk; a loss of fat from the face, arms, and legs may also occur.

Nursing Implications Inform patients of the possibility of a fatal abacavir hypersensitivity reaction and the signs and symptoms (see Warnings and Patient Information)

Additional Information The Patient Medication Guide, which includes written manufacturer information, should be dispensed to the patient with each new prescription and refill; a Warning Card describing the hypersensitivity reaction should be given to the patient to carry with them

Dosage Forms Tablet: Abacavir 300 mg [as abacavir sulfate], lamivudine 150 mg, and zidovudine 300 mg

References

Center for Disease Control and Prevention, "Guidelines for Using Antiretroviral Agents Among HIV-Infected Adults and Adolescents. Recommendations of the Panel on Clinical Practices for Treatment of HIV," *MMWR*, 2002, 51(RR-7):1-55.

Panel on Clinical Practices for Treatment of HIV Infection, "Guidelines for the Use of Antiretroviral Agents in HIV-Infected Adults and Adolescents," February 4, 2002, http://www.aidsinfo.nih.gov.

Saez-Llorens X, Nelson RP, Emmanuel P, et al, "A Randomized, Double-Blind Study of Triple Nucleoside Therapy of Abacavir, Lamivudine, and Zidovudine Versus Lamivudine and Zidovudine in Previously Treated Human Immunodeficiency Virus Type 1-Infected Children," *Pediatrics*, 2001, 107(1), URL: http://www.pediatrics.org/cgi/content/full/107/1/e4.

Yuen GJ, Lou Y, Thompson NF, et al, "Abacavir/Lamivudine/Zidovudine as a Combined Formulation Tablet: Bioequivalence Compared With Each Component Administered Concurrently and the Effect of Food on Absorption," *J Clin Pharmacol*, 2001, 41(3):277-88.

♦ **Abacavir, Zidovudine, and Lamivudine** *see* Abacavir, Lamivudine, and Zidovudine *on page 32*

♦ **Abbokinase®** *see* Urokinase *on page 1127*

♦ **ABC, 3TC, and AZT** *see* Abacavir, Lamivudine, and Zidovudine *on page 32*

♦ **ABC, 3TC, and ZDV** *see* Abacavir, Lamivudine, and Zidovudine *on page 32*

♦ **Abelcet®** *see* Amphotericin B Lipid Complex *on page 100*

♦ **Abenol® (Can)** *see* Acetaminophen *on page 36*

♦ **ABLC** *see* Amphotericin B Lipid Complex *on page 100*

♦ **Absorbine Jr.® Antifungal [OTC]** *see* Tolnaftate *on page 1102*

♦ **ABT-378/Ritonavir** *see* Lopinavir and Ritonavir *on page 688*

Acarbose (AY car bose)

U.S. Brand Names Precose®

Canadian Brand Names Prandase®

Therapeutic Category Antidiabetic Agent, Oral; Antidiabetic Agent, Alpha-glucosidase Inhibitor

Generic Available No

Use Management of type II diabetes mellitus (noninsulin-dependent, NIDDM) when hyperglycemia cannot be managed by diet alone; may be used concomitantly with metformin, a sulfonylurea, or insulin to improve glycemic control

Pregnancy Risk Factor B

Contraindications Hypersensitivity to acarbose or any component; diabetic ketoacidosis; cirrhosis; patients with inflammatory bowel disease, colonic ulceration, partial intestinal obstruction, or patients predisposed to intestinal obstruction; patients who have chronic intestinal diseases associated with marked disorders of digestion or absorption; patients who have conditions that may deteriorate as a result of increased gas formation in the intestine

Warnings Dose-related elevations in serum transaminases occurred in 15% of acarbose-treated patients in long-term studies; these elevations were asymptomatic, reversible, more common in females, and not associated with other evidence of liver dysfunction; acarbose serum levels are proportionately higher in patients with renal dysfunction (S_{cr} >2 mg/dL); until long term clinical studies are completed, use in renally-compromised patients is not recommended

Precautions Hypoglycemia may occur when used in combination with sulfonylureas or insulin; oral glucose (absorption is not affected by acarbose) should be used instead of sucrose (table sugar) for the treatment of mild to moderate hypoglycemia

Adverse Reactions

Central nervous system: Headache, vertigo, drowsiness

Dermatologic: Urticaria, erythema

Endocrine & metabolic: Hypoglycemia

Gastrointestinal: Abdominal pain, diarrhea, flatulence

Hepatic: Elevated liver enzymes

Neuromuscular & skeletal: Weakness

Drug Interactions Drugs that produce hyperglycemia (eg, diuretics, corticosteroids, phenothiazines, thyroid products, estrogens, oral contraceptives, phenytoin, nicotinic acid, sympathomimetics, calcium channel blocking drugs, rifampin, and isoniazid) may lead to a loss of glycemic control; intestinal adsorbents; digestive enzyme preparations; decreases bioavailability of digoxin resulting in decreased serum levels

Mechanism of Action Competitive inhibitor of pancreatic α-glucosidases, resulting in delayed hydrolysis of ingested complex carbohydrates and disaccharides and (Continued)

Acarbose *(Continued)*

absorption of glucose; dose-dependent reduction in postprandial serum insulin and glucose peaks; inhibits the metabolism of sucrose to glucose and fructose

Pharmacodynamics Average decrease in fasting blood sugar: 20-30 mg/dL

Pharmacokinetics

Absorption: <2% absorbed as active drug

Metabolism: Metabolized exclusively within the GI tract, principally by intestinal bacteria and by digestive enzymes; 13 metabolites have been identified

Bioavailability: Low systemic bioavailability of parent compound

Elimination: Fraction absorbed as intact drug is almost completely excreted in urine

Usual Dosage Oral:

Adolescents and Adults: Dosage must be individualized on the basis of effectiveness and tolerance; do not exceed the maximum recommended dose (use slow titration to prevent or minimize GI effects):

Initial: 25 mg 3 times/day; increase in 25 mg/day increments in 2-4 week intervals to maximum dose

Maximum dose:

Patients ≤60 kg: 50 mg 3 times/day

Patients >60 kg: 100 mg 3 times/day

Dosing adjustment in renal impairment: See Warnings

Administration Oral: Administer with first bite of each main meal

Monitoring Parameters Fasting blood glucose; hemoglobin A_{1c}; liver enzymes every 3 months for the first year of therapy and periodically thereafter

Reference Range Target range:

Blood glucose: Fasting and preprandial: 80-120 mg/dL; bedtime: 100-140 mg/dL

Glycosylated hemoglobin (hemoglobin A_{1c}): <7%

Additional Information Acarbose has been used successfully to treat postprandial hypoglycemia in children with Nissen fundoplications. Six children (4-25 months) initially received 12.5 mg before each bolus feeding of formula containing complex carbohydrates. The dosage was increased in 12.5 mg increments (dosage range: 12.5-50 mg per dose) until postprandial serum glucose was stable ≥60 mg/dL. Most commonly reported side effects were flatulence, abdominal distension, and diarrhea (Ng, 2001).

Dosage Forms Tablet: 25 mg, 50 mg, 100 mg

References

DeFronzo RA, "Pharmacologic Therapy for Type 2 Diabetes Mellitus," *Ann Intern Med*, 1999, 131(4):281-303.

Ng DD, Ferry RJ Jr, Kelly A, et al, "Acarbose Treatment of Postprandial Hypoglycemia in Children After Nissen Fundoplication," *J Pediatr*, 2001, 139(6):877-9.

♦ **Accolate**® *see Zafirlukast on page 1160*

♦ **AccuNeb**™ *see Albuterol on page 54*

♦ **Accutane**® *see Isotretinoin on page 632*

♦ **Acephen**® **[OTC]** *see Acetaminophen on page 36*

Acetaminophen *(a seet a MIN oh fen)*

Related Information

Acetaminophen Toxicity Nomogram *on page 1403*

Carbohydrate and Alcohol Content of Liquid Medications for Use in Patients Receiving Ketogenic Diets *on page 1431*

OTC Cough & Cold Preparations, Pediatric *on page 1225*

Overdose and Toxicology *on page 1388*

U.S. Brand Names Acephen® [OTC]; Aspirin Free Anacin® Maximum Strength; Cetafen® [OTC]; Cetafen Extra® [OTC]; Feverall® [OTC]; Genapap® [OTC]; Genapap®, Children [OTC]; Genapap® Extra Strength [OTC]; Genapap®, Infant [OTC]; Genebs® [OTC]; Genebs® Extra Strength [OTC]; Infantaire® [OTC]; Liquiprin® for Children [OTC]; Mapap® [OTC]; Mapap®, Children's [OTC]; Mapap® Extra Strength [OTC]; Mapap®, Infants [OTC]; Redutemp® [OTC]; Silapap®, Children's [OTC]; Silapap®, Infant's [OTC]; Tylenol® [OTC]; Tylenol® Arthritis Pain [OTC]; Tylenol®, Children's [OTC]; Tylenol® Extra Strength [OTC]; Tylenol®, Infants [OTC]; Tylenol®, Junior Strength [OTC]; Tylenol® Sore Throat [OTC]; Valorin [OTC]; Valorin Extra [OTC]

Canadian Brand Names Abenol®; Apo®-Acetaminophen; Atasol®; Pediatrix; Tempra®

Synonyms APAP; N-Acetyl-P-Aminophenol; Paracetamol

Therapeutic Category Analgesic, Non-narcotic; Antipyretic

Generic Available Yes

Use Treatment of mild to moderate pain and fever; does not have antirheumatic or systemic anti-inflammatory effects

Pregnancy Risk Factor B

Contraindications Hypersensitivity to acetaminophen or any component

Warnings May cause severe hepatic toxicity with overdose. Some elixir preparations (Children Genapap® elixir) contain sodium benzoate; benzoic acid (benzoate) is a metabolite of benzyl alcohol; large amounts of benzyl alcohol (≥99 mg/kg/day) have been associated with a potentially fatal toxicity ("gasping syndrome") in neonates; the "gasping syndrome" consists of metabolic acidosis, respiratory distress, gasping respirations, CNS dysfunction (including convulsions, intracranial hemorrhage), hypotension and cardiovascular collapse; avoid use of acetaminophen products containing sodium benzoate in neonates; *in vitro* and animal studies have shown that benzoate displaces bilirubin from protein binding sites

Precautions Some products (eg, chewable tablets) contain aspartame which is metabolized to phenylalanine and must be avoided (or used with caution) in patients with phenylketonuria.

G-6-PD deficiency: Although several case reports of acetaminophen-associated hemolytic anemia have been reported in patients with G-6-PD deficiency, a direct cause and effect relationship has not been well established (concurrent illnesses such as fever or infection may precipitate hemolytic anemia in patients with G-6-PD deficiency); therefore, acetaminophen is generally thought to be safe when given in therapeutic doses to patients with G-6-PD deficiency.

Adverse Reactions
Dermatologic: Rash
Hematologic: Blood dyscrasias (neutropenia, pancytopenia, leukopenia)
Hepatic: Hepatic necrosis with overdose
Renal: Renal injury with chronic use
Miscellaneous: Hypersensitivity reactions (rare)

Drug Interactions Cytochrome P450 isoenzyme CYP1A2 substrate (minor), CYP2A6, CYP2C9, CYP2D6, CYP2E1 and CYP3A3/4 isoenzyme substrate
Enzyme inducers (barbiturates, carbamazepine, phenytoin, rifampin), carmustine (with high dose acetaminophen), isoniazid, alcohol (especially chronic use) can increase hepatotoxicity; rifampin may decrease acetaminophen's therapeutic effect; anticholinergic agents (scopolamine) may effect GI absorption; acetaminophen may increase the clearance of lamotrigine; acetaminophen may increase zidovudine concentration and toxicity

Food Interactions Rate of absorption may be decreased when given with food high in carbohydrates

Mechanism of Action Inhibits the synthesis of prostaglandins in the CNS and peripherally blocks pain impulse generation; produces antipyresis from inhibition of hypothalamic heat-regulating center

Pharmacokinetics
Protein binding: 20% to 50%
Metabolism: At normal therapeutic dosages the parent compound is metabolized in the liver to sulfate and glucuronide metabolites, while a small amount is metabolized by microsomal mixed function oxidases to a highly reactive intermediate (N-acetyl-imidoquinone) which is conjugated with glutathione and inactivated; at toxic doses (as little as 4 g in a single day) glutathione can become depleted, and conjugation becomes insufficient to meet the metabolic demand causing an increase in N-acetyl-imidoquinone concentration, which is thought to cause hepatic cell necrosis.
Half-life:
Neonates: 2-5 hours
Adults: 1-3 hours
Time to peak serum concentration: 10-60 minutes after normal oral doses, but may be delayed in acute overdoses

Usual Dosage
Neonates: Oral, rectal: 10-15 mg/kg/dose every 6-8 hours as needed
International Evidence-Based Group for Neonatal Pain recommendations (Anand, 2001; Anand, 2002):
Preterm infants 28-32 weeks:
Oral: 10-12 mg/kg/dose every 6-8 hours; maximum daily dose: 40 mg/kg/day
Rectal: 20 mg/kg/dose every 12 hours; maximum daily dose: 40 mg/kg/day
Preterm infants 32-36 weeks and term infants <10 days:
Oral: 10-15 mg/kg/dose every 6 hours; maximum daily dose: 60 mg/kg/day
Rectal: Loading dose: 30 mg/kg; then 15 mg/kg/dose every 8 hours; maximum daily dose: 60 mg/kg/day
Term infants ≥10 days:
Oral: 10-15 mg/kg/dose every 4-6 hours; maximum daily dose: 90 mg/kg/day
Rectal: Loading dose: 30 mg/kg; then 20 mg/kg/dose every 6-8 hours; maximum daily dose: 90 mg/kg/day

(Continued)

Acetaminophen *(Continued)*

Infants and Children:

Oral: 10-15 mg/kg/dose every 4-6 hours as needed; do **not** exceed 5 doses in 24 hours; alternatively, the following doses may be used. See table.

Acetaminophen Dosing (Oral)*

Weight (lbs)	Age	Dosage (mg)
6-11	0-3 mo	40
12-17	4-11 mo	80
18-23	1-2 y	120
24-35	2-3 y	160
36-47	4-5 y	240
48-59	6-8 y	320
60-71	9-10 y	400
72-95	11 y	480

*Manufacturer's recommendations; use of weight to select dose is preferred; if weight is not available, then use age

Rectal: 10-20 mg/kg/dose every 4-6 hours as needed. **Note:** Although the perioperative use of high-dose rectal acetaminophen (eg, 25-45 mg/kg/dose) has been investigated in several studies, its routine use remains controversial; optimal doses and dosing frequency to ensure efficacy and safety have not yet been established; further studies are needed (see Buck, 2001).

Children ≥12 years and Adults: Oral, rectal: 325-650 every 4-6 hours or 1000 mg 3-4 times/day; do **not** exceed 4 g/day

Administration Oral: Administer with food to decrease GI upset; shake suspension well before use; do not crush or chew extended release products

Reference Range Acute ingestions: Toxic concentration with probable hepatotoxicity: >200 µg/mL at 4 hours or 50 µg/mL at 12 hours after ingestion of overdose

Patient Information Avoid alcohol; do not take longer than 10 days without physician's advice

Additional Information Drops contain saccharin

Acetaminophen (15 mg/kg/dose given orally every 6 hours for 24 hours) did **not** relieve the intraoperative or the immediate postoperative pain associated with neonatal circumcision; some benefit was seen 6 hours after circumcision (see Howard, 1994).

There is currently no scientific evidence to support alternating acetaminophen with ibuprofen in the treatment of fever (see Mayoral, 2000).

Dosage Forms Most commonly available concentrations for nonsolid dosage forms are **bolded** when more than one concentration is available

Caplet (Genapap® Extra Strength, Genebs® Extra Strength, Tylenol® Extra Strength): 500 mg

Caplet, extended release (Tylenol® Arthritis Pain): 650 mg

Capsule (Mapap® Extra Strength): 500 mg

Drops: See Solution, oral **drops**; suspension, oral **drops**

Elixir: 160 mg/5 mL (5 mL, 10 mL, 20 mL, 120 mL, 240 mL, 500 mL, 3780 mL)

Children Genapap®: 160 mg/5 mL (120 mL) [contains sodium benzoate; cherry and grape flavors]

Children's Silapap®: 160 mg/5 mL (120 mL, 240 mL, 480 mL)

Gelcap (Genapap® Extra Strength, Tylenol® Extra Strength): 500 mg

Geltab (Tylenol® Extra Strength): 500 mg

Liquid, oral: **160 mg/5 mL** (120 mL, 240 mL, 480 mL, 3870 mL); 500 mg/15 mL (240 mL)

Redutemp®: 500 mg/15 mL (120 mL)

Tylenol® Sore Throat: 500 mg/15 mL (240 mL) [cherry and honey lemon flavors]

Solution, oral **drops**: 100 mg/mL (15 mL, 30 mL) [droppers are marked at 0.4 mL (40 mg) and at 0.8 mL (80 mg)]

Infant Genapap®: 80 mg/0.8 mL (15 mL)

Infantaire®, Infant's Silapap®: 80 mg/0.8 mL (15 mL, 30 mL)

Liquiprin® for Children: 80 mg/0.8 mL (30 mL)

Suppository, rectal: 80 mg, 120 mg, 325 mg, 650 mg

Acephen®: 120 mg, 325 mg, 650 mg

Feverall®: 80 mg, 120 mg, 325 mg

Mapap®: 120 mg, 650 mg

Suspension, oral: 160 mg/5 mL (120 mL)

Children's Mapap®: 160 mg/5 mL (120 mL) [cherry, grape, and bubblegum flavors]

Children's Tylenol®: 160 mg/5 mL (120 mL, 240 mL) [cherry, grape, and bubblegum flavors]

Suspension, oral **drops**: 100 mg/mL (15 mL, 30 mL) [droppers are marked at 0.4 mL (40 mg) and at 0.8 mL (80 mg)]

Infants Mapap®: 80 mg/0.8 mL (15 mL, 30 mL) [cherry flavor]

Infants Tylenol®: 80 mg/0.8 mL (15 mL, 30 mL) [cherry and grape flavors]

Syrup, oral: 160 mg/5 mL (120 mL)

Tablet: 160 mg, 325 mg, 500 mg

Aspirin Free Anacin® Maximum Strength, Cetafen Extra®, Genapap® Extra Strength, Genebs® Extra Strength, Mapap® Extra Strength, Redutemp®, Tylenol® Extra Strength, Valorin Extra: 500 mg

Cetafen®, Genapap®, Genebs®, Tylenol®, Valorin: 325 mg

Mapap® 160 mg, 325 mg

Tablet, chewable: 80 mg, 160 mg

Children Genapap®, Children's Mapap®: 80 mg [contains 3 mg phenylalanine (as aspartame)/tablet; fruit and grape flavors]

Children's Tylenol®: 80 mg [bubblegum flavor contains 6 mg phenylalanine (as aspartame)/tablet; fruit and grape flavors contain 3 mg phenylalanine (as aspartame)/tablet]

Junior Strength Tylenol®: 160 mg [contains 6 mg phenylalanine (as aspartame)/tablet; fruit and grape flavors]

References

American Academy of Pediatrics: Committee on Drugs, "Acetaminophen Toxicity in Children," *Pediatrics*, 2001, 108(4):1020-4.

Anand KJ and International Evidence-Based Group for Neonatal Pain, "Consensus Statement for the Prevention and Management of Pain in the Newborn," *Arch Pediatr Adolesc Med*, 2001, 155(2):173-80.

Anand KJ, Chair, International Evidence-Based Group for Neonatal Pain, personal correspondence, April 2002.

Buck ML, "Perioperative Use of High-Dose Rectal Acetaminophen," *Pediatr Pharm*, 2001, 7(9), http://www.medscape.com/viewarticle/415082.

Howard CR, Howard FM, and Weitzman ML, "Acetaminophen Analgesia in Neonatal Circumcision: The Effect on Pain," *Pediatrics*, 1994, 93(4):641-646.

Mayoral CE, Marino RV, Rosenfeld W, et al, "Alternating Antipyretics: Is This An Alternative?" *Pediatrics*, 2000, 105(5):1009-12.

Acetaminophen and Codeine (a seet a MIN oh fen & KOE deen)

Related Information

Carbohydrate and Alcohol Content of Liquid Medications for Use in Patients Receiving Ketogenic Diets *on page 1431*

Overdose and Toxicology *on page 1388*

U.S. Brand Names Capital® and Codeine; Phenaphen® With Codeine; Tylenol® With Codeine

Canadian Brand Names Emtec-30; Lenoltec; Triatec-8; Triatec-8 Strong; Triatec-30

Synonyms Codeine and Acetaminophen

Therapeutic Category Analgesic, Narcotic

Generic Available Yes

Use Relief of mild to moderate pain

Restrictions C-III; C-V

Pregnancy Risk Factor C

Contraindications Hypersensitivity to acetaminophen, codeine phosphate, or any component (see Warnings)

Warnings Some tablets contain metabisulfite which may cause allergic reactions in susceptible individuals. Tylenol® With Codeine elixir contains sodium benzoate; benzoic acid (benzoate) is a metabolite of benzyl alcohol; large amounts of benzyl alcohol (≥99 mg/kg/day) have been associated with a potentially fatal toxicity ("gasping syndrome") in neonates; the "gasping syndrome" consists of metabolic acidosis, respiratory distress, gasping respirations, CNS dysfunction (including convulsions, intracranial hemorrhage), hypotension and cardiovascular collapse; avoid use of acetaminophen and codeine products containing sodium benzoate in neonates; *in vitro* and animal studies have shown that benzoate displaces bilirubin from protein binding sites

Precautions Use with caution in patients with hypersensitivity reactions to other phenanthrene derivative opioid agonists (morphine, hydrocodone, hydromorphone, levorphanol, oxycodone, oxymorphone) or respiratory disease/compromise.

G-6-PD deficiency: Although several case reports of acetaminophen-associated hemolytic anemia have been reported in patients with G-6-PD deficiency, a direct cause and effect relationship has not been well established (concurrent illnesses such as fever or infection may precipitate hemolytic anemia in patients with G-6-PD deficiency); therefore, acetaminophen is generally thought to be safe when given in therapeutic doses to patients with G-6-PD deficiency.

(Continued)

Acetaminophen and Codeine *(Continued)*

Adverse Reactions
Acetaminophen:
Dermatologic: Rash
Hematologic: Blood dyscrasias (neutropenia, pancytopenia, leukopenia)
Hepatic: Hepatic necrosis with overdose
Renal: Renal injury with chronic use
Miscellaneous: Hypersensitivity reactions (rare)
Codeine:
Cardiovascular: Palpitations, hypotension, bradycardia, peripheral vasodilation
Central nervous system: CNS depression, dizziness, drowsiness, sedation, elevated intracranial pressure
Dermatologic: Pruritus
Endocrine & metabolic: Antidiuretic hormone release
Gastrointestinal: Nausea, vomiting, constipation, biliary tract spasm
Genitourinary: Urinary retention
Ocular: Miosis
Respiratory: Respiratory depression
Miscellaneous: Histamine release, physical and psychological dependence with prolonged use

Drug Interactions See Acetaminophen *on page 36* and Codeine *on page 301*
Food Interactions Rate of absorption of acetaminophen may be decreased when given with food high in carbohydrates
Mechanism of Action See individual monographs for Acetaminophen *on page 36* and Codeine *on page 301*
Pharmacokinetics See individual monographs for Acetaminophen *on page 36* and Codeine *on page 301*
Usual Dosage Oral (doses should be titrated to appropriate analgesic effect):
Children: Analgesic: 0.5-1 mg codeine/kg/dose every 4-6 hours
3-6 years: 5 mL 3-4 times/day as needed
7-12 years: 10 mL 3-4 times/day as needed
>12 years: 15 mL every 4 hours as needed
Adults: 1-2 tablets every 4 hours; maximum dose: 12 tablets/24 hours
Administration Oral: Administer with food to decrease GI upset; shake suspension well before use
Patient Information Codeine may be habit-forming; avoid abrupt discontinuation after prolonged use; may cause drowsiness and impair ability to perform activities requiring mental alertness or physical coordination; avoid alcohol
Nursing Implications Observe patient for excessive sedation, respiratory depression
Additional Information Tylenol® With Codeine elixir contains saccharin
Dosage Forms
Capsule (C-III) (Phenaphen® With Codeine): #3: Acetaminophen 325 mg and codeine phosphate 30 mg
Elixir, oral (C-V): Acetaminophen 120 mg and codeine phosphate 12 mg per 5 mL (5 mL, 10 mL, 12.5 mL, 15 mL, 120 mL, 480 mL, 3840 mL) [contains 7% alcohol]
Tylenol® With Codeine: Acetaminophen 120 mg and codeine phosphate 12 mg per 5 mL (480 mL) [contains 7% alcohol and sodium benzoate; cherry flavor]
Suspension, oral (C-V) (Capital® and Codeine): Acetaminophen 120 mg and codeine phosphate 12 mg per 5 mL (480 mL) [alcohol free; fruit punch flavor]
Tablet (C-III):
#2: Acetaminophen 300 mg and codeine phosphate 15 mg
#3 (Tylenol® With Codeine): Acetaminophen 300 mg and codeine phosphate 30 mg [contains metabisulfite]
#4 (Tylenol® With Codeine): Acetaminophen 300 mg and codeine phosphate 60 mg [contains metabisulfite]

♦ **Acetaminophen and Hydrocodone** *see* Hydrocodone and Acetaminophen *on page 571*
♦ **Acetaminophen and Oxycodone** *see* Oxycodone and Acetaminophen *on page 847*
♦ **Acetaminophen and Propoxyphene** *see* Propoxyphene and Acetaminophen *on page 951*
♦ **Acetaminophen Toxicity Nomogram** *see page 1403*

AcetaZOLAMIDE *(a set a ZOLE a mide)*
Related Information
Antiepileptic Drugs *on page 1374*
U.S. Brand Names Diamox®; Diamox Sequels®
Canadian Brand Names Apo®-Acetazolamide

Therapeutic Category Anticonvulsant, Miscellaneous; Carbonic Anhydrase Inhibitor; Diuretic, Carbonic Anhydrase Inhibitor

Generic Available Yes

Use Reduce elevated intraocular pressure in glaucoma; diuretic; adjunct to the treatment of refractory seizures; prevent acute altitude sickness; treatment of centrencephalic epilepsies; reduce CSF production in hydrocephalus

Pregnancy Risk Factor C

Contraindications Hypersensitivity to acetazolamide, any component, or other sulfonamides; patients with hepatic disease or insufficiency; decreased serum sodium and/or potassium; adrenocortical insufficiency; hyperchloremic acidosis; or severe renal disease

Warnings Tolerance to antiepileptic effects may require dosage adjustment

Precautions Use with caution in patients with respiratory acidosis, COPD, diabetes mellitus, and gout; reduce dosage in patients with renal impairment

Adverse Reactions

Cardiovascular: Cyanosis

Central nervous system: Drowsiness, fatigue, vertigo, fever, seizures, dizziness, depression, malaise

Dermatologic: Rash, erythema multiforme, photosensitivity, Stevens-Johnson syndrome

Endocrine & metabolic: Hypokalemia, hyperchloremic metabolic acidosis, hyperglycemia

Gastrointestinal: GI irritation, anorexia, nausea, vomiting, xerostomia, melena, dysgeusia, metallic taste, black stools

Genitourinary: Dysuria, polyuria

Hematologic: Bone marrow suppression, thrombocytopenia, hemolytic anemia, pancytopenia, agranulocytosis

Hepatic: Hepatic insufficiency

Neuromuscular & skeletal: Paresthesia, muscle weakness

Ocular: Myopia

Renal: Renal calculi, phosphaturia, renal colic

Respiratory: Hyperpnea

Drug Interactions Increases lithium excretion; may decrease the rate of excretion of other drugs such as procainamide, flecainide, quinidine, and tricyclic antidepressants; may increase the excretion of salicylates and phenobarbital; may inactivate methenamine in the urine; may increase cyclosporine levels; may increase the risk of developing osteomalacia in patients receiving phenytoin or phenobarbital; topiramate may increase risk of nephrolithiasis and paresthesia; salicylates increase acetazolamide serum levels resulting in CNS toxicity; ammonium chloride increases plasma concentration of nonionized acetazolamide; increased toxicity with propofol (cardiorespiratory instability)

Food Interactions Avoid natural licorice (causes sodium and water retention and increases potassium loss)

Stability After reconstitution, acetazolamide injection is stable for 12 hours at room temperature and for 1 week when refrigerated; physically incompatible with parenteral multivitamins

Mechanism of Action Competitive, reversible inhibition of the enzyme carbonic anhydrase resulting in increased renal excretion of sodium, potassium, bicarbonate, and water and decreased formation of aqueous humor; also inhibits carbonic anhydrase in CNS to retard abnormal and excessive discharge from CNS neurons

Pharmacodynamics

Onset of action:

Capsule, extended release: 2 hours

Tablet: 1-1.5 hours

I.V.: 2 minutes

Maximum effect:

Capsule, extended release: 3-6 hours

Tablet: 1-4 hours

I.V.: 15 minutes

Duration:

Capsule, extended release: 18-24 hours

Tablet: 8-12 hours

I.V.: 4-5 hours

Pharmacokinetics

Absorption: Appears to be dose dependent; erratic with daily doses >10 mg/kg

Distribution: Into erythrocytes, kidneys, and breast milk (breast milk to plasma ratio of 0.25 has been reported); crosses the blood-brain barrier and the placenta

Protein binding: 95%

Half-life: 2.4-5.8 hours

(Continued)

AcetaZOLAMIDE *(Continued)*

Time to peak serum concentration: Tablet: 2-4 hours

Elimination: 70% to 100% of an I.V. or tablet dose and 47% of an extended release capsule excreted unchanged in urine within 24 hours

Dialysis: 20% to 50% removed by hemodialysis

Usual Dosage

Children:

Glaucoma:

Oral: 8-30 mg/kg/day or 300-900 mg/m^2/day divided every 8 hours

I.V.: 20-40 mg/kg/day divided every 6 hours, not to exceed 1 g/day

Edema: Oral, I.V.: 5 mg/kg/dose or 150 mg/m^2/dose once daily

Epilepsy: Oral: 4-16 mg/kg/day in 1-4 divided doses, not to exceed 30 mg/kg/day or 1 g/day; **extended release capsule is not recommended for treatment of epilepsy**

Adults:

Glaucoma:

Chronic simple (open-angle): Oral: 250 mg 1-4 times/day or 500 mg sustained release capsule twice daily

Secondary, acute (closed-angle): I.V.: 250-500 mg, may repeat in 2-4 hours to a maximum of 1 g/day

Edema: Oral, I.V.: 250-375 mg/day

Epilepsy: Oral: 4-16 mg/kg/day in 1-4 divided doses, not to exceed 30 mg/kg/day or 1 g/day; **extended release capsule is not recommended for treatment of epilepsy**

Altitude sickness: Oral: 250 mg every 8-12 hours or 500 mg extended release capsules every 12-24 hours; therapy should begin 24-48 hours before and continued during ascent and for at least 48 hours after arrival at the high altitude

Urine alkalinization: Oral: 5 mg/kg/dose repeated 2-3 times over 24 hours

Dosing interval in renal impairment: Children and Adults:

Cl$_{cr}$ 10-50 mL/minute: Administer every 12 hours

Cl$_{cr}$ <10 mL/minute: Avoid use

Administration

Oral: Administer with food to decrease GI upset; tablet may be crushed and suspended in cherry or chocolate syrup to disguise the bitter taste of the drug (See Extemporaneous Preparations)

Parenteral:

I.V.: Reconstitute with at least 5 mL SWI to provide a solution containing not more than 100 mg/mL; maximum concentration: 100 mg/mL; maximum rate of I.V. infusion: 500 mg/minute

I.M.: Not generally recommended as the drug's alkaline pH makes it very painful

Monitoring Parameters Serum electrolytes, periodic hematologic determinations

Test Interactions May cause false-positive results for urinary protein with Albustix®, Labstix®, Albutest®, Bumintest®

Patient Information Do not crush or chew long-acting capsule; may cause dry mouth. May rarely cause photosensitivity reactions (eg, exposure to sunlight may cause severe sunburn, skin rash, redness, or itching); avoid direct exposure to sunlight

Additional Information Sodium content of 500 mg injection: 2.049 mEq

Extended release capsules are indicated only for use for the adjunctive treatment of open-angle or secondary glaucoma and the prevention of high altitude sickness; avoid using extended release capsules for anticonvulsant or diuretic therapy

Acetazolamide has been used with questionable efficacy to slow the progression of hydrocephalus in neonates and infants who may not be good candidates for surgery. I.V. or oral doses of 5 mg/kg/dose every 6 hours increased by 25 mg/kg/day to a maximum of 100 mg/kg/day, if tolerated, have been used. Furosemide was used in combination with acetazolamide (Libenson, 1999).

Dosage Forms

Capsule, sustained release (Diamox Sequels®): 500 mg

Injection, powder for reconstitution, as sodium: 500 mg

Tablet: 125 mg, 250 mg

Diamox®: 250 mg

Extemporaneous Preparations

A 25 mg/mL suspension may be made by crushing twelve 250 mg tablets and mixing with 120 mL of a 1:1 mixture of Ora-Sweet® and Ora-Plus® or a 1:1 mixture of Ora-Sweet® SF and Ora-Plus®. The resulting suspension is stable for 60 days refrigerated (Allen, 1996).

A 25 mg/mL suspension may be made by crushing one hundred 250 mg tablets; add 100 mL flavor/purified water; add a mixture of 10 g Veegum (already mixed with 200 mL purified water), 300 mL 1% methylcellulose and 300 mL syrup; qsad to

1000 mL with flavor/purified water and 10 mL paraben concentrate (methylparaben 120 mg, propylparaben 12 mg, propylene glycol qsad to 100 mL); stable 79 days refrigerated (Alexander, 1991).

Allen LV and Erickson MA, "Stability of Acetazolamide, Allopurinol, Azathioprine, Clonazepam, and Flucytosine in Extemporaneously Compounded Oral Liquids," *Am J Health Sys Pharm*, 1996, 53:1944-9.

Alexander KS, Haribhakti RP, and Parker GA, "Stability of Acetazolamide in Suspension Compounded From Tablets," *Am J Hosp Pharm*, 1991, 48(6):1241-4.

References
Libenson MH, Kaye EM, Rosman NP, et al, "Acetazolamide and Furosemide for Posthemorrhagic Hydro-cephalus of the Newborn," *Pediatr Neurol*, 1999, 20(3):185-91.

Reiss WG and Oles KS, "Acetazolamide in the Treatment of Seizures," *Ann Pharmacother*, 1996, 30(5):514-9.

Shinnar S, Gammon K, Bergman EW Jr, et al, "Management of Hydrocephalus in Infancy: Use of Acetazolamide and Furosemide to Avoid Cerebrospinal Fluid Shunts," *J Pediatr*, 1985, 107(1):31-7.

♦ **Acetoxyl® (Can)** *see* Benzoyl Peroxide *on page 165*
♦ **Acetoxymethylprogesterone** *see* MedroxyPROGESTERone *on page 712*

Acetylcholine (a se teel KOE leen)
U.S. Brand Names Miochol-E®
Therapeutic Category Cholinergic Agent, Ophthalmic; Ophthalmic Agent, Miotic
Generic Available No
Use Produces complete miosis in cataract surgery, keratoplasty, iridectomy and other anterior segment surgery where rapid miosis is required
Pregnancy Risk Factor C
Contraindications Hypersensitivity to acetylcholine chloride or any component; acute iritis and acute inflammatory disease of the anterior chamber
Warnings Open under aseptic conditions only
Precautions Systemic effects rarely occur, but can cause problems for patients with acute CHF, bronchial asthma, peptic ulcer, hyperthyroidism, GI spasm, and urinary tract obstruction
Adverse Reactions
Cardiovascular: Transient bradycardia and hypotension
Central nervous system: Headache
Ocular: Iris atrophy, temporary lens opacities (attributed to osmotic effect of 5% mannitol present in preparation)
Respiratory: Dyspnea
Miscellaneous: Diaphoresis
Drug Interactions Flurbiprofen decreases effectiveness; sodium nitrate antagonizes acetylcholine's effects
Stability Prepare solution immediately before use; do not use solution which is not clear and colorless
Mechanism of Action Causes contraction of the sphincter muscles of the iris, resulting in miosis and contraction of the ciliary muscle, leading to accommodation
Pharmacodynamics
Onset of action: Miosis occurs promptly
Duration: ~10-20 minutes
Usual Dosage Ophthalmic: Adults: Instill 0.5-2 mL of 1% injection (5-20 mg)
Administration Ophthalmic: Instill into anterior chamber before or after securing one or more sutures; instillation should be gentle and parallel to the iris face and tangential to the pupil border; in cataract surgery, acetylcholine should be used only after delivery of the lens
Dosage Forms Powder for suspension, intraocular, as chloride: 1% 1:100 [10 mg/mL] (2 mL)

Acetylcysteine (a se teel SIS teen)
U.S. Brand Names Mucomyst®; Mucosil™
Canadian Brand Names Parvolex®
Synonyms Mercapturic Acid; NAC; N-Acetylcysteine; N-Acetyl-L-Cysteine
Therapeutic Category Antidote, Acetaminophen; Mucolytic Agent
Generic Available Yes
Use Adjunctive therapy in patients with abnormal or viscid mucous secretions in bronchopulmonary diseases, pulmonary complications of surgery, and cystic fibrosis; diagnostic bronchial studies; antidote for acute acetaminophen toxicity; enema to treat bowel obstruction due to meconium ileus or its equivalent
Pregnancy Risk Factor B
Contraindications Hypersensitivity to acetylcysteine or any component
(Continued)

Acetylcysteine *(Continued)*

Warnings Since increased bronchial secretions may develop after inhalation, percussion, postural drainage and suctioning should follow

Precautions If bronchospasm occurs, administer a bronchodilator; discontinue acetylcysteine if bronchospasm progresses

Adverse Reactions
Cardiovascular: Tachycardia, hypotension, hypertension (after large oral doses)
Central nervous system: Drowsiness, chills
Dermatologic: Generalized urticaria, rash
Gastrointestinal: Stomatitis, nausea, vomiting, hemoptysis
Hepatic: Mild elevations in liver function tests have occurred after oral therapy
Respiratory: Bronchospasm, rhinorrhea
Miscellaneous: Unpleasant odor during administration

Drug Interactions May potentiate the effects of nitrates; adsorbed by activated charcoal

Stability Store opened vials in the refrigerator; use within 96 hours; contact with rubber, copper, iron, and cork may inactivate the drug; the light purple color of solution does **not** affect its activity

Mechanism of Action Exerts mucolytic action through its free sulfhydryl group which opens up the disulfide bonds in the mucoproteins thus lowering the viscosity. The exact mechanism of action in acetaminophen toxicity is unknown. It may act by maintaining or restoring glutathione levels or by acting as an alternative substrate for conjugation with the toxic metabolite.

Pharmacodynamics
Onset of action: Upon inhalation, mucus liquefaction occurs maximally within 5-10 minutes
Duration of mucus liquefaction: More than 1 hour

Pharmacokinetics
Protein binding: ~50%
Half-life:
Reduced acetylcysteine: 2 hours
Total acetylcysteine: 5.5 hours
Time to peak serum concentration: 1-2 hours

Usual Dosage
Acetaminophen poisoning: Children and Adults: Oral: 140 mg/kg; followed by 17 doses of 70 mg/kg every 4 hours; repeat dose if emesis occurs within 1 hour of administration; therapy should continue until all doses are administered even though the acetaminophen plasma level has dropped below the toxic range
Inhalation:
Infants: 1-2 mL of 20% solution or 2-4 mL of 10% solution until nebulized, given 3-4 times/day
Children: 3-5 mL of 20% solution or 6-10 mL of 10% solution until nebulized, given 3-4 times/day
Adolescents: 5-10 mL of 10% to 20% solution until nebulized, given 3-4 times/day
Note: Patients should receive an aerosolized bronchodilator 10-15 minutes prior to acetylcysteine
Intratracheal: Children and Adults: 1-2 mL of 10% to 20% solution every 1-4 hours as needed
Meconium ileus equivalent: Children and Adults (varying regimens have been reported): Oral, Rectal Irrigation: 5-30 mL of 10% to 20% solution 3-6 times/day for at least 24 hours and symptom improvement

Administration
Oral: For treatment of acetaminophen overdosage, administer as a 5% solution; dilute the 20% solution 1:3 with a cola, orange juice, or other soft drink; use within 1 hour of preparation
Oral inhalation: May be administered either undiluted (both 10% and 20%) or diluted in NS

Monitoring Parameters When used in acetaminophen overdose, determine acetaminophen level as soon as possible, but no sooner than 4 hours after ingestion (to ensure peak levels have been obtained) (see Acetaminophen Serum Level Nomogram *on page 1403* in the appendix); liver function tests

Patient Information Clear airway by coughing deeply before aerosol treatment

Nursing Implications Assess patient for nausea, vomiting, and skin rash following oral administration for treatment of acetaminophen poisoning; intermittent aerosol treatments are commonly given when patient arises, before meals, and just before retiring at bedtime

Additional Information I.V. route is investigational in the U.S.; contact a poison control center for more information

Dosage Forms Solution, as sodium: 10% [100 mg/mL] (4 mL, 10 mL, 30 mL); 20% [200 mg/mL] (4 mL, 10 mL, 30 mL, 100 mL)

References

Hanly JG and Fitzgerald MX, "Meconium Ileus Equivalent in Older Patients With Cystic Fibrosis," *Br Med J (Clin Res Ed)*, 1983, 286(6375):1411-3.

Walson PD and Groth JF Jr, "Acetaminophen Hepatotoxicity After Prolonged Ingestion," *Pediatrics*, 1993, 91(5):1021-2.

- **Acetylsalicylic Acid** *see* Aspirin *on page 134*
- **Aciclovir** *see* Acyclovir *on page 45*
- **Acilac (Can)** *see* Lactulose *on page 649*
- **ACT** *see* Dactinomycin *on page 335*
- **ACT® [OTC]** *see* Fluoride *on page 500*
- **Act-D** *see* Dactinomycin *on page 335*
- **ACTH** *see* Corticotropin *on page 307*
- **Acticin®** *see* Permethrin *on page 885*
- **Actidose-Aqua® [OTC]** *see* Charcoal *on page 250*
- **Actidose® With Sorbitol [OTC]** *see* Charcoal *on page 250*
- **Actifed® Cold and Allergy [OTC]** *see* Triprolidine and Pseudoephedrine *on page 1122*
- **Actigall™** *see* Ursodiol *on page 1129*
- **Actinomycin D** *see* Dactinomycin *on page 335*
- **Actiq®** *see* Fentanyl *on page 479*
- **Activase®** *see* Alteplase *on page 67*
- **Activated Carbon** *see* Charcoal *on page 250*
- **Activated Charcoal** *see* Charcoal *on page 250*
- **Activated Dimethicone** *see* Simethicone *on page 1020*
- **Activated Ergosterol** *see* Ergocalciferol *on page 445*
- **Activated Methylpolysiloxane** *see* Simethicone *on page 1020*
- **Activated Protein C, Human Recombinant** *see* Drotrecogin Alfa (Activated) *on page 420*
- **Acular®** *see* Ketorolac *on page 641*
- **Acular® P.F.** *see* Ketorolac *on page 641*
- **ACV** *see* Acyclovir *on page 45*
- **Acycloguanosine** *see* Acyclovir *on page 45*

Acyclovir (ay SYE kloe veer)

Related Information

Carbohydrate and Alcohol Content of Liquid Medications for Use in Patients Receiving Ketogenic Diets *on page 1431*

U.S. Brand Names Zovirax®

Canadian Brand Names Alti-Acyclovir; Apo®-Acyclovir; Gen-Acyclovir; Nu-Acyclovir; ratio-Acyclovir

Synonyms Aciclovir; ACV; Acycloguanosine

Therapeutic Category Antiviral Agent, Oral; Antiviral Agent, Parenteral; Antiviral Agent, Topical

Generic Available Yes (capsule)

Use Treatment of initial and prophylaxis of recurrent mucosal and cutaneous herpes simplex (HSV 1 and HSV 2) infections; herpes simplex encephalitis; herpes zoster infections; varicella-zoster infections in healthy, nonpregnant persons >13 years of age, children >12 months of age who have a chronic skin or lung disorder or are receiving long-term aspirin therapy, and immunocompromised patients

Pregnancy Risk Factor C

Contraindications Hypersensitivity to acyclovir, valacyclovir, or any component

Warnings HSV and VZV with reduced susceptibility to acyclovir have been isolated from immunocompromised patients, especially with advanced HIV infection; renal failure, in some cases resulting in death, has occurred with acyclovir

Precautions Use with caution in patients with renal disease, dehydration, underlying neurologic disease, and in patients with hypoxia, hepatic, or electrolyte abnormalities; dosage should be reduced in patients with renal impairment

Adverse Reactions

Central nervous system: Headache, lethargy, delirium, coma, dizziness, seizures, pain, insomnia, fever, hallucinations, aggressive behavior, ataxia

Dermatologic: Skin rash, pruritus, alopecia, erythema multiforme, urticaria, photosensitivity, Stevens-Johnson syndrome, angioedema

Gastrointestinal: Nausea, vomiting, diarrhea

(Continued)

Acyclovir *(Continued)*

Hematologic: Bone marrow suppression, neutropenia, thrombotic thrombocytopenic purpura/hemolytic uremic syndrome

Hepatic: Elevated liver enzymes, hepatitis, jaundice, hyperbilirubinemia

Local: Phlebitis at injection site, tissue necrosis upon extravasation, local pain and stinging with topical use

Neuromuscular & skeletal: Tremulousness, myalgia, paresthesia

Renal: Nephrotoxicity, hematuria, elevated BUN and serum creatinine

Respiratory: Sore throat

Miscellaneous: Diaphoresis, anaphylaxis

Drug Interactions Zidovudine (neurotoxicity); probenecid decreases renal clearance of acyclovir

Food Interactions Food does not appear to affect absorption

Stability Incompatible with blood products and protein-containing solutions; reconstituted 50 mg/mL solution should be used within 12 hours; do not refrigerate reconstituted solutions as they may precipitate

Mechanism of Action Inhibits DNA synthesis and viral replication by competing with deoxyguanosine triphosphate for viral DNA polymerase and by incorporation into viral DNA

Pharmacokinetics

Absorption: Oral: 15% to 30%

Distribution: Widely distributed throughout the body including brain, kidney, lungs, liver, spleen, muscle, uterus, vagina, and the CSF; CSF acyclovir concentration is 50% of serum concentration; crosses the placenta; excreted into breast milk; V_d:

Neonates to 3 months of age: 28.8 L/1.73 m^2

Children 1-2 years: 31.6 L/1.73 m^2

Children 2-7 years: 42 L/1.73 m^2

Protein binding: <30%

Half-life, terminal phase:

Neonates: 4 hours

Children 1-12 years: 2-3 hours

Adults: 2-3.5 hours (with normal renal function)

Time to peak serum concentration: Oral: Within 1.5-2 hours

Elimination: Primary route is the kidney with 30% to 90% of a dose excreted unchanged in the urine; requires dosage adjustment with renal impairment; hemodialysis removes ~60% of a dose while removal by peritoneal dialysis is to a much lesser extent; supplemental dose recommended after hemodialysis

Usual Dosage

Children and Adults: Oral:

Genital herpes simplex virus (HSV), first infection: 1000 mg/day in 5 divided doses **or** 1200 mg/day in 3 divided doses for 7-10 days; maximum dose in children: 80 mg/kg/day in 3-5 divided doses

Genital HSV infection recurrence: 1000 mg/day in 5 divided doses **or** 1200 mg/day in 3 divided doses or 1600 mg/day in 2 divided doses for 5 days; maximum dose in children: 80 mg/kg/day in 2-5 divided doses

Recurrent genital HSV: Chronic suppressive therapy for frequent recurrences: 800-1000 mg/day in 2-5 divided doses; maximum dose in children: 80 mg/kg/day in 2-5 divided doses

HSV in immunocompromised host: 1000 mg/day in 3-5 divided doses for 7-14 days; maximum dose in children: 80 mg/kg/day in 3-5 divided doses

Prophylaxis of HSV in immunocompromised HSV-seropositive patient: 600-1000 mg/day in 3-5 divided doses during risk period; maximum dose in children: 80 mg/kg/day in 3-5 divided doses

Zoster in immunocompetent host: 4000 mg/day in 5 divided doses for 5-7 days; maximum dose in children: 80 mg/kg/day in 5 divided doses

Herpes zoster in immunocompromised patients:

Children: 250-600 mg/m^2/dose 4-5 times/day

Adults: 800 mg every 4 hours (5 times/day) for 7-10 days; prophylaxis: 400 mg 5 times/day

Varicella zoster (chickenpox) in immunocompetent host: 80 mg/kg/day in 4 divided doses for 5 days; maximum daily dose: 3200 mg/day; start treatment within the first 24 hours of rash onset

Prophylaxis of CMV infection in immunocompromised host: 800-3200 mg/day in 1-4 divided doses during risk period; maximum dose in children: 80 mg/kg/day in 3-4 divided doses

Premature neonates: HSV infection: I.V.: 20 mg/kg/day divided every 12 hours for 14-21 days

Neonates: HSV infection: I.V.: 1500 mg/m^2/day divided every 8 hours **or** 30 mg/kg/day divided every 8 hours for 14-21 days. In one study (Kimberlin, 2001), 88 neonates with a gestational age >32 weeks and weight ≥1200 g received I.V. acyclovir dosages >30 mg/kg/day for 21 days to treat neonatal CNS and disseminated HSV disease. Survival rate for patients treated with acyclovir dosages of 60 mg/kg/day divided every 8 hours for 21 days was statistically significantly higher than that for patients treated with 30 mg/kg/day for 10 days.

Children and Adults: I.V. (dosage for obese patients should be based on ideal body weight):

HSV infection: 750 mg/m^2/day divided every 8 hours **or** 15 mg/kg/day divided every 8 hours for 5-7 days

HSV in immunocompromised host:
Children <1 year: 15-30 mg/kg/day divided every 8 hours for 7-14 days
Children ≥1 year: 750-1500 mg/m^2/day divided every 8 hours or 15-30 mg/kg/day divided every 8 hours for 7-14 days

Prophylaxis of HSV in immunocompromised HSV-seropositive patients: 750 mg/m^2/day divided every 8 hours during risk period

HSV encephalitis: 1500 mg/m^2/day divided every 8 hours **or** 30 mg/kg/day divided every 8 hours for 14-21 days

Varicella or zoster in immunocompromised host or zoster in immunocompetent host:
Children <1 year: 30 mg/kg/day divided every 8 hours for 7-10 days
Children ≥1 year: 1500 mg/m^2/day divided every 8 hours or 30 mg/kg/day divided every 8 hours for 7-10 days

Prophylaxis of CMV infection in immunocompromised host: 1500 mg/m^2/day divided every 8 hours during risk period

Prophylaxis of bone marrow transplant recipients:
Autologous patients who are HSV-seropositive: 250 mg/m^2/dose every 8 hours
Autologous patients who are CMV seropositive: 500 mg/m^2/dose every 8 hours; for clinically symptomatic CMV infection, consider replacing acyclovir with ganciclovir

Children and Adults: Topical: Apply ½" ribbon of ointment for a 4" square surface area every 3 hours (6 times/day) for 7 days

Dosing interval in renal impairment:

Neonates: I.V.:
S_{cr} 0.8-1.1 mg/dL: Administer 20 mg/kg/dose every 12 hours
S_{cr} 1.2-1.5 mg/dL: Administer 20 mg/kg/dose every 24 hours
S_{cr} >1.5 mg/dL: Administer 10 mg/kg/dose every 24 hours

Children ≥6 months and Adults:
Oral:

Usual Dose	Creatinine Clearance	Adjusted Dose
200 mg 5 times/day	Cl_{cr} <10 mL/minute	Administer 200 mg q12h
800 mg 5 times/day	Cl_{cr} 10-25 mL/minute	Administer 800 mg q8h
	Cl_{cr} <10 mL/minute	Administer 800 mg q12h

I.V.:
Cl_{cr} 25-50 mL/minute: Administer normal dose every 12 hours
Cl_{cr} 10-25 mL/minute: Administer normal dose every 24 hours
Cl_{cr} <10 mL/minute: 50% decrease in dose, administer every 24 hours

Administration

Oral: May administer with food; shake suspension well before use

Parenteral: Reconstitute vial for injection with paraben-free SWI; administer by slow I.V. infusion over at least 1 hour at a final concentration not to exceed 7 mg/mL since rapid infusions can cause nephrotoxicity with crystalluria and renal tubular damage; in patients who require fluid restriction, a concentration of up to 10 mg/mL has been infused; concentration >10 mg/mL increases the risk of phlebitis

Monitoring Parameters Urinalysis, BUN, serum creatinine, I & O; liver enzymes, CBC; neutrophil count at least twice weekly in neonates receiving acyclovir 60 mg/kg/day I.V.

Nursing Implications Maintain adequate hydration and urine output the first 2 hours after I.V. infusion to decrease the risk of nephrotoxicity; check infusion site for phlebitis; avoid extravasation

Additional Information Sodium content of 1 g: 4.2 mEq

Dosage Forms

Capsule: 200 mg
Infusion, as sodium [premixed in NS]: 5 mg/mL (100 mL, 200 mL)
Injection, powder for reconstitution, as sodium: 500 mg; 1000 mg
Injection, solution, as sodium [preservative free]: 50 mg/mL (10 mL, 20 mL)
(Continued)

Acyclovir *(Continued)*

Ointment, topical: 5% (3 g, 15 g)
Suspension, oral: 200 mg/5 mL (473 mL) [banana flavor]
Tablet: 400 mg, 800 mg

References

American Academy of Pediatrics Committee on Infectious Diseases, "The Use of Oral Acyclovir in Otherwise Healthy Children With Varicella," *Pediatrics*, 1993, 91(3):674-6.

Desparmet J, Meistelman C, Barre J, et al, "Continuous Epidural Infusion of Bupivacaine for Postoperative Pain Relief in Children," *Anesthesiology*, 1987, 67(1):108-10.

Dunkle LM, Arvin AM, Whitley RJ, et al, "A Controlled Trial of Acyclovir for Chickenpox in Normal Children," *N Engl J Med*, 1991, 325(22):1539-44.

Englund JA, Fletcher CV, and Balfour HH Jr, "Acyclovir Therapy in Neonates," *J Pediatr*, 1991, 119(1 Pt 1):129-35.

Kimberlin DW, Lin CY, Jacobs RF, et al, "Safety and Efficacy of High-Dose Intravenous Acyclovir in the Management of Neonatal Herpes Simplex Virus Infections," *Pediatrics*, 2001, 108(2):230-8.

Meyers JD, Reed EC, Shepp DH, et al, "Acyclovir for Prevention of Cytomegalovirus Infection and Disease After Allogenic Marrow Transplantation," *N Engl J Med*, 1988, 318(2):70-5.

Novelli VM, Marshall WC, Yeo J, et al, "High-Dose Oral Acyclovir for Children at Risk of Disseminated Herpes Virus Infections," *J Infect Dis*, 1985, 151(2):372.

♦ **Adalat® CC** *see NIFEdipine on page 811*

♦ **Adamantanamine** *see Amantadine on page 73*

♦ **Adderall®** *see Dextroamphetamine and Amphetamine on page 361*

♦ **Adderall XR™** *see Dextroamphetamine and Amphetamine on page 361*

♦ **ADEKs®** *see page 1213*

♦ **Adenine Arabinoside** *see Vidarabine on page 1147*

♦ **Adenocard®** *see Adenosine on page 48*

Adenosine *(a DEN oh seen)*

Related Information

Adult ACLS Algorithm, Narrow-Complex Supraventricular Tachycardia *on page 1190*
Adult ACLS Algorithm, Tachycardia Overview *on page 1189*
CPR Pediatric Drug Dosages *on page 1175*
Pediatric ALS Algorithm, Tachycardia - Rapid Rhythm and Adequate Perfusion *on page 1181*
Pediatric ALS Algorithm, Tachycardia - Rapid Rhythm and Evidence of Poor Perfusion *on page 1182*

U.S. Brand Names Adenocard®
Synonyms 9-Beta-D-ribofuranosyladenine
Therapeutic Category Antiarrhythmic Agent, Miscellaneous
Generic Available No

Use Treatment of paroxysmal supraventricular tachycardia (PSVT); used in adult ACLS algorithms for narrow-complex tachycardias, stable narrow-complex supraventricular tachycardias, and wide-complex tachycardias that are supraventricular in origin; used in PALS algorithms for probable supraventricular tachycardia; investigationally used as a continuous infusion for the treatment of primary pulmonary hypertension in adults and persistent pulmonary hypertension of the newborn (PPHN) (see Additional Information)

Pregnancy Risk Factor C

Contraindications Hypersensitivity to adenosine or any component; second and third degree A-V block or sick sinus syndrome unless pacemaker placed

Warnings Heart block, including transient or prolonged asystole may occur as well as other arrhythmias; episodes of asystole or other arrhythmias may be fatal; if arrhythmia is not due to re-entry pathway through A-V node or sinus node (ie, atrial fibrillation, flutter, or tachycardia or ventricular tachycardia), adenosine will not terminate the arrhythmia but can produce transient ventriculoatrial or A-V block; possible mutagenic effects

Precautions Bronchoconstriction may occur in asthmatics (avoid use in patients with bronchospasm or bronchoconstriction); use with caution in patients with underlying dysfunction of sinus or A-V node, obstructive lung disease, and those taking digoxin or verapamil; initial adenosine dose should be significantly decreased in patients receiving dipyridamole

Adverse Reactions

Cardiovascular: Flushing, arrhythmias, palpitations, chest pain, bradycardia, heart block, minimal hemodynamic disturbances, hypotension (<1%)
Central nervous system: Irritability, headaches, lightheadedness, dizziness
Gastrointestinal: Nausea, metallic taste
Respiratory: Dyspnea, hyperventilation, bronchoconstriction in asthmatics

Drug Interactions Dipyridamole potentiates effects of adenosine (dose of adenosine should be significantly reduced); methylxanthines (aminophylline, theophylline, caffeine) antagonize adenosine's effects so that larger doses of adenosine or an alternative agent may be required; carbamazepine may increase heart block; digoxin and verapamil may cause ventricular fibrillation (rare cases reported)

Stability Do **not** refrigerate, precipitation may occur; contains no preservatives, discard unused portion

Mechanism of Action Slows conduction time through the A-V node, interrupting the re-entry pathways through the A-V node, restoring normal sinus rhythm

Pharmacodynamics

Onset of action: Rapid

Duration: Very brief

Pharmacokinetics

Metabolism: Removed from systemic circulation primarily by vascular endothelial cells and erythrocytes (by cellular uptake); rapidly metabolized intracellularly; phosphorylated by adenosine kinase to adenosine monophosphate (AMP) which is then incorporated into high-energy pool; intracellular adenosine is also deaminated by adenosine deaminase to inosine; inosine can be metabolized to hypoxanthine, then xanthine and finally to uric acid.

Half-life: <10 seconds

Usual Dosage Note: Adequate controlled studies in pediatric patients have not been conducted.

Manufacturer's recommendations: Rapid I.V.:

Neonates, Infants, Children, and Adolescents weighing <50 kg: Initial dose: 0.05-0.1 mg/kg; if not effective within 1-2 minutes, increase dose by 0.05-0.1 mg/kg increments every 1-2 minutes to a maximum single dose of 0.3 mg/kg or until termination of PSVT

Children and Adolescents weighing ≥50 kg and Adults: 6 mg, if not effective within 1-2 minutes, 12 mg may be given; may repeat 12 mg bolus if needed

Alternative pediatric dosing:

Neonates: Rapid I.V.: Initial dose: 0.05 mg/kg; if not effective within 2 minutes, increase dose by 0.05 mg/kg increments every 2 minutes to a maximum dose of 0.25 mg/kg or until termination of PSVT

Infants and Children: **PALS dose for treatment of SVT**: Rapid I.V.; I.O.: Initial: 0.1 mg/kg (maximum: 6 mg); if not effective, give 0.2 mg/kg (maximum: 12 mg)

Administration Parenteral: For rapid bolus I.V. use, administer over 1-2 seconds at peripheral I.V. site closest to patient's heart (I.V. administration into lower extremities may result in therapeutic failure or requirement of higher doses); follow each bolus with NS flush (infants and children: 5-10 mL; adults: 20 mL); if given peripherally in adults, elevate the extremity for 10-20 seconds after the NS flush. To administer doses <600 mcg (0.2 mL of commercial product), a dilution with NS (final concentration: 300 mcg/mL) may be made. **Note:** Preliminary results in adults suggest adenosine may be administered via a **central line** at lower doses (eg, Adults: Initial dose: 3 mg); FDA approved labeling for pediatric patients weighing <50 kg states that doses listed may be administered either peripherally or centrally (further studies are needed)

Monitoring Parameters Continuous EKG, heart rate, blood pressure, respirations

Nursing Implications Be alert for dyspnea, shortness of breath, and possible exacerbation of asthma

Additional Information Not effective in atrial flutter, atrial fibrillation, or ventricular tachycardia; short duration of action is an advantage as adverse effects are usually rapidly self-limiting; effects may be prolonged in patients with denervated transplanted hearts. Individualize treatment of prolonged adverse effects: Give I.V. fluids for hypotension, aminophylline/theophylline may antagonize effects.

Limited information is available regarding the use of adenosine for the treatment of persistent pulmonary hypertension of the newborn (PPHN); efficacy, optimal dose, and duration of therapy is not established; a randomized, masked, placebo-controlled pilot study of 18 term infants with PPHN used initial doses of 25 mcg/kg/minute (n=9); after 30 minutes, doses were increased to 50 mcg/kg/minute if no improvement in PaO_2 was observed; all patients received study drug via central line into the right atrium (inserted via the umbilical vein); significant improvement in oxygenation was observed in 4 of 9 newborns receiving 50 mcg/kg/minute; hypotension or tachycardia were not observed; further studies are needed (Kondur, 1996).

Adenosine is also available as Adenoscan®, which is used in adults as an adjunct to thallium-201 myocardial perfusion scintigraphy; see package insert for further information on this use.

Dosage Forms Injection, solution [preservative free] (Adenocard®): 3 mg/mL (2 mL, 4 mL)

References

Eubanks AP and Artman M, "Administration of Adenosine to a Newborn of 26 Weeks' Gestation," *Pediatr Cardiol*, 1994, 15(3):157-8.

(Continued)

Adenosine *(Continued)*

"Guidelines 2000 for Cardiopulmonary Resuscitation and Emergency Cardiovascular Care, Part 6: Advanced Cardiovascular Life Support, The American Heart Association in Collaboration With the International Liaison Committee on Resuscitation," *Circulation*, 2000, 102(8 Suppl):I86-171.

"Guidelines 2000 for Cardiopulmonary Resuscitation and Emergency Cardiovascular Care, Part 10: Pediatric Advanced Life Support, The American Heart Association in Collaboration With the International Liaison Committee on Resuscitation," *Circulation*, 2000, 102(8 Suppl): I291-342.

Konduri GG, Garcia DC, Kazzi NJ, et al, "Adenosine Infusion Improves Oxygenation in Term Infants With Respiratory Failure," *Pediatrics*, 1996, 97(3):295-300.

McIntosh-Yellin NL, Drew BJ, and Scheinman MM, "Safety and Efficacy of Central Intravenous Bolus Administration of Adenosine for Termination of Supraventricular Tachycardia," *J Am Coll Cardiol*, 1993, 22(3):741-5.

Paul T and Pfammatter JP, "Adenosine: An Effective and Safe Antiarrhythmic Drug in Pediatrics," *Pediatr Cardiol*, 1997, 18(2):118-26.

Sherwood MC, Lau KC, and Sholler GF, "Adenosine in the Management of Supraventricular Tachycardia in Children," *J Paediatr Child Health*, 1998, 34(1):53-6.

Till J, Shinebourne EA, Rigby ML, et al, "Efficacy and Safety in the Treatment of Supraventricular Tachycardia in Infants and Children," *Br Heart J*, 1989, 62(3):204-11.

Zeigler V, "Adenosine in the Pediatric Population: Nursing Implications," *Pediatr Nurs*, 1991, 17(6):600-2.

- **ADH** *see* Vasopressin *on page 1136*
- **Adoxa™** *see* Doxycycline *on page 415*
- **ADR** *see* DOXOrubicin *on page 413*
- **Adrenalin®** *see* Epinephrine *on page 439*
- **Adrenaline** *see* Epinephrine *on page 439*
- **Adrenocorticotropic Hormone** *see* Corticotropin *on page 307*
- **Adriamycin PFS®** *see* DOXOrubicin *on page 413*
- **Adriamycin RDF®** *see* DOXOrubicin *on page 413*
- **Adrucil®** *see* Fluorouracil *on page 503*
- **Adsorbent Charcoal** *see* Charcoal *on page 250*
- **Adult ACLS Algorithm, Asystole** *see page 1187*
- **Adult ACLS Algorithm, Bradycardia** *see page 1188*
- **Adult ACLS Algorithm, Cardiac Arrest** *see page 1183*
- **Adult ACLS Algorithm, Comprehensive ECC** *see page 1184*
- **Adult ACLS Algorithm, Narrow-Complex Supraventricular Tachycardia** *see page 1190*
- **Adult ACLS Algorithm, Pulseless Electrical Activity** *see page 1186*
- **Adult ACLS Algorithm, Stable Ventricular Tachycardia** *see page 1191*
- **Adult ACLS Algorithm, Synchronized Cardioversion** *see page 1192*
- **Adult ACLS Algorithm, Tachycardia Overview** *see page 1189*
- **Adult ACLS Algorithm, V. Fib and Pulseless VT** *see page 1185*
- **Adult and Adolescent HIV** *see page 1327*
- **Advair™ Diskus®** *see* Fluticasone and Salmeterol *on page 514*
- **Advil® [OTC]** *see* Ibuprofen *on page 588*
- **Advil®, Children's [OTC]** *see* Ibuprofen *on page 588*
- **Advil®, Infants' Concentrated Drops [OTC]** *see* Ibuprofen *on page 588*
- **Advil®, Junior [OTC]** *see* Ibuprofen *on page 588*
- **Advil® Migraine [OTC]** *see* Ibuprofen *on page 588*
- **Aerius® (Can)** *see* Desloratadine *on page 351*
- **AeroBid®** *see* Flunisolide *on page 497*
- **AeroBid®-M** *see* Flunisolide *on page 497*
- **Afrin® [OTC]** *see* Oxymetazoline *on page 849*
- **Afrin® Extra Moisturizing [OTC]** *see* Oxymetazoline *on page 849*
- **Afrin® Original [OTC]** *see* Oxymetazoline *on page 849*
- **Afrin® Severe Congestion [OTC]** *see* Oxymetazoline *on page 849*
- **Afrin® Sinus [OTC]** *see* Oxymetazoline *on page 849*
- **Aftate® Antifungal [OTC]** *see* Tolnaftate *on page 1102*
- **Agenerase®** *see* Amprenavir *on page 106*
- **Agoral® Maximum Strength Laxative [OTC]** *see* Senna *on page 1014*
- **AHF** *see* Antihemophilic Factor (Human) *on page 116*
- **AHF (Recombinant)** *see* Antihemophilic Factor (Recombinant) *on page 119*
- **AHG** *see* Antihemophilic Factor (Human) *on page 116*
- **A-hydroCort®** *see* Hydrocortisone *on page 573*
- **Airomir (Can)** *see* Albuterol *on page 54*
- **AK-Con™** *see* Naphazoline *on page 795*
- **AK-Dilate®** *see* Phenylephrine *on page 892*
- **AK-Nefrin®** *see* Phenylephrine *on page 892*

- **Akne-Mycin®** *see Erythromycin on page 448*
- **AK-Pentolate®** *see Cyclopentolate on page 319*
- **AK-Poly-Bac®** *see Bacitracin and Polymyxin B on page 157*
- **AK-Pred®** *see PrednisoLONE on page 925*
- **AK-Spore H.C.® [DSC]** *see Neomycin, (Bacitracin) Polymyxin B, and Hydrocortisone on page 802*
- **AK-Sulf®** *see Sulfacetamide on page 1048*
- **AK-T-Caine™** *see Tetracaine on page 1073*
- **AKTob®** *see Tobramycin on page 1097*
- **AK-Tracin®** *see Bacitracin on page 156*
- **AK-Trol®** *see Dexamethasone, Neomycin, and Polymyxin B on page 357*
- **Alavert™ [OTC]** *see Loratadine on page 692*
- **Albalon®** *see Naphazoline on page 795*

Albendazole (al BEN da zole)

U.S. Brand Names Albenza®
Therapeutic Category Anthelmintic
Generic Available No
Use Treatment of parenchymal neurocysticercosis due to active lesions caused by larval forms of *Taenia solium*; treatment of cystic hydatid disease of the liver, lung, and peritoneum caused by the larval form of *Echinococcus granulosus*; active against *Ascaris lumbricoides* (roundworm), *Ancylostoma duodenale* and *Necator americanus* (hookworm), *Enterobius vermicularis* (pinworm), *Clonorchis sinensis* (Chinese liver fluke), *Trichuris trichiura* (whipworm), and *Capillaria philippinensis*

Pregnancy Risk Factor C
Contraindications Hypersensitivity to albendazole, any component, or the benzimidazole class of compounds

Warnings Fatalities due to granulocytopenia or pancytopenia associated with the use of albendazole have been reported; women of childbearing age should only begin treatment after a negative pregnancy test and should be cautioned against becoming pregnant during and for at least one month after treatment cessation with albendazole since it may cause harm to fetus.

Precautions Use with caution in patients with hepatic impairment or decreased total leukocyte count; discontinue albendazole if significant elevation of liver enzymes occur; may restart therapy when liver enzymes decrease to pretreatment values; corticosteroids should be administered 1-2 days before initiating albendazole therapy in patients with neurocysticercosis to minimize inflammatory reactions and should be followed by concurrent steroid and anticonvulsant therapy for the first week of therapy to prevent cerebral hypertension. Albendazole may induce further retinal damage in patients having retinal lesions with neurocysticercosis.

Adverse Reactions
Central nervous system: Headache, dizziness, vertigo, elevated intracranial pressure, meningeal signs, fever, seizures
Dermatologic: Rash, urticaria, alopecia
Gastrointestinal: Abdominal pain, nausea, vomiting
Hematologic: Leukopenia, pancytopenia, thrombocytopenia, granulocytopenia, agranulocytosis
Hepatic: Elevated liver enzymes, hepatotoxicity
Renal: Acute renal failure
Miscellaneous: Hypersensitivity reactions, migration of *Ascaris* through mouth and nose

Drug Interactions Cytochrome P450 isoenzyme CYP1A2 inducer; isoenzyme CYP1A2 substrate (minor) and CYP3A4 substrate (major)
Dexamethasone, cimetidine, and praziquantel increase albendazole sulfoxide (active metabolite) concentration

Food Interactions Bioavailability is increased when taken with a fatty meal
Stability Store at room temperature
Mechanism of Action Binds to β-tubulin in parasite cells inhibiting tubulin polymerization which results in the loss of cytoplasmic microtubules and inhibition of glucose uptake

Pharmacokinetics
Absorption: Poorly absorbed from the GI tract
Distribution: Widely distributed throughout the body including urine, bile, liver, cyst wall, cyst fluid, and CSF
Protein binding: 70%
Metabolism: Extensive first-pass metabolism; hepatic metabolism to albendazole sulfoxide, an active metabolite
Half-life: Albendazole sulfoxide: 8-12 hours
(Continued)

Albendazole *(Continued)*

Time to peak serum concentration: 2-5 hours for the metabolite
Elimination: Biliary

Usual Dosage Children and Adults: Oral:

Neurocysticercosis: (patients should receive appropriate corticosteroid and anticonvulsant therapy as required):
<60kg: 15 mg/kg/day in 2 divided doses (maximum: 800 mg/day) for 8-30 days
≥60kg: 400 mg twice daily for 8-30 days

Hydatid disease:
<60kg: 15 mg/kg/day in 2 divided doses (maximum: 800 mg/day) for 1-6 months
≥60kg: 400 mg twice daily for 1-6 months

Ancylostoma caninum, ascariasis (roundworm), hookworm, trichuriasis (whipworm): 400 mg as a single dose

Capillariasis: 400 mg once daily for 10 days

Clonorchis sinensis (Chinese liver fluke): 10 mg/kg/day once daily for 7 days

Cutaneous larva migrans: 400 mg once daily for 3 days

Enterobius vermicularis (pinworm): 400 mg as a single dose; repeat in 2 weeks

Filariasis (*Mansonella perstans*): 400 mg twice daily for 10 days

Trichinosis (*Trichinella spiralis*): 400 mg twice daily for 8-14 days

Visceral larva migrans: 400 mg twice daily for 5 days

Administration Oral: Administer with food

Monitoring Parameters Monitor liver function tests, CBC at start of each cycle and every 2 weeks during therapy

Dosage Forms Tablet, film coated: 200 mg

References

Baranwal AK, Singhi PD, Khandelwal N, et al, "Albendazole Therapy in Children With Focal Seizures and Single Small Enhancing Computerized Tomographic Lesions: A Randomized, Placebo-Controlled, Double Blind Trial," *Pediatr Infect Dis J*, 1998, 17(8):696-700.

Jung H, Sanchez M, Gonzalez-Astiazaran A, et al, "Clinical Pharmacokinetics of Albendazole in Children With Neurocysticercosis," *Am J Ther*, 1997, 4(1):23-6.

Paul I, Gnanamani G, and Nallam NR, "Intestinal Helminth Infections Among School Children in Visakhapatnam," *Indian J Pediatr*, 1999, 66(5):669-73.

Pengsaa K, Sirivichayakul C, Pojjaroen-anant C, et al, "Albendazole Treatment for *Giardia intestinalis* Infections in School Children," *Southeast Asian J Trop Med Public Health*, 1999, 30(1):78-83.

♦ **Albenza®** *see* Albendazole *on page 51*

♦ **Albert® Docusate (Can)** *see* Docusate *on page 402*

♦ **Albert® Glyburide (Can)** *see* GlyBURIDE *on page 540*

♦ **Albert® Pentoxifylline (Can)** *see* Pentoxifylline *on page 884*

♦ **Albumarc®** *see* Albumin *on page 52*

Albumin *(al BYOO min)*

U.S. Brand Names Albumarc®; Albuminar®; Albutein®; Buminate®; Plasbumin®

Canadian Brand Names Plasbumin®-5; Plasbumin®-25

Synonyms Albumin Human; Normal Human Serum Albumin; Normal Serum Albumin (Human); Salt Poor Albumin

Therapeutic Category Blood Product Derivative; Plasma Volume Expander

Generic Available Yes

Use Treatment of hypovolemia; plasma volume expansion and maintenance of cardiac output in the treatment of certain types of shock or impending shock; hypoproteinemia resulting in generalized edema or decreased intravascular volume (eg, hypoproteinemia associated with acute nephrotic syndrome, premature neonates)

Note: PALS and Neonatal Resuscitation 2000 Guidelines recommend isotonic crystalloid solutions (eg, NS or LR) as initial volume expansion; albumin is used less frequently due to limited supply, potential risk of infections, and an association with an increase in mortality (identified by meta-analyses); few studies in these analyses included children, so no firm conclusions in pediatric patients can be made

Pregnancy Risk Factor C

Contraindications Hypersensitivity to albumin or any component; patients with severe anemia or cardiac failure

Warnings Use 25% concentration with extreme caution and infuse slowly in preterm neonates, due to increased risk of IVH (from rapid expansion of intravascular volume). Some products (eg, Albumarc®, Albuminar®, Buminate®) contain natural rubber latex (in certain components of the product packaging) which may cause allergic reactions in susceptible individuals; avoid use in patients with allergy to latex

Precautions Rapid infusion of albumin solutions may cause vascular overload. Do not administer albumin to burn patients for the first 24 hours after the burn (capillary exudation of albumin will occur); use with caution in patients with hepatic or renal failure (added protein load) and in patients who require sodium restriction; monitor for signs of hypervolemia

Due to the occasional shortage of 5% human albumin, 5% solutions may at times be prepared by diluting 25% human albumin with NS or with D_5W (if sodium load is a concern); however, **do not use sterile water** to dilute albumin solutions, as this may result in hypotonic-associated hemolysis which can be fatal

Adverse Reactions

Cardiovascular: Precipitation of CHF or pulmonary edema, hypertension, tachycardia, hypervolemia, hypotension due to hypersensitivity reaction

Central nervous system: Fever, chills

Dermatologic: Rash

Gastrointestinal: Nausea, vomiting

Stability Use within 4 hours after opening vial, do not use if turbid or contains a deposit; do not use SWI to dilute albumin (see Precautions)

Mechanism of Action Provides increase in intravascular oncotic pressure and causes mobilization of fluids from interstitial into intravascular space

Pharmacodynamics Duration of volume expansion: ~24 hours

Pharmacokinetics Half-life: 21 days

Usual Dosage 5% should be used in hypovolemic or intravascularly depleted patients; 25% should be used in patients with fluid or sodium restrictions (eg, patients with hypoproteinemia and generalized edema). Dose depends on condition of patient: I.V.:

Hypoproteinemia: Neonates, Infants, Children: 0.5-1 g/kg/dose; may repeat every 1-2 days; up to 1.5 g/kg/day has been added to hyperalimentation solutions; see Administration

Hypovolemia:

Neonates: Usual dose: 0.5 g/kg/dose (10 mL/kg/dose of 5% albumin); range: 0.25-0.5 g/kg/dose (5-10 mL/kg/dose of 5% albumin)

Infants and Children: 0.5-1 g/kg/dose (10-20 mL/kg/dose of 5% albumin); may repeat as needed; maximum dose: 6 g/kg/day (120 mL/kg/day of 5% albumin); see Administration

Adults: 25 g; no more than 250 g should be administered within 48 hours

Administration Parenteral: I.V.: Too rapid infusion may result in vascular overload

Albumarc®: May administer via the administration set provided (in-line 15 micron filter) or via any administration set with a 15 micron filter

Albuminar®: May administer via the administration set provided (in-line 60 micron filter) or via any administration set; use of filter is optional; size of filter may vary according to institutional policy. Method of filter sterilization used by manufacturer includes 0.2 micron filter; however, aggregates may form under storage, shipping, and handling. Administration via very small filter will not damage product, but will slow flow rate.

Albutein®: May administer via the administration set provided (in-line 50 micron filter) or via any administration set; use of filter is optional; size of filter may vary according to institutional policy. Method of production includes passage through 0.22 micron filter. May administer via filter as small as 0.22 microns.

Buminate®: Administer via the administration set provided (in-line 15 micron filter) or via any filtered administration set; use ≥5 micron filter to ensure adequate flow rate

Plasbumin®: May administer with or without an I.V. filter; filter as small as 0.22 microns may be used

Hypoproteinemia: Infuse over 2-4 hours; for neonates, dose may be added to hyperalimentation fluid and infused over 24 hours; **Note:** Hyperalimentation fluid containing >25 g/L of albumin is more likely to occlude 0.22 micron in-line filters; but hyperalimentation solutions containing albumin in concentrations as low as 10.8 g/L have also occluded 0.22 micron filters; use ≥5 micron filter to ensure adequate flow rate; addition of albumin to hyperalimentation solutions may increase potential for growth of bacteria or fungi.

Hypovolemia: Rate of infusion depends on severity of hypovolemia and patient's symptoms; usually infuse dose over 30-60 minutes (faster infusion rates may be clinically necessary)

Maximum rates of I.V. infusion after initial volume replacement:

5%: 2-4 mL/minute

25%: 1 mL/minute

To prepare 5% albumin from 25%, see Precautions.

Monitoring Parameters Observe for signs of hypervolemia, pulmonary edema, cardiac failure, vital signs, I & O, Hgb, Hct, urine specific gravity

Nursing Implications Albumin administration must be completed within 6 hours after entering container, provided that administration is begun within 4 hours of entering the container

Additional Information In certain conditions (eg, hypoproteinemia with generalized edema, nephrotic syndrome), doses of albumin may be followed with I.V. furosemide: 0.5-1 mg/kg/dose. Both 5% and 25% albumin contain 130-160 mEq of sodium/L; osmolarity: 5% albumin = 300 mOsm/L; 25% albumin = 1500 mOsm/L

(Continued)

Albumin (Continued)

Dosage Forms

Injection, solution, as human: 5% [50 mg/mL] (50 mL, 250 mL, 500 mL); 25% [250 mg/mL] (50 mL, 100 mL)

Albumarc®: 5% [50 mg/mL] (250 mL, 500 mL); 25% [250 mg/mL] (50 mL, 100 mL)

Albuminar®: 5% [50 mg/mL] (250 mL, 500 mL, 1000 mL); 25% [250 mg/mL] (20 mL, 50 mL, 100 mL)

Albutein®, Buminate®: 5% [50 mg/mL] (250 mL, 500 mL); 25% [250 mg/mL] (20 mL, 50 mL, 100 mL)

Plasbumin®: 5% [50 mg/mL] (50 mL, 250 mL, 500 mL); 20% [200 mg/mL] (50 mL); 25% [250 mg/mL] (20 mL, 50 mL, 100 mL)

References

"Guidelines 2000 for Cardiopulmonary Resuscitation and Emergency Cardiovascular Care, Part 10: Pediatric Advanced Life Support, The American Heart Association in Collaboration With the International Liaison Committee on Resuscitation," *Circulation*, 2000, 102(8 Suppl):I306.

"Guidelines 2000 for Cardiopulmonary Resuscitation and Emergency Cardiovascular Care, Part 11: Neonatal Resuscitation, The American Heart Association in Collaboration With the International Liaison Committee on Resuscitation," *Circulation*, 2000, 102(8 Suppl):I352.

♦ **Albuminar®** *see Albumin on page 52*

♦ **Albumin Human** *see Albumin on page 52*

♦ **Albutein®** *see Albumin on page 52*

Albuterol (al BYOO ter ole)

Related Information

Asthma Guidelines *on page 1376*

Carbohydrate and Alcohol Content of Liquid Medications for Use in Patients Receiving Ketogenic Diets *on page 1431*

U.S. Brand Names AccuNeb™; Proventil®; Proventil® HFA; Proventil® Repetabs®; Ventolin®; Ventolin® HFA; Volmax®; VoSpire ER™

Canadian Brand Names Airomir; Alti-Salbutamol; Apo®-Salvent; Gen-Salbutamol; PMS-Salbutamol; ratio-Inspra-Sal; ratio-Salbutamol; Rhoxal-salbutamol; Salbu-2; Salbu-4; Ventolin® Diskus; Ventrodisk

Synonyms Salbutamol

Therapeutic Category Adrenergic Agonist Agent; Antiasthmatic; Beta$_2$-Adrenergic Agonist Agent; Bronchodilator; Sympathomimetic

Generic Available Yes

Use Prevention and relief of bronchospasm in patients with reversible airway obstruction due to asthma or COPD; prevention of exercise-induced bronchospasm

Pregnancy Risk Factor C

Contraindications Hypersensitivity to albuterol, any component, or adrenergic amine

Warnings Inhaled albuterol can produce paradoxical bronchospasm; discontinue therapy immediately if this occurs. Excessive or prolonged use can lead to tolerance; excessive use has also been associated with deaths, possibly due to cardiac arrest. Outbreaks of lower respiratory tract colonization and infection have been attributed to contaminated multidose albuterol bottles (see Administration).

Precautions Use with caution in patients with hyperthyroidism, diabetes mellitus; cardiovascular disorders including coronary insufficiency or hypertension

Adverse Reactions

Cardiovascular: Tachycardia, palpitations, hypertension, chest pain

Central nervous system: Nervousness, CNS stimulation, hyperactivity and insomnia occur more frequently in younger children than adults; dizziness, lightheadedness, drowsiness, headache

Dermatologic: Angioedema, urticaria

Endocrine & metabolic: Hypokalemia

Gastrointestinal: GI upset, xerostomia, heartburn, vomiting, nausea, unusual taste, hoarseness (inhalation only)

Genitourinary: Dysuria

Neuromuscular & skeletal: Tremor, weakness, muscle cramping

Respiratory: Irritation of oropharynx, coughing, paradoxical bronchospasm (oral inhalation only)

Miscellaneous: Diaphoresis (increased)

Drug Interactions Action of albuterol is antagonized by beta-adrenergic blocking agents such as propranolol; cardiovascular effects are potentiated in patients also receiving MAO inhibitors or tricyclic antidepressants; concomitant administration of sympathomimetics may result in enhanced cardiovascular effects

Food Interactions Caffeinated beverages may increase side effects of albuterol

Stability Liquid, tablets, and oral inhalation solutions are stable at room temperature; compatible with cromolyn and ipratropium nebulizer solutions

Mechanism of Action Relaxes bronchial smooth muscle by action on beta$_2$-receptors with little effect on heart rate

Pharmacodynamics

Nebulization/oral inhalation:

Peak bronchodilation: Within 0.5-2 hours nebulization

Duration: 2-5 hours

Oral:

Peak bronchodilatation: 2-3 hours

Duration: 4-6 hours

Extended release tablets: Duration: Up to 12 hours

Pharmacokinetics

Metabolism: By the liver to an inactive sulfate

Half-life:

Oral: 2.7-5 hours

Inhalation: 3.8 hours

Elimination: 30% appears in urine as unchanged drug

Usual Dosage

Acute asthma exacerbation (NIH guidelines):

Nebulization:

Children: 0.15 mg/kg (minimum dose: 2.5 mg) every 20 minutes for 3 doses then 0.15-0.3 mg/kg (not to exceed 10 mg) every 1-4 hours as needed or 0.5 mg/kg/hour by continuous infusion

Note: Continuous nebulized albuterol at 0.3 mg/kg/hour has also been used safely in the treatment of severe status asthmaticus in children; continuous nebulized doses of 3 mg/kg/hour ± 2.2 mg/kg/hour (Katz, 1993) in children whose mean age was 20.7 months resulted in no cardiotoxicity; the optimal dosage for continuous nebulization remains to be determined

Adults: 2.5-5 mg every 20 minutes for 3 doses then 2.5-10 mg every 1-4 hours as needed or 10-15 mg/hour by continuous infusion

Inhalation: MDI: 90 mcg/spray:

Children: 4-8 puffs every 20 minutes for 3 doses then every 1-4 hours

Adults: 4-8 puffs every 20 minutes for up to 4 hours then every 1-4 hours as needed

Maintenance therapy (nonacute):

Oral:

Children 2-6 years: 0.1-0.2 mg/kg/dose 3 times/day; maximum dose not to exceed 4 mg 3 times/day

Children 6-12 years: 2 mg/dose 3-4 times/day; Repetabs®: 4 mg 2 times/day (maximum daily dosage: 24 mg)

Children >12 years to Adults: 2-4 mg/dose 3-4 times/day; Repetabs®: 4-8 mg 2 times/day (maximum daily dosage: 32 mg)

Inhalation: MDI: 90 mcg/spray:

Children <12 years: 1-2 inhalations 4 times/day

Children ≥12 years to Adults: 1-2 inhalations every 4-6 hours; maximum 12 inhalations/day

Exercise-induced bronchospasm: Children ≥12 years to Adults: 2 inhalations 15-30 minutes before exercising

Inhalation: Children and Adults: Nebulization: See dosage table; administer every 4-6 hours

Albuterol Nebulization Dosage
(Maintenance Therapy– Non-Acute)

Age	Dose (by weight)	0.5% Solution (mL/kg)	0.083% Solution (mL/kg)	AccuNeb™† (mg as sulfate)
Children <12 y	0.15-0.25 mg/kg (maximum: 5 mg)*	0.01-0.05 (maximum: 1 mL)*	0.06-0.3 (maximum: 6 mL)*	0.75-1.5 mg
Children 12 y - Adults	2.5 mg	0.5 mL	3 mL	1.5 mg

*Doses >2.5 mg have been associated with a higher frequency of adverse systemic effects.

†AccuNeb™ has not been studied in the treatment of acute bronchospasm; a more concentrated form may be necessary for treatment in acute bronchospasm especially in children ≥6 years.

Administration

Inhalation: Nebulization: Using 0.5% solution, dilute dosage in 1-2 mL NS (0.083% solution and AccuNeb™ do not require further dilution); adjust nebulizer flow to deliver dosage over 5-15 minutes; avoid contact of the dropper tip (multidose (Continued)

Albuterol *(Continued)*

bottle) with any surface, including the nebulizer reservoir and associated ventilator equipment (see Warnings)

Oral: Administer with food; do not crush or chew extended release tablets (Repetabs® or Volmax®)

Oral inhalation: Prime the inhaler (before first use or if it has not been used for more than 2 weeks) by releasing 4 test sprays into the air away from the face; shake well before use; use spacer for children <8 years of age

Monitoring Parameters Serum potassium, heart rate, pulmonary function tests, respiratory rate; arterial or capillary blood gases (if patient's condition warrants)

Patient Information Do not exceed recommended dosage; may cause dry mouth; rinse mouth with water following each inhalation to help with dry throat and mouth; if more than one inhalation is necessary, wait at least 1 full minute between inhalations; notify physician if palpitations, tachycardia, chest pain, muscle tremors, dizziness, headache, flushing, or if breathing difficulty persists; limit caffeinated beverages; to prevent medication build-up or blockage in the inhaler, the actuator, with the canister removed, should be washed and air-dried once weekly

Dosage Forms

Aerosol for oral inhalation: 90 mcg/spray (17 g)
   Proventil®: 90 mcg/spray (17 g)
   Ventolin®: 90 mcg/spray (17 g)
Aerosol for oral inhalation, as sulfate:
   Proventil® HFA: 90 mcg/dose (6.7 g) [chlorofluorocarbon free]
   Ventolin® HFA: 90 mcg/dose (18 g) [chlorofluorocarbon free]
Solution for inhalation, as sulfate: 0.083% [0.83 mg/mL] (3 mL); 0.5% [5 mg/mL] (0.5 mL, 20 mL)
   AccuNeb™: 0.75 mg/3 mL [0.63 mg albuterol/3 mL] (5 vials/pouch); 1.5 mg/3 mL [1.25 mg albuterol/3 mL] (5 vials/pouch)
   Proventil®: 0.083% [0.83 mg/mL] (3 mL); 0.5% [5 mg/mL] (20 mL)
Syrup, as sulfate: 2 mg/5 mL (120 mL, 480 mL) [strawberry flavor]
   Ventolin®: 2 mg/5 mL (480 mL) [alcohol and sugar free; strawberry flavor] [DSC]
Tablet, as sulfate: 2 mg, 4 mg
Tablet, extended release, as sulfate:
   Proventil®, Repetabs®: 4 mg
   Volmax®: 4 mg, 8 mg
   VoSpire ER™: 4 mg, 8 mg

References

"Guidelines for the Diagnosis and Management of Asthma. NAEPP Expert Panel Report 2," July 1997, www.nhlbi.nih.gov/guidelines/asthma/asthgdln.pdf.

Katz RW, Kelly HW, Crowley MR, et al, "Safety of Continuous Nebulized Albuterol for Bronchospasm in Infants and Children," *Pediatrics*, 1993, 92(5):666-69.

"National Asthma Education and Prevention Program. Expert Panel Report: Guidelines for the Diagnosis and Management of Asthma Update on Selected Topics--2002," *J Allergy Clin Immunol*, 2002, 110(5 Suppl):S141-219.

O'Callaghan C, Milner AD, and Swarbrick A, "Nebulized Salbutamol Does Have a Protective Effect on Airways in Children Under One Year Old," *Arch Dis Child*, 1988, 63(5):479-83.

Papo MC, Frank J, and Thompson AE, "A Prospective, Randomized Study of Continuous Versus Intermittent Nebulized Albuterol for Severe Status Asthmaticus in Children," *Crit Care Med*, 1993, 21(10):1479-86.

Rachelefsky GS and Siegel SC, "Asthma in Infants and Children - Treatment of Childhood Asthma: Part II," *J Allergy Clin Immunol*, 1985, 76(3):409-25.

Schuh S, Parkin P, Rajan A, et al, "High- Versus Low-Dose, Frequently Administered, Nebulized Albuterol in Children With Severe, Acute Asthma," *Pediatrics*, 1989, 83(4):513-8.

Schuh S, Reider MJ, Canny G, et al, "Nebulized Albuterol in Acute Childhood Asthma: Comparison of Two Doses," *Pediatrics*, 1990, 86(4):509-13.

♦ **Alcaine®** *see* Proparacaine *on page 946*

♦ **Alcohol** *see* Ethyl Alcohol *on page 465*

♦ **Alcomicin® (Can)** *see* Gentamicin *on page 533*

♦ **Aldactazide®** *see* Hydrochlorothiazide and Spironolactone *on page 570*

♦ **Aldactone®** *see* Spironolactone *on page 1037*

Aldesleukin *(al des LOO kin)*

U.S. Brand Names Proleukin®

Synonyms Epidermal Thymocyte Activating Factor; ETAF; IL-2; Interleukin-2; Lymphocyte Mitogenic Factor; NSC-373364; T-Cell Growth Factor; TCGF; Thymocyte Stimulating Factor

Therapeutic Category Antineoplastic Agent, Miscellaneous; Biological Response Modulator

Generic Available No

Use Treatment of metastatic renal cell carcinoma and metastatic melanoma; for investigational use in tumors known to have a response to immunotherapy such as colorectal cancer and non-Hodgkin's lymphoma (alone or in combination with lymphokine-activated killer cells); investigational treatment of Kaposi's sarcoma in combination with zidovudine and acute myelogenous leukemia (AML)

Pregnancy Risk Factor C

Contraindications Hypersensitivity to aldesleukin or any component; abnormal thallium stress test or pulmonary function tests; organ allografts (due to increased risk of rejection); **retreatment** in patients who have experienced sustained ventricular tachycardia (≥5 beats), cardiac rhythm disturbances not controlled or unresponsive to management, recurrent chest pain with EKG changes (consistent with angina or MI), intubation required >72 hours, pericardial tamponade; renal dysfunction requiring dialysis >72 hours, coma or toxic psychosis lasting >48 hours, repetitive or difficult to control seizures, bowel ischemia/perforation, and GI bleeding requiring surgery

Warnings High-dose aldesleukin therapy is associated with capillary leak syndrome (CLS) resulting in hypotension and reduced organ perfusion (occurring within 2-12 hours after start of treatment) which may be severe and fatal; CLS may be associated with cardiac arrhythmias, angina, MI, respiratory insufficiency requiring intubation, GI bleeding or infarction, renal insufficiency, edema, and mental status changes; therapy should be restricted to patients with normal cardiac and pulmonary functions as defined by thallium stress and formal pulmonary function testing; hold aldesleukin administration in patients developing moderate to severe lethargy or somnolence as continued administration may result in coma; may exacerbate disease symptoms in patients with clinically unrecognized or untreated CNS metastases; thoroughly evaluate and treat all patients with CNS metastases prior to therapy

Precautions Use with extreme caution in patients with normal thallium stress tests and pulmonary functions tests who have a history of prior cardiac or pulmonary disease; intensive aldesleukin treatment is associated with impaired neutrophil function (reduced chemotaxis) and with an increased risk of disseminated infection (particularly with *Staphylococcus aureus*) including sepsis and bacterial endocarditis; patients with indwelling central lines are particularly at increased risk of infection; treat pre-existing bacterial infections prior to initiation of aldesleukin therapy; standard supportive care during high-dose aldesleukin treatment includes acetaminophen to relieve fever and chills and an H_2 antagonist to reduce the risk of GI ulceration and/or bleeding; aldesleukin may exacerbate autoimmune disease; closely monitor for thyroid abnormalities or other potentially autoimmune phenomena; use with caution in patients with known seizure disorders

Adverse Reactions Many adverse effects of aldesleukin are dosage and schedule dependent; greater toxicity occurs with high dose, bolus administration and the least toxicity with low dose, subcutaneous administration

Cardiovascular: Hypotension (dose-limiting, possibly fatal), sinus tachycardia, arrhythmias, edema, angina, MI, CHF, capillary leak syndrome

Central nervous system: Confusion, drowsiness, transient memory loss, dizziness, cognitive changes, fatigue, chills, malaise, somnolence, disorientation, headaches, insomnia, paranoid delusion, seizures, coma, fever, pain

Dermatologic: Macular erythematous rash, pruritus, erythema, exfoliative dermatitis, dry skin, alopecia, petechiae, purpura, vitiligo

Endocrine & metabolic: Hypomagnesemia, hypocalcemia, hypokalemia, hypophosphatemia, hyponatremia, hypoglycemia, hyperglycemia, hypermagnesemia, hypercalcemia, hyperkalemia, hyperphosphatemia, hypernatremia, thyroid dysfunction

Gastrointestinal: Nausea, vomiting, diarrhea, stomatitis, GI bleeding, anorexia, weight gain, pancreatitis

Hematologic: Anemia, thrombocytopenia, leukopenia, eosinophilia

Hepatic: Transient elevations of bilirubin and liver enzymes, jaundice, ascites, decreased clotting factors

Neuromuscular & skeletal: Weakness, rigors, arthralgia, myalgia

Renal: Oliguria, proteinuria, transient elevation in BUN, hematuria

Respiratory: Congestion, dyspnea, pleural effusion, pulmonary edema

Miscellaneous: Allergic reactions

Drug Interactions Corticosteroids may decrease efficacy; increased CNS depression when administered concomitantly with other sedating agents; increased toxicity when administered concomitantly with other potentially nephrotoxic, myelotoxic, cardiotoxic, or hepatotoxic agents; increased hypotensive effects with antihypertensives or beta-blocking agents; acute reactions including fever, chills, nausea, vomiting, pruritus, rash, diarrhea, hypotension, edema, and oliguria with iodinated contrast media (may occur within 4 weeks to several months after aldesleukin administration); hypersensitivity reactions have been reported when combined with dacarbazine, cis-platinum, tamoxifen, and interferon-alfa; exacerbation of autoimmune and inflammatory disorders and myocardial injury when used in combination with interferon-alfa

(Continued)

Aldesleukin (Continued)

Stability Store in refrigerator; do not freeze; reconstituted solution is stable 48 hours in refrigerator or at room temperature; since aldesleukin contains no preservatives, refrigerated storage of the reconstituted solution is preferred; reconstituted solution packaged in tuberculin syringes for S.C. administration are stable 14 days refrigerated and 6 hours at room temperature; compatible **only** with D_5W; incompatible with sodium chloride solutions; do not mix with other medications

Stability of Aldesleukin Related to Final Concentration

Infusion Duration	Final Concentration of Aldesleukin (mcg/mL)				Stability at Room Temperature (h)
	1-30	31-69	70-100	>100	
Short I.V. infusion (15 minutes)	Add albumin*	Not necessary to add albumin	Due to poor stability; **AVOID** use at this concentration	Not necessary to add albumin	48 h
Continuous I.V. infusion (24 h) at room temperature	Add albumin*	Not necessary to add albumin	Due to poor stability; **AVOID** use at this concentration	Not necessary to add albumin	48 h
Continuous I.V. infusion via CADD pump†	Add albumin*	Add albumin*	Due to poor stability; **AVOID** use at this concentration	Not necessary to add albumin	6 d†

*To improve stability, albumin must be added to a final concentration of 0.1% (1 mg/mL); albumin must be added first to D_5W followed by the reconstituted aldesleukin solution

†Continuous infusion via CADD pump or similar infusion device raises aldesleukin temperature to ≥32°C (89°F)

Mechanism of Action Aldesleukin, a human recombinant interleukin-2 product, promotes proliferation, differentiation, and recruitment of T and B cells, natural killer cells, and thymocytes; also causes cytolytic activity in some lymphocytes and subsequent interactions between lymphokine-activated killer cells and tumor-infiltrating lymphocytes; causes multiple immunological effects including activation of cellular immunity with lymphocytosis, eosinophilia, and thrombocytopenia; production of cytokines (including tumor necrosis factor, interleukin-1), and inhibition of tumor growth

Pharmacokinetics

Absorption: Oral: Not absorbed

Distribution: Primarily into plasma, lymphocytes, lungs, liver, kidney, and spleen

V_d: Adults: 4-7 L

Metabolism: Metabolized to amino acids in the cells lining the proximal convoluted tubules of the kidney

Bioavailability: I.M.: 30% to 37%

Half-life:

Children:

Distribution: 14 ± 6 minutes

Elimination: 51 ± 11 minutes

Adults:

Distribution: 6-27 minutes

Elimination: 85 minutes

Time to peak serum concentration: S.C.: 2-3 hours

Clearance: Adults: 7.2-16.1 L/hour

Usual Dosage A wide variety of dosages have been or are currently under investigation (refer to individual protocols):

AML: Children: (Investigational use only, Sievers, 1998): Continuous I.V. infusion: 9 million international units (9×10^6 international units) daily for 4 days; repeat 4 days later with 1.6 million international units (1.6×10^6 international units) daily for 10 days

Metastatic renal cell carcinoma and metastatic melanoma: Adults:

I.V.:

Initial: Treatment consists of two 5-day treatment cycles separated by a rest period: 600,000 international units/kg (0.037 mg/kg) every 8 hours for a total of 14 doses; followed by a rest period of 9 days, then repeat the 14-dose regimen; these two cycles constitute one course of therapy

Retreatment: Each treatment course should be separated by a rest period of at least 7 weeks from the date of completion; patients should be evaluated for response approximately 4 weeks after completion of a course of therapy and again immediately prior to the scheduled start of the next treatment course

S.C.: (Investigational): 11 million international units (11×10^6 international units) daily for 4 days per week for 4 consecutive weeks; repeat every 6 weeks, or alternatively, 18 million international units (18×10^6 international units) daily for 5 days followed by a 2-day rest period, then 9 million international units (9 x 10⁶ international units) for 2 days, followed by 18 million international units (18 x 10⁶ international units) daily for 3 days

Dosage modification for toxicity: In high-dose therapy, see manufacturer's guidelines (or refer to specific protocol for recommendations) for holding and restarting therapy; hold or interrupt a dose, **do not dose reduce**

Administration Parenteral:

I.V.: Reconstitute with 1.2 mL SWI (swirl, do not shake); resulting concentration is 1.1 mg/mL [18 million (18 x 10⁶) international units/mL]; further dilute dosage in D₅W to a final concentration between 30-70 mcg/mL (0.49-1.1 million international units/mL) and infuse over 15 minutes; for continuous infusions, dilute in D₅W maintaining the same final concentration; final dilutions <30 mcg/mL or >70 mcg/mL have shown increased variability in drug stability and bioactivity; addition of albumin has been used to improve stability if final dilution concentrations <30 mcg/mL are necessary; when continuous infusion is via devices which expose aldesleukin to temperatures higher than room temperature (≥32°C/89.6°F) (eg, CADD pump or similar infusion device), drug stability is also altered; see Stability for more detailed information; do not use in-line filter when administering

S.C.: Reconstituted solution may be administered subcutaneously without further dilution (**Note:** Subcutaneous administration is a non-FDA approved route)

Monitoring Parameters Baseline chest x-ray, pulmonary function tests and thallium stress study; CBC with differential, platelet counts, electrolytes, BUN, serum creatinine, hepatic enzymes, vital signs, weight, pulse oximetry, arterial blood gases (if pulmonary symptoms), fluid intake and output

Nursing Implications See Warnings and Precautions

Additional Information
1 Cetus Unit = 6 international units
1 Roche Unit (Teceleukin) = 3 international units
1.1 mg = 18 x 10⁶ international units or 3 x 10⁶ Cetus units

Dosage Forms Injection, powder for reconstitution, lyophilized: 22 x 10⁶ international units (1.3 mg) [18 x 10⁶ international units/mL] [1.1 mg/mL]

References
Sievers EL, Lange BJ, Sondel PM, et al, "Feasibility, Toxicity, and Biologic Response of Interleukin-2 After Consolidation Chemotherapy for Acute Myelogenous Leukemia: A Report From the Children's Cancer Group," *J Clin Oncol*, 1998, 16(3):914-9.

Whittington R and Faulds D, "Interleukin-2: A Review of Its Pharmacological Properties and Therapeutic Use in Patients With Cancer," *Drugs*, 1993, 46(3):446-514.

◆ **Aldurazyme®** *see* Laronidase *on page 658*
◆ **Aler-Dryl [OTC]** *see* DiphenhydrAMINE *on page 393*
◆ **Aleve® [OTC]** *see* Naproxen *on page 796*
◆ **Alfenta®** *see* Alfentanil *on page 59*

Alfentanil (al FEN ta nil)

Related Information
Narcotic Analgesics Comparison *on page 1223*
Overdose and Toxicology *on page 1388*

U.S. Brand Names Alfenta®

Therapeutic Category Analgesic, Narcotic; General Anesthetic

Generic Available Yes

Use Analgesia; analgesia adjunct; anesthetic agent

Restrictions C-II

Pregnancy Risk Factor C (D if used for prolonged periods or high doses at term)

Contraindications Hypersensitivity to alfentanil hydrochloride or any component; increased intracranial pressure; severe respiratory depression

Warnings Rapid I.V. infusion may result in skeletal muscle and chest wall rigidity → impaired ventilation → respiratory distress/arrest; inject slowly over 3-5 minutes; nondepolarizing skeletal muscle relaxant may be required

Precautions Use with caution in patients with bradycardia

Adverse Reactions
Cardiovascular: Bradycardia, peripheral vasodilation, hypotension
Central nervous system: Drowsiness, dizziness, sedation, CNS depression, elevated intracranial pressure
Dermatologic: Pruritus
Endocrine & metabolic: Antidiuretic hormone release
Gastrointestinal: Nausea, vomiting, constipation, biliary tract spasm
Genitourinary: Urinary tract spasm
Neuromuscular & skeletal: Skeletal muscle and chest wall rigidity especially following rapid I.V. administration
Ocular: Miosis
(Continued)

Alfentanil *(Continued)*

Respiratory: Respiratory depression, apnea, respiratory arrest

Miscellaneous: Histamine release, physical and psychological dependence with prolonged use

Drug Interactions Cytochrome P450 isoenzyme CYP3A3/4 substrate

CNS depressants, phenothiazines, tricyclic antidepressants may potentiate the adverse effects of opiate agonists; use with benzodiazepines may cause vasodilation, hypotension, and delay recovery; cimetidine may decrease and erythromycin may significantly decrease alfentanil clearance; chronic beta-blocker therapy may potentiate alfentanil-induced bradycardia; propofol may increase serum concentrations of alfentanil

Mechanism of Action Binds with stereospecific receptors at many sites within the CNS, increases pain threshold, alters pain reception, inhibits ascending pain pathways

Pharmacodynamics

Onset of action: Within 5 minutes

Duration: <15-20 minutes

Pharmacokinetics

Distribution: V_d beta:

Newborns, premature: 1 L/kg

Children: 0.163-0.48 L/kg

Adults: 0.46 L/kg

Protein binding:

Neonates: 67%

Adults: 88% to 92%

Bound to alpha$_1$-acid glycoprotein

Metabolism: Hepatic

Half-life, elimination:

Newborns, premature: 320-525 minutes

Children: 40-60 minutes

Adults: 83-97 minutes

Usual Dosage Doses should be titrated to appropriate effects; wide range of doses is dependent upon desired degree of analgesia/anesthesia

Neonates, Infants, and Children <12 years: Dose not established; A high percent of newborn infants receiving alfentanil (prior to procedures) at doses of 9-15 mcg/kg (mean dose: 11.7 mcg/kg) developed chest wall rigidity; 9 out of 20 newborns (45%) developed mild or moderate rigidity that did not affect ventilation, while 4 out of 20 (20%) had severe rigidity interfering with respiration for ~5-10 minutes; use of a skeletal muscle relaxant to prevent chest wall rigidity is recommended; however,

Alfentanil: Adult Dosing

Indication	Approximate Duration of Anesthesia (min)	Induction Period (Initial Dose) (mcg/kg)	Maintenance Period (Increments/ Infusion)	Total Dose (mcg/kg)	Effects
Incremental injection	≤30	8-20	3-5 mcg/kg or 0.5-1 mcg/kg/min	8-40	Spontaneously breathing or assisted ventilation when required.
	30-60	20-50	5-15 mcg/kg	Up to 75	Assisted or controlled ventilation required. Attenuation of response to laryngoscopy and intubation.
Continuous infusion	>45	50-75	0.5-3 mcg/kg/min; average infusion rate: 1-1.5 mcg/kg/min	Dependent on duration of procedure	Assisted or controlled ventilation required. Some attenuation of response to intubation and incision, with intraoperative stability.
Anesthetic induction	>45	130-245	0.5-1.5 mcg/kg/min or general anesthetic	Dependent on duration of procedure	Assisted or controlled ventilation required. Administer slowly (over 3 minutes). Concentration of inhalation agents reduced by 30% to 50% for initial hour.

smaller alfentanil doses may be required in newborns. Further studies are needed to determine appropriate doses of alfentanil in pediatric patients.

Adults: Use lean body weight for patients who weigh >20% over ideal body weight; see table on previous page.

Administration Parenteral: I.V.: Inject slowly over 3-5 minutes or by I.V. continuous infusion; maximum concentration: 80 mcg/mL

Monitoring Parameters Respiratory rate, blood pressure, heart rate, neurological status (for degree of analgesia/anesthesia)

Nursing Implications Alfentanil may produce more hypotension compared to fentanyl, therefore, be sure to administer slowly and ensure patient has adequate hydration; may be habit-forming; avoid abrupt discontinuation after prolonged use

Dosage Forms Injection, solution, as hydrochloride [preservative free]: 500 mcg/mL (2 mL, 5 mL, 10 mL, 20 mL)

References

Davis PJ, Killian A, Stiller RL, et al, "Pharmacokinetics of Alfentanil in Newborn Premature Infants and Older Children," *Dev Pharmacol Ther*, 1989, 13(1):21-7.

Marlow N, Weindling AM, Van Peer A, et al, "Alfentanil Pharmacokinetics in Preterm Infants," *Arch Dis Child*, 1990, 65(4 Spec No):349-51.

Meistelman C, Saint-Maurice C, Lepaul M, et al, "A Comparison of Alfentanil Pharmacokinetics in Children and Adults," *Anesthesiology*, 1987, 66(1):13-6.

Pokela ML, Ryhanen PT, Koivisto ME, et al, "Alfentanil-Induced Rigidity in Newborn Infants," *Anesth Analg*, 1992, 75(2):252-7.

Alglucerase (al GLOO ser ase)

U.S. Brand Names Ceredase®

Synonyms Glucocerebrosidase

Therapeutic Category Enzyme, Glucocerebrosidase; Gaucher's Disease, Treatment Agent

Generic Available No

Use Long-term enzyme replacement in patients with confirmed Type I Gaucher disease who exhibit one or more of the following conditions: Moderate to severe anemia; thrombocytopenia and bleeding tendencies; bone disease; hepatomegaly or splenomegaly; growth retardation related to Gaucher disease

Pregnancy Risk Factor C

Contraindications Hypersensitivity to alglucerase or any component

Precautions Alglucerase is prepared from pooled human placental tissue that may contain the causative agents of some viral diseases; the risk of contamination from slowly active or latent viruses is believed to be remote due to steps taken in the manufacturing process; observe for signs of early virilization in males <10 years of age

Adverse Reactions

Central nervous system: Fever, chills, fatigue

Endocrine & metabolic: Early virilization (males <10 years)

Gastrointestinal: Abdominal discomfort, nausea, vomiting, diarrhea, oral ulcerations

Local: Discomfort, burning, and edema at the site of injection

Neuromuscular: Weakness, backache

Miscellaneous: Hypersensitivity reactions

Drug Interactions No information available at this time

Stability When diluted to 100-200 mL with NS, resultant solution is stable up to 18 hours when stored at 2°C to 8°C

Mechanism of Action Glucocerebrosidase is an enzyme prepared from human placental tissue. Gaucher's disease is an inherited metabolic disorder caused by the defective activity of beta-glucosidase and the resultant accumulation of glucosyl ceramide laden macrophages in the liver, bone, and spleen. Alglucerase acts by replacing the missing enzyme associated with Gaucher's disease.

Pharmacodynamics

Onset of significant improvement in symptoms:

Hepatosplenomegaly and hematologic abnormalities: Occurs within 6 months

Improvement in bone mineralization: Noted at 80-104 weeks of therapy

Pharmacokinetics

Distribution: V_d: 0.05-0.28 L/kg

Half-life, elimination: ~4-10 minutes

Usual Dosage Children, Adolescents, and Adults: I.V. infusion: Dosage varies with the severity of disease; the recommended dosage ranges from 1.15 units/kg 3 times/ week to 60 units/kg administered as frequently as once weekly or as infrequently as every 4 weeks; a common low-dose high-frequency protocol is 30 units/kg/month divided into 3 infusions weekly; after a response is firmly established, the dosage may be progressively lowered at periods of 3-6 months

(Continued)

Alglucerase *(Continued)*

Administration Parenteral: Dilute to a final volume of 100-200 mL NS and infuse I.V. over 1-2 hours; an in-line filter should be used; do not shake solution as it denatures the enzyme

Monitoring Parameters CBC, platelets, liver function tests

Dosage Forms Injection, solution: 10 units/mL (5 mL); 80 units/mL (5 mL)

References
Barton NW, Brady RO, Dambrosia JM, et al, "Replacement Therapy for Inherited Enzyme Deficiency - Macrophage-Targeted Glucocerebrosidase for Gaucher's Disease," *N Engl J Med*, 1991, 324(21):1464-70.

- ◆ **Alka-Mints® [OTC]** *see* Calcium Supplements *on page 200*
- ◆ **Alka-Seltzer® Gas Relief [OTC]** *see* Simethicone *on page 1020*
- ◆ **Alkeran®** *see* Melphalan *on page 716*
- ◆ **Allegra®** *see* Fexofenadine *on page 483*
- ◆ **Allerdryl® (Can)** *see* DiphenhydrAMINE *on page 393*
- ◆ **Allerfrim® [OTC]** *see* Triprolidine and Pseudoephedrine *on page 1122*
- ◆ **Allergen®** *see* Antipyrine and Benzocaine *on page 122*
- ◆ **AllerMax® [OTC]** *see* DiphenhydrAMINE *on page 393*
- ◆ **Allernix (Can)** *see* DiphenhydrAMINE *on page 393*
- ◆ **Allerphed® [OTC]** *see* Triprolidine and Pseudoephedrine *on page 1122*
- ◆ **Allersol®** *see* Naphazoline *on page 795*

Allopurinol *(al oh PURE i nole)*

Related Information
Tumor Lysis Syndrome, Management *on page 1315*

U.S. Brand Names Aloprim™; Zyloprim®

Canadian Brand Names Apo®-Allopurinol

Therapeutic Category Antigout Agent; Uric Acid Lowering Agent

Generic Available Yes (tablet)

Use Prevention of attacks of gouty arthritis and nephropathy; also used in treatment of secondary hyperuricemia which may occur during treatment of tumors or leukemia; prevention of recurrent calcium oxalate calculi

Pregnancy Risk Factor C

Contraindications Hypersensitivity to allopurinol or any component

Warnings Do not use to treat asymptomatic hyperuricemia; monitor liver function and complete blood counts before initiating therapy and periodically

Precautions Reduce dosage in renal impairment; discontinue drug at the first sign of rash; risk of skin rash may be increased in patients receiving amoxicillin or ampicillin; risk of hypersensitivity may be increased in patients receiving thiazides and possibly ACE inhibitors

Adverse Reactions
Cardiovascular: (reported with I.V. administration) Hypotension, flushing, hypertension, bradycardia, heart failure
Central nervous system: Drowsiness, fever, headache, chills, somnolence, agitation
Dermatologic: Pruritic maculopapular rash, exfoliative dermatitis, erythema multiforme, alopecia
Gastrointestinal: GI irritation, dyspepsia, nausea, vomiting, diarrhea, abdominal pain, gastritis
Genitourinary: Hematuria
Hematologic: Leukocytosis, leukopenia, thrombocytopenia, eosinophilia, bone marrow suppression
Hepatic: Hepatitis, elevated liver enzymes, hepatomegaly, hyperbilirubinemia, jaundice
Local: Local injection site reaction
Neuromuscular & skeletal: Peripheral neuropathy, paresthesia, neuritis, arthralgia, myoclonus
Ocular: Cataracts, optic neuritis
Renal: Renal impairment
Respiratory: Epistaxis; (reported with I.V. administration) apnea, hyperpnea, ARDS
Vascular: Necrotizing angiitis, vasculitis

Drug Interactions Inhibits metabolism of azathioprine and mercaptopurine; use with ampicillin or amoxicillin may increase the incidence of skin rash; may increase myelosuppressive effects of cyclophosphamide; large doses may decrease theophylline clearance; increased risk of hypersensitivity reactions when coadministered with ACE inhibitors and thiazide diuretics; decreased allopurinol effectiveness when coadministered with uricosuric agents; increases kidney stone formation when taken with large doses of vitamin C; aluminum hydroxide antacids decrease allopurinol's absorption; increases chlorpropamide effects; may increase risk of osteomalacia in patients receiving phenytoin or phenobarbital; prolongs the half-life of oral anticoagulants; may increase cyclosporine serum levels

Stability Reconstituted parenteral solution should be stored at room temperature; do not refrigerate; use within 10 hours of preparation; physically **incompatible** when mixed with or infused through the same line with the following: Amikacin, amphotericin B, carmustine, cefotaxime, chlorpromazine, cimetidine, clindamycin, cytarabine, dacarbazine, daunorubicin, diphenhydramine, doxorubicin, doxycycline, droperidol, floxuridine, gentamicin, haloperidol, hydroxyzine, idarubicin, imipenem-cilastatin, mechlorethamine, meperidine, metoclopramide, methylprednisolone sodium succinate, minocycline, nalbuphine, netilmicin, ondansetron, prochlorperazine, promethazine, sodium bicarbonate, streptozocin, tobramycin, vinorelbine

Mechanism of Action Decreases the production of uric acid by inhibiting the action of xanthine oxidase, an enzyme that converts hypoxanthine to xanthine and xanthine to uric acid

Pharmacodynamics Decrease in serum uric acid occurs in 1-2 days with a nadir achieved in 1-3 weeks

Pharmacokinetics

Absorption: Oral: ~80% from the GI tract

Distribution: Into breast milk; breast milk to plasma ratio: 0.9-1.4

Protein binding: <1%

Metabolism: ~75% of drug metabolized to active metabolites, chiefly oxypurinol

Half-life:

Parent: 1-3 hours

Oxypurinol metabolite: 18-30 hours in patients with normal renal function

Time to peak serum concentration: Within 2-6 hours

Dialysis: Allopurinol and oxypurinol are dialyzable

Usual Dosage

Prevention of acute uric acid nephropathy in myeloproliferative neoplastic disorders (beginning 1-2 days before chemotherapy): Daily doses >300 mg should be administered in divided doses:

Children ≤10 years:

I.V.: 200 mg/m²/day in 1-3 divided doses; maximum dose: 600 mg/day

Oral: 10 mg/kg/day in 2-3 divided doses or 200-300 mg/m²/day in 2-4 divided doses; maximum dose: 800 mg/day

Alternative:

<6 years: 150 mg/day in 3 divided doses

6-10 years: 300 mg/day in 2-3 divided doses

Children >10 years and Adults:

I.V.: 200-400 mg/m²/day in 1-3 divided doses; maximum: 600 mg/day

Oral: 600-800 mg/day in 2-3 divided doses

Gout: Children >10 years and Adults: Oral:

Mild: 200-300 mg/day

Severe: 400-600 mg/day

Recurrent calcium oxalate stones: Children >10 years and Adults: Oral: 200-300 mg daily in divided or single daily dosage

Dosing adjustment in renal impairment:

Cl_{cr} >50 mL/minute: No dosage change

Cl_{cr} 10-50 mL/minute: Reduce dosage to 50% of recommended

Cl_{cr} <10 mL/minute: Reduce dosage to 30% of recommended

Administration

Oral: Administer after meals with plenty of fluid

Parenteral: Reconstitute 500 mg vial with 25 mL SWI; prior to administration, further dilute with D_5W or NS to a maximum concentration of 6 mg/mL; rate of infusion is dependent upon the volume of infusate (in research studies, 100-300 mg doses were infused over 30 minutes)

Monitoring Parameters CBC, liver function tests, renal function, serum uric acid; 24-hour urinary urate (when treating calcium oxalate stones)

Reference Range

Uric acid: Male: 3.0-7.0 mg/dL; Female: 2.0-6.0 mg/dL

Urinary urate excretion: Male: <800 mg/day; Female: <750 mg/day

Patient Information Report any skin rash, painful urination, blood in urine, irritation of the eyes, or swelling of lips or mouth; avoid alcohol; drink plenty of fluids; may cause drowsiness and and impair ability to perform activities requiring mental alertness or physical coordination

Dosage Forms

Injection, as sodium (Aloprim™): 500 mg

Tablet (Zyloprim®): 100 mg, 300 mg

(Continued)

Allopurinol (Continued)

Extemporaneous Preparations

A 20 mg/mL suspension may be made by crushing eight 300 mg tablets and mixing with 120 mL of either a 1:1 mixture of Ora-Sweet® and Ora-Plus® or a 1:1 mixture of Ora-Sweet® SF and Ora-Plus®. The resulting suspension is stable for 60 days refrigerated (Allen, 1996).

A 20 mg/mL suspension may be made by crushing one 100 mg tablet; wet crushed tablet with small amount of 1% methylcellulose then add syrup NF to a final volume of 5 mL; stable 56 days refrigerated (Dressman, 1983).

Allen LV and Erickson MA, "Stability of Acetazolamide, Allopurinol, Azathioprine, Clonazepam, and Flucytosine in Extemporaneously Compounded Oral Liquids," *Am J Health Sys Pharm*, 1996, 53:1944-9.

Dressman JB and Poust RI, "Stability of Allopurinol and of Five Antineoplastics in Suspension," *Am J Hosp Pharm*, 1983, 40(4):616-8.

References

Bennett WM, Aronoff GR, Golper TA, et al, *Drug Prescribing in Renal Failure*, Philadelphia, PA: American College of Physicians, 1987.

Krakoff IH and Murphy ML, "Hyperuricemia in Neoplastic Disease in Children: Prevention With Allopurinol, A Xanthine Oxidase Inhibitor" *Pediatrics*, 1968, 41(1):52-6.

♦ **Almora®** [OTC] *see* Magnesium Supplements *on page 701*
♦ **Alocril™** *see* Nedocromil *on page 798*
♦ **Aloe Vesta® 2-n-1 Antifungal** [OTC] *see* Miconazole *on page 759*
♦ **Alophen®** [OTC] *see* Bisacodyl *on page 173*
♦ **Aloprim™** *see* Allopurinol *on page 62*
♦ **Alora®** *see* Estradiol *on page 456*
♦ **Alphanate®** *see* Antihemophilic Factor (Human) *on page 116*
♦ **Alphatrex®** *see* Betamethasone *on page 169*

Alprazolam (al PRAY zoe lam)

Related Information

Carbohydrate and Alcohol Content of Liquid Medications for Use in Patients Receiving Ketogenic Diets *on page 1431*
Overdose and Toxicology *on page 1388*
Serotonin Syndrome *on page 1420*

U.S. Brand Names Alprazolam Intensol®; Xanax®; Xanax XR®

Canadian Brand Names Alti-Alprazolam; Apo®-Alpraz; Gen-Alprazolam; Novo-Alprazol; Nu-Alprax

Therapeutic Category Antianxiety Agent; Benzodiazepine

Generic Available Yes (immediate release tablet)

Use Treatment of generalized anxiety disorder (GAD); symptoms of anxiety (short-term treatment); anxiety associated with depression; management of panic disorder, with or without agoraphobia

Restrictions C-IV

Pregnancy Risk Factor D

Contraindications Hypersensitivity to alprazolam, any component, or other benzodiazepines; severe uncontrolled pain, narrow-angle glaucoma, severe respiratory depression, pre-existing CNS depression; not to be used in pregnancy or lactation or in patients taking certain medications (see Drug Interactions)

Warnings Withdrawal symptoms including seizures have occurred 18 hours to 3 days after abrupt discontinuation; when discontinuing therapy, decrease daily dose by no more than 0.5 mg every 3 days; reduce dose in patients with significant hepatic disease

Precautions Safety and effectiveness have not been established in children <18 years of age

Adverse Reactions

Central nervous system: Drowsiness, dizziness, confusion, sedation, fatigue, headache, ataxia, somnolence, dysarthria, memory impairment, depression

Gastrointestinal: Xerostomia, constipation, diarrhea, nausea, vomiting, appetite increased or decreased, weight gain or weight loss

Ocular: Blurred vision

Miscellaneous: Physical and psychological dependence with prolonged use

Drug Interactions Cytochrome P450 isoenzyme CYP3A3/4 substrate

Enzyme inducers may increase metabolism of alprazolam; CNS depressants including alcohol may enhance CNS effects; cimetidine, erythromycin, fluvoxamine, fluoxetine, nefazodone, propoxyphene, and oral contraceptives may decrease the metabolism of alprazolam (monitor for increased adverse effects); Delavirdine, ritonavir, ketoconazole, or itraconazole may decrease the metabolism of alprazolam and significantly increase alprazolam levels; concurrent use of delavirdine, ritonavir, ketoconazole, or itraconazole with alprazolam is not recommended. Alprazolam may increase plasma concentrations of imipramine (by 31%) and desipramine (by 20%); clinical significance not known, monitor patients

Food Interactions Extended release tablet: A high-fat meal eaten ≤2 hours before the dose may increase peak concentrations by ~25%. A high-fat meal eaten immediately before the dose may decrease the time to peak concentrations by about 33%. A high-fat meal eaten ≥1 hour after the dose may increase the time to peak concentrations by about 33%. The extent of absorption (AUC) is not affected by food.

Mechanism of Action Depresses all levels of the CNS, including the limbic and reticular formation, by binding to the benzodiazepine site on the gamma-aminobutyric acid (GABA) receptor complex and modulating GABA, which is a major inhibitory neurotransmitter in the brain

Pharmacokinetics

Absorption: Oral:

Immediate release tablet: Rapidly and well absorbed

Extended release tablet: Rate of absorption is increased following night time dosing (versus morning dosing)

Distribution: 0.9-1.2 L/kg; distributes into breast milk

Protein binding: 80%

Metabolism: Extensive in the liver, primarily via cytochrome P450 isoenzyme CYP3A; major metabolites: alpha-hydroxy-alprazolam (about half as active as alprazolam), 4-hydroxyalprazolam (active), and a benzophenone metabolite (inactive). **Note:** Active metabolites are not likely to contribute to pharmacologic effects due to low levels of activity and low concentrations.

Bioavailability: Similar for extended and immediate release tablets (~90%)

Half-life: Adults: 6.3-26.9 hours; mean: 11.2 hours

Time to peak serum concentration: Immediate release tablet: Within 1-2 hours

Elimination: Excretion of metabolites and parent compound in urine

Usual Dosage Oral: **Note:** Titrate dose to effect; use lowest effective dose

Children <18 years: Immediate release: Dose not established; investigationally in children 7-16 years of age (n=13), initial doses of 0.005 mg/kg or 0.125 mg/dose were given 3 times/day for situational anxiety and increments of 0.125-0.25 mg/dose were used to increase doses to maximum of 0.02 mg/kg/dose or 0.06 mg/kg/day; a range of 0.375-3 mg/day was needed (see Pfefferbaum, 1987). **Note:** A more recent study in 17 children (8-17 years of age) with overanxious disorder or avoidant disorders used initial daily doses of 0.25 mg for children <40 kg and 0.5 mg for those >40 kg. The dose was titrated at 2-day intervals to a maximum of 0.04 mg/kg/day. Required doses ranged from 0.5-3.5 mg/day with a mean of 1.6 mg/day. Based on clinical global ratings, alprazolam appeared to be better than placebo, however, this difference was **not** statistically significant (see Simeon, 1992); further studies are needed.

Adults:

Anxiety: Immediate release: Initial: 0.25-0.5 mg 3 times/day; titrate dose upward as needed every 3-4 days; maximum dose: 4 mg/day given in divided doses

Panic disorder:

Immediate release: Initial: 0.5 mg 3 times/day; titrate dose upward as needed every 3-4 days in increments ≤1 mg/day; mean dose used in controlled trials: 5-6 mg/day; maximum dose: 10 mg/day (rarely required)

Extended release: Initial: 0.5-1 mg once daily; titrate dose upward as needed every 3-4 days in increments ≤1 mg/day; usual dose: 3-6 mg/day; maximum dose: 10 mg/day (rarely required)

Switching from immediate release to extended release: Administer the same total daily dose, but give once daily; if effect is not adequate, titrate dose as above

Administration Oral:

Immediate release tablet: Administer with food to decrease GI upset

Extended release tablet: Administer once daily, preferably in the morning; do not crush, chew, or break; swallow whole

Monitoring Parameters CNS status, respiratory rate

Patient Information May cause drowsiness and impair ability to perform activities requiring mental alertness or physical coordination; may be habit-forming; avoid abrupt discontinuation after prolonged use; avoid alcohol; limit caffeine; may cause dry mouth

Nursing Implications Assist with ambulation during beginning of therapy; allow patient to rise slowly to avoid fainting

Additional Information If used for an extended period of time, long-term usefulness of alprazolam should be periodically re-evaluated for an individual patient.

Dosage Forms

Solution, oral (Alprazolam Intensol®): 1 mg/mL (30 mL)

Tablet (Xanax®): 0.25 mg, 0.5 mg, 1 mg, 2 mg

(Continued)

Alprazolam *(Continued)*

Tablet, extended release (Xanax XR®): 0.5 mg, 1 mg, 2 mg, 3 mg

References

Bernstein GA, Garfinkel BD, and Borchardt CM, "Comparative Studies of Pharmacotherapy for School Refusal," *J Am Acad Child Adolesc Psychiatry*, 1990, 29(5):773-81.

DeVane CL, Hill M, and Antal EJ, "Therapeutic Drug Monitoring of Alprazolam in Adolescents With Asthma," *Ther Drug Monit*, 1998, 20(3):257-60.

Pfefferbaum B, Overall JE, Boren HA, et al, "Alprazolam in the Treatment of Anticipatory and Acute Situational Anxiety in Children With Cancer," *J Am Acad Child Adolesc Psychiatry*, 1987, 26(4):532-5.

Simeon JG and Ferguson HB, "Alprazolam Effects in Children With Anxiety Disorders," *Can J Psychiatry*, 1987, 32(7):570-4.

Simeon JG, Ferguson HB, Knott V, et al, "Clinical, Cognitive, and Neurophysiological Effects of Alprazolam in Children and Adolescents With Overanxious and Avoidant Disorders," *J Am Acad Child Adolesc Psychiatry*, 1992, 31(1):29-33.

♦ **Alprazolam Intensol**® *see Alprazolam on page 64*

Alprostadil (al PROS ta dill)

U.S. Brand Names Prostin VR Pediatric®
Canadian Brand Names Caverject®; Muse® Pellet
Synonyms PGE$_1$; Prostaglandin E$_1$
Therapeutic Category Prostaglandin
Generic Available Yes [Injection (500 mcg/mL)]
Use Temporary maintenance of patency of ductus arteriosus in neonates with ductal-dependent congenital heart disease until surgery can be performed. These defects include cyanotic (eg, pulmonary atresia, pulmonary stenosis, tricuspid atresia, Fallot's tetralogy, transposition of the great vessels) and acyanotic (eg, interruption of aortic arch, coarctation of aorta, hypoplastic left ventricle) heart disease.

Investigationally used for the treatment of pulmonary hypertension in infants and children with congenital heart defects with left-to-right shunts

Adult males: Diagnosis and treatment of erectile dysfunction (see Additional Information)

Pregnancy Risk Factor X
Contraindications Hypersensitivity to alprostadil or any component; respiratory distress syndrome or persistent fetal circulation
Warnings Apnea occurs in 10% to 12% of neonates with congenital heart defects (especially in those weighing <2 kg at birth) and usually appears during the first hour of drug infusion
Precautions Use cautiously in neonates with bleeding tendencies; if hypotension or pyrexia occurs, the infusion rate should be reduced until symptoms subside; severe hypotension, apnea, or bradycardia requires drug discontinuation with cautious reinstitution at a lower dose; tissue necrosis may occur with extravasation of concentrated solutions (due to high osmolality)
Adverse Reactions
Cardiovascular: Systemic hypotension, flushing, bradycardia, rhythm disturbances, tachycardia, edema
Central nervous system: Seizure-like activity, fever
Endocrine & metabolic: Hypocalcemia, hypoglycemia, hypokalemia, hyperkalemia
Gastrointestinal: Diarrhea, gastric-outlet obstruction secondary to antral hyperplasia (occurrence related to duration of therapy and cumulative dose)
Hematologic: Inhibition of platelet aggregation
Neuromuscular & skeletal: Cortical proliferation of long bones (cortical hyperostosis) has been seen with long-term infusions (incidence and severity are related to duration of therapy and cumulative dose); **Note:** Cortical hyperostosis may present with clinical symptoms that mimic cellulitis or osteomyelitis (eg, symptomatic bone tenderness, soft tissue swelling)
Respiratory: Respiratory depression, apnea
Miscellaneous: Pretibial and soft tissue swelling, swelling of upper and lower extremities
Stability Compatible in D$_5$W, D$_{10}$W, and saline solutions; refrigerate ampuls at 2°C to 8°C. Avoid direct contact of undiluted alprostadil with the plastic walls of volumetric infusion chambers because the drug will interact with the plastic and create a hazy solution; discard solution and volumetric chamber if this occurs.
Mechanism of Action Causes vasodilation by means of direct effect on vascular and ductus arteriosus smooth muscle
Pharmacodynamics
Maximum effect:
Acyanotic congenital heart disease: Usual: 1.5-3 hours; range: 15 minutes to 11 hours
Cyanotic congenital heart disease: Usual: ~30 minutes
Duration: Ductus arteriosus will begin to close within 1-2 hours after drug is stopped

Pharmacokinetics

Metabolism: ~70% to 80% metabolized by oxidation during a single pass through the lungs; metabolite (13,14 dihydro-PGE_1) is active and has been identified in neonates

Half-life: 5-10 minutes; since the half-life is so short, the drug must be administered by continuous infusion

Elimination: Metabolites excreted in urine

Usual Dosage

Neonates and Infants: 0.05-0.1 mcg/kg/minute; with therapeutic response, rate is reduced to lowest effective dosage; with unsatisfactory response, rate is increased gradually; maintenance: 0.01-0.4 mcg/kg/minute

PGE_1 is usually given at an infusion rate of 0.1 mcg/kg/minute; but it is often possible to reduce the dosage to $1/2$ or even $1/10$ without losing the therapeutic effect. The mixing schedule is shown in the table.

Add 1 Ampul (500 mcg) to:	Concentration (mcg/mL)	Infusion Rate to Deliver 0.1 mcg/kg/min		
		mL/kg/min	mL/kg/h	mL/kg/24 h
250 mL	2	0.05	3	72
100 mL	5	0.02	1.2	28.8
50 mL	10	0.01	0.6	14.4
25 mL	20	0.005	0.3	7.2

Administration Parenteral: I.V. continuous infusion into a large vein or alternatively through an umbilical artery catheter placed at the ductal opening; maximum concentration listed (per package insert) for I.V. infusion: 20 mcg/mL; has also been administered via continuous infusion into the right pulmonary artery for investigational treatment of pulmonary hypertension in infants and children with congenital heart defects with left-to-right shunts; rate of infusion (mL/hour) = dose (mcg/kg/minute) x weight (kg) x 60 minutes/hour divided by the concentration (mcg/mL)

Monitoring Parameters Arterial pressure, respiratory rate, heart rate, temperature, pO_2; monitor for gastric obstruction in patients receiving PGE_1 for longer than 120 hours; x-rays may be needed to assess cortical hyperostosis in patients receiving prolonged PGE_1 therapy

Nursing Implications Prepare fresh solution every 24 hours; flushing of arm or face may indicate misplacement of intra-arterial catheter and infusion of drug into subclavian or carotid artery; reposition catheter

Additional Information Therapeutic response is indicated by an increase in systemic blood pressure and pH in those with restricted systemic blood flow and acidosis, or by an increase in oxygenation (pO_2) in those with restricted pulmonary blood flow. Most cases of bone changes occurred 4-6 weeks after starting alprostadil, but it has occurred as early as 9 days; cortical hyperostosis usually resolves over 6-12 months after stopping PGE_1 therapy

Alprostadil is also available as Caverject® injection, Edex® injection, and Muse® Pellet (urethral) for the diagnosis and treatment of erectile dysfunction in adult males; see package inserts for further information for this use.

Dosage Forms Injection, solution (Prostin VR Pediatric®): 500 mcg/mL (1 mL)

References

Kaufman MB and El-Chaar GM, "Bone and Tissue Changes Following Prostaglandin Therapy in Neonates," *Ann Pharmacother*, 1996, 30(3):269-74, 277.

Lewis AB, Freed MD, Heymann MA, et al, "Side Effects of Therapy With Prostaglandin E₁ in Infants With Critical Congenital Heart Disease," *Circulation*, 1981, 64(5):893-8.

Peled N, Dagan O, Babyn P, et al, "Gastric-Outlet Obstruction Induced by Prostaglandin Therapy in Neonates," *N Engl J Med*, 1992, 327(8):505-10.

Weesner KM, "Hemodynamic Effects of Prostaglandin E₁ in Patients With Congenital Heart Disease and Pulmonary Hypertension," *Cathet Cardiovasc Diagn*, 1991, 24(1):10-5.

Woo K, Emery J, and Peabody J, "Cortical Hyperostosis: A Complication of Prolonged Prostaglandin Infusion in Infants Awaiting Cardiac Transplantation," *Pediatrics*, 1994, 93(3):417-20.

◆ **Altamist [OTC]** *see* Sodium Chloride *on page 1027*

Alteplase (AL te plase)

Related Information

Antithrombotic Therapy in Children *on page 1316*

U.S. Brand Names Activase®; CathFlo™ Activase®

Synonyms Alteplase, Recombinant; Tissue Plasminogen Activator, Recombinant; t-PA

Therapeutic Category Thrombolytic Agent; Thrombotic Occlusion (Central Venous Catheter), Treatment Agent

Generic Available No

(Continued)

Alteplase (Continued)

Use

Activase®: Thrombolytic agent used in treatment of acute MI, acute ischemic stroke, and acute massive pulmonary embolism

CathFlo™ Activase®: Treatment of occluded central venous catheters

Pregnancy Risk Factor C

Contraindications Hypersensitivity to alteplase or any component (see Additional Information)

Contraindications for use in the treatment of acute MI or pulmonary embolism: Active internal bleeding; known bleeding diathesis; history of CVA; intracranial neoplasm, arteriovenous malformation, or aneurysm; recent intracranial or intraspinal surgery or trauma; severe uncontrolled hypertension

Contraindications for use in the treatment of acute ischemic stroke: Active internal bleeding; known bleeding diathesis (including but not limited to: Current use of oral anticoagulants or an INR >1.7 or PT >15 seconds, use of heparin within 48 hours before the onset of stroke and an elevated aPTT at presentation, platelet count <100,000/mm³); evidence of intracranial hemorrhage on pretreatment evaluation; history of intracranial hemorrhage; suspicion of subarachnoid hemorrhage; recent (within 3 months) intracranial or intraspinal surgery, serious head trauma, or previous stroke; intracranial neoplasm, arteriovenous malformation, or aneurysm; seizure at the onset of stroke; uncontrolled hypertension at time of treatment (eg, adults with blood pressures of >185 mm Hg systolic or >110 mm Hg diastolic)

Warnings Activase®: May cause bleeding (internal, superficial, or surface bleeding); concurrent use of heparin anticoagulation may increase bleeding; monitor all potential bleeding sites. Avoid I.M. injections and nonessential handling of patient; carefully perform venipunctures and only when necessary. If an arterial puncture is required, use vessel in an upper extremity that can be manually compressed. Stop alteplase (and heparin) if serious bleeding occurs (effects of heparin can be reversed by protamine). Do not exceed recommended doses; do not use doses of 150 mg to treat acute MI as this dose has been associated with an increase in intracranial hemorrhage.

Risks from alteplase may be increased in the following conditions (risks versus benefits should be weighed carefully before use): Recent major surgery (eg, organ biopsy, previous puncture of noncompressible vessels, coronary artery bypass graft, obstetrical delivery), recent trauma, recent GI or GU bleeding, current use of oral anticoagulants, cerebrovascular disease, diabetic hemorrhagic retinopathy or other hemorrhagic ophthalmic conditions, hypertension (eg, adults with systolic BP ≥175 mm Hg and/or diastolic BP ≥110 mm Hg), patients with an increased risk of left heart thrombus (eg, mitral stenosis with atrial fibrillation), acute pericarditis, subacute bacterial endocarditis, hemostatic defects including ones caused by severe renal or hepatic dysfunction, significant hepatic dysfunction, pregnancy, septic thrombophlebitis or occluded AV cannula at seriously infected site, advanced age (eg, >75 years old), any other condition in which bleeding would be a significant risk or would be especially difficult to manage due to its location.

Cholesterol embolism may occur (rare). Risk of stroke in acute MI patients who are at low risk for death from cardiac causes and who present with high blood pressure, may be greater than the survival benefit from thrombolytic therapy. Reperfusion arrhythmias may occur following coronary thrombolysis. In patients with pulmonary embolism, alteplase has not been proven to adequately treat underlying DVT; possible reembolization from DVT may occur.

Acute ischemic stroke: Risks of alteplase therapy may be increased in patients with major early signs of infarct on CT and in those with severe neurological deficit at presentation (risks versus benefits should be weighed carefully); treatment of patients >3 hours after onset of symptoms and those with rapidly improving symptoms or minor neurological deficit is not recommended.

Precautions

Activase®: Use with caution if drug is readministered; discontinue immediately if anaphylactoid reaction occurs. For treatment of acute ischemic stroke, frequent monitoring and control of blood pressure during and after alteplase administration is recommended. For systemic use, pretreatment lab studies should include platelet count, PT/PTT, fibrinogen, fibrin degradation products, plasminogen, antithrombin III, protein S, protein C.

CathFlo™ Activase®: Consider other causes of central venous catheter occlusion (eg, mechanical failure, constriction by a suture, catheter malposition, and drug precipitates or lipid deposits within the lumen of the catheter) before use; do not use vigorous suction when determining catheter occlusion (vascular wall damage or collapse of soft-walled catheters may occur); avoid excessive pressure when instilling alteplase into an occluded catheter (catheter may rupture or clot may become dislodged and enter the circulation). The use of CathFlo™ Activase® has not been evaluated in patients who are at risk for bleeding; use with caution in patients with active internal bleeding or those who have had any of the following within 48 hours: Surgery, puncture of noncompressible vessels, obstetrical delivery, or percutaneous biopsy of viscera or deep tissues; use with caution in patients with thrombocytopenia, hemostatic defects including ones caused by severe renal or hepatic dysfunction, any condition in which bleeding would be a significant risk or would be especially difficult to manage due to its location, or those who are at a high risk for embolic complications (eg, venous thrombosis in the region of the catheter). Discontinue CathFlo™ Activase® and withdraw from catheter if serious bleeding in a critical location occurs. Use with caution in patients with known or suspected catheter infection (use of CathFlo™ Activase® in these patients may release a localized infection in the catheter into the systemic circulation).

Use of >2 doses of CathFlo™ Activase® has not been studied. Use in infants and children <2 years of age or <10 kg body weight has not been studied. The relative efficacy and relative rates of adverse effects of CathFlo™ Activase® in pediatric patients (or in those ≥10 kg and <30 kg) could not be determined in present clinical trials, due to an insufficient number of patients enrolled.

Adverse Reactions Note: Adverse reactions listed below have been reported with systemic use. Major adverse events after intracatheter use include: Sepsis, GI bleeding, and venous thrombosis; injection site hemorrhage in a patient with pre-existing thrombocytopenia has also been reported.

Cardiovascular: Hypotension; reperfusion arrhythmias (following coronary thrombolysis)

Central nervous system: Fever, intracranial hemorrhage, cerebral hemorrhage

Dermatologic: Bruising (1%), rash, urticaria (rare)

Gastrointestinal: GI bleeding (5%), nausea, vomiting

Genitourinary: GU bleeding (4%)

Hematologic: Surface bleeding, internal bleeding

Local: Bleeding at catheter puncture site; bruising and inflammation with extravasation

Respiratory: Epistaxis (<1%), laryngeal edema (rare)

Miscellaneous: Anaphylactoid reaction (rare)

Drug Interactions Anticoagulants (warfarin, heparin) and drugs that affect platelet function (aspirin, NSAIDs, dipyridamole, abciximab) may increase the risk of bleeding. Aspirin and heparin have been given concurrently with and after alteplase infusions in patients with acute MI or pulmonary embolism (careful monitoring for bleeding is recommended). However, the concurrent use of aspirin or heparin with alteplase within the first 24 hours after the onset of symptoms of stroke was prohibited in the major stroke trial; therefore, safety of the use of these agents with alteplase in patients with acute ischemic stroke is unknown. Antifibrinolytic agents (aminocaproic acid) may decrease effectiveness.

Stability

Activase®: Store lyophilized product at room temperature [not to exceed 86°F (30°C)] or under refrigeration; protect from excessive light exposure during extended storage. Reconstitute vials with supplied diluent (SWI); do not reconstitute with bacteriostatic water for injection; use large bore needle and syringe to reconstitute 50 mg vial and accompanying transfer device to reconstitute 100 mg vial (100 mg vial does not contain vacuum); swirl gently, do not shake; final concentration after reconstitution: 1 mg/mL; reconstituted solution must be used within 8 hours (manufacturer's recommendations).

The 1 mg/mL solution may be diluted further (immediately before use) with an equal volume of NS or D_5W to yield a final concentration of 0.5 mg/mL; swirl gently, do not shake to dilute; diluted solutions are stable for 8 hours at room temperature. Dilutions to concentrations <0.5 mg/mL are not recommended for routine clinical use; dilutions <0.5 mg/mL using D_5W or SWI will result in a precipitate; an immediate formation of a precipitate following dilution of alteplase with D_5W to 0.16 mg/mL has been reported (Frazin, 1990); after reconstitution to 1 mg/mL, alteplase may be further diluted with NS to concentrations as low as 0.2 mg/mL without precipitation (Frazin, 1990); do not dilute <0.2 mg/mL; after reconstitution to 1 mg/mL, further dilution with NS to target concentrations of 0.05 mg/mL, 0.025 mg/mL, and 0.01 mg/mL resulted in <90% recovery of active alteplase (data on file at Genetech).

Do not add other medications to alteplase solutions. Alteplase is incompatible with bacteriostatic water, dobutamine, dopamine, heparin, morphine, and nitroglycerin infusions; physically compatible with lidocaine, metoprolol, and propranolol when administered via Y site.

Solutions of 0.5 mg/mL, 1 mg/mL, and 2 mg/mL in SWI retained ≥94% of fibrinolytic activity at 48 hours when stored at 2°C in plastic syringes; these solutions

(Continued)

Alteplase *(Continued)*

retained ≥90% of fibrinolytic activity when stored in plastic syringes at -25°C or -70°C for 7 or 14 days, thawed at room temperature and then stored at 2°C for 48 hours (see Davis, 2000). Solutions of 1 mg/mL in SWI were stable for 22 weeks in plastic syringes when stored at -30°C and for ~1 month in glass vials when stored at -20°C; bioactivity remained unchanged for 6 months in propylene containers when stored at -20°C and for 2 weeks in glass vials when stored at -70°C (see review by Generali, 2001).

CathFlo™ Activase®: Store lyophilized product at refrigerated temperature [2°C to 8°C (36°F to 46°C)]; protect from excessive light exposure during extended storage. Reconstitute vial with 2.2 mL of SWI; do not reconstitute with bacteriostatic water for injection; allow vial to stand undisturbed so large bubbles may dissipate; swirl gently, do not shake; complete dissolution occurs within 3 minutes; final concentration after reconstitution: 1 mg/mL; reconstituted solution must be used within 8 hours when stored at 2°C to 30°C (36°F to 81°F); discard any unused solution (solution does not contain preservatives); do not add other medications to CathFlo™ Activase® solutions

Mechanism of Action A naturally-occurring serine protease (enzyme) that initiates local fibrinolysis by binding to fibrin in a thrombus (clot) and directly activating entrapped plasminogen to plasmin; plasmin degrades fibrin, fibrinogen, and other procoagulant proteins into soluble fragments

Pharmacokinetics

Distribution: Initial: Approximates plasma volume; distribution into breast milk is unknown

Metabolism: In the liver

Half-life: Adults:

Initial: <5 minutes

Terminal: 72 minutes

Clearance: Plasma: Adults: 380-570 mL/minute

Usual Dosage

Neonates, Infants, and Children:

Occluded I.V. catheters: Intracatheter:

Chest, 2001 dosing recommendations:

Central venous catheter: **Dose listed is per lumen; for multilumen catheters, treat one lumen at a time:** [Note: Some institutions use lower doses (eg, 0.25 mg/0.5 mL) in neonates and infants <3 months]

Patients ≤10 kg: 0.5 mg diluted in NS to a volume equal to the internal volume of the lumen; instill in each lumen over 1-2 minutes; leave in lumen for 1-2 hours, then **aspirate out of catheter, do not infuse into patient**; flush catheter with NS

Patients >10 kg: 1 mg in 1 mL of NS; use a volume equal to the internal volume of the lumen; maximum: 2 mg in 2 mL per lumen; instill in each lumen over 1-2 minutes; leave in lumen for 1-2 hours; then **aspirate out of catheter, do not infuse into patient**; flush catheter with NS

S.C. port:

Patients ≤10 kg: 0.5 mg diluted with NS to 3 mL

Patients >10 kg: 2 mg diluted with NS to 3 mL

Manufacturer's recommendations (CathFlo™ Activase®):

Central venous catheter:

Patients ≥10 kg to <30 kg: Use a 1 mg/mL concentration; instill a volume equal to 110% of the internal lumen volume of the catheter; do no exceed 2 mg in 2 mL; may instill a second dose if catheter remains occluded after 2-hour dwell time (see Administration)

Patients ≥30 kg: 2 mg in 2 mL; may instill second dose if catheter remains occluded ofter 2-hour dwell time (see Administration)

Systemic thromboses: I.V. (**Note:** Dose must be titrated to effect): *Chest*, 2001 recommendations: 0.1-0.6 mg/kg/hour for 6 hours (some patients may require longer or shorter duration of therapy). **Note:** The optimal dose for various thrombotic conditions is not established in pediatric patients; most published papers consist of case reports; few prospective pediatric studies have been conducted; several studies have used the following doses (see Levy, 1991 and Weiner, 1998). **Note:** Bleeding complications were associated with doses in the higher range.

Initial: 0.1 mg/kg/hour for 6 hours; monitor patient closely for bleeding, monitor fibrinogen levels; if no response after 6 hours, increase infusion by 0.1 mg/kg/hour at 6-hour intervals to a maximum of 0.5 mg/kg/hour; maintain fibrinogen >100 mg/dL (**Note:** Some centers maintain fibrinogen >150 mg/dL in newborns); duration of therapy is based on clinical response

Low-dose (local) infusion for occluded catheters: Note: No pediatric studies have compared local to systemic thrombolytic therapy; therefore, there is no evidence to suggest that local infusions are superior. The pediatric patients' small vessel size may increase the chance of local damage to blood vessels and formation of a new thrombus; however, local infusion may be appropriate for catheter related thromboses if the catheter is already in place (See *Chest*, 2001). Various "low-dose" regimens have been used; the following dosing recommendations are based on Doyle, 1992 and Anderson, 1991:

Initial: 0.01 mg/kg/hour for 6 hours; if no response after 6 hours, increase infusion by 0.01 mg/kg/hour at 6-hour intervals to a maximum of 0.05 mg/kg/hour; monitor patient closely; systemic fibrinolysis (decreased plasma fibrinogen levels) or bleeding has been reported in some neonates and infants receiving 0.05 mg/kg/hour; duration of therapy is based on clinical response

Adults:
  Acute MI: I.V. (**Note:** Alteplase should be administered as soon as possible after symptom onset):
    Accelerated infusion:
      Patients >67 kg: Total dose: 100 mg given in 3 divided doses as follows: Infuse 15 mg I.V. bolus over 1-2 minutes, then infuse 50 mg over the next 30 minutes, then 35 mg over the next 60 minutes. Maximum total dose: 100 mg
      Patients ≤67 kg: Infuse 15 mg I.V. bolus over 1-2 minutes, then infuse 0.75 mg/kg (maximum: 50 mg) over the next 30 minutes, then 0.5 mg/kg (maximum 35 mg) over the next 60 minutes. Maximum total dose: 100 mg
    3-hour infusion:
      Patients ≥65 kg: Total dose: 100 mg given as follows: Infuse 60 mg over the first hour with 6-10 mg given as an I.V. bolus, then infuse 20 mg/hour for 2 hours
      Patients <65 kg: Total dose: 1.25 mg/kg given over 3 hours as described above
  Acute ischemic stroke: I.V. (**Note:** Alteplase therapy should only be started within 3 hours after the onset of symptoms of stroke and after exclusion of intracranial hemorrhage by CT scan or other sensitive diagnostic imaging method): Total dose: 0.9 mg/kg (maximum: 90 mg) given over 1 hour as follows: Infuse 10% of total dose (0.09 mg/kg) I.V. bolus over 1 minute, then infuse the rest of the total dose (0.81 mg/kg) over 60 minutes
  Pulmonary embolism: I.V.: 100 mg infused over 2 hours
  Occluded central venous catheter: Intracatheter: Manufacturer's recommendations (CathFlo™ Activase®): Patients ≥30 kg: 2 mg in 2 mL; may instill second dose if catheter remains occluded after 2-hour dwell time (see Administration); **Note:** A recent study using escalating doses of 0.5 mg, 1 mg, and 2 mg (60 minute dwell time) found that 86.2% of catheters were cleared with the 0.5 mg dose (see Davis, 2000).

Administration

Parenteral: Activase®: I.V.: May administer at a final concentration of 1 mg/mL or may dilute and administer as 0.5 mg/mL (see Stability). Prepare bolus dose using one of the following methods: 1) Remove bolus dose from reconstituted vial using syringe and needle; for 50 mg vial: do not prime syringe with air, insert needle into vial stopper; for 100 mg vial, insert needle away from puncture mark created by transfer device; 2) Remove bolus dose from a port on the infusion line after priming; 3) Program an infusion pump to deliver the bolus at the beginning of the infusion. Administer the remaining dose as follows: From 50 mg vial: Use polyvinyl chloride I.V. bag or glass vial and infusion set; from 100 mg vial: Use same puncture site made by transfer device to insert spike end of infusion set and infuse from vial.

CathFlo™ Activase®: Intracatheter: Instill the appropriate dose into the occluded catheter (see Usual Dosage); leave in lumen; evaluate catheter function (by attempting to aspirate blood) after 30 minutes; if catheter is functional, aspirate 4-5 mL of blood out of catheter to remove drug and residual clot, then gently flush catheter with NS; if catheter is still occluded, leave alteplase in lumen and evaluate catheter function after 120 minutes of dwell time; if catheter is functional, aspirate 4-5 mL of blood out of catheter and gently flush with NS; if catheter remains occluded after 120 minutes of dwell time, a second dose may be instilled by repeating the above administration procedure.

Monitoring Parameters

Systemic use: Blood pressure; temperature; CBC, reticulocyte, platelet count; fibrinogen level, plasminogen, fibrin/fibrinogen degradation products, D-dimer, PT, PTT, antithrombin III, protein C; urinalysis, signs of bleeding
Intracatheter use: Catheter function (by attempting to aspirate blood); temperature, signs of sepsis, GI bleeding, bleeding at injection site, and venous thrombosis

Nursing Implications Extravasation may cause bruising or inflammation; monitor infusion site for patency of I.V.; if extravasation occurs, discontinue infusion at site of (Continued)

Alteplase *(Continued)*

extravasation and apply local treatment; avoid I.M. injections; assess patient for bleeding

Additional Information

Activase® and CathFlo™ Activase® also contain L-arginine, polysorbate 80, and phosphoric acid (for pH adjustment).

Advantages of alteplase include: Low immunogenicity, short half-life, direct activation of plasminogen, and a strong and specific affinity for fibrin. Failure of thrombolytic agents in newborns/neonates may occur due to the low plasminogen concentrations (~50% to 70% of adult levels); supplementing plasminogen (via administration of fresh frozen plasma) may possibly help. Osmolality of 1 mg/mL solution is ~215 mOsm/kg.

Appropriate intracatheter use of alteplase for the treatment of occluded central venous catheters is not expected to cause systemic pharmacologic effects; in adults, if a 2 mg dose is administered I.V. (instead of being instilled into the catheter), the serum concentration of alteplase would be expected to return to normal endogenous levels within 30 minutes.

Dosage Forms

Injection, powder for reconstitution, lyophilized, recombinant:

Activase®: 50 mg [29 million units]; 100 mg [58 million units]

CathFlo™ Activase®: 2 mg

References

Anderson BJ, Keeley SR, and Johnson ND, "Caval Thrombolysis in Neonates Using Low Doses of Recombinant Human Tissue-Type Plasminogen Activator," *Anaesth Intensive Care*, 1991, 19(1):22-7.

Andrew M, Brooker L, Leaker M, et al, "Fibrin Clot Lysis by Thrombolytic Agents is Impaired in Newborns Due to a Low Plasminogen Concentration," *Thromb Haemost*, 1992, 68(3):325-30.

Cada DJ, Levien T, and Baker DE, "Alteplase," *Hospital Pharmacy*, 2002, 37(2): 148-54.

Choi SN, Massicotte MP, Marzinotto V, et al, "The Use of Alteplase to Restore Patency of Central Venous Lines in Pediatric Patients: A Cohort Study," *J Pediatr*, 2001, 139(1):152-6.

Davis SN, Vermeulen L, Banton J, et al, "Activity and Dosage of Alteplase Dilution for Clearing Occlusions of Venous-Access Devices," *Am J Health Syst Pharm*, 2000, 57(11):1039-45.

Doyle E, Britto J, Freeman J, et al, "Thrombolysis With Low Dose Tissue Plasminogen Activator," *Arch Dis Child*, 1992, 67(12):1483-4.

Farnoux C, Camard O, Pinquier D, et al, "Recombinant Tissue-Type Plasminogen Activator Therapy of Thrombosis in 16 Neonates," *J Pediatr*, 1998, 133(1):137-40.

Frazin BS, "Maximal Dilution of Activase," *Am J Hosp Pharm*, 1990, 47(5):1016.

Generali J and Cada DJ, "Alteplase (t-PA) Bolus: Occluded Catheters," *Hospital Pharmacy*, 2001, 36(1):93-103.

Kothari SS, Varma S, and Wasir S, "Thrombolytic Therapy in Infants and Children," *Am Heart J*, 1994, 127(3):651-7.

Levy M, Benson LN, Burrows PE, et al, "Tissue Plasminogen Activator for the Treatment of Thromboembolism in Infants and Children," *J Pediatr*, 1991, 118(3):467-72.

Monagle P, Michelson AD, Bovill E, et al, "Antithrombotic Therapy in Children," *Chest*, 2001, 119(1 Suppl):344S-370S.

Nowak-Gottl U, Auberger K, Halimeh S, et al, "Thrombolysis in Newborns and Infants," *Thromb Haemost*, 1999, 82 (Suppl 1):112-6.

Ponec D, Irwin D, Haire WD, et al, "Recombinant Tissue Plasminogen Activator (Alteplase) for Restoration of Flow in Occluded Central Venous Access Devices: A Double-Blind Placebo-Controlled Trial - The Cardiovascular Thrombolytic to Open Occluded Lines (COOL) Efficacy Trial," *J Vasc Intern Radiol*, 2001, 12(8):951-5.

Weiner GM, Castle VP, DiPietro MA, et al, "Successful Treatment of Neonatal Arterial Thromboses With Recombinant Tissue Plasminogen Activator," *J Pediatr*, 1998, 133(1):133-6.

- **Alti-MPA (Can)** *see* MedroxyPROGESTERone *on page 712*
- **Altinac™** *see* Tretinoin *on page 1111*
- **Alti-Nadolol (Can)** *see* Nadolol *on page 788*
- **Alti-Nortriptyline (Can)** *see* Nortriptyline *on page 822*
- **Alti-Ranitidine (Can)** *see* Ranitidine *on page 972*
- **Alti-Salbutamol (Can)** *see* Albuterol *on page 54*
- **Alti-Sotalol (Can)** *see* Sotalol *on page 1032*
- **Alti-Sulfasalazine (Can)** *see* Sulfasalazine *on page 1055*
- **Alti-Timolol (Can)** *see* Timolol *on page 1095*
- **Alti-Trazodone (Can)** *see* Trazodone *on page 1110*
- **Alti-Verapamil (Can)** *see* Verapamil *on page 1144*
- **Altocor™** *see* Lovastatin *on page 697*

Aluminum Acetate (a LOO mi num AS e tate)
U.S. Brand Names Bluboro® [OTC]; Domeboro® [OTC]; Pedi-Boro® [OTC]
Synonyms Burow's Solution
Therapeutic Category Topical Skin Product
Generic Available Yes
Use Astringent wet dressing for relief of inflammatory conditions of the skin and to reduce weeping that may occur in dermatitis
Pregnancy Risk Factor C
Contraindications Use with topical collagenase
Precautions Do not use plastic or other impervious material to prevent evaporation
Adverse Reactions Local: Irritation
Usual Dosage Children and Adults: Topical: Soak the affected area in the solution 2-4 times/day for 15-30 minutes or apply wet dressing soaked in the solution 2-4 times/day for 30-minute treatment periods; rewet dressing with solution every few minutes to keep it moist
Administration Topical: Keep away from eyes, external use only; one tablet dissolved in 12 ounces of water makes a modified Burow's solution equivalent to a 1:40 dilution, 2 tablets: 1:20 dilution, 4 tablets: 1:10 dilution; one powder packet dissolved in a pint of water makes a modified Burow's solution equivalent to a 1:40 dilution
Dosage Forms Aluminum sulfate and calcium acetate [forms aluminum acetate when mixed]:
  Powder for topical solution (Bluboro®, Domeboro®, Pedi-Boro®): 1 packet/16 ounces of water = 1:40 solution = Modified Burow's Solution
  Tablet for topical solution, effervescent (Domeboro®): 1 tablet/12 ounces of water = 1:40 solution = Modified Burow's Solution

- **Aluminum Carbonate** *see* Antacid Preparations *on page 112*
- **Aluminum Carbonate Gel** *see* Antacid Preparations *on page 112*
- **Aluminum Hydroxide** *see* Antacid Preparations *on page 112*
- **Aluminum Hydroxide and Magnesium Hydroxide** *see* Antacid Preparations *on page 112*
- **Aluminum Hydroxide and Magnesium Trisilicate** *see* Antacid Preparations *on page 112*
- **Aluminum Hydroxide Gel** *see* Antacid Preparations *on page 112*
- **Aluminum Hydroxide, Magnesium Hydroxide, and Simethicone** *see* Antacid Preparations *on page 112*
- **Aluminum Sucrose Sulfate, Basic** *see* Sucralfate *on page 1046*
- **Alupent®** *see* Metaproterenol *on page 726*

Amantadine (a MAN ta deen)
U.S. Brand Names Symmetrel®
Canadian Brand Names Endantadine®; PMS-Amantadine
Synonyms Adamantanamine
Therapeutic Category Anti-Parkinson's Agent; Antiviral Agent, Oral
Generic Available Yes
Use Prophylaxis and treatment of influenza A viral infection; symptomatic and adjunct treatment of parkinsonism
Pregnancy Risk Factor C
Contraindications Hypersensitivity to amantadine hydrochloride or any component
Warnings Deaths due to amantadine overdose have been reported with the lowest lethal dose being 1 gram. Drug overdose has resulted in cardiac (ie, arrhythmia, tachycardia, hypertension), respiratory, renal, or central nervous system toxicity.
Precautions Use with caution in patients with liver disease, epilepsy, history of recurrent eczematoid dermatitis, uncontrolled psychosis, and in patients receiving CNS
(Continued)

Amantadine *(Continued)*

stimulant drugs; may increase seizure activity or EEG disturbances in patients with pre-existing seizure disorders; neuroleptic malignant syndrome has been reported in patients undergoing dosage reduction or withdrawal of amantadine; modify dosage in patients with renal impairment; may need to modify dose in patients with active seizure disorders, CHF, peripheral edema, and orthostatic hypotension

Adverse Reactions

Cardiovascular: Orthostatic hypotension, edema

Central nervous system: Dizziness, confusion, headache, insomnia, difficulty in concentrating, anxiety, restlessness, irritability, hallucinations, seizures, suicide ideation, neuroleptic malignant syndrome

Dermatologic: Livedo reticularis

Gastrointestinal: Nausea, vomiting, xerostomia, anorexia, constipation

Genitourinary: Urinary retention

Drug Interactions Additive anticholinergic effects in patients receiving drugs with anticholinergic activity; additive CNS stimulant effect with CNS stimulants

Mechanism of Action As an antiviral, blocks the uncoating of influenza A virus preventing penetration of virus into host and inhibits M_2 protein in the assembly of progeny virions; antiparkinsonian activity may be due to its blocking the reuptake of dopamine into presynaptic neurons and causing direct stimulation of postsynaptic receptors

Pharmacokinetics

Absorption: Well absorbed from the GI tract

Half-life, patients with normal renal function: 10-28 hours

Time to peak serum concentration: 1-4 hours

Elimination: 80% to 90% excreted unchanged in the urine by glomerular filtration and tubular secretion

Dialysis: 0% to 5% removed by hemodialysis; no supplemental dose needed after hemodialysis or peritoneal dialysis

Usual Dosage Oral:

Children: Influenza A prophylaxis and treatment:

1-9 years: 5 mg/kg/day in 1-2 divided doses; maximum dose: 150 mg/day

≥10-12 years: 5 mg/kg/day in 1-2 divided doses; maximum dose: 200 mg/day

Note: After first influenza A virus vaccine dose, amantadine prophylaxis may be administered for up to 6 weeks, or until 2 weeks after the second dose of vaccine; administer a 10-day course of therapy following exposure; for symptomatic treatment, administer within 24-48 hours of symptom onset with usual duration of therapy between 2-5 days or for 24-48 hours after patient becomes asymptomatic

Alternative dosage for influenza A prophylaxis: Children >20 kg and Adults: 100 mg/day in 1-2 divided doses

Adults:

Parkinson's disease: 100 mg twice daily

Influenza A viral infection: 200 mg/day in 1-2 divided doses

Prophylaxis: Minimum 10-day course of therapy following exposure, or continue for 2-3 weeks after influenza A virus vaccine is given

Dosing interval in renal impairment: Adults:

Cl_{cr} 30-50 mL/minute: Administer 100 mg/day

Cl_{cr} 15-29 mL/minute: Administer 100 mg every other day

Cl_{cr} <15 mL/minute: Administer 200 mg every 7 days

Monitoring Parameters Renal function; monitor for signs of neurotoxicity

Patient Information May cause drowsiness and impair ability to perform activities requiring mental alertness or physical coordination; do not abruptly discontinue therapy, may precipitate a parkinsonian crisis; avoid alcohol; may cause dry mouth

Nursing Implications If insomnia occurs, the last daily dose should be taken several hours before retiring

Dosage Forms

Capsule, as hydrochloride: 100 mg

Syrup, as hydrochloride: 50 mg/5 mL (480 mL)

Symmetrel®: 50 mg/5 mL (480 mL) [raspberry flavor]

Tablet, as hydrochloride (Symmetrel®): 100 mg

References

Strong DK, Eisenstat DD, Bryson SM, et al, "Amantadine Neurotoxicity in a Pediatric Patient With Renal Insufficiency," *DICP*, 1991, 25(11):1175-7.

♦ **A-Methapred**® *see* MethylPREDNISolone *on page 747*
♦ **Amethocaine** *see* Tetracaine *on page 1073*
♦ **Amethopterin** *see* Methotrexate *on page 737*
♦ **Ametop**™ **(Can)** *see* Tetracaine *on page 1073*
♦ **Amibid LA** *see* Guaifenesin *on page 550*
♦ **Amicar**® *see* Aminocaproic Acid *on page 80*

Amifostine (am i FOS teen)

U.S. Brand Names Ethyol®
Therapeutic Category Antidote, Cisplatin; Cytoprotective Agent
Generic Available No
Use Cytoprotective agent which scavenges free radicals and binds to reactive drug derivatives due to radiation therapy, cisplatin, carboplatin, cyclophosphamide, ifosfamide, carmustine, melphalan, and mechlorethamine to selectively protect normal tissues against toxicity due to these agents; reduction of moderate to severe xerostomia from radiation treatment of the head and neck where the radiation port includes a substantial portion of the parotid glands
Pregnancy Risk Factor C
Contraindications Hypersensitivity to amifostine, aminothiol compounds, or any component; patients who are hypotensive or dehydrated
Warnings Due to limited experience and the possibility of amifostine interference with antineoplastic efficacy, amifostine should not be administered to patients in settings where chemotherapy can produce a significant survival benefit or cure, except in the context of a clinical study. Monitor serum calcium levels in patients at risk of hypocalcemia (eg, those patients receiving multiple doses of amifostine, patients with nephrotic syndrome).
Precautions Use with caution in patients with pre-existing cardiovascular or cerebrovascular conditions such as ischemic heart disease, arrhythmias, CHF, history of stroke or transient ischemic attacks; may cause hypotension; use special caution in situations where concomitant antihypertensive therapy cannot be interrupted 24 hours prior to starting amifostine or in patients in whom the adverse effects of nausea/vomiting may be more likely to have serious consequences
Adverse Reactions
Cardiovascular: Transient hypotension (62%; incidence is higher in patients with head and neck cancer, esophageal cancer, non-small cell lung cancer, prior neck irradiation, or hypercalcemia), flushing, warm sensation
Central nervous system: Chills, fever, dizziness, somnolence, hiccups, anxiety, malaise
Dermatologic: Rash
Endocrine & metabolic: Hypocalcemia, hypomagnesemia
Gastrointestinal: Nausea, vomiting, metallic taste in mouth
Genitourinary: Urinary retention (reversible)
Respiratory: Sneezing
Drug Interactions Antihypertensive agents may potentiate the hypotensive effects of amifostine
Stability When 500 mg amifostine is reconstituted with 9.7 mL of NS, the resultant solution is stable for 5 hours at room temperature or up to 24 hours if refrigerated; amifostine solutions diluted to 5-40 mg/mL in NS are chemically stable for 5 hours at room temperature or 24 hours if refrigerated; decreased stability in low pH conditions; incompatible with acyclovir, amphotericin B, chlorpromazine, cisplatin, ganciclovir, hydroxyzine, prochlorperazine
Mechanism of Action Amifostine is a prodrug that is converted by the plasma membrane-bound enzyme alkaline phosphatase to the active free sulfhydryl compound WR-1065, which is further oxidized to a symmetrical disulfide (WR-33278) or to mixed disulfides. The active drug scavenges free radicals, donates hydrogen ions to free radicals, and binds to active derivatives of antineoplastic agents, thus preventing the alkylation of nucleic acid. Selective protection of normal tissue is demonstrated by:
1) decreased alkaline phosphatase activity in tumor cells,
2) decreased vascularity of tumors, and
3) lower pH in tumor tissues due to the predominance of anaerobic metabolism (WR-1065 requires a pH in the range of 6.6-8.2 for uptake into tissues)
Pharmacokinetics
Distribution: V_d: Adults: 6.4 L; unmetabolized prodrug is largely confined to the intravascular compartment; active metabolite is distributed into normal tissues with high concentrations in bone marrow, GI mucosa, skin, liver, and salivary glands
Protein binding: 4%
Metabolism: Amifostine (phosphorylated prodrug) is hydrolyzed by alkaline phosphatase to an active free sulfhydryl compound (WR-1065)
(Continued)

Amifostine *(Continued)*

Half-life:
  Children: 9.3 minutes
  Adults: 8 minutes
Elimination: Metabolites excreted in urine

Usual Dosage I.V. (refer to individual protocols):
  Children: Limited data available on use in pediatric patients; dosing based on a prior clinical phase I trial and single case reports: 740 mg/m^2 once daily administered 30 minutes prior to chemotherapy; doses as high as 600 mg/m^2/dose administered 15 minutes prior to and 2 hours after chemotherapy (total of 1200 mg/m^2/day) have been used in phase I trials in patients treated with ifosfamide, carboplatin, and etoposide chemotherapy; repeat amifostine doses may be required when using a cytotoxic agent with a long half-life or long infusion time
  Adults: 910 mg/m^2 once daily administered 30 minutes prior to chemotherapy; reduce dose to 740 mg/m^2 in patients who have a higher incidence of hypotension
    Reduction of moderate to severe xerostomia from radiation of the head and neck: 200 mg/m^2 once daily starting 15-30 minutes prior to standard fraction radiation therapy

Administration Parenteral: I.V.: Reconstituted amifostine dose must be further diluted with NS to a final volume of 50 mL (adults) or a final concentration of 5-40 mg/mL (children). Administer amifostine doses >740 mg/m^2 as an I.V. intermittent infusion over 15 minutes since the 15-minute infusion is better tolerated than a more prolonged infusion. Administer 200 mg/m^2 dose as a 3-minute infusion. Amifostine should be interrupted if the blood pressure decreases significantly from baseline or if the patient develops symptoms related to decreased cerebral or cardiovascular perfusion. Patients experiencing decreased blood pressure should receive a rapid infusion of NS and be kept supine or placed in the Trendelenburg position. Amifostine can be restarted if the blood pressure returns to the baseline level.

Monitoring Parameters Baseline blood pressure followed by a blood pressure reading every 3-5 minutes during the 15-minute infusion; monitor electrolytes, urinalysis, serum calcium, serum magnesium; monitor I & O

Nursing Implications Pretreat patient with antiemetics; patients should be well hydrated prior to amifostine infusion; patients taking antihypertensive medications should discontinue therapy 24 hours before administration of amifostine; begin chemotherapy or radiation therapy 15 minutes after completion of amifostine

Dosage Forms Injection, powder for reconstitution: 500 mg

References
Adamson PC, Balis FM, Belasco JE, et al, "A Phase I Trial of Amifostine (WR-2721) and Melphalan in Children With Refractory Cancer," *Cancer Res*, 1995, 55(18): 4069-72.

Fouladi M, Stempak D, Gammon J, et al, "Phase I Trial of a Twice-Daily Regimen of Amifostine With Ifosfamide, Carboplatin, and Etoposide Chemotherapy in Children With Refractory Carcinoma," *Cancer*, 2001, 92(4):914-23.

Schuchter LM, "Guidelines for the Administration of Amifostine," *Semin Oncol*, 1996, 23(4 Suppl 8):40-3.

Shaw LM, Bonner H, and Lieberman R, "Pharmacokinetic Profile of Amifostine," *Semin Oncol*, 1996, 23(4 Suppl 8):18-22.

Amikacin *(am i KAY sin)*

Related Information
  Blood Level Sampling Time Guidelines *on page 1386*
  Overdose and Toxicology *on page 1388*

U.S. Brand Names Amikin®

Therapeutic Category Antibiotic, Aminoglycoside

Generic Available Yes

Use Treatment of documented gram-negative enteric infection resistant to gentamicin and tobramycin; amikacin is usually effective against *Pseudomonas, Klebsiella, Enterobacter, Serratia, Proteus,* and *E. coli;* documented infection of mycobacterial organisms susceptible to amikacin

Pregnancy Risk Factor D

Contraindications Hypersensitivity to amikacin sulfate or any component (see Warnings); cross-sensitivity may exist with other aminoglycosides

Warnings Aminoglycosides are associated with significant nephrotoxicity or ototoxicity; the ototoxicity is directly proportional to the amount of drug given and the duration of treatment. Tinnitus or vertigo are indications of vestibular injury and impending bilateral irreversible deafness. Risk of nephrotoxicity increases when used concurrently with other potentially nephrotoxic drugs; renal damage is usually reversible. Aminoglycosides can cause fetal harm when administered to a pregnant woman, and have been associated with several reports of total irreversible bilateral congenital deafness in pediatric patients exposed *in utero.* Some products contain sulfites which may cause allergic reactions in susceptible individuals.

Precautions Use with caution in neonates (due to renal immaturity that results in a prolonged half-life); patients with pre-existing renal impairment, auditory or vestibular impairment, hypocalcemia, myasthenia gravis, and in conditions which depress neuromuscular transmission; dose and/or frequency of administration must be modified in patients with renal impairment

Adverse Reactions
Central nervous system: Fever, headache, dizziness, drowsiness, ataxia, vertigo
Dermatologic: Rash
Gastrointestinal: Nausea, vomiting
Hematologic: Eosinophilia, anemia, leukopenia
Neuromuscular & skeletal: Neuromuscular blockade, tremor, paresthesia, weakness, gait instability
Otic: Ototoxicity
Renal: Nephrotoxicity

Drug Interactions Extended-spectrum penicillins (decrease serum amikacin concentration in patients with renal failure); loop diuretics may potentiate the ototoxicity of the aminoglycosides; amphotericin, vancomycin, acyclovir, cisplatin, or cephalosporins may increase nephrotoxicity; may potentiate the effects of neuromuscular blocking agents and general anesthetics; indomethacin may increase serum amikacin concentrations

Mechanism of Action Inhibits protein synthesis in susceptible bacteria by binding to ribosomal subunits

Pharmacokinetics
Distribution: Primarily into extracellular fluid (highly hydrophilic); 12% of serum concentration penetrates into bronchial secretions; poor penetration into the blood-brain barrier even when meninges are inflamed; V_d is increased in neonates and patients with edema, ascites, fluid overload; V_d is decreased in patients with dehydration; crosses the placenta
Half-life:
Infants:
Low birth weight, 1-3 days of age: 7 hours
Full-term >7 days: 4-5 hours
Children: 1.6-2.5 hours
Adolescents: 1.5 ± 1 hour
Adults: 2-3 hours
Anuria: 28-86 hours; half-life and clearance are dependent on renal function
Time to peak serum concentration:
I.M.: Within 45-120 minutes
I.V.: Within 30 minutes following a 30-minute infusion
Elimination: 94% to 98% is excreted unchanged in the urine via glomerular filtration within 24 hours
Dialysis: Dialyzable (50% to 100%); supplemental dose recommended after hemodialysis or peritoneal dialysis

Usual Dosage I.M., I.V. (dosage should be based on an estimate of ideal body weight except in neonates; neonatal dosage should be based on actual weight unless the patient has hydrocephalus or hydrops fetalis):

Neonates:
0-4 weeks, <1200 g: 7.5 mg/kg/dose every 18-24 hours
Postnatal age ≤7 days:
1200-2000 g: 7.5 mg/kg/dose every 12 hours
>2000 g: 7.5-10 mg/kg/dose every 12 hours
Postnatal age >7 days:
1200-2000 g: 7.5-10 mg/kg/dose every 8-12 hours
>2000 g: 10 mg/kg/dose every 8 hours
Infants and Children: 15-22.5 mg/kg/day divided every 8 hours; some consultants recommend initial doses of 30 mg/kg/day divided every 8 hours in patients who may require larger doses; see **Note**
Treatment for nontuberculous mycobacterial infection: 15-30 mg/kg/day divided every 12-24 hours as part of a multiple drug regimen; maximum dose: 1.5 g/day
Adults: 15 mg/kg/day divided every 8-12 hours; maximum: 1.5 g/day
Treatment of *M. avium* complex infection: 7.5-15 mg/kg/day divided every 12-24 hours as part of a multiple drug regimen
Dosing interval in renal impairment: Loading dose: 5-7.5 mg/kg; subsequent dosages and frequency of administration are best determined by measurement of serum levels and assessment of renal insufficiency
Note: Some patients may require larger or more frequent doses if serum levels document the need (ie, cystic fibrosis or febrile granulocytopenic patients)

Administration Parenteral: Administer by I.M. or slow intermittent I.V. infusion over 30 minutes at a final concentration not to exceed 10 mg amikacin/mL. Administer other (Continued)

Amikacin (Continued)

antibiotics such as penicillins and cephalosporins at least 1 hour before or after an amikacin dose.

Monitoring Parameters Urinalysis, urine output, BUN, serum creatinine, peak and trough serum amikacin concentrations; be alert to ototoxicity

Not all infants and children who receive aminoglycosides require monitoring of serum aminoglycoside concentrations. Indications for use of aminoglycoside serum concentration monitoring include:

- treatment course >5 days
- patients with decreased or changing renal function
- patients with poor therapeutic response
- infants <3 months of age
- atypical body constituency (obesity, expanded extracellular fluid volume)
- clinical need for higher doses or shorter intervals (eg, cystic fibrosis, burns, endocarditis, meningitis, critically ill patients, relatively resistant organisms)
- patients on hemodialysis or chronic ambulatory peritoneal dialysis
- signs of nephrotoxicity or ototoxicity
- concomitant use of other nephrotoxic agents

Reference Range

Peak: 20-30 µg/mL

Trough: <10 µg/mL

Patient Information Report loss of hearing, ringing or roaring in the ears, or feeling of fullness in head

Nursing Implications Aminoglycoside levels measured from blood taken from Silastic® central catheters can sometimes give falsely elevated readings; peak serum levels should be drawn 30 minutes after the end of a 30-minute infusion; trough levels are drawn within 30 minutes before the next dose; provide optimal patient hydration

Dosage Forms

Infusion, as sulfate [premixed in NS]: 5 mg/mL (100 mL)

Injection, solution, as sulfate: 50 mg/mL (2 mL); 62.5 mg/mL (8 mL); 250 mg/mL (2 mL, 4 mL) [contains sulfites]

References

Kenyon CF, Knoppert DC, Lee SK, et al, "Amikacin Pharmacokinetics and Suggested Dosage Modifications for the Preterm Infant," *Antimicrob Agents Chemother*, 1990, 34(2):265-8.

Public Health Service Task Force on Prophylaxis and Therapy for *Mycobacterium avium* Complex, "Recommendations on Prophylaxis and Therapy for Disseminated *Mycobacterium avium* Complex Disease in Patients Infected With the Human Immunodeficiency Virus," *N Engl J Med*, 1993, 329(12):898-904.

Starke JR and Correa AG, "Management of Mycobacterial Infection and Disease in Children," *Pediatr Infect Dis J*, 1995, 14(6):455-69.

Vogelstein B, Kowarski A, and Lietman PS, "The Pharmacokinetics of Amikacin in Children," *J Pediatr*, 1977, 91(2):333-9.

♦ **Amikin®** *see* Amikacin *on page 76*

Amiloride (a MIL oh ride)

U.S. Brand Names Midamor®

Therapeutic Category Antihypertensive Agent; Diuretic, Potassium Sparing

Generic Available Yes

Use Management of edema associated with CHF, hepatic cirrhosis, and hyperaldosteronism; hypertension; primary hyperaldosteronism; hypokalemia induced by kaliuretic diuretics

Pregnancy Risk Factor B

Contraindications Hypersensitivity to amiloride or any component; hyperkalemia; anuria

Warnings Due to potential severe hyperkalemia, amiloride should be discontinued in diabetic patients for at least 3 days prior to glucose tolerance testing; discontinue if serum potassium >5.5 mEq/L

Precautions Use with caution in patients with dehydration, electrolyte imbalance, metabolic or respiratory acidosis, diabetes (particularly those with nephropathy), hyponatremia, impaired renal function, or hepatic dysfunction; patients receiving potassium or other potassium-sparing diuretics; use with caution and modify dosage in patients with decreased renal function

Adverse Reactions

Cardiovascular: Angina, orthostatic hypotension, arrhythmia, palpitations

Central nervous system: Headache, dizziness, encephalopathy, vertigo, nervousness, mental confusion, insomnia, depression, somnolence

Dermatologic: Skin rash, pruritus, alopecia

Endocrine & metabolic: Hyperkalemia, hyperchloremic metabolic acidosis, dehydration, hyponatremia, gynecomastia

Gastrointestinal: Nausea, anorexia, diarrhea, vomiting, abdominal pain, appetite changes, constipation, GI bleeding, xerostomia, heartburn, flatulence, dyspepsia

Genitourinary: Impotence, dysuria, urinary frequency, bladder spasms

Hematologic: Aplastic anemia, neutropenia

Hepatic: Abnormal liver function

Neuromuscular & skeletal: Weakness, muscle cramps, joint and back pain, paresthesia, tremors

Ocular: Visual disturbances, elevated intraocular pressure

Otic: Tinnitus

Renal: Polyuria

Respiratory: Cough, dyspnea, nasal congestion, shortness of breath

Drug Interactions Potassium, other potassium-sparing diuretics, cyclosporine, tacrolimus, and ACE inhibitors (eg, captopril) may additively increase the serum potassium; may decrease digoxin clearance and attenuate its inotropic effect; decreases lithium clearance; decreased diuresis and antihypertensive effects with concomitant NSAID use

Food Interactions Avoid natural licorice (causes sodium and water retention and increases potassium loss) and salt substitutes; food decreases absorption to ~30%

Mechanism of Action Acts directly on the distal renal tubule to inhibit sodium-potassium ion exchange; decreases sodium reabsorption in the distal tubule by inhibiting cellular sodium transport mechanisms such as the conductive sodium influx pathway and possibly the sodium-hydrogen ion exchange system; also inhibits hydrogen ion secretion; its diuretic activity is **independent** of aldosterone.

Pharmacodynamics
Onset of action: 2 hours

Maximum effect: 6-10 hours

Duration: 24 hours

Pharmacokinetics
Absorption: 50%

Distribution: Adults: V_d: 350-380 L

Metabolism: No active metabolites

Half-life: Adults:

Normal renal function: 6-9 hours

End stage renal disease: 21-144 hours

Elimination: Unchanged drug, equally in urine and feces

Usual Dosage Oral:

Children 6-20 kg: 0.625 mg/kg/day once daily; maximum dose: 10 mg/day

Children >20 kg and Adults: 5-10 mg/day; maximum dose: 20 mg/day

Dosing adjustment in renal impairment:

Cl_{cr} 10-50 mL/minute: Administer at 50% of normal dose

Cl_{cr} <10 mL/minute: Avoid use

Administration Oral: Administer with food or milk

Monitoring Parameters Serum potassium, sodium, creatinine, BUN, blood pressure, fluid balance

Test Interactions May falsely elevate serum digoxin levels done by radioimmunoassay

Patient Information Report to your physician any muscle cramps, weakness, nausea, or dizziness; may cause drowsiness and impair ability to perform activities requiring mental alertness or physical coordination; may cause dry mouth

Additional Information Studies utilizing aerosolized amiloride (5 mmol/L in 0.3% saline) in adult cystic fibrosis patients (Tomkiewicz, 1993) have suggested that inhaled amiloride is capable of improving the rheologic properties of the abnormally thickened mucus by increasing mucus sodium content

Dosage Forms Tablet, as hydrochloride: 5 mg

Extemporaneous Preparations A 1 mg/mL oral liquid may be prepared from crushed tablets added to a small quantity of sterile water to which glycerin (final concentration of 40% w/v) is added; sterile water is then added in sufficient quantity to make the desired volume; stable 21 days when refrigerated

Fawcett JP, Woods DJ, Ferry DG, et al, "Stability of Amiloride Hydrochloride Oral Liquids Prepared From Tablets and Powder," *Aust J Hosp Pharm*, 1995, 25:10-23.

References
Tomkiewicz RP, App, EM, Zayas JG, et al, "Amiloride Inhalation Therapy in Cystic Fibrosis. Influence on Ion Content, Hydration, and Rheology of Sputum," *Am Rev Resp Dis*, 1993, 148:1002-7.

♦ **2-Amino-6-mercaptopurine** *see* Thioguanine *on page 1083*

♦ **Aminobenzylpenicillin** *see* Ampicillin *on page 103*

Aminocaproic Acid (a mee noe ka PROE ik AS id)

Related Information
Carbohydrate and Alcohol Content of Liquid Medications for Use in Patients Receiving Ketogenic Diets *on page 1431*

U.S. Brand Names Amicar®

Therapeutic Category Hemostatic Agent

Generic Available Yes (injection and syrup)

Use Treatment of excessive bleeding resulting from systemic hyperfibrinolysis, urinary fibrinolysis, or traumatic ocular hyphema

Pregnancy Risk Factor C

Contraindications Hypersensitivity to aminocaproic acid or any component (see Warnings); disseminated intravascular coagulation; evidence of an intravascular clotting process; use of factor IX concentrate or anti-inhibitor coagulant concentrate

Warnings Aminocaproic acid may accumulate in patients with decreased renal function; intrarenal obstruction may occur secondary to glomerular capillary thrombosis or clots in the renal pelvis and ureters; do not use in hematuria of upper urinary tract origin unless benefits outweigh potential risks; inhibition of fibrinolysis may promote clotting or thrombosis.

Injection contains benzyl alcohol which may cause allergic reactions in susceptible individuals; large amounts of benzyl alcohol (≥99 mg/kg/day) have been associated with a potentially fatal toxicity ("gasping syndrome") in neonates; the "gasping syndrome" consists of metabolic acidosis, respiratory distress, gasping respirations, CNS dysfunction (including convulsions, intracranial hemorrhage), hypotension and cardiovascular collapse; avoid use of injection in neonates; *in vitro* and animal studies have shown that benzoate, a metabolite of benzyl alcohol, displaces bilirubin from protein-binding sites

Precautions Use with caution in patients with cardiac, renal or hepatic disease; adjust dosage in patients with oliguria or end-stage renal disease; use with caution in patients at risk for veno-occlusive disease of the liver

Adverse Reactions
Cardiovascular: Hypotension, bradycardia and arrhythmias (following rapid I.V. administration)
Central nervous system: Dizziness, headache, malaise, seizures, confusion
Dermatologic: Rash
Endocrine & metabolic: Hyperkalemia
Gastrointestinal: GI irritation, nausea, cramps, diarrhea
Hematologic: Decreased platelet function, agranulocytosis, leukopenia
Neuromuscular & skeletal: Myopathy, acute rhabdomyolysis, weakness
Ocular: Glaucoma, watery eyes
Otic: Tinnitus, deafness
Renal: Renal failure
Respiratory: Nasal congestion, dyspnea, pulmonary embolism

Drug Interactions Increased risk of thrombosis with oral contraceptives, estrogens, and factor IX

Mechanism of Action Competitively inhibits activation of plasminogen thereby reducing fibrinolysin, without inhibiting lysis of clot

Pharmacodynamics Onset of action: Inhibition of fibrinolysis: Within 1-72 hours (onset shortened substantially if loading dose is used)

Pharmacokinetics
Distribution: Widely distributes through intravascular and extravascular compartments
Metabolism: Hepatic metabolism is minimal
Bioavailability: Oral: 100%
Half-life: 1-2 hours
Elimination: 40% to 60% excreted as unchanged drug in the urine within 12 hours

Usual Dosage
Children:
Oral, I.V.: Loading dose: 100-200 mg/kg; maintenance: 100 mg/kg/dose every 6 hours; maximum daily dose: 30 g
or as an alternative: I.V. loading dose: 100 mg/kg or 3 g/m^2 followed by a continuous infusion of 33.3 mg/kg/hour or 1 g/m^2/hour; total dosage should not exceed 18 g/m^2/day
Traumatic hyphema: Oral, I.V.: 100 mg/kg/dose every 4 hours (maximum dose: 5 g/dose; maximum daily dose: 30 g/day)
Adults:
Oral: For the treatment of acute bleeding syndromes due to elevated fibrinolytic activity, give 5 g during first hour, followed by 1-1.25 g/hour for about 8 hours or until bleeding stops; daily dose should not exceed 30 g

I.V.: Give 4-5 g during first hour followed by continuous infusion at the rate of 1-1.25 g/hour, continue for 8 hours or until bleeding stops

Dosing adjustment in renal impairment: Oliguria or ESRD: Reduce dose to 25% of normal

Administration

Oral: May administer without regard to food

Parenteral: Maximum concentration for I.V. administration: 20 mg/mL; administer single doses over at least 1 hour

Monitoring Parameters Fibrinogen, fibrin split products, serum creatinine kinase (long-term therapy); serum potassium (may be elevated by aminocaproic acid, especially if the patient has impaired renal function)

Reference Range Therapeutic concentration: >130 µg/mL (concentration necessary for inhibition of fibrinolysis)

Nursing Implications Rapid I.V. injection (IVP) should be avoided since hypotension, bradycardia, and arrhythmias may result

Dosage Forms

Injection: 250 mg/mL (20 mL) [contains 0.9% benzyl alcohol]

Syrup: 250 mg/mL (480 mL) [raspberry flavor]

Tablet: 500 mg

References

McGetrick JJ, Jampol LM, Goldberg MP, et al, "Aminocaproic Acid Decreases Secondary Hemorrhage After Traumatic Hyphema," *Arch Ophthalmol*, 1983, 101(7):1031-3.

♦ **Aminohydroxypropylidene Diphosphonate** *see Pamidronate on page 853*

Aminophylline (am in OFF i lin)

Related Information

Asthma Guidelines *on page 1376*

Overdose and Toxicology *on page 1388*

Theophylline *on page 1076*

Synonyms Theophylline Ethylenediamine

Therapeutic Category Antiasthmatic; Bronchodilator; Respiratory Stimulant; Theophylline Derivative

Generic Available Yes

Use Bronchodilator in reversible airway obstruction due to asthma or COPD; increase diaphragmatic contractility; neonatal idiopathic apnea of prematurity

Pregnancy Risk Factor C

Contraindications Hypersensitivity to aminophylline or any component; uncontrolled arrhythmias

Adverse Reactions See Theophylline *on page 1076*

Drug Interactions Cytochrome P450 isoenzyme CYP1A2, CYP2E1 (minor), and CYP3A3/4 substrate

Decreases adenosine, benzodiazepines, and pancuronium effects; decreases zafirlukast serum levels; increases lithium clearance; increases CNS side effects with ephedrine; increases risk of cardiac arrhythmias with halothane; for medications which change aminophylline (theophylline) clearance, see tables on next page.

Food Interactions Food does not appreciably affect absorption; avoid extremes of dietary protein and carbohydrate intake; limit charcoal-broiled foods and caffeinated beverages

Mechanism of Action See Theophylline *on page 1076*

Pharmacokinetics Aminophylline is the ethylenediamine salt of theophylline, pharmacokinetic parameters are those of **theophylline**; fraction available: 80% (eg, 100 mg aminophylline = 80 mg theophylline); see Theophylline *on page 1076*

Usual Dosage All dosages based upon **aminophylline**; dose should be based on ideal body weight

Neonates:

Apnea of prematurity: Oral, I.V.:

Loading dose: 5 mg/kg

Maintenance: Initial: 5 mg/kg/day every 12 hours; increased dosages may be indicated as liver metabolism matures (usually >30 days of life); monitor serum levels to determine appropriate dosages

Theophylline levels should be initially drawn after 3 days of therapy; repeat levels are indicated 3 days after each increase in dosage or weekly if on a stabilized dosage

Infants, Children, and Adults: Treatment of acute bronchospasm: I.V.: Loading dose (in patients not currently receiving aminophylline or theophylline): 6 mg/kg (based on aminophylline) given I.V. over 20-30 minutes

(Continued)

Aminophylline *(Continued)*

Approximate I.V. maintenance dosages are based upon **continuous infusions**; intermittent dosing (often used in children <6 months of age) may be determined by multiplying the hourly infusion rate by 24 hours and dividing by the desired number of doses/day (usually in 3-4 doses/day)

6 weeks to 6 months: 0.5 mg/kg/hour
6 months to 1 year: 0.6-0.7 mg/kg/hour
1-9 years: 1-1.2 mg/kg/hour
9-12 years and young adult smokers: 0.9 mg/kg/hour
12-16 years: 0.7 mg/kg/hour
Adults (healthy, nonsmoking): 0.7 mg/kg/hour
Older patients and patients with cor pulmonale, patients with CHF or liver failure: 0.25 mg/kg/hour
Oral dose: See Theophylline *on page 1076*, (consider mg theophylline available when using aminophylline products)
Dosage should be adjusted according to serum level measurements during the first 12- to 24-hour period. See table on next page.

Clinical Factors Reported to Affect Theophylline Clearance

Decreased Theophylline Level	Increased Theophylline Level
Smoking (cigarettes, marijuana)	Acute pulmonary edema
High protein/low carbohydrate diet	Cessation of smoking (after chronic use)
Charcoal broiled beef	Cor pulmonale
	Congestive heart failure
	Hypothyroidism
	Fever (≥102° for 24 hours or more, or lesser temperature elevations for longer periods)
	Hepatic cirrhosis/acute hepatitis
	Renal failure in infants <3 mo of age
	Sepsis with multisystem organ failure
	Shock
	Viral illness

Medications Affecting Theophylline Clearance Resulting in Either Increased or Decreased Serum Levels

Decreased Theophylline Level	Increased Theophylline Level
Aminoglutethimide	Alcohol
Carbamazepine	Allopurinol (>600 mg/day)
Isoproterenol (I.V.)	Beta-blockers
Isoniazid*	Calcium channel blockers
Ketoconazole	Cimetidine
Loop diuretics*	Ciprofloxacin
Nevirapine	Clarithromycin
Phenobarbital	Corticosteroids
Phenytoin	Disulfiram
Rifampin	Ephedrine
Ritonavir	Erythromycin
Sulfinpyrazone	Esmolol
Sympathomimetics	Influenza virus vaccine
	Interferon, human recombinant alpha 2-a and 2-b
	Isoniazid*
	Loop diuretics*
	Methotrexate
	Mexiletine
	Oral contraceptives
	Propafenone
	Propranolol
	Tacrine
	Thiabendazole
	Thyroid hormones
	Troleandomycin (TAO®)
	Verapamil
	Zileuton

*Both increased and decreased theophylline levels have been reported.

Administration

Oral: May be administered without regard to meals

Parenteral: Do not administer I.M. (I.M. administration causes intense pain); dilute with I.V. fluid to a concentration of 1 mg/mL and infuse over 20-30 minutes; maximum concentration: 25 mg/mL; maximum rate of infusion: 0.36 mg/kg/minute, and not to exceed 25 mg/minute

Guidelines for Drawing Theophylline Serum Levels

Dosage Form	Time to Draw Level*
I.V. bolus	30 min after end of 30-min infusion
I.V. continuous infusion	12-24 h after initiation of infusion
P.O. liquid, fast-release formulation	Peak: 1 h postdose after at least 1 day of therapy Trough: Just before a dose after at least 1 day of therapy

*The time to achieve steady-state serum levels is prolonged in patients with longer half-lives (eg, premature neonates, infants, and adults with cardiac or liver failure (see theophylline half-life table). In these patients, serum theophylline levels should be drawn after 48-72 hours of therapy; serum levels may need to be done prior to steady-state to assess the patient's current progress or evaluate potential toxicity.

Monitoring Parameters Serum theophylline levels, heart rate, respiratory rate, number and severity of apnea spells (when used for apnea of prematurity); arterial or capillary blood gases (if applicable); pulmonary function tests

Reference Range Therapeutic: For asthma 10-20 µg/mL; for neonatal apnea 6-13 µg/mL (serum levels are reduced for neonatal apnea due to decreased binding of theophylline to fetal albumin resulting in a greater amount of free "active" theophylline)

Dosage Forms Theophylline (anhydrous) equivalent listed in brackets:
Injection, solution: 25 mg/mL [19.7 mg/mL] (10 mL, 20 mL)
Liquid, oral: 105 mg/5 mL [90 mg/5 mL] (10 mL, 500 mL) [apricot flavor]
Tablet: 100 mg [79 mg]; 200 mg [158 mg]

References
Bhatt-Mehta V and Schumacher RE, "Treatment of Apnea of Prematurity," *Paediatr Drugs*, 2003, 5(3):195-210.
"National Asthma Education and Prevention Program. Expert Panel Report: Guidelines for the Diagnosis and Management of Asthma Update on Selected Topics--2002," *J Allergy Clin Immunol*, 2002, 110(5 Suppl):S141-219.

♦ **5-Aminosalicylic Acid** see Mesalamine on page 723
♦ **Aminoxin® [OTC]** see Pyridoxine on page 964

Amiodarone (a MEE oh da rone)
Related Information
Adult ACLS Algorithm, Narrow-Complex Supraventricular Tachycardia on page 1190
Adult ACLS Algorithm, Stable Ventricular Tachycardia on page 1191
Adult ACLS Algorithm, V. Fib and Pulseless VT on page 1185
CPR Pediatric Drug Dosages on page 1175
Pediatric ALS Algorithm, Pulseless Arrest on page 1180
Pediatric ALS Algorithm, Tachycardia - Rapid Rhythm and Adequate Perfusion on page 1181
Pediatric ALS Algorithm, Tachycardia - Rapid Rhythm and Evidence of Poor Perfusion on page 1182
U.S. Brand Names Cordarone®; Pacerone®
Canadian Brand Names Alti-Amiodarone; Gen-Amiodarone; Novo-Amiodarone; Rhoxal-amiodarone
Therapeutic Category Antiarrhythmic Agent, Class III
Generic Available Yes
Use
Oral: Management of life-threatening ventricular arrhythmias [eg, recurrent ventricular fibrillation (VF) or recurrent hemodynamically unstable ventricular tachycardia (VT)] unresponsive to other therapy

I.V.: Initiation of management and prophylaxis of frequently recurrent VF and hemodynamically unstable VT unresponsive to other therapy; VF and VT in patients requiring amiodarone who are not able to take oral therapy

Note: Also has been used to treat supraventricular arrhythmias unresponsive to other therapy. A benzyl alcohol free and polysorbate free injectable product is available from the manufacturer via orphan drug status or compassionate use for acute treatment and prophylaxis of life-threatening ventricular tachycardia or ventricular fibrillation (see Dosage Forms)

Pregnancy Risk Factor D
(Continued)

Amiodarone *(Continued)*

Contraindications Hypersensitivity to amiodarone or any component (see Warnings); severe sinus node dysfunction; marked sinus bradycardia, second and third degree A-V block; cardiogenic shock; bradycardia-induced syncope, except if pacemaker is placed

Warnings Not considered first-line antiarrhythmic due to high incidence of toxicity; 75% of patients experience adverse effects with large doses. Discontinuation is required in 5% to 20% of patients. Pulmonary and hepatic toxicities may be fatal (see Adverse Reactions); reserve for use in life-threatening arrhythmias refractory to other therapy. Optic neuropathy and/or optic neuritis resulting in visual impairment may occur at any time and can progress to permanent blindness; prompt ophthalmic exam is recommended if visual impairment occurs; re-evaluate amiodarone therapy if optic neuropathy or neuritis occurs. Hypotension with I.V. product occurs in about 16% of patients and may be associated with infusion rate. Bradycardia and AV block may occur; temporary pacemaker should be available when I.V. product is used in patients with known predisposition to bradycardia or AV block. Patients should be hospitalized for initiation of therapy and loading dose administration.

Injectable products (Cordarone® and generic) contain polysorbate (Tween®) 80 and benzyl alcohol; benzyl alcohol may cause allergic reactions in susceptible individuals; large amounts of benzyl alcohol (≥99 mg/kg/day) have been associated with a potentially fatal toxicity ("gasping syndrome") in neonates; the "gasping syndrome" consists of metabolic acidosis, respiratory distress, gasping respirations, CNS dysfunction (including convulsions, intracranial hemorrhage), hypotension and cardiovascular collapse; use amiodarone products containing benzyl alcohol with caution in neonates (see also Precautions); a benzyl alcohol free and polysorbate free injection is available (see Dosage Forms); *in vitro* and animal studies have shown that benzoate, a metabolite of benzyl alcohol, displaces bilirubin from protein binding sites

Precautions Amiodarone HCl contains 37% iodine by weight; avoid use during pregnancy and while breast-feeding (fetal/neonatal goiters, hypothyroidism, and possible cerebral damage may occur); use with caution and monitor closely in patients with thyroid disease (**Note:** Oral amiodarone has caused dose-related thyroid tumors in rats). May worsen or precipitate arrhythmias; when possible, hypokalemia and hypomagnesemia should be corrected prior to I.V. amiodarone use due to increased risk for torsade de pointes. Serious drug interactions may occur (see Drug Interactions).

Safety and efficacy of amiodarone have not been established in pediatric patients. I.V. amiodarone has been shown to leach out plasticizers [eg, DEHP or di-(2-ethylhexyl)phthalate] from I.V. tubing, including polyvinyl chloride tubing. In immature animals, exposure to DEHP may adversely affect the development of the male reproductive tract. In order to decrease the potential exposure of infants to plasticizers, consider the use of bolus dosing in 1 mg/kg aliquots as described by Perry, 1996; see Usual Dosage. See also http://www.fda.gov/medwatch/safety/2001/safety01.htm#cordar.

Adverse Reactions

Cardiovascular: Proarrhythmia (including torsade de pointes), atropine-resistant bradycardia, heart block, sinus arrest, myocardial depression, CHF, paroxysmal ventricular tachycardia, cardiogenic shock, hypotension (**Note:** In adults, I.V. daily doses >2100 mg are associated with a greater risk of hypotension.)

Central nervous system (20% to 40% incidence): Lack of coordination, fatigue, malaise, abnormal gait, dizziness, headache, insomnia, nightmares, ataxia, behavioral changes, fever

Dermatologic: Discoloration of skin (slate blue), photosensitivity, rash, angioedema

Endocrine & metabolic: Hypothyroidism (or less commonly hyperthyroidism, see Additional Information), hyperglycemia, elevated triglycerides

Gastrointestinal: Nausea, vomiting, anorexia, constipation

Genitourinary: Sterile epididymitis

Hematologic: Coagulation abnormalities, thrombocytopenia; neutropenia, pancytopenia, hemolytic anemia, aplastic anemia

Hepatic: Elevated liver enzymes, severe hepatic toxicity (potentially fatal), elevated bilirubin, elevated serum ammonia

Local: Phlebitis (with I.V. formulation; concentration dependent)

Neuromuscular & skeletal: Paresthesia, tremor, peripheral neuropathy (rare)

Ocular: Corneal microdeposits, halos or blurred vision (10% incidence), photophobia, optic neuropathy, optic neuritis, visual impairment, permanent blindness (**Note:** Asymptomatic corneal microdeposits alone do not require dose reduction or discontinuation)

Respiratory (potentially fatal): Interstitial pneumonitis, hypersensitivity pneumonitis, pulmonary fibrosis (may present with cough, fever, dyspnea, malaise, chest x-ray changes); adult respiratory distress syndrome following surgery

Drug Interactions Cytochrome P450 isoenzyme CYP3A3/4 substrate; isoenzyme CYP2C9, CYP2D6, and CYP3A3/4 inhibitor

Amiodarone inhibits P450 enzymes and may increase plasma concentrations of digoxin, cyclosporine, flecainide, lidocaine, methotrexate, theophylline, procainamide, quinidine, warfarin, and phenytoin resulting in toxicities. **Note:** Dosage reduction of these agents and follow-up serum concentration monitoring are recommended (eg, a 50% dosage reduction in digoxin, 30% dosage reduction in flecainide, and a 30% to 50% dosage reduction in warfarin have been recommended).

Combined use of amiodarone with beta-blockers, digitalis glycosides, or calcium channel blockers may result in bradycardia, sinus arrest and heart block; use with class I antiarrhythmics may cause ventricular arrhythmias; amiodarone and general anesthetics may result in bradycardia, hypotension, heart block; use with fentanyl may cause bradycardia, hypotension, decreased cardiac output; combined use of amiodarone with lovastatin or simvastatin may result in an increased risk of myopathy or rhabdomyolysis (dosage reduction of lovastatin or simvastatin is recommended); amiodarone may inhibit the metabolism of dextromethorphan; phenytoin, rifampin and cholestyramine may decrease and cimetidine may increase amiodarone serum levels. Protease inhibitors may increase the serum concentration of amiodarone; monitor patients receiving concomitant indinavir closely; concurrent use of amiodarone with ritonavir or nelfinavir is not recommended.

The herbal medicine St John's wort (*Hypericum perforatum*) may significantly decrease concentrations of amiodarone and is **not** recommended for concurrent use. Concomitant use with antiarrhythmic agents or other drugs that prolong the QT interval may cause arrhythmias; reserve the combined use of amiodarone with other antiarrhythmic agents for life-threatening ventricular arrhythmias in patients who do not completely respond to a single agent; carefully evaluate the risks and benefits of concurrent use of any drug known to prolong the QT interval. **Note:** Due to the long half-life of amiodarone, drug interactions may potentially occur even after discontinuation of amiodarone.

Food Interactions Food increases rate and extent of oral absorption (high fat meal increased AUC by a mean of 2.3 times); grapefruit juice increases oral absorption

Stability
Storage: Tablets and I.V. product should be kept at room temperature and protected from light during storage; injection should also be protected from excessive heat; there is no need to protect diluted solutions from light during I.V. administration

Compatibility: Injection is compatible in D_5W at concentrations of 1-6 mg/mL for 24 hours in glass or polyolefin bottles and for 2 hours in polyvinyl chloride bags; although amiodarone adsorbs to polyvinyl chloride tubing, all clinical studies used polyvinyl chloride tubing and the recommended doses take adsorption into account, therefore, in adults, polyvinyl chloride tubing is recommended; amiodarone I.V. in D_5W is **not** compatible with aminophylline, cefamandole, cefazolin, mezlocillin, heparin, or sodium bicarbonate when administered together at the Y-site (a precipitate will occur)

Mechanism of Action A class III antiarrhythmic agent which inhibits adrenergic stimulation, prolongs the action potential and refractory period in myocardial tissue; decreases A-V conduction and sinus node function; possesses vasodilatory and negative inotropic effects

Pharmacodynamics
Onset of action: Oral: 2-3 days to 1-3 weeks after starting therapy; I.V.: (electrophysiologic effects) within hours; antiarrhythmic effects: 2-3 days to 1-3 weeks; mean onset of effect may be shorter in children vs adults and in patients receiving I.V. loading doses

Maximum effect: Oral: 1 week to 5 months

Duration of effects after discontinuation of oral therapy: Variable, 2 weeks to months: Children: less than a few weeks; adults: several months

Pharmacokinetics
Absorption: Oral: Slow and incomplete

Distribution: Amiodarone and its active metabolite cross the placenta; both distribute to breast milk in concentrations higher than maternal plasma concentrations

I.V.: Rapid redistribution with a decrease to 10% of peak values within 30-45 minutes after completion of infusion

V_{dss}: I.V. single dose in adults: Mean range: 40-84 L/kg

V_d: Oral dose in adults: 66 L/kg: range: 18-148 L/kg

Protein binding: >96%

Metabolism: In the liver and possibly the GI tract via cytochrome P450 enzymes; the major metabolite N-desethylamiodarone is active

Bioavailability: Oral: ~50% (range: 35% to 65%)

(Continued)

Amiodarone (Continued)

Half-life:
  Amiodarone:
    Single dose in adults: Mean: 58 days (range 15-142 days)
    Oral chronic therapy in adults: Mean range: 40-55 days (range: 26-107 days)
    I.V. single dose in adults: Mean range: 20-47 days
    Half-life is shortened in children vs adults
  N-desethylamiodarone (active metabolite):
    Single dose in adults: Mean: 36 days (range 14-75 days)
    Oral chronic therapy in adults: Mean: 61 days
Elimination: Via biliary excretion; possible enterohepatic recirculation; <1% excreted unchanged in urine
Dialysis: Nondialyzable (parent and metabolite)

Usual Dosage

Infants and Children:
  Oral: **Note:** Calculate dose using body surface area for children <1 year of age:
  Loading dose: 10-15 mg/kg/day or 600-800 mg/1.73 m^2/day in 1-2 divided doses/day for 4-14 days or until adequate control of arrhythmia or prominent adverse effects occur; dosage should then be reduced to 5 mg/kg/day or 200-400 mg/1.73 m^2/day given once daily for several weeks; if arrhythmia does not recur, reduce to lowest effective dosage possible; usual daily minimal dose: 2.5 mg/kg; maintenance doses may be given for 5 of 7 days/week.
  Note: A more aggressive dosing regimen was used in neonates and infants (n=50; mean age: 1 ± 1.5 months) <9 months of age, treated for various types of SVT; 90% of patients at discharge and 100% of patients within 3 months of discharge were free of tachycardia; however, patients who received a higher loading dose (20 mg/kg/day in 2 divided doses) were more likely to have a prolongation of the corrected QT interval (see Etheridge, 2001); further studies are needed.

  I.V., I.O.:
    PALS dose for treatment of pulseless VF or VT: 5 mg/kg rapid I.V. bolus or I.O.
    PALS dose for treatment of perfusing tachycardias: Loading dose: 5 mg/kg I.V. over 20-60 minutes or I.O.; may repeat up to maximum dose: 15 mg/kg/day.
    Note: Routine use with drugs that prolong the QT interval is **not** recommended; monitor for hypotension.

    I.V.: Limited data is available. Four retrospective studies (Figa, 1994; Raja, 1994; Soult, 1995; Celiker, 1998) used I.V. loading doses of 5 mg/kg. Loading doses were administered over 1 hour in three of these studies to treat various life-threatening tachyarrhythmias including junctional ectopic tachycardia after cardiac surgery (in conjunction with atrial pacing). Soult 1995 used I.V. amiodarone for short-term treatment of paroxysmal supraventricular tachycardia (PSVT) and administered the loading dose via slow I.V. bolus over 5 minutes. For continuous infusion, Figa 1994 and Celiker 1998 used initial maintenance doses of 5 mcg/kg/minute (7.2 mg/kg/day) which was increased incrementally until the desired effect was seen or a maximum dose of 15 mcg/kg/minute (21.6 mg/kg/day) was reached. The mean effective dose in the study by Figa 1994 (n=30) was 9.5 mcg/kg/minute (13.7 mg/kg/day) and in Celiker 1998 (n=12) was 10 ± 4.7 mcg/kg/minute (range: 5-15 mcg/kg/minute).
    A multicenter study (Perry, 1996; n=40; mean age 5.4 years with 24 of 40 children <2 years of age) used an I.V. loading dose of 5 mg/kg that was divided into five 1 mg/kg aliquots, with each aliquot given over 5-10 minutes. Additional 1-5 mg/kg doses could be administered 30 minutes later in a similar fashion if needed. The mean loading dose was 6.3 mg/kg. A maintenance dose (continuous infusion of 10-15 mg/kg/day) was administered to 21 of the 40 patients. Further studies are needed.

Adults:
  ACLS dose for cardiac arrest due to pulseless VT or VF: I.V.: Initial: 300 mg diluted in 20-30 mL D_5W or NS given rapid I.V. push; supplemental bolus doses of 150 mg rapid I.V. infusion may be given for recurring VF or pulseless VT; maximum total dose: 2.2 g/24 hours
  Ventricular arrhythmias:
    Oral: Loading dose: 800-1600 mg/day divided in 1-2 doses/day for 1-3 weeks, then 600-800 mg/day in 1-2 doses/day for 1 month; maintenance: 400 mg/day; lower doses are recommended for supraventricular arrhythmias.
    I.V.: Loading dose: ~1000 mg delivered over 24 hours as follows: 150 mg given over 10 minutes (at a rate of 15 mg/minute) followed by 360 mg given over 6 hours (at a rate of 1 mg/minute); follow with maintenance dose: 540 mg given over the next 18 hours (at a rate of 0.5 mg/minute); after the first 24 hours the maintenance dose is continued at 0.5 mg/minute; additional supplemental

bolus doses of 150 mg infused over 10 minutes may be given for breakthrough VF or hemodynamically unstable VT; maintenance dose infusion may be increased to control arrhythmia; maximum daily dose: 2 g

Atrial fibrillation (see Goldschlager, 2000):

Oral: Loading dose: 600-800 mg/day divided in 2 doses/day for 2-4 weeks, then 400 mg/day; at 3-6 months, dose may be reduced further to 100-300 mg/day based on clinical efficacy and adverse effects; usual maintenance: 200 mg/day; **Note:** some patients may require higher maintenance doses or increased maintenance doses for short periods of time for breakthrough arrhythmias; some patients can be maintained with 200 mg/day given for 5 of 7 days/week

Transition from I.V. to oral therapy: Optimal initial daily dose depends on I.V. dose administered and oral bioavailability; use the following as a guide for an initial daily dose, assuming patient received 0.5 mg/minute for the listed duration of I.V. infusion:

<1 week infusion: 800-1600 mg/day

1-3 week infusion: 600-800 mg/day

>3 week infusion: 400 mg/day

Dosing adjustment in renal impairment: No adjustment necessary

Administration

Oral: Administer at same time in relation to meals; do not administer with grapefruit juice

I.V.: Injection must be diluted before I.V. use. Adults: Usual dilutions: First loading infusion: 150 mg in 100 mL D_5W (1.5 mg/mL) for infusion over 10 minutes; then 900 mg in 500 mL D_5W (1.8 mg/mL) to deliver rest of dose; administer via central venous catheter, if possible; increased phlebitis may occur with peripheral infusions >3 mg/mL in D_5W, but concentrations ≤2.5 mg/mL may be less irritating; the use of a central venous catheter with concentrations >2 mg/mL for infusions >1 hour is recommended; maximum concentration for infusion: 6 mg/mL; use glass or poly-olefin bottles for infusions >2 hours; the use of polyvinyl chloride tubing is recommended in adults (see Stability); must be infused via volumetric infusion device; drop size of I.V. solution may be reduced and underdosage may occur if drop counter infusion sets are used; use in-line filter during administration; adults: Do not exceed 30 mg/minute initial infusion rate; infants and children: See Usual Dosage I.V.

Monitoring Parameters Heart rate and rhythm, blood pressure, EKG, chest x-ray, pulmonary function tests, thyroid function tests (see Additional Information), serum glucose, triglycerides, liver enzymes, ophthalmologic exams including fundoscopy and slit-lamp examinations, physical signs and symptoms of thyroid dysfunction (lethargy, edema of hands and feet, weight gain or loss), and pulmonary toxicity (dyspnea, cough; oxygen saturation, blood gases)

Reference Range Therapeutic: Chronic oral dosing: 1-2.5 mg/L (SI: 2-4 μmol/L) (parent); desethyl metabolite (active) is present in equal concentration to parent drug; serum levels may not be of great value for predicting toxicity and efficacy; toxicity may occur even at therapeutic concentrations

Patient Information Avoid grapefruit juice and the herbal medicine, St John's wort. Notify physician if persistent dry cough, shortness of breath, or decreased vision occurs. May discolor skin to a slate blue color. May cause photosensitivity reactions (eg, exposure to sunlight may cause severe sunburn, skin rash, redness, or itching); avoid exposure to sunlight and artificial light sources (sunlamps, tanning booth/bed); wear protective clothing, wide-brimmed hats, sunglasses, and lip sunscreen (SPF ≥15); use a sunscreen [broad-spectrum sunscreen or physical sunscreen (preferred) or sunblock with SPF ≥15]; contact physician if reaction occurs.

Nursing Implications Ambulation of patient may be impaired due to adverse effects; due to possible infusion rate-related hypotension, the I.V. infusion rate should be carefully monitored

Additional Information Intoxication with amiodarone necessitates EKG monitoring; bradycardia may be atropine resistant, I.V. isoproterenol or cardiac pacemaker may be required; hypotension, cardiogenic shock, heart block, QT prolongation and hepatotoxicity may also be seen; patients should be monitored for several days following overdose due to long half-life

I.V. product is used for acute treatment; the duration of I.V. treatment is usually 48-96 hours, however, in adults, infusions may be used cautiously for 2-3 weeks; there is limited experience with administering infusions for >3 weeks

Use of amiodarone 300 mg I.V. in adults with cardiac arrest (out-of-hospital) due to refractory ventricular arrhythmias improved the rate of survival to hospital admission (see Kudenchuk, 1999). In a randomized, double blind, placebo controlled trial in adults with shock-resistant ventricular fibrillation (out-of-hospital), I.V. amiodarone [initial dose: 5 mg/kg; second dose (if needed): 2.5 mg/kg] resulted in higher rates of (Continued)

Amiodarone *(Continued)*

survival to hospital admission as compared to I.V. lidocaine [initial dose: 1.5 mg/kg; second dose (if needed): 1.5 mg/kg] (see Dorian, 2002).

Thyroid function tests: Amiodarone partially inhibits the peripheral conversion of thyroxine (T_4) to triiodothyronine (T_3); serum T_4 and reverse triiodothyronine (RT_3) concentrations may be increased and serum T_3 may be decreased; most patients remain clinically euthyroid, however, clinical hypothyroidism or hyperthyroidism may occur

Dosage Forms

Injection, solution, as hydrochloride: 50 mg/mL (3 mL, 18 mL) [contains benzyl alcohol and polysorbate (Tween®) 80]

Cordarone®: 50 mg/mL (3 mL) [contains benzyl alcohol and polysorbate (Tween®) 80]

Amio-Aqueous®: 15 mg/mL (10 mL) [benzyl alcohol free and polysorbate free; contains an aqueous acetate buffer; available via orphan drug status or compassionate use from the manufacturer Academic Pharmaceuticals, Inc (847) 735-1170]

Tablet, scored, as hydrochloride: 200 mg

Cordarone®: 200 mg

Pacerone®: 200 mg, 400 mg

Extemporaneous Preparations

A 5 mg/mL oral suspension can be made from tablets; two stability studies using different vehicles exist; a 5 mg/mL oral suspension made with simple syrup NF containing methylcellulose 1% (50:50, v/v) was stable for 42 days at room temperature (25°C) and 91 days under refrigeration (4°C) in both glass and plastic prescription bottles (Nahata, 1997); label "shake well" and "protect from light"

Five 200 mg tablets were crushed in a mortar; the vehicle (either a 1:1 mixture of Ora-Sweet® and Ora-Plus® or a 1:1 mixture of Ora-Sweet® SF and Ora-Plus®) was adjusted to a pH between 6-7 using a sodium bicarbonate solution (5 g/100 mL of distilled water). A small amount of the vehicle was added to the mortar to make a uniform paste; geometric amounts of the vehicle were added while mixing to **almost** the desired volume; suspension was transferred to a graduate and qsad to 200 mL while mixing. Suspensions prepared in both vehicles were stable for 42 days at room temperature (25°C) and 91 days under refrigeration (4°C) in plastic prescription bottles (Nahata 1999); label "shake well" and "protect from light"

Neither of these 2 studies determined microbial growth; extended storage under refrigeration is recommended

Nahata MC, "Stability of Amiodarone in an Oral Suspension Stored Under Refrigeration and at Room Temperature," *Ann Pharmacother*, 1997, 31(7-8):851-2.

Nahata MC, Morosco RS, and Hipple TF, "Stability of Amiodarone in Extemporaneous Oral Suspensions Prepared From Commercially Available Vehicles," *J Ped Pharmacy Practice*, 1999, 4(4):186-9.

References

Celiker A, Ceviz N, and Ozme S, "Effectiveness and Safety of Intravenous Amiodarone in Drug-Resistant Tachyarrhythmias of Children," *Acta Paediatr Jpn*, 1998, 40(6):567-72.

Coumel P and Fidelle J, "Amiodarone in the Treatment of Cardiac Arrhythmias in Children: One Hundred Thirty-Five Cases," *Am Heart J*, 1980, 100(6 Pt 2):1063-9.

Dorian P, Cass D, Schwartz B, et al, "Amiodarone as Compared With Lidocaine for Shock-Resistant Ventricular Fibrillation," *N Engl J Med*, 2002, 346(12):884-90.

Drago F, Mazza A, Guccione P, et al, "Amiodarone Used Alone or in Combination With Propranolol: A Very Effective Therapy for Tachyarrhythmias in Infants and Children," *Pediatr Cardiol*, 1998, 19(6):445-9.

Etheridge SP, Craig JE, and Compton SJ, "Amiodarone is Safe and Highly Effective Therapy for Supraventricular Tachycardia in Infants," *Am Heart J*, 2001, 141(1):105-10.

Figa FH, Gow RM, Hamilton RM, et al, "Clinical Efficacy and Safety of Intravenous Amiodarone in Infants and Children," *Am J Cardiol*, 1994, 74(6):573-7.

Garson A Jr, Gillette PC, McVey P, et al, "Amiodarone Treatment of Critical Arrhythmias in Children and Young Adults," *J Am Coll Cardiol*, 1984, 4(4):749-55.

Goldschlager N, Epstein AE, Naccarelli G, et al, "Practical Guidelines for Clinicians Who Treat Patients With Amiodarone," *Arch Intern Med*, 2000, 160(12):1741-8.

"Guidelines 2000 for Cardiopulmonary Resuscitation and Emergency Cardiovascular Care, Part 6: Advanced Cardiovascular Life Support, The American Heart Association in Collaboration With the International Liasion Committee on Resuscitation," *Circulation*, 2000, 102(8 Suppl):I86-171.

"Guidelines 2000 for Cardiopulmonary Resuscitation and Emergency Cardiovascular Care, Part 10: Pediatric Advanced Life Support, The American Heart Association in Collaboration With the International Liaison Committee on Resuscitation," *Circulation*, 2000, 102(8 Suppl): I291-342.

Kudenchuk PJ, Cobb LA, Copass MK, et al, "Amiodarone for Resuscitation After Out-of-Hospital Cardiac Arrest Due to Ventricular Fibrillation," *N Engl J Med*, 1999, 341(12):871-8.

Paul T and Guccione P, "New Antiarrhythmic Drugs in Pediatric Use: Amiodarone," *Pediatr Cardiol*, 1994, 15(3):132-8.

Perry JC, Fenrich AL, Hulse JE, et al, "Pediatric Use of Intravenous Amiodarone: Efficacy and Safety in Critically Ill Patients From a Multicenter Protocol," *J Am Coll Cardiol*, 1996, 27(5):1246-50.

Raja P, Hawker RE, Chaikitpinyo A, et al, "Amiodarone Management of Junctional Ectopic Tachycardia After Cardiac Surgery in Children," *Br Heart J*, 1994, 72(3):261-5.

Shahar E, Barzilay Z, Frand M, et al, "Amiodarone in Control of Sustained Tachyarrhythmias in Children With Wolff-Parkinson-White Syndrome," *Pediatrics*, 1983, 72(6):813-6.

Shuler CO, Case CL, and Gillette PC, "Efficacy and Safety of Amiodarone in Infants," *Am Heart J*, 1993, 125(5 Pt 1):1430-2.

Soult JA, Munoz M, Lopez JD, et al, "Efficacy and Safety of Intravenous Amiodarone for Short-Term Treatment of Paroxysmal Supraventricular Tachycardia in Children," *Pediatr Cardiol*, 1995, 16(1):16-9.

♦ **Amitone® [OTC]** *see* Calcium Supplements *on page 200*

Amitriptyline (a mee TRIP ti leen)

Related Information

Comparison of Adverse Effects of Antidepressants *on page 1210*

Comparison of Usual Adult Dosage and Mechanism of Action of Antidepressants *on page 1209*

Drugs and Breast-Feeding *on page 1404*

Overdose and Toxicology *on page 1388*

Serotonin Syndrome *on page 1420*

U.S. Brand Names Elavil®

Canadian Brand Names Apo®-Amitriptyline; Levate®; PMS-Amitriptyline

Therapeutic Category Antidepressant, Tricyclic; Antimigraine Agent

Generic Available Yes (tablet)

Use Treatment of various forms of depression, often in conjunction with psychotherapy; analgesic for certain chronic and neuropathic pain; migraine prophylaxis

Pregnancy Risk Factor C

Contraindications Hypersensitivity to amitriptyline (cross-sensitivity with other tricyclics may occur) or any component; narrow-angle glaucoma; use of MAO inhibitors within 14 days (potentially fatal reactions may occur, see Drug Interactions); concurrent use of cisapride; use during acute recovery phase after MI

Warnings Do not discontinue abruptly in patients receiving high doses chronically

Precautions Use with caution in patients with cardiac conduction disturbances, cardiovascular disease, seizure disorders, narrow-angle glaucoma, increased intraocular pressure, history of urinary retention or bowel obstruction, hepatic or renal dysfunction, hyperthyroidism or those receiving thyroid hormone replacement; degree of sedation, anticholinergic effects, and risk of orthostatic hypotension are very high relative to other antidepressants

Adverse Reactions Anticholinergic effects may be pronounced; moderate to marked sedation can occur (tolerance to these effects usually occurs)

Cardiovascular: Postural hypotension, arrhythmias, tachycardia, sudden death

Central nervous system: Sedation, fatigue, anxiety, confusion, insomnia, impaired cognitive function, seizures; extrapyramidal symptoms are possible

Dermatologic: Photosensitivity, urticaria, rash

Endocrine & metabolic: Rarely SIADH

Gastrointestinal: Xerostomia, constipation, decrease of lower esophageal sphincter tone, GE reflux, increased appetite, weight gain

Genitourinary: Urinary retention, discoloration of urine (blue-green)

Hematologic: Rarely agranulocytosis, leukopenia, eosinophilia

Hepatic: Elevated liver enzymes, cholestatic jaundice

Neuromuscular & skeletal: Tremor, weakness

Ocular: Blurred vision, increased intraocular pressure

Miscellaneous: Allergic reactions

Drug Interactions Cytochrome P450 isoenzyme CYP1A2, CYP2C9, CYP2C19, CYP2D6 and CYP3A3/4 substrate

Amitriptyline may decrease the effects of clonidine and guanethidine; with clonidine, hypertensive crisis may occur following discontinuation of clonidine; amitriptyline may increase the effects of CNS depressants (including alcohol), adrenergic agents (epinephrine, isoproterenol), anticholinergic agents and warfarin. With MAO inhibitors, hyperpyrexia, tachycardia, hypertension, confusion, seizures, and death have been reported. The herbal medicine St John's wort (*Hypericum perforatum*) may increase serious side effects; its use is **not** recommended. Cimetidine, fluoxetine, and methylphenidate may decrease the metabolism and phenobarbital, carbamazepine, and rifampin may increase the metabolism of amitriptyline; amitriptyline may potentiate the cardiac effects of cisapride (do not administer concurrently); concurrent use of high-dose TCAs and ritonavir may cause the serotonin syndrome

Food Interactions Riboflavin dietary requirements may be increased; increased dietary fiber may decrease drug effect

Stability Protect injection and Elavil® 10 mg tablets from light; store injection at <40°C (preferably 15°C to 30°C)

(Continued)

Amitriptyline (Continued)

Mechanism of Action Increases the synaptic concentration of serotonin and/or norepinephrine in the CNS by inhibition of their reuptake by the presynaptic neuronal membrane

Pharmacodynamics Onset of action: Therapeutic antidepressant effects begin in 7-21 days; maximum effects may not occur for ≥2 weeks and as long as 4-6 weeks

Pharmacokinetics

Absorption: Oral: Rapid, well absorbed

Distribution: Crosses placenta; enters breast milk

Protein binding: >90%

Metabolism: In the liver to nortriptyline (active), hydroxy derivatives and conjugated derivatives

Half-life, adults: 9-25 hours (15-hour average)

Time to peak serum concentration: Within 4 hours

Elimination: Renal excretion of 18% as unchanged drug; small amounts eliminated in feces by bile

Dialysis: Nondialyzable

Usual Dosage

Chronic pain management: Children: Oral: Initial: 0.1 mg/kg at bedtime, may advance as tolerated over 2-3 weeks to 0.5-2 mg/kg at bedtime

Depressive disorders: Oral:

Children: Investigationally initial doses of 1 mg/kg/day given in 3 divided doses with increases to 1.5 mg/kg/day have been reported in a small number of children (n=9) 9-12 years of age; clinically, doses up to 3 mg/kg/day (5 mg/kg/day if monitored closely) have been proposed

Adolescents: Initial: 25-50 mg/day; may give in divided doses; increase gradually to 100 mg/day in divided doses; maximum dose: 200 mg/day

Migraine prophylaxis: Children: Limited studies exist; one small study (n=24; mean age: 8 years; range: 6-12 years) used increasing doses over 5 days to reach a final dose of 1.5 mg/kg/day; effectiveness was seen in 19 of 24 patients, but 5 children dropped out of the trial due to adverse effects (see Sorge, 1982). A recent large open-label trial in 192 children (mean age 12 ± 3 years) with >3 headaches/month (61% with migraine, 8% with migraine with aura, and 10% with tension-type headaches) used an initial dose of 0.25 mg/kg/day given before bedtime; doses were increased every 2 weeks by 0.25 mg/kg/day to a final dose of 1 mg/kg/day; patients also used appropriate abortive medications and lifestyle adjustments; at initial re-evaluation (mean: 67 days after initiation of therapy), the mean number of headaches per month significantly decreased from 17.1 to 9.2; the mean duration of headaches decreased from 11.5 to 6.3 hours; continued improvement was observed at follow-up visits; minimal adverse effects were reported. **Note:** Mean final dose was 0.99 ± 0.23 mg/kg; range: 0.16-1.7 mg/kg/day; EKGs were obtained on children receiving >1 mg/kg/day or in those describing a cardiac side effect (see Hershey, 2000). Further studies are needed.

Adults:

Oral: 30-100 mg/day single dose at bedtime or in divided doses; dose may be gradually increased up to 300 mg/day; once symptoms are controlled, decrease gradually to lowest effective dose

I.M.: 20-30 mg 4 times/day

Administration

Oral: May administer with food to decrease GI upset

Parenteral: Administer by I.M. route only; do not administer I.V.

Monitoring Parameters Heart rate, blood pressure, mental status, weight

Reference Range Note: Plasma levels do not always correlate with clinical effectiveness

Therapeutic:

Amitriptyline plus nortriptyline (active metabolite): 100-250 ng/mL (SI: 360-900 nmol/L)

Nortriptyline 50-150 ng/mL (SI: 190-570 nmol/L)

Toxic: >500 ng/mL (SI: >1800 nmol/L)

Patient Information Avoid alcohol and the herbal medicine St John's wort; limit caffeine intake; may cause drowsiness and impair ability to perform activities requiring mental alertness or physical coordination; may cause dry mouth; do not discontinue abruptly; may discolor urine to a blue-green color. May cause photosensitivity reactions (eg, exposure to sunlight may cause severe sunburn, skin rash, redness, or itching); avoid exposure to sunlight and artificial light sources (sunlamps, tanning booth/bed); wear protective clothing, wide-brimmed hats, sunglasses, and lip sunscreen (SPF ≥15); use a sunscreen [broad-spectrum sunscreen or physical sunscreen (preferred) or sunblock with SPF ≥15]; contact physician if reaction occurs.

Additional Information Due to promotion of weight gain with amitriptyline, other antidepressants (ie, imipramine or desipramine) may be preferred in heavy or obese children and adolescents

Dosage Forms

Injection, solution, as hydrochloride (Elavil®): 10 mg/mL (10 mL)

Tablet, as hydrochloride (Elavil®): 10 mg, 25 mg, 50 mg, 75 mg, 100 mg, 150 mg

References

Elser JM and Woody RC, "Migraine Headache in the Infant and Young Child," *Headache*, 1990, 30(6):366-8.

Hershey AD, Powers SW, Bentti AL, et al, "Effectiveness of Amitriptyline in the Prophylactic Management of Childhood Headaches," *Headache*, 2000, 40(7):539-49.

Kashani JH, Shekim WO, and Reid JC, "Amitriptyline in Children With Major Depressive Disorder: A Double-Blind Crossover Pilot Study," *J Am Acad Child Psychiatry*, 1984, 23(3):348-51.

Levy HB, Harper CR, and Weinberg WA, "A Practical Approach to Children Failing in School," *Pediatr Clin North Am*, 1992, 39(4):895-928.

Sorge F, Barone P, Steardo L, et al, "Amitriptyline as a Prophylactic for Migraine in Children," *Acta Neurol (Napoli)*, 1982, 4(5):362-7.

♦ **AmLactin® [OTC]** *see* Lactic Acid and Ammonium Hydroxide *on page 647*

Amlodipine (am LOE di peen)

U.S. Brand Names Norvasc®

Therapeutic Category Antianginal Agent; Antihypertensive Agent; Calcium Channel Blocker

Generic Available No

Use Treatment of hypertension and angina

Pregnancy Risk Factor C

Contraindications Hypersensitivity to amlodipine or any component

Warnings May increase frequency, duration, and severity of angina or precipitate acute MI during initiation of therapy or dosage increase (particularly in patients with severe obstructive coronary artery disease)

Precautions Use with caution in patients with CHF or severe aortic stenosis; use with caution and reduce the dose in patients with severe hepatic impairment; acute hypotension may rarely occur

Adverse Reactions

Cardiovascular system: Peripheral edema, flushing, palpitations; rarely: hypotension, arrhythmia, chest pain, syncope, peripheral ischemia, vasculitis; MI (rare)

Central nervous system: Headache, dizziness, somnolence, fatigue; less common: vertigo, insomnia, abnormal dreams, nervousness, depression, anxiety

Dermatologic: Rash, pruritus, erythema multiforme, angioedema

Endocrine & Metabolic: Sexual dysfunction, gynecomastia, hyperglycemia

Gastrointestinal: Nausea, abdominal pain, dyspepsia, anorexia, constipation, diarrhea, dysphagia, pancreatitis, vomiting, xerostomia, weight gain, weight loss; gingival hyperplasia (may be less than with nifedipine)

Hematologic: Thrombocytopenia, leukopenia, purpura

Hepatic: Jaundice, elevated liver enzymes

Neuromuscular & skeletal: Muscle cramps, asthenia, arthralgia, myalgia, paresthesia, peripheral neuropathy, hypoesthesia, tremor

Ocular: Diplopia, abnormal vision, eye pain, conjunctivitis

Otic: Tinnitus

Respiratory: Dyspnea, epistaxis

Miscellaneous: Diaphoresis, hypersensitivity reactions, thirst

Drug Interactions Cytochrome P450 isoenzyme CYP3A4 substrate

Azole antifungal agents may inhibit the metabolism of amlodipine and result in an increase in amlodipine serum concentrations or effect; calcium may decrease the pharmacologic effect of calcium channel blockers; rifampin may decrease amlodipine serum concentrations; amlodipine may (or may not) increase cyclosporine serum concentrations (conflicting studies exist)

Food Interactions Food does not affect the bioavailability of amlodipine. Grapefruit juice increased amlodipine peak serum concentrations by 15% and AUC by 16% in one single dose study (Josefsson, 1996); however, repeated daily ingestion of grapefruit juice did **not** affect amlodipine pharmacokinetics in another single-dose amlodipine study (Vincent, 2000); multiple dose amlodipine-grapefruit juice interaction studies are needed. Avoid natural licorice (causes sodium and water retention and increases potassium loss)

Mechanism of Action Inhibits calcium ions from entering the "slow channels" or select voltage-sensitive areas of vascular smooth muscle and myocardium during depolarization; produces a relaxation of coronary vascular smooth muscle and coronary vasodilation; increases myocardial oxygen delivery in patients with vasospastic angina

(Continued)

Amlodipine *(Continued)*

Pharmacodynamics Antihypertensive effects: Duration: ≥24 hours with chronic daily dosing

Pharmacokinetics

Absorption: Oral: Well absorbed

Distribution: Distribution into breast milk is unknown

Mean V_d: Adults: 21 L/kg

Protein binding: 93%

Metabolism: In the liver with 90% metabolized to inactive metabolites

Bioavailability: 64% to 90%

Half-life: Terminal: 30-50 hours

Time to peak serum concentrations: 6-12 hours

Elimination: 10% of unchanged drug and 60% of metabolites are excreted in the urine

Clearance: May be decreased in patients with hepatic insufficiency or moderate to severe heart failure

Dialysis: Not dialyzable

Usual Dosage Oral:

Children: Hypertension:

Limited information exists; only 3 prospective studies are available. In one study, 21 hypertensive children (mean age: 13.1 years; range: 6-17 years) received the following initial daily doses of amlodipine based on weight groups: Children <50 kg: 0.05 mg/kg/day; children 50-70 kg: 2.5 mg daily; children >70 kg: 5 mg daily; mean initial dose: 0.07 ± 0.04 mg/kg/day; doses were increased by 25% to 50% (rounded to the nearest 2.5 mg) every 5-7 days to a maximum of 0.5 mg/kg/day, as needed to control blood pressure; the mean required dose was almost twice as high for children <13 years of age (0.29 ± 0.13 mg/kg/day) compared to children ≥13 years of age (0.16 ± 0.11 mg/kg/day) (see Tallian, 1999).

In a small randomized crossover trial, amlodipine was compared to nifedipine or felodipine in 11 hypertensive children (mean age: 16 years; range: 9-17 years); amlodipine was administered once daily as a liquid preparation (tablets dissolved in water immediately prior to administration); an initial daily dose of 0.1 mg/kg/day (maximum: 5 mg daily) was increased by 50% to 100% after 1 week to a maximum of 10 mg/day, as needed for blood pressure control; mean initial dose: 0.09 ± 0.01 mg/kg/day; mean required dose: 0.12 mg/kg/day (Rogan, 2000). A third prospective study used fixed mg doses, rather than dosing on a mg/kg basis (Pfammatter, 1998).

Four retrospective studies used a variety of initial amlodipine doses ranging from 0.05-0.13 mg/kg/day; mean required dose after dosage titration (for all aged patients) ranged from 0.15-0.17 mg/kg/day (Khattak, 1998; Silverstein 1999; Flynn JT, et al, *Am J Hypertens*, 2000, 13(10):1061-6; Parker 2002). Two of these studies noted a relationship between dose and age, with younger patients requiring higher mg/kg/day doses. Several retrospective studies used twice daily dosing in younger children, but it is unknown whether this reflects altered pharmacokinetics or physician prescribing habits. Further pediatric studies are needed.

Adults:

Hypertension: Initial: 2.5-5 mg once daily; use initial dose of 2.5 mg once daily in patients who are small, fragile, or elderly, and when adding amlodipine to other antihypertensive therapy; in general, titrate dose over 7-14 days to fully assess effects; usual dose: 5 mg once daily; maximum dose: 10 mg once daily

Angina: 5-10 mg; use lower dose for patients with hepatic impairment and in the elderly

Dosing adjustment in renal impairment: Not needed; patients may receive the usual initial dose

Dosing adjustment in hepatic impairment: Adults: Initial: 2.5 mg once daily

Administration Oral: May be administered without regard to food; use caution if administered with grapefruit juice (see Food Interactions)

Monitoring Parameters Blood pressure, liver enzymes

Patient Information Do not discontinue abruptly; report unrelieved headache, vomiting, palpitations, peripheral or facial swelling, weight gain, or respiratory changes; may cause dizziness or drowsiness and impair ability to perform activities requiring mental alertness or physical coordination; may cause dry mouth

Dosage Forms Available as amlodipine besylate; mg strength refers to amlodipine

Tablet: 2.5 mg, 5 mg, 10 mg

Extemporaneous Preparations A 1 mg/mL oral suspension made from tablets and two different vehicles (a 1:1 mixture of simple syrup and 1% methylcellulose or a 1:1 mixture of OraPlus® and OraSweet®) was stable for 56 days at room temperature (25°C) and 91 days under refrigeration (4°C) when stored in amber plastic prescription bottles; grind fifty 5 mg tablets in a mortar into a fine powder; add a small amount of the vehicle and mix well to form a uniform paste; mix while adding the vehicle in geometric proportions to **almost** 250 mL; transfer to a calibrated bottle and qsad with vehicle to 250 mL. Microbial growth was not determined in this study; extended storage under refrigeration is recommended to minimize microbial contamination. Label "shake well" and "refrigerate"

Nahata MC, Morosco RS, and Hipple TF, "Stability of Amlodipine Besylate in Two Liquid Dosage Forms," *J Am Pharm Assoc*, 1999, 39(3):375-7.

References

Flynn JT and Pasko DA, "Calcium Channel Blockers: Pharmacology and Place in Therapy of Pediatric Hypertension," *Pediatr Nephrol*, 2000, 15(3-4):302-16.

Flynn JT, Smoyer WE, and Bunchman TE, "Treatment of Hypertensive Children With Amlodipine," *Am J Hypertens*, 2000, 13(10):1061-6.

Josefsson M, Zackrisson AL, and Ahlner J, "Effect of Grapefruit Juice on the Pharmacokinetics of Amlodipine in Healthy Volunteers," *Eur J Clin Pharmacol*, 1996, 51(2):189-93.

Khattak S, Rogan JW, Saunders EF, et al, "Efficacy of Amlodipine in Pediatric Bone Marrow Transplant Patients," *Clin Pediatr (Phila)*, 1998, 37(1):31-5.

Parker ML, Robinson RF, and Nahata MC, "Amlodipine Therapy in Pediatric Patients With Hypertension," *J Am Pharm Assoc*, 2002, 42(1):114-7.

Pfammatter JP, Clericetti-Affolter C, Truttmann AC, et al, "Amlodipine Once-Daily in Systemic Hypertension," *Eur J Pediatr*, 1998, 157(8):618-21.

Rogan JW, Lyszkiewicz DA, Blowey D, et al, "A Randomized Prospective Crossover Trial of Amlodipine in Pediatric Hypertension," *Pediatr Nephrol*, 2000, 14(12):1083-7.

Silverstein DM, Palmer J, Baluarte HJ, et al, "Use of Calcium-Channel Blockers in Pediatric Renal Transplant Recipients," *Pediatr Transplant*, 1999, 3(4):288-92.

Tallian KB, Nahata MC, Turman MA, et al, "Efficacy of Amlodipine in Pediatric Patients With Hypertension," *Pediatr Nephrol*, 1999, 13(4):304-10.

Vincent J, Harris SI, Foulds G, et al, "Lack of Effect of Grapefruit Juice on the Pharmacokinetics and Pharmacodynamics of Amlodipine," *Br J Clin Pharmacol*, 2000, 50(5):455-63.

♦ **Ammens® Medicated Deodorant [OTC]** *see Zinc Oxide on page 1167*

♦ **Ammonapse** *see Sodium Phenylbutyrate on page 1028*

Ammonium Chloride (a MOE nee um KLOR ide)

Synonyms NH$_4$Cl

Therapeutic Category Metabolic Alkalosis Agent; Urinary Acidifying Agent

Generic Available Yes

Use Diuretic or systemic and urinary acidifying agent; treatment of hypochloremia

Pregnancy Risk Factor C

Contraindications Hypersensitivity to ammonium chloride or any component; severe hepatic and renal dysfunction; patients with primary respiratory acidosis

Adverse Reactions

Cardiovascular: Bradycardia

Central nervous system: Mental confusion, coma, headache

Dermatologic: Rash

Endocrine & metabolic: Metabolic acidosis secondary to hyperchloremia

Gastrointestinal: GI irritation

Local: Pain at site of injection

Respiratory: Hyperventilation

Drug Interactions Chlorpropamide's effects may be enhanced due to decreased urinary excretion; may decrease flecainide levels due to increased urinary excretion; systemic acidosis may occur when used with spironolactone

Mechanism of Action Its dissociation to ammonium and chloride ions increases acidity by increasing free hydrogen ion concentration which combines with bicarbonate ion to form CO_2 and water; the net result is the replacement of bicarbonate ions by chloride ions

Pharmacokinetics

Metabolism: In the liver

Elimination: In urine

Usual Dosage

The following equations represent different methods of chloride or alkalosis correction utilizing either the serum HCO$_3^-$, the serum Cl$^-$ or the base excess: Children and Adults: I.V. (**Note:** Ammonium chloride is an alternative treatment and should be used only after sodium and potassium chloride supplementation has been optimized.):

Correction of refractory hypochloremic metabolic alkalosis: mEq NH$_4$Cl = 0.5 L/kg x wt in kg x [serum HCO$_3^-$ - 24] mEq/L; give ½ of ⅔ of the calculated dose, then re-evaluate

Correction of hypochloremia: mEq NH$_4$Cl = 0.2 L/kg x wt in kg x [103 - serum Cl$^-$] mEq/L, give ½ to ⅔ of calculated dose, then re-evaluate

Correction of alkalosis via base excess method: mEq NH$_4$Cl = 0.3 L/kg x wt in kg x base excess (mEq/L), give ½ to ⅔ of calculated dose, then re-evaluate

Children: I.V.: 75 mg/kg/day in 4 divided doses for urinary acidification; maximum daily dose: 6 g

(Continued)

Ammonium Chloride *(Continued)*

Adults: I.V.: 1.5 g/dose every 6 hours

Administration
Parenteral: Dilute to 0.2 mEq/mL and infuse I.V. over 3 hours; maximum concentration: 0.4 mEq/mL; maximum rate of infusion: 1 mEq/kg/hour

Monitoring Parameters Serum electrolytes, serum ammonia

Nursing Implications Rapid I.V. injection may increase the likelihood of ammonia toxicity

Dosage Forms Injection, solution: 26.75% [267.5 mg/mL, 5 mEq/mL] (20 mL)

♦ **Ammonium Hydroxide and Lactic Acid** *see* Lactic Acid and Ammonium Hydroxide *on page 647*

♦ **Ammonium Lactate** *see* Lactic Acid and Ammonium Hydroxide *on page 647*

♦ **Ammonium Molybdate** *see* Trace Metals *on page 1106*

Amoxicillin *(a moks i SIL in)*

Related Information
Carbohydrate and Alcohol Content of Liquid Medications for Use in Patients Receiving Ketogenic Diets *on page 1431*
Endocarditis Prophylaxis *on page 1321*

U.S. Brand Names Amoxil®; Moxilin®; Trimox®

Canadian Brand Names Apo®-Amoxi; Gen-Amoxicillin; Lin-Amox; Novamoxin®; Nu-Amoxi

Synonyms Amoxycillin; *p*-Hydroxyampicillin

Therapeutic Category Antibiotic, Penicillin

Generic Available Yes

Use Treatment of otitis media, sinusitis, and infections involving the respiratory tract, skin, and urinary tract due to susceptible *H. influenzae, N. gonorrhoeae, E. coli, P. mirabilis, E. faecalis,* streptococci, and nonpenicillinase-producing staphylococci; treatment of Lyme disease in children <8 years of age; prophylaxis of bacterial endocarditis; prophylaxis of postexposure inhalational anthrax

Pregnancy Risk Factor B

Contraindications Hypersensitivity to amoxicillin, penicillin, or any component

Warnings Epstein-Barr virus infection, acute lymphocytic leukemia or cytomegalovirus infection increases risk for amoxicillin-induced maculopapular rash

Precautions In patients with renal dysfunction, doses and/or frequency of administration should be modified in response to the degree of renal impairment; use with caution in patients with history of cephalosporin allergy; chewable tablets contain aspartame which is metabolized to phenylalanine and must be used with caution in patients with phenylketonuria

Adverse Reactions
Central nervous system: Fever
Dermatologic: Rash, exfoliative dermatitis, Stevens-Johnson syndrome, urticaria
Gastrointestinal: Diarrhea, nausea, vomiting, pseudomembranous colitis
Hematologic: Anemia, neutropenia, eosinophilia, thrombocytopenia, prolongation of bleeding time
Miscellaneous: Superinfection, hypersensitivity reactions, serum sickness, vasculitis, anaphylaxis

Drug Interactions Probenecid (increases serum amoxicillin concentration); allopurinol may increase frequency for amoxicillin rash; decreases oral contraceptive efficacy

Food Interactions Food does not interfere with absorption

Stability Suspensions are stable for 14 days at room temperature or if refrigerated; refrigeration is preferred

Mechanism of Action Interferes with bacterial cell wall synthesis during active multiplication by binding to one or more of the penicillin-binding proteins, causing cell wall death and resultant bactericidal activity against susceptible bacteria

Pharmacokinetics
Absorption: Oral: Rapid and nearly complete (74% to 92% of a single dose is absorbed)
Distribution: Into liver, lungs, prostate, muscle, middle ear effusions, maxillary sinus secretions, bile, and into ascitic and synovial fluids; excreted into breast milk
Protein binding: 17% to 20%, lower in neonates
Metabolism: Partial
Half-life:
Neonates, full-term: 3.7 hours
Infants and children: 1-2 hours
Adults with normal renal function: 0.7-1.4 hours

Patients with Cl$_{cr}$ <10 mL/minute: 7-21 hours
Time to peak serum concentration:
  Capsule: Within 2 hours
  Suspension: Neonates: 3-4.5 hours; children: 1 hour
Elimination: Renal excretion (80% unchanged drug)
Dialysis: Moderately dialyzable (20% to 50%); ~30% removed by 3-hour hemodialysis; supplemental dose is recommended after hemodialysis

Usual Dosage Oral:

Neonates and Infants: ≤3 months: 20-30 mg/kg/day in divided doses every 12 hours
Infants >3 months and Children: 25-50 mg/kg/day in divided doses every 8 hours or 25-50 mg/kg/day in divided doses every 12 hours
  Acute otitis media due to highly resistant strains of *S. pneumoniae*: 80-90 mg/kg/day divided every 12 hours
  Uncomplicated gonorrhea:
    <2 years, probenecid is contraindicated in this age group
    ≥2 years: 50 mg/kg plus probenecid 25 mg/kg as a single dose
  Endocarditis prophylaxis: 50 mg/kg 1 hour before procedure, not to exceed adult dose
  Postexposure inhalational anthrax prophylaxis:
    <40 kg: 45 mg/kg/day in divided doses every 8 hours
    ≥40 kg: 500 mg every 8 hours
Adults: 250-500 mg every 8 hours or 500-875 mg tablets twice daily; maximum dose: 2-3 g/day
  Uncomplicated gonorrhea: 3 g plus probenecid 1 g as a single dose
  Endocarditis prophylaxis: 2 g 1 hour before procedure

Dosing interval in renal impairment:
Cl$_{cr}$ 10-30 mL/minute: Administer every 12 hours
Cl$_{cr}$ <10 mL/minute: Administer every 24 hours

Administration Oral: May be administered on an empty or full stomach; may be mixed with formula, milk, or juice; shake suspension well before use

Monitoring Parameters With prolonged therapy, monitor renal, hepatic, and hematologic function periodically; monitor for diarrhea

Additional Information Appearance of a rash should be carefully evaluated to differentiate a nonallergic amoxicillin rash from a hypersensitivity reaction. Amoxicillin rash occurs in 5% to 10% of children receiving amoxicillin and is a generalized dull, red, maculopapular rash, generally appearing 3-14 days after the start of therapy. It normally begins on the trunk and spreads over most of the body. It may be most intense at pressure areas, elbows, and knees. Incidence of amoxicillin rash is higher in patients with viral infections, cytomegalovirus infections, infectious mononucleosis, lymphocytic leukemia, or patients with hyperuricemia who are receiving allopurinol.

Dosage Forms

Capsule, as trihydrate: 250 mg, 500 mg
  Amoxil®, Moxilin®, Trimox®: 250 mg, 500 mg
Powder for oral suspension, as trihydrate: 125 mg/5 mL (80 mL, 100 mL, 150 mL); 250 mg/5 mL (100 mL, 150 mL)
  Amoxil®: 125 mg/5 mL (80 mL, 150 mL) [strawberry flavor]; 200 mg/5 mL (5 mL, 50 mL, 75 mL, 100 mL) [bubblegum flavor]; 250 mg/5 mL (100 mL, 150 mL) [bubblegum flavor]; 400 mg/5 mL (5 mL, 50 mL, 75 mL, 100 mL) [bubblegum flavor]
  Moxilin®: 250 mg/5 mL (100 mL, 150 mL)
  Trimox®: 125 mg/5 mL (80 mL, 100 mL, 150 mL); 250 mg/5 mL (80 mL, 100 mL, 150 mL)
Powder for suspension, oral **drops**, as trihydrate (Amoxil®): 50 mg/mL (15 mL, 30 mL) [strawberry flavor]
Tablet, chewable, as trihydrate: 125 mg, 200 mg, 250 mg, 400 mg
  Amoxil®: 200 mg [contains 1.82 mg phenylalanine/tablet (as aspartame); cherry-banana-peppermint flavor], 400 mg [contains 3.64 mg phenylalanine (as aspartame); cherry-banana-peppermint flavor]
Tablet, film coated, as trihydrate: 500 mg, 875 mg
  Amoxil®: 500 mg, 875 mg

References

Boguniewicz M and Leung DY, "Hypersensitivity Reactions to Antibiotics Commonly Used in Children," *Pediatr Infect Dis J*, 1995, 14(3):221-31.

Canafax, DM, Yuan Z, Chonmaitree T, et al, "Amoxicillin Middle Ear Fluid Penetration and Pharmacokinetics in Children with Acute Otitis Media," *Pediatr Infect Dis J*, 1998, 17(2):149-56.

CDC and Johns Hopkins Working Group on Civilian Biodefense, "Commentary on Non-Labeled Dosing of Oral Amoxicillin in Adults and Pediatrics for Post-Exposure Inhalational Anthrax," December 10, 2001, http://www.fda.gov/cder/drugprepare/amox-anthrax.htm.

Dajani AS, Taubert KA, Wilson WW, et al, "Prevention of Bacterial Endocarditis. Recommendations by the American Heart Association," *JAMA*, 1997, 277(22):1794-1801.

Amoxicillin and Clavulanic Acid
(a moks i SIL in & klav yoo LAN ic AS id)

Related Information
Carbohydrate and Alcohol Content of Liquid Medications for Use in Patients Receiving Ketogenic Diets *on page 1431*

U.S. Brand Names Augmentin®; Augmentin ES-600™; Augmentin XR™

Canadian Brand Names Alti-Amoxi-Clav®; Apo®-Amoxi-Clav; Clavulin®; ratio-Amox-iClav

Synonyms Clavulanic Acid and Amoxicillin

Therapeutic Category Antibiotic, Beta-lactam and Beta-lactamase Combination; Antibiotic, Penicillin

Generic Available Yes (excludes extended release)

Use Infections caused by susceptible organisms involving the lower respiratory tract, otitis media, sinusitis, skin and skin structure, and urinary tract; spectrum same as amoxicillin in addition to beta-lactamase producing *M. catarrhalis, H. influenzae, N. gonorrhoeae,* and *S. aureus* (not MRSA)

Pregnancy Risk Factor B

Contraindications Hypersensitivity to amoxicillin, clavulanic acid, penicillins, or any component; history of amoxicillin/clavulanic acid-associated cholestatic jaundice or hepatic dysfunction

Warnings Epstein-Barr virus infection, acute lymphocytic leukemia or cytomegalovirus infection increase the risk for amoxicillin-induced maculopapular rash. Pseudomembranous colitis has been reported; prolonged use may result in superinfection

Precautions Use with caution in patients with history of cephalosporin hypersensitivity; in patients with renal dysfunction, doses and/or frequency of administration should be modified in response to the degree of renal impairment. The "BID" formulation may contain aspartame which is metabolized to phenylalanine and must be avoided or used with caution in patients with phenylketonuria.

Adverse Reactions
Central nervous system: Headache, agitation
Dermatologic: Rash, urticaria, exfoliative dermatitis, Stevens-Johnson syndrome
Gastrointestinal: Nausea, vomiting, abdominal pain, pseudomembranous colitis; incidence of diarrhea (9%) is higher than with amoxicillin alone
Genitourinary: Vaginal candidiasis
Hepatic: Elevated AST, ALT, alkaline phosphatase, and bilirubin
Miscellaneous: Superinfection, hypersensitivity reactions, serum sickness, vasculitis, anaphylaxis

Drug Interactions Probenecid (increases serum amoxicillin concentration), allopurinol (may increase incidence of rash); amoxicillin and clavulanic acid may reduce the efficacy of oral contraceptives

Stability Reconstituted oral suspension should be refrigerated; discard unused suspension after 10 days; store tablets, chewable tablets, and powder for oral suspension at room temperature

Mechanism of Action Clavulanic acid binds and inhibits beta-lactamases that inactivate amoxicillin resulting in amoxicillin having an expanded spectrum of activity; amoxicillin interferes with bacterial cell wall synthesis by binding to one or more of the penicillin-binding proteins and causing cell wall death

Pharmacokinetics
Absorption: Both amoxicillin and clavulanate are well absorbed
Distribution: Both widely distributed into lungs, pleural, peritoneal, synovial, and ascitic fluid as well as bone, gynecologic tissue, and middle ear fluid; crosses the placenta; excreted in breast milk
Protein binding:
Amoxicillin: 17% to 20%
Clavulanate: 25%
Metabolism: Clavulanic acid: Metabolized in the liver
Half-life of both agents in adults with normal renal function: ~1 hour; amoxicillin pharmacokinetics are not affected by clavulanic acid
Time to peak serum concentration: Within 2 hours
Elimination: Amoxicillin: 60% to 80%; excreted unchanged in the urine
Dialysis: ~30% of amoxicillin removed by 3-hour hemodialysis; supplemental dose recommended after hemodialysis (do **not** use extended release tablets)

Usual Dosage Oral (dosing based on amoxicillin component):
Neonates and Infants <3 months: 30 mg/kg/day divided every 12 hours using the 125 mg/5 mL suspension
Children <40 kg: 20-40 mg (amoxicillin component)/kg/day in divided doses every 8 hours **or** 25-45 mg (amoxicillin component)/kg/day divided every 12 hours using either 200 mg/5 mL or 400 mg/5 mL suspension, or 200 mg, 400 mg chewable tablet formulation

Multidrug-resistant pneumococcal otitis media: 80-90 mg/kg/day divided every 12 hours (use a 7:1 "BID" formulation or Augmentin ES-600™)

Note: Children <40 kg should not receive the 250 mg film-coated tablets which contain a higher dose of clavulanic acid than the 250 mg chewable tablets.

Children ≥16 years and Adults:

Acute bacterial sinusitis: Extended release tablet: 2000 mg every 12 hours for 10 days

Community-acquired pneumonia: 2000 mg every 12 hours for 7-10 days

Adults:

Less severe infection: 250 mg every 8 hours or 500 mg every 12 hours

More severe infections and respiratory tract infections: 500 mg every 8 hours or 875 mg every 12 hours

Dosing interval in renal impairment:

Cl_{cr} <30 mL/minute: Do not use 875 mg tablet or extended release tablet

Cl_{cr} 10-30 mL/minute: Administer 250-500 mg every 12 hours

Cl_{cr} <10 mL/minute: Administer 250-500 mg every 24 hours

Administration Oral: Administer at the start of a meal to decrease the frequency or severity of GI side effects; do not administer with a high fat meal (clavulanate absorption is decreased); may mix with milk, formula, or juice; shake suspension well before use

Monitoring Parameters With prolonged therapy, monitor renal, hepatic, and hematologic function periodically

Test Interactions May interfere with urinary glucose determinations using Clinitest®

Patient Information Adverse GI effects may occur less frequently if taken with food. Report persistent diarrhea to physician.

Additional Information Since both the 250 mg and 500 mg tablets contain the same amount of clavulanic acid, two 250 mg tablets are not equivalent to one 500 mg tablet. Four 250 mg tablets or two 500 mg tablets are **not** equivalent to a single 1000 mg extended release tablet.

Appearance of a rash should be carefully evaluated to differentiate a nonallergic amoxicillin rash from a hypersensitivity reaction. Amoxicillin rash occurs in 5% to 10% of children receiving amoxicillin and is a generalized dull, red, maculopapular rash, generally appearing 3-14 days after the start of therapy. It normally begins on the trunk and spreads over most of the body. It may be most intense at pressure areas, elbows, and knees. Incidence of amoxicillin rash is higher in patients with viral infections, *Salmonella* infections, lymphocytic leukemia, or patients with hyperuricemia who are receiving allopurinol.

Dosage Forms Amoxicillin as trihydrate and clavulanic acid as potassium:

Powder for oral suspension: 200: Amoxicillin 200 mg and clavulanic acid 28.5 mg per 5 mL (100 mL) [contains phenylalanine]; 400: Amoxicillin 400 mg and clavulanic acid 57 mg per 5 mL (100 mL) [contains phenylalanine]

125: Amoxicillin 125 mg and clavulanic acid 31.25 mg per 5 mL (75 mL, 100 mL, 150 mL) [contains 0.16 mEq potassium/5 mL; banana flavor]

200: Amoxicillin 200 mg and clavulanic acid 28.5 mg per 5 mL (50 mL, 75 mL, 100 mL) [contains 7 mg phenylalanine (as aspartame) and 0.14 mEq potassium per 5 mL; orange-raspberry flavor] ["BID" formulation]

250: Amoxicillin 250 mg and clavulanic acid 62.5 mg per 5 mL (75 mL, 100 mL, 150 mL) [contains 0.32 mEq potassium/5 mL; orange flavor]

400: Amoxicillin 400 mg and clavulanic acid 57 mg per 5 mL (50 mL, 75 mL, 100 mL) [contains 7 mg phenylalanine (as aspartame) and 0.29 mEq potassium per 5 mL; orange-raspberry flavor] ["BID" formulation]

ES-600™: Amoxicillin 600 mg and clavulanic acid 42.9 mg per 5 mL (50 mL, 75 mL, 100 mL, 150 mL) [contains 7 mg phenylalanine (as aspartame) and 0.23 mEq potassium per 5 mL; orange-raspberry flavor] ["BID" formulation]

Tablet: 500: Amoxicillin 500 mg and clavulanic acid 125 mg; 875: Amoxicillin 875 mg and clavulanic acid 125 mg

250: Amoxicillin 250 mg and clavulanic acid 125 mg [contains 0.63 mEq potassium/tablet]

500: Amoxicillin 500 mg and clavulanic acid 125 mg [contains 0.63 mEq potassium/tablet]

875: Amoxicillin 875 mg and clavulanic acid 125 mg [contains 0.63 mEq potassium/tablet] ["BID" formulation]

Tablet, chewable: 200: Amoxicillin 200 mg and clavulanic acid 28.5 mg [contains phenylalanine]; 400: Amoxicillin 400 mg and clavulanic acid 57 mg [contains phenylalanine]

125: Amoxicillin 125 mg and clavulanic acid 31.25 mg [contains 0.16 mEq potassium/tablet; lemon-lime flavor]

(Continued)

Amoxicillin and Clavulanic Acid *(Continued)*

200: Amoxicillin 200 mg and clavulanic acid 28.5 mg [contains 2.1 mg phenylalanine (as aspartame) and 0.14 mEq potassium per tablet; cherry-banana flavor] ["BID" formulation]

250: Amoxicillin 250 mg and clavulanic acid 62.5 mg [contains 0.32 mEq potassium/tablet; lemon-lime flavor]

400: Amoxicillin 400 mg and clavulanic acid 57 mg [contains 4.2 mg phenylalanine (as aspartame) and 0.29 mEq potassium per tablet; cherry-banana flavor] ["BID" formulation]

Tablet, extended release (Augmentin XR™): Amoxicillin 1000 mg and clavulanic acid 62.5 mg [contains 0.32 mEq potassium and 1.27 mEq sodium per tablet]

References

Gan VN, Kusmiesz H, Shelton S, et al, "Comparative Evaluation of Loracarbef and Amoxicillin-Clavulanate for Acute Otitis Media," *Antimicrob Agents Chemother*, 1991, 35(5):967-71.

Hoberman A, Paradise JL, Burch DJ, et al, "Equivalent Efficiency and Reduced Occurrence of Diarrhea From a New Formulation of Amoxicillin/Clavulanate Potassium (Augmentin®) for Treatment of Acute Otitis Media in Children," *Pediatr Infect Dis J*, 1997, 16(5):463-70.

Reed MD, "Clinical Pharmacokinetics of Amoxicillin and Clavulanate," *Pediatr Infect Dis J*, 1996, 15(10):949-54.

Thoene DE and Johnson CE, "Pharmacotherapy of Otitis Media," *Pharmacotherapy*, 1991, 11(3):212-21.

Todd PA and Benfield P, "Amoxicillin/Clavulanic Acid. An Update of Its Antibacterial Activity, Pharmacokinetic Properties and Therapeutic Use," *Drugs*, 1990, 39(2):264-307.

♦ **Amoxil®** *see* Amoxicillin *on page 94*

♦ **Amoxycillin** *see* Amoxicillin *on page 94*

♦ **Amphetamine and Dextroamphetamine** *see* Dextroamphetamine and Amphetamine *on page 361*

♦ **Amphocin®** *see* Amphotericin B (Conventional) *on page 98*

Amphotericin B (Conventional)

(am foe TER i sin bee con VEN sha nal)

U.S. Brand Names Amphocin®; Fungizone®

Therapeutic Category Antifungal Agent, Systemic; Antifungal Agent, Topical

Generic Available Yes (powder)

Use Treatment of severe systemic infections and meningitis caused by susceptible fungi such as *Candida* species, *Histoplasma capsulatum, Cryptococcus neoformans, Aspergillus* species, *Mucor* species, *Blastomyces dermatitidis, Torulopsis glabrata, Sporothrix schenckii, Paracoccidioides brasiliensis,* and *Coccidioides immitis*; fungal peritonitis; irrigant for bladder fungal infections; treatment of amebic meningoencephalitis caused by *Naegleria fouleri*; topically for cutaneous and mucocutaneous candidal infections

Pregnancy Risk Factor B

Contraindications Hypersensitivity to amphotericin or any component

Warnings I.V. amphotericin is used primarily for the treatment of patients with progressive and potentially fatal fungal infections; not to be used for common clinically inapparent forms of fungal disease; anaphylaxis has been reported with amphotericin B-containing drugs; facilities for cardiopulmonary resuscitation should be available during administration due to the possibility of anaphylactic reaction

Precautions Due to the nephrotoxic potential of amphotericin, other nephrotoxic drugs should be avoided

Adverse Reactions

Cardiovascular: Hypotension, hypertension, cardiac arrhythmias, flushing

Central nervous system: Fever, chills, and headache are the most common adverse effects reported with amphotericin B infusion; delirium, seizures, malaise

Endocrine & metabolic: Hypokalemia, hypomagnesemia

Gastrointestinal: Anorexia, nausea, vomiting, steatorrhea, weight loss

Hematologic: Anemia, leukopenia, thrombocytopenia

Hepatic: Acute hepatic failure, jaundice

Local: Phlebitis

Renal: Renal tubular acidosis, renal failure (oliguria, azotemia, elevated serum creatinine)

Respiratory: Wheezing, hypoxemia

Miscellaneous: Anaphylactoid reaction

Adverse effects due to intrathecal amphotericin:

Central nervous system: Headache, pain along lumbar nerves, arachnoiditis

Gastrointestinal: Nausea, vomiting

Genitourinary: Urinary retention

Neuromuscular & skeletal: Paresthesia, leg and back pain, foot drop

Ocular: Vision changes

Drug Interactions Nephrotoxic drugs may cause additive toxic effects; corticosteroids may increase potassium depletion caused by amphotericin; may predispose patients receiving cardiac glycosides or skeletal muscle relaxants to toxicity secondary to hypokalemia; imidazole derivatives (eg, miconazole, fluconazole, ketoconazole) may antagonize the effect and induce fungal resistance to amphotericin; may increase toxicity of flucytosine by increasing cellular uptake and/or impairing its renal excretion; may potentiate renal toxicity, bronchospasm, and hypotension of antineoplastic agents

Stability Reconstitute only with SWI without preservatives, not bacteriostatic water; benzyl alcohol, sodium chloride, or other electrolyte solutions may cause precipitation; can be diluted in D_5W, $D_{10}W$, up to $D_{20}W$; for I.V. infusion, an in-line filter (>1 micron mean pore diameter) may be used; irrigating solutions should be diluted in sterile water; short-term exposure (<24 hours) to light during I.V. infusion does **not** appreciably affect potency

Mechanism of Action Binds to ergosterol altering cell membrane permeability in susceptible fungi and causing leakage of cell components with subsequent cell death

Pharmacokinetics

Absorption: Poor oral absorption

Distribution: Minimal amounts enter the aqueous humor, bile, amniotic fluid, pericardial fluid, pleural fluid, and synovial fluid; poor CSF penetration

Protein binding: 90%

Half-life: Increased in small neonates and young infants

Initial: 15-48 hours

Terminal phase: 15 days

Elimination: 2% to 4% of dose eliminated in urine unchanged; ~40% eliminated over 7-day period and may be detected in urine for up to 8 weeks after discontinued use

Dialysis: Poorly dialyzed

Usual Dosage Medication errors, including deaths, have resulted from confusion between lipid-based forms of amphotericin (Abelcet®, Amphotec®, AmBisome®) and conventional amphotericin B for injection; conventional amphotericin B for injection doses should not exceed 1.5 mg/kg/day

Neonates, Infants, and Children:

I.V.: Test dose: 0.1 mg/kg/dose to a maximum of 1 mg; infuse over 20-60 minutes; an alternative method to the 0.1 mg/kg test dose is to initiate therapy with 0.25 mg/kg amphotericin administered over 6 hours; frequent observation of the patient and assessment of vital signs during the first several hours of the infusion is recommended

Initial therapeutic dose: If the 0.1 mg/kg test dose is tolerated without the occurrence of serious adverse effects, a therapeutic dose of 0.4 mg/kg can be given the same day as the test dose

The daily dose can then be gradually increased, usually in 0.25 mg/kg increments on each subsequent day until the desired daily dose is reached; in critically ill patients, more rapid dosage acceleration (up to 0.5 mg/kg increments on each subsequent day) may be warranted

Maintenance dose: 0.25-1 mg/kg/day given once daily; infuse over 2-6 hours; rapidly progressing disease may require short-term use of doses to 1.5 mg/kg/day; once therapy has been established, amphotericin B can be administered on an every-other-day basis at 1-1.5 mg/kg/dose

Intrathecal, intraventricular, or intracisternal (preferably into the lateral ventricles through a cisternal Ommaya reservoir): 25-100 mcg every 48-72 hours; increase to 500 mcg as tolerated

Adults:

I.V.: Test dose: 1 mg infused over 20-30 minutes

Initial therapeutic dose (if the test dose is tolerated): 0.25 mg/kg

The daily dose can then be gradually increased, usually in 0.25 mg/kg increments on each subsequent day until the desired daily dose is reached

Maintenance dose: 0.25-1 mg/kg/day once daily, infuse over 2-6 hours; or 1-1.5 mg/kg/dose every other day; do not exceed 1.5 mg/kg/day

Intrathecal, intraventricular, or intracisternal (preferably into the lateral ventricles through a cisternal Ommaya reservoir): 25-100 mcg every 48-72 hours; increase to 500 mcg as tolerated

Children and Adults:

Bladder irrigation: 5-15 mg amphotericin/100 mL of sterile water irrigation solution at 100-300 mL/day. Fluid is instilled into the bladder; the catheter is clamped for 60-120 minutes and the bladder drained. Perform irrigation 3-4 times/day for 2-5 days.

Dialysate: 1-4 mg/L of peritoneal dialysis fluid either with or without low-dose I.V. amphotericin B therapy

Topical: Apply to affected areas 2-4 times/day

(Continued)

Amphotericin B (Conventional) *(Continued)*

Note: Amphotericin B has been administered intranasally to reduce the frequency of invasive aspergillosis in neutropenic patients; 7 mg amphotericin B in 7 mL sterile water was placed in a De Vilbiss atomizer and the aerosolized solution was instilled intranasally to each nostril 4 times/day delivering an average of 5 mg amphotericin/day

Dosing adjustment in renal impairment: Dosage adjustments are not necessary with pre-existing renal impairment; if decreased renal function is due to amphotericin, the daily dose can be decreased by 50% or the dose can be given every other day. Therapy may be held until serum creatinine concentrations begin to decline.

Administration Parenteral: Amphotericin is administered by I.V. infusion over 2-3 hours (range: 1-6 hours) at a final concentration not to exceed 0.1 mg/mL through a peripheral venous catheter; in patients unable to tolerate a large fluid volume, amphotericin B at a final concentration not to exceed 0.5 mg/mL in D_5W or $D_{10}W$ may be administered through a central venous catheter

Monitoring Parameters BUN and serum creatinine levels should be determined every other day while therapy is increased and at least weekly thereafter; serum potassium and magnesium should be monitored closely; monitor electrolytes, liver function, hematocrit, CBC regularly; monitor I & O; monitor for signs of hypokalemia (muscle weakness, cramping, drowsiness, EKG changes, etc); blood pressure, temperature, pulse, respiration

Patient Information Amphotericin cream may slightly discolor skin and stain clothing; personal hygiene is very important to help reduce the spread and recurrence of lesions; avoid covering topical applications with occlusive bandages; most skin lesions require 1-3 weeks of therapy

Nursing Implications Cardiovascular collapse has been reported after rapid amphotericin injection; may premedicate patients who experience mild adverse reactions with acetaminophen and diphenhydramine 30 minutes prior to the amphotericin infusion. Meperidine and ibuprofen may help to reduce fevers and chills. Hydrocortisone can be added to the infusion solution to reduce febrile and other systemic reactions. Heparin 1 unit per 1 mL of infusion solution can be added to reduce phlebitis.

Additional Information A study by Harbarth, et al, reported that 29% of patients who experienced moderate to severe nephrotoxicity during conventional amphotericin B treatment had 3 or more risk factors which included body weight ≥90 kg, male sex, mean daily amphotericin B dosage ≥35 mg, chronic kidney disease, or concomitant use of amikacin or cyclosporine. Amphotericin B-induced nephrotoxicity may be minimized by sodium loading with 10-15 mL/kg of NS infused prior to each amphotericin B dose or pentoxifylline, and avoiding use of other nephrotoxic agents

Dosage Forms

Cream (Fungizone®): 3% (20 g)

Lotion (Fungizone®): 3% (30 mL)

Injection, powder for reconstitution, lyophilized (Amphocin®, Fungizone®): 50 mg [contains sodium desoxycholate]

References

The Ad Hoc Advisory Panel on Peritonitis Management. "Continuous Ambulatory Peritoneal Dialysis (CAPD) Peritonitis Treatment Recommendations: 1989 Update," *Perit Dial Int*, 1989, 9(4):247-56.

Benson JM and Nahata MC, "Pharmacokinetics of Amphotericin B in Children," *Antimicrob Agents Chemother*, 1989, 33(11):1989-93.

Bianco JA, Almgren J, Kern DL, et al, "Evidence That Oral Pentoxifylline Reverses Acute Renal Dysfunction in Bone Marrow Transplant Recipients Receiving Amphotericin B and Cyclosporine," *Transplantation*, 1991, 51(4):925-7.

Branch RA, "Prevention of Amphotericin B-Induced Renal Impairment. A Review on the Use of Sodium Supplementation," *Arch Intern Med*, 1988, 148(11):2389-94.

Harbarth S, Pestotnik SL, Lloyd JF, et al, "The Epidemiology of Nephrotoxicity Associated With Conventional Amphotericin B Therapy," *Am J Med*, 2001, 111(7):528-34.

Jeffery GM, Beard ME, Ikram RB, et al, "Intranasal Amphotericin B Reduces the Frequency of Invasive Aspergillosis in Neutropenic Patients," *Am J Med*, 1991, 90(6):685-92.

Kintzel PE and Smith GH, "Practical Guidelines for Preparing and Administering Amphotericin B," *Am J Hosp Pharm*, 1992, 49(5):1156-64.

Koren G, Lau A, Klein J, et al, "Pharmacokinetics and Adverse Effects of Amphotericin B in Infants and Children," *J Pediatr*, 1988, 113(3):559-63.

Amphotericin B Lipid Complex

(am foe TER i sin bee LIP id KOM pleks)

U.S. Brand Names Abelcet®

Synonyms ABLC

Therapeutic Category Antifungal Agent, Systemic

Generic Available No

Use Treatment of aspergillosis or invasive fungal infections in patients who are refractory to or intolerant of conventional amphotericin B therapy (refractory to or intolerant is defined as renal dysfunction with a serum creatinine ≥1.5 mg/dL that develops during therapy, or disease progression after a total dose of conventional amphotericin

B of at least 10 mg/kg). This indication is primarily based on results of emergency studies for the treatment of aspergillosis; may be useful in the treatment of hepatosplenic candidiasis and cryptococcal meningitis.

Pregnancy Risk Factor B

Contraindications Hypersensitivity to amphotericin B, dimyristoylphosphatidylcholine (DMPC) and dimyristoylphosphatidylglycerol (DMPG) which are two phospholipids in the formulation, or any component

Warnings Anaphylaxis has been reported with amphotericin B-containing drugs; facilities for cardiopulmonary resuscitation should be available during administration due to the possibility of anaphylactic reaction

Precautions Due to the nephrotoxic potential of amphotericin B, other nephrotoxic drugs should be avoided

Adverse Reactions
Cardiovascular: Hypotension, cardiac arrest, arrhythmias, flushing
Central nervous system: Headache; transient chills and fever during infusion of the drug are the most common effects reported with ABLC
Dermatologic: Rash, pruritus
Endocrine & metabolic: Hypokalemia, bilirubinemia, hypomagnesemia
Gastrointestinal: Diarrhea, abdominal pain
Hematologic: Thrombocytopenia, leukopenia, anemia
Renal: Renal tubular acidosis, elevated serum creatinine (occurs to a lesser degree than with conventional amphotericin B), azotemia, oliguria
Respiratory: Dyspnea, respiratory failure
Miscellaneous: Anaphylactoid and other allergic reactions

Drug Interactions Nephrotoxic drugs may cause additive nephrotoxic effects; corticosteroids may increase potassium depletion caused by amphotericin; may predispose patients receiving cardiac glycosides or skeletal muscle relaxants to toxicity secondary to hypokalemia; may increase myelotoxicity and nephrotoxicity of zidovudine; imidazole derivatives (eg, miconazole, fluconazole, ketoconazole) may antagonize the effect and induce fungal resistance to amphotericin; may increase toxicity of flucytosine by increasing cellular uptake and/or impairing its renal excretion; may potentiate renal toxicity, bronchospasm, and hypotension of antineoplastic agents

Stability Prior to admixture, refrigerate vial and protect from light; diluted ABLC infusion solution in D_5W is stable up to 48 hours refrigerated and an additional 6 hours at room temperature. Do not freeze. Do not dilute with saline solutions or mix with other drugs or electrolytes.

Mechanism of Action Binds to ergosterol altering cell membrane permeability in susceptible fungi and causing leakage of cell components with subsequent cell death

Pharmacokinetics Exhibits nonlinear kinetics; volume of distribution and clearance from blood increases with increasing dose
Distribution: High tissue concentration found in the liver, spleen, and lung
Half-life, terminal: 173 hours
Elimination: 0.9% of dose excreted in urine over 24 hours; effects of hepatic and renal impairment on drug disposition are unknown
Dialysis: ABLC is not hemodialyzable

Usual Dosage Children and Adults: I.V.: 2.5-5 mg/kg given as a once daily infusion
Dosing adjustment in renal failure: Renal toxicity is dose dependent; there are no firm guidelines for dose adjustment based on lab test results (serum creatinine levels).

Administration Parenteral: I.V.: Prior to administration, assure serum potassium is >3.2 mEq/L; do not use an in-line filter less than 5 microns; administer at a rate of 2.5 mg/kg/hour (over 2 hours) at a final concentration of 1 mg/mL in D_5W. A maximum concentration of 2 mg/mL may be used in fluid-restricted patients

Monitoring Parameters BUN, serum creatinine, liver function tests, serum electrolytes, CBC; vital signs, I & O; monitor for signs of hypokalemia (muscle weakness, cramping, drowsiness, EKG changes, etc)

Nursing Implications If infusion time exceeds 2 hours, mix the contents by gently rotating the infusion bag every 2 hours.

Additional Information Management of side effects is similar to conventional amphotericin B. [See Amphotericin B (Conventional) *on page 98* for suggested management guidelines of side effects.]

Dosage Forms Injection, suspension: 5 mg/mL (10 mL, 20 mL)

References

De Marie S, "Clinical Use of Liposomal and Lipid-Complexed Amphotericin B," *J Antimicrob Chemother*, 1994, 33(5):907-16.

Kline S, Larsen TA, Fieber L, et al, "Limited Toxicity of Prolonged Therapy With High Doses of Amphotericin B Lipid Complex," *Clin Infect Dis*, 1995, 21(5):1154-8.

Amphotericin B Liposome (am foe TER i sin bee LYE po som)

U.S. Brand Names AmBisome®

Synonyms L-AmB

Therapeutic Category Antifungal Agent, Systemic

Generic Available No

Use Treatment of aspergillosis, candidiasis, or cryptococcosis in patients who are refractory to or intolerant of conventional amphotericin B therapy (refractory to or intolerant is defined as renal dysfunction with a serum creatinine ≥1.5 mg/dL that develops during therapy, or disease progression after a total dose of conventional amphotericin B of at least 10 mg/kg); empiric therapy for presumed fungal infection in febrile, neutropenic bone marrow transplant patients or febrile, neutropenic acute nonlymphocytic leukemia patients after an unsuccessful trial of antibiotics; treatment of suspected or proven fungal infections in patients with renal impairment

Pregnancy Risk Factor B

Contraindications Hypersensitivity to amphotericin B or any component

Warnings Anaphylaxis has been reported with amphotericin B-containing drugs; facilities for cardiopulmonary resuscitation should be available during administration due to the possibility of anaphylactic reaction

Precautions Due to the nephrotoxic potential of amphotericin B, other nephrotoxic drugs should be avoided

Adverse Reactions

Cardiovascular: Hypotension, arrhythmias, chest pain, cardiac arrest, vasodilatation

Central nervous system: Headache, transient chills or rigors (18%), fever (17%), anxiety, insomnia, dizziness, hallucinations

Dermatologic: Pruritus, rash, diaphoresis

Endocrine & metabolic: Hypokalemia, bilirubinemia, hypomagnesemia, hyperglycemia, hypocalcemia

Gastrointestinal: Diarrhea, nausea, vomiting

Hematologic: Anemia, thrombocytopenia

Hepatic: Elevated ALT, AST, and alkaline phosphatase

Renal: Renal tubular acidosis, elevated serum creatinine and BUN (19%; occurs to a lesser degree than with conventional amphotericin B), oliguria, hematuria

Respiratory: Dyspnea, respiratory failure, cough

Miscellaneous: Anaphylactoid and other allergic reactions

Drug Interactions Nephrotoxic drugs may cause additive nephrotoxic effects; corticosteroids may increase potassium depletion caused by amphotericin; may predispose patients receiving cardiac glycosides or skeletal muscle relaxants to toxicity secondary to hypokalemia; may result in acute pulmonary toxicity in patients simultaneously receiving leukocyte transfusions; ketoconazole, fluconazole may induce fungal resistance to amphotericin B; may increase toxicity of flucytosine by increasing cellular uptake and/or impairing its renal excretion; may potentiate renal toxicity, bronchospasm and hypotension of antineoplastic agents

Stability Store unopened vials under refrigeration; reconstituted drug is stable for 24 hours under refrigeration. Do not dilute with saline solutions or mix with other drugs or electrolytes since this may cause precipitation of AmBisome®. AmBisome® is stable when further diluted to a concentration of 0.2-2 mg/mL in D_5W, $D_{10}W$, $D_{20}W$, and $D_{25}W$ (see table)

AmBisome® Stability

	Solution	Temperature	Stability
D_5W	2 mg/mL	2°C to 8°C	14 days
	0.2 mg/mL	2°C to 8°C	11 days
	0.2-2 mg/mL	23°C to 27°C	24 hours
$D_{10}W$	0.2-2 mg/mL	2°C to 8°C	48 hours
$D_{20}W$	2 mg/mL	2°C to 8°C	48 hours
$D_{25}W$	2 mg/mL	2°C to 8°C	48 hours

Pharmacokinetics Exhibits nonlinear kinetics (greater than proportional increase in serum concentration with an increase in dose)

Distribution: V_d: 0.1-0.16 L/kg

Half-life (terminal): 100-153 hours

Usual Dosage Children and Adults: I.V.: 3-5 mg/kg/day given as a once daily infusion; doses as high as 6 mg/kg/day have been used in patients with documented *Aspergillus* infection

Administration Parenteral: I.V.: Do not use in-line filter less than 1 micron to administer AmBisome®. Flush line with D_5W prior to infusion; infusion of diluted AmBisome® should start within 6 hours of preparation; infuse over 2 hours; infusion time may be reduced to 1 hour in patients who tolerate the treatment; AmBisome® may be diluted with D₅W, D₁₀W, or D₂₀W to a final concentration of 1-2 mg/mL; lower concentrations (0.2-0.5 mg/mL) may be administered to infants and small children to provide sufficient volume for infusion

Monitoring Parameters BUN, serum creatinine, liver function tests, serum electrolytes, CBC, vital signs, I & O; monitor for signs of hypokalemia (muscle weakness, cramping, drowsiness, EKG changes)

Nursing Implications Management of side effects is similar to conventional amphotericin B. [See Amphotericin B (Conventional) *on page 98* for suggested management guidelines of side effects.]

Dosage Forms Injection, powder for reconstitution: 50 mg

References

Emminger W, Graninger W, Emminger-Schmidmeir W, et al, "Tolerance of High Doses of Amphotericin B by Infusion of a Liposomal Formulation in Children With Cancer," *Ann Hematol*, 1994, 68:27-31.

Ringden O, Andstrom E, Remberger M, et al, "Safety of Liposomal Amphotericin B (AmBisome®) In 187 Transplant Recipients Treated With Cyclosporin," *Bone Marrow Transplant*, 1994, 14 Suppl 5:S10-4.

Walsh TJ, Finberg RW, Arndt C, et al, "Liposomal Amphotericin B for Empirical Therapy in Patients With Persistent Fever and Neutropenia," *N Engl J Med*, 1999, 340:764-71.

Ampicillin (am pi SIL in)

Related Information

Carbohydrate and Alcohol Content of Liquid Medications for Use in Patients Receiving Ketogenic Diets *on page 1431*

Endocarditis Prophylaxis *on page 1321*

U.S. Brand Names Marcillin®; Principen®

Canadian Brand Names Apo®-Ampi; Novo-Ampicillin; Nu-Ampi

Synonyms Aminobenzylpenicillin

Therapeutic Category Antibiotic, Penicillin

Generic Available Yes

Use Treatment of susceptible bacterial infections caused by streptococci, pneumococci, enterococci, nonpenicillinase-producing staphylococci, *Listeria*, meningococci, some strains of *H. influenzae*, *P. mirabilis*, *Salmonella*, *Shigella*, *E. coli*, *Enterobacter*, and *Klebsiella*; initial empiric treatment of neonates with suspected bacterial sepsis or meningitis used in combination with an aminoglycoside or cefotaxime; endocarditis prophylaxis

Pregnancy Risk Factor B

Contraindications Hypersensitivity to ampicillin (penicillins) or any component

Warnings Epstein-Barr virus infection, acute lymphocytic leukemia or cytomegalovirus infection increases risk for ampicillin-induced maculopapular rash

Precautions Dosage adjustment may be necessary in patients with renal impairment (Cl_cr <10-15 mL/minute); use with caution in patients allergic to cephalosporins

Adverse Reactions

Central nervous system: Seizures, headache, dizziness, drug fever

Dermatologic: Rash, urticaria, exfoliative dermatitis, Stevens-Johnson syndrome

Gastrointestinal: Diarrhea (20%), nausea, vomiting, glossitis, pseudomembranous enterocolitis, oral candidiasis

Hematologic: Eosinophilia, hemolytic anemia, thrombocytopenia, neutropenia, prolongation of bleeding time

Renal: Interstitial nephritis

Miscellaneous: Anaphylaxis, hypersensitivity reactions, serum sickness, vasculitis, superinfection

Drug Interactions Estrogen-containing oral contraceptives (decreases contraceptive effectiveness), aminoglycosides, probenecid (increases ampicillin serum levels), chloroquine (decreases bioavailability of ampicillin), allopurinol (possible increased frequency of ampicillin rash)

Food Interactions Food decreases rate and extent of absorption

Stability Oral suspension is stable for 14 days under refrigeration; reconstituted solutions for I.M. or direct I.V. should be used within 1 hour; solutions for I.V. infusion will be inactivated by dextrose at room temperature; if dextrose-containing solutions are to be used as a diluent, the resultant solution will only be stable for 2 hours vs 8 hours in solutions containing NS

Mechanism of Action Interferes with bacterial cell wall synthesis by binding to one or more penicillin-binding proteins during active multiplication; inhibits the final transpeptidation step of peptidoglycan synthesis causing cell wall death and resultant bactericidal activity against susceptible bacteria

Pharmacokinetics

Absorption: Oral: 50%

Distribution: Into bile; penetration into CSF occurs with inflamed meninges only; low excretion into breast milk

(Continued)

Ampicillin *(Continued)*

Protein binding:
   Neonates: 10%
   Adults: 15% to 18%
Half-life:
   Neonates:
      2-7 days: 4 hours
      8-14 days: 2.8 hours
      15-30 days: 1.7 hours
   Children and Adults: 1-1.8 hours
   Anuric patients: 8-20 hours
Time to peak serum concentration: Oral: Within 1-2 hours
Elimination: ~90% of drug excreted unchanged in urine within 24 hours; excreted in bile
Dialysis: ~40% is removed by hemodialysis

Usual Dosage

Children: Oral: 50-100 mg/kg/day divided every 6 hours; maximum dose: 2-3 g/day
Adults: Oral: 250-500 mg every 6 hours
Neonates: I.M., I.V.:
   Postnatal age ≤7 days:
      ≤2000 g: 50 mg/kg/day divided every 12 hours; meningitis: 100 mg/kg/day divided every 12 hours
      >2000 g: 75 mg/kg/day divided every 8 hours; meningitis: 150 mg/kg/day divided every 8 hours
      Group B streptococcal meningitis: 200 mg/kg/day divided every 8 hours
   Postnatal age >7 days:
      <1200 g: 50 mg/kg/day divided every 12 hours; meningitis: 100 mg/kg/day divided every 12 hours
      1200-2000 g: 75 mg/kg/day divided every 8 hours; meningitis: 150 mg/kg/day divided every 8 hours
      >2000 g: 100 mg/kg/day divided every 6 hours; meningitis: 200 mg/kg/day divided every 6 hours
      Group B streptococcal meningitis: 300 mg/kg/day divided every 6 hours
Infants and Children: I.M., I.V.: 100-200 mg/kg/day divided every 6 hours; meningitis: 200-400 mg/kg/day divided every 6 hours; maximum dose: 12 g/day
   Endocarditis prophylaxis:
      50 mg/kg within 30 minutes before procedure (dental, oral, respiratory tract, or esophageal procedures); maximum dose: 2 g
      50 mg/kg (maximum dose: 2 g) plus gentamicin 1.5 mg/kg (maximum dose: 120 mg) within 30 minutes of starting the procedure; 25 mg/kg 6 hours later (for high-risk patients undergoing genitourinary and GI tract procedures)
Adults: I.M., I.V.: 500 mg to 3 g every 6 hours; maximum dose: 14 g/day
   Endocarditis prophylaxis:
      2 g within 30 minutes before procedure (dental, oral, respiratory tract, or esophageal procedures)
      2 g plus gentamicin 1.5 mg/kg (maximum dose: 120 mg) within 30 minutes of starting the procedure; 1 g 6 hours later (for high-risk patients undergoing genitourinary and GI tract procedures)
Adults: I.M., I.V.: 500 mg to 3 g every 4-6 hours
Dosing interval in renal impairment: Adults:
   Cl_{cr} 10-30 mL/minute: Administer every 6-12 hours
   Cl_{cr} <10 mL/minute: Administer every 12 hours

Administration

Oral: Administer with water 1-2 hours prior to food on an empty stomach; shake suspension well before using
Parenteral: Ampicillin may be administered IVP over 3-5 minutes at a rate not to exceed 100 mg/minute or I.V. intermittent infusion over 15-30 minutes; final concentration for I.V. administration should not exceed 100 mg/mL (IVP) or 30 mg/mL (I.V. intermittent infusion)

Monitoring Parameters With prolonged therapy monitor renal, hepatic, and hematologic function periodically; observe for change in bowel frequency

Test Interactions False-positive urinary glucose (Benedict's solution, Clinitest®); + Coombs' [direct]

Nursing Implications Ampicillin and gentamicin should not be mixed in the same I.V. tubing or administered concurrently

Additional Information Appearance of a rash should be carefully evaluated to differentiate a nonallergic ampicillin rash from a hypersensitivity reaction. Ampicillin rash occurs in 5% to 10% of children receiving ampicillin and is a generalized dull red, maculopapular rash, generally appearing 3-14 days after the start of therapy. It normally begins on the trunk and spreads over most of the body. It may be most intense at pressure areas, elbows, and knees. Incidence of ampicillin rash is higher in patients with viral infections, infectious mononucleosis, lymphocytic leukemia, or patients with hyperuricemia who are receiving allopurinol.

Sodium content of suspension (250 mg/5 mL, 5 mL): 10 mg (0.4 mEq)
Sodium content of 1 g: 66.7 mg (3 mEq)

Dosage Forms

Capsule, as trihydrate: 250 mg, 500 mg
Marcillin®: 500 mg
Principin®: 250 mg, 500 mg
Injection, powder for reconstitution, as sodium: 125 mg, 250 mg, 500 mg, 1 g, 2 g, 10 g
Powder for oral suspension, as trihydrate (Principin®): 125 mg/5 mL (100 mL, 200 mL); 250 mg/5 mL (100 mL, 200 mL)

References

Boguniewicz M and Leung DY, "Hypersensitivity Reactions to Antibiotics Commonly Used in Children," *Pediatr Infect Dis J*, 1995, 14(3):221-31.

Brown RD, Campoli-Richards DM, "Antimicrobial Therapy in Neonates, Infants, and Children," *Clin Pharmacokinet*, 1989, 17(Suppl 1):105-15.

Ampicillin and Sulbactam (am pi SIL in & SUL bak tam)

U.S. Brand Names Unasyn®

Synonyms Sulbactam and Ampicillin

Therapeutic Category Antibiotic, Beta-lactam and Beta-lactamase Combination; Antibiotic, Penicillin

Generic Available No

Use Treatment of susceptible bacterial infections involved with skin and skin structure, intra-abdominal infections, gynecological infections; spectrum is that of ampicillin plus organisms producing beta-lactamases such as *S. aureus*, *H. influenzae*, *E. coli*, *Klebsiella*, *Acinetobacter*, *Enterobacter*, and anaerobes

Pregnancy Risk Factor B

Contraindications Hypersensitivity to ampicillin, sulbactam, any component, or penicillins

Warnings Epstein-Barr virus infection, acute lymphocytic leukemia or cytomegalovirus infection increases risk for ampicillin-induced maculopapular rash; not FDA approved for children <12 years of age

Precautions Modify dosage in patients with renal impairment; use with caution in patients allergic to cephalosporins

Adverse Reactions
Cardiovascular: Chest pain
Central nervous system: Fatigue, malaise, headache, chills, dizziness, seizures
Dermatologic: Rash (2%), itching, urticaria, exfoliative dermatitis, Stevens-Johnson syndrome
Gastrointestinal: Diarrhea (3%), nausea, vomiting, candidiasis, flatulence, pseudomembranous colitis, hairy tongue
Genitourinary: Dysuria, hematuria
Hematologic: Decreased WBC, neutrophils, platelets, hemoglobin, and hematocrit
Hepatic: Elevated liver enzymes
Local: Pain at injection site (I.M.: 16%, I.V.: 3%), thrombophlebitis (3%)
Renal: Elevated BUN, elevated serum creatinine
Miscellaneous: Hypersensitivity reactions, anaphylaxis, serum sickness, vasculitis, superinfection

Drug Interactions Probenecid (decreased elimination of ampicillin and sulbactam); allopurinol (possible increased frequency of ampicillin rash); efficacy of oral contraceptives may be reduced

Stability Ampicillin/sulbactam infusion solution is stable for 8 hours in NS at room temperature; incompatible when mixed with aminoglycosides

Mechanism of Action Sulbactam has very little antibacterial activity by itself. The addition of sulbactam, a beta-lactamase inhibitor, to ampicillin extends the spectrum of ampicillin to include beta-lactamase producing organisms; ampicillin acts by inhibiting bacterial cell wall synthesis during the stage of active multiplication

Pharmacokinetics
Distribution: Into bile, blister and tissue fluids; poor penetration into CSF with uninflamed meninges; higher concentrations attained with inflamed meninges
Protein binding:
Ampicillin: 28%
Sulbactam: 38%
Half-life: Ampicillin and sulbactam are similar: 1-1.8 hours and 1-1.3 hours, respectively in patients with normal renal function
(Continued)

Ampicillin and Sulbactam *(Continued)*

Elimination: ~75% to 85% of both drugs are excreted unchanged in urine within 8 hours following administration

Usual Dosage Unasyn® (ampicillin/sulbactam) is a combination product; each 3 g vial contains 2 g of ampicillin and 1 g of sulbactam. Dosage recommendations are based on the **ampicillin** component.

I.M., I.V.:
  Infants ≥1 month: 100-150 mg ampicillin/kg/day divided every 6 hours
    Meningitis: 200-300 mg ampicillin/kg/day divided every 6 hours
  Children: 100-200 mg ampicillin/kg/day divided every 6 hours
    Meningitis: 200-400 mg ampicillin/kg/day divided every 6 hours; maximum dose: 8 g ampicillin/day
  Adults: 1-2 g ampicillin every 6-8 hours; maximum dose: 12 g ampicillin/day
Dosing interval in renal impairment:
  Cl_{cr} 15-29 mL/minute: Administer every 12 hours
  Cl_{cr} 5-14 mL/minute: Administer every 24 hours

Administration Parenteral: May be administered by slow I.V. injection over 10-15 minutes at a final concentration for administration not to exceed 45 mg Unasyn® (30 mg ampicillin and 15 mg sulbactam)/mL or by intermittent infusion over 15-30 minutes

Monitoring Parameters With prolonged therapy monitor hematologic, renal, and hepatic function; observe for change in bowel frequency

Test Interactions False-positive urinary glucose levels (Benedict's solution, Clinitest®); positive Coombs' [direct]

Additional Information Sodium content of 1.5 g (1 g ampicillin plus 0.5 g sulbactam): 5 mEq

Dosage Forms Injection, powder for reconstitution, as ampicillin sodium and sulbactam sodium: 1.5 g [ampicillin 1 g and sulbactam 0.5 g]; 3 g [ampicillin 2 g and sulbactam 1 g]; 15 g [ampicillin 10 g and sulbactam 5 g] (bulk package)

References

Dajani AS, "Sulbactam/Ampicillin in Pediatric Infections," *Drugs*, 1988, 35(Suppl 7):35-8.

Goldfarb J, Aronoff SC, Jaffé A, et al, "Sultamicillin in the Treatment of Superficial Skin and Soft Tissue Infections in Children," *Antimicrob Agents Chemother*, 1987, 31(4):663-4.

Kulhanjian J, Dunphy MG, Hamstra S, et al, "Randomized Comparative Study of Ampicillin/Sulbactam vs Ceftriaxone for Treatment of Soft Tissue and Skeletal Infections in Children," *Pediatr Infect Dis J*, 1989, 8(9):605-10.

Syriopoulou V, Bitsi M, Theodoridis C, et al, "Clinical Efficacy of Sulbactam/Ampicillin in Pediatric Infections Caused by Ampicillin-Resistant or Penicillin-Resistant Organisms," *Rev Infect Dis*, 1986, 8(Suppl 5):S630-3.

Amprenavir *(am PRE na veer)*

Related Information

Adult and Adolescent HIV *on page 1327*
Pediatric HIV *on page 1323*

U.S. Brand Names Agenerase®

Therapeutic Category Antiretroviral Agent; HIV Agents (Anti-HIV Agents); Protease Inhibitor

Generic Available No

Use Treatment of HIV infection in combination with other antiretroviral agents (Note: HIV regimens consisting of **three** antiretroviral agents are strongly recommended)

Pregnancy Risk Factor C

Contraindications Hypersensitivity to amprenavir or any component; concurrent therapy with astemizole, cisapride, dihydroergotamine, ergonovine, ergotamine, methylergonovine, pimozide, midazolam, or triazolam; due to the high amount of propylene glycol, amprenavir oral **solution** is contraindicated in infants and children <4 years, pregnancy, renal or hepatic failure, and in patients receiving disulfiram or metronidazole

Warnings Amprenavir is a potent CYP3A4 isoenzyme inhibitor that interacts with numerous drugs. Due to potential serious and/or life-threatening drug interactions, some drugs are contraindicated (see Contraindications and Drug interactions) and the following drugs require concentration monitoring if coadministered with amprenavir: amiodarone, systemic lidocaine, tricyclic antidepressants, and quinidine. Concurrent use with rifampin, hormonal contraceptives, or certain cholesterol-lowering agents (lovastatin, simvastatin) is **not** recommended.

Amprenavir oral solution contains a high amount of propylene glycol and should only be used when the capsules or other protease inhibitors are not options; women and certain ethnic groups (Native Americans, Eskimos, Asians) may have a decreased capacity to metabolize propylene glycol and therefore, may be at a higher risk for adverse effects of propylene glycol; patients with renal or hepatic impairment are also at higher risk for adverse effects of propylene glycol (use oral solution with caution);

when using the oral solution, monitor patients for propylene glycol adverse effects (see Monitoring Parameters); change patient to capsule formulation as soon as patient is able to take capsules.

Severe and life-threatening skin reactions (eg, Stevens-Johnson syndrome) may occur; discontinue amprenavir in patients who develop severe or life-threatening rashes or in patients with moderate rashes and systemic symptoms. Spontaneous bleeding episodes have been reported in patients with hemophilia type A and B receiving protease inhibitors. New onset diabetes mellitus, exacerbations of diabetes, and hyperglycemia have been reported in HIV-infected patients receiving protease inhibitors. Acute hemolytic anemia has been reported.

Precautions Use with caution in patients with diabetes mellitus, sulfonamide allergy (amprenavir is a sulfonamide), or hemophilia. Use with caution and decrease the dose in patients with hepatic impairment. Capsules and oral solution contain high amounts of vitamin E; additional supplements of vitamin E should be avoided. Fat redistribution and accumulation [ie, central obesity, peripheral wasting, facial wasting, breast enlargement, dorsocervical fat enlargement (buffalo hump), and cushingoid appearance] have been observed in patients receiving antiretroviral agents (causal relationship not established).

Adverse Reactions Note: Percent incidence of adverse reactions are similar in adult and pediatric patients; percent incidence listed reflects combination antiretroviral therapy (but not concurrent therapy with ritonavir; see package insert)

Central nervous system: Depression or mood disorders (9% to 16%), headache, fatigue

Dermatologic: Rash (22% incidence; usually mild to moderate, maculopapular, some pruritic; median onset: 11 days, range: 7-73 days); severe or life-threatening rash, including Stevens-Johnson syndrome (1% of patients, 4% of patients who develop a rash)

Endocrine & metabolic: Hyperglycemia (45% to 53%), hypertriglyceridemia (41% to 56%), hypercholesterolemia (7% to 13%), new onset diabetes, exacerbation of diabetes mellitus, fat redistribution and accumulation (see Precautions)

Gastrointestinal: Nausea (43% to 74%), vomiting (24% to 34%), diarrhea (39% to 60%), taste disorders (2% to 10%)

Hematologic: Acute hemolytic anemia (rare, one case reported), spontaneous bleeding in hemophiliacs

Hepatic: Elevated liver enzymes

Neuromuscular & skeletal: Paresthesia (perioral or peripheral)

Drug Interactions Cytochrome P450 isoenzyme CYP3A4 substrate and inhibitor

Amprenavir may inhibit the metabolism of the following drugs and cause serious or life-threatening adverse effects: Astemizole, cisapride, dihydroergotamine, ergotamine, midazolam, and triazolam (concurrent therapy with these drugs and amprenavir is contraindicated); **Note:** If amprenavir and ritonavir capsules are used concurrently, flecainide and propafenone are also contraindicated; amprenavir may increase the toxic effects of amiodarone, lidocaine, quinidine, warfarin, cyclosporine, tacrolimus, rapamycin, and tricyclic antidepressants (serum concentration monitoring of these drugs is necessary); amprenavir may increase the serum concentration of bepridil and result in life-threatening cardiac arrhythmias (use with caution; monitor closely); amprenavir significantly increases the AUC of rifabutin by 193% (rifabutin dose should be decreased by at least $1/2$ the recommended dose when used in combination with amprenavir); amprenavir may increase the AUC of ketoconazole and zidovudine and decrease the AUC of indinavir and saquinavir; amprenavir may increase serum concentrations or toxicity of diltiazem, nifedipine, alprazolam, clorazepate, diazepam, flurazepam, itraconazole, dapsone, erythromycin, loratadine, sildenafil, carbamazepine, pimozide, and cholesterol-lowering agents (concurrent use of lovastatin or simvastatin is **not** recommended; concurrent use of atorvastatin may increase risk of myopathy and rhabdomyolysis; use lowest possible dose of atorvastatin and carefully monitor patient; consider use of pravastatin or fluvastatin for concurrent use with amprenavir)

Rifampin significantly reduces amprenavir plasma concentrations (AUC of amprenavir is decreased by about 90%) and should **not** be used concurrently; hormonal contraceptives (eg, ethinyl estradiol/norethindrone) decrease amprenavir serum concentrations and should **not** be used concurrently (nonhormonal contraception is recommended); methadone may decrease the serum concentrations of amprenavir (consider alternative antiretroviral agent); amprenavir may decrease plasma concentrations of methadone (increase in methadone dosage may be required); amprenavir may decrease serum concentrations of delavirdine and result in a loss of virological response and possible delavirdine resistance (concomitant use of amprenavir and delavirdine is **not** recommended); the herbal medicine St John's wort (*Hypericum perforatum*) may significantly decrease concentrations of amprenavir and (Continued)

Amprenavir *(Continued)*

is **not** recommended for concurrent use; efavirenz decreases amprenavir concentrations by 39%; saquinavir decreases amprenavir AUC by 32%; dexamethasone may decrease amprenavir serum concentrations (use with caution); nevirapine, phenobarbital, phenytoin, or carbamazepine may decrease amprenavir concentrations; abacavir, clarithromycin, indinavir, ketoconazole, or zidovudine may increase the AUC of amprenavir; nelfinavir may increase the trough concentrations of amprenavir; cimetidine, lopinavir/ritonavir, or ritonavir may increase amprenavir concentrations [**Note:** Amprenavir dose of capsules should be decreased when used in combination with ritonavir capsules (see Usual Dosage)]; use of amprenavir oral solution with ritonavir oral solution is not recommended (see paragraph below)

Antacids or didanosine (buffered formulations) should be given at least 1 hour before or after amprenavir; vitamin E supplements should be avoided (amprenavir products contain high amounts of vitamin E); alcohol may interact with the high amount of propylene glycol in the oral solution and should be avoided; concomitant use of ritonavir oral solution with amprenavir oral solution is not recommended due to the large amounts of propylene glycol in amprenavir oral solution and ethanol in ritonavir oral solution [**Note:** Propylene glycol and ethanol (alcohol) may compete for the same metabolic pathway]

Food Interactions A high fat meal may decrease mean AUC by 14%

Stability Capsules and solution: Store at room temperature; do not refrigerate

Mechanism of Action A protease inhibitor which acts on an enzyme (protease) late in the HIV replication process after the virus has entered into the cell's nucleus; amprenavir binds to the protease activity site and inhibits the activity of the enzyme, thus preventing cleavage of viral polyprotein precursors (gag-pol protein precursors) into individual functional proteins found in infectious HIV; this results in the formation of immature, noninfectious viral particles

Pharmacokinetics

Distribution: V_d (apparent): Adults: 430 L

Protein binding: 90%; high affinity binding protein: alpha$_1$ acid glycoprotein

Metabolism: In the liver via cytochrome P450 CYP3A4 isoenzyme system; glucuronide conjugation of oxidized metabolites also occurs

Bioavailability: Absolute bioavailability not established; oral solution is 14% less bioavailable than capsules (do not interchange on a mg per mg basis)

Half-life: Adults: 7.1-10.6 hours

Time to peak serum concentration (single dose): 1-2 hours

Elimination: Minimal excretion of unchanged drug in urine (<3%) and feces; 75% of dose excreted as metabolites via biliary tract into feces and 14% excreted as metabolites in urine

Usual Dosage Oral (use in combination with other antiretroviral agents): **Note:** Due to differences in bioavailability, capsules and solution are **not** interchangeable on a mg per mg basis:

Neonates, Infants, and Children <4 years:

Capsules: Not approved for use

Solution: Contraindicated due to potential toxicity from propylene glycol

Children 4-12 years and Adolescents 13-16 years with a body weight <50 kg:

Capsules: 20 mg/kg twice daily or 15 mg/kg 3 times/day; maximum: 2400 mg/day

Solution: 22.5 mg/kg (1.5 mL/kg) twice daily or 17 mg/kg (1.1 mL/kg) 3 times/day; maximum: 2800 mg/day

Note: Concomitant therapy of amprenavir oral solution with ritonavir oral solution is not recommended (see Drug Interactions)

Adolescents 13-16 years with a body weight ≥50 kg and Adults:

Capsules: 1200 mg twice daily

Solution: 1400 mg twice daily

Adults: Concomitant therapy with ritonavir: Capsules: Amprenavir 1200 mg (with ritonavir 200 mg) once daily or amprenavir 600 mg (with ritonavir 100 mg) twice daily

Dosing adjustment in hepatic impairment: Adults:

Capsules:

Child-Pugh score 5-8: 450 mg twice daily

Child-Pugh score 9-12: 300 mg twice daily

Solution:

Child-Pugh score 5-8: 513 mg (34 mL) twice daily

Child-Pugh score 9-12: 342 mg (23 mL) twice daily

Administration May be administered without regard to meals; avoid administration with high fat meals; do not administer concurrently with antacids

Monitoring Parameters Signs and symptoms of rash or adverse effects; serum glucose, triglycerides, cholesterol, liver enzymes, CBC with differential, CD4 cell count, viral load; patients treated with amprenavir oral solution need to be monitored for adverse effects of propylene glycol, such as hyperosmolality, lactic acidosis, seizures, stupor, tachycardia, renal toxicity, and hemolysis

Patient Information Inform your physician if you have a sulfa allergy; amprenavir is not a cure for HIV; notify physician immediately if rash develops; some medicines should not be taken with amprenavir; report the use of other medications, nonprescription medications, and herbal or natural products to your physician and pharmacist; avoid the herbal medicine St John's wort and vitamin E supplements; take amprenavir every day as prescribed; do not change dose or discontinue without physician's advice; if a dose is missed, take it as soon as possible, then return to normal dosing schedule; if a dose is skipped, do not double the next dose; avoid alcohol and ritonavir oral solution if taking amprenavir oral solution

HIV medications may cause changes in body fat, including an increase in fat in the upper back and neck, breasts, and trunk; a loss of fat from the face, arms, and legs may also occur.

Additional Information To increase amprenavir solubility, propylene glycol has been added to the oral solution. **Note:** The recommended pediatric (twice daily) dose of the oral solution delivers 1650 mg/kg/day of propylene glycol; the acceptable amount of propylene glycol (when used as an excipient) is not known; treatment of overdose of the oral solution should include monitoring and management of propylene glycol adverse effects including acid-base abnormalities (see Monitoring Parameters); hemodialysis for removal of propylene glycol may be needed.

To increase amprenavir bioavailability, d-alpha tocopherol polyethylene glycol 1000 succinate (a form of vitamin E) has been added in significant concentrations to the product formulations; vitamin E content: 150 mg capsule: 109 international units; oral solution: 46 international units/mL. **Note:** The recommended pediatric dose of the oral solution delivers 138 international units/kg/day of vitamin E; this significantly exceeds the pediatric RDA of 10 international units. The recommended adult dose in capsule form delivers 1744 international units/day of vitamin E; this significantly exceeds the adult RDA of 30 international units. Long-term effects of high dose vitamin E are not well defined; high doses of vitamin E may worsen blood coagulation defects of vitamin K deficiency that are caused by malabsorption or from anticoagulant therapy.

Dosage Forms

Capsule: 50 mg, 150 mg

Solution, oral: 15 mg/mL (240 mL) [grape bubblegum peppermint flavor]

References

Adkins JC and Faulds D, "Amprenavir," *Drugs*, 1998, 55(6):837-42.

Center for Disease Control and Prevention, "Guidelines for Using Antiretroviral Agents Among HIV-Infected Adults and Adolescents. Recommendations of the Panel on Clinical Practices for Treatment of HIV," *MMWR*, 2002, 51(RR-7):1-55.

Collura JM and Kraus DM, "New Pediatric Antiretroviral Agents," *J Pediatr Health Care*, 2000, 14(4):183-90.

Panel on Clinical Practices for Treatment of HIV Infection, "Guidelines for the Use of Antiretroviral Agents in HIV-Infected Adults and Adolescents," February 4, 2002, http://www.aidsinfo.nih.gov.

Piscitelli SC, Burstein AH, Chaitt D, et al, "Indinavir Concentrations and St. John's Wort," *Lancet*, 2000, 355(9203):547-8.

Sadler BM, Hanson CD, Chittick GE, et al, "Safety and Pharmacokinetics of Amprenavir (141W94), a Human Immunodeficiency Virus (HIV) Type 1 Protease Inhibitor, Following Oral Administration of Single Doses to HIV-Infected Adults," *Antimicrob Agents Chemother*, 1999, 43(7):1686-92.

Working Group on Antiretroviral Therapy and Medical Management of HIV-Infected Children, "Guidelines for the Use of Antiretroviral Agents in Pediatric HIV Infection," December 14, 2001, http://www.aidsinfo.nih.gov.

Working Group on Antiretroviral Therapy and Medical Management of HIV-Infected Children, "Guidelines for the Use of Antiretroviral Agents in Pediatric HIV Infection. Hyperlink Supplement I: Pediatric Antiretroviral Drug Information," December 14, 2001, http://www.aidsinfo.nih.gov.

♦ **Amrinone** *see* Inamrinone *on page 601*

Amyl Nitrate, Sodium Nitrate, and Sodium Thiosulfate

(SYE a nide AN tee dote kit)

Therapeutic Category Antidote, Cyanide

Generic Available No

Use Treatment agents for cyanide poisoning

Pregnancy Risk Factor Sodium thiosulfate, sodium nitrite, and amyl nitrite: C

Contraindications Hypersensitivity to amyl nitrite, sodium nitrite, sodium thiosulfate, or any component

Warnings Excessive methemoglobin results when sodium nitrite dosage is exceeded; use only enough sodium nitrite to achieve a satisfactory clinical response; avoid methemoglobin levels >30%; patients with malignancy and G6PD deficiency have increased sensitivity to the methemoglobin-generating activities of sodium nitrite

Precautions When cyanide poisoning is related to smoke inhalation, if possible, the patient should be at pressure in a hyperbaric chamber before the kit is administered; (Continued)

Amyl Nitrate, Sodium Nitrate, and Sodium Thiosulfate
(Continued)

the methemoglobin initially produced by sodium nitrite injection may otherwise exacerbate concomitant carbon monoxide poisoning that has already severely diminished oxygen-carrying capacity in red cells

Adverse Reactions Reactions listed are those of sodium nitrite; see individual monographs for Amyl Nitrite *on page 111* and Sodium Thiosulfate *on page 1030*

Cardiovascular: Tachycardia, syncope, cyanosis, hypotension (associated with rapid infusion), flushing

Central nervous system: Dizziness, headache

Gastrointestinal: Nausea, vomiting

Miscellaneous: Methemoglobin formation

Drug Interactions Sodium nitrite antagonizes acetylcholine, epinephrine, and histamine effects; sodium nitrite potentiates hypotensive effects and/or anticholinergic effects of tricyclic antidepressants, antihistamines, and meperidine and related CNS depressants; also see Amyl Nitrite *on page 111*

Stability Sodium nitrite is stable at room temperature; do not mix with other medications; see individual monographs Amyl Nitrite *on page 111* and Sodium Thiosulfate *on page 1030*

Mechanism of Action Amyl nitrite and sodium nitrite promote the formation of methemoglobin which binds with cyanide to form cyanomethemoglobin (nontoxic); sodium thiosulfate, by providing an extra sulfur group to the enzyme rhodanese, increases the rate of detoxification of cyanide

Usual Dosage Administer in sequential order:

Amyl nitrite: Infants, Children, and Adults: Inhale vapors from 1 ampul continuously for 15-30 seconds, followed by a rest for 15 seconds (this interrupted schedule is important because continuous use of amyl nitrite may prevent adequate oxygenation); reapply until sodium nitrite can be administered

Sodium nitrite: I.V.:

Infants and Children ≤25 kg: See table

Variation of Sodium Nitrite and Sodium Thiosulfate Dose With Hemoglobin Concentration*

Hemoglobin (g/dL)	Initial Dose Sodium Nitrite (mg/kg)	Initial Dose Sodium Nitrite 3% (mL/kg)	Initial Dose Sodium Thiosulfate 25% (mL/kg)
7	5.8	0.19	0.95
8	6.6	0.22	1.10
9	7.5	0.25	1.25
10	8.3	0.27	1.35
11	9.1	0.30	1.50
12	10.0	0.33	1.65
13	10.8	0.36	1.80
14	11.6	0.39	1.95

*Adapted from Berlin DM Jr, "The Treatment of Cyanide Poisoning in Children," *Pediatrics*, 1970, 46:793.

Follow immediately with sodium thiosulfate

Children >25 kg, Adolescents, and Adults: 300 mg; follow immediately with sodium thiosulfate

Sodium thiosulfate: I.V.:

Infants and Children ≤25 kg: See table

Children >25 kg, Adolescents, and Adults: 12.5 g

Patients should be watched for at least 24-48 hours; if signs of poisoning reappear, injection of both sodium nitrite and sodium thiosulfate should be repeated, but each in $1/2$ of the original dose; even if the patient is asymptomatic, repeat $1/2$ doses of both sodium nitrite and sodium thiosulfate may be given for prophylactic purposes 2 hours after the first injection

Administration

Inhalation: **Amyl nitrite:** Crush ampul in cloth and hold under patient's nares for 15-30 seconds; remove for 15 seconds; repeat

Parenteral: I.V.:

Sodium nitrite: Administer undiluted at a rate of 2.5-5 mL/minute

Sodium thiosulfate: Administer undiluted over at least 10 minutes; rapid administration may cause hypotension

Monitoring Parameters Blood cyanide levels, methemoglobin levels, arterial blood gases, oxygen saturation, vital signs

Reference Range Symptoms associated with blood cyanide levels:
Flushing and tachycardia: 0.5-1 µg/mL
Obtundation: 1-2.5 µg/mL
Coma and respiratory depression: >2.5 µg/mL
Death: >3 µg/mL

Dosage Forms Kit (Cyanide Antidote Package):
Injection, solution: Sodium nitrite 300 mg/10 mL (2 ampuls); sodium thiosulfate 12.5 g/50 mL (2 ampuls)
Inhalant: Amyl nitrite 0.3 mL (12 crushable ampuls)

Amyl Nitrite (AM il NYE trite)

Synonyms Isoamyl Nitrite

Therapeutic Category Antidote, Cyanide; Vasodilator, Coronary

Generic Available Yes

Use Coronary vasodilator in angina pectoris; an adjunct in treatment of cyanide poisoning

Pregnancy Risk Factor C

Contraindications Hypersensitivity to nitrates or any component; severe anemia; recent head trauma or cerebral hemorrhage; glaucoma; hyperthyroidism; recent MI

Warnings Postural hypotension with episodes of dizziness, weakness, or syncope may occur after inhalation; may cause harm to the fetus if administered to a pregnant woman (may significantly decrease systemic blood pressure and blood flow)

Precautions Use with great caution in patients with increased intracranial pressure or low systolic blood pressure; tolerance to coronary vasodilator effects may occur (to minimize tolerance, use lowest effective initial dose and alternate with another coronary vasodilator); high doses of nitrates may cause methemoglobinemia (especially in patients with methemoglobin reductase deficiency or other metabolic abnormalities)

Adverse Reactions
Cardiovascular: Postural hypotension; cutaneous flushing of head, neck, and clavicular area; tachycardia; palpitations; vasodilation; syncope
Central nervous system: Headache, dizziness, restlessness
Dermatologic: Skin rash (contact dermatitis)
Gastrointestinal: Nausea, vomiting
Hematologic: Hemolytic anemia
Neuromuscular & skeletal: Weakness
Ocular: Elevated intraocular pressure
Miscellaneous: Tolerance to coronary vasodilator effects may occur

Drug Interactions Alcohol (may increase side effects and cause severe hypotension or cardiovascular collapse); medications that cause hypotension may increase the postural hypotensive effects of amyl nitrite

Stability Store in cool place, protect from light; flammable, avoid exposure to heat or flame

Mechanism of Action Vasodilator (vascular smooth muscle relaxant) which decreases afterload and improves myocardial blood supply via coronary artery vasodilation; antidote for cyanide poisoning: promotes formation of methemoglobin which combines with cyanide molecule to form cyanmethemoglobin (nontoxic)

Pharmacodynamics
Onset of action: Within 30 seconds
Duration: 3-5 minutes

Pharmacokinetics
Absorption: Inhalation: Readily absorbed through respiratory tract
Metabolism: In the liver to form inorganic nitrates (less potent)
Half-life:
Amyl nitrite: <1 hour
Methemoglobin: 1 hour
Elimination: Renal; ~33%

Usual Dosage Nasal inhalation:
Children and Adults: Cyanide poisoning: Inhale the vapor from a 0.3 mL crushed ampul every minute for 15-30 seconds until I.V. sodium nitrite infusion is available
Adults: Angina: 1-6 inhalations from 1 crushed ampul; may repeat in 3-5 minutes

Administration Give by nasal inhalation with patient in recumbent or seated position; crush ampul in woven covering between finger and hold under patient's nostrils

Monitoring Parameters Blood pressure; with treatment for cyanide poisoning: methemoglobin levels, arterial blood gas

Patient Information Remain seated or lying down during administration because of possible hypotension and dizziness; do not get up suddenly after use; avoid alcohol; if angina pain is not relieved after 2 doses, seek immediate medical attention
(Continued)

Amyl Nitrite *(Continued)*

Nursing Implications To facilitate recovery from symptoms of postural hypotension, place patient in head-down position; may also use measures such as deep breathing and movement of extremities

Additional Information Amyl nitrite has been used to treat penile erections after urological surgery (eg, circumcisions in adults) and has been used to change the intensity of heart murmurs to aid in their diagnosis

Dosage Forms Vapor for nasal inhalation [crushable glass perles]: 0.3 mL (ampuls)

♦ **Anaprox®** *see* Naproxen *on page 796*

♦ **Anaprox® DS** *see* Naproxen *on page 796*

♦ **Anaspaz®** *see* Hyoscyamine *on page 585*

♦ **Anbesol® [OTC]** *see* Benzocaine *on page 163*

♦ **Anbesol® Baby [OTC]** *see* Benzocaine *on page 163*

♦ **Anbesol® Maximum Strength [OTC]** *see* Benzocaine *on page 163*

♦ **Ancef®** *see* Cefazolin *on page 225*

♦ **Ancobon®** *see* Flucytosine *on page 491*

♦ **Andehist NR Drops** *see* Carbinoxamine and Pseudoephedrine *on page 214*

♦ **Andehist NR Syrup** *see* Brompheniramine and Pseudoephedrine *on page 182*

♦ **Andriol® (Can)** *see* Testosterone *on page 1070*

♦ **Androderm®** *see* Testosterone *on page 1070*

♦ **AndroGel®** *see* Testosterone *on page 1070*

♦ **Andropository (Can)** *see* Testosterone *on page 1070*

♦ **Anectine® [DSC]** *see* Succinylcholine *on page 1044*

♦ **Anestacon®** *see* Lidocaine *on page 671*

♦ **Aneurine** *see* Thiamine *on page 1081*

♦ **Anexate® (Can)** *see* Flumazenil *on page 495*

♦ **Anexsia®** *see* Hydrocodone and Acetaminophen *on page 571*

♦ **Anhydrous Glucose** *see* Dextrose *on page 366*

♦ **Ansaid®** *see* Flurbiprofen *on page 510*

♦ **Ansamycin** *see* Rifabutin *on page 983*

Antacid Preparations (ant AS id prep a RAE shuns)

Related Information

Calcium Supplements *on page 200*

Carbohydrate and Alcohol Content of Liquid Medications for Use in Patients Receiving Ketogenic Diets *on page 1431*

Magnesium Supplements *on page 701*

Sodium Bicarbonate *on page 1025*

U.S. Brand Names AlternaGel® [OTC]; Gaviscon® [OTC]; Maalox® Fast Release [OTC]; Maalox® Max [OTC]; Maalox® Quick Dissolve [OTC]; Maalox® TC [OTC]; Mylanta® CalciTabs [OTC]; Mylanta® Extra Strength [OTC]; Mylanta® Supreme [OTC]; Riopan® Plus [OTC]; Titralac® [OTC]; Tums® [OTC]

Available Salts Aluminum Carbonate; Aluminum Carbonate Gel; Aluminum Hydroxide; Aluminum Hydroxide and Magnesium Hydroxide; Aluminum Hydroxide and Magnesium Trisilicate; Aluminum Hydroxide Gel; Aluminum Hydroxide, Magnesium Hydroxide, and Simethicone; Hydroxide and Magnesium Carbonate

Therapeutic Category Antacid; Gastrointestinal Agent, Gastric or Duodenal Ulcer Treatment

Generic Available Yes

Use Adjunct for the relief of peptic ulcer pain and to promote healing of peptic ulcers; relief of stomach upset associated with hyperacidity; prevention of stress ulcer bleeding; treatment of duodenal ulcer and gastroesophageal reflux disease. Aluminum hydroxide is also used to reduce phosphate absorption in hyperphosphatemia; calcium carbonate is used to treat calcium deficiency and to bind phosphate; magnesium oxide is used to treat hypomagnesemia.

Contraindications Magnesium-containing antacids should not be used in patients with a creatinine clearance <30 mL/minute

Warnings Use aluminum-containing antacids with caution in patients with: Decreased bowel motility and dehydration, gastric outlet obstruction, renal failure, and in patients who have an upper GI hemorrhage; use magnesium-containing products with caution in patients with renal impairment; use sodium-containing antacids with caution in patients on low-sodium diets, and in patients with CHF, edema, renal failure, or hepatic failure; some tablets contain tartrazine which may cause allergic reactions in susceptible individuals

Precautions Maalox® Quick Dissolve tablets contain aspartame which is metabolized to phenylalanine and must be avoided or used with caution in patients with phenylketonuria.

Adverse Reactions

Aluminum-containing antacids:

Central nervous system: Dementia, encephalopathy, malaise, seizures, confusion, coma

Endocrine & metabolic: Hypophosphatemia, hyperaluminemia, osteoporosis

Gastrointestinal: Constipation, anorexia

Genitourinary: Urinary calculi

Neuromuscular & skeletal: Muscle weakness, osteomalacia

Calcium-containing antacids:

Endocrine & metabolic: Milk-alkali syndrome (hypercalcemia, metabolic alkalosis), hypophosphatemia

Gastrointestinal: Constipation, flatulence, nausea

Magnesium-containing antacids:

Endocrine & metabolic: Hypermagnesemia, fluid and electrolyte imbalance

Gastrointestinal: Laxative effects, diarrhea

Sodium-containing antacids:

Cardiovascular: Fluid retention

Endocrine & metabolic: Metabolic alkalosis, sodium overload

Gastrointestinal: Flatulence

Drug Interactions Aluminum-, calcium-, or magnesium-containing antacids (decrease tetracycline and quinolone absorption); antacids decrease absorption of delavirdine, itraconazole, ketoconazole, iron, digoxin, phenytoin, indomethacin, chlorpromazine; increased absorption of buffered or enteric-coated aspirin; aluminum hydroxide (decreased absorption of isoniazid); sucralfate antacids (may impair binding of sucralfate to ulcerated mucosa)

Food Interactions Aluminum-containing antacids (except aluminum phosphate) form insoluble salts with dietary phosphorus decreasing phosphorus absorption

Stability Avoid freezing aluminum hydroxide and magnesium hydroxide

Mechanism of Action Neutralizes gastric acidity increasing gastric pH; inhibits proteolytic activity of pepsin when gastric pH is increased >4; binds bile salts

Pharmacodynamics

Duration: Dependent on gastric emptying time

Fasting state: 20-60 minutes

1 hour after meals: May be up to 3 hours

Usual Dosage Oral: Aluminum/magnesium hydroxide combination (for extra strength or concentrated suspension, use half the volume of the stated dose):

Peptic ulcer disease:

Infants: 1-2 mL/kg/dose 1-3 hours after meals and at bedtime

Children: 5-15 mL/dose every 3-6 hours or 1-3 hours after meals and at bedtime

Adults: 15-45 mL every 3-6 hours or 1-3 hours after meals and at bedtime

Prophylaxis against GI bleeding:

Neonates: 1 mL/kg every 4 hours as needed

Infants: 2-5 mL/dose every 1-2 hours, titrate to gastric pH >3.5

Children: 5-15 mL/dose every 1-2 hours, titrate to gastric pH >3.5

Adults: 30-60 mL every 1-2 hours, titrate to gastric pH >3.5

Hyperphosphatemia:

Children: Use $Al(OH)_3$ or aluminum carbonate gel product only: 50-150 mg/kg/day (as aluminum hydroxide gel) divided every 4-6 hours; titrate to normal serum phosphorus level

Adults: 30-40 mL of $Al(OH)_3$ 3-4 times/day between meals and at bedtime

Administration Oral: Thoroughly chew tablets before swallowing; shake suspensions well before use; administer prior to meals when stomach acidity is highest

Monitoring Parameters GI complaints, stool frequency; serum phosphate concentrations in patients on hemodialysis receiving chronic aluminum-containing antacid therapy; serum calcium, phosphate, and bicarbonate in patients receiving large doses of calcium carbonate; serum electrolytes in patients with renal impairment receiving magnesium-containing antacids

Patient Information Antacids may impair or increase absorption of many drugs, do not take oral medications within 1-2 hours of an antacid dose unless specifically instructed to do so

Additional Information Antacid products containing alginic acid form a viscous solution that serves as a protective barrier for the esophagus against reflux of gastric contents.

Dosage Forms See tables on pages 114 and 115.

Gelcap (Mylanta®): Calcium carbonate 550 mg and magnesium hydroxide 125 mg

(Continued)

Antacid Preparations *(Continued)*

Antacid Preparations

Generic/Therapeutic Groupings Brand Names	Al(OH)₃*	Mg(OH)₂*	CaCO₃*	Other Content	Sodium† (mEq)	ANC‡ (mEq)	How Supplied
Aluminum hydroxide gel	320			Saccharin, sorbitol	<0.1	10	Suspension
	300				0.08	9	Tablet
	600				0.13	16	Tablet
AlternaGel®	600			Saccharin, sorbitol	<0.13	16	Suspension
Aluminum/magnesium hydroxide							
Maalox® Fast Release liquid	500	450		Simethicone 40 mg, saccharin, sorbitol (sugar-free)	0.05	29	Suspension
Mylanta®	200	200		Simethicone 20 mg	0.03	12.7	Suspension
Mylanta® Extra Strength	400	400		Simethicone 40 mg	0.05	25.4	Suspension
Riopan® Plus				Magaldrate 540 mg, simethicone 40 mg	0.013	15	Suspension

Suspension:
AlternaGel®: Aluminum hydroxide 600 mg/5 mL (360 mL)
Gaviscon®: Aluminum hydroxide 31.7 mg/5 mL and magnesium carbonate 119.3 mg/5 mL (360 mL)
Maalox® Fast Release Liquid: Aluminum hydroxide 500 mg/5 mL, magnesium hydroxide 450 mg/5 mL, simethicone 40 mg/5 mL (355 mL)
Maalox® Max: Aluminum hydroxide 400 mg/5 mL, magnesium hydroxide 400 mg/5 mL and simethicone 40 mg/5 mL (355 mL)
Maalox® TC: Aluminum hydroxide 600 mg/5 mL and magnesium hydroxide 300 mg/5 mL (355 mL)
Mylanta®: Aluminum hydroxide 200 mg/5 mL, magnesium hydroxide 200 mg/5 mL, simethicone 20 mg/5 mL (150 mL, 360 mL, 720 mL) [original, cherry, mint, and lemon flavors]
Mylanta® Extra Strength: Aluminum hydroxide 400 mg/5 mL, magnesium hydroxide 400 mg/5 mL and simethicone 40 mg/5 mL (150 mL, 360 mL, 720 mL) [original, cherry, and mint flavors]

Antacid Preparations (continued)

Generic/Therapeutic Groupings Brand Names	Al(OH)$_3$*	Mg(OH)$_2$*	CaCO$_3$*	Other Content	Sodium† (mEq)	ANC‡ (mEq)	How Supplied
Aluminum hydroxide/magnesium carbonate							
Gaviscon®	31.7			Magnesium carbonate 119.3 mg, sodium alginate, EDTA, saccharin, sorbitol, parabens	0.57	4	Suspension
Aluminum hydroxide/magnesium trisilicate							
Gaviscon®	80			Magnesium trisilicate 20 mg, alginic acid, sodium bicarbonate	0.8	0.5	Tablet/chewable
Calcium carbonate tablets							
Tums®			500		≤0.087	10	Tablet/chewable
Tums E-X® Extra Strength			750		≤0.087		Tablet/chewable
Tums® Ultra			1000	Sodium ≤4 mg			Tablet/chewable
Calcium carbonate suspension			1250		<0.217		Suspension
Titralac® Plus			420	Simethicone 21 mg	≤0.001	7.5	Tablet

*Liquids in mg per 5 mL; capsules and tablets in mg.
†mEq of sodium per tablet, capsule, or 5 mL of liquid (23 mg = 1 mEq sodium)
‡ANC = Acid neutralizing capacity per tablet, capsule, or 5 mL of liquid.

Mylanta® Supreme: Calcium carbonate 400 mg/5 mL and magnesium hydroxide 135 mg/5 mL (30 mL, 360 mL, 720 mL) [cherry and mint flavors]
Riopan® Plus: Magaldrate 540 mg/5 mL and simethicone 40 mg/5 mL (360 mL)
Riopan® Plus Double Strength: Magaldrate 1080 mg/5 mL and simethicone 40 mg/5 mL (360 mL)

Tablet, chewable:
Gaviscon®: Aluminum hydroxide 80 mg and magnesium trisilicate 20 mg
Gaviscon® Extra Strength: Aluminum hydroxide 160 mg and magnesium carbonate 105 mg
Maalox® Quick Dissolve: Calcium carbonate 600 mg [contains 0.5 mg phenylalanine (as aspartame); lemon, wildberry, wintergreen, and assorted flavors]
Mylanta® CalciTabs Extra Strength: Calcium carbonate 750 mg [contains tartrazine]
Mylanta® CalciTabs Ultra: Calcium carbonate 1000 mg [contains tartrazine]
Mylanta® Children's Chewable: Calcium carbonate 400 mg
Titralac®: Calcium carbonate 420 mg
Titralac® Extra Strength: Calcium carbonate 750 mg
Titralac® Plus: Calcium carbonate 420 mg and simethicone 21 mg
Tums®: Calcium carbonate 500 mg
(Continued)

115

Antacid Preparations *(Continued)*

Tums® E-X Extra Strength: Calcium carbonate 750 mg
Tums® Ultra: Calcium carbonate 1000 mg

References

Nord KS, "Peptic Ulcer Disease in the Pediatric Population," *Pediatr Clin North Am*, 1988, 35(1):117-140.

♦ **Antibiotic® Ear** *see* Neomycin, (Bacitracin) Polymyxin B, and Hydrocortisone *on page 802*
♦ **Antidigoxin Fab Fragments** *see* Digoxin Immune Fab *on page 383*
♦ **Antidiuretic Hormone** *see* Vasopressin *on page 1136*
♦ **Antiepileptic Drugs** *see page 1374*

Antihemophilic Factor (Human)

(an tee hee moe FIL ik FAK tor HYU man)

U.S. Brand Names Alphanate®; Hemofil® M; Humate-P®; Koate®-DVI; Monarc® M; Monoclate-P®
Synonyms AHF; AHG; Factor VIII
Therapeutic Category Antihemophilic Agent; Blood Product Derivative
Generic Available Yes

Antihemophilic Factor (Human) [Factor VIII (Human)] Products

Note: Source of all products is pooled human plasma

Product	Preparation and Purification Methods	Viral Inactivation	Stabilizers and Excipients
Alphanate®	• Cryoprecipitation • Fractional solubilization • Affinity chromatography (heparin/argose)	• Organic solvent/detergent treatment • Heat treatment (dry; 80°C x 72 hours)	• Albumin (human)* • Calcium • Glycine • Heparin • Histidine • Imidazole • Arginine • Polyethylene glycol • Polysorbate 80 • Sodium • Tri-n-butyl phosphate
Hemofil® M	• Method M process • Immunoaffinity chromatography using murine monoclonal antibody • Ion exchange chromatography	• Organic solvent/detergent treatment	• Albumin (human)* • Polyethylene glycol* • Histidine* • Glycine* • Mouse protein • Tri-n-butyl phosphate • Octoxynol 9
Humate-P®†	• Purified from cold insoluble fraction of fresh-frozen plasma	• Heat treatment in aqueous solution (pasteurization; 60°C x 10 hours)	• Albumin (human) • Glycine • Sodium citrate • Sodium chloride • Other proteins • von Willebrand factor (clinically significant amounts)
Koate®-DVI	• Purified from cold insoluble fraction of fresh-frozen plasma • Gel permeation chromatography	• Organic solvent/detergent treatment • Heat treatment (dry; in lyophilized form in final container; 80°C x 72 hours)	• Albumin (human) • Polyethylene glycol • Glycine • Polysorbate 80 • Tri-n-butyl phosphate • Calcium • Aluminum • Histidine
Monarc® M	• Method M process • Immunoaffinity chromatography using murine monoclonal antibody • Ion exchange chromatography	• Organic solvent/detergent treatment	• Albumin (human)* • Polyethylene glycol* • Histidine* • Glycine* • Mouse protein • Tri-n-butyl phosphate • Octoxynol 9
Monoclate-P®	• Immunoaffinity chromatography using murine monoclonal antibody	• Heat treatment in aqueous solution (pasteurization; 60°C x 10 hours)	• Albumin (human)* • Sodium (300-450 millimoles/L) • Calcium chloride • Mannitol • Histidine • Hydrochloric acid and/or sodium hydroxide (pH adjustment) • Mouse protein

*Listed as a stabilizer in the product's package insert
†Antihemophilic factor/von Willebrand factor complex (human)

Use Prevention and control of hemorrhagic episodes in patients with hemophilia A in whom a deficiency of activity in factor VIII has been demonstrated; perioperative management of patients with hemophilia A; can provide therapeutic effects in patients with acquired factor VIII inhibitors <10 Bethesda units/mL

Humate-P®: Also indicated for the control of hemorrhagic episodes in patients with severe von Willebrand disease, and in mild and moderate von Willebrand disease where desmopressin is suspected or known to be inadequate

Pregnancy Risk Factor C

Contraindications

All products: Hypersensitivity to any component (see Warnings and previous table)
Antihemophilic factor, human (Method M, monoclonal purified); Hemofil® M; Monarc® M; Monoclate-P®: Hypersensitivity to mouse protein

Warnings Hemofil® M and Monarc® M contain natural rubber latex (in certain components of the product packaging) which may cause allergic reactions in susceptible individuals; avoid use in patients with allergy to latex

Precautions Human antihemophilic factor is prepared from pooled plasma and even with heat treated or other viral attenuated processes, the risk of viral transmission (ie, viral hepatitis, HIV, parvovirus B19, and theoretically, Creutzfeldt-Jacob disease agent) is not totally eradicated. Hepatitis B vaccination is recommended for all patients receiving human antihemophilic factor and hepatitis A vaccination is recommended for seronegative patients. [**Note:** The use of recombinant antihemophilic factor products (such as Bioclate™, Helixate®, Helixate® FS, Kogenate®, Kogenate® FS, Recombinate™, or ReFacto®) substantially decreases the risk of viral transmission because these products are biosynthetically prepared.] Progressive anemia and hemolysis may occur in individuals with blood groups A, B, and AB who receive large or frequent doses of human antihemophilic factor due to trace amounts of blood group A and B isohemagglutinins (see Monitoring Parameters).

Formation of factor VIII inhibitors (neutralizing antibodies to AHF human) may occur (see Adverse Reactions); monitor patients appropriately (see Monitoring Parameters). Allergic-type hypersensitivity reactions are possible; discontinue therapy immediately if urticaria, hives, hypotension, tightness of the chest, wheezing, dyspnea, faintness, or anaphylaxis develop. Products vary by preparation method (see table); final formulations contain human albumin

Adverse Reactions

Cardiovascular: Flushing, tachycardia, fever, chills, chest tightness

Central nervous system: Headache, lethargy, somnolence, dizziness, nervousness

Dermatologic: Urticaria, rash, pruritus

Gastrointestinal: Nausea, vomiting, GI upset; unusual taste (one patient)

Local: Injection site reactions, stinging; phlebitis

Neuromuscular & skeletal: Paresthesia

Ocular: Blurred vision

Miscellaneous: Allergic vasomotor reactions, edema, development of inhibitor antibodies (3% to 52%); inhibitor antibodies are IgG immunoglobulins that neutralize the activity of factor VIII; an increase of inhibitor antibody concentration is seen at 2-7 days, with peak concentrations at 1-3 weeks after therapy. Children <5 years of age are greatest risk; higher doses of AHF may be needed if antibody is present; if antibody concentration is >10 Bethesda units/mL, patients may not respond to larger doses and alternative treatment modalities may be needed (see Additional Information).

Stability

Storage: Store unopened vials under refrigeration 2°C to 8°C (36°F to 46°F); avoid freezing (to prevent damage to diluent vial)

Alphanate®: May also be stored at room temperature (≤30°C or 86°F) for up to 2 months

Hemofil® M: May also be stored at room temperature (≤30°C or 86°F)

Humate-P®, Monoclate-P®: May also be stored at room temperature (≤30°C or 86°F) for up to 6 months

Koate®-DVI: May also be stored at room temperature (≤25°C or 77°F) for up to 6 months

Monarc® M: May also be stored at room temperature (≤30°C or 86°F) for up to 12 months

Reconstitution: If refrigerated, the dried concentrate and diluent should be warmed to room temperature before reconstitution; see individual product labeling for specific reconstitution guidelines; gently agitate or rotate vial after adding diluent, do not shake vigorously (**Note:** For Koate®-DVI: Swirl vigorously without creating excessive foaming); use filter needle provided by manufacturer to draw product into syringe; use one filter needle per vial; do **not** refrigerate after reconstitution (precipitation may occur); administer within 3 hours after reconstitution; **Note:** Use plastic syringes, since AHF may stick to the surface of glass syringes

Mechanism of Action Factor VIII is a protein in normal plasma which is necessary for clot formation and maintenance of hemostasis; it activates factor X in conjunction with activated factor IX; activated factor X converts prothrombin to thrombin, which converts fibrinogen to fibrin and with factor XIII forms a stable clot

(Continued)

Antihemophilic Factor (Human) *(Continued)*

Pharmacodynamics Maximum effect: 1-2 hours

Pharmacokinetics

Distribution: Does not readily cross the placenta

Half-life: 4-24 hours; mean = 12 hours (biphasic)

Usual Dosage Children and Adults: I.V.: Individualize dosage based on coagulation studies performed prior to and during treatment at regular intervals:

Hemophilia A: For every 1 international unit per kg body weight of AHF (human) administered, factor VIII level should increase by 2%; calculated dosage should be adjusted to the actual vial size

Formula to calculate dosage required, based on desired increase in factor VIII (% of normal) **(Note:** This formula assumes that the patient's baseline AHF level is <1%): International units required = Body weight (kg) x 0.5 x desired increase in factor VIII (international units/dL or % of normal)

Hospitalized patients: 20-50 units/kg/dose; may be higher for special circumstances. Dose can be given every 12-24 hours and more frequently in special circumstances.

Hemophilia A with high titer of inhibitor antibody: 50-75 units/kg/hour has been given

General dosing guidelines (consult individual product labeling for specific dosage recommendations):

Minor Hemorrhage (required peak postinfusion AHF level: 20% to 40%): 10-20 international units/kg; repeat every 12-24 hours for 1-3 days until bleeding is resolved or healing achieved; mild superficial or early hemorrhages may respond to a single dose

Moderate hemorrhage (required peak postinfusion AHF level: 30% to 60%): 15-30 international units/kg; repeat every 12-24 hours for ≥3 days until pain and disability are resolved

Alternatively (to achieve peak postinfusion AHF level: 50%) Initial: 25 international units/kg; maintenance: 10-15 international units/kg every 8-12 hours

Severe/life-threatening hemorrhage (required peak postinfusion AHF level: 60% to 100%): 30-50 international units/kg; repeat every 8-24 hours until threat is resolved

Alternatively (to achieve peak postinfusion AHF level: 80% to 100%): 40-50 international units/kg; maintenance: 20-25 international units/kg every 8-12 hours

Minor surgery (required peak postinfusion AHF level: Range 30% to 80%): 15-40 international units/kg; dose is highly dependent upon procedure and specific product recommendations; for some procedures, a single dose plus oral antifibrinolytic therapy within 1 hour is sufficient; in other procedures, may repeat dose every 12-24 hours as needed

Major surgery (required peak pre- and postsurgery AHF level: 80% to 100%): 40-50 international units/kg; repeat every 8-24 hours depending on state of healing

Prophylaxis: May also be given on a regular schedule to prevent bleeding

von Willebrand disease (Humate-P®):

For every 1 international unit per kg body weight of factor VIII administered, von Willebrand factor: ristocetin cofactor (vWF:RCof) level should increase by approximately 3.5-4 international units/dL

Type 1, mild (if desmopressin is not appropriate): Major hemorrhage:

Loading dose: 40-60 international units/kg

Maintenance dose: 40-50 international units/kg every 8-12 hours for 3 days, keeping vWF:RCof nadir >50%; follow with 40-50 international units/kg daily for up to 7 days

Type 1, moderate or severe:

Minor hemorrhage: 40-50 international units/kg for 1-2 doses

Major hemorrhage:

Loading dose: 50-75 international units/kg

Maintenance dose: 40-60 international units/kg every 8-12 hours for 3 days keeping vWF:RCof nadir >50%; follow with 40-60 international units/kg daily for up to 7 days

Types 2 (all variants) and 3:

Minor hemorrhage: 40-50 international units/kg for 1-2 doses

Major hemorrhage:

Loading dose: 60-80 international units/kg

Maintenance dose: 40-60 international units/kg every 8-12 hours for 3 days, keeping vWF:RCof nadir >50%; follow with 40-60 international units/kg daily for up to 7 days

Administration Parenteral: I.V. administration only; see Stability for reconstitution and dosage preparation; administer through a separate line, do not mix with drugs or other I.V. fluids.

Maximum rate of administration is product dependent:

Alphanate®, Hemofil M, Monarc® M: 10 mL/minute

Humate-P®: 4 mL/minute

Monoclate-P®: 2 mL/minute

Koate®-DVI: Total dose may be given over 5-10 minutes; adjust administration rate based on patient response

Monitoring Parameters Bleeding; heart rate and blood pressure (before and during I.V. administration); AHF levels prior to and during treatment; monitor for development of inhibitor antibodies by clinical observation (eg, inadequate control of bleeding with adequate doses) and laboratory tests (eg, inhibitor level, Bethesda assay); in patients with blood groups A, B, or AB who receive large or frequent doses, monitor Hct, direct Coombs' test, and signs of intravascular hemolysis

Reference Range

Plasma antihemophilic factor level:

Normal range: 50% to 150%

Level to prevent spontaneous hemorrhage: 5%

Required peak postinfusion AHF activity in blood (as % of normal or units/dL plasma):

Early hemarthrosis, muscle bleed, or oral bleed: 20% to 40%

More extensive hemarthrosis, muscle bleed, or hematoma: 30% to 60%

Life-threatening bleeds (such as head injury, throat bleed, severe abdominal pain): 80% to 100%

Minor surgery, including tooth extraction: 60% to 80%

Major surgery: 80% to 100% (pre- and postoperative)

Patient Information This medication can only be given intravenously. Stop taking antihemophilic factor human and notify physician immediately if any of the following signs or symptoms of an allergic (hypersensitivity) reaction occur: Itching, hives, low blood pressure, tightness in chest, wheezing, or anaphylaxis. Wear identification indicating that you have a hemophilic condition.

Nursing Implications Reduce rate of administration or temporarily discontinue if patient experiences tachycardia or any other adverse reaction; hypersensitivity reactions (eg, hives, chest tightness, itching, wheezing, dyspnea, faintness, hypotension, anaphylaxis) may occur (see Precautions)

Additional Information One international unit of AHF is equal to the factor VIII activity present in 1 mL of normal human plasma. If bleeding is not controlled with adequate dose, test for the presence of factor VIII inhibitor; larger doses of AHF may be therapeutic with inhibitor titers <10 Bethesda units/mL; it may not be possible or practical to control bleeding if inhibitor titers >10 Bethesda units/mL (due to the very large AHF doses required); other treatments [eg, antihemophilic factor (porcine), factor IX complex concentrates, recombinant factor VIIa, or anti-inhibitor coagulant complex] may be needed in patients with inhibitor titers >10 Bethesda units/mL.

Dosage Forms Injection, powder for reconstitution, human [single-dose vial]: Exact potency labeled on each vial in international units

References

Liesner RJ, "Prophylaxis in Haemophilic Children," *Blood Coagul Fibrinolysis*, 1997, 8(Suppl 1):S7-10.

Scharrer I, Bray GL, and Neutzling O, "Incidence of Inhibitors in Haemophilia A Patients--A Review of Recent Studies of Recombinant and Plasma-Derived Factor VIII Concentrates," *Haemophilia*, 1999, 5(3):145-54.

Shord SS and Lindley CM, "Coagulation Products and Their Uses," *Am J Health Syst Pharm*, 2000, 57(15):1403-20.

Antihemophilic Factor (Recombinant)

(an tee hee moe FIL ik FAK tor ree KOM be nant)

U.S. Brand Names Helixate® FS; Kogenate® FS; Recombinate™; ReFacto®

Synonyms AHF (Recombinant); Factor VIII (Recombinant); rAHF

Therapeutic Category Antihemophilic Agent

Generic Available No

Use Prevention and control of hemorrhagic episodes in patients with hemophilia A in whom a deficiency of activity in factor VIII has been demonstrated; perioperative management of patients with hemophilia A; can provide therapeutic effects in patients with acquired factor VIII inhibitors <10 Bethesda units/mL; **Note:** AHF recombinant is not indicated for the treatment of von Willebrand disease

Pregnancy Risk Factor C

Contraindications

All products: Hypersensitivity to any component (see Warnings and table on next page)

Helixate® FS; Kogenate® FS: Hypersensitivity to mouse or hamster protein

Recombinate™; ReFacto®: Hypersensitivity to mouse, hamster, or bovine protein

(Continued)

Antihemophilic Factor (Recombinant) *(Continued)*

Antihemophilic Factor (Recombinant) [Factor VIII (Recombinant)] Products

Product	Synthesis	Purification Methods	Stabilizers and Excipients
Helixate® FS	• Recombinant DNA technology • Baby Hamster Kidney (BHK) cells • Human Plasma Protein Solution (HPPS) and recombinant insulin in cell culture medium	• Solvent/detergent virus inactivation • Ion exchange chromatography • Monoclonal antibody immunoaffinity chromatography • Other chromatographic steps	• Sucrose* • Glycine* • Histidine* • Calcium chloride • Sodium • Chloride • Polysorbate-80 • Imidazole • Tri-n-butyl-phosphate • Copper
Kogenate® FS	• Recombinant DNA technology • Baby Hamster Kidney (BHK) cells • Human Plasma Protein Solution (HPPS) and recombinant insulin in cell culture medium	• Solvent/detergent virus inactivation • Ion exchange chromatography • Monoclonal antibody immunoaffinity chromatography • Other chromatographic steps	• Sucrose* • Glycine* • Histidine* • Calcium chloride • Sodium • Chloride • Polysorbate-80 • Imidazole • Tri-n-butyl phosphate • Copper
Recombinate™	• Recombinant DNA technology • Chinese Hamster Ovary (CHO) cell line	• Column chromatography • Monoclonal antibody immunoaffinity chromatography	• Albumin (human)* • Calcium* • Polyethylene glycol* • Sodium* • Histidine* • Polysorbate-80* • von Willebrand factor* (insignificant amounts)
ReFacto®	• Recombinant DNA technology • Chinese Hamster Ovary (CHO) cell line • Human Serum Albumin and recombinant insulin in cell culture medium	• Chromatography	• Sodium chloride • Sucrose • L-histadine • Calcium chloride • Polysorbate-80

*Listed as a stabilizer in the product's package insert

Warnings Recombinate™ contains natural rubber latex (in certain components of the product packaging) which may cause allergic reactions in susceptible individuals; avoid use in patients with allergy to latex.

Precautions Formation of factor VIII inhibitors (neutralizing antibodies to AHF recombinant) may occur; antibody formation may occur at any time, but is more common in young children with severe hemophilia during the first years of therapy, or in patients at any age who received little prior therapy with factor VIII; monitor patients appropriately (see Monitoring Parameters). Allergic type hypersensitivity reactions are theoretically possible; discontinue therapy immediately if urticaria, hives, hypotension, tightness of the chest, wheezing or anaphylaxis develop. Products vary by preparation method (see table). Recombinate™ formulation is stabilized using human albumin; Helixate® FS, Kogenate® FS, and ReFacto® formulations are stabilized using sucrose

Adverse Reactions

Cardiovascular: Flushing, vasodilation, fever, chills, chest discomfort, hypotension (slight), mildly elevated blood pressure, angina pectoris, tachycardia

Central nervous system: Mild fatigue, dizziness, headache, lethargy, asthenia, somnolence, depersonalization

Dermatologic: Urticaria, rash, pruritus

Gastrointestinal: Nausea, vomiting, diarrhea, sore throat, unusual taste, constipation, anorexia

Hepatic: Elevated aminotransferase, elevated bilirubin

Local: Injection site reactions (burning, pruritus, erythema)

Neuromuscular & skeletal: Muscle weakness

Ocular: Abnormal vision

Respiratory: Epistaxis, rhinitis, dyspnea, cough

Miscellaneous: Cold feet, adenopathy, allergic reactions, anaphylaxis, permanent venous catheter access complications, diaphoresis, elevated CPK, development of inhibitor antibodies; inhibitor antibodies are IgG immunoglobulins that neutralize the activity of factor VIII; higher doses of AHF recombinant may be needed if antibody is present; if antibody concentration is >10 Bethesda units/mL, patients may not respond to larger doses and alternative treatment modalities may be needed (see Additional Information)

Stability

Storage: Store unopened vials under refrigeration 2°C to 8°C (36°F to 46°F); avoid freezing

Helixate® FS, Kogenate® FS: May also be stored at room temperature (≤25°C or 77°F) for up to 2 months. Avoid extreme exposure to light during storage (store drug in carton before use)

Recombinate™: May also be stored at room temperature (≤30°C or 86°F)

ReFacto®: May also be stored at room temperature (≤25°C or 77°F) for up to 3 months; avoid prolonged exposure to light during storage

Reconstitution: If refrigerated, the dried concentrate and diluent should be warmed to room temperature before reconstitution; see individual product labeling for specific reconstitution guidelines; gently agitate or rotate vial after adding diluent, do not shake vigorously; use filter needle provided by manufacturer to draw product into syringe; do **not** refrigerate after reconstitution; administer within 3 hours after reconstitution; **Note:** Use plastic syringes, since rAHF may stick to the surface of glass syringes

Mechanism of Action Antihemophilic factor (recombinant) has the same biological activity as AHF (factor VIII) derived from human plasma; factor VIII is a protein in normal plasma which is necessary for clot formation and maintenance of hemostasis; factor VIII activates factor X in conjunction with activated factor IX; activated factor X converts prothrombin to thrombin, which converts fibrinogen to fibrin, and with factor XIII forms a stable clot

Pharmacokinetics Half-life: Mean: 13-16 hours

Usual Dosage Neonates, Infants, Children, and Adults: I.V.: Individualize dosage based on coagulation studies performed prior to treatment and at regular intervals during treatment; for every 1 international unit per kg body weight of rAHF administered, factor VIII level should increase by 2%; calculated dosage should be adjusted to the actual vial size

Formula to calculate dosage required, based on desired increase in factor VIII (% of normal) (**Note:** This formula assumes that the patient's baseline AHF level is <1%): International units required = body weight (kg) x 0.5 x desired increase in factor VIII (international units/dL or % of normal)

General dosing guidelines (consult individual product labeling for specific dosage recommendations):

Minor hemorrhage (required peak postinfusion AHF level: 20% to 40%): 10-20 international units/kg; repeat every 12-24 hours for 1-3 days until bleeding is resolved or healing achieved; mild, superficial, or early hemorrhages may respond to a single dose

Moderate hemorrhage (required peak post-infusion AHF level: 30% to 60%): 15-30 international units/kg, repeat every 12-24 hours for 3-4 days until pain and disability are resolved

Severe/life-threatening hemorrhage:

Helixate® FS, Kogenate® FS (required peak post-infusion AHF level: 80% to 100%): Initial: 40-50 international units/kg; maintenance: 20-25 international units/kg every 8-12 hours

Recombinate™, ReFacto® (required peak post-infusion AHF level: 60% to 100%): 30-50 international units/kg; repeat every 8-24 hours until threat is resolved

Minor surgery (required peak post-infusion AHF level: range: 30% to 80%): 15-40 international units/kg; dose is highly dependent upon procedure and specific product recommendations; for some procedures, a single dose plus oral antifibrinolytic therapy within 1 hour is sufficient; in other procedures, may repeat dose in 12-24 hours as needed

Major surgery:

Helixate® FS, Kogenate® FS (required peak pre- and post-surgery AHF level: 100%): 50 international units/kg; may repeat every 6-12 hours initially and until healing complete (10-14 days); intensity of regimen is dependent on type of surgery and postoperative care

Recombinate™, ReFacto® (required peak pre- and post-surgery AHF level: 80% to 100%): 40-50 international units/kg; repeat every 8-24 hours depending on state of healing

Prophylaxis: May also be given on a regular schedule to prevent bleeding

Administration Parenteral: I.V. administration only; see Stability for reconstitution and dosage preparation; total dose may be administered over 5-10 minutes; maximum rate of infusion: 10 mL/minute; adjust administration rate based on patient response; for Helixate® FS, Kogenate® FS, and ReFacto®, use sterile administration set provided by manufacturer

Monitoring Parameters Bleeding; heart rate and blood pressure (before and during I.V. administration); AHF levels prior to and during treatment; monitor for the development of inhibitor antibodies by clinical observations (eg, inadequate control of bleeding with adequate doses) and laboratory tests (eg, inhibitor level, Bethesda assay)

(Continued)

Antihemophilic Factor (Recombinant) *(Continued)*

Reference Range
Plasma antihemophilic factor level:
Normal range: 50% to 150%
Level to prevent spontaneous hemorrhage: 5%
Required peak post-infusion AHF activity in blood (as % of normal or units/dL plasma):
Early hemarthrosis, muscle bleed, or oral bleed: 20% to 40%
More extensive hemarthrosis, muscle bleed, or hematoma: 30% to 60%
Life-threatening bleeds (such as head injury, throat bleed, severe abdominal pain): 80% to 100%
Minor surgery, including tooth extraction: 60% to 80%
Major surgery: 80% to 100% (pre- and postoperative)

Patient Information This medication can only be given intravenously. Stop taking antihemophilic factor recombinant and notify physician immediately if any of the following signs or symptoms of an allergic (hypersensitivity) reaction occur: Itching, hives, low blood pressure, tightness of the chest, wheezing, or anaphylaxis. Wear identification indicating that you have a hemophilic condition.

Nursing Implications Reduce rate of administration, or temporarily discontinue, if patient experiences any adverse reactions; hypersensitivity reactions (eg, hives, chest tightness, itching, wheezing, hypotension) are possible

Additional Information One international unit of rAHF is equal to the factor VIII activity present in 1 mL of fresh pooled human plasma. If bleeding is not controlled with adequate dose, test for the presence of factor VIII inhibitor; larger doses of rAHF may be therapeutic with inhibitor titers <10 Bethesda units/mL; it may not be possible or practical to control bleeding if inhibitor titers >10 Bethesda units/mL (due to the very large rAHF doses required); other treatments [eg, antihemophilic factor (porcine), factor IX complex concentrates, recombinant factor VIIa, or anti-inhibitor coagulant complex] may be needed in patients with inhibitor titers >10 Bethesda units/mL

Dosage Forms
Injection, powder for reconstitution, lyophilized, recombinant [preservative free, single dose vial] (approximate factor VIII activity per vial):
Helixate® FS, Kogenate® FS: 250 international units/vial, 500 international units/vial, 1000 international units/vial [contains 28 mg sucrose/vial; exact potency labeled on each vial]
Recombinate™: 250 international units/vial, 500 international units/vial, 1000 international units/vial [contains 12.5 mg human albumin/mL; exact potency labeled on each vial]
ReFacto®: 250 international units/vial, 500 international units/vial, 1000 international units/vial, 2000 international units/vial [contains 12 mg sucrose/vial]

References
Abshire TC, Brackmann HH, Scharrer I, et al, "Sucrose Formulated Recombinant Human Antihemophilic Factor VIII is Safe and Efficacious for Treatment of Hemophilia A in Home Therapy. International Kogenate-FS Study Group," *Thromb Haemost*, 2000, 83(6):811-6.
Bray GL, Gomperts ED, Courter S, et al, "A Multicenter Study of Recombinant Factor VIII (Recombinate): Safety, Efficacy, and Inhibitor Risk in Previously Untreated Patients With Hemophilia A. The Recombinate Study Group," *Blood*, 1994, 83(9):2428-35.
Kelly KM, Butler RB, Farace L, et al, "Superior In Vivo Response of Recombinant Factor VIII Concentrate in Children With Hemophilia A," *J Pediatr*, 1997, 130(4):537-40.
Liesner RJ, "Prophylaxis in Haemophilic Children," *Blood Coagul Fibrinolysis*, 1997, 8(Suppl 1):S7-10.
Scharrer I, Bray GL, and Neutzling O, "Incidence of Inhibitors in Haemophilia A Patients - A Review of Recent Studies of Recombinant and Plasma-Derived Factor VIII Concentrates," *Haemophilia*, 1999, 5(3):145-54.
Shord SS and Lindley CM, "Coagulation Products and Their Uses," *Am J Health Syst Pharm*, 2000, 57(15):1403-20.
Schwartz RS, Abildgaard CF, Aledort LM, et al, "Human Recombinant DNA-Derived Antihemophilic Factor (Factor VIII) in the Treatment of Hemophilia A. Recombinant Factor VIII Study Group," *N Engl J Med*, 1990, 323(26):1800-5.

◆ **Antiphogistine Rub A-535 Capsaicin (Can)** *see* Capsaicin *on page 206*

Antipyrine and Benzocaine *(an tee PYE reen & BEN zoe kane)*
U.S. Brand Names Allergen®; Auralgan®; Auroto®
Synonyms Benzocaine and Antipyrine
Therapeutic Category Otic Agent, Analgesic; Otic Agent, Cerumenolytic
Generic Available Yes
Use Temporary relief of pain and reduction of inflammation associated with acute congestive and serous otitis media, swimmer's ear, otitis externa; facilitates ear wax removal
Contraindications Hypersensitivity to antipyrine, benzocaine, or any component; perforated tympanic membrane

Warnings Use of otic anesthetics may mask symptoms of a fulminating middle ear infection (acute otitis media); not intended for prolonged use

Adverse Reactions
Hematologic: Methemoglobinemia
Local: Burning, stinging, tenderness, edema
Miscellaneous: Hypersensitivity reactions

Usual Dosage Infants, Children, and Adults: Otic: Fill ear canal; moisten cotton pledget, place in external ear, repeat every 1-2 hours until pain and congestion is relieved; for ear wax removal instill drops 3-4 times/day for 2-3 days

Dosage Forms
Solution, otic: Antipyrine 5.4% and benzocaine 1.4% (10 mL, 15 mL)
Allergen®, Auroto®: Antipyrine 5.4% and benzocaine 1.4% (15 mL)
Auralgan®: Antipyrine 5.4% and benzocaine 1.4% (10 mL)

References
Rodriguez LF, Smolik LM, and Zbehlik AJ, "Benzocaine-Induced Methemoglobinemia: Report of a Severe Reaction and Review of the Literature," *Ann Pharmacother*, 1994, 28(5):643-9.

♦ **Antithrombotic Therapy in Children** see page 1316

Antithymocyte Globulin (Equine) (LIM foe site i MYUN GLOB yoo lin)

U.S. Brand Names Atgam®

Synonyms Antithymocyte Globulin (equine); ATG; Horse Antihuman Thymocyte Gamma Globulin

Therapeutic Category Immunosuppressant Agent

Generic Available No

Use Prevention and/or treatment of allograft rejection; treatment of moderate to severe aplastic anemia in patients not considered suitable candidates for bone marrow transplantation; prevention of graft-vs-host disease following bone marrow transplantation

Pregnancy Risk Factor C

Contraindications Hypersensitivity to ATG, thimerosal, any component, or other equine gamma globulins; severe, unremitting leukopenia and/or thrombocytopenia

Warnings Should only be used by physicians experienced in immunosuppressive therapy or management of renal transplant patients; adequate laboratory and supportive medical resources must be readily available in the facility for patient management. Anaphylaxis (symptoms can include hypotension, respiratory distress, pain in the chest, rash, and tachycardia) may occur at any time during ATG therapy. Epinephrine and oxygen should be readily available to treat anaphylaxis.

Adverse Reactions
Cardiovascular: Hypotension, hypertension, tachycardia, edema
Central nervous system: Seizures, fever, headache, chills
Dermatologic: Rash, pruritus, urticaria
Gastrointestinal: Diarrhea, nausea, stomatitis
Hematologic: Leukopenia, thrombocytopenia, hemolysis, anemia
Local: Thrombophlebitis
Neuromuscular & skeletal: Arthralgia; pain in the chest, flank, or back; weakness
Renal: Acute renal failure
Respiratory: Dyspnea
Miscellaneous: Lymphadenopathy, serum sickness, night sweats; anaphylaxis may be indicated by hypotension or respiratory distress

Stability Store in refrigerator; dilute in ½NS or NS; when diluted to concentrations up to 4 mg/mL, ATG infusion solution is stable for 24 hours; use of dextrose solution is not recommended; precipitation can occur in solutions with a low salt concentration (ie, D_5W)

Mechanism of Action May involve elimination of antigen-reactive T-lymphocytes (killer cells) in peripheral blood or alteration of T-cell function

Pharmacokinetics
Distribution: Poor into lymphoid tissues; binds to circulating lymphocytes, granulocytes, platelets, bone marrow cells
Half-life, plasma: 1.5-12 days
Elimination: ~1% of dose excreted in urine

Usual Dosage Intradermal skin test is recommended prior to administration of the initial dose of ATG; use 0.1 mL of a 1:1000 dilution of ATG in NS; observe the skin test every 15 minutes for 1 hour; a local reaction ≥10 mm diameter with a wheal or erythema or both should be considered a positive skin test
(Continued)

Antithymocyte Globulin (Equine) *(Continued)*

I.V.:
Children:
Aplastic anemia protocol: 10-20 mg/kg/day for 8-14 days, or 40 mg/kg/day once daily over 4 hours for 4 days; then give 10-30 mg/kg/dose every other day for 7 more doses
Cardiac allograft: 10 mg/kg/day for 7 days or as per protocol
Renal allograft: 5-25 mg/kg/day or as per protocol
Children and Adults:
Rejection prevention: 15 mg/kg/day for 14 days, then give every other day for 7 more doses; initial dose should be administered within 24 hours before or after transplantation
Rejection treatment: 10-15 mg/kg/day for 14 days, then give every other day for 7 more doses

Administration Parenteral: Administer via central line; use of high flow veins will minimize the occurrence of phlebitis and thrombosis; administer by slow I.V. infusion through a 0.2-1 micron in-line filter over 4-8 hours at a final concentration not to exceed 4 mg ATG/mL

Monitoring Parameters Lymphocyte profile; CBC with differential and platelet count, vital signs during administration, renal function test

Nursing Implications Patient may need to be pretreated with an antipyretic, antihistamine, and/or corticosteroid to prevent chills, fever, itching, and erythema

Dosage Forms Injection, solution: 50 mg/mL (5 mL)

References

Rosenfeld SJ, Kimball J, Vining D, et al, "Intensive Immunosuppression With Antithymocyte Globulin and Cyclosporine as Treatment for Severe Acquired Aplastic Anemia," *Blood*, 1995, 85(11):3058-65.

Whitehead B, James I, Helms P, et al, "Intensive Care Management of Children Following Heart and Heart-Lung Transplantation," *Intensive Care Med*, 1990, 16(7):426-30.

- ◆ **Antitumor Necrosis Factor-Alpha** *see* Infliximab *on page 608*
- ◆ **Antivenin Polyvalent [Equine]** *see* Crotalidae Polyvalent Antivenin (Equine) *on page 313*
- ◆ **Antivert®** *see* Meclizine *on page 710*
- ◆ **Antizol®** *see* Fomepizole *on page 517*
- ◆ **Anucort™ HC** *see* Hydrocortisone *on page 573*
- ◆ **Anusol® [OTC]** *see* Hemorrhoidal Preparations *on page 556*
- ◆ **Anusol-HC®** *see* Hydrocortisone *on page 573*
- ◆ **Anusol® HC-1™ [OTC]** *see* Hemorrhoidal Preparations *on page 556*
- ◆ **Anusol® HC-1 [OTC]** *see* Hydrocortisone *on page 573*
- ◆ **Anzemet®** *see* Dolasetron *on page 403*
- ◆ **APAP** *see* Acetaminophen *on page 36*
- ◆ **APD** *see* Pamidronate *on page 853*
- ◆ **Aphedrid™ [OTC]** *see* Triprolidine and Pseudoephedrine *on page 1122*
- ◆ **A.P.L.®** *see* Chorionic Gonadotropin *on page 269*
- ◆ **Apo®-Acetaminophen (Can)** *see* Acetaminophen *on page 36*
- ◆ **Apo®-Acetazolamide (Can)** *see* AcetaZOLAMIDE *on page 40*
- ◆ **Apo®-Acyclovir (Can)** *see* Acyclovir *on page 45*
- ◆ **Apo®-Allopurinol (Can)** *see* Allopurinol *on page 62*
- ◆ **Apo®-Alpraz (Can)** *see* Alprazolam *on page 64*
- ◆ **Apo®-Amitriptyline (Can)** *see* Amitriptyline *on page 89*
- ◆ **Apo®-Amoxi (Can)** *see* Amoxicillin *on page 94*
- ◆ **Apo®-Amoxi-Clav (Can)** *see* Amoxicillin and Clavulanic Acid *on page 96*
- ◆ **Apo®-Ampi (Can)** *see* Ampicillin *on page 103*
- ◆ **Apo®-Atenol (Can)** *see* Atenolol *on page 137*
- ◆ **Apo®-Azathioprine (Can)** *see* Azathioprine *on page 149*
- ◆ **Apo®-Baclofen (Can)** *see* Baclofen *on page 158*
- ◆ **Apo®-Beclomethasone (Can)** *see* Beclomethasone *on page 160*
- ◆ **Apo®-Benztropine (Can)** *see* Benztropine *on page 166*
- ◆ **Apo®-Bisacodyl (Can)** *see* Bisacodyl *on page 173*
- ◆ **Apo®-Buspirone (Can)** *see* BusPIRone *on page 191*
- ◆ **Apo®-Capto (Can)** *see* Captopril *on page 207*
- ◆ **Apo®-Carbamazepine (Can)** *see* Carbamazepine *on page 209*
- ◆ **Apo®-Carbamazepine CR (Can)** *see* Carbamazepine *on page 209*
- ◆ **Apo®-Cefaclor (Can)** *see* Cefaclor *on page 223*
- ◆ **Apo®-Cefadroxil (Can)** *see* Cefadroxil *on page 224*
- ◆ **Apo®-Cefuroxime (Can)** *see* Cefuroxime *on page 242*

- Apo®-Cephalex (Can) *see* Cephalexin *on page 244*
- Apo®-Cetirizine (Can) *see* Cetirizine *on page 249*
- Apo®-Chlorhexadine (Can) *see* Chlorhexidine Gluconate *on page 257*
- Apo®-Chlorpromazine (Can) *see* ChlorproMAZINE *on page 263*
- Apo®-Cimetidine (Can) *see* Cimetidine *on page 272*
- Apo®-Clonazepam (Can) *see* Clonazepam *on page 292*
- Apo®-Clonidine (Can) *see* Clonidine *on page 294*
- Apo®-Clorazepate (Can) *see* Clorazepate *on page 296*
- Apo®-Cloxi (Can) *see* Cloxacillin *on page 298*
- Apo®-Cromolyn (Can) *see* Cromolyn *on page 311*
- Apo®-Cyclobenzaprine (Can) *see* Cyclobenzaprine *on page 318*
- Apo®-Desipramine (Can) *see* Desipramine *on page 349*
- Apo®-Desmopressin (Can) *see* Desmopressin *on page 352*
- Apo®-Diazepam (Can) *see* Diazepam *on page 369*
- Apo®-Diclo (Can) *see* Diclofenac *on page 374*
- Apo®-Diclo Rapide (Can) *see* Diclofenac *on page 374*
- Apo®-Diclo SR (Can) *see* Diclofenac *on page 374*
- Apo®-Diltiaz (Can) *see* Diltiazem *on page 388*
- Apo®-Diltiaz CD (Can) *see* Diltiazem *on page 388*
- Apo®-Diltiaz SR (Can) *see* Diltiazem *on page 388*
- Apo®-Dimenhydrinate (Can) *see* DimenhyDRINATE *on page 390*
- Apo®-Dipivefrin (Can) *see* Dipivefrin *on page 396*
- Apo®-Dipyridamole FC (Can) *see* Dipyridamole *on page 397*
- Apo®-Divalproex (Can) *see* Valproic Acid and Derivatives *on page 1131*
- Apo®-Doxepin (Can) *see* Doxepin *on page 411*
- Apo®-Doxy (Can) *see* Doxycycline *on page 415*
- Apo®-Doxy Tabs (Can) *see* Doxycycline *on page 415*
- Apo®-Erythro Base (Can) *see* Erythromycin *on page 448*
- Apo®-Erythro E-C (Can) *see* Erythromycin *on page 448*
- Apo®-Erythro-ES (Can) *see* Erythromycin *on page 448*
- Apo®-Erythro-S (Can) *see* Erythromycin *on page 448*
- Apo®-Famotidine (Can) *see* Famotidine *on page 473*
- Apo®-Fluconazole (Can) *see* Fluconazole *on page 488*
- Apo®-Flunisolide (Can) *see* Flunisolide *on page 497*
- Apo®-Fluoxetine (Can) *see* Fluoxetine *on page 505*
- Apo®-Flurazepam (Can) *see* Flurazepam *on page 509*
- Apo®-Flurbiprofen (Can) *see* Flurbiprofen *on page 510*
- Apo®-Folic (Can) *see* Folic Acid *on page 516*
- Apo®-Furosemide (Can) *see* Furosemide *on page 526*
- Apo®-Gabapentin (Can) *see* Gabapentin *on page 527*
- Apo®-Gain (Can) *see* Minoxidil *on page 768*
- Apo®-Glyburide (Can) *see* GlyBURIDE *on page 540*
- Apo®-Haloperidol (Can) *see* Haloperidol *on page 554*
- Apo®-Haloperidol LA (Can) *see* Haloperidol *on page 554*
- Apo®-Hydralazine (Can) *see* HydrALAZINE *on page 568*
- Apo®-Hydro (Can) *see* Hydrochlorothiazide *on page 569*
- Apo®-Hydroxyzine (Can) *see* HydrOXYzine *on page 584*
- Apo®-Ibuprofen (Can) *see* Ibuprofen *on page 588*
- Apo®-Imipramine (Can) *see* Imipramine *on page 597*
- Apo®-Indomethacin (Can) *see* Indomethacin *on page 606*
- Apo®-Ipravent (Can) *see* Ipratropium *on page 620*
- Apo®-Ketoconazole (Can) *see* Ketoconazole *on page 639*
- Apo®-Ketorolac (Can) *see* Ketorolac *on page 641*
- Apo®-Ketorolac Injectable (Can) *see* Ketorolac *on page 641*
- Apo®-Labetalol (Can) *see* Labetalol *on page 645*
- Apo®-Lactulose (Can) *see* Lactulose *on page 649*
- Apo®-Levobunolol (Can) *see* Levobunolol *on page 665*
- Apo®-Lisinopril (Can) *see* Lisinopril *on page 682*
- Apo®-Lithium (Can) *see* Lithium *on page 684*
- Apo®-Loperamide (Can) *see* Loperamide *on page 687*
- Apo®-Loratadine (Can) *see* Loratadine *on page 692*
- Apo®-Lorazepam (Can) *see* Lorazepam *on page 695*

- ♦ Apo®-Lovastatin (Can) *see* Lovastatin *on page 697*
- ♦ Apo®-Megestrol (Can) *see* Megestrol *on page 714*
- ♦ Apo®-Metformin (Can) *see* Metformin *on page 729*
- ♦ Apo®-Methotrexate (Can) *see* Methotrexate *on page 737*
- ♦ Apo®-Methyldopa (Can) *see* Methyldopa *on page 741*
- ♦ Apo®-Metoclop (Can) *see* Metoclopramide *on page 749*
- ♦ Apo®-Metoprolol (Can) *see* Metoprolol *on page 752*
- ♦ Apo®-Metronidazole (Can) *see* Metronidazole *on page 754*
- ♦ Apo®-Midazolam (Can) *see* Midazolam *on page 761*
- ♦ Apo®-Misoprostol (Can) *see* Misoprostol *on page 769*
- ♦ Apo®-Nadol (Can) *see* Nadolol *on page 788*
- ♦ Apo®-Napro-Na (Can) *see* Naproxen *on page 796*
- ♦ Apo®-Napro-Na DS (Can) *see* Naproxen *on page 796*
- ♦ Apo®-Naproxen (Can) *see* Naproxen *on page 796*
- ♦ Apo®-Naproxen SR (Can) *see* Naproxen *on page 796*
- ♦ Apo®-Nifed (Can) *see* NIFEdipine *on page 811*
- ♦ Apo®-Nifed PA (Can) *see* NIFEdipine *on page 811*
- ♦ Apo®-Nitrofurantoin (Can) *see* Nitrofurantoin *on page 814*
- ♦ Apo®-Nizatidine (Can) *see* Nizatidine *on page 819*
- ♦ Apo®-Nortriptyline (Can) *see* Nortriptyline *on page 822*
- ♦ Apo®-Pentoxifylline SR (Can) *see* Pentoxifylline *on page 884*
- ♦ Apo®-Pen VK (Can) *see* Penicillin V Potassium *on page 877*
- ♦ Apo®-Piroxicam (Can) *see* Piroxicam *on page 910*
- ♦ Apo®-Prazo (Can) *see* Prazosin *on page 924*
- ♦ Apo®-Prednisone (Can) *see* PredniSONE *on page 928*
- ♦ Apo®-Primidone (Can) *see* Primidone *on page 931*
- ♦ Apo®-Procainamide (Can) *see* Procainamide *on page 934*
- ♦ Apo®-Prochlorperazine (Can) *see* Prochlorperazine *on page 938*
- ♦ Apo®-Propranolol (Can) *see* Propranolol *on page 952*
- ♦ Apo®-Quin-G (Can) *see* Quinidine *on page 967*
- ♦ Apo®-Quinidine (Can) *see* Quinidine *on page 967*
- ♦ Apo®-Ranitidine (Can) *see* Ranitidine *on page 972*
- ♦ Apo®-Salvent (Can) *see* Albuterol *on page 54*
- ♦ Apo®-Sertraline (Can) *see* Sertraline *on page 1016*
- ♦ Apo®-Sotalol (Can) *see* Sotalol *on page 1032*
- ♦ Apo®-Sucralate (Can) *see* Sucralfate *on page 1046*
- ♦ Apo®-Sulfatrim (Can) *see* Sulfamethoxazole and Trimethoprim *on page 1052*
- ♦ Apo®-Sulin (Can) *see* Sulindac *on page 1058*
- ♦ Apo®-Tetra (Can) *see* Tetracycline *on page 1074*
- ♦ Apo®-Theo LA (Can) *see* Theophylline *on page 1076*
- ♦ Apo®-Thioridazine (Can) *see* Thioridazine *on page 1085*
- ♦ Apo®-Timol (Can) *see* Timolol *on page 1095*
- ♦ Apo®-Timop (Can) *see* Timolol *on page 1095*
- ♦ Apo®-Trazodone (Can) *see* Trazodone *on page 1110*
- ♦ Apo®-Trazodone D (Can) *see* Trazodone *on page 1110*
- ♦ Apo®-Triazo (Can) *see* Triazolam *on page 1116*
- ♦ Apo®-Trihex (Can) *see* Trihexyphenidyl *on page 1118*
- ♦ Apo®-Trimethoprim (Can) *see* Trimethoprim *on page 1120*
- ♦ Apo®-Verap (Can) *see* Verapamil *on page 1144*
- ♦ Apo®-Warfarin (Can) *see* Warfarin *on page 1156*
- ♦ Apo®-Zidovudine (Can) *see* Zidovudine *on page 1163*
- ♦ APPG *see* Penicillin G Procaine *on page 876*

Aprepitant (ap RE pi tant)

U.S. Brand Names Emend®

Therapeutic Category Antiemetic; Substance P/Neurokinin 1 (NK$_1$) Receptor Antagonist

Generic Available No

Use Prevention of acute and delayed chemotherapy-induced emesis when used as an adjunctive agent with a 5-HT$_3$ antagonist and a corticosteroid

Pregnancy Risk Factor B

Contraindications Hypersensitivity to aprepitant or any component; concurrent use with pimozide, terfenadine, astemizole, or cisapride

Warnings Aprepitant has a potential to significantly interact with many medications (see Drug Interactions); potential increased serum levels of pimozide, terfenadine, astemizole, or cisapride could result in serious or life-threatening adverse effects; concomitant use with warfarin may result in clinically significant decrease in INR; patients on warfarin should have INR monitored closely, particularly at 7-10 days following initiation of 3-day aprepitant therapy. The efficacy of oral contraceptives may also be reduced during treatment with aprepitant; alternative methods of birth control should be used during aprepitant therapy.

Precautions Aprepitant is a moderate cytochrome P450 isoenzyme CYP3A4 inhibitor; use with caution in patients receiving medications metabolized by CYP3A4 as a reduction in metabolism and consequent elevation of serum levels may occur. Use with caution and monitor use closely in patients receiving docetaxel, paclitaxel, etoposide, irinotecan, ifosfamide, imatinib, vinorelbine, vinblastine, and vincristine as they are known to be metabolized by CYP3A4 isoenzymes

Adverse Reactions

Cardiovascular: Hypertension, hypotension, MI, tachycardia

Central nervous system: Confusion, depression, anxiety, headache, insomnia, dizziness, fatigue, fever

Dermatologic: Rash, alopecia, urticaria, angioedema, Stevens-Johnson syndrome (rare)

Endocrine & metabolic: Anorexia, hyperglycemia, hypokalemia, weight loss, hyponatremia

Gastrointestinal: Abdominal pain, constipation, diarrhea, epigastric discomfort, gastritis, heartburn, nausea, vomiting, dysgeusia, dyspepsia, dysphagia, flatulence, taste disturbance, vocal disturbance, pharyngitis, increased salivation

Genitourinary: Dysuria

Hematologic: Anemia, thrombocytopenia, neutropenia

Hepatic: Elevated serum transaminases

Neuromuscular & skeletal: Weakness, myalgia, muscle pain

Otic: Tinnitus

Renal: Renal insufficiency

Respiratory: Hiccups, cough, dyspnea, pneumonitis, respiratory insufficiency

Drug Interactions Cytochrome P450 isoenzyme CYP3A4 substrate, moderate inhibitor, and inducer; CYP2C9 inducer

Aprepitant induces the metabolism of warfarin, tolbutamide, and other drugs known to be metabolized by CYP2C9; decreases AUC of oral contraceptives which may result in reduced efficacy; increases serum levels of medications primarily metabolized by CYP3A4 such as pimozide, terfenadine, astemizole, cisapride, docetaxel, paclitaxel, etoposide, irinotecan, ifosfamide, imatinib, vinorelbine, vinblastine, and vincristine; increases serum levels of pimozide, terfenadine, astemizole, and cisapride (see Contraindications); increases AUC for corticosteroids (reduce the oral dexamethasone dose by 50%, I.V. methylprednisolone dose by 25%, and oral methylprednisolone dose by 50%); increases serum level of midazolam and potentially other benzodiazepines; CYP3A4 inhibitors (ketoconazole, itraconazole, nefazodone, troleandomycin, clarithromycin, ritonavir, nelfinavir) may significantly increase aprepitant serum levels; CYP3A4 inducers (rifampin, carbamazepine, and phenytoin) may reduce aprepitant serum levels; diltiazem increases aprepitant serum levels; when concomitantly used with paroxetine, serum levels of both agents are reduced

Stability Store capsules at room temperature.

Mechanism of Action Aprepitant is a selective high-affinity antagonist of human substance P/neurokinin 1 receptors. Antiemetic activity is via central action with little or no affinity for serotonin, dopamine, and corticosteroid receptors.

Pharmacokinetics

Distribution: V_d: Adults: 70 L

Protein binding: >95%

Metabolism: Extensive hepatic metabolism primarily by CYP3A4 with minor metabolism by CYP1A2 and CYP2C19

Bioavailability: 60% to 65%

Half-life: Adults: 9-13 hours

Time to peak serum concentration: 4 hours

Elimination:

Clearance: Adults: 62-90 mL/minute

Usual Dosage Oral: Adults: 125 mg one hour prior to chemotherapy followed by 80 mg once daily for the next two days. Use in combination with a 5-HT$_3$ antagonist and a corticosteroid.

Note: Aprepitant has only been studied in a three-day regimen combined with a corticosteroid and 5-HT$_3$ antagonist. Efficacy as a single agent or for prolonged treatment has not been demonstrated.

Dosage adjustment in renal impairment: No dosage adjustment needed

(Continued)

Aprepitant *(Continued)*

Dosage adjustment in hepatic impairment: No dosage adjustment needed in mild to moderate hepatic insufficiency; the pharmacokinetic profile of aprepitant in severe hepatic insufficiency (Child-Pugh score >9) has not be studied

Administration Oral: May be administered without regard to food, one hour prior to chemotherapy on the first day of treatment and in the morning on the subsequent next two days.

Patient Information Aprepitant may react with many other medications; report all medication use including OTC and herbal products to your physician; due to potential decrease effectiveness of oral contraceptives, alternative contraceptive methods should be used during therapy

Dosage Forms

Capsule: 80 mg, 125 mg [available in unit-dose packs of 5, or bulk bottles]
Combination unit-dose pack: 80 mg (2s) and 125 mg (1s)

♦ **Apresoline®** **(Can)** *see* HydrALAZINE *on page 568*

♦ **Aprodine®** [OTC] *see* Triprolidine and Pseudoephedrine *on page 1122*

Aprotinin *(a proe TYE nin)*

U.S. Brand Names Trasylol®

Therapeutic Category Hemostatic Agent

Generic Available No

Use Prophylactic use to reduce perioperative blood loss and the need for blood transfusion in patients undergoing cardiopulmonary bypass in the course of coronary artery bypass graft surgery (CABG); in selected repeat cases of primary CABG surgery where the risk of bleeding is especially high or where transfusion is unavailable or unacceptable

Pregnancy Risk Factor B

Contraindications Hypersensitivity to aprotinin or any component

Warnings Patients with a previous exposure to aprotinin (particularly when re-exposure is within 6 months) are at an increased risk for hypersensitivity reactions including anaphylactic or anaphylactoid reactions; pretreatment with an antihistamine and H_2-blocker before administration of the loading dose is recommended in these patients; delay the addition of aprotinin into the pump prime solution until the loading dose has safely been administered.

Precautions All patients treated with aprotinin should first receive a test dose at least 10 minutes before the loading dose to assess the potential for allergic reactions

Adverse Reactions

Cardiovascular: Atrial fibrillation, MI, heart failure, atrial flutter, ventricular tachycardia, cerebral embolism, cerebrovascular events, chest pain, hypotension, pericardial effusion, pulmonary hypertension

Central nervous system: Fever, mental confusion, seizures, agitation, dizziness, anxiety

Endocrine & metabolic: Hyperglycemia, hypokalemia, acidosis

Gastrointestinal: Nausea, vomiting, constipation, diarrhea, GI hemorrhage

Hematologic: Hemolysis, anemia, thrombosis

Hepatic: Liver damage, jaundice

Local: Phlebitis

Neuromuscular & skeletal: Arthralgia

Renal: Decreased renal function

Respiratory: Dyspnea, bronchoconstriction, pulmonary edema, apnea, increased cough

Miscellaneous: Anaphylaxis (see Warnings)

Drug Interactions Decreases effects of fibrinolytic agents such as streptokinase or anistreplase; decreases effects of captopril; prolonged activated clotting time when used with heparin

Stability Store between 2°C to 25°C (36°F to 77°F); do not freeze; do not mix with other medications; incompatible with corticosteroids, heparin, amino acids, and fat emulsion

Mechanism of Action Aprotinin, a serine protease inhibitor, modulates the systemic inflammatory response associated with cardiopulmonary bypass surgery; inhibits plasmin, kallikrein, and platelet activation producing antifibrinolytic effects; is a weak inhibitor of plasma pseudocholinesterase; inhibits the contact phase activation of coagulation and preserves adhesive platelet glycoproteins making them resistant to damage from increased circulating plasmin or mechanical injury occurring during bypass

Pharmacokinetics

Metabolism: Aprotinin is slowly degraded by lysosomal enzymes

Half-life, elimination: 150 minutes; terminal elimination: 10 hours

Elimination: <10% excreted unchanged in the urine

Usual Dosage I.V.: Test dose: All patients should receive a test dose at least 10 minutes prior to the loading dose to assess the potential for allergic reactions

Infants and Children: No conclusive dosage regimen has been established; variable dosage recommendations in the literature. Test dose: (dosage not well documented in studies) 0.1 mg/kg (maximum: 1.4 mg) has been used. Two of the more common recommendations follow (see References for other recommendations):

Body surface area: ≤1.16 m^2:
  240 mg/m^2 loading dose
  240 mg/m^2 into pump prime volume
  56 mg/m^2/hour continuous infusion during surgery

Body surface area: >1.16 m^2:
  280 mg/m^2 loading dose
  280 mg/m^2 into pump prime volume
  70 mg/m^2/hour continuous infusion during surgery

Alternative (based upon body weight only):
  30,000 Kallikrein inhibitor units/kg (4.2 mg/kg) loading dose
  30,000 Kallikrein inhibitor units/kg (4.2 mg/kg) into pump prime volume
  30,000 Kallikrein inhibitor units/kg/hour (4.2 mg/kg/hour) continuous infusion

Adults: Test dose: 1 mL (1.4 mg)

Regimen A (standard dose):
  2 million Kallikrein inhibitor units (280 mg) loading dose
  2 million Kallikrein inhibitor units (280 mg) into pump prime volume
  500,000 Kallikrein inhibitor units/hour (70 mg/hour) continuous infusion during surgery

Regimen B (low dose):
  1 million Kallikrein inhibitor units (140 mg) loading dose
  1 million Kallikrein inhibitor units (140 mg) into pump prime volume
  250,000 Kallikrein inhibitor units/hour (35 mg/hour) continuous infusion during surgery

Administration Parenteral: For I.V. use only; all I.V. doses should be administered through a central line; infuse test dose over at least 10 minutes; infuse loading dose over 20-30 minutes with patient in the supine position; add pump priming dose while recirculating the priming fluid of the cardiopulmonary bypass circuit

Monitoring Parameters Bleeding times, PT, activated clotting time, platelet count, CBC, Hct, Hgb, and fibrinogen degradation products

Test Interactions Aprotinin prolongs whole blood clotting time of heparinized blood as determined by the Hemochrom® method or similar surface activation methods; patients may require additional heparin even in the presence of activated clotting time levels that appear to represent adequate anticoagulation

Dosage Forms Injection, solution: 1.4 mg/mL [10,000 Kallikrein inhibitor units/mL] (100 mL, 200 mL)

References

Boldt J, "Endothelial-Related Coagulation in Pediatric Surgery," *Ann Thorac Surg*, 1998, 65(6 Suppl):S56-9.

Carrel TP, Schwanda M, Vogt P, et al, "Aprotinin in Pediatric Cardiac Operations: A Benefit in Complex Malformations and With High-Dose Regimen Only," *Ann Thorac Surg*, 1998, 66(1):153-8.

Miller BE, Tosone SR, Tam VK, et al, "Hematologic and Economic Impact of Aprotinin in Reoperative Pediatric Cardiac Operations," *Ann Thorac Surg*, 1998, 66(2):535-41.

Penkoske P, Entwistle LM, Marchak BE, et al, "Aprotinin in Children Undergoing Repair of Congenital Heart Defects," *Ann Thorac Surg*, 1995, 60(6 Suppl):S529-32.

Spray TL, "Use of Aprotinin in Pediatric Organ Transplantation," *Ann Thorac Surg*, 1998, 65(6 Suppl):S71-3.

♦ **Aranesp**™ *see* Darbepoetin Alfa *on page 341*

♦ **Aredia**® *see* Pamidronate *on page 853*

Arginine (AR ji neen)

U.S. Brand Names R-Gene®

Therapeutic Category Diagnostic Agent, Growth Hormone Function; Metabolic Alkalosis Agent; Urea Cycle Disorder (UCD) Treatment Agent

Generic Available No

Use Pituitary function test (growth hormone); management of severe, uncompensated, metabolic alkalosis (pH ≥7.55) **after** optimizing therapy with sodium or potassium chloride supplements; treatment agent for urea cycle disorders

Contraindications Hypersensitivity to arginine or any component; renal or hepatic failure

Precautions Arginine hydrochloride is metabolized to nitrogen-containing products for excretion; the temporary effect of a high nitrogen load on the kidneys should be evaluated; accumulation of excess arginine may result in an overproduction of nitric oxide, leading to vasodilation and hypotension; each 1 mEq chloride delivers 1 mEq hydrogen; monitor acid base balance closely, particularly in neonates

Adverse Reactions

Cardiovascular: Flushing (after rapid I.V. administration), hypotension

Central nervous system: Headache (after rapid I.V. administration)

Endocrine & metabolic: Hyperglycemia, hyperkalemia, metabolic acidosis

Gastrointestinal: Nausea, vomiting, abdominal pain, bloating

Local: Venous irritation, severe tissue necrosis with extravasation

Miscellaneous: Elevated serum gastrin concentration

Drug Interactions Estrogen-progesterone combinations, spironolactone (potentially fatal hyperkalemia has been reported in patients with hepatic disease)

Mechanism of Action Stimulates pituitary release of growth hormone and prolactin and pancreatic release of glucagon and insulin; patients with impaired pituitary function have lower or no increase in plasma concentrations of growth hormone after administration of arginine. Arginine hydrochloride has been used for treatment of hypochloremic metabolic alkalosis due to its high chloride content. Arginine becomes an essential amino acid in ASL deficiency due to a decrease in the conversion of argininosuccinate to arginine; in other urea cycle disorders, arginine is used not only to increase its serum concentration but also to prevent the breakdown of endogenous protein.

Pharmacokinetics

Absorption: Oral: Well absorbed

Time to peak serum concentration: Within 2 hours

Usual Dosage I.V.:

Growth hormone reserve test:

Children: 500 mg/kg over 30 minutes

Adults: 300 mL over 30 minutes

Treatment of urea cycle disorders: Neonates, Infants, Children, and Adults:

Argininosuccinic acid lyase (ASL) or argininosuccinic acid synthetase (ASS) disorders or pending definitive diagnosis: 600 mg/kg as a loading dose followed by 600 mg/kg/day as a continuous infusion

Carbamyl phosphate synthetase (CPS) or ornithine transcarbamylase (OTC) disorder: 200 mg/kg as a loading dose followed by 200 mg/kg/day as a continuous infusion

Intermittent hyperammonemic crisis in patients with urea cycle disorders: Neonates, Infants, Children, and Adults:

ASL or ASS: 0.6 g/kg or 12 g/m^2 loading dose followed by 0.6 g/kg/day or 12 g/m^2/day continuous infusion

CPS or OTC: 0.2 g/kg or 4 g/m^2 loading dose followed by 0.2 g/kg/day or 4 g/m^2/day continuous infusion

Metabolic alkalosis: Infants, Children, and Adults: Arginine hydrochloride dose (g) = weight (kg) x 0.1 x [HCO$_3^-$ - 24] where HCO$_3^-$ = the patient's serum bicarbonate concentration in mEq/L; give $1/2$ to $2/3$ of calculated dose and re-evaluate

Note: Arginine hydrochloride is an alternative treatment for uncompensated metabolic alkalosis after sodium chloride and potassium chloride supplementation have been optimized

To correct hypochloremia: Infants, Children, and Adults: Arginine hydrochloride dose (mEq) = 0.2 x weight (kg) x [103 - Cl$^-$] where Cl$^-$ = the patient's serum chloride concentration in mEq/L; give $1/2$ to $2/3$ of calculated dose and re-evaluate

Note: Arginine hydrochloride should never be used as initial therapy for chloride supplementation but as an alternative in the patient who is unresponsive to sodium chloride or potassium chloride supplementation.

Administration Parenteral: May be infused without further dilution; maximum rate of I.V. infusion: 1 g/kg/hour (4.75 mEq/kg/hour) (maximum dose: 60 g/hour = 285 mEq over 1 hour); administration through a central line is recommended; infuse loading doses for urea cycle disorders over 90 minutes

Monitoring Parameters Acid-base status (arterial or capillary blood gases), serum electrolytes, BUN, glucose, plasma growth hormone concentrations (when evaluating growth hormone reserve), plasma ammonia and amino acids (when treating urea cycle disorders)

Reference Range If intact pituitary function, human growth hormone levels should rise after arginine administration to 10-30 ng/mL (control range: 0-6 ng/mL)

Nursing Implications I.V. infiltration of arginine hydrochloride may cause necrosis and phlebitis; prolongation of the infusion may diminish the stimulus to the pituitary gland and nullify the test

Additional Information When treating urea cycle disorders, sodium bicarbonate use may be necessary to neutralize the acidifying effects of arginine HCl.

Dosage Forms Injection, solution, as hydrochloride: 10% (300 mL) [contains 0.475 mEq chloride/mL]

References
Batshaw ML, MacArthur RB, and Tuchman M, "Alternative Pathway Therapy for Urea Cycle Disorders: Twenty Years Later," *J Pediatr*, 2001, 138(1 Suppl):S46-54.

Bushinsky DA and Gennari FJ, "Life-Threatening Hyperkalemia Induced by Arginine," *Ann Intern Med*, 1978, 89(5 Pt 1):632-4.

Summar M, "Current Strategies for the Management of Neonatal Urea Cycle Disorders," *J Pediatr*, 2001, 138(1 Suppl):S30-9.

- ♦ **8-Arginine Vasopressin** *see* Vasopressin *on page 1136*
- ♦ **Aristocort®** *see* Triamcinolone *on page 1112*
- ♦ **Aristocort® A** *see* Triamcinolone *on page 1112*
- ♦ **Aristocort® Forte** *see* Triamcinolone *on page 1112*
- ♦ **Aristospan®** *see* Triamcinolone *on page 1112*
- ♦ **ASA** *see* Aspirin *on page 134*
- ♦ **5-ASA** *see* Mesalamine *on page 723*
- ♦ **Asacol®** *see* Mesalamine *on page 723*
- ♦ **Asaphen (Can)** *see* Aspirin *on page 134*
- ♦ **Asaphen E.C. (Can)** *see* Aspirin *on page 134*

Ascorbic Acid (a SKOR bik AS id)

U.S. Brand Names C-500-GR™ [OTC]; Cecon® [OTC]; Cenolate®; Cevi-Bid® [OTC]; C-Gram [OTC]; Citraderm® [OTC]; Dull-C® [OTC]; Vita-C® [OTC]

Canadian Brand Names Proflavanol C™; Revitalose C-1000®

Synonyms Vitamin C

Therapeutic Category Nutritional Supplement; Urinary Acidifying Agent; Vitamin, Water Soluble

Generic Available Yes

Use Prevention and treatment of scurvy; urinary acidification; dietary supplementation; prevention and reduction in the severity of colds

Pregnancy Risk Factor A (C if used in doses above RDA recommendation)

Contraindications Hypersensitivity to ascorbic acid or any component (see Warnings); large doses during pregnancy

Warnings Cenolate® injection contains sulfites which may cause allergic reactions in susceptible individuals

Precautions Some products contain aspartame which is metabolized to phenylalanine and must be avoided (or used with caution) in patients with phenylketonuria.

Adverse Reactions
Cardiovascular: Flushing
Central nervous system: Faintness, dizziness, headache, fatigue
Gastrointestinal: Nausea, vomiting, heartburn, diarrhea
Renal: Hyperoxaluria

Drug Interactions Aspirin, iron, oral contraceptives (increases estrogen levels), decreased warfarin effect

Stability Injectable form should be stored under refrigeration (2°C to 8°C); protect oral dosage forms from light; ascorbic acid solution is rapidly oxidized

Mechanism of Action Necessary for collagen formation and tissue repair in the body; involved in some oxidation-reduction reactions as well as many other metabolic reactions

Pharmacodynamics Reversal of scurvy symptoms: 2 days to 3 weeks

Pharmacokinetics
Absorption: Oral: Readily absorbed; absorption is an active process and is thought to be dose-dependent
(Continued)

Ascorbic Acid *(Continued)*

Distribution: Widely distributed

Protein binding: 25%

Metabolism: In the liver by oxidation and sulfation

Elimination: In urine; there is an individual specific renal threshold for ascorbic acid; when blood levels are high, ascorbic acid is excreted in urine, whereas when the levels are subthreshold very little if any ascorbic acid is excreted into urine

Usual Dosage Oral, I.M., I.V., S.C.:

Recommended adequate intake (AI):

0-6 months: 40 mg

6-12 months: 50 mg

Recommended daily allowance (RDA):

1-3 years: 15 mg

4-8 years: 25 mg

9-13 years: 45 mg

14-18 years: Males: 75 mg, females: 65 mg

19 years to Adults: Males: 90 mg, females: 75 mg

Children:

Scurvy: 100-300 mg/day in divided doses

Urinary acidification: 500 mg every 6-8 hours

Dietary supplement (variable): 35-100 mg/day

Adults:

Scurvy: 100-250 mg 1-2 times/day

Urinary acidification: 4-12 g/day in 3-4 divided doses

Dietary supplement (variable): 50-200 mg/day

Prevention and treatment of cold: 1-3 g/day

Children and Adults: To increase iron excretion during deferoxamine administration: 100-200 mg/day during deferoxamine therapy

Administration

Oral: May be administered without regard to meals

Parenteral: Use only in circumstances when the oral route is not possible; I.M. preferred parenteral route due to improved utilization; for I.V. use dilute in equal volume D_5W or NS, and infuse over at least 10 minutes

Reference Range

Normal levels: 10-20 µg/mL

Scurvy: <1-1.5 µg/mL

Test Interactions False-positive urinary glucose with cupric sulfate reagent, false-negative urinary glucose with glucose oxidase method, false-negative amine-dependent stool occult blood test

Additional Information Sodium content of 1 g: ~5 mEq

Dosage Forms

Capsule: 500 mg, 1000 mg

C-500-GR™: 500 mg

Capsule, timed release: 500 mg

Crystals (Vita-C®): 4 g/teaspoonful (100 g)

Injection, solution: 250 mg/mL (2 mL, 30 mL); 500 mg/mL (50 mL)

Cenolate®: 500 mg/mL (1 mL, 2 mL) [contains sodium hydrosulfite]

Powder (Dull-C®): 4 g/teaspoonful (100 g, 500 g)

Solution, oral (Cecon®): 90 mg/mL (50 mL)

Tablet: 100 mg, 250 mg, 500 mg, 1000 mg

C-Gram: 1000 mg

Tablet, chewable: 100 mg, 250 mg, 500 mg [some products may contains aspartame]

Tablet, timed release: 500 mg, 1000 mg, 1500 mg

Cevi-Bid®: 500 mg

References

"Dietary Reference Intakes for Vitamin C, Vitamin E, Selenium, and Carotenoids. A Report of the Panel on Dietary Antioxidants and Related Compounds Food and Nutrition Board, Institute of Medicine," National Academy of Sciences, Washington, DC: National Academy Press, 2000.

♦ **Ascriptin®** [OTC] *see* Aspirin *on page 134*

♦ **Ascriptin® Arthritis Pain** [OTC] *see* Aspirin *on page 134*

♦ **Ascriptin® Enteric** [OTC] *see* Aspirin *on page 134*

♦ **Ascriptin® Extra Strength** [OTC] *see* Aspirin *on page 134*

♦ **ASN-ase** *see* Asparaginase *on page 132*

Asparaginase *(a SPIR a ji nase)*

Related Information

Emetogenic Potential of Single Chemotherapeutic Agents *on page 1286*

U.S. Brand Names Elspar®

Canadian Brand Names Kidrolase®

Synonyms A-ase; ASN-ase; Colaspase; LASP

Therapeutic Category Antineoplastic Agent, Miscellaneous

Generic Available No

Use In combination therapy for the treatment of acute lymphocytic leukemia, lymphoma

Pregnancy Risk Factor C

Contraindications Hypersensitivity to *E. coli*, asparaginase, or any component (if a reaction to Elspar® occurs, obtain investigational *Erwinia* preparation from McKesson BioServices at (301) 762-0069 or pegaspargase from Gentiva Health Services at (888) 276-2217 is another alternative - use with caution); pancreatitis

Warnings The FDA currently recommends that procedures for proper handling and disposal of antineoplastic agents be considered; be prepared to treat anaphylaxis at each administration

Precautions Use with caution in patients with impaired renal function; discontinue asparaginase at the first sign of renal failure or pancreatitis

Adverse Reactions

Cardiovascular: Hypotension, edema

Central nervous system: Fever, drowsiness, seizures, chills, malaise, lethargy, coma, headache, stroke, confusion, dizziness, hallucinations

Dermatologic: Rash, pruritus, urticaria

Endocrine & metabolic: Hyperglycemia, transient diabetes mellitus, hyperammonemia, hyperuricemia, hypoalbuminemia; decreased thyroxine and thyroxine-binding globulin concentration

Gastrointestinal: Vomiting, pancreatitis, nausea, anorexia, abdominal cramps

Hematologic: Leukopenia, coagulation abnormalities (prolonged thrombin, PT, and partial prothrombin times), reduced fibrinogen

Hepatic: Hepatotoxicity (elevated liver enzymes, hyperbilirubinemia)

Renal: Azotemia

Respiratory: Coughing, laryngeal edema, bronchospasm

Miscellaneous: Hypersensitivity reactions (incidence in children is 20% with *E. coli* asparaginase and <5% with *Erwinia* asparaginase); anaphylaxis

Drug Interactions Methotrexate (decreased antineoplastic effect if given prior to methotrexate); vincristine (increases toxicity if given concomitantly); prednisone (increases hyperglycemic effect)

Stability Refrigerate; no loss in potency was noted after storage for 1 week at room temperature, however, the manufacturer recommends that reconstituted solutions should be discarded after 8 hours since there is no preservative; discard immediately if solution becomes cloudy; use of a 0.2 micron filter may result in some loss of potency

Mechanism of Action Inhibits protein synthesis by deaminating asparagine and depriving tumor cells of this essential amino acid

Pharmacokinetics

Absorption: Not absorbed from GI tract, therefore requires parenteral administration

Distribution: Asparaginase not detected in CSF but CSF asparagine is depleted

Half-life:

E. coli L-asparaginase: 24-36 hours

Patients who have had a hypersensitivity reaction to asparaginase have a decreased half-life

Erwinia L-asparaginase: Significantly shorter than for the *E. coli*-derived product; mean half-life *Erwinia* L-asparaginase: 10-15 hours

Elimination: Clearance is unaffected by age, renal function, or hepatic function

Usual Dosage Children and Adults: Refer to individual protocols

Perform intradermal sensitivity testing with 2 units of asparaginase before the initial dose and when a week or more has elapsed between doses:

I.M. (preferred): 6000-10,000 units/m²/dose 3 times/week for 3 weeks for combination therapy; high-dose I.M. regimen of 25,000 units/m²/dose once weekly for 9 doses has also been used

I.V.: 1000 units/kg/day for 10 days for combination therapy or 200 units/kg/day for 28 days if combination therapy is inappropriate

Administration

I.M.: Maximum 2 mL volume is recommended for I.M. injections; if the volume to be administered is >2 mL, use multiple injection sites

I.V.: Must be infused over a minimum of 30 minutes

Monitoring Parameters Vital signs during administration, CBC, urinalysis, amylase, liver enzymes, bilirubin, prothrombin time, renal function tests, urine glucose, blood glucose

Patient Information Notify physician if fever, sore throat, painful/burning urination, bruising, bleeding, or shortness of breath occurs

(Continued)

Asparaginase *(Continued)*

Nursing Implications I.M. route is associated with a more delayed, less severe anaphylactoid reaction compared to the I.V. route; patients should be observed for one hour following an I.M. injection for signs of severe hypersensitivity; appropriate agents for maintenance of an adequate airway and treatment of a hypersensitivity reaction (antihistamine, epinephrine, oxygen, I.V. corticosteroids) should be readily available

Dosage Forms Injection, powder for reconstitution: 10,000 units/vial

References

Asselin BL, Whitin JC, Coppola DJ, et al, "Comparative Pharmacokinetic Studies of Three Asparaginase Preparations," *J Clin Oncol*, 1993, 11(9):1780-6.

Clavell LA, Gelber RD, Cohen HJ, et al, "Four-Agent Induction and Intensive Asparaginase Therapy for Treatment of Childhood Acute Lymphoblastic Leukemia," *N Engl J Med*, 1986, 315(11):657-63.

Nesbit M, Chard R, Evans A, et al, "Evaluation of Intramuscular Versus Intravenous Administration of L-Asparaginase in Childhood Leukemia," *Am J Pediatr Hematol Oncol*, 1979, 1(1):9-13.

Ortega JA, Nesbit ME Jr, and Donaldson MH, "L-Asparaginase, Vincristine, and Prednisone for Induction of First Remission in Acute Lymphocytic Leukemia," *Cancer Res*, 1977, 37(2):535-40.

♦ **Aspercin [OTC]** *see* Aspirin *on page 134*

♦ **Aspercin Extra [OTC]** *see* Aspirin *on page 134*

♦ **Aspergum® [OTC]** *see* Aspirin *on page 134*

Aspirin *(AS pir in)*

Related Information

Antithrombotic Therapy in Children *on page 1316*
Drugs and Breast-Feeding *on page 1404*
Overdose and Toxicology *on page 1388*

U.S. Brand Names Ascriptin® [OTC]; Ascriptin® Arthritis Pain [OTC]; Ascriptin® Enteric [OTC]; Ascriptin® Extra Strength [OTC]; Aspercin [OTC]; Aspercin Extra [OTC]; Aspergum® [OTC]; Bayer® Aspirin [OTC]; Bayer® Aspirin Extra Strength [OTC]; Bayer® Aspirin Regimen Adult Low Strength [OTC]; Bayer® Aspirin Regimen Adult Low Strength With Calcium [OTC]; Bayer® Aspirin Regimen, Children's [OTC]; Bayer® Aspirin Regimen Regular Strength [OTC]; Bayer® Plus Extra Strength [OTC]; Bufferin® [OTC]; Bufferin® Arthritis Strength [OTC]; Bufferin® Extra Strength [OTC]; Easprin®; Ecotrin® [OTC]; Ecotrin® Adult Low Strength [OTC]; Ecotrin® Maximum Strength [OTC]; Halfprin® [OTC]; St. Joseph Pain Reliever [OTC]; ZORprin®

Canadian Brand Names Asaphen; Asaphen E.C.; Entrophen®; Novasen

Synonyms Acetylsalicylic Acid; ASA

Therapeutic Category Analgesic, Non-narcotic; Anti-inflammatory Agent; Antiplatelet Agent; Antipyretic; Nonsteroidal Anti-inflammatory Drug (NSAID), Oral; Salicylate

Generic Available Yes

Use Treatment of mild to moderate pain, inflammation and fever; adjunctive treatment of Kawasaki disease; prevention of vascular mortality during suspected acute MI; prevention of recurrent MI; prevention of MI in patients with angina; prevention of recurrent stroke and mortality following TIA or stroke; management of rheumatoid arthritis, rheumatic fever, osteoarthritis, and gout (high dose); adjunctive therapy in revascularization procedures (coronary artery bypass graft, percutaneous transluminal coronary angioplasty, carotid endarterectomy)

Pregnancy Risk Factor C (D if full-dose aspirin in 3rd trimester)

Contraindications Hypersensitivity to salicylates, any component, or other NSAIDs; bleeding disorders; hepatic failure

Warnings Do not use aspirin in children <16 years of age for chickenpox or flu symptoms due to the association with Reye's syndrome

Precautions Use with caution in patients with impaired renal function, erosive gastritis, peptic ulcer, gout, platelet and bleeding disorders

Adverse Reactions

Dermatologic: Rash, urticaria
Gastrointestinal: Nausea, vomiting, GI distress, GI bleeding, ulcers
Hematologic: Inhibition of platelet aggregation
Hepatic: Hepatotoxicity
Otic: Tinnitus
Renal: Interstitial nephritis, renal papillary necrosis
Respiratory: Bronchospasm

Drug Interactions Aspirin may increase methotrexate serum levels and may displace valproic acid from binding sites which can result in toxicity; aspirin may increase free (unbound) buspirone concentrations; use of warfarin, heparin, low molecular weight heparins, urokinase, streptokinase, alteplase, and platelet inhibitors (eg, dipyridamole) with aspirin may cause an increase in bleeding; use of NSAIDs with aspirin may cause an increase in GI adverse effects and a possible decrease in serum concentration of NSAIDs; aspirin may antagonize effects of probenecid; aspirin, especially high doses, may decrease the antihypertensive effects of ACE inhibitors; buffered preparations may decrease the oral absorption of tetracycline or ketoconazole, therefore, administer 3-4 hours apart

Food Interactions Aspirin may increase the renal excretion of vitamin C and may decrease serum folate levels; some suggest increasing the dietary intake of foods that are high in vitamin C and folic acid

Stability Keep suppositories in refrigerator, do not freeze; hydrolysis of aspirin occurs upon exposure to water or moist air, resulting in salicylate and acetate; acetate possesses a vinegar-like odor; do not use if a strong odor is present

Mechanism of Action Inhibits prostaglandin synthesis, acts on the hypothalamus heat-regulating center to reduce fever, blocks prostaglandin synthetase action which prevents formation of the platelet-aggregating substance thromboxane A_2

Pharmacokinetics

Absorption: From the stomach and small intestine

Distribution: Readily distributes into most body fluids and tissues; hydrolyzed to salicylate (active) by esterases in the GI mucosa, red blood cells, synovial fluid and blood

Metabolism: Primarily by hepatic microsomal enzymes

Half-life: 15-20 minutes; metabolic pathways are saturable such that salicylate half-life is dose-dependent ranging from 3 hours at lower doses (300-600 mg), 5-6 hours (after 1 g) and 10 hours with higher doses

Time to peak serum concentration: Salicylate: ~1-2 hours; may be delayed with controlled or timed-release preparations

Elimination: Renal as salicylate and conjugated metabolites

Dialysis: Dialyzable: 50% to 100%

Usual Dosage

Children:

Analgesic and antipyretic: Oral, rectal: 10-15 mg/kg/dose every 4-6 hours; maximum dose: 4 g/day

Anti-inflammatory: Oral: Initial: 60-90 mg/kg/day in divided doses; usual maintenance: 80-100 mg/kg/day divided every 6-8 hours; monitor serum concentrations

Antiplatelet effects: Adequate pediatric studies have not been performed; pediatric dosage is derived from adult studies and clinical experience and is not well established; suggested doses have ranged from 3-5 mg/kg/day to 5-10 mg/kg/day given as a single daily dose. Doses are rounded to a convenient amount (eg, $1/2$ of 80 mg tablet).

Mechanical prosthetic heart valves: 6-20 mg/kg/day given as a single daily dose (used in combination with an oral anticoagulant in children who have systemic embolism despite adequate oral anticoagulation therapy (INR 2.5-3.5) and used in combination with low-dose anticoagulation (INR 2-3) and dipyridamole when full-dose oral anticoagulation is contraindicated)

Blalock-Taussig shunts: 3-5 mg/kg/day given as a single daily dose

Kawasaki disease: Oral: 80-100 mg/kg/day divided every 6 hours; monitor serum concentrations; after fever resolves: 3-5 mg/kg/day once daily; in patients without coronary artery abnormalities, give lower dose for at least 6-8 weeks or until ESR and platelet count are normal; in patients with coronary artery abnormalities, low-dose aspirin should be continued indefinitely

Adults:

Analgesic and antipyretic: Oral, rectal: 325-1000 mg every 4-6 hours up to 4 g/day

Anti-inflammatory: Oral: Initial: 2.4-3.6 g/day in divided doses; usual maintenance: 3.6-5.4 g/day; monitor serum concentrations

Suspected acute MI: Oral: Initial: 160-162.5 mg as soon as MI is suspected; then 160-162.5 mg once daily for 30 days post MI; then consider further aspirin treatment

MI prophylaxis: Oral: 75-325 mg once daily (continue indefinitely)

Prevention of stroke following ischemic stroke or TIA: Oral: 50-325 mg once daily (continue indefinitely)

Administration Oral: Administer with water, food, or milk to decrease GI upset. Do not crush or chew controlled release, timed release, or enteric coated tablets; these preparations should be swallowed whole

Monitoring Parameters Serum salicylate concentration with chronic use

Reference Range

Therapeutic levels:

Anti-inflammatory effect: 150-300 µg/mL

Analgesic and antipyretic effect: 30-50 µg/mL

Timing of serum samples: Peak levels usually occur 2 hours after normal doses but may occur 6-24 hours after acute toxic ingestion.

Salicylate serum concentrations correlate with the pharmacological actions and adverse effects observed. See table on next page.

(Continued)

Aspirin *(Continued)*

Serum Salicylate: Clinical Correlations

Serum Salicylate Concentration (μg/mL)	Desired Effects	Adverse Effects/Intoxication
~100	Antiplatelet Antipyresis Analgesia	GI intolerance and bleeding, hypersensitivity, hemostatic defects
150-300	Anti-inflammatory	Mild salicylism
250-400	Treatment of rheumatic fever	Nausea/vomiting, hyperventilation, salicylism, flushing, sweating, thirst, headache, diarrhea, and tachycardia
>400-500		Respiratory alkalosis, hemorrhage, excitement, confusion, asterixis, pulmonary edema, convulsions, tetany, metabolic acidosis, fever, coma, cardiovascular collapse, renal and respiratory failure

Test Interactions False-negative results for glucose oxidase urinary glucose tests (Clinistix®); false-positives using the cupric sulfate method (Clinitest®); interferes with Gerhardt test, VMA determination; 5-HIAA, xylose tolerance test and T_3 and T_4

Patient Information Watch for bleeding gums or signs of GI bleeding, (bright red blood in emesis or stool, coffee ground-like emesis, black tarry stools); notify physician if ringing in the ears, persistent GI pain, or GI bleeding occurs

Dosage Forms

Caplet, buffered:
  Ascriptin® Arthritis Pain: 325 mg [contains aluminum hydroxide, calcium carbonate, and magnesium hydroxide]
  Ascriptin® Extra Strength: 500 mg [contains aluminum hydroxide, calcium carbonate, and magnesium hydroxide]
Gelcap:
  Bayer® Aspirin: 325 mg
  Bayer® Aspirin Extra Strength: 500 mg
Gum (Aspergum®): 227 mg
Suppository, rectal: 60 mg, 120 mg, 125 mg, 200 mg, 300 mg, 325 mg, 600 mg, 650 mg
Tablet: 325 mg, 500 mg
  Aspercin: 325 mg
  Aspercin Extra, Bayer® Aspirin Extra Strength: 500 mg
  Bayer® Aspirin: 325 mg [film coated]
Tablet, buffered:
  Ascriptin®: 325 mg [contains aluminum hydroxide, calcium carbonate, and magnesium hydroxide]
  Bayer® Plus Extra Strength: 500 mg [contains calcium carbonate]
  Bufferin®: 325 mg [contains citric acid]
  Bufferin® Arthritis Strength, Bufferin® Extra Strength: 500 mg [contains citric acid]
Tablet, chewable: 81 mg
  Children's Bayer® Aspirin Regimen, St. Joseph Pain Reliever: 81 mg
Tablet, controlled release (ZORprin®): 800 mg
Tablet, enteric coated: 81 mg, 162 mg, 325 mg, 500 mg, 650 mg, 975 mg
  Ascriptin® Enteric, Bayer® Aspirin Regimen Adult Low Strength, Ecotrin® Adult Low Strength, St. Joseph Pain Reliever: 81 mg
  Bayer® Aspirin Regimen Adult Low Strength With Calcium: 81 mg [contains 250 mg calcium carbonate]
  Bayer® Aspirin Regimen Regular Strength, Ecotrin®: 325 mg
  Easprin®: 975 mg
  Ecotrin® Maximum Strength: 500 mg
  Halfprin®: 81 mg, 162 mg

References

Hathaway WE, "Use of Antiplatelet Agents in Pediatric Hypercoagulable States," *Am J Dis Child*, 1984, 138(3):301-4.

Monagle P, Michelson AD, Bovill E, et al, "Antithrombotic Therapy in Children," *Chest*, 2001, 119(1 Suppl):344S-370S.

Pickering LK, ed, *2000 Red Book, Report of the Committee on Infectious Diseases*, 25th ed, Elk Grove Village IL: American Academy of Pediatrics, 2000, 360-3.

♦ **Aspirin and Oxycodone** *see* Oxycodone and Aspirin *on page 848*
♦ **Aspirin Free Anacin® Maximum Strength** *see* Acetaminophen *on page 36*

- **Astelin®** *see* Azelastine *on page 151*
- **Asthma Guidelines** *see page 1376*
- **Astramorph/PF™** *see* Morphine Sulfate *on page 778*
- **Atarax®** *see* HydrOXYzine *on page 584*
- **Atasol® (Can)** *see* Acetaminophen *on page 36*

Atenolol (a TEN oh lole)

Related Information
Overdose and Toxicology *on page 1388*

U.S. Brand Names Tenormin®

Canadian Brand Names Apo®-Atenolol; Gen-Atenolol; Novo-Atenol; Nu-Atenol; PMS-Atenolol; Rhoxal-atenolol; Tenolin

Therapeutic Category Antianginal Agent; Antihypertensive Agent; Beta-Adrenergic Blocker

Generic Available Yes (tablet)

Use Treatment of hypertension, alone or in combination with other agents; management of angina pectoris; antiarrhythmic; post-MI patients; acute alcohol withdrawal

Pregnancy Risk Factor D

Contraindications Hypersensitivity to atenolol or any component; pulmonary edema, cardiogenic shock, bradycardia, heart block, or uncompensated CHF

Warnings Abrupt withdrawal of the drug should be avoided; drug should be discontinued over 1-2 weeks

Precautions Use with caution and modify dosage in patients with renal impairment; use with caution in patients with CHF, bronchospastic disease, diabetes mellitus, and hyperthyroidism. Patients who have a history of anaphylactic hypersensitivity reactions to various substances may be more reactive while receiving beta-blockers; these patients may not be responsive to the normal doses of epinephrine used to treat hypersensitivity reactions.

Adverse Reactions
Cardiovascular: Bradycardia, hypotension, second or third degree A-V block, CHF, chest pain, edema, Raynaud's phenomenon
Central nervous system: Dizziness, fatigue, lethargy, headache, nightmares, insomnia, confusion, mental impairment
Gastrointestinal: Constipation, nausea, diarrhea
Respiratory: Wheezing and dyspnea have occurred with higher doses (eg, >100 mg/day in adults)

Drug Interactions Catecholamine-depleting drugs, such as reserpine, may have additive effects (hypotension, bradycardia); hypotensive agents, diuretics, cardiac glycosides, amiodarone, calcium channel blockers, agents that slow AV conduction, and myocardial depressant general anesthetics may have additive effects with beta-blockers; abrupt withdrawal of clonidine while receiving beta-blockers may result in an exaggerated hypertensive crisis; NSAIDs may decrease the antihypertensive effects of beta-blockers; atenolol (especially at higher doses) may reverse the therapeutic effects of theophylline

Mechanism of Action Competitively blocks response to beta-adrenergic stimulation; selectively blocks beta$_1$-receptors with little or no effect on beta$_2$-receptors except at high doses; does not possess membrane stabilizing or intrinsic sympathomimetic (partial agonist) activities

Pharmacodynamics
Beta-blocking effect:
Onset of action: Oral: ≤1 hour
Maximum effect:
Oral: 2-4 hours
I.V.: ≤5 minutes
Duration:
Oral: ≥24 hours
I.V.: 12 hours
Antihypertensive effect:
Duration: Oral: 24 hours

Pharmacokinetics
Absorption: Incomplete from the GI tract; ~50% absorbed
Distribution: Does not cross the blood-brain barrier; low lipophilicity
Protein binding: Low (6% to 16%)
Half-life, beta:
Neonates: Mean: 16 hours, up to 35 hours
Children 5-16 years of age: Mean: 4.6 hours; range: 3.5-7 hours; children >10 years of age may have longer half-life (>5 hours) compared to children 5-10 years of age (<5 hours)
Adults: 6-7 hours
(Continued)

Atenolol (Continued)

Prolonged half-life with renal dysfunction
Time to peak serum concentration: Oral: Within 2-4 hours
Elimination: 40% as unchanged drug in urine, 50% in feces
Dialysis: Moderately dialyzable (20% to 50%)

Usual Dosage

Oral:
Children: Initial: 0.8-1 mg/kg/dose given daily; range: 0.8-1.5 mg/kg/day; maximum dose: 2 mg/kg/day; do not exceed adult maximum dose of 100 mg/day
Adults:
Initial: 25-50 mg/dose given daily; usual dose: 50-100 mg/dose given daily
Maximum dose: Hypertension: 100 mg given daily; angina: 200 mg given daily
See table for oral dosing interval in renal impairment.

Creatinine Clearance	Maximum Oral Dose	Frequency of Administration
15-35 mL/min	50 mg or 1 mg/kg/dose	Daily
<15 mL/min	50 mg or 1 mg/kg/dose	Every other day

I.V.: Adults: For early treatment of MI: 5 mg slow I.V. over 5 minutes; may repeat in 10 minutes; if both doses are tolerated, may start oral atenolol 50 mg every 12 hours for 6-9 days post MI

Administration

Oral: May be administered without regard to food
Parenteral: Administer by slow I.V. injection at a rate not to exceed 1 mg/minute; the injection can be administered undiluted or diluted with a compatible I.V. solution

Monitoring Parameters Blood pressure, heart rate, EKG, fluid intake and output, daily weight, respiratory rate

Patient Information Abrupt withdrawal of the drug should be avoided

Additional Information In diabetic patients, atenolol may potentiate hypoglycemia and mask signs and symptoms of hypoglycemia; limited data suggests that atenolol may have a shorter half-life and faster clearance in patients with Marfan syndrome. Higher doses (2 mg/kg/day divided every 12 hours) have been used in patients with Marfan syndrome (6-22 years of age) to decrease aortic root growth rate and prevent aortic dissection or rupture; further studies are needed.

Dosage Forms

Injection, solution (Tenormin®): 0.5 mg/mL (10 mL)
Tablet: 25 mg, 50 mg, 100 mg

Extemporaneous Preparations

A 2 mg/mL atenolol oral liquid compounded from tablets and a commercially available oral diluent was found to be stable for up to 40 days when stored at 5°C or 25°C (Garner, 1994)

Stability of a 2 mg/mL atenolol oral liquid compounded from tablets and several different vehicles was studied at room temperature in amber prescription bottles. The 2 mg/mL atenolol oral liquid in Ora-Sweet® SF was stable for 90 days; in a vehicle of simple syrup, the preparation was stable for approximately 3 weeks; when formulated in Ora-Sweet® however, the preparation was stable for <1 week (Patel, 1997)

Garner SS, Wiest DB, and Reynolds ER, "Stability of Atenolol in an Extemporaneously Compounded Oral Liquid," *Am J Hosp Pharm*, 1994, 51(4):508-11.

Patel D, Doski DH, and Desai A, "Short-Term Stability of Atenolol in Oral Liquid Formulations," *Int J Pharmaceut Compd*, 1997, 1:437-9.

References

Buck ML, Wiest D, Gillette PC, et al, "Pharmacokinetics and Pharmacodynamics of Atenolol in Children," *Clin Pharmacol Ther*, 1989, 46(6):629-33.

Case CL, Trippel DL, and Gillette PC, "New Antiarrhythmic Agents in Pediatrics," *Pediatr Clin North Am*, 1989, 36(5):1293-320.

Trippel DL and Gillette PC, "Atenolol in Children With Supraventricular Tachycardia," *Am J Cardiol*, 1989, 64(3):233-6.

Trippel DL and Gillette PC, "Atenolol in Children With Ventricular Arrhythmias," *Am Heart J*, 1990, 119(6):1312-6.

♦ **ATG** see Antithymocyte Globulin (Equine) on page 123

♦ **Atgam®** see Antithymocyte Globulin (Equine) on page 123

♦ **Ativan®** see Lorazepam on page 695

Atomoxetine (AT oh mox e teen)

U.S. Brand Names Strattera™
Synonyms LY139603; Tomoxetine
Therapeutic Category Norepinephrine Reuptake Inhibitor, Selective

Generic Available No

Use Treatment of attention deficit/hyperactivity disorder (ADHD); has been used investigationally to treat depression

Pregnancy Risk Factor C

Contraindications Hypersensitivity to atomoxetine or any component; concurrent use or use within 14 days of MAO inhibitors; narrow-angle glaucoma

Warnings Allergic reactions (including rash, urticaria, and angioneurotic edema) may occur. Suppression of growth may occur with long-term use in children (monitor carefully; consider interruption of therapy in children who are not growing or gaining weight appropriately).

Precautions May cause increased heart rate or blood pressure, use with caution in patients with hypertension, tachycardia, or other cardiovascular or cerebrovascular disease; may cause orthostatic hypotension, use with caution in patients with conditions that predispose to hypotension; may cause urinary retention or hesitancy, use with caution in patients with a history of urinary retention or bladder outlet obstruction; use with caution and reduce the dose in patients with hepatic dysfunction; use with caution in patients who are cytochrome P450 CYP2D6 poor metabolizers; use with caution and modify dose in patients receiving strong CYP2D6 inhibitors (see Drug Interactions and Usual Dosage). Safety and efficacy have not been established in children <6 years of age; safety and efficacy of long-term use have not been established.

Adverse Reactions Note: Adverse reactions reported to be increased in poor metabolizers of CYP2D6 substrates include: Decreased appetite, insomnia, sedation, depression, tremor, early morning awakening, pruritus, and mydriasis

Cardiovascular: Palpitations, tachycardia, hypertension, orthostatic hypotension, chest pain

Central nervous system: Headache, insomnia, fatigue, lethargy, irritability, somnolence, dizziness, mood swings, abnormal dreams, sleep disorder, pyrexia, rigors, crying, aggression, sedation, depression, early morning awakening

Dermatologic: Dermatitis, pruritus

Endocrine & metabolic: Weight loss, dysmenorrhea, decreased libido, menstruation disorders, hot flashes

Gastrointestinal: Xerostomia, abdominal pain, vomiting, decreased appetite, dyspepsia, diarrhea, flatulence, constipation, nausea

Genitourinary: Sexual dysfunction

Neuromuscular & skeletal: Paresthesia, myalgia, tremor

Ocular: Mydriasis

Renal: Urinary retention, urinary hesitation, difficulty in micturition

Respiratory: Cough, rhinorrhea, sinus headache

Miscellaneous: Increased diaphoresis, sinusitis, ear infection, influenza, hypersensitivity reactions, urticaria, angioedema

Drug Interactions Cytochrome P450 isoenzyme CYP2D6 and CYP2C19 (minor) substrate

Concurrent use or use within 2 weeks of MAO inhibitors may cause serious and potentially fatal reactions, eg, hyperthermia, rigidity, myoclonus, mental status changes, autonomic instability, neuroleptic malignant syndrome (combined use is contraindicated). Atomoxetine may potentiate cardiovascular effects of albuterol and sympathomimetic or pressor agents (use atomoxetine with caution and monitor patients closely); atomoxetine may increase midazolam serum concentrations (monitor patients). Cytochrome P450 CYP2D6 inhibitors (eg, paroxetine, fluoxetine, quinidine) may increase atomoxetine concentrations in extensive metabolizers (atomoxetine dosage reduction may be needed; see Usual Dosage).

Food Interactions A high fat meal decreases the rate, but not the extent of absorption.

Stability Store at room temperature of 25°C (77°F).

Mechanism of Action Enhances norepinephrine activity by selectively inhibiting norepinephrine reuptake; little to no activity at other neuronal reuptake pumps or receptor sites

Pharmacokinetics

Absorption: Oral: Rapid

Distribution: V_d: Adults: I.V.: 0.85 L/kg

Protein binding: 98%, primarily albumin

Metabolism: Extensive in the liver, primarily by oxidative metabolism via cytochrome P450 CYP2D6 to 4-hydroxyatomoxetine (major metabolite regardless of CYP2D6 status, active, equipotent to atomoxetine) with subsequent glucuronidation; also metabolized via CYP2C19 to N-desmethylatomoxetine (active, minimal activity);

Note: CYP2D6 poor metabolizers have atomoxetine AUCs that are ~10-fold higher and peak concentrations that are ~5-fold greater than extensive metabolizers; 4-hyroxyatomoxetine plasma concentrations are very low (extensive metabolizers: (Continued)

139

Atomoxetine *(Continued)*

1% of atomoxetine concentrations; poor metabolizers: 0.1% of atomoxetine concentrations)

Bioavailability: Extensive metabolizers: 63%; poor metabolizers: 94%

Half-life: Adults:

Atomoxetine: Extensive metabolizers: 5.2 hours; poor metabolizers: 21.6 hours

4-hydroxyatomoxetine: Extensive metabolizers: 6-8 hours

N-desmethlyatomoxetine: Extensive metabolizers: 6-8 hours; poor metabolizers: 34-40 hours

Elimination: Urine: <3% is excreted unchanged; 80% excreted as 4-hydroxyatomoxetine glucuronide; feces: <17%

Usual Dosage Oral:

Children and Adolescents ≤70 kg: Initial: 0.5 mg/kg/day; increase after a minimum of 3 days to approximately 1.2 mg/kg/day; may administer once daily in the morning or divide into two doses and administer in the morning and late afternoon/early evening. Maximum daily dose: 1.4 mg/kg/day or 100 mg/day, whichever is less. **Note:** Doses >1.2 mg/kg/day have not been shown to provide additional benefit.

Note: In patients receiving strong CYP2D6 inhibitors (eg, paroxetine, fluoxetine, quinidine), maintain the above listed initial dose for 4 weeks; increase dose to 1.2 mg/kg/day only if clinically needed and the initial dose is well tolerated; do not exceed 1.2 mg/kg/day

Children and Adolescents >70 kg and Adults: Initial: 40 mg/day; increase after a minimum of 3 days to approximately 80 mg/day; may administer once daily in the morning or divide into two doses and administer in morning and late afternoon/early evening. May increase (if needed) to 100 mg/day in 2-4 additional weeks

Note: In patients receiving strong CYP2D6 inhibitors (eg, paroxetine, fluoxetine, quinidine), maintain the above listed initial dose for 4 weeks; increase dose to 80 mg/day only if clinically needed and the initial dose is well tolerated; do not exceed 80 mg/day

Dosage adjustment in renal impairment: No adjustment needed

Dosage adjustment in hepatic impairment:

Moderate hepatic insufficiency (Child-Pugh class B): All doses should be reduced to 50% of normal

Severe hepatic insufficiency (Child-Pugh class C): All doses should be reduced to 25% of normal

Administration Oral: May be administered without regard to food.

Monitoring Parameters Weight, height (in children), blood pressure, heart rate

Patient Information Inform physician if you have allergies, narrow-angle glaucoma (an eye disease), current or past liver problems, or high or low blood pressure; report problems with rapid or irregular heartbeats. Some medicines should not be taken with atomoxetine; report the use of other medications, nonprescription medications, and herbal or natural products to your physician and pharmacist. If a dose is missed, take it as soon as possible, but do not take more than the prescribed total daily amount in any 24-hour period. May cause dizziness and impair ability to perform activities requiring mental alertness or physical coordination; may cause weight loss; may cause decreased growth in children; may make it difficult to urinate; may cause dry mouth

Additional Information Atomoxetine hydrochloride is the R(-) isomer. Therapy may be discontinued without being tapered. Total daily doses >150 mg/day and single doses >120 mg/dose have not been systematically evaluated. Medications used to treat ADHD should be part of a total treatment program that may include other components such as psychological, educational, and social measures. If used for an extended period of time, long-term usefulness of atomoxetine should be periodically re-evaluated for the individual patient.

Dosage Forms Available as atomoxetine hydrochloride; mg strength refers to atomoxetine

Capsule: 10 mg, 18 mg, 25 mg, 40 mg, 60 mg

References

Biderman J, Heiligenstein JH, Faries DE, at al, "Efficacy of Atomoxetine Versus Placebo in School-Age Girls With Attention-Deficit/Hyperactivity Disorder," *Pediatrics,* 2002, 110(6), http://www.pediatrics.org/cgi/content/full/110/6/e75.

Kratochvil CJ, Heiligenstein JH, Dittmann R, et al, "Atomoxetine and Methylphenidate Treatment in Children With ADHD: A Prospective, Randomized, Open-Label trial," *J Am Acad Child Adolesc Psychiatry,* 2002, 41(7):776-84.

Michelson D, Allen AJ, Busner J, et al, "Once-Daily Atomoxetine Treatment for Children and Adolescents With Attention Deficit Hyperactivity Disorder: A Randomized, Placebo-Controlled Study," *Am J Psychiatry,* 2002, 159(11):1896-901.

Michelson D, Faries D, Wernicke J, et al, "Atomoxetine in the Treatment of Children and Adolescents With Attention-Deficit/Hyperactivity Disorder: A Ramdomized, Placebo-Controlled, Dose-Response Study," *Pediatrics,* 2001, 108(5), http://www.pediatrics.org.cgi/content/full/108/5/e83.

Spencer T, Heiligenstein JH, Biederman J, et al, "Results From 2 Proof-of-Concept, Placebo-Controlled Studies of Atomoxetine in Children With Attention-Deficit/Hyperactivity Disorder," *J Clin Psychiatry*, 2002, 63(12):1140-7.

Wernicke JF and Kratochvil CJ, "Safety Profile of Atomoxetine in the Treatment of Children and Adolescents With ADHD," *J Clin Psychiatry*, 2002, 63(Suppl 12):50-5.

Atovaquone (a TOE va kwone)

U.S. Brand Names Mepron®

Synonyms Hydroxy-1,4-naphthoquinone

Therapeutic Category Antiprotozoal

Generic Available No

Use Second-line treatment of mild to moderate *Pneumocystis carinii* pneumonia (PCP) in patients intolerant of trimethoprim/sulfamethoxazole (TMP/SMX); mild to moderate PCP is defined as an alveolar-arterial oxygen diffusion gradient ≤45 mm Hg and PaO_2 ≥60 mm Hg on room air; patients intolerant of TMP/SMX are defined as having a significant rash (ie, Stevens-Johnson-like syndrome), neutropenia, or hemolysis; prevention of PCP in patients who are intolerant to TMP/SMX; treatment of babesiosis

Pregnancy Risk Factor C

Contraindications Hypersensitivity to atovaquone or any component (see Warnings)

Warnings Clinical experience with atovaquone has been limited to patients with mild to moderate PCP; treatment of more severe episodes of PCP has not been systematically studied

Suspension contains benzyl alcohol which may cause allergic reactions in susceptible individuals; large amounts of benzyl alcohol (≥99 mg/kg/day) have been associated with a potentially fatal toxicity ("gasping syndrome") in neonates; the "gasping syndrome" consists of metabolic acidosis, respiratory distress, gasping respirations, CNS dysfunction (including convulsions, intracranial hemorrhage), hypotension and cardiovascular collapse; avoid use in neonates; *in vitro* and animal studies have shown that benzoate, a metabolite of benzyl alcohol, displaces bilirubin from protein binding sites

Precautions For patients who have difficulty taking atovaquone with food or who have chronic diarrhea, stomach or intestinal problems which may result in drug malabsorption, parenteral therapy with other agents should be considered since a low serum atovaquone concentration could lead to treatment failure

Adverse Reactions

Central nervous system: Fever, headache, insomnia, dizziness, pain

Dermatologic: Maculopapular rash, erythema multiforme, pruritus

Endocrine & metabolic: Hyponatremia

Gastrointestinal: Nausea, vomiting, diarrhea, abdominal pain, constipation, anorexia, elevated amylase

Hematologic: Rare: Neutropenia, anemia

Hepatic: Elevated hepatic enzymes, cholestasis

Respiratory: Cough, sinusitis

Miscellaneous: Diaphoresis

Drug Interactions Rifampin may decrease plasma atovaquone concentration; since atovaquone is highly protein bound, it may compete for protein binding sites with other highly protein-bound agents like warfarin (however, there have been no drug-drug interactions of this type reported to date)

Food Interactions Administration with food increases bioavailability of atovaquone suspension 1.4-fold over that achieved in a fasting state or up to 3-fold with a high fat meal

Stability Store at room temperature; do not freeze

Mechanism of Action The mechanism of action against *Pneumocystis carinii* has not been fully elucidated; in *Plasmodium* species, atovaquone selectively inhibits the mitochondrial electron-transport system at the cytochrome bc_1 complex resulting in depletion of dihydroorotate dehydrogenase and ultimately resulting in the inhibition of nucleic acid and adenosine triphosphate synthesis

Pharmacokinetics

Absorption: Oral:

Infants and Children <2 years of age: Decreased absorption

Adults: Oral suspension: Absorption is enhanced 1.4-fold with food; decreased absorption with single doses exceeding 750 mg

Distribution: V_{dss}: 0.6 L/kg; CSF concentration is <1% of the plasma concentration

Protein binding: >99%

Bioavailability: Suspension (administered with food): 47%

Half-life, elimination:

Children (4 months to 12 years): 60 hours (range: 31-163 hours)

Adults: 2.9 days

Adults with AIDS: 2.2 days

(Continued)

Atovaquone *(Continued)*

Time to peak serum concentration: Dual peak serum concentrations at 1 to 8 hours and at 24 to 96 hours after dose due to enterohepatic cycling

Elimination: ~94% is recovered as unchanged drug in feces; 0.6% excreted in urine

Usual Dosage Oral:

Children:

Treatment: Dose of 40 mg/kg/day divided twice daily (maximum dose: 1500 mg/day) may be necessary to attain comparable plasma concentrations associated with the successful treatment of PCP as seen in adults.

Prophylaxis of *Pneumocystis carinii* pneumonia:

1-3 months of age and >24 months of age: 30 mg/kg/day once daily (maximum dose: 1500 mg/day)

4-24 months of age: 45 mg/kg/day once daily (maximum dose: 1500 mg/day)

Babesiosis: 40 mg/kg/day divided twice daily (maximum dose: 1500 mg/day) with azithromycin 12 mg/kg/day once daily for 7-10 days

Adolescents 13-16 years and Adults:

Treatment: 750 mg/dose twice daily for 21 days

Prophylaxis of *Pneumocystis carinii* pneumonia: 1500 mg once daily

Babesiosis: 750 mg/dose twice daily for 7-10 days with azithromycin 1000 mg once daily for 3 days then 500 mg once daily for 7 days

Administration Oral: Administer with food or a high-fat meal; shake suspension well before using

Monitoring Parameters CBC with differential, liver enzymes, serum chemistries, serum amylase

Additional Information The suspension contains the inactive ingredient poloxamer 188

Dosage Forms Suspension, oral: 750 mg/5 mL (5 mL, 210 mL) [contains benzyl alcohol; citrus flavor]

References

Centers for Disease Control and Prevention, "2001 USPHS/IDSA Guidelines for the Prevention of Opportunistic Infections in Persons Infected With Human Immunodeficiency Virus," November 28, 2001, http://www.aidsinfo.nih.gov

Haile LG and Flaherty JF, "Atovaquone: A Review," *Ann Pharmacother*, 1993, 27(12):1488-94.

Hughes W, Dorenbaum A, Yogev R, et al, "Phase I Safety and Pharmacokinetics Study of Micronized Atovaquone Human Immunodeficiency Virus-Infected Infants and Children. Pediatric AIDS Clinical Trials Group," *Antimicrob Agents Chemother*, 1998, 42(6):1315-8.

Hughes W, Leoung G, Kramer F, et al, "Comparison of Atovaquone (566C80) With Trimethoprim-Sulfamethoxazole to Treat *Pneumocystis carinii* Pneumonia in Patients With AIDS," *N Engl J Med*, 1993, 328(21):1521-7.

Atracurium *(a tra KYOO ree um)*

U.S. Brand Names Tracrium®

Therapeutic Category Neuromuscular Blocker Agent, Nondepolarizing; Skeletal Muscle Relaxant, Paralytic

Generic Available Yes

Use Eases endotracheal intubation as an adjunct to general anesthesia and relaxes skeletal muscle during surgery or mechanical ventilation

Pregnancy Risk Factor C

Contraindications Hypersensitivity to atracurium besylate or any component

Warnings Reduce initial dosage and inject slowly (over 1-2 minutes) in patients in whom substantial histamine release would be potentially hazardous (eg, patients with clinically important cardiovascular disease); maintenance of an adequate airway and respiratory support is critical; avoid use of preservative-containing formulation in

Clinical Conditions Affecting Neuromuscular Blockade

Potentiation	Antagonism
Electrolyte abnormalities	Alkalosis
Severe hyponatremia	Hypercalcemia
Severe hypocalcemia	Demyelinating lesions
Severe hypokalemia	Peripheral neuropathies
Hypermagnesemia	Diabetes mellitus
Neuromuscular diseases	
Acidosis	
Acute intermittent porphyria	
Renal failure	
Hepatic failure	

neonates; certain clinical conditions may result in potentiation or antagonism of neuromuscular blockade, see table on previous page.

Increased sensitivity in patients with myasthenia gravis, Eaton-Lambert syndrome; resistance to neuromuscular blockade in burn patients (>30% of body) for period of 5-70 days postinjury; resistance in patients with muscle trauma, denervation, immobilization, infection, chronic treatment with atracurium. When used in conjunction with anesthetics, bradycardia may be more common with atracurium than with other neuromuscular blocking agents; it has no clinically significant effects on heart rate to counteract the bradycardia produced by anesthetics.

Precautions Due to potential histamine release, use with caution in patients in whom histamine release may be hazardous (eg, cardiovascular disease, asthma); patients with severe electrolyte disorders; patients with myasthenia gravis

Adverse Reactions
Cardiovascular: Effects are minimal and transient
Dermatologic: Erythema, itching, urticaria
Respiratory: Wheezing, bronchial secretions (increased)

Drug Interactions See table.

Potential Drug Interactions

Potentiation	Antagonism
Inhalation anesthetics	Calcium
Desflurane, sevoflurane, enflurane and	Carbamazepine
isoflurane > halothane > nitrous	Phenytoin
oxide	Steroids (chronic administration)
Antibiotics	Theophylline
Aminoglycosides, polymyxins,	Anticholinesterases*
clindamycin, vancomycin, tetracycline	Neostigmine, pyridostigmine,
Magnesium	edrophonium, echothiophate
Antiarrhythmics	ophthalmic solution
Quinidine, procainamide, bretylium, and	Caffeine
possibly lidocaine	Azathioprine
Diuretics	
Furosemide, mannitol, thiazides	
Amphotericin B (secondary to hypokalemia)	
Local anesthetics	
Dantrolene (directly depresses skeletal muscle)	
Beta blockers	
Calcium channel blockers	
Ketamine	
Lithium	
Succinylcholine (when administered prior to nondepolarizing neuromuscular-blocking agent)	
Cyclosporine	

*Can prolong the effects of acetylcholine

Stability Refrigerate; stable at room temperature for 14 days; unstable in alkaline solutions; compatible with D_5W, D_5NS, and NS; do not dilute in LR

Mechanism of Action Blocks neural transmission at the myoneural junction by binding with cholinergic receptor sites

Pharmacodynamics
Onset of action: I.V.: 1-4 minutes
Maximum effect: Within 3-5 minutes
Duration: Recovery begins in 20-35 minutes when anesthesia is balanced

Pharmacokinetics
Distribution: V_d:
Infants: 0.21 L/kg
Children: 0.13 L/kg
Adults: 0.1 L/kg
Metabolism: Some metabolites are active; undergoes rapid nonenzymatic degradation (Hofmann elimination) in the bloodstream; additional metabolism occurs via ester hydrolysis
Half-life: Elimination:
Infants: 20 minutes
(Continued)

Atracurium (Continued)

Children: 17 minutes
Adults: 16 minutes
Elimination: Clearance:
Infants: 7.9 mL/kg/minute
Children: 6.8 mL/kg/minute
Adults: 5.3 mL/kg/minute

Usual Dosage I.V.:
Neonates, Infants, and Children ≤2 years:
0.3-0.4 mg/kg initially followed by maintenance doses of 0.3-0.4 mg/kg as needed to maintain neuromuscular blockade
or
Continuous infusion: 0.6-1.2 mg/kg/hour or 10-20 mcg/kg/minute
Children >2 years to Adults:
0.4-0.5 mg/kg then 0.08-0.1 mg/kg 20-45 minutes after initial dose to maintain neuromuscular block
or
Continuous infusion: 0.4-0.8 mg/kg/hour or 6.7-13 mcg/kg/minute (range: 2-15 mcg/kg/minute)

Dosage adjustment in hepatic or renal impairment: Not necessary

Dosage adjustment with enflurane or isoflurane: Reduce dosage by 33%

Dosage adjustment with induced hypothermia (cardio-bypass surgery): Reduce dosage by 50%

Administration Parenteral: May be administered without further dilution by rapid I.V. injection; for continuous infusions, dilute to a maximum concentration of 0.5 mg/mL (more concentrated solutions have reduced stability, ie, <24 hours at room temperature); not for I.M. injection due to tissue irritation

Monitoring Parameters Muscle twitch response to peripheral nerve stimulation, heart rate, blood pressure

Additional Information Neuromuscular blockade may be reversed with neostigmine; atropine or glycopyrrolate should be available to treat excessive cholinergic effects from neostigmine

Dosage Forms
Injection, as besylate: 10 mg/mL (5 mL, 10 mL)
Injection, as besylate [preservative free]: 10 mg/mL (5 mL)

References
Martin LD, Bratton SL, and O'Rourke PP, "Clinical Uses and Controversies of Neuromuscular Blocking Agents in Infants and Children," Crit Care Med, 1999, 27(7):1358-68.

♦ Atrial Fibrillation / Atrial Flutter see page 1193

Atropine (A troe peen)

Related Information
Adult ACLS Algorithm, Asystole on page 1187
Adult ACLS Algorithm, Bradycardia on page 1188
Adult ACLS Algorithm, Pulseless Electrical Activity on page 1186
Asthma Guidelines on page 1376
Compatibility of Medications Mixed in a Syringe on page 1412
CPR Pediatric Drug Dosages on page 1175
Overdose and Toxicology on page 1388
Pediatric ALS Algorithm, Bradycardia on page 1179

U.S. Brand Names Atropine-Care®; Atropisol®; Isopto® Atropine; Ocu-Tropine®; Sal-Tropine™

Canadian Brand Names Dioptic's Atropine Solution; Minim's Atropine Solution

Therapeutic Category Antiasthmatic; Anticholinergic Agent; Anticholinergic Agent, Ophthalmic; Antidote, Organophosphate Poisoning; Antispasmodic Agent, Gastrointestinal; Bronchodilator; Ophthalmic Agent, Mydriatic

Generic Available Yes

Use Preoperative medication to inhibit salivation and secretions; treatment of sinus bradycardia; treatment of asystole and pulseless electrical activity (adults); management of peptic ulcer; reversal of the muscarinic effects of cholinergic agents such as neostigmine and pyridostigmine; treatment of exercise-induced bronchospasm; antidote for organophosphate or carbamate pesticide poisoning; used to produce mydriasis and cycloplegia for examination of the retina and optic disk and accurate measurement of refractive errors; treatment of uveitis

Pregnancy Risk Factor C

Contraindications Hypersensitivity to atropine sulfate or any component; narrow-angle glaucoma; tachycardia; thyrotoxicosis; obstructive disease of the GI tract; obstructive uropathy

Precautions Use with caution in children with spastic paralysis or brain damage; children are at increased risk for rapid rise in body temperature due to suppression of sweat gland activity; paradoxical hyperexcitability may occur in children given large doses; infants with Down's syndrome have both increased sensitivity to cardiac effects and mydriasis

Adverse Reactions
Cardiovascular: Tachycardia, palpitations
Central nervous system: Fatigue, delirium, headache, restlessness, ataxia
Dermatologic: Dry hot skin
Gastrointestinal: Impaired GI motility
Neuromuscular & skeletal: Tremor
Ocular: Blurred vision

Drug Interactions Additive effects when administered with other anticholinergic agents; may alter response to beta-adrenergic blockers

Mechanism of Action Blocks the action of acetylcholine at parasympathetic sites in smooth muscle, secretory glands, and the CNS; increases cardiac output, dries secretions, antagonizes histamine and serotonin

Pharmacodynamics
Inhibition of salivation:
Onset of action:
Oral: 30-60 minutes
I.M.: 30 minutes
Maximum effect:
Oral: 2 hours
I.M.: 1-1.6 hours
Duration: Oral, I.M.: Up to 4 hours
Increased heart rate:
Onset of action:
Oral: 30 minutes to 2 hours
I.M.: 5-40 minutes
Maximum effect:
Oral: 1-2 hours
I.M.: 20 minutes to 1 hour
I.V.: 2-4 minutes
Bronchodilation: Oral Inhalation:
Onset of action: 15 minutes
Maximum effect: 15 minutes to 1.5 hours

Pharmacokinetics
Absorption: Well absorbed from all dosage forms
Distribution: Widely distributes throughout the body; crosses the placenta; trace amounts appear in breast milk; crosses the blood-brain barrier
Protein binding: 20%
Metabolism: In the liver
Half-life: Adults: 2-3 hours
Elimination: Both metabolites and unchanged drug (30% to 50%) are excreted into urine

Usual Dosage Note: Doses <0.1 mg have been associated with paradoxical brady-cardia

Neonates, Infants and Children:
Preanesthetic: Oral, I.M., I.V., S.C.:
<5 kg: 0.02 mg/kg/dose 30-60 minutes preop then every 4-6 hours as needed; use of a minimum dosage of 0.1 mg in neonates <5 kg will result in dosages >0.02 mg/kg; there is no documented minimum dosage in this age group
>5 kg: 0.01-0.02 mg/kg/dose to a maximum 0.4 mg/dose 30-60 minutes preop; minimum dose: 0.1 mg
Bradycardia: I.V., intratracheal, I.O.: 0.02 mg/kg, minimum dose 0.1 mg, maximum single dose: 0.5 mg in children and 1 mg in adolescents; may repeat in 5 minutes; maximum total dose of 1 mg in children or 2 mg in adolescents. (**Note:** For intratracheal administration, must be diluted; see Administration.) When treating bradycardia in neonates, reserve use for those patients unresponsive to improved oxygenation and epinephrine.

Children:
Bronchospasm: Inhalation: 0.03-0.05 mg/kg/dose 3-4 times/day; maximum: 2.5 mg/dose
Refraction: Ophthalmic:
Infants <1 year: Instill 1 drop of 0.25% solution 3 times/day for 3 days before the procedure
Children: 1-5 years: Instill 1 drop of 0.5% solution 3 times/day for 3 days before the procedure

(Continued)

Atropine *(Continued)*

Children >5 years or Children with dark irides: Instill 1 drop of 1% solution 3 times/day for 3 days before the procedure

Organophosphate or carbamate poisoning: I.V.: 0.02-0.05 mg/kg every 10-20 minutes until atropine effect (dry flushed skin, tachycardia, mydriasis, fever) is observed then every 1-4 hours for at least 24 hours

Uveitis: Ophthalmic: Instill 1 drop of 0.5% solution 1-3 times daily

Adults (doses <0.5 mg have been associated with paradoxical bradycardia):

Asystole and slow pulseless electrical activity: I.V.: 1 mg; may repeat every 3-5 minutes as needed to a total dose of 0.04 mg/kg

Preanesthetic: Oral, I.M., I.V., S.C.: 0.4-0.6 mg 30-60 minutes preop

Bradycardia: I.V.: 0.5-1 mg every 5 minutes, not to exceed a total of 2 mg or 0.04 mg/kg

Bronchospasm: Inhalation: 0.025-0.05 mg/kg/dose every 4-6 hours as needed; maximum: 2.5 mg/dose

Organophosphate or carbamate poisoning: I.V.: 1-2 mg/dose every 10-20 minutes until atropine effect (dry flushed skin, tachycardia, mydriasis, fever) is observed then every 1-4 hours for at least 24 hours; up to 50 mg in first 24 hours and 2 g over several days may be given in cases of severe intoxication

Refraction: Ophthalmic: Instill 1-2 drops of 1% solution before the procedure

Uveitis: Ophthalmic: Instill 1-2 drops of 1% solution up to 4 times/day

Administration

Intratracheal: Dilute with NS to a total volume of 3-5 mL followed by several positive-pressure ventilations

Parenteral: Administer undiluted by rapid I.V. injection; slow injection may result in paradoxical bradycardia

Oral: Administer without regard to food

Ophthalmic: Due to the discontinuance of 0.5% ophthalmic solutions commercially, 0.5% and 0.25% solutions may be prepared by dilution of 1% atropine ophthalmic solution with artificial tears; a 1:1 dilution for 0.5% and a 1:4 dilution for 0.25%; instill solution into conjunctival sac of affected eye(s); avoid contact of bottle tip with eye or skin

Monitoring Parameters Heart rate

Dosage Forms

Injection, solution, as sulfate: 0.1 mg/mL (5 mL, 10 mL); 0.4 mg/mL (1 mL, 20 mL); 0.5 mg/mL (1 mL); 1 mg/mL (1 mL)

Ointment, ophthalmic, as sulfate (Ocu-Tropine®): 1% (3.5 g)

Solution, ophthalmic, as sulfate: 1% (5 mL, 15 mL)

Atropine-Care®: 1% (2 mL)

Atropisol®: 1% (1 mL)

Isopto® Atropine: 1% (5 mL, 15 mL)

Tablet, as sulfate (Sal-Tropine™): 0.4 mg

References

"Guidelines 2000 for Cardiopulmonary Resuscitation and Emergency Cardiovascular Care. Part 10: Pediatric Advanced Life Support. The American Heart Association in Collaboration With the International Liaison Committee on Resuscitation," *Circulation*, 2000, 102(8 Suppl):I291-342.

◆ **Atropine and Diphenoxylate** *see* Diphenoxylate and Atropine *on page 395*

◆ **Atropine-Care®** *see* Atropine *on page 144*

◆ **Atropine, Hyoscyamine, Scopolamine, and Phenobarbital** *see* Hyoscyamine, Atropine, Scopolamine, and Phenobarbital *on page 587*

◆ **Atropisol®** *see* Atropine *on page 144*

◆ **Atrovent®** *see* Ipratropium *on page 620*

◆ **A/T/S®** *see* Erythromycin *on page 448*

Attapulgite *(at a PULL gite)*

U.S. Brand Names Diasorb® [OTC]

Therapeutic Category Antidiarrheal

Generic Available Yes

Use Treatment of uncomplicated diarrhea

Pregnancy Risk Factor B

Contraindications Hypersensitivity to attapulgite or any component

Warnings Not to be used for self-medication for diarrhea >48 hours or in the presence of high fever in infants and children <3 years of age; do not use for diarrhea associated with pseudomembranous enterocolitis or in diarrhea caused by toxigenic bacteria

Adverse Reactions

Gastrointestinal: Constipation

Respiratory: Pneumoconiosis (from inhalation of the powder chronically as it contains large amounts of silica)

Drug Interactions May inhibit GI absorption of promazine, digoxin, clindamycin, tetracycline, and penicillamine

Mechanism of Action Controls diarrhea because of its absorbent action

Usual Dosage Adequate controlled clinical studies documenting the efficacy of attapulgite are lacking; its usage and dosage has been primarily empiric; the following are manufacturer's recommended dosages

Oral: Give after each bowel movement
Children:
3-6 years: 300-750 mg/dose; maximum dose: 7 doses/day or 2250 mg/day
6-12 years: 600-1500 mg/dose; maximum dose: 7 doses/day or 4500 mg/day
Children >12 years and Adults: 1200-3000 mg/dose; maximum dose: 8 doses/day or 9000 mg/day

Administration May be administered without regard to meals; shake liquid preparation well before use

Patient Information Do not exceed maximum number of doses per day; drink plenty of fluids; contact your physician if diarrhea persists more than 48 hours or if fever develops in children <3 years of age

Additional Information Kaopectate®, Kaopectate® Advanced Formula, Children's Kaopectate®, and Kaopectate® Maximum Strength have been reformulated. Previously, Kaopectate® contained attapulgite. The new formulation contains only bismuth subsalicylate. Bismuth salicylate has significant contraindications, particularly in children with influenza and chickenpox. Please refer to bismuth monograph for product information. During the transition period, the older formulation may still be available, read product label closely.

Dosage Forms
Liquid, oral **concentrate**: Activated attapulgite 600 mg/15 mL (120 mL, 180 mL, 240 mL); activated attapulgite 750 mg/15 mL (120 mL, 360 mL)
Diasorb®: 750 mg/5 mL (120 mL) [sugar free; cola flavor]

♦ **Augmentin®** *see* Amoxicillin and Clavulanic Acid *on page 96*

♦ **Augmentin ES-600™** *see* Amoxicillin and Clavulanic Acid *on page 96*

♦ **Augmentin XR™** *see* Amoxicillin and Clavulanic Acid *on page 96*

♦ **Auralgan®** *see* Antipyrine and Benzocaine *on page 122*

Auranofin (au RANE oh fin)

U.S. Brand Names Ridaura®

Therapeutic Category Gold Compound

Generic Available No

Use Management of active stage of classic or definite rheumatoid or psoriatic arthritis in patients who do not respond to or tolerate other agents; adjunctive or alternative therapy for pemphigus

Pregnancy Risk Factor C

Contraindications Hypersensitivity to auranofin or any component; renal disease; history of blood dyscrasias; CHF; exfoliative dermatitis; necrotizing enterocolitis; urticaria, eczema, SLE, bone marrow aplasia, pulmonary fibrosis; history of severe toxicity resulting from previous exposure to other heavy metals; patients who have recently received radiation therapy

Warnings Explain the possibility of adverse reactions before initiating therapy; signs of gold toxicity include decrease in hemoglobin, leukocytes, granulocytes and platelets, proteinuria, hematuria, pruritus, stomatitis or persistent diarrhea; advise patients to report any symptoms of toxicity; therapy should be discontinued if platelet count falls to <100,000/mm^3

Precautions Use with caution and modify dose in patients with renal impairment

Adverse Reactions
Central nervous system: Confusion, hallucinations, seizures
Dermatologic: Dermatitis, pruritus, alopecia, chrysiasis, rash, angioedema, photosensitivity
Gastrointestinal: Diarrhea, loose stools, stomatitis, abdominal cramping, metallic taste, glossitis, ulcerative enterocolitis, GI hemorrhage, gingivitis, dysphagia
Hematologic: Thrombocytopenia, aplastic anemia, eosinophilia, leukopenia
Hepatic: Elevated liver enzymes, jaundice, hepatitis
Neuromuscular & skeletal: Peripheral neuropathy
Ocular: Conjunctivitis, iritis, corneal ulcers
Renal: Proteinuria, hematuria, nephrotic syndrome
Respiratory: Interstitial pneumonitis, fibrosis, gold bronchitis
(Continued)

Auranofin (Continued)

Drug Interactions Possible increase of phenytoin serum levels (1 case reported); penicillamine, antimalarials, hydroxychloroquine, cytotoxic drugs, or immunosuppressive agents

Mechanism of Action Unknown, acts principally via immunomodulating effects and by decreasing lysosomal enzyme release; may alter cellular mechanisms by inhibiting sulfhydryl systems

Pharmacodynamics Onset of action: Therapeutic response may not be seen for 3-4 months after start of therapy

Pharmacokinetics
Absorption: Oral: Only about 20% to 25% of gold in a dose is absorbed
Protein binding: 60%
Half-life: 21-31 days (half-life dependent upon single or multiple dosing)
Time to peak serum concentration: Within 2 hours
Elimination: 60% of absorbed gold is eliminated in urine while the remainder is eliminated in feces

Usual Dosage Oral:
Children: Initial: 0.1 mg/kg/day in 1-2 divided doses; usual maintenance: 0.15 mg/kg/day in 1-2 divided doses; maximum dose: 0.2 mg/kg/day in 1-2 divided doses
Adults: 6 mg/day in 1-2 divided doses; after 3 months may be increased to 9 mg/day in 3 divided doses; if still no response after 3 months at 9 mg/day, discontinue drug

Dosing adjustment in renal impairment:
Cl_{cr} 50-80 mL/minute: Reduce dose to 50%
Cl_{cr} <50 mL/minute: Avoid use

Monitoring Parameters CBC with differential, platelet count, urinalysis, baseline renal and liver function tests

Reference Range Gold: Normal: 0-0.1 µg/mL (SI: 0-0.0064 µmol/L); Therapeutic: 1-3 µg/mL (SI: 0.06-0.18 µmol/L); Urine <0.1 µg/24 hours

Test Interactions May enhance the response to a tuberculin skin test

Patient Information Notify your physician of pruritus, sore mouth, indigestion, metallic taste; observe careful oral hygiene. May cause photosensitivity reactions (eg, exposure to sunlight may cause severe sunburn, skin rash, redness, or itching); avoid exposure to sunlight and artificial light sources (sunlamps, tanning booth/bed); wear protective clothing, wide-brimmed hats, sunglasses, and lip sunscreen (SPF ≥15); use a sunscreen [broad-spectrum sunscreen or physical sunscreen (preferred) or sunblock with SPF ≥15]; contact physician if reaction occurs.

Additional Information Metallic taste may indicate stomatitis

Dosage Forms Capsule: 3 mg [gold 29%]

♦ **Aurolate®** *see* Gold Sodium Thiomalate *on page 545*

Aurothioglucose (aur oh thye oh GLOO kose)

U.S. Brand Names Solganal®
Therapeutic Category Gold Compound
Generic Available No
Use Management of active stage of classic or definite rheumatoid or psoriatic arthritis in patients that do not respond to or tolerate other agents
Pregnancy Risk Factor C

Contraindications Hypersensitivity to aurothioglucose or any component; renal disease; history of blood dyscrasias; CHF; exfoliative dermatitis; necrotizing enterocolitis; urticaria, eczema, SLE, bone marrow aplasia, pulmonary fibrosis; history of severe toxicity resulting from previous exposure to other heavy metals; patients who have recently received radiation therapy

Warnings Explain the possibility of adverse reactions before initiating therapy; signs of gold toxicity include: decrease in hemoglobin, leukocytes, granulocytes and platelets; proteinuria, hematuria, pruritus, stomatitis, persistent diarrhea, rash, or metallic taste; advise patients to report any symptoms of toxicity; therapy should be discontinued if platelet count <100,000/mm³, WBC <4000/mm³, or granulocytes <1500/mm³

Adverse Reactions
Central nervous system: Confusion, hallucinations, seizures, encephalitis, EEG abnormalities, fever
Dermatologic: Alopecia, urticaria, mild to severe dermatitis, pruritus, chrysiasis, exfoliative dermatitis, photosensitivity
Gastrointestinal: Diarrhea, stomatitis, glossitis, metallic taste, gingivitis, ulcerative enterocolitis
Genitourinary: Vaginitis
Hematologic: Eosinophilia, leukopenia, thrombocytopenia, aplastic anemia
Hepatic: Hepatitis, jaundice, elevated liver enzymes
Neuromuscular & skeletal: Peripheral neuropathy

Ocular: Conjunctivitis, corneal ulcers, iritis

Renal: Hematuria, proteinuria, nephrotic syndrome, glomerulitis

Respiratory: Interstitial pneumonitis, fibrosis, gold bronchitis, pharyngitis, pulmonary fibrosis

Miscellaneous: Anaphylactic shock, allergic reaction

Drug Interactions Increased toxicity with penicillamine, antimalarials, hydroxychloroquine, cytotoxic agents, and immunosuppressants

Mechanism of Action Unknown, may decrease prostaglandin synthesis or may alter cellular mechanisms by inhibiting sulfhydryl systems; may decrease lysosomal enzyme release

Pharmacokinetics

Absorption: I.M.: Erratic and slow

Distribution: Crosses the placenta; appears in breast milk

Protein binding: 95% to 99%

Metabolism: Unknown

Half-life: 3-27 days (single dose); 14-40 days (third dose); up to 168 days (11th dose)

Time to peak serum concentration: Within 4-6 hours

Elimination: Majority ultimately excreted in urine (70%) and the remainder in feces (30%)

Usual Dosage I.M. (doses should initially be given at weekly intervals):

Children: Initial: 0.25 mg/kg/dose first week; increase by 0.25 mg/kg/dose increments with each weekly dose; maintenance: 0.75-1 mg/kg/dose weekly not to exceed 25 mg/dose to a total of 20 doses, then every 2-4 weeks

Adults: 10 mg first week; 25 mg second and third week; then 50 mg/week until 800 mg to 1 g cumulative dose has been given; if improvement occurs without adverse reactions, give 25-50 mg every 2-3 weeks, then every 3-4 weeks

Administration Parenteral: Deep I.M. injection into the upper outer quadrant of the gluteal region; vial should be thoroughly shaken before withdrawing a dose. Do not administer I.V.

Monitoring Parameters CBC with differential, platelet count, urinalysis, baseline renal and liver function tests

Reference Range Gold: Normal: 0-0.1 µg/mL (SI: 0-0.0064 µmol/L); Therapeutic: 1-3 µg/mL (SI: 0.06-0.18 µmol/L); Urine <0.1 µg/24 hours

Patient Information Notify physician of pruritus, sore mouth, indigestion, metallic taste; observe careful oral hygiene. May cause photosensitivity reactions (eg, exposure to sunlight may cause severe sunburn, skin rash, redness, or itching); avoid exposure to sunlight and artificial light sources (sunlamps, tanning booth/bed); wear protective clothing, wide-brimmed hats, sunglasses, and lip sunscreen (SPF ≥15); use a sunscreen [broad-spectrum sunscreen or physical sunscreen (preferred) or sunblock with SPF ≥15]; contact physician if reaction occurs.

Dosage Forms Injection, suspension: 50 mg/mL [gold 50%] (10 mL)

♦ **Auroto**® see Antipyrine and Benzocaine on page 122

♦ **Avandia**® see Rosiglitazone on page 999

♦ **Aventyl**® **HCl** see Nortriptyline on page 822

♦ **Avinza**™ see Morphine Sulfate on page 778

♦ **Avita**® see Tretinoin on page 1111

♦ **Axid**® see Nizatidine on page 819

♦ **Axid**® **AR [OTC]** see Nizatidine on page 819

♦ **Aygestin**® see Norethindrone on page 821

♦ **Ayr**® **Baby Saline [OTC]** see Sodium Chloride on page 1027

♦ **Ayr**® **Saline [OTC]** see Sodium Chloride on page 1027

♦ **Ayr**® **Saline Mist [OTC]** see Sodium Chloride on page 1027

♦ **Azactam**® see Aztreonam on page 154

Azathioprine (ay za THYE oh preen)

U.S. Brand Names Imuran®

Canadian Brand Names Alti-Azathioprine; Apo®-Azathioprine; Gen-Azathioprine

Therapeutic Category Antineoplastic Agent, Adjuvant; Immunosuppressant Agent

Generic Available Yes

Use Adjunct with other agents in prevention of transplant rejection; used as an immunosuppressant in a variety of autoimmune diseases such as SLE, severe rheumatoid arthritis unresponsive to other agents, and nephrotic syndrome

Pregnancy Risk Factor D

Contraindications Hypersensitivity to azathioprine or any component; pregnancy and lactation

(Continued)

Azathioprine *(Continued)*

Warnings Chronic immunosuppression increases the risk of neoplasia, particularly lymphoma and skin cancers; mutagenic potential in both men and women; may cause irreversible bone marrow suppression

Precautions Use with caution in patients with liver disease, renal impairment, and those with cadaveric kidneys; modify dosage in patients with renal impairment; reduce dosage to 25% to 33% of usual dosage in patients receiving allopurinol and azathioprine concurrently; discontinue azathioprine therapy in patients with hepatic veno-occlusive disease

Adverse Reactions

Central nervous system: Fever, chills

Dermatologic: Alopecia, erythematous or maculopapular rash

Gastrointestinal: Nausea, vomiting, anorexia, diarrhea, aphthous stomatitis, pancreatitis

Hematologic: Bone marrow depression (leukopenia, thrombocytopenia, anemia)

Hepatic: Hepatotoxicity, jaundice, hepatic veno-occlusive disease

Neuromuscular & skeletal: Arthralgias

Ocular: Retinopathy

Miscellaneous: Rare hypersensitivity reactions which include myalgias, rigors, dyspnea, hypotension, serum sickness, rash

Drug Interactions Allopurinol inhibits the metabolic pathway of azathioprine by inhibiting xanthine oxidase and blocking the conversion of mercaptopurine to inactive products which increases azathioprine's effects; nondepolarizing neuromuscular blockers (decreased blockade); captopril or enalapril in combination with azathioprine has resulted in severe anemia

Stability Reconstituted 10 mg/mL injection is stable for 24 hours at room temperature; stable in neutral or acid solutions, but is hydrolyzed to mercaptopurine in alkaline solutions

Mechanism of Action Antagonizes purine metabolism and may inhibit synthesis of DNA, RNA, and proteins; may also interfere with cellular metabolism and inhibit mitosis

Pharmacokinetics

Distribution: Crosses the placenta

Protein binding: ~30%

Metabolism: Extensive by hepatic xanthine oxidase to 6-mercaptopurine (active)

Bioavailability: ~50%

Half-life:

Parent: 12 minutes

6-mercaptopurine: 0.7-3 hours; with anuria: 50 hours

Elimination: Small amount eliminated as unchanged drug; metabolites eliminated eventually in the urine

Dialysis: Slightly dialyzable (5% to 20%)

Usual Dosage Children and Adults:

Transplantation: Oral, I.V.: Initial: 2-5 mg/kg/dose once daily; maintenance: 1-3 mg/kg/dose once daily

Lupus nephritis: Oral: 2-3 mg/kg/dose once daily

Rheumatoid arthritis: Oral: 1 mg/kg/dose once daily for 6-8 weeks; increase by 0.5 mg/kg every 4 weeks until response or up to 2.5 mg/kg/day

Dosing interval in renal impairment:

Cl_{cr} 10-50 mL/minute: Administer every 36 hours or administer 75% of dose once daily

Cl_{cr} <10 mL/minute: Administer every 48 hours or administer 50% of dose once daily

Administration

Oral: Administer with food to decrease GI upset

Parenteral: Administer IVP over 5 minutes at a concentration not to exceed 10 mg/mL; or may be further diluted with NS or D_5W and administered by intermittent infusion over 15-60 minutes

Monitoring Parameters CBC, platelet counts, creatinine, total bilirubin, alkaline phosphatase, liver function tests

Patient Information Response in rheumatoid arthritis may not occur for up to 2-3 months; inform physician of persistent sore throat, unusual bleeding or bruising, or fatigue

Dosage Forms

Injection, powder for reconstitution, lyophilized, as sodium: 100 mg

Tablet: 50 mg

Extemporaneous Preparations A 50 mg/mL suspension compounded from one-hundred twenty 50 mg tablets comminuted to a fine powder in a mortar with 40 mL of a 1:1 mixture of Ora-Sweet® and Ora-Plus® added and mixed to a fine paste, and then adding the 1:1 mixture of Ora-Sweet® and Ora-Plus® to a total volume of 120 mL, was stable for 60 days at 5°C and 25°C when protected from light. Label "shake well before using" and "protect from light."

Allen LV Jr and Erickson MA, "Stability of Acetazolamide, Allopurinol, Azathioprine, Clonazepam, and Flucytosine in Extemporaneously Compounded Oral Liquids," *Am J Health Syst Pharm*, 1996, 53(16):1944-9.

References

American College of Rheumatology Ad Hoc Committee on Clinical Guidelines, "Guidelines for Monitoring Drug Therapy in Rheumatoid Arthritis," *Arthritis Rheum*, 1996, 39(5):723-31.

Baum D, Bernstein D, Starnes VA, et al, "Pediatric Heart Transplantation at Stanford: Results of a 15-Year Experience," *Pediatrics*, 1991, 88(2):203-14.

Leichter HE, Sheth KJ, Gerlach MJ, et al, "Outcome of Renal Transplantation in Children Aged 1-5 and 6-18 Years," *Child Nephrol Urol*, 1992, 12(1):1-5.

Azelastine (a ZEL as teen)

U.S. Brand Names Astelin®; Optivar™

Therapeutic Category Antiallergic, Ophthalmic; Antihistamine, Nasal

Generic Available No

Use

Nasal: Treatment of the symptoms of seasonal allergic rhinitis (SAR), perennial allergic rhinitis (PAR)

Ophthalmic: Treatment of itching of the eye associated with allergic conjunctivitis

Pregnancy Risk Factor C

Contraindications Hypersensitivity to azelastine or any component

Warnings Ophthalmic solution not for use in contact lens-related irritation; preservative in ophthalmic solution may be absorbed by soft contact lenses; wait at least 10 minutes after instillation before inserting soft contact lenses

Precautions Use with caution in asthmatics; patients with hepatic or renal dysfunction may require lower doses

Adverse Reactions

Cardiovascular: Flushing, hypertension, tachycardia

Central nervous system: Drowsiness, headache, somnolence, fatigue, vertigo, depression, nervousness, hypoesthesia

Dermatologic: Contact dermatitis, eczema, hair and follicle infection, furunculosis

Endocrine & metabolic: Weight gain

Gastrointestinal: Nausea, xerostomia, bitter taste, glossitis, ulcerative stomatitis, aphthous stomatitis, constipation, abdominal pain

Genitourinary: Urinary frequency, hematuria

Neuromuscular & skeletal: Myalgia, hyperkinesia

Ocular: Conjunctivitis, watery eyes, eye pain, transient eye burning/stinging (ophthalmic use)

Respiratory: Nasal burning, paroxysmal sneezing, rhinitis, epistaxis, bronchospasm, coughing, throat burning, laryngitis (nasal use)

Drug Interactions May cause additive sedation when concomitantly administered with other CNS depressant medications

Stability Stable 3 months after opening

Mechanism of Action Competes with histamine for H_1-receptor sites on effector cells in the blood vessels and respiratory tract; reduces hyper-reactivity of the airways; increases the motility of bronchial epithelial cilia, improving mucociliary transport

Pharmacodynamics

Onset of action: 30 minutes to 1 hour

Maximum effect: 3 hours

Duration: 12 hours

Pharmacokinetics

Protein binding: 88%

Metabolism: Metabolized by cytochrome P450 enzyme system; active metabolite desmethylazelastine

Bioavailability: After intranasal administration: 40%

Half-life, elimination: 22 hours

Time to peak serum concentration: 2-3 hours

Usual Dosage

Intranasal:

Children 5-12 years: 1 spray each nostril twice daily

Children ≥12 years and Adults: 2 sprays each nostril twice daily

Ophthalmic: Children ≥3 years and Adults: Instill 1 drop into each affected eye twice daily

Administration

Intranasal: Before use, the child-resistant screw cap on the bottle should be replaced with the pump unit and the delivery system should be primed with 4 sprays or until a

(Continued)

Azelastine *(Continued)*

fine mist appears; when 3 or more days have elapsed since the last use, the pump should be reprimed with 2 sprays or until a fine mist appears

Ophthalmic: Apply finger pressure to lacrimal sac during and for 1-2 minutes after instillation to decrease risk of systemic effects; avoid contact of bottle tip with skin or eye

Patient Information May cause drowsiness and impair ability to perform activities requiring mental alertness or physical coordination; may cause dry mouth

Dosage Forms

Solution, nasal, as hydrochloride (Astelin®): 1 mg/mL [137 mcg/spray] (17 mL)

Solution, ophthalmic, as hydrochloride (Optivar™): 0.05% (3 mL, 6 mL)

References

McNeely W and Wiseman LR, "Intranasal Azelastine. A Review of Its Efficacy in the Management of Allergic Rhinitis," *Drugs*, 1988, 56(1):91-114.

♦ **Azidothymidine** *see* Zidovudine *on page 1163*

♦ **Azidothymidine, Abacavir, and Lamivudine** *see* Abacavir, Lamivudine, and Zidovudine *on page 32*

♦ **Azidothymidine, Lamivudine and Abacavir** *see* Abacavir, Lamivudine, and Zidovudine *on page 32*

Azithromycin *(az ith roe MYE sin)*

Related Information

Carbohydrate and Alcohol Content of Liquid Medications for Use in Patients Receiving Ketogenic Diets *on page 1431*

Endocarditis Prophylaxis *on page 1321*

U.S. Brand Names Zithromax®; Zithromax® TRI-PAK™; Zithromax® Z-PAK®

Therapeutic Category Antibiotic, Macrolide

Generic Available No

Use Treatment of mild to moderate upper and lower respiratory tract infections, community-acquired pneumonia, infections of the skin and skin structure, acute otitis media, and urethritis and cervicitis due to susceptible strains of *C. trachomatis*, *N. gonorrhoeae*, *M. catarrhalis*, *H. influenzae*, *S. aureus*, *S. pneumoniae*, *Mycoplasma pneumoniae*, *M. avium* complex, *C. psittaci*, and *C. pneumoniae*; treatment of babesiosis; endocarditis prophylaxis

Pregnancy Risk Factor B

Contraindications Hypersensitivity to azithromycin, erythromycin, any component, or macrolide antibiotics

Warnings Oral azithromycin should not be used to treat pneumonia that is considered inappropriate for outpatient oral therapy; may mask or delay symptoms of incubating gonorrhea or syphilis so appropriate culture and susceptibility tests should be performed prior to initiating azithromycin; pseudomembranous colitis has been reported with use of macrolide antibiotics; patients who experience allergic reactions to azithromycin may require prolonged periods of observation and symptomatic treatment possibly due to the drug's long tissue half-life

Precautions Use with caution in patients with impaired hepatic function and patients with severe renal impairment (Cl_{cr} <10 mL/minute)

Adverse Reactions

Cardiovascular: Palpitations, chest pain, ventricular arrhythmias, hypotension

Central nervous system: Headache, dizziness, agitation, nervousness, insomnia, fever, fatigue, seizures

Dermatologic: Rash, pruritus, angioedema, photosensitivity, Stevens-Johnson syndrome, toxic epidermal necrolysis

Gastrointestinal: Diarrhea (6%), nausea (2%), abdominal pain (2.5%), vomiting, anorexia, pseudomembranous colitis, pancreatitis, oral candidiasis

Genitourinary: Vaginitis

Hematologic: Anemia, leukopenia, thrombocytopenia

Hepatic: Elevated hepatic enzymes, cholestatic jaundice

Local: Pain at injection site, inflammation

Otic: Ototoxicity

Renal: Nephritis, acute renal failure

Miscellaneous: Anaphylaxis

Drug Interactions Cytochrome P450 isoenzyme CYP3A3/4 substrate; CYP3A3/4 isoenzyme inhibitor (mild)

Aluminum- and magnesium-containing antacids decrease azithromycin peak serum levels by 24%; monitor patients receiving azithromycin and drugs known to interact with erythromycin (ie, theophylline, cisapride, anticoagulants) since there are still very few studies examining drug-drug interactions with azithromycin; azithromycin may increase levels of tacrolimus, phenytoin, ergot alkaloids, alfentanil, astemizole, terfenadine, bromocriptine, carbamazepine, cyclosporine, digoxin, disopyramide, and triazolam; avoid use with pimozide due to risk of cardiotoxicity; nelfinavir may increase azithromycin serum levels (monitor for azithromycin side effects)

Food Interactions Presence of food does not affect bioavailability of the tablet formulation, oral suspension, or the 1 g suspension regimen

Stability Store intact vials of injection, dry powder for oral suspension, and tablets at room temperature.

Oral suspension: After reconstitution, multiple dose oral suspension may be stored for 10 days at room temperature or in the refrigerator.

Injection: After reconstituting 500 mg vial at a concentration of 100 mg/mL, solution is stable for 24 hours at room temperature. If solution is further diluted with a compatible diluent to a 1-2 mg/mL concentration, this solution is stable for 24 hours at room temperature or 7 days if refrigerated.

Mechanism of Action Inhibits bacterial RNA-dependent protein synthesis by binding to the 50S ribosomal subunit which results in the blockage of transpeptidation

Pharmacokinetics

Absorption: Oral: Rapid from the GI tract

Distribution: Extensive tissue distribution into skin, lungs, bone, prostate, cervix; CSF concentrations are low; crosses the placenta

Protein binding: 7% to 50% (concentration-dependent and dependent on alpha$_1$-acid glycoprotein levels)

Metabolism: In the liver to inactive metabolites

Bioavailability: Capsule, tablet, oral suspension: 34% to 52%

Half-life, terminal: 68 hours

Time to peak serum concentration: Oral: 2-3 hours

Elimination: 50% of dose is excreted unchanged in bile; 6% of dose is excreted unchanged in urine

Usual Dosage

Oral:

Children ≥6 months:

Respiratory tract infections: 10 mg/kg on day 1 (maximum dose: 500 mg/day) followed by 5 mg/kg/day once daily on days 2-5 (maximum dose: 250 mg/day)

Otitis media:

Single dose regimen: 30 mg/kg as a single dose (maximum dose: 1500 mg)

Three-day regimen: 10 mg/kg once daily for 3 days (maximum dose: 500 mg/day)

Five-day regimen: 10 mg/kg on day 1 (maximum dose: 500 mg), followed by 5 mg/kg once daily on days 2-5 (maximum dose: 250 mg/day)

Children ≥2 years: Pharyngitis, tonsillitis: 12 mg/kg/day once daily for 5 days (maximum dose: 500 mg/day)

Children:

Chancroid: Single 20 mg/kg dose (maximum dose: 1 g)

Uncomplicated chlamydial urethritis or cervicitis: Single 10 mg/kg dose (maximum dose: 1 g)

Primary prevention of disseminated MAC: 5 mg/kg/day once daily (maximum dose: 250 mg/day) or 20 mg/kg (maximum dose: 1200 mg) once weekly given alone or in combination with rifabutin

Treatment and secondary prevention of disseminated MAC: 5 mg/kg/day once daily (maximum dose: 250 mg/day) in combination with ethambutol, with or without rifabutin

Babesiosis: 12 mg/kg/day once daily for 7-10 days with oral atovaquone 40 mg/kg/day divided twice daily

Endocarditis prophylaxis: 15 mg/kg/dose 1 hour before procedure

Adolescents ≥16 years and Adults:

Respiratory tract, skin and soft tissue infections: 500 mg on day 1 followed by 250 mg/day once daily on days 2-5

Alternative regimen for bacterial exacerbation of COPD: 500 mg once daily for 3 days

Chancroid or nongonococcal urethritis and cervicitis due to *C. trachomatis*: Single 1 g dose

Urethritis and cervicitis due to *N. gonorrhoeae*: Single 2 g dose

Prevention of disseminated MAC: 1200 mg once weekly alone or in combination with rifabutin

Treatment and secondary prevention of disseminated MAC: 500 mg once daily in combination with ethambutol, with or without rifabutin

I.V.: Adolescents ≥16 years and Adults: 500 mg once daily for 2 days followed by a switch to oral azithromycin therapy

(Continued)

Azithromycin *(Continued)*

Administration

Oral: Shake suspension well before use; oral suspension, tablet, or the 1 g suspension regimen formulation may be administered with or without food; do not administer with antacids that contain aluminum or magnesium; azithromycin 1 g oral suspension for a single dose regimen should be prepared by mixing contents of 1 packet with approximately 60 mL of water. Have the patient drink the entire contents immediately; add an additional 60 mL of water, mix, and drink.

Parenteral: Administer infusion at a final concentration of 1 mg/mL over 3 hours; for a 2 mg/mL concentration, infuse over 1 hour; do not infuse over a period of less than 60 minutes

Monitoring Parameters Liver function tests, WBC with differential; monitor patients receiving azithromycin and drugs known to interact with erythromycin (ie, theophylline, digoxin, anticoagulants, triazolam) since there are still very few studies examining drug-drug interactions with azithromycin

Patient Information Report any symptoms of chest pain, heart palpitations, and yellowing of skin or eyes. May cause photosensitivity reactions (eg, exposure to sunlight may cause severe sunburn, skin rash, redness, or itching); avoid exposure to sunlight and artificial light sources (sunlamps, tanning booth/bed); wear protective clothing, wide-brimmed hats, sunglasses, and lip sunscreen (SPF ≥15); use a sunscreen [broad-spectrum sunscreen or physical sunscreen (preferred) or sunblock with SPF ≥15]; contact physician if reaction occurs.

Dosage Forms

Injection, powder for reconstitution, as dihydrate: 500 mg

Powder for oral suspension, as dihydrate: 100 mg/5 mL (15 mL); 200 mg/5 mL (15 mL, 22.5 mL, 30 mL); 1 g [single dose packet] [contains sucrose]

Tablet, film-coated, as dihydrate: 250 mg, 500 mg, 600 mg

Tablet, unit dose pack, as dihydrate:

Zithromax® TRI-PAK™: 500 mg (3s)

Zithromax® Z-PAK®: 250 mg (6s)

References

Drew RH and Gallis HA, "Azithromycin-Spectrum of Activity, Pharmacokinetics, and Clinical Applications," *Pharmacotherapy*, 1992, 12(3):161-73.

Foulds G, Shepard RM, and Johnson RB, "The Pharmacokinetics of Azithromycin in Human Serum and Tissues," *J Antimicrob Chemother*, 1990, 25(Suppl A):73-82.

Hammerschlag MR, Golden NH, Oh MK, et al, "Single Dose of Azithromycin for the Treatment of Genital Chlamydial Infections in Adolescents," *J Pediatr*, 1993, 122(6):961-5.

Nahata MC, Koranyi KI, Gadgil SD, et al, "Pharmacokinetics of Azithromycin After Oral Administration of Multiple Doses of Suspension," *Antimicrob Agents Chemother*, 1993, 37(2):314-16.

Starke JR and Correa AG, "Management of Mycobacterial Infection and Disease in Children," *Pediatr Infect Dis J*, 1995, 14(6):455-69.

"2001 USPHS/IDSA Guidelines for the Prevention of Opportunistic Infections in Persons Infected With Human Immunodeficiency Virus. USPHS/IDSA Prevention of Opportunistic Working Group," November 28, 2001, http://http://www.aidsinfo.nih.gov.

- ◆ **Azmacort®** *see* Triamcinolone *on page 1112*
- ◆ **Azo-Gesic® [OTC]** *see* Phenazopyridine *on page 887*
- ◆ **Azo-Standard® [OTC]** *see* Phenazopyridine *on page 887*
- ◆ **AZT** *see* Zidovudine *on page 1163*
- ◆ **AZT, Abacavir, and 3TC** *see* Abacavir, Lamivudine, and Zidovudine *on page 32*
- ◆ **AZT, Abacavir, and Lamivudine** *see* Abacavir, Lamivudine, and Zidovudine *on page 32*
- ◆ **AZT, ABC, and 3TC** *see* Abacavir, Lamivudine, and Zidovudine *on page 32*
- ◆ **AZT and 3TC** *see* Lamivudine and Zidovudine *on page 652*
- ◆ **Azthreonam** *see* Aztreonam *on page 154*

Aztreonam *(AZ tree oh nam)*

U.S. Brand Names Azactam®

Synonyms Azthreonam

Therapeutic Category Antibiotic, Miscellaneous

Generic Available No

Use Treatment of patients with documented multidrug resistant aerobic gram-negative infection in which beta-lactam therapy is contraindicated; used for UTI, lower respiratory tract infections, septicemia, skin/skin structure infections, intra-abdominal infections and gynecological infections caused by susceptible *Enterobacteriaceae*, *E. coli*, *K. pneumoniae*, *P. mirabilis*, *S. marcescens*, *Citrobacter* species, *H. influenzae*, and *P. aeruginosa*

Pregnancy Risk Factor B

Contraindications Hypersensitivity to aztreonam or any component

Warnings Check for hypersensitivity to other beta-lactams (hypersensitivity reactions to aztreonam have occurred rarely in patients with a history of penicillin or cephalosporin hypersensitivity); prolonged use may result in superinfection

Precautions Use with caution and reduce dose in patients with renal impairment

Adverse Reactions

Cardiovascular: Hypotension, transient EKG changes

Central nervous system: Seizures, confusion, fever

Dermatologic: Rash, toxic epidermal necrolysis, urticaria, pruritus

Gastrointestinal: Diarrhea, nausea, vomiting, abdominal pain, pseudomembranous colitis

Hematologic: Eosinophilia, leukopenia, neutropenia, thrombocytopenia, anemia

Hepatic: Elevated liver enzymes, hepatitis, jaundice

Local: Pain at injection site, thrombophlebitis, swelling at injection site

Renal: Elevated BUN and serum creatinine

Miscellaneous: Anaphylaxis

Drug Interactions Avoid antibiotics that induce beta-lactamase production (cefoxitin, imipenem); probenecid and furosemide increases aztreonam serum levels

Stability Reconstituted solution is stable 48 hours at room temperature and 7 days when refrigerated; incompatible when mixed with nafcillin, metronidazole, or cephradine

Mechanism of Action Binds to penicillin-binding protein 3 which produces filamentation of the bacterium inhibiting bacterial cell wall synthesis and causing cell wall destruction

Pharmacokinetics

Absorption: I.M.: Well absorbed

Distribution: Widely distributed into body tissues, cerebrospinal fluid, bronchial secretions, peritoneal fluid, bone, and breast milk; crosses the placenta

V_d:

Neonates: 0.26-0.36 L/kg

Children: 0.2-0.29 L/kg

Adults: 0.2 L/kg

Protein binding: 56%

Half-life:

Neonates:

<7 days, ≤2.5 kg: 5.5-9.9 hours

<7 days, >2.5 kg: 2.6 hours

1 week to 1 month: 2.4 hours

Children 2 months to 12 years: 1.7 hours

Children with cystic fibrosis: 1.3 hours

Adults: 1.3-2.2 hours (half-life prolonged in renal failure)

Time to peak serum concentration: Within 60 minutes after an I.M. dose

Elimination: 60% to 70% excreted unchanged in the urine and partially excreted in feces

Dialysis: Moderately dialyzable

Hemodialysis: 27% to 58% in 4 hours

Peritoneal dialysis: 10% with a 6-hour dwell time

Usual Dosage I.M., I.V.:

Neonates:

Postnatal age ≤7 days:

≤2000 g: 60 mg/kg/day divided every 12 hours

>2000 g: 90 mg/kg/day divided every 8 hours

Postnatal age >7 days:

<1200 g: 60 mg/kg/day divided every 12 hours

1200-2000 g: 90 mg/kg/day divided every 8 hours

>2000 g: 120 mg/kg/day divided every 6 hours

Children >1 month: 90-120 mg/kg/day divided every 6-8 hours

Cystic fibrosis: 50 mg/kg/dose every 6-8 hours (ie, up to 200 mg/kg/day); maximum dose: 8 g/day

Adults:

Urinary tract infection: 500 mg to 1 g every 8-12 hours

Moderately severe systemic infections: 1 g I.V. or I.M. or 2 g I.V. every 8-12 hours

Severe systemic or life-threatening infections (especially if caused by *Pseudomonas aeruginosa*): I.V.: 2 g every 6-8 hours; maximum dose: 8 g/day

Dosing adjustment in renal impairment:

Cl_{cr} 10-30 mL/minute: Reduce dose by 50%; give at the usual interval

Cl_{cr} <10 mL/minute: Reduce dose by 75%; give at the usual interval

Administration Parenteral:

I.V.: Administer by IVP over 3-5 minutes at a maximum concentration of 66 mg/mL or by intermittent infusion over 20-60 minutes at a final concentration not to exceed 20 mg/mL

(Continued)

Aztreonam *(Continued)*

I.M.: Deep I.M. injection into a large muscle mass such as ths upper outer quadrant of the gluteus maximus or lateral part of the thigh

Monitoring Parameters Periodic liver function test

Test Interactions False positive urine glucose (Clinitest®), positive Coombs' test

Dosage Forms

Infusion [premixed]: 1 g (50 mL); 2 g (50 mL)

Injection, powder for reconstitution: 500 mg, 1 g, 2 g [contains arginine]

References

Bosso JA and Black PG, "The Use of Aztreonam in Pediatric Patients: A Review," *Pharmacotherapy*, 1991, 11(1):20-5.

Stutman HR, Chartrand SA, Tolentino T, et al, "Aztreonam Therapy for Serious Gram-Negative Infections in Children," *Am J Dis Child*, 1986, 140(11):1147-51.

- ♦ **Azulfidine®** *see* Sulfasalazine *on page 1055*
- ♦ **Azulfidine® EN-tabs®** *see* Sulfasalazine *on page 1055*
- ♦ **Babee Cof Syrup [OTC]** *see* Dextromethorphan *on page 365*
- ♦ **Babee® Teething [OTC]** *see* Benzocaine *on page 163*
- ♦ **Baby Gasz [OTC]** *see* Simethicone *on page 1020*
- ♦ **Bacid® [OTC]** *see* Lactobacillus acidophilus and Lactobacillus bulgaricus *on page 648*
- ♦ **Baciguent® [OTC]** *see* Bacitracin *on page 156*
- ♦ **Baci-IM®** *see* Bacitracin *on page 156*

Bacitracin *(bas i TRAY sin)*

U.S. Brand Names AK-Tracin®; Baciguent® [OTC]; Baci-IM®

Therapeutic Category Antibiotic, Ophthalmic; Antibiotic, Topical; Antibiotic, Miscellaneous

Generic Available Yes

Use Treatment of pneumonia and empyema caused by susceptible staphylococci; prevention or treatment of superficial skin infections or infections of the eye caused by susceptible organisms; due to its toxicity, use of bacitracin systemically or as an irrigant should be limited to situations where less toxic alternatives would not be effective; treatment of antibiotic-associated colitis

Pregnancy Risk Factor C

Contraindications Hypersensitivity to bacitracin or any component; I.M. use is contraindicated in patients with renal impairment

Warnings I.M. use may cause renal failure due to tubular and glomerular necrosis; do **not** administer intravenously because severe thrombophlebitis occurs; bacitracin may be absorbed from denuded areas and irrigation sites

Precautions Prolonged use may result in overgrowth of nonsusceptible organisms

Adverse Reactions

Cardiovascular: Hypotension, tightness of chest

Central nervous system: Pain

Dermatologic: Rash, itching

Gastrointestinal: Anorexia, nausea, vomiting, diarrhea, rectal itching and burning

Hematologic: Blood dyscrasias

Renal: With I.M. use: Renal tubular and glomerular necrosis, azotemia, renal failure

Miscellaneous: Diaphoresis, edema of lips and face

Drug Interactions Nephrotoxic drugs (increase toxicity), neuromuscular blocking agents and anesthetics (increase neuromuscular blockade)

Stability Sterile powder should be stored in the refrigerator; once reconstituted, bacitracin is stable for 1 week under refrigeration (2°C to 8°C); incompatible with diluents containing parabens

Mechanism of Action Inhibits bacterial cell wall synthesis by preventing transfer of mucopeptides into the growing cell wall

Pharmacokinetics

Absorption: Poor from mucous membranes and intact skin; rapid following I.M. administration

Protein binding: Minimally bound to plasma proteins

Time to peak serum concentration: I.M.: Within 1-2 hours

Elimination: Slow elimination into the urine with 10% to 40% of a dose excreted within 24 hours

Usual Dosage

I.M. (not recommended):

Infants:

≤2.5 kg: 900 units/kg/day in 2-3 divided doses

>2.5 kg: 1000 units/kg/day in 2-3 divided doses

Children: 800-1200 units/kg/day divided every 8 hours

Adults: 10,000-25,000 units/dose every 6 hours; not to exceed 100,000 units/day
Children and Adults:

Topical: Apply 1-5 times/day

Ophthalmic ointment: Instill ¼" to ½" ribbon directly into conjunctival sac(s) every 3-4 hours; reduce frequency of administration as the infection is brought under control to 1-3 times/day

Irrigation, solution: 50-100 units/mL in NS, LR, or sterile water for irrigation; soak sponges in solution for topical compresses 1-5 times/day or as needed during surgical procedures

Antibiotic-associated colitis: Adults: Oral: 25,000 units every 6 hours for 7-10 days

Administration

Ophthalmic: Do not use topical ointment in the eyes; avoid contact of tube tip with skin or eye

Parenteral: For I.M. administration, pH of urine should be kept above 6 by using sodium bicarbonate; bacitracin sterile powder should be dissolved in NS injection containing 2% procaine hydrochloride; administer I.M. injection into the upper outer quadrant of the buttocks; alternate injection sites

Monitoring Parameters I.M.: Urinalysis, renal function tests

Patient Information Ophthalmic ointment may cause blurred vision; topical bacitracin should not be used for longer than 1 week unless directed by a physician

Dosage Forms

Injection, powder for reconstitution (Baci-IM®): 50,000 units

Ointment, ophthalmic (AK-Tracin®): 500 units/g (3.5 g)

Ointment, topical: 500 units/g (0.9 g, 15 g, 30 g, 120 g, 454 g)

Baciguent®: 500 units/g (15 g, 30 g)

References

Kelly CP, Pothoulakis C, and LaMont JT, "*Clostridium difficile* Colitis," *N Engl J Med*, 1994, 330(4):257-62.

Bacitracin and Polymyxin B (bas i TRAY sin & pol i MIKS in bee)

U.S. Brand Names AK-Poly-Bac®; Betadine® First Aid Antibiotics + Moisturizer [OTC]; Polysporin® Ophthalmic; Polysporin® Topical [OTC]

Canadian Brand Names LID-Pack®; Optimyxin®; Optimyxin Plus®; Polycidin® Ophthalmic Ointment

Synonyms Polymyxin B and Bacitracin

Therapeutic Category Antibiotic, Ophthalmic; Antibiotic, Topical

Generic Available Yes

Use Treatment of superficial infections involving the conjunctiva and/or cornea caused by susceptible organisms; prevent infection in minor cuts, scrapes and burns

Pregnancy Risk Factor C

Contraindications Hypersensitivity to polymyxin, bacitracin, or any component

Precautions Prolonged use may result in overgrowth of nonsusceptible organisms

Adverse Reactions

Local: Rash, itching, burning, edema

Ocular: Conjunctival erythema

Miscellaneous: Anaphylactoid reactions

Pharmacokinetics Absorption: Insignificant from intact skin or mucous membrane

Usual Dosage Children and Adults:

Ophthalmic: Instill ¼" to ½" directly into conjunctival sac(s) every 3-4 hours depending on severity of the infection

Topical: Apply a small amount of ointment or dusting of powder to the affected area 1-3 times/day

Administration Ophthalmic: Do not use topical ointment in the eyes; avoid contact of tube tip with skin or eye

Patient Information Do not use longer than 1 week unless directed by physician; ophthalmic ointment may cause blurred vision

Dosage Forms

Ointment, ophthalmic (AK-Poly-Bac®, Polysporin®): Bacitracin 500 units and polymyxin B sulfate 10,000 units per g (3.5 g)

Ointment, topical: Bacitracin 500 units and polymyxin B sulfate 10,000 units per g in white petrolatum (15 g, 30 g)

Betadine® First Aid Antibiotics + Moisturizer: Bacitracin 500 units and polymyxin B sulfate 10,000 units per g (14 g)

Polysporin®: Bacitracin 500 units and polymyxin B sulfate 10,000 units per g (15 g, 30 g)

Powder, topical (Polysporin®): Bacitracin 500 units and polymyxin B sulfate 10,000 units per g (10 g)

♦ **Bacitracin, Neomycin, and Polymyxin B** *see* Neomycin, Polymyxin B, and Bacitracin *on page 804*

• **Bacitracin, Neomycin, Polymyxin B, and Hydrocortisone** *see* Neomycin, (Bacitracin) Polymyxin B, and Hydrocortisone *on page 802*

Baclofen (BAK loe fen)

U.S. Brand Names Lioresal®

Canadian Brand Names Apo®-Baclofen; Gen-Baclofen; Liotec; Nu-Baclo; PMS-Baclofen

Therapeutic Category Skeletal Muscle Relaxant, Nonparalytic

Generic Available Yes (tablets)

Use Treatment of cerebral spasticity, reversible spasticity associated with multiple sclerosis or spinal cord lesions; intrathecal use for the management of spasticity in patients who are unresponsive to oral baclofen or experience intolerable CNS side effects; treatment of trigeminal neuralgia; adjunctive treatment of tardive dyskinesia

Pregnancy Risk Factor C

Contraindications Hypersensitivity to baclofen or any component

Warnings Should not be used when spasticity is used to maintain posture or balance; due to the life-threatening complications of intrathecal use, physicians must be adequately trained in its use; physostigmine should be available to reverse life-threatening central nervous side effects (eg, respiratory depression); injection for intrathecal use is not recommended or intended for I.V., I.M., S.C. or epidural administration; abrupt withdrawal of oral baclofen has been reported to precipitate hallucinations and/or seizures. Abrupt discontinuation of intrathecal baclofen regardless of the cause, has resulted in sequelae that include high fever, altered mental status, exaggerated rebound spasticity, and muscle rigidity, that in rare cases, has advanced to rhabdomyolysis, multiple organ system failure, and death. Early symptoms of withdrawal include: Return of baseline spasticity, pruritus, hypotension, and paresthesias. Clinical characteristics of advanced withdrawal may resemble autonomic dysreflexia, sepsis, malignant hyperthermia, neuroleptic-malignant syndrome, and other conditions associated with hypermetabolic state or widespread rhabdomyolysis. Patients at increased risk include spinal cord injuries at T-6 or above, patients with communication difficulties, and history of withdrawal symptoms from oral baclofen. If restoration of intrathecal baclofen is delayed, oral baclofen or benzodiazepine treatment may be used as a temporary measure.

Precautions Use with caution in patients with seizure disorder, impaired renal function, peptic ulcer disease, stroke, ovarian cysts, psychotic disorders, autonomic dysreflexia (intrathecal therapy)

Adverse Reactions

Cardiovascular: Hypotension, cardiovascular collapse (with intrathecal therapy), chest pain, palpitations

Central nervous system: Drowsiness, fatigue, vertigo, dizziness, psychiatric disturbances, insomnia, slurred speech, headache, hypotonia, ataxia, life-threatening CNS depression (with intrathecal use)

Dermatologic: Rash, pruritus

Gastrointestinal: Nausea, constipation, anorexia, dysgeusia, diarrhea, abdominal pain, xerostomia

Genitourinary: Impotence, urinary frequency, nocturia

Renal: Hematuria

Respiratory: Respiratory failure (with intrathecal administration), dyspnea

Miscellaneous: Diaphoresis

Drug Interactions Increased CNS depression when administered with other CNS depressants (eg, opiates, alcohol, benzodiazepines), tricyclic antidepressants; MAO inhibitors; baclofen may decrease lithium's effect

Mechanism of Action Inhibits the transmission of both monosynaptic and polysynaptic reflexes at the spinal cord level, possibly by hyperpolarization of primary afferent fiber terminals, with resultant relief of muscle spasticity

Pharmacodynamics

Oral: Muscle relaxation effects require 3-4 days and maximal clinical effects are not seen for 5-10 days

Intrathecal:

Bolus:

Onset of action: 30 minutes to 1 hour

Maximum effect: 4 hours

Duration: 4-8 hours

Continuous intrathecal infusion:

Onset of action: 6-8 hours

Maximum activity: 24-48 hours

Pharmacokinetics

Oral:

Absorption: Rapid; absorption from the GI tract is thought to be dose dependent

Protein binding: 30%
Metabolism: Minimal in the liver (15%)
Half-life: 2.5-4 hours
Time to peak serum concentration: Oral: Within 2-3 hours
Elimination: 85% of dose excreted in urine and feces as unchanged drug
Intrathecal:
Half-life, CSF elimination: 1.5 hours
Clearance, CSF: 30 mL/hour

Usual Dosage
Oral:
Children:
2-7 years: Initial: 10-15 mg/day divided every 8 hours; titrate dose every 3 days in increments of 5-15 mg/day to a maximum of 40 mg/day
≥8 years: Titrate dosage as above to a maximum of 60 mg/day
Adults: 5 mg 3 times/day, may increase 5 mg/dose every 3 days to a maximum of 80 mg/day
Intrathecal: Children and Adults:
Screening dosage: 50 mcg for 1 dose and observe for 4-8 hours; very small children may receive 25 mcg; if ineffective, a repeat dosage increased by 50% (eg, 75 mcg) may be repeated in 24 hours; if still suboptimal, a third dose increased by 33% (eg, 100 mcg) may be repeated in 24 hours; patients who do not respond to 100 mcg intrathecally should not be considered for continuous chronic administration via an implantable pump
Maintenance dose: Continuous infusion: Initial: Depending upon the screening dosage and its duration:
If the screening dose duration >8 hours: Daily dose = effective screening dose
If the screening dose duration <8 hours: Daily dose = **twice** effective screening dose
Continuous infusion dose mcg/hour = daily dose divided by 24 hours
Note: Further adjustments in infusion rate may be done every 24 hours as needed; for spinal cord-related spasticity, increase in 10% to 30% increments/24 hours; for spasticity of cerebral origin, increase in 5% to 10% increments/24 hours
Average daily dose:
Children ≤12 years: 100-300 mcg/day (4.2-12.5 mcg/hour); doses as high as 1000 mcg/day have been used
Children >12 years and Adults: 300-800 mcg/day (12.5-33 mcg/hour); doses as high as 2000 mcg/day have been used

Administration
Oral: Administer with food or milk
Parenteral: Intrathecal: Test dosage: Use dilute concentration (50 mcg/mL) and inject over at least 1 minute; for maintenance infusion via implantable infusion pump, concentrations of 500-2000 mcg/mL may be used; do not abruptly discontinue intrathecal baclofen administration (see Warnings)

Monitoring Parameters Muscle rigidity, spasticity (decrease in number and severity of spasms), modified Ashworth score

Patient Information Avoid alcohol and other CNS depressants; may cause drowsiness and impair ability to perform activities requiring mental alertness or physical coordination; may cause dry mouth; do not abruptly discontinue therapy

Dosage Forms
Injection, solution, intrathecal [preservative free]: 0.05 mg/mL (1 mL); 0.5 mg/mL (20 mL); 2 mg/mL (5 mL)
Tablet: 10 mg, 20 mg

Extemporaneous Preparations
A 5 mg/mL suspension may be made by crushing thirty 20 mg tablets; levigate with a small amount of glycerin to form a paste. Add simple syrup incrementally to a total volume of 120 mL; shake well; refrigerate; stable 35 days (Johnson, 1993)
A 10 mg/mL oral suspension may be made by crushing one hundred twenty 10 mg tablets; gradually add 60 mL Ora-Sweet® or Ora-Plus® and mix until a uniform paste, then add more vehicle to make a total volume of 120 mL; refrigerate; shake well; stable 60 days (Allen, 1996)

Allen LV Jr and Erickson MA 3rd, "Stability of Baclofen, Captopril, Diltiazem Hydrochloride, Dipyridamole, and Flecainide Acetate in Extemporaneously Compounded Oral Liquids," *Am J Health Syst Pharm*, 1996, 53(18):2179-84.
Johnson CE and Hart SM, "Stability of an Extemporaneously Compounded Baclofen Oral Liquid," *Am J Hosp Pharm*, 1993, 50(11):2353-5.

♦ **BactoShield® CHG [OTC]** *see* Chlorhexidine Gluconate *on page 257*
♦ **Bactrim™** *see* Sulfamethoxazole and Trimethoprim *on page 1052*
♦ **Bactrim™ DS** *see* Sulfamethoxazole and Trimethoprim *on page 1052*

- **Bactroban®** *see* Mupirocin *on page 783*
- **Bactroban® Nasal** *see* Mupirocin *on page 783*
- **Baking Soda** *see* Sodium Bicarbonate *on page 1025*
- **BAL in Oil®** *see* Dimercaprol *on page 391*
- **Balmex® [OTC]** *see* Zinc Oxide *on page 1167*
- **Balminil® Decongestant (Can)** *see* Pseudoephedrine *on page 958*
- **Balminil DM E (Can)** *see* Guaifenesin and Dextromethorphan *on page 553*
- **Balminil Expectorant (Can)** *see* Guaifenesin *on page 550*
- **Balnetar® (Can)** *see* Coal Tar *on page 299*
- **Bancap HC®** *see* Hydrocodone and Acetaminophen *on page 571*
- **Band-Aid® Hurt-Free™ Antiseptic Wash [OTC]** *see* Lidocaine *on page 671*
- **Banophen® [OTC]** *see* DiphenhydrAMINE *on page 393*
- **Bausch & Lomb® Computer Eye Drops [OTC]** *see* Glycerin *on page 543*
- **Bayer® Aspirin [OTC]** *see* Aspirin *on page 134*
- **Bayer® Aspirin Extra Strength [OTC]** *see* Aspirin *on page 134*
- **Bayer® Aspirin Regimen Adult Low Strength [OTC]** *see* Aspirin *on page 134*
- **Bayer® Aspirin Regimen Adult Low Strength With Calcium [OTC]** *see* Aspirin *on page 134*
- **Bayer® Aspirin Regimen, Children's [OTC]** *see* Aspirin *on page 134*
- **Bayer® Aspirin Regimen Regular Strength [OTC]** *see* Aspirin *on page 134*
- **Bayer® Plus Extra Strength [OTC]** *see* Aspirin *on page 134*
- **BayRho-D® Full-Dose** *see* Rh₀(D) Immune Globulin *on page 978*
- **BayRho-D® Mini-Dose** *see* Rh₀(D) Immune Globulin *on page 978*
- **Baza® Antifungal [OTC]** *see* Miconazole *on page 759*
- **BCNU** *see* Carmustine *on page 217*
- **B Complex** *see page 1213*
- **B-D™ Glucose [OTC]** *see* Dextrose *on page 366*
- **Bebulin® VH** *see* Factor IX Complex (Human) *on page 471*

Beclomethasone (be kloe METH a sone)

Related Information
Asthma Guidelines *on page 1376*
Estimated Comparative Daily Dosages for Inhaled Corticosteroids *on page 1382*

U.S. Brand Names Beconase® [DSC]; Beconase® AQ; QVAR® 40 mcg; QVAR® 80 mcg; Vancenase® AQ 84 mcg [DSC]; Vancenase® Pockethaler® [DSC]; Vanceril® [DSC]

Canadian Brand Names Apo®-Beclomethasone; Gen-Beclo; Nu-Beclomethasone; Propaderm®; Rivanase AQ

Therapeutic Category Adrenal Corticosteroid; Antiasthmatic; Anti-inflammatory Agent; Corticosteroid, Inhalant (Oral); Corticosteroid, Intranasal; Glucocorticoid

Generic Available No

Use
Oral inhalation: Long-term (chronic) control of persistent bronchial asthma; **NOT** indicated for the relief of acute bronchospasm. Also used to help reduce or discontinue oral corticosteroid therapy for asthma.
Intranasal: Management of seasonal or perennial rhinitis and nasal polyposis

Pregnancy Risk Factor C

Contraindications Hypersensitivity to beclomethasone or any component; primary treatment of status asthmaticus or other acute episodes of bronchial asthma where intensive treatment is needed

Warnings Fatalities have occurred due to adrenal insufficiency in asthmatic patients during and after switching from systemic corticosteroids to aerosol steroids; several months may be required for full recovery of the adrenal glands; patients receiving higher doses of systemic corticosteroids (eg, adults receiving ≥20 mg of prednisone per day) may be at greater risk; during this period of adrenal suppression, aerosol steroids do **not** provide the systemic corticosteroid needed to treat patients requiring stress doses (ie, patients with major stress such as trauma, surgery, or infections). When used at high doses hypothalamic - pituitary - adrenal (HPA) suppression may occur; use with inhaled or systemic corticosteroids (even alternate-day dosing) may increase risk of HPA suppression; withdrawal and discontinuation of corticosteroids should be done carefully. Switching from systemic corticosteroids to inhalation may unmask allergic conditions (such as eczema, conjunctivitis, and rhinitis) that were previously suppressed by systemic steroids. Immunosuppression may occur

Precautions Avoid using higher than recommended dosages; suppression of HPA function, suppression of linear growth, or hypercorticism (Cushing's syndrome) may occur; use with extreme caution in patients with respiratory tuberculosis, untreated systemic infections, or ocular herpes simplex. Rare cases of increased IOP, glaucoma, or cataracts may occur.

Adverse Reactions

Central nervous system: Headache

Endocrine & metabolic: Potential adrenal suppression, dysmenorrhea

Gastrointestinal: Xerostomia, sore throat, pharyngitis

Local: Growth of *Candida* in the mouth, throat, or nares

Neuromuscular & skeletal: Growth velocity suppression (reported in asthmatic children receiving oral inhalation 2 puffs 4 times/day)

Respiratory: Cough, sneezing, hoarseness; irritation and burning of the nasal mucosa, nasal ulceration, epistaxis, rhinorrhea, nasal congestion (intranasal use)

Drug Interactions Cytochrome P450 isoenzyme CYP3A substrate

Interactions similar to other corticosteroids may potentially occur

Stability Do not store near heat or open flame; store QVAR® so inhaler rests on concave end of canister (with plastic actuator on top); use Vanceril® within 6 months after removal from moisture protective package

Mechanism of Action Controls the rate of protein synthesis, depresses the migration of polymorphonuclear leukocytes and fibroblasts, reverses capillary permeability, and stabilizes lysosomal membranes at the cellular level to prevent or control inflammation

Pharmacodynamics

Onset of action:

Oral inhalation: Within 1-2 days in some patients; usually within 1-2 weeks

Nasal inhalation: Within a few days up to 2 weeks

Maximum effect: Oral inhalation: 3-4 weeks

Pharmacokinetics

Absorption: Inhalation: Readily absorbed; quickly hydrolyzed by pulmonary esterases prior to absorption; oral: 90%

Distribution: 10% to 25% of inhaled dose reaches respiratory tract (50% with QVAR®); secreted into breast milk

Protein binding: 87%

Metabolism: In the liver via cytochrome P450 isoenzyme CYP3A to 3 major metabolites: Beclomethasone-17-monopropionate (17-BMP), beclomethasone-21-monopropionate (21-BMP), and beclomethasone (BOH); most active metabolite is 17-BMP

Half-life: Biphasic: Initial 3 hours; terminal: 15 hours

Elimination: Primary route of excretion is via feces; 12% to 15% of oral dose excreted in urine as metabolites

Usual Dosage

Aqueous inhalation, nasal:

Beconase® AQ:

Children 6-12 years: Initial: 1 inhalation in each nostril twice daily; may increase if needed to 2 inhalations in each nostril twice daily; once symptoms are adequately controlled, decrease dose to 1 inhalation in each nostril twice daily

Children ≥12 years and Adults: 1-2 inhalations in each nostril twice daily

Vancenase® AQ 84 mcg: Children ≥6 years and Adults: 1-2 inhalations in each nostril once daily

Intranasal (Vancenase®, Beconase®):

Children 6-12 years: 1 inhalation in each nostril 3 times/day

Children ≥12 years and Adults: 1 inhalation in each nostril 2-4 times/day or 2 inhalations each nostril twice daily; usual maximum maintenance: 1 inhalation in each nostril 3 times/day

Oral inhalation (doses should be titrated to the lowest effective dose once asthma is controlled):

Vanceril®:

Children 6-12 years: 1-2 inhalations 3-4 times/day (alternatively: 2-4 inhalations twice daily); maximum dose: 10 inhalations/day

Children ≥12 years and Adults: 2 inhalations 3-4 times/day (alternatively: 4 inhalations twice daily); maximum dose: 20 inhalations/day; patients with severe asthma: Initial: 12-16 inhalations/day (divided 3-4 times/day); dose should be adjusted downward according to patient's response

QVAR®

Children 5-11 years: Initial: 40 mcg twice daily; maximum dose: 80 mcg twice daily

Children ≥12 years and Adults:

No previous inhaled corticosteroids: Initial: 40-80 mcg twice daily; maximum dose: 320 mcg twice daily

Previous inhaled corticosteroid use: Initial: 40-160 mcg twice daily; maximum dose: 320 mcg twice daily

(Continued)

Beclomethasone *(Continued)*

Note: Therapeutic ratio between QVAR® and other beclomethasone inhalers has not been established; when switching to QVAR®, monitor patients for efficacy and adverse effects (see Additional Information)

NIH Asthma Guidelines (NAEPP, 2002; NIH, 1997) [give in divided doses]:

CFC formulation (eg, Vanceril®):

Children ≤12 years:
"Low" dose: 84-336 mcg/day (42 mcg/puff: 2-8 puffs/day)
"Medium" dose: 336-672 mcg/day (42 mcg/puff: 8-16 puffs/day)
"High" dose: >672 mcg/day (42 mcg/puff: >16 puffs/day)

Children >12 years and Adults:
"Low" dose: 168-504 mcg/day (42 mcg/puff: 4-12 puffs/day)
"Medium" dose: 504-840 mcg/day (42 mcg/puff: 12-20 puffs/day)
"High" dose: >840 mcg/day (42 mcg/puff: >20 puffs/day)

HFA formulation (eg, QVAR®):

Children ≤12 years:
"Low" dose: 80-160 mcg/day (40 mcg/puff: 2-4 puffs/day or 80 mcg/puff: 1-2 puffs/day)
"Medium" dose: 160-320 mcg/day (40 mcg/puff: 4-8 puffs/day or 80 mcg/puff: 2-4 puffs/day)
"High" dose: >320 mcg/day (40 mcg/puff: >8 puffs/day or 80 mcg/puff: >4 puff/day)

Children >12 years and Adults:
"Low" dose: 80-240 mcg/day (40 mcg/puff: 2-6 puffs/day or 80 mcg/puff: 1-3 puffs/day)
"Medium" dose: 240-480 mcg/day (40 mcg/puff: 6-12 puffs/day or 80 mcg/puff: 3-6 puffs/day)
"High" dose: >480 mcg/day (40 mcg/puff: >12 puffs/day or 80 mcg/puff: 6 puffs/day)

Administration

Nasal inhalation: Shake container well before use; gently blow nose to clear nasal passages before administration; occlude one nostril with finger while carefully inserting nasal applicator into other nostril to administer dose

Oral inhalation: Use a spacer device for children <8 years of age; shake container well before use (all products except QVAR®)

Monitoring Parameters Check mucous membranes for signs of fungal infection; monitor growth in pediatric patients

Patient Information Notify physician if condition being treated persists or worsens; do not decrease dose or discontinue without physician approval; may cause dry mouth; avoid spraying in eyes; avoid exposure to chicken pox or measles; if exposed, seek medical advice without delay; discard canister when labeled number of metered doses (sprays) have been used. QVAR® may taste differently and have a different feeling during inhalation compared to other inhalers containing chlorofluorocarbons (CFCs).

Oral inhalant: Rinse mouth after inhalation to decrease chance of oral candidiasis; report sore mouth or mouth lesions to physician

Additional Information

Oral inhalation: If bronchospasm with wheezing occurs after use, a fast-acting bronchodilator may be used.

QVAR®: Does not contain chlorofluorocarbons (CFCs), uses hydrofluoroalkane (HFA) as the propellant; is a solution formulation (other beclomethasone inhalers are suspension aerosols); uses smaller-size particles which results in a higher percent of drug delivered to the respiratory tract and lower recommended doses than other products. An open-label, randomized, multicenter, 12-month study in 300 asthmatic children 5-11 years of age indicated that QVAR® provided long-term control of asthma at approximately half the dose compared with a CFC propelled beclomethasone MDI and spacer (see Pederson, 2002). Further studies are needed to define therapeutic ratio between QVAR® and other beclomethasone inhalers.

Aqueous beclomethasone nasal spray (42 mcg/inhalation; 2 sprays in each nostril twice daily for 4 weeks, followed by 1 spray in each nostril twice daily) may be useful in reducing adenoidal hypertrophy and nasal airway obstruction in children 5-11 years of age (Demain, 1995)

Dosage Forms

Aerosol for nasal inhalation, as dipropionate:
Beconase®: 42 mcg/inhalation (6.7 g) [80 metered doses]; (16.8 g) [200 metered doses] [DSC]
Vancenase® Pockethaler: 42 mcg/inhalation (7 g) [200 metered doses] [DSC]

Aerosol for oral inhalation, as dipropionate:
QVAR® 40 mcg: 40 mcg/inhalation (7.3 g) [100 metered doses]
QVAR® 80 mcg: 80 mcg/inhalation (7.3 g) [100 metered doses]
Vanceril®: 42 mcg/inhalation (16.8 g) [200 metered doses] [DSC]
Suspension, nasal spray, aqueous, as dipropionate:
Beconase® AQ: 42 mcg/inhalation (25 g) [180 metered doses]
Vancenase® AQ 84 mcg: 84 mcg/inhalation (19 g) [120 metered doses] [DSC]

References

Demain JG and Goetz DW, "Pediatric Adenoidal Hypertrophy and Nasal Airway Obstruction: Reduction With Aqueous Nasal Beclomethasone," *Pediatrics*, 1995, 95(3):355-64.

Expert Panel Report 2, "Guidelines for the Diagnosis and Management of Asthma," *Clinical Practice Guidelines*, National Institutes of Health, National Heart, Lung, and Blood Institute, NIH Publication No. 94-4051, April, 1997.

Kobayashi RH, Tinkelman DG, Reese ME, et al, "Beclomethasone Dipropionate Aqueous Nasal Spray for Seasonal Allergic Rhinitis in Children," *Ann Allergy*, 1989, 62(3):205-8.

"National Asthma Education and Prevention Program. Expert Panel Report: Guidelines for the Diagnosis and Management of Asthma Update on Selected Topics--2002," *J Allergy Clin Immunol*, 2002, 110(5 Suppl):S141-219.

Pedersen S, Warner J, Wahn U, et al, "Growth, Systemic Safety, and Efficacy During 1 Year of Asthma Treatment With Different Beclomethasone Dipropionate Formulations: An Open-Label, Randomized Comparison of Extra Fine and Conventional Aerosols in Children," *Pediatrics*, 2002, 109(6), http://www.pediatrics.org/cgi/content/full/109/6/e92.

Tinkelman DG, Reed CE, Nelson HS, et al, "Aerosol Beclomethasone Dipropionate Compared With Theophylline as Primary Treatment of Chronic, Mild to Moderately Severe Asthma in Children," *Pediatrics*, 1993, 92(1):64-77.

Wyatt R, Waschek J, Weinberger M, et al, "Effects of Inhaled Beclomethasone Dipropionate and Alternate-Day Prednisone on Pituitary-Adrenal Function in Children With Chronic Asthma," *N Engl J Med*, 1978, 299(25):1387-92.

- ◆ **Beconase® [DSC]** *see* Beclomethasone *on page 160*
- ◆ **Beconase® AQ** *see* Beclomethasone *on page 160*
- ◆ **Benadryl® Allergy [OTC]** *see* DiphenhydrAMINE *on page 393*
- ◆ **Benadryl® Cream [OTC]** *see* DiphenhydrAMINE *on page 393*
- ◆ **Benadryl® Dye-Free Allergy [OTC]** *see* DiphenhydrAMINE *on page 393*
- ◆ **Benadryl® Extra Strength Cream [OTC]** *see* DiphenhydrAMINE *on page 393*
- ◆ **Benadryl® Extra Strength Spray [OTC]** *see* DiphenhydrAMINE *on page 393*
- ◆ **Benadryl® Gel [OTC]** *see* DiphenhydrAMINE *on page 393*
- ◆ **Benadryl® Gel Extra Strength [OTC]** *see* DiphenhydrAMINE *on page 393*
- ◆ **Benadryl® Injection** *see* DiphenhydrAMINE *on page 393*
- ◆ **Benadryl® Itch Relief [OTC]** *see* DiphenhydrAMINE *on page 393*
- ◆ **Benadryl® Spray [OTC]** *see* DiphenhydrAMINE *on page 393*
- ◆ **Benoxyl® (Can)** *see* Benzoyl Peroxide *on page 165*
- ◆ **Bentyl®** *see* Dicyclomine *on page 376*
- ◆ **Bentylol® (Can)** *see* Dicyclomine *on page 376*
- ◆ **Benuryl™ (Can)** *see* Probenecid *on page 933*
- ◆ **Benylin® Adult [OTC]** *see* Dextromethorphan *on page 365*
- ◆ **Benylin® DM-E (Can)** *see* Guaifenesin and Dextromethorphan *on page 553*
- ◆ **Benylin® E Extra Strength (Can)** *see* Guaifenesin *on page 550*
- ◆ **Benylin® Expectorant [OTC]** *see* Guaifenesin and Dextromethorphan *on page 553*
- ◆ **Benylin® Pediatric [OTC]** *see* Dextromethorphan *on page 365*
- ◆ **Benzac®** *see* Benzoyl Peroxide *on page 165*
- ◆ **Benzac® AC** *see* Benzoyl Peroxide *on page 165*
- ◆ **Benzac® AC Wash** *see* Benzoyl Peroxide *on page 165*
- ◆ **Benzac® W** *see* Benzoyl Peroxide *on page 165*
- ◆ **Benzac® W Wash** *see* Benzoyl Peroxide *on page 165*
- ◆ **Benzagel®** *see* Benzoyl Peroxide *on page 165*
- ◆ **Benzagel® Wash** *see* Benzoyl Peroxide *on page 165*
- ◆ **Benzashave®** *see* Benzoyl Peroxide *on page 165*
- ◆ **Benzathine Benzylpenicillin** *see* Penicillin G Benzathine *on page 874*
- ◆ **Benzathine Penicillin G** *see* Penicillin G Benzathine *on page 874*
- ◆ **Benzazoline** *see* Tolazoline [DSC] *on page 1100*
- ◆ **Benzene Hexachloride** *see* Lindane *on page 677*
- ◆ **Benzhexol** *see* Trihexyphenidyl *on page 1118*

Benzocaine (BEN zoe kane)

U.S. Brand Names Americaine® [OTC]; Americaine® Anesthetic Lubricant; Anbesol® [OTC]; Anbesol® Baby [OTC]; Anbesol® Maximum Strength [OTC]; Babee® Teething [OTC]; Benzodent® [OTC]; Chiggerex® [OTC]; Chiggertox® [OTC]; Cylex® [OTC]; Detane® [OTC]; Foille® [OTC]; Foille® Medicated First Aid [OTC]; Foille® Plus [OTC]; (Continued)

Benzocaine *(Continued)*

HDA Toothache® [OTC]; Hurricaine®; Lanacane® [OTC]; Mycinettes® [OTC]; Orabase®-B [OTC]; Orajel® [OTC]; Orajel® Baby [OTC]; Orajel® Baby Nighttime [OTC]; Orajel® Maximum Strength [OTC]; Orasol® [OTC]; Solarcaine® [OTC]; Trocaine® [OTC]; Zilactin®-B [OTC]; Zilactin® Baby [OTC]

Synonyms Ethyl Aminobenzoate

Therapeutic Category Analgesic, Topical; Local Anesthetic, Oral; Local Anesthetic, Topical

Generic Available Yes

Use Temporary relief of pain associated with pruritic dermatosis, pruritus, minor burns, toothache, minor sore throat pain, canker sores, hemorrhoids, rectal fissures; anesthetic lubricant for passage of catheters and endoscopic tubes

Pregnancy Risk Factor C

Contraindications Hypersensitivity to benzocaine, other ester-type local anesthetics, or any component (see Warnings); secondary bacterial infection of area; perforated tympanic membrane (otic formulations only)

Warnings Some products contain tartrazine and benzyl alcohol which may cause allergic reactions in susceptible individuals; large amounts of benzyl alcohol (≥99 mg/kg/day) have been associated with a potentially fatal toxicity ("gasping syndrome") in neonates; the "gasping syndrome" consists of metabolic acidosis, respiratory distress, gasping respirations, CNS dysfunction (including convulsions, intracranial hemorrhage), hypotension and cardiovascular collapse; avoid use of injection in neonates. *In vitro* and animal studies have shown that benzoate, a metabolite of benzyl alcohol, displaces bilirubin from protein-binding sites.

Adverse Reactions

Cardiovascular: Edema

Dermatologic: Angioedema, urticaria

Genitourinary: Urethritis

Hematologic: Methemoglobinemia in infants

Local: Contact dermatitis, burning, stinging, tenderness

Mechanism of Action Blocks both the initiation and conduction of nerve impulses from sensory nerves by decreasing the neuronal membrane's permeability to sodium ions, which results in inhibition of depolarization with resultant blockade of conduction

Pharmacokinetics

Absorption: Poor after topical administration to intact skin, but well absorbed from mucous membranes and traumatized skin

Metabolism: Hydrolyzed in plasma and to a lesser extent in the liver by cholinesterase

Elimination: Excretion of the metabolites in urine

Usual Dosage Children and Adults:

Mucous membranes: Dosage varies depending on area to be anesthetized and vascularity of tissues

Oral mouth/throat preparations: Do not administer for >2 days or in children <2 years of age, unless directed by a physician; refer to specific package labeling

Otic: 4-5 drops into ear canal; may repeat every 1-2 hours as needed

Topical: Apply to affected area as needed

Administration

Mucous membranes: Apply to mucous membrane; do not eat for 1 hour after application to oral mucosa

Otic: After instilling into external ear canal, insert cotton pledget into ear canal

Topical: Apply evenly; do not apply to deep or puncture wounds or to serious burns

Patient Information Do not eat for 1 hour after application to oral mucosa; do not chew gum while mouth or throat is anesthetized due to potential biting trauma; do not overuse; do not apply to infected areas or to large areas of broken skin

Dosage Forms

Aerosol, topical spray **for skin disorders**:

Americaine®: 20% (20 mL, 120 mL)

Foille®: 5% (97.5 mL) [contains 0.63% chloroxylenol]

Foille® Plus: 5% (105 mL) [contains 57.33% alcohol and 0.63% chloroxylenol]

Hurricaine®: 20% (60 mL) [cherry flavor]

Solarcaine®: 20% (90 mL, 120 mL, 135 mL) [contains 0.13% alcohol and triclosam]

Cream, topical **for skin disorders**: 5% (30 g, 454 g)

Lanacane®: 20% (30 g)

Gel, oral, **mouth and throat preparations**:

Anbesol®: 6.3% (7.5 g)

Anbesol® Baby, Detane®, Orajel® Baby: 7.5% (7.5 g, 10 g, 15 g)

Anbesol® Maximum Strength, Orajel® Maximum Strength: 20% (6 g, 7.5 g, 10 g)

HDA Toothache®: 6.5% (15 mL) [contains benzyl alcohol]

Hurricaine®: 20% (5 g, 30 g) [wild cherry, pina colada, watermelon, and mint flavors]

Orabase-B®: 20% (7 g)

Orajel®, Orajel® Baby Nighttime, Zilactin®-B, Zilactin® Baby: 10% (6 g, 7.5 g, 10 g)

Gel, topical **for mucus membranes** (Americaine® Anesthetic Lubricant): 20% (2.5 g, 28 g) [contains 0.1% benzethonium chloride]

Liquid, oral, **mouth and throat preparations**:

Anbesol®, Orasol®: 6.3% (9 mL, 15 mL, 30 mL)

Anbesol® Maximum Strength: 20% (9 mL, 14 mL)

Hurricaine®: 20% (30 mL) [wild cherry and pina colada flavors]

Orajel®: 10% (13 mL) [contains tartrazine]

Orajel® Baby: 7.5% (13 mL)

Orajel® Maximum Strength: 20% (13 mL) [contains tartrazine]

Liquid, topical **for skin disorders** (Chiggertox®): 2% (30 mL)

Lotion, oral, **mouth and throat preparations** (Babee® Teething): 2.5% (15 mL)

Lozenges, **mouth and throat preparations**:

Cylex®, Mycinettes®: 15 mg [Cylex® contains 5 mg cetylpyridinium chloride]

Trocaine®: 10 mg

Ointment, oral, **mouth and throat preparations** (Benzodent®): 20% (30 g)

Ointment, topical **for skin disorders**:

Chiggerex®: 2% (52 g)

Foille® Medicated First Aid: 5% (3.5 g, 28 g) [contains 0.1% chloroxylenol, benzyl alcohol; corn oil base]

Paste, **mouth and throat preparations** (Orabase® B): 20% (7 g)

♦ **Benzocaine and Antipyrine** see Antipyrine and Benzocaine on page 122

♦ **Benzodent® [OTC]** see Benzocaine on page 163

Benzoyl Peroxide (BEN zoe il peer OKS ide)

U.S. Brand Names Benzac®; Benzac® AC; Benzac® AC Wash; Benzac® W; Benzac® W Wash; Benzagel®; Benzagel® Wash; Benzashave®; Brevoxyl®; Brevoxyl® Cleansing; Brevoxyl® Wash; Clearplex® [OTC]; Clinac™ BPO; Del Aqua®; Desquam-E®; Desquam-X®; Exact® Acne Medication [OTC]; Fostex® BPO [OTC]; Loroxide® [OTC]; Neutrogena® Acne Mask [OTC]; Neutrogena® On The Spot® Acne Treatment [OTC]; Oxy 10® Balanced Medicated Face Wash [OTC]; Oxy 10® Balance Spot Treatment [OTC]; Palmer's® Skin Success Acne [OTC]; PanOxyl®; PanOxyl®-AQ; PanOxyl® Aqua Gel; PanOxyl® Bar [OTC]; Seba-Gel™; Triaz®; Triaz® Cleanser; Zapzyt® [OTC]

Canadian Brand Names Acetoxyl®; Benoxyl®; Oxyderm™; Solugel®

Therapeutic Category Acne Products; Topical Skin Product

Generic Available Yes (except cream and soap)

Use Adjunctive treatment of mild to moderate acne vulgaris

Pregnancy Risk Factor C

Contraindications Hypersensitivity to benzoyl peroxide, benzoic acid, or any component

Warnings Discontinue if burning, swelling, or undue dryness occurs

Precautions For external use only; may bleach colored fabrics; avoid contact with eyes, eyelids, lips, mucous membranes, and highly inflamed or denuded skin

Adverse Reactions

Dermatologic: Contact dermatitis

Local: Irritation, stinging, dryness, peeling, erythema

Mechanism of Action Releases free-radical oxygen which oxidizes bacterial proteins in the sebaceous follicles decreasing the number of anaerobic bacteria and irritating free fatty acids; exerts a keratolytic activity and a comedolytic effect

Pharmacokinetics

Absorption: ~5% through the skin

Metabolism: Major metabolite is benzoic acid

Elimination: In the urine as benzoate

Usual Dosage Children and Adults: Topical: Apply sparingly 1-3 times/day; initially apply for 15 minutes; length of exposure, strength, and frequency of application are increased as tolerated

Administration Topical: Shake lotion before using; cleanse skin before applying; for external use only; avoid contact with eyes and mucous membranes

Additional Information Granulation may indicate effectiveness; gels are more penetrating than creams and last longer than creams or lotions

Dosage Forms

Cream, topical:

Benzashave®: 5% (120 g); 10% (120 g)

Exact® Acne Medication: 5% (18 g)

(Continued)

Benzoyl Peroxide *(Continued)*

Neutrogena® Acne Mask: 5% (60 g)
Neutrogena® On The Spot® Acne Treatment: 2.5% (22.5 g)
Gel, topical: 2.5% (60 g); 5% (45 g, 60 g, 90 g); 10% (45 g, 60 g, 90 g)
  Benzac®: 5% (60 g); 10% (60 g) [contains 12% alcohol]
  Benzac® AC: 2.5% (60 g); 5% (60 g); 10% (60 g) [water based]
  Benzac® W: 2.5% (60 g); 5% (60 g); 10% (60 g) [water based]
  Benzagel®: 5% (45 g); 10% (45 g)
  Benzagel® Wash: 10% (60 g) [water based]
  Brevoxyl®: 4% (43 g, 90 g); 8% (43 g, 90 g)
  Clearplex®: 5% (45 g); 10% (45 g)
  Clinac™ BPO: 7% (45 g)
  Desquam-E®: 2.5% (42.5 g); 5% (42.5 g); 10% (42.5 g) [emollient gel; water based]
  Desquam-X®: 5% (42.5 g, 90 g); 10% (42.5 g, 90 g)
  Fostex® BPO: 10% (45 g)
  Oxy 10® Balance Spot Treatment: 5% (30 g); 10% (30 g)
  PanOxyl®: 5% (57 g, 113 g); 10% (57 g, 113 g) [alcohol based]
  PanOxyl® AQ: 2.5% (57 g, 113 g); 5% (57 g, 113 g); 10% (57 g, 113 g) [water based]
  PanOxyl® Aqua Gel: 10% (42.5 g)
  Seba-Gel™: 5% (60 g, 90 g); 10% (60 g, 90 g)
  Triaz®: 3% (42.5 g); 6% (42.5 g); 10% (42.5 g)
  Triaz® Cleanser: 3% (170 g, 340 g); 6% (170 g, 340 g); 10% (170 g, 340 g)
  Zapzyt®: 10% (30 g)
Liquid, topical: 2.5% (240 mL); 5% (120 mL, 150 mL, 240 mL); 10% (150 mL, 240 mL)
  Benzac® AC Wash: 2.5% (240 mL); 5% (240 mL); 10% (240 mL) [water based]
  Benzac® W Wash: 5% (240 mL); 10% (240 mL) [water based]
  Del-Aqua®: 5% (45 mL); 10% (45 mL)
  Desquam-X®: 5% (150 mL)
  Oxy-10® Balance Medicated Face Wash: 10% (240 mL)
Lotion, topical: 5% (30 mL); 10% (30 mL)
  Brevoxyl® Cleansing: 4% (297 g); 8% (297 g) [in a lathering vehicle]
  Brevoxyl® Wash: 4% (170 g); 8% (170 g) [in a lathering vehicle]
  Fostex® BPO: 10% (150 mL)
  Loroxide®: 5.5% (26 mL)
  Palmer's® Skin Success Acne: 10% (30 mL) [contains vitamin E]
Soap, topical [bar]:
  Desquam-X®: 10% (113 g)
  Fostex® BPO: 10% (113 g)
  PanOxyl® Bar: 5% (113 g); 10% (113 g)

References
Winston MH and Shalita AR, "Acne Vulgaris: Pathogenesis and Treatment," *Pediatr Clin North Am*, 1991, 38(4):889-903.

Benztropine *(BENZ troe peen)*

Related Information
Overdose and Toxicology *on page 1388*
U.S. Brand Names Cogentin®
Canadian Brand Names Apo®-Benztropine
Therapeutic Category Anticholinergic Agent; Antidote, Drug-induced Dystonic Reactions; Anti-Parkinson's Agent
Generic Available Yes (tablet)
Use Adjunctive treatment of parkinsonism; also used in treatment of drug-induced extrapyramidal effects (except tardive dyskinesia) and acute dystonic reactions
Pregnancy Risk Factor C
Contraindications Hypersensitivity to benztropine mesylate or any component; children <3 years of age; patients with narrow-angle glaucoma, pyloric or duodenal obstruction, stenosing peptic ulcers; bladder neck obstructions; achalasia; myasthenia gravis
Precautions Use with caution in hot weather or during exercise; may cause anhydrosis and hyperthermia; increased risk of hyperthermia in alcoholics, patients with CNS disease, and with prolonged outdoor exposure
Adverse Reactions
Cardiovascular: Tachycardia, orthostatic hypotension, ventricular fibrillation, palpitations
Central nervous system: Drowsiness, nervousness, hallucinations, coma
Dermatologic: Dry skin
Endocrine & metabolic: Decreased flow of breast milk
Gastrointestinal: Nausea, vomiting, xerostomia, constipation, dry throat, dysphagia

Neuromuscular & skeletal: Weakness
Ocular: Blurred vision, mydriasis, elevated intraocular pain
Respiratory: Dry nose
Miscellaneous: Diaphoresis (decreased)

Drug Interactions As an anticholinergic, benztropine may potentiate the CNS depressant effects of CNS depressants; may inhibit the therapeutic response to neuroleptics; central and/or peripheral anticholinergic syndrome can occur when administered with amantadine, rimantadine, narcotic analgesics, phenothiazides, TCAs, quinidine, and antihistamines

Mechanism of Action Thought to partially block striatal cholinergic receptors to help balance cholinergic and dopaminergic activity

Pharmacodynamics
Onset of action:
Oral: Within 1 hour
Parenteral: Within 15 minutes
Duration: 6-48 hours

Usual Dosage
Drug-induced extrapyramidal reaction: Oral, I.M., I.V.:
Children >3 years: 0.02-0.05 mg/kg/dose 1-2 times/day; use in children <3 years should be reserved for life-threatening emergencies
Adults: 1-4 mg/dose 1-2 times/day
Acute dystonia: Adults: I.M., I.V.: 1-2 mg as a single dose
Parkinsonism: Adults: Oral: 0.5-6 mg/day in 1-2 divided doses; begin with 0.5 mg/day; increase in 0.5 mg increments at 5- to 6-day intervals to achieve the desired effect

Administration
Oral: Administer with food to decrease GI upset
Parenteral: I.V. route should be reserved for situations when oral or I.M. are not appropriate

Patient Information May causes drowsiness and impair ability to perform activities requiring mental alertness or physical coordination; may cause dry mouth.

Dosage Forms
Injection, solution, as mesylate: 1 mg/mL (2 mL)
Tablet, as mesylate: 0.5 mg, 1 mg, 2 mg

♦ **Benzylpenicillin Benzathine** *see* Penicillin G Benzathine *on page 874*

Benzylpenicilloyl-polylysine (BEN zil pen i SIL oyl pol i LIE seen)

U.S. Brand Names Pre-Pen®

Synonyms Penicilloyl-polylysine; PPL

Therapeutic Category Diagnostic Agent, Penicillin Allergy Skin Test

Generic Available No

Use Adjunct in assessing the risk of administering penicillin (penicillin or benzylpenicillin) in patients with a history of clinical penicillin hypersensitivity

Pregnancy Risk Factor C

Contraindications Patients known to be extremely hypersensitive to penicillin

Warnings PPL test alone has a sensitivity rate of 76% and does not identify those patients who react to a minor antigenic determinant; does not appear to reliably predict the occurrence of late reactions and patients at risk for anaphylaxis can be missed; PPL test alone is estimated to miss 3% to 6% of penicillin-allergic patients who are at risk for serious or fatal reactions

Adverse Reactions
Dermatologic: Erythema, urticaria
Local: Pruritus, wheal, edema
Miscellaneous: Systemic allergic reactions occur rarely

Drug Interactions Antihistamines, tricyclic antidepressants, and sympathomimetic agents may affect skin response

Stability Store in refrigerator; discard if left at room temperature for longer than 1 day

Mechanism of Action Elicits IgE antibodies which produce type I accelerated urticarial reactions to penicillins

Usual Dosage Children and Adults:
Scratch test: Use scratch technique with a 20-gauge needle to make 3-5 mm non-bleeding scratch on epidermis, apply a small drop of solution to scratch, rub in gently with applicator or toothpick. A positive reaction consists of a pale wheal surrounding the scratch site which develops within 10 minutes and ranges from 5-15 mm or more in diameter.
Intradermal test: Use intradermal test with a tuberculin syringe with a 26- to 30-gauge short bevel needle; a dose of 0.01-0.02 mL is injected intradermally. A control of NS should be injected at least 1½" from the PPL test site. Most skin responses to the intradermal test will develop within 5-15 minutes.
(Continued)

Benzylpenicilloyl-polylysine *(Continued)*

Interpretation:
(-) Negative: No reaction
(+/-) Equivocal: Wheal only slightly larger than original bleb with or without erythematous flare and larger than control site
(+) Positive: Itching and marked increase in size of original bleb
Control site should not exhibit any reaction

Administration Parenteral: PPL is administered by a scratch technique or by intradermal injection. For initial testing, PPL should always be applied via the scratch technique on the inner volar surface of the forearm. Do not administer intradermally to patients who have positive reactions to a scratch test.

Intradermal test: Administer on the upper, outer arm at least several inches below the deltoid muscle

Nursing Implications Always use scratch test for initial testing

Additional Information Hydroxyzine and diphenhydramine should be discontinued for at least 4 days and astemizole for 6-8 weeks before skin testing

Dosage Forms Injection, solution: 0.25 mL

References

Boguniewicz M and Leung DYM, "Hypersensitivity Reactions to Antibiotics Commonly Used in Children," *Pediatr Infect Dis J*, 1995, 14(3):221-31.

Beractant *(ber AKT ant)*

U.S. Brand Names Survanta®

Synonyms Bovine Lung Surfactant; Natural Lung Surfactant

Therapeutic Category Lung Surfactant

Generic Available No

Use Prevention and treatment of respiratory distress syndrome (RDS) in premature infants

Prophylactic therapy: Infants with body weight <1250 g who are at risk for developing or with evidence of surfactant deficiency

Rescue therapy: Treatment of infants with RDS confirmed by x-ray and requiring mechanical ventilation

Warnings Rapidly affects oxygenation and lung compliance and should be restricted to a highly supervised use in a clinical setting with immediate availability of clinicians experienced with intubation and ventilatory management of premature infants. If transient episodes of bradycardia and decreased oxygen saturation occur, discontinue the dosing procedure and initiate measures to alleviate the condition; produces rapid improvements in lung oxygenation and compliance that may require immediate reductions in ventilator settings and FiO_2.

Precautions Use of beractant in infants <600 g birth weight or >1750 g birth weight has not been evaluated

Adverse Reactions During the dosing procedure:
Cardiovascular: Transient bradycardia, vasoconstriction, hypotension, hypertension, pallor
Respiratory: Oxygen desaturation, endotracheal tube blockage, hypocarbia, hypercarbia, apnea, pulmonary air leaks, pulmonary interstitial emphysema, pulmonary hemorrhage
Miscellaneous: Increased probability of post-treatment nosocomial sepsis

Stability Refrigerate; protect from light; prior to administration warm by standing at room temperature for 20 minutes or hold in hand for 8 minutes; artificial warming methods should **not** be used; unused, unopened vials warmed to room temperature may be returned to the refrigerator within 8 hours of warming only once

Mechanism of Action Replaces deficient or ineffective endogenous lung surfactant in neonates with respiratory distress syndrome (RDS) or in neonates at risk of developing RDS. Surfactant prevents the alveoli from collapsing during expiration by lowering surface tension between air and alveolar surfaces.

Usual Dosage Intratracheal: Neonates:
Prophylactic treatment: Give 4 mL/kg as soon as possible; as many as 4 doses may be administered during the first 48 hours of life, no more frequently than 6 hours apart. The need for additional doses is determined by evidence of continuing respiratory distress or if the infant is still intubated and requiring at least 30% inspired oxygen to maintain a PaO_2 ≤80 torr.

Rescue treatment: Give 4 mL/kg as soon as the diagnosis of RDS is made; may repeat if needed, no more frequently than every 6 hours to a maximum of 4 doses

Administration Intratracheal: For intratracheal administration only. Do not shake; if settling occurs during storage, gently swirl. Suction infant prior to administration; inspect solution to verify complete mixing of the suspension. Administer intratracheally by instillation through a 5-French end-hole catheter inserted into the infant's endotracheal tube. Administer the dose in four 1 mL/kg aliquots. Each quarter-dose is instilled over 2-3 seconds; each quarter-dose is administered with the infant in a different position; slightly downward inclination with head turned to the right, then repeat with head turned to the left; then slightly upward inclination with head turned to the right, then repeat with head turned to the left.

Monitoring Parameters Continuous heart rate and transcutaneous O$_2$ saturation should be monitored during administration; frequent ABG sampling is necessary to prevent postdosing hyperoxia and hypocarbia.

Dosage Forms Suspension for inhalation: 25 mg/mL (4 mL, 8 mL)

♦ **Beta-2® (Can)** *see* Isoetharine [DSC] *on page 628*

♦ **Betaderm (Can)** *see* Betamethasone *on page 169*

♦ **Betadine® First Aid Antibiotics + Moisturizer [OTC]** *see* Bacitracin and Polymyxin B *on page 157*

♦ **9-Beta-D-ribofuranosyladenine** *see* Adenosine *on page 48*

♦ **Betagan® Liquifilm®** *see* Levobunolol *on page 665*

Betaine Anhydrous (BAY tayne an HY drus)

U.S. Brand Names Cystadane®

Therapeutic Category Homocystinuria, Treatment Agent

Generic Available No

Use Treatment of homocystinuria

Pregnancy Risk Factor C

Contraindications Hypersensitivity to betaine or any component

Adverse Reactions Gastrointestinal: Nausea, vomiting, diarrhea, GI distress

Mechanism of Action Betaine reduces homocysteine blood concentrations by acting as a methyl group donor in the remethylation of homocysteine to methionine

Usual Dosage Oral:
Children <3 years: 100 mg/kg/day divided into 2 doses; increase at weekly intervals in 100 mg/kg/day increments
Children ≥3 years and Adults: 3 g twice daily; doses up to 20 g/day have been needed to control homocysteine plasma concentrations in some patients

Administration Oral: Shake bottle lightly before opening; measure prescribed amount with provided measuring scoop and dissolve in 4-6 ounces of water, juice, milk, or formula; administer immediately; do not use if powder does not completely dissolve or gives a colored solution

Monitoring Parameters Plasma homocysteine concentration (should be low or undetectable)

Additional Information Orphan drug; may only be obtained by contacting Chronimed Inc at 1-800-900-4267; vitamin B$_6$, vitamin B$_{12}$, and folate have been helpful in the management of homocystinuria and are often used in conjunction

Dosage Forms Powder for oral solution: 1 g/scoop (1 scoop = 1.7 mL) (180 g)

♦ **Betaject™ (Can)** *see* Betamethasone *on page 169*

♦ **Betaloc® (Can)** *see* Metoprolol *on page 752*

♦ **Betaloc® Durules® (Can)** *see* Metoprolol *on page 752*

Betamethasone (bay ta METH a sone)

Related Information
Corticosteroids Comparison, Topical *on page 1212*

U.S. Brand Names Alphatrex®; Betatrex®; Beta-Val®; Celestone®; Celestone® Phosphate; Celestone® Soluspan®; Diprolene®; Diprolene® AF; Diprosone® [DSC]; Luxiq®; Maxivate®

Canadian Brand Names Betaderm; Betaject™; Betnesol®; Betnovate®; Celestoderm®-EV/2; Celestoderm®-V; Diprolene® Glycol; Ectosone; Prevex® B; Taro-Sone®; Topilene®; Topisone®; Valisone® Scalp Lotion

Synonyms Flubenisolone

Therapeutic Category Adrenal Corticosteroid; Anti-inflammatory Agent; Corticosteroid, Systemic; Corticosteroid, Topical; Glucocorticoid

Generic Available Yes

Use Anti-inflammatory; immunosuppressant agent; corticosteroid replacement therapy
Topical: Inflammatory dermatoses such as psoriasis, seborrheic or atopic dermatitis, neurodermatitis, inflammatory phase of xerosis, late phase of allergic dermatitis or irritant dermatitis; Foam: Inflammatory and pruritic symptoms of scalp dermatoses responsive to corticosteroids

Pregnancy Risk Factor C

Contraindications Hypersensitivity to betamethasone or any component; systemic fungal infections
(Continued)

Betamethasone *(Continued)*

Precautions Use with caution in patients with hypothyroidism, cirrhosis, ulcerative colitis; use topical products sparingly in children, systemic effects may be seen; **Note:** Due to the high incidence of developing adrenal suppression, Diprosone® cream, ointment, and lotion, and Diprolene® AF cream are not recommended for use in children ≤12 years of age (see Additional Information)

Adverse Reactions

Cardiovascular: Edema, hypertension

Central nervous system: Convulsions, vertigo, confusion, headache

Dermatologic: Thin fragile skin, hyperpigmentation or hypopigmentation, acne, impaired wound healing, skin atrophy (bruising, shininess, telangiectasia, thinness, loss of skin markings), erythema, rash, dry skin

Endocrine & metabolic: Cushingoid state, sodium retention, pituitary-adrenal axis suppression, growth suppression, glucose intolerance, hypokalemia

Gastrointestinal: Peptic ulcer, nausea, vomiting

Local: Burning, itching, stinging, sterile abscess

Neuromuscular & skeletal: Muscle weakness, osteoporosis, fractures

Ocular: Cataracts, glaucoma

Drug Interactions Cytochrome P450 isoenzyme CYP3A substrate

Barbiturates, phenytoin and rifampin will decrease corticosteroid effects; salicylates; NSAIDs; diuretics (potassium depleting); caffeine and alcohol may increase risk for GI ulcer; with systemic use: Live virus vaccines (increase risk of viral infection), vaccines may have decreased effects

Food Interactions Systemic use of corticosteroids may require a diet with increased potassium, vitamins A, B_6, C, D, folate, calcium, zinc, and phosphorus and decreased sodium

Stability Foam canister is flammable; store at controlled room temperature; avoid fire, flame, heat; do not store at >120°F (49°C)

Mechanism of Action Controls the rate of protein synthesis, depresses the migration of polymorphonuclear leukocytes and fibroblasts, reverses capillary permeability, and causes lysosomal stabilization at the cellular level to prevent or control inflammation

Pharmacokinetics

Protein binding: 64%

Metabolism: Hepatic

Elimination: <5% of dose excreted renally as unchanged drug; small amounts eliminated via biliary tract

Usual Dosage Base dosage on severity of disease and patient response

I.M.:

Children: Use lowest dose listed as initial dose for adrenocortical insufficiency (physiologic replacement); 0.0175-0.125 mg base/kg/day divided every 6-12 hours **or** 0.5-7.5 mg base/m²/day divided every 6-12 hours

Adolescents and Adults: 0.6-9 mg/day divided every 12-24 hours

Oral:

Children: Use lowest dose listed as initial dose for adrenocortical insufficiency (physiologic replacement); 0.0175-0.25 mg/kg/day divided every 6-8 hours **or** 0.5-7.5 mg/m²/day divided every 6-8 hours

Adolescents and Adults: 2.4-4.8 mg/day in 2-4 doses; range: 0.6-7.2 mg/day

Topical:

Children and Adults: Apply thin film 1-3 times/day (see Precautions and Additional Information)

Adolescents ≥13 years and Adults:

Diprolene® AF cream: Apply thin film 1-2 times/day; maximum: 45 g of cream/week

Diprosone® cream and ointment: Apply thin film once daily; twice daily application may be needed in some cases

Diprosone® lotion: Apply a few drops and massage gently into skin twice daily (in morning and at night)

Adolescents ≥16 years and Adults: Luxiq® foam: Apply twice daily (in morning and at night)

Administration

Oral: Administer with food to decrease GI effects

Parenteral: Do not administer injectable suspension I.V.; shake injectable suspension before use

Topical: Apply sparingly, rub in gently until it disappears; do not apply to face or inguinal areas; not for use on broken skin or in areas of infection

Foam: Invert can, dispense small amount of foam onto saucer or other cool surface; foam will melt upon contact with warm skin (do not dispense directly into hands); use fingers to apply small amounts of foam to affected scalp area; rub in gently until it disappears; avoid fire, flame, or smoking during use; contents of can are flammable and under pressure

Test Interactions Skin tests

Patient Information

Systemic use: Avoid alcohol and caffeine

Topical use: Avoid contact with eyes; do not use occlusive dressings or other corticosteroid-containing products unless directed by physician

Additional Information Medium to high potency topical corticosteroid; long-acting corticosteroid with minimal or no sodium-retaining potential

Several recent studies conducted in children ≤12 years of age with atopic dermatitis demonstrated a high incidence of adrenal suppression when topical betamethasone products were applied twice daily for 2-3 weeks. Adrenal suppression occurred in: 10 of 43 (23%) evaluable patients (2-12 years of age) using Diprosone® cream 0.05%; 15 of 53 (28%) evaluable patients (6 months to 12 years of age) using Diprosone® ointment 0.05%; 11 of 15 (73%) evaluable patients (6-12 years of age) using Diprosone® lotion 0.05%; and 19 of 60 (32%) evaluable patients (3 months to 12 years of age) using Diprolene® AF cream 0.05%. A higher percent incidence of adrenal suppression was noted in younger children and infants (see product package inserts). Pediatric patients may be more susceptible to adrenal suppression and other systemic side effects of topical corticosteroids, due to their larger skin surface area to body weight ratio. The smallest effective dose of topical corticosteroids should be used in pediatric patients.

Dosage Forms

Cream, topical, as **dipropionate**: 0.05% (15 g, 45 g, 60 g)

Alphatrex®, Diprosone® [DSC]: 0.05% (15 g, 45 g)

Maxivate®: 0.05% (45 g)

Cream, topical, as **dipropionate augmented** (Diprolene®, Diprolene® AF): 0.05% (15 g, 50 g) [emollient base]

Cream, topical, as **valerate** (Betatrex®, Beta-Val®): 0.1% (15 g, 45 g)

Foam, topical, as **valerate** (Luxiq®): 0.12% (50 g, 100 g) [contains 60.4% alcohol]

Gel, topical, as **dipropionate augmented** (Diprolene®): 0.05% (15 g, 50 g)

Injection, solution, as **sodium phosphate** (Celestone® Phosphate): 4 mg/mL [equivalent to 3 mg/mL betamethasone base] (5 mL)

Injection, suspension, as **sodium phosphate and acetate** (Celestone® Soluspan®): 6 mg/mL [3 mg betamethasone as betamethasone sodium phosphate and 3 mg betamethasone acetate per mL] (5 mL)

Lotion, topical, as **dipropionate**: 0.05% (20 mL, 30 mL, 60 mL)

Alphatrex®, Maxivate®: 0.05% (60 mL)

Diprosone®: 0.05% (20 mL, 60 mL) [DSC]

Lotion, topical, as **dipropionate augmented** (Diprolene® AF): 0.05% (30 mL, 60 mL)

Lotion, topical, as **valerate** (Betatrex®, Beta-Val®): 0.1% (60 mL)

Ointment, topical, as **dipropionate**: 0.05% (15 g, 45 g)

Alphatrex®, Maxivate: 0.05% (45 g)

Diprosone®: 0.05% (15 g, 45 g) [DSC]

Ointment, topical, as **dipropionate augmented**: 0.05% (15 g, 45 g, 50 g)

Diprolene®: 0.05% (15 g, 50 g)

Ointment, topical, as **valerate** (Betatrex®): 0.1% (15 g, 45 g)

Syrup, as **base** (Celestone®): 0.6 mg/5 mL (120 mL)

Tablet, as **base** (Celestone®): 0.6 mg

♦ **Betapace®** *see* Sotalol *on page 1032*

♦ **Betapace AF™** *see* Sotalol *on page 1032*

♦ **Betasept® [OTC]** *see* Chlorhexidine Gluconate *on page 257*

♦ **Betatar® [OTC]** *see* Coal Tar *on page 299*

♦ **Betatrex®** *see* Betamethasone *on page 169*

♦ **Beta-Val®** *see* Betamethasone *on page 169*

♦ **Betaxin® (Can)** *see* Thiamine *on page 1081*

Bethanechol (be THAN e kole)

U.S. Brand Names Urecholine®

Canadian Brand Names Duvoid®; Myotonachol®; PMS-Bethanechol

Therapeutic Category Cholinergic Agent

Generic Available Yes

Use Treatment of nonobstructive urinary retention and retention due to neurogenic bladder; gastroesophageal reflux

Pregnancy Risk Factor C

Contraindications Hypersensitivity to bethanechol chloride or any component; do not use in patients with mechanical obstruction of the GI or GU tract; do not use in patients with hyperthyroidism, peptic ulcer, bronchial asthma, or cardiac disease (Continued)

Bethanechol *(Continued)*

Adverse Reactions

Cardiovascular: Hypotension, cardiac arrest, flushed skin (vasomotor response)

Central nervous system: Headache

Gastrointestinal: Abdominal cramps, diarrhea, nausea, vomiting, salivation

Genitourinary: Urinary frequency

Hepatic: Elevated liver enzymes, elevated bilirubin

Ocular: Miosis, lacrimation

Respiratory: Bronchial constriction

Miscellaneous: Diaphoresis

Drug Interactions Ganglionic blockers may cause a critical fall in blood pressure; additive effects with other cholinergic agents; quinidine, and procainamide decrease the effects of bethanechol; anticholinergic agents (atropine, antihistamines, TCAs, phenothiazine) may decrease bethanechol's effects

Mechanism of Action Stimulates cholinergic receptors in the smooth muscle of the urinary bladder and GI tract resulting in increased peristalsis, increased GI and pancreatic secretions, bladder muscle contraction, and increased ureteral peristaltic waves

Pharmacodynamics

Onset of action: Oral: 30-90 minutes

Duration: Oral: Up to 6 hours

Pharmacokinetics

Absorption: Oral: Variable

Metabolic fate and excretion have not been determined

Usual Dosage Oral:

Children:

Abdominal distention or urinary retention: 0.6 mg/kg/day divided 3-4 times/day

Gastroesophageal reflux: 0.1-0.2 mg/kg/dose or 3 mg/m^2/dose given 30 minutes to 1 hour before each meal to a maximum of 4 times/day

Adults: 10-50 mg 2-4 times/day

Administration Oral: Administer on an empty stomach to reduce nausea and vomiting

Patient Information Dizziness, lightheadedness, or fainting may occur especially when getting up from a lying position

Dosage Forms Tablet, as chloride: 5 mg, 10 mg, 25 mg, 50 mg

Extemporaneous Preparations

A 1 mg/mL solution may be made by crushing twelve 10 mg tablets; add sterile water in increments to a total volume of 120 mL; shake well; refrigerate; stable for 30 days (Schlatter, 1997).

A 5 mg/mL suspension may be made by crushing twelve 50 mg tablets; add to a total volume of 120 mL of a 1:1 mixture of Ora-Plus®:Ora-Sweet® or Ora-Plus®:Ora-Sweet® SF; stable 60 days refrigerated; label "shake well" and protect from light (Allen, 1998).

Allen LV Jr and Erickson MA, "Stability of Bethanechol Chloride, Pyrazinamide, Quinidine Sulfate, Rifampin, and Tetracycline Hydrochloride in Extemporaneously Compounded Oral Liquids," *Am J Health Syst Pharm*, 1998, 55(17):1804-9.

Schlatter JL and Saulnier JL, "Bethanechol Chloride Oral Solutions: Stability and Use in Infants," *Ann Pharmacother*, 1997, 31(3):294-6.

- ◆ **Betimol®** *see* Timolol *on page 1095*
- ◆ **Betnesol® (Can)** *see* Betamethasone *on page 169*
- ◆ **Betnovate® (Can)** *see* Betamethasone *on page 169*
- ◆ **Biaxin®** *see* Clarithromycin *on page 285*
- ◆ **Biaxin® XL** *see* Clarithromycin *on page 285*
- ◆ **Bicillin® L-A** *see* Penicillin G Benzathine *on page 874*
- ◆ **Bicitra®** *see* Citrate and Citric Acid *on page 282*
- ◆ **BiCNU®, Gliadel®** *see* Carmustine *on page 217*
- ◆ **Biltricide®** *see* Praziquantel *on page 923*
- ◆ **Biobase™ (Can)** *see* Ethyl Alcohol *on page 465*
- ◆ **Biobase-G™ (Can)** *see* Ethyl Alcohol *on page 465*
- ◆ **Biocef®** *see* Cephalexin *on page 244*
- ◆ **Biofed [OTC]** *see* Pseudoephedrine *on page 958*
- ◆ **BioQuin® Durules™ (Can)** *see* Quinidine *on page 967*
- ◆ **Bio-Statin®** *see* Nystatin *on page 827*

Biotin (BYE oh tin)

U.S. Brand Names Biotin® Forte [OTC]; d-Biotin [OTC]; Meribin® [OTC]

Therapeutic Category Biotinidase Deficiency, Treatment Agent; Nutritional Supplement; Vitamin, Water Soluble

Generic Available Yes

Use Treatment of primary biotinidase deficiency; nutritional biotin deficiency; component of the vitamin B complex

Contraindications Hypersensitivity to biotin or any component

Food Interactions Large amounts of raw egg whites prevent biotin absorption

Mechanism of Action A member of the B-complex group of vitamins; biotin is required for various metabolic functions such as gluconeogenesis, lipogenesis, fatty acid biosynthesis, propionate metabolism, and the catabolism of branched-chain amino acids; there are 9 known biotin-dependent enzymes; the enzyme biotinidase regenerates biotin in the body and is also required for the release of dietary protein-bound biotin.

Biotinidase deficiency is an autosomal recessively inherited metabolic disorder characterized by deficient activity of the enzyme in serum. Children with the disorder usually exhibit seizures, hypotonia, ataxia, skin rash, alopecia, metabolic ketoacidosis, and organic aciduria.

Usual Dosage Oral:

RDA: Infants, Children, and Adults: There is no official RDA, however 100-200 mcg/day is considered adequate

Biotinidase deficiency: Neonates, Infants, Children, and Adults: 5-10 mg once daily

Biotin deficiency: Children and Adults: 5-20 mg once daily

Administration Oral: May be administered without regard to meals

Reference Range Serum biotinidase activity

Dosage Forms

Capsule (Meribin®): 5 mg

Tablet: 300 mcg

Biotin® Forte: 3 mg, 5 mg

d-Biotin: 2.5 mg, 10 mg

References

McVoy JR, Levy HL, Lawler M, et al, "Partial Biotinidase Deficiency: Clinical and Biochemical Features," 1990, J Pediatr, 116(1):78-83.

Salbert BA, Pellock JM, and Wolf B, "Characterization of Seizures Associated With Biotinidase Deficiency," Neurology, 1993, 43(7):1351-5.

Wastell HJ, Bartlett K, Dale G, et al, "Biotinidase Deficiency: A Survey of 10 Cases," Arch Dis Child, 1988, 63(10):1244-9.

♦ **Biotin® Forte [OTC]** see Biotin on page 173

♦ **Bisac-Evac® [OTC]** see Bisacodyl on page 173

Bisacodyl (bis a KOE dil)

U.S. Brand Names Alophen® [OTC]; Bisac-Evac® [OTC]; Bisacodyl Uniserts® [OTC]; Dulcolax® [OTC]; Femilax™ [OTC]; Fleet® Bisacodyl Enema [OTC]; Fleet® Stimulant Laxative [OTC]; Modane® Tablets [OTC]

Canadian Brand Names Apo®-Bisacodyl

Therapeutic Category Laxative, Stimulant

Generic Available Yes

Use Treatment of constipation; colonic evacuation prior to procedures or examination

Pregnancy Risk Factor C

Contraindications Hypersensitivity to bisacodyl or any component; do not use in patients with abdominal pain, appendicitis, obstruction, nausea or vomiting; not to be used during pregnancy or lactation

Warnings Stimulant laxatives are habit-forming; long-term use may result in laxative dependence and loss of normal bowel function.

Precautions Bisacodyl tannex powder for preparation as a rectal solution should be used with caution in patients with ulceration of the colon

Adverse Reactions

Endocrine & metabolic: Electrolyte and fluid imbalance (metabolic acidosis or alkalosis, hypocalcemia)

Gastrointestinal: Abdominal cramps, nausea, vomiting, diarrhea, rectal burning, proctitis (rare)

Food Interactions Administration within 1 hour of ingesting antacids, alkaline material, milk, or dairy products will cause premature dissolution of the enteric coating and resultant gastric irritation

Stability Store enteric-coated tablets and rectal suppositories at <30°C.

(Continued)

Bisacodyl *(Continued)*

Mechanism of Action Stimulates peristalsis by directly irritating the smooth muscle of the intestine, possibly the colonic intramural plexus; alters water and electrolyte secretion producing net intestinal fluid accumulation and laxation

Pharmacodynamics Onset of action:
Oral: Within 6-10 hours
Rectal: 15-60 minutes

Pharmacokinetics
Absorption: Oral, rectal: <5% absorbed systemically
Metabolism: In the liver
Elimination: Conjugated metabolites excreted in breast milk, bile, and urine

Usual Dosage
Bisacodyl (Dulcolax®) tablet: Oral:
Children 3-12 years: 5-10 mg or 0.3 mg/kg/day as a single dose
Children ≥12 years and Adults: 5-15 mg/day as a single dose; maximum dose: 30 mg
Bisacodyl (Dulcolax®) suppository: Rectal:
Children:
<2 years: 5 mg/day as a single dose
2-11 years: 5-10 mg/day as a single dose
Children ≥12 years and Adults: 10 mg/day as a single dose

Administration Oral: Administer on an empty stomach with water; patient should swallow tablet whole; do not break or chew enteric-coated tablet; do not administer within 1 hour of ingesting antacids, alkaline material, milk, or dairy products

Patient Information Should not be used regularly for more than 1 week

Additional Information In a randomized prospective study of 70 patients, bisacodyl tablets were given orally once daily in the morning for 2 days before colonoscopy to 19 patients (dose for children <5 years: 5 mg; 5-12 years: 10 mg; >12 years: 15 mg) with a Fleet® enema given on the morning of the procedure without any dietary restriction. Results showed that bisacodyl without dietary restriction provided unsatisfactory colon cleansing.

Dosage Forms
Enema, suspension (Fleet® Bisacodyl Enema): 10 mg/30 mL
Suppository, rectal (Bisac-Evac™, Bisacodyl Uniserts®, Dulcolax®): 10 mg
Tablet, enteric coated (Alophen®, Bisac-Evac™, Dulcolax®, Femilax™, Fleet® Stimulant Laxative, Modane®): 5 mg

References
BaKer SS, Liptak GS, Colletti RB, et al, "Constipation in Infants and Children: Evaluation and Treatment," 2000, www.naspgn.org/constipation.
Dahshan A, Lin CH, Peters J, et al, "A Randomized, Prospective Study to Evaluate the Efficacy and Acceptance of Three Bowel Preparations for Colonoscopy in Children," *Am J Gastroenterol*, 1999, 94(12):3497-501.

♦ **Bisacodyl Uniserts® [OTC]** *see* Bisacodyl *on page 173*

Bismuth *(BIZ muth)*

U.S. Brand Names Colo-Fresh™ [OTC]; Devrom®; Diotame® [OTC]; Kaopectate® [OTC]; Kaopectate®, Children's (Reformulation) [OTC]; Kaopectate® Extra Strength [OTC]; Pepto-Bismol® [OTC]; Pepto-Bismol® Maximum Strength [OTC]

Synonyms BSS

Therapeutic Category Antidiarrheal; Gastrointestinal Agent, Gastric or Duodenal Ulcer Treatment

Generic Available Yes

Use Symptomatic treatment of mild, nonspecific diarrhea including traveler's diarrhea; chronic infantile diarrhea; adjunctive treatment of *Helicobacter pylori*-associated antral gastritis

Pregnancy Risk Factor C (D in 3rd trimester)

Contraindications Hypersensitivity to bismuth, salicylates, or any component; do not use subsalicylate in patients with influenza or chickenpox because of risk of Reye's syndrome; history of severe GI bleeding or coagulopathy

Warnings Subsalicylate should be used with caution if patient is taking aspirin, due to additive toxicity; use with caution in children <3 years of age and those with viral illness; be aware of salicylate content when prescribing for use in children

Precautions May interfere with radiologic examinations of GI tract as bismuth is radiopaque

Adverse Reactions
Central nervous system: Anxiety, confusion, slurred speech, headache, mental depression
Gastrointestinal: Impaction (infants and debilitated patients), grayish-black stools, darkened tongue

Neuromuscular & skeletal: Muscle spasms, weakness

Otic: Tinnitus, loss of hearing

Drug Interactions Decreases absorption of tetracycline; increases toxicity of aspirin (due to absorption of salicylate), warfarin, hypoglycemics

Mechanism of Action Adsorbs extra water in large intestine, as well as toxins; forms a protective coat on the intestinal mucosa; appears to have antisecretory (salicylate moiety) and antimicrobial effects (bismuth moiety) against bacterial and viral pathogens

Pharmacokinetics

Absorption: Bismuth is minimally absorbed (<1%) across the GI tract while salicylate salt is readily absorbed (80%)

Distribution: Salicylate: V_d: 170 mL/kg

Protein binding, plasma: Bismuth and salicylate: >90%

Metabolism: Bismuth salts undergo chemical dissociation after oral administration; salicylate is extensively metabolized in the liver

Half-life:

Bismuth: Terminal: 21-72 days

Salicylate: Terminal: 2-5 hours

Elimination:

Bismuth: Renal, biliary

Salicylate: Only 10% excreted unchanged in urine

Usual Dosage Oral: Bismuth subsalicylate: **(bismuth subsalicylate liquid dosages expressed in mL of 262 mg/15 mL concentration):**

Nonspecific diarrhea: 100 mg/kg/day divided into 5 equal doses for 5 days (maximum: 4.19 g/day) **or**

Children: Up to 8 doses/24 hours:

3-6 years: $1/3$ tablet or 5 mL every 30 minutes to 1 hour as needed

6-9 years: $2/3$ tablet or 10 mL every 30 minutes to 1 hour as needed

9-12 years: 1 tablet or 15 mL every 30 minutes to 1 hour as needed

Adults: 2 tablets or 30 mL every 30 minutes to 1 hour as needed up to 8 doses/24 hours

Chronic infantile diarrhea:

2-24 months: 2.5 mL every 4 hours

24-48 months: 5 mL every 4 hours

48-70 months: 10 mL every 4 hours

Prevention of traveler's diarrhea: Adults: 2.1 g/day or 2 tablets 4 times/day before meals and at bedtime

Helicobacter pylori-associated antral gastritis: Dosage in children is not well established, the following dosages have been used [in conjunction with ampicillin and metronidazole or (in adults) tetracycline and metronidazole]:

Children ≤10 years: 15 mL (262 mg) 4 times/day for 6 weeks

Children >10 years and Adults: 30 mL of 262 mg/15 mL solution or two 262 mg tablets 4 times/day for 6 weeks

Dosing adjustment in renal impairment: Avoid use in patients with renal failure

Administration Oral: Shake liquid well before using; chew tablets or allow to dissolve in mouth before swallowing

Test Interactions Bismuth absorbs x-rays and may interfere with diagnostic procedures of GI tract

Patient Information May darken stools; if diarrhea persists for more than 2 days, consult a physician; may turn tongue black

Additional Information Bismuth subsalicylate: 262 mg = 130 mg nonaspirin salicylate; 525 mg = 236 mg nonaspirin salicylate

Dosage Forms

Caplet, as **subgallate** (Devrom®): 200 mg

Liquid, as **subsalicylate:** 262 mg/15 mL (240 mL, 360 mL, 480 mL); 525 mg/15 mL (240 mL, 360 mL)

Children's Kaopectate®: 87 mg/5 mL (180 mL) [cherry flavor]

Diotame®: 262 mg/15 mL (30 mL)

Kaopectate®: 262 mg/15 mL (240 mL) [regular and peppermint flavor]

Kaopectate® Extra Strength: 525 mg/15 mL (240 mL) [peppermint flavor]

Pepto-Bismol®: 262 mg/15 mL (120 mL, 240 mL, 360 mL, 480 mL) [wintergreen flavor]

Pepto-Bismol® Maximum Strength: 525 mg/15 mL (120 mL, 240 mL, 360 mL) [wintergreen flavor]

Tablet, as **subgallate** (Colo-Fresh™): 324 mg

Tablet, chewable, as **subgallate** (Devrom®): 200 mg

Tablet, chewable, as **subsalicylate** (Diotame®, Pepto-Bismol®): 262 mg

References

Drumm B, Sherman P, Karmali M, et al, "Treatment of *Campylobacter pylori*-associated Antral Gastritis in Children With Bismuth Subsalicylate and Ampicillin," *J Pediatr*, 1988, 113(5):908-12.

(Continued)

Bismuth *(Continued)*

Soriano-Brucher HE, Avendano P, O'Ryan M, et al, "Use of Bismuth Subsalicylate in Acute Diarrhea in Children," *Rev Infect Dis*, 1990, 12(Suppl 1):S51-5.

Walsh JH and Peterson WL, "The Treatment of *Helicobacter pylori* Infection in the Management of Peptic Ulcer Disease," *N Engl J Med*, 1995, 333(15):984-91.

♦ **Bistropamide** *see* Tropicamide *on page 1125*

Bitolterol *(bye TOLE ter ole)*

Related Information

Asthma Guidelines *on page 1376*

U.S. Brand Names Tornalate® [DSC]

Therapeutic Category Adrenergic Agonist Agent; Antiasthmatic; Beta$_2$-Adrenergic Agonist Agent; Bronchodilator; Sympathomimetic

Use Prevention and treatment of bronchial asthma and bronchospasm

Pregnancy Risk Factor C

Contraindications Hypersensitivity to bitolterol or any component

Warnings Excessive use may result in cardiac arrest and death

Precautions Use with caution in patients with unstable vasomotor symptoms, diabetes, hyperthyroidism, prostatic hypertrophy or a history of seizures, cardiovascular disorders such as coronary artery disease, arrhythmias, and hypertension; do not use concurrently with other sympathomimetic bronchodilators

Adverse Reactions

Cardiovascular: Flushing of face, hypertension, pounding heartbeat, chest pain, arrhythmias, tachycardia

Central nervous system: Dizziness, lightheadedness, nervousness, insomnia

Gastrointestinal: Xerostomia, nausea, unpleasant taste, mouth and throat irritation

Neuromuscular & skeletal: Tremors, hyperkinesia, paresthesia

Respiratory: Bronchial irritation, coughing, paradoxical bronchospasm

Drug Interactions Bitolterol decreases the effects of beta-adrenergic blockers (eg, propranol); inhaled ipratropium may increase duration of bronchodilation; nifedipine may increase FEV$_1$; increased toxicity with MAO inhibitors, tricyclic antidepressants, sympathomimetic agents, inhaled anesthetics (eg, enflurane)

Stability Solution for nebulization should not be mixed with cromolyn sodium or acetylcysteine; stability when mixed with other nebulized drugs has not been established

Mechanism of Action Bitolterol, a prodrug, undergoes hydrolysis in the lungs to the active agent, colterol. Colterol selectively stimulates beta$_2$-adrenergic receptors in the lungs producing bronchial smooth muscle relaxation. Colterol possesses minor beta$_1$ activity.

Pharmacodynamics

Onset of action: After oral inhalation: 3-5 minutes

Maximum effect: 0.5-2 hours

Duration: 4-8 hours

Pharmacokinetics Since blood levels of colterol (active drug) are too low to be measured by currently available assay methods, the pharmacokinetics of this agent following inhalation are not known.

Usual Dosage Children >12 years and Adults:

Bronchospasm: Oral inhalation: 2 inhalations at an interval of at least 1-3 minutes, followed by a third inhalation if needed

Prevention of bronchospasm: Oral inhalation: 2 inhalations every 8 hours; maximum daily dosage: 3 inhalations every 6 hours or 2 inhalations every 4 hours

Intermittent nebulization: 1 mg (0.5 mL) [range: 0.5-1.5 mg (0.25-0.75 mL)] every 8 hours; treatments may be increased to four times daily, however, the interval between treatments should **not** be less than 4 hours; a dosage of 2 mg (1 mL) may be used in severely obstructed patients; maximum daily dosage: 8 mg (4 mL)

Continuous flow nebulization: 2.5 mg (1.25 mL) 3 times/day [range: 1.5-3.5 mg (0.75-1.75 mL)]; maximum daily dosage 14 mg (7 mL); treatments should be at least 4 hours apart

Administration

Oral inhalation: Shake canister well before use; administer pressurized inhalation during the second half of inspiration, as the airways are open and the aerosol distribution is more extensive. If more than one inhalation per dose is necessary, wait at least 1 full minute between inhalations; the second inhalation is best delivered after 10 minutes. Administer every 8 hours rather than 3 times/day, to promote less variation in peak and trough serum levels

Nebulization: Dilute with NS to a total volume of 2-4 mL prior to use; after adding to nebulizer reservoir, swirl contents gently; the patient should breathe deeply until the nebulizer chamber is empty (approximately 5-15 minutes)

Monitoring Parameters Assess lung sounds, heart rate, respiratory rate, peak flow; arterial or capillary blood gases (if patient's condition warrants)

Patient Information Do not exceed recommended dosage, excessive use may lead to adverse effects or loss of effectiveness; may cause dry mouth; may cause nervousness, restlessness, and insomnia; if these effects continue after dosage reduction, notify physician; also notify physician if palpitations, tachycardia, chest pain, muscle tremors, dizziness, headache, flushing, or if breathing difficulty persists

Dosage Forms

Aerosol for oral inhalation, as mesylate: 0.8% [370 mcg/metered spray, 300 inhalations] (15 mL) [DSC]

Solution for oral inhalation, as mesylate: 0.2% (10 mL, 30 mL, 60 mL) [DSC]

References

"National Asthma Education and Prevention Program. Expert Panel Report: Guidelines for the Diagnosis and Management of Asthma Update on Selected Topics--2002," *J Allergy Clin Immunol*, 2002, 110(5 Suppl):S141-219.

♦ **Blenoxane®** *see* Bleomycin *on page 177*

Bleomycin (blee oh MYE sin)

Related Information

Emetogenic Potential of Single Chemotherapeutic Agents *on page 1286*

U.S. Brand Names Blenoxane®

Synonyms BLM

Therapeutic Category Antineoplastic Agent, Antibiotic

Generic Available Yes

Use Palliative treatment of squamous cell carcinoma, testicular carcinoma, and germ cell tumors; Hodgkin's lymphoma, non-Hodgkin's lymphoma, renal carcinoma, and soft tissue sarcoma; sclerosing agent to control malignant effusions

Pregnancy Risk Factor D

Contraindications Hypersensitivity to bleomycin sulfate or any component

Warnings The FDA currently recommends that procedures for proper handling and disposal of antineoplastic agents be considered. Occurrence of pulmonary fibrosis is higher in elderly patients and in those receiving a total cumulative dose >400 units; pulmonary toxicity has occurred at a total dosage <200 units or 250 units/m^2 in younger patients; pulmonary irradiation and use of supplemental oxygen increase the chance for developing toxic pulmonary reactions in patients previously treated with bleomycin; a severe idiosyncratic reaction consisting of hypotension, mental confusion, fever, chills, and wheezing is possible.

Precautions Use with caution in patients with renal or pulmonary impairment; dosage modification is recommended in patients with renal impairment; dosage modification may be necessary in patients with a 20% decrease from baseline in FEV_1, FVC, or DL_{co}; administer test dose to lymphoma patients prior to starting therapy

Adverse Reactions

Cardiovascular: Cerebrovascular accident, hypotension, Raynaud's phenomenon

Central nervous system: Fever, chills, malaise

Dermatologic: Hyperpigmentation, hyperkeratosis of hands and nails, rash, alopecia, desquamation

Gastrointestinal: Stomatitis, vomiting, anorexia, mild nausea

Hematologic: Thrombocytopenia, leukopenia

Local: Phlebitis

Respiratory: Interstitial pneumonitis (10%), pulmonary fibrosis (cumulative lifetime dose should not exceed 400 units or 250 units/m^2 in younger patients), dyspnea, tachypnea, nonproductive cough, rales

Miscellaneous: Anaphylactoid reactions

Drug Interactions Phenytoin (decreases phenytoin concentrations), cisplatin (decreases bleomycin clearance), bleomycin may decrease digoxin absorption; concurrent use with amphotericin B products may increase nephrotoxicity and risk for hypotension and bronchospasm

Stability Refrigerate; intact vials are stable 28 days at room temperature; reconstituted solution is stable for 24 hours at room temperature; incompatible with amino acid solutions, ascorbic acid, cefazolin, furosemide, diazepam, hydrocortisone, mitomycin, nafcillin, penicillin G, aminophylline, copper; dilution in dextrose solutions may result in a 10% loss of activity within 24 hours

Mechanism of Action Inhibits synthesis of DNA; binds to DNA leading to single- and double-strand breaks by a Fe^{++}-O_2-catalyzed free radical reaction

Pharmacokinetics

Distribution: Into skin, lungs, kidneys, peritoneum, and lymphatics

Protein binding: <10%

Half-life: Dependent upon renal function

Children: 2.1-3.5 hours

Adults, with normal renal function: 2-3 hours

Time to peak serum concentration: I.M.: Within 30-60 minutes

(Continued)

Bleomycin *(Continued)*

Elimination: 60% to 70% of a dose excreted in the urine as active drug

Dialysis: Not removed by hemodialysis

Usual Dosage Refer to individual protocol

Children and Adults:

I.M., I.V., S.C.:

Test dose for lymphoma patients: 1-2 units of bleomycin for the first 2 doses; monitor vital signs every 15 minutes; wait a minimum of 1 hour before administering remainder of dose

Treatment: 10-20 units/m² (0.25-0.5 units/kg) 1-2 times/week in combination regimens or once every 2-4 weeks

Germ cell tumors: 15 units/m²/dose once weekly for 3 weeks per regimen

Hodgkin's disease: 10 units/m²/dose on days 1 and 15 of cycle

I.V. continuous infusion: 15-20 units/m²/day over 24 hours for 3-5 days

Adults: Intracavitary injection for pleural effusion: 15-60 units (dose generally does not exceed 1 unit/kg); drug is diluted with 50-100 mL of NS and is instilled into the pleural cavity via a thoracostomy tube

Dosing adjustment in renal impairment:

Cl_{cr} 25-50 mL/minute: Reduce dose by 25%

Cl_{cr} <25 mL/minute: Reduce dose by 50% to 75%

Administration Parenteral:

I.V.: Administer I.V. slowly over at least 10 minutes (no greater than 1 unit/minute) at a concentration not to exceed 3 units/mL; bleomycin for I.V. continuous infusion can be further diluted in NS (preferred) or D_5W; administration by continuous infusion may produce less severe pulmonary toxicity

I.M., S.C.: 15 units/mL concentration may be used for I.M., S.C. administration

Monitoring Parameters Pulmonary function tests (total lung volume, FEV_1, FVC, DL_{co}), renal function tests, chest x-ray; vital signs and temperature initially; CBC with differential and platelet count

Patient Information Report any coughing, shortness of breath, or wheezing to physician

Nursing Implications Fever and chills can occur 2-6 hours following parenteral administration; pretreatment with acetaminophen, antihistamine, and hydrocortisone may decrease the severity of fever and chills

Dosage Forms Injection, powder for reconstitution, as sulfate: 15 units, 30 units (1 unit = 1 mg)

References

Alberts DS, Chen HS, Liu R, et al, "Bleomycin Pharmacokinetics in Man. I. Intravenous Administration," *Cancer Chemother Pharmacol*, 1978, 1(3):177-81.

Berg SL, Grisell DL, Delaney TF, et al, "Principles of Treatment of Pediatric Solid Tumors," *Pediatr Clin North Am*, 1991, 38(2):249-67.

♦ **Bleph®-10** *see Sulfacetamide on page 1048*

♦ **BLM** *see Bleomycin on page 177*

♦ **Blocadren®** *see Timolol on page 1095*

♦ **Blood Level Sampling Time Guidelines** *see page 1386*

♦ **Bluboro® [OTC]** *see Aluminum Acetate on page 73*

♦ **Bonamine™ (Can)** *see Meclizine on page 710*

♦ **Bonine® [OTC]** *see Meclizine on page 710*

♦ **Botox®** *see Botulinum Toxin Type A on page 178*

Botulinum Toxin Type A *(BOT yoo lin num TOKS in type aye)*

U.S. Brand Names Botox®

Synonyms *Clostridium botulinum* Toxin Type A; Oculinum®

Therapeutic Category Muscle Contracture, Treatment; Ophthalmic Agent, Toxin

Generic Available No

Use Treatment of strabismus and blepharospasm associated with dystonia (including benign essential blepharospasm or VII nerve disorders); treatment of dynamic muscle contracture in pediatric cerebral palsy patients (orphan drug); treatment of cervical dystonia

Pregnancy Risk Factor C

Contraindications Hypersensitivity to botulinum A toxin or any component; infection at the site of injection

Warnings The European formulation of botulinum A toxin (Dysport®) is not equivalent in potency to Botox®; the Dysport®:Botox® equivalency ratio is ~3:1 or 4:1, respectively; patients treated for cervical dystonia may experience dysphagia which rarely may result in dyspnea, aspiration, and pneumonia

Precautions Presence of antibodies to botulinum toxin type A may reduce the effectiveness of therapy; to minimize the development of antibodies, keep the dose of botulinum toxin type A as low as possible. Reduced blinking from botulinum toxin type A injection of the orbicularis muscle can lead to corneal exposure, persistent epithelial defect, and corneal ulceration, especially in patients with VII nerve disorders; carefully test corneal sensation in eyes previously operated upon. Avoid injection into the lower lid area to avoid ectropion, and vigorously treat any epithelial defect (this may require protective drops, ointment, therapeutic soft contact lenses, or closure of the eye by patching). Retrobulbar hemorrhages sufficient to compromise retinal circulation have occurred from needle penetrations into the orbit; have appropriate instruments to decompress the orbit accessible; ocular (globe) penetrations by needles have also occurred (an ophthalmoscope to diagnose this condition should be available).

Use with caution in patients with peripheral motor neuropathic diseases (eg, amyotrophic lateral sclerosis or motor neuropathy) or neuromuscular junction disorders (eg, myasthenia gravis or Lambert-Eaton syndrome) as these patients may be at increased risk for development of significant systemic side effects including severe dysphagia and respiratory compromise; use cautiously if there is inflammation present at the proposed injection site or when excessive weakness or atrophy is present in the target muscles

Adverse Reactions

Cardiovascular: Arrhythmia, MI (rare)

Central nervous system: Fever

Dermatologic: Rash, keratitis, pruritus, erythema multiforme, psoriasiform eruption

Gastrointestinal: Dysphagia (particularly after treatment of cervical dystonia), dyspepsia, xerostomia

Local: Pain, bruising at injection site

Neuromuscular & skeletal: Weakness, temporary loss of function

Ocular: Dry eyes, lagophthalmos, ptosis, photophobia, vertical deviation, tearing, diplopia, eyelid edema, spatial disorientation, blepharospasm, ectropion, entropion, retrobulbar hemorrhage

Drug Interactions Effects of botulinum toxin may be potentiated by aminoglycoside antibiotics, or any other drug that interferes with neuromuscular transmission

Stability Store lyophilized product in refrigerator at 2°C to 8°C (36°F to 46°F); administer within 4 hours after reconstitution; reconstituted solution may be stored in the refrigerator (2°C to 8°C/36°F to 46°F) until administered

Mechanism of Action Botulinum A toxin is a neurotoxin produced by *Clostridium botulinum*, a spore-forming anaerobic bacillus; it blocks neuromuscular conduction by binding to receptor sites on motor nerve terminals, entering the nerve terminals and inhibiting the release of acetylcholine. When injected intramuscularly at therapeutic doses, it produces a localized chemical denervation muscle paralysis. When the muscle is chemically denervated, it atrophies and may develop extrajunctional acetylcholine receptors. There is evidence that the nerve can sprout and reinnervate the muscle, with the weakness being reversible. Following several weeks of paralysis, alignment of the eye is measurably changed, despite return of innervation to the injected muscle.

Pharmacodynamics

Strabismus:

Onset of action: 1-2 days after injection

Duration of paralysis: 2-6 weeks

Blepharospasm:

Onset of action: 3 days after injection

Maximum effect: 1-2 weeks

Duration of paralysis: 3 months

Spasticity associated with cerebral palsy

Onset of action: Several days

Duration of paralysis: 3-8 months

Usual Dosage I.M.:

Strabismus:

Children 2 months to 12 years:

Horizontal or vertical deviations <20 prism diopters: 1.25 units into any one muscle

Horizontal or vertical deviations 20-25 prism diopters: 1-2.5 units into any one muscle

Persistent VI nerve palsy of ≥1 month duration: 1-1.25 units into the medial rectus muscle

Children ≥12 years and Adults:

Horizontal or vertical deviations <20 prism diopters: 1.25-2.5 units into any one muscle

Horizontal or vertical deviations 20-50 prism diopters: 2.5-5 units into any one muscle

(Continued)

Botulinum Toxin Type A *(Continued)*

Persistent VI nerve palsy of ≥1 month duration: 1.25-2.5 units into the medial rectus muscle

Note: Re-examine patient 7-14 days after each injection to assess effects; dosage may be increased up to twofold of the previously administered dose; do not exceed 25 units as a single injection for any one muscle

Blepharospasm: Adults: Initial: 1.25-2.5 units injected into the medial and lateral pretarsal orbicularis oculi of the upper lid and into the lateral pretarsal orbicularis oculi of the lower lid; dose may be increased up to 2.5-5 units at repeat treatment sessions; do not exceed 5 units per injection or cumulative dose of 200 units in a 30-day period

Spasticity associated with cerebral palsy: Children >18 months to Adolescents: Small muscle: 1-2 units/kg; large muscle: 3-6 units/kg; maximum dose per injection site: 50 units; maximum dose for any one visit: 12 units/kg, up to 400 units; no more than 400 units should be administered during a 3-month period

Cervical dystonia: Adults: Initial and sequential doses should be individualized related to the patient's head and neck position, localization of pain, muscle hypertrophy, and patient response; mean dosage used in research trials: 236 units (range: 198-300 units) divided among affected muscles; limit total dose into sternocleidomastoid muscles to ≤100 units

Administration Parenteral: For I.M. administration only by individuals understanding the relevant neuromuscular and orbital anatomy and any alterations to the anatomy due to prior surgical procedures and standard electromyographic techniques; reconstitute vial with preservative-free NS to obtain an optimal injection volume of 0.1 mL; suggested diluent volumes and resulting concentrations: 1 mL (10 units/0.1 mL); 2 mL (5 units/0.1 mL), 4 mL (2.5 units/0.1 mL) or 8 mL (1.25 units/0.1 mL); gently swirl as botulinum toxin type A is denatured by violent agitation

Patient Information Patients with blepharospasm may have been extremely sedentary for a long time; sedentary patients should be cautioned to resume activity slowly and carefully following injection; may cause dry mouth

Dosage Forms Injection, powder for reconstitution, lyophilized: 100 units *Clostridium botulinum* toxin type A

References

Scott AB, Magoon EH, McNeer KW, et al, "Botulinum Treatment of Childhood Strabismus," *Ophthalmology*, 1990, 97(11):1434-8.

Russman BS, Tilton A, and Gormley ME Jr, "Cerebral Palsy: A Rational Approach to a Treatment Protocol, and the Role of Botulinum Toxin in Treatment," *Muscle Nerve Suppl*, 1997, 6:S181-S193.

♦ **Boudreaux's® Butt Paste [OTC]** *see* Zinc Oxide *on page 1167*
♦ **Bovine Lung Surfactant** *see* Beractant *on page 168*
♦ **Bovine Lung Surfactant** *see* Calfactant *on page 205*
♦ **Breathe Right® Saline [OTC]** *see* Sodium Chloride *on page 1027*
♦ **Breonesin® [OTC] [DSC]** *see* Guaifenesin *on page 550*
♦ **Brethine®** *see* Terbutaline *on page 1069*

Bretylium *(bre TIL ee um)*

Therapeutic Category Antiarrhythmic Agent, Class III

Generic Available Yes

Use Ventricular tachycardia or ventricular fibrillation; other serious ventricular arrhythmias resistant to lidocaine

Note: Bretylium has been removed from the 2000 Adult ACLS and PALS Guidelines due to the limited supply, high incidence of adverse effects (eg, hypotension), and availability of safer agents; studies of its use in children are lacking and effectiveness in treatment of VT has not been demonstrated

Pregnancy Risk Factor C

Contraindications Hypersensitivity to bretylium or any component; digitalis intoxication-induced arrhythmias

Precautions Hypotension; patients with fixed cardiac output (severe pulmonary hypertension or aortic stenosis) may experience severe hypotension due to decrease in peripheral resistance without ability to increase cardiac output; reduce dose in renal failure patients

Adverse Reactions

Cardiovascular: Hypotension (incidence 50% to 75%), transient initial hypertension, increase in PVCs, bradycardia, flushing, syncope

Central nervous system: Vertigo, confusion, anxiety, lethargy, hyperthermia

Dermatologic: Rash

Gastrointestinal: Nausea and vomiting with rapid I.V. administration; rarely diarrhea, abdominal pain

Local: Muscle atrophy and necrosis with repeated I.M. injections at same site

Ocular: Conjunctivitis
Renal: Renal impairment
Respiratory: Nasal congestion
Miscellaneous: Hiccups, diaphoresis

Drug Interactions Other antiarrhythmic agents may potentiate or antagonize cardiac effects, toxic effects may be additive; the pressor effects of catecholamines may be enhanced by bretylium; may potentiate digitalis toxicity; methylphenidate may antagonize effects of bretylium

Mechanism of Action Class III antiarrhythmic; after an initial release of norepinephrine at the peripheral adrenergic nerve terminals, bretylium inhibits further release by postganglionic nerve endings in response to sympathetic nerve stimulation

Pharmacodynamics
Onset of antiarrhythmic action:
I.M.: Up to 2 hours
I.V.: Within 6-20 minutes
Maximum effect: Within 6-9 hours

Pharmacokinetics
Protein binding: 1% to 6%
Half-life, adults: 7-11 hours; increases with decreased renal function
Elimination: Unchanged in urine

Usual Dosage Note: Bretylium has been removed from the 2000 Adult ACLS and PALS Guidelines (see Note in Use section); if it is used, patients should undergo defibrillation/cardioversion before and after bretylium doses as necessary

Children: (**Note:** Dose not well established; the following dose has been recommended):
I.M.: 2-5 mg/kg as a single dose
I.V.: 5 mg/kg/dose, may repeat every 10-20 minutes as needed to a total dose of 30 mg/kg
1992 PALS guidelines for treatment of ventricular fibrillation **(see note in Use section):** Initial: 5 mg/kg, then attempt electrical defibrillation; repeat with 10 mg/kg and then reattempt electrical defibrillation if ventricular fibrillation persists; may repeat as needed to a total dose of 30 mg/kg
Maintenance dose: I.M., I.V.: 5 mg/kg every 6-8 hours; maximum dose: 40 mg/kg/day

Adults **(see note in Use section):**
Immediately life-threatening ventricular arrhythmias, ventricular fibrillation, unstable ventricular tachycardia:
Initial dose: I.V.: 5 mg/kg (undiluted) over 1 minute; if arrhythmia persists, give 10 mg/kg (undiluted) over 1 minute and repeat as necessary (usually at 15- to 30-minute intervals) up to a total dose of 30-35 mg/kg
Maintenance dose (for continuous suppression):
I.V. (diluted): 5-10 mg/kg every 6 hours
I.V. continuous infusion (diluted): 1-2 mg/minute (little experience with doses >40 mg/kg/day)
Other ventricular arrhythmias:
Initial dose: I.M., I.V.: 5-10 mg/kg, may repeat every 1-2 hours if arrhythmia persists; give I.V. dose (diluted) over 8-10 minutes
Maintenance dose:
I.M.: 5-10 mg/kg every 6-8 hours
I.V. (diluted): 5-10 mg/kg every 6 hours
I.V. continuous infusion (diluted): 1-2 mg/minute (little experience with doses >40 mg/kg/day)

Dosing interval in renal impairment:
Cl_{cr} 10-50 mL/minute: Administer 25% to 50% of normal dose
Cl_{cr} <10 mL/minute: Administer 25% of normal dose or use alternative agent

Administration Parenteral:
I.M.: Not recommended for ventricular fibrillation; no more than 5 mL should be injected I.M. per site (adults); rotate injection sites
I.V.:
Life-threatening situations: May administer undiluted I.V. push over <30 seconds
Nonlife-threatening situations: Dilute to 10 mg/mL and administer slow I.V. push over at least 8 minutes

Monitoring Parameters EKG, heart rate, rhythm, blood pressure

Nursing Implications Avoid extravasation

Additional Information Change patient to oral antiarrhythmic agent as soon as possible (when indicated) for maintenance therapy

Dosage Forms
Injection, solution, as tosylate: 50 mg/mL (10 mL)
(Continued)

Bretylium *(Continued)*

Injection, solution, as tosylate [premixed in D₅W]: 2 mg/mL (250 mL); 4 mg/mL (250 mL)

References

Emergency Cardiac Care Committee and Subcommittees, American Heart Association, "Guidelines for Cardiopulmonary Resuscitation and Emergency Cardiac Care, III: Adult Advanced Cardiac Life Support," and "VI: Pediatric Advanced Life Support," *JAMA*, 1992, 268(16):2199-241 and 2262-75.

"Guidelines 2000 for Cardiopulmonary Resuscitation and Emergency Cardiovascular Care, Part 6: Advanced Cardiovascular Life Support, The American Heart Association in Collaboration With the International Liaison Committee on Resuscitation," *Circulation*, 2000, 102(8 Suppl):I86-171.

"Guidelines 2000 for Cardiopulmonary Resuscitation and Emergency Cardiovascular Care, Part 10: Pediatric Advanced Life Support, The American Heart Association in Collaboration With the International Liaison Committee on Resuscitation," *Circulation*, 2000, 102(8 Suppl): I291-342.

- ♦ **Brevibloc®** *see Esmolol on page 453*
- ♦ **Brevital® Sodium** *see Methohexital on page 736*
- ♦ **Brevoxyl®** *see Benzoyl Peroxide on page 165*
- ♦ **Brevoxyl® Cleansing** *see Benzoyl Peroxide on page 165*
- ♦ **Brevoxyl® Wash** *see Benzoyl Peroxide on page 165*
- ♦ **Bricanyl® [DSC] (Can)** *see Terbutaline on page 1069*
- ♦ **Brioschi® [OTC]** *see Sodium Bicarbonate on page 1025*
- ♦ **Bromanate® [OTC]** *see Brompheniramine and Pseudoephedrine on page 182*
- ♦ **Bromfed® [OTC]** *see Brompheniramine and Pseudoephedrine on page 182*
- ♦ **Bromfed-PD® [OTC]** *see Brompheniramine and Pseudoephedrine on page 182*
- ♦ **Bromfenex®** *see Brompheniramine and Pseudoephedrine on page 182*
- ♦ **Bromfenex® PD** *see Brompheniramine and Pseudoephedrine on page 182*

Brompheniramine and Pseudoephedrine

(brome fen IR a meen & soo doe e FED rin)

Related Information
OTC Cough & Cold Preparations, Pediatric *on page 1225*

U.S. Brand Names Andehist NR Syrup; Bromanate® [OTC]; Bromfed® [OTC]; Bromfed-PD® [OTC]; Bromfenex®; Bromfenex® PD; Dimetapp® Elixir Cold & Allergy, Children's; Rondec® Syrup

Synonyms Pseudoephedrine and Brompheniramine

Therapeutic Category Antihistamine/Decongestant Combination

Generic Available Yes

Use Temporary relief of nasal congestion, running nose, sneezing, and itchy, watery eyes; also promotes nasal or sinus drainage

Pregnancy Risk Factor C

Contraindications Hypersensitivity to brompheniramine, pseudoephedrine, or any component; MAO inhibitor therapy, severe hypertension, severe coronary artery disease

Precautions Use with caution in patients with mild-moderate hypertension, heart disease, arrhythmias, diabetes mellitus, thyroid disease, asthma, glaucoma, and prostatic hypertrophy

Adverse Reactions See individual monograph for Pseudoephedrine *on page 958*.
Brompheniramine component only:
  Cardiovascular: Palpitations
  Central nervous system: Paradoxical excitability, drowsiness, dizziness, headache, fever, nervousness, depression
  Dermatologic: Rash, photosensitivity, angioedema
  Gastrointestinal: Nausea, anorexia, xerostomia, appetite increase, weight gain, diarrhea, abdominal pain
  Hepatic: Hepatitis
  Neuromuscular & skeletal: Myalgia, paresthesia
  Respiratory: Bronchospasm, epistaxis, thickening of bronchial secretions

Drug Interactions See individual monograph for Pseudoephedrine *on page 958*.
Brompheniramine component only: May cause additive sedation with other CNS depressants; may cause additive anticholinergic effects with other anticholinergic agents; MAO inhibitors

Pharmacodynamics See individual monograph for Pseudoephedrine *on page 958*.
Brompheniramine component only:
  Maximum effect: Maximal clinical effects seen within 3-9 hours
  Duration: Varies with formulation

Pharmacokinetics See individual monograph for Pseudoephedrine *on page 958*.
Brompheniramine component only:
  Metabolism: Extensive by the liver
  Half-life: 12-34 hours

Time to peak serum concentration: Oral: Within 2-5 hours
Elimination: In urine as inactive metabolites

Usual Dosage Oral:

Manufacturer's recommendations:

Children's Dimetapp® Elixir Cold & Allergy:
Children 6-12 years: 10 mL (pseudoephedrine 30 mg) every 4 hours
Children >12 years and Adults: 20 mL (pseudoephedrine 60 mg) every 4 hours

Rondec® Syrup:
Children 2-6 years: 2.5 mL (pseudoephedrine 22.5 mg) 4 times/day
Children >6 years and Adults: 5 mL (pseudoephedrine 45 mg) 4 times/day

Alternative pediatric dosing: May dose according to the pseudoephedrine component:
Infants and Children <2 years: 4 mg/kg/day in divided doses every 6 hours
Children 2-5 years: 15 mg every 6 hours; maximum dose: 60 mg/24 hours
Children 6-12 years: 30 mg every 6 hours or extended release product 60 mg every 12 hours; maximum dose: 120 mg/24 hours
Children >12 years and Adults: 30-60 mg every 6 hours or extended release product 120 mg every 12 hours; maximum dose: 240 mg/24 hours

Administration Oral: Administer with food

Test Interactions False-positive test for amphetamines by EMIT assay

Patient Information May cause drowsiness and impair ability to perform activities requiring mental alertness or physical coordination. May cause photosensitivity reactions (eg, exposure to sunlight may cause severe sunburn, skin rash, redness, or itching); avoid direct exposure to sunlight

Dosage Forms

Capsule, extended release:
Bromfed®, Bromfenex®: Brompheniramine maleate 12 mg and pseudoephedrine **hydrochloride** 120 mg
Bromfed-PD®, Bromfenex® PD: Brompheniramine maleate 6 mg and pseudoephedrine **hydrochloride** 60 mg

Elixir:
Bromanate®: Brompheniramine maleate 1 mg and pseudoephedrine **sulfate** 15 mg per 5 mL (120 mL, 240 mL, 480 mL) [alcohol free; grape flavor]
Children's Dimetapp® Elixir Cold & Allergy: Brompheniramine maleate 1 mg and pseudoephedrine **hydrochloride** 15 mg per 5 mL (240 mL) [alcohol and sugar free; grape flavor]

Syrup (Andehist NR, Rondec® Syrup): Brompheniramine maleate 4 mg and pseudoephedrine **sulfate** 45 mg per 5 mL (473 mL) [raspberry flavor]

- **Broncho® Saline [OTC]** *see* Sodium Chloride *on page 1027*
- **Bronkometer® (Can)** *see* Isoetharine [DSC] *on page 628*
- **Bronkosol® (Can)** *see* Isoetharine [DSC] *on page 628*
- **Brontex®** *see* Guaifenesin and Codeine *on page 551*
- **BSS** *see* Bismuth *on page 174*

Budesonide (byoo DES oh nide)

Related Information
Asthma Guidelines *on page 1376*
Estimated Comparative Daily Dosages for Inhaled Corticosteroids *on page 1382*

U.S. Brand Names Entocort™ EC; Pulmicort® Respules®; Pulmicort® Turbuhaler®; Rhinocort® [DSC]; Rhinocort® Aqua™

Canadian Brand Names Gen-Budesonide AQ

Therapeutic Category Adrenal Corticosteroid; Antiasthmatic; Anti-inflammatory Agent; Corticosteroid, Inhalant (Oral); Corticosteroid, Intranasal; Corticosteroid, Oral; Glucocorticoid

Generic Available No

Use

Intranasal:
Children and Adults: Management of seasonal or perennial allergic rhinitis
Adults: Nonallergic perennial rhinitis

Nebulization: Children 12 months to 8 years: Maintenance therapy and prophylaxis of bronchial asthma; **not** indicated for the relief of acute bronchospasm

Oral: Treatment of mild to moderate active Crohn's disease of the ileum and/or ascending colon

Oral inhalation: Long-term (chronic) control of persistent bronchial asthma; **NOT** indicated for the relief of acute bronchospasm; also indicated in bronchial asthma patients requiring oral corticosteroids (inhalation may decrease or eliminate need for oral steroids over time)

Pregnancy Risk Factor Pulmicort® Respules® and Turbuhaler®: B; all other products: C
(Continued)

Budesonide *(Continued)*

Contraindications Hypersensitivity to budesonide or any component; Pulmicort® Respules® and Pulmicort® Tubuhaler®: Primary treatment of status asthmaticus or other acute episodes of bronchial asthma where intensive treatment is needed

Warnings

Oral inhalation and nebulization: Fatalities have occurred due to adrenal insufficiency in asthmatic patients during and after switching from systemic corticosteroids to aerosol steroids; several months may be required for full recovery of the adrenal glands; patients receiving ≥20 mg of prednisone per day may be at higher risk; during this period of adrenal suppression, aerosol steroids do **not** provide the systemic corticosteroid needed to treat patients requiring stress doses (ie, patients with major stress such as trauma, surgery, or infections); when used at high doses, hypothalamic-pituitary-adrenal (HPA) suppression may occur; use with inhaled or systemic corticosteroids (even alternate-day dosing) may increase risk of HPA suppression; withdrawal and discontinuation of corticosteroids should be done carefully. Immunosuppression may occur.

Oral: HPA axis suppression may occur; patients may require supplementation with a systemic glucocorticosteroid in stress situations or if undergoing surgery; adrenal suppression may occur when switching patients from systemic corticosteroids to oral budesonide (due to lower bioavailability); withdrawal and discontinuation of systemic corticosteroids should be done carefully (monitoring of adrenocorticoid function may be needed). Immunosuppression may occur.

Precautions Avoid using higher than recommended dosages; suppression of HPA function, suppression of linear growth, or hypercorticism (Cushing's syndrome) may occur. Use of oral, inhaled, nebulized, or nasal budesonide in place of systemic corticosteroids may unmask allergies (eg, eczema, rhinitis) that were previously controlled by the systemic corticosteroids. Use oral budesonide with caution in patients with hypertension, tuberculosis, osteoporosis, diabetes mellitus, peptic ulcer disease, glaucoma, cataracts, or a family history of glaucoma or diabetes mellitus; use oral budesonide with caution and consider dosage reduction in patients with hepatic cirrhosis. Use inhaled budesonide with extreme caution in patients with respiratory tuberculosis, untreated systemic infections, or ocular herpes simplex. Rare cases of increased IOP, glaucoma, or cataracts may occur with inhaled corticosteroids.

Adverse Reactions

Cardiovascular: Facial edema

Central nervous system: Nervousness, migraine, insomnia, fatigue, dizziness, headache

Dermatologic: Rash, pruritus, contact dermatitis

Endocrine & metabolic: Adrenal suppression, hypokalemia, Cushingoid state

Gastrointestinal: Xerostomia, dysgeusia, GI irritation, nausea, weight gain, abdominal pain, vomiting, diarrhea

Local: Nasal irritation, burning, or ulceration; pharyngitis; growth of *Candida* in the mouth, throat, or nares

Neuromuscular & skeletal: Growth suppression, fracture, myalgia, arthralgia

Ocular: Conjunctivitis

Otic: Otitis media

Respiratory: Cough, epistaxis, wheezing, decreased sense of smell, hoarseness, respiratory infection, rhinitis, sinusitis

Drug Interactions Cytochrome P450 isoenzyme CYP3A4 substrate

Ketoconazole, itraconazole, cimetidine, erythromycin, ritonavir, indinavir, saquinavir, or other CYP3A4 inhibitors may increase budesonide serum concentrations (monitor for signs of hypercorticoidism with oral budesonide; consider reduction of oral budesonide dose); interactions similar to other corticosteroids may potentially occur; since dissolution of the coating of the oral capsules is pH dependent (see Additional Information), absorption of budesonide capsules may be altered by drugs that change the gastrointestinal pH

Food Interactions A high-fat meal delays the time to peak concentration by 2.5 hours, but does not affect the extent of oral absorption; grapefruit juice significantly increases oral absorption

Stability

Capsule: Store at room temperature in a tightly closed container

Intranasal inhaler: Use within 6 months after opening; avoid storage in high humidity; do not store or use by heat or open flame

Nebulization: Store Respules® upright at room temperature (68°F to 77°F); do not refrigerate or freeze; do not mix with other medications; after foil packet has been opened, Respules® are stable for 2 weeks when protected from light; return unused Respules® to foil packet to protect from light; use opened Respules® promptly

Oral inhaler: Keep clean and dry; store at room temperature 68°F to 77°F

Mechanism of Action Controls the rate of protein synthesis, depresses the migration of polymorphonuclear leukocytes and fibroblasts, reverses capillary permeability, and stabilizes lysosomal membranes at the cellular level to prevent or control inflammation

Pharmacodynamics Clinical effects are due to direct local effect, rather than systemic absorption

Onset of action:

Oral inhalation; intranasal inhaler: Within 24 hours

Intranasal spray (Rhinocort® Aqua™): Within 10 hours

Nebulization (control of asthma symptoms): Within 2-8 days

Maximum effect:

Intranasal: Inhaler: 3-7 days; spray: 2 weeks

Nebulization: 4-6 weeks

Oral inhalation: 1-2 weeks or more

Duration after discontinuation: Intranasal: Several days

Pharmacokinetics

Absorption:

Intranasal:

Inhaler: 20% of dose delivered reaches systemic circulation

Spray: 34% of dose delivered reaches systemic circulation

Oral inhalation: 39% of the metered dose is systemically available

Distribution: V_d:

Children 4-6 years: 3 L/kg

Adults: ~200 L or 2.2-3.9 L/kg

Protein binding: 85% to 90%

Metabolism: Extensively metabolized by the liver via cytochrome P450 CYP3A isoenzyme to 2 major metabolites: 16α-hydroxyprednisolone and 6β-hydroxybudesonide; both are <1% as active as parent

Bioavailability:

Nebulization: Children 4-6 years: 6%; **Note:** AUC of single 1 mg dose was comparable to a single 2 mg dose in healthy adults

Oral: ~10% (large first pass effect); **Note:** Oral bioavailability is 2.5-fold higher in patients with hepatic cirrhosis

Half-life:

Children: 4-6 years: 2.3 hours (after nebulization)

Children 10-14 years: 1.5 hours

Adults: 2-3.6 hours

Time to peak serum concentration: Oral: 30-600 minutes

Elimination: 60% to 66% of dose renally excreted as metabolites; no unchanged drug found in urine

Clearance:

Children 4-6 years: 0.5 L/minute (~50% greater than healthy adults after weight adjustment)

Adults: 0.9-1.8 L/minute

Usual Dosage

Intranasal: Children ≥6 years and Adults:

Rhinocort®: Initial: 8 sprays (4 sprays/nostril) per day (256 mcg/day), given as either 2 sprays in each nostril in the morning and evening or as 4 sprays in each nostril in the morning; after symptoms decrease (usually by 3-7 days), reduce dose slowly every 2-4 weeks to the smallest effective dose

Rhinocort® Aqua™ (32 mcg/spray): Initial: 2 sprays (1 spray/nostril) once daily (64 mcg/day); dose may be increased if needed

Maximum dose:

Children <12 years: 4 sprays (2 sprays/nostril) once daily (128 mcg/day)

Children ≥12 years and Adults: 8 sprays (4 sprays/nostril) once daily (256 mcg/day)

Nebulization: Pulmicort® Respules®: Doses should be titrated to the lowest effective dose once asthma is controlled:

Manufacturer's recommendations: Children 12 months to 8 years:

Previously treated with bronchodilators alone: Initial: 0.25 mg twice daily or 0.5 mg once daily; maximum dose: 0.5 mg/day

Previously treated with inhaled corticosteroids: Initial: 0.25 mg twice daily or 0.5 mg once daily; maximum dose: 1 mg/day

Previously treated with oral corticosteroids: Initial: 0.5 mg twice daily or 1 mg once daily; maximum dose: 1 mg/day

Symptomatic children not responding to nonsteroidal asthma medications: Initial: 0.25 mg once daily may be considered

(Continued)

Budesonide *(Continued)*

Oral:

Children: A retrospective study of 62 children (mean age: 14.1 ± 2.5 years; range: 9.5-18 years) used oral budesonide in doses of 0.45 mg/kg/day (maximum dose: 9 mg/day) for the treatment of mild to moderate Crohn's disease (see Levine, 2002); further studies are needed

Adults: 9 mg once daily in the morning for ≤8 weeks; safety and efficacy of use >8 weeks has not been established; may repeat the 8-week course for recurring episodes of active Crohn's disease; may taper dose to 6 mg once daily for 2 weeks prior to discontinuation; **Note:** When switching patients from oral prednisolone to oral budesonide, do not stop prednisolone abruptly; prednisolone taper should begin at the same time that budesonide is started

Oral inhalation: Note: Doses should be titrated to the lowest effective dose once asthma is controlled; Manufacturer's recommendations:

Children ≥6 years:

Previously treated with bronchodilators alone or with inhaled corticosteroids: Initial: 200 mcg (1 puff) twice daily; maximum dose: 400 mcg (2 puffs) twice daily

Treated with oral corticosteroids: Initial: 400 mcg (2 puffs) twice daily (maximum dose)

Adults:

Previously treated with bronchodilators alone: Initial: 200-400 mcg (1-2 puffs) twice daily; maximum dose: 400 mcg (2 puffs) twice daily

Treated with inhaled corticosteroids: Initial: 200-400 mcg (1-2 puffs) twice daily; maximum dose: 800 mcg (4 puffs) twice daily

Treated with oral corticosteroids: Initial: 400-800 mcg (2-4 puffs) twice daily; maximum dose: 800 mcg (4 puffs) twice daily

NIH Asthma Guidelines (NAEPP, 2002):

Nebulization [give once daily or in divided doses twice daily]:

Children ≤12 years:

"Low" dose: 0.5 mg/day

"Medium" dose: 1 mg/day

"High" dose: 2 mg/day daily

Oral inhalation [give in divided doses twice daily]:

Children ≤12 years:

"Low" dose: 200-400 mcg/day (1-2 inhalations/day)

"Medium" dose: 400-800 mcg/day (2-4 inhalations/day)

"High" dose: >800 mcg/day (>4 inhalations/day)

Children >12 years and Adults:

"Low" dose: 200-600 mcg/day (1-3 inhalations/day)

"Medium" dose: 600-1200 mcg/day (3-6 inhalations/day)

"High" dose: >1200 mcg/day (>6 inhalations/day)

Dosage adjustment in moderate to severe liver dysfunction: Oral: Monitor for signs and symptoms of hypercorticism; consider dosage reduction

Administration

Intranasal inhaler and intranasal spray: Clear nasal passage by blowing nose prior to use

Intranasal inhaler: Shake well before each use

Intranasal spray: Shake gently before use

Nebulization: Shake gently with a circular motion before use. Administer only with a compressed air driven jet nebulizer; do not use an ultrasonic nebulizer; use adequate flow rates and administer via appropriate size face mask or mouthpiece; avoid exposure of nebulized medication to eyes

Oral: May be administered without regard to meals; do not chew, crush, break, or open capsule; swallow whole; do not administer with grapefruit juice

Oral inhaler: Do **not** shake inhaler; do not use inhaler with a spacer

Monitoring Parameters Monitor growth in pediatric patients; inhalation and intranasal: Check mucous membranes for signs of fungal infection

Patient Information Notify physician if condition being treated persists or worsens; do not decrease dose or discontinue without physician approval; avoid exposure to chicken pox or measles; if exposed, seek medical advice without delay; may cause dry mouth

Nebulization: Rinse mouth after treatment and wash face after using face mask to decrease chance of oral candidiasis and steroid effects on skin

Oral: Avoid grapefruit juice and grapefruit

Oral inhaler: Rinse mouth after inhalation to decrease chance of oral candidiasis; report sore mouth or mouth lesions to physician. A red mark will appear on the indicator window of the Pulmicort Turbuhaler® when 20 doses are left.

Additional Information If bronchospasm with wheezing occurs after use of oral inhaler, a fast-acting bronchodilator may be used. Pulmicort Turbuhaler® delivers budesonide as a fine powder. Children and adolescents (n=18; 6-15 years) receiving budesonide nebulizations of 1 and 2 mg twice daily showed a significant reduction in urinary cortisol excretion; this reduction was not seen when patients were dosed at 1 mg/day (maximum recommended dose). Long-term effects of chronic use of budesonide nebulization on immunological or developmental processes of upper airways, mouth, and lung are unknown.

Budesonide capsules (Entocort™ EC) contain granules in an ethylcellulose matrix; the granules are coated with a methacrylic acid polymer to protect from dissolution in the stomach; the coating dissolves at a pH >5.5 (duodenal pH); the ethylcellulose matrix controls the release of drug in a time-dependent manner (until the drug reaches the ileum and ascending colon)

Dosage Forms

Capsule (Entocort™ EC): 3 mg

Powder for oral inhalation (Pulmicort® Turbuhaler®): 200 mcg/inhalation (104 g) [delivers ~160 mcg/inhalation; 200 metered doses]

Suspension for nasal inhalation (Rhinocort®): 50 mcg/inhalation (7 g) [delivers ~32 mcg/inhalation; 200 metered doses] [DSC]

Suspension for oral inhalation (Pulmicort® Respules®): 0.25 mg/2 mL (30 doses); 0.5 mg/2 mL (30 doses)

Suspension, nasal spray (Rhinocort® Aqua™): 32 mcg/spray (8.6 g) [120 metered sprays]

References

"Budesonide (Entocort™ EC) for Crohn's Disease," *Med Lett Drugs Ther*, 2002, 44(1122):6-8.

Expert Panel Report 2, "Guidelines for the Diagnosis and Management of Asthma," *Clinical Practice Guidelines*, National Institutes of Health, National Heart, Lung, and Blood Institute, NIH Publication No. 94-4051, April, 1997.

Levine A, Broide E, Stein M, et al, "Evaluation of Oral Budesonide for Treatment of Mild and Moderate Exacerbations of Crohn's Disease in Children," *J Pediatr*, 2002, 140(1):75-80.

"National Asthma Education and Prevention Program. Expert Panel Report: Guidelines for the Diagnosis and Management of Asthma Update on Selected Topics--2002," *J Allergy Clin Immunol*, 2002, 110(5 Suppl):S141-219.

Szefler SJ, "A Review of Budesonide Inhalation Suspension in the Treatment of Pediatric Asthma," *Pharmacotherapy*, 2001, 21(2):195-206.

♦ **Bufferin® [OTC]** *see Aspirin on page 134*

♦ **Bufferin® Arthritis Strength [OTC]** *see Aspirin on page 134*

♦ **Bufferin® Extra Strength [OTC]** *see Aspirin on page 134*

Bumetanide (byoo MET a nide)

U.S. Brand Names Bumex®

Canadian Brand Names Burinex®

Therapeutic Category Antihypertensive Agent; Diuretic, Loop

Generic Available Yes

Use Management of edema secondary to CHF or hepatic or renal disease including nephrotic syndrome; may also be used alone or in combination with antihypertensives in the treatment of hypertension

Pregnancy Risk Factor C

Contraindications Hypersensitivity to bumetanide or any component; anuria or increasing azotemia; hepatic coma; severe electrolyte depletion (until condition is improved or corrected)

Warnings Loop diuretics are potent diuretics; excess amounts can lead to profound diuresis with fluid and electrolyte loss; close medical supervision and dose evaluation is required. Injection contains benzyl alcohol which may cause allergic reactions in susceptible individuals; large amounts of benzyl alcohol (≥99 mg/kg/day) have been associated with a potentially fatal toxicity ("gasping syndrome") in neonates; the "gasping syndrome" consists of metabolic acidosis, respiratory distress, gasping respirations, CNS dysfunction (including convulsions, intracranial hemorrhage), hypotension and cardiovascular collapse; *in vitro* and animal studies have shown that benzoate, a metabolite of benzyl alcohol, displaces bilirubin from protein binding sites; avoid or use injection cautiously in neonates. *In vitro* studies using pooled sera from critically ill neonates have also shown bumetanide to be a potent displacer of bilirubin; avoid use in neonates at risk for kernicterus; increased risk of ototoxicity with rapid I.V. administration, renal impairment, excessive doses, and concurrent use of other ototoxins

Precautions Use with caution in patients with cirrhosis; allergy to sulfonamides may result in cross hypersensitivity to bumetanide

Adverse Reactions

Cardiovascular: Hypotension, chest pain

Central nervous system: Dizziness, headache, encephalopathy, vertigo

(Continued)

Bumetanide *(Continued)*

Dermatologic: Rash, pruritus, urticaria

Endocrine & metabolic: Hyperglycemia, hypokalemia, hypochloremia, hypomagnesemia, hyponatremia, hyperuricemia

Gastrointestinal: Cramps, nausea, vomiting, diarrhea, abdominal pain, xerostomia

Hematologic: Thrombocytopenia (rare)

Hepatic: Elevated liver enzymes

Neuromuscular & skeletal: Weakness, muscle cramps, arthritic pain

Otic: Ototoxicity (with rapid I.V. administration)

Renal: Decreased uric acid excretion, elevated serum creatinine, azotemia

Drug Interactions Decreased blood pressure when used with other antihypertensive agents and ACE inhibitors (may need to decrease dose of one or both agents); indomethacin and probenecid may decrease bumetanide's effect; decreased lithium excretion; ototoxic drugs (aminoglycoside antibiotics, cisplatin); cholestyramine may decrease absorption

Stability Store at room temperature; light sensitive, may discolor when exposed to light

Mechanism of Action Inhibits reabsorption of sodium and chloride in the ascending loop of Henle and proximal renal tubule, interfering with the chloride-binding cotransport system, thus causing increased excretion of water, sodium, chloride, magnesium, calcium, and phosphate

Pharmacodynamics

Onset of action:

Oral, I.M.: Within 30-60 minutes

I.V.: Within a few minutes

Maximum effect:

Oral, I.M.: 1-2 hours

I.V.: 15-30 minutes

Duration:

Oral: 4-6 hours

I.V.: 2-3 hours

Pharmacokinetics

Distribution: V_d: Neonates and infants: 0.26-0.39 L/kg

Protein binding: 95%

Neonates: 97%

Metabolism: Partial metabolism occurs in the liver

Bioavailability: 72% to 96%

Half-life:

Premature and full term neonates: 6 hours (range up to 15 hours)

Infants <2 months: 2.5 hours

Infants 2-6 months: 1.5 hours

Adults: 1-1.5 hours

Time to peak serum concentration: 0.5-2 hours

Elimination: Unchanged drug excreted in urine (45%); biliary/fecal (2%)

Clearance:

Preterm and full term neonates: 0.2-1.1 mL/minute/kg

Infants <2 months: 2.17 mL/minute/kg

Infants 2-6 months: 3.8 mL/minute/kg

Adults: 2.9 ± 0.2 mL/minute/kg

Usual Dosage

Oral, I.M., I.V.:

Neonates (see Warnings): 0.01-0.05 mg/kg/dose every 24-48 hours

Infants and Children: 0.015-0.1 mg/kg/dose every 6-24 hours (maximum dose: 10 mg/day)

Adults:

Edema:

Oral: 0.5-2 mg/dose (maximum dose: 10 mg/day) 1-2 times/day

I.M., I.V.: 0.5-1 mg/dose; may repeat in 2-3 hours for up to 2 doses if needed (maximum dose: 10 mg/day)

Continuous I.V. infusion: 0.9-1 mg/hour

Hypertension: Oral: 0.5 mg daily (range: 1-4 mg/day, maximum dose: 5 mg/day); for larger doses, divide into 2-3 doses daily

Administration

Oral: Administer with food to decrease GI irritation

Parenteral: Administer without additional dilution by direct I.V. injection over 1-2 minutes; for intermittent I.V. infusion, dilute in D_5W, LR, or NS and infuse over 5 minutes; for continuous infusion, dilute in D_5W to a final concentration of 0.024 mg/mL

Monitoring Parameters Blood pressure, serum electrolytes, renal function, urine output

Patient Information May cause dry mouth

Additional Information Patients with impaired hepatic function must be monitored carefully, often requiring reduced doses; larger doses may be necessary in patients with impaired renal function to obtain the same therapeutic response; 1 mg bumetanide approximately equivalent in potency to 40 mg furosemide

Dosage Forms

Injection, solution: 0.25 mg/mL (2 mL, 4 mL, 10 mL) [contains 1% benzyl alcohol]
Tablet (Bumex®): 0.5 mg, 1 mg, 2 mg

References

Wells TG, "The Pharmacology and Therapeutics of Diuretics in the Pediatric Patient," *Pediatr Clin North Am*, 1990, 37(2):463-504.

♦ **Bumex®** *see* Bumetanide *on page 187*

♦ **Buminate®** *see* Albumin *on page 52*

♦ **Buphenyl®** *see* Sodium Phenylbutyrate *on page 1028*

Bupivacaine (byoo PIV a kane)

U.S. Brand Names Marcaine®; Marcaine® Spinal; Sensorcaine®; Sensorcaine-MPF®

Therapeutic Category Local Anesthetic, Injectable

Generic Available Yes

Use Local anesthetic (injectable) for peripheral nerve block, infiltration, sympathetic block, caudal or epidural block, retrobulbar block

Pregnancy Risk Factor C

Contraindications Hypersensitivity to bupivacaine hydrochloride, other amide-type anesthetics, or any component (see Warnings); not recommended for I.V. regional anesthesia (Bier block); obstetrical paracervical block anesthesia (use is associated with fetal bradycardia and death); 0.75% concentration in obstetrical anesthesia

Warnings Convulsions due to systemic toxicity leading to cardiac arrest have been reported, presumably following unintentional I.V. injection; some products contain sulfites which may cause allergic reactions in susceptible individuals; **do not use solutions containing preservatives for caudal or epidural block.** Infants are at greater risk for bupivacaine toxicity because α_1-acid-glycoprotein, the major serum protein to which bupivacaine is bound, is lower in infants compared with older children; use epidural infusions with caution in infants and monitor more closely; increased toxicity may be minimized by limiting the duration of infusion to ≤48 hours (McCloskey, 1992). Reduce epidural infusion dosage in patients with seizure disorders or at increased risk for seizures (eg, electrolyte imbalance) (Berde, 1992).

Precautions Use with caution in patients with liver disease and impaired cardiovascular function; when used for epidural anesthesia, a smaller test dose is recommended to evaluate the patient's response

Adverse Reactions

Cardiovascular: Cardiac arrest, hypotension, bradycardia, palpitations
Central nervous system: Headache, restlessness, anxiety, dizziness, seizures
Dermatologic: Pruritus, angioneurotic edema
Gastrointestinal: Nausea, vomiting
Neuromuscular & skeletal: Weakness
Ocular: Blurred vision
Otic: Tinnitus
Respiratory: Apnea, sneezing
Miscellaneous: Hypersensitivity reactions

Drug Interactions Interactions relate to use in combination with epinephrine; see Epinephrine monograph

Stability Store at room temperature; solutions containing epinephrine should be protected from light; bupivacaine 0.4375 mg/mL when mixed with epinephrine 0.6875 mcg/mL and fentanyl 1.25 mcg/mL is stable refrigerated for 20 days and at room temperature for 48 hours; bupivacaine 625 mcg/mL or 1250 mcg/mL mixed with morphine sulfate 100 mcg/mL or 500 mcg/mL in NS is stable for 72 hours at room temperature

Mechanism of Action Blocks both the initiation and conduction of nerve impulses by decreasing the neuronal membrane's permeability to sodium ions, which results in inhibition of depolarization with resultant blockade of conduction

Pharmacodynamics

Onset of anesthetic action: Dependent on total dose, concentration, and route administered, but generally occurs within 4-10 minutes
Duration: 1.5-8.5 hours (depending upon route of administration)

Pharmacokinetics

Distribution: V_d:
Infants: 3.9 ± 2 L/kg
Children: 2.7 ± 0.2 L/kg
Protein binding: 84% to 95%
(Continued)

Bupivacaine *(Continued)*

Metabolism: In the liver
Half-life (age-dependent):
Neonates: 8.1 hours
Adults: 2.7 hours
Time to peak serum concentration: Caudal, epidural, or peripheral nerve block: 30-45 minutes
Elimination: Small amounts (~6%) excreted in urine unchanged
Clearance:
Infants: 7.1 ± 3.2 mL/kg/minute
Children: 10 ± 0.7 mL/kg/minute

Usual Dosage Dose varies with procedure, depth of anesthesia, vascularity of tissues, duration of anesthesia and condition of patient

Caudal block (with or without epinephrine, **preservative free**):
Children: 1-3.7 mg/kg
Adults: 15-30 mL of 0.25% or 0.5%
Epidural block, **preservative free** (other than caudal block):
Children: 1.25 mg/kg/dose
Adults: 10-20 mL of 0.25%, 0.5%, or 0.75%
Peripheral nerve block: 5 mL dose of 0.25% or 0.5% (12.5-25 mg); maximum dose: 400 mg/day
Sympathetic nerve block: 20-50 mL of 0.25% (no epinephrine) solution
Continuous epidural (caudal or lumbar) infusion (limited information in neonates, infants, and children):
Loading dose: 2-2.5 mg/kg (0.8-1 mL/kg of 0.25% bupivacaine)
Infusion dose: See table

Bupivacaine Infusion Dose

Age	Dose	Dose (using 0.25% solution)	Dose (using 0.125% solution)	Dose (using 0.05% solution)
Neonates and Infants ≤4 months	0.2-0.25 mg/kg/h	0.08-0.1 mL/kg/h	0.16-0.2 mL/kg/h	0.4-0.5 mL/kg/h
Infants >4 months and Children	0.4-0.5 mg/kg/h	0.16-0.2 mL/kg/h	0.32-0.4 mL/kg/h	0.8-1 mL/kg/h
Adults	5-20 mg/h	2-8 mL/h	4-16 mL/h	10-40 mL/h

Administration Solutions containing preservatives should not be used for epidural or caudal blocks; for epidural infusion, may use undiluted or diluted with preservative free NS

Reference Range Toxicity: 2-4 mcg/mL (however, some experts have suggested that the rate of rise of the serum level is more predictive of toxicity than the actual value; Scott, 1975)

Patient Information May experience temporary loss of sensation and motor activity, usually in the lower half of the body following caudal or lumbar epidural anesthesia

Additional Information For epidural infusion, lower dosages of bupivacaine may be effective when used in combination with narcotic analgesics

Dosage Forms

Injection, solution, as hydrochloride [preservative free]: 0.25% [2.5 mg/mL] (20 mL, 30 mL, 50 mL); 0.5% [5 mg/mL] (20 mL, 30 mL); 0.75% [7.5 mg/mL] (20 mL, 30 mL)
Marcaine®: 0.25% [2.5 mg/mL] (10 mL, 30 mL, 50 mL); 0.5% [5 mg/mL] (10 mL, 30 mL); 0.75% [7.5 mg/mL] (10 mL, 30 mL)
Marcaine® Spinal: 0.75% [7.5 mg/mL] (2 mL)
Sensorcaine®-MPF: 0.25% [2.5 mg/mL] (10 mL, 30 mL); 0.5% [5 mg/mL] (10 mL, 30 mL); 0.75% [7.5 mg/mL] (10 mL, 30 mL)
Injection, solution, as hydrochloride [with preservative]: 0.25% [2.5 mg/mL] (10 mL, 30 mL, 50 mL); 0.5% [5 mg/mL] (10 mL, 30 mL, 50 mL); 0.75% [7.5 mg/mL] (10 mL, 30 mL)
Marcaine®, Sensorcaine®: 0.25% [2.5 mg/mL] (50 mL); 0.5% [5 mg/mL] (50 mL) [contains 1 mg/mL methylparaben]
Injection, solution, **with epinephrine 1:200,000**, as hydrochloride [preservative free]:
Marcaine®: 0.25% [2.5 mg/mL] (10 mL, 30 mL, 50 mL); 0.5% [5 mg/mL] (3 mL, 10 mL, 30 mL); 0.75% [7.5 mg/mL] (30 mL) [contains 0.5 mg/mL sodium metabisulfite]
Sensorcaine®-MPF: 0.25% [2.5 mg/mL] (10 mL, 30 mL); 0.5% [5 mg/mL] (5 mL, 10 mL, 30 mL) [contains 0.5 mg/mL sodium metabisulfite]

Injection, solution, **with epinephrine 1:200,000**, as hydrochloride [with preservative] (Marcaine®, Sensorcaine®): 0.25% [2.5 mg/mL] (50 mL); 0.5% [5 mg/mL] (50 mL) [contains 1 mg/mL methylparaben and 0.5 mg/mL sodium metabisulfite]

References

Berde CB, "Convulsions Associated With Pediatric Regional Anesthesia," *Anesth Analg*, 1992, 75(2):164-6.

Desparmet J, Meistelman C, Barre J, et al, "Continuous Epidural Infusion of Bupivacaine for Postoperative Pain Relief in Children," *Anesthesiology*, 1987, 67(1):108-10.

Luz G, Innerhofer P, Bachmann B, et al, "Bupivacaine Plasma Concentrations During Continuous Epidural Anesthesia in Infants and Children," *Anesth Analg*, 1996, 82(2):231-4.

McCloskey JJ, Haun SE, and Deshpande JK, "Bupivacaine Toxicity Secondary to Continuous Caudal Epidural Infusion in Children," *Anesth Analg*, 1992, 75(2):287-90.

Scott DB, "Evaluation of Clinical Tolerance of Local Anaesthetic Agents," *Br J Anaesth*, 1975, 47:328-31.

♦ **Burinex® (Can)** *see* Bumetanide *on page 187*
♦ **Burnamycin [OTC]** *see* Lidocaine *on page 671*
♦ **Burn Jel [OTC]** *see* Lidocaine *on page 671*
♦ **Burn-O-Jel [OTC]** *see* Lidocaine *on page 671*
♦ **Burow's Solution** *see* Aluminum Acetate *on page 73*
♦ **BuSpar®** *see* BusPIRone *on page 191*
♦ **Buspirex (Can)** *see* BusPIRone *on page 191*

BusPIRone (byoo SPYE rone)

Related Information
Serotonin Syndrome *on page 1420*
U.S. Brand Names BuSpar®
Canadian Brand Names Apo®-Buspirone; Buspirex; Gen-Buspirone; Lin-Buspirone; Novo-Buspirone; Nu-Buspirone; PMS-Buspirone
Therapeutic Category Antianxiety Agent
Generic Available Yes
Use Management of anxiety disorders
Pregnancy Risk Factor B
Contraindications Hypersensitivity to buspirone or any component
Warnings Do not use concurrently with MAO inhibitors or within 10 days of MAO inhibitors as significant increases in blood pressure may occur
Precautions Use with caution in patients with hepatic or renal dysfunction; use in severe hepatic or renal impairment is not recommended; buspirone does not prevent or treat withdrawal from benzodiazepines or sedative/hypnotic drugs
Adverse Reactions
Cardiovascular: Chest pain, tachycardia
Central nervous system: Dizziness, lightheadedness, headache, fatigue, restlessness, confusion, insomnia, nightmares, sedation (about $1/3$ of that with benzodiazepines), disorientation, excitement, fever, drowsiness (more common with ≥20 mg/day), akathisia; possible psychotic deterioration has been reported (two pediatric cases, see Soni, 1992)
Dermatologic: Rash, urticaria
Gastrointestinal: Nausea, vomiting, diarrhea, flatulence, xerostomia
Hematologic: Rare: Leukopenia, eosinophilia, thrombocytopenia
Neuromuscular & skeletal: Muscle weakness, numbness
Ocular: Blurred vision
Otic: Tinnitus
Drug Interactions Cytochrome P450 isoenzyme CYP3A4 substrate
Use with MAO inhibitors may cause significant increases in blood pressure; alcohol or other CNS depressants may increase CNS adverse effects; buspirone may increase haloperidol levels; buspirone may displace digoxin from serum proteins; fluoxetine; use with warfarin may increase PT; erythromycin, itraconazole, ketoconazole, nefazodone, diltiazem, verapamil, or other inhibitors of CYP3A4 may increase buspirone plasma concentrations (the dose of buspirone should be reduced); when used with diazepam, buspirone may increase nordiazepam serum concentrations; aspirin may increase and flurazepam may decrease free (unbound) buspirone concentrations; rifampin, phenytoin, phenobarbital, carbamazepine, dexamethasone, or other inducers of CYP3A4 may decrease serum concentrations of buspirone (dosage adjustment of buspirone may be needed)
Food Interactions Food may delay oral absorption, decrease the first-pass metabolism effect and increase oral bioavailability; grapefruit juice may greatly increase buspirone concentrations
Stability Protect from light; store at room temperature
Mechanism of Action Decreases the spontaneous firing of serotonin-containing neurons in the CNS by selectively binding to and acting as agonist at presynaptic CNS serotonin 5-HT₁A receptors; possesses partial agonist activity (mixed agonist/
(Continued)

BusPIRone *(Continued)*

antagonist) at postsynaptic 5-HT$_2$A receptors; does not bind to benzodiazepine-GABA receptors; binds to dopamine$_2$ receptors; may have other effects on other neurotransmitter systems; buspirone is "anxiolytic-select" and does not possess the anticonvulsant, muscle relaxant, or sedative effects of the benzodiazepines; little potential for abuse, tolerance, or withdrawal reactions

Pharmacodynamics

Onset of action: Within 2 weeks

Maximum effect: 3-4 weeks, up to 4-6 weeks

Pharmacokinetics

Absorption: Rapid and complete, but bioavailability is limited by extensive first-pass effect; only 1.5% to 13% (mean 4%) of the oral dose reaches the systemic circulation unchanged

Protein binding: 86%

Metabolism: In the liver by oxidation (by cytochrome P450 isoenzyme CYP3A4) to several metabolites including 1-pyrimidinyl piperazine (about $\frac{1}{4}$ as active as buspirone)

Half-life: Adults: Mean: 2-3 hours; increased with renal or liver dysfunction

Elimination: 29% to 63% excreted in urine (primarily as metabolites)

Usual Dosage Oral:

Children and Adolescents: Anxiety disorders: Limited information is available; dose is not well established. One pilot study of 15 children, 6-14 years of age (mean 10 years), with mixed anxiety disorders, used initial doses of 5 mg daily; doses were individualized with increases in increments of 5 mg/day every week as needed to a maximum dose of 20 mg/day divided into 2 doses; the mean dose required: 18.6 mg/day (Simeon, 1994). Some authors (Carrey, 1996 and Kutcher, 1992), based on their clinical experience, recommend higher doses (eg, 15-30 mg/day in 2 divided doses). An open-label study in 25 prepubertal inpatients (mean age: 8 ± 1.8 years; range: 5-11 years) with anxiety symptoms and moderately aggressive behavior used initial doses of 5 mg daily; doses were titrated upwards (over 3 weeks) by 5-10 mg every 3 days to a maximum dose of 50 mg/day; doses >5 mg/day were administered in 2 divided doses/day; buspirone was discontinued in 25% of the children due to increased aggression and agitation or euphoric mania; mean optimal dose (n=19): 28 mg/day; range: 10-50 mg/day; median: 30 mg/day (Pfeffer, 1997). Two placebo-controlled 6-week trials in children and adolescents (n=559; age: 6-17 years) with generalized anxiety disorder studied doses of 7.5-30 mg twice daily (15-60 mg/day); no significant differences between buspirone and placebo with respect to generalized anxiety disorder symptoms were observed (see package insert).

Adults: Initial: 7.5 mg twice daily; increase in increments of 5 mg/day every 2-3 days as needed to a maximum of 60 mg/day; usual dose: 20-30 mg/day in 2 or 3 divided doses; **Note:** For patients receiving concomitant therapy with cytochrome P450 CYP3A4 inhibitors, a lower dose of buspirone is recommended (eg, 2.5 mg twice daily for patients receiving erythromycin; 2.5 mg daily for patients receiving itraconazole or nefazodone); with further dosage adjustments based on clinical assessment

Dosing adjustment in renal impairment:

Mild to moderate renal dysfunction: Dose reductions not required

Patients with anuria: Reduce dose by 25% to 50%; further studies are needed

Administration Oral: Administer in a consistent manner in relation to food (ie, either always with food or always without food); may administer with food to decrease GI upset; use caution if administered with grapefruit juice; avoid large amounts of grapefruit juice (see Food Interactions)

Monitoring Parameters Mental status, signs and symptoms of anxiety, liver and renal function

Patient Information Avoid alcohol and large amounts of grapefruit juice; may cause drowsiness and impair ability to perform activities requiring mental alertness or physical coordination; may cause dry mouth

Additional Information Not appropriate for "as needed" (prn) use or for brief, situational anxiety; buspirone is equipotent to diazepam on a milligram to milligram basis in the treatment of anxiety; however, unlike diazepam, the onset of buspirone is delayed (see Pharmacodynamics)

Dosage Forms

Tablet, as hydrochloride: 5 mg, 7.5 mg, 10 mg, 15 mg, 30 mg

BuSpar®: 5 mg, 10 mg, 15 mg, 30 mg

References

Carrey NJ, Wiggins DM, and Milin RP, "Pharmacological Treatment of Psychiatric Disorders in Children and Adolescents," *Drugs*, 1996, 51(5):750-9.

Hanna GL, Feibusch EL, and Albright KJ, "Buspirone Treatment of Anxiety, Associated With Pharyngeal Dysphagia in a Four-Year Old," *J Child Adolesc Psychopharmacol*, 1997, 7(2):137-43.

Kutcher SP, Reiter S, Gardner DM, et al, "The Pharmacotherapy of Anxiety Disorders in Children and Adolescents," *Psychiatr Clin North Am*, 1992, 15(1):41-67.

Pfeffer CR, Jiang H, and Domeshek LJ, "Buspirone Treatment of Psychiatrically Hospitalized Prepubertal Children With Symptoms of Anxiety and Moderately Severe Aggression," *J Child Adolesc Psychopharmacol*, 1997, 7(3):145-55.

Simeon JG, Knott VJ, DuBois C, et al, "Buspirone Therapy of Mixed Anxiety Disorders in Childhood and Adolescence: A Pilot Study," *J Child Adolesc Psychopharmacol*, 1994, 4(3):159-70.

Soni P and Weintraub AL, "Buspirone-Associated Mental Status Changes," *J Am Acad Child Adolesc Psychiatry*, 1992, 31(6):1098-9.

Busulfan (byoo SUL fan)

Related Information
Emetogenic Potential of Single Chemotherapeutic Agents *on page 1286*

U.S. Brand Names Busulfex®; Myleran®

Synonyms 1,4-Butanediol Dimethanesulfonate

Therapeutic Category Antineoplastic Agent, Alkylating Agent

Generic Available No

Use Chronic myelogenous leukemia (CML); component of marrow-ablative conditioning regimen prior to bone marrow transplantation (BMT) for refractory leukemias, lymphomas, and pediatric solid tumors

Pregnancy Risk Factor D

Contraindications Hypersensitivity to busulfan or any component; failure to respond to previous courses; should not be used in pregnancy or lactation

Warnings The FDA currently recommends that procedures for proper handling and disposal of antineoplastic agents be considered; discontinue busulfan if lung toxicity develops; busulfan is potentially carcinogenic; malignant tumors and acute leukemias have been reported in patients who received busulfan; busulfan is associated with ovarian failure including failure to achieve puberty in females

Profound myelosuppression with severe granulocytopenia, thrombocytopenia, and anemia are the most frequent serious adverse events occurring when high-dose busulfan is used as a conditioning regimen. Seizures have been reported in patients receiving high-dose busulfan. Prophylactic anticonvulsant therapy should be initiated prior to high-dose busulfan therapy. High busulfan AUC values (>1500 µM•minute) may be associated with an increased risk of developing hepatic veno-occlusive disease (HVOD). Patients who have received prior radiation therapy, ≥3 cycles of chemotherapy, or prior progenitor cell transplant may be at increased risk for developing HVOD. Of the patients who developed HVOD, it was fatal in 40% of the cases.

Precautions May induce severe bone marrow hypoplasia; reduce dosage in patients with bone marrow suppression; use with extreme caution in patients who have recently received other myelosuppressive drugs or radiation therapy; use with caution in patients with a history of seizure disorder, head trauma, or when receiving other epileptogenic drugs

Adverse Reactions
Cardiovascular: Cardiac tamponade (reported in a small number of thalassemia patients who received busulfan and cyclophosphamide as part of a BMT conditioning regimen), edema, tachycardia

Central nervous system: Dizziness, seizures, fever, chills, insomnia, confusion, hallucinations

Dermatologic: Hyperpigmentation, alopecia, rash, urticaria

Endocrine & metabolic: Addisonian-like syndrome (hyperpigmentation, wasting, hypotension), hyperuricemia, gynecomastia, testicular atrophy, amenorrhea, sterility, hyperglycemia, hypomagnesemia, hypokalemia

Gastrointestinal: Nausea, vomiting, mucositis, diarrhea, abdominal pain, constipation, ileus, anorexia, pancreatitis

Genitourinary: Hemorrhagic cystitis

Hematologic: Myelosuppression with nadirs of 14-21 days for leukopenia and thrombocytopenia; anemia, aplastic anemia, thrombosis

Hepatic: Hepatic impairment, hepatic veno-occlusive disease (7.7% to 12% with high-dose busulfan), hyperbilirubinemia, hepatocellular necrosis, ascites

Ocular: Blurred vision, subcapsular cataracts, corneal thinning

Respiratory: Pulmonary fibrosis (may occur 4 months to 10 years after initiation of therapy), dyspnea

Drug Interactions Cytochrome P450 isoenzyme CYP3A3/4 substrate

Thioguanine (may increase hepatotoxicity); itraconazole (may decrease busulfan clearance by 25% and increase busulfan toxicity); phenytoin lowers busulfan plasma AUC by 15%; acetaminophen may decrease busulfan clearance

Food Interactions No clear or firm data on the effect of food on busulfan bioavailability

Stability Store tablets at room temperature. Store intact ampuls in the refrigerator; diluted busulfan solution is stable for up to 8 hours at room temperature; infusion
(Continued)

Busulfan *(Continued)*

must be completed within that 8 hour time frame. If diluted in NS, the solution is stable for 12 hours if refrigerated, but the infusion must be completed within that 12-hour time frame.

Mechanism of Action Interferes with the normal function of DNA by alkylation of intracellular nucleophiles and cross-linking the strands of DNA

Pharmacokinetics

Absorption: Oral: 70% absorbed

Distribution: Crosses into CSF, saliva, placenta, and liver

V_d: Children: 0.64 L/kg

Protein binding: 32% to 55%

Metabolism: Extensive in the liver by conjugation with glutathione

Half-life:

Children: 2.5 hours

Adults: 2.3-2.6 hours

Time to peak serum concentration: Oral: Within 1-2 hours

Elimination: 10% to 50% excreted in urine as metabolites, 1% excreted unchanged in urine within 24 hours; total plasma clearance rate is 2-4 times higher in children than in adults

Clearance:

Children: 3.37 mL/minute/kg

Adults: 2.52 mL/minute/kg (range: 1.49-4.31 mL/minute/kg)

Usual Dosage Refer to individual protocols; dose should be based on ideal body weight:

Children:

Oral:

Remission induction of CML: 0.06-0.12 mg/kg once daily **or** 1.8-4.6 mg/m²/day once daily; titrate dose to maintain a leukocyte count >40,000/mm³; discontinue busulfan if counts fall to ≤20,000/mm³

BMT marrow-ablative conditioning regimen: 1 mg/kg/dose every 6 hours for 16 doses

Hematopoietic stem cell transplant regimen: Children ≤6 years: 40 mg/m²/dose every 6 hours for 16 doses

I.V.: High-dose BMT or peripheral blood progenitor cell transplantation conditioning regimen: Dose based on actual body weight:

≤12 kg: 1.1 mg/kg/dose every 6 hours for 16 doses over 4 consecutive days

>12 kg: 0.8 mg/kg/dose every 6 hours for 16 doses over 4 consecutive days

Dosage adjustment based on therapeutic drug monitoring:

Adjusted dose (mg) = Actual dose (mg) x target AUC (μM•minute) / actual AUC (μM•minute)

Target AUC = 1125 μM•minute

Adults:

Oral:

Remission induction of CML: 4-8 mg/day or 0.06 mg/kg/day

Maintenance dose: Controversial; range is from 1-4 mg/day to 2 mg/week; reduce dose in proportion to the decrease in leukocyte count or discontinue busulfan when the leukocyte count falls to ≤20,000/mm³

I.V.: High-dose BMT conditioning regimen: 0.8 mg/kg/dose every 6 hours for 16 doses over 4 consecutive days

I.V. dose for obese patients: Dose should be based on adjusted ideal body weight (AIBW)

AIBW = Ideal body weight (IBW) + 0.25 x (actual weight - IBW)

Administration

Oral: May be administered without regard to meals. To facilitate ingestion of high doses, insert multiple tablets into clear gelatin capsules for administration.

Parenteral: Filter busulfan using 5 micron syringe filter provided, using one filter per ampul. If using the syringe filter in the forward flow direction, allow for ~0.16 mL of residual busulfan to remain in the filter. Dilute busulfan injection with either NS or D_5W to a final concentration of ≥0.5 mg/mL (diluent volume should be 10 times the volume of busulfan injection); infuse over 2 hours through a central venous catheter; flush line before and after each infusion with D_5W or NS. Do **not** use polycarbonate syringes or filters.

Monitoring Parameters CBC with differential and platelet count, hemoglobin, liver function tests, bilirubin, alkaline phosphatase; monitor busulfan plasma concentration

Patient Information Report any difficulty in breathing, cough, fever, sore throat, bleeding or bruising to physician. Report any signs of abrupt weakness, fatigue, anorexia, weight loss, nausea, vomiting, and melanoderma. Female patients of child-bearing potential should avoid becoming pregnant during and for one month following therapy.

Additional Information One method used to prevent seizures during high-dose busulfan (~4 mg/kg/day for 4 days) is to initiate a standard loading dose of phenytoin (15 mg/kg) 1 day prior to starting busulfan therapy followed by a maintenance dose adjusted to maintain a therapeutic phenytoin concentration until 24 hours after the final busulfan dose

"Juvenile type" chronic myelogenous leukemia which typically occurs in young children and is associated with the absence of Philadelphia chromosome responds poorly to busulfan.

Dosage Forms
Injection, solution (Busulfex®): 6 mg/mL (10 mL) [contains 33% w/w dimethylacetamide and 67% w/w polyethylene glycol]
Tablet, scored (Myleran®): 2 mg

Extemporaneous Preparations A 2 mg/mL oral suspension can be prepared in a vertical flow hood using simple syrup; crush one-hundred twenty 2 mg tablets into a fine powder in a mortar; levigate with a small amount of simple syrup and mix to make a uniform paste; mix while adding simple syrup in geometric portions to almost 120 mL; pour contents into a graduated cylinder; rinse mortar and pestle with simple syrup, transfer to the graduated cylinder, and qsad with vehicle to 120 mL. Transfer contents of the graduated cylinder into an amber prescription bottle. Preparation is stable for 30 days when stored under refrigeration; label "shake well" and "caution chemotherapy"
Allen LV, "Busulfan Oral Suspension," *US Pharmacist*, 1990, 15:94-5.

References
Bolinger AM, Zangwill AB, Slattery JT, et al, "An Evaluation of Engraftment, Toxicity and Busulfan Concentration in Children Receiving Bone Marrow Transplantation for Leukemia or Genetic Disease," *Bone Marrow Transplant*, 2000, 25(9):925-30.
Heard BE and Cooke RA, "Busulphan Lung," *Thorax*, 1968, 23(2):187-93.
Ozkaynak MF, Weinberg K, Kohn D, et al, "Hepatic Veno-Occlusive Disease Post-Bone Marrow Transplantation in Children Conditioned With Busulfan and Cyclophosphamide: Incidence, Risk Factors, and Clinical Outcome," *Bone Marrow Transplant*, 1991, 7(6):467-74.
Regazzi MB, Locatelli F, Buggia I, et al, "Disposition of High Dose Busulfan in Pediatric Patients Undergoing Bone Marrow Transplantation," *Clin Pharmacol Ther*, 1993, 54(1):45-52.
Vassal G, Gouyette A, Hartmann O, et al, "Pharmacokinetics of High-Dose Busulfan in Children," *Cancer Chemother Pharmacol*, 1989, 24(6):386-90.

♦ **Busulfex®** *see* Busulfan *on page 193*
♦ **1,4-Butanediol Dimethanesulfonate** *see* Busulfan *on page 193*
♦ **BW-430C** *see* Lamotrigine *on page 653*
♦ **C-500-GR™ [OTC]** *see* Ascorbic Acid *on page 131*
♦ **Cafcit®** *see* Caffeine *on page 195*
♦ **Cafergor® (Can)** *see* Ergotamine *on page 447*
♦ **Cafergot®** *see* Ergotamine *on page 447*

Caffeine (KAF een, SIT rated)

Related Information
Overdose and Toxicology *on page 1388*

U.S. Brand Names Cafcit®

Available Salts Caffeine Citrate; Caffeine Sodium Benzoate

Therapeutic Category Central Nervous System Stimulant, Nonamphetamine; Diuretic; Respiratory Stimulant

Generic Available Yes (caffeine sodium benzoate injection)

Use
Treatment of idiopathic apnea of prematurity **(caffeine citrate)**
Emergency stimulant in acute circulatory failure; diuretic; treatment of spinal puncture headaches **(caffeine sodium benzoate)**

Pregnancy Risk Factor C

Contraindications Hypersensitivity to caffeine or any component; sodium benzoate salt form in neonates (see Warnings)

Warnings Do not interchange the caffeine citrate salt formulation with the caffeine sodium benzoate formulation; sodium benzoate has been associated with a potentially fatal toxicity ("gasping syndrome") in neonates; the "gasping syndrome" consists of metabolic acidosis, respiratory distress, gasping respirations, CNS dysfunction (including convulsions, intracranial hemorrhage), hypotension and cardiovascular collapse; *in vitro* and animal studies have shown that benzoate also displaces bilirubin from protein-binding sites; avoid use of products containing sodium benzoate in neonates. During a Cafcit® double-blind, placebo-controlled study, 6 of 85 patients developed necrotizing enterocolitis (NEC); 5 of these 6 patients had received caffeine citrate; although no causal relationship has been established, neonates who receive caffeine citrate should be closely monitored for the development of NEC. Caffeine serum levels should be closely monitored to optimize therapy and prevent serious toxicity.
(Continued)

Caffeine *(Continued)*

Precautions Use with caution in patients with a history of peptic ulcer, impaired renal or hepatic function, seizure disorders, or cardiovascular disease; avoid in patients with symptomatic cardiac arrhythmias

Adverse Reactions

Cardiovascular: Cardiac arrhythmias, tachycardia, extrasystoles

Central nervous system: Insomnia, restlessness, agitation, irritability, hyperactivity, jitteriness, headache, nervousness, anxiety

Endocrine & metabolic: Hypoglycemia, hyperglycemia

Gastrointestinal: Nausea, vomiting, gastric irritation, necrotizing enterocolitis, GI hemorrhage

Genitourinary: Increased urine output

Neuromuscular & skeletal: Muscle tremors or twitches

Drug Interactions Cytochrome P450 isoenzyme CYP1A2, CYP2E1, and CYP3A3/4 substrate

Enhances the positive cardiac inotropic and chronotropic effects of beta-adrenergic agonists; cimetidine, ketoconazole, fluconazole, mexiletine, and phenylpropanolamine may impair caffeine metabolism (increase serum levels); caffeine decreases the hemodynamic effect of adenosine; phenobarbital and phenytoin may increase caffeine elimination (lower serum levels)

Stability Caffeine citrate: Injection and oral solution contain no preservatives; injection is chemically stable for at least 24 hours at room temperature when diluted to 10 mg/mL (as caffeine citrate) with D_5W, $D_{50}W$, Intralipid® 20%, and Aminosyn® 8.5%; also compatible with dopamine (600 mcg/mL), calcium gluconate 10%, heparin (1 unit/mL), and fentanyl (10 mcg/mL) at room temperature for 24 hours

Mechanism of Action Increases levels of 3'5' cyclic AMP by inhibiting phosphodiesterase; CNS stimulant which increases medullary respiratory center sensitivity to carbon dioxide, stimulates central inspiratory drive, and improves skeletal muscle contraction (diaphragmatic contractility); prevention of apnea may occur by competitive inhibition of adenosine

Pharmacokinetics

Distribution: V_d:

Neonates: 0.8-0.9 L/kg

Children >9 months to Adults: 0.6 L/kg

Protein binding: 17%

Metabolism: Interconversion between caffeine and theophylline has been reported in preterm neonates (caffeine levels are ~25% of measured theophylline after theophylline administration and ~3% to 8% of caffeine would be expected to be converted to theophylline)

Half-life:

Neonates: 72-96 hours (range: 40-230 hours)

Infants >9 months, Children, and Adults: 5 hours

Time to peak serum concentration: Oral: Within 30 minutes to 2 hours

Elimination:

Neonates ≤1 month: 86% excreted unchanged in urine

Infants >1 month and Adults: Extensively liver metabolized to a series of partially demethylated xanthines and methyluric acids

Clearance:

Neonates: 8.9 mL/hour/kg (range: 2.5-17)

Adults: 94 mL/hour/kg

Usual Dosage

Apnea of prematurity: **Caffeine citrate:** Neonates: Oral, I.V.:

Loading dose: 10-20 mg/kg as caffeine citrate (5-10 mg/kg as caffeine base). If theophylline has been administered to the patient within the previous 3 days, a full or modified loading dose (50% to 75% of a loading dose) may be given (caffeine is a significant metabolite of theophylline in the newborn; see Pharmacokinetics).

Maintenance dose: 5 mg/kg/day as caffeine citrate (2.5 mg/kg/day as caffeine base) once daily starting 24 hours after the loading dose. Maintenance dose is adjusted based on patient's response (efficacy and adverse effects), and serum caffeine concentrations.

Stimulant/diuretic: **Caffeine sodium benzoate:** Adults: I.M., I.V.: 500 mg as a single dose

Treatment of spinal puncture headache: **Caffeine sodium benzoate:** Adults: I.V.: 500 mg as a single dose; may repeat in 4 hours if headache unrelieved (see Administration)

Administration

Oral: May be administered without regard to feedings or meals; may administer injectable formulation (caffeine citrate) orally

Parenteral:

Caffeine citrate: Infuse loading dose over at least 30 minutes; maintenance dose may be infused over at least 10 minutes; may administer without dilution or diluted with D_5W to 10 mg caffeine citrate/mL

Caffeine sodium benzoate: I.V. as slow direct injection; for spinal headaches, dilute in 1000 mL NS and infuse over 1 hour; follow with 1000 mL NS, infuse over 1 hour; administer I.M. undiluted

Monitoring Parameters Heart rate, number and severity of apnea spells, serum caffeine levels

Reference Range

Therapeutic: Apnea of prematurity: 8-20 µg/mL

Potentially toxic: >20 µg/mL

Toxic: >50 µg/mL

Dosage Forms

Injection, solution, as **caffeine citrate** [preservative free] (Calcit®): 20 mg/mL (3 mL) [equivalent to 10 mg/mL caffeine base]

Injection, solution, as **caffeine sodium benzoate:** 125 mg/mL (2 mL)

Solution, oral, as **caffeine citrate** (Calcit®): 20 mg/mL (3 mL) [equivalent to 10 mg/mL caffeine base]

Extemporaneous Preparations An oral solution of 20 mg/mL caffeine citrate, prepared from 10 g caffeine (anhydrous) combined with 10 g citric acid USP and 1000 mL SWI is stable for 3 months refrigerated (Nahata, 1987).

An oral solution 20 mg/mL caffeine citrate may be made by dissolving 5 g anhydrous caffeine and 5 g citric acid USP in 250 mL SWI. Stir solution until completely clear; add 2:1 simple syrup:cherry syrup mixture to a final volume of 500 mL; stable refrigerated 90 days (Eisenberg, 1984).

Eisenberg MG and Kang N, "Stability of Citrated Caffeine Solutions for Injectable and Enteral Use," *Am J Hosp Pharm*, 1984, 41(11):2405-6.

Nahata MC and Roberts DL, "Formulation of Caffeine Injection for I.V. Administration," *Am J Hosp Pharm*, 1987, 44(6):1308, 1312.

References

Bhatt-Mehta V and Schumacher RE, "Treatment of Apnea of Prematurity," *Paediatr Drugs*, 2003, 5(3):195-210.

Erenberg A, Leff RD, Haack DG, et al, "Caffeine Citrate for the Treatment of Apnea of Prematurity: A Double-Blind, Placebo-Controlled Study," *Pharmacotherapy*, 2000, 20(6):644-52.

Kriter KE and Blanchard J, "Management of Apnea in Infants," *Clin Pharm*, 1989, 8(8):577-87.

♦ **Caffeine Citrate** *see* Caffeine *on page 195*

♦ **Caffeine Sodium Benzoate** *see* Caffeine *on page 195*

Calamine Lotion (KAL a myne loe shun)

Therapeutic Category Topical Skin Product

Generic Available Yes

Use Employed primarily as an astringent, protectant, and soothing agent for conditions such as poison ivy, poison oak, poison sumac, sunburn, insect bites, or minor skin irritations

Precautions For external use only

Adverse Reactions

Dermatologic: Rash

Local: Irritation

Usual Dosage Topical: Apply 1-4 times/day as needed; reapply after bathing

Administration Topical: Shake well before using; avoid contact with the eyes; do not use on open wounds or burns

Additional Information Active ingredients: Calamine, zinc oxide

Dosage Forms

Lotion, topical:

Calamine, USP: Calamine 8%, zinc oxide 8%, glycerin 2% and bentonite magma in calcium hydroxide solution (120 mL, 180 mL, 240 mL, 480 mL)

Calamine, USP, phenolated: Calamine 8%, zinc oxide 8%, glycerin 2%, bentonite magma, and phenol 1% in calcium hydroxide solution (120 mL, 180 mL)

♦ **Calan®** *see* Verapamil *on page 1144*

♦ **Calan® SR** *see* Verapamil *on page 1144*

♦ **Calcarb 600 [OTC]** *see* Calcium Supplements *on page 200*

♦ **Calci-Chew® [OTC]** *see* Calcium Supplements *on page 200*

♦ **Calciferol™** *see* Ergocalciferol *on page 445*

♦ **Calcijex®** *see* Calcitriol *on page 199*

♦ **Calcimar® (Can)** *see* Calcitonin *on page 198*

♦ **Calci-Mix® [OTC]** *see* Calcium Supplements *on page 200*

Calcitonin (kal si TOE nin)

U.S. Brand Names Miacalcin®

Canadian Brand Names Calcimar®; Caltine®; Miacalcin® NS

Therapeutic Category Antidote, Hypercalcemia

Generic Available No

Use Treatment of Paget's disease of bone and as adjunctive therapy for hypercalcemia; also used in postmenopausal osteoporosis and osteogenesis imperfecta

Pregnancy Risk Factor C

Contraindications Hypersensitivity to calcitonin, salmon protein, or gelatin diluent

Precautions A skin test should be performed prior to initiating therapy; the skin test is 0.1 mL of 10 unit/mL calcitonin injection in NS (must be prepared) injected intradermally; observe injection site for 15 minutes for wheal or significant erythema

Adverse Reactions

Cardiovascular: Flushing of the face, edema

Central nervous system: Dizziness, headache, chills

Dermatologic: Rash

Gastrointestinal: Nausea, vomiting, diarrhea, anorexia, metallic taste

Local: Inflammatory reactions at the injection site

Neuromuscular & skeletal: Weakness, tingling of palms and soles, back and joint pain

Renal: Diuresis

Respiratory: Shortness of breath, nasal congestion, epistaxis, nasal sores, and sore bridge of nose (nasal spray)

Stability

Injection: Store under refrigeration; stable for up to 2 weeks at room temperature

Nasal spray: Store unopened bottle under refrigeration; once the pump has been activated, store at room temperature; stable at room temperature for 30 days

Mechanism of Action Calcitonin directly inhibits osteoclastic bone resorption; promotes the renal excretion of calcium, phosphate, sodium, magnesium and potassium by decreasing tubular reabsorption; increases the jejunal secretion of water, sodium, potassium, and chloride

Pharmacodynamics

Hypercalcemia:

Onset of action:

I.M., S.C.: 15 minutes

I.V.: Immediate

Maximum effect: I.M., S.C.: 4 hours

Duration:

I.M., S.C.: 8-24 hours

I.V.: 30 minutes to 12 hours

Pharmacokinetics

Absorption: Intranasal: Rapidly but highly variable and lower than I.M. administration

Metabolism: Rapidly in the kidneys, blood, and peripheral tissues

Half-life, elimination: Intranasal: 43 minutes

Time to peak serum concentration: Intranasal: 31-39 minutes

Elimination: As inactive metabolites in urine

Clearance: Salmon calcitonin: 3.1 mL/kg/minute

Usual Dosage Dosage for children not established; Adults:

Paget's disease:

I.M., S.C.: Initial: 100 units/day; maintenance dose: 50 units/day or 50-100 units every 1-3 days

Intranasal: 200-400 units (1-2 sprays) per day

Hypercalcemia: Initial: I.M., S.C.: 4 units/kg every 12 hours; may increase up to 8 units/kg every 12 hours to a maximum of every 6 hours

Osteogenesis imperfecta: I.M., S.C.: 2 units/kg 3 times/week

Postmenopausal osteoporosis:

I.M., S.C.: 100 units/day

Intranasal: 200 units (1 spray) per day

Administration

Intranasal: Alternate spray into each nostril daily

Parenteral: Do not exceed 2 mL volume per injection site; may be administered S.C. or I.M.

Monitoring Parameters Serum electrolytes and calcium; alkaline phosphatase and 24-hour urine collection for hydroxyproline excretion (Paget's disease); serum calcium

Reference Range Therapeutic: <19 pg/mL (SI: 19 ng/L) basal, depending on the assay

Patient Information Nasal spray: Notify physician if you develop significant nasal irritation; alternate nostrils; in treatment of postmenopausal osteoporosis, maintain adequate vitamin D intake and supplemental calcium

Dosage Forms
Injection, solution, salmon calcitonin: 200 units/mL (2 mL)
Solution, intranasal spray, salmon calcitonin: 200 units/activation [0.09 mL/dose] (2 mL glass bottle with pump)

♦ **Cal-Citrate® [OTC]** *see* Calcium Supplements *on page 200*

Calcitriol (kal si TRYE ole)

U.S. Brand Names Calcijex®; Rocaltrol®

Synonyms 1,25 dihydroxycholecalciferol

Therapeutic Category Rickets, Treatment Agent; Vitamin D Analog; Vitamin, Fat Soluble

Generic Available Yes (capsule)

Use Management of secondary hyperparathyroidism and resultant metabolic bone disease in patients with moderate to severe chronic renal failure not yet on dialysis; management of hypocalcemia and resultant metabolic bone disease in patients on chronic renal dialysis; management of hypocalcemia in patients with hypoparathyroidism and pseudohypoparathyroidism

Pregnancy Risk Factor C

Contraindications Hypersensitivity to calcitriol or any component; hypercalcemia; vitamin D toxicity; abnormal sensitivity to the effects of vitamin D

Precautions Excessive calcitriol therapy induces hypercalcemia and possible hypercalciuria; monitor serum calcium levels closely

Adverse Reactions Effects primarily associated with hypercalcemia
Cardiovascular: Elevated blood pressure, cardiac arrhythmias
Central nervous system: Somnolence, headache, hyperthermia, apathy
Dermatologic: Pruritus
Endocrine & metabolic: Hypercholesterolemia, hypercalcemia, polydipsia
Gastrointestinal: Nausea, vomiting, constipation, anorexia, xerostomia, pancreatitis, metallic taste, weight loss
Genitourinary: Nocturia
Hepatic: Elevated liver enzymes
Neuromuscular & skeletal: Myalgia, bone pain, weakness
Ocular: Calcific conjunctivitis, photophobia
Renal: Polyuria, uremia, albuminuria, nephrocalcinosis, UTIs
Respiratory: Rhinorrhea
Miscellaneous: Hypersensitivity reactions, dehydration

Drug Interactions May antagonize the effects of calcium channel blockers by increasing serum calcium levels; may be associated with digoxin toxicity by increasing calcium levels; an additive increase in calcium levels due to decreased calcium excretion by thiazide diuretics; magnesium-containing antacids (potential development of hypermagnesemia); cholestyramine, colestipol, orlistat, and excessive use of mineral oil decrease absorption; ketoconazole may inhibit both the synthetic and catabolic enzymes of calcitriol; corticosteroids decrease calcium absorption counteracting the calcitriol function of increasing calcium absorption

Stability Protect from light and heat

Mechanism of Action Promotes absorption of calcium in the intestines and retention via the kidneys thereby increasing calcium levels in the serum; decreases excessive serum phosphatase levels, parathyroid hormone levels, and decreases bone resorption

Pharmacodynamics Oral:
Onset of action: 2 hours
Maximum effect: 10 hours
Duration: 3-5 days

Pharmacokinetics
Metabolism: Primarily to 1,24,25-trihydroxycholecalciferol and 1,24,25-trihydroxy ergocalciferol
Half-life: 4-6 hours
Time to peak serum concentration: Oral: 3-6 hours
Elimination: Principally in bile and feces

Usual Dosage Individualize dosage to maintain calcium levels of 9-10 mg/dL; successful treatment requires the patient to receive adequate but not excessive calcium supplementation
Management of hypocalcemia in patients with chronic renal failure:
Hemodialysis patients:
I.V.:
Children: 0.01-0.05 mcg/kg 3 times/week
(Continued)

Calcitriol *(Continued)*

Adults: 0.5 mcg (0.01 mcg/kg) 3 times/week; may increase dosage by 0.25-0.5 mcg increments at 2- to 4-week intervals until an optimal response is achieved; range: 0.5-3 mcg (0.01-0.05 mcg/kg)

Oral:

Children: 0.25-2 mcg/day

Adults: 0.25 mcg; may increase in 0.25 mcg increments at 4- to 8-week intervals; range: 0.5-1 mcg/day

Nonhemodialysis patients: Moderate to severe renal failure (Cl_{cr} 15-55 mL/minute; corrected for surface area in children): Oral:

Children <3 years: 0.01-0.015 mcg/kg once daily

Children ≥3 years and Adults: 0.25 mcg/day (maximum dose: 0.5 mcg/day)

Hypoparathyroidism/pseudohypoparathyroidism: Oral (evaluate dosage at 2- to 4-week intervals):

Children:

<1 year: 0.04-0.08 mcg/kg once daily

1-5 years: 0.25-0.75 mcg once daily

Children >6 years and Adults: 0.5-2 mcg once daily

Vitamin D-dependent rickets: Children and Adults: Oral: 1 mcg once daily

Vitamin D-resistant rickets (familial hypophosphatemia): Children and Adults: Oral: Initial: 0.015-0.02 mcg/kg once daily; maintenance: 0.03-0.06 mcg/kg once daily; maximum dose: 2 mcg once daily

Hypocalcemia in premature infants: Oral: 1 mcg once daily for 5 days

Hypocalcemic tetany in premature infants: I.V.: 0.05 mcg/kg once daily for 5-12 days

Administration

Oral: When administering small doses from the liquid-filled capsules, consider the following concentration for Rocaltrol®:

0.25 mcg capsule = 0.25 mcg per 0.17 mL

0.5 mcg capsule = 0.5 mcg per 0.17 mL

Parenteral: May be administered undiluted as a bolus dose I.V. through the catheter at the end of hemodialysis

Monitoring Parameters Serum calcium and phosphorus levels at least twice weekly at the onset of therapy and after each dosage adjustment; weekly for 12 weeks, then monthly after stabilization of dosage; magnesium, 24-hour urinary calcium; alkaline phosphatase; baseline parathyroid hormone and every 3-4 months in predialysis patients

Patient Information May cause dry mouth; follow diet and calcium supplementation instructions carefully

Dosage Forms

Capsule (Rocaltrol®): 0.25 mcg, 0.5 mcg

Injection (Calcijex®): 1 mcg/mL (1 mL); 2 mcg/mL (1 mL)

Solution, oral (Rocaltrol®): 1 mcg/mL (15 mL)

- ♦ **Calcium Acetate** *see Calcium Supplements on page 200*
- ♦ **Calcium Carbonate** *see Calcium Supplements on page 200*
- ♦ **Calcium Chloride** *see Calcium Supplements on page 200*
- ♦ **Calcium Citrate** *see Calcium Supplements on page 200*
- ♦ **Calcium Disodium Edathamil** *see Edetate Calcium Disodium on page 424*
- ♦ **Calcium Disodium Edetate** *see Edetate Calcium Disodium on page 424*
- ♦ **Calcium Disodium Versenate®** *see Edetate Calcium Disodium on page 424*
- ♦ **Calcium Edetate** *see Edetate Calcium Disodium on page 424*
- ♦ **Calcium EDTA** *see Edetate Calcium Disodium on page 424*
- ♦ **Calcium Glubionate** *see Calcium Supplements on page 200*
- ♦ **Calcium Gluconate** *see Calcium Supplements on page 200*
- ♦ **Calcium Lactate** *see Calcium Supplements on page 200*
- ♦ **Calcium Phosphate, Tribasic** *see Calcium Supplements on page 200*

Calcium Supplements *(KAL see um SUP la ments)*

Related Information

Antacid Preparations *on page 112*

Carbohydrate and Alcohol Content of Liquid Medications for Use in Patients Receiving Ketogenic Diets *on page 1431*

CPR Pediatric Drug Dosages *on page 1175*

Extravasation Treatment *on page 1240*

U.S. Brand Names Alka-Mints® [OTC]; Amitone® [OTC]; Calcarb 600 [OTC]; Calci-Chew® [OTC]; Calci-Mix® [OTC]; Cal-Citrate® [OTC]; Cal-lac® [OTC]; Cal-Mint [OTC]; Caltrate® 600 [OTC]; Chooz® [OTC]; Citracal® [OTC]; Citracal® Liquitab [OTC]; Flor-ical® [OTC]; Maalox® Max Quick Dissolve [OTC]; Maalox® Quick Dissolve [OTC];

Mallamint® [OTC]; Mylanta® Calci Tabs Extra Strength [OTC]; Mylanta® Calci Tabs Ultra [OTC]; Mylanta®, Children's [OTC]; Nephro-Calci® [OTC]; Os-Cal® 500 [OTC]; Oysco® [OTC]; Oyst-Cal 500 [OTC]; PhosLo® Posture® [OTC]; Rolaids® [OTC]; Rolaids® Extra Strength [OTC]; Titralac® [OTC]; Titralac® Extra Strength [OTC]; Tums® [OTC]; Tums® 500 [OTC]; Tums® E-X [OTC]; Tums® Ultra® [OTC]

Available Salts Calcium Acetate; Calcium Carbonate; Calcium Chloride; Calcium Citrate; Calcium Glubionate; Calcium Gluconate; Calcium Lactate; Calcium Phosphate, Tribasic

Therapeutic Category Antacid; Antidote, Hydrofluoric Acid; Calcium Salt; Electrolyte Supplement, Oral; Electrolyte Supplement, Parenteral

Generic Available Yes

Use Treatment and prevention of calcium depletion; relief of acid indigestion, heartburn; emergency treatment of hypocalcemic tetany; treatment of hypermagnesemia, cardiac disturbances of hyperkalemia, hypocalcemia, or calcium channel blocking agent toxicity; topical treatment of hydrofluoric acid burns; control of hyperphosphatemia in endstage renal failure

Pregnancy Risk Factor C

Contraindications Hypersensitivity to calcium formulation (see Warnings); hypercalcemia, renal calculi, ventricular fibrillation

Warnings Some products may contain tartrazine which may cause allergic reactions in susceptible individuals

Precautions Use cautiously in patients with sarcoidosis, respiratory failure, acidosis, renal or cardiac disease; avoid too rapid I.V. administration; avoid extravasation; use with caution in digitalized patients; some products may contain aspartame which is metabolized to phenylalanine and must be avoided in patients with phenylketonuria.

Adverse Reactions
Cardiovascular: Vasodilation, hypotension, bradycardia, cardiac arrhythmias, ventricular fibrillation, syncope
Central nervous system: Headache, mental confusion, dizziness, lethargy, coma
Dermatologic: Erythema
Endocrine & metabolic: Hypercalcemia, milk-alkali syndrome, hypophosphatemia, hypercalciuria, hypomagnesemia
Gastrointestinal: Constipation, nausea, vomiting, xerostomia, elevated serum amylase
Local: Tissue necrosis (I.V. administration)
Neuromuscular & skeletal: Muscle weakness

Drug Interactions May potentiate digoxin toxicity; may antagonize the effects of calcium channel blockers (eg, verapamil); when administered orally, calcium decreases the absorption of tetracycline, atenolol, iron, quinolone antibiotics, alendronate, sodium fluoride, and zinc; high doses of calcium with thiazide diuretics may result in milk-alkali syndrome and hypercalcemia; decreases potassium-binding ability of polystyrene sulfonate

Food Interactions Do not give orally with bran, foods high in oxalates, or whole grain cereals which may decrease calcium absorption

Stability Incompatible with bicarbonates, phosphates, and sulfates

Mechanism of Action Moderates nerve and muscle performance via action potential excitation threshold regulation; neutralizes acidity of stomach (carbonate salt); combines with dietary phosphate to form insoluble calcium phosphate which is excreted in feces and reduces phosphate absorption (acetate and carbonate salts)

Usual Dosage Note: Multiple salt forms of calcium exist; close attention must be paid to the salt form when ordering and administering calcium; incorrect selection or

Elemental Calcium Content of Calcium Salts

Calcium Salt	Elemental Calcium (mg/1 g of salt form)	mEq calcium per gram	Approximate Equivalent Doses (mg of calcium salt)
Calcium acetate	250	12.7	354
Calcium carbonate	400	20	225
Calcium chloride	270	13.5	330
Calcium citrate	211	10.6	425
Calcium glubionate	64	3.2	1400
Calcium gluconate	90	4.5	1000
Calcium lactate	130	6.5	700
Calcium phosphate, tribasic	390	19.3	233

(Continued)

Calcium Supplements *(Continued)*

substitution of one salt for another without proper dosage adjustment may result in serious over- or underdosing.

Oral: **Note:** For comparison information of calcium salts, see table on previous page.

Recommended daily allowance (RDA): Dosage is in terms of elemental calcium:
<6 months: 400 mg/day
6-12 months: 600 mg/day
1-10 years: 800 mg/day
11-24 years: 1200 mg/day
Adults >24 years: 800 mg/day

Adequate intake (1997 National Academy of Science Recommendations): **Dosage is in terms of elemental calcium:**
0-6 months: 210 mg/day
7-12 months: 270 mg/day
1-3 years: 500 mg/day
4-8 years: 800 mg/day
9-18 years: 1300 mg/day
19-50 years: 1000 mg/day
>50 years: 1200 mg/day

Hypocalcemia (dose depends on clinical condition and serum calcium level): **Oral:**
Dose expressed in mg of **elemental calcium:**
Neonates: 50-150 mg/kg/day in 4-6 divided doses; not to exceed 1 g/day
Children: 45-65 mg/kg/day in 4 divided doses
Adults: 1-2 g or more per day in 3-4 divided doses
Dose expressed in mg of **calcium gluconate:**
Neonates: 500-1500 mg/kg/day in 4-6 divided doses
Infants and Children: 500-725 mg/kg/day in 3-4 divided doses
Adults: 10-20 g daily in 3-4 divided doses
Dose expressed in mg of **calcium glubionate:**
Neonates: 1200 mg/kg/day in 4-6 divided doses
Infants and Children: 600-2000 mg/kg/day in 4 divided doses up to a maximum of 9 g/day
Adults: 6-18 g/day in divided doses
Dose expressed in mg of **calcium lactate:**
Neonates and Infants: 400-500 mg/kg/day divided every 4-6 hours
Children: 500 mg/kg/day divided every 6-8 hours; maximum daily dose 9 g
Adults: 1.5-3 g divided every 8 hours

Hypocalcemia: I.V.:
Dosage expressed in mg of **calcium chloride:**
Manufacturer's recommendations: Children: 2.7-5 mg/kg/dose every 4-6 hours
Alternative pediatric dosing: Neonates, Infants, and Children: 10-20 mg/kg/dose, repeat every 4-6 hours if needed
Adults: 500 mg to 1 g/dose every 6 hours
Dose expressed in mg of **calcium gluconate:**
Neonates: 200-800 mg/kg/day as a continuous infusion or in 4 divided doses
Infants and Children: 200-500 mg/kg/day as a continuous infusion or in 4 divided doses
Adults: 2-15 g/day as a continuous infusion or in divided doses

Cardiac arrest in the presence of hyperkalemia or hypocalcemia, magnesium toxicity, or calcium antagonist toxicity: I.V., I.O.:
Dosage expressed in mg of **calcium chloride:**
Neonates, Infants, and Children: 20 mg/kg; may repeat in 10 minutes if necessary
Adults: 2-4 mg/kg; may repeat in 10 minutes if necessary
Dosage expressed in mg of **calcium gluconate:**
Neonates, Infants, and Children: 60-100 mg/kg/dose (maximum 3 g/dose)
Adults: 500-800 mg (maximum 3 g/dose)

Hypocalcemia secondary to citrated blood infusion: I.V.: Give 0.45 mEq **elemental** calcium for each 100 mL citrated blood infused

Tetany: I.V.:
Dose expressed in mg of **calcium chloride:**
Neonates, Infants, and Children: 10 mg/kg over 5-10 minutes; may repeat after 6 hours or follow with an infusion with a maximum dose of 200 mg/kg/day
Adults: 1 g over 10-30 minutes; may repeat after 6 hours
Dose expressed in mg of **calcium gluconate:**
Neonates: 100-200 mg/kg/dose; may follow with 500 mg/kg/day in 3-4 divided doses or as a continuous infusion
Infants and Children: 100-200 mg/kg/dose over 5-10 minutes; may repeat after 6 hours or follow with an infusion of 500 mg/kg/day

Adults: 1-3 g may be administered until therapeutic response occurs

Antacid (calcium carbonate): See Antacid Preparations *on page 112*

Treatment of hyperphosphatemia in end stage renal failure: Oral:

Dose expressed in mg of **calcium acetate:** Adults: 1334 mg (two 667 mg capsules) with each meal; may increase up to 2668 mg (four 667 mg capsules) with each meal

Dose expressed in mg of **calcium carbonate:** Children and Adults: 1 g with each meal; increase as needed; range: 4-7 g/day

Hydrofluoric acid (HF) burns (HF concentration <20%): Topical: Various topical calcium preparations have been used anecdotally for treatment of dermal exposure to HF solutions; both calcium gluconate and carbonate at concentrations ranging from 2.5% to 33% have been used: Massage calcium gluconate gel or slurry into exposed area for 15 minutes; topical calcium preparations must be compounded (see Extemporaneous Preparations)

Administration

Oral: Administer with plenty of fluids with or following meals; for phosphate binding, administer on an empty stomach before meals to optimize effectiveness

Parenteral:

I.V.: For direct I.V. injection infuse at a maximum rate of 50-100 mg/minute of calcium salt (gluconate or chloride)

I.V. infusion: Dilution and infusion rates are dependent upon the salt form; dilute with I.V. fluid to a final concentration listed below

Salt form (dilution; rate of infusion)

Calcium **chloride:** 20 mg/mL; 45-90 mg/kg over 1 hour; 0.6-1.2 mEq/kg over 1 hour

Calcium **gluconate:** 50 mg/mL; 120-240 mg/kg over 1 hour; 0.6-1.2 mEq/kg over 1 hour

Do not inject calcium salts I.M. or administer S.C. since severe necrosis and sloughing may occur; extravasation of calcium can result in severe necrosis and tissue sloughing. Do not use scalp vein or small hand or foot veins for I.V. administration. Not for endotracheal administration.

Monitoring Parameters Serum calcium (ionized calcium preferred if available, see Additional Information), phosphate, magnesium, heart rate, EKG

Reference Range

Calcium: Newborns: 7.0-12.0 mg/dL; 0-2 years: 8.8-11.2 mg/dL; 2 years to adults: 9.0-11.0 mg/dL

Calcium, ionized, whole blood: 4.4-5.4 mg/dL

Patient Information May cause dry mouth

Additional Information Due to a poor correlation between the serum ionized calcium (free) and total serum calcium, particularly in states of low albumin or acid/base imbalances, direct measurement of ionized calcium is recommended. If ionized calcium is unavailable, in low albumin states, the corrected **total** serum calcium may be estimated by this equation (assuming a normal albumin of 4 g/dL); corrected total calcium = total serum calcium + 0.8 (4 - measured serum albumin)

Dosage Forms

Calcium acetate:

Gelcap (PhosLo®): 667 mg [equivalent to 169 mg elemental calcium]

Injection, solution: 0.5 mEq/mL (10 mL, 50 mL, 100 mL)

Tablet (PhosLo®): 667 mg [equivalent to 169 mg elemental calcium]

Calcium carbonate:

Capsule: 1500 mg [equivalent to 600 mg elemental calcium]

Calci-Mix®: 1250 mg [equivalent to 500 mg elemental calcium]

Florical®: 364 mg [equivalent to 145.6 mg elemental caclium; contains 8.3 mg sodium fluoride]

Suspension, oral: 1250 mg/5 mL (5 mL, 500 mL) [equivalent to 500 mg elemental calcium; mint flavor]

Tablet: 650 mg [equivalent to 260 mg elemental calcium], 1500 mg [equivalent to 600 mg elemental calcium]

Calcarb 600, Caltrate® 600, Nephro-Calci®: 1500 mg [equivalent to 600 mg elemental calcium]

Florical®: 364 mg [equivalent to 145 mg elemental calcium; contains 8.3 mg sodium fluoride]

Os-Cal® 500, Oysco®, Oyst-Cal 500: 1250 mg [equivalent to 500 mg elemental calcium]

Tablet, chewable: 500 mg [equivalent to 200 mg elemental calcium]; 650 mg [equivalent to 260 mg elemental calcium]; 750 mg [equivalent to 300 mg elemental calcium]; 1000 mg [equivalent to 400 mg elemental calcium]

Alka-Mints®: 850 mg [equivalent to 340 mg elemental calcium; assorted and spearmint flavors]

Amitone®: 350 mg [equivalent to 140 mg elemental calcium; spearmint flavor]

(Continued)

Calcium Supplements *(Continued)*

Calci-Chew®: 1250 mg [equivalent to 500 mg elemental calcium; cherry, lemon, and orange flavors]

Cal-Mint: 650 mg [equivalent to 260 mg elemental calcium; mint flavor]

Children's Mylanta®: 400 mg [equivalent to 160 mg elemental calcium; bubblegum flavor]

Chooz®: 500 mg [equivalent to 200 mg elemental calcium]

Maalox® Quick Dissolve: 600 mg [equivalent to 222 mg elemental calcium; contains 0.5 mg phenylalanine (as aspartame)/tablet; lemon, wild berry; wintergreen, and assorted flavors]

Maalox® Max Quick Dissolve: 1000 mg [equivalent to 370 mg elemental calcium; contains 0.9 mg phenylalanine (as aspartame)/tablet; lemon, wild berry, wintergreen, and assorted flavors]

Mallamint®: 420 mg [equivalent to 168 mg elemental calcium]

Mylanta® Calci Tabs Extra Strength: 750 mg [equivalent to 300 mg elemental calcium; contains tartrazine; cool mint and fruit medley flavors]

Mylanta® Calci Tabs Ultra: 1000 mg [equivalent to 400 mg elemental calcium; contains tartrazine; cool mint and fruit medley flavors]

Os-Cal® 500: 1250 mg [equivalent to 500 mg elemental calcium; Bavarian cream flavor]

Rolaids®: 550 mg [equivalent to 220 mg elemental calcium; contains 110 mg magnesium hydroxide (equivalent to 45 mg elemental magnesium); original, cherry, and spearmint flavors]

Rolaids® Extra Strength: 675 mg [equivalent to 271 mg elemental calcium; contains 135 mg magnesium hydroxide; fruit flavor (contains tartrazine) and freshmint flavor]

Titralac™: 420 mg [equivalent to 168 mg elemental calcium; sugar free; mint flavor]

Titralac™ Extra Strength: 750 mg [equivalent to 300 mg elemental calcium; sugar free; mint flavor]

Tums®: 500 mg [equivalent to 200 mg elemental calcium; assorted fruit and peppermint flavors]

Tums® 500: 1250 mg [equivalent to 500 mg elemental calcium; assorted fruit and peppermint flavors]

Tums® E-X: 750 mg [equivalent to 300 mg elemental calcium; assorted fruit, tropical assorted fruit, wintergreen, and assorted berry flavors; sugar free orange cream flavor]

Tums® Ultra®: 1000 mg [equivalent to 400 mg elemental calcium; assorted mint, assorted fruit, and tropical assorted berry flavors]

Calcium chloride:

Injection, solution: 10% [100 mg/mL] (10 mL) [equivalent to 27.2 mg elemental calcium/mL; 1.4 mEq calcium/mL]

Calcium citrate:

Tablet:

Cal-Citrate®: 250 mg [equivalent to 53 mg elemental calcium]

Citracal®: 950 mg [equivalent to 200 mg elemental calcium]

Tablet, effervescent (Citracal® Liquitab): 2376 mg [equivalent to 500 mg elemental calcium; contains 6 mg phenylalanine (as aspartame)/tablet; citrus flavor]

Calcium glubionate:

Syrup: 1.8 g/5 mL (480 mL) [equivalent to 115 mg elemental calcium/5 mL; 1.2 mEq calcium/mL]

Calcium gluconate:

Injection, solution: 10% [100 mg/mL] (10 mL, 50 mL, 100 mL, 200 mL) [equivalent to 9 mg elemental calcium/mL; 0.46 mEq calcium/mL]

Tablet: 500 mg [equivalent to 45 mg elemental calcium], 650 mg [equivalent to 58.5 mg elemental calcium], 975 mg [equivalent to 87.75 mg elemental calcium]

Calcium lactate:

Capsule (Cal-lac®): 500 mg [equivalent to 96 mg elemental calcium]

Tablet: 325 mg [equivalent to 42.25 mg elemental calcium], 650 mg [equivalent to 84.5 mg elemental calcium]

Calcium phosphate, tribasic:

Tablet (Posture®): 1565.2 mg [equivalent to 600 mg elemental calcium; sugar free]

Extemporaneous Preparations

Calcium gluconate gel: Crush 3.5 g calcium gluconate tablets into a fine powder; add to 5 oz tube of water-soluble surgical lubricant (eg, K-Y® Jelly) or add 3.5 g calcium gluconate injection to 5 oz of water-soluble surgical lubricant (calcium carbonate may be substituted; do not use calcium chloride due to potential for irritation)

Calcium carbonate slurry: 32.5% slurry can be prepared by triturating ten 650 mg tablets into a fine powder and adding 20 mL of water-soluble lubricant gel (eg, K-Y® Jelly)

References

Baker SS, Cochran WJ, Flores CA, et al, "American Academy of Pediatrics. Committee on Nutrition: Calcium Requirements of Infants, Children, and Adolescents," *Pediatrics*, 1999, 104(5):1152-7.

"Dietary Reference Intakes for Calcium, Phosphorus, Magnesium, Vitamin D, and Fluoride. Standing Committee on the Scientific Evaluation of Dietary Reference Intakes, Food and Nutrition Board, Institute of Medicine," National Academy of Sciences, Washington, DC: National Academy Press, 1997.

"Guidelines 2000 for Cardiopulmonary Resuscitation and Emergency Cardiovascular Care. Part 10: Pediatric Advanced Life Support. The American Heart Association in Collaboration With the International Liaison Committee on Resuscitation," *Circulation*, 2000, 102(8 Suppl):I291-342.

NIH Consensus Conference, "Optimal Calcium Intake," *JAMA*, 1994, 272(24):1942-8.

♦ **Caldecort® [OTC]** *see* Hydrocortisone *on page 573*

Calfactant (cal FAC tant)

U.S. Brand Names Infasurf®

Synonyms Bovine Lung Surfactant

Therapeutic Category Lung Surfactant

Generic Available No

Use Prevention and treatment of respiratory distress syndrome (RDS) in premature infants

Prophylactic therapy: Infants <29 weeks at significant risk for RDS

Treatment: Infants ≤72 hours of age with RDS (confirmed by clinical and radiologic findings and requiring endotracheal intubation)

Warnings Rapidly affects oxygenation and lung compliance and should be restricted to a highly supervised use in a clinical setting with immediate availability of clinicians experienced with intubation and ventilatory management of premature infants; if transient episodes of bradycardia and decreased oxygen saturation occur, discontinue the dosing procedure and initiate measures to alleviate the condition; produces rapid improvement in lung oxygenation and compliance that may require immediate reductions in ventilator settings and FiO_2; for intratracheal administration only

Precautions Transient episodes of reflux of calfactant into the endotracheal tube, cyanosis, bradycardia, or airway obstruction have occurred during dosing procedures; such episodes may require stopping administration and taking appropriate measures to alleviate the condition before resuming therapy

Adverse Reactions Most adverse reactions occur during the dosing procedure

Cardiovascular: Bradycardia, cyanosis

Respiratory: Airway obstruction, pneumothorax, pulmonary hemorrhage, apnea

Stability Refrigerate; protect from light; unopened, unused warmed vials of calfactant may be returned to refrigerator within 24 hours for future use; repeated warming to room temperature should be avoided

Mechanism of Action Replaces deficient or ineffective endogenous lung surfactant in neonates with RDS or in neonates at risk of developing RDS; surfactant prevents the alveoli from collapsing during expiration by lowering surface tension between air and alveolar surfaces

Usual Dosage Intratracheal: Neonates: 3 mL/kg every 12 hours up to a total of 3 doses; repeat doses have been administered as early as 6 hours after the previous dose for a total of up to four doses (if the infant was still intubated and required at least 30% inspired oxygen to maintain a PaO_2 ≤80 torr)

Administration Intratracheal: Gently swirl to redisperse suspension; do not shake; administer dosage divided into two aliquots of 1.5 mL/kg each into the endotracheal tube; after each instillation, reposition the infant with either the right or left side dependent; administration is made while ventilation is continued over 20-30 breaths for each aliquot, with small bursts timed only during the inspiratory cycles; a pause followed by evaluation of the respiratory status and repositioning should separate the two aliquots; calfactant dosage has also been divided into four equal aliquots and administered with repositioning in four different positions (prone, supine, right and left lateral)

Monitoring Parameters Continuous heart rate and transcutaneous O_2 saturation should be monitored during administration; frequent ABG sampling is necessary to prevent postdosing hyperoxia and hypocarbia

Dosage Forms Suspension, intratracheal [preservative free]: 35 mg/mL (6 mL)

References

Hudak ML, Martin DJ, Egan EA, et al, "A Multicenter Randomized Masked Comparison Trail of Synthetic Surfactant Versus Calf Lung Surfactant Extract in the Prevention of Neonatal Respiratory Distress Syndrome," *Pediatrics*, 1997, 100(1):39-50.

Bloom BT, Kattwinkel J, Hall RT, et al, "Comparison of Infasurf® (Calf Lung Surfactant Extract) to Survanta® (Beractant) in the Treatment and Prevention of Respiratory Distress Syndrome," *Pediatrics*, 1997, 100(1):31-8.

- ◆ **Cal-lac® [OTC]** *see* Calcium Supplements *on page 200*
- ◆ **Cal-Mint [OTC]** *see* Calcium Supplements *on page 200*
- ◆ **Caltine® (Can)** *see* Calcitonin *on page 198*
- ◆ **Caltrate® 600 [OTC]** *see* Calcium Supplements *on page 200*
- ◆ **Camphorated Tincture of Opium** *see* Paregoric *on page 864*
- ◆ **Camptosar®** *see* Irinotecan *on page 621*
- ◆ **Camptothecin-11** *see* Irinotecan *on page 621*
- ◆ **Canasa™** *see* Mesalamine *on page 723*
- ◆ **Cancidas®** *see* Caspofungin *on page 221*
- ◆ **Candistatin® (Can)** *see* Nystatin *on page 827*
- ◆ **Canesten® Topical (Can)** *see* Clotrimazole *on page 297*
- ◆ **Canesten® Vaginal (Can)** *see* Clotrimazole *on page 297*
- ◆ **Cankaid® [OTC]** *see* Carbamide Peroxide *on page 212*
- ◆ **Capex™** *see* Fluocinolone *on page 498*
- ◆ **Capital® and Codeine** *see* Acetaminophen and Codeine *on page 39*
- ◆ **Capoten®** *see* Captopril *on page 207*
- ◆ **Capsagel® [OTC]** *see* Capsaicin *on page 206*
- ◆ **Capsagel® Extra Strength [OTC]** *see* Capsaicin *on page 206*
- ◆ **Capsagel® Maximum Strength [OTC]** *see* Capsaicin *on page 206*

Capsaicin (kap SAY sin)

U.S. Brand Names Capsagel® [OTC]; Capsagel® Extra Strength [OTC]; Capsagel® Maximum Strength [OTC]; Capsin® [OTC]; Rid-a-Pain-HP® [OTC]; TheraPatch® Warm [OTC]; Zostrix® [OTC]; Zostrix®-HP [OTC]; Zostrix® Sports [OTC]

Canadian Brand Names Antiphlogistine Rub A-535 Capsaicin

Therapeutic Category Analgesic, Topical; Topical Skin Product

Generic Available Yes

Use Topical treatment of pain associated with postherpetic neuralgia, rheumatoid arthritis, osteoarthritis, diabetic neuropathy, and postsurgical pain; also used for treatment of pain associated with psoriasis, chronic neuralgias unresponsive to other forms of therapy, and intractable pruritus

Contraindications Hypersensitivity to capsaicin or any component

Warnings Avoid contact with eyes, mucous membrane, or with damaged or irritated skin

Precautions Since warm water or excessive sweating may intensify the localized burning sensation after capsaicin application, the affected area should not be tightly bandaged or exposed to direct sunlight or a heat lamp

Adverse Reactions
Dermatologic: Erythema
Local: Itching, burning, or stinging sensation
Respiratory: Cough

Mechanism of Action Induces release of substance P, the principal chemomediator of pain impulses from the periphery to the CNS, from peripheral sensory neurons. After repeated application, capsaicin depletes the neuron of substance P and prevents reaccumulation.

Pharmacodynamics
Onset of action: Pain relief is usually seen within 14-28 days of regular topical application; maximal response may require 4-6 weeks of continuous therapy
Duration: Several hours

Usual Dosage Children ≥2 years and Adults: Topical: Apply to affected area at least 3-4 times/day; application frequency less than 3-4 times/day prevents the total depletion, inhibition of synthesis, and transport of substance P resulting in decreased clinical efficacy and increased local discomfort

Administration Topical: Should not be applied to wounds or damaged skin; avoid eye and mucous membrane exposure

Patient Information For external use only. Avoid washing treated areas for 30 minutes after application

Nursing Implications Wash hands with soap and water after applying to avoid spreading cream to eyes or other sensitive areas of the body

Additional Information In patients with severe and persistent local discomfort, pretreatment with topical lidocaine 5% ointment or concurrent oral analgesics for the first 2 weeks of therapy have been effective in alleviating the initial burning sensation and enabling continuation of topical capsaicin

Dosage Forms
Cream, topical: 0.025% (60 g); 0.075% (60 g)
Rid-a-Pain-HP®: 0.075% (45 g)

Zostrix®: 0.025% (60 g)
Zostrix®-HP: 0.075% (60 g)
Zostrix® Sports: 0.075% (30 g)
Gel, topical:
Capsagel®: 0.025% (60 g)
Capsagel® Extra Strength: 0.05% (60 g)
Capsagel® Maximum Strength: 0.075% (30 g, 60 g)
Lotion, topical (Capsin®): 0.025% (59 mL); 0.075% (59 mL)
Patch, topical (TheraPatch® Warm): 0.09% (7s)

References

Bernstein JE, Korman NJ, Bickers DR, et al, "Topical Capsaicin Treatment of Chronic Postherpetic Neuralgia," *J Am Acad Dermatol*, 1989, 21(2 Pt 1):265-70.

♦ **Capsin® [OTC]** *see* Capsaicin *on page 206*

Captopril (KAP toe pril)

U.S. Brand Names Capoten®

Canadian Brand Names Alti-Captopril; Apo®-Capto; Gen-Captopril; Novo-Captopril; Nu-Capto®; PMS-Captopril®

Therapeutic Category Angiotensin-Converting Enzyme (ACE) Inhibitor; Antihypertensive Agent

Generic Available Yes

Use Management of hypertension; treatment of CHF; in post-MI patients, improves survival in clinically stable patients with left-ventricular dysfunction

Pregnancy Risk Factor C (1st trimester); D (may cause injury and death to the developing fetus when used during the second and third trimester of pregnancy)

Contraindications Hypersensitivity to captopril, any component, or other ACE inhibitors

Warnings Serious adverse effects including angioedema, anaphylactoid reactions, neutropenia, agranulocytosis, proteinuria, hypotension, and hepatic failure may occur (see Adverse Reactions); risk of neutropenia is increased 15 fold to 1 per 500 in patients with renal dysfunction, and increased to 3.7% in patients with both collagen vascular disease and renal dysfunction

Precautions Use with caution and modify dosage in patients with renal impairment, especially those with severe renal artery stenosis; elevated BUN and serum creatinine may occur in these patients after decrease in blood pressure with captopril; dosage reduction of captopril or discontinuation of concurrent diuretic may be needed; control of blood pressure while maintaining adequate renal perfusion may not be possible in some of these patients. Use with caution in patients with collagen vascular disease and in patients with volume depletion.

Adverse Reactions

Cardiovascular: Hypotension, tachycardia

Central nervous system: Headache, dizziness, fatigue, insomnia, fever

Dermatologic: Rash, angioedema. **Note:** The relative risk of angioedema with ACE inhibitors is higher within the first 30 days of use (compared to >1 year of use), for Black Americans (compared to Whites), for lisinopril or enalapril (compared to captopril), and for patients previously hospitalized within 30 days (Brown, 1996).

Endocrine & metabolic: Hyperkalemia

Gastrointestinal: Ageusia

Hematologic: Neutropenia, agranulocytosis, eosinophilia

Hepatic: Cholestatic jaundice, fulminant hepatic necrosis (rare, but potentially fatal)

Respiratory: Cough, dyspnea; **Note:** An isolated dry cough lasting >3 weeks was reported in 7 of 42 pediatric patients (17%) receiving ACE inhibitors (see von Vigier, 2000)

Renal: Elevated BUN and serum creatinine, proteinuria, oliguria

Drug Interactions Cytochrome P450 isoenzyme CYP2D6 substrate

Captopril plus potassium supplements or potassium-sparing diuretics may cause an additive hyperkalemic effect; captopril plus indomethacin or NSAIDs may result in a reduced antihypertensive response to captopril

Food Interactions Absorption of captopril may be reduced by food; long-term use of captopril may result in a zinc deficiency which can result in a decrease in taste perception; zinc supplements may be used; limit salt substitutes or potassium-rich diet; avoid natural licorice (causes sodium and water retention and increases potassium loss)

Stability Unstable in aqueous solutions

Mechanism of Action Competitive inhibitor of angiotensin-converting enzyme (ACE); prevents conversion of angiotensin I to angiotensin II, a potent vasoconstrictor; results in lower levels of angiotensin II which causes an increase in plasma renin activity and a reduction in aldosterone secretion

(Continued)

Captopril *(Continued)*

Pharmacodynamics
Onset of action: Decrease in blood pressure within 15 minutes
Maximum effect: 60-90 minutes; may require several weeks of therapy before full hypotensive effect is seen
Duration: Dose-related

Pharmacokinetics
Absorption: 60% to 75%
Distribution: 7 L/kg
Protein binding: 25% to 30%
Metabolism: 50% metabolized
Half-life:
Infants with CHF: 3.3 hours; range: 1.2-12.4 hours
Children: 1.5 hours; range: 0.98-2.3 hours
Normal adults (dependent upon renal and cardiac function): 1.9 hours
Adults with CHF: 2.1 hours
Anuria: 20-40 hours
Time to peak serum concentration: Within 1-2 hours
Elimination: 95% excreted in urine in 24 hours

Usual Dosage Note: Dosage must be titrated according to patient's response; use lowest effective dose; lower doses (~½ of those listed) should be used in patients who are sodium and water depleted due to diuretic therapy; Oral:

Newborns and premature Neonates: Initial: 0.01 mg/kg/dose every 8-12 hours; titrate dose
Neonates: Initial: 0.05-0.1 mg/kg/dose every 8-24 hours; titrate dose up to 0.5 mg/kg/dose given every 6-24 hours
Infants: Initial: 0.15-0.3 mg/kg/dose; titrate dose upward to maximum of 6 mg/kg/day in 1-4 divided doses; usual required dose: 2.5-6 mg/kg/day
Children: Initial: 0.3-0.5 mg/kg/dose; titrate upward to maximum of 6 mg/kg/day in 2-4 divided doses
Older Children: Initial: 6.25-12.5 mg/dose every 12-24 hours; titrate upward to maximum of 6 mg/kg/day in 2-4 divided doses
Adolescents and Adults: Initial: 12.5-25 mg/dose given every 8-12 hours; increase by 25 mg/dose to maximum of 450 mg/day

Dosing adjustment in renal impairment:
Cl_{cr} 10-50 mL/minute: Administer 75% of dose
Cl_{cr} <10 mL/minute: Administer 50% of dose

Administration Oral: Administer on an empty stomach 1 hour before meals or 2 hours after meals

Monitoring Parameters Blood pressure, BUN, serum creatinine, renal function, urine dipstick for protein, WBC with differential, serum potassium

Patient Information Limit alcohol; notify physician if swelling of face, lips, tongue, difficulty in breathing, or persistent cough occurs; do not use salt substitute (potassium-containing) without physician advice

Nursing Implications Discontinue if angioedema occurs; monitor blood pressure for hypotension within 1-3 hours after first dose or after a new higher dose

Additional Information Severe hypotension may occur in patients who are sodium and/or volume depleted

Dosage Forms Tablet: 12.5 mg, 25 mg, 50 mg, 100 mg

Extemporaneous Preparations
Captopril has limited stability in aqueous preparations. The addition of an antioxidant [sodium ascorbate (using an injectable product) or ascorbic acid (using tablets)] has been shown to increase the stability of captopril in solution; captopril (1 mg/mL) in syrup with methylcellulose is stable for 7 days stored either at 4°C or 22°C. Captopril (1 mg/mL) in distilled water (no additives) is stable for 14 days if stored at 4°C and 7 days if stored at 22°C; captopril (1 mg/mL) with sodium ascorbate (5 mg/mL) in distilled water is stable for 56 days at 4°C and 14 days at 22°C (Nahata, 1994); captopril (1 mg/mL) with ascorbic acid (5 mg/mL) in distilled water is stable for 56 days at 4°C and 28 days at 22°C (Nahata, 1994a); captopril (1 mg/mL) in an undiluted syrup containing preservatives is stable for 30 days at 5°C in amber glass containers (Lye, 1997).
Captopril (0.75 mg/mL) in cherry syrup is stable for only 2 days in amber clear plastic containers stored at room temperature or under refrigeration; captopril (0.75 mg/mL) in either a 1:1 mixture of Ora-Sweet® and Ora-Plus® or a 1:1 mixture of Ora-Sweet® SF and Ora-Plus® is stable for 10 days or less depending on the storage temperature (see Allen, 1996).
Powder papers can also be made; powder papers are stable for 12 weeks when stored at room temperature (Taketomo, 1990).

Allen LV and Erickson MA, "Stability of Baclofen, Captopril, Diltiazem Hydrochloride, Dipyridamole, and Flecainide Acetate in Extemporaneously Compounded Oral Liquids," *Am J Health Sys Pharm*, 1996, 53(18):2179-84.

Lye MY, Yow KL, Lim LY, et al, "Effects of Ingredients on Stability of Captopril in Extemporaneously Prepared Oral Liquids," *Am J Health Syst Pharm*, 1997, 54(21):2483-7.

Nahata MC, Morosco RS, and Hipple TF, "Stability of Captopril in Three Liquid Dosage Forms," *Am J Hosp Pharm*, 1994, 51(1):95-6.

Nahata MC, Morosco RS, and Hipple TF, "Stability of Captopril in Liquid Containing Ascorbic Acid or Sodium Ascorbate," *Am J Hosp Pharm*, 1994a, 51(13):1707-8.

Taketomo CK, Chu SA, Cheng MH, et al, "Stability of Captopril in Powder Papers Under Three Storage Conditions," *Am J Hosp Pharm*, 1990, 47(8):1799-801.

References
Brown NJ, Ray WA, Snowden M, et al, "Black Americans Have an Increased Rate of Angiotensin-Converting Enzyme Inhibitor-Associated Angioedema," *Clin Pharmacol Ther*, 1996, 60(1):8-13.

Friedman WF and George BL, "New Concepts and Drugs in the Treatment of Congestive Heart Failure," *Pediatr Clin North Am*, 1984, 31(6):1197-227.

Levy M, Koren G, Klein J, et al, "Captopril Pharmacokinetics, Blood Pressure Response and Plasma Renin Activity in Normotensive Children With Renal Scarring," *Dev Pharmacol Ther*, 1991, 16(4):185-93.

Mirkin BL and Newman TJ, "Efficacy and Safety of Captopril in the Treatment of Severe Childhood Hypertension: Report of the International Collaborative Study Group," *Pediatrics*, 1985, 75(6):1091-100.

Pereira CM, Tam YK, Collins-Nakai RL, "The Pharmacokinetics of Captopril in Infants With Congestive Heart Failure," *Ther Drug Monit*, 1991, 13(3):209-14.

von Vigier RO, Mozzettini S, Truttmann AC, et al, "Cough is Common in Children Prescribed Converting Enzyme Inhibitors," *Nephron*, 2000, 84(1):98.

♦ **Carac**™ *see Fluorouracil on page 503*

♦ **Carafate**® *see Sucralfate on page 1046*

Carbamazepine (kar ba MAZ e peen)

Related Information
Antiepileptic Drugs *on page 1374*
Blood Level Sampling Time Guidelines *on page 1386*
Carbohydrate and Alcohol Content of Liquid Medications for Use in Patients Receiving Ketogenic Diets *on page 1431*
Overdose and Toxicology *on page 1388*
Serotonin Syndrome *on page 1420*

U.S. Brand Names Carbatrol®; Epitol®; Tegretol®; Tegretol®-XR

Canadian Brand Names Apo®-Carbamazepine; Apo®-Carbamazepine CR; Gen-Carbamazepine CR; Novo-Carbamaz; Nu-Carbamazepine®; PMS-Carbamazepine; Taro-Carbamazepine Chewable

Synonyms CBZ

Therapeutic Category Anticonvulsant, Miscellaneous

Generic Available Yes (except extended release capsule and extended release tablet)

Use Prophylaxis of generalized tonic-clonic, partial (especially complex partial), and mixed partial or generalized seizure disorder; to relieve pain in trigeminal neuralgia or diabetic neuropathy; treatment of bipolar disorders

Pregnancy Risk Factor D

Contraindications Hypersensitivity to carbamazepine or any component; patients with a history of bone marrow suppression; cross-sensitivity with tricyclic antidepressants may occur; concomitant therapy with MAO inhibitors

Warnings Potentially fatal blood cell abnormalities have been reported following treatment; early detection of hematologic change is important; advise patients of early signs and symptoms which are: fever, sore throat, mouth ulcers, infections, easy bruising, petechial or purpuric hemorrhage

Substitution of Tegretol® with generic carbamazepine has resulted in decreased carbamazepine levels and increased seizure activity, as well as increased carbamazepine levels and toxicity. Monitoring of carbamazepine serum concentrations is mandatory when patients are switched from any product to another.

Precautions MAO inhibitors should be discontinued for a minimum of 14 days before carbamazepine is begun; administer with caution to patients with history of cardiac disease, hepatic disease, renal failure, or history of hypersensitivity reactions to other anticonvulsants (eg, phenobarbital, phenytoin); hepatic failure (rare) and multi-organ hypersensitivity reactions may occur (see Adverse Reactions); consider discontinuation of carbamazepine if any evidence of hypersensitivity occurs; higher peak concentrations occur with the suspension, so treatment is initiated with lower amounts per dose and increased slowly to avoid adverse effects

Adverse Reactions
Cardiovascular: Edema, CHF, syncope, dysrhythmias, heart block
(Continued)

Carbamazepine (Continued)

Central nervous system: Sedation, dizziness, drowsiness, fatigue, slurred speech, ataxia, confusion

Dermatologic: Rash, Stevens-Johnson syndrome, photosensitivity

Endocrine & metabolic: SIADH, hyponatremia

Gastrointestinal: Nausea, diarrhea, vomiting, abdominal cramps, pancreatitis

Genitourinary: Urinary retention

Hematologic: Neutropenia (can be transient), aplastic anemia, agranulocytosis, thrombocytopenia

Hepatic: Elevated liver enzymes, jaundice, hepatitis; hepatic failure (very rare)

Ocular: Nystagmus, diplopia, blurred vision

Miscellaneous: Multi-organ hypersensitivity reactions (rare): Reactions may include vasculitis, lymphadenopathy, fever, rash, lymphoma-like symptoms, arthralgia, eosinophilia, leukopenia, elevated liver enzymes, hepato-splenomegaly

Drug Interactions Cytochrome P450 isoenzyme CYP2C8 and CYP3A3/4 substrate; isoenzyme CYP1A2, CYP2C, and CYP3A3/4 inducer

Clarithromycin, erythromycin, isoniazid, danazol, fluoxetine, ketoconazole, itraconazole, propoxyphene, verapamil, diltiazem, and cimetidine may inhibit hepatic metabolism of carbamazepine with resultant increase of carbamazepine serum concentrations and toxicity; carbamazepine may induce the metabolism of warfarin, cyclosporine, doxycycline, oral or subdermal contraceptives (consider alternative or back-up methods of contraception), phenytoin, theophylline, ritonavir, saquinavir, delavirdine, benzodiazepines, ethosuximide, valproic acid, lamotrigine, tiagabine, topiramate, midazolam, corticosteroids, teniposide, etoposide, doxorubicin, vincristine, methotrexate, and thyroid hormones; use with lithium may increase neurotoxic side effects; ritonavir and cefixime may affect the metabolism of carbamazepine; administration of Tegretol® suspension in combination with liquid chlorpromazine or thioridazine results in an orange rubbery precipitate

Food Interactions Extended release capsules (Carbatrol®): A high fat meal may increase the rate of absorption, reduce time to peak concentration (from 24 hours to 14 hours), and increase peak concentrations, but does not effect extent of absorption (AUC)

Grapefruit juice increases the oral bioavailability of carbamazepine by an average of 40%

Stability Store tablets in dry place, protect from moisture

Mechanism of Action May depress activity in the nucleus ventralis of the thalamus or decrease synaptic transmission or decrease summation of temporal stimulation leading to neural discharge, by limiting influx of sodium ions across cell membrane; other unknown mechanisms; stimulates the release of ADH and potentiates its action in promoting reabsorption of water; chemically related to tricyclic antidepressants; in addition to anticonvulsant effects, carbamazepine has anticholinergic, antineuralgic, antidiuretic, muscle relaxant and antiarrhythmic properties

Pharmacokinetics

Absorption: Slowly from the GI tract

Distribution: V_d:

Neonates: 1.5 L/kg

Children: 1.9 L/kg

Adults: 0.59-2 L/kg

Protein binding: 75% to 90%, bound to alpha$_1$-acid glycoprotein and nonspecific binding sites on albumin; protein binding may be decreased in newborns

Metabolism: Induces liver enzymes to increase metabolism and shorten half-life over time; metabolized in the liver by cytochrome P450 3A4 to active epoxide metabolite; ratio of serum epoxide to carbamazepine concentrations may be higher in patients receiving polytherapy (vs monotherapy) and in infants (vs older children); boys may have faster carbamazepine clearances and may, therefore, require higher mg/kg/day doses of carbamazepine compared to girls of similar age and weight

Bioavailability, oral: 75% to 85%; relative bioavailability of extended release tablet to suspension: 89%

Half-life:

Initial: 25-65 hours

Multiple dosing:

Children: 8-14 hours

Adults: 12-17 hours

Time to peak serum concentration: Unpredictable, within 4-8 hours

Chronic administration:

Suspension: 1.5 hours

Tablet: 4-5 hours

Extended release tablet: 3-12 hours

Elimination: 1% to 3% excreted unchanged in urine

Usual Dosage Dosage must be adjusted according to patient's response and serum concentrations. Administer tablets (chewable or conventional) in 2-3 divided doses daily and suspension in 4 divided doses daily. (See Additional Information for investigational oral loading dose and rectal maintenance dose information.) Oral: Epilepsy:

Children:

<6 years: Initial: 10-20 mg/kg/day divided twice or 3 times daily as tablets or 4 times/day as suspension; increase dose every week until optimal response and therapeutic levels are achieved; maintenance dose: Divide into 3-4 doses daily (tablets or suspension); maximum recommended dose: 35 mg/kg/day

6-12 years: Initial: 100 mg twice daily (tablets or extended release tablets) or 50 mg of suspension 4 times/day (200 mg/day); increase by up to 100 mg/day at weekly intervals using a twice daily regimen of extended release tablets or 3-4 times daily regimen of other formulations until optimal response and therapeutic levels are achieved; usual maintenance: 400-800 mg/day; maximum recommended dose: 1000 mg/day

Note: Children <12 years who receive ≥400 mg/day of carbamazepine may be converted to extended release capsules (Carbatrol®) using the same total daily dosage divided twice daily

Children >12 years and Adults: Initial: 200 mg twice daily (tablets, extended release tablets, or extended release capsules) or 100 mg of suspension 4 times/day (400 mg daily); increase by up to 200 mg/day at weekly intervals using a twice daily regimen of extended release tablets or capsules, or a 3-4 times/day regimen of other formulations until optimal response and therapeutic levels are achieved; usual dose: 800-1200 mg/day

Maximum recommended doses:

Children 12-15 years: 1000 mg/day

Children >15 years: 1200 mg/day

Adults: 1600 mg/day; however, some patients have required up to 1.6-2.4 g/day

Dosing adjustment in renal impairment: Cl_{cr} <10 mL/minute: Administer 75% of recommended dose; monitor serum levels

Administration

Oral: Administer with food to decrease GI upset; avoid administration with grapefruit juice; extended release capsules (Carbatrol®) may be taken without regard to meals; suspension dosage should be administered on a 3-4 times/day schedule vs tablet (conventional or chewable) which can be administered 2-4 times/day; extended release (XR) tablets should be dosed twice daily; do not crush or chew XR tablets; examine XR tablets for cracks or chips; do not use damaged XR tablets or XR tablets without a release portal; chewable tablet should be chewed well and swallowed. Swallow extended release capsules whole or open and sprinkle contents on small amount of soft food (eg, 1 teaspoonful of applesauce); swallow sprinkle/food mixture immediately; do not chew; do not store for later use; drink fluids after dose to make sure mixture is completely swallowed

Suspension: Tegretol® should not be administered with diluents or other liquid medicines due to the possibility of a component interaction (see Drug Interactions); shake suspension well before use

Monitoring Parameters CBC with platelet count, liver function tests, serum drug concentration; observe patient for excessive sedation especially when instituting or increasing therapy

Reference Range Therapeutic: 4-12 µg/mL (SI: 17-51 µmol/L). Patients who require higher levels [8-12 µg/mL (SI: 34-51 µmol/L)] should be carefully monitored. Side effects (especially CNS) occur commonly at higher levels. If other anticonvulsants (enzyme inducers) are given, therapeutic range is 4-8 µg/mL (SI: 17-34 µmol/L) due to increase in unmeasured active epoxide metabolite.

Test Interactions Carbamazepine may interfere with a serum immunoassay for tricyclic antidepressants; false-positive qualitative serum tricyclic antidepressant drug screen results have been reported in patients with carbamazepine intoxication (see Matos, 2000)

Patient Information Avoid alcohol and grapefruit juice. May cause drowsiness and impair ability to perform activities requiring mental alertness or physical coordination. Report fever, sore throat, infection, mouth ulcers, easy bruising, bleeding, loss of appetite, nausea, vomiting, or yellow skin or eyes to physician. The tablet coating of Tegretol®-XR tablet is not absorbed and may appear in the stool. May cause photosensitivity reactions (eg, exposure to sunlight may cause severe sunburn, skin rash, redness, or itching); avoid exposure to sunlight and artificial light sources (sunlamps, tanning booth/bed); wear protective clothing, wide-brimmed hats, sunglasses, and lip sunscreen (SPF ≥15); use a sunscreen [broad-spectrum sunscreen or physical sunscreen (preferred) or sunblock with SPF ≥15]; contact physician if reaction occurs. (Continued)

Carbamazepine *(Continued)*

Additional Information Carbamazepine is not effective in absence, myoclonic, akinetic, or febrile seizures; exacerbation of certain seizure types have been seen after initiation of carbamazepine therapy in children with mixed seizure disorders

Investigationally, loading doses of the suspension (10 mg/kg for children <12 years of age and 8 mg/kg for children >12 years) were given (via NG or ND tubes followed by 5-10 mL of water to flush through tube) to PICU patients with frequent seizures/status; 5 of 6 patients attained mean plasma concentrations of 4.3 mcg/mL and 7.3 mcg/mL at 1 and 2 hours postload; concurrent enteral feeding or ileus may delay absorption of loading dose (Miles, 1990)

Carbamazepine suspension may be administered rectally as maintenance doses, if oral therapy is not possible (**Note:** Rectally administered carbamazepine is not useful in status epilepticus due to its slow absorption); when using carbamazepine suspension rectally, administer the same total daily dose, but give in small, diluted, multiple doses; dilute the oral suspension with an equal volume of water; if defecation occurs within the first 2 hours, repeat the dose (see Graves, 1987)

A recent study (Relling, 2000) demonstrated that enzyme-inducing antiepileptic drugs (AEDs) (carbamazepine, phenobarbital, and phenytoin) increased systemic clearance of antileukemic drugs (teniposide and methotrexate) and were associated with a worse event-free survival, CNS relapse, and hematologic relapse, (ie, lower efficacy), in B-lineage ALL children receiving chemotherapy; the authors recommend using nonenzyme-inducing AEDs in patients receiving chemotherapy for ALL.

Dosage Forms

Capsule, extended release (Carbatrol®): 200 mg, 300 mg

Suspension, oral (Tegretol®): 100 mg/5 mL (450 mL) [citrus-vanilla flavor]

Tablet (Epitol®, Tegretol®): 200 mg

Tablet, chewable (Tegretol®): 100 mg

Tablet, extended release (Tegretol® XR): 100 mg, 200 mg, 400 mg

References

Gilman JT, "Carbamazepine Dosing for Pediatric Seizure Disorders: The Highs and Lows," *DICP*, 1991, 25(10):1109-12.

Graves NM and Kriel RL, "Rectal Administration of Antiepileptic Drugs in Children," *Pediatr Neurol*, 1987, 3(6):321-6.

Korinthenberg R, Haug C, and Hannak D, "The Metabolization of Carbamazepine to CBZ-10,11 Epoxide in Children From the Newborn Age to Adolescence," *Neuropediatrics*, 1994, 25(4):214-6.

Matos ME, Burns MM, and Shannon MW, "False-Positive Tricyclic Antidepressant Drug Screen Results Leading to the Diagnosis of Carbamazepine Intoxication," *Pediatrics*, 2000, 105(5), http://www.pediatrics.org/cgi/content/full/105/5/e66.

Liu H and Delgado MR, "Influence of Sex, Age, Weight, and Carbamazepine Dose on Serum Concentrations, Concentration Ratios, and Level/Dose Ratios of Carbamazepine and Its Metabolites," *Ther Drug Monit*, 1994, 16(5):469-76.

Miles MV, Lawless ST, Tennison MB, et al, "Rapid Loading of Critically Ill Patients With Carbamazepine Suspension," *Pediatrics*, 1990, 86(2):263-6.

Relling MV, Pui CH, Sandlund JT, et al, "Adverse Effect of Anticonvulsants on Efficacy of Chemotherapy for Acute Lymphoblastic Leukaemia," *Lancet*, 2000, 356(9226):285-90.

Carbamide Peroxide *(KAR ba mide per OKS ide)*

U.S. Brand Names Cankaid® [OTC]; Debrox® [OTC]; E•R•O [OTC]; Gly-Oxide® [OTC]; Mollifene® [OTC]; Murine® Ear [OTC]; Orajel® Perioseptic Spot Treatment [OTC]

Synonyms Urea Peroxide

Therapeutic Category Otic Agent, Cerumenolytic

Generic Available Yes

Use

Oral: Relief of minor inflammation of gums, oral mucosal surfaces and lips including canker sores and dental irritation; adjunct in oral hygiene

Otic: Emulsify and disperse ear wax

Pregnancy Risk Factor C

Contraindications Hypersensitivity to carbamide peroxide or any component; otic preparation should not be used in patients with a perforated tympanic membrane or following otic surgery; ear drainage, ear pain, or rash in the ear; dizziness; oral preparation should not be used for self medication in children <3 years of age

Warnings With prolonged use of oral carbamide peroxide, there is a potential for overgrowth of opportunistic organisms, damage to periodontal tissues, delayed wound healing

Adverse Reactions

Central nervous system: Dizziness

Dermatologic: Rash

Local: Irritation, tenderness, pain, redness

Stability Protect from heat and direct light

Mechanism of Action Carbamide peroxide releases hydrogen peroxide which serves as a source of nascent oxygen upon contact with catalase; deodorant action is probably due to inhibition of odor-causing bacteria; softens impacted cerumen due to its foaming action

Pharmacodynamics Onset of action: Otic: Slight disintegration of hard ear wax in 24 hours

Usual Dosage

Oral: Children and Adults:

Gel: Massage on affected area 4 times/day for up to 7 days

Solution: Apply several drops undiluted to affected area of the mouth 4 times/day after meals and at bedtime for up to 7 days, expectorate after 2-3 minutes; as an adjunct to oral hygiene after brushing, swish 10 drops for 2-3 minutes, then expectorate

Otic: Solution:

Children <12 years: Individualize the dose according to patient size; 3 drops (range: 1-5 drops) twice daily for up to 4 days

Children ≥12 years and Adults: Instill 5-10 drops twice daily for up to 4 days

Administration

Oral: Apply undiluted solution with an applicator or cotton swab to the affected area after meals and at bedtime; or place drops on the tongue, mix with saliva, swish in the mouth for several minutes, then expectorate. Patient should not rinse mouth or drink fluids for 5 minutes after oral administration.

Otic: Instill drops into the external ear canal; keep drops in ear for several minutes by keeping head tilted or placing cotton in ear. Gently irrigate ear canal with warm water to remove loosened cerumen.

Patient Information Contact physician if dizziness or otic redness, rash, irritation, tenderness, pain, drainage or discharge develop; do not use in the eye

Nursing Implications Drops foam on contact with ear wax

Dosage Forms

Solution, oral: 10% (60 mL)

Cankaid®: 10% (22 mL) [in anhydrous glycerol]

Gly-Oxide®: 10% (15 mL, 60 mL) [in glycerin]

Orajel® Perioseptic Spot Treatment: 15% (13.3 mL) [in anhydrous glycerin]

Solution, otic: 6.5% (15 mL)

Debrox®: 6.5% (15 mL, 30 mL) [in propylene glycol]

E•R•O, Mollifene®, Murine® Ear: 6.5% (15 mL)

◆ **Carbatrol®** *see* Carbamazepine *on page 209*

Carbenicillin (kar ben i SIL in)

U.S. Brand Names Geocillin®

Synonyms Carindacillin

Therapeutic Category Antibiotic, Penicillin (Antipseudomonal)

Generic Available No

Use Treatment of urinary tract infections, asymptomatic bacteriuria, or prostatitis caused by susceptible strains of *Pseudomonas aeruginosa*, *E. coli*, indole-positive *Proteus*, and *Enterobacter*

Pregnancy Risk Factor B

Contraindications Hypersensitivity to carbenicillin, any component, or penicillins

Warnings Oral carbenicillin should be limited to treatment of urinary tract infections

Precautions Use with caution in patients with history of cephalosporin hypersensitivity; do not use in patients with severe renal impairment (Cl_{cr} <10 mL/minute) since drug concentration in urine is reduced and inadequate for treatment of UTIs

Adverse Reactions

Dermatologic: Rash, urticaria, pruritus

Gastrointestinal: Nausea, vomiting, diarrhea, abdominal cramps, furry tongue

Genitourinary: Vaginitis

Hematologic: Eosinophilia, hemolytic anemia, neutropenia, leukopenia, thrombocytopenia

Hepatic: Elevated liver enzymes, hepatotoxicity

Drug Interactions Probenecid, lithium

Mechanism of Action Interferes with bacterial cell wall synthesis during active multiplication

Pharmacokinetics

Absorption: Oral: 30% to 40%; in patients with normal renal function, serum concentrations of carbenicillin following oral absorption are inadequate for the treatment of systemic infections

Protein binding: 50%

(Continued)

Carbenicillin *(Continued)*

Half-life:
    Neonates:
        <7 days, ≤2.5 kg: 4 hours
        <7 days, >2.5 kg: 2.7 hours
    Children: 0.8-1.8 hours
    Adults: 1-1.5 hours; prolonged to 10-20 hours with renal insufficiency
Time to peak serum concentration: Within 30-120 minutes
Elimination: Carbenicillin and its metabolites are excreted in the urine; ~80% to 99% of the dose is excreted unchanged in the urine
Dialysis: Moderately dialyzable (20% to 50%)

Usual Dosage Oral:
Children: 30-50 mg/kg/day divided every 6 hours; maximum dose: 2-3 g/day
Adults:
    Urinary tract infections: 1-2 tablets every 6 hours
    Prostatitis: 2 tablets every 6 hours

Administration Oral: Administer with water

Monitoring Parameters Renal, hepatic, and hematologic function tests

Test Interactions False-positive urine or serum proteins; false-positive urine glucose (Clinitest®)

Patient Information Tablets have a bitter taste

Additional Information Sodium content of 382 mg tablet: 23 mg (1 mEq)

Dosage Forms Tablet, film coated, as indanyl sodium: 382 mg [base]

Carbinoxamine and Pseudoephedrine

(kar bi NOKS a meen & soo doe e FED rin)

U.S. Brand Names Andehist NR Drops; Palgic® D; Palgic® DS; Rondec® Drops; Rondec® Tablets; Rondec-TR® Tablets

Synonyms Pseudoephedrine and Carbinoxamine

Therapeutic Category Antihistamine/Decongestant Combination

Generic Available Yes

Use Temporary relief of nasal congestion, running nose, sneezing, itching of nose or throat, and itchy, watery eyes due to the common cold, hay fever, or other respiratory allergies

Pregnancy Risk Factor C

Contraindications Hypersensitivity to carbinoxamine, pseudoephedrine, or any component; severe hypertension or coronary artery disease, MAO inhibitor therapy, GI or GU obstruction, narrow-angle glaucoma

Precautions Use with caution in patients with mild to moderate hypertension, heart disease, diabetes, asthma, thyroid disease, or prostatic hypertrophy

Adverse Reactions
Cardiovascular: Hypertension, tachycardia, arrhythmias, edema, palpitations
Central nervous system: Sedation, CNS stimulation, headache, seizures, drowsiness, fatigue, nervousness, depression
Dermatologic: Angioedema, photosensitivity, rash
Gastrointestinal: Nausea, vomiting, xerostomia, anorexia, diarrhea, heart burn
Genitourinary: Dysuria
Hepatic: Hepatitis
Neuromuscular & skeletal: Weakness, myalgia, paresthesia
Ocular: Diplopia
Respiratory: Bronchospasm, epistaxis
Renal: Polyuria

Drug Interactions May produce severe hypertensive episodes when used with MAO inhibitors; may inhibit hypotensive effects of beta-adrenergic blocking agents; additive effects with other sympathomimetics, sedatives, alcohol, barbiturates, and other CNS depressants

Mechanism of Action Carbinoxamine competes with histamine for H_1-receptor sites on effector cells in the GI tract, blood vessels, and respiratory tract; pseudoephedrine directly stimulates alpha-adrenergic receptors of respiratory mucosa causing vasoconstriction; directly stimulates beta-adrenergic receptors causing bronchial relaxation, increased heart rate and contractility

Usual Dosage Oral:
Children: May dose according to pseudoephedrine component: 4 mg/kg/day **or** the carbinoxamine component: 0.2-0.4 mg/kg/day
Alternative dosing (manufacturer's recommendation):
    Drops:
        1-3 months: 1/4 dropperful (0.25 mL) 4 times/day
        3-6 months: 1/2 dropperful (0.5 mL) 4 times/day

6-9 months: ³/₄ dropperful (0.75 mL) 4 times/day
9-18 months: 1 dropperful (1 mL) 4 times/day
Syrup:
  1-3 months: 1.25 mL every 4 hours
  >3-6 months: 5 mL every 4 hours
  >6-9 months: 3.75 mL every 4 hours
  >9-18 months: 3.75-5 mL every 4 hours
  >18 months to 6 years: 5 mL every 4 hours
  ≥6 years and Adults: 10 mL every 4 hours
Tablet: Children >6 years and Adults: 1 tablet 4 times/day
Extended release tablet:
  Children ≥6-12 years: ¹/₂ tablet every 12 hours
  Children >12 years and Adults: 1 tablet every 12 hours

Administration Oral: Do not crush or chew extended release tablets

Patient Information May cause drowsiness or impair ability to perform activities requiring mental alertness or physical coordination; may cause blurred vision; may also cause CNS excitation and difficulty sleeping; may cause dry mouth; avoid alcohol. May rarely cause photosensitivity reactions (eg, exposure to sunlight may cause severe sunburn, skin rash, redness, or itching); avoid direct exposure to sunlight

Dosage Forms
Solution, oral **drops**:
  Andehist NR: Carbinoxamine maleate 1 mg and pseudoephedrine hydrochloride 15 mg per mL (30 mL) [alcohol and sugar free; raspberry flavor]
  Rondec® Drops: Carbinoxamine maleate 1 mg and pseudoephedrine hydrochloride 15 mg per mL (30 mL) [alcohol free; cherry flavor]
Syrup (Palgic® DS): Carbinoxamine maleate 2 mg and pseudoephedrine hydrochloride 15 mg per 5 mL (480 mL) [alcohol and sugar free; strawberry-pineapple flavor]
Tablet, film-coated (Rondec® Tablets): Carbinoxamine maleate 4 mg and pseudoephedrine hydrochloride 60 mg
Tablet, sustained release:
  Palgic® D: Carbinoxamine maleate 8 mg and pseudoephedrine hydrochloride 90 mg
  Rondec-TR® Tablets: Carbinoxamine maleate 8 mg and pseudoephedrine hydrochloride 120 mg

♦ **Carbohydrate and Alcohol Content of Liquid Medications for Use in Patients Receiving Ketogenic Diets** *see page 1431*
♦ **Carbolith™ (Can)** *see Lithium on page 684*

Carboplatin (KAR boe pla tin)

Related Information
Emetogenic Potential of Single Chemotherapeutic Agents *on page 1286*

U.S. Brand Names Paraplatin®

Synonyms CBDCA

Therapeutic Category Antineoplastic Agent, Alkylating Agent

Generic Available No

Use Treatment of ovarian carcinoma; treatment of small cell lung cancer, squamous cell carcinoma of the esophagus; solid tumors of the bladder, cervix and testes; pediatric brain tumor, neuroblastoma, bony and soft tissue sarcomas, germ cell tumors, and high-dose therapy with stem cell/bone marrow transplants

Pregnancy Risk Factor D

Contraindications Hypersensitivity to carboplatin, cisplatin, any component, other platinum-containing compounds, or mannitol; severe bone marrow suppression or excessive bleeding

Warnings The FDA currently recommends that procedures for proper handling and disposal of antineoplastic agents be considered. When carboplatin is dosed using AUC as the endpoint, note that the calculated dose is the dose administered, not the dose based on body surface area

Precautions Bone marrow suppression, which may be severe, and vomiting are dose-related; high doses have also resulted in severe abnormalities of liver function; reduce dosage in patients with bone marrow suppression and impaired renal function (creatinine clearance values <60 mL/minute)

Adverse Reactions
Cardiovascular: Hypotension
Central nervous system: Pain
Dermatologic: Urticaria, rash, alopecia, pruritus, erythema
Endocrine & metabolic: Electrolyte abnormalities such as hypocalcemia, hypokalemia, hypomagnesemia
(Continued)

Carboplatin *(Continued)*

Gastrointestinal: Nausea, vomiting, diarrhea, anorexia, hemorrhagic colitis, mucositis, constipation, metallic taste

Hematologic: Neutropenia, leukopenia, thrombocytopenia (platelet count reaches a nadir between 14-21 days), anemia

Hepatic: Abnormal liver function tests

Neuromuscular & skeletal: Peripheral neuropathy, weakness

Otic: Tinnitus, hearing loss at high tones

Renal: Nephrotoxicity, elevated BUN and serum creatinine, hematuria

Respiratory: Bronchospasm, interstitial pneumonia

Miscellaneous: Anaphylactic-like reactions

Drug Interactions Aminoglycosides (increased ototoxicity and nephrotoxicity); nephrotoxic drugs (increased renal toxicity); decreases phenytoin serum levels

Stability Store unopened vials at room temperature; protect from light; after reconstitution, solutions are stable for 8 hours; 2 mg/mL solutions diluted in D_5W for infusion are stable for 24 hours; 7 mg/mL solutions diluted in NS for infusion are stable for 24 hours; aluminum reacts with carboplatin resulting in a precipitate and loss of potency

Mechanism of Action Platination of DNA results in possible cross-linking and interference with the function of DNA

Pharmacokinetics

Distribution: V_d: 16 L/kg

Protein binding: 0%; however, platinum is 30% protein bound

Half-life: Patients with Cl_{cr} >60 mL/minute: 2.5-5.9 hours

Elimination: ~60% to 80% is excreted renally

Usual Dosage I.V. (refer to individual protocols):

Infants and Children <3 years or ≤12 kg: Various protocols calculate dosage on the basis of body weight rather than body surface area

Children:

Solid tumor: 560 mg/m² once every 4 weeks

Sarcoma (bony/soft tissue): 400 mg/m²/day for 2 days

Brain tumor: 175 mg/m² once weekly for 4 weeks with a 2-week recovery period between courses; dose is then adjusted on platelet count and neutrophil count values; courses should not be repeated until the platelet count is ≥100,000/mm³ and the neutrophil count is ≥2000/mm³

Bone marrow transplant preparative regimen: 500 mg/m²/day for 3 days

Retinoblastoma: Subconjunctival injection of carboplatin for intraocular retinoblastoma has been administered using 1-2 mL of a 10 mg/mL solution per dose to affected eye(s)

Alternative carboplatin dosing: Some investigators calculate pediatric carboplatin doses using a modified Calvert formula: Dosing based on target AUC (modified Calvert formula for use in children): Total dose (mg) = [Target AUC (mg/mL/minute)] x [GFR (mL/minute) + (0.36 x body weight in kilograms)]

Note: Calvert formula was based on using chromic edetate (^{51}Cr-EDTA) plasma clearance to establish GFR. Some clinicians have recommended that methods for estimating Cl_{cr} not be substituted for GFR since carboplatin dosing based on such estimates may not be predictive.

Note: The dose of carboplatin calculated is TOTAL mg DOSE not mg/m²

Adults:

Single agent: 360 mg/m² once every 4 weeks; dose is then adjusted on platelet count and neutrophil count values; courses should not be repeated until the platelet count is ≥100,000/mm³ and the neutrophil count is ≥2000/mm³

Calvert formula: See table

Calvert Formula for Carboplatin Dosing in Adults
Total dose (mg) = Target AUC (mg/mL/minute) x (GFR [mL/minute] + 25)

Single Agent Carboplatin/No Prior Chemotherapy	Total dose (mg): 6-8 (GFR + 25)
Single Agent Carboplatin/Prior Chemotherapy	Total dose (mg): 4-6 (GFR + 25)
Combination Chemotherapy/No Prior Chemotherapy	Total dose (mg): 4.5-6 (GFR + 25)
Combination Chemotherapy/Prior Chemotherapy	Use a target AUC value <5 for the initial cycle

Dosing adjustment in renal impairment: Adults: Calvert formula (dosing adjustment for renal impairment is implied with this formula):

Total dose (mg) = [Target AUC (mg/mL/minute)] x [GFR (mL/minute) + 25]

Note: The dose of carboplatin calculated is TOTAL mg DOSE not mg/m²; target AUC will vary depending upon: Number of agents in the regimen and treatment status (ie, previously untreated or treated)

Administration Parenteral: Administer by I.V. intermittent infusion over 15 minutes to 1 hour, or by continuous infusion (continuous infusion regimens may be less toxic than the bolus route); reconstituted carboplatin 10 mg/mL should be further diluted to a final concentration of 0.5-2 mg/mL with D₅W or NS for administration

Monitoring Parameters CBC with differential and platelet count, serum electrolytes, urinalysis, creatinine clearance, liver function tests

Nursing Implications Needle or intravenous administration sets containing aluminum parts should not be used in the administration or preparation of carboplatin (aluminum can interact with carboplatin resulting in precipitate formation and loss of potency)

Dosage Forms Injection, powder for reconstitution, lyophilized: 50 mg, 150 mg, 450 mg

References
Abramson DH, Frank CM, and Dunkel IJ, "A Phase I/II Study of Subconjunctival Carboplatin for Intraocular Retinoblastoma," *Ophthalmology*, 1999, 106(10):1947-50.

Cairo MS, "The Use of Ifosfamide, Carboplatin, and Etoposide in Children With Solid Tumors," *Semin Oncol*, 1995, 22(3 Suppl 7):23-7.

Lovett D, Kelsen D, Eisenberger M, et al, "A Phase II Trial of Carboplatin and Vinblastine in the Treatment of Advanced Squamous Cell Carcinoma of the Esophagus," *Cancer*, 1991, 67(2):354-6.

Newell DR, Pearson AD, Balmanno K, et al, "Carboplatin Pharmacokinetics in Children: The Development of a Pediatric Dosing Formula. The United Kingdom Children's Cancer Study Group," *J Clin Oncol*, 1993, 11(12):2314-23.

Zeltzer PM, Epport K, Nelson MD Jr, et al, "Prolonged Response to Carboplatin in an Infant With Brain Stem Glioma," *Cancer*, 1991, 67(1):43-7.

♦ **Cardizem®** *see Diltiazem on page 388*

♦ **Cardizem® CD** *see Diltiazem on page 388*

♦ **Cardizem® LA** *see Diltiazem on page 388*

♦ **Cardizem® SR** *see Diltiazem on page 388*

♦ **Carimune™** *see Immune Globulin (Intravenous) on page 598*

♦ **Carindacillin** *see Carbenicillin on page 213*

♦ **Carmol® Scalp** *see Sulfacetamide on page 1048*

Carmustine (kar MUS teen)

Related Information
Emetogenic Potential of Single Chemotherapeutic Agents *on page 1286*

U.S. Brand Names BiCNU®, Gliadel®

Synonyms BCNU

Therapeutic Category Antineoplastic Agent, Alkylating Agent (Nitrosourea)

Generic Available No

Use

Injection: Treatment of brain tumors, multiple myeloma, Hodgkin's disease, and non-Hodgkin's lymphomas; some activity in malignant melanoma, lung and colon cancer

Wafer (implant): Adjunct to surgery in patients with high grade malignant glioma or in patients with recurrent glioblastoma multiforme

Pregnancy Risk Factor D

Contraindications Hypersensitivity to carmustine or any component

Warnings The FDA currently recommends that procedures for proper handling and disposal of antineoplastic agents be considered. Bone marrow suppression, notably thrombocytopenia and leukopenia, may lead to bleeding and overwhelming infection in an already compromised patient; myelosuppressive effects will last for at least 6 weeks after a dose, do not give courses more frequently than every 6 weeks because the toxicity is cumulative; pulmonary toxicity is more common in patients receiving a cumulative dose >1400 mg/m², patients with recent mediastinal irradiation, and in patients with a past history of lung disease; delayed-onset pulmonary fibrosis has occurred up to 17 years after carmustine treatment in children and adolescents; acute leukemia has been reported in patients receiving long-term carmustine.

Cases of intracerebral mass effect unresponsive to corticosteroids, including one case leading to brain herniation, have been reported. Monitor patients receiving Gliadel® implant for seizures, intracranial infections, abnormal wound healing, and brain edema. Carmustine injection diluent contains absolute alcohol which can cause an "alcohol flushing syndrome" in susceptible patients; use with caution in patients with aldehyde dehydrogenase-2 deficiency.

Precautions Administer with caution to patients with depressed platelet, leukocyte or erythrocyte counts and in patients with renal or hepatic impairment; dosage reduction (Continued)

Carmustine *(Continued)*

is recommended in patients with compromised bone marrow function (decreased leukocyte and platelet counts)

Adverse Reactions

Cardiovascular: Flushing; high dose (≥300 mg/m^2) can produce hypotension, tachycardia, confusion, chest pain

Central nervous system: Ataxia, dizziness, seizures, fever, headache

Dermatologic: Dermatitis, hyperpigmentation, alopecia, rash

Gastrointestinal: Nausea, vomiting, diarrhea, esophagitis, anorexia, mucositis, metallic taste

Hematologic: Myelosuppression (leukopenia, thrombocytopenia) with nadir at 28 days, anemia

Hepatic: Hepatotoxicity, elevated liver enzymes and serum bilirubin, jaundice, veno-occlusive disease with high doses

Local: Pain and thrombophlebitis at injection site, burning sensation

Ocular: Retinitis, optic neuritis

Renal: Renal failure, azotemia

Respiratory: Pulmonary fibrosis, cough, dyspnea, tachypnea

Drug Interactions Cimetidine (potentiates myelosuppressive effects); may potentiate hepatotoxicity with high doses of acetaminophen; may decrease serum digoxin and phenytoin levels; metronidazole (disulfiram reaction)

Stability Store vial in refrigerator; protect from light and heat; discard vial if oily film is found on the bottom of the vial; reconstituted solution is stable for 8 hours at room temperature, 24 hours when refrigerated, or 48 hours when refrigerated after further dilution in D$_5$W or NS in a glass bottle to a concentration of 0.2 mg/mL; incompatible with sodium bicarbonate; adsorption of carmustine to plastics and polyvinyl chloride-based infusion containers has been documented. Store Gliadel® wafers at or below -20°C (-4°F).

Mechanism of Action Inhibits key enzymatic reactions involved with DNA synthesis; carbamoylation of amine groups on proteins; interferes with the normal function of DNA by alkylation and forms DNA-protein cross-links

Pharmacokinetics

Distribution: Readily crosses the blood-brain barrier since it is highly lipid soluble; CSF:plasma ratio >90%; distributes into breast milk

Protein binding: 75%

Metabolism: Denitrosation through action of microsomal enzymes; some enterohepatic circulation occurs

Half-life, terminal: 20-70 minutes (active metabolites may persist for days)

Elimination: ~60% to 70% excreted as metabolites in the urine and 6% to 10% excreted as CO$_2$ by the lungs

Usual Dosage

I.V. infusion (refer to individual protocols):

Children: 200-250 mg/m^2 every 4-6 weeks as a single dose; next dose is to be determined based on clinical and hematologic response to the previous dose (a repeat course should not be given until platelets are >100,000/mm^3 and leukocytes are >4000/mm^3)

BMT-conditioning agent: 300-600 mg/m^2 over at least 2 hours or may be divided into 2 doses administered 12 hours apart or 100 mg/m^2 every 12 hours for 6 doses

Adults: 150-200 mg/m^2 every 6 weeks as a single dose or divided into 75-100 mg/m^2/dose on 2 successive days; next dose is to be determined based on clinical and hematologic response to the previous dose (a repeat course should not be given until platelets are >100,000/mm^3 and leukocytes are >4000/mm^3)

Intracranial implant (wafer): Adults: Place 8 wafers (total dose: 61.6 mg) in the resection cavity; should the size and shape not accommodate 8 wafers, the maximum number of wafers as allowed should be placed

Administration Parenteral: Reconstitute 100 mg vial with 3 mL sterile dehydrated (absolute) alcohol followed by addition of 27 mL SWI. Further dilute the 3.3 mg of carmustine per mL solution with NS or D$_5$W in a glass or polyolefin container to a final concentration of 0.2-1 mg/mL and administer by I.V. infusion over 1-2 hours to prevent vein irritation; rapid I.V. carmustine infusion may result in flushing, hypotension, and agitation; carmustine has also been administered over 15-45 minutes diluted in 100-250 mL D$_5$W with monitoring for vein irritation; burning sensation and pain at I.V. site can be decreased with reduction of infusion rate and further dilution of solution or placing ice pack on I.V. site; flush line before and after carmustine administration to ensure vein patency

Monitoring Parameters CBC with differential and platelet count; pulmonary function, liver function, and renal function tests; monitor blood pressure and infusion site during administration

Patient Information Report occurrence of fever, sore throat, unusual bleeding or bruising to physician; may discolor skin brown; women of childbearing potential should avoid becoming pregnant while on carmustine therapy

Nursing Implications Must administer in glass containers; do not mix or administer with solutions containing sodium bicarbonate; accidental skin contact may cause transient burning and brown discoloration of the skin

Additional Information Myelosuppressive effects:

WBC: Moderate (nadir: 5-6 weeks)

Platelets: Severe (nadir: 4-5 weeks)

Dosage Forms

Injection, powder for reconstitution (BiCNU®): 100 mg [packaged with 3 mL of absolute alcohol as diluent]

Wafer (Gliadel®): 7.7 mg (8s)

References

Aronin PA, Mahaley MS Jr, Rudnick SA, et al, "Prediction of BCNU Pulmonary Toxicity in Patients With Malignant Gliomas," *N Engl J Med*, 1980, 303(4):183-8.

Colvin M, Hartner J and Summerfield M, "Stability of Carmustine in the Presence of Sodium Bicarbonate," *Am J Hosp Pharm*, 1980, 37(5):677-8.

Dunkel IJ, Garvin JH Jr, Goldman S, et al, "High Dose Chemotherapy With Autologous Bone Marrow Rescue for Children With Diffuse Pontine Brain Stem Tumors. Children's Cancer Group," *J Neurooncol*, 1998, 37(1):67-73.

O'Driscoll BR, Hasleton PS, Taylor PM, et al, "Active Lung Fibrosis Up to 17 Years After Chemotherapy With Carmustine (BCNU) in Childhood," *N Engl J Med*, 1990, 323(6):378-82.

Carnitine (KAR ni teen)

Related Information

Carbohydrate and Alcohol Content of Liquid Medications for Use in Patients Receiving Ketogenic Diets *on page 1431*

U.S. Brand Names Carnitor®

Synonyms L-carnitine; Levocarnitine

Therapeutic Category Nutritional Supplement

Generic Available Yes

Use Treatment of primary or secondary carnitine deficiency; prevention and treatment of carnitine deficiency (injection) in patients undergoing dialysis for end stage renal disease (ESRD)

Pregnancy Risk Factor B

Contraindications Hypersensitivity to carnitine or any component

Precautions Use with caution in patients with seizure disorders; both new onset seizure activity and increased frequency of seizures have been reported; chronic administration of high doses of oral carnitine in patients with severely compromised renal function or ESRD on dialysis may result in accumulation of potentially toxic metabolites, trimethylamine and trimethylamine-N-oxide; monitor use in these patients closely

Adverse Reactions

Central nervous system: Myasthenia (in uremic patients on D,L-carnitine not L-carnitine), dizziness, fever, depression, seizures

Gastrointestinal: Nausea, vomiting, abdominal cramps, diarrhea, gastritis

Neuromuscular & skeletal: Weakness, paresthesia, myasthenia (mild)

Miscellaneous: Body odor (dose-related), allergic reactions

Drug Interactions Valproic acid, sodium benzoate; D,L-carnitine sold in health food stores as vitamin B_T, competitively inhibits L-carnitine

Stability Protect from light

Mechanism of Action Endogenous substance required in energy metabolism; facilitates long chain fatty acid entry into the mitochondria; modulates intracellular coenzyme A homeostasis; carnitine deficiency exists when there is insufficient carnitine to buffer toxic acyl-Co A compounds; secondary carnitine deficiency may be a consequence of inborn errors of metabolism

Pharmacokinetics

Metabolism: Major metabolites: Trimethylamine, trimethylamine-N-oxide and acylcarnitine

Half-life, terminal: Adults: 17.4 hours

Bioavailability:

Tablet: 15.1% ± 5.3%

Solution: 15.9% ± 4.9%

Time to peak serum concentration: Oral: 3.3 hours

Elimination: Renal excretion of free and conjugated metabolites (acylcarnitine)

Clearance: 4 L/hour

(Continued)

Carnitine *(Continued)*

Usual Dosage

Primary carnitine deficiency:

Oral:

Children: 50-100 mg/kg/day divided 2-3 times/day, maximum 3 g/day; dosage must be individualized based upon patient response; higher dosages have been used

Adults: 330-990 mg/dose 2-3 times/day; maximum: 3 g/day

I.V.: Children and Adults: 50 mg/kg as a loading dose, followed (in severe cases) by 50 mg/kg/day infusion; maintenance: 50 mg/kg/day divided every 4-6 hours, increase as needed to a maximum of 300 mg/kg/day

ESRD patients on hemodialysis: Adults: I.V.: Predialysis carnitine levels below normal (30-60 µmol): 10-20 mg/kg after each dialysis session; maintenance doses as low as 5 mg/kg may be used after 3-4 weeks of therapy depending upon response (carnitine level)

Supplement to parenteral nutrition: I.V.: Neonates: 10-20 mg/kg/day in parenteral nutrition solution

Administration

Oral: Dilute in beverages or liquid food; administer with meals; consume slowly

Parenteral: May be administered by direct I.V. infusion over 2-3 minutes or as a continuous infusion diluted to 0.5-8 mg/mL in LR or NS

Monitoring Parameters Serum triglycerides, fatty acids, and carnitine levels

Reference Range Plasma free carnitine level: >20 µmol/L; plasma total carnitine level 30-60 µmol/L; to evaluate for carnitine deficiency determine the plasma acylcarnitine/free carnitine ratio (A/F ratio)

A/F ratio = [plasma total carnitine - free carnitine] divided by free carnitine

Normal plasma A/F ratio = 0.25; in carnitine deficiency A/F ratio >0.4

Additional Information Routine prophylactic use of carnitine in children receiving valproic acid to avoid carnitine deficiency and hepatotoxicity is probably not indicated

Dosage Forms

Capsule: 250 mg

Injection, solution (Carnitor®): 200 mg/mL (5 mL)

Liquid (Carnitor®): 100 mg/mL (120 mL) [cherry flavor]

Tablet: 500 mg

Carnitor®: 330 mg

References

Bonner CM, De Brie KL, Hug G, et al, "Effects of Parenteral L-Carnitine Supplementation on Fat Metabolism and Nutrition in Premature Neonates," *J Pediatr*, 1995, 126(2):287-92.

Borum PR, "Carnitine in Neonatal Nutrition," *J Child Neurol*, 1995, 10(Suppl 2):S25-31.

Helms RA, Mauer EC, and Hay WW Jr, "Effect of Intravenous L-Carnitine on Growth Parameters and Fat Metabolism During Parenteral Nutrition in Neonates," *JPEN J Parenter Enteral Nutr*, 1990, 14(5):448-53.

♦ **Carnitor®** *see* Carnitine *on page 219*

♦ **Carrington Antifungal [OTC]** *see* Miconazole *on page 759*

♦ **Cartia XT™** *see* Diltiazem *on page 388*

♦ **Casanthranol and Docusate** *see* Docusate and Casanthranol *on page 402*

Cascara Sagrada *(kas KAR a sah GRAH dah)*

Therapeutic Category Laxative, Stimulant

Generic Available Yes

Use Temporary relief of constipation; sometimes used with milk of magnesia ("black and white" mixture)

Pregnancy Risk Factor C

Contraindications Nausea, vomiting, abdominal pain, fecal impaction, intestinal obstruction, GI bleeding, appendicitis, CHF

Warnings Long-term use may result in laxative dependence

Adverse Reactions

Cardiovascular: Faintness

Endocrine & metabolic: Electrolyte and fluid imbalance

Gastrointestinal: Abdominal cramps, nausea, diarrhea, benign pigmentation of the colonic mucosa (with prolonged use)

Genitourinary: Discoloration of urine (reddish, pink, or brown)

Stability Protect from light and heat

Mechanism of Action Direct chemical irritation of the intestinal mucosa resulting in an increased rate of colonic motility and change in fluid and electrolyte secretion

Pharmacodynamics Onset of action: 6-10 hours

Pharmacokinetics

Absorption: Oral: Small amount from small intestine

Metabolism: In the liver

Usual Dosage Oral (**aromatic** fluid extract):
Infants: 1.25 mL/day as a single dose (range: 0.5-2 mL) as needed
Children 2-11 years: 2.5 mL/day as a single dose (range: 1-3 mL) as needed
Children ≥12 years and Adults: 5 mL/day (range: 2-6 mL) as needed at bedtime

Administration Oral: Administer on an empty stomach at bedtime; drink plenty of fluids

Patient Information Should not be used regularly for more than 1 week; may discolor urine reddish, pink, or brown

Additional Information Cascara sagrada fluid extract is 5 times more potent than cascara sagrada aromatic fluid extract

Dosage Forms Solution, aromatic fluid-extract: 5 mL, 120 mL, 473 mL [licorice flavor]

Caspofungin (kas poe FUN jin)

U.S. Brand Names Cancidas®

Therapeutic Category Antifungal Agent, Echinocandin; Antifungal Agent, Systemic

Generic Available No

Use Treatment of invasive aspergillosis in patients who are refractory to or intolerant of other therapies (ie, amphotericin B, lipid formulations of amphotericin B, and/or itraconazole); candidemia, intra-abdominal abscess, peritonitis, and pleural space infection caused by susceptible *Candida* species; esophageal candidiasis

Pregnancy Risk Factor C

Contraindications Hypersensitivity to caspofungin or any component

Warnings Transient elevations of alanine transaminase (ALT) and aspartate transaminase (AST) have been reported with concomitant use of caspofungin and cyclosporine (avoid concurrent use of cyclosporine).

Precautions Use with caution and modify dose in patients with moderate hepatic impairment; use with caution and modify dose in patients on concurrent drugs which induce drug clearance such as efavirenz, nevirapine, phenytoin, dexamethasone, carbamazepine, or rifampin (see Drug Interactions)

Adverse Reactions
Cardiovascular: Facial swelling, peripheral edema
Central nervous system: Chills, fever, headache, insomnia
Dermatologic: Rash, pruritus, erythema
Endocrine & metabolic: Hypokalemia, hypercalcemia
Gastrointestinal: Diarrhea, vomiting, nausea, abdominal pain
Hematologic: Eosinophilia, anemia, decreased hemoglobin, neutropenia
Hepatic: Elevated alkaline phosphatase, ALT, AST, serum bilirubin; hepatic impairment
Local: Phlebitis, thrombophlebitis
Neuromuscular & skeletal: Tremor, paresthesia, myalgia
Renal: Elevated creatinine, proteinuria, hematuria
Respiratory: Bronchospasm, dyspnea
Miscellaneous: Anaphylaxis, flu-like syndrome, ARDS

Drug Interactions Decreases blood concentration of tacrolimus (monitor tacrolimus blood concentrations); cyclosporine may increase caspofungin concentrations (see Warnings); rifampin may decrease caspofungin trough concentrations by 30% (adjust caspofungin daily dose; eg, in adults, increase caspofungin dose to 70 mg/day); efavirenz, nevirapine, phenytoin, dexamethasone, or carbamazepine may decrease caspofungin concentration (adjust caspofungin daily dose)

Stability Store lyophilized vial in refrigerator at 2°C to 8°C (36°F to 46°F); reconstitute 50 mg or 70 mg vial with the appropriate volume of NS (consult manufacturer's prescribing information for details); reconstituted solution may be stored in the refrigerator for 1 hour prior to preparation of the infusion solution; final infusion solution may be stored at room temperature (≤25°C or ≤77°F) for 24 hours or for 48 hours in the refrigerator; caspofungin is not stable in dextrose-containing solutions

Mechanism of Action Inhibits synthesis of beta (1,3)-D-glucan, an essential cell wall component of susceptible fungi

Pharmacokinetics
Protein binding: 97% to albumin
Metabolism: Via hydrolysis and N-acetylation in the liver; undergoes spontaneous chemical degradation to an open-ring peptide and hydrolysis to amino acids
Half-life: Adults: Beta (distribution): 9-11 hours; terminal: 40-50 hours; beta phase half-life is 32% to 43% lower in pediatric patients than in adult patients
Elimination: 35% of dose excreted in feces, 41% of dose excreted in urine; 1.4% of dose excreted unchanged in urine
Dialysis: Not dialyzable

Usual Dosage I.V.: Safety and efficacy in pediatric patients has not been established
Children 2-11 years: Loading dose: 70 mg/m²/day on day 1, maximum dose: 70 mg; followed by 50 mg/m²/day, maximum dose: 50 mg, once daily thereafter
(Continued)

Caspofungin *(Continued)*

Children >12 years, Adolescents and Adults: Loading dose: 70 mg on day 1, followed by 50 mg once daily thereafter; 70 mg daily dose has been administered and well tolerated in patients not clinically responding to the daily 50 mg dose; may need to adjust dose in patients receiving a concomitant enzyme inducer

Esophageal candidiasis: 50 mg once daily

Patients receiving concomitant enzyme inducer:

Patients receiving rifampin: 70 mg caspofungin once daily

Patients receiving carbamazepine, dexamethasone, phenytoin, nevirapine, or efavirenz: May require an increase in caspofungin dose to 70 mg once daily

Dosing adjustment in renal impairment: No adjustment needed

Dosing adjustment in hepatic impairment:

Mild hepatic impairment (Child-Pugh score 5 to 6): No dosage adjustment necessary

Moderate hepatic impairment (Child-Pugh score 7 to 9): Decrease daily dose by 30%

Administration Parenteral: I.V.: Administer by slow I.V. infusion over 1 hour at a maximum concentration of 0.47 mg/mL diluted in NS, LR, 0.45% sodium chloride, or 0.225% sodium chloride injection. Do not mix or coinfuse with other medications. **Do not use** diluents containing dextrose.

Monitoring Parameters Periodic liver function tests, serum potassium, CBC, hemoglobin

Nursing Implications Infuse slowly over 1 hour; possible histamine-related reactions have been reported (monitor during infusion)

Dosage Forms Injection, powder for reconstitution, as acetate: 50 mg, 70 mg

References

Walsh TJ, Adamson PC, Seibel NL, et al, "Pharmacokinetics (PK) of Caspofungin (CAS) in Pediatric Patients (#M-896)," 42nd Interscience Conference on Antimicrobial Agents and Chemotherapy, San Diego, CA, Sept 27-30, 2002.

Castor Oil *(KAS tor oyl)*

U.S. Brand Names Emulsoil® [OTC]; Neoloid® [OTC]; Purge® [OTC]

Synonyms Oleum Ricini

Therapeutic Category Laxative, Stimulant

Generic Available Yes

Use Preparation for rectal or bowel examination or surgery; rarely used to relieve constipation; also applied to skin as emollient and protectant

Pregnancy Risk Factor X

Contraindications Hypersensitivity to castor oil; nausea, vomiting, abdominal pain, fecal impaction, GI bleeding, appendicitis, CHF, menstruation, dehydration

Warnings Long-term use may result in laxative dependence

Adverse Reactions

Central nervous system: Dizziness

Endocrine & metabolic: Electrolyte disturbance, dehydration

Gastrointestinal: Abdominal cramps, nausea, diarrhea

Stability Protect from heat (emulsion should be protected from freezing)

Mechanism of Action Acts primarily in the small intestine; hydrolyzed to ricinoleic acid which reduces net absorption of fluid and electrolytes and stimulates peristalsis

Pharmacodynamics Onset of action: Oral: Within 2-6 hours

Usual Dosage Oral:

Castor oil:

Infants <2 years: 1-5 mL or 15 mL/m²/dose as a single dose

Children 2-11 years: 5-15 mL as a single dose

Children ≥12 years and Adults: 15-60 mL as a single dose

Emulsified castor oil:

Infants: 2.5-7.5 mL/dose

Children:

<2 years: 5-15 mL/dose

2-11 years: 7.5-30 mL/dose

Children ≥12 years and Adults: 30-60 mL/dose

Administration Oral: Do not administer at bedtime because of rapid onset of action; chill or administer with milk, juice or carbonated beverage to improve palatability; administer on an empty stomach; castor oil emulsions should be shaken well before use

Monitoring Parameters I & O, serum electrolytes, stool frequency

Dosage Forms

Emulsion, oral:

Emulsoil®: 95% (60 mL)

Neoloid®: 36.4% (118 mL) [mint flavor]

Liquid, oral: 100% (60 mL, 120 mL, 480 mL)
Purge®: 95% (30 mL, 60 mL) [lemon flavor]

Cefaclor (SEF a klor)

Related Information
Carbohydrate and Alcohol Content of Liquid Medications for Use in Patients Receiving Ketogenic Diets on page 1431
U.S. Brand Names Ceclor®; Ceclor® CD
Canadian Brand Names Apo®-Cefaclor; Novo-Cefaclor; Nu-Cefaclor; PMS-Cefaclor
Therapeutic Category Antibiotic, Cephalosporin (Second Generation)
Generic Available Yes
Use Infections caused by susceptible organisms including Staph aureus, S. pneumoniae, and H. influenzae; treatment of otitis media, sinusitis, and infections involving the respiratory tract, skin and skin structure, bone and joint; treatment of urinary tract infections caused by E. coli, Klebsiella, and Proteus mirabilis
Pregnancy Risk Factor B
Contraindications Hypersensitivity to cefaclor, any component, or cephalosporins
Warnings Prolonged use may result in superinfection; do not use in patients with immediate-type hypersensitivity reactions to penicillin
Precautions Use with caution in patients with impaired renal function, history of colitis, or history of penicillin hypersensitivity; modify dosage in patients with severe renal impairment
Adverse Reactions
Dermatologic: Rash, urticaria, pruritus
Gastrointestinal: Nausea, vomiting, diarrhea
Hematologic: Eosinophilia, neutropenia
Hepatic: Elevated liver enzymes, cholestatic jaundice
Miscellaneous: Serum sickness-like reaction (estimated incidence ranges from 0.024% to 0.2% per drug course); majority of reactions have occurred in children <5 years of age with symptoms of rash and arthralgia, often occurring during the second or third exposure
Drug Interactions Probenecid (increased cefaclor concentration); magnesium- or aluminum-containing antacids administered with cefaclor extended-release tablet (decreased cefaclor absorption)
Food Interactions
Capsules and suspension: Food or milk delays and decreases peak concentration
Extended release tablets: Food increases extent of absorption and peak concentrations
Stability Refrigerate suspension after reconstitution; discard after 14 days
Mechanism of Action Inhibits bacterial cell wall synthesis by binding to one or more of the penicillin-binding proteins and interfering with the final transpeptidation step of peptidoglycan synthesis resulting in cell wall death
Pharmacokinetics
Absorption: Oral: Well absorbed; acid stable
Distribution: Distributes into tissues and fluids including bone, pleural and synovial fluid; crosses the placenta; appears in breast milk
Protein binding: 25%
Half-life: 30-60 minutes (prolonged with renal impairment)
Time to peak serum concentration:
Capsule: 60 minutes
Suspension: 45 minutes
Tablet, extended release: 1.5-2.7 hours
(Continued)

Cefaclor *(Continued)*

Elimination: Most of dose (80%) excreted unchanged in urine

Dialysis: Moderately dialyzable (20% to 50%)

Usual Dosage Oral:

Children >1 month: 20-40 mg/kg/day divided every 8-12 hours; maximum dose: 2 g/day (twice daily option is for treatment of otitis media or pharyngitis)

Adults: 250-500 mg every 8 hours or daily dose can be given in 2 divided doses (twice daily option is for treatment of otitis media or pharyngitis)

Acute bronchitis: 500 mg extended release tablet every 12 hours for 7 days

Pharyngitis and/or tonsillitis: 375 mg extended release tablet every 12 hours for 10 days

Uncomplicated skin and skin structure infection: 375 mg extended release tablet every 12 hours for 7-10 days

Dosing adjustment in renal impairment: Cl_{cr} <10 mL//minute: Administer 50% of dose

Administration Oral:

Capsule, suspension: Administer 1 hour before or 2 hours after a meal; shake suspension well before use

Extended release tablet: Administer with food; do not crush, cut, or chew tablet

Monitoring Parameters With prolonged therapy, monitor CBC and stool frequency periodically

Test Interactions Positive Coombs' [direct], false-positive urine glucose (Clinitest®), false ↑ of serum or urine creatinine

Dosage Forms

Capsule (Ceclor®): 250 mg, 500 mg

Powder for oral suspension (Ceclor®): 125 mg/5 mL (75 mL, 150 mL); 187 mg/5 mL (100 mL); 250 mg/5 mL (75 mL, 150 mL); 375 mg/5 mL (50 mL, 100 mL) [strawberry flavor]

Tablet, extended release (Ceclor® CD): 375 mg, 500 mg

References

Boguniewicz M and Leung DYM, "Hypersensitivity Reactions to Antibiotics Commonly Used in Children," *Pediatr Infect Dis J*, 1995, 14(3):221-31.

Hyslop DL, "Cefaclor Safety Profile: A Ten Year Review," *Clin Ther*, 1988, 11(Suppl A):83-94.

Levine LR, "Quantitative Comparison of Adverse Reactions to Cefaclor vs Amoxicillin in a Surveillance Study," *Pediatr Infect Dis*, 1985, 4(4):358-61.

Cefadroxil *(sef a DROKS il mon o HYE drate)*

Related Information

Carbohydrate and Alcohol Content of Liquid Medications for Use in Patients Receiving Ketogenic Diets *on page 1431*

U.S. Brand Names Duricef®

Canadian Brand Names Apo®-Cefadroxil; Novo-Cefadroxil

Therapeutic Category Antibiotic, Cephalosporin (First Generation)

Generic Available Yes

Use Treatment of susceptible bacterial infections including group A beta-hemolytic streptococcal pharyngitis or tonsillitis; skin and soft tissue infections caused by streptococci or staphylococci; urinary tract infections caused by *Klebsiella*, *E. coli*, and *Proteus mirabilis*

Pregnancy Risk Factor B

Contraindications Hypersensitivity to cefadroxil, any component, or cephalosporins

Warnings Prolonged use may result in superinfection; do not use in patients with immediate-type hypersensitivity reaction to penicillin

Precautions Use with caution in patients who are hypersensitive to penicillin; modify dosage in patients with renal impairment

Adverse Reactions

Dermatologic: Rash

Gastrointestinal: Nausea, vomiting, diarrhea, pseudomembranous colitis

Genitourinary: Vaginitis

Hematologic: Transient neutropenia

Drug Interactions Probenecid may decrease renal tubular secretion and increase cefadroxil serum concentrations

Food Interactions Concomitant administration with food, infant formula, or cow's milk does **not** significantly affect absorption

Stability Refrigerate suspension after reconstitution; discard after 14 days

Mechanism of Action Interferes with bacterial cell wall synthesis during active replication, causing cell wall death and resultant bactericidal activity against susceptible bacteria

Pharmacokinetics

Absorption: Oral: Rapid; well absorbed from GI tract

Distribution: V_d: 0.31 L/kg; crosses the placenta; appears in breast milk
Protein binding: 20%
Half-life: 1-2 hours; 20-24 hours in renal failure
Time to peak serum concentration: Within 70-90 minutes
Elimination: >90% of dose excreted unchanged in urine within 24 hours

Usual Dosage Oral:

Infants and Children: 30 mg/kg/day divided twice daily up to a maximum of 2 g/day
Adolescents and Adults: 1-2 g/day in 1-2 divided doses; maximum dose for adults: 4 g/day

Dosing interval in renal impairment:

Cl_{cr} 10-25 mL/minute: Administer every 24 hours
Cl_{cr} <10 mL/minute: Administer every 36 hours

Administration Oral: May be administered without regard to food; administration with food may decrease nausea or vomiting; shake suspension well before use

Monitoring Parameters Stool frequency, resolution of infection

Test Interactions Positive Coombs' [direct], false-positive with urinary glucose tests using cupric sulfate (Clinitest®, Benedict's solution)

Patient Information Report persistent diarrhea; entire course of medication (eg, 10-14 days) should be taken to ensure eradication of organism

Dosage Forms

Capsule, as monohydrate: 500 mg
Powder for oral suspension, as monohydrate: 250 mg/5 mL (50 mL, 100 mL); 500 mg/5 mL (50 mL, 75 mL, 100 mL) [orange-pineapple flavor]
Tablet, as monohydrate: 1 g

♦ **Cefadyl® (Can)** see Cephapirin [DSC] on page 246

Cefazolin (sef A zoe lin)

Related Information

Endocarditis Prophylaxis on page 1321

U.S. Brand Names Ancef®; Kefzol® [DSC]

Therapeutic Category Antibiotic, Cephalosporin (First Generation)

Generic Available Yes

Use Treatment of respiratory tract, skin and skin structure, urinary tract, biliary tract, bone and joint infections and septicemia due to susceptible gram-positive cocci (except enterococcus); some gram-negative bacilli including *E. coli*, *Proteus*, and *Klebsiella* may be susceptible; perioperative prophylaxis; bacterial endocarditis prophylaxis for dental and upper respiratory procedures

Pregnancy Risk Factor B

Contraindications Hypersensitivity to cefazolin sodium, any component, or cephalosporins

Warnings Prolonged use may result in superinfection; do not use in patients with immediate-type hypersensitivity reactions to penicillin

Precautions Use with caution in patients with a history of colitis or in patients with a history of hypersensitivity to penicillins; modify dosage in patients with renal impairment

Adverse Reactions

Central nervous system: Fever, CNS irritation, seizures
Dermatologic: Rash, urticaria, pruritus
Gastrointestinal: Nausea, vomiting, diarrhea, pseudomembranous colitis
Hematologic: Leukopenia, thrombocytopenia, eosinophilia
Hepatic: Transient elevation of liver enzymes
Local: Thrombophlebitis
Miscellaneous: Anaphylaxis

Drug Interactions Probenecid may decrease renal tubular secretion and increase cefazolin serum concentrations; nephrotoxic agents

Stability Reconstituted solution is stable for 24 hours at room temperature or 96 hours when refrigerated; thawed solutions of the commercially available frozen cefazolin injections are stable for 48 hours at room temperature or 10 days when refrigerated

Mechanism of Action Inhibits bacterial cell wall synthesis by binding to one or more of the penicillin-binding proteins and interfering with the final transpeptidation step of peptidoglycan synthesis resulting in cell wall death

Pharmacokinetics

Distribution: Crosses the placenta; small amounts appear in breast milk; CSF penetration is poor; penetrates bone and synovial fluid well; distributes into bile
Protein binding: 74% to 86%
Metabolism: Hepatic is minimal
Half-life:
Neonates: 3-5 hours
(Continued)

Cefazolin *(Continued)*

Adults: 90-150 minutes (prolonged with renal impairment)
Time to peak serum concentration:
I.M.: Within 0.5-2 hours
I.V.: Within 5 minutes
Elimination: 80% to 100% excreted unchanged in urine
Dialysis: Moderately dialyzable (20% to 50%)

Usual Dosage I.M., I.V.:
Neonates:
Postnatal age ≤7 days: 40 mg/kg/day divided every 12 hours
Postnatal age >7 days:
≤2000 g: 40 mg/kg/day divided every 12 hours
>2000 g: 60 mg/kg/day divided every 8 hours
Infants and Children: 50-100 mg/kg/day divided every 8 hours; maximum dose: 6 g/day
Bacterial endocarditis prophylaxis for dental and upper respiratory procedures in penicillin allergic patients (see Precautions): 25 mg/kg 30 minutes before procedure; maximum dose: 1 g
Adults: 0.5-2 g every 6-8 hours; maximum dose: 12 g/day
Bacterial endocarditis prophylaxis for dental and upper respiratory procedures in penicillin allergic patients (see Precautions): 1 g 30 minutes before procedure
Perioperative prophylaxis: 1 g 30-60 minutes prior to surgery; 0.5-1 g every 8 hours for 24 hours postoperatively depending on the procedure
Dosing interval in renal impairment:
Cl_{cr} 10-30 mL/minute: Administer every 12 hours
Cl_{cr} <10 mL/minute: Administer every 24 hours

Administration Parenteral:
I.V.: Cefazolin may be administered IVP over 3-5 minutes at a maximum concentration of 100 mg/mL or I.V. intermittent infusion over 10-60 minutes at a final concentration for I.V. administration of 20 mg/mL. In fluid-restricted patients, a concentration of 138 mg/mL has been administered IVP.
I.M.: Deep I.M. injection into a large muscle mass. May dilute vial using SWI to a final concentration between 225-330 mg/mL (see package insert)

Monitoring Parameters Renal function periodically when used in combination with other nephrotoxic drugs, hepatic function tests, and CBC

Test Interactions False-positive urine glucose using Clinitest®, positive Coombs' [direct], false ↑ serum or urine creatinine

Additional Information Sodium content of 1 g: 2 mEq

Dosage Forms
Infusion, as sodium [premixed in D_5W, frozen]: 500 mg (50 mL); 1 g (50 mL)
Injection, powder for reconstitution, as sodium: 500 mg, 1 g, 10 g, 20 g
Ancef®, Kefzol® [DSC]: 1 g, 10 g

References
Dajani AS, Taubert KA, Wilson WW, et al, "Prevention of Bacterial Endocarditis. Recommendations by the American Heart Association," *JAMA*, 1997, 277(22):1794-801.
Pickering LK, O'Connor DM, Anderson D, et al, "Clinical and Pharmacologic Evaluation of Cefazolin in Children," *J Infect Dis* 1973, 128(Suppl):S407-1.
Robinson DC, Cookson TL, and Grisafe JA, "Concentration Guidelines for Parenteral Antibiotics in Fluid-Restricted Patients," *Drug Intell Clin Pharm*, 1987, 21(12):985-9.

Cefdinir *(SEF di ner)*

U.S. Brand Names Omnicef®
Therapeutic Category Antibiotic, Cephalosporin (Third Generation)
Generic Available No
Use Infections caused by susceptible organisms including *S. pneumoniae* (penicillin-susceptible strains only; inadequate activity against resistant pneumococcus), *H. influenzae* (including beta-lactamase-producing strains), *M. catarrhalis* (including beta-lactamase-producing strains), *S. aureus*, and *S. pyogenes*; treatment of infections involving the respiratory tract, skin and skin structure, and otitis media
Pregnancy Risk Factor B
Contraindications Hypersensitivity to cefdinir, any component, or cephalosporins
Warnings Pseudomembranous colitis has been reported with cefdinir; prolonged use may result in superinfection; serum sickness-like reactions have been reported with signs and symptoms occurring after a few days of therapy and resolving a few days after drug discontinuation.
Precautions Use with caution in patients with impaired renal function, history of colitis, or in penicillin-sensitive patients; modify dosage in patients with severe renal impairment

Adverse Reactions

Central nervous system: Headache, hyperactivity, insomnia, somnolence, seizures

Dermatologic: Rash, pruritus, diaper rash, Stevens-Johnson syndrome

Gastrointestinal: Diarrhea, nausea, vomiting, abdominal pain, pseudomembranous colitis, dyspepsia

Genitourinary: Vaginitis, microhematuria

Hematologic: Leukopenia, neutropenia, hemolytic anemia, eosinophilia, thrombocytopenia

Hepatic: Elevated AST, ALT, alkaline phosphatase; cholestatic jaundice, prolonged PT

Renal: Elevated BUN/serum creatinine

Miscellaneous: Serum sickness-like reactions, anaphylaxis

Drug Interactions Probenecid increases cefdinir serum levels; aluminum- or magnesium-containing antacids decrease cefdinir absorption by 40%; iron decreases cefdinir absorption by 80%

Food Interactions Total absorption is not affected by food.

Stability Store at room temperature; reconstituted suspension stable for 10 days at room temperature

Mechanism of Action Inhibits bacterial cell wall synthesis by binding to one or more of the penicillin-binding proteins resulting in disruption of cell wall synthesis and cell lysis

Pharmacokinetics

Absorption: High-fat meal decreases extent of absorption by 10%

Distribution: Penetrates into blister fluid, middle ear fluid, tonsils, sinus, and lung tissues

V_d:

Children 6 months to 12 years: 0.67 L/kg

Adults: 0.35 L/kg

Protein binding: 60% to 70%

Bioavailability:

Capsules: 16% to 21%

Suspension: 25%

Half-life, elimination: 1.7 (± 0.6) hours with normal renal function

Time to peak serum concentration: 2-4 hours

Elimination: 11.6% to 18.4% of a dose is excreted unchanged in urine

Dialysis: ~63% is removed by hemodialysis

Usual Dosage Oral:

Infants and Children (≥6 months to 12 years):

Otitis media or pharyngitis/tonsillitis: 14 mg/kg/day divided every 12 hours for 5-10 days or 14 mg/kg/day once daily for 10 days; maximum: 600 mg/day

Skin and skin structure infection: 14 mg/kg/day divided twice daily for 10 days; maximum: 600 mg/day

Acute maxillary sinusitis: 14 mg/kg/day divided every 12 hours for 10 days or 14 mg/kg/day once daily for 10 days; maximum: 600 mg/day

Children >12 years and Adults:

Acute exacerbations of chronic bronchitis or pharyngitis/tonsillitis: 600 mg once daily for 10 days or 300 mg every 12 hours for 5-10 days

Skin and skin structure infection or community-acquired pneumonia: 300 mg every 12 hours for 10 days

Acute maxillary sinusitis: 600 mg once daily for 10 days or 300 mg every 12 hours for 10 days

Dosing adjustment in renal impairment: Cl_{cr} <30 mL/minute:

Children ≥6 months to 12 years: 7 mg/kg/dose once daily

Adults: 300 mg once daily

Patients receiving hemodialysis: 300 mg or 7 mg/kg/dose starting at the conclusion of each hemodialysis session with subsequent doses every other day

Administration Oral: May administer with or without food; administer with food if stomach upset occurs; administer cefdinir at least 2 hours before or after antacids or iron supplements; shake suspension well before use

Monitoring Parameters Evaluate renal function before and during therapy; with prolonged therapy, monitor coagulation tests, CBC, and liver function test periodically

Test Interactions Positive Coombs' [direct]; may produce false-positive reaction to urine glucose with Clinitest®; may produce false-positive reaction for ketones in the urine with tests using nitroprusside

Patient Information Report persistent diarrhea to physician; may discolor stools red if taken with iron

Additional Information Oral suspension contains 2.86 g of sucrose per teaspoon.

Dosage Forms

Capsule: 300 mg

(Continued)

Cefdinir *(Continued)*

Powder for oral suspension: 125 mg/5 mL (60 mL, 100 mL) [strawberry flavor]

References
Klein JO and McCracken GH Jr, "Summary: Role of a New Oral Cephalosporin, Cefdinir, for Therapy of Infections of Infants and Children," *Pediatr Infect Dis J*, 2000, 19(12 Suppl):S181-3.

Cefepime *(SEF e pim)*

U.S. Brand Names Maxipime®

Therapeutic Category Antibiotic, Cephalosporin (Fourth Generation)

Generic Available No

Use Treatment of lower respiratory tract infections, cellulitis, other skin and soft tissue infections, and urinary tract infections; empiric monotherapy in febrile neutropenia; considered a fourth generation cephalosporin because it is active against aerobic gram-negative bacteria, including *Pseudomonas aeruginosa*, active against some gram-negative bacteria that are resistant to third-generation cephalosporins, and more active than third-generation cephalosporins against gram-positive bacteria such as *Staphylococcus aureus*

Pregnancy Risk Factor B

Contraindications Hypersensitivity to cefepime, any component, or cephalosporins

Warnings Modify dosage in patients with severe renal impairment; prolonged use may result in superinfection; use with caution in patients with penicillin hypersensitivity; do not use in patients with immediate-type hypersensitivity reactions to penicillin

Adverse Reactions

Central nervous system: Headache, lightheadedness, fever, encephalopathy

Dermatologic: Maculopapular rash, pruritus, urticaria

Gastrointestinal: Dyspepsia, diarrhea, nausea, vomiting, pseudomembranous colitis

Hematologic: Neutropenia after extended therapy, transient leukopenia and thrombocytopenia, agranulocytosis, eosinophilia, anemia

Hepatic: Transient elevations in LFTs

Local: Phlebitis

Ocular: Blurred vision

Renal: Elevated BUN, elevated serum creatinine

Miscellaneous: Anaphylaxis including anaphylactic shock

Drug Interactions Probenecid decreases the clearance of cefepime; aminoglycosides increase nephrotoxic potential

Stability Store vial at room temperature and protect from light; incompatible with metronidazole, vancomycin, aminoglycosides, and aminophylline

Mechanism of Action Inhibits bacterial cell wall synthesis by binding to one or more of the penicillin-binding proteins; inhibits the final transpeptidation step of peptidoglycan synthesis in bacterial cell walls

Pharmacokinetics

Distribution: V_d:

Children (2 months to 6 years): 0.32-0.35 L/kg

Adults: 14-20 L; penetrates into inflammatory fluid at concentrations ~80% of serum levels and into bronchial mucosa at levels ~60% of plasma levels; excreted in breast milk at very low concentrations

Protein binding: 16% to 19%

Metabolism: Very little

Half-life:

Children 2 months to 6 years: 1.77-1.96 hours

Adults: 2 hours

Elimination: At least 85% eliminated as unchanged drug in urine

Dialysis: 45% to 68% removed by hemodialysis

Usual Dosage I.M., I.V.:

Children 2 months to 16 years, ≤40 kg in weight: 50 mg/kg/dose every 12 hours

Febrile neutropenic patients: 50 mg/kg/dose every 8 hours

Cefepime has been studied in 12 cystic fibrosis patients (ages 4-41 years) with bronchopulmonary infection at a dose of 50 mg/kg/dose every 8 hours (maximum dose: 2 g/dose every 8 hours); cefepime was as effective as cefotaxime in 90 children <15 years of age who were randomized to receive cefepime 50 mg/kg/dose every 8 hours (n=43) or cefotaxime 50 mg/kg/dose every 6 hours (n=47) for the treatment of bacterial meningitis

Adults: 1-2 g every 12 hours; high doses or more frequent administration may be required in pseudomonal infections

UTIs: 500 mg every 12 hours

Empiric monotherapy in febrile neutropenia: 2 g every 8 hours

Administration Parenteral:

I.V.: Cefepime may be administered by I.V. intermittent infusion over 20-30 minutes; final concentration for I.V. administration should not exceed 40 mg/mL in D_5W, NS,

D$_{10}$W, D$_5$/NS, or D$_5$/LR; in clinical trials, cefepime was administered by direct I.V. injection over 3-5 minutes at a final concentration of 100 mg/mL for mild to moderate infections

I.M.: Deep I.M. injection. May dilute vial using SWI, NS, D$_5$W, or 0.5% or 1% lidocaine to a final concentration of 280 mg/mL (see package insert)

Dosing Adjustment in Renal Impairment, Adults

Cl$_{cr}$ (mL/min)	Infection		
	Mild to Moderate	Moderate to Severe	Severe
30-60	0.5-1 g I.M./I.V. every 24 hours	1-2 g I.V. every 24 hours	2 g I.V. every 24 hours
11-29	0.5 g I.M./I.V. every 24 hours	0.5-1 g I.V. every 24 hours	1 g I.V. every 24 hours
≤10	0.25 g I.M./I.V. every 24 hours	0.25-0.5 g I.V. every 24 hours	0.5 g I.V. every 24 hours

Monitoring Parameters With prolonged therapy, monitor renal and hepatic function periodically; number and type of stools/day for diarrhea; CBC with differential

Test Interactions Positive Coombs' [direct]; may falsely elevate creatinine values when Jaffé reaction is used; may cause false-positive results in urine glucose tests when using Clinitest®; false-positive urinary proteins and steroids

Patient Information Report side effects such as diarrhea, dyspepsia, headache, blurred vision, and lightheadedness to your physician

Nursing Implications Do not admix with aminoglycosides

Dosage Forms Injection, powder for reconstitution, as hydrochloride: 500 mg, 1 g, 2 g

References

Arguedas AG, Stutman HR, Zaleska M, et al, "Cefepime. Pharmacokinetics and Clinical Response in Patients With Cystic Fibrosis," *Am J Dis Child*, 1992, 146(7):797-802.

Blumer JL, Reed MD, Lemon E, et al, "Pharmacokinetics (PK) of Cefepime in Pediatric Patients Administered Single and Multiple 50 mg/kg Doses Every 8 Hours by the Intravenous (I.V.) or Intramuscular (I.M.) Route," 34th Interscience Conference on Antimicrobial Agents and Chemotherapy, 1994, Orlando, Fl. Abs. A69.

Saez-Llorens X, Castano E, Garcia R, et al, "Prospective Randomized Comparison of Cefepime and Cefotaxime for Treatment of Bacterial Meningitis in Infants and Children", *Antimicrob Agents Chemother*, 1995, 39(4):937-40.

Wynd MA and Paladino JA, "Cefepime: A Fourth-Generation Parenteral Cephalosporin," *Ann Pharmacother*, 1996, 30(12):1414-24.

Cefixime [DSC] (sef IKS eem)

U.S. Brand Names Suprax® [DSC]

Therapeutic Category Antibiotic, Cephalosporin (Third Generation)

Generic Available No

Use Treatment of urinary tract infections, otitis media, respiratory infections due to susceptible organisms including *S. pneumoniae* and *pyogenes*, *H. influenzae*, *M. catarrhalis*, and many *Enterobacteriaceae*; documented poor compliance with other oral antimicrobials; outpatient therapy of serious soft tissue or skeletal infections due to susceptible organisms; single-dose oral treatment of uncomplicated cervical/urethral gonorrhea due to *N. gonorrhoeae*; treatment of shigellosis in areas with a high rate of resistance to TMP-SMX

Pregnancy Risk Factor B

Contraindications Hypersensitivity to cefixime, any component, or cephalosporins

Warnings Prolonged use may result in superinfection; do not use in patients with immediate-type hypersensitivity reactions to penicillin

Precautions Use with caution in patients hypersensitive to penicillin, patients with impaired renal function, and patients with a history of colitis; modify dosage in patients with renal impairment

Adverse Reactions

Central nervous system: Headache, fever, dizziness, fatigue

Dermatologic: Skin rash, urticaria, pruritus

Gastrointestinal: Nausea, diarrhea (up to 15% of children), abdominal pain, pseudo-membranous colitis

Genitourinary: Vaginitis

Hematologic: Eosinophilia, thrombocytopenia, leukopenia

Hepatic: Transient elevation of liver enzymes

Renal: Transient elevation of BUN and serum creatinine

Drug Interactions Probenecid (increases cefixime concentration); cefixime may increase carbamazepine serum concentrations

Food Interactions Food delays the time to reach peak concentrations

Stability After reconstitution, suspension may be stored for 14 days at room temperature

(Continued)

Cefixime [DSC] *(Continued)*

Mechanism of Action Inhibits bacterial cell wall synthesis by binding to one or more of the penicillin-binding proteins; inhibits the final transpeptidation step of peptidoglycan synthesis resulting in cell wall death

Pharmacokinetics

Absorption: Oral: 40% to 50%

Distribution: Into bile, sputum, middle ear fluid; crosses the placenta

Protein binding: 65%

Half-life:

Normal renal function: 3-4 hours

Renal failure: Up to 11.5 hours

Time to peak serum concentration: Within 2-6 hours; peak serum concentrations are 15% to 50% higher for the oral suspension versus tablets

Elimination: 50% of absorbed dose excreted as active drug in urine and 10% in bile

Dialysis: 10% removed by hemodialysis

Usual Dosage Oral:

Infants and Children: 8 mg/kg/day divided every 12-24 hours; maximum dose: 400 mg/day

Treatment of acute UTI: 16 mg/kg/day divided every 12 hours on day 1, then 8 mg/kg/day every 24 hours for 13 days

Prophylaxis after sexual victimization: 8 mg/kg in a single dose (maximum dose: 400 mg) **plus** azithromycin 20 mg/kg in a single dose (maximum dose: 1 g); also begin or complete hepatitis B virus immunization and consider prophylaxis for trichomoniasis and bacterial vaginosis

Adolescents and Adults: 400 mg/day divided every 12-24 hours

Uncomplicated cervical/urethral gonorrhea due to *N. gonorrhoeae*: 400 mg as a single dose plus azithromycin 1 g orally in a single dose **or** doxycycline 100 mg orally twice daily for 7 days

Prophylaxis after sexual victimization: 400 mg in a single dose **plus** azithromycin 1 g orally in a single dose **or** doxycycline 100 mg orally twice daily for 7 days **plus** metronidazole 2 g orally in a single dose **plus** hepatitis B virus immunization if not fully immunized plus consider prophylaxis for HIV depending on circumstances

Dosing adjustment in renal impairment:

Cl_{cr} 21-60 mL/minute: Administer 75% of the standard dose

Cl_{cr} <20 mL/minute: Administer 50% of the standard dose

Administration Oral: May be administered with or without food; administer with food to decrease GI distress; shake suspension well before use

Monitoring Parameters With prolonged therapy, monitor renal and hepatic function periodically; number and type of stools/day for diarrhea

Test Interactions False-positive reaction for urine glucose using Clinitest®; false-positive urine ketones using tests with nitroprusside

Patient Information Report problems with diarrhea

Additional Information Otitis media should be treated with the suspension since it results in higher peak blood levels than the tablet

Dosage Forms

Powder for oral suspension, as anhydrous: 100 mg/5 mL (50 mL, 75 mL, 100 mL) [strawberry flavor] [DSC]

Tablet, film coated, scored, as anhydrous: 400 mg [DSC]

References

Ashkenazi S, Amir J, Waisman Y, et al, "A Randomized, Double-Blind Study Comparing Cefixime and Trimethoprim-Sulfamethoxazole in the Treatment of Childhood Shigellosis," *J Pediatr*, 1993, 123(5):817-21.

"2002 Guidelines for the Treatment of Sexually Transmitted Diseases. Centers for Disease Control and Prevention," *MMWR Morb Mortal Wkly Rep*, 2002, 51(RR-6):1-80.

Hoberman A, Wald ER, Hickey RW, et al, "Oral Versus Initial Intravenous Therapy for Urinary Tract Infections in Young Febrile Children," *Pediatrics*, 1999, 104(1 Pt 1):79-86.

Johnson CE, Carlin SA, Super DM, et al, "Cefixime Compared With Amoxicillin for Treatment of Acute Otitis Media," *J Pediatr*, 1991, 119(1):117-22.

♦ **Cefizox**® *see* Ceftizoxime *on page 239*

♦ **Cefobid**® *see* Cefoperazone *on page 230*

Cefoperazone *(sef oh PER a zone)*

U.S. Brand Names Cefobid®

Therapeutic Category Antibiotic, Cephalosporin (Third Generation)

Generic Available No

Use Treatment of susceptible bacterial infections, mainly respiratory tract, skin and skin structure, urinary tract and sepsis; as a third generation cephalosporin, cefoperazone has activity against gram-negative bacilli (eg, *E. coli*, *Klebsiella*, and *Haemophilus*)

but variable activity against *Streptococcus* and *Staphylococcus* species; it has activity against *Pseudomonas aeruginosa*, but less than ceftazidime

Pregnancy Risk Factor B

Contraindications Hypersensitivity to cefoperazone, any component, or cephalosporins

Warnings Modify dosage in patients who have both severe renal impairment and hepatic dysfunction; prolonged use may result in superinfection; do not use in patients with immediate-type hypersensitivity reactions to penicillin

Precautions Use with caution in patients who are hypersensitive to penicillins

Adverse Reactions
Dermatologic: Rash
Gastrointestinal: Nausea, vomiting, diarrhea, pseudomembranous colitis
Hematologic: Bleeding, bruising, positive Coombs' test
Local: Pain and induration at I.M. injection site, phlebitis

Drug Interactions Disulfiram-like reaction may occur if taken with alcohol; concomitant use of anticoagulants or other agents that affect blood clotting may increase the risk of severe hemorrhage

Food Interactions Cefoperazone may decrease vitamin K synthesis by suppressing GI flora; vitamin K deficiency may occur and result in an increased risk of hemorrhage; patients at risk include those with malabsorption states (eg, cystic fibrosis) or poor nutritional status; monitor prothrombin time and administer vitamin K as needed

Stability Reconstituted solution and I.V. infusion in NS or D_5W are stable for 24 hours at room temperature, 5 days when refrigerated or 3 weeks when frozen; after freezing, thawed solution is stable for 48 hours at room temperature or 10 days when refrigerated; do not refreeze, do not mix with aminoglycosides

Mechanism of Action Interferes with bacterial cell wall synthesis during active replication, causing cell wall death and resultant bactericidal activity against susceptible bacteria

Pharmacokinetics
Protein binding: Concentration dependent and nonlinear; range: 82% to 93%
Half-life:
Neonates (low birth weight): 6-10 hours
Adults: 2 hours; half-life increases with hepatic disease or biliary obstruction
Time to peak serum concentration:
I.M.: Within 1-2 hours
I.V.: Within 15-20 minutes (serum levels 2-3 times the serum levels following I.M. administration)
Elimination: Excreted primarily in the bile (70% to 75%); 20% to 30% recovered unchanged in urine within 12 hours

Usual Dosage I.M., I.V.:
Neonates: 50 mg/kg/dose every 12 hours
Infants and Children: 100-150 mg/kg/day divided every 8-12 hours; up to 12 g/day
Adults: 2-4 g/day in divided doses every 12 hours; maximum dose: 12 g/day divided every 6-12 hours; 16 g/day has been given via continuous infusion to severely immunocompromised patients
Maximum dose with impaired hepatic function and/or biliary obstruction: 4 g/day
Maximum dose with combined hepatic and renal dysfunction: 1-2 g/day

Administration Parenteral:
I.M.: For concentrations ≥250 mg/mL, may dilute using SWI and 2% lidocaine to make final concentration of 0.5% lidocaine (see package insert)
Intermittent I.V.: Administer over 15-30 minutes at a maximum concentration of 50 mg/mL
I.V. continuous infusion: Infuse at a concentration of 2-25 mg/mL

Monitoring Parameters Prothrombin time; number and type of stools/day for diarrhea; resolution of infection

Test Interactions False-positive with urinary glucose tests using cupric sulfate (Clinitest®, Benedict's solution)

Patient Information Avoid alcohol

Nursing Implications Monitor for coagulation abnormalities and diarrhea

Additional Information Sodium content of 1 g cefoperazone sodium: 1.5 mEq (34 mg); chemical structure contains the N-methylthiotetrazole side chain which may be responsible for the increased risk of bleeding and the disulfiram-like reaction with alcohol

Dosage Forms
Injection, powder for reconstitution, as sodium: 1 g, 2 g, 10 g

♦ **Cefotan®** see Cefotetan on page 233

Cefotaxime (sef oh TAKS eem)

U.S. Brand Names Claforan®

Therapeutic Category Antibiotic, Cephalosporin (Third Generation)

Generic Available Yes

Use Treatment of susceptible lower respiratory tract, skin and skin structure, bone and joint, intra-abdominal and genitourinary tract infections; treatment of a documented or suspected meningitis due to susceptible organisms such as *H. influenzae* and *N. meningitidis*; indicated for *Neisseria gonorrhoeae* infections (including uncomplicated cervical and urethral gonorrhea and gonorrhea pelvic inflammatory disease); non-pseudomonal gram-negative rod infection in a patient at risk of developing aminoglycoside-induced nephrotoxicity and/or ototoxicity; infection due to an organism whose susceptibilities clearly favor cefotaxime over cefuroxime or an aminoglycoside

Pregnancy Risk Factor B

Contraindications Hypersensitivity to cefotaxime, any component, or cephalosporins

Warnings Prolonged use may result in superinfection; do not use in patients with immediate-type hypersensitivity reactions to penicillin; cefotaxime rapid bolus injection (over <1 minute through a central venous catheter) has been associated with potentially life-threatening arrhythmias

Precautions Use with caution in patients with history of penicillin hypersensitivity, impaired renal function, or history of colitis; modify dosage in patients with Cl_{cr} <20 mL/minute

Adverse Reactions

Cardiovascular: Arrhythmias

Central nervous system: Fever, headache

Dermatologic: Rash, pruritus

Gastrointestinal: Antibiotic-associated pseudomembranous colitis, diarrhea, nausea, vomiting

Hematologic: Transient neutropenia, thrombocytopenia, eosinophilia, leukopenia

Hepatic: Transient elevation of liver enzymes

Local: Phlebitis, pain at injection site

Renal: Transient elevation of BUN and serum creatinine

Drug Interactions Probenecid (increases cefotaxime concentration)

Stability Reconstituted solution is stable for 24 hours at room temperature and 10 days when refrigerated

Mechanism of Action Inhibits bacterial cell wall synthesis by binding to one or more of the penicillin-binding proteins; inhibits the final transpeptidation step of peptidoglycan synthesis resulting in cell wall death

Pharmacokinetics

Distribution: Into bronchial secretions, middle ear effusions, bone, bile; penetration into CSF when meninges are inflamed; crosses the placenta; appears in breast milk

Protein binding: 31% to 50%

Metabolism: Partially metabolized in the liver to active metabolite, desacetylcefotaxime

Half-life:

Cefotaxime:

Neonates, premature: <1 week: 5-6 hours

Neonates, full-term: <1 week: 2-3.4 hours; 1-4 weeks: 2 hours

Children: 1.5 hours

Adults: 1-1.5 hours (prolonged with renal and/or hepatic impairment)

Desacetylcefotaxime: Adults: 1.5-1.9 hours (prolonged with renal impairment)

Time to peak serum concentration: I.M.: Within 30 minutes

Elimination: 40% to 60% of a dose excreted as unchanged drug and 24% excreted as desacetylcefotaxime in the urine

Dialysis: Moderately dialyzable (20% to 50%)

Usual Dosage I.M., I.V.:

Neonates: 0-4 weeks: <1200 g: 100 mg/kg/day divided every 12 hours

Postnatal age ≤7 days:

1200-2000 g: 100 mg/kg/day divided every 12 hours

>2000 g: 100-150 mg/kg/day divided every 8-12 hours

Postnatal age >7 days:

1200-2000 g: 150 mg/kg/day divided every 8 hours

>2000 g: 150-200 mg/kg/day divided every 6-8 hours

Infants and Children 1 month to 12 years:

<50 kg: 100-200 mg/kg/day divided every 6-8 hours

Meningitis: 200 mg/kg/day divided every 6 hours; 225-300 mg/kg/day divided every 6-8 hours has been used to treat invasive pneumococcal meningitis

≥50 kg: Moderate to severe infection: 1-2 g every 6-8 hours; life-threatening infection: 2 g/dose every 4 hours; maximum dose: 12 g/day

Children >12 years and Adults: 1-2 g every 6-8 hours (up to 12 g/day)
Dosing adjustment in renal impairment: Cl$_{cr}$ <20 mL/minute: Reduce dose by 50%
Administration Parenteral:
I.V.: Cefotaxime may be administered IVP over 3-5 minutes at a maximum concentration of 100 mg/mL or I.V. intermittent infusion over 15-30 minutes at a final concentration of 20-60 mg/mL; in fluid-restricted patients, a concentration of 150 mg/mL may be administered IVP; rapid IVP over <1 minute may cause arrhythmias (see Warnings)

I.M.: Deep I.M. injection into a large muscle mass such as the upper outer quadrant of the gluteus maximus. Doses as large as 2 g should be divided and administered at 2 different sites. May dilute vial using SWI to a final concentration between 230-330 mg/mL (see package insert).

Monitoring Parameters With prolonged therapy, monitor renal, hepatic, and hematologic function periodically; number and type of stools/day for diarrhea

Test Interactions Positive Coombs' [direct]

Additional Information Sodium content of 1 g: 2.2 mEq

Dosage Forms
Infusion, as sodium [premixed in D$_5$W, frozen]: 1 g (50 mL); 2 g (50 mL)
Injection, powder for reconstitution, as sodium: 500 mg, 1 g, 2 g, 10 g, 20 g

References
Spritzer R, Kamp HJ, Dzoljic G, et al, "Five Years of Cefotaxime Use in a Neonatal Intensive Care Unit," *Pediatr Infect Dis J*, 1990, 9(2):92-6.

Cefotetan (SEF oh tee tan)

U.S. Brand Names Cefotan®
Therapeutic Category Antibiotic, Cephalosporin (Second Generation)
Generic Available No
Use Treatment of susceptible lower respiratory tract, skin and skin structure, bone and joint, genitourinary tract, sepsis, gynecologic, and intra-abdominal infections; active against anaerobes including *Bacteroides* species of GI tract, gram-negative enteric bacilli including *E. coli*, *Klebsiella*, and *Proteus*; active against many strains of *N. gonorrhoeae*; inactive against *Enterobacter* sp.; perioperative prophylaxis
Pregnancy Risk Factor B
Contraindications Hypersensitivity to cefotetan, any component, or cephalosporins
Warnings Prolonged use may result in superinfection; do not use in patients with immediate-type hypersensitivity reactions to penicillin
Precautions Use with caution and modify dosage in patients with renal impairment; use with caution in patients with history of colitis or penicillin hypersensitivity
Adverse Reactions
Central nervous system: Seizures, fever
Dermatologic: Rash, pruritus, urticaria
Gastrointestinal: Diarrhea, nausea, vomiting, pseudomembranous colitis
Hematologic: Neutropenia, leukopenia, thrombocytopenia, eosinophilia, hemolytic anemia, bleeding, prolongation of PT
Hepatic: Elevated serum AST, ALT, alkaline phosphatase, LDH
Local: Phlebitis, pain at the injection site, edema
Renal: Elevated BUN, elevated serum creatinine
Drug Interactions Alcohol (disulfiram-like reaction), anticoagulants (may increase the risk of hemorrhage)
Stability Reconstituted solution is stable for 24 hours at room temperature and 96 hours when refrigerated; thawed solutions of the commercially available frozen cefotetan injections are stable for 48 hours at room temperature or 21 days when refrigerated; do not refreeze; incompatible with aminoglycosides, heparin, and tetracycline
Mechanism of Action Inhibits bacterial cell wall synthesis by binding to one or more of the penicillin-binding proteins; inhibits the final transpeptidation step of peptidoglycan synthesis resulting in cell wall death
Pharmacokinetics
Absorption: I.M.: Completely absorbed
Distribution: Distributes into tissues and fluids including gallbladder, kidney, skin, tonsils, uterus, sputum, prostatic and peritoneal fluids; poor penetration into CSF; cross the placenta; small amounts appear in breast milk
Protein binding: 76% to 91%
Half-life: 3.5 hours, prolonged in patients with impaired renal function (up to 10 hours)
Time to peak serum concentration: I.M.: Within 1.5-3 hours
Elimination: 49% to 81% excreted as unchanged drug in urine, 20% of dose is excreted in bile
Dialysis: <10% removed by hemodialysis
Usual Dosage I.M., I.V.: Safety and efficacy in children have not been established
Children: 40-80 mg/kg/day divided every 12 hours; up to 6 g/day
(Continued)

Cefotetan *(Continued)*

Adolescents and Adults: 2-4 g/day divided every 12 hours; maximum dose: 6 g/day
Urinary tract infections: 1-2 g/day divided every 12-24 hours
Perioperative prophylaxis: I.V.: 1-2 g 30-60 minutes prior to procedure
Pelvic inflammatory disease: I.V.: 2 g every 12 hours continued for 24-48 hours after significant clinical improvement is demonstrated **plus** doxycycline 100 mg I.V. or orally every 12 hours for 14 days

Dosing interval in renal impairment:
Cl_{cr} 10-30 mL/minute: Administer every 24 hours
Cl_{cr} <10 mL/minute: Administer every 48 hours

Administration Parenteral:
IVP: Administer over 3-5 minutes at a maximum concentration of 100 mg/mL
I.V. intermittent: Infuse over 20-60 minutes at a concentration of 10-40 mg/mL
I.M.: Deep I.M. injection into a large muscle mass such as the upper outer quadrant of the gluteus maximus. May dilute vial using SWI, NS, or 0.5% or 1% lidocaine to a final concentration of 375-471.5 mg/mL (see package insert)

Monitoring Parameters Prothrombin time, renal function tests; number and type of stools/day for diarrhea

Test Interactions Positive Coombs' [direct], false-positive urine glucose (Clinitest®), falsely elevated serum or urinary creatinine (Jaffé reaction)

Patient Information Avoid alcohol

Additional Information Sodium content of 1 g: 3.5 mEq; chemical structure contains a methyltetrazolethiol side chain which may be responsible for the disulfiram-like reaction with alcohol and increased risk of bleeding

Dosage Forms
Infusion, as disodium [premixed in dextrose, frozen]: 1 g (50 mL); 2 g (50 mL)
Injection, powder for reconstitution, as disodium: 1 g, 2 g, 10 g

References
Martin C, Thomachot L, and Albanese J, "Clinical Pharmacokinetics of Cefotetan," *Clin Pharmacokinet,* 1994, 26(4):248-58.

Cefoxitin *(se FOKS i tin)*

U.S. Brand Names Mefoxin®

Therapeutic Category Antibiotic, Cephalosporin (Second Generation)

Generic Available Yes

Use Treatment of susceptible lower respiratory tract, skin and skin structure, bone and joint, genitourinary tract, sepsis, gynecologic, and intra-abdominal infections; active against anaerobes including *Bacteroides* species of the GI tract, gram-negative enteric bacilli including *E. coli, Klebsiella,* and *Proteus*; active against many strains of *N. gonorrhoeae*; inactive against *Enterobacter* sp.; perioperative prophylaxis

Pregnancy Risk Factor B

Contraindications Hypersensitivity to cefoxitin, any component, or cephalosporins

Warnings Prolonged use may result in superinfection; high doses in children have been associated with an increased incidence of eosinophilia and elevation of serum AST; safety and efficacy in infants <3 months have not been established; do not use in patients with immediate-type hypersensitivity reactions to penicillin

Precautions Use with caution and modify dosage in patients with renal impairment; use with caution in patients with history of colitis or penicillin hypersensitivity

Adverse Reactions
Central nervous system: Fever, headache
Dermatologic: Rash, pruritus, exfoliative dermatitis
Gastrointestinal: Pseudomembranous colitis, diarrhea, nausea, vomiting
Hematologic: Transient leukopenia, thrombocytopenia, neutropenia, anemia, eosinophilia
Hepatic: Transient elevation of liver enzymes, AST, ALT, and alkaline phosphatase
Local: Thrombophlebitis, pain at injection site
Renal: Transient elevation of BUN and serum creatinine

Drug Interactions Probenecid (increases serum concentration of cefoxitin)

Stability Reconstituted solution is stable for 24 hours at room temperature and for 1 week under refrigeration; thawed solutions of the commercially available frozen cefoxitin injections are stable for 24 hours at room temperature or 5 days when refrigerated

Mechanism of Action Inhibits bacterial cell wall synthesis by binding to one or more of the penicillin-binding proteins; inhibits the final transpeptidation step of peptidoglycan synthesis resulting in cell wall death

Pharmacokinetics

Distribution: Distributes into tissues and fluids including ascitic, pleural, bile, and synovial fluids; poor penetration into CSF even with inflamed meninges; crosses the placenta; small amounts appear in breast milk

Protein binding: 65% to 79%

Half-life:

Infants (10-53 days of age): 1.4 hours

Adults: 45-60 minutes, increases significantly with renal insufficiency

Time to peak serum concentration: I.M.: Within 20-30 minutes

Elimination: Rapidly excreted as unchanged drug (85%) in the urine

Dialysis: Moderately dialyzable (20% to 50%)

Usual Dosage I.M., I.V.:

Neonates: 90-100 mg/kg/day divided every 8 hours

Infants ≥3 months and Children:

Mild-moderate infection: 80-100 mg/kg/day divided every 6-8 hours

Severe infection: 100-160 mg/kg/day divided every 4-6 hours; maximum dose: 12 g/day

Perioperative prophylaxis: 30-40 mg/kg 30-60 minutes prior to surgery followed by 30-40 mg/kg/dose every 6 hours for no more than 24 hours after surgery depending on the procedure

Adolescents and Adults: 1-2 g every 6-8 hours (I.M. injection is painful); maximum dose: 12 g/day

Pelvic inflammatory disease: I.V.: 2 g every 6 hours continued for 24-48 hours after significant clinical improvement is demonstrated **plus** doxycycline 100 mg I.V. or orally every 12 hours for 14 days

Perioperative prophylaxis: 1-2 g 30-60 minutes prior to surgery followed by 1-2 g every 6-8 hours for no more than 24 hours after surgery depending on the procedure

Dosing interval in renal impairment:

Cl_{cr} 30-50 mL/minute: Administer every 8-12 hours

Cl_{cr} 10-30 mL/minute: Administer every 12-24 hours

Cl_{cr} <10 mL/minute: Administer every 24-48 hours

Administration Parenteral:

IVP: Administer over 3-5 minutes at a maximum concentration of 200 mg/mL

I.V. intermittent infusion: Administer over 10-60 minutes at a final concentration not to exceed 40 mg/mL

I.M.: Deep I.M. injection into a large muscle mass such as the upper outer quadrant of the gluteus maximus. May dilute vial using SWI or 0.5% or 1% lidocaine to a final concentration of 400 mg/mL (see package insert)

Monitoring Parameters Renal function periodically when used in combination with other nephrotoxic drugs; liver function and hematologic function tests; number and type of stools/day for diarrhea

Test Interactions Positive Coombs' [direct]; false-positive urine glucose (Clinitest®), false ↑ in serum or urine creatinine

Additional Information Sodium content of 1 g: 2.3 mEq

Dosage Forms

Infusion, as sodium [premixed in D_5W, frozen]: 1 g (50 mL); 2 g (50 mL)

Injection, powder for reconstitution, as sodium: 1 g, 2 g, 10 g

References

Feldman WE, Moffitt S, and Sprow N, "Clinical and Pharmacokinetic Evaluation of Parenteral Cefoxitin in Infants and Children," *Antimicrob Agents Chemother*, 1980, 17(4):669-74.

Regazzi MB, Chirico G, Cristiani D, et al, "Cefoxitin in Newborn Infants. A Clinical and Pharmacokinetic Study," *Eur J Clin Pharmacol*, 1983, 25(4):507-9.

Cefpodoxime (sef pode OKS eem)

Related Information

Carbohydrate and Alcohol Content of Liquid Medications for Use in Patients Receiving Ketogenic Diets on page 1431

U.S. Brand Names Vantin®

Therapeutic Category Antibiotic, Cephalosporin (Third Generation)

Generic Available No

Use Treatment of susceptible acute, community-acquired pneumonia caused by *S. pneumoniae* or nonbeta-lactamase producing *H. influenzae*; alternative regimen for acute uncomplicated gonorrhea caused by *N. gonorrhoeae*; uncomplicated skin and skin structure infections caused by *S. aureus* or *S. pyogenes*; acute otitis media caused by *S. pneumoniae*, *H. influenzae*, or *M. catarrhalis*; pharyngitis or tonsillitis; and uncomplicated urinary tract infections caused by *E. coli*, *Klebsiella*, and *Proteus*; inactive against *Pseudomonas* and *Enterobacter* spp.

Pregnancy Risk Factor B

(Continued)

Cefpodoxime *(Continued)*

Contraindications Hypersensitivity to cefpodoxime, any component, or cephalosporins

Warnings Prolonged use may result in superinfection; do not use in patients with immediate-type hypersensitivity reactions to penicillin

Precautions Use with caution in patients with history of penicillin hypersensitivity, impaired renal function, and patients with a history of colitis; modify dosage in patients with renal impairment

Adverse Reactions

Central nervous system: Headache

Dermatologic: Rash

Gastrointestinal: Nausea (3.8%), vomiting, abdominal pain, diarrhea (7.1%), pseudo-membranous colitis

Genitourinary: Vaginal fungal infections (3.3%)

Hematologic: Eosinophilia, leukocytosis, thrombocytosis, decrease in hemoglobin or hematocrit, leukopenia, prolonged PT and PTT

Hepatic: Transient elevation in AST, ALT, bilirubin

Renal: Elevated BUN, elevated serum creatinine

Drug Interactions Antacids and H_2-receptor antagonists (reduce absorption and serum concentration of cefpodoxime); probenecid (inhibits renal excretion of cefpodoxime)

Food Interactions Food increases oral bioavailability

Stability After reconstitution, suspension may be stored in refrigerator for 14 days

Mechanism of Action Inhibits bacterial cell wall synthesis by binding to one or more of the penicillin-binding proteins; inhibits the final transpeptidation step of peptidoglycan synthesis resulting in cell wall death

Pharmacokinetics

Absorption: Enhanced in the presence of food or low gastric pH

Distribution: Good tissue penetration, including lung and tonsils; penetrates into pleural fluid; poor penetration into CSF; small amounts appear in breast milk

Protein binding: 18% to 23%

Metabolism: Following oral administration, cefpodoxime proxetil is de-esterified in the GI tract to the active metabolite, cefpodoxime

Bioavailability: Oral: 50%

Half-life: 2.2 hours (prolonged with renal impairment)

Time to peak serum concentration: Within 2-3 hours

Elimination: Primarily by the kidney with 80% of absorbed dose excreted unchanged in urine in 24 hours

Usual Dosage Oral:

Infants >6 months and Children to 12 years: 10 mg/kg/day divided every 12 hours; maximum dose: 800 mg/day

Adolescents and Adults: 100-400 mg/dose every 12 hours

Uncomplicated gonorrhea: 200 mg as a single dose

Dosing adjustment in renal impairment: Cl_{cr} <30 mL/minute: Administer every 24 hours; patients on hemodialysis, administer dose 3 times/week

Dosing adjustment in hepatic impairment: Not necessary in patient with cirrhosis

Administration Oral:

Tablet: Administer with food

Suspension: May administer with or without food; shake suspension well before use

Monitoring Parameters Observe patient for diarrhea; with prolonged therapy, monitor renal function periodically

Test Interactions Positive Coombs' [direct]

Dosage Forms

Powder for oral suspension, as proxetil: 50 mg/5 mL (100 mL); 100 mg/5 mL (100 mL) [lemon creme flavor]

Tablet, film coated, as proxetil: 100 mg, 200 mg

References

Borin MT, "A Review of the Pharmacokinetics of Cefpodoxime Proxetil," *Drugs*, 1991, 42(Suppl 3):13-21.

Fujii R, "Clinical Trials of Cefpodoxime Proxetil Suspension in Pediatrics," *Drugs*, 1991, 42(Suppl 3):57-60.

Mendelman PM, Del-Beccaro MA, McLinn SE, et al, "Cefpodoxime Proxetil Compared With Amoxicillin-Clavulanate for the Treatment of Otitis Media," *J Pediatr*, 1992, 121(3):459-65.

Cefprozil *(sef PROE zil)*

Related Information

Carbohydrate and Alcohol Content of Liquid Medications for Use in Patients Receiving Ketogenic Diets *on page 1431*

U.S. Brand Names Cefzil®

Therapeutic Category Antibiotic, Cephalosporin (Second Generation)

Generic Available No

Use Infections caused by susceptible organisms including *S. pneumoniae*, *H. influenzae*, *M. catarrhalis*, *S. aureus*, *S. pyogenes*; treatment of infections involving the respiratory tract, skin and skin structure, and otitis media

Pregnancy Risk Factor B

Contraindications Hypersensitivity to cefprozil, any component, or cephalosporins

Warnings Prolonged use may result in superinfection; do not use in patients with immediate-type hypersensitivity reactions to penicillin

Oral suspension contains sodium benzoate; benzoic acid (benzoate) is a metabolite of benzyl alcohol; large amounts of benzyl alcohol ($\geq$99 mg/kg/day) have been associated with a potentially fatal toxicity ("gasping syndrome") in neonates; the "gasping syndrome" consists of metabolic acidosis, respiratory distress, gasping respirations, CNS dysfunction (including convulsions, intracranial hemorrhage), hypotension and cardiovascular collapse; use oral suspension containing sodium benzoate with caution in neonates; *in vitro* and animal studies have shown that benzoate displaces bilirubin from protein binding sites

Precautions Use with caution in patients with impaired renal function, history of colitis, or in penicillin-sensitive patients; modify dosage in patients with severe renal impairment; some products (eg, oral suspension) contain aspartame which is metabolized to phenylalanine and must be used with caution in patients with phenylketonuria.

Adverse Reactions
Central nervous system: Headache, hyperactivity, insomnia, confusion, dizziness
Dermatologic: Rash, pruritus, diaper rash
Gastrointestinal: Diarrhea, nausea, vomiting, abdominal pain
Genitourinary: Vaginitis
Hematologic: Decrease in leukocyte and platelet count, eosinophilia
Hepatic: Elevated AST, ALT, and alkaline phosphatase; cholestatic jaundice; prolonged PT
Renal: Elevated BUN and serum creatinine
Miscellaneous: Serum sickness-like reactions

Drug Interactions Probenecid increases cefprozil serum levels

Food Interactions Total absorption is not affected by food

Stability Refrigerate suspension after reconstitution; discard after 14 days

Mechanism of Action Inhibits bacterial cell wall synthesis by binding to one or more of the penicillin-binding proteins resulting in disruption of cell wall synthesis and cell lysis

Pharmacokinetics
Absorption: Oral: Well absorbed (95%)
Distribution: Low excretion into breast milk
Protein binding: 35% to 45%
Bioavailability: 94%
Half-life, elimination: 1.3 hours (normal renal function)
Time to peak serum concentration: 1.5 hours (fasting state)
Elimination: 61% excreted unchanged in urine
Dialysis: ~55% is removed by hemodialysis

Usual Dosage Oral:
Infants >6 months and Children to 12 years:
Otitis media: 30 mg/kg/day divided every 12 hours; maximum dose: 1 g/day
Children 2-12 years:
Pharyngitis/tonsillitis: 15 mg/kg/day divided every 12 hours; maximum dose: 1 g/day
Skin and skin structure infection: 20 mg/kg once daily
Children >12 years and Adults: 250-500 mg every 12 hours or 500 mg every 24 hours
Dosing adjustment in renal impairment: Cl_{cr} <30 mL/minute: Reduce dose by 50%

Administration Oral: May administer with or without food; administer with food if stomach upset occurs; chilling improves flavor of suspension (do not freeze); shake suspension well before use

Monitoring Parameters Evaluate renal function before and during therapy; with prolonged therapy, monitor coagulation tests, CBC, and liver function tests periodically

Test Interactions Positive Coombs' [direct]; may produce false-positive reaction for urine glucose with Clinitest®

Patient Information Report persistent diarrhea to physician

Additional Information Suspension also contains FD&C red No. 3, glycine, carboxymethylcellulose, and sucrose

Dosage Forms
Powder for oral suspension, as anhydrous: 125 mg/5 mL (50 mL, 75 mL, 100 mL) [contains 28 mg phenylalanine (as aspartame)/5 mL and sodium benzoate; (Continued)

Cefprozil *(Continued)*

bubblegum flavor]; 250 mg/5 mL (50 mL, 75 mL, 100 mL) [contains 28 mg phenylal-anine (as aspartame)/5 mL and sodium benzoate; bubblegum flavor]

Tablet, film coated, as anhydrous: 250 mg, 500 mg

References

Arguedas AG, Zaleska M, Stutman HR, et al, "Comparative Trial of Cefprozil vs Amoxicillin Clavulanate Potassium in the Treatment of Children With Acute Otitis Media With Effusion," *Pediatr Infect Dis J*, 1991, 10(5):375-80.

Barriere SL, "Review of *In Vitro* Activity, Pharmacokinetic Characteristics, Safety, and Clinical Efficacy of Cefprozil, a New Oral Cephalosporin," *Ann Pharmacother*, 1993, 27(9):1082-9.

Lowery N, Kearns GL, Young RA, et al, "Serum Sickness-Like Reactions Associated With Cefprozil Therapy," *J Pediatr*, 1994, 125(2):325-8.

Ceftazidime *(SEF tay zi deem)*

U.S. Brand Names Ceptaz®; Fortaz®; Tazicef®; Tazidime®

Therapeutic Category Antibiotic, Cephalosporin (Third Generation)

Generic Available No

Use Treatment of infections of the respiratory tract, urinary tract, skin and skin struc-ture, intra-abdominal, osteomyelitis, sepsis, and meningitis caused by susceptible gram-negative aerobic organisms such as Enterobacteriaceae and *Pseudomonas*; pseudomonal infection in patient at risk of developing aminoglycoside-induced neph-rotoxicity and/or ototoxicity; empiric therapy for febrile, granulocytopenic patients

Pregnancy Risk Factor B

Contraindications Hypersensitivity to ceftazidime, any component, or cephalosporins

Warnings Prolonged use may result in superinfection; do not use in patients with immediate-type hypersensitivity reactions to penicillin

Precautions Use with caution and modify dosage in patients with impaired renal function; use with caution in patients with history of colitis or patients with penicillin hypersensitivity

Adverse Reactions

Central nervous system: Fever, headache, dizziness, coma

Dermatologic: Rash, pruritus, urticaria

Gastrointestinal: Pseudomembranous colitis, diarrhea, nausea, vomiting, candidiasis

Hematologic: Transient leukopenia, thrombocytopenia, eosinophilia, thrombocytosis, hemolytic anemia

Hepatic: Transient elevation of liver enzymes, jaundice, hyperbilirubinemia

Local: Phlebitis, pain at injection site

Neuromuscular & skeletal: Myoclonia

Renal: Transient elevation of BUN and serum creatinine, renal impairment

Miscellaneous: Anaphylaxis

Drug Interactions Probenecid decreases renal clearance of ceftazidime; aminoglyco-sides may increase risk of nephrotoxicity

Stability Reconstituted solution is stable for 24 hours at room temperature and 10 days when refrigerated; incompatible with sodium bicarbonate; potentially incompat-ible with aminoglycosides

Mechanism of Action Bactericidal antibiotic with a mechanism similar to that of penicillins by binding to one or more of the penicillin-binding proteins; inhibits muco-peptide synthesis in the bacterial cell wall

Pharmacokinetics

Distribution: Widely distributed throughout the body including bone, bile, skin, CSF (diffuses into CSF at higher concentrations when the meninges are inflamed), endometrium, heart, pleural and lymphatic fluids; distributes into breast milk

Protein binding: 17%

Half-life:

Neonates <23 days: 2.2-4.7 hours

Adults: 1-2 hours (prolonged with renal impairment)

Time to peak serum concentration: I.M.: Within 60 minutes

Elimination: By glomerular filtration with 80% to 90% of the dose excreted as unchanged drug in urine within 24 hours

Dialysis: Dialyzable (50% to 100%)

Usual Dosage I.M., I.V.:

Neonates: 0-4 weeks: <1200 g: 100 mg/kg/day divided every 12 hours

Postnatal age ≤7 days:

1200-2000 g: 100 mg/kg/day divided every 12 hours

>2000 g: 100-150 mg/kg/day divided every 8-12 hours

Postnatal age >7 days: ≥1200 g: 150 mg/kg/day divided every 8 hours

Infants and Children 1 month to 12 years: 100-150 mg/kg/day divided every 8 hours; maximum dose: 6 g/day

Meningitis: 150 mg/kg/day divided every 8 hours; maximum dose: 6 g/day

Adults: 1-2 g every 8-12 hours

Urinary tract infections: 250-500 mg every 12 hours

Dosing interval in renal impairment:
Cl_{cr} 30-50 mL/minute: Administer every 12 hours
Cl_{cr} 10-30 mL/minute: Administer every 24 hours
Cl_{cr} <10 mL/minute: Administer every 24-48 hours

Administration Parenteral: Any carbon dioxide bubbles that may be present in the withdrawn solution should be expelled prior to injection

IVP: Administer over 3-5 minutes at a maximum concentration of 180 mg/mL

I.V. intermittent infusion: Administer over 15-30 minutes at a final concentration ≤40 mg/mL

I.M.: Deep I.M. injection into a large muscle mass such as the upper outer quadrant of the gluteus maximus or lateral part of the thigh. May dilute vial using SWI or 0.5% or 1% lidocaine to a final concentration of 280 mg/mL (see package insert)

Monitoring Parameters Renal function periodically when used in combination with aminoglycosides; with prolonged therapy also monitor hepatic and hematologic function periodically; number and type of stools/day for diarrhea

Test Interactions Positive Coombs' [direct], false-positive urine glucose (Clinitest®)

Additional Information Sodium content of 1 g: 2.3 mEq

Dosage Forms
Infusion, as sodium [premixed in dextrose, frozen] (Fortaz®): 1 g (50 mL); 2 g (50 mL)
Injection, powder for reconstitution:
Ceptaz®: 1 g, 2 g, 10 g [contains L-arginine]
Fortaz®: 500 mg, 1 g, 2 g, 6 g [contains sodium carbonate]
Tazicef®, Tazidime®: 1 g, 2 g, 6 g, [contains sodium carbonate]

References
McCracken GH Jr, Threlkeld N, and Thomas ML, "Pharmacokinetics of Ceftazidime in Newborn Infants," *Antimicrob Agents Chemother,* 1984, 26(4):583-4.
Robinson DG, Cookson TL, and Frisafe JA, "Concentration Guidelines for Parenteral Antibiotics in Fluid-Restricted Patients," *Drug Intell Clin Pharm,* 1987, 21(12):985-9.

♦ **Ceftin®** *see* Cefuroxime *on page 242*

Ceftizoxime (sef ti ZOKS eem)

U.S. Brand Names Cefizox®

Therapeutic Category Antibiotic, Cephalosporin (Third Generation)

Generic Available No

Use Treatment of susceptible bacterial infections, mainly respiratory tract, skin and skin structure, bone and joint, urinary tract and sepsis; as a third generation cephalosporin, ceftizoxime has activity against gram-negative enteric bacilli (eg, *E. coli, Klebsiella*), and cocci (eg, *Neisseria*), and variable activity against gram-positive cocci (*Staphylococcus* and *Streptococcus*); ceftizoxime has some anaerobic coverage but is less active against *B. fragilis* than cefoxitin; also indicated for *Neisseria gonorrhoeae* infections (including uncomplicated cervical and urethral gonorrhea and gonorrhea pelvic inflammatory disease), and *Haemophilus influenzae* meningitis

Pregnancy Risk Factor B

Contraindications Hypersensitivity to ceftizoxime, any component, or cephalosporins

Warnings Prolonged use may result in superinfection; do not use in patients with immediate-type hypersensitivity reaction to penicillin

Precautions Use with caution in patients who are hypersensitive to penicillins; use with caution and modify dosage in patients with renal impairment

Adverse Reactions
Central nervous system: Fever
Dermatologic: Rash, pruritus
Gastrointestinal: Diarrhea, occasionally nausea and vomiting
Genitourinary: Vaginitis (rare)
Hematologic: Positive Coombs' test, eosinophilia, thrombocytosis (transient); rarely: anemia, leukopenia, neutropenia, thrombocytopenia
Hepatic: Elevated bilirubin; transient elevation of AST, ALT, alkaline phosphatase
Local: Pain, burning at injection site
Neuromuscular & skeletal: Numbness
Renal: Transient elevations of BUN and serum creatinine

Drug Interactions Probenecid may decrease renal tubular secretion and increase ceftizoxime serum concentrations

Stability Reconstituted solution is stable for 24 hours at room temperature and 96 hours when refrigerated; for I.V. infusion in NS or D_5W solution is stable for 24 hours at room temperature, 96 hours when refrigerated or 12 weeks when frozen; after freezing, thawed solution is stable for 24 hours at room temperature or 10 days when refrigerated; do not refreeze; do not mix with aminoglycosides
(Continued)

Ceftizoxime *(Continued)*

Mechanism of Action Interferes with bacterial cell wall synthesis during active replication, causing cell wall death and resultant bactericidal activity against susceptible bacteria

Pharmacokinetics
Distribution: V_d: 0.35-0.5 L/kg; penetrates CSF
Protein binding: 30%
Half-life: 1.6 hours, increases to 25 hours when Cl_{cr} falls to <10 mL/minute
Time to peak serum concentration: I.M.: Within 0.5-1 hour
Elimination: Excreted unchanged in urine
Dialysis: Moderately dialyzable (20% to 50%)

Usual Dosage I.M., I.V.:
Infants ≥6 months and Children: 150-200 mg/kg/day divided every 6-8 hours; maximum dose: 12 g/24 hours
Adults: 1-2 g every 8-12 hours
Life-threatening infections: Up to 2 g every 4 hours or 4 g every 8 hours
Uncomplicated gonorrhea: I.M.: 1 g (single dose)
Dosing interval in renal impairment:
Cl_{cr} 50-80 mL/minute: Administer every 8-12 hours
Cl_{cr} 10-50 mL/minute: Administer every 36-48 hours
Cl_{cr} <10 mL/minute: Administer every 48-72 hours

Administration Parenteral:
I.V. intermittent infusion: Administer over 30 minutes; usual dilution: 1 g/50 mL, doses >1 g are usually diluted to 100 mL
I.V. direct (bolus) injection: Administer slowly over 3-5 minutes at a concentration of 95 mg/mL

Test Interactions May falsely elevate creatine values when Jaffé reaction is used; may cause false-positive urinary glucose tests using cupric sulfate (Clinitest®, Benedict's solution)

Additional Information Sodium content of 1 g ceftizoxime: 60 mg (2.6 mEq); ceftizoxime does not cover *Chlamydia trachomatis* infections and must, therefore, be used with appropriate antichlamydial agents when treating pelvic inflammatory disease if *C. trachomatis* is suspected

Dosage Forms
Infusion, as sodium [preservative free; premixed in D_5W, frozen]: 1 g (50 mL); 2 g (50 mL)
Injection, powder for reconstitution, as sodium [preservative free]: 500 mg [DSC], 1 g, 2 g, 10 g

Ceftriaxone *(sef trye AKS one)*

U.S. Brand Names Rocephin®
Therapeutic Category Antibiotic, Cephalosporin (Third Generation)
Generic Available No
Use Treatment of sepsis, meningitis, infections of the lower respiratory tract, skin and skin structure, bone and joint, intra-abdominal and urinary tract due to susceptible organisms; as a third generation cephalosporin, ceftriaxone has activity against gram-negative aerobic bacteria (ie, *H. influenzae*, Enterobacteriaceae, *Neisseria*), and variable activity against gram-positive cocci; considered inactive against *Pseudomonas aeruginosa* and *C. trachomatis*; documented or suspected infection due to susceptible organisms in home care patients and patients without I.V. line access; treatment of documented or suspected gonococcal infection or chancroid; emergency room management of patients at high risk for bacteremia, periorbital or buccal cellulitis, salmonellosis or shigellosis and pneumonia of unestablished etiology (<5 years of age); treatment of resistant acute otitis media; in children with acute otitis media who are unable to take oral antibiotics

Pregnancy Risk Factor B
Contraindications Hypersensitivity to ceftriaxone sodium, any component, or cephalosporins; do not use in hyperbilirubinemic neonates, particularly those who are premature since ceftriaxone is reported to displace bilirubin from albumin binding sites increasing the risk for kernicterus
Warnings Prolonged use may result in superinfection with yeasts, enterococci, *B. fragilis*, or *P. aeruginosa*; do not use in patients with immediate-type hypersensitivity reactions to penicillin
Precautions Use with caution in patients with gallbladder, biliary tract, liver, or pancreatic disease; or in patients with history of colitis or penicillin hypersensitivity
Adverse Reactions
Central nervous system: Fever, chills, headache, dizziness
Dermatologic: Rash, pruritus

Gastrointestinal: Diarrhea, nausea, vomiting, sludging in the gallbladder, cholelithiasis, pseudomembranous colitis

Genitourinary: Vaginitis, casts in urine

Hematologic: Eosinophilia, leukopenia, anemia, thrombocytopenia, thrombocytosis, bleeding, neutropenia

Hepatic: Transient elevation in liver enzymes, jaundice, elevation in serum bilirubin

Local: Pain at injection site

Renal: Elevated BUN and serum creatinine

Drug Interactions High-dose probenecid (decreases elimination half-life of ceftriaxone); aminoglycosides may increase risk of nephrotoxicity

Stability Reconstituted solution (100 mg/mL) is stable for 3 days at room temperature and 10 days when refrigerated; reconstituted solution (250 mg/mL) is stable for 24 hours at room temperature and 3 days when refrigerated

Mechanism of Action Inhibits bacterial cell wall synthesis by binding to one or more of the penicillin-binding proteins; inhibits the final transpeptidation step of peptidoglycan synthesis resulting in cell wall death

Pharmacokinetics

Distribution: Widely distributed throughout the body including gallbladder, lungs, bone, bile, CSF (diffuses into the CSF at higher concentrations when the meninges are inflamed); crosses the placenta

Protein binding: 85% to 95%

Half-life:

Neonates:

1-4 days: 16 hours

9-30 days: 9 hours

Adults: 5-9 hours (with normal renal and hepatic function)

Time to peak serum concentration: I.M.: Within 1-2 hours

Elimination: Unchanged in the urine (33% to 65%) by glomerular filtration and in feces via bile

Dialysis: Not dialyzable (0% to 5%)

Usual Dosage I.M., I.V.:

Neonates:

Postnatal age ≤7 days: 50 mg/kg/day given every 24 hours

Postnatal age >7 days:

≤2000 g: 50 mg/kg/day given every 24 hours

>2000 g: 50-75 mg/kg/day given every 24 hours

Gonococcal prophylaxis: 25-50 mg/kg as a single dose (dose not to exceed 125 mg)

Gonococcal infection: 25-50 mg/kg/day (maximum dose: 125 mg) given every 24 hours for 7 days, up to 10-14 days if meningitis is documented

Note: Use cefotaxime in place of ceftriaxone in hyperbilirubinemic neonates

Infants and Children: 50-75 mg/kg/day divided every 12-24 hours

Meningitis: 80-100 mg/kg/day divided every 12-24 hours; loading dose of 75 mg/kg may be administered at the start of therapy; maximum dose: 4 g/day

Chemoprophylaxis for high-risk contacts of patients with invasive meningococcal disease:

≤12 years: I.M.: 125 mg in a single dose

>12 years: I.M.: 250 mg in a single dose

Uncomplicated gonococcal infections, sexual assault, and STD prophylaxis: I.M.: 125 mg in a single dose

Complicated gonococcal infections: I.M., I.V.:

<45 kg:

Peritonitis, arthritis, or bacteremia: 50 mg/kg/day once daily for 7 days; maximum dose: 1 g/day

Conjunctivitis: 50 mg/kg (maximum dose: 1 g) in a single dose

Meningitis or endocarditis: 50 mg/kg/day divided every 12 hours for 10-14 days (meningitis), for 28 days (endocarditis); maximum dose: 2 g/day

>45 kg:

Disseminated gonococcal infections: 1 g/day once daily for 7 days

Meningitis: 1-2 g/dose every 12 hours for 10-14 days

Endocarditis: 1-2 g/dose every 12 hours for 28 days

Conjunctivitis: I.M.: 1 g in a single dose

Chancroid: I.M.: 50 mg/kg as a single dose (maximum dose: 250 mg)

Acute epididymitis: I.M.: 250 mg in a single dose

Acute otitis media: 50 mg/kg in a single dose (maximum dose: 1 g)

Persistent or relapsing acute otitis media: 50 mg/kg once daily for 3 days (maximum dose: 1 g/day)

Adults: 1-2 g every 12-24 hours depending on the type and severity of the infection; maximum dose: 4 g/day

Dosing interval in renal impairment: No change necessary with dose ≤2 g/day

(Continued)

Ceftriaxone *(Continued)*

Administration Parenteral:

IVP: Administer over 2-4 minutes at a maximum concentration of 40 mg/mL. Rapid IVP injection over 5 minutes of a 2 g dose resulted in tachycardia, restlessness, diaphoresis, and palpitations in an adult patient

I.V. intermittent infusion: Administer over 10-30 minutes; final concentration for I.V. administration should not exceed 40 mg/mL

I.M. injection: May be diluted with SWI or 1% lidocaine to a final concentration of 250 mg/mL or may be concentrated by using the manufacturer's recommended diluent volume of 1% lidocaine with a resultant concentration of 350 mg/mL; administer I.M. injections deep into a large muscle mass

Monitoring Parameters CBC with differential, platelet count, PT, renal and hepatic function tests periodically; number and type of stools/day for diarrhea

Test Interactions False-positive urine glucose with Clinitest®; may falsely elevate serum or urinary creatinine values when a manual Jaffé method is used

Additional Information Sodium content of 1 g: 3.6 mEq

Dosage Forms

Infusion, as sodium [premixed in dextrose, frozen]: 1 g (50 mL); 2 g (50 mL)

Injection, powder for reconstitution, as sodium: 250 mg, 500 mg, 1 g, 2 g, 10 g

References

Bradley JS, Compogiannis LS, Murray WE, et al, "Pharmacokinetics and Safety of Intramuscular Injection of Concentrated Ceftriaxone in Children," *Clin Pharm*, 1992, 11(11):961-4.

Centers for Disease Control and Prevention, "2002 Guidelines for Treatment of Sexually Transmitted Diseases," *MMWR Morb Mortal Wkly Rep*, 2002, 51(RR-6):1-80.

Committee on Adolescence, American Academy of Pediatrics, "Sexual Assault and the Adolescent," *Pediatrics*, 1994, 94(5):761-5.

Dowell SF, Butler JC, Giebink GS, et al, "Acute Otitis Media: Management and Surveillance in an era of Pneumococcal Resistance--A Report From the Drug-Resistant *Streptococcus pneumoniae* Therapeutic Working Group," *Pediatr Infect Dis J*, 1999, 18(1):1-9.

Richards DM, Heel RC, Brogden RN, et al, "Ceftriaxone: A Review of Its Antibacterial Activity, Pharmacological Properties and Therapeutic Use," *Drugs*, 1984, 27(6):469-527.

Cefuroxime *(se fyoor OKS eem)*

Related Information

Carbohydrate and Alcohol Content of Liquid Medications for Use in Patients Receiving Ketogenic Diets *on page 1431*

U.S. Brand Names Ceftin®; Kefurox® [DSC]; Zinacef®

Canadian Brand Names Apo®-Cefuroxime

Therapeutic Category Antibiotic, Cephalosporin (Second Generation)

Generic Available Yes (tablet and powder for injection)

Use A second generation cephalosporin useful in infections caused by susceptible staphylococci, group B streptococci, pneumococci, *H. influenzae* (type A and B), *E. coli*, *Enterobacter*, and *Klebsiella*; treatment of susceptible infections of the upper and lower respiratory tract, otitis media, acute bacterial maxillary sinusitis, urinary tract, skin and soft tissue, bone and joint, and sepsis

Pregnancy Risk Factor B

Contraindications Hypersensitivity to cefuroxime, any component, or cephalosporins

Warnings Prolonged use may result in superinfection; patients with renal or hepatic impairment, poor nutritional state, patients previously stabilized on anticoagulant therapy, or who have received a prolonged course of antimicrobial therapy are at risk for developing a fall in prothrombin activity. Monitor prothrombin time and consider administering vitamin K if indicated. Safety and efficacy in infants <3 months of age have not been established; do not use in patients with immediate-type hypersensitivity reactions to penicillin

Precautions Use with caution and modify dosage in patients with renal impairment; use with caution in patients with history of colitis or history of penicillin hypersensitivity

Adverse Reactions

Central nervous system: Fever, headache, dizziness, vertigo, seizures

Dermatologic: Rash, pruritus, erythema multiforme, diaper rash, urticaria

Gastrointestinal: Nausea, vomiting, diarrhea, stomach cramps, GI bleeding, antibiotic-associated colitis, stomatitis

Genitourinary: Vaginitis

Hematologic: Hemolytic anemia, transient neutropenia and leukopenia, decreased hemoglobin and hematocrit, eosinophilia, increased prothrombin time

Hepatic: Transient elevation in liver enzymes, hepatitis, cholestasis

Local: Pain at injection site, thrombophlebitis

Renal: Elevated BUN and serum creatinine

Miscellaneous: Anaphylaxis

Drug Interactions Probenecid (increases serum cefuroxime concentration); aminoglycosides may increase risk of nephrotoxicity

Food Interactions Food and milk increase bioavailability and peak levels

Stability Reconstituted injectable solution (100 mg/mL) or injectable suspension (200-220 mg/mL) is stable for 24 hours at room temperature or 48 hours when refrigerated; reconstituted oral suspension can be stored in the refrigerator or at room temperature; discard after 10 days

Mechanism of Action Inhibits bacterial cell wall synthesis by binding to one or more of the penicillin-binding proteins; inhibits the final transpeptidation step of peptidoglycan synthesis resulting in cell wall death

Pharmacokinetics

Absorption: Oral: Increased when given with or shortly after food or infant formula

Distribution: Into bronchial secretions, synovial and pericardial fluid, kidneys, heart, liver, bone and bile; penetrates into CSF with inflamed meninges; crosses the placenta; excreted into breast milk

Protein binding: 33% to 50%

Bioavailability: Oral cefuroxime axetil tablets: 37% to 52%; cefuroxime axetil suspension is less bioavailable than the tablet (91% of the AUC for tablets)

Half-life:

Neonates:

≤3 days: 5.1-5.8 hours

6-14 days: 2-4.2 hours

3-4 weeks: 1-1.5 hours

Adults: 1-2 hours (prolonged in renal impairment)

Time to peak serum concentration:

Oral: 2-3 hours

I.M.: Within 15-60 minutes

Elimination: Primarily 66% to 100% as unchanged drug in urine by both glomerular filtration and tubular secretion

Dialysis: Dialyzable

Usual Dosage

I.M., I.V.:

Neonates: 50-100 mg/kg/day divided every 12 hours

Children: 75-150 mg/kg/day divided every 8 hours; maximum dose: 6 g/day

Meningitis: Not recommended (doses of 200-240 mg/kg/day divided every 6-8 hours have been used); maximum dose: 9 g/day

Adults: 750 mg to 1.5 g/dose every 8 hours

Oral: **Cefuroxime axetil film-coated tablets and oral suspension are not bioequivalent and are not substitutable on a mg/mg basis**

Infants ≥3 months and Children to 12 years:

Pharyngitis, tonsillitis: Suspension: 20 mg/kg/day (maximum dose: 500 mg/day) in 2 divided doses

Acute otitis media, acute bacterial maxillary sinusitis, impetigo:

Suspension: 30 mg/kg/day (maximum dose: 1 g/day) in 2 divided doses

Tablet: 250 mg every 12 hours

Adolescents and Adults: 250-500 mg twice daily

Uncomplicated urinary tract infection: 125-250 mg every 12 hours

Uncomplicated gonorrhea: Single 1 g dose

Early Lyme disease: 500 mg twice daily for 20 days

Dosing interval in renal impairment:

Cl_{cr} 10-20 mL/minute: Administer every 12 hours

Cl_{cr} <10 mL/minute: Administer every 24 hours

Administration

Oral: Cefuroxime axetil suspension must be administered with food; shake suspension well before use; tablets may be administered with or without food; administer with food to decrease GI upset; avoid crushing the tablet due to its bitter taste

Parenteral:

IVP: Administer over 3-5 minutes at a maximum concentration of 100 mg/mL

I.V. intermittent infusion: Administer over 15-30 minutes at a final concentration for administration ≤30 mg/mL; in fluid restricted patients, a concentration of 137 mg/mL may be administered

I.M.: I.M. injection is less painful when administered as an injectable suspension rather than a solution (see Stability), and is less painful when administered into the buttock rather than the thigh

Monitoring Parameters With prolonged therapy, monitor renal, hepatic, and hematologic function periodically; number and type of stools/day for diarrhea; and prothrombin time

Test Interactions Positive Coombs' [direct]; false-positive urine glucose with Clinitest®

Additional Information Sodium content of 1 g: 2.4 mEq

(Continued)

Cefuroxime *(Continued)*

Dosage Forms

Infusion, as **sodium** [premixed iso-osmotic solution] (Zinacef®): 750 mg (50 mL); 1.5 g (50 mL)

Injection, powder for reconstitution, as **sodium** (Kefurox® [DSC], Zinacef®): 750 mg, 1.5 g, 7.5 g

Powder for oral suspension, as **axetil** (Ceftin®): 125 mg/5 mL (100 mL); 250 mg/5 mL (50 mL, 100 mL) [contains sucrose; tutti-frutti flavor]

Tablet, film coated, as **axetil**: 250 mg

Ceftin®: 125 mg [DSC], 250 mg, 500 mg

References

de Louvois J, Mulhall A, and Hurley R, "Cefuroxime in the Treatment of Neonates," *Arch Dis Child*, 1982, 57(1):59-62.

Gooch WM 3rd, Blair E, Puopolo A, et al, "Effectiveness of Five Days of Therapy With Cefuroxime Axetil Suspension for Treatment of Acute Otitis Media," *Pediatr Infect Dis J*, 1996, 15(2):157-64.

Nelson JD, "Cefuroxime: A Cephalosporin With Unique Applicability to Pediatric Practice," *Pediatr Infect Dis*, 1983, 2(5):394-6.

Thoene DE and Johnson CE, "Pharmacotherapy of Otitis Media," *Pharmacotherapy*, 1991, 11(3):212-21.

♦ **Cefzil®** *see* Cefprozil *on page 236*

♦ **Celestoderm®-EV/2 (Can)** *see* Betamethasone *on page 169*

♦ **Celestoderm®-V (Can)** *see* Betamethasone *on page 169*

♦ **Celestone®** *see* Betamethasone *on page 169*

♦ **Celestone® Phosphate** *see* Betamethasone *on page 169*

♦ **Celestone® Soluspan®** *see* Betamethasone *on page 169*

♦ **CellCept®** *see* Mycophenolate *on page 785*

♦ **Celontin®** *see* Methsuximide *on page 740*

♦ **Cenestin (Can)** *see* Estrogens (Conjugated/Equine) *on page 459*

♦ **Cenolate®** *see* Ascorbic Acid *on page 131*

♦ **Cepacol® Maximum Strength [OTC]** *see* Dyclonine *on page 422*

♦ **Cepacol Viractin® [OTC]** *see* Tetracaine *on page 1073*

Cephalexin *(sef a LEKS in)*

Related Information

Carbohydrate and Alcohol Content of Liquid Medications for Use in Patients Receiving Ketogenic Diets *on page 1431*

Endocarditis Prophylaxis *on page 1321*

U.S. Brand Names Biocef®; Keflex®; Keftab®

Canadian Brand Names Apo®-Cephalex; Novo-Lexin®; Nu-Cephalex®

Therapeutic Category Antibiotic, Cephalosporin (First Generation)

Generic Available Yes

Use Treatment of susceptible bacterial infections, including those caused by group A beta-hemolytic *Streptococcus*, *Staphylococcus*, *Klebsiella pneumoniae*, *E. coli*, and *Proteus mirabilis*; not active against enterococci; used to treat susceptible infections of the respiratory tract, skin and skin structure, bone, genitourinary tract, and otitis media

Pregnancy Risk Factor B

Contraindications Hypersensitivity to cephalexin, any component, or cephalosporins

Warnings Prolonged use may result in GI or genitourinary superinfection; do not use in patients with immediate-type hypersensitivity reactions to penicillin

Precautions Use with caution and modify dosage in patients with renal impairment; use with caution in patients with history of colitis or history of penicillin hypersensitivity

Adverse Reactions

Central nervous system: Dizziness, headache, fatigue, fever

Dermatologic: Rash

Gastrointestinal: Nausea, vomiting, pseudomembranous colitis, diarrhea, cramps

Hematologic: Transient neutropenia, anemia, eosinophilia

Hepatic: Transient elevation in liver enzymes

Drug Interactions Probenecid increases serum concentration of cephalexin

Food Interactions Food may delay absorption

Stability Refrigerate suspension after reconstitution; discard after 14 days

Mechanism of Action Inhibits bacterial cell wall synthesis by binding to one or more of the penicillin-binding proteins; inhibits the final transpeptidation step of peptidoglycan synthesis resulting in cell wall death

Pharmacokinetics

Absorption: Delayed in young children and may be decreased up to 50% in neonates

Distribution: Into tissues and fluids including bone, pleural and synovial fluid; crosses the placenta; appears in breast milk

Protein binding: 6% to 15%

Half-life:
  Neonates: 5 hours
  Children 3-12 months: 2.5 hours
  Adults: 0.5-1.2 hours (prolonged with renal impairment)
Time to peak serum concentration: Oral: Within 60 minutes
Elimination: 80% to 100% of dose excreted as unchanged drug in urine within 8 hours
Dialysis: Moderately dialyzable (20% to 50%)

Usual Dosage Oral:
  Children: 25-100 mg/kg/day divided every 6-8 hours; maximum dose: 4 g/day
  Adults: 250-500 mg every 6 hours; maximum dose: 4 g/day
  Dosing interval in renal impairment:
    Cl_{cr} 10-40 mL/minute: Administer every 8-12 hours
    Cl_{cr} <10 mL/minute: Administer every 12-24 hours

Administration Oral: Administer on an empty stomach (ie, 1 hour prior to, or 2 hours after meals); administer with food if GI upset occurs; shake suspension well before use

Monitoring Parameters With prolonged therapy, monitor renal, hepatic, and hematologic function periodically; number and type of stools/day for diarrhea

Test Interactions False-positive urine glucose with Clinitest®; positive Coombs' [direct]; false ↑ serum or urine creatinine

Dosage Forms
  Capsule, as **monohydrate**: 250 mg, 500 mg
    Biocef®: 500 mg
    Keflex®: 250 mg, 500 mg
  Powder for oral suspension, as **monohydrate**: 125 mg/5 mL (100 mL, 200 mL); 250 mg/5 mL (100 mL, 200 mL) [mixed berry flavor]
  Tablet, as **hydrochloride** (Keftab®): 500 mg
  Tablet, film coated, as **monohydrate**: 250 mg, 500 mg

Cephalothin (sef A loe thin)

Therapeutic Category Antibiotic, Cephalosporin (First Generation)
Generic Available Yes
Use Treatment of respiratory tract, skin and skin structure, urinary tract, bone and joint infections, endocarditis, and septicemia due to susceptible gram-positive cocci (except enterococcus); some gram-negative bacilli including *E. coli*, *Proteus*, and *Klebsiella* may be susceptible; perioperative prophylaxis
Pregnancy Risk Factor B
Contraindications Hypersensitivity to cephalothin, any component, or cephalosporins
Warnings Prolonged use may result in superinfection; do not use in patients with immediate-type hypersensitivity reactions to penicillin
Precautions Use with caution in patients with a history of colitis or in patients with a history of hypersensitivity to penicillins; modify dosage in patients with renal impairment

Adverse Reactions
  Central nervous system: Dizziness, headache, fever
  Dermatologic: Rash, urticaria, pruritus
  Gastrointestinal: Nausea, vomiting, diarrhea, dyspepsia, pseudomembranous colitis
  Hematological: Hemolytic anemia, granulocytopenia, eosinophilia, thrombocytopenia, prolonged PT, bleeding
  Hepatic: Transient elevation in AST and alkaline phosphatase
  Local: Severe phlebitis (especially with doses >6 g/day for longer than 3 days), thrombophlebitis, pain and induration at injection site
  Renal: Elevated BUN and serum creatinine, nephrotoxicity

Drug Interactions Probenecid decreases renal clearance of cephalothin; aminoglycosides may increase risk of nephrotoxicity
Stability Reconstituted solution is stable for 12-24 hours at room temperature and 96 hours when refrigerated; thawed solution of the commercially available frozen cephalothin injection is stable for 12 hours at room temperature or 7 days when refrigerated
Mechanism of Action Inhibits bacterial cell wall synthesis by binding to one or more of the penicillin-binding proteins and interfering with the final transpeptidation step of peptidoglycan synthesis

Pharmacokinetics
  Distribution: Widely distributed throughout the body but with poor penetration into CSF and bile; crosses the placenta
  Protein binding: 65% to 80%
  Metabolism: 10% to 40% metabolized in the liver and kidneys to desacetylcephalothin (active metabolite)
(Continued)

Cephalothin *(Continued)*

Half-life:
Neonates <7 days: 90-120 minutes
Adults with normal renal function: 30-60 minutes (cephalothin) and 12 minutes (desacetylcephalothin)
Time to peak serum concentration: I.M.: Within 30 minutes
Elimination: 50% to 75% of a dose is excreted in the urine as unchanged drug

Usual Dosage
Neonates: I.V.:
Postnatal age ≤7 days:
≤2000 g: 40 mg/kg/day divided every 12 hours
>2000 g: 60 mg/kg/day divided every 8 hours
Postnatal age >7 days:
<1200 g: 40 mg/kg/day divided every 12 hours
1200-2000 g: 60 mg/kg/day divided every 8 hours
>2000 g: 80 mg/kg/day divided every 6 hours
Children: I.M., I.V.: 80-150 mg/kg/day divided every 4-6 hours; maximum dose: 12 g/day
Perioperative prophylaxis: I.V.: 20-30 mg/kg 30-60 minutes prior to surgery and 20-30 mg/kg every 6 hours for no more than 24 hours after surgery depending on the procedure
Adults: I.M., I.V.: 500 mg to 2 g every 4-6 hours; maximum dose: 12 g/day
Perioperative prophylaxis: I.V.: 1-2 g 30-60 minutes prior to surgery and 1-2 g every 6 hours for no more than 24 hours after surgery depending on the procedure

Dosing interval in renal impairment:
Cl_{cr} 10-50 mL/minute: Administer every 6-8 hours
Cl_{cr} <10 mL/minute: Administer every 12 hours

Administration Parenteral:
IVP: Administer over 3-5 minutes at a maximum concentration of 100 mg/mL
I.V. intermittent infusion: Administer over 30-60 minutes at a final concentration for I.V. administration ≤100 mg/mL

Monitoring Parameters Periodic renal function tests when used in combination with other nephrotoxic drugs, hepatic function tests, platelet count and CBC with differential; number and type of stools/day for diarrhea

Test Interactions False-positive urine glucose, using Clinitest®, positive Coombs' [direct], false ↑ serum or urine creatinine

Nursing Implications Monitor patient for vein irritation

Additional Information Sodium content of 1 g: 2.8 mEq

Dosage Forms
Infusion, as sodium [premixed in $D_{1.1}W$, frozen]: 2 g (50 mL)
Infusion, as sodium [premixed in $D_{3.5}W$, frozen]: 1 g (50 mL)

References
Pickering LK, O'Connor DM, Anderson D, et al, "Comparative Evaluation of Cefazolin and Cephalothin in Children," *J Pediatr*, 1974, 85(6):842-7.

Cephapirin [DSC] (sef a PYE rin)

Canadian Brand Names Cefadyl®

Therapeutic Category Antibiotic, Cephalosporin (First Generation)

Generic Available No

Use Treatment of respiratory tract, skin and skin structure, urinary tract, bone and joint infections, endocarditis and septicemia due to susceptible gram-positive cocci (except enterococcus); some gram-negative bacilli including *E. coli*, *Proteus*, and *Klebsiella*, may be susceptible; perioperative prophylaxis

Pregnancy Risk Factor B

Contraindications Hypersensitivity to cephapirin sodium, any component, or cephalosporins

Warnings Prolonged use may result in superinfection; safety and efficacy in infants <3 months of age have not been established; do not use in patients with immediate-type hypersensitivity reactions to penicillin

Precautions Use with caution in patients with a history of colitis or in patients with a history of hypersensitivity to penicillins; modify dosage in patients with renal impairment

Adverse Reactions
Central nervous system: Fever
Dermatologic: Rash, urticaria
Gastrointestinal: Diarrhea, pseudomembranous colitis
Hematologic: Neutropenia, eosinophilia, leukopenia, thrombocytopenia
Hepatic: Elevated AST, ALT, alkaline phosphatase, and bilirubin; jaundice
Local: Thrombophlebitis, pain on injection

Renal: Nephrotoxicity, acute interstitial nephritis, elevated BUN, elevated serum creatinine

Drug Interactions Probenecid decreases renal clearance of cephapirin; aminoglycosides may increase risk of nephrotoxicity

Stability Reconstituted solution is stable for 12 hours at room temperature and 10 days when refrigerated; after freezing, thawed solution is stable for 12 hours at room temperature or 10 days when refrigerated

Mechanism of Action Inhibits bacterial cell wall synthesis by binding to one or more of the penicillin-binding proteins and interfering with the final transpeptidation step of peptidoglycan synthesis

Pharmacokinetics

Distribution: Widely distributed to tissues and fluids including heart, bone, pericardial, pleural and synovial fluid; crosses the placenta; only small amounts distribute into CSF and breast milk

Protein binding: 44% to 50%

Metabolism: Partially metabolized in the liver, kidneys, and plasma to desacetylcephapirin (active metabolite)

Half-life: 21-48 minutes (adults with normal renal function); desacetylcephapirin: 26 minutes

Time to peak serum concentration: I.M.: Within 30 minutes

Elimination: 30% to 70% excreted as unchanged drug in urine

Dialysis: 23% of a dose is removed by hemodialysis

Usual Dosage I.M., I.V.:

Infants >3 months of age and Children: 40-80 mg/kg/day divided every 6 hours; maximum dose: 12 g/day

Adults: 500 mg to 1 g every 6 hours up to 12 g/day

Perioperative prophylaxis: 1-2 g 30-60 minutes prior to surgery and 1-2 g every 6 hours for no more than 24 hours after surgery depending on the procedure

Dosing interval in renal impairment:

Cl_{cr} 10-50 mL/minute: Administer every 6-8 hours

Cl_{cr} <10 mL/minute: Administer every 12 hours

Administration Parenteral:

IVP: Administer over 3-5 minutes at a maximum concentration of 100 mg/mL

I.V. intermittent infusion: Administer over 30 minutes; maximum cephapirin concentration that can be administered to fluid-restricted patients is 200 mg/mL

Monitoring Parameters Periodic renal and hepatic function tests, CBC with differential, platelet count; number and type of stools/day for diarrhea

Test Interactions False-positive urine glucose using Clinitest®; positive Coombs' [direct]; false ↑ serum or urine creatinine

Nursing Implications Monitor patient for vein irritation

Additional Information Sodium content of 1 g: 2.4 mEq

Dosage Forms Powder for injection, as sodium: 1 g [DSC]

References
Khan AJ and Pryles CV, "Clinical and Pharmacological Evaluation of Cephapirin Sodium (BL-P-1322) in Infants and Children (Cephapirin in Pediatric Patients)," *Curr Ther Res Clin Exp*, 1973, 15(4):198-204.

Cephradine (SEF ra deen)

Related Information

Carbohydrate and Alcohol Content of Liquid Medications for Use in Patients Receiving Ketogenic Diets *on page 1431*

U.S. Brand Names Velosef®

Therapeutic Category Antibiotic, Cephalosporin (First Generation)

Generic Available Yes

Use Treatment of susceptible bacterial infections, including skin and skin structure infections caused by *Streptococcus* or *Staphylococcus*; urinary tract infections caused by *Klebsiella, E. coli*, and *Proteus mirabilis*; respiratory tract infections caused by group A beta-hemolytic streptococci and *Streptococcus pneumoniae*; otitis media caused by group A beta-hemolytic streptococci, *Streptococcus pneumoniae*, or *H. influenzae*

Pregnancy Risk Factor B

Contraindications Hypersensitivity to cephradine, any component, or cephalosporins

Warnings Prolonged use may result in superinfection; do not use in patients with immediate-type hypersensitivity reaction to penicillin

Precautions Use with caution in patients with a history of penicillin hypersensitivity; reduce dose in patients with renal impairment

Adverse Reactions

Dermatologic: Rash

Gastrointestinal: Diarrhea, nausea, vomiting, pseudomembranous colitis

Genitourinary: Vaginitis

(Continued)

Cephradine *(Continued)*

Hematologic: Transient neutropenia, eosinophilia, leukopenia
Hepatic: Elevated liver enzymes, elevated bilirubin
Neuromuscular & skeletal: Arthralgia
Renal: Elevated BUN and serum creatinine

Drug Interactions Probenecid may decrease renal tubular secretion and increase cephradine serum concentrations

Food Interactions Food will decrease the rate, but not the extent of oral absorption

Stability Oral suspension: Stable for 7 days at room temperature, or 14 days at 2°C to 8°C after reconstitution

Mechanism of Action Interferes with bacterial cell wall synthesis during active replication, causing cell wall death and resultant bactericidal activity against susceptible bacteria

Pharmacokinetics

Absorption: Well absorbed from GI tract
Distribution: V_d: 0.25 L/kg; crosses the placenta; appears in breast milk
Protein binding: 6% to 20%
Half-life: Adults: 0.7-2 hours; Children: 1 hour; half-life increases with renal dysfunction
Time to peak serum concentration: Oral: Within 1-2 hours
Elimination: Excreted unchanged in the urine (80% to 90%) via glomerular filtration and tubular secretion

Usual Dosage Oral:

Infants ≥9 months and children:
Usual: 25-50 mg/kg/day in divided doses every 6-12 hours
Otitis media: 75-100 mg/kg/day in divided doses every 6-12 hours
Maximum dose: 4 g/day
Adults: Oral: 250-500 mg every 6-12 hours

Dosing adjustment in renal impairment:

Cl_{cr} 10-50 mL/minute: Administer 50% of dose given at normal interval
Cl_{cr} <10 mL/minute: Administer 25% of dose given at normal interval
or
Cl_{cr} 25-50 mL/minute: Administer normal dose every 12 hours
Cl_{cr} 10-25 mL/minute: Administer normal dose every 24 hours
Cl_{cr} <10 mL/minute: Administer normal dose every 36 hours

Administration Oral: May be administered without regard to food; shake suspension well before use

Monitoring Parameters Periodic renal and hepatic function tests; number and type of stools/day for diarrhea; resolution of infection

Test Interactions False-positive Coombs' test; may falsely elevate creatinine values when Jaffé reaction is used; may cause false-positive results in urine glucose tests using cupric sulfate (Benedict's solution, Clinitest®)

Patient Information Report persistent diarrhea; entire course of medication (eg, 10-14 days) should be taken to ensure eradication of organism

Additional Information Efficacy not established for twice daily dosing in infants <9 months of age; parenteral product no longer available in the United States

Dosage Forms

Capsule: 250 mg, 500 mg
Powder for oral suspension: 250 mg/5 mL (100 mL, 200 mL) [fruit flavor]

References

Donowitz GR and Mandell GL, "Drug Therapy. Beta-Lactam Antibiotics (1)," *N Engl J Med*, 1988, 318(7):419-26.
Donowitz GR and Mandell GL, "Drug Therapy. Beta-Lactam Antibiotics (2)," *N Engl J Med*, 1988, 318(8):490-500.
Gustaferro CA and Steckelberg JM, "Cephalosporin Antimicrobial Agents and Related Compounds," *Mayo Clin Proc*, 1991, 66(10):1064-73.
Smith GH, "Oral Cephalosporins in Perspective," *DICP*, 1990, 24(1):45-51.

♦ **Ceta-Plus**® *see* Hydrocodone and Acetaminophen *on page 571*

Cetirizine (se TI ra zeen)
U.S. Brand Names Zyrtec®
Canadian Brand Names Apo®-Cetirizine; Reactine™
Synonyms P-071; UCB-P071
Therapeutic Category Antihistamine
Generic Available No
Use Treatment of perennial and seasonal allergic rhinitis; chronic idiopathic urticaria
Pregnancy Risk Factor B
Contraindications Hypersensitivity to cetirizine, hydroxyzine, or any component
Warnings Doses >10 mg/day may cause significant drowsiness
Precautions Use with caution in patients with hepatic or renal dysfunction
Adverse Reactions
 Cardiovascular: Palpitations, tachycardia, hypertension
 Central nervous system: Headache, drowsiness, somnolence, fatigue, dizziness, depression, confusion, vertigo, ataxia, syncope
 Dermatologic: Rash, photosensitivity, pruritus
 Gastrointestinal: Diarrhea, flatulence, constipation, xerostomia, dyspepsia, abdominal pain, pharyngitis, taste loss, taste perversion, anorexia
 Genitourinary: Dysuria, cystitis, polyuria, urinary incontinence, dysmenorrhea, vaginitis
 Hepatic: Transient hepatic enzyme elevation
 Neuromuscular & skeletal: Paresthesias, hyperkinesia, hypertonia, tremor, leg cramps
 Otic: Tinnitus, ototoxicity, earache (<2%)
 Respiratory: Cough, epistaxis, bronchospasm
Drug Interactions Cytochrome P450 isoenzyme CYP3A4 substrate
 Increased cetirizine toxicity: CNS depressants, anticholinergics; theophylline may decrease cetirizine clearance with potential increased toxicity
Stability Store at room temperature; protect syrup from light
Mechanism of Action Cetirizine, a metabolite of hydroxyzine, competes with histamine for H_1-receptor sites on effector cells in the GI tract, blood vessels, and respiratory tract
Pharmacodynamics
 Onset of action: 20-60 minutes
 Duration: 24 hours
Pharmacokinetics
 Absorption: Well absorbed from the GI tract
 Distribution: V_d:
  Children: 0.7 L/kg
  Adults: 0.5-0.8 L/kg
 Protein binding: 93%
 Metabolism: Exact fate is unknown, limited hepatic metabolism
 Half-life:
  Children: 6.2 hours
  Adults: 7.4-9 hours
  Adults with mild-moderate renal failure: 19-21 hours
 Time to peak serum concentration: 1 hour
 Elimination: 60% to 70% excreted unchanged in urine
 Dialysis: <10% removed during hemodialysis
Usual Dosage Oral:
 Children 6-12 months: 2.5 mg once daily
 Children 12-23 months: Initial: 2.5 mg once daily; dosage may be increased to 2.5 mg twice daily
 Children 2-5 years: 2.5 mg/day; may be increased to a maximum of 5 mg/day given either as a single dose or divided into 2 doses
 Children ≥6 years to Adults: 5-10 mg/day as a single dose or divided into 2 doses
 Dosage adjustment in renal or hepatic impairment:
  Children <6 years: Cetirizine use not recommended
  Children 6-11 years: <2.5 mg once daily
  Children ≥12 and Adults:
   Cl_{cr} 11-31 mL/minute, hemodialysis, or hepatic impairment: 5 mg once daily
   Cl_{cr} <11 mL/minute, not on dialysis: Cetirizine use not recommended
Administration Oral: Administer without regard to food
Patient Information May cause drowsiness and impair ability to perform activities requiring mental alertness or physical coordination; may cause dry mouth. May cause photosensitivity reactions (eg, exposure to sunlight may cause severe sunburn, skin rash, redness, or itching); avoid exposure to sunlight and artificial light sources
(Continued)

Cetirizine *(Continued)*

(sunlamps, tanning booth/bed); wear protective clothing, wide-brimmed hats, sunglasses, and lip sunscreen (SPF ≥15); use a sunscreen [broad-spectrum sunscreen or physical sunscreen (preferred) or sunblock with SPF ≥15]; contact physician if reaction occurs.

Dosage Forms

Syrup, as hydrochloride: 5 mg/5 mL (120 mL, 480 mL) [banana-grape flavor]

Tablet, film-coated, as hydrochloride: 5 mg, 10 mg

- ◆ **Cevi-Bid® [OTC]** *see* Ascorbic Acid *on page 131*
- ◆ **CG** *see* Chorionic Gonadotropin *on page 269*
- ◆ **C-Gram [OTC]** *see* Ascorbic Acid *on page 131*
- ◆ **Charcadole® (Can)** *see* Charcoal *on page 250*
- ◆ **Charcadole®, Aqueous (Can)** *see* Charcoal *on page 250*
- ◆ **Charcadole® TFS (Can)** *see* Charcoal *on page 250*
- ◆ **CharcoAid G® [OTC]** *see* Charcoal *on page 250*

Charcoal *(CHAR kole)*

U.S. Brand Names Actidose-Aqua® [OTC]; Actidose® With Sorbitol [OTC]; CharcoAid G® [OTC]; Charcoal Plus® DS [OTC]; Charcocaps® [OTC]; EZ-Char™ [OTC]; Kerr Insta-Char® [OTC]; Liqui-Char® [OTC]

Canadian Brand Names Charcadole®; Charcadole®, Aqueous; Charcadole® TFS

Synonyms Activated Carbon; Activated Charcoal; Adsorbent Charcoal; Liquid Antidote; Medicinal Carbon; Medicinal Charcoal

Therapeutic Category Antidiarrheal; Antidote, Adsorbent; Antiflatulent

Generic Available Yes

Use Emergency treatment in poisoning by drugs and chemicals (see Additional Information); repetitive doses for GI dialysis in drug overdose to enhance the elimination of certain drugs (eg, theophylline, phenobarbital, carbamazepine, dapsone, quinine) and in uremia to adsorb various waste products

Pregnancy Risk Factor C

Contraindications Patients with an unprotected airway (eg, depressed CNS state without endotracheal intubation); patients at increased risk and severity of aspiration (eg, ingestion of hydrocarbon with a high potential for aspiration); patients at risk of GI perforation or hemorrhage due to medical conditions, recent surgery, or other pathology; **Note:** Ingestion of a corrosive (caustic) substance is **not** a contraindication if charcoal is used for coingested systemic toxin. Charcoal is not effective for cyanide, mineral acids, caustic alkalis, organic solvents, iron, ethanol, methanol or lithium poisonings; do not use charcoal with sorbitol in patients with fructose intolerance; charcoal with sorbitol is not recommended in children <1 year of age

Warnings If charcoal in sorbitol is administered, doses should be limited to prevent excessive fluid and electrolyte losses

Precautions When using ipecac with charcoal, induce vomiting with ipecac before administering activated charcoal since charcoal adsorbs ipecac syrup; charcoal may cause vomiting which is hazardous in petroleum distillate and caustic ingestions; charcoal (especially in multiple doses) may adsorb maintenance medications and place the patient at risk for exacerbation of concomitant disorders

Adverse Reactions

Gastrointestinal: Vomiting (**Note:** Use of charcoal with sorbitol may increase rate of emesis), constipation, intestinal obstruction, black stools; diarrhea if product contains sorbitol

Ocular: Corneal abrasions if spilled into eyes

Miscellaneous: Aspiration may cause tracheal obstruction in infants, but usually not a major problem in adults; aspiration pneumonitis, bronchiolitis obliterans, and ARDS have been reported following aspiration of charcoal; however, these problems may be due to the aspiration of gastric contents and not charcoal per se

Food Interactions Milk, ice cream, sherbet, or marmalade may reduce charcoal's effectiveness; chocolate or fruit syrup do not appear to reduce efficacy

Stability Adsorbs gases from air; store in closed container

Mechanism of Action Adsorbs toxic substances or irritants, thus inhibiting GI absorption; for select drugs, increases drug clearance by interfering with enterohepatic recycling or causing dialysis across intestinal membrane; adsorbs intestinal gas; the addition of sorbitol results in hyperosmotic laxative action causing catharsis

Pharmacodynamics In studies using adult human volunteers: Mean **reduction** in drug absorption following a single dose of activated charcoal:

All size doses of activated charcoal:

Given within 30 minutes after ingestion: 69.1% reduction

Given at 60 minutes after ingestion: 34.4% reduction

50 g activated charcoal:
Given within 30 minutes after ingestion: 88.6% reduction
Given at 60 minutes after ingestion: 37.3% reduction

Pharmacokinetics
Absorption: Not absorbed from the GI tract
Metabolism: Not metabolized
Elimination: Excreted as charcoal in feces

Usual Dosage Oral:
Acute poisoning:
Single dose: Charcoal with sorbitol (**Note:** The use of repeated oral charcoal with sorbitol doses is not recommended):
Infants <1 year: Not recommended
Children 1-12 years: 1-2 g/kg or 25-50 g or approximately 5-10 times the weight of the ingested poison on a gram-to-gram basis; 1 g adsorbs 100-1000 mg of poison; in young children sorbitol should be repeated **no more** than 1-2 times/day
Adolescents and Adults: 30-100 g
Single dose: Charcoal in water (a cathartic such as sorbitol should be added in appropriate doses):
Infants <1 year: 1 g/kg
Children 1-12 years: 1-2 g/kg or 25-50 g
Adolescents and Adults: 30-100 g or 1-2 g/kg
Multiple dose: Charcoal in water (doses are repeated until clinical observations of toxicity subside and serum drug concentrations have returned to a subtherapeutic range or until the development of absent bowel sounds or ileus; use only one dose of cathartic daily):
Infants <1 year: 1 g/kg every 4-6 hours
Children 1-12 years: 1-2 g/kg or 15-30 g every 2-6 hours
Adolescents and Adults: 25-60 g or 1-2 g/kg every 2-6 hours
Gastric dialysis: Adults: 20-50 g every 6 hours for 1-2 days

Administration Oral: Administer as soon as possible after ingestion, preferably within 1 hour for greatest effect; shake well before use; do not mix with milk, ice cream, sherbet, or marmalade; may be mixed with chocolate or fruit syrup to increase palatability; instruct patient to drink slowly, rapid administration may increase frequency of vomiting; if patient has persistent vomiting, multiple doses may be administered as a continuous enteral infusion

Monitoring Parameters Fluid status, sorbitol intake, number of stools, electrolytes if increase in stools or diarrhea occurs; continually assess for active bowel sounds in patients receiving multiple dose activated charcoal

Patient Information Charcoal causes the stools to turn black

Nursing Implications Charcoal slurries that are too concentrated may clog airways, if aspirated

Additional Information 5-6 tablespoonfuls of activated charcoal powder is approximately equal to 30 g; minimum dilution of 240 mL water per 20-30 g activated charcoal should be mixed as an aqueous slurry; multiple dose activated charcoal has been shown to be effective in increasing the elimination of certain drugs (carbamazepine, theophylline, phenobarbital) even after these drugs have been absorbed

The Position Statement on single-dose activated charcoal by The American Academy of Clinical Toxicology and The European Association of Poisons Centres and Clinical Toxicologists (AACT and EAPCCT, 1997) does not advocate **routine** use of single dose activated charcoal in the treatment of poisoned patients; scientific literature supports the use of activated charcoal within 1 hour of toxin ingestion, when it will be more likely to produce benefit. Therefore, this publication states that activated charcoal may be considered up to 1 hour following ingestion of a potentially toxic amount of poison; the use of activated charcoal may be considered greater than 1 hour following ingestion, but there are no studies to support or exclude its use. Furthermore, based on current literature, the routine administration of a cathartic with activated charcoal is not recommended; when cathartics are used, only a single dose should be administered so as to decrease adverse effects (AACT and EAPCCT, 1997a).

Dosage Forms
Capsule, activated (Charcocaps®): 260 mg
Granules, activated (CharcoAid® G): 15 g (120 mL)
Liquid, activated, aqueous base:
Actidose-Aqua®: 15 g (72 mL); 25 g (120 mL); 50 g (240 mL)
Kerr Insta-Char®: 25 g (120 mL) [cherry flavor]; 50 g (240 mL) [cherry or unflavored]
Liqui-Char®: 15 g (75 mL); 25 g (120 mL); 30 g (120 mL) [DSC]; 50 g (240 mL)
Liquid, activated, with sorbitol:
Actidose® With Sorbitol, Liqui-Char®: 25 g (120 mL); 50 g (240 mL)
(Continued)

Charcoal *(Continued)*

Kerr Insta-Char®: 25 g (120 mL); 50 g (240 mL) [cherry flavor]
Pellets for suspension, activated (EZ-Char™): 25 g
Powder for suspension, activated: 125 g, 500 g, 2500 g
Tablets, enteric coated, activated (Charcoal Plus® DS): 250 mg

References

Burns MM, "Activated Charcoal as the Sole Intervention for Treatment After Childhood Poisoning," *Curr Opin Pediatr*, 2000, 12(2):166-71.

Farley TA, "Severe Hypernatremic Dehydration After Use of an Activated Charcoal-Sorbitol Suspension," *J Pediatr*, 1986, 109(4):719-22.

"Position Statement and Practice Guidelines on the Use of Multi-dose Activated Charcoal in the Treatment of Acute Poisoning. American Academy of Clinical Toxicology; European Association of Poisons Centres and Clinical Toxicologists," *J Toxicol Clin Toxicol*, 1999, 37(6):731-51.

"Position Statement: Cathartics. American Academy of Clinical Toxicology; European Association of Poisons Centres and Clinical Toxicologists," *J Toxicol Clin Toxicol*, 1997a, 35(7):743-52.

"Position Statement: Single-Dose Activated Charcoal. American Academy of Clinical Toxicology; European Association of Poisons Centres and Clinical Toxicologists," *J Toxicol Clin Toxicol*, 1997, 35(7):721-41.

Shannon M, "Ingestion of Toxic Substances by Children," *N Engl J Med*, 2000, 342(3):186-91.

♦ **Charcoal Plus® DS [OTC]** *see* Charcoal *on page 250*
♦ **Charcocaps® [OTC]** *see* Charcoal *on page 250*
♦ **Chemet®** *see* Succimer *on page 1043*
♦ **Cheracol®** *see* Guaifenesin and Codeine *on page 551*
♦ **Cheracol D® [OTC]** *see* Guaifenesin and Dextromethorphan *on page 553*
♦ **Cheracol® Plus [OTC]** *see* Guaifenesin and Dextromethorphan *on page 553*
♦ **Chiggerex® [OTC]** *see* Benzocaine *on page 163*
♦ **Chiggertox® [OTC]** *see* Benzocaine *on page 163*
♦ **Chloral** *see* Chloral Hydrate *on page 252*

Chloral Hydrate *(KLOR al HYE drate)*

Related Information

Carbohydrate and Alcohol Content of Liquid Medications for Use in Patients Receiving Ketogenic Diets *on page 1431*

Preprocedure Sedatives in Children *on page 1367*

U.S. Brand Names Aquachloral® Supprettes®; Somnote™

Canadian Brand Names PMS-Chloral Hydrate

Synonyms Chloral; Hydrated Chloral; Trichloroacetaldehyde Monohydrate

Therapeutic Category Hypnotic; Sedative

Generic Available Yes (syrup)

Use Short-term sedative and hypnotic (<2 weeks), sedative/hypnotic prior to nonpainful therapeutic or diagnostic procedures (eg, EEG, CT scan, MRI, ophthalmic exam, dental procedure)

Restrictions C-IV

Pregnancy Risk Factor C

Contraindications Hypersensitivity to chloral hydrate or any component (see Warnings); hepatic or renal impairment; severe cardiac disease. Oral forms are also contraindicated in patients with gastritis, esophagitis, or gastric or duodenal ulcers.

Warnings Deaths and permanent neurologic injury from respiratory compromise have been reported in children sedated with chloral hydrate; respiratory obstruction may occur in children with tonsillar and adenoidal hypertrophy, obstructive sleep apnea, and Leigh's encephalopathy, and in ASA class III children; depressed levels of consciousness may occur; chloral hydrate should **not** be administered for sedation by nonmedical personnel or in a nonsupervised medical environment; sedation with chloral hydrate requires careful patient monitoring (see Monitoring Parameters) (Cote, 2000); animal studies suggest that chloral hydrate may depress the genioglossus muscle and other airway-maintaining muscles in patients who are already at risk for life-threatening airway obstruction (eg, obstructive sleep apnea); alternative sedative agents should be considered for these patients (see Hershenson, 1984).

Trichloroethanol (TCE), an active metabolite of chloral hydrate, is a carcinogen in mice; there is no data in humans. The 325 mg suppositories contain tartrazine which may cause allergic reactions in susceptible individuals. Syrup contains sodium benzoate; benzoic acid (benzoate) is a metabolite of benzyl alcohol; large amounts of benzyl alcohol (≥99 mg/kg/day) have been associated with a potentially fatal toxicity ("gasping syndrome") in neonates; the "gasping syndrome" consists of metabolic acidosis, respiratory distress, gasping respirations, CNS dysfunction (including convulsions, intracranial hemorrhage), hypotension and cardiovascular collapse; use chloral hydrate products containing sodium benzoate with caution in neonates; *in vitro* and animal studies have shown that benzoate displaces bilirubin from protein binding sites

Precautions Use with caution in neonates, drug and metabolites may accumulate with repeated use; prolonged use in neonates is associated with direct hyperbilirubinemia [active metabolite (TCE) competes with bilirubin for glucuronide conjugation in the liver]; use with caution in patients with porphyria. Tolerance to hypnotic effect develops, therefore, not recommended for use >2 weeks; taper dosage to avoid withdrawal with prolonged use. Avoid use in patients with moderate to severe renal failure (Cl_{cr} <50 mL/minute).

Adverse Reactions

Central nervous system: Disorientation, sedation, excitement (paradoxical), dizziness, fever, headache, ataxia

Dermatologic: Rash, urticaria

Gastrointestinal: Gastric irritation, nausea, vomiting, diarrhea, flatulence

Hematologic: Leukopenia, eosinophilia

Respiratory: Respiratory depression when combined with other sedatives or narcotics

Miscellaneous: Physical and psychological dependence with prolonged use

Drug Interactions May potentiate effects of warfarin, CNS depressants, alcohol; vasodilation reaction (flushing, tachycardia, etc) may occur with concurrent use of alcohol; concomitant use of furosemide (I.V.) may result in flushing, sweating, and blood pressure changes; chloral hydrate may increase the conversion of cyclophosphamide and ifosfamide to active metabolites and may increase toxicity

Stability Sensitive to light; exposure to air causes volatilization; store in light-resistant, airtight container at room temperature; do not refrigerate

Mechanism of Action Central nervous system depressant effects are primarily due to its active metabolite trichloroethanol, mechanism unknown; in neonates, chloral hydrate itself may play a role in the immediate sedative effects; **Note:** Chloral hydrate does not interfere with EEG results (unlike barbiturates and benzodiazepines)

Pharmacodynamics

Onset of action: 10-20 minutes

Maximum effect: Within 30-60 minutes

Duration: 4-8 hours

Pharmacokinetics

Absorption: Oral, rectal: Well absorbed

Distribution: Crosses the placenta; distributes to breast milk

Protein binding: Trichloroethanol: 35% to 40%; trichloroacetic acid: ~94% (may compete with bilirubin for albumin binding sites)

Metabolism: Rapidly metabolized by alcohol dehydrogenase to trichloroethanol (active metabolite); trichloroethanol undergoes glucuronidation in the liver; variable amounts of chloral hydrate and trichloroethanol are metabolized in liver and kidney to trichloroacetic acid (inactive)

Half-life:

Chloral hydrate: Infants: 1 hour

Trichloroethanol (active metabolite):

Neonates: Range: 8.5-66 hours

Half-life decreases with increasing postconceptional age (PCA):

Preterm infants (PCA 31-37 weeks): Mean half-life: 40 hours

Term infants (PCA 38-42 weeks): Mean half-life: 28 hours

Older children (PCA 57-708 weeks): Mean half-life: 10 hours

Adults: 8-11 hours

Trichloroacetic acid: Adults: 67.2 hours

Elimination: Metabolites excreted in urine; small amounts excreted in feces via bile

Dialysis: Dialyzable (50% to 100%)

Usual Dosage Oral, rectal:

Neonates: 25 mg/kg/dose for sedation prior to a procedure; **Note:** Repeat doses should be used with great caution, as drug and metabolites accumulate with repeated use; toxicity has been reported after 3 days in a preterm neonate and after 7 days in a term neonate receiving chloral hydrate 40-50 mg/kg every 6 hours

Infants and Children:

Sedation, anxiety: 25-50 mg/kg/day divided every 6-8 hours, maximum dose: 500 mg/dose

Prior to EEG: 25-50 mg/kg/dose 30-60 minutes prior to EEG; may repeat in 30 minutes to a total maximum of 100 mg/kg or 1 g total for infants and 2 g total for children

Hypnotic: 50 mg/kg; maximum dose: 2 g/dose/day

Sedation, nonpainful procedure: 50-75 mg/kg/dose 30-60 minutes prior to procedure; may repeat 30 minutes after initial dose if needed, to a total maximum dose of 120 mg/kg or 1 g total for infants and 2 g total for children

Adults:

Sedation, anxiety: 250 mg 3 times/day

Hypnotic: 500-1000 mg at bedtime or 30 minutes prior to procedure, not to exceed 2 g/24 hours

(Continued)

Chloral Hydrate *(Continued)*

Dosing adjustment in renal impairment:
Cl_{cr} ≥50 mL/minute: No dosage adjustment needed
Cl_{cr} <50 mL/minute: Avoid use

Administration Oral: Minimize unpleasant taste and gastric irritation by administering with water, infant formula, fruit juice, or ginger ale; do not crush capsule, contains drug in liquid form with unpleasant taste

Monitoring Parameters Level of sedation; vital signs and O_2 saturation with doses used for sedation prior to procedure

Test Interactions False-positive urine glucose using Clinitest® method; may interfere with fluorometric urine catecholamine and urinary 17-hydroxycorticosteroid tests

Patient Information May cause drowsiness and impair ability to perform activities requiring mental alertness or physical coordination; avoid alcohol and other CNS depressants; may be habit-forming; avoid abrupt discontinuation after prolonged use

Nursing Implications May cause irritation of skin and mucous membranes

Additional Information Not an analgesic; osmolality of 500 mg/5 mL syrup is approximately 3500 mOsm/kg

Dosage Forms

Capsule (Somnote™): 500 mg

Suppository, rectal (Aquachloral® Supprettes®): 325 mg [contains tartrazine]; 650 mg

Syrup: 500 mg/5 mL (480 mL) [contains <0.4% alcohol and sodium benzoate; orange flavor]

References

American Academy of Pediatrics, Committee on Drugs and Committee on Environmental Health, "Use of Chloral Hydrate for Sedation in Children," *Pediatrics*, 1993, 92(3):471-3.

Buck ML, "Chloral Hydrate Use During Infancy," *Neonatal Pharmacology Quarterly*, 1992, 1(1):31-7.

Cote CJ, Karl HW, Notterman DA, et al, "Adverse Sedation Events in Pediatrics: Analysis of Medications Used for Sedation," *Pediatrics*, 2000, 106(4):633-44.

Hershenson M, Brouillette RT, Olsen E, et al, "The Effect of Chloral Hydrate on Genioglossus and Diaphragmatic Activity," *Pediatr Res*, 1984, 18(6):516-9.

Mayers DJ, Hindmarsh KW, Gorecki DK, et al, "Sedative/Hypnotic Effects of Chloral Hydrate in the Neonate: Trichloroethanol or Parent Drug?" *Dev Pharmacol Ther*, 1992, 19(2-3):141-6.

Mayers DJ, Hindmarsh KW, Sankaran K, et al, "Chloral Hydrate Disposition Following Single-Dose Administration to Critically Ill Neonates and Children," *Dev Pharmacol Ther*, 1991, 16(2):71-7.

Steinberg AD, "Should Chloral Hydrate be Banned?" *Pediatrics*, 1993, 92(3)442-6.

Chlorambucil *(klor AM byoo sil)*

Related Information

Emetogenic Potential of Single Chemotherapeutic Agents *on page 1286*

U.S. Brand Names Leukeran®

Therapeutic Category Antineoplastic Agent, Alkylating Agent (Nitrogen Mustard)

Generic Available No

Use Treatment of chronic lymphocytic leukemia (CLL), Hodgkin's and non-Hodgkin's lymphoma; breast and ovarian carcinoma, testicular carcinoma, choriocarcinoma; Waldenström's macroglobulinemia, and nephrotic syndrome unresponsive to conventional therapy

Pregnancy Risk Factor D

Contraindications Hypersensitivity to chlorambucil or any component; cross hypersensitivity (skin rash) may occur with other alkylating agents; previous resistance

Warnings The FDA currently recommends that procedures for proper handling and disposal of antineoplastic agents be considered. Chlorambucil can severely suppress bone marrow function; affects human fertility; carcinogenic in humans and probably mutagenic and teratogenic as well; chromosomal damage has been documented; secondary AML may be associated with chronic therapy.

Precautions Use with caution in patients with seizure disorder and bone marrow suppression; children with nephrotic syndrome may have an increased risk of seizures; reduce initial dosage if patient has received radiation therapy, myelosuppressive drugs or has a depressed baseline leukocyte or platelet count within the previous 4 weeks

Adverse Reactions

Central nervous system: Seizures, fever, agitation, irritability, hyperactivity, confusion, ataxia, hallucinations

Dermatologic: Rash, pruritus, erythema multiforme, toxic epidermal necrolysis, urticaria, angioneurotic edema

Endocrine & metabolic: Hyperuricemia, menstrual cramps, amenorrhea

Gastrointestinal: Nausea, vomiting, abdominal pain, stomatitis, diarrhea

Genitourinary: Oligospermia, azoospermia

Hematologic: Leukopenia, thrombocytopenia, anemia, lymphocytopenia, neutropenia

Hepatic: Hepatotoxicity, jaundice

Neuromuscular & skeletal: Tremor, muscular twitching, weakness, myoclonia, peripheral neuropathy

Respiratory: Pulmonary fibrosis, interstitial pneumonia

Drug Interactions Phenobarbital (possible increased chlorambucil toxicity)

Food Interactions Avoid acidic foods, hot foods, and spices; increased bioavailability when administered with food

Mechanism of Action Interferes with DNA replication and RNA transcription by alkylation and cross-linking the strands of DNA; immunosuppressive activity due to suppression of lymphocytes

Pharmacokinetics

Absorption: Oral: 70% to 80% from GI tract

Distribution: To liver, ascitic fluid, fat; extensively bound to plasma and tissue proteins; crosses the placenta

Protein binding: ~99%

Metabolism: In the liver to an active metabolite, phenylacetic acid mustard

Bioavailability: 56% to 100% (increased when taken with food)

Half-life: Chlorambucil: 1.5 hours; phenylacetic acid mustard: 2.5 hours

Time to peak serum concentration: Within 1 hour

Elimination: 60% excreted in urine within 24 hours principally as metabolites; <1% excreted as unchanged drug in urine

Dialysis: Probably not dialyzable

Usual Dosage Oral (refer to individual protocols):

Children:

General short courses: 0.1-0.2 mg/kg/day or 4.5 mg/m²/day once daily for 3-6 weeks for remission induction (usual: 4-10 mg/day); maintenance therapy: 0.03-0.1 mg/kg/day (usual: 2-4 mg/day)

Nephrotic syndrome: 0.1-0.2 mg/kg/day every day for 5-12 weeks with low dose prednisone

CLL:

Biweekly regimen: Initial: 0.4 mg/kg/dose every 2 weeks; increase dose by 0.1 mg/kg every 2 weeks until a response occurs and/or myelosuppression occurs

Monthly regimen: Initial: 0.4 mg/kg every 4 weeks, increase dose by 0.2 mg/kg every 4 weeks until a response occurs and/or myelosuppression occurs

Malignant lymphomas:

Non-Hodgkin's lymphoma: 0.1 mg/kg/day

Hodgkin's: 0.2 mg/kg/day

Adults: 0.1-0.2 mg/kg/day or 3-6 mg/m²/day once daily for 3-6 weeks, then adjust dose on basis of blood counts

Administration Oral: Administer with food; do not administer with acidic foods, hot foods, and spices

Monitoring Parameters Liver function tests, CBC with differential, hemoglobin, leukocyte and platelet counts, serum uric acid

Patient Information Notify physician if fever, sore throat, skin rash, seizures, amenorrhea, unusual lumps/masses, or bleeding occurs; avoid acidic foods, hot foods, and spices

Additional Information Myelosuppressive effects:

WBC: Moderate

Platelets: Moderate

Onset (days): 7

Nadir (days): 14-21

Dosage Forms Tablet, sugar coated: 2 mg

Extemporaneous Preparations A 2 mg/mL suspension was stable for 7 days when refrigerated and compounded as follows: Pulverize sixty 2 mg tablets; levigate with a small amount of glycerin; add 20 mL Cologel® and levigate until a uniform mixture is obtained; add a 2:1 simple syrup/cherry syrup mixture to make a total volume of 60 mL; label "refrigerate" and "shake well before use"

Dressman JB and Poust RI, "Stability of Allopurinol and of Five Antineoplastics in Suspension," *Am J Hosp Pharm*, 1983, 40(4):616-8.

References

Baluarte HJ, Hiner L, and Gruskin AB, "Chlorambucil Dosage in Frequently Relapsing Nephrotic Syndrome: A Controlled Clinical Trial," *J Pediatr*, 1978, 92(2):295-8.

Williams SA, Makker SP, and Grupe WE, "Seizures: A Significant Side Effect of Chlorambucil Therapy in Children," *J Pediatr*, 1978, 93(3):516-8.

Chloramphenicol (klor am FEN i kole)

Related Information

Blood Level Sampling Time Guidelines *on page 1386*

Drugs and Breast-Feeding *on page 1404*

U.S. Brand Names Chloromycetin®; Chloromycetin® Sodium Succinate; Chloroptic®

Canadian Brand Names Diochloram®; Pentamycetin®

(Continued)

Chloramphenicol *(Continued)*

Therapeutic Category Antibacterial, Otic; Antibiotic, Ophthalmic; Antibiotic, Otic; Antibiotic, Miscellaneous

Generic Available Yes

Use Treatment of serious infections due to organisms resistant to other less toxic antibiotics or when its penetrability into the site of infection is clinically superior to other antibiotics to which the organism is sensitive; useful in infections caused by *Bacteroides*, *H. influenzae*, *Neisseria meningitidis*, *S. pneumoniae*, *Salmonella*, and *Rickettsia*

Pregnancy Risk Factor C

Contraindications Hypersensitivity to chloramphenicol or any component

Warnings Serious and fatal blood dyscrasias have occurred after both short-term and prolonged therapy; should not be used when less potentially toxic agents are effective; prolonged use may result in superinfection; breast-feeding is not recommended

Precautions Use with caution in patients with G-6-PD deficiency, impaired renal or hepatic function and in neonates; monitor serum concentrations and CBC in all patients; reduce dose in patients with hepatic and renal impairment

Adverse Reactions

Cardiovascular: Cardiotoxicity (left ventricular dysfunction), gray baby syndrome (see Additional Information)

Central nervous system: Nightmares, headache

Dermatologic: Rash

Gastrointestinal: Diarrhea, stomatitis, enterocolitis, vomiting, nausea

Hematologic: Bone marrow suppression, aplastic anemia, neutropenia, thrombocytopenia, hemolysis in patients with G-6-PD deficiency, anemia (see Additional Information)

Hepatic: Hepatitis-pancytopenia syndrome

Neuromuscular & skeletal: Peripheral neuropathy

Ocular: Optic neuritis

Miscellaneous: Anaphylaxis

Drug Interactions Cytochrome P450 isoenzyme CYP2C9 inhibitor

Chloramphenicol inhibits the metabolism of chlorpropamide, phenytoin, cyclosporine, tacrolimus, oral anticoagulants; phenobarbital and rifampin may decrease concentration of chloramphenicol; phenytoin may increase chloramphenicol concentration

Food Interactions May decrease intestinal absorption of vitamin B_{12}; may have increased dietary need for riboflavin, pyridoxine, and vitamin B_{12}

Stability Store ophthalmic solution in the refrigerator; reconstituted parenteral solution (100 mg/mL) is stable for 30 days at room temperature

Mechanism of Action Reversibly binds to 50S ribosomal subunits of susceptible organisms preventing amino acids from being transferred to growing peptide chains thus inhibiting protein synthesis

Pharmacokinetics

Distribution: Readily crosses the placenta; appears in breast milk; distributes to most tissues and body fluids; good CSF and brain penetration

CSF concentration with uninflamed meninges: 21% to 50% of plasma concentration

CSF concentration with inflamed meninges: 45% to 89% of plasma concentration

Protein binding: 60%

Metabolism: Extensive in the liver (90%) to inactive metabolites, principally by glucuronidation; chloramphenicol sodium succinate must be hydrolyzed by esterases to active base.

Half-life:

Neonates:

1-2 days: 24 hours

10-16 days: 10 hours

Adults: 1.6-3.3 hours (prolonged with hepatic insufficiency)

Elimination: 5% to 15% excreted as unchanged drug in urine and 4% excreted in bile; in neonates, 6% to 80% of the dose may be excreted unchanged in urine

Dialysis: Slightly dialyzable (5% to 20%)

Usual Dosage

Neonates: Initial loading dose: I.V. (I.M. administration is not recommended): 20 mg/kg (the first maintenance dose should be given 12 hours after the loading dose)

Maintenance dose: Postnatal age:

≤7 days: 25 mg/kg/day once every 24 hours

>7 days, ≤2000 g: 25 mg/kg/day once every 24 hours

>7 days, >2000 g: 50 mg/kg/day divided every 12 hours

Meningitis: I.V.: Infants and Children: Maintenance dose: 75-100 mg/kg/day divided every 6 hours

Other infections: I.V.:

Infants and Children: 50-75 mg/kg/day divided every 6 hours; maximum daily dose: 4 g/day

Adults: 50 mg/kg/day in divided doses every 6 hours; maximum daily dose: 4 g/day

Dosing adjustment in renal and/or hepatic impairment: Dose reduction should be based upon serum chloramphenicol concentrations

Children and Adults:

Ophthalmic: Apply 1-2 drops or small amount of ointment every 3-6 hours; increase interval between applications after 48 hours

Otic: Place 2-3 drops into the affected ear 3 times/day

Topical: Gently rub into the affected area 3-4 times/day

Administration

Ophthalmic: Solution: Avoid contact of tube or bottle tip with skin or eye; reconstitute powder with sterile water to make a final concentration of 0.5%, 0.25%, or 0.16% chloramphenicol; apply finger pressure to lacrimal sac during and for 1-2 minutes after instillation to decrease risk of absorption and systemic effects

Otic: Apply topically to external ear

Parenteral:

IVP: Administer over 5 minutes at a maximum concentration of 100 mg/mL

I.V. intermittent infusion: Administer over 15-30 minutes at a final concentration for administration ≤20 mg/mL

Monitoring Parameters CBC with reticulocyte and platelet counts, hematocrit, serum iron level, iron-binding capacity, periodic liver and renal function tests, serum drug concentration

Reference Range

Meningitis:

Peak: 15-25 µg/mL

Trough: 5-15 µg/mL

Other infections:

Peak: 10-20 µg/mL

Trough: 5-10 µg/mL

Nursing Implications Draw peak levels 90 minutes after the end of a 30-minute infusion; trough levels should be drawn just prior to the next dose

Additional Information Sodium content of 1 g injection: 2.25 mEq

Three major toxicities associated with chloramphenicol include:

Aplastic anemia, an idiosyncratic reaction which can occur with any route of administration; usually occurs 3 weeks to 12 months after initial exposure to chloramphenicol; incidence: 1 in 40,000 cases

Bone marrow suppression is thought to be dose-related with serum concentrations >25 mcg/mL and reversible once chloramphenicol is discontinued; anemia and neutropenia may occur during the first week of therapy

Gray baby syndrome is characterized by circulatory collapse, hypothermia, cyanosis, acidosis, abdominal distention, myocardial depression, coma, and death; reaction appears to be associated with serum levels ≥50 mcg/mL; may result from drug accumulation in patients with impaired hepatic or renal function; may occur after 3-4 days of therapy or within hours of initiating therapy

Dosage Forms

Injection, powder for reconstitution, as sodium succinate (Chloromycetin® Sodium Succinate): 1 g

Powder for ophthalmic solution (Chloromycetin®): 25 mg/vial [packaged with 15 mL sterile water diluent]

Solution, ophthalmic (Chloroptic®): 0.5% [5 mg/mL] (2.5 mL, 7.5 mL)

References

Nahata MC and Powell DA, "Bioavailability and Clearance of Chloramphenicol After Intravenous Chloramphenicol Succinate," *Clin Pharmacol Ther*, 1981, 30(3):368-72.

♦ **ChloraPrep® [OTC]** *see* Chlorhexidine Gluconate *on page 257*

Chlorhexidine Gluconate (klor HEKS i deen GLOO koe nate)

U.S. Brand Names BactoShield® CHG [OTC]; Betasept® [OTC]; ChloraPrep® [OTC]; Chlorostat® [OTC]; Dyna-Hex® [OTC]; Hibiclens® [OTC]; 3M™ Avagard™ [OTC]; Peridex®; PerioGard®; Stat Touch 2® [OTC] [DSC]

Canadian Brand Names Apo®-Chlorhexadine; Hibidil® 1:2000; ORO-Clense; Spec-troGram 2™

Therapeutic Category Antibacterial, Topical; Antibiotic, Oral Rinse

Generic Available Yes (oral liquid)

Use Skin cleanser for surgical scrub; cleanser for skin wounds; germicidal hand rinse; antibacterial dental rinse to reduce plaque formation and control gingivitis; prophylactic dental rinse to prevent oral infections in immunocompromised patients, particularly bone marrow transplant patients receiving cytotoxic therapy; and short-term (Continued)

Chlorhexidine Gluconate *(Continued)*

substitute for toothbrushing in situations where the patient is unable to tolerate mechanical stimulation of the gums

Pregnancy Risk Factor B

Contraindications Hypersensitivity to chlorhexidine gluconate or any component; do not use as a preoperative skin preparation of the face or head (except Hibiclens® liquid) as serious, permanent eye injury has occurred when chlorhexidine gluconate enters and remains in the eye during surgery.

Warnings For topical use only; there have been several case reports of anaphylaxis following disinfection with chlorhexidine; a case of bradycardic episodes after breast-feeding in a 2 day old infant whose mother used chlorhexidine gluconate topically on her breasts to prevent mastitis has been reported

Precautions Staining of oral surfaces, teeth, restorations, and dorsum of tongue may occur and may be visible as soon as 1 week after therapy begins; staining is more pronounced when there is a heavy accumulation of unremoved plaque and when teeth fillings have rough surfaces; stain does not have clinically adverse effect, but because removal may not be possible, patients with frontal restoration should be advised of the potential permanency of the stain; avoid contact with meninges; corneal injury has been associated with direct eye contact (see Contraindications); deafness has been associated with direct instillation into the middle ear through a perforated eardrum

Adverse Reactions

Dermatologic: Skin irritation

Gastrointestinal: Tongue irritation, minor irritation and superficial desquamation of oral mucosa (particularly among children), increased tartar on teeth, staining of oral surfaces (mucosa, teeth, and dorsum of tongue; see Warnings), dysgeusia, transient parotiditis; toothache (chip)

Ocular: Corneal damage (see Precautions)

Otic: Deafness (see Precautions)

Respiratory: Nasal congestion, shortness of breath

Miscellaneous: Edema of face, anaphylactoid reactions

Drug Interactions When combined with nystatin, *in vitro*, the minimum inhibitory concentrations (MIC) of susceptible organisms, were increased to both agents.

Stability Store away from heat and direct light; do not freeze

Mechanism of Action The bactericidal effect of chlorhexidine is a result of the binding of this cationic molecule to negatively charged bacterial cell walls and extramicrobial complexes. At low concentrations, this causes an alteration of bacterial cell osmotic equilibrium and leakage of potassium and phosphorous resulting in a bacteriostatic effect. At high concentrations of chlorhexidine, the cytoplasmic contents of the bacterial cell precipitate and result in cell death. Chlorhexidine is active against gram-positive and gram-negative organisms, facultative anaerobes, anaerobes, and yeast.

Pharmacokinetics

Absorption: ~30% of chlorhexidine is retained in the oral cavity following rinsing and is slowly released into the oral fluids; chlorhexidine is poorly absorbed from the GI tract and is not absorbed topically through intact skin

Serum concentrations: Detectable levels are not present in the plasma 12 hours after administration

Elimination: Primarily through the feces (~90%); <1% excreted in the urine

Usual Dosage

Oral rinse (Peridex® or PerioGard®) (see Administration: Oral):

Children and Adults: 15 mL twice daily

Immunocompromised patient: 10-15 mL, 2-3 times/day

Cleanser: Children and Adults: Apply 5 mL per scrub or hand wash; apply 25 mL per body wash or hair wash

Administration

Oral rinse: Precede use of solution by flossing and brushing teeth, completely rinse toothpaste from mouth; swish undiluted oral rinse around in mouth for 30 seconds, then expectorate; caution patient not to swallow the medicine; avoid eating for 2-3 hours after treatment.

Topical:

Surgical scrub: Scrub 3 minutes and rinse thoroughly, wash for an additional 3 minutes

Hand wash: Wash for 15 seconds and rinse

Hand rinse: Rub vigorously for 15 seconds

Body wash: Wet body and/or hair, apply, rinse thoroughly, repeat.

Monitoring Parameters Improvement in gingival inflammation and bleeding; development of teeth or denture discoloration; dental prophylaxis to remove stains at regular intervals of no greater than 6 months.

Test Interactions If chlorhexidine is used as a disinfectant before midstream urine collection, a false-positive urine protein may result (when using dipstick method based upon a pH indicator color change).

Patient Information

Oral rinse: Use after tooth brushing; do not swallow, do not rinse after use; may cause reduced taste perception which is reversible; may cause discoloration of teeth which may be removed with professional dental cleaning; notify dentist or physician if difficulty breathing or flushing or swelling of face occurs

Topical administration is for external use only; if accidentally enters eyes or ears, rinse out promptly and thoroughly with water

Dosage Forms

Liquid, oral rinse: 0.12% (480 mL)

Peridex®: 0.12% (480 mL) [contains 11.6% alcohol]

PerioGard®: 0.12% (480 mL) [contains 11.6% alcohol; mint flavor]

Liquid, topical, surgical scrub:

BactoShield® CHG: 2% (120 mL, 480 mL, 750 mL, 1000 mL, 3800 mL); 4% (120 mL, 480 mL, 750 mL, 1000 mL, 3800 mL) [contains isopropyl alcohol]

Betasept®: 4% (120 mL, 240 mL, 480 mL, 960 mL, 3840 mL) [contains isopropyl alcohol]

ChloraPrep®: 2% (0.67 mL) [contains 70% isopropyl alcohol; prefilled applicator]

Chlorostat®: 2% (360 mL, 3840 mL) [contains isopropyl alcohol]

Dyna-Hex: 2% (120 mL, 960 mL, 3840 mL); 4% (120 mL, 960 mL, 3840 mL)

Hibiclens®: 4% (15 mL, 120 mL, 240 mL, 480 mL, 960 mL, 3840 mL) [contains isopropyl alcohol]

3M™ Avagard™: 1% (500 mL) [contains ethyl alcohol and moisturizers]

Stat Touch 2®: 2% (946 mL, 3800 mL) [DSC]

Sponge/brush (BactoShield® CHG, Hibiclens®): 4% (each) [contains isopropyl alcohol]

References

Quinn MW and Bini RM, "Bradycardia Associated With Chlorhexidine Spray," *Arch Dis Child*, 1989, 64(6):892-3.

Yong D, Parker FC, and Foran SM, "Severe Allergic Reactions and Intra-Urethral Chlorhexidine Gluconate," *Med J Aust*, 1995, 162(5):257-8.

♦ **2-Chlorodeoxyadenosine** *see* Cladribine *on page 284*
♦ **Chloromycetin®** *see* Chloramphenicol *on page 255*
♦ **Chloromycetin® Sodium Succinate** *see* Chloramphenicol *on page 255*
♦ **Chloroptic®** *see* Chloramphenicol *on page 255*

Chloroquine (KLOR oh kwin)

U.S. Brand Names Aralen®

Therapeutic Category Amebicide; Antimalarial Agent

Generic Available Yes (tablet)

Use Suppression or chemoprophylaxis of malaria in chloroquine-sensitive areas; treatment of uncomplicated or mild-moderate malaria due to susceptible *Plasmodium* species, except chloroquine-resistant *Plasmodium falciparum*; extraintestinal amebiasis; rheumatoid arthritis; discoid lupus erythematosus, scleroderma, pemphigus

Pregnancy Risk Factor C

Contraindications Hypersensitivity to chloroquine or any component; retinal or visual field changes; patients with psoriasis

Precautions Use with caution in patients with liver disease, G-6-PD deficiency, or in conjunction with hepatotoxic drugs

Adverse Reactions

Cardiovascular: Hypotension, EKG changes

Central nervous system: Fatigue, personality changes, headache, confusion, agitation, psychotic episodes, seizures

Dermatologic: Pruritus, hair bleaching, skin eruptions, exfoliative dermatitis

Gastrointestinal: Anorexia, nausea, vomiting, diarrhea, stomatitis, weight loss

Hematologic: Blood dyscrasias (neutropenia, aplastic anemia, thrombocytopenia)

Neuromuscular & skeletal: Peripheral neuropathy, neuromyopathy, myalgia

Ocular: Retinopathy, blurred vision, corneal opacity, photophobia

Otic: Tinnitus, deafness

Drug Interactions Intradermally administered rabies vaccine; cimetidine increases levels of chloroquine; urinary acidifiers increase the elimination of chloroquine

Stability Protect from light

Mechanism of Action Binds to and inhibits DNA and RNA polymerase; interferes with metabolism and hemoglobin utilization by parasites; inhibits prostaglandin effects

Pharmacokinetics

Absorption: Oral: Rapid

(Continued)

Chloroquine *(Continued)*

Distribution: Widely distributed in body tissues including eyes, heart, kidneys, liver, and lungs where retention is prolonged; crosses the placenta; appears in breast milk

Protein binding: 50% to 65%

Metabolism: Partial hepatic

Half-life: 3-5 days

Time to peak serum concentration: Oral: Within 1-2 hours

Elimination: ~70% of dose excreted unchanged in urine; acidification of the urine increases elimination of drug; small amounts of drug may be present in urine months following discontinuation of therapy

Dialysis: Minimally removed by hemodialysis

Usual Dosage (Dosage expressed in terms of base):

Oral:

Suppression or prophylaxis of malaria:

Children: Administer 5 mg base/kg/week on the same day each week (not to exceed 300 mg base/dose); begin 1-2 weeks prior to exposure; continue for 4 weeks after leaving endemic area; if suppressive therapy is not begun prior to exposure, double the initial loading dose to 10 mg base/kg and give in 2 divided doses 6 hours apart, followed by the usual dosage regimen

Adults: 300 mg/week (base) on the same day each week; begin 1-2 weeks prior to exposure; continue for 4 weeks after leaving endemic area; if suppressive therapy is not begun prior to exposure, double the initial loading dose to 600 mg base and give in 2 divided doses 6 hours apart, followed by the usual dosage regimen

Acute attack:

Children: 10 mg base/kg (maximum dose: 600 mg base) stat, then 5 mg base/kg (maximum dose: 300 mg base) 6 hours later and then 5 mg base/kg/day (maximum daily dose: 300 mg base) once daily for 2 days

Adults: 600 mg base/dose one time, then 300 mg base/dose 6 hours later, and then 300 mg base/dose once daily for 2 days

Extraintestinal amebiasis:

Children: 10 mg base/kg once daily for 2-3 weeks (up to 300 mg base/day)

Adults: 600 mg base/day for 2 days followed by 300 mg base/day for at least 2-3 weeks

Rheumatoid arthritis: Adults: 150 mg base once daily

I.M.:

Severe malaria when oral therapy is not feasible:

Children: 5 mg base/kg (maximum dose: 200 mg base); dose may be repeated in 6 hours; maximum dose: 10 mg base/kg in a 24-hour period

Adults: 200 mg base every 6 hours

Administration

Oral: Administer with meals to decrease GI upset; chloroquine phosphate tablets have also been mixed with chocolate syrup or enclosed in gelatin capsules to mask the bitter taste

Parenteral: Cautious administration of frequent small doses by I.M. or S.C. injection in children with severe malaria may reduce risk of severe adverse effects (eg, 2.5 mg base/kg every 4 hours not to exceed 10 mg base/kg in a 24-hour period)

Monitoring Parameters Periodic CBC, examination for muscular weakness and ophthalmologic examination in patients receiving prolonged therapy

Patient Information Report any visual disturbances, muscular weakness, or difficulty in hearing or ringing in the ears; tablets are bitter tasting

Dosage Forms

Injection, solution, as **hydrochloride**: 50 mg/mL **[40 mg base/mL]** (5 mL)

Tablet, as **phosphate**: 250 mg **[150 mg base]**

Aralen®: 500 mg **[300 mg base]**; film coated]

Extemporaneous Preparations A 15 mg chloroquine phosphate/mL suspension (equivalent to 9 mg chloroquine base/mL) is made by pulverizing three Aralen® 500 mg phosphate = 300 mg base/tablet, levigating with 15 mL of a 1:1 vehicle of Ora-Sweet® and Ora-Plus®, and adding vehicle by geometric proportion, levigating until a uniform mixture is obtained; qsad to 100 mL with vehicle, stable for up to 60 days when stored at 5°C or 25°C and protected from light. Label "shake well before using" and "protect from light."

Allen LV Jr and Erickson MA, "Stability of Alprazolam, Chloroquine Phosphate, Cisapride, Enalapril Maleate, and Hydralazine Hydrochloride in Extemporaneously Compounded Oral Liquids," *Am J Health Syst Pharm*, 1998, 55(18):1915-20.

References

Wyler DJ, "Malaria Chemoprophylaxis for the Traveler," *N Engl J Med*, 1993, 329(1):31-7.

♦ **Chlorostat®** [OTC] *see* Chlorhexidine Gluconate *on page 257*

Chlorothiazide (klor oh THYE a zide)

Related Information
Carbohydrate and Alcohol Content of Liquid Medications for Use in Patients Receiving Ketogenic Diets *on page 1431*

U.S. Brand Names Diuril®

Therapeutic Category Antihypertensive Agent; Diuretic, Thiazide

Generic Available Yes (tablet)

Use Management of mild to moderate hypertension; edema associated with CHF, pregnancy, or nephrotic syndrome

Pregnancy Risk Factor C

Contraindications Hypersensitivity to chlorothiazide or any component; cross-sensitivity with other thiazides or sulfonamides; do not use in anuric patients

Warnings The injection must not be administered subcutaneously or I.M.

Precautions Use with caution in patients with severe renal disease, impaired hepatic function, moderate-high cholesterol concentrations, and in patients with high triglycerides

Adverse Reactions
Cardiovascular: Hypotension, arrhythmia, weak pulse
Central nervous system: Dizziness, vertigo, headache, fever
Dermatologic: Rash, photosensitivity
Endocrine & metabolic: Hypokalemia, hypochloremic alkalosis, hyperglycemia, hyperlipidemia, hyperuricemia
Gastrointestinal: Anorexia, nausea, vomiting, cramping, diarrhea, pancreatitis, constipation
Hematologic: Rarely blood dyscrasias, thrombocytopenia
Hepatic: Intrahepatic cholestasis
Neuromuscular & skeletal: Muscle weakness, paresthesia
Ocular: Blurred vision
Renal: Prerenal azotemia, hematuria

Drug Interactions NSAIDs with chlorothiazide may result in decreased antihypertensive effect; additive potassium losses with steroids, loop diuretics and amphotericin B; decreases lithium clearance; increases hypersensitivity reactions to allopurinol; increases hyperglycemia with diazoxide; decreased absorption of chlorothiazide when administered with cholestyramine; milk-alkali syndrome with high calcium dosages

Food Interactions Avoid natural licorice (causes sodium and water retention and increases potassium loss); may need to decrease sodium and calcium, may need to increase potassium, zinc, magnesium, and riboflavin in diet

Stability Reconstituted injection is stable for 24 hours at room temperature

Mechanism of Action Inhibits sodium reabsorption in the distal tubules causing increased excretion of sodium, chloride, potassium, bicarbonate, magnesium, phosphate, calcium (transiently) and water

Pharmacodynamics
Diuresis: Onset of action: Oral: Within 2 hours
Duration:
Oral: ~6-12 hours
I.V.: 2 hours

Pharmacokinetics
Absorption: Oral: Poor (~10% to 20%); dose dependent
Distribution: Breast milk to plasma ratio: 0.05
Half-life: Adults: 45-120 minutes
Time to peak serum concentration: Within 4 hours
Elimination: Excreted unchanged in urine

Usual Dosage I.V. dosage in infants and children has not been established. The following I.V. dosages in infants and children are based upon anecdotal reports. Lower dosing regimens have been extrapolated from oral dosing recommendations as 10% to 20% of an oral dose is absorbed.

Neonates and Infants <6 months:
Oral: 20-40 mg/kg/day in 2 divided doses; maximum: 375 mg/day
I.V.: 2-8 mg/kg/day in 2 divided doses; doses up to 20 mg/kg/day have been used
Infants >6 months and Children:
Oral: 20 mg/kg/day in 2 divided doses; maximum: 1 g/day
I.V.: 4 mg/kg/day divided in 1-2 doses; doses up to 20 mg/kg/day have been used
Adults:
Oral: 500 mg to 2 g/day divided in 1-2 doses
I.V.:100-500 mg/day divided in 1-2 doses
(Continued)

Chlorothiazide (Continued)

Administration

Oral: Administer with food; shake suspension well before use

Parenteral: Dilute 500 mg vial with 18 mL SWI (resulting in 27.8 mg/mL concentration); administer by direct I.V. infusion over 3-5 minutes or infusion over 30 minutes in dextrose or NS; avoid extravasation of parenteral solution since it is extremely irritating to tissues

Monitoring Parameters
Serum electrolytes (sodium, potassium, chloride, and bicarbonate), glucose, uric acid, triglycerides

Patient Information
May cause photosensitivity reactions (eg, exposure to sunlight may cause severe sunburn, skin rash, redness, or itching); avoid exposure to sunlight and artificial light sources (sunlamps, tanning booth/bed); wear protective clothing, wide-brimmed hats, sunglasses, and lip sunscreen (SPF ≥15); use a sunscreen [broad-spectrum sunscreen or physical sunscreen (preferred) or sunblock with SPF ≥15]; contact physician if reaction occurs.

Dosage Forms

Injection, powder for reconstitution, lyophilized, as sodium: 500 mg

Suspension, oral: 250 mg/5 mL (237 mL) [contains 0.5% alcohol]

Tablet: 250 mg, 500 mg

Chlorpheniramine (klor fen IR a meen)

Related Information

OTC Cough & Cold Preparations, Pediatric on page 1225

Overdose and Toxicology on page 1388

U.S. Brand Names Chlor-Trimeton® [OTC]; Polaramine® [DSC]

Canadian Brand Names Chlor-Tripolon®

Therapeutic Category Antihistamine

Generic Available Yes

Use Perennial and seasonal allergic rhinitis and other allergic symptoms including urticaria

Pregnancy Risk Factor B

Contraindications Hypersensitivity to chlorpheniramine maleate or any component; narrow-angle glaucoma, bladder neck obstruction, symptomatic prostatic hypertrophy, stenosing peptic ulcer, pyloroduodenal obstruction

Precautions Use with caution in patients with asthma; young children may be more susceptible to side effects and CNS stimulation

Adverse Reactions

Cardiovascular: Palpitations

Central nervous system: Drowsiness, vertigo, headache, excitability (children may be at increased risk for developing CNS stimulation), nervousness, fatigue, dizziness, depression

Dermatologic: Dermatitis, photosensitivity, angioedema

Gastrointestinal: Nausea, xerostomia, diarrhea, abdominal pain, appetite increase, weight gain

Genitourinary: Urinary retention

Neuromuscular & skeletal: Weakness, arthralgia, paresthesia

Ocular: Diplopia, blurred vision

Renal: Polyuria

Respiratory: Thickening of bronchial secretions, pharyngitis, epistaxis

Drug Interactions Cytochrome P450 isoenzyme CYP2D6 substrate

May cause additive sedation when concomitantly administered with other CNS depressant medications

Mechanism of Action Competes with histamine for H_1-receptor sites on effector cells in the GI tract, blood vessels, and respiratory tract

Pharmacodynamics

Onset of action: Oral: 6 hours

Duration: Oral: 24 hours

Pharmacokinetics (Data from chlorpheniramine maleate)

Distribution: V_d:

Children: 3.8 L/kg

Adults: 2.5-3.2 L/kg

Protein binding: 69% to 72%

Metabolism: Substantial metabolism in GI mucosa and on first pass through liver

Bioavailability: Chlorpheniramine:

Solution: 35% to 60%

Tablet: 25% to 45%

Half-life:

Children: Average: 9.6-13.1 hours (range: 5.2-23.1 hours)

Adults: 12-43 hours

Time to peak serum concentration: Oral (solution and conventional tablets): 2-6 hours

Elimination: 35% excreted in 48 hours

Usual Dosage

Chlorpheniramine maleate: Oral:

Children <12 years: Oral: 0.35 mg/kg/day in divided doses every 4-6 hours or as an alternative

2-5 years: 1 mg every 4-6 hours

6-11 years: 2 mg every 4-6 hours, not to exceed 12 mg/day or timed release 8 mg every 12 hours

Children ≥12 years and Adults: 4 mg every 4-6 hours, not to exceed 24 mg/day or timed release 8-12 mg every 12 hours

Dexchlorpheniramine maleate: Oral:

Children 2-5 years: 0.5 mg every 4-6 hours, not to exceed 3 mg/day

Children 6-11 years: 1 mg every 4-6 hours, not to exceed 6 mg/day **or** as timed release tablets: 4 mg once daily at bedtime

Children ≥12 years and Adults: 2 mg every 4-6 hours **or** as timed release tablets: 4-6 mg at bedtime or every 8-10 hours; not to exceed 12 mg/day

Administration Oral: Administer with food to decrease GI distress; do not crush or chew timed release tablets

Patient Information May cause drowsiness and impair ability to perform activities requiring mental alertness or physical coordination; may cause dry mouth. May cause photosensitivity reactions (eg, exposure to sunlight may cause severe sunburn, skin rash, redness, or itching); avoid direct exposure to sunlight

Dosage Forms

Syrup, as **dexchlorpheniramine maleate**: 2 mg/5 mL (480 mL, 3840 mL) [contains 6% alcohol; orange flavor]

Tablet, as **chlorpheniramine maleate** (Chlor-Trimeton®): 4 mg

Tablet, timed release, as **chlorpheniramine maleate** (Chlor-Trimeton®): 8 mg, 12 mg

Tablet, timed release, as **dexchlorpheniramine maleate**: 4 mg, 6 mg

ChlorproMAZINE (klor PROE ma zeen)

Related Information

Carbohydrate and Alcohol Content of Liquid Medications for Use in Patients Receiving Ketogenic Diets *on page 1431*

Compatibility of Medications Mixed in a Syringe *on page 1412*

Drugs and Breast-Feeding *on page 1404*

Overdose and Toxicology *on page 1388*

Prochlorperazine *on page 938*

U.S. Brand Names Thorazine®

Canadian Brand Names Apo®-Chlorpromazine; Largactil®; Novo-Chlorpromazine

Therapeutic Category Antiemetic; Antipsychotic Agent; Phenothiazine Derivative

Generic Available Yes

Use Treatment of nausea and vomiting, schizophrenia, Tourette's syndrome, mania, acute intermittent porphyria, restlessness and apprehension prior to surgery, intractable hiccups (adults), severe behavioral problems (children); used as an adjunct in the treatment of tetanus

Pregnancy Risk Factor C

Contraindications Hypersensitivity to chlorpromazine hydrochloride or any component (see Warnings); cross-sensitivity with other phenothiazines may exist; avoid use in patients with narrow-angle glaucoma, bone marrow suppression, severe liver or cardiac disease

Warnings Significant hypotension may occur, especially when the drug is administered parenterally; injection and oral concentrate contain sulfites which may cause allergic reactions in susceptible individuals

Extended release capsules and multiple dose vial of injection contain benzyl alcohol which may cause allergic reactions in susceptible individuals; syrup contains sodium benzoate and tablets contain benzoic acid; benzoic acid (benzoate) is a metabolite of benzyl alcohol; large amounts of benzyl alcohol (≥99 mg/kg/day) have been associated with a potentially fatal toxicity ("gasping syndrome") in neonates; the "gasping syndrome" consists of metabolic acidosis, respiratory distress, gasping respirations, CNS dysfunction (including convulsions, intracranial hemorrhage), hypotension and cardiovascular collapse; use chlorpromazine products containing benzyl alcohol, benzoic acid, or sodium benzoate with caution in neonates; *in vitro* and animal studies have shown that benzoate displaces bilirubin from protein binding sites

Precautions Use with caution in patients with cardiovascular, renal, or hepatic disease; chronic respiratory diseases (especially in children); seizures; significant medical disorders or children with acute illnesses

(Continued)

ChlorproMAZINE (Continued)

Adverse Reactions

Cardiovascular: Hypotension (especially with I.V. use), orthostatic hypotension, tachycardia, arrhythmias

Central nervous system: Sedation, drowsiness, restlessness, anxiety, extrapyramidal reactions, pseudoparkinsonian signs and symptoms, tardive dyskinesia, neuroleptic malignant syndrome, seizures, altered central temperature regulation

Dermatologic: Hyperpigmentation, pruritus, rash, photosensitivity; oral solution or injection may cause contact dermatitis (avoid contact with skin)

Endocrine & metabolic: Amenorrhea, galactorrhea, gynecomastia

Gastrointestinal: Xerostomia, constipation, GI upset, weight gain

Genitourinary: Impotence, urinary retention

Hematologic: Agranulocytosis, leukopenia (usually in patients with large doses for prolonged periods), thrombocytopenia, hemolytic anemia, eosinophilia

Hepatic: Cholestatic jaundice (rare)

Local: Thrombophlebitis

Ocular: Retinal pigmentation, blurred vision

Miscellaneous: Anaphylactoid reactions

Drug Interactions

Cytochrome P450 isoenzyme CYP1A2, CYP2D6, and CYP3A3/4 substrate; isoenzyme CYP2D6 inhibitor

Additive effects with other CNS depressants; epinephrine may cause hypotension in patients receiving chlorpromazine due to phenothiazine-induced alpha-adrenergic blockade and unopposed epinephrine beta$_2$ action; thiazide diuretics may increase the orthostatic hypotension of phenothiazines; chlorpromazine may increase valproic acid, phenytoin, and haloperidol serum concentrations; use with propranolol will result in an increase in plasma concentrations of both chlorpromazine and propranolol; chlorpromazine may decrease the effects of oral anticoagulants; absorption of chlorpromazine may be decreased if administered concomitantly with aluminum- or magnesium-containing antacids; liquid preparations of chlorpromazine will form an orange rubbery precipitate if mixed with or administered simultaneously with carbamazepine suspension; may interact with metyrapone and reduce test effectiveness; may interact with tranexamic acid

Food Interactions

Increases riboflavin elimination and may induce depletion; some may recommend increasing riboflavin in diet; may also decrease absorption of vitamin B$_{12}$; undiluted oral concentrate may precipitate when mixed with tube feeding; brown precipitate may occur when chlorpromazine is mixed with caffeine-containing liquids

Stability

Protect oral dosage forms from light; discard solution if markedly discolored; diluted injection (1 mg/mL) with NS stored in 5 mL vials remains stable for 30 days

Mechanism of Action

Blocks postsynaptic mesolimbic dopaminergic receptors in the brain; exhibits a strong alpha-adrenergic blocking effect and depresses the release of hypothalamic and hypophyseal hormones

Pharmacodynamics

Onset of action:

Oral tablet: 30-60 minutes

Rectal suppository: >60 minutes

Antipsychotic effects: Gradual, may take up to several weeks

Maximum antipsychotic effect: 6 weeks to 6 months

Duration:

Oral tablets: 4-6 hours

Rectal suppository: 3-4 hours

Pharmacokinetics

Absorption: Oral: Rapid and virtually complete; large first-pass effect due to metabolism during absorption in the GI mucosa

Distribution: Widely distributed into most body tissues and fluids; crosses blood-brain barrier and placenta; appears in breast milk; V$_d$: 8-160 L/kg (adults)

Protein binding: 90% to 99%

Metabolism: Extensively in the liver by demethylation (followed by glucuronide conjugation) and amine oxidation

Bioavailability: Oral: ~32%

Half-life, biphasic:

Initial:

Children: 1.1 hours

Adults: ~2 hours

Terminal:

Children: 7.7 hours

Adults: ~30 hours

Elimination: <1% excreted in urine as unchanged drug within 24 hours

Dialysis: Not dialyzable (0% to 5%)

Usual Dosage

Neonates: Neonatal abstinence syndrome (withdrawal from maternal narcotic use): I.M. and Oral: Initial: I.M.: 0.5-0.7 mg/kg/dose given every 6 hours; change to oral after ~4 days, decrease dose gradually over 2-3 weeks. **Note:** Chlorpromazine is rarely used for neonatal abstinence syndrome due to adverse effects such as hypothermia and eosinophilia. Other agents (eg, phenobarbital or a 25-fold dilution of tincture of opium) are preferred.

Infants ≥6 months and Children:

Schizophrenia/psychoses:

Oral: 0.5-1 mg/kg/dose every 4-6 hours; older children may require 200 mg/day or higher

I.M., I.V.: 0.5-1 mg/kg/dose every 6-8 hours

Maximum recommended doses:

Children <5 years (<22.7 kg): 40 mg/day

Children 5-12 years (22.7-45.5 kg): 75 mg/day

Nausea and vomiting:

Oral: 0.5-1 mg/kg/dose every 4-6 hours as needed

I.M., I.V.: 0.5-1 mg/kg/dose every 6-8 hours; maximum recommended doses:

Children <5 years (<22.7 kg): 40 mg/day

Children 5-12 years (22.7-45.5 kg): 75 mg/day

Rectal: 1 mg/kg/dose every 6-8 hours as needed

Adults:

Schizophrenia/psychoses:

Oral: Range: 30-800 mg/day in 1-4 divided doses, initiate at lower doses and titrate as needed; usual dose is 200 mg/day; some patients may require 1-2 g/day

I.M., I.V.: 25 mg initially, may repeat (25-50 mg) in 1-4 hours, gradually increase to a maximum of 400 mg/dose every 4-6 hours until patient controlled; usual dose 300-800 mg/day

Nausea and vomiting:

Oral: 10-25 mg every 4-6 hours

I.M., I.V.: 25-50 mg every 4-6 hours

Rectal: 50-100 mg every 6-8 hours

Administration

Oral: Administer with water, food, or milk to decrease GI upset. Swallow sustained release capsule whole, do not chew or crush. Dilute oral concentrate solution in water, tomato or fruit juice, milk, simple syrup, orange syrup, carbonated beverages, applesauce, or pudding just before administration; patient should consume entire mixture of drug/liquid or drug/food immediately; do not store for further use; do not mix undiluted oral concentrate with tube feeding (see Food Interactions). Do not administer chlorpromazine liquid preparations simultaneously with carbamazepine suspension (see Drug Interactions).

Parenteral: Do not administer S.C. (tissue damage and irritation may occur); for direct I.V. injection: Dilute with NS to a maximum concentration of 1 mg/mL, administer slow I.V. at a rate not to exceed 0.5 mg/minute in children and 1 mg/minute in adults

Monitoring Parameters Periodic eye exam with prolonged therapy; blood pressure with parenteral administration; CBC with differential

Reference Range Relationship of plasma concentration to clinical response is not well established

Therapeutic: 50-300 ng/mL (SI: 157-942 nmol/L)

Toxic: >750 ng/mL (SI: >2355 nmol/L)

Test Interactions False-positives for phenylketonuria, amylase, uroporphyrins, urobilinogen; possible false-negative pregnancy urinary test

Patient Information May cause drowsiness and impair ability to perform activities requiring mental alertness or physical coordination; may cause dry mouth; avoid alcohol. May cause photosensitivity reactions (eg, exposure to sunlight may cause severe sunburn, skin rash, redness, or itching); avoid exposure to sunlight and artificial light sources (sunlamps, tanning booth/bed); wear protective clothing, wide-brimmed hats, sunglasses, and lip sunscreen (SPF ≥15); use a sunscreen [broad-spectrum sunscreen or physical sunscreen (preferred) or sunblock with SPF ≥15]; contact physician if reaction occurs.

Nursing Implications Avoid contact of oral solution or injection with skin (may cause contact dermatitis; use of rubber gloves is recommended)

Additional Information Although chlorpromazine has been used in combination with meperidine and promethazine as a premedication ("lytic cocktail"), this combination may have a higher rate of adverse effects compared to alternative sedatives/analgesics (see AAP, 1995). Use decreased doses in elderly or debilitated patients; dystonic reactions may be more common in patients with hypocalcemia; extrapyramidal reactions may be more common in pediatric patients, especially those with dehydration or (Continued)

ChlorproMAZINE *(Continued)*

acute illnesses (viral or CNS infections); avoid rectal administration in immunocompromised patients.

Dosage Forms

Capsule, sustained action, as **hydrochloride**: 30 mg, 75 mg, 150 mg [contains benzyl alcohol]

Injection, solution, as **hydrochloride**: 25 mg/mL (1 mL, 2 mL) [contains sodium bisulfite and sodium sulfite] (10 mL) [contains 2% benzyl alcohol, sodium bisulfite, and sodium sulfite]

Solution, oral **concentrate**, as **hydrochloride**: 30 mg/mL (120 mL); 100 mg/mL (240 mL) [contains 0.068% alcohol, sodium bisulfite, and sodium sulfite]

Suppository, rectal, as **base**: 25 mg, 100 mg

Syrup, as **hydrochloride**: 10 mg/5 mL (120 mL) [contains sodium benzoate; orange-custard flavor]

Tablet, as **hydrochloride:** 10 mg, 25 mg, 50 mg, 100 mg, 200 mg [contains benzoic acid]

References

American Academy of Pediatrics Committee on Drugs, "Reappraisal of Lytic Cocktail/Demerol®, Phenergan®, and Thorazine® (DPT) for the Sedation of Children," *Pediatrics*, 1995, 95(4):598-602.

Furlanut M, Benetello P, Baraldo M, et al, "Chlorpromazine Disposition in Relation to Age in Children," *Clin Pharmacokinet*, 1990, 18(4):329-31.

♦ **Chlor-Trimeton® [OTC]** *see* Chlorpheniramine *on page 262* *see* Chlorpheniramine *on page 262*

♦ **Chlor-Tripolon® (Can)** *see* Chlorpheniramine *on page 262*

Chlorzoxazone *(klor ZOKS a zone)*

U.S. Brand Names Parafon Forte® DSC; Remular® S

Canadian Brand Names Strifon Forte®

Therapeutic Category Skeletal Muscle Relaxant, Nonparalytic

Generic Available Yes

Use Symptomatic treatment of muscle spasm and pain associated with acute musculoskeletal conditions

Pregnancy Risk Factor C

Contraindications Hypersensitivity to chlorzoxazone or any component; impaired liver function

Warnings Serious (including fatal) hepatocellular toxicity has been reported rarely

Adverse Reactions

Cardiovascular: Tachycardia, tightness in chest, flushing of face, syncope

Central nervous system: Drowsiness, dizziness, lightheadedness, headache, paradoxical stimulation, ataxia

Dermatologic: Rash, urticaria, petechiae, angioneurotic edema, erythema multiforme

Gastrointestinal: Nausea, vomiting, diarrhea, GI bleeding (rare), stomach cramps

Genitourinary: Discoloration of urine (orange or purple-red)

Hematologic: Anemia, granulocytopenia, eosinophilia

Hepatic: Hepatitis

Neuromuscular & skeletal: Paresthesia, trembling

Ocular: Burning of eyes

Respiratory: Shortness of breath

Miscellaneous: Hiccups

Drug Interactions Cytochrome P450 isoenzyme CYP2E1 substrate

May cause additive sedation when concomitantly administered with other CNS depressant medications

Food Interactions Watercress may decrease chlorzoxazone clearance

Mechanism of Action Acts on the spinal cord and subcortical levels by depressing polysynaptic reflexes

Pharmacodynamics

Onset of action: Within 60 minutes

Duration: 3-4 hours

Pharmacokinetics

Absorption: Oral: Readily

Metabolism: Extensive in the liver by glucuronidation

Half-life: ~60 minutes

Elimination: In urine as conjugates

Usual Dosage Oral:

Children: 20 mg/kg/day or 600 mg/m^2/day in 3-4 divided doses

Adults: 250-750 mg 3-4 times/day

Administration Oral: Administer with food

Monitoring Parameters Periodic liver function tests

Patient Information May color urine orange or purple-red; may cause drowsiness and impair ability to perform activities requiring mental alertness or physical coordination; notify physician if experiencing fever, rash, anorexia, right upper quadrant pain, dark urine, or jaundice

Dosage Forms
Caplet (Parafon Forte® DSC): 500 mg
Tablet: 500 mg
Remular®: 250 mg

♦ **Cholac®** see Lactulose on page 649

Cholestyramine Resin (koe LES tir a meen REZ in)

U.S. Brand Names LoCHOLEST®; LoCHOLEST® Light; Prevalite®; Questran®; Questran® Light

Canadian Brand Names Novo-Cholamine; Novo-Cholamine Light; PMS-Cholestyramine

Therapeutic Category Antilipemic Agent

Generic Available Yes

Use Adjunct in the management of primary hypercholesterolemia; pruritus associated with elevated levels of bile acids; diarrhea associated with excess fecal bile acids; pseudomembraneous colitis

Pregnancy Risk Factor C

Contraindications Hypersensitivity to cholestyramine or any component; avoid using in complete biliary obstruction or biliary atresia

Precautions Use with caution in patients with constipation or recent abdominal surgery (see Additional Information); Prevalite®, LoCHOLEST® Light, and Questran® Light contain aspartame which is metabolized to phenylalanine and must be avoided (or used with caution) in patients with phenylketonuria.

Adverse Reactions
Dermatologic: Rash
Endocrine & metabolic: Hyperchloremic acidosis
Gastrointestinal: Constipation, nausea, vomiting, abdominal distention and pain, steatorrhea, malabsorption of fat-soluble vitamins
Genitourinary: Increased urinary calcium excretion
Hematologic: Hypoprothrombinemia
Local: Irritation of perianal area, skin, or tongue

Drug Interactions May decrease oral absorption of digitalis glycosides, warfarin, thyroid hormones, thiazide diuretics, propranolol, phenobarbital, amiodarone, methotrexate, NSAIDs, and other drugs by binding to the drug in the intestine (administer medications at least 1 hour before or at least 4-6 hours after cholestyramine)

Food Interactions Cholestyramine (especially high doses or long-term therapy) may decrease the absorption of fat-soluble vitamins (vitamins A, D, E, and K), folic acid, calcium, iron, zinc, and magnesium; deficiencies may occur including hypoprothrombinemia and increased bleeding from vitamin K deficiency; supplementation of vitamins A, D, E, and K, folic acid, and iron may be required with high-dose, long-term therapy (administer vitamins or mineral supplements at least 1 hour before or at least 4-6 hours after cholestyramine)

Mechanism of Action Forms a nonabsorbable complex with bile acids in the intestine, releasing chloride ions in the process; inhibits enterohepatic reuptake of intestinal bile salts and thereby increases the fecal loss of bile salt-bound low density lipoprotein cholesterol

Pharmacodynamics
Maximum effect on serum cholesterol levels: Within 4 weeks

Pharmacokinetics
Absorption: Not absorbed from the GI tract
Elimination: Forms an insoluble complex with bile acids which is excreted in feces

Usual Dosage Oral (dosages are expressed in terms of anhydrous resin):
Children: 240 mg/kg/day in 3 divided doses; need to titrate dose depending on indication
Hypercholesterolemia (**Note:** Doses >8 g/day may not provide additional significant cholesterol-lowering effects, but may increase adverse effects): Some centers use the following doses (see Sprecher, 1996):
Children ≤10 years: Initial: 2 g/day; titrate dose based on efficacy and tolerance; range: 1-4 g/day
Children >10 years and Adolescents: Initial: 2 g/day; titrate dose based on efficacy and tolerance, up to 8 g/day
Note: Lipid-lowering effects are better if dose is administered as a single daily dose with the evening meal (single daily morning doses are less effective); if patients cannot tolerate once daily dosing, the dose/day may be divided into 2 doses and

(Continued)

Cholestyramine Resin *(Continued)*

administered with the morning and evening meals; may also be administered in 3 divided doses/day (Daniels, 2002)

Adults: 3-4 g 3-4 times/day to a maximum of 16-32 g/day in 2-4 divided doses

Administration Oral: Administer at mealtime; do not administer the powder in its dry form; just prior to administration, mix with 2-6 ounces of water, noncarbonated liquid, or applesauce; to minimize binding of concomitant medications, administer other drugs including vitamins or mineral supplements at least 1 hour before or at least 4-6 hours after cholestyramine

Monitoring Parameters Serum cholesterol, serum triglycerides; with prolonged use, prothrombin time, liver enzymes, CBC, electrolytes; number of stools/day

Nursing Implications Maintain adequate oral fluid intake to avoid constipation; with high-dose, long-term therapy, use of daily multivitamin with iron and folic acid is recommended

Additional Information Overdose may result in GI obstruction; intestinal obstruction has been reported in patients with recent abdominal surgery (see Tonstad, 1996)

Dosage Forms

Powder for oral suspension:

LoCHOLEST®: 4 g of resin/9 g of powder (9 g packets, 378 g can) [strawberry flavor]

LoCHOLEST® Light: 4 g of resin/5.7 g powder (5.7 g packets, 239 g can) [contains 22.4 mg phenylalanine (as aspartame)/5.7 g; strawberry flavor]

Prevalite®: 4 g of resin/5.5 g of powder (5.5 g packets, 231 g can) [contains 14.1 mg phenylalanine (as aspartame)/5.5 g; orange flavor]

Questran®: 4 g of resin/9 g powder (9 g packets, 378 g can)

Questran® Light: 4 g of resin/5 g powder (5 g packets, 210 g can) [contains 16.8 mg phenylalanine (as aspartame)/5 g]

References

Daniels SR, personal communication, May 2002.

McCrindle BW, O'Neill MB, Cullen-Dean G, et al, "Acceptability and Compliance With Two Forms of Cholestyramine in the Treatment of Hypercholesterolemia in Children: A Randomized, Crossover Trial," *J Pediatr*, 1997, 130(2):266-73.

Sprecher DL and Daniels SR, "Rational Approach to Pharmacologic Reduction of Cholesterol Levels in Children," *J Pediatr*, 1996, 129(1):4-7.

Tonstad S, Knudtzon J, Sivertsen M, et al, "Efficacy and Safety of Cholestyramine Therapy in Peripubertal and Prepubertal Children With Familial Hypercholesterolemia," *J Pediatr*, 1996, 129(1):42-9.

Choline Magnesium Trisalicylate

(KOE leen mag NEE zhum trye sa LIS i late)

Related Information

Overdose and Toxicology *on page 1388*

U.S. Brand Names Tricosal®; Trilisate®

Therapeutic Category Analgesic, Non-narcotic; Anti-inflammatory Agent; Antipyretic; Nonsteroidal Anti-inflammatory Drug (NSAID), Oral; Salicylate

Generic Available Yes

Use Management of osteoarthritis, rheumatoid arthritis, and other arthritides; treatment of acute painful shoulder, mild to moderate pain, and fever

Pregnancy Risk Factor C (D in 3rd trimester)

Contraindications Hypersensitivity to salicylates, any component, or other nonacetylated salicylates

Warnings Avoid use in patients with suspected varicella or influenza (salicylates have been associated with Reye's syndrome in children <16 years of age when used to treat symptoms of chickenpox or the flu)

Precautions Use with extreme caution in patients with impaired renal function, erosive gastritis or peptic ulcer

Adverse Reactions

Dermatologic: Rash, pruritus, urticaria

Gastrointestinal: Nausea, vomiting, GI distress, ulceration

Hepatic: Hepatotoxicity

Otic: Tinnitus

Respiratory: Pulmonary edema

Drug Interactions Antacids may decrease salicylate concentration; salicylates may increase hypoprothrombinemic effect of warfarin

Mechanism of Action Inhibits prostaglandin synthesis; acts on the hypothalamus heat-regulating center to reduce fever; blocks the generation of pain impulses

Pharmacokinetics

Absorption: From stomach and small intestine

Distribution: Readily distributes into most body fluids and tissues; crosses the placenta; appears in breast milk

Protein binding: 90% to 95%

Metabolism: Hepatic microsomal enzyme system

Half-life: Dose-dependent, ranging from 2-3 hours at low doses to 30 hours at high doses

Time to peak serum concentration:
Solution: 20-35 minutes
Tablet: Within ~2 hours

Elimination: 10% excreted as unchanged drug

Usual Dosage Oral (based on **total salicylate content**):
Children: 30-60 mg/kg/day given in 3-4 divided doses
Adults: 500 mg to 1.5 g 1-3 times/day

Administration Oral: Administer with food or milk to decrease GI upset; liquid may be mixed with fruit juice just before drinking; do not administer with antacids

Monitoring Parameters Serum salicylate levels; serum magnesium with high doses or in patients with decreased renal function

Reference Range
Salicylate blood levels for anti-inflammatory effect: 150-300 µg/mL
Analgesia and antipyretic effect: 30-50 µg/mL

Test Interactions False-negative results for Clinistix® urine test; false-positive results with Clinitest®

Patient Information Avoid alcohol; notify physician if ringing in ears or persistent GI pain occurs

Additional Information Salicylate salts do not inhibit platelet aggregation and, therefore, should not be substituted for aspirin in the prophylaxis of thrombosis (ie, for aspirin's antiplatelet effects)

Dosage Forms See table.

Choline Magnesium Trisalicylate

Brand Name	Dosage Form	Labeled Strength (Total Salicylate)	Choline Salicylate	Magnesium Salicylate
Trilisate® [cherry cordial flavor]	Liquid	500 mg/5 mL	293 mg/5 mL	362 mg/5 mL
Trilisate®, Tricosal®	Tablet	500 mg	293 mg	362 mg
Trilisate®, Tricosal®	Tablet	750 mg	440 mg	544 mg
Trilisate®, Tricosal®	Tablet	1000 mg	587 mg	725 mg

References
Berde C, Ablin A, Glazer J, et al, "American Academy of Pediatrics Report of the Subcommittee on Disease-Related Pain in Childhood Cancer," Pediatrics, 1990, 86(5 Pt 2):818-25.

♦ **Chooz®** [OTC] see Calcium Supplements on page 200

Chorionic Gonadotropin (kor ee ON ik goe NAD oh troe pin)

U.S. Brand Names A.P.L.®; Novarel™; Pregnyl®; Profasi®

Synonyms CG; hCG

Therapeutic Category Gonadotropin; Ovulation Stimulator

Generic Available Yes

Use Treatment of hypogonadotropic hypogonadism; prepubertal cryptorchidism; induce ovulation

Pregnancy Risk Factor X

Contraindications Hypersensitivity to chorionic gonadotropin or any component (see Warnings); precocious puberty, prostatic carcinoma or similar neoplasms

Warnings hCG is **not** effective in the treatment of obesity. Pregnyl® contains benzyl alcohol which may cause allergic reactions in susceptible individuals; large amounts of benzyl alcohol (≥99 mg/kg/day) have been associated with a potentially fatal toxicity ("gasping syndrome") in neonates; the "gasping syndrome" consists of metabolic acidosis, respiratory distress, gasping respirations, CNS dysfunction (including convulsions, intracranial hemorrhage), hypotension and cardiovascular collapse; avoid use of Pregnyl® in neonates. In vitro and animal studies have shown that benzoate, a metabolite of benzyl alcohol, displaces bilirubin from protein-binding sites.

Precautions Use with caution in patients with asthma, seizure disorders, migraine, cardiac or renal disease; may induce precocious puberty

Adverse Reactions
Cardiovascular: Edema
(Continued)

Chorionic Gonadotropin *(Continued)*

Central nervous system: Irritability, restlessness, depression, fatigue, headache, aggressive behavior

Endocrine & metabolic: Gynecomastia, precocious puberty

Local: Pain at the injection site

Neuromuscular & skeletal: Premature closure of epiphyses

Stability Following reconstitution with provided diluent, stable for 30-90 days (depending upon preparation) when stored at 2°C to 15°C

Mechanism of Action Stimulates production of gonadal steroid hormones by causing production of androgen by the testis; as a substitute for luteinizing hormone (LH) to stimulate ovulation

Pharmacokinetics

Half-life, biphasic:
Initial: 11 hours
Terminal: 23 hours
Elimination: Excreted unchanged in urine within 3-4 days

Usual Dosage Children: I.M. (many regimens have been described):

Prepubertal cryptorchidism:
1000-2000 units/m²/dose 3 times/week for 3 weeks or 4000 units 3 times/week for 3 weeks
or
5000 units every second day for 4 injections
or
500 units 3 times/week for 4-6 weeks

Hypogonadotropic hypogonadism:
500-1000 units 3 times/week for 3 weeks, followed by the same dose twice weekly for 3 weeks
or
1000-2000 units 3 times/week
or
4000 units 3 times/week for 6-9 months; reduce dosage to 2000 units 3 times/week for additional 3 months

Induction of ovulation: 5000-10,000 units the day following the last dose of menotropins

Administration Parenteral: Administer I.M. only

Reference Range Depends on application and methodology; <3 milli international units/mL (SI: <3 units/L) usually normal (nonpregnant)

Dosage Forms

Injection, powder for reconstitution [packaged with diluent; diluent contains benzyl alcohol]:
A.P.L.®: 5000 units, 10,000 units, 20,000 units
Novarel™: 10,000 units [diluent also contains mannitol]
Pregnyl®, Profasi®: 10,000 units

♦ **Chromium Chloride** *see* Trace Metals *on page 1106*

♦ **Chronovera® (Can)** *see* Verapamil *on page 1144*

Cidofovir *(si DOF o veer)*

U.S. Brand Names Vistide®

Synonyms HPMPC

Therapeutic Category Antiviral Agent, Parenteral

Generic Available No

Use Treatment of cytomegalovirus (CMV) retinitis in patients with acquired immunodeficiency syndrome; antiviral agent with activity against ganciclovir-resistant CMV, foscarnet-resistant CMV, acyclovir-resistant HSV or VZV, and adenovirus

Pregnancy Risk Factor C

Contraindications Hypersensitivity to cidofovir or any component; history of clinically severe hypersensitivity to probenecid or other sulfa-containing medications; patients with a serum creatinine >1.5 mg/dL, creatinine clearance ≤55 mL/minute, urine protein ≥100 mg/dL (≥2 plus proteinuria); patients who are receiving other nephrotoxic agents; direct intraocular injection

Warnings Safety and efficacy have not been established in children; due to risk of long-term carcinogenicity and reproductive toxicity, administration of cidofovir to children warrants extreme caution. Prepare admixture in a Class II laminar flow hood, administer, and dispose according to guidelines issued for cytotoxic drugs. Acute renal failure resulting in dialysis and/or contributing to death has been reported to occur after as few as one or two cidofovir doses; neutropenia and ocular hypotony have been reported in association with cidofovir treatment.

Precautions Modify dose in patients with changing renal function due to dose-dependent nephrotoxicity. Cidofovir administration must be accompanied by oral probenecid and NS I.V. prehydration to reduce possible nephrotoxicity.

Adverse Reactions

Cardiovascular: Hypotension, pallor, syncope, tachycardia, cardiomyopathy, edema, hypertension

Central nervous system: Headache, agitation, dizziness, fever, chills, amnesia, confusion, seizures, insomnia, personality/mood disorder, hallucinations, anxiety, somnolence, malaise

Dermatologic: Alopecia, rash, acne, skin discoloration, pruritus, urticaria

Endocrine & metabolic: Metabolic acidosis, hyperglycemia, hyperlipidemia, hypocalcemia, hypokalemia, dehydration, hypomagnesemia, hyponatremia, hypophosphatemia

Gastrointestinal: Nausea, vomiting, diarrhea, anorexia, abdominal pain, constipation, dyspepsia, gastritis, abnormal taste, stomatitis, colitis, cholangitis, pancreatitis, dysphagia

Genitourinary: Glycosuria, urinary incontinence, hematuria, proteinuria

Hematologic: Neutropenia (not dose-related; occurs in up to 24% of AIDS patients), thrombocytopenia, anemia

Hepatic: Hepatomegaly, elevated SGOT and SGPT

Neuromuscular & skeletal: Weakness, paresthesia, skeletal pain, peripheral neuropathy

Ocular: Amblyopia, conjunctivitis, iritis, uveitis, decreased intraocular pressure, ocular hypotony, retinal detachment

Renal: Tubular damage (dose-dependent), elevated BUN and serum creatinine, Fanconi-like syndrome

Respiratory: Asthma, bronchitis, coughing, dyspnea, pharyngitis, pneumonia, rhinitis, sinusitis

Miscellaneous: Diaphoresis, allergic reactions

Drug Interactions Aminoglycosides, amphotericin B, foscarnet, vancomycin, I.V. pentamidine and NSAIDs increase nephrotoxicity (cidofovir is contraindicated in patients who are receiving other nephrotoxic drugs); probenecid may decrease zidovudine clearance (temporarily discontinue zidovudine or decrease its dose by 50% on the days of cidofovir administration only); probenecid reduces the risk of cidofovir-induced nephrotoxicity by decreasing its concentration in proximal tubular cells; ganciclovir ocular implant (increased toxicity)

Stability Store vials at room temperature; cidofovir admixture is stable for 24 hours under refrigeration.

Mechanism of Action Cidofovir is converted to cidofovir diphosphate which is the active intracellular metabolite; suppresses CMV replication by selective inhibition of viral DNA polymerase; incorporation of cidofovir into the growing viral DNA chain results in reduction in the rate of viral DNA synthesis

Pharmacokinetics

Distribution: V_d: 0.54 L/kg; does not cross significantly into the CSF

Protein binding: <6%

Metabolism: Cidofovir is phosphorylated intracellularly to the active metabolite cidofovir diphosphate

Half-life: ~2.6 hours (cidofovir); 17 hours (cidofovir diphosphate)

Elimination: Renal tubular secretion and glomerular filtration

Renal clearance without probenecid: 130-170 mL/minute/1.73 m^2

Renal clearance with probenecid: 70-125 mL/minute/1.73 m^2

Usual Dosage I.V.: Administration of cidofovir must be accompanied by concomitant oral probenecid and I.V. NS hydration

Children: **Note:** Limited information regarding cidofovir use in pediatric patients is currently available in the literature; some centers have used doses of 1 mg/kg/dose 3 times/week or 5 mg/kg/dose once weekly for 3 weeks then every 2 weeks for the treatment of adenovirus infection after bone marrow transplantation. Oral probenecid 1.25 g/m^2/dose is administered 3 hours prior to and 1 hour and 8 hours after completion of each 1-hour cidofovir infusion. NS bolus equal to 3 times the maintenance fluid is administered for 1 hour before cidofovir infusion and 1 hour after, then decrease to 2 times the maintenance fluid for the subsequent 2 hours.

Adults: Cytomegalovirus (CMV) retinitis: Administer 2 g probenecid orally 3 hours prior to each cidofovir dose and 1 g at 2 and 8 hours after completion of the cidofovir infusion (total probenecid dose: 4 g); infuse one liter NS over 1-2 hours prior to the cidofovir infusion; may administer second liter of NS over 1-3 hours with or immediately after the cidofovir infusion if tolerated

Induction: 5 mg/kg/dose once weekly for 2 consecutive weeks

Maintenance: 5 mg/kg/dose once every other week

Dosing adjustment in renal impairment: If the serum creatinine increases by 0.3-0.4 mg/dL above baseline, reduce the cidofovir dose to 3 mg/kg; discontinue (Continued)

Cidofovir *(Continued)*

cidofovir therapy for increases ≥0.5 mg/dL above baseline or development of ≥3+ proteinuria.

Administration Do **not** administer by direct intraocular injection due to risk of iritis, ocular hypotony, and permanent visual impairment.
Parenteral: Administer by I.V. infusion over 1 hour. Dilute in 100 mL NS or D$_5$W or to a final concentration not to exceed 8 mg/mL.

Monitoring Parameters Monitor renal function (BUN, serum creatinine), urinalysis (urine glucose and protein), CBC with differential (neutrophil count), electrolytes (calcium, magnesium, phosphorus, uric acid), liver function tests (SGOT/SGPT), intraocular pressure and visual acuity

Patient Information Cidofovir is not a cure for CMV retinitis; regular follow-up ophthalmologic exams and careful monitoring of renal function are necessary; report any rash immediately to your physician; use contraception during and for 3 months following treatment

Nursing Implications Administration of probenecid with a meal may decrease associated nausea; acetaminophen and antihistamines may ameliorate hypersensitivity reactions. Handle and dispose of cidofovir according to guidelines issued for cytotoxic drugs. Maintain adequate patient hydration.

Dosage Forms Injection, solution, as dihydrate [preservative free]: 75 mg/mL (5 mL)

References

Izadifar-legrand F, Berrebi D, Faye A, et al, "Early Diagnosis of Adenovirus Infection and Treatment With Cidofovir After Bone Marrow Transplantation in Children," *Blood*, 1999, 94:341a.

Lalezari JP, Holland GN, Kramer F, et al, "Randomized, Controlled Study of the Safety and Efficacy of Intravenous Cidofovir for the Treatment of Relapsing Cytomegalovirus Retinitis in Patients With AIDS," *J Acquir Immune Defic Syndr Hum Retrovirol*, 1998, 17(4):339-44.

Legrand F, Berrebi D, Houhou N, et al, "Early Diagnosis of Adenovirus Infection and Treatment With Cidofovir After Bone Marrow Transplantation in Children," *Bone Marrow Transplant*, 2001, 27(6):621-6.

Ribaud P, Scieux C, Freymuth F, et al, "Successful Treatment of Adenovirus Disease With Intravenous Cidofovir in an Unrelated Stem-Cell Transplant Recipient," *Clinical Infectious Diseases*, 1999, 28(3):690-1.

♦ **Cilastatin and Imipenem** *see* Imipenem and Cilastatin *on page 595*

♦ **Ciloxan®** *see* Ciprofloxacin *on page 274*

Cimetidine *(sye MET i deen)*

Related Information
Carbohydrate and Alcohol Content of Liquid Medications for Use in Patients Receiving Ketogenic Diets *on page 1431*

U.S. Brand Names Tagamet®; Tagamet®-HB [OTC]; Tagamet®-HB 200 [OTC]

Canadian Brand Names Apo®-Cimetidine; Gen-Cimetidine; Novo-Cimetidine; Nu-Cimet®; PMS-Cimetidine

Therapeutic Category Gastrointestinal Agent, Gastric or Duodenal Ulcer Treatment; Histamine H$_2$ Antagonist

Generic Available Yes

Use Short-term treatment of active duodenal ulcers and benign gastric ulcers; long-term prophylaxis of duodenal ulcer; gastric hypersecretory states; gastroesophageal reflux (GERD); prevention of upper GI bleeding in critically ill patients; over-the-counter (OTC) formulation for relief of acid indigestion, heartburn, or sour stomach

Pregnancy Risk Factor B

Contraindications Hypersensitivity to cimetidine or any component (see Warnings)

Warnings Rapid I.V. administration may cause hypotension or cardiac arrhythmias. Injection (8 mL vial) contains benzyl alcohol which may cause allergic reactions in susceptible individuals; large amounts of benzyl alcohol (≥99 mg/kg/day) have been associated with a potentially fatal toxicity ("gasping syndrome") in neonates; the "gasping syndrome" consists of metabolic acidosis, respiratory distress, gasping respirations, CNS dysfunction (including convulsions, intracranial hemorrhage), hypotension and cardiovascular collapse; avoid use of injection containing benzyl alcohol in neonates. *In vitro* and animal studies have shown that benzoate, a metabolite of benzyl alcohol, displaces bilirubin from protein-binding sites.

Precautions Modify dosage in patients with renal and/or hepatic impairment; multiple drug interactions exist requiring dose modifications of other medications or cimetidine (see Drug Interactions)

Adverse Reactions
Cardiovascular: Bradycardia, hypotension, cardiac arrhythmias (after rapid I.V. administration), tachycardia
Central nervous system: Dizziness, mental confusion, agitation, headache, psychosis, drowsiness, fever
Dermatologic: Rash
Endocrine & metabolic: Gynecomastia
Gastrointestinal: Mild diarrhea, nausea, vomiting

Hematologic: Neutropenia, agranulocytosis, thrombocytopenia
Hepatic: Elevated AST and ALT
Neuromuscular & skeletal: Myalgia
Renal: Elevated serum creatinine

Drug Interactions Cytochrome P450 isoenzyme CYP1A2, CYP2C9, CYP2C19, CYP2D6, CYP3A3/4, and CYP2C18 inhibitor; isoenzyme CYP3A3/4 substrate

Cimetidine reduces the hepatic metabolism of drugs metabolized by the cytochrome P450 pathway which may result in decreased elimination of lidocaine, diazepam, theophylline, phenytoin, gabapentin, metronidazole, triamterene, procainamide, quinidine, propranolol, carbamazepine, chloroquine, lomustine, warfarin, flecainide, and tricyclic antidepressants; antacids, metoclopramide, and anticholinergics may reduce the absorption of cimetidine; cimetidine may decrease the absorption of iron, melphalan, indomethacin, ketoconazole, tetracyclines, delavirdine, and possibly fluconazole; cimetidine may decrease digoxin serum levels; may increase diltiazem, flecainide, praziquantel, tacrolimus, cyclosporin, nevirapine, mexiletine, and pentoxifylline serum levels; cimetidine decreases the renal clearance of zalcitabine and zidovudine; potentiates myelosuppressive effects of carmustine; may increase didanosine absorption

Food Interactions Limit xanthine-containing foods and beverages

Stability Protect from light; store at room temperature; do not refrigerate the injection since precipitation may occur (can be redissolved by warming without degradation); stable in parenteral nutrition solutions for up to 7 days when protected from light

Mechanism of Action Competitive inhibition of histamine at H_2-receptors of the gastric parietal cells resulting in reduced gastric acid secretion

Pharmacokinetics

Distribution: Crosses the placenta; breast milk to plasma ratio: 4.6-11.76
Protein binding: 13% to 25%
Bioavailability: 60% to 70%
Half-life:
Neonates: 3.6 hours
Children: 1.4 hours
Adults with normal renal function: 2 hours
Time to peak serum concentration: Oral: Within 1-2 hours
Elimination: Principally as unchanged drug by the kidney; some excretion in bile and feces

Usual Dosage

Neonates: Oral, I.M., I.V.: 5-10 mg/kg/day in divided doses every 8-12 hours
Infants: Oral, I.M., I.V.: 10-20 mg/kg/day divided every 6-12 hours
Children: Oral, I.M., I.V.: 20-40 mg/kg/day in divided doses every 6 hours
Adults:
Short-term treatment of active ulcers:
Oral: 300 mg 4 times/day or 800 mg at bedtime or 400 mg twice daily for up to 8 weeks
I.M., I.V.: 300 mg every 6 hours or 150 mg single dose followed by 37.5 mg/hour by continuous infusion; adjust dosage to maintain an intragastric pH ≥5 or acid secretory rate of <10 mEq/hour; (average dose 160 mg/hour; range: 40-600 mg/hour)
Duodenal ulcer prophylaxis: Oral: 400-800 mg at bedtime
Gastric hypersecretory conditions: Oral, I.M., I.V.: 300-600 mg every 6 hours; dosage not to exceed 2.4 g/day
GERD: Oral: 800 mg twice daily or 400 mg 4 times/day for 12 weeks
Acid indigestion, heartburn, sour stomach relief (OTC use): Oral: 100 mg right before or up to 30 minutes before a meal; no more than 2 tablets per day
Prevention of upper GI bleeding: Continuous I.V. infusion of 50 mg/hour

Dosing interval in renal impairment using 5-10 mg/kg/dose in children or 300 mg in adults (titrate dose to gastric pH and Cl_{cr}):
Cl_{cr} >40 mL/minute: Administer every 6 hours
Cl_{cr} 20-40 mL/minute: Administer every 8 hours or reduce dose by 25%
Cl_{cr} <20 mL/minute: Administer every 12 hours or reduce dose by 50%
Hemodialysis: Administer after dialysis and every 12 hours during the interdialysis period

Dosing adjustment in hepatic impairment: Reduce dosage in severe liver disease

Administration

Oral: Administer with food; do not administer with antacids
Parenteral: Can be administered as a slow I.V. push over 15 minutes (minimum 5 minutes; rapid administration has been associated with hypotension and cardiac arrhythmias) at a concentration not to exceed 15 mg/mL; or preferably as an I.V. intermittent or I.V. continuous infusion. Intermittent infusions are administered over 15-30 minutes at a final concentration not to exceed 6 mg/mL; for patients with an
(Continued)

Cimetidine *(Continued)*

active bleed, preferred method of administration is continuous infusion; may be administered intramuscularly

Monitoring Parameters Blood pressure and heart rate with I.V. push administration; CBC; gastric pH

Patient Information Avoid excessive amount of coffee and aspirin; when self medicating, if symptoms of heartburn, acid indigestion, or sour stomach persist after 2 weeks of continuous use of the drug, consult a clinician; notify your physician if taking other medications (multiple drug interactions exist)

Dosage Forms

Infusion, as hydrochloride [premixed in NS: 300 mg (50 mL)]

Injection, solution, as hydrochloride: 150 mg/mL (2 mL, 8 mL) [8 mL size contains benzyl alcohol]

Liquid, oral (Tagamet®-HB 200): 200 mg/20 mL (355 mL) [cool mint flavor]

Liquid, oral, as hydrochloride: 300 mg/5 mL (240 mL, 480 mL) [contains 2.8% alcohol; mint-peach flavor]

Tablet: 200 mg [OTC], 300 mg, 400 mg, 800 mg

Tagamet®-HB: 200 mg

Tagamet®: 300 mg, 400 mg

References

Lambert J, Mobassaleh M, and Grand RJ, "Efficacy of Cimetidine for Gastric Acid Suppression in Pediatric Patients," *J Pediatr*, 1992, 120(3):474-8.

Lloyd CW, Martin WJ, Taylor BD, et al, "Pharmacokinetics and Pharmacodynamics of Cimetidine and Metabolites in Critically Ill Children," *J Pediatr*, 1985, 107(2):295-300.

Lloyd CW, Martin WJ, and Taylor BD, "The Pharmacokinetics of Cimetidine and Metabolites in a Neonate," *Drug Intell Clin Pharm*, 1985, 19(3):203-5.

Somogyi A and Gugler R, "Clinical Pharmacokinetics of Cimetidine," *Clin Pharmacokinet*, 1983, 8(6):463-95.

♦ **Cipro®** *see* Ciprofloxacin on page 274

Ciprofloxacin *(sip roe FLOKS a sin)*

U.S. Brand Names Ciloxan®; Cipro®; Cipro® XR

Therapeutic Category Antibiotic, Ophthalmic; Antibiotic, Quinolone

Generic Available No

Use Treatment of documented or suspected pseudomonal infection of the respiratory or urinary tract, skin and soft tissue, bone and joint, eye and ear; documented multidrug-resistant, aerobic gram-negative bacilli, some gram-positive staphylococci, and *Mycobacterium tuberculosis*; documented infectious diarrhea due to *Campylobacter jejuni*, *Shigella*, or *Salmonella*; osteomyelitis caused by susceptible organisms in which parenteral therapy is not feasible; pulmonary exacerbation of cystic fibrosis; initial therapy or postexposure prophylaxis for anthrax infection; used ophthalmically for treatment of corneal ulcers and conjunctivitis due to susceptible organisms; extended release tablet is used for the treatment of uncomplicated UTI

Pregnancy Risk Factor C

Contraindications Hypersensitivity to ciprofloxacin, any component, or other quinolones; not recommended for use in pregnant women or during breast-feeding

Warnings Not recommended in children <18 years of age; ciprofloxacin has caused arthropathy with erosions of the cartilage in weight bearing joints of immature animals; green discoloration of teeth in newborns has been reported; Achilles tendonitis and tendon rupture have been reported with fluoroquinolones; prolonged use may result in superinfection; CNS stimulation may occur resulting in tremors, restlessness, confusion, and very rarely hallucinations or convulsive seizures

Serious and fatal reactions including cardiac arrest, seizure, status epilepticus, and respiratory failure have been reported in patients receiving ciprofloxacin and theophylline concurrently. Serum theophylline levels should be monitored and dosage adjustments made when concomitant use cannot be avoided. Severe hypersensitivity reactions, including anaphylaxis, have been reported in patients receiving quinolones. If an allergic reaction occurs, discontinue drug immediately.

Precautions Use with caution in patients with seizure disorders or renal impairment; modify dosage in patients with renal impairment

Adverse Reactions

Central nervous system: Headache, restlessness, dizziness, confusion, seizures, insomnia, hallucinations, agitation

Dermatologic: Rash, photosensitivity, pruritus, urticaria

Gastrointestinal: Nausea, diarrhea, vomiting, GI bleeding, abdominal pain, pseudomembranous colitis

Genitourinary: Crystalluria

Hematologic: Anemia, eosinophilia, neutropenia

Hepatic: Elevated liver enzymes

Local: With I.V.: Phlebitis, burning, pain, erythema, and swelling (occurs more frequently with infusion time <30 minutes)

Neuromuscular & skeletal: Arthralgia, joint and back pain, tremor, joint stiffness, arthritis, tendonitis

Renal: Elevated BUN and serum creatinine, acute renal failure, interstitial nephritis

Miscellaneous: Anaphylaxis

Drug Interactions Cytochrome P450 isoenzyme CYP1A2 inhibitor

Magnesium-, aluminum- or calcium-containing antacids and sucralfate decrease ciprofloxacin absorption by up to 90% if given at the same time; antacids in didanosine formulation chelate ciprofloxacin and decrease its absorption (administer ciprofloxacin 2 hours before or 6 hours after antacids and didanosine); probenecid decreases renal clearance of ciprofloxacin and can increase ciprofloxacin concentrations; ciprofloxacin decreases theophylline, warfarin, and cyclosporine clearance; NSAID (increase CNS stimulation)

Food Interactions Dairy foods (milk, yogurt) and mineral supplements decrease ciprofloxacin concentrations; avoid concomitant administration with dairy products, mineral supplements, or with calcium-fortified juices; ciprofloxacin increases caffeine concentrations; use caution with xanthine-containing foods and beverages

Stability Premixed bags: Out of overwrap stability: 14 days at room temperature; reconstituted oral suspension: Stable for 14 days when stored at room temperature or refrigerated; store tablets, intact injection vial, ophthalmic solution/ointment, and oral suspension prior to reconstitution at room temperature; protect from intense light; protect from freezing

Mechanism of Action Inhibits DNA-gyrase in susceptible organisms; inhibits relaxation of supercoiled DNA and promotes breakage of double-stranded DNA

Pharmacokinetics

Absorption: Oral: Well absorbed

Distribution: Widely distributed into body tissues and fluids with high concentration in bile, urine, sputum, stool, lungs, liver, skin, muscle, and bone; low concentration in CSF; crosses the placenta; appears in breast milk

Protein binding: 16% to 43%

Metabolism: Partially in the liver to active metabolites

Bioavailability: Oral: 50% to 85%; younger CF patients have a lower bioavailability of 68% versus CF patients >13 years of age with bioavailability of 95%

Half-life:

Infants: 2.73 hours

Children:

1-5 years: 1.28 hours

6-12 years: 2.5-2.6 hours

Adults with normal renal function: 3-5 hours

Time to peak serum concentration: Oral: Immediate release tablet: Within 0.5-2 hours; Extended release tablet: 1-2.5 hours

Elimination: 30% to 50% excreted as unchanged drug in urine; 20% to 40% excreted in feces primarily from biliary excretion

Clearance: After I.V.:

CF child: 0.84 L/hour/kg

Adult: 0.5-0.6 L/hour/kg

Dialysis: Only small amounts of ciprofloxacin are removed by dialysis (<10%)

Usual Dosage

Neonates: I.V. ciprofloxacin has been used in 23 neonates at doses ranging from 7-40 mg/kg/day divided every 12 hours (Schaad, 1995)

Children:

Oral: 20-30 mg/kg/day in 2 divided doses; maximum dose: 1.5 g/day

I.V.: 20-30 mg/kg/day divided every 12 hours; maximum dose: 800 mg/day

Anthrax:

Initial treatment: I.V.: 20-30 mg/kg/day divided every 12 hours for 60 days; maximum dose: 800 mg/day (substitute oral antibiotics for I.V. antibiotics as soon as clinical condition improves)

Postexposure prophylaxis: Oral: 20-30 mg/kg/day divided every 12 hours for 60 days; maximum dose: 1000 mg/day

Cystic fibrosis:

Oral: 40 mg/kg/day divided every 12 hours; maximum dose: 2 g/day

I.V.: 30 mg/kg/day divided every 8-12 hours; maximum dose: 1.2 g/day

Adults:

Oral: 250-750 mg every 12 hours, depending on severity of infection and susceptibility

Uncomplicated UTI/acute cystitis: Extended release tablet: 500 mg every 24 hours for 3 days

Chemoprophylaxis regimen for high-risk contacts of invasive meningococcal disease: 500 mg as a single dose

(Continued)

Ciprofloxacin *(Continued)*

Uncomplicated gonorrhea: 500 mg as a single dose

Chancroid: 500 mg twice daily for 3 days

Anthrax infection postexposure prophylaxis: 500 mg every 12 hours for 60 days

I.V.: 200-400 mg every 12 hours depending on severity of infection

Treatment of anthrax infection: 400 mg every 12 hours for 60 days (substitute oral antibiotics for I.V. antibiotics as soon as clinical condition improves)

Ophthalmic: Instill 1-2 drops into the affected eye(s) every 2 hours while awake for 2 days, then 1-2 drops every 4 hours while awake for the next 5 days **or** instill $1/2$" ointment ribbon 3 times/day for 2 days, then twice daily for the next 5 days

Treatment of corneal ulcers: Instill 2 drops every 15 minutes for the first 6 hours, then 2 drops every 30 minutes for the remainder of the first day; on the second day, 2 drops every hour; then 2 drops every 4 hours thereafter

Dosing interval in renal impairment: Cl_{cr} <30 mL/minute: Administer every 18-24 hours

Administration

Oral: Administer immediate release tablets 2 hours after a meal; may administer with food to minimize GI upset; extended release tablet and oral suspension may be administered with or without food; to prepare oral suspension, pour the microcapsules (small bottle) completely into the large bottle of diluent - DO NOT ADD WATER TO THE SUSPENSION. Shake suspension vigorously before use. Avoid antacid use. Drink plenty of fluids to maintain proper hydration and urine output

Parenteral: Administer by slow I.V. infusion over 60 minutes to reduce the risk of venous irritation (burning, pain, erythema, and swelling); final concentration for administration should not exceed 2 mg/mL

Ophthalmic:

Ointment: Instill ointment in the lower conjunctival sac

Solution: Apply finger pressure to lacrimal sac during and for 1-2 minutes after instillation to decrease risk of absorption and systemic effects

Monitoring Parameters Monitor renal, hepatic, and hematopoietic function periodically; number and type of stools/day for diarrhea. Patients receiving concurrent ciprofloxacin and theophylline should have serum levels of theophylline monitored; monitor INR in patients receiving warfarin; patients receiving concurrent ciprofloxacin and cyclosporine should have cyclosporine levels monitored

Reference Range Avoid peak serum concentrations >5 µg/mL

Patient Information Do not chew microcapsules of the oral suspension; do not split, crush, or chew extended release tablet; avoid caffeine; may cause dizziness or lightheadedness and impair ability to perform activities requiring mental alertness or physical coordination; notify physician if tendon pain or swelling occurs; remove contact lenses prior to administration of ophthalmic solution and ointment. May cause photosensitivity reactions (eg, exposure to sunlight may cause severe sunburn, skin rash, redness, or itching); avoid exposure to sunlight and artificial light sources (sunlamps, tanning booth/bed); wear protective clothing, wide-brimmed hats, sunglasses, and lip sunscreen (SPF ≥15); use a sunscreen [broad-spectrum sunscreen or physical sunscreen (preferred) or sunblock with SPF ≥15]; contact physician if reaction occurs.

Nursing Implications Do not administer antacids with or within 4 hours of a ciprofloxacin dose; ensure adequate patient hydration to prevent crystalluria

Dosage Forms

Infusion, as **lactate** [premixed in D_5W] (Cipro®): 200 mg (100 mL); 400 mg (200 mL)

Injection, solution, as **lactate** (Cipro®): 10 mg/mL (40 mL)

Ointment, ophthalmic, as **hydrochloride** (Ciloxan®): 3.33 mg/g [0.3% base] (3.5 g)

Solution, ophthalmic, as **hydrochloride** (Ciloxan®): 3.33 mg/mL [0.3% base] (2.5 mL, 5 mL, 10 mL) [contains benzalkonium chloride]

Suspension, oral, as **base** (Cipro®): 5% (50 mg/mL) (100 mL); 10% (100 mg/mL) (100 mL) [microcapsules for suspension; packaged with diluent; strawberry flavor]

Tablet, film coated, as **hydrochloride** (Cipro®): 100 mg, 250 mg, 500 mg, 750 mg

Tablet, extended release, film coated (Cipro® XR): 500 mg [equivalent to ciprofloxacin hydrochloride 287.5 mg and ciprofloxacin base 212.6 mg]

References

Campoli-Richards DM, Monk JP, Price A, et al, "Ciprofloxacin: A Review of Its Antibacterial Activity, Pharmacokinetic Properties and Therapeutic Use," *Drugs*, 1988, 35(4):373-447.

Inglesby TV, Henderson DA, Bartlett JG, et al, "Anthrax as a Biological Weapon: Medical and Public Health Management. Working Group on Civilian Biodefense," *JAMA*, 1999, 281(18):1735-45.

Rodriguez WJ, and Wiedermann BL, "The Role of Newer Oral Cephalosporins, Fluoroquinolones, and Macrolides in the Treatment of Pediatric Infections," *Adv Pediatr Infect Dis*, 1994, 9:125-59.

Rubio TT, Miles MV, Lettieri JT, et al, "Pharmacokinetic Disposition of Sequential Intravenous/Oral Ciprofloxacin in Pediatric Cystic Fibrosis Patients with Acute Pulmonary Exacerbation," *Pediatr Infect Dis J*, 1997, 16:112-7

Schaad UB, abdus Salam M, Aujard Y, et al, "Use of Fluoroquinolones in Pediatrics: Consensus Report of an International Society of Chemotherapy Commission," *Pediatr Infect Dis J*, 1995, 14(1):1-9.

Ciprofloxacin and Hydrocortisone
(sip roe FLOKS a sin & hye droe KOR ti sone)

Related Information
Ciprofloxacin *on page 274*
Hydrocortisone *on page 573*

U.S. Brand Names Cipro® HC Otic

Therapeutic Category Antibiotic/Corticosteroid, Otic

Generic Available No

Use Treatment of acute bacterial otitis externa due to susceptible strains of *S. aureus*, *P. aeruginosa*, or *Proteus mirabilis*

Contraindications Hypersensitivity to ciprofloxacin, hydrocortisone, any component, or other quinolones; patients with perforated tympanic membrane; patients with viral infections of the external ear canal

Adverse Reactions
Central nervous system: Headache
Dermatologic: Pruritus, fungal dermatitis, rash, urticaria, alopecia
Neuromuscular & skeletal: Paresthesia, hypoesthesia
Respiratory: Cough

Usual Dosage Children ≥1 year and Adults: Otic: Instill 3 drops into the affected ear(s) twice daily for 7 days

Administration Otic: Warm suspension by holding bottle in hand prior to instillation; shake well before use; patient should lie with affected ear upward and maintain position for 30-60 seconds after suspension is instilled into the ear canal

Dosage Forms Suspension, otic: Ciprofloxacin hydrochloride 0.2% base and hydrocortisone 1% (10 mL) [contains benzyl alcohol]

♦ **Cipro® HC Otic** *see Ciprofloxacin and Hydrocortisone on page 277*

♦ **Cipro® XR** *see Ciprofloxacin on page 274*

Cisapride *U.S. - Available Via Limited-Access Protocol Only* (SIS a pride)

Related Information
Carbohydrate and Alcohol Content of Liquid Medications for Use in Patients Receiving Ketogenic Diets *on page 1431*

U.S. Brand Names Propulsid®

Therapeutic Category Gastrointestinal Agent, Prokinetic

Generic Available No

Use Treatment of nocturnal symptoms of gastroesophageal reflux disease (GERD), also demonstrated effectiveness for gastroparesis, refractory constipation, and nonulcer dyspepsia in patients failing other therapies (see Warnings)

Pregnancy Risk Factor C

Contraindications Hypersensitivity to cisapride or any component; GI hemorrhage, mechanical obstruction, GI perforation, or other situations when GI motility stimulation is dangerous; patients with CHF, renal failure, multisystem organ failure, and COPD; patients at risk for developing or who have hypokalemia, hypocalcemia, or hypomagnesemia (eg, severe dehydration, vomiting, diarrhea, malnutrition, or receiving chronic diuretic therapy); patients with a known family history of congenital long-QT syndrome; prolonged QT intervals (QT_c >450), ventricular arrhythmias, ischemic heart disease, sinus node dysfunction, clinically significant bradycardia, and second or third degree AV block; patients receiving medications known to prolong the QT interval such as quinidine, procainamide, sotalol, amitriptyline (and other tricyclic antidepressants), maprotiline, phenothiazines, sertindole, astemizole, bepridil, or sparfloxacin, (see Warnings and Drug Interactions); serious cardiac arrhythmias including ventricular tachycardia, ventricular fibrillation, torsade de pointes, and QT prolongations have been reported in patients taking medications which inhibit cytochrome P450 3A4; some of these events have been fatal; do not coadminister with ketoconazole, itraconazole, fluconazole, miconazole, erythromycin, clarithromycin, nefazodone, delavirdine, indinavir, nelfinavir, ritonavir, saquinavir, or troleandomycin; do not coadminister with grapefruit juice

Warnings Serious cardiac arrhythmias including ventricular tachycardia, ventricular fibrillation, torsade de pointes, and QT prolongation have been reported in patients receiving cisapride; more than 270 cases have been reported including 70 fatalities; 85% of these cases occurred in patients with known risk factors (see Contraindications); for this reason, cisapride is available only for use in patients with severely debilitating conditions who meet specific criteria for a limited-access program directly through PRA International; for more information contact them at 877-795-4247

Precautions Use with caution in neonates, particularly if premature due to a potential increased risk of serious cardiac arrhythmias; decreased cisapride clearance found in (Continued)

Cisapride *U.S. - Available Via Limited-Access Protocol Only (Continued)*

neonates may result in increased serum levels; a 12-lead EKG (measuring QT intervals) should be done in all patients before beginning therapy

Adverse Reactions

Cardiovascular: Sinus tachycardia, QT interval prolongation, serious cardiac arrhythmias (see Warnings and Contraindications)

Central nervous system: Headache, insomnia, anxiety, nervousness, confusion

Dermatologic: Rash, pruritus

Endocrine & metabolic: Hypoglycemia with acidosis, hyperglycemia

Gastrointestinal: Diarrhea, abdominal pain, nausea, flatulence, dyspepsia, constipation, xerostomia

Genitourinary: Vaginitis (rare), urinary frequency

Hematologic: Thrombocytopenia, leukopenia, aplastic anemia, pancytopenia, hemolytic anemia, methemoglobinemia

Hepatic: Hepatitis, elevated liver enzymes

Neuromuscular & skeletal: Arthralgia, tremor

Respiratory: Rhinitis, sinusitis, cough, apnea

Miscellaneous: Positive ANA

Drug Interactions Cytochrome P450 isoenzyme CYP3A3/4 substrate

Decreased absorption of digoxin; decreased effect with atropine

Increased effect/toxicity of warfarin, diazepam (increased levels); increased bioavailability of cisapride with cimetidine and ranitidine use

Concomitant administration with ketoconazole has resulted in markedly elevated cisapride plasma concentrations and prolonged QT intervals on the EKG. These prolonged intervals have rarely been associated with serious ventricular arrhythmias and torsade de pointes; some of these adverse reactions have been fatal. Since the interaction is due to a decrease in cytochrome P450 metabolism induced by ketoconazole, it is expected that similar reactions would occur with itraconazole, miconazole, fluconazole, troleandomycin, delavirdine, indinavir, erythromycin, clarithromycin, nefazodone, nelfinavir, amprenavir, ritonavir, and saquinavir; see Contraindications and Food Interactions

Food Interactions Do not use grapefruit juice which increases cisapride bioavailability

Mechanism of Action A GI prokinetic agent which enhances the release of acetylcholine at the myenteric plexus. *In vitro* studies have shown cisapride to have serotonin-4 receptor agonistic properties; it has no dopamine receptor blocking activity and, therefore, no extrapyramidal side effects or central antiemetic activity. It increases lower esophageal sphincter pressure, increases the amplitude of peristalsis, accelerates gastric emptying, improves antroduodenal coordination, increases colonic motility, and enhances cecal and ascending colonic emptying.

Pharmacodynamics Onset of action: 0.5-1 hour

Pharmacokinetics

Distribution: Breast milk to plasma ratio: 0.045

Protein binding: 98%

Metabolism: Extensive in liver via cytochrome P450 isoenzyme CYP 3A3/4 to norcisapride, which is eliminated in urine and feces

Bioavailability: 40% to 50%

Half-life: 7-10 hours

Elimination: <10% of dose excreted into feces and urine

Usual Dosage Oral:

Neonates: 0.15-0.2 mg/kg/dose 3-4 times/day; maximum dose: 0.8 mg/kg/day

Infants and Children: 0.15-0.3 mg/kg/dose 3-4 times/day; maximum dose: 10 mg/dose

Adults: Initial: 10 mg 4 times/day at least 15 minutes before meals and at bedtime; in some patients the dosage will need to be increased to 20 mg to obtain a satisfactory result

Dosage adjustment in liver dysfunction: Reduce daily dosage by 50%

Administration Oral: Administer 15 minutes before meals or feeding

Monitoring Parameters EKG (prior to beginning therapy), serum electrolytes in patients on diuretic therapy (prior to beginning therapy and periodically thereafter); see Contraindications

Patient Information May cause dry mouth.

Dosage Forms

Suspension: 1 mg/mL (450 mL) [cherry cream flavor]

Tablet: 10 mg, 20 mg

References

Cucchiara S, Staiano A, Boccieri A, et al, "Effects of Cisapride on Parameters of Oesophageal Motility and on the Prolonged Intraoesophageal pH Test in Infants With Gastro-Oesophageal Reflux Disease," *Gut*, 1990, 31(1):21-5.

Hill SL, Evangelista KJ, Pizzi AM, et al, "Proarrhythmia Associated With Cisapride in Children," *Pediatrics*, 1998, 101(6):1053-6.

Khongphatthanayothin A, Lane J, Thomas D, et al, "Effects of Cisapride on QT Interval in Children," *J Pediatr*, 1998, 133(1):51-6.

Lander A, "The Risks and Benefits of Cisapride in Premature Neonates, Infants and Children," *Arch Dis Child*, 1998, 79:469-71.

Lewin AB, Bryant RM, Fenrich AL, et al, "Cisapride-Induced QT Interval," *J Pediatr*, 1996, 128(2):279-81.

Tolia V, "Long-Term Use of Cisapride in Premature Neonates of <34 Weeks Gestational Age," *J Pediatr Gastroenterol Nutr*, 1990, 11:420-2.

Van Eygen M and Van Ravensteyn H, "Effect of Cisapride on Excessive Regurgitation in Infants," *Clin Ther*, 1989, 11(5):669-77.

Cisatracurium (sis a tra KYOO ree um)

U.S. Brand Names Nimbex®

Therapeutic Category Neuromuscular Blocker Agent, Nondepolarizing; Skeletal Muscle Relaxant, Paralytic

Generic Available No

Use Eases endotracheal intubation as an adjunct to general anesthesia and relaxes skeletal muscle during surgery or mechanical ventilation

Pregnancy Risk Factor B

Contraindications Hypersensitivity to cisatracurium or any component (see Warnings)

Warnings Maintenance of an adequate airway and respiratory support is critical. Due to its intermediate onset of action, cisatracurium is not recommended for rapid sequence intubation; certain clinical conditions may result in potentiation or antagonism of neuromuscular blockade, see table.

10 mL multiple use vials contain benzyl alcohol as a preservative; benzyl alcohol may cause allergic reactions in susceptible individuals; large amounts of benzyl alcohol (≥99 mg/kg/day) have been associated with a potentially fatal toxicity ("gasping syndrome") in neonates; the "gasping syndrome" consists of metabolic acidosis, respiratory distress, gasping respirations, CNS dysfunction (including convulsions, intracranial hemorrhage), hypotension and cardiovascular collapse; avoid use of vials containing benzyl alcohol in neonates; *in vitro* and animal studies have shown that benzoate, a metabolite of benzyl alcohol, displaces bilirubin from protein-binding sites

Increased sensitivity in patients with myasthenia gravis, Eaton-Lambert syndrome, resistance to neuromuscular blockade in burn patients (>30% of body) for period of 5-70 days postinjury; resistance to neuromuscular blockade in patients with muscle trauma, denervation, immobilization, infection

Precautions Certain clinical conditions may result in potentiation or antagonism of neuromuscular blockade, see table.

Clinical Conditions Affecting Neuromuscular Blockade

Potentiation	Antagonism
Electrolyte abnormalities	Alkalosis
Severe hyponatremia	Hypercalcemia
Severe hypocalcemia	Demyelinating lesions
Severe hypokalemia	Peripheral neuropathies
Hypermagnesemia	Diabetes mellitus
Neuromuscular diseases	
Acidosis	
Acute intermittent porphyria	
Renal failure	
Hepatic failure	

Adverse Reactions

Cardiovascular: Rarely mild histamine release, cardiovascular effects are minimal and transient

Dermatologic: Rash

Respiratory: Bronchospasm

Miscellaneous: Hypersensitivity reactions including anaphylaxis

Drug Interactions See table on next page.

Stability Protect from light; refrigerate; once removed from refrigerator, stable 21 days even if re-refrigerated; unstable in alkaline solutions; **compatible** with D_5W, D_5NS, and NS; do not dilute in LR; **incompatible** for Y-site administration with propofol or

(Continued)

Cisatracurium *(Continued)*

ketorolac; **compatible** for Y-site administration with sufentanil, alfentanil, fentanyl, midazolam, and droperidol.

Potential Drug Interactions

Potentiation	Antagonism
Inhalation anesthetics	Calcium
Desflurane, sevoflurane, enflurane and	Carbamazepine
isoflurane > halothane > nitrous	Phenytoin
oxide	Steroids (chronic administration)
Antibiotics	Theophylline
Aminoglycosides, polymyxins,	Anticholinesterases*
clindamycin, vancomycin, tetracycline	Neostigmine, pyridostigmine,
Magnesium	edrophonium, echothiophate
Antiarrhythmics	ophthalmic solution
Quinidine, procainamide, bretylium, and	Caffeine
possibly lidocaine	Azathioprine
Diuretics	
Furosemide, mannitol, thiazides	
Amphotericin B (secondary to hypokalemia)	
Local anesthetics	
Dantrolene (directly depresses skeletal muscle)	
Beta blockers	
Calcium channel blockers	
Ketamine	
Lithium	
Succinylcholine (when administered prior to nondepolarizing neuromuscular-blocking agent)	
Cyclosporine	

*Can prolong the effects of acetylcholine

Mechanism of Action Blocks neural transmission at the myoneural junction by binding with cholinergic receptor sites

Pharmacodynamics

Onset of action: I.V.: Within 2-3 minutes

Maximum effect: Within 3-5 minutes

Duration: Dose dependent, 35-45 minutes after a single 0.1 mg/kg dose; recovery begins in 20-35 minutes when anesthesia is balanced; recovery is attained in 90% of patients in 25-93 minutes

Pharmacokinetics

Distribution: V_d: Adults: 0.16 L/kg

Metabolism: Some metabolites are active; 80% of drug clearance is via a rapid nonenzymatic degradation (Hofmann elimination) in the bloodstream; additional metabolism occurs via ester hydrolysis

Half-life: 22-31 minutes

Elimination: <10% of dose excreted as unchanged drug in urine

Clearance:

  Children: 5.9 mL/kg/minute

  Adults: 5.1 mL/kg/minute

Usual Dosage I.V.:

Children 2-12 years: Initial: 0.1 mg/kg followed by maintenance dose of 0.03 mg/kg as needed to maintain neuromuscular blockade

Children >12 years to Adults: Initial: 0.15-0.2 mg/kg followed by maintenance dose of 0.03 mg/kg 40-65 minutes later or as needed to maintain neuromuscular blockade

Continuous infusion:

  Children ≥2 years: 1-4 mcg/kg/minute

  Adults: 1-3 mcg/kg/minute

Note: There may be wide interpatient variability in dosage (range 0.5-10 mcg/kg/minute in adults) which may increase and decrease over time; optimize patient dosage by utilizing a peripheral nerve stimulator

Administration Parenteral: May be administered without further dilution by rapid I.V. injection over 5-10 seconds; for continuous infusions, dilute to a concentration of 0.1-0.4 mg/mL in D₅W or NS; not for I.M. injection due to tissue irritation

Monitoring Parameters Muscle twitch response to peripheral nerve stimulation, heart rate, blood pressure

Additional Information Neuromuscular blocking potency is 3 times that of atracurium; maximum block is up to 2 minutes longer than for equipotent doses of atracurium; laudanosine, a metabolite without neuromuscular blocking activity has been associated with hypotension and seizure activity in animal studies.

Dosage Forms Injection, solution, as besylate: 2 mg/mL (5 mL, 10 mL); 10 mg/mL (20 mL) [contains benzyl alcohol]

References
Martin LD, Bratton SL, and O'Rourke PP, "Clinical Uses and Controversies of Neuromuscular Blocking Agents in Infants and Children," *Crit Care Med*, 1999, 27(7):1358-68.

Cisplatin (SIS pla tin)

Related Information
Emetogenic Potential of Single Chemotherapeutic Agents *on page 1286*
Extravasation Treatment *on page 1240*

U.S. Brand Names Platinol®-AQ

Synonyms CDDP

Therapeutic Category Antineoplastic Agent, Alkylating Agent

Generic Available Yes

Use Treatment of testicular, ovarian, and breast cancer; advanced bladder cancer, osteosarcoma, Hodgkin's and non-Hodgkin's lymphoma, head or neck cancer, cervical cancer, lung cancer, brain tumors, neuroblastoma; used alone or in combination with other agents

Pregnancy Risk Factor D

Contraindications Hypersensitivity to cisplatin, platinum-containing agents, or any component; pre-existing renal impairment, hearing impairment, and myelosuppression; pregnancy

Warnings The FDA currently recommends that procedures for proper handling and disposal of antineoplastic agents be considered. Cumulative renal toxicity may be severe; dose-related toxicities include myelosuppression, nausea and vomiting; ototoxicity, especially pronounced in children, is manifested by tinnitus or loss of high frequency hearing and occasionally, deafness

Precautions All patients should receive adequate hydration prior to and for 24 hours after cisplatin administration with a sodium chloride-containing I.V. solution to promote chloruresis, with or without mannitol and/or furosemide, to ensure good urine output and decrease the chance of nephrotoxicity; reduce dosage in renal impairment and in infants <6 months of age due to their decreased renal function and renal tubular secretion; serum magnesium, as well as electrolytes, should be monitored before and within 48 hours after cisplatin therapy. Patients who are magnesium-depleted should receive replacement therapy before the start of cisplatin.

Adverse Reactions
Cardiovascular: Bradycardia, arrhythmias, Raynaud's phenomenon
Central nervous system: Seizures, encephalopathy
Dermatologic: Mild alopecia
Endocrine & metabolic: Hypomagnesemia, hypocalcemia, hypokalemia, hypophosphatemia, hyperuricemia
Gastrointestinal: Nausea and vomiting occur in 76% to 100% of patients and is dose-related
Hematologic: Myelosuppression
Hepatic: Elevated liver enzymes
Local: Phlebitis, tissue sloughing and necrosis if infiltrated
Neuromuscular & skeletal: Peripheral neuropathy (related to cumulative doses >200 mg/m^2)
Ocular: Papilledema, optic neuritis
Otic: Ototoxicity (especially pronounced in children; hearing loss in the high-frequency range is related to a cumulative dose of cisplatin >400 mg/m^2)
Renal: Nephrotoxicity (damage to the proximal tubules), azotemia, elevated BUN and serum creatinine
Miscellaneous: Anaphylactoid reactions (bronchoconstriction, tachycardia, hypotension, facial edema)

Drug Interactions Aminoglycosides, amphotericin B, and other nephrotoxic drugs (increase risk of nephrotoxicity); loop diuretics, aminoglycosides (potentiate ototoxicity); synergistic antineoplastic activity with cytarabine, 5-fluorouracil, etoposide; reduces renal elimination of methotrexate

Stability Reconstituted powder for injection is stable for 20 hours at room temperature; do not refrigerate reconstituted solution since precipitation may occur; protect from light; incompatible with sodium bicarbonate; do not infuse in solutions containing <0.2% sodium chloride; stable when combined with mannitol (12.5-50 g mannitol/L)
(Continued)

Cisplatin *(Continued)*

Mechanism of Action Platination of DNA leads to reactive intermediates that bind to DNA and form intrastrand and interstrand DNA cross-links

Pharmacokinetics

Distribution: I.V.: Rapid tissue distribution; CSF unbound platinum concentration: 40% of the plasma concentration

Protein binding: >90%; only the free (unbound) platinum and parent drug are cytotoxic

Metabolism: Undergoes nonenzymatic metabolism

Half-life, terminal: Children:

Free drug: 1.3 hours

Total platinum: 44 hours

Elimination: ~50% of dose excreted in urine within 5 days in an inactive form

Dialysis: Minimally removed by hemodialysis

Usual Dosage Children and Adults: I.V. (refer to individual protocols): **TO PREVENT POSSIBLE OVERDOSE, VERIFY ANY CISPLATIN DOSE EXCEEDING 120 mg/m^2 PER COURSE:**

Intermittent dosing schedule: 37-75 mg/m^2 once every 2-3 weeks or 50-100 mg/m^2 over 4-6 hours, once every 21-28 days

Daily dosing schedule: 15-20 mg/m^2/day for 5 days every 3-4 weeks

Osteogenic sarcoma or neuroblastoma: 60-100 mg/m^2 on day 1 every 3-4 weeks

Recurrent brain tumors: 60 mg/m^2 once daily for 2 consecutive days every 3-4 weeks

Bone marrow/blood cell transplantation: Continuous infusion: High dose: 55 mg/m^2/day for 72 hours; total dose = 165 mg/m^2

Dosing adjustment in renal impairment:

Cl$_{cr}$ 10-50 mL/minute: Administer 75% of dose

Cl$_{cr}$ <10 mL/minute: Administer 50% of dose

Administration Parenteral: I.V.: Administer according to protocol; rate of administration has varied from a 15- to 20-minute infusion, 1 mg/minute infusion, 6- to 8-hour infusion or 24-hour infusion; rapid I.V. injection may be associated with increased nephrotoxicity or ototoxicity compared to a slower I.V. infusion

Monitoring Parameters Renal function tests (serum creatinine, BUN, Cl$_{cr}$), electrolytes (particularly magnesium, calcium, potassium), hearing test, neurologic exam (with high dose), liver function tests periodically, CBC with differential and platelet count, urine output, urinalysis

Nursing Implications Needles, syringes, catheters, or I.V. administration sets that contain aluminum parts should not be used for administration of drug; methods to prevent nephrotoxicity include prehydration, diuresis with mannitol, and administration of sodium chloride containing I.V. solutions to promote chloruresis. Adequate hydration and urinary output should be maintained for 24 hours after administration. Extravasation may cause tissue sloughing and necrosis; care should be taken to avoid extravasation. Infiltration of cisplatin infusions with concentrations >0.5 mg/mL may result in a more severe tissue toxicity.

Additional Information Myelosuppressive effects:

WBC: Mild

Platelets: Mild

Onset (days): 10

Nadir (days): 18-23

Recovery (days): 21-40

Dosage Forms

Injection, aqueous solution [preservative free]: 1 mg/mL (50 mL, 100 mL, 200 mL)

Platinol®-AQ: 1 mg/mL (50 mL, 100 mL)

References

Costello MA, Dominick C, and Clerico A, "A Pilot Study of 5-Day Continuous Infusion of High-Dose Cisplatin and Pulsed Etoposide in Childhood Solid Tumors," *Am J Pediatr Hematol Oncol*, 1988, 10:103-8.

Reece PA, Stafford I, Abbott RL, et al, "Two-Versus 24-Hour Infusion of Cisplatin: Pharmacokinetic Considerations," *J Clin Oncol*, 1989, 7(2):270-5.

- ◆ **13-*cis*-Retinoic Acid** *see* Isotretinoin *on page 632*
- ◆ **Citracal® [OTC]** *see* Calcium Supplements *on page 200*
- ◆ **Citracal® Liquitab [OTC]** *see* Calcium Supplements *on page 200*
- ◆ **Citraderm® [OTC]** *see* Ascorbic Acid *on page 131*

Citrate and Citric Acid *(SIT rate & SIT rik AS id)*

Related Information

Carbohydrate and Alcohol Content of Liquid Medications for Use in Patients Receiving Ketogenic Diets *on page 1431*

U.S. Brand Names Bicitra®; Cytra-2; Cytra-3®; Cytra-K®; Oracit®; Polycitra®; Polycitra K®; Polycitra-LC®; Urocit®-K

Synonyms Citrate/Citric Acid; Citric Acid and Citrate; Shohl's Solution, Modified

Therapeutic Category Alkalinizing Agent, Oral

Generic Available No

Use Treatment of metabolic acidosis; alkalinizing agent in conditions where long-term maintenance of an alkaline urine is desirable

Potassium citrate: Prevention of uric acid nephrolithiasis, prevention of calcium renal stones in patients with hypocitraturia; urinary alkalizer when sodium citrate is contraindicated

Pregnancy Risk Factor C

Contraindications Hypersensitivity to citrate, citric acid, or any component; patients receiving sodium-restricted diet (sodium salts); severe renal impairment with oliguria, azotemia, or anuria; untreated Addison's disease, acute dehydration, heat cramps, severe myocardial damage, hyperkalemia (potassium salts); Urocit®-K (wax matrix tablet) is contraindicated in patients with delayed gastric emptying, intestinal obstruction, or stricture, patients receiving anticholinergic medications and in patients with peptic ulcer disease

Warnings Conversion to bicarbonate may be impaired in patients with hepatic failure, in shock, or who are severely ill. Some products contain sodium benzoate; benzoic acid (benzoate) is a metabolite of benzyl alcohol; large amounts of benzyl alcohol (≥99 mg/kg/day) have been associated with a potentially fatal toxicity ("gasping syndrome") in neonates; the "gasping syndrome" consists of metabolic acidosis, respiratory distress, gasping respirations, CNS dysfunction (including convulsions, intracranial hemorrhage), hypotension and cardiovascular collapse; avoid use of sodium benzoate containing products in neonates; *in vitro* and animal studies have shown that benzoate displaces bilirubin from protein binding sites

Precautions Use sodium salts with caution in patients with CHF, hypertension, pulmonary edema; may predispose patient to urolithiasis

Adverse Reactions

Central nervous system: Tetany

Endocrine & metabolic: Metabolic alkalosis, hypernatremia (if sodium salt used), hypocalcemia, hyperkalemia (if potassium salt used)

Gastrointestinal: Diarrhea, nausea, vomiting, stenotic or ulcerative lesions (wax matrix tablets)

Drug Interactions

Decreased effect/levels of chlorpropamide, lithium, methenamine, methotrexate, salicylates, and tetracycline due to urinary alkalinization

Increased toxicity/levels of amphetamines, flecainide, ephedrine, pseudoephedrine, quinidine, and quinine due to urinary alkalinization

Potassium-sparing diuretics, salt substitutes, captopril, and enalapril may result in increased serum potassium (potassium-containing salt forms only)

Mechanism of Action Citrate salts are oxidized in the body to form bicarbonate

Usual Dosage Oral (dilute in water or juice):

Infants and Children: 2-3 mEq/kg/day in divided doses 3-4 times/day **or** 5-15 mL with water after meals and at bedtime

Adults:

Solution: 15-30 mL with water after meals and at bedtime

Wax matrix tablet (Urocit®-K): 30-60 mEq/day in divided doses 3-4 times/day

Administration Oral: Dilute with water or juice and administer after meals; do not crush or chew wax matrix tablets (Urocit®-K)

Monitoring Parameters Serum sodium, bicarbonate, potassium, urine pH

Dosage Forms

Crystals for oral solution:

Cytra-K: Potassium citrate monohydrate 3300 mg and citric acid monohydrate 1002 mg per packet (100s) **[equivalent to 2 mEq/mL potassium and 2 mEq/mL bicarbonate; fruit flavor]**

Polycitra® K: Potassium citrate monohydrate 3300 mg and citric acid monohydrate 1002 mg per packet (100s) **[equivalent to 2 mEq/mL potassium and 2 mEq/mL bicarbonate; sugar free]**

Solution, oral:

Bicitra®, Cytra-2: Sodium citrate dihydrate 500 mg and citric acid monohydrate 334 mg per 5 mL (480 mL) **[equivalent to 1 mEq/mL sodium and 1 mEq/mL bicarbonate; grape flavor]**

Cytra-K: Potassium citrate monohydrate 1100 mg, and citric acid monohydrate 334 mg per 5 mL (480 mL) **[equivalent to 2 mEq/mL potassium and 2 mEq/mL bicarbonate; alcohol and sugar free; contains sodium benzoate; cherry flavor]**

Oracit®: Sodium citrate 490 mg and citric acid 640 mg per 5 mL (15 mL, 30 mL, 480 mL, 4000 mL) **[equivalent to 1 mEq/mL sodium and 1 mEq/mL bicarbonate]**

(Continued)

Citrate and Citric Acid *(Continued)*

Polycitra-K®: Potassium citrate monohydrate 1100 mg and citric acid monohydrate 334 per 5 mL (480 mL) **[equivalent to 2 mEq/mL potassium and 2 mEq/mL bicarbonate**; alcohol and sugar free]

Syrup:

Cytra-3: Potassium citrate monohydrate 550 mg and sodium citrate dihydrate 500 mg per 5 mL (480 mL) **[equivalent to 1 mEq/mL sodium, 1 mEq/mL potassium, and 2 mEq/mL bicarbonate**; alcohol free; contains sodium benzoate; raspberry flavor]

Polycitra®: Potassium citrate monohydrate 550 mg, sodium citrate dihydrate 500 mg, and citric acid monohydrate 334 mg per 5 mL (480 mL) **[equivalent to 1 mEq/mL sodium, 1 mEq/mL potassium, and 2 mEq/mL bicarbonate**; alcohol free]

Polycitra-LC®: Potassium citrate monohydrate 550 mg, sodium citrate dihydrate 500 mg, and citric acid monohydrate 334 mg per 5 mL (480 mL) **[equivalent to 1 mEq/mL sodium, 1 mEq/mL potassium, and 2 mEq/mL bicarbonate**; alcohol and sugar free]

Tablet, extended release, as potassium citrate (Urocit®-K): 5 mEq [540 mg], 10 mEq [1080 mg]

- ◆ **Citrate/Citric Acid** *see* Citrate and Citric Acid *on page 282*
- ◆ **Citrate of Magnesia (Magnesium Citrate)** *see* Magnesium Supplements *on page 701*
- ◆ **Citric Acid and Citrate** *see* Citrate and Citric Acid *on page 282*
- ◆ **Citrovorum Factor** *see* Leucovorin *on page 660*
- ◆ **CL-65336** *see* Tranexamic Acid *on page 1109*

Cladribine *(KLA dri been)*

U.S. Brand Names Leustatin®

Synonyms 2-CdA; 2-Chlorodeoxyadenosine

Therapeutic Category Antineoplastic Agent, Antimetabolite (Purine)

Generic Available Yes

Use Treatment of hairy cell leukemia, chronic myeloid leukemia, and chronic lymphocytic leukemia; cladribine has activity in the treatment of Langerhans cell histiocytosis (LCH), non-Hodgkin's lymphomas, T-cell lymphomas, relapsed acute lymphocytic leukemia and relapsed acute myeloid leukemia

Pregnancy Risk Factor D

Contraindications Hypersensitivity to cladribine or any component

Warnings The FDA currently recommends that procedures for proper handling and disposal of antineoplastic agents be considered. Serious neurological toxicity has been reported in patients who received cladribine by continuous infusion at high doses (0.4-0.8 mg/kg/day or >16 mg/m^2/day); neurologic toxicity appears to be dose-related. Severe neurologic toxicity has been reported rarely with standard dosing regimens. Acute nephrotoxicity has been observed with cladribine doses of 0.4-0.8 mg/kg/day, especially in patients concurrently receiving other nephrotoxic agents.

Precautions Dose-limiting toxicity is myelosuppression; use with caution in patients with pre-existing hematologic or immunologic abnormalities; prophylactic administration of allopurinol should be considered in patients receiving cladribine due to the potential for hyperuricemia secondary to tumor lysis; appropriate antibiotic therapy should be administered promptly in patients exhibiting signs and symptoms of neutropenia and infection.

Adverse Reactions

Cardiovascular: Edema, tachycardia

Central nervous system: Fever (69%), fatigue (45%), headache, dizziness, insomnia, malaise, irreversible neurologic toxicity (paraparesis/quadriparesis) at high doses (0.4-0.8 mg/kg/day or >16 mg/m^2/day)

Dermatologic: Pruritus, erythema, rash

Gastrointestinal: Constipation, abdominal pain, nausea, vomiting, decreased appetite, diarrhea

Hematologic: Myelosuppression (prolonged pancytopenia), thrombocytopenia, aplastic anemia, hemolytic anemia

Hepatic: Reversible, mild elevations of bilirubin and transaminase levels

Local: Injection site reactions, pain

Neuromuscular & skeletal: Myalgia, trunk pain

Renal: Acute nephrotoxicity reported at high doses (rare)

Respiratory: Abnormal breath sounds, cough, shortness of breath

Stability Refrigerate unopened vials (2°C to 8°C/36°F to 46°F); protect from light. Solutions should be administered immediately after the initial dilution or stored in the refrigerator (2°C to 8°C) for ≤8 hours. **The use of D$_5$W as a diluent is not recommended due to increased degradation of cladribine;** should not be mixed with other intravenous drugs or additives or infused simultaneously via a common intravenous line. Diluted solution of cladribine in NS is stable for 24 hours at room temperature under normal room light in polyvinyl chloride infusion containers.

Mechanism of Action A purine nucleoside analogue; prodrug which enters the cells through a transport system and is activated via phosphorylation by deoxycytidine kinase to a 5'-triphosphate derivative. This active form incorporates into DNA resulting in inhibition of DNA synthesis and early chain termination. The induction of strand breaks results in a drop in the cofactor nicotinamide adenine dinucleotide and disruption of cell metabolism. ATP is depleted to deprive cells of an important source of energy. Cladribine kills both resting as well as dividing cells.

Pharmacokinetics
Distribution: V$_d$:
Children: 305 L/m^2
Adults: 0.5-9 L/kg (53-160 L/m^2)
CSF: Plasma concentration ratio: 18.2%
Protein binding: 20%
Bioavailability: S.C.: 100%
Half-life: 19.7 hours ± 3.4 hours
Elimination: 21% to 44% renally excreted

Usual Dosage I.V.: (refer to individual protocols):
Children:
Hairy cell leukemia: 0.09 mg/kg/day continuous infusion for 7 days
AML:
<3 years: 0.3 mg/kg/day over 2 hours daily for 5 days
≥3 years: 9 mg/m^2/day over 2 hours daily for 5 days or 8.9 mg/m^2/day over 24 hours for 5 days
Langerhans cell histiocytosis: 5-7 mg/m^2/day for 5 days; repeat every 21-28 days; do not administer if platelet count <100,000
Adults: 0.09-0.1 mg/kg/day continuous infusion for 7 consecutive days

Administration Parenteral: I.V.: **Single daily infusion:** May administer diluted in NS as an intermittent infusion or continuous infusion; administer through a 0.22 micron in-line filter

Monitoring Parameters CBC with differential and platelet count; creatinine clearance before initial dose; periodic renal and hepatic function tests

Nursing Implications Cladribine I.V. solution for administration should be inspected visually for particulates. A precipitate may occur at low temperatures and may be resolubilized at room temperature or by shaking the solution vigorously.

Dosage Forms Injection, solution [preservative free]: 1 mg/mL (10 mL)

References
Kearns CM, Biakley RL, Santane VM, et al, "Pharmacokinetics of Cladribine (2-Chlorodeoxyadenosine) in Children with Acute Leukemia," *Cancer Research*, 1994, 54:1235-39.
Larson RA, et al, "Dose Escalation Trial of Cladribine Using 5 Daily I.V. Infusions in Patients with Advanced Hematologic Malignancies," *J Clin Oncol*, 1996, 14(1):188-95.
Liliemark J, "The Clinical Pharmacokinetics of Cladribine," *Clin Pharmacokinet*, 1997, 32:120-131.
Rodriguez-Galindo C, Kelly P, Jeng M, et al, "Treatment of Children With Langerhans Cell Histiocytosis With 2-Chlorodeoxyadenosine," *Am J Hematol*, 2002, 69(3):179-84.
Stine KC, Saylors RL, Williams LL, et al, "2-Chlorodeoxyadenosine (2-CDA) for the Treatment of Refractory or Recurrent Langerhans Cell Histiocytosis (LCH) in Pediatric Patients," *Med Pediatr Oncol*, 1997, 29:288-92.

♦ **Claforan®** *see Cefotaxime on page 232*
♦ **Clarinex®** *see Desloratadine on page 351*

Clarithromycin (kla RITH roe mye sin)

Related Information
Carbohydrate and Alcohol Content of Liquid Medications for Use in Patients Receiving Ketogenic Diets *on page 1431*
Endocarditis Prophylaxis *on page 1321*

U.S. Brand Names Biaxin®; Biaxin® XL

Therapeutic Category Antibiotic, Macrolide

Generic Available No

Use Treatment of upper and lower respiratory tract infections, acute otitis media, and infections of the skin and skin structure due to susceptible strains of *S. aureus, S. pyogenes, S. pneumoniae, H. influenzae, M. catarrhalis, Mycoplasma pneumoniae, C. trachomatis,* and *Legionella* species; prophylaxis and treatment of *Mycobacterium avium* complex (MAC) disease in patients with advanced HIV infection; treatment of *Helicobacter pylori* infection; prophylaxis of bacterial endocarditis in penicillin-allergic patients

Pregnancy Risk Factor C
(Continued)

Clarithromycin *(Continued)*

Contraindications Hypersensitivity to clarithromycin, any component, erythromycin, or any macrolide antibiotics; concomitant administration of terfenadine, astemizole, pimozide, or cisapride with clarithromycin may result in QT interval prolongation, ventricular tachycardia, ventricular fibrillation, hypotension, palpitations, cardiac arrest, and death

Warnings Safety and efficacy of clarithromycin have not been established in children <6 months of age; pseudomembranous colitis has been reported with use of clarithromycin

Precautions Use with caution in patients with hepatic or renal impairment; reduce dosage or prolong dosing interval in patients with severe renal impairment with or without coexisting hepatic impairment

Adverse Reactions

Central nervous system: Headache, hallucinations

Dermatologic: Pruritus, rash, Stevens-Johnson syndrome

Gastrointestinal: Diarrhea, nausea, vomiting, abdominal pain, pseudomembranous colitis, dysgeusia, stomatitis; incidence of adverse GI effects (diarrhea, nausea, vomiting, dyspepsia, abdominal pain) is lower (13%) compared to erythromycin treated patients (32%)

Hematologic: Elevated prothrombin time, decreased WBC

Hepatic: Elevated liver enzymes, hyperbilirubinemia

Otic: Hearing loss

Renal: Elevated BUN and serum creatinine

Drug Interactions Cytochrome P450 isoenzyme CYP3A3/4 substrate; CYP1A2 and CYP3A3/4 isoenzyme inhibitor

Clarithromycin has been shown to increase serum **theophylline** levels by as much as 20%; **carbamazepine** levels have been shown to increase after a single dose of clarithromycin; hepatic metabolism of terfenadine, astemizole, pimozide, and cisapride are reduced by clarithromycin (see Contraindications); increases serum level of digoxin, cyclosporine, tacrolimus, ergot alkaloids, omeprazole, lovastatin, simvastatin, and triazolam; potentiates the effects of warfarin; fluconazole and ritonavir increase serum level of clarithromycin; efavirenz decreases clarithromycin levels while increasing the levels of its metabolite

Food Interactions Food may delay the rate but not the extent of oral absorption

Stability Reconstituted oral suspension should **not** be refrigerated because it might gel; microencapsulated particles of clarithromycin in suspension are stable for 14 days when stored at room temperature

Mechanism of Action Inhibits bacterial RNA-dependent protein synthesis by binding to the 50S ribosomal subunit; the 14-hydroxy metabolite of clarithromycin is twice as active as the parent compound

Pharmacokinetics

Absorption: Rapid from the GI tract; food delays onset of absorption and formation of active metabolite, but does not affect the extent of tablet absorption; in pediatric patients, coadministration of the suspension with food did not significantly alter the extent of clarithromycin absorption or formation of the 14-OH metabolite

Distribution: Widely distributed throughout the body with tissue concentrations higher than serum concentrations

Protein binding: 65% to 70%

Metabolism: In the liver to active and inactive metabolites; undergoes extensive first-pass metabolism

Bioavailability: 50% to 68%

Half-life: Dose-dependent, prolonged with renal dysfunction

Clarithromycin:
250 mg dose: 3-4 hours
500 mg dose: 5-7 hours
14-hydroxy metabolite:
250 mg dose: 5-6 hours
500 mg dose: 7 hours

Time to peak serum concentration: 1-4 hours

Elimination: After a 250 mg dose, 20% is excreted unchanged in urine, 10% to 15% is excreted as active metabolite 14-OH clarithromycin, and 4% is excreted in feces

Usual Dosage Oral:

Infants and Children:

Acute otitis media: 15 mg/kg/day divided every 12 hours for 10 days

Respiratory, skin and skin structure infections: 15 mg/kg/day divided every 12 hours for 7-14 days

Prophylaxis for bacterial endocarditis: 15 mg/kg 1 hour before procedure

Prophylaxis for first episode of MAC with the following CD4+ T-lymphocyte counts (see next page): 15 mg/kg/day divided every 12 hours; maximum dose: 1 g/day

Children <12 months: <750 cells/μL
1-2 years: <500 cells/μL
2-6 years: <75 cells/μL
≥6 years: <50 cells/μL

Prophylaxis for recurrence of MAC: 15 mg/kg/day divided every 12 hours; maximum dose: 1 g/day (use in combination with ethambutol and with or without rifabutin)

Adolescents and Adults: Immediate-release tablet: 250 mg every 12 hours for 7-14 days for all indications except sinusitis and chronic bronchitis due to *H. influenzae*; for these indications, 500 mg every 12 hours for 7-14 days

Prophylaxis for bacterial endocarditis: 500 mg 1 hour before procedure

Prophylaxis for first episode of MAC in patients with CD4+ T-lymphocyte count <50 cells/μL: 500 mg twice daily

Prophylaxis for recurrence of MAC: 500 mg twice daily in combination with ethambutol and with or without rifabutin

Helicobacter pylori (combination therapy with omeprazole or with bismuth subsalicylate, tetracycline, and an H_2-receptor antagonist): 250 mg twice daily up to 500 mg 3 times/day

Adolescents and Adults: Extended-release tablet: Two 500 mg tablets for 7 days for chronic bronchitis and community-acquired pneumonia; two 500 mg tablets for 14 days for sinusitis

Dosing adjustment in renal impairment: Cl_{cr} <30 mL/minute: Decrease dose by 50% and administer once or twice daily

Administration Oral: May administer immediate-release tablet or oral suspension with or without meals; extended-release tablet must be administered with food; do not crush or chew extended-release tablet; may administer with milk; shake suspension well before use

Monitoring Parameters Monitor serum concentration of other drugs in patients receiving clarithromycin and drugs known to interact with erythromycin (ie, theophylline, digoxin, anticoagulants, triazolam) since there are still very few studies examining drug-drug interactions with clarithromycin; liver function tests; hearing (in patients receiving long-term treatment with clarithromycin); observe for changes in bowel frequency

Dosage Forms
Granules for oral suspension (Biaxin®): 125 mg/5 mL (50 mL, 100 mL); 250 mg/5 mL (50 mL, 100 mL) [fruit punch flavor]
Tablet, film coated (Biaxin®): 250 mg, 500 mg
Tablet, film coated, extended release (Biaxin® XL): 500 mg

References
Aspin MM, Hoberman A, McCarty J, et al, "Comparative Study of the Safety and Efficacy of Clarithromycin and Amoxicillin-Clavulanate in the Treatment of Acute Otitis Media in Children," *J Pediatr*, 1994, 125(1):136-41.

Guay DR and Craft JC, "Overview of the Pharmacology of Clarithromycin Suspension in Children and a Comparison With That in Adults," *Pediatr Infect Dis J*, 1993, 12(12 Suppl 3):S106-11.

Husson RN, Ross LA, Sandelli S, et al, "Orally Administered Clarithromycin for the Treatment of Systemic *Mycobacterium avium* Complex Infection in Children With Acquired Immunodeficiency Syndrome," *J Pediatr*, 1994, 124(5 Pt 1):807-14.

Kaplan JE, Masur H, and Holmes KK, "Guidelines for Preventing Opportunistic Infections Among HIV-Infected Persons - 2002 Recommendations of the USPHS and IDSA," *MMWR*, 2002, 51(RR-8):1-46.

Neu HC, "The Development of Macrolides: Clarithromycin in Perspective," *J Antimicrob Chemother*, 1991, 27(Suppl A):1-9.

Clemastine (KLEM as teen)

Related Information
Carbohydrate and Alcohol Content of Liquid Medications for Use in Patients Receiving Ketogenic Diets *on page 1431*
Drugs and Breast-Feeding *on page 1404*
(Continued)

Clemastine *(Continued)*

U.S. Brand Names Tavist® Allergy [OTC]

Synonyms Meclastine; Mecloprodin

Therapeutic Category Antihistamine

Generic Available Yes

Use Perennial and seasonal allergic rhinitis and other allergic symptoms including urticaria

Pregnancy Risk Factor C

Contraindications Hypersensitivity to clemastine or any component; narrow-angle glaucoma; patients receiving MAO inhibitors

Precautions Use with caution in patients with stenosing peptic ulcer, GI or GU obstruction, asthma, or prostatic hypertrophy

Adverse Reactions

Cardiovascular: Bradycardia, edema, palpitations

Central nervous system: Drowsiness, fatigue, headache, dizziness, vertigo, ataxia, CNS stimulation (more common in children)

Dermatologic: Rash, angioedema, photosensitivity

Gastrointestinal: Nausea, vomiting, xerostomia, gastritis, appetite increase, weight gain, diarrhea, abdominal pain

Hepatic: Hepatitis

Neuromuscular & skeletal: Arthralgia, myalgia, paresthesia

Respiratory: Shortness of breath, pharyngitis, bronchospasm, epistaxis

Drug Interactions Increased toxicity (CNS depression or excessive anticholinergic activity): CNS depressants, MAO inhibitors, tricyclic antidepressants, phenothiazines

Mechanism of Action Competes with histamine for H_1-receptor sites on effector cells in the GI tract, blood vessels, and respiratory tract

Pharmacodynamics

Onset of action: 2 hours after administration

Maximum effect: 5-7 hours

Duration: 10-12 hours

Pharmacokinetics

Absorption: Oral: Well absorbed

Distribution: Breast milk to plasma ratio: 0.25-0.5

Metabolism: In the liver

Time to peak serum concentration: 2-4 hours

Elimination: Majority of an oral dose eliminated in the urine

Usual Dosage Oral:

Infants and Children <6 years: 0.05 mg/kg/day as **clemastine base** or 0.335-0.67 mg/day clemastine fumarate (0.25-0.5 mg base/day) divided into two or three doses; maximum daily dosage: 1.34 mg (1 mg base)

Children 6-12 years: 0.67-1.34 mg clemastine fumarate (0.5-1 mg base) twice daily; do not exceed 4.02 mg/day (3 mg/day base)

Children ≥12 years and Adults: 1.34 mg clemastine fumarate (1 mg base) twice daily to 2.68 mg (2 mg base) 3 times/day; do not exceed 8.04 mg/day (6 mg base)

Administration Oral: Administer with food

Monitoring Parameters Look for a reduction of rhinitis, urticaria, eczema, pruritus, or other allergic symptoms

Patient Information Avoid alcohol; may cause drowsiness and impair ability to perform activities requiring mental alertness or physical coordination; may cause dry mouth. May rarely cause photosensitivity reactions (eg, exposure to sunlight may cause severe sunburn, skin rash, redness, or itching); avoid direct exposure to sunlight

Dosage Forms

Syrup, as fumarate [RX]: 0.67 mg/5 mL (120 mL) [0.5 mg/base/5 mL; contains 5.5% alcohol]

Tablet, as fumarate: 1.34 mg [1 mg base; OTC], 2.68 mg [2 mg base; RX]

Tavist® Allergy: 134 mg [1 mg base]

- **Cleocin®** *see* Clindamycin *on page 289*
- **Cleocin HCl®** *see* Clindamycin *on page 289*
- **Cleocin Pediatric®** *see* Clindamycin *on page 289*
- **Cleocin Phosphate®** *see* Clindamycin *on page 289*
- **Cleocin T®** *see* Clindamycin *on page 289*
- **Climara®** *see* Estradiol *on page 456*
- **Clinac™ BPO** *see* Benzoyl Peroxide *on page 165*
- **Clindagel™** *see* Clindamycin *on page 289*

Clindamycin (klin da MYE sin)
Related Information
Carbohydrate and Alcohol Content of Liquid Medications for Use in Patients Receiving Ketogenic Diets *on page 1431*
Endocarditis Prophylaxis *on page 1321*

U.S. Brand Names Cleocin®; Cleocin HCl®; Cleocin Pediatric®; Cleocin Phosphate®; Cleocin T®; Clindagel™; Clindets®

Canadian Brand Names Alti-Clindamycin; Dalacin® C; Dalacin® T; Dalacin® Vaginal

Therapeutic Category Acne Products; Antibiotic, Anaerobic; Antibiotic, Miscellaneous

Generic Available Yes

Use Useful agent against most aerobic gram-positive staphylococci and streptococci (except enterococci); useful against *Fusobacterium*, *Bacteroides* species and *Actinomyces* for treatment of respiratory tract infections, skin and soft tissue infections, sepsis, intra-abdominal infections, and infections of the female pelvis and genital tract; bacterial endocarditis prophylaxis for dental and upper respiratory procedures in penicillin-allergic patients; treatment of babesiosis; used topically in treatment of acne vulgaris; used intravaginally for treatment of bacterial vaginosis

Pregnancy Risk Factor B

Contraindications Hypersensitivity to clindamycin, lincomycin, or any component (see Warnings); previous pseudomembranous colitis, hepatic impairment, regional enteritis or ulcerative colitis

Warnings Can cause severe and possibly fatal colitis characterized by severe persistent diarrhea, severe abdominal cramps and possibly, the passage of blood and mucus; discontinue drug if significant diarrhea occurs. Antiperistaltic agents such as opiates or diphenoxylate with atropine may prolong and worsen the condition.

Capsule contains tartrazine which may cause allergic reactions in susceptible individuals. Injection contains benzyl alcohol which may cause allergic reactions in susceptible individuals; large amounts of benzyl alcohol ($\geq$99 mg/kg/day) have been associated with a potentially fatal toxicity ("gasping syndrome") in neonates; the "gasping syndrome" consists of metabolic acidosis, respiratory distress, gasping respirations, CNS dysfunction (including convulsions, intracranial hemorrhage), hypotension and cardiovascular collapse; use clindamycin injection products containing benzyl alcohol with caution in neonates; *in vitro* and animal studies have shown that benzoate, a metabolite of benzyl alcohol, displaces bilirubin from protein binding sites

Precautions Use with caution and modify dosage in patients with severe renal and/or hepatic impairment

Adverse Reactions
Cardiovascular: Hypotension, cardiac arrest (with rapid I.V. administration); arrhythmia due to QT_c prolongation

Dermatologic: Urticaria, rash, Stevens-Johnson syndrome, dry skin, erythema, pruritus

Gastrointestinal: Diarrhea, nausea, vomiting, pseudomembranous colitis, esophagitis

Genitourinary: Vaginal candidiasis, vaginitis

Hematologic: Eosinophilia, granulocytopenia, thrombocytopenia

Hepatic: Elevated liver enzymes

Local: Sterile abscess at I.M. injection site; thrombophlebitis, erythema, pain, swelling

Renal: Rare: Renal dysfunction

Drug Interactions Cytochrome P450 isoenzyme CYP3A3/4 substrate
Clindamycin may increase the neuromuscular blocking action of tubocurarine, pancuronium

Stability Do **not** refrigerate the reconstituted oral solution because it will thicken; oral solution stable for 2 weeks at room temperature following reconstitution; I.V. clindamycin is incompatible with aminophylline, tobramycin

Mechanism of Action Reversibly binds to 50S ribosomal subunits preventing peptide bond formation thus inhibiting bacterial protein synthesis; bacteriostatic or bactericidal depending on drug concentration, infection site, and organism

Pharmacokinetics
Absorption:
Oral: 90% of clindamycin hydrochloride is rapidly absorbed; clindamycin palmitate must be hydrolyzed in the GI tract before it is active

Topical: ~10% absorbed systemically

Distribution: No significant levels are seen in CSF, even with inflamed meninges; crosses the placenta; distributes into breast milk, saliva, ascites fluid, pleural fluid, bone, and bile

Protein binding: 94%

Bioavailability: Oral: ~90%

(Continued)

Clindamycin *(Continued)*

Half-life:
  Neonates:
    Premature: 8.7 hours
    Full-term: 3.6 hours
  Infants 1 month to 1 year: 3 hours
  Children and Adults with normal renal function: 2-3 hours
Time to peak serum concentration:
  Oral: Within 60 minutes
  I.M.: Within 1-3 hours
Elimination: Most of the drug is eliminated by hepatic metabolism; 10% of an oral dose excreted in urine and 3.6% excreted in feces as active drug and metabolites
Dialysis: Not dialyzable (0% to 5%)

Usual Dosage
Neonates: I.M., I.V.:
  Postnatal age ≤7 days:
    ≤2000 g: 10 mg/kg/day divided every 12 hours
    >2000 g: 15 mg/kg/day divided every 8 hours
  Postnatal age >7 days:
    <1200 g: 10 mg/kg/day divided every 12 hours
    1200-2000 g: 15 mg/kg/day divided every 8 hours
    >2000 g: 20-30 mg/kg/day divided every 6-8 hours
Infants and Children:
  Oral: 10-30 mg/kg/day divided every 6-8 hours; maximum dose: 1.8 g/day
  I.M., I.V.: 25-40 mg/kg/day divided every 6-8 hours; maximum dose: 4.8 g/day
  Bacterial endocarditis prophylaxis for dental and upper respiratory procedures in penicillin allergic patients:
    Oral: 20 mg/kg 1 hour before procedure **or** I.V.: 20 mg/kg 30 minutes before procedure; maximum dose: 600 mg
  Babesiosis: Oral: 20-40 mg/kg/day divided every 8 hours for 7 days plus quinine
Children and Adults: Topical: Apply a thin film twice daily
Adolescents and Adults:
  Oral: 150-450 mg/dose every 6-8 hours; maximum dose: 1.8 g/day
  I.M., I.V.: 1.2-1.8 g/day in 2-4 divided doses; maximum dose: 4.8 g/day
  Vaginal: One full applicator (100 mg) inserted intravaginally once daily before bedtime for seven consecutive days
  Bacterial endocarditis prophylaxis for dental and upper respiratory procedures in penicillin allergic patients:
    Oral: 600 mg 1 hour before procedure **or** I.V.: 600 mg 30 minutes before procedure
  Pelvic inflammatory disease: 900 mg I.V. every 8 hours for 24-48 hours after significant clinical improvement, followed by 600 mg orally 3 times/day to complete a 14-day course
  Babesiosis:
    I.V.: 1.2 g twice daily plus quinine
    or
    Oral: 600 mg 3 times/day for 7 days plus quinine
Dosing interval in renal/hepatic impairment: Reduce dosage in patients with severe renal or hepatic impairment

Administration
Intravaginal: Do not use for topical therapy, instillation in the eye, or oral administration
Oral: Capsule should be taken with a full glass of water to avoid esophageal irritation; shake oral solution well before use; may administer with or without meals
Parenteral: Administer by I.V. intermittent infusion over at least 10-60 minutes, at a rate **not** to exceed 30 mg/minute; hypotension and cardiopulmonary arrest have been reported following rapid I.V. administration; final concentration for administration should not exceed 18 mg/mL
Topical: Do not use intravaginally, instill in the eye, or administer orally; shake lotion well before use

Monitoring Parameters Observe for changes in bowel frequency; during prolonged therapy monitor CBC with differential, platelet count, hepatic and renal function tests periodically

Patient Information Report any severe diarrhea immediately; clindamycin vaginal cream (oil-based) may weaken latex condoms for up to 72 hours after completing therapy

Dosage Forms
Capsule, as **hydrochloride** (Cleocin HCl®): 75 mg [contains tartrazine], 150 mg [contains tartrazine], 300 mg

Cream, vaginal, as **phosphate** (Cleocin®): 2% (40 g) [packaged with 7 disposable applicators]

Gel, topical, as **phosphate**: 1% (30 g, 60 g)
Cleocin T®: 1% [10 mg/g] (30 g, 60 g)
Clindagel™: 1% [10 mg/g] (42 g, 77 g)

Granules for oral solution, as **palmitate** (Cleocin® Pediatric): 75 mg/5 mL (100 mL) [cherry flavor]

Infusion, as **phosphate** [premixed in D₅W] (Cleocin Phosphate®): 300 mg (50 mL); 600 mg (50 mL); 900 mg (50 mL)

Injection, solution, as **phosphate** (Cleocin Phosphate®): 150 mg/mL (2 mL, 4 mL, 6 mL, 60 mL) [contains benzyl alcohol]

Lotion, as **phosphate** (Cleocin T®): 1% (60 mL)

Solution, topical, as **phosphate** (Cleocin T®): 1% (30 mL, 60 mL) [contains 50% v/v isopropyl alcohol]

Suppositories, vaginal, as **phosphate** (Cleocin®): 100 mg (3s)

Swabs, topical: 1% (60s)
Clindets®: 1% (69s)
Cleocin T®: 1% (60s)

References
Dajani AS, Taubert KA, Wilson W, et al, "Prevention of Bacterial Endocarditis. Recommendations by the American Heart Association," *JAMA*, 1997, 277(22):1794-801.

♦ **Clindets®** see Clindamycin on page 289

♦ **Clinoril®** see Sulindac on page 1058

Clofazimine (kloe FA zi meen)
U.S. Brand Names Lamprene®
Therapeutic Category Antibiotic, Miscellaneous; Leprostatic Agent
Generic Available No
Use Treatment of dapsone-resistant lepromatous leprosy (*Mycobacterium leprae*); multibacillary dapsone-sensitive leprosy; erythema nodosum leprosum; **Note:** Clofazimine has been associated with an adverse outcome in the treatment of MAC disease and should not be used
Pregnancy Risk Factor C
Contraindications Hypersensitivity to clofazimine or any component
Precautions Well tolerated when administered in dosages ≤100 mg/day; dosages >100 mg/day should be used for as short a duration as possible; use with caution in patients with GI problems; patients with abdominal pain, colic, nausea, vomiting, or diarrhea during clofazimine therapy may require a dosage adjustment or discontinuation of therapy
Adverse Reactions
Central nervous system: Dizziness, drowsiness, fatigue, headache, fever
Dermatologic: Discoloration of the skin and conjunctiva (pink to brownish-black), dry skin, rash, pruritus, acneiform eruptions, erythema multiforme, phototoxicity
Endocrine & metabolic: Hyperglycemia
Gastrointestinal: Constipation, abdominal pain, diarrhea, nausea, anorexia, vomiting, bowel obstruction, GI bleeding, dysgeusia
Hepatic: Hepatitis, jaundice
Ocular: Irritation of the eyes
Neuromuscular & skeletal: Peripheral neuropathy
Drug Interactions Isoniazid increases clofazimine plasma and urinary concentration and decreases clofazimine skin concentration
Food Interactions Food increases the extent of absorption
Stability Protect from moisture
Mechanism of Action Binds preferentially to mycobacterial DNA at the guanine base to inhibit mycobacterial growth; also has some anti-inflammatory activity through an unknown mechanism
Pharmacokinetics
Absorption: Oral: 45% to 70% slowly absorbed
Distribution: Remains in tissues for prolonged periods and distributes into fatty tissues of the reticuloendothelial system, mesenteric lymph nodes, adrenal glands, liver, bile, spleen, small intestine, lungs, muscles, bone, skin, breast milk; does not appear to penetrate into the CSF
Metabolism: In the liver to three metabolites
Half-life:
Terminal: 8 days
Tissue: 70 days
Elimination: Principally in feces; only negligible amounts excreted unchanged in the urine; small amounts excreted in sputum, saliva, and sweat

(Continued)

Clofazimine *(Continued)*

Usual Dosage Oral:

Children: Leprosy: 1 mg/kg/day every 24 hours in combination with dapsone and rifampin

Adults:

Dapsone-resistant leprosy: 50-100 mg once daily in combination with one or more antileprosy drugs for 2 years; then alone 50-100 mg/day

Dapsone-sensitive multibacillary leprosy: 50-100 mg once daily in combination with two or more antileprosy drugs for at least 2 years and continue until negative skin smears are obtained, then institute single-drug therapy with appropriate agent

Erythema nodosum leprosum: 100-200 mg/day for up to 3 months or longer then taper dose to 100 mg/day when possible

Administration Oral: Administer with meals or milk to maximize absorption

Monitoring Parameters GI complaints, periodic liver function tests

Patient Information May discolor skin, conjunctiva, tears, sweat, urine, feces, and nasal secretions to a pink to brownish-black color; skin discoloration reversal may take several months after discontinuation of clofazimine

Nursing Implications Clofazimine-induced dry skin may be relieved by applying petrolatum or an emollient lotion containing 25% urea to the affected areas

Dosage Forms Capsule: 50 mg

References

Chesney PJ, "New Concepts for Antimicrobial Use in Opportunistic Infections," *Semin Pediatr Infect Dis*, 1991, 2(1):67-73.

Garrelts JC, "Clofazimine: A Review of Its Use in Leprosy and *Mycobacterium avium* Complex Infection," *DICP*, 1991, 25(5):525-31.

Kaplan JE, Masur H, and Holmes KK, "Guidelines for Preventing Opportunistic Infections Among HIV-Infected Persons - 2002 Recommendations of the USPHS and IDSA," *MMWR*, 2002, 51(RR-8):1-46.

♦ **Clonapam (Can)** *see* Clonazepam *on page 292*

Clonazepam *(kloe NA ze pam)*

Related Information

Antiepileptic Drugs *on page 1374*

Overdose and Toxicology *on page 1388*

U.S. Brand Names Klonopin®

Canadian Brand Names Alti-Clonazepam; Apo®-Clonazepam; Clonapam; Gen-Clonazepam; Novo-Clonazepam; Nu-Clonazepam; PMS-Clonazepam; Rho-Clonazepam; Rivotril®

Therapeutic Category Anticonvulsant, Benzodiazepine; Benzodiazepine

Generic Available Yes

Use Alone or as an adjunct in the treatment of absence (petit mal), petit mal variant (Lennox-Gastaut), infantile spasms, akinetic, and myoclonic seizures; panic disorder with or without agoraphobia

Restrictions C-IV

Pregnancy Risk Factor D

Contraindications Hypersensitivity to clonazepam, any component, or other benzodiazepines; severe liver disease, acute narrow-angle glaucoma

Precautions Use with caution in patients with chronic respiratory disease, hepatic disease, or impaired renal function; abrupt discontinuance may precipitate withdrawal symptoms, status epilepticus or seizures (withdraw gradually when discontinuing therapy; see Additional Information); worsening of seizures may occur when clonazepam is added to patients with multiple seizure types

Adverse Reactions

Cardiovascular: Hypotension

Central nervous system: Drowsiness, changes in behavior or personality, aggression, vertigo, confusion, depression, memory impairment, decreased concentration, headache, ataxia, hypotonia

Dermatologic: Rash

Gastrointestinal: Nausea, xerostomia, vomiting, diarrhea, constipation, anorexia, hypersalivation

Hematologic: Thrombocytopenia, anemia, leukopenia, eosinophilia

Neuromuscular & skeletal: Tremor, choreiform movements

Ocular: Nystagmus, blurred vision

Respiratory: Bronchial hypersecretion, respiratory depression

Miscellaneous: Physical and psychological dependence

Drug Interactions Cytochrome P450 isoenzyme CYP3A3/4 substrate

CNS depressants or alcohol increase sedation; phenytoin, carbamazepine, rifampin, or barbiturates increase clonazepam clearance; drugs that inhibit cytochrome P450 isoenzyme CYP3A3/4 may increase levels and effects of clonazepam (monitor for altered benzodiazepine response); concurrent use with valproic acid may result in absence status

Mechanism of Action Suppresses the spike-and-wave discharge in absence seizures by depressing nerve transmission in the motor cortex; depresses all levels of the CNS, including the limbic and reticular formation, by binding to the benzodiazepine site on the gamma-aminobutyric acid (GABA) receptor complex and modulating GABA, which is a major inhibitory neurotransmitter in the brain

Pharmacodynamics

Onset of action: 20-60 minutes

Duration:

Infants and young children: Up to 6-8 hours

Adults: Up to 12 hours

Pharmacokinetics

Absorption: Oral: Well absorbed

Distribution: V_d: Adults: 1.5-4.4 L/kg

Protein binding: 85%

Metabolism: Extensively metabolized in the liver; undergoes nitroreduction to 7-aminoclonazepam, followed by acetylation to 7-acetamidoclonazepam; nitroreduction and acetylation are via cytochrome P450 enzyme system; metabolites undergo glucuronide and sulfate conjugation

Bioavailability: 90%

Half-life:

Children: 22-33 hours

Adults: Usual: 30-40 hours; range: 19-50 hours

Elimination: Metabolites excreted as glucuronide or sulfate conjugates; <2% excreted unchanged in urine

Usual Dosage Oral:

Seizure disorders:

Infants and Children <10 years or 30 kg:

Initial daily dose: 0.01-0.03 mg/kg/day (maximum initial dose: 0.05 mg/kg/day) given in 2-3 divided doses; increase by no more than 0.5 mg every third day until seizures are controlled or adverse effects seen

Maintenance dose: 0.1-0.2 mg/kg/day divided 3 times/day; not to exceed 0.2 mg/kg/day

Children ≥10 years (>30 kg) and Adults:

Initial daily dose not to exceed 1.5 mg given in 3 divided doses; may increase by 0.5-1 mg every third day until seizures are controlled or adverse effects seen

Maintenance dose: 0.05-0.2 mg/kg/day; do not exceed 20 mg/day

Panic disorder: Adolescents ≥18 years and Adults: Initial: 0.25 mg twice daily; increase in increments of 0.125-0.25 mg twice daily every 3 days; target dose: 1 mg/day; maximum dose: 4 mg/day

Administration Oral: May administer with food or water to decrease GI distress

Monitoring Parameters Long-term use: CBC with differential, platelets, liver enzymes

Reference Range Relationship between serum concentration and seizure control is not well established; measurement at random times postdose may contribute to this problem; predose concentrations are recommended

Proposed therapeutic levels: 20-80 ng/mL

Potentially toxic concentration: >80 ng/mL

Patient Information Avoid alcohol; limit caffeine; may cause drowsiness and impair ability to perform activities requiring mental alertness or physical coordination; may be habit-forming; avoid abrupt discontinuation after prolonged use; may cause dry mouth

Additional Information Ethosuximide or valproic acid may be preferred for treatment of absence (petit mal) seizures. Clonazepam-induced behavioral disturbances may be more frequent in mentally handicapped patients. When discontinuing therapy in children, the clonazepam dose may be safely reduced by ≤0.04 mg/kg/week and discontinued when the daily dose is ≤0.04 mg/kg/day. When discontinuing therapy in adults treated for panic disorder, the clonazepam dose may be decreased by 0.125 mg twice daily every 3 days, until the drug is completely withdrawn. Treatment of panic disorder for >9 weeks has not been studied; long-term usefulness of clonazepam for the treatment of panic disorder should be re-evaluated periodically.

Dosage Forms Tablet: 0.5 mg, 1 mg, 2 mg

Extemporaneous Preparations A 0.1 mg/mL oral liquid can be made using 3 different vehicles (cherry syrup; a 1:1 mixture of Ora-Sweet® and Ora-Plus®; or a 1:1 mixture of Ora-Sweet® SF and Ora-Plus®); crush six 2 mg tablets into a fine powder in a mortar; add 10 mL of the vehicle and mix to make a uniform paste; mix while adding the vehicle in geometric portions to **almost** 120 mL; transfer to a calibrated bottle and qsad with vehicle to 120 mL; preparation is stable for 60 days when stored in amber

(Continued)

Clonazepam *(Continued)*

prescription bottles in the dark at room temperature (25°C) or under refrigeration (5°C); label "shake well" and "protect from light"

Allen LV and Erickson MA, "Stability of Acetazolamide, Allopurinol, Azathioprine, Clonazepam, and Flucytosine in Extemporaneously Compounded Oral Liquids," *Am J Health Syst Pharm*, 1996, 53(16):1944-9.

References

Sugai K, "Seizures With Clonazepam: Discontinuation and Suggestions for Safe Discontinuation Rates in Children," *Epilepsia*, 1993, 34(6):1089-97.

Walson PD and Edge JH, "Clonazepam Disposition in Pediatric Patients," *Ther Drug Monit*, 1996, 18(1):1-5.

Clonidine *(KLOE ni deen)*

U.S. Brand Names Catapres®; Catapres-TTS®; Duraclon™

Canadian Brand Names Apo®-Clonidine; Dixarit®; Novo-Clonidine®; Nu-Clonidine®

Therapeutic Category Adrenergic Agonist Agent; Alpha-Adrenergic Agonist; Analgesic, Non-narcotic (Epidural); Antihypertensive Agent

Generic Available Yes (tablet)

Use Management of hypertension; aid in the diagnosis of pheochromocytoma and growth hormone deficiency; used for heroin withdrawal and smoking cessation therapy in adults; alternate agent for the treatment of attention-deficit/hyperactivity disorder (ADHD); adjunct in the treatment of neuropathic pain; epidural form is used in combination with opiates for relief of severe pain in cancer patients whose pain was not relieved by opiates alone

Pregnancy Risk Factor C

Contraindications Hypersensitivity to clonidine hydrochloride or any component; epidural injection is contraindicated in patients receiving anticoagulation therapy and in patients with a bleeding diathesis or an infection at the injection site. Administration of epidural clonidine above the C_4 dermatome is contraindicated.

Warnings Do not abruptly discontinue as rapid increase in blood pressure and symptoms of sympathetic overactivity (such as increased heart rate, tremors, agitation, anxiety, insomnia, sweating, palpitations) may occur; if need to discontinue, taper dose gradually over more than 1 week. EKG abnormalities and 4 cases of sudden cardiac death have been reported in children receiving clonidine with methylphenidate; reduce dose of methylphenidate by 40% when used concurrently with clonidine; consider EKG monitoring. Epidural clonidine is not recommended for perioperative, obstetrical, or postpartum pain [due to the risk of hemodynamic instability] (hypotension, bradycardia)], in patients with severe cardiovascular disease, or those who are hemodynamically unstable.

Precautions Dosage modification is required in patients with renal impairment; use with caution in cerebrovascular disease, coronary insufficiency, renal impairment, sinus node dysfunction; monitor patients for signs of depression (especially those with a history of affective disorders)

Adverse Reactions

Cardiovascular: Raynaud's phenomenon, hypotension, bradycardia, palpitations, tachycardia, CHF, rebound hypertension if discontinued abruptly

Central nervous system: Drowsiness, sedation, headache, dizziness, fatigue, insomnia, anxiety, depression

Dermatologic: Rash, local skin reactions with patch

Endocrine & metabolic: Sodium and water retention, parotid pain

Gastrointestinal: Constipation, anorexia, xerostomia

Respiratory: Respiratory depression and ventilatory abnormalities with high epidural doses

Drug Interactions Use with methylphenidate may potentially increase EKG effects (see Warnings); tricyclic antidepressants antagonize hypotensive effects of clonidine; beta-blockers may potentiate bradycardia in patients receiving clonidine and may increase the rebound hypertension seen with clonidine withdrawal; discontinue beta-blocker several days before clonidine is tapered off; CNS depressants and alcohol may increase sedative effects; use with opiates may increase hypotension; epidural clonidine may prolong the effects of epidural local anesthetics

Food Interactions Avoid natural licorice (causes sodium and water retention and increases potassium loss)

Stability Epidural injection: Discard unused portion of vial (injection is preservative free); do not use with preservative

Mechanism of Action Stimulates alpha$_2$-adrenoreceptors in the brain stem, thus activating an inhibitory neuron, resulting in reduced sympathetic outflow, producing a decrease in vasomotor tone and heart rate

Epidural use: Prevents pain signal transmission to the brain and produces analgesia at presynaptic and postjunctional alpha$_2$-adrenoreceptors in the spinal cord

Pharmacodynamics Antihypertensive effects: Oral:
Onset of action: 30-60 minutes
Maximum effect: Within 2-4 hours
Duration: 6-10 hours

Pharmacokinetics
Distribution: V_d: Adults: 2.1 L/kg
Protein binding: 20% to 40%
Metabolism: Hepatic to inactive metabolites
Bioavailability, oral: 75% to 95%
Half-life, serum:
Neonates: 44-72 hours
Children: 8-12 hours
Adults:
Normal renal function: 6-20 hours
Renal impairment: 18-41 hours
Half-life, CSF: Adults: 1.3 ± 0.5 hours
Elimination: 65% excreted in urine (32% unchanged) and 22% excreted in feces via enterohepatic recirculation
Dialysis: Not dialyzable (0% to 5%)

Usual Dosage
Children:
Hypertension: Oral: Initial: 5-10 mcg/kg/day in divided doses every 8-12 hours; increase gradually, if needed, to 5-25 mcg/kg/day in divided doses every 6 hours; maximum dose: 0.9 mg/day
ADHD: Oral: Initial: 0.05 mg/day, increase every 3-7 days by 0.05 mg/day to 3-5 mcg/kg/day given in divided doses 3-4 times/day; usual maximum dose: 0.3-0.4 mg/day. **Note:** Some centers use doses as high as 8 mcg/kg/day or 0.5 mg/day (see Hunt, 1990).
Clonidine tolerance test (test of growth hormone release from the pituitary): Oral: 0.15 mg/m^2 or 4 mcg/kg as a single dose
Analgesia: Epidural (continuous infusion): Reserved for cancer patients with severe intractable pain, unresponsive to other analgesics or epidural or spinal opiates: Initial: 0.5 mcg/kg/hour; adjust with caution, based on clinical effect; usual range: 0.5-2 mcg/kg/hour; do not exceed adult doses
Neuropathic pain: Oral: Some centers use the following doses (see Galloway, 2000): Initial: 2 mcg/kg/dose every 4-6 hours; increase incrementally over several days; range: 2-4 mcg/kg/dose every 4-6 hours; may also be given as transdermal (see Transdermal)
Transdermal: Children may be switched to the transdermal delivery system after oral therapy is titrated to an optimal and stable dose; a transdermal dose approximately equivalent to the total oral daily dose may be used (see Hunt, 1990; see Administration)
Adults:
Hypertension:
Oral: Initial dose: 0.1 mg twice daily, usual maintenance dose: 0.2-1.2 mg/day in 2-4 divided doses; maximum recommended dose: 2.4 mg/day
Transdermal: Applied once weekly as transdermal delivery system; initial therapy with 0.1 mg/24 hours applied once every 7 days; adjust dosage based on response; hypotensive action may not begin until 2-3 days after initial application
Analgesia: Epidural (continuous infusion): Initial: 30 mcg/hour; titrate to clinical effect; usual maximum dose: 40 mcg/hour

Administration
Epidural: Dilute the 500 mcg/mL product with preservative free NS to a final concentration of 100 mcg/mL prior to use; visually inspect for particulate matter and discoloration prior to administration (whenever permitted by container and solution)
Oral: May be administered without regard to meals
Transdermal: Patches should be applied at bedtime to a clean, hairless area of the upper arm or chest; rotate patch sites weekly in adults; in children, the patch may need to be changed more frequently (eg, every 3-5 days); **Note:** Transdermal patch is a membrane-controlled system; do **not** cut the patch to deliver partial doses; rate of drug delivery, reservoir contents, and adhesion may be affected if cut; if partial dose is needed, surface area of patch can be blocked proportionally using adhesive bandage (see Lee, 1997)

Monitoring Parameters Blood pressure, heart rate; consider EKG monitoring in patients with history of heart disease or concurrent use of medications affecting cardiac conduction; with epidural administration: Blood pressure, heart rate; pulse oximetry with large bolus doses; monitor infusion pump and catheter tubing for obstruction or dislodgment throughout the course of therapy to decrease risk of inadvertent abrupt discontinuation
(Continued)

Clonidine *(Continued)*

Patient Information Avoid alcohol; may cause drowsiness and impair ability to perform activities requiring mental alertness or physical coordination; do not stop drug abruptly; may cause dry mouth

Nursing Implications Counsel patient/parent about compliance and danger of withdrawal reaction if doses are missed or drug is discontinued

Additional Information Epidural clonidine may be more effective in the treatment of neuropathic pain compared to somatic or visceral pain; clonidine-induced symptomatic bradycardia may be treated with atropine

Dosage Forms

Injection, epidural solution, as hydrochloride [preservative free] (Duraclon™): 100 mcg/mL (10 mL); 500 mcg/mL (10 mL)

Patch, transdermal [7-day duration]:
Catapres-TTS®-1: 0.1 mg/day (4s)
Catapres-TTS®-2: 0.2 mg/day (4s)
Catapres-TTS®-3: 0.3 mg/day (4s)

Tablet, as hydrochloride (Catapres®): 0.1 mg, 0.2 mg, 0.3 mg

Extemporaneous Preparations A 0.1 mg/mL oral suspension compounded from tablets is stable for 28 days when stored in amber glass bottles and refrigerated (4°C); thirty 0.2 mg tablets are crushed in a glass mortar and ground to a fine powder; 2 mL Purified Water USP is slowly added, and triturated to make a fine paste; Simple Syrup, NF is slowly added in 15 mL increments and triturated; qsad 60 mL; shake well before use

Levinson ML and Johnson CE, "Stability of an Extemporaneously Compounded Clonidine Hydrochloride Oral Liquid," *Am J Hosp Pharm*, 1992, 49(1):122-5.

References

Chafin CC, Hovinga CA,and Phelps SJ, "Clonidine in the Treatment of Attention Deficit Hyperactivity Disorder," *Journal of Pediatric Pharmacy Practice*, 1999, 4(6):308-15.

Galloway KS and Yaster M, "Pain and Symptom Control in Terminally Ill Children," *Pediatr Clin North Am*, 2000, 47(3):711-46.

Hart-Santora D and Hart LL, "Clonidine in Attention Deficit Hyperactivity Disorder," *Ann Pharmacother*, 1992, 26(1):37-9.

Hunt RD, Capper L, and O'Connell P, "Clonidine in Child and Adolescent Psychiatry," *J Child Adol Psychpharm*, 1990, 1(1):87-102.

Hunt RD, Minderaa RB, and Cohen DJ, "The Therapeutic Effect of Clonidine in Attention Deficit Disorder With Hyperactivity: A Comparison With Placebo and Methylphenidate," *Psychopharmacol Bull*, 1986, 22(1):229-35.

Lee NA and Anderson PO, "Giving Partial Doses of Transdermal Patches," *Am J Health Syst Pharm*, 1997, 54(15):1759-60.

Rocchini AP, "Childhood Hypertension: Etiology, Diagnosis, and Treatment," *Pediatr Clin North Am*, 1984, 31(6):1259-73.

Sinaiko AR, "Pharmacologic Management of Childhood Hypertension," *Pediatr Clin North Am*, 1993, 40(1):195-212.

Clorazepate *(klor AZ e pate)*

Related Information

Antiepileptic Drugs *on page 1374*
Overdose and Toxicology *on page 1388*

U.S. Brand Names Gen-XENE®; Tranxene® SD™; Tranxene® SD™-Half Strength; Tranxene® T-Tab®

Canadian Brand Names Apo®-Clorazepate; Novo-Clopate®

Therapeutic Category Anticonvulsant, Benzodiazepine; Benzodiazepine; Sedative

Generic Available Yes

Use Treatment of generalized anxiety and panic disorders; management of alcohol withdrawal; adjunct anticonvulsant in management of partial seizures

Restrictions C-IV

Pregnancy Risk Factor D

Contraindications Hypersensitivity to clorazepate dipotassium or any component; cross-sensitivity with other benzodiazepines may exist; avoid using in patients with pre-existing CNS depression, severe uncontrolled pain, or narrow-angle glaucoma

Warnings Abrupt discontinuation may cause withdrawal symptoms or seizures

Precautions Use with caution in patients with hepatic or renal disease

Adverse Reactions

Cardiovascular: Hypotension
Central nervous system: Drowsiness, dizziness, confusion, amnesia, nervousness, headache, depression, ataxia, insomnia, fatigue, irritability, slurred speech
Dermatologic: Rash
Gastrointestinal: Nausea, xerostomia
Hematologic: Reduced hematocrit (with long-term use)
Neuromuscular & skeletal: Tremor
Ocular: Blurred vision, diplopia

Miscellaneous: Physical and psychological dependence with long-term use; long-term use may also be associated with renal or hepatic injury

Drug Interactions Cytochrome P450 isoenzyme CYP3A3/4 substrate

Cimetidine or other hepatic enzyme inhibitors may decrease hepatic clearance, monitor for altered benzodiazepine response; concurrent use of clorazepate with ritonavir is not recommended

Stability Unstable in water

Mechanism of Action Depresses all levels of the CNS, including the limbic and reticular formation, by binding to the benzodiazepine site on the gamma-aminobutyric acid (GABA) receptor complex and modulating GABA, which is a major inhibitory neurotransmitter in the brain

Pharmacokinetics

Absorption: Rapidly decarboxylated to desmethyldiazepam (active) in acidic stomach prior to absorption

Distribution: Crosses the placenta

Metabolism: In the liver to oxazepam (active)

Half-life, adults:

Desmethyldiazepam: 48-96 hours

Oxazepam: 6-8 hours

Time to peak serum concentration: Oral: Within 1 hour

Elimination: Primarily in urine

Usual Dosage Oral:

Anticonvulsant:

Children: Initial dose: 0.3 mg/kg/day; maintenance dose: 0.5-3 mg/kg/day divided 2-4 times/day

or

Children 9-12 years: Initial: 3.75-7.5 mg/dose twice daily; increase dose by 3.75 mg at weekly intervals, not to exceed 60 mg/day in 2-3 divided doses

Children >12 years and Adults: Initial: Up to 7.5 mg/dose 2-3 times/day; increase dose by 7.5 mg at weekly intervals; usual dose: 0.5-1 mg/kg/day; not to exceed 90 mg/day (up to 3 mg/kg/day has been used)

Anxiety: Adults: 7.5-15 mg 2-4 times/day, or given as single dose of 15-22.5 mg at bedtime

Alcohol withdrawal: Adults: Initial: 30 mg, then 15 mg 2-4 times/day on first day; maximum daily dose: 90 mg; gradually decrease dose over subsequent days

Administration Oral: May administer with food or water to decrease GI upset

Monitoring Parameters Excessive CNS depression, respiratory rate, and cardiovascular status; with prolonged use: CBC, liver enzymes, renal function

Reference Range Therapeutic: 0.12-1 µg/mL (SI: 0.36-3.01 µmol/L)

Patient Information Avoid alcohol; may cause drowsiness and impair ability to perform activities requiring mental alertness or physical coordination; may be habit-forming; avoid abrupt discontinuation after prolonged use; may cause dry mouth

Dosage Forms

Tablet, as dipotassium (Gen-XENE®, Tranxene®-T-Tab®): 3.75 mg, 7.5 mg, 15 mg

Tablet, extended release, as dipotassium:

Tranxene® SD™: 22.5 mg

Tranxene® SD™-Half Strength: 11.25 mg

References

Fenichel GM, *Clinical Pediatric Neurology: A Signs and Symptoms Approach*, 2nd ed, Philadelphia, PA: WB Saunders Co, 1993.

Fujii T, Okuno T, Go T, et al, "Clorazepate Therapy for Intractable Epilepsy," *Brain Dev*, 1987, 9(3):288-91.

Mimaki T, Tagawa T, Ono J, et al, "Antiepileptic Effect and Serum Levels of Clorazepate on Children With Refractory Seizures," *Brain Dev*, 1984, 6(6):539-44.

♦ *Clostridium botulinum* **Toxin Type A** *see* Botulinum Toxin Type A *on page 178*

♦ **Clotrimaderm (Can)** *see* Clotrimazole *on page 297*

Clotrimazole (kloe TRIM a zole)

U.S. Brand Names Cruex® Prescription Strength Cream [OTC]; Gyne-Lotrimin® [OTC]; Gyne-Lotrimin® 3 [OTC]; Lotrimin®; Lotrimin AF® [OTC]; Mycelex®; Mycelex®-7 [OTC]

Canadian Brand Names Canesten® Topical; Canesten® Vaginal; Clotrimaderm; Trivagizole-3®

Therapeutic Category Antifungal Agent, Oral Nonabsorbed; Antifungal Agent, Topical; Antifungal Agent, Vaginal

Generic Available Yes

Use Treatment of susceptible fungal infections, including oropharyngeal candidiasis, dermatophytoses, superficial mycoses, cutaneous candidiasis, as well as vulvovaginal candidiasis; limited data suggests that the use of clotrimazole troches may be effective for prophylaxis against oropharyngeal candidiasis in neutropenic patients

(Continued)

Clotrimazole *(Continued)*

Pregnancy Risk Factor B (topical); C (troches)

Contraindications Hypersensitivity to clotrimazole or any component

Warnings Clotrimazole troches should not be used for treatment of systemic fungal infection

Precautions Safety and effectiveness of clotrimazole lozenges (troches) in children <3 years of age have not been established

Adverse Reactions

Dermatologic: Erythema, pruritus, urticaria, skin fissures, blistering

Gastrointestinal: Nausea and vomiting may occur in patients on clotrimazole troches; lower abdominal cramps may occur in patients receiving clotrimazole vaginal tablets

Hepatic: Abnormal liver function tests (causal relationship between troches and elevated LFTs not clearly established)

Local: Mild burning, irritation, stinging of skin or vaginal area

Mechanism of Action Binds to phospholipids in the fungal cell membrane altering cell wall permeability resulting in loss of essential intracellular elements

Pharmacokinetics

Absorption: Negligible through intact skin when administered topically; 3% to 10% of an intravaginal dose is absorbed

Distribution: Following oral/topical administration, clotrimazole is present in saliva for up to 3 hours following 30 minutes of dissolution time in the mouth

Usual Dosage

Children >3 years and Adults:

Topical/Oral: 10 mg troche dissolved slowly 5 times/day

Topical: Apply twice daily

Children >12 years and Adults: Vaginal: 100 mg/day at bedtime for 7 days or 200 mg/day at bedtime for 3 days or 500 mg single dose; or 5 g (= 1 applicatorful) of 1% vaginal cream daily at bedtime for 7-14 days

Administration

Oral: Dissolve lozenge (troche) in mouth over 15-30 minutes

Topical: Apply sparingly and rub gently into the cleansed, affected area and surrounding skin; do not apply to the eye

Vaginal: Wash hands before using. Insert full applicator into vagina gently and expel cream, or insert tablet into vagina. Wash applicator with soap and water following use. Remain lying down for 30 minutes following administration.

Monitoring Parameters Periodic liver function tests during oral therapy with clotrimazole lozenges

Patient Information Vaginal cream and tablet are oil-based and may weaken latex condoms and diaphragms; avoid intercourse during therapy. Do not use tampons until therapy is complete.

Dosage Forms

Combination pack: Vaginal tablet 200 mg (3s) and vaginal cream 1%

Gyne-Lotrimin® 3: Vaginal tablet 200 mg (3s) and vaginal cream 1%

Mycelex®-7: Vaginal tablet 100 mg (7s) and vaginal cream 1%

Cream, topical: 1% (15 g, 30 g, 45 g)

Cruex® Prescription Strength Cream: 1% (15 g)

Lotrimin®: 1% (15 g, 30 g, 45 g)

Lotrimin AF®: 1% (12 g, 24 g)

Cream, vaginal: 1% (45 g); 2% (21 g)

Gyne-Lotrimin®: 1% (45 g)

Gyne-Lotrimin® 3: 2% (21g)

Mycelex®-7: 1% (45 g)

Lotion, topical:

Lotrimin®: 1% (30 mL)

Lotrimin® AF: 1% (20 mL)

Solution, topical: 1% (10 mL, 30 mL)

Lotrimin®: 1% (10 mL, 30 mL)

Lotrimin® AF: 1% (10 mL)

Tablet, vaginal: (Gyne-Lotrimin® 3): 200 mg (3s)

Troche (Mycelex®): 10 mg

Cloxacillin *(kloks a SIL in)*

Related Information

Carbohydrate and Alcohol Content of Liquid Medications for Use in Patients Receiving Ketogenic Diets *on page 1431*

U.S. Brand Names Cloxapen®; Tegopen®

Canadian Brand Names Apo®-Cloxi; Novo-Cloxin®; Nu-Cloxi®

Therapeutic Category Antibiotic, Penicillin (Antistaphylococcal)
Generic Available Yes
Use Treatment of susceptible bacterial infections of the respiratory tract, skin and skin structure, bone and joint caused by penicillinase-producing staphylococci
Pregnancy Risk Factor B
Contraindications Hypersensitivity to cloxacillin, any component, or penicillins
Precautions Use with caution in patients with a history of cephalosporin hypersensitivity
Adverse Reactions
    Central nervous system: Fever
    Dermatologic: Rash
    Gastrointestinal: Nausea, vomiting, diarrhea
    Hematologic: Eosinophilia, leukopenia, neutropenia, thrombocytopenia, agranulocytosis
    Hepatic: Hepatotoxicity
    Renal: Hematuria, elevated BUN and serum creatinine
    Miscellaneous: Serum sickness-like reactions
Drug Interactions Probenecid (increases serum cloxacillin concentration)
Food Interactions Food decreases extent of absorption
Stability Refrigerate oral solution after reconstitution; discard after 14 days; stable for 3 days at room temperature
Mechanism of Action Inhibits bacterial cell wall synthesis by binding to one or more of the penicillin-binding proteins; inhibits the final transpeptidation step of peptidoglycan synthesis resulting in cell wall death
Pharmacokinetics
    Absorption: Oral: ~50%
    Distribution: Into pleural and synovial fluid, bone, liver, and kidneys; poor penetration into CSF; crosses the placenta; appears in breast milk
    Protein binding: 90% to 98%
    Metabolism: Significant in the liver to active and inactive metabolites
    Half-life: 30-90 minutes (prolonged with renal impairment and in neonates)
    Time to peak serum concentration: Oral: Within 0.5-2 hours
    Elimination: In the urine and through the bile
    Dialysis: Not dialyzable (0% to 5%)
Usual Dosage Oral:
    Children >1 month: 50-100 mg/kg/day in divided doses every 6 hours; up to a maximum of 4 g/day
    Adults: 250-500 mg every 6 hours
Administration Oral: Administer 1 hour before or 2 hours after meals; shake suspension well before use
Monitoring Parameters CBC with differential, platelet count, urinalysis, BUN, serum creatinine, and liver enzymes
Test Interactions False-positive urine and serum proteins
Additional Information
    Sodium content of 250 mg capsule: 0.6 mEq
    Sodium content of 5 mL of 125 mg/5 mL solution, oral: 0.48 mEq
Dosage Forms
    Capsule, as sodium: 250 mg, 500 mg
    Powder for oral suspension, as sodium: 125 mg/5 mL (100 mL, 200 mL)

♦ **Cloxapen®** *see* Cloxacillin *on page 298*

Coal Tar (KOLE tar)

U.S. Brand Names Betatar® [OTC]; Cutar® [OTC]; Denorex® [OTC]; Denorex® Extra Strength [OTC]; DHS™ Tar [OTC]; DHS™ Targel [OTC]; Estar® [OTC]; MG 217® [OTC]; MG 217® Medicated Tar [OTC]; Neutrogena® T/Gel [OTC]; Oxipor® VHC [OTC]; Pentrax® [OTC]; Polytar® [OTC]; Psorigel® [OTC]; Tegrin® [OTC]; Zetar® [OTC]
Canadian Brand Names Balnetar®; SpectroTar Skin Wash™; Targel®
Synonyms LCD
Therapeutic Category Antipsoriatic Agent, Topical; Antiseborrheic Agent, Topical
Generic Available Yes
Use Topically for controlling dandruff, seborrheic dermatitis, or psoriasis
Contraindications Hypersensitivity to coal tar or any ingredient in the formulation
Warnings Due to a potential carcinogenic risk, do not use around the rectum or in the genital area or groin
Precautions Do not apply to acutely inflamed skin; avoid exposure to sunlight for at least 24 hours
(Continued)

Coal Tar *(Continued)*

Adverse Reactions Dermatologic: Dermatitis, folliculitis, irritation, acneiform eruption, photosensitivity

Drug Interactions Tetracyclines, phenothiazines, tretinoin, and sulfonamides also have phototoxic potential

Mechanism of Action Reduces the number and size of epidermal cells produced

Usual Dosage Children and Adults: Topical:

Bath: 60-90 mL of a 5% to 20% solution or 15-25 mL of 30% lotion is added to bath water; soak 5-20 minutes, then pat dry; use once daily to once every 3 days

Shampoo: Apply twice weekly for the first 2 weeks then once weekly or more often if needed

Skin: Apply to the affected area 1-4 times/day; decrease frequency to 2-3 times/week once condition has been controlled

Atopic dermatitis: 2% to 5% coal tar cream may be applied once daily or every other day to reduce inflammation

Scalp psoriasis: Tar oil bath or coal tar solution may be painted sparingly to the lesions 3-12 hours before each shampoo

Psoriasis of the body, arms, legs: Apply at bedtime; if thick scales are present, use product with salicylic acid and apply several times during the day

Administration Topical:

Bath: Add appropriate amount of coal tar to lukewarm bath water and mix thoroughly

Shampoo: Rub shampoo onto wet hair and scalp, rinse thoroughly; repeat; leave on 5 minutes; rinse thoroughly

Patient Information Avoid contact with eyes, genital, or rectal area; coal tar preparations frequently stain the skin and hair; shake suspension well before use. May cause photosensitivity reactions (eg, exposure to sunlight may cause severe sunburn, skin rash, redness, or itching); avoid exposure to sunlight and artificial light sources (sunlamps, tanning booth/bed); wear protective clothing, wide-brimmed hats, sunglasses, and lip sunscreen (SPF ≥15); use a sunscreen [broad-spectrum sunscreen or physical sunscreen (preferred) or sunblock with SPF ≥15]; contact physician if reaction occurs.

Dosage Forms

Emulsion, topical (Cutar®): 7.5% coal tar solution (180 mL, 3840 mL)

Gel, shampoo:

Betatar®: 5% coal tar solution (240 mL) [green apple scent]

DHS™ Targel: 2.9% coal tar solution (240 mL) [equivalent to 0.5% coal tar]

Gel, topical:

Estar®: 5% coal tar (90 g)

Psorigel®: 7.5% coal tar solution (120 g)

Lotion, topical:

MG 217®: 5% coal tar solution (120 mL) [equivalent to 1% coal tar]

Oxipor® VHC: 25% coal tar solution (60 mL, 120 mL)

Ointment, topical (MG 217®): 10% coal tar solution (107 g, 430 g) [equivalent to 2% coal tar]

Shampoo:

Denorex®: 9% coal tar solution (120 mL, 240 mL, 360 mL) [equivalent to 1.8% coal tar; available with or without conditioner; mountain fresh scent]

Denorex® Extra Strength: 12.5% coal tar solution (240 mL, 360 mL) [available with or without conditioner]

DHS™ Tar: 2.9% coal tar solution (120 mL, 240 mL, 480 mL) [equivalent to 0.5% coal tar]

MG 217® Medicated Tar: 15% coal tar solution (120 mL, 240 mL, 480 mL) [equivalent to 3% coal tar]

Neutrogena® T/Gel: 2% coal tar extract (132 mL) [alcohol free]

Pentrax®: 5% coal tar (120 mL, 240 mL)

Polytar®: 0.5% coal tar (177 mL, 355 mL)

Tegrin®: 7% coal tar solution (210 mL) [equivalent to 1% coal tar; available with or without conditioner]

Zetar®: 1% coal tar (180 mL)

Soap (Polytar®): 0.5% coal tar (113 g)

References

Greaves MW, Weinstein GD, "Treatment of Psoriasis," *N Engl J Med*, 1995, 332(9):581-8.

Hanifin JM, "Atopic Dermatitis in Infants and Children," *Pediatr Clin North Am*, 1991, 38(4):763-89.

Cocaine *(koe KANE)*

Related Information

Drugs and Breast-Feeding *on page 1404*

Laboratory Detection of Drugs in Urine *on page 1400*

Therapeutic Category Analgesic, Topical; Local Anesthetic, Topical

Generic Available Yes

Use Topical anesthesia for mucous membranes

Restrictions C-II

Pregnancy Risk Factor C (X if nonmedical use)

Contraindications Hypersensitivity to cocaine or any component; systemic use

Precautions Use with caution in patients with hypertension, severe cardiovascular disease, thyrotoxicosis, and in infants; use with caution in patients with severely traumatized mucosa in the region of intended application

Adverse Reactions

Cardiovascular: Hypertension, tachycardia, cardiac arrhythmias

Central nervous system: Restlessness, nervousness, euphoria, excitement, hallucinations, seizures

Gastrointestinal: Vomiting

Neuromuscular & skeletal: Tremor

Ocular: Topical: Sloughing of the corneal epithelium, ulceration of the cornea

Respiratory: Tachypnea

Drug Interactions Cytochrome P450 isoenzyme CYP3A3/4 substrate

MAO inhibitors, inhalational anesthetics, levodopa, methyldopa, sympathomimetics and ethanol may increase risk of cardiac arrhythmias; CNS stimulants; beta-adrenergic blocking agents; cholinesterase inhibitors

Stability Store in well closed, light-resistant containers

Mechanism of Action Blocks both the initiation and conduction of nerve impulses by decreasing the neuronal membrane's permeability to sodium ions. This results in inhibition of depolarization with resultant blockade of conduction; interferes with the uptake of norepinephrine by adrenergic nerve terminals producing vasoconstriction.

Pharmacodynamics Following topical administration to mucosa:

Onset of action: Within 1 minute

Maximum effect: Within 5 minutes

Duration: ≥30 minutes, depending upon route and dosage administered

Pharmacokinetics

Absorption: Well absorbed through mucous membranes; absorption is limited by drug-induced vasoconstriction and enhanced by inflammation

Distribution: V_d: ~2 L/kg; appears in breast milk (see Additional Information)

Metabolism: In the liver; major metabolites are ecgonine methyl ester and benzoyl ecgonine

Half-life: 75 minutes

Elimination: Primarily in urine as metabolites and unchanged drug (<10%); cocaine metabolites may appear in the urine of neonates for up to 5 days after birth due to maternal cocaine use shortly before birth

Usual Dosage Topical application (ear, nose, throat, bronchoscopy): Concentrations of 1% to 4% are used; use lowest effective dose; do not exceed 1 mg/kg; patient tolerance, anesthetic technique, vascularity of tissue, and area to be anesthetized will determine dose needed. Solutions >4% are not recommended due to increased risk and severity of systemic toxicities.

Administration Topical: Use only on mucous membranes of the oral, laryngeal, and nasal cavities; do not use on extensive areas of broken skin; do not apply commercially available products to the eye (an extemporaneously prepared ophthalmic product must be made)

Monitoring Parameters Heart rate, blood pressure, respiratory rate, temperature

Additional Information Repeated ophthalmic applications to the eye may cause cornea to become clouded or pitted, therefore, NS should be used to irrigate and protect cornea during surgery; not for injection; cocaine intoxication of infants who are receiving breast milk from their mothers abusing cocaine has been reported

Dosage Forms

Powder, as hydrochloride: 5 g, 25 g

Solution, topical, as hydrochloride: 4% [40 mg/mL] (4 mL, 10 mL); 10% [100 mg/mL] (4 mL, 10 mL)

References

Chasnoff IJ, Lewis DE, and Squires L, "Cocaine Intoxication in Breast-Fed Infants," *Pediatrics*, 1987, 80(6):836-8.

Greenglass EJ, "The Adverse Effects of Cocaine on the Developing Human," Yaffe SJ and Arana JV, eds, *Pediatric Pharmacology: Therapeutic Principles in Practice*, 2nd ed, Philadelphia, PA: WB Saunders Co, 1992, 598-604.

Codeine (KOE deen)

Related Information

Compatibility of Medications Mixed in a Syringe *on page 1412*

Laboratory Detection of Drugs in Urine *on page 1400*

Narcotic Analgesics Comparison *on page 1223*

Overdose and Toxicology *on page 1388*

(Continued)

Codeine (Continued)

Synonyms Methylmorphine

Therapeutic Category Analgesic, Narcotic; Antitussive; Cough Preparation

Generic Available Yes

Use Treatment of mild to moderate pain; antitussive in lower doses (for nonproductive cough)

Restrictions C-II

Pregnancy Risk Factor C (D if used for prolonged periods or in high doses at term)

Contraindications Hypersensitivity to codeine or any component (see Warnings)

Warnings Some preparations contain sulfites which may cause allergic reactions in susceptible individuals; do not discontinue abruptly after prolonged use

Precautions Use with caution in patients with hypersensitivity reactions to other phenanthrene derivative opioid agonists (morphine, hydrocodone, hydromorphone, levorphanol, oxycodone, oxymorphone); respiratory diseases including: asthma, emphysema, COPD or severe liver or renal insufficiency

Adverse Reactions

Cardiovascular: Palpitations, bradycardia, peripheral vasodilation, hypotension due to vasodilation from histamine release

Central nervous system: CNS depression, elevated intracranial pressure, dizziness, drowsiness, sedation

Dermatologic: Pruritus from histamine release

Endocrine & metabolic: Antidiuretic hormone release

Gastrointestinal: Nausea, vomiting, constipation, biliary tract spasm

Genitourinary: Urinary tract spasm

Ocular: Miosis

Respiratory: Respiratory depression

Miscellaneous: Physical and psychological dependence, histamine release

Drug Interactions Cytochrome P450 isoenzyme CYP2D6 and CYP3A3/4 substrate; isoenzyme CYP2D6 inhibitor

CNS depressants, phenothiazines, tricyclic antidepressants may potentiate the adverse effects of codeine

Mechanism of Action Binds to opiate receptors in the CNS, causing inhibition of ascending pain pathways, altering the perception of and response to pain; causes cough suppression by direct central action in the medulla; produces generalized CNS depression

Pharmacodynamics

Onset of action:

Oral: 30-60 minutes

I.M.: 10-30 minutes

Maximum effect:

Oral: 60-90 minutes

I.M.: 30-60 minutes

Duration: 4-6 hours

Pharmacokinetics

Absorption: Oral: Adequate

Distribution: Crosses the placenta; appears in breast milk

Protein binding: 7%

Metabolism: Hepatic to morphine (active); undergoes hydroxylation and O-demethylation via cytochrome P450 isoenzyme CYP2D6 and demethylation via CYP3A3/4

Bioavailability: 60% to 70%

Half-life: 2.5-3.5 hours

Elimination: 3% to 16% in urine as unchanged drug, norcodeine, and free and conjugated morphine

Usual Dosage Doses should be titrated to appropriate analgesic effect; when changing routes of administration, note that oral dose is $^2/_3$ as effective as parenteral dose

Analgesic: Oral, I.M., S.C.:

Children: 0.5-1 mg/kg/dose every 4-6 hours as needed; maximum dose: 60 mg/dose

Adults: Usual: 30 mg/dose; range: 15-60 mg every 4-6 hours as needed

Antitussive: Oral (for nonproductive cough):

Infants and Children <2 years: Not recommended

Children ≥2 years: 1-1.5 mg/kg/day in divided doses every 4-6 hours as needed:

Alternatively dose according to age:

2-5 years: 2.5-5 mg every 4-6 hours as needed; maximum dose: 30 mg/day

6-12 years: 5-10 mg every 4-6 hours as needed; maximum dose: 60 mg/day

Children >12 years and Adults: 10-20 mg/dose every 4-6 hours as needed; maximum dose: 120 mg/day

Dosing adjustment in renal impairment:
Cl_{cr} 10-50 mL/minute: Administer 75% of dose
Cl_{cr} <10 mL/minute: Administer 50% of dose

Administration
Oral: Administer with food or water to decrease nausea and GI upset
Parenteral: I.M., S.C.: Not intended for I.V. use due to large histamine release and cardiovascular effects

Monitoring Parameters Respiratory rate, heart rate, blood pressure, pain relief

Patient Information Increase fluid and fiber intake to avoid constipation; avoid alcohol; may cause drowsiness and impair ability to perform activities requiring mental alertness or physical coordination; may be habit-forming; avoid abrupt discontinuation after prolonged use

Nursing Implications Observe patient for excessive sedation and respiratory depression; implement safety measures; may need to assist with ambulation

Additional Information Not recommended for use for cough control in patients with a productive cough; equianalgesic doses: 120 mg codeine phosphate I.M. approximately equals morphine 10 mg I.M.

Dosage Forms
Injection, solution, as **phosphate**: 15 mg/mL (2 mL); 30 mg/mL (2 mL) [contains sodium metabisulfite]
Solution, oral, as **phosphate**: 15 mg/5 mL (5 mL, 500 mL) [strawberry flavor]
Tablet, as **phosphate**: 30 mg, 60 mg
Tablet, as **sulfate**: 15 mg, 30 mg, 60 mg

♦ **Codeine and Acetaminophen** see Acetaminophen and Codeine on page 39
♦ **Codeine and Glycerol Guaiacolate** see Guaifenesin and Codeine on page 551
♦ **Codeine and Guaifenesin** see Guaifenesin and Codeine on page 551
♦ **Codeine and Promethazine** see Promethazine and Codeine on page 942
♦ **Codeine, Promethazine, and Phenylephrine** see Promethazine, Phenylephrine, and Codeine on page 945
♦ **CO Fluoxetine (Can)** see Fluoxetine on page 505
♦ **Cogentin®** see Benztropine on page 166
♦ **Co-Gesic®** see Hydrocodone and Acetaminophen on page 571
♦ **Colace® [OTC]** see Docusate on page 402
♦ **Colaspase** see Asparaginase on page 132
♦ **Colax-C® (Can)** see Docusate on page 402

Colchicine (KOL chi seen)

Canadian Brand Names ratio-Colchicine

Therapeutic Category Antigout Agent; Anti-inflammatory Agent

Generic Available Yes

Use Treatment of acute gouty arthritis attacks and prevention of recurrences of such attacks; management of familial Mediterranean fever

Pregnancy Risk Factor D

Contraindications Hypersensitivity to colchicine or any component; severe renal, GI disease, or cardiac disorders

Warnings Patients who become pregnant while receiving colchicine therapy may be at greater risk of producing trisomic offspring

Precautions Use with caution and modify dosage in patients with renal impairment

Adverse Reactions
Dermatologic: Rash, alopecia
Endocrine & metabolic: Azoospermia, hypothyroidism, metabolic acidosis
Gastrointestinal: Nausea, vomiting, diarrhea, abdominal pain, steatorrhea, paralytic ileus
Hematologic: Agranulocytosis, aplastic anemia, leukopenia
Hepatic: Elevated liver enzymes
Local: Irritation if extravasation occurs
Neuromuscular & skeletal: Myopathy, peripheral neuropathy
Renal: Hematuria, renal failure

Drug Interactions Colchicine may decrease absorption of Vitamin B_{12}

Food Interactions May need low purine diet during acute gouty attack

Stability I.V. colchicine is incompatible with dextrose or I.V. solutions with preservatives; protect from light

Mechanism of Action Decreases leukocyte motility, phagocytosis in joints and lactic acid production, thereby reducing the deposition of urate crystals that perpetuates the inflammatory response; inhibits secretion of serum amyloid A protein

Pharmacodynamics Onset of action:
Oral: Relief of pain and inflammation occurs after 24-48 hours
(Continued)

Colchicine (Continued)

I.V.: 6-12 hours

Pharmacokinetics

Distribution: Concentrates in leukocytes, kidney, spleen, and liver; does not distribute in heart, skeletal muscle, and brain

Metabolism: Partially deacetylated in the liver

Half-life, terminal: 9.3-10.6 hours

Time to peak serum concentration: Oral: Within 30-120 minutes then declines for 2 hours before increasing again due to enterohepatic recycling

Elimination: Primarily in the feces via bile; 10% to 20% excreted in urine

Dialysis: Not dialyzable (0% to 5%)

Usual Dosage

Prophylaxis of familial Mediterranean fever: Oral:

Children:

≤5 years: 0.5 mg/day

>5 years: 1-1.5 mg/day in 2-3 divided doses

Adults: 1-2 mg/day in 2-3 divided doses

Gouty arthritis: Acute attacks: Adults:

Oral: Initial: 0.5-1.2 mg, then 0.5-0.6 mg every 1-2 hours or 1-1.2 mg every 2 hours until relief or GI side effects occur to a maximum total dose of 8 mg

I.V.: Initial: 1-3 mg, then 0.5 mg every 6 hours until response, **not to exceed 4 mg/ week**; if pain recurs, it may be necessary to administer a daily dose of 1-2 mg for several days, however, do not give more colchicine by any route for at least 7 days after a full course of I.V. therapy (4 mg); transfer to oral colchicine in a dose similar to that being given I.V.

Prophylaxis of recurrent attacks: Oral: 0.5-0.6 mg every day or every other day

Dosing adjustment in renal impairment: Cl_{cr} <10 mL/minute: Decrease dose by 50%

Administration

Oral: Administer with water and maintain adequate fluid intake

Parenteral: Administer I.V. over 2-5 minutes into tubing of free-flowing I.V. with compatible fluid

Monitoring Parameters CBC with differential, urinalysis, and renal function test

Test Interactions May cause false-positive results in urine tests for erythrocytes or hemoglobin

Patient Information If taking for acute gouty attacks, discontinue if pain is relieved or if nausea, vomiting or diarrhea occur; avoid alcohol

Nursing Implications Severe local irritation can occur if inadvertently administered S.C. or I.M.; extravasation can cause tissue irritation

Dosage Forms

Injection, solution: 0.5 mg/mL (2 mL)

Tablet: 0.6 mg

References

Levy M, Spino M, and Read SE, "Colchicine: A State-of-the-Art Review," *Pharmacotherapy*, 1991, 11(3):196-211.

Majeed HA, Carroll JE, Khuffash FA, et al, "Long-term Colchicine Prophylaxis in Children With Familial Mediterranean Fever (Recurrent Hereditary Polyserositis)," *J Pediatr*, 1990, 116(6):997-9.

♦ Cold-Eeze® [OTC] *see* Zinc Supplements *on page 1167*

Colfosceril [DSC] (kole FOS er il)

U.S. Brand Names Exosurf® Neonatal [DSC]

Synonyms Dipalmitoylphosphatidylcholine; DPPC; Synthetic Lung Surfactant

Therapeutic Category Lung Surfactant

Generic Available No

Use Neonatal respiratory distress syndrome (RDS):

Prophylactic therapy: Infants at risk for developing RDS with body weight <1350 g; infants with evidence of pulmonary immaturity with body weight >1350 g

Rescue therapy: Treatment of infants with RDS based on respiratory distress not attributable to any other causes and chest radiographic findings consistent with RDS

Warnings This drug may rapidly affect oxygenation and lung compliance. If chest expansion improves substantially the ventilator peak inspiratory pressure setting should be reduced immediately. Hyperoxia and hypocarbia (hypocarbia can decrease blood flow to the brain) may occur requiring appropriate ventilator adjustments.

Adverse Reactions Respiratory: Pulmonary hemorrhage, apnea, mucous plugging, decrease in transcutaneous O_2 >20%

Stability Reconstituted suspension is stable 12 hours after reconstitution; **do not refrigerate**

Mechanism of Action Replaces deficient or ineffective endogenous lung surfactant in neonates with RDS or in neonates at risk of developing RDS; reduces surface tension and stabilizes the alveoli from collapsing

Pharmacokinetics Absorption: Following intratracheal administration, colfosceril is absorbed from the alveolus; catabolized and reutilized for further synthesis and secretion in lung tissue

Usual Dosage Intratracheal: Neonates:

Prophylactic treatment: Give 5 mL/kg as soon as possible; the second and third doses should be administered at 12 and 24 hours later to those infants remaining on ventilators

Rescue treatment: Give 5 mL/kg as soon as the diagnosis of RDS is made. The second 5 mL/kg dose should be administered 12 hours later

Administration Reconstitute with 8 mL preservative SWI; each mL contains 13.5 mg colfosceril; if the suspension appears to separate, gently swirl vial to resuspend contents; do not use if persistent large flakes or particulates appear

Intratracheal: For intratracheal administration only. Suction infant prior to administration; inspect solution to verify complete mixing of the suspension. Administer via sideport on the special endotracheal tube adapter without interrupting mechanical ventilation. Administer the dose in two 2.5 mL/kg aliquots. Each half-dose is instilled slowly over 1-2 minutes in small bursts with each inspiration. After the first 2.5 mL/kg dose turn the infants head and torso 45° right for 30 seconds, then return to the midline position and administer the second dose as above. Following the second dose, turn the infant's head and torso 45° to the left for 30 seconds and return the infant to the midline position.

Monitoring Parameters Continuous EKG and transcutaneous O_2 saturation should be monitored during administration; frequent ABG sampling is necessary to prevent postdosing hyperoxia and hypocarbia.

Dosage Forms Powder for intratracheal suspension, as palmitate: 108 mg (10 mL) [DSC]

Colistimethate (koe lis ti METH ate)

U.S. Brand Names Coly-Mycin® M

Synonyms Colistin (Polymyxin E); Colistin Sodium Methanesulfonate

Therapeutic Category Antibiotic, Miscellaneous

Generic Available Yes

Use Treatment of gram-negative infections due to susceptible *Pseudomonas aeruginosa*, *Enterobacter aerogenes*, *Escherichia coli*, and *Klebsiella pneumoniae*; not indicated for infections due to *Proteus* or *Neisseria* species. Parenteral use of colistimethate has mainly been replaced by less toxic antibiotics. Reserved for life-threatening infections caused by organisms resistant to the preferred drugs. Used as inhalation therapy in cystic fibrosis patients for treatment of initial colonization and management of chronic colonization with *P. aeruginosa*

Pregnancy Risk Factor C

Contraindications Hypersensitivity to colistimethate or any component

Warnings Colistimethate can cause serious nephrotoxicity or neurotoxicity; neurotoxic reactions may be manifested by circumoral paresthesia, numbness, tingling of the extremities, pruritus, vertigo, dizziness, and slurring of speech. Dosage reduction may alleviate symptoms. Nephrotoxicity is dose-dependent and reversible if the antibiotic is discontinued. Avoid concurrent or sequential use of other nephrotoxic and neurotoxic drugs, particularly bacitracin, kanamycin, streptomycin, paromomycin, polymyxin B, tobramycin, neomycin, gentamicin, and amikacin. Neuromuscular blockade resulting in respiratory arrest has been reported in patients with neuromuscular disease (ie, myasthenia gravis) and patients receiving neuromuscular blocking agents [see Drug Interactions]; impaired renal function increases the possibility of apnea and neuromuscular blockade. Pseudomembranous colitis has been reported with colistimethate.

Precautions Use with caution and modify dosage in patients with impaired renal function

Adverse Reactions

Central nervous system: Slurred speech, dizziness, vertigo, fever, ataxia, mental confusion, seizures

Dermatologic: Pruritus, urticaria, rash

Gastrointestinal: GI upset

Local: Pain at injection site

Neuromuscular & skeletal: Paresthesia, muscle weakness, peripheral neuropathy

Renal: Elevated BUN, creatinine; decreased urine output; hematuria; albuminuria; nephrotoxicity

Respiratory: Apnea; respiratory distress; bronchospasm, cough (with inhaled colistimethate)

(Continued)

Colistimethate (Continued)

Drug Interactions Neuromuscular blocking agents, aminoglycosides, general anesthetics, polymyxin B, and sodium citrate potentiate the neuromuscular blocking effect; cephalothin, aminoglycosides, amphotericin B, vancomycin, and polymyxin B may potentiate nephrotoxicity (avoid concomitant use with colistimethate) (see Warnings)

Stability Store vial at room temperature; reconstituted solution is stable for 7 days when stored in the refrigerator or at room temperature.

Mechanism of Action Hydrolyzed to colistin which acts as a cationic detergent damaging the bacterial cytoplasmic membrane of gram-negative organisms causing leakage of intracellular substances and cell death

Pharmacokinetics

Absorption: Not absorbed from the GI tract, mucous membranes, or intact skin

Distribution: Widely distributed to body tissues; does not penetrate into CSF, synovial, pleural, or pericardial fluids; crosses the placenta

V_d: Adults: 0.09 ± 0.03 L/kg

Protein binding: 50%

Half-life:

Children: 2-3 hours

Adolescents and adults with cystic fibrosis: 3.5 ± 1 hour

Time to peak serum concentration: I.M.: ~2 hours

Elimination: Primarily in urine as unchanged drug

Usual Dosage Children, Adolescents, and Adults: Dosage should be based on an estimate of ideal body weight: **dosage expressed in terms of colistin:**

I.M., I.V.: 2.5-5 mg/kg/day divided every 6-12 hours

I.V.: Cystic fibrosis: 5-8 mg/kg/day divided every 8 hours; maximum dose: 160 mg/dose

Inhalation: 75 mg in NS (4 mL total volume) via nebulizer twice daily

Dosing adjustment in renal impairment: Parenteral: Adults:

S_{cr} 1.3-1.5 mg/dL: 2.5-3.8 mg/kg/day divided every 12 hours

S_{cr} 1.6-2.5 mg/dL: 2.5 mg/kg/day divided every 12-24 hours

S_{cr} 2.6-4 mg/dL: 1.5 mg/kg/dose every 36 hours

Administration

Parenteral: Reconstitute vial with 2 mL SWI resulting in a concentration of 75 mg colistin/mL; swirl gently to avoid frothing. Administer by I.M., direct I.V. injection over 3-10 minutes, intermittent infusion over 30 minutes, or by continuous I.V. infusion. For continuous I.V. infusion, one-half of the total daily dose is administered by direct I.V. injection over 3-10 minutes followed 1-2 hours later by the remaining one-half of the total daily dose diluted in a compatible I.V. solution infused over 22-23 hours. The final concentration for administration should be based on the patient's fluid needs.

Inhalation: Further dilute dose to a total volume of 4 mL in NS and administer via nebulizer.

Monitoring Parameters Renal function tests, urine output; for inhalation therapy: Pre- and post-treatment spirometry

Patient Information May impair ability to perform activities requiring mental alertness or physical coordination

Nursing Implications May premedicate with a bronchodilator to reduce the potential of bronchospasm when administering inhaled colistimethate

Dosage Forms Injection, powder for reconstitution, as sodium: 150 mg colistin base

References

Beringer P, "The Clinical Use of Colistin in Patients With Cystic Fibrosis," *Curr Opin Pulm Med*, 2001, 7(6):434-40.

Cunningham S, Prasad A, Collyer L, et al, "Bronchoconstriction Following Nebulised Colistin in Cystic Fibrosis," *Arch Dis Child*, 2001, 84(5):432-3.

+ **Colistin (Polymyxin E)** *see* Colistimethate *on page 305*

+ **Colistin Sodium Methanesulfonate** *see* Colistimethate *on page 305*

+ **Colocort™** *see* Hydrocortisone *on page 573*

+ **Colo-Fresh™ [OTC]** *see* Bismuth *on page 174*

+ **Colonic Lavage Solution** *see* Polyethylene Glycol-Electrolyte Solution *on page 914*

+ **Coly-Mycin® M** *see* Colistimethate *on page 305*

+ **CoLyte®** *see* Polyethylene Glycol-Electrolyte Solution *on page 914*

+ **Combantrin™ (Can)** *see* Pyrantel Pamoate *on page 960*

+ **Combivir®** *see* Lamivudine and Zidovudine *on page 652*

+ **Comparison of Adverse Effects of Antidepressants** *see page 1210*

+ **Comparison of Usual Adult Dosage and Mechanism of Action of Antidepressants** *see page 1209*

+ **Compatibility of Medications Mixed in a Syringe** *see page 1412*

♦ **Compazine®** *see* Prochlorperazine *on page 938*
♦ **Compound F** *see* Hydrocortisone *on page 573*
♦ **Compound S** *see* Zidovudine *on page 1163*
♦ **Compound S, Abacavir, and 3TC** *see* Abacavir, Lamivudine, and Zidovudine *on page 32*
♦ **Compound S, Abacavir, and Lamivudine** *see* Abacavir, Lamivudine, and Zidovudine *on page 32*
♦ **Compound S, ABC, and 3TC** *see* Abacavir, Lamivudine, and Zidovudine *on page 32*
♦ **Compound W® [OTC]** *see* Salicylic Acid *on page 1002*
♦ **Compound W® One Step Wart Remover [OTC]** *see* Salicylic Acid *on page 1002*
♦ **Compoz® Nighttime Sleep Aid [OTC]** *see* DiphenhydrAMINE *on page 393*
♦ **Compro™** *see* Prochlorperazine *on page 938*
♦ **Concerta®** *see* Methylphenidate *on page 744*
♦ **Congest (Can)** *see* Estrogens (Conjugated/Equine) *on page 459*
♦ **Conjugated Estrogens** *see* Estrogens (Conjugated/Equine) *on page 459*
♦ **Constilac®** *see* Lactulose *on page 649*
♦ **Constulose®** *see* Lactulose *on page 649*
♦ **Contac® Cold 12 Hour Relief Non Drowsy (Can)** *see* Pseudoephedrine *on page 958*
♦ **Copegus™** *see* Ribavirin *on page 981*
♦ **Copper Sulfate** *see* Trace Metals *on page 1106*
♦ **Cordarone®** *see* Amiodarone *on page 83*
♦ **Corgard®** *see* Nadolol *on page 788*
♦ **CortaGel® Maximum Strength [OTC]** *see* Hydrocortisone *on page 573*
♦ **Cortaid® Intensive Therapy [OTC]** *see* Hydrocortisone *on page 573*
♦ **Cortaid® Maximum Strength [OTC]** *see* Hydrocortisone *on page 573*
♦ **Cortaid® Sensitive Skin With Aloe [OTC]** *see* Hydrocortisone *on page 573*
♦ **Cortamed® (Can)** *see* Hydrocortisone *on page 573*
♦ **Cortate® (Can)** *see* Hydrocortisone *on page 573*
♦ **Cortef®** *see* Hydrocortisone *on page 573*
♦ **Cortenema® (Can)** *see* Hydrocortisone *on page 573*
♦ **Corticool® [OTC]** *see* Hydrocortisone *on page 573*
♦ **Corticosteroids Comparison, Systemic** *see page 1211*
♦ **Corticosteroids Comparison, Topical** *see page 1212*

Corticotropin (kor ti koe TROE pin)

Related Information
  Antiepileptic Drugs *on page 1374*
U.S. Brand Names H.P. Acthar® Gel
Synonyms ACTH; Adrenocorticotropic Hormone; Corticotropin, Repository
Therapeutic Category Adrenal Corticosteroid; Diagnostic Agent, Adrenocortical Insufficiency; Infantile Spasms, Treatment
Generic Available No
Use Infantile spasms; diagnostic aid in adrenocortical insufficiency; acute exacerbations of multiple sclerosis; severe muscle weakness in myasthenia gravis
Pregnancy Risk Factor C
Contraindications Hypersensitivity to corticotropin, porcine proteins, or any component; scleroderma, osteoporosis, systemic fungal infections, ocular herpes simplex, peptic ulcer, hypertension, CHF
Warnings May mask signs of infection; do not administer live vaccines; long-term therapy in children may retard bone growth; acute adrenal insufficiency may occur with abrupt withdrawal after chronic use or with stress
Precautions Use with caution in patients with hypothyroidism, cirrhosis, thromboembolic disorders, seizure disorders or renal insufficiency
Adverse Reactions
  Cardiovascular: Hypertension
  Central nervous system: Seizures, mood swings, headache, pseudotumor cerebri
  Dermatologic: Skin atrophy, bruising, hyperpigmentation, acne, hirsutism
  Endocrine & metabolic: Amenorrhea, sodium and water retention, Cushing's syndrome, hyperglycemia, bone growth suppression, hypokalemia
  Gastrointestinal: Abdominal distention, ulcerative esophagitis, pancreatitis
  Neuromuscular & skeletal: Muscle wasting
  Miscellaneous: Hypersensitivity reactions, including anaphylaxis
  (Continued)

Corticotropin *(Continued)*

Drug Interactions NSAIDs (increase risk of ulcers, increase clearance of NSAIDs), loop diuretics, thiazide diuretics, amphotericin B (increases potassium wasting), antidiabetic agents (may require increased doses due to hyperglycemic activity of adrenal glucocorticoids), live virus vaccines (increase risk of viral infection), vaccines may have decreased effect

Food Interactions May increase renal loss of potassium, calcium, zinc, and vitamin C; may need to increase dietary intake or give supplements

Stability Store repository injection (gel) in the refrigerator; warm gel before administration

Mechanism of Action Stimulates the adrenal cortex to secrete adrenal steroids (including hydrocortisone, cortisone), androgenic substances, and a small amount of aldosterone. Exact mechanism of action for treatment of infantile spasms is unknown, but may be an independent antiepileptic effect (unrelated to stimulation of release of adrenocorticosteroids). One theory is that ACTH suppresses corticotropin-releasing hormone (CRH). CRH is an excitatory neuropeptide that has a greater potency in infants. Infants with infantile spasms may have increased CRH activity. ACTH may decrease CRH release and, therefore, decrease infantile spasms.

Pharmacodynamics
Maximum effect on cortisol levels: I.M., S.C. (gel): 3-12 hours
Duration: Repository (gel): 10-25 hours, up to 3 days

Pharmacokinetics
Absorption: I.M. (repository): Over 8-16 hours
Half-life: 15 minutes
Elimination: In urine

Usual Dosage
Children: I.M.: Gel (repository) formulation:
Anti-inflammatory/immunosuppressant: 0.8 units/kg/day or 25 units/m²/day divided every 12-24 hours
Infantile spasms: Various regimens have been used. Some neurologists recommend low-dose ACTH (5-40 units/day) for short periods (1-6 weeks), while others recommend larger doses of ACTH (40-160 units/day) for long periods of treatment (3-12 months)
A prospective, single-blind study (Hrachovy, 1994) found no major difference in effectiveness between high-dose long-duration versus low-dose short-duration ACTH therapy. Hypertension, however, occurred more frequently in the high-dose group. Further studies comparing long-term outcomes are needed. Low-dose regimen used in this study:
Initial: 20 units/day for 2 weeks, if patient responds, taper and discontinue over a 1-week period; if patient does not respond, increase dose to 30 units/day for 4 weeks then taper and discontinue over a 1-week period
Usual dose: 20-40 units/day or 5-8 units/kg/day in 1-2 divided doses; range: 5-160 units/day
Adults: I.M.: Gel (repository) formulation:
Acute exacerbation of multiple sclerosis: 80-120 units/day in divided doses for 2-3 weeks
Diagnostic purposes: 25 units
Anti-inflammatory/immunosuppressant: 40-80 units every 24-72 hours

Administration Parenteral: Gel should be administered I.M. only

Monitoring Parameters Electrolytes, glucose, blood pressure, height, and weight; for infantile spasms, monitor seizure frequency, type, and duration

Test Interactions Skin tests

Patient Information Do not abruptly discontinue the medication; tell your physician you are using this drug if you are going to have skin tests, immunizations, surgery, emergency treatment, or if you have a serious infection or injury

Additional Information Cosyntropin is preferred over corticotropin for diagnostic test of adrenocortical insufficiency (cosyntropin is less allergenic and test is shorter in duration); oral prednisone (2 mg/kg/day) was as effective as I.M. ACTH gel (20 units/day) in controlling infantile spasms; corticotropin zinc hydroxide (Cortrophin® Zinc) and corticotropin aqueous (Acthar®) have been discontinued by the manufacturer

Dosage Forms Injection, repository (H.P. Acthar® Gel): 80 units/mL (5 mL)

References
Haines ST and Casto DT, "Treatment of Infantile Spasms," *Ann Pharmacother*, 1994, 28(6):779-91.
Hrachovy RA and Frost JD Jr, "Infantile Spasms," *Pediatr Clin North Am*, 1989, 36(2):311-29.
Hrachovy RA, Frost JD Jr, and Glaze DG, "High-Dose, Long-Duration Versus Low-Dose, Short-Duration Corticotropin Therapy for Infantile Spasms," *J Pediatr*, 1994, 124(5 Pt 1):803-6.
Hrachovy RA, Frost JD Jr, Kellaway P, et al, "Double-Blind Study of ACTH vs Prednisone Therapy in Infantile Spasms," *J Pediatr*, 1983, 103(4):641-5.

♦ **Corticotropin, Repository** *see* Corticotropin *on page 307*

♦ **Cortifoam**® *see* Hydrocortisone *on page 573*
♦ **Cortimyxin**® **(Can)** *see* Neomycin and Polymyxin B *on page 802*
♦ **Cortimyxin**® **(Can)** *see* Neomycin, (Bacitracin) Polymyxin B, and Hydrocortisone *on page 802*
♦ **Cortisol** *see* Hydrocortisone *on page 573*

Cortisone (KOR ti sone)

Related Information
Corticosteroids Comparison, Systemic *on page 1211*

Therapeutic Category Adrenal Corticosteroid; Anti-inflammatory Agent; Corticosteroid, Systemic; Glucocorticoid

Generic Available Yes

Use Management of adrenocortical insufficiency

Pregnancy Risk Factor D

Contraindications Hypersensitivity to cortisone, any component, or corticosteroids; serious infections, except septic shock or tuberculous meningitis; systemic fungal or viral infections

Warnings May retard bone growth; acute adrenal insufficiency may occur with abrupt withdrawal after long-term therapy or with stress

Precautions Use with caution in patients with hypothyroidism, cirrhosis, hypertension, CHF, ulcerative colitis, thromboembolic disorders, osteoporosis, peptic ulcer, diabetes mellitus, seizure disorders; avoid using higher than recommended dosages; suppression of hypothalamic - pituitary - adrenal function, suppression of linear growth, or hypercorticism (Cushing's syndrome) may occur

Adverse Reactions
Cardiovascular: Edema, hypertension
Central nervous system: Vertigo, seizures, headache, psychoses, pseudotumor cerebri
Dermatologic: Acne, skin atrophy
Endocrine & metabolic: Cushing's syndrome, pituitary-adrenal axis suppression, growth suppression, glucose intolerance, hypokalemia, alkalosis, weight gain
Gastrointestinal: Peptic ulcer, nausea, vomiting
Neuromuscular & skeletal: Muscle weakness, osteoporosis, fractures
Ocular: Cataracts, glaucoma

Drug Interactions Cytochrome P450 isoenzyme CYP3A3/4 substrate
Barbiturates, phenytoin, rifampin, salicylates, estrogens, NSAID, diuretics (potassium depleting), anticholinesterase agents, warfarin; caffeine and alcohol may increase risk for GI ulcer; live virus vaccines (increase risk of viral infection); vaccines may have decreased effects

Food Interactions Systemic use of corticosteroids may require a diet with increased potassium, vitamins A, B_6, C, D, folate, calcium, zinc, phosphorus, and decreased sodium

Mechanism of Action Controls the rate of protein synthesis, depresses the migration of polymorphonuclear leukocytes and fibroblasts, reverses capillary permeability, and stabilizes lysosomal membranes at the cellular level to prevent or control inflammation

Pharmacodynamics
Maximum effect: Oral: Within 2 hours
Duration: 30-36 hours

Pharmacokinetics
Distribution: Crosses the placenta; appears in breast milk; distributes to muscles, liver, skin, intestines, and kidneys
Metabolism: In the liver to inactive metabolites
Half-life: 30 minutes
Elimination: In bile and urine

Usual Dosage Depends upon the condition being treated and the response of the patient. Supplemental doses may be warranted during times of stress in the course of withdrawing therapy. Oral:
Children:
Anti-inflammatory or immunosuppressive: 2.5-10 mg/kg/day or 20-300 mg/m²/day in divided doses every 6-8 hours
Physiologic replacement: 0.5-0.75 mg/kg/day or 20-25 mg/m²/day in divided doses every 8 hours
Adults: 20-300 mg/day divided every 12-24 hours

Administration Oral: Administer with meals, food, or milk to decrease GI effects

Monitoring Parameters Long-term use: Electrolytes, glucose, blood pressure, height, weight

Test Interactions Skin tests
(Continued)

Cortisone *(Continued)*

Patient Information Do not discontinue or reduce dose without physician's approval; limit caffeine; avoid alcohol

Nursing Implications Taper dose gradually with long-term use

Additional Information Insoluble in water

Dosage Forms Tablet, as acetate: 5 mg, 10 mg, 25 mg

- ◆ **Cortisporin®** *see* Neomycin, (Bacitracin) Polymyxin B, and Hydrocortisone *on page 802*
- ◆ **Cortizone®-5 [OTC]** *see* Hydrocortisone *on page 573*
- ◆ **Cortizone®-10 [OTC]** *see* Hydrocortisone *on page 573*
- ◆ **Cortizone®-10 Plus [OTC]** *see* Hydrocortisone *on page 573*
- ◆ **Cortizone®-10 Quick Shot [OTC]** *see* Hydrocortisone *on page 573*
- ◆ **Cortizone® for Kids [OTC]** *see* Hydrocortisone *on page 573*
- ◆ **Cortoderm (Can)** *see* Hydrocortisone *on page 573*
- ◆ **Cortrosyn®** *see* Cosyntropin *on page 310*
- ◆ **Cosmegen®** *see* Dactinomycin *on page 335*

Cosyntropin (koe sin TROE pin)

U.S. Brand Names Cortrosyn®

Synonyms Synacthen; Tetracosactide

Therapeutic Category Adrenal Corticosteroid; Diagnostic Agent, Adrenocortical Insufficiency

Generic Available No

Use Diagnostic test to differentiate primary adrenal from secondary (pituitary) adrenocortical insufficiency; used in the diagnosis of congenital adrenal hyperplasia

Pregnancy Risk Factor C

Contraindications Hypersensitivity to cosyntropin or any component

Precautions Use with caution in patients with pre-existing allergic disease or a history of allergic reactions to corticotropin

Adverse Reactions

Dermatologic: Pruritus, flushing

Endocrine & metabolic: Decreased carbohydrate tolerance; increased requirements for insulin or oral hypoglycemic agents in diabetics; activation of latent diabetes mellitus

Miscellaneous: Hypersensitivity reactions, including anaphylaxis

Drug Interactions Cortisone, hydrocortisone, estrogens, spironolactone

Stability Reconstituted solution is stable for 24 hours at room temperature and 21 days when refrigerated; when diluted in NS or D_5W, I.V. infusion is stable for 12 hours at room temperature

Mechanism of Action Stimulates the adrenal cortex to secrete adrenal steroids (including hydrocortisone, cortisone), androgenic substances, and a small amount of aldosterone

Pharmacodynamics I.M., I.V.:

Onset of action: Plasma cortisol levels rise in healthy individuals in 5 minutes

Maximum effect: Plasma cortisol levels usually peak at 45-60 minutes after the cosyntropin dose

Pharmacokinetics Metabolism: Unknown

Usual Dosage Diagnostic test doses:

Adrenocortical insufficiency: I.M., I.V.:

Preterm neonates: Dose not well defined; Korte 1996 used physiologic doses of cosyntropin (0.1 mcg/kg) to test adrenal function in VLBW infants [mean weight 900 g; mean gestational age 27 weeks (range: 23-32 weeks)]; only 36% of infants responded; increasing the dose to 0.2 mcg/kg resulted in 67% of the infants responding, but sensitivity of the test was decreased. Cole 1999 used cosyntropin doses of 3.5 mcg/kg to test adrenal function in 44 preterm infants [mean birthweight 823 g; mean gestational age 26.2 weeks; mean postmenstrual age 30.1 weeks] during inhaled beclomethasone therapy.

Neonates: 0.015 mg/kg/dose

Children ≤2 years: 0.125 mg

Children >2 years and Adults: 0.25 mg

When greater cortisol stimulation is needed, an I.V. infusion may be used: Children >2 years and Adults: 0.25 mg administered over 4-8 hours (usually 6 hours)

Congenital adrenal hyperplasia evaluation: 1 mg/m²/dose up to a maximum of 1 mg

Administration Parenteral:

I.V. push: Administer in 2-5 mL of NS over 2 minutes

I.V. infusion (Children >2 years and Adults): Dose may be added to dextrose or NS solution and administered over 4-8 hours (at a rate of approximately 0.04 mg/hour for 6 hours)

Reference Range Plasma cortisol concentrations should be measured immediately before and exactly 30 minutes after the dose; dose should be given in the early morning; normal morning baseline cortisol >5 µg/dL (SI: >138 nmol/L); normal response 30 minutes after cosyntropin injection: an increase in serum cortisol concentration of ≥7 µg/dL (SI: ≥193 nmol/L) or peak response >18 µg/dL (SI: >497 nmol/L).

Nursing Implications Patient should not receive corticosteroids or spironolactone the day prior to and the day of the test

Additional Information Each 0.25 mg of cosyntropin is equivalent to 25 units of corticotropin.

Dosage Forms Injection, powder for reconstitution: 0.25 mg

References

Cole CH, Shah B, Abbasi S, et al, "Adrenal Function in Premature Infants During Inhaled Beclomethasone Therapy," J Pediatr, 1999, 135(1):65-70.

Korte C, Styne D, Merritt TA, et al, "Adrenocortical Function in the Very Low Birth Weight Infant: Improved Testing Sensitivity and Association With Neonatal Outcome," J Pediatr, 1996, 128(2):257-63.

♦ **Cotazym® [DSC]** see Pancrelipase on page 856
♦ **Cotazym-S® [DSC]** see Pancrelipase on page 856
♦ **Co-Trimoxazole** see Sulfamethoxazole and Trimethoprim on page 1052
♦ **Coumadin®** see Warfarin on page 1156
♦ **Covera® (Can)** see Verapamil on page 1144
♦ **Covera-HS®** see Verapamil on page 1144
♦ **CPM** see Cyclophosphamide on page 321
♦ **CPR Pediatric Drug Dosages** see page 1175
♦ **CPT-11** see Irinotecan on page 621
♦ **Creomulsion® Cough [OTC]** see Dextromethorphan on page 365
♦ **Creomulsion® for Children [OTC]** see Dextromethorphan on page 365
♦ **Creon®** see Pancrelipase on page 856
♦ **Creo-Terpin® [OTC]** see Dextromethorphan on page 365
♦ **Critic-Aid Skin Care® [OTC]** see Zinc Oxide on page 1167
♦ **Crixivan®** see Indinavir on page 604
♦ **CroFab™** see Crotalidae Polyvalent Immune Fab (Ovine) on page 314
♦ **Crolom®** see Cromolyn on page 311
♦ **Cromoglycic Acid** see Cromolyn on page 311

Cromolyn (KROE moe lin)

Related Information
Asthma Guidelines on page 1376

U.S. Brand Names Crolom®; Gastrocrom®; Intal®; Nasalcrom® [OTC]; Opticrom®

Canadian Brand Names Apo®-Cromolyn; Nu-Cromolyn

Synonyms Cromoglycic Acid; Disodium Cromoglycate; DSCG

Therapeutic Category Antiasthmatic; Inhalation, Miscellaneous

Generic Available Yes (solution for inhalation, ophthalmic drops)

Use
Oral inhalation and nebulization: Prophylactic agent used for long-term (chronic) control of persistent asthma (see Additional Information); **NOT** indicated for the relief of acute bronchospasm; also used for the prevention of allergen- or exercise-induced bronchospasm

Intranasal: Management of seasonal or perennial allergic rhinitis

Ophthalmologic: Vernal conjunctivitis, vernal keratoconjunctivitis, and vernal keratitis

Systemic: Mastocytosis, food allergy, and treatment of inflammatory bowel disease

Pregnancy Risk Factor B

Contraindications Hypersensitivity to cromolyn or any component; primary treatment of status asthmaticus

Warnings Cromolyn is a prophylactic drug with no benefit for acute situations; rare but severe anaphylactic reactions can occur; discontinue if eosinophilic pneumonia occurs

Precautions Use with caution and decrease dose in patients with renal and hepatic impairment; use inhalation aerosol with caution in patients with coronary artery disease or history of cardiac arrhythmias (due to propellants); use with caution when tapering the dose or withdrawing the drug since symptoms may reoccur; patients should not wear contact lenses during treatment with ophthalmic solution.

Oral cromolyn increased mortality in neonatal rats when administered at ~9 times the maximum recommended daily dose for infants, but not at ~3 times the maximum (Continued)

Cromolyn (Continued)

recommended daily dose; use of oral cromolyn in infants and children <2 years is not recommended and should be reserved for patients with severe mastocytosis in whom potential benefits clearly outweigh the risks.

Adverse Reactions

Central nervous system: Dizziness, headache

Dermatologic: Rash, urticaria, angioedema

Gastrointestinal: Nausea, vomiting, diarrhea, xerostomia, unpleasant taste (inhalation aerosol)

Local: Nasal burning

Neuromuscular & skeletal: Arthralgia

Ocular (topical): Ocular stinging, lacrimation

Respiratory: Coughing, wheezing, sneezing, nasal congestion, throat irritation, eosinophilic pneumonia, pulmonary infiltrates, hoarseness

Stability Protect from direct light and heat; nebulization solution is compatible with beta agonists, anticholinergic solutions, acetylcysteine and NS; incompatible with alkaline solutions, calcium and magnesium salts; store oral concentrate ampuls in foil pouch until ready for use

Mechanism of Action Prevents the mast cell release of histamine, leukotrienes and slow-reacting substance of anaphylaxis by inhibiting degranulation after contact with antigens

Pharmacodynamics Not effective for immediate relief of symptoms in acute asthmatic attacks; must be used at regular intervals for 2-4 weeks to be effective

Pharmacokinetics

Absorption:

Oral: 0.5% to 2%

Inhalation: ~8% of dose reaches the lungs upon inhalation of the powder and is well absorbed

Half-life: 80-90 minutes

Time to peak serum concentration: Within 15 minutes after inhalation

Elimination: Equally excreted unchanged in urine and feces (via bile); small amounts after inhalation are exhaled

Usual Dosage

Inhalation:

For chronic control of asthma, taper frequency to the lowest effective dose (ie, 4 times/day to 3 times/day to twice daily):

Nebulization solution: Children >2 years and Adults: Initial: 20 mg 4 times/day; usual dose: 20 mg 3-4 times/day

Metered spray:

Children 5-12 years: Initial: 2 inhalations 4 times/day; usual dose: 1-2 inhalations 3-4 times/day

Children ≥12 years and Adults: Initial: 2 inhalations 4 times/day; usual dose: 2-4 inhalations 3-4 times/day

Prevention of allergen- or exercise-induced bronchospasm: Administer 10-15 minutes prior to exercise or allergen exposure but no longer than 1 hour before:

Nebulization solution: Children >2 years and Adults: Single dose of 20 mg

Metered spray: Children >5 years and Adults: Single dose of 2 inhalations

NIH Asthma Guidelines (NAEPP, 2002):

Nebulization solution: Children and Adults: 20 mg 3-4 times/day

Metered spray:

Children ≤12 years: 1-2 inhalations 3-4 times/day

Children >12 years and Adults: 2-4 inhalations 3-4 times/day

Intranasal: Children ≥2 years and Adults: 1 spray in each nostril 3-4 times/day; maximum dose: 1 spray in each nostril 6 times/day

Ophthalmic: Children >4 years and Adults: Instill 1-2 drops 4-6 times/day

Oral:

Systemic mastocytosis:

Neonates and Preterm Infants: Not recommended

Infants and Children <2 years: Not recommended; reserve use for patients with severe disease in whom potential benefits outweigh risks (see Precautions); 20 mg/kg/day in 4 divided doses; may increase in patients 6 months to 2 years of age if benefits not seen after 2-3 weeks; do not exceed 30 mg/kg/day

Children 2-12 years: 100 mg 4 times/day; not to exceed 40 mg/kg/day

Children >12 years and Adults: 200 mg 4 times/day

Food allergy and inflammatory bowel disease:

Infants and Children <2 years: Not recommended

Children 2-12 years: Initial dose: 100 mg 4 times/day; may double the dose if effect is not satisfactory within 2-3 weeks; not to exceed 40 mg/kg/day

Children >12 years and Adults: Initial dose: 200 mg 4 times/day; may double the dose if effect is not satisfactory within 2-3 weeks; up to 400 mg 4 times/day

Once desired effect is achieved, dose may be tapered to lowest effective dose

Administration

Oral concentrate: Open ampul and squeeze contents into glass of water; stir well; administer at least 30 minutes before meals and at bedtime; do not mix with juice, milk, or food

Oral inhalation: Shake canister gently before use; do not immerse canister in water

Nasal inhalation: Clear nasal passages by blowing nose prior to use

Monitoring Parameters Asthma: Periodic pulmonary function tests; signs and symptoms of disease state when tapering dose

Patient Information May cause dry mouth. Cromolyn is not effective for the immediate relief of symptoms in acute asthmatic attacks; must be used at regular intervals for 2-4 weeks to be effective for asthma control. Cromolyn nasal spray is not effective for the immediate relief of nasal allergies; must be used at regular intervals for 1-2 weeks for optimal control of nasal allergies; to prevent nasal allergy symptoms, start using product 1-2 weeks before contact with the cause of allergies.

Additional Information The 2002 Expert Panel Report of the National Asthma Education and Prevention Program (NAEPP, 2002) no longer recommends cromolyn for initial treatment of persistent asthma in children; inhaled corticosteroids are the preferred agents; cromolyn is considered an alternative medication for the treatment of mild persistent asthma in children. Inhalation aerosol contains fluorocarbon propellants. Reserve systemic use in children <2 years of age for severe disease; avoid systemic use in premature infants.

Dosage Forms

Solution for nebulization, as sodium (Intal®): 10 mg/mL (2 mL)

Solution, nasal spray, as sodium (Nasalcrom® [OTC]): 40 mg/mL (13 mL) [5.2 mg/metered spray; 100 metered sprays]; (26 mL) [5.2 mg/metered spray; 200 metered sprays]

Solution, ophthalmic, as sodium (Crolom®, Opticrom®): 4% (2.5 mL, 10 mL)

Solution, oral **concentrate**, as sodium (Gastrocrom®): 100 mg/5 mL ampul (96s)

Solution for oral inhalation, as sodium (Intal®): 800 mcg/inhalation (8.1 g) [112 metered inhalations; 56 metered doses]; (14.2 g) [200 metered inhalations; 100 metered doses]

References

Expert Panel Report 2, "Guidelines for the Diagnosis and Management of Asthma," *Clinical Practice Guidelines*, National Institutes of Health, National Heart, Lung, and Blood Institute, NIH Publication No. 94-4051, April, 1997.

"National Asthma Education and Prevention Program. Expert Panel Report: Guidelines for the Diagnosis and Management of Asthma Update on Selected Topics--2002," *J Allergy Clin Immunol*, 2002, 110(5 Suppl):S141-219.

Crotalidae Polyvalent Antivenin (Equine)

(an tee VEN in (kroe TAL ih die) pol i VAY lent)

U.S. Brand Names Antivenin Polyvalent [Equine]

Synonyms Crotaline Antivenin, Polyvalent (Equine Origin); North and South American Antisnake-bite Serum; Snake (Pit Vipers) Antivenin

Therapeutic Category Antivenin

Generic Available No

Use Neutralization of venoms of North and South American crotalids: rattlesnake, copperhead, cottonmouth, tropical moccasins, fer-de-lance, bushmaster

Pregnancy Risk Factor C

Contraindications Not effective against the venoms of coral snakes

Warnings Desensitization may need to be performed on patients with positive skin test reaction or history of sensitivity to equine serum

Precautions Patients with a negative skin test may still react when antivenin is administered; skin test should not be performed unless antivenin is to be used. If patient has a positive history for allergy and a positive skin test, antivenin administration may be dangerous. Risk of administering antivenin must be weighed against the risk of withholding it

Adverse Reactions

Cardiovascular: Flushing, cyanosis, shock, edema of the face

Central nervous system: Apprehension

Dermatologic: Urticaria

Gastrointestinal: Vomiting

Neuromuscular & skeletal: Muscle weakness, peripheral neuritis

Respiratory: Dyspnea, cough

Miscellaneous: Anaphylaxis, serum sickness (dose-related; occurs in 83% of patients receiving more than 8 vials)

(Continued)

Crotalidae Polyvalent Antivenin (Equine) *(Continued)*

Stability Avoid storage temperatures >37°C; reconstituted solutions should be used within 48 hours

Usual Dosage The initial dose of antivenin should be administered as soon as possible to be most effective (within 4 hours after the bite). Intradermal sensitivity test should be performed prior to administering antivenin; see Additional Information.

Children and Adults: I.V.:
 Minimal envenomation: 20-40 mL
 Moderate envenomation: 50-90 mL
 Severe envenomation: 100-150 mL
 See table.

Dosage Based on Severity of Clinical Picture

	Clinical Severity	# of Vials
Minimal	Symptoms confined to bite area; absent of insignificant systemic symptoms	0
Mild	Edema progressing slowly; bite site reveals small amount of ecchymosis; only systemic sign is metallic taste	5
Moderate	Tissue damage beyond immediate bite area; moderate laboratory changes; perioral fasciculation; paresthesias	10
Severe	Tissue damage to entire extremity; major systemic symptoms; significant laboratory abnormalities	>15

Gold BS and Barish RA, "Venomous Snakebites: Current Concepts in Diagnosis, Treatment, and Management," *Emerg Med Clin North Am*, 1992, 10(2):249-67.

Additional doses of antivenin are based on clinical response to the initial dose. If swelling continues to progress, symptoms increase in severity, hypotension occurs, or decrease in hematocrit appears, an additional 10-50 mL should be administered.

Administration Parenteral: Antivenin may be administered I.M. into a large muscle mass for minimal envenomation. I.V. administration of antivenin is preferred for moderate to severe envenomation or in the presence of shock; for I.V. infusion, prepare a 1:1 to 1:10 dilution of reconstituted antivenin in NS or D_5W; infuse the initial 5-10 mL dilution over 3-5 minutes while carefully observing the patient for signs and symptoms of sensitivity reactions. If no reaction occurs, continue infusion at a safe I.V. fluid delivery rate.

Monitoring Parameters Vital signs, hematocrit, hemoglobin; platelet count, prothrombin time; signs and symptoms of allergy, anaphylaxis, and serum sickness

Nursing Implications Do not inject into a finger or toe; immediate sensitivity reactions usually occur within 30 minutes after administration; if an immediate reaction occurs, temporarily discontinue antivenin, administer epinephrine, corticosteroid, and/or an antihistamine; then reinstate infusion at a slower rate after control of the reaction; serum-sickness reaction may occur 5-24 days after a dose

Additional Information Intradermal skin test: 0.02-0.03 mL of a 1:10 dilution of antivenin in NS. If the patient has a history of equine serum sensitivity, administer a 1:100 or greater dilution skin test. Test site is read after 5-30 minutes.

Dosage Forms Injection, powder for reconstitution, lyophilized serum: Equine origin: [With 10 mL SWI diluent]

Crotalidae Polyvalent Immune Fab (Ovine)

(kroe TAL ih die pol i VAY lent i MYUN fab (OE vine))

U.S. Brand Names CroFab™

Synonyms Crotalid Antivenom Ovine Fab, Polyvalent

Therapeutic Category Antivenin

Generic Available No

Use Neutralization of venoms of North American crotalids: Western diamondback rattlesnake, Eastern diamondback rattlesnake, Mojave rattlesnake, and cottonmouth or water moccasin

Pregnancy Risk Factor C

Contraindications Hypersensitivity to *Crotalidae* polyvalent immune Fab (ovine), papaya, papain, chymopapain, or any component

Warnings Recurrent coagulopathy characterized by decreased fibrinogen and platelets and elevated PT has occurred in 50% of patients studied but was only observed in patients who had experienced coagulation abnormalities during their initial treatment. Recurrent coagulopathy may persist >1-2 weeks. Evaluate patients for the need for repeat dosing.

Precautions Use with caution in patients with hypersensitivity to the pineapple enzyme bromelain, dust mite allergens, or latex allergens. *Crotalidae* polyvalent immune Fab (ovine) contains mercury in the form of ethyl mercury from thimerosal; although there is limited toxicologic data available on ethyl mercury, developing fetuses and very young children are the most susceptible to neurologic and renal toxicities associated with methyl mercury exposure. Carefully monitor all patients receiving antivenin for signs and symptoms of an anaphylactic reaction, acute allergic reaction, delayed allergic reactions (ie, serum sickness, rash, fever, myalgia, arthralgia) and infusion-related reactions. Use with caution if administering a repeat course for a subsequent envenomation episode since patients may become sensitized to the foreign protein. Skin testing is not indicated.

Adverse Reactions
Cardiovascular: Chest pain, hypotension
Central nervous system: Chills, nervousness
Dermatologic: Rash, urticaria, pruritus, erythema
Gastrointestinal: Nausea, anorexia
Hematologic: Coagulation disorder (thrombocytopenia, hypofibrinogenemia, elevated PT)
Neuromuscular & skeletal: Myalgia, paresthesia
Respiratory: Dyspnea, wheezing, cough
Miscellaneous: Serum sickness, allergic reaction

Stability Store vials at 2°C to 8°C; do not freeze; reconstitute vial with 10 mL SWI and mix by continuous gentle swirling; further dilute the number of vials needed for dose in 250 mL NS and continue to mix by gently swirling; use reconstituted and diluted product within 4 hours

Mechanism of Action Antivenom composed of purified Fab fragment of IgG specific to indigenous snake species; binds and neutralizes venom toxins; facilitates their distribution away from target tissues and their elimination from the body

Pharmacodynamics
Onset of action: Within 4 hours
Duration: 6-18 hours

Pharmacokinetics
Distribution: V_d: Adults: 110 mL/kg
Half-life: 18 hours

Usual Dosage The initial dose of antivenin should be administered as soon as possible (within 6 hours after the crotalid snakebite). Skin testing prior to administering antivenin is not required.

Children and Adults: I.V.:
Initial: 4-6 vials
Observe patient for 1 hour following the completion of the first dose. If initial control is not achieved after the first dose, an additional 4-6 vials may be repeated until initial control of the envenomation syndrome has been achieved.
After initial control has been established: 2 vials every 6 hours for up to 18 hours (3 doses); an additional 2 vial dose may be administered if deemed necessary based on clinical response

Administration Parenteral: I.V. administration only; infuse dose in 250 mL NS; initial: Infuse slowly over the first 10 minutes at 25-50 mL/hour along with careful observation for any allergic reaction; if no reaction occurs, may increase to 250 mL/hour until total dose is infused

Monitoring Parameters Vital signs, PT, hematocrit, hemoglobin, platelet count, fibrin split products, fibrinogen level; signs and symptoms of allergy, anaphylaxis, and serum sickness

Patient Information Notify physician if rash, pruritus, urticaria, bruising, or bleeding occurs; bruising and bleeding may occur for up to one week or longer following initial treatment

Nursing Implications Immediate sensitivity reactions usually occur within 30 minutes after administration; if an immediate reaction occurs, temporarily discontinue CroFab™, administer epinephrine, I.V. antihistamine, and/or albuterol

Dosage Forms
Injection: Each vial contains up to 1 g of total protein, a maximum of 0.11 mg of mercury, and not less than the indicated number of mouse LD_{50} neutralizing units:
C. atrox (Western diamondback rattlesnake): 1350 units
C. adamanteus (Eastern diamondback rattlesnake): 800 units
C. scutulatus (Mojave rattlesnake): 5210 units
A. piscivorus (cottonmouth and water moccasin): 460 units

References
Clark RF, Williams SR, Nordt SP, et al, "Successful Treatment of Crotalid-Induced Neurotoxicity With a New Polyspecific Crotalid Fab Antivenom," *Ann Emerg Med*, 1997, 30(1):54-7.
Dart RC and McNally J, "Efficacy, Safety, and Use of Snake Antivenoms in the United States," *Ann Emerg Med*, 2001, 37(2):181-8.

♦ **Crotalid Antivenom Ovine Fab, Polyvalent** *see Crotalidae* Polyvalent Immune Fab (Ovine) *on page 314*

♦ **Crotaline Antivenin, Polyvalent (Equine Origin)** *see Crotalidae* Polyvalent Antivenin (Equine) *on page 313*

Crotamiton (kroe TAM i tonn)

U.S. Brand Names Eurax®
Therapeutic Category Scabicidal Agent
Generic Available No
Use Treatment of scabies (*Sarcoptes scabiei*) in infants and children
Pregnancy Risk Factor C
Contraindications Hypersensitivity to crotamiton or any component; patients who manifest a primary irritation response to topical medications
Precautions Avoid contact with face, eyes, mucous membranes, and urethral meatus; do not apply to acutely inflamed or raw skin
Adverse Reactions
  Dermatologic: Pruritus, contact dermatitis
  Local: Irritation
Mechanism of Action Mechanism for scabicidal activity is unknown
Usual Dosage Scabicide: Topical: Infants, Children, and Adults: Apply over entire body below the head; apply once daily for 2 days followed by a cleansing bath 48 hours after the last application; treatment may be repeated after 7-10 days if mites appear
Administration Topical: Wash thoroughly and scrub away loose scales, then towel dry; apply a thin layer and gently massage drug onto skin of the entire body from the neck to the toes (with special attention to skin folds, creases, and interdigital spaces); since scabies can affect the head, scalp, and neck in infants and young children, apply to head, neck, and body of this age group; do not apply to the face, eyes, mouth, mucous membranes, or urethral meatus; shake lotion well before use
Patient Information For topical use only; all contaminated clothing and bed linen should be washed to avoid reinfestation
Additional Information Treatment may be repeated after 7-10 days if live mites are still present
Dosage Forms
  Cream: 10% (60 g)
  Lotion: 10% (60 mL, 480 mL)
References
Eichenfield LF, Honig PJ, "Blistering Disorders in Childhood," *Pediatr Clin North Am*, 1991, 38(4):959-76.
Hogan DJ, Schachner L, Tanglertsampan C, "Diagnosis and Treatment of Childhood Scabies and Pediculosis," *Pediatr Clin North Am*, 1991, 38(4):941-57.

♦ **Cruex® Prescription Strength Cream [OTC]** *see* Clotrimazole *on page 297*

♦ **Crystalline Penicillin** *see* Penicillin G (Parenteral/Aqueous) *on page 875*

♦ **Crystal Violet** *see* Gentian Violet *on page 537*

♦ **CsA** *see* CycloSPORINE *on page 324*

♦ **CTX** *see* Cyclophosphamide *on page 321*

♦ **Cupric Chloride** *see* Trace Metals *on page 1106*

♦ **Cuprimine®** *see* Penicillamine *on page 872*

♦ **Curosurf®** *see* Poractant Alfa *on page 917*

♦ **Cutar® [OTC]** *see* Coal Tar *on page 299*

♦ **Cutivate®** *see* Fluticasone *on page 511*

♦ **CyA** *see* CycloSPORINE *on page 324*

Cyanocobalamin (sye an oh koe BAL a min)

U.S. Brand Names LA-12®; Nascobal®
Canadian Brand Names Scheinpharm B12
Synonyms Vitamin B$_{12}$
Therapeutic Category Nutritional Supplement; Vitamin, Water Soluble
Generic Available Yes
Use Pernicious anemia; vitamin B$_{12}$ deficiency; increased B$_{12}$ requirements due to pregnancy, thyrotoxicosis, hemorrhage, malignancy, liver or kidney disease; nutritional supplement
Pregnancy Risk Factor A (C if dose exceeds RDA recommendation)
Contraindications Hypersensitivity to cyanocobalamin, any component (see Warnings), or cobalt; patients with hereditary optic nerve atrophy
Warnings Vitamin B$_{12}$ deficiency for >3 months results in irreversible degenerative CNS lesions; vegetarian diets may result in vitamin B$_{12}$ deficiency. Injection may contain benzyl alcohol which may cause allergic reactions in susceptible individuals;

large amounts of benzyl alcohol (≥99 mg/kg/day) have been associated with a potentially fatal toxicity ("gasping syndrome") in neonates; the "gasping syndrome" consists of metabolic acidosis, respiratory distress, gasping respirations, CNS dysfunction (including convulsions, intracranial hemorrhage), hypotension and cardiovascular collapse; avoid use of benzyl alcohol containing injections in neonates; *in vitro* and animal studies have shown that benzoate, a metabolite of benzyl alcohol, displaces bilirubin from protein-binding sites. Intranasal therapy is only for use in patients who are in remission following injectable treatment.

Precautions Serum potassium concentrations should be monitored early as severe hypokalemia has occurred after the conversion of megaloblastic anemia to normal erythropoiesis

Adverse Reactions

Cardiovascular: Peripheral vascular thrombosis
Dermatologic: Itching, urticaria, exanthema
Endocrine & metabolic: Hypokalemia
Gastrointestinal: Diarrhea
Respiratory: Rhinitis (nasal gel)
Miscellaneous: Allergic reactions

Drug Interactions

Decreased absorption of cyanocobalamin from GI tract: aminoglycoside antibiotics, colchicine, extended release potassium products, aminosalicylic acid, phenytoin, and phenobarbital; antagonism of hematopoietic response to cyanocobalamin: chloramphenicol; chemical degradation of cyanocobalamin: large doses of ascorbic acid

Stability Clear pink to red solutions are stable at room temperature; protect from light; **incompatible** with chlorpromazine, phytonadione, prochlorperazine, warfarin, ascorbic acid, dextrose, heavy metals, oxidizing or reducing agents

Mechanism of Action Coenzyme for various metabolic functions, including fat and carbohydrate metabolism and protein synthesis, used in cell replication and hematopoiesis

Pharmacodynamics Onset of action:

Megaloblastic anemia: I.M.:
Conversion of megaloblastic to normoblastic erythroid hyperplasia within bone marrow: 8 hours
Increased reticulocytes: 2-5 days
Complicated vitamin B_{12} deficiency: I.M., S.C.: Resolution of:
Psychiatric sequelae: 24 hours
Thrombocytopenia: 10 days
Granulocytopenia: 2 weeks

Pharmacokinetics

Absorption: Oral: Drug is absorbed from the terminal ileum in the presence of calcium; for absorption to occur, gastric "intrinsic factor" must be present to transfer the compound across the intestinal mucosa
Distribution: Principally stored in the liver, also stored in the kidneys and adrenals
Protein binding: Bound to transcobalamin II
Metabolism: Converted in the tissues to active coenzymes methylcobalamin and deoxyadenosylcobalamin
Bioavailability: Oral: Pernicious anemia: 1.2%
Time to peak serum concentration:
I.M., S.C.: 30 minutes to 2 hours
Intranasal: 1.6 hours
Elimination: 50% to 98% unchanged in the urine

Usual Dosage

Recommended daily allowance (RDA): Oral:
Children: 0.3-2 mcg
Adults: 2 mcg
Adults, pregnancy: 2.2 mcg
Adults, lactation: 2.6 mcg
Adults, vegetarians: 6 mcg
Pernicious anemia:
Neonates and infants (congenital; if evidence of neurologic involvement): I.M., S.C.: 1000 mcg/day for at least 2 weeks; maintenance: 50 mcg/month
Children: I.M., S.C.: 30-50 mcg/day for 2 or more weeks (to a total dose of 1000 mcg); maintenance: 100 mcg monthly
Adults: I.M., S.C.: 100 mcg/day for 6-7 days; if improvement, give same dose on alternate days for 7 doses; then every 3-4 days for 2-3 weeks
Maintenance:
I.M., S.C.: 100 mcg/month
Intranasal: 500 mcg once weekly
Oral: 1000-2000 mcg/day
(Continued)

Cyanocobalamin *(Continued)*

Vitamin B$_{12}$ deficiency:

Children (dosage in children not well established): I.M., S.C.: 0.2 mcg/kg for 2 days followed by 1000 mcg/day for 2-7 days followed by 100 mcg/week for a month; for malabsorptive causes of B$_{12}$ deficiency, monthly maintenance doses of 100 mcg have been recommended or as an alternative 100 mcg/day for 10-15 days (total dose of 1-1.5 mg), then once or twice weekly for several months; may taper to 60 mcg every month

Adults:

Uncomplicated: Initial:

Oral: 1000-2000 mcg/day

I.M. or deep S.C.: 100 mcg/day for 5-10 days, followed by 100-200 mcg monthly until remission is complete **or** as an alternative: 100 mcg/day for 7 days, followed by 100 mcg every other day for 2 weeks, followed by 100 mcg every 3-4 days until remission is complete

Complicated (severe anemia, CHF, thrombocytopenia with bleeding, severe neurologic damage or granulocytopenia with infection): Initial: I.M. or deep S.C.: 1000 mcg with I.M. and I.V. folic acid 15 mg as single doses, followed by 1000 mcg/day plus oral folic acid 5 mg/day for 1 week; **Note:** Oral cyanocobalamin therapy is **not** indicated for treatment of complicated deficiency

Maintenance:

I.M., deep S.C.: 100-200 mcg monthly

Oral: 1000-2000 mcg/day

Note: Low initial B$_{12}$ doses combined with potassium supplementation (as needed) may prevent a hypokalemia seen in patients with severe deficiency

Dosage adjustment in renal impairment: Increased dosage may be required in vitamin B$_{12}$-deficient patients

Administration

Oral: Not generally recommended for treatment of severe vitamin B$_{12}$ deficiency due to poor oral absorption (lack of intrinsic factor); oral administration may be used in less severe deficiencies and maintenance therapy; may be administered without regard to food

Parenteral: I.M. or deep S.C.: Avoid I.V. administration due to a more rapid system elimination with resulting decreased utilization

Intranasal: Administer at least one hour before or after ingestion of hot foods or liquids; hot foods can cause nasal secretions and a resulting loss of medication

Monitoring Parameters Serum potassium, erythrocyte and reticulocyte count, hemoglobin, hematocrit, serum B$_{12}$ level

Reference Range Serum vitamin B$_{12}$ levels: Normal: 200-900 pg/mL; vitamin B$_{12}$ deficiency: <200 pg/mL; megaloblastic anemia: <100 pg/mL

Dosage Forms

Gel, intranasal (Nascobal®): 500 mcg/0.1 mL (2.3 mL)

Injection, solution: 1000 mcg/mL (1 mL, 10 mL, 30 mL) [products may contain benzyl alcohol]

LA-12®: 1000 mcg/mL (30 mL)

Lozenge [OTC]: 100 mcg, 250 mcg, 500 mcg

Tablet [OTC]: 50 mcg, 100 mcg, 250 mcg, 500 mcg, 1000 mcg, 5000 mcg

Tablet, extended release [OTC]: 1500 mcg

Tablet, sublingual [OTC]: 2500 mcg

References

Lane LA and Rojas-Fernandez C, "Treatment of Vitamin B(12)-Deficiency Anemia: Oral Versus Parenteral Therapy," *Ann Pharmacother*, 2002, 36(7):1268-72.

Rasmussen SA, Fernhoff PM, and Scanlon KS, "Vitamin B$_{12}$ Deficiency in Children and Adolescents," *J Pediatr*, 2001, 138(1):10-7.

Cyclobenzaprine *(sye kloe BEN za preen)*

U.S. Brand Names Flexeril®

Canadian Brand Names Apo®-Cyclobenzaprine; Flexitec; Gen-Cyclobenzaprine; Novo-Cycloprine®; Nu-Cyclobenzaprine

Therapeutic Category Skeletal Muscle Relaxant, Nonparalytic

Generic Available Yes

Use Treatment of muscle spasm associated with acute painful musculoskeletal conditions; supportive therapy in tetanus

Pregnancy Risk Factor B

Contraindications Hypersensitivity to cyclobenzaprine or any component; hyperthyroidism, acute recovery phase of MI, CHF, arrhythmias, heart block; do not use concomitantly or within 14 days of MAO inhibitors

Warnings Abrupt withdrawal after prolonged administration may result in nausea, headache, and malaise; not effective in the treatment of spasticity due to cerebral or spinal cord disease; avoid use in patients with moderate to severe hepatic dysfunction

Precautions Use with caution in patients with urinary retention, angle-closure glaucoma and patients receiving anticholinergic medications; use with caution and reduce dosage in patients with mildly impaired liver function

Adverse Reactions
Cardiovascular: Tachycardia, hypotension, arrhythmias, edema of face/lips, syncope, palpitations
Central nervous system: Drowsiness, headache, dizziness, fatigue, nervousness, confusion, anorexia, seizures, ataxia, vertigo, insomnia, psychosis, anxiety, agitation, hallucinations
Dermatologic: Rash, pruritus, urticaria
Gastrointestinal: Dyspepsia, nausea, constipation, xerostomia, vomiting, diarrhea, paralytic ileus, dysgeusia, stomach cramps, flatulence, tongue edema
Genitourinary: Urinary frequency or retention
Hepatic: Hepatitis, cholestasis, jaundice
Neuromuscular & skeletal: Weakness, muscle twitching, tremors, paresthesia
Ocular: Diplopia
Otic: Tinnitus
Miscellaneous: Hypersensitivity reactions, angioedema

Drug Interactions Cytochrome P450 isoenzyme CYP1A2, CYP2D6, CYP3A3/4 substrate
MAO inhibitors; additive effects with sedatives, alcohol, anticholinergic agents, and other CNS depressants; due to close chemical and physiologic relationship to tricyclic antidepressants, cyclobenzaprine may share some of the same drug interactions; may increase risk of seizures with tramadol; may decrease antihypertensive effects of guanethidine

Stability Store at room temperature

Mechanism of Action Centrally-acting skeletal muscle relaxant pharmacologically related to tricyclic antidepressants; reduces tonic somatic motor activity influencing both alpha and gamma motor neurons

Pharmacodynamics
Onset of action: Within 1 hour
Duration: 12-24 hours

Pharmacokinetics
Absorption: Oral: Complete
Metabolism: Hepatic
Bioavailability: 33% to 55%
Half-life: Adults: 18 hours (range 8-37 hours)
Time to peak serum concentration: Within 3-8 hours
Elimination: Primarily renal as inactive metabolites and in the feces (via bile) as unchanged drug; may undergo enterohepatic recycling
Clearance: Adults: 0.7 L/minute

Usual Dosage Oral:
Children: Dosage has not been established
Adolescents and Adults: 5 mg 3 times/day; may increase to 10 mg 3 times/day; usage for more than 2-3 weeks is not recommended
Dosage adjustment in hepatic impairment:
Mild: 5 mg 3 times/day
Moderate to severe: Use not recommended

Administration Oral: May be administered without regard to meals

Monitoring Parameters Relief of muscle spasms and pain; improvement in physical activities

Patient Information Avoid alcohol; may cause drowsiness and impair ability to perform activities requiring mental alertness or physical coordination; may cause dry mouth

Dosage Forms
Tablet, as hydrochloride: 10 mg
Flexeril®: 5 mg, 10 mg [film coated]

♦ **Cyclogyl®** see Cyclopentolate on page 319
♦ **Cyclomen® (Can)** see Danazol on page 336
♦ **Cyclomydril®** see Cyclopentolate and Phenylephrine on page 320

Cyclopentolate (sye kloe PEN toe late)
U.S. Brand Names AK-Pentolate®; Cyclogyl®; Cylate®; Ocu-Pentolate®
Canadian Brand Names Diopentolate®
Therapeutic Category Anticholinergic Agent, Ophthalmic; Ophthalmic Agent, Mydriatic
(Continued)

Cyclopentolate *(Continued)*

Generic Available Yes

Use Diagnostic procedures requiring mydriasis and cycloplegia

Pregnancy Risk Factor C

Contraindications Hypersensitivity to cyclopentolate or any component; narrow-angle glaucoma

Warnings Use of cyclopentolate has been associated with psychotic reactions and behavioral disturbances in pediatric patients; increased susceptibility to these effects has been reported in young infants, young children, and in children with spastic paralysis or brain damage, particularly with concentrations >1%; observe neonates and infants closely for at least 30 minutes after administration; may cause transient elevation of intraocular pressure

Adverse Reactions Central nervous system and cardiovascular reactions most commonly seen in children after receiving 2% solution:

Cardiovascular: Tachycardia, hypertension

Central nervous system: Psychotic and behavioral disturbances manifested by ataxia, restlessness, hallucinations, psychosis, hyperactivity, seizures, incoherent speech

Local: Burning sensation

Ocular: Elevated intraocular pressure, loss of visual accommodation

Miscellaneous: Allergic reactions

Mechanism of Action Prevents the muscle of the ciliary body and the sphincter muscle of the iris from responding to cholinergic stimulation, causing mydriasis and cycloplegia

Pharmacodynamics

Maximum effect:

Cycloplegia: 15-60 minutes

Mydriasis: Within 15-60 minutes, with recovery taking up to 24 hours

Usual Dosage Ophthalmic:

Neonates and Infants: See Cyclopentolate and Phenylephrine *on page 320* (preferred agent for use in neonates and infants due to lower cyclopentolate concentration and reduced risk for systemic reactions)

Children: 1 drop of 0.5% or 1% in eye followed by 1 drop of 0.5% or 1% in 5 minutes, if necessary, approximately 40-50 minutes before procedure

Adults: 1 drop of 1% followed by another drop in 5 minutes; approximately 40-50 minutes prior to the procedure, may use 2% solution in heavily pigmented iris

Administration Ophthalmic: Instill drops into conjunctival sac of affected eye(s); avoid contact of bottle tip with skin or eye; to avoid excessive systemic absorption, finger pressure should be applied on the lacrimal sac during and for 1-2 minutes following application

Patient Information May cause blurred vision and increased sensitivity to light

Additional Information Pilocarpine ophthalmic drops applied after the examination may reduce recovery time to 3-6 hours

Dosage Forms

Solution, ophthalmic, as hydrochloride: 1% (2 mL, 5 mL, 15 mL)

Ak-Pentolate®, Cylate®, Ocu-Pentolate®: 1% (2 mL, 15 mL)

Cyclogyl®: 0.5% (15 mL); 1% (2 mL, 5 mL, 15 mL); 2% (2 mL, 5 mL, 15 mL)

Cyclopentolate and Phenylephrine

(sye kloe PEN toe late & fen il EF rin)

U.S. Brand Names Cyclomydril®

Synonyms Phenylephrine and Cyclopentolate

Therapeutic Category Adrenergic Agonist Agent, Ophthalmic; Anticholinergic Agent, Ophthalmic; Ophthalmic Agent, Mydriatic

Generic Available No

Use Diagnostic procedures requiring mydriasis and cycloplegia; preferred agent for use in neonates and infants

Pregnancy Risk Factor C

Contraindications Hypersensitivity to cyclopentolate, phenylephrine, or any component; narrow-angle glaucoma or untreated anatomically narrow angles

Warnings Use of cyclopentolate has been associated with psychotic reactions and behavioral disturbances in pediatric patients; increased susceptibility to these effects has been reported in young infants, young children, and in children with spastic paralysis or brain damage, particularly with concentrations >1%; observe neonates and infants closely for at least 30 minutes after administration; may cause transient elevation of intraocular pressure

Precautions Use with caution in patient's with Down's syndrome, cardiovascular disease, hypertension, and hyperthyroidism; feeding intolerance may follow ophthalmic use of this product in neonates and infants; withhold feedings for 4 hours after examination

Adverse Reactions

Cardiovascular: Tachycardia, hypertension

Central nervous system: Psychotic and behavioral disturbances manifested by ataxia, restlessness, hallucinations, psychosis, hyperactivity, seizures, incoherent speech, hyperpyrexia

Gastrointestinal: Feeding intolerance, decreased gastric motility

Genitourinary: Urinary retention

Local: Burning sensation

Ocular: Elevated intraocular pressure, loss of visual accommodation, transient stinging, browache, photophobia, lacrimation, superficial punctate keratitis

Miscellaneous: Allergic reactions

Drug Interactions May interfere with the ocular antihypertensive action of carbachol, pilocarpine, or ophthalmic cholinesterase inhibitors

Stability Store at room temperature

Mechanism of Action See individual monographs for Cyclopentolate *on page 319* and Phenylephrine *on page 892*

Pharmacodynamics Onset of action and duration of effect are partially dependent upon eye pigment; dark eyes have a prolonged onset of action and shorter duration than blue eyes

Onset of action: 15-60 minutes

Duration: 4-12 hours

Usual Dosage Ophthalmic:

Neonates, Infants, Children, and Adults: Instill 1 drop into the eye every 5-10 minutes, for up to 3 doses, approximately 40-50 minutes before the examination

Administration Ophthalmic: Instill drops into conjunctival sac of affected eye(s); avoid contact of bottle tip with skin or eye; to avoid excessive systemic absorption, finger pressure should be applied on the lacrimal sac during and for 1-2 minutes following application

Patient Information May cause blurred vision and increased sensitivity to light

Nursing Implications Do not repeat dosage within at least 4 hours, but preferably 24 hours, after initial treatment to prevent drug accumulation and potential systemic toxicity; see Warnings

Additional Information Cyclomydril® is the preferred agent for use in neonates and infants because lower concentrations of both cyclopentolate and phenylephrine provide optimal dilation while minimizing the systemic side effects noted with a higher concentration of each agent used alone

Dosage Forms Solution, ophthalmic: Cyclopentolate hydrochloride 0.2% and phenylephrine hydrochloride 1% (2 mL, 5 mL)

Cyclophosphamide (sye kloe FOS fa mide)

Related Information

Drugs and Breast-Feeding *on page 1404*

Emetogenic Potential of Single Chemotherapeutic Agents *on page 1286*

U.S. Brand Names Cytoxan®; Neosar®

Canadian Brand Names Procytox®

Synonyms CPM; CTX; CYT

Therapeutic Category Antineoplastic Agent, Alkylating Agent (Nitrogen Mustard)

Generic Available Yes (tablets)

Use Treatment of Hodgkin's disease, malignant lymphomas, multiple myeloma, leukemias, sarcomas, mycosis fungoides, neuroblastoma, ovarian carcinoma, breast carcinoma, a variety of other tumors; conditioning regimen for bone marrow transplantation; nephrotic syndrome, lupus erythematosus, severe rheumatoid arthritis, and rheumatoid vasculitis

Pregnancy Risk Factor D

Contraindications Hypersensitivity to cyclophosphamide or any component

Warnings The FDA currently recommends that procedures for proper handling and disposal of antineoplastic agents be considered; cyclophosphamide is potentially carcinogenic and mutagenic; it may impair fertility or cause sterility and birth defects

Precautions Use with caution in patients with bone marrow suppression and impaired renal or hepatic function; modify dosage in patients with renal impairment or compromised bone marrow function. Patients with compromised bone marrow function may require a 33% to 50% reduction in initial dose.

Adverse Reactions

Cardiovascular: Cardiotoxicity with high-dose therapy, pericardial effusion, CHF

Dermatologic: Alopecia, rash, pigmentation of skin, nail changes, Stevens-Johnson syndrome (rare), toxic epidermal necrolysis (rare)

(Continued)

Cyclophosphamide *(Continued)*

Endocrine & metabolic: Hypokalemia, amenorrhea, SIADH, hyperuricemia, hyperkalemia, hyponatremia, oligospermia, sterility (interferes with oogenesis and spermatogenesis) which may be irreversible

Gastrointestinal: Nausea, vomiting, dysgeusia, anorexia, diarrhea, mucositis

Genitourinary: Hemorrhagic cystitis (5% to 10%)

Hematologic: Leukopenia nadir at 8-15 days, hemolytic anemia, thrombocytopenia, hypothrombinemia

Hepatic: Dose-related hepatotoxicity, jaundice

Renal: Nephrotoxicity

Respiratory: Interstitial pulmonary fibrosis, nasal stuffiness

Drug Interactions Cytochrome P450 isoenzyme CYP2B6, CYP2D6, and CYP3A3/4 substrate

Allopurinol (increases myelotoxicity of cyclophosphamide); phenobarbital, phenytoin, and chloral hydrate may increase conversion of cyclophosphamide to active metabolites; chloramphenicol, phenothiazines, imipramine may inhibit the metabolism of cyclophosphamide (increased bone marrow suppression); cyclophosphamide may prolong the neuromuscular blocking activity of succinylcholine

Stability Reconstituted I.V. solution is stable for 24 hours at room temperature or 6 days if refrigerated

Mechanism of Action Interferes with the normal function of DNA by alkylation and cross-linking the strands of DNA, and by possible protein modification

Pharmacokinetics

Absorption: 75% to 95% with low doses

Distribution: Crosses the placenta; appears in breast milk; distributes throughout the body including the brain and CSF, but not in concentrations high enough to treat meningeal leukemia

Protein binding: 20%; metabolite: 60%

Metabolism: Inactive prodrug must undergo hydroxylation to form active alkylating mustards; further oxidation leads to formation of inactive metabolites

Half-life: Range 3-12 hours

Children: 4 hours

Adults: 6-8 hours

Time to peak serum concentration: Oral: Within 1 hour

Elimination: In urine as unchanged drug (<20%) and as metabolites (85% to 90%)

Dialysis: Moderately dialyzable (20% to 50%)

Usual Dosage Refer to individual protocols

Children and Adults with no hematologic problems:

Induction:

Oral, I.V.: Children: 2-8 mg/kg or 60-250 mg/m^2/day

I.V.: 40-50 mg/kg (1.5-1.8 g/m^2) in divided doses over 2-5 days

Maintenance:

Oral: Children: 2-5 mg/kg or 50-150 mg/m^2 twice weekly

Oral: Adults: 1-5 mg/kg/day

I.V.: 10-15 mg/kg (350-550 mg/m^2) every 7-10 days or 3-5 mg/kg (110-185 mg/m^2) twice weekly

Children:

SLE: I.V.: 500-750 mg/m^2 every month; maximum dose: 1 g/m^2

JRA/vasculitis: I.V.: 10 mg/kg every 2 weeks

BMT conditioning regimen: I.V.: 50 mg/kg/day once daily for 3-4 days

Nephrotic syndrome: Oral: 2-3 mg/kg/day every day for up to 12 weeks when corticosteroids are unsuccessful

Dosing adjustment in renal impairment:

Cl$_{cr}$ >10 mL/minute: Administer 100% of normal dose

Cl$_{cr}$ ≤10 mL/minute: Administer 75% of normal dose

Administration

Oral: Administer with food only if GI distress occurs

Parenteral: May administer IVP, I.V. intermittent, or continuous infusion at a final maximum concentration for administration of 20-25 mg/mL; usually administered as a single bolus dose or in fractionated doses over 2-3 days. Most protocols use a 30-60 minute infusion time; doses >1800 mg/m^2 need to be infused over a longer period (ie, 4- or 6-hour infusions)

Monitoring Parameters CBC with differential and platelet count, ESR, BUN, urinalysis, serum electrolytes, serum creatinine, urine specific gravity, urine output

Test Interactions Positive Coombs' [direct]

Patient Information Maintain high fluid intake and urine output. Report any difficulty or pain with urination, unusual bleeding or bruising, persistent fever or sore throat, blood in urine or stool, skin rash, or yellowing of skin or eyes. You may be more susceptible to infection; avoid crowds and unnecessary exposure to infection.

Nursing Implications Encourage adequate hydration and frequent voiding to help prevent hemorrhagic cystitis; before initiating cyclophosphamide therapy, verify that urine specific gravity is <1.010 and that urine output is >100 mL/m²/hour (or 3 mL/kg/hour)

Additional Information Aggressive hydration using fluid containing at least 0.45% sodium chloride at 125 mL/m²/hour, frequent emptying of the bladder, and concurrent administration of mesna are used to reduce the potential of hemorrhagic cystitis (use mesna with cyclophosphamide doses >1 g/m²/day; doses ≤1 g/m²/day may not require use of mesna)

Myelosuppressive effects:
WBC: Moderate
Platelets: Moderate
Onset (days): 7
Nadir (days): 8-14
Recovery (days): 21

Dosage Forms
Injection, powder for reconstitution, as anhydrous:
Cytoxan®: 100 mg, 200 mg, 500 mg, 1 g, 2 g [contains 75 mg mannitol per 100 mg cyclophosphamide]
Neosar®: 100 mg, 200 mg, 500 mg, 1 g, 2 g [contains 82 mg sodium bicarbonate per 100 mg cyclophosphamide]
Tablet, as anhydrous (Cytoxan®): 25 mg, 50 mg

Extemporaneous Preparations To make a 2 mg/mL oral elixir, reconstitute a 200 mg vial with aromatic elixir, withdraw the solution, and add sufficient aromatic elixir to make a final volume of 100 mL in a graduate; store in amber glass; stable for 14 days in the refrigerator
Brook D, Davis RE, and Bequette RJ, "Chemical Stability of Cyclophosphamide in Aromatic Elixir USP," *Am J Hosp Pharm*, 1973, 30:618-20.

References
Bostrom BC, Weisdorf DJ, Kim TH, et al, "Bone Marrow Transplantation for Advanced Acute Leukemia: A Pilot Study of High-Energy Total Body Irradiation, Cyclophosphamide and Continuous Infusion Etoposide," *Bone Marrow Transplant*, 1990, 5(2):83-9.
McCune WJ, Golbus J, Zeldes W, et al, "Clinical and Immunologic Effects of Monthly Administration of Intravenous Cyclophosphamide in Severe Systemic Lupus Erythematosus," *N Engl J Med*, 1988, 318(22):1423-31.

CycloSERINE (sye kloe SER een)

U.S. Brand Names Seromycin® Pulvules®

Therapeutic Category Antibiotic, Miscellaneous; Antitubercular Agent

Generic Available No

Use Adjunctive treatment in pulmonary or extrapulmonary tuberculosis; treatment of acute urinary tract infections caused by *E. coli* or *Enterobacter* species when less toxic conventional therapy has failed or is contraindicated

Pregnancy Risk Factor C

Contraindications Hypersensitivity to cycloserine or any component; epilepsy, depression, severe anxiety or psychosis, severe renal insufficiency, chronic alcoholism

Precautions Dosage must be adjusted in patients with renal impairment

Adverse Reactions
Cardiovascular: Cardiac arrhythmias, CHF
Central nervous system: Drowsiness, headache, dizziness, vertigo, seizures, confusion, psychosis, paresis, coma, anxiety, nervousness, depression, personality changes
Dermatologic: Rash, photosensitivity
Endocrine & metabolic: Vitamin B_{12} deficiency, folate deficiency
Hepatic: Elevated liver enzymes
Neuromuscular & skeletal: Tremor, dysarthria

Drug Interactions Cycloserine inhibits metabolism of phenytoin; alcohol may increase risk of seizures; ethionamide, isoniazid (additive neurotoxicity with cycloserine)

Food Interactions May increase vitamin B_{12} and folic acid dietary requirements

Mechanism of Action Inhibits bacterial cell wall synthesis by competing with amino acid (D-alanine) for incorporation into the bacterial cell wall

Pharmacokinetics
Absorption: ~70% to 90% from the GI tract
Distribution: Crosses the placenta; appears in breast milk, bile, sputum, synovial fluid and CSF
Protein binding: Not plasma protein bound
Half-life: Patients with normal renal function: 10 hours
Time to peak serum concentration: Within 3-4 hours
(Continued)

CycloSERINE (Continued)

Elimination: 60% to 70% of an oral dose excreted unchanged in urine by glomerular filtration within 72 hours, small amounts excreted in feces, remainder is metabolized

Usual Dosage Oral:

Tuberculosis:

Children: 10-20 mg/kg/day divided every 12 hours up to 1000 mg/day

Adults: Initial: 250 mg every 12 hours for 14 days, then give 500 mg to 1 g/day in 2 divided doses

Urinary tract infection: Adults: 250 mg every 12 hours for 14 days

Dosing adjustment in renal impairment:

Cl_{cr} 10-50 mL/minute: Administer every 24 hours

Cl_{cr} <10 mL/minute: Administer every 36-48 hours

Administration Oral: May administer without regard to meals

Monitoring Parameters Periodic renal, hepatic, hematological tests, and plasma cycloserine concentrations

Reference Range Adjust dosage to maintain blood cycloserine concentrations <30 μg/mL

Patient Information May cause drowsiness and impair ability to perform activities requiring mental alertness or physical coordination; avoid alcohol. May cause photosensitivity reactions (eg, exposure to sunlight may cause severe sunburn, skin rash, redness, or itching); avoid exposure to sunlight and artificial light sources (sunlamps, tanning booth/bed); wear protective clothing, wide-brimmed hats, sunglasses, and lip sunscreen (SPF ≥15); use a sunscreen [broad-spectrum sunscreen or physical sunscreen (preferred) or sunblock with SPF ≥15]; contact physician if reaction occurs.

Nursing Implications Some of the neurotoxic effects may be relieved or prevented by the concomitant administration of pyridoxine; sedatives may be effective in reducing anxiety or tremor

Dosage Forms Capsule: 250 mg

CycloSPORINE (SYE kloe spor een)

Related Information

Blood Level Sampling Time Guidelines *on page 1386*

Carbohydrate and Alcohol Content of Liquid Medications for Use in Patients Receiving Ketogenic Diets *on page 1431*

Drugs and Breast-Feeding *on page 1404*

U.S. Brand Names Gengraf™; Neoral®; Restasis™; Sandimmune®

Canadian Brand Names Rhoxal-cyclosporine

Synonyms CsA; CyA; Cyclosporine A

Therapeutic Category Immunosuppressant Agent

Generic Available Yes

Use Immunosuppressant used with corticosteroids to prevent organ rejection in patients with kidney, liver, lung, heart, and bone marrow transplants; treatment of nephrotic syndrome in patients with documented focal glomerulosclerosis when corticosteroids and cyclophosphamide are unsuccessful; severe psoriasis; severe rheumatoid arthritis not responsive to methotrexate alone; severe autoimmune disease that is resistant to corticosteroids and other therapy; prevention and treatment of graft-versus-host disease in bone marrow transplant patients

Ophthalmic emulsion: Increase tear production in patients with moderate to severe keratoconjunctivitis sicca-associated ocular inflammation

Pregnancy Risk Factor C

Contraindications Hypersensitivity to cyclosporine or any component (ie, polyoxyl 35 castor oil is an ingredient of the parenteral formulation and polyoxyl 40 hydrogenated castor oil is an ingredient of the cyclosporine capsules and solution for microemulsion). AAP considers cyclosporine to be contraindicated during breast-feeding. Concurrent therapy with PUVA or UVB, methotrexate, coal tar, or radiation therapy for use in patients with psoriasis; presence of uncontrolled hypertension, abnormal renal function, or malignancies in treatment of psoriasis or rheumatoid arthritis. Ophthalmic emulsion is contraindicated in patients with active ocular infections.

Warnings Immunosuppression with cyclosporine may result in an increased susceptibility to infection and an increased risk of malignancy (lymphomas, lymphoproliferative disorders and squamous cell carcinoma); closely monitor and be prepared to treat anaphylaxis in patients receiving I.V. cyclosporine; serious nephrotoxicity, hepatotoxicity, hypertension, and/or seizures may occur in children receiving cyclosporine; **monitor renal function and adjust dosage to avoid toxicity or possible organ rejection via cyclosporine blood or plasma concentration monitoring.**

Transplant patients: Cyclosporine may cause significant hyperkalemia and hyperuricemia. May cause seizures, particularly if used with high-dose corticosteroids. Predisposing factors associated with neurological disorders include hypertension, hypomagnesemia, hypocholesterolemia, high-dose corticosteroids, high cyclosporine serum concentration, and graft-versus-host disease.

Precautions Close monitoring and dosage adjustment is required in patients with renal and hepatic impairment. Use caution when changing dosage forms since products cannot be used interchangeably.

Adverse Reactions

Cardiovascular: Hypertension, flushing, edema, arrhythmia

Central nervous system: Seizures, headache, confusion, fever, anxiety, lethargy, dizziness, depression

Dermatologic: Hirsutism, gingival hyperplasia, acne, hypertrichosis, pruritus

Endocrine & metabolic: Hyperkalemia, hypomagnesemia, hyperuricemia, hyperchloremic metabolic acidosis, gynecomastia, hyperlipidemia (in patients receiving I.V. cyclosporine)

Gastrointestinal: Abdominal discomfort, diarrhea, nausea, vomiting, anorexia, pancreatitis, hiccups, peptic ulcer, weight loss

Hematologic: Leukopenia, anemia, thrombocytopenia

Hepatic: Hepatotoxicity (elevated liver enzymes, hyperbilirubinemia)

Neuromuscular & skeletal: Myositis, tremor, paresthesia, leg cramps, weakness

Ocular: Ophthalmic preparation: Ocular burning, hyperemia, eye pain, pruritus, stinging

Otic: Tinnitus, hearing loss

Renal: Nephrotoxicity (elevated BUN and serum creatinine)

Respiratory: Sinusitis, cough, dyspnea

Miscellaneous: Lymphoproliferative disorder, increased susceptibility to infection, sensitivity to temperature extremes, anaphylaxis in patients receiving I.V. cyclosporine (reaction includes flushing of the face, respiratory distress with dyspnea and wheezing, hypotension, tachycardia), flu-like symptoms

Drug Interactions Cytochrome P450 isoenzyme CYP3A3/4 substrate

Ketoconazole, itraconazole, amiodarone, fluconazole, azithromycin, clarithromycin, allopurinol, erythromycin, tacrolimus, diltiazem, verapamil, and methylprednisolone increase cyclosporine concentration by inhibiting hepatic metabolism; acyclovir, amphotericin B, aminoglycosides, NSAIDs, sulfamethoxazole and trimethoprim, melphalan, ciprofloxacin, tacrolimus, and vancomycin may increase nephrotoxicity of cyclosporine; erythromycin and metoclopramide increase cyclosporine absorption; phenytoin and octreotide decrease cyclosporine bioavailability; phenytoin, phenobarbital, carbamazepine, primidone, ticlopidine, rifabutin, rifampin, trimethoprim, and nafcillin decrease cyclosporine concentration by increasing hepatic metabolism of cyclosporine; decreases clearance of digoxin, prednisolone; potassium-sparing diuretics increase risk of hyperkalemia; lovastatin, simvastatin, and cimetidine may increase cyclosporine concentration; the herbal medicine St John's wort (*Hypericum perforatum*) may significantly decrease concentrations of cyclosporine; live vaccines may be less effective (avoid vaccination during therapy); cyclosporine increases plasma levels of methotrexate; cyclosporine increases AUC of doxorubicin

Food Interactions Grapefruit and grapefruit juice may affect cyclosporine metabolism resulting in increased cyclosporine concentrations

Stability Do **not** store oral solution or oral solution for emulsion in the refrigerator; store oral solutions in original container only and use contents within 2 months after opening; store ampuls and ophthalmic emulsion-containing vials at room temperature; protect from light; I.V. cyclosporine prepared in NS is stable 6 hours in a polyvinyl chloride container or 12 hours in a glass container; I.V. cyclosporine diluted in D_5W to a final concentration of 2 mg/mL is stable for 24 hours in glass or polyvinyl chloride containers; I.V. cyclosporine may bind to the plastic tubing in I.V. administration sets and to polyvinyl chloride bags. Polyoxyethylated castor oil (Cremophor El®) surfactant in cyclosporine injection may leach phthalate from polyvinyl chloride containers such as bags and tubing.

Mechanism of Action Inhibition of production and release of interleukin II and inhibits interleukin II-induced activation of resting T lymphocytes

Pharmacokinetics

Absorption: Oral:

Cyclosporine (non-modified) solution or soft gelatin capsule: Erratically and incompletely absorbed; dependent on the presence of food, bile acids, and GI motility; larger oral doses of cyclosporine are needed in pediatric patients vs adults due to a shorter bowel length resulting in limited intestinal absorption

Cyclosporine (modified) solution in a microemulsion or soft gelatin capsule in a microemulsion: Erratically and incompletely absorbed; increased absorption, up to 30% when compared to cyclosporine (non-modified); absorption is less

(Continued)

CycloSPORINE *(Continued)*

dependent on food intake, bile, or GI motility when compared to cyclosporine (non-modified)

Distribution: Widely distributed in tissues and body fluids including the liver, pancreas, and lungs; crosses the placenta; excreted into breast milk

V_{dss}: 4-6 L/kg in renal, liver, and marrow transplant recipients (slightly lower values in cardiac transplant patients; children <10 years of age have higher values)

Protein binding: 90% to 98% of dose binds to blood lipoproteins

Metabolism: Undergoes extensive first-pass metabolism following oral administration; extensively metabolized by the cytochrome P450 system in the liver; forms at least 25 metabolites

Bioavailability:

Cyclosporine (non-modified): Dependent on patient population and transplant type (<10% in adult liver transplant patients and as high as 89% in renal patients). The bioavailability of Sandimmune® capsules and oral solution are equivalent; bioavailability of oral solution is ~30% of the I.V. solution.

Children: 28% (range: 17% to 42%); with gut dysfunction commonly seen in BMT recipients, oral bioavailability is further reduced

Cyclosporine (modified): Bioavailability of Neoral® capsules and oral solution are equivalent:

Children: 43% (range: 30% to 68%)

Adults: 23% greater than with Sandimmune® in renal transplant patients, 50% greater in liver transplant patients

Half-life: May be prolonged in patients with hepatic impairment and lower in pediatric patients due to a higher metabolic rate

Cyclosporine (non-modified): Biphasic

Alpha phase: 1.4 hours

Terminal phase: 6-24 hours

Cyclosporine (modified): 8.4 hours (range: 5-18 hours)

Time to peak serum concentration:

Cyclosporine (non-modified): 2-6 hours; some patients have a second peak at 5-6 hours

Cyclosporine (modified): 1.5-2 hours (in renal transplant patients)

Elimination: Primarily biliary with 6% of the dose excreted in urine as unchanged drug (0.1%) and metabolites; clearance is more rapid in pediatric patients than in adults

Usual Dosage Children and Adults (oral dosage is ~3 times the I.V. dosage):

Transplantations:

I.V.: Cyclosporine (non-modified):

Initial: 5-6 mg/kg/dose (⅓ the oral dose) administered 4-12 hours prior to organ transplantation

Maintenance: 2-10 mg/kg/day in divided doses every 8-24 hours; patients should be switched to oral cyclosporine as soon as possible; cyclosporine doses should be adjusted to maintain whole blood HPLC trough concentrations in the reference range

Oral: Cyclosporine (non-modified):

Initial: 14-18 mg/kg/dose administered 4-12 hours prior to organ transplantation; lower initial doses of 10-14 mg/kg/day have been used for renal transplants

Maintenance, postoperative: 5-15 mg/kg/day divided every 12-24 hours; maintenance dose is usually tapered to 3-10 mg/kg/day

When using non-modified formulation, cyclosporine levels may increase in liver transplant patients when the T-tube is closed; may need to decrease dose

Oral: Cyclosporine (modified): Based on the organ transplant population:

Initial: Same as the initial dose for solution or soft gelatin capsule

or

Renal: 9 mg/kg/day (range: 6-12 mg/kg/day) divided every 12 hours

Liver: 8 mg/kg/day (range: 4-12 mg/kg/day) divided every 12 hours

Heart: 7 mg/kg/day (range: 4-10 mg/kg/day) divided every 12 hours

Note: A 1:1 ratio conversion from Sandimmune® to Neoral® has been recommended initially; however, lower doses of Neoral® may be required after conversion to prevent overdose. Total daily doses should be adjusted based on the cyclosporine trough blood concentration and clinical assessment of organ rejection. Cyclosporine blood trough levels should be determined prior to conversion. After conversion to Neoral®, cyclosporine trough levels should be monitored every 4-7 days. **Neoral® and Sandimmune® are not bioequivalent and cannot be used interchangeably.**

Focal segmental glomerulosclerosis: Oral: Initial: 3 mg/kg/day divided every 12 hours

Rheumatoid arthritis: Oral: Cyclosporine (modified): Initial: 2.5 mg/kg/day divided every 12 hours; may increase dose by 0.5-0.75 mg/kg/day if insufficient response is seen after 8 weeks of treatment; maximum dose: 4 mg/kg/day

Psoriasis: Oral: Cyclosporine (modified): Initial: 2.5 mg/kg/day divided every 12 hours; may increase dose by 0.5 mg/kg/day if insufficient response is seen after 4 weeks of treatment; maximum dose: 4 mg/kg/day

Autoimmune diseases: Oral: 1-3 mg/kg/day

Ophthalmic: Children ≥16 years and Adults: Instill one drop in affected eye(s) every 12 hours

Administration

Oral: Administer consistently at the same time twice daily; use oral syringe, glass dropper, or glass container (not plastic or styrofoam cup); to improve palatability, oral solution may be mixed with milk, chocolate milk, orange juice, or apple juice that is at room temperature; dilution of Neoral® with milk can be unpalatable; stir well and drink at once; do not allow to stand before drinking; rinse with more diluent to ensure that the total dose is taken; after use, dry outside of glass dropper, do not rinse with water or other cleaning agents

Parenteral: May administer by I.V. intermittent infusion or continuous infusion; for intermittent infusion, administer over 2-6 hours at a final concentration not to exceed 2.5 mg/mL. Anaphylaxis has been reported with I.V. use. Patients should be continuously monitored for at least the first 30 minutes of the infusion, and should be monitored frequently thereafter

Ophthalmic: Invert vial prior to use to obtain a uniform emulsion. Avoid contact of vial tip with skin or eye; remove contact lenses prior to administration; lenses may be inserted 15 minutes after instillation. May be used with artificial tears; separate administration by at least 15 minutes.

Monitoring Parameters Blood/serum drug concentration (trough), renal and hepatic function tests, serum electrolytes, lipid profile, blood pressure, heart rate

Reference Range Reference ranges are method dependent and specimen dependent; use the same analytical method consistently; trough levels should be obtained immediately prior to next dose

Therapeutic: Not well defined, dependent on organ transplanted, time after transplant, organ function, and cyclosporine toxicity. Empiric therapeutic concentration ranges for trough cyclosporine concentrations:

Kidney: 100-200 ng/mL (serum, RIA)

BMT: 100-250 ng/mL (serum, RIA)

Heart: 100-200 ng/mL (serum, RIA)

Liver: 100-400 ng/mL (blood, HPLC)

Method dependent (optimum cyclosporine trough concentrations):

Serum, RIA: 150-300 ng/mL; 50-150 ng/mL (late post-transplant period)

Whole blood, RIA: 250-800 ng/mL; 150-450 ng/mL (late post-transplant period)

Whole blood, HPLC: 100-500 ng/mL

Test Interactions Cyclosporine adsorbs to silicone; specific whole blood assay for cyclosporine may be falsely elevated if sample is drawn from the same central venous line through which dose was administered (even if flush has been administered and/or dose was given hours before); cyclosporine metabolites cross-react with radioimmunoassay and fluorescence polarization immunoassay

Patient Information Avoid the herbal medicine St John's wort; take dose at the same time each day; do not allow diluted oral solution to stand before drinking; do not change brands of cyclosporine unless directed by your physician. Patients with psoriasis should avoid excessive sun exposure. Notify physician of severe headache; persistent nausea, vomiting; muscle pain or cramping; unusual swelling of extremities; chest pain or rapid heartbeat.

Nursing Implications Adequate airway, supportive measures, epinephrine and I.V. steroids for treating anaphylaxis should be present when I.V. cyclosporine is administered

Additional Information Diltiazem has been used to prevent cyclosporine nephrotoxicity, reduce the frequency of delayed graft function when administered before and after surgery, and used to treat the mild hypertension that occurs in most patients after transplantation; diltiazem increases cyclosporine blood concentration by delaying its clearance resulting in decreased dosage requirements for cyclosporine

Dosage Forms

Capsule, soft gel, modified: 25 mg, 100 mg [contains castor oil and ethanol]

Gengraf™: 25 mg, 100 mg [contains alcohol, castor oil, and propylene glycol]

Neoral®: 25 mg, 100 mg [contains dehydrated alcohol, corn oil, polyoxyl 40 hydrogenated castor oil, and propylene glycol]

Capsule, soft gel, non-modified (Sandimmune®): 25 mg, 100 mg [contains dehydrated alcohol and corn oil]

Emulsion, ophthalmic [preservative free, single-use vial] (Restasis™): 0.05% (0.4 mL) [contains glycerin, castor oil, polysorbate 80, carbomer 1342; 32 vials/box]

Injection, solution, non-modified (Sandimmune®): 50 mg/mL (5 mL) [contains alcohol and Cremophor EL (polyoxyethylated castor oil)]

(Continued)

CycloSPORINE (Continued)

Solution, oral, modified (Neoral®): 100 mg/mL (50 mL) [contains dehydrated alcohol, corn oil, polyoxyl 40 hydrogenated castor oil, and propylene glycol]

Solution, oral, non-modified (Sandimmune®): 100 mg/mL (50 mL) [contains alcohol and olive oil]

References

Burckart GJ, Canafax DM, and Yee GC, "Cyclosporine Monitoring," *Drug Intell Clin Pharm*, 1986, 20(9):649-52.

Holt DW, Mueller EA, Kovarik JM, et al, "Sandimmune® Neoral® Pharmacokinetics: Impact of the New Oral Formulation," *Transplant Proc*, 1995, 27(1):1434-7.

Lin CY and Lee SF, "Comparison of Pharmacokinetics Between CsA Capsules and Sandimmune® Neoral® in Pediatric Patients," *Transplant Proc*, 1994, 26(5):2973-4.

Niese D, "A Double-Blind Randomized Study of Sandimmune® Neoral® vs Sandimmune® in New Renal Transplant Recipients: Results After 12 Months," *Transplant Proc*, 1995, 27(2):1849-56.

Taesch S, Niese D, and Mueller EA, "Sandimmune® Neoral®, A New Oral Formulation of Cyclosporine With Improved Pharmacokinetic Characteristics: Safety and Tolerability in Renal Transplant Patients," *Transplant Proc*, 1994, 26(6):3147-9.

Wandstrat TL, Schroeder TJ, and Myre SA, "Cyclosporine Pharmacokinetics in Pediatric Transplant Recipients," *Ther Drug Monit*, 1989, 11(5):493-6.

Yee GC, "Recent Advances in Cyclosporine Pharmacokinetics," *Pharmacotherapy*, 1991, 11(5):130S-134S.

- ◆ **Cyclosporine A** *see* CycloSPORINE *on page 324*
- ◆ **Cyklokapron®** *see* Tranexamic Acid *on page 1109*
- ◆ **Cylate®** *see* Cyclopentolate *on page 319*
- ◆ **Cylert®** *see* Pemoline *on page 870*
- ◆ **Cylex® [OTC]** *see* Benzocaine *on page 163*

Cyproheptadine (si proe HEP ta deen)

Related Information

Overdose and Toxicology *on page 1388*

U.S. Brand Names Periactin®

Therapeutic Category Antihistamine

Generic Available Yes

Use Perennial and seasonal allergic rhinitis and other allergic symptoms including urticaria; appetite stimulant (useful in the management of anorexia nervosa); prophylactic treatment of cluster and migraine headaches; spasticity associated with spinal cord damage associated with spasticity

Pregnancy Risk Factor B

Contraindications Hypersensitivity to cyproheptadine or any component; narrow-angle glaucoma, bladder neck obstruction, acute asthmatic attack, stenosing peptic ulcer, GI tract obstruction, those on MAO inhibitors

Adverse Reactions

Cardiovascular: Tachycardia, palpitations, edema

Central nervous system: Sedation, CNS stimulation, seizures, fatigue, headache, nervousness, depression

Dermatologic: Photosensitivity, rash, angioedema

Gastrointestinal: Appetite stimulation, xerostomia, nausea, diarrhea, abdominal pain

Hematologic: Hemolytic anemia, leukopenia, thrombocytopenia

Hepatic: Hepatitis

Neuromuscular & skeletal: Myalgia, paresthesia, arthralgia

Respiratory: Bronchospasm, epistaxis, pharyngitis

Miscellaneous: Allergic reactions

Drug Interactions MAO inhibitors; enhances sedative effects of other CNS depressants; enhances anticholinergic effects of other anticholinergic agents

Mechanism of Action A potent antihistamine and serotonin antagonist, competes with histamine for H_1-receptor sites on effector cells in the GI tract, blood vessels, and respiratory tract

Pharmacokinetics

Absorption: Well absorbed

Metabolism: Extensively by conjugation

Elimination: >50% excreted in urine (primarily as metabolites); approximately 25% excreted in feces

Usual Dosage Oral:

Allergic conditions:

Children: 0.25 mg/kg/day or 8 mg/m^2/day in 2-3 divided doses **or**

2-6 years: 2 mg every 8-12 hours (not to exceed 12 mg/day)

7-14 years: 4 mg every 8-12 hours (not to exceed 16 mg/day)

Adults: 4-20 mg/day divided every 8 hours (not to exceed 0.5 mg/kg/day)

Appetite stimulation (anorexia nervosa): Children >13 years and Adults: 2 mg 4 times/day; may be increased gradually over a 3-week period to 8 mg 4 times/day

Cluster headaches: Adults: 4 mg 4 times/day
Migraine headaches:
Children: 4 mg 2-3 times/day
Adults: 4-8 mg 3 times/day
Spasticity associated with spinal cord damage: Children ≥12 years and Adults: 4 mg at bedtime; increase by a 4 mg dose every 3-4 days; average daily dose: 16 mg in divided doses; not to exceed 36 mg/day

Dosage adjustment in hepatic impairment: Reduce dosage in patients with significant hepatic dysfunction

Administration Oral: Administer with food or milk

Test Interactions Diagnostic antigen skin tests; ↑ amylase (S); ↓ fasting glucose (S)

Patient Information May cause drowsiness and impair ability to perform activities requiring mental alertness or physical coordination; may cause dry mouth. May rarely cause photosensitivity reactions (eg, exposure to sunlight may cause severe sunburn, skin rash, redness, or itching); avoid direct exposure to sunlight

Dosage Forms
Syrup, as hydrochloride: 2 mg/5 mL (473 mL) [contains 5% alcohol; mint flavor]
Tablet, as hydrochloride (Periactin®): 4 mg

References
Gracies JM, Nance P, Elovic E, et al, "Traditional Pharmacological Treatments for Spasticity. Part II: General and Regional Treatments," *Muscle Nerve Suppl*, 1997, 6:S92-120.

♦ **Cystadane®** *see* Betaine Anhydrous *on page 169*
♦ **Cystagon®** *see* Cysteamine *on page 329*

Cysteamine (sis TEE a meen)

U.S. Brand Names Cystagon®

Therapeutic Category Cystinosis, Treatment Agent

Generic Available No

Use Management of nephropathic cystinosis

Pregnancy Risk Factor C

Contraindications Hypersensitivity to cysteamine, penicillamine, or any component

Warnings Leukocyte cystine levels should be monitored during oral cysteamine therapy; cysteamine should be given in the lowest doses possible to achieve adequate leukocyte cystine depletion; toxicity can be reduced by initiating therapy with a slowly increasing dose schedule (See Usual Dosage)

Precautions Use with caution in patients with a history of blood dyscrasias, gastric or duodenal ulcer, or neurologic disorder

Adverse Reactions
Cardiovascular: Hypertension
Central nervous system: Somnolence, encephalopathy, headache, seizures, ataxia, confusion, dizziness, jitteriness, nervousness, impaired cognition, emotional changes, hallucinations, nightmares, fever, lethargy
Dermatologic: Urticaria, rash
Endocrine & metabolic: Dehydration
Gastrointestinal: Bad breath, abdominal pain, dyspepsia, constipation, gastroenteritis, duodenitis, duodenal ulceration, vomiting, anorexia, diarrhea
Hematologic: Anemia, leukopenia
Hepatic: Abnormal liver enzymes
Neuromuscular & skeletal: Tremor, hyperkinesia
Otic: Decreased hearing

Mechanism of Action Reacts with cystine in the lysosome to convert it to cysteine and to a cysteine-cysteamine mixed disulfide, both of which can then exit the lysosome in patients with cystinosis, an inherited defect of lysosomal transport

Pharmacokinetics
Absorption: Rapid
Protein binding: 10% to 18%
Half-life: 1 hour

Usual Dosage Oral:
Children <12 years: Initial: 10 mg/kg/day divided into 4 doses; increase by 10 mg/kg/day every 3 weeks to a maximum of 90 mg/kg/day (average effective dose: 50-60 mg/kg/day) **or** 0.16-0.32 g/m²/day divided into 4 doses; increasing every 3 weeks to a maximum of 1.3 g/m²/day
Children ≥12 years and Adults (>110 lb): 2 g/day in 4 divided doses; dosage may be increased gradually to 1.95 g/m²/day

Administration Oral: Contents of capsule may be sprinkled over food

Monitoring Parameters Blood counts and liver enzymes during therapy; blood pressure; monitor leukocyte cystine measurements to determine adequate dosage and compliance (measure 5-6 hours after administration)
(Continued)

Cysteamine (Continued)

Reference Range Leukocyte cystine: <1 nmol of half-cystine/mg protein

Patient Information May cause drowsiness or impair ability to perform activities requiring mental alertness or physical coordination

Dosage Forms Capsule, as bitartrate: 50 mg, 150 mg

Cysteine (SIS teen)

Therapeutic Category Nutritional Supplement

Generic Available Yes

Use Supplement to crystalline amino acid solutions, in particular the specialized pediatric formulas (eg, Aminosyn® PF, TrophAmine®) to meet the intravenous amino acid nutritional requirements of infants receiving parenteral nutrition (PN)

Contraindications Hypersensitivity to cysteine or any component; patients with hepatic coma or metabolic disorders involving impaired nitrogen utilization

Warnings Metabolic acidosis has occurred in infants related to the "hydrochloride" component of cysteine; each 1 mmol cysteine (175 mg) delivers 1 mEq chloride and 1 mEq hydrogen ion; to balance the extra hydrochloride ions and prevent acidosis, addition to the PN solution of a 1 mEq acetate electrolyte salt for each mmol (175 mg) of cysteine may be needed; each 40 mg cysteine (equal to every 1 g amino acid when used in the recommended ratio) adds 0.228 mEq chloride and hydrogen

Precautions Use with caution in patients with renal dysfunction and hepatic insufficiency

Adverse Reactions

Central nervous system: Fever

Endocrine & metabolic: Metabolic acidosis (see Warnings)

Gastrointestinal: Nausea

Renal: Elevated BUN, azotemia

Stability Avoid excessive heat, do not freeze; when combined with parenteral amino acid solutions, cysteine is relatively unstable; it is intended to be added immediately prior to administration to the patient; infusion of the admixture should begin within 1 hour of mixing or refrigerated until use; stable 24 hours in PN solution; opened vials must be used within 4 hours of entry

Mechanism of Action Cysteine is a sulfur-containing amino acid synthesized from methionine via the transulfuration pathway. It is a precursor of the tripeptide glutathione and also of taurine. Newborn infants have a relative deficiency of the enzyme necessary to affect this conversion. Cysteine may be considered an essential amino acid in infants.

Usual Dosage I.V.: Neonates and Infants: Added as a fixed ratio to crystalline amino acid solution: 40 mg cysteine per g of amino acids; dosage will vary with the daily amino acid dosage (eg, 0.5-2.5 g/kg/day amino acids would result in 20-100 mg/kg/day cysteine); individual doses of cysteine of 0.8-1 mmol/kg/day have also been added directly to the daily PN solution; the duration of treatment relates to the need for PN; patients on chronic PN therapy have received cysteine until 6 months of age and in some cases until 2 years of age

Administration Parenteral: Use only after dilution into PN solution; dilute with amino acid solution in a ratio of 40 mg cysteine to 1 g amino acid: eg, 500 mg cysteine is added to 12.5 g (250 mL) of 5% amino acid solution

Monitoring Parameters BUN, ammonia, electrolytes, pH, acid-base balance, serum creatinine, liver function tests, growth curve

Additional Information Addition of cysteine to PN solutions enhances the solubility of calcium and phosphate by lowering the overall pH of the solution

Dosage Forms Injection, solution, as hydrochloride: 50 mg/mL [~0.285 mmol/mL] (10 mL)

♦ **Cystospaz®** see Hyoscyamine on page 585

♦ **Cystospaz-M®** see Hyoscyamine on page 585

♦ **CYT** see Cyclophosphamide on page 321

Cytarabine (sye TARE a been)

Related Information

Emetogenic Potential of Single Chemotherapeutic Agents on page 1286

U.S. Brand Names Cytosar-U®

Synonyms Arabinosylcytosine; Ara-C; Cytosine Arabinoside

Therapeutic Category Antineoplastic Agent, Antimetabolite

Generic Available Yes

Use Used in combination regimens for the treatment of leukemias, meningeal leukemia, Hodgkin's lymphoma, and non-Hodgkin's lymphoma

Pregnancy Risk Factor D

Contraindications Hypersensitivity to cytarabine or any component

Warnings The FDA currently recommends that procedures for proper handling and disposal of antineoplastic agents be considered. Must monitor for drug toxicity; drug toxicity includes bone marrow suppression with leukopenia, thrombocytopenia, and anemia along with nausea, vomiting, diarrhea, abdominal pain, oral ulceration, and hepatic dysfunction; irreversible cerebellar toxicity may occur with a cumulative dose ≥ 30 g/m^2; cytarabine is potentially mutagenic and carcinogenic.

Precautions Marked bone marrow suppression necessitates dosage reduction or a reduction in the number of days of administration; with severe hepatic dysfunction, dosage may need to be reduced

Adverse Reactions
  Cardiovascular: Cardiomegaly, chest pain, pericarditis
  Central nervous system: Headache, malaise, confusion, seizures, fever, irritability, cerebral and cerebellar dysfunction (somnolence, personality changes, coma, ataxia)
  Dermatologic: Alopecia, rash
  Endocrine & metabolic: Hyperuricemia
  Gastrointestinal: Nausea, vomiting, oral and anal inflammation with ulceration, anorexia, diarrhea, GI hemorrhage, mucositis
  Hematologic: Myelosuppression (leukopenia, thrombocytopenia, anemia)
  Hepatic: Hepatic dysfunction, jaundice, elevated serum bilirubin and liver enzymes
  Local: Thrombophlebitis
  Neuromuscular & skeletal: Myalgia, bone pain, peripheral neuropathy, weakness, gait disturbances
  Ocular: Conjunctivitis, hemorrhagic conjunctivitis, corneal toxicity, photophobia, blurred vision
  Respiratory: Syndrome of sudden respiratory distress progressing to pulmonary edema and diffuse interstitial pneumonitis have been reported with high-dose regimens
  Miscellaneous: Ara-C syndrome (fever, myalgia, bone pain, rash, conjunctivitis, malaise occurring 6-12 hours after administration); headache and vomiting with I.T. administration; anaphylactoid reaction

Drug Interactions Decreases digoxin oral tablet absorption

Stability Reconstituted solutions containing 20-100 mg/mL cytarabine are stable for 48 hours at room temperature; I.T. Ara-C is compatible with methotrexate and hydrocortisone mixed in the same syringe; physically incompatible with fluorouracil, heparin

Mechanism of Action Converted intracellularly to the active metabolite cytarabine triphosphate; inhibits DNA polymerase by competing with deoxycytidine triphosphate resulting in inhibition of DNA synthesis; incorporated into DNA chain resulting in termination of chain elongation; cell cycle-specific for the S-phase of cell division

Pharmacokinetics
  Distribution: Penetrates the CSF in limited amounts, crosses the placenta
  Protein binding: 13%
  Metabolism: Deactivated by cytidine deaminase primarily in the liver, but also in kidneys, GI mucosa, and granulocytes
  Half-life, terminal: 1-3 hours
  Elimination: ~80% of dose excreted in urine as metabolites within 24 hours; 10% excreted in urine as unchanged drug

Usual Dosage Children and Adults (refer to individual protocols):
  Induction remission:
    I.V.: 200 mg/m^2/day for 5 days at 2-week intervals as a single agent; in combination chemotherapy, 100-200 mg/m^2/day for 5- to 10-day therapy course every 2-4 weeks, or every day until remission, given as an I.V. continuous drip or in 2 divided doses/day
    I.T.: 5-75 mg/m^2 every 2-7 days until CNS findings normalize
  Maintenance remission:
    I.V.: 70-200 mg/m^2/day for 2-5 days at monthly intervals
    I.M., S.C.: 1-1.5 mg/kg single dose for maintenance at 1- to 4-week intervals
    I.T.: 5-75 mg/m^2 every 2-7 days until CNS findings normalize **or**
      <1 year: 20 mg
      1-2 years: 30 mg
      2-3 years: 50 mg
      >3 years: 70 mg
  High-dose regimen: Refractory leukemias or refractory non-Hodgkin's lymphoma: I.V. infusion: 3 g/m^2/dose every 12 hours for up to 12 doses

Administration Parenteral: May administer S.C., I.M., IVP, I.V. infusion, or I.T. at a concentration not to exceed 100 mg/mL
    High-dose regimens or for use in neonates: Diluents containing benzyl alcohol should not be used to reconstitute the drug; high-dose regimens (dose >1 g/m^2)

(Continued)

Cytarabine *(Continued)*

are usually administered by I.V. infusion over 2 hours or longer, or as an I.V. continuous infusion

IVP: May administer over 15 minutes; rapid administration is associated with greater neurotoxicity

I.T. administration: Reconstitute with preservative free NS, Elliotts B solution, or preservative free LR solution; use preservative free injection formulation for I.T. use; filter through a 0.22 micron filter; the volume to be given I.T. is in the range of 3-10 mL and should correspond to an equivalent volume of CSF removed; antiemetic therapy should be administered prior to intrathecal doses of cytarabine

S.C. administration: Rotate injection sites to thigh, abdomen, and flank regions; avoid repeated administration to a single site

Monitoring Parameters Liver function tests, CBC with differential and platelet count, serum creatinine, BUN, serum uric acid; signs of neurotoxicity

Patient Information Notify physician of any fever, sore throat, bleeding, or bruising

Nursing Implications Administer corticosteroid eye drops for prophylaxis of conjunctivitis around-the-clock prior to, during, and for 2-7 days after high-dose Ara-C; pyridoxine has been administered on days of high-dose Ara-C therapy for prophylaxis of CNS toxicity

Additional Information Myelosuppressive effects:

WBC: Severe

Platelets: Severe

Onset (days): 4-7

Nadir (days): 14-18

Recovery (days): 21-28

Dosage Forms Injection, powder for reconstitution: 100 mg, 500 mg, 1 g, 2 g

References

Baker WJ, Royer GL, and Weiss RB, "Cytarabine and Neurologic Toxicity," *J Clinical Oncology*, 1991, 9(4):679-93.

Grossman L, Baker MA, Sutton DM, et al, "Central Nervous System Toxicity of High-Dose Cytosine Arabinoside," *Med Pediatr Oncol*, 1983, 11(4):246-50.

- ◆ **Cytochrome P450 Enzymes and Drug Metabolism** *see page 1230*
- ◆ **Cytomel®** *see* Liothyronine *on page 680*
- ◆ **Cytosar-U®** *see* Cytarabine *on page 330*
- ◆ **Cytosine Arabinoside** *see* Cytarabine *on page 330*
- ◆ **Cytotec®** *see* Misoprostol *on page 769*
- ◆ **Cytovene®** *see* Ganciclovir *on page 530*
- ◆ **Cytoxan®** *see* Cyclophosphamide *on page 321*
- ◆ **Cytra-2** *see* Citrate and Citric Acid *on page 282*
- ◆ **Cytra-3®** *see* Citrate and Citric Acid *on page 282*
- ◆ **Cytra-K®** *see* Citrate and Citric Acid *on page 282*
- ◆ **D-3-Mercaptovaline** *see* Penicillamine *on page 872*
- ◆ **d4T** *see* Stavudine *on page 1039*
- ◆ **D₅W** *see* Dextrose *on page 366*
- ◆ **D₁₀W** *see* Dextrose *on page 366*
- ◆ **D₂₅W** *see* Dextrose *on page 366*
- ◆ **D₃₀W** *see* Dextrose *on page 366*
- ◆ **D₄₀W** *see* Dextrose *on page 366*
- ◆ **D₅₀W** *see* Dextrose *on page 366*
- ◆ **D₆₀W** *see* Dextrose *on page 366*
- ◆ **D₇₀W** *see* Dextrose *on page 366*

Dacarbazine *(da KAR ba zeen)*

Related Information

Emetogenic Potential of Single Chemotherapeutic Agents *on page 1286*

U.S. Brand Names DTIC-Dome®

Synonyms DIC; Imidazole Carboxamide

Therapeutic Category Antineoplastic Agent, Miscellaneous

Generic Available Yes

Use Treatment of malignant melanoma, Hodgkin's disease, soft-tissue sarcomas (fibrosarcomas, rhabdomyosarcoma), islet cell carcinoma, medullary carcinoma of the thyroid, and neuroblastoma

Pregnancy Risk Factor C

Contraindications Hypersensitivity to dacarbazine or any component

Warnings The FDA currently recommends that procedures for proper handling and disposal of antineoplastic agents be considered. Hematopoietic depression is common; hepatic necrosis is also possible; dacarbazine has been reported to cause sterility and is mutagenic and teratogenic in rats

Precautions Use with caution in patients with bone marrow suppression, renal and/or hepatic impairment; dosage reduction may be necessary in patients with renal or hepatic insufficiency; avoid extravasation of the drug

Adverse Reactions
Cardiovascular: Facial flushing, hypotension
Central nervous system: Malaise, headache, fever, seizure
Dermatologic: Alopecia, rash, photosensitivity
Gastrointestinal: Anorexia, nausea, vomiting, metallic taste
Hematologic: Myelosuppression (nadir: 2-4 weeks): Leukopenia, thrombocytopenia
Hepatic: Hepatotoxicity, hepatic vein thrombosis, hepatocellular necrosis
Local: Pain and burning at infusion site, thrombophlebitis
Neuromuscular & skeletal: Myalgia, paresthesia
Ocular: Blurred vision
Respiratory: Sinus congestion
Miscellaneous: Flu-like syndrome, anaphylactic reactions

Drug Interactions Phenytoin, phenobarbital may induce dacarbazine metabolism

Stability Store in refrigerator; intact vials are stable for 4 weeks at room temperature; protect dacarbazine solutions from light; reconstituted dacarbazine solution 10 mg/mL is stable for 72 hours when refrigerated or 8 hours at room temperature; drug decomposition has occurred if the solution turns pink; dacarbazine is incompatible with hydrocortisone sodium succinate

Mechanism of Action Alkylating agent which forms methyldiazonium ions that attack nucleophilic groups in DNA; inhibits DNA, RNA, and protein synthesis by cross-linking DNA strands

Pharmacokinetics
Distribution: Distributes to the liver; very little distribution into CSF with CSF concentrations ~14% of plasma concentrations
V_{dss}: Adults: 17 L/m^2
Protein binding: Minimal, 5%
Metabolism: N-demethylated in the liver by microsomal enzymes; metabolites may also have an antineoplastic effect
Half-life, biphasic: Initial: 20-40 minutes; terminal: 5 hours (in patients with normal renal/hepatic function)
Elimination: ~30% to 50% of dose excreted in urine by tubular secretion, 15% to 25% is excreted in urine as unchanged drug

Usual Dosage I.V. (refer to individual protocols):
Children:
Pediatric solid tumors: 200-470 mg/m^2/day over 5 days every 21-28 days
Pediatric neuroblastoma: 800-900 mg/m^2 as a single dose on day 1 of therapy every 3-4 weeks in combination therapy
Hodgkin's disease: 375 mg/m^2 on days 1 and 15 of treatment course, repeat every 28 days
Adults:
Malignant melanoma: 2-4.5 mg/kg/day for 10 days, repeat in 4 weeks or may use 250 mg/m^2/day for 5 days, repeat in 3 weeks
Hodgkin's disease: 150 mg/m^2/day for 5 days, repeat every 4 weeks or 375 mg/m^2 on day 1, repeat in 15 days of each 28-day cycle in combination with other agents

Administration Parenteral: Reconstitute vial for IVP doses with at least 2 mL of D$_5$W or NS; administer dose diluted in 5-10 mL D$_5$W or NS by slow IVP over 2-3 minutes or by I.V. infusion over 15-120 minutes at a concentration not to exceed 10 mg/mL

Monitoring Parameters CBC with differential, erythrocytes and platelet count; liver function tests

Patient Information Restrict intake of food for 4-6 hours prior to dacarbazine dose to decrease vomiting; flu-like symptoms (ie, malaise, fever, myalgia) may occur 1 week after infusion. May cause photosensitivity reactions (eg, exposure to sunlight may cause severe sunburn, skin rash, redness, or itching); avoid exposure to sunlight and artificial light sources (sunlamps, tanning booth/bed); wear protective clothing, wide-brimmed hats, sunglasses, and lip sunscreen (SPF ≥15); use a sunscreen [broad-spectrum sunscreen or physical sunscreen (preferred) or sunblock with SPF ≥15]; contact physician if reaction occurs.

Nursing Implications Avoid extravasation; use a D$_5$W or NS flush before and after a dacarbazine infusion; local pain, burning sensation, and irritation at the injection site may be relieved by local application of hot packs, slowing the I.V. rate and further dilution in I.V. fluid
(Continued)

Dacarbazine *(Continued)*

Dosage Forms
Injection, powder for reconstitution: 200 mg, 500 mg
DTIC-Dome®: 100 mg, 200 mg

References
Berg SL, Grisell DL, DeLaney TF, et al, "Principles of Treatment of Pediatric Solid Tumors," *Pediatr Clin North Am*, 1991, 38(2):249-67.

Finklestein JZ, Albo V, Ertel I, et al, "5-(3,3-Dimethyl-l-triazeno) imidazole-4-carboxamide (NSC-45388) in the Treatment of Solid Tumors in Children," *Cancer Chemother Rep*, 1975, 59(2 Pt 1):351-7.

Mutz ID and Urban CE, "Dimethyl-triazeno-imidazole-carboxamide (DTIC) in Combination Chemotherapy for Childhood Neuroblastoma," *Wien Klin Wochenschr*, 1978, 90(24):867-70.

Daclizumab (da CLI zoo mab)

U.S. Brand Names Zenapax®

Synonyms HAT Antibody; Humanized Anti-CD25 mo Ab; Humanized Anti-interleukin-2 Receptor mo Ab; Humanized Anti-Tac mo Ab

Therapeutic Category Immunosuppressant Agent

Generic Available No

Use In combination with an immunosuppressive regimen, including cyclosporine and corticosteroids, for prophylaxis of acute organ rejection in patients receiving renal transplants; daclizumab has also been studied in pediatric bone marrow patients; steroid-refractory graft-versus-host disease

Pregnancy Risk Factor C

Contraindications Hypersensitivity to daclizumab or any component

Warnings Should only be used by physicians experienced in immunosuppressive therapy or management of transplant patients; adequate laboratory and supportive medical resources must be readily available in the facility for patient management; may result in an increased susceptibility to infection or an increased risk for developing lymphoproliferative disorders. Severe hypersensitivity reactions have been reported rarely; medications for the management of severe allergic reactions should be available for immediate use.

Adverse Reactions
Cardiovascular: Edema, hypertension (48% in pediatric patients), hypotension, tachycardia, thrombosis, chest pain

Central nervous system: Headache, dizziness, insomnia, depression, anxiety, fever, chills

Dermatologic: Impaired wound healing, acne, pruritus, rash, hirsutism

Endocrine & metabolic: Dehydration (frequency may be higher for pediatric patients than for adults), diabetes mellitus

Gastrointestinal: Constipation, nausea, diarrhea (36%), vomiting (32%), abdominal pain, abdominal distention

Genitourinary: Oliguria, dysuria

Hematologic: Bleeding

Neuromuscular & skeletal: Tremors, back pain, arthralgia, myalgia

Ocular: Blurred vision

Renal: Renal tubular necrosis, hematuria

Respiratory: Atelectasis, congestion, hypoxia, pharyngitis, pleural effusion

Miscellaneous: Diaphoresis; incidence of anti-daclizumab antibodies (children: 34%)

Stability Refrigerate; do not shake or freeze; protect from direct light; diluted daclizumab solution is stable for 24 hours if refrigerated or for 4 hours at room temperature; discard solution if colored or if particulate matter is present

Mechanism of Action A humanized IgG1 monoclonal antibody produced by recombinant DNA technology that binds specifically to the alpha subunit (p55 alpha, CD25, or Tac subunit) of the human high affinity interleukin-2 receptor (IL-2R) on the surface of activated lymphocytes inhibiting IL-2 binding; inhibits IL-2 mediated activation of lymphocytes which is involved in allograft rejection

Pharmacokinetics Daclizumab serum levels appeared to be somewhat lower in pediatric renal transplant patients than in adult transplant patients administered the same 1 mg/kg dosing regimen
Distribution: V_d: Adults: ~6 L
Half-life:
Children: 13 days
Adults: 20 days

Usual Dosage I.V. (refer to individual protocols): Children and Adults:
Initial dose: 1 mg/kg given no more than 24 hours before transplantation, followed by 1 mg/kg/dose administered every 14 days for a total of 5 doses; maximum dose: 100 mg

Steroid-refractory graft-versus-host disease: 0.5-1.5 mg/kg as a single dose administered for transient response (repeat doses have been given 11-48 days following the initial dose)

Dosing interval in renal impairment: No dosage adjustment necessary

Administration Parenteral: Daclizumab dose should be diluted in 50 mL NS solution. In fluid-restricted patients, a final concentration of 1 mg/mL can be administered over 15 minutes. When mixing the solution, gently invert the bag to avoid foaming; do not shake. Daclizumab solution should be administered within 4 hours of preparation if stored at room temperature; infuse over a 15-minute period via a peripheral or central vein. Do not mix or infuse other medications through the same I.V. line.

Monitoring Parameters CBC with differential, vital signs, immunologic monitoring of T cells, renal function tests, serum glucose

Reference Range Serum trough levels: 5-10 µg/mL

Patient Information Women of childbearing potential should avoid becoming pregnant while on daclizumab. Use an effective form of contraception before beginning therapy, during therapy, and for 4 months following daclizumab treatment.

Dosage Forms Injection, solution [preservative free]: 5 mg/mL (5 mL)

References
Vincenti F, Kirkman R, Light S, et al, "Interleukin-2-Receptor Blockade With Daclizumab to Prevent Acute Rejection in Renal Transplantation. Daclizumab Triple Therapy Study Group," *N Engl J Med*, 1998, 338(3):161-5.

Dactinomycin (dak ti noe MYE sin)

Related Information
Emetogenic Potential of Single Chemotherapeutic Agents *on page 1286*

U.S. Brand Names Cosmegen®

Synonyms ACT; Act-D; Actinomycin D

Therapeutic Category Antineoplastic Agent, Antibiotic

Generic Available No

Use Management (either alone or in combination with other treatment modalities) of Wilms' tumor, rhabdomyosarcoma, neuroblastoma, retinoblastoma, Ewing's sarcoma, trophoblastic neoplasms, testicular tumors and uterine sarcomas

Pregnancy Risk Factor C

Contraindications Hypersensitivity to dactinomycin or any component; patients with chickenpox or herpes zoster; avoid in infants <6 months of age since the incidence of adverse effects is increased in infants

Warnings The FDA currently recommends that procedures for proper handling and disposal of antineoplastic agents be considered. Dactinomycin is extremely irritating to tissues. If extravasation occurs during I.V. use, severe damage to soft tissue may occur leading to pain, swelling, ulceration, and necrosis.

Precautions Use with caution in patients with hepatobiliary dysfunction or in patients who have received radiation therapy; reduce dosage in patients receiving concurrent radiation therapy and in patients with hepatobiliary dysfunction; avoid administering live virus vaccinations after dactinomycin

Adverse Reactions
Central nervous system: Fatigue, fever
Dermatologic: Alopecia, erythema, hyperpigmentation of skin, desquamation, acne, maculopapular rash
Endocrine & metabolic: Hypocalcemia, hyperuricemia
Gastrointestinal: Anorexia, vomiting, diarrhea, stomatitis, proctitis, nausea
Hematologic: Myelosuppression (nadir: 2-3 weeks), leukopenia, thrombocytopenia, anemia
Hepatic: Hepatitis, hepatic veno-occlusive disease, elevated liver enzymes
Local: Soft tissue damage with extravasation
Miscellaneous: Anaphylactoid reaction, immunosuppression

Drug Interactions Dactinomycin potentiates the effects of radiation therapy; enflurane, halothane (increased hepatotoxicity); decreased effectiveness of vaccines given following dactinomycin

Stability Binds to cellulose filters, therefore, avoid in-line filtration; adsorbs to glass and plastic so dactinomycin should not be given by continuous or intermittent infusion; use of a diluent containing preservatives for reconstitution may result in a precipitate; any unused portion of the reconstituted 0.5 mg/mL solution should be discarded after 24 hours

Mechanism of Action Binds to the guanine portion of DNA intercalating between guanine and cytosine base pairs blocking replication and transcription of the DNA template; causes topoisomerase-mediated single-strand breaks in DNA

Pharmacokinetics
Distribution: Concentrates in nucleated cells and bone marrow; crosses the placenta; poor penetration into CSF (CSF:plasma ratio is <10%); distributes into submaxillary gland, liver, and kidney
Half-life: 3.5 hours (using radioimmunoassay)
Time to peak serum concentration: I.V.: Within 2-5 minutes
(Continued)

Dactinomycin *(Continued)*

Elimination: ~10% of dose excreted as unchanged drug in urine; 15% recovered in feces; 50% appears in bile

Usual Dosage Dosage should be based on body surface area in obese or edematous patients

Children >6 months and Adults: I.V. (refer to individual protocols): 15 mcg/kg/day or 400-600 mcg/m^2/day (maximum dose: 500 mcg/day) for 5 days, may repeat every 3-6 weeks; or 2.5 mg/m^2 given in divided doses over 1 week; or 0.75-2 mg/m^2 as a single dose given at intervals of 3-6 weeks has been used

Administration Parenteral: I.V.: For I.V. administration only; since drug is extremely irritating to tissues, **do not give I.M. or S.C.**; avoid extravasation; use a D$_5$W or NS flush before and after a dactinomycin dose to ensure venous patency; administer by slow IVP over a few minutes at a concentration not to exceed 500 mcg/mL into the side-port of a freely flowing I.V. infusion; if extravasation occurs, apply cold compresses to the site

Monitoring Parameters CBC with differential and platelet count, liver function tests and renal function tests

Patient Information Notify physician if fever, sore throat, bleeding, or bruising occurs

Dosage Forms Injection, powder for reconstitution, lyophilized: 0.5 mg [contains 20 mg mannitol]

References

Berg SL, Grisell DL, DeLaney TF, et al, "Principles of Treatment of Pediatric Solid Tumors," *Pediatr Clin North Am*, 1991, 38(2):249-67.

Berkowitz RS and Goldstein DP, "Gestational Trophoblastic Disease," *Cancer*, 1995, 76(10 Suppl):2079-85.

Carli M, Pastore G, Perilongo G, et al, "Tumor Response and Toxicity After Single High-Dose Versus Standard Five-Day Divided Dose Dactinomycin in Childhood Rhabdomyosarcoma," *J Clin Oncol*, 1988, 6(4):654-8.

◆ **Dalacin® C (Can)** *see* Clindamycin *on page 289*

◆ **Dalacin® T (Can)** *see* Clindamycin *on page 289*

◆ **Dalacin® Vaginal (Can)** *see* Clindamycin *on page 289*

◆ **Dalmane®** *see* Flurazepam *on page 509*

◆ **d-Alpha Tocopherol** *see* Vitamin E *on page 1152*

Danazol *(DA na zole)*

U.S. Brand Names Danocrine®

Canadian Brand Names Cyclomen®

Therapeutic Category Androgen

Generic Available Yes

Use Treatment of endometriosis amenable to hormonal management; fibrocystic breast disease; hereditary angioedema (see also Additional Information)

Pregnancy Risk Factor X

Contraindications Hypersensitivity to danazol or any component; pregnancy; undiagnosed abnormal genital bleeding; breast-feeding; porphyria; markedly impaired renal, hepatic, or cardiac function

Warnings Exposure to danazol in utero may result in androgenic effects on the female fetus; clitoral hypertrophy, labial fusion, urogenital sinus defect, vaginal atresia, and ambiguous genitalia have been reported; a sensitive test capable of determining early pregnancy is recommended immediately prior to initiation of therapy; nonhormonal method of contraception should be used during treatment if indicated. Thromboembolism, thrombotic, and thrombophlebitic events have been reported (including life-threatening or fatal stroke). Long-term use has been associated with peliosis hepatis and hepatic adenoma; these conditions may be complicated by acute, potentially life-threatening intra-abdominal hemorrhage; monitor liver function. Danazol has been associated with benign intracranial hypertension (pseudotumor cerebri); monitor for early signs and symptoms including papilledema, headache, nausea, vomiting, and visual disturbances. May increase risk of atherosclerosis and CAD due to decreased HDL and possible increase LDL. May cause nonreversible androgenic effects; patients should be watched closely for signs of androgenic effects.

Precautions Use with caution in patients with seizure disorders, migraine headaches, or conditions influenced by edema

Adverse Reactions

Cardiovascular: Edema, benign intracranial hypertension (rare), flushing, hypertension, diaphoresis, thromboembolism

Central nervous system: Nervousness, emotional lability, depression, dizziness, fainting, fever (rare), headache, sleep disorders, anxiety (rare), chills (rare), seizures (rare), stroke, Guillain-Barré syndrome

Dermatologic: Acne, seborrhea, mild hirsutism, hair loss, rashes (maculopapular, vestibular, papular, purpuric, and petechial), erythema multiforme, pruritus, urticaria, photosensitivity (rare)

Endocrine & metabolic: Weight gain, menstrual irregularities (spotting, altered timing of cycle), amenorrhea, clitoral hypertrophy (rare), breast size reduction, nipple discharge, semen abnormalities (changes in volume, viscosity, sperm count, and motility), libido changes, glucose intolerance, decreased HDL, increased LDL

Gastrointestinal: Nausea, vomiting, gastroenteritis, pancreatitis (rare), appetite changes (rare), bleeding gums (rare), constipation

Genitourinary: Vaginal dryness, vaginal irritation, pelvic pain

Hematologic: Eosinophilia, erythrocytosis (reversible), leukocytosis, leukopenia, thrombocytosis, polycythemia, thrombocytopenia

Hepatic: Peliosis hepatis, hepatic adenoma, cholestatic jaundice, elevated liver enzymes

Neuromuscular & skeletal: Back pain, carpal tunnel syndrome (rare), extremity pain, joint pain, joint swelling, muscle cramps, neck pain, paresthesias, spasms, weakness, tremor

Ocular: Cataracts (rare), visual disturbances

Renal: Hematuria

Respiratory: Nasal congestion (rare)

Miscellaneous: Voice alterations (hoarseness, sore throat, instability, deepening of pitch)

Drug Interactions Cytochrome P450 isoenzyme CYP3A3/4 enzyme inhibitor

Increases effects of warfarin; increases serum concentrations of carbamazepine, cyclosporine, and tacrolimus; may increase risk of myopathy or rhabdomyolysis with HMG-CoA reductase inhibitors

Food Interactions Food delays time to peak serum level; high-fat meal increases plasma concentration

Stability Store at room temperature.

Mechanism of Action Danazol, a synthetic steroid analog, has strong antigonadotropic properties. It inhibits the mid-cycle surge of LH and FSH from the pituitary resulting in suppression of ovarian steroidogenesis. Danazol does not have any progestational or estrogenic properties but does exhibit weak anabolic and androgenic effects. Through its inactivation of the pituitary-ovarian axis, regression and atrophy of normal and ectopic endometrial tissue occurs. Danazol decreases the rate of growth of abnormal breast tissue and reduces attacks associated with hereditary angioedema by increasing levels of C4 component of complement.

Pharmacodynamics

Endometriosis:

Onset of action: 3 weeks

Fibrocystic breast disease:

Onset of action: 1 month

Maximum effect: 4-6 months

Duration: Symptoms recur in 50% of patients within one year after discontinuation of treatment

Pharmacokinetics

Absorption: Well absorbed

Metabolism: Extensive hepatic metabolism to inactive metabolites

Half-life: Adults: 4.5 hours

Time to peak serum concentration: 2 hours

Usual Dosage Adolescents and Adults: Oral: **Note:** Begin treatment during menstruation or obtain appropriate tests to ensure patient is not pregnant:

Endometriosis:

Mild case: 100-200 mg twice daily for 3-6 months; may be continued up to 9 months if necessary

Moderate to severe case: 400 mg twice daily for 3-6 months; may be continued up to 9 months if necessary

Note: A gradual downward titration to a dose sufficient to maintain amenorrhea may be considered depending upon the patient's response

Fibrocystic breast disease: 50-200 mg twice daily

Hereditary angioedema: Initial: 200 mg 2-3 times/day depending upon the patient's response; after a favorable response is obtained, decrease the dosage by 50% or less at intervals of 1-3 months or longer. If an attack occurs, the daily dosage may be increased by up to 200 mg.

Administration Oral: Avoid administration with fatty meals.

Monitoring Parameters Liver function tests, symptomatology and site of disease; serum glucose (if diabetic); HDL and LDL cholesterol; signs and symptoms of pseudotumor cerebri; androgenic effects

(Continued)

Danazol *(Continued)*

Test Interactions Danazol may interfere with laboratory determinations for testosterone, androstenedione, and dehydroepiandrosterone.

Patient Information Do not discontinue without consulting prescriber; therapy may take up to several months for full benefit depending upon the purpose of treatment. Report any prodromal symptoms of hepatitis (fatigue, weakness, nausea, vomiting, dark urine, or yellowing of eyes); avoid becoming pregnant while taking this medicine and for several months after stopping; use an effective form of birth control. This medication may alter hypoglycemic requirements; diabetics should monitor serum glucose closely. May cause photosensitivity reactions (eg, exposure to sunlight may cause severe sunburn, skin rash, redness, or itching); avoid direct exposure to sunlight.

Additional Information Danazol has seen limited use for treatment of ITP in children refractory to steroids. Ten children, 2.5-17 years of age were treated with 20-30 mg/kg/day in divided doses (maximum: 800 mg/day). Treatment was tapered off after patients responded to therapy (Weinblatt, 1988). Danazol has also been evaluated in hemophilia A in a randomized, double-blind placebo-controlled crossover trial in 19 children. Children <15 years received 150 mg/day and >15 years received 300 mg/day for 3 months. Factor VIII:C levels were increased (Mehta, 1992).

Dosage Forms Capsule: 50 mg, 100 mg, 200 mg

References

Mehta J, Singhal S, Kamath MV, et al, "A Randomized Placebo-Controlled Double-Blind Study of Danazol in Hemophilia A," *Acta Haematol*, 1992, 88(1):14-6.

Weinblatt ME, Kochen J, and Ortega J, "Danazol for Children With Immune Thrombocytopenic Purpura," *Am J Dis Child*, 1988, 142(12):1317-9.

♦ **Danocrine®** *see Danazol on page 336*

♦ **Dantrium®** *see Dantrolene on page 338*

Dantrolene *(DAN troe leen)*

U.S. Brand Names Dantrium®

Therapeutic Category Antidote, Malignant Hyperthermia; Hyperthermia, Treatment; Skeletal Muscle Relaxant, Nonparalytic

Generic Available No

Use Treatment of spasticity associated with upper motor neuron disorders such as spinal cord injury, stroke, cerebral palsy, or multiple sclerosis; also used as treatment of malignant hyperthermia

Pregnancy Risk Factor C

Contraindications Hypersensitivity to dantrolene or any component; active hepatic disease; should not be administered where spasticity is used to maintain posture or balance

Warnings May cause hepatotoxicity; overt hepatitis has been most frequently observed between the third and twelfth month of therapy and with doses ≥800 mg/day; hepatic injury appears to be greater in females and in patients >35 years of age

Precautions Use with caution in patients with impaired cardiac or pulmonary function or history of previous liver disease

Adverse Reactions

Cardiovascular/respiratory: Pleural effusion with pericarditis, tachycardia

Central nervous system: Seizures, drowsiness, dizziness, lightheadedness, confusion, headache, fatigue, speech disturbances, mental depression, chills, fever

Dermatologic: Rash, acne-like rash, pruritus, urticaria, abnormal hair growth

Gastrointestinal: Diarrhea, nausea, vomiting, severe constipation, GI bleeding, abdominal cramps, dysphagia

Genitourinary: Urinary retention or frequency, urinary incontinence

Hepatic: Hepatitis

Local: Phlebitis

Neuromuscular & skeletal: Muscle weakness, myalgia, backache

Ocular: Visual disturbances, excessive tearing

Renal: Hematuria

Drug Interactions Use with verapamil may result in hyperkalemia and myocardial depression; estrogen increases incidence of hepatotoxicity when used concomitantly; additive CNS depressive effects with other CNS depressants; increased toxicity with MAO inhibitors, phenothiazines, clindamycin, warfarin, clofibrate, and tolbutamide

Stability Protect from light; use reconstituted injection within 6 hours; incompatible with dextrose, NS, or bacteriostatic water for injection; precipitates when placed in glass containers for infusion

Mechanism of Action Acts directly on skeletal muscle by interfering with release of calcium ion from the sarcoplasmic reticulum; prevents or reduces the increase in myoplasmic calcium ion concentration that activates the acute catabolic processes associated with malignant hyperthermia

Pharmacokinetics
Absorption: Oral: 35%
Metabolism: Extensive
Half-life:
Children: 7.3 hours
Adults: 8.7 hours
Elimination: 25% excreted in urine as metabolites and unchanged drug; 45% to 50% excreted in feces via bile

Usual Dosage
Spasticity: Oral:
Children: Initial: 0.5 mg/kg/dose twice daily, increase frequency to 3-4 times/day at 4- to 7-day intervals, then increase dose by 0.5 mg/kg to a maximum of 3 mg/kg/dose 2-4 times/day up to 400 mg/day
Adults: 25 mg/day to start, increase frequency to 2-4 times/day, then increase dose by 25 mg every 4-7 days to a maximum of 100 mg 2-4 times/day or 400 mg/day
Hyperthermia: Children and Adults:
Preoperative prophylaxis:
Oral: 4-8 mg/kg/day in 4 divided doses given 1-2 days prior to surgery for those patients at risk; to prevent recurrence, administer last dosage 3-4 hours before scheduled surgery
I.V.: 2.5 mg/kg 1¼ hours before surgery and infused over 1 hour; additional doses may be needed during surgery especially for prolonged surgery
Crisis: I.V.: 1 mg/kg; may repeat as needed to a maximum cumulative dose of 10 mg/kg; if physiologic and metabolic abnormalities reappear, repeat regimen
Postcrisis follow-up: Oral: 4-8 mg/kg/day in 4 divided doses for 1-3 days; I.V. dantrolene may be used when oral therapy is not practical; individualize dosage beginning with 1 mg/kg or more as the clinical situation dictates

Administration
Oral: Contents of capsule may be mixed with juice or liquid
Parenteral: Reconstitute by adding 60 mL SWI (**not bacteriostatic water for injection**), resultant concentration 0.333 mg/mL; administer by rapid I.V. injection; for infusion, do **not** further dilute with NS or dextrose; place solution in plastic container for continuous infusion

Monitoring Parameters Baseline and periodic liver function tests; temperature (hyperthermia use)

Patient Information Avoid alcohol; may cause drowsiness and impair ability to perform activities requiring mental alertness or physical coordination

Nursing Implications Avoid extravasation since dantrolene is a tissue irritant

Dosage Forms
Capsule, as sodium: 25 mg, 50 mg, 100 mg
Injection, powder for reconstitution, lyophilized, as sodium: 20 mg [contains 3 g mannitol]

Extemporaneous Preparations A 5 mg/mL suspension may be made by adding five 100 mg capsules to a citric acid solution (150 mg citric acid powder in 10 mL water) and then adding syrup to a total volume of 100 mL; shake well; stable 2 days in refrigerator
Nahata MC and Hipple TF, *Pediatric Drug Formulations*, 4th ed, Cincinnati, OH: Harvey Whitney Books Co, 2000.

Dapsone (DAP sone)

Synonyms Diaminodiphenylsulfone
Therapeutic Category Antibiotic, Sulfone; Leprostatic Agent
Generic Available Yes
Use Treatment of leprosy due to susceptible strains of *M. leprae*; treatment of dermatitis herpetiformis; prophylaxis against *Pneumocystis carinii* pneumonia (PCP) in patients who cannot tolerate sulfamethoxazole and trimethoprim or aerosolized pentamidine; prophylaxis against toxoplasmic encephalitis in patients who cannot tolerate sulfamethoxazole and trimethoprim

Pregnancy Risk Factor C

Contraindications Hypersensitivity to dapsone or any component; patients with severe anemia

Precautions Use with caution in patients with G-6-PD deficiency, methemoglobin reductase deficiency or hemoglobin M; in patients receiving drugs capable of inducing hemolysis; hypersensitivity to other sulfonamides

Adverse Reactions
Cardiovascular: Tachycardia
(Continued)

Dapsone *(Continued)*

Central nervous system: Psychotic episodes, hallucinations, insomnia, vertigo, irritability, headache, fever, uncoordinated speech

Dermatologic: Exfoliative dermatitis, erythema multiforme, toxic epidermal necrolysis, urticaria, morbilliform reactions, erythema nodosum, photosensitivity

Endocrine & metabolic: Hyperkalemia, hypoalbuminemia

Gastrointestinal: Nausea, vomiting, abdominal pain, anorexia

Hematologic: Hemolytic anemia, methemoglobinemia, leukopenia, agranulocytosis, aplastic anemia, neutropenia

Hepatic: Hepatitis, cholestatic jaundice; elevated alkaline phosphatase, AST, bilirubin, and LDH

Neuromuscular & skeletal: Muscle weakness, peripheral neuropathy

Ocular: Blurred vision

Otic: Tinnitus

Renal: Acute tubular necrosis, nephrotic syndrome, albuminuria

Miscellaneous: Lupus erythematosus, mononucleosis-like syndrome

Drug Interactions Cytochrome P450 isoenzyme CYP2C9, CYP2E1, and CYP3A3/4 substrate

Didanosine (decreases dapsone absorption); rifampin (decreases dapsone concentrations); trimethoprim (increases dapsone concentration); pyrimethamine, nitrofurantoin, primaquine (increase risk of hematologic side effects)

Food Interactions Do not administer with antacids, alkaline foods, or alkaline drugs (may decrease dapsone absorption)

Stability Protect from light

Mechanism of Action Dapsone is a sulfone antimicrobial. The mechanism of action of the sulfones is similar to that of the sulfonamides. Sulfonamides are competitive antagonists of para-aminobenzoic acid (PABA) and inhibit folic acid synthesis in susceptible organisms.

Pharmacokinetics

Absorption: Oral: 86% to 100%

Distribution: Distributes into skin, muscle, kidneys, liver, sweat, sputum, tears, and bile; distributes into breast milk

Protein binding: 50% to 90%

Metabolism: Acetylated and hydroxylated in the liver

Half-life:

Children: 15.1 hours

Adults: 13-83 hours (mean: 20-30 hours)

Time to peak serum concentration: Within 2-8 hours

Elimination: 5% to 20% of dose excreted in urine as unchanged drug; 70% to 85% excreted in urine as metabolites; small amount excreted in feces

Usual Dosage Oral:

Children ≥1 month of age:

Prophylaxis for first episode of opportunistic disease due to *Toxoplasma gondii*: 2 mg/kg or 15 mg/m^2 (maximum dose: 25 mg) once daily in combination with pyrimethamine 1 mg/kg once daily and leucovorin 5 mg every 3 days

Primary and secondary PCP prophylaxis (see **Note** in Additional Information): 2 mg/kg/day once daily (maximum dose: 100 mg/day), or 4 mg/kg/dose once weekly (maximum dose: 200 mg)

Children:

Leprosy: 1-2 mg/kg/day given once daily in combination therapy; maximum dose: 100 mg/day

Adults:

Leprosy: 50-100 mg once daily; combination therapy with one or more antileprosy drugs is recommended to avoid dapsone resistance

Dermatitis herpetiformis: Initial: 50 mg once daily; maintenance dosage range: 25-400 mg/day

PCP treatment: 100 mg once daily in combination with trimethoprim

Primary and secondary PCP prophylaxis: 50 mg twice daily; or dapsone 50 mg once daily plus pyrimethamine 50 mg orally every week plus leucovorin 25 mg orally every week; or dapsone 200 mg orally plus pyrimethamine 75 mg orally plus leucovorin 25 mg orally every week

Toxoplasma gondii prophylaxis: 50 mg once daily plus pyrimethamine 50 mg orally every week, plus leucovorin 25 mg orally every week

Administration Oral: Administer with water

Monitoring Parameters CBC with differential, platelet count, hemoglobin, hematocrit, liver function tests, and urinalysis

Patient Information Notify physician if fever, sore throat, pallor, fatigue, rash, purpura, or jaundice occurs. May cause photosensitivity reactions (eg, exposure to sunlight may cause severe sunburn, skin rash, redness, or itching); avoid exposure to sunlight and artificial light sources (sunlamps, tanning booth/bed); wear protective clothing, wide-brimmed hats, sunglasses, and lip sunscreen (SPF ≥15); use a sunscreen [broad-spectrum sunscreen or physical sunscreen (preferred) or sunblock with SPF ≥15]; contact physician if reaction occurs.

Additional Information Note: Guidelines for prophylaxis of *Pneumocystis carinii* pneumonia: Initiate PCP prophylaxis in the following patients: In all HIV-exposed children at 4-6 weeks of age and continue through the first year of life or until HIV infection has been reasonably excluded; children 1-5 years of age with CD4+ count <500 or CD4+ percentage <15%; children 6-12 years of age with CD4+ count <200 or CD4+ percentage <15%; adolescents and adults with CD4+ count <200 or oropharyngeal candidiasis. Folinic acid (leucovorin) should be given if bone marrow suppression occurs.

Dosage Forms Tablet, scored: 25 mg, 100 mg

Extemporaneous Preparations A 2 mg/mL oral suspension can be made using a 1:1 mixture of Ora-Sweet® and Ora-Plus®; crush eight 25 mg tablets into a fine powder in a mortar; add a small amount of vehicle and mix to make a uniform paste; mix while adding the vehicle in geometric portions to almost 100 mL; transfer to a calibrated bottle and qsad with vehicle to 100 mL; preparation is stable for 90 days when stored at room temperature or under refrigeration; label "shake well"

Jacobus Pharmaceutical Company (609) 921-7447 makes a 2 mg/mL proprietary liquid formulation available under an IND for the prophylaxis of *Pneumocystis carinii* pneumonia

Nahata MC, Morosco RS, and Trowbridge JM, "Stability of Dapsone in Two Oral Liquid Dosage Forms," *Ann Pharmacother*, 2000, 34(7-8):848-50.

References

Barnett ED, Pelton SI, Mirochnick M, et al, "Dapsone for Prevention of *Pneumocystis* Pneumonia in Children With Acquired Immunodeficiency Syndrome," *Pediatr Infect Dis J*, 1994, 13(1):72-4.

Kaplan JE, Masur H, and Holmes KK, "Guidelines for Preventing Opportunistic Infections Among HIV-Infected Persons - 2002 Recommendations of the USPHS and IDSA," *MMWR*, 2002, 51(RR-8):1-46.

Mirochnick M, Michaels M, Clarke D, et al, "Pharmacokinetics of Dapsone in Children," *J Pediatr*, 1993, 122(5 Pt 1):806-9.

Stavola JJ and Noel GJ, "Efficacy and Safety of Dapsone Prophylaxis Against *Pneumocystis carinii* Pneumonia in Human Immunodeficiency Virus-Infected Children," *Pediatr Infect Dis J*, 1993, 12(8):644-7.

♦ **Daraprim**® *see* Pyrimethamine *on page 965*

Darbepoetin Alfa (dar be POE e tin AL fa)

U.S. Brand Names Aranesp™

Synonyms NESP; Novel Erythropoiesis Stimulating Protein

Therapeutic Category Colony-Stimulating Factor; Erythropoiesis Stimulating Protein

Generic Available No

Use Treatment of anemia associated with chronic renal failure or chemotherapy (non-myeloid malignancies)

Pregnancy Risk Factor C

Contraindications Hypersensitivity to darbepoetin alfa or any component; uncontrolled hypertension

Factors Limiting Response to Darbepoetin Alfa

Factor	Mechanism
Iron deficiency	Limits hemoglobin synthesis
Blood loss/hemolysis	Counteracts darbepoetin alfa-stimulated erythropoiesis
Infection/inflammation	Inhibits iron transfer from storage to bone marrow
	Suppresses erythropoiesis through activated macrophages
Aluminum overload	Inhibits iron incorporation into heme protein
Bone marrow replacement Hyperparathyroidism Metastatic, neoplastic disease	Limits bone marrow volume
Folic acid/vitamin B_{12} deficiency	Limits hemoglobin synthesis
Patient compliance	Self administered darbepoetin alfa or iron therapy

Warnings Due to an association of cardiovascular events, including death, in patients with CRF with higher hemoglobin and/or higher rates of rise of hemoglobin, the hemoglobin should not exceed 12 g/dL and the rate of rise of hemoglobin should not (Continued)

Darbepoetin Alfa *(Continued)*

exceed 1 g/dL in any 2-week period. Blood pressure should be controlled adequately before initiation of darbepoetin alfa therapy; since blood pressure may rise during therapy, close blood pressure monitoring is recommended. Seizures have occurred during therapy; monitor closely for premonitory neurologic symptoms during the first several months of therapy.

Precautions See table on previous page.

Use with caution in patients with porphyria or a history of seizures. Darbepoetin alfa is not intended for patients who require acute corrections of anemia and is not a substitute for emergency blood transfusion. Allow sufficient time (an interval of 4-6 weeks) to determine the patient's response to a particular dosage (see Warnings regarding rapid responsiveness); patients with CRF not yet requiring dialysis may require lower maintenance doses.

Assessment of iron stores and therapeutic iron supplementation is essential to optimal darbepoetin alfa therapy. Iron supplementation is necessary to provide for increased requirements during expansion of the red cell mass secondary to marrow stimulation, unless iron stores are already in excess. Optimal iron stores are demonstrated by a transferrin saturation of 20% or more and a serum ferritin of 100-150 mcg/L.

Adverse Reactions

Cardiovascular: Hypertension, hypotension, edema, tachycardia, chest pain, cardiac arrhythmia, cardiac arrest, CHF, MI, TIA/CVA, venous thrombosis

Central nervous system: Fatigue, dizziness, headache, seizure, fever

Dermatologic: Pruritus, rash

Gastrointestinal: Nausea, diarrhea, vomiting, abdominal pain, constipation

Hematologic: Neutropenia

Local: Pain, irritation at injection site (S.C. injection)

Neuromuscular & skeletal: Myalgia, arthralgia, back pain, limb pain

Respiratory: Cough, dyspnea, bronchitis, upper respiratory infection, pulmonary embolism

Miscellaneous: Hypersensitivity reactions, flu-like symptoms, sepsis

Stability Refrigerate; stable 7 days at room temperature; protect from light; contains no preservatives; discard after entry; may dilute with NS or bacteriostatic NS in a 1:10 ratio at the time of administration; dilution stable for 24 hours refrigerated; do not dilute with other solutions or medications

Mechanism of Action Darbepoetin alfa, manufactured by recombinant DNA technology, has the same effects as endogenous erythropoietin (EPO). It differs slightly from recombinant human erythropoietin in containing 5 N-linked oligosaccharide chains instead of 3. EPO induces erythropoiesis by stimulating the division and differentiation of committed erythroid progenitor cells. It induces the release of reticulocytes from the bone marrow into the bloodstream, where they mature to erythrocytes (dose response relationship) resulting in an increase in reticulocyte counts followed by a rise in hematocrit and hemoglobin levels. There is normally an inverse correlation between the plasma EPO level and the hemoglobin concentration (only when the hemoglobin concentration is <10.5 g/dL).

Pharmacodynamics

Onset of action: Several days

Maximum effect: 4-6 weeks

Pharmacokinetics

Absorption: S.C.: Slow and rate-limiting

Distribution: V_d:

Children: 51.6 mL/kg (range: 21-73 mL/kg)

Adults: 52.4 ± 6.6 mL/kg

Bioavailability: S.C.: CRF patients: ~37% (range: 30% to 50%)

Half-life:

Children:

I.V.: Terminal: 22.1 hours (range: 12-30 hours)

S.C.: Terminal: 42.8 hours (range: 16-86 hours)

Adults:

I.V.: Terminal: 25.3 ± 7.3 hours

S.C.: Terminal: 49 ± 12.7 hours

Time to peak serum concentration: S.C.: 34 hours (range: 24-72 hours)

Elimination:

Clearance: I.V.:

Children: 2.29 mL/hour/kg (range: 1.6-3.5 mL/hour/kg)

Adults: 1.6 ± 1.0 mL/hour/kg

Usual Dosage Dosing schedules need to be individualized by treatment indication and patient response. Careful monitoring of patients receiving the drug is recommended. See "Darbepoetin Alfa Dosage Adjustments" table. Darbepoetin alfa may be ineffective if other factors such as iron or B_{12}/folate deficiency limit marrow response.

Anemia in chronic renal failure: Adults: I.V., S.C.: 0.45 mcg/kg/dose once weekly

Note: Allow at least 4 weeks to determine full effects of the new regimen. For many patients, the appropriate maintenance dose may be less than the initial dose. Patients not receiving hemodialysis may be particularly sensitive and require lower doses. S.C. dosing every two weeks has been effective in some patients.

Anemia associated with chemotherapy in patients with non-myeloid malignancies: Adults: S.C.: 2.25 mcg/kg/dose once weekly

Note: Adjust dosage depending upon response; if indicated dosage may be increased to a maximum of 4.5 mcg/kg/dose; allow at least 6 weeks of therapy before increasing the dosage

Darbepoetin Alfa Dosage Adjustments

Target hemoglobin range	9-12 g/dL; not to exceed 12 g/dL
Increase dose (not more frequently than once monthly)	By 25% when hemoglobin does not increase by 1 g/dL after 4 weeks of therapy **and** hemoglobin is below target range
Reduce dose	By 25% when hemoglobin increases >1 g/dL in any 2-week period or when hemoglobin >12 g/dL
Stop therapy	When hemoglobin continues to increase after dosage reduction; reinstate therapy at a 25% lower dose after the hemoglobin begins to decrease

Conversion From Epoetin Alfa to Darbepoetin Alfa (I.V. or S.C.)*
(maintain the same route of administration for the conversion)

Previous Weekly Epoetin Alfa Dose (units/week)	Weekly Darbepoetin Alfa Dosage (mcg/week†)
<2500	6.25
2500-4999	12.5
5000-10,999	25
11,000-17,999	40
18,000-33,999	60
34,000-89,999	100
≥90,000	200

*1 mcg darbepoetin alfa is equivalent to 200 units epoetin alfa.

†Due to the longer serum half-life of darbepoetin alfa, when converting from epoetin alfa, administer darbepoetin alfa once weekly if the patient was receiving epoetin alfa 2-3 times weekly and administer darbepoetin alfa once every two weeks if the patient was receiving epoetin alfa once weekly.

Administration Parenteral: Do not shake as this may denature the glycoprotein rendering the drug biologically inactive. I.V.: Infuse over 1-3 minutes

Test	Initial Phase Frequency	Maintenance Phase Frequency
Hemoglobin	Weekly	2-4 times/month
Blood pressure	3 times/week	3 times/week
Serum ferritin	Monthly	Quarterly
Transferrin saturation	Monthly	Quarterly
Serum chemistries*	Regularly per routine	Regularly per routine
Reticulocyte count	Baseline prior to starting therapy	After 10 days of therapy

*Including CBC with differential, creatinine, BUN, potassium, phosphorus

(Continued)

Darbepoetin Alfa *(Continued)*

Monitoring Parameters

Careful monitoring of blood pressure is indicated; problems with hypertension have been noted especially in renal failure patients treated with darbepoetin alfa. See table on previous page.

Hemoglobin should be determined weekly until stabilization within the target range (9-12 g/dL), and weekly for at least 2-6 weeks after a dose increase.

Patient Information Frequent blood tests are needed to determine the correct dose; notify physician if any severe headache develops; due to increased risk of seizure activity in CRF patients during the first 90 days of therapy, avoid potentially hazardous activities (eg, driving) during this period

Additional Information Optimal response is achieved when iron stores are maintained with supplemental iron if necessary; evaluate iron stores prior to and during therapy; injection with polysorbate solution is not available in U.S.

Dosage Forms Injection, solution, with human albumin [preservative free]: 25 mcg/mL (1 mL); 40 mcg/mL (1 mL); 60 mcg/mL (1 mL); 100 mcg/mL (1 mL); 200 mcg/mL (1 mL)

References

Joy MS, "Darbepoetin Alfa: A Novel Erythropoiesis-Stimulating Protein," *Ann Pharmacother*, 2002, 36(7):1183-92.

Lerner G, Kale AS, Warady BA, et al, "Pharmacokinetics of Darbepoetin Alfa in Pediatric Patients With Chronic Kidney Disease," *Pediatr Nephrol*, 2002, 17(11):933-7.

- ◆ **Darvocet-N® 50** *see* Propoxyphene and Acetaminophen *on page 951*
- ◆ **Darvocet-N® 100** *see* Propoxyphene and Acetaminophen *on page 951*
- ◆ **Darvon®** *see* Propoxyphene *on page 950*
- ◆ **Darvon-N®** *see* Propoxyphene *on page 950*
- ◆ **Daunomycin** *see* DAUNOrubicin *on page 344*

DAUNOrubicin *(daw noe ROO bi sin)*

Related Information

Extravasation Treatment *on page 1240*

U.S. Brand Names Cerubidine®

Synonyms Daunomycin; DNR; Rubidomycin

Therapeutic Category Antineoplastic Agent, Anthracycline; Antineoplastic Agent, Antibiotic

Generic Available Yes

Use In combination with other agents in the treatment of leukemias (ALL, AML)

Pregnancy Risk Factor D

Contraindications Hypersensitivity to daunorubicin or any component; CHF, left ventricular ejection fraction <30% to 40%, or arrhythmias; pre-existing bone marrow suppression

Warnings The FDA currently recommends that procedures for proper handling and disposal of antineoplastic agents be considered; I.V. use only; severe local tissue necrosis will result if extravasation occurs; irreversible myocardial toxicity may occur as total dosage approaches 550 mg/m² in adults, 400 mg/m² in patients receiving chest radiation, 300 mg/m² in children ≥2 years of age, or 10 mg/kg in children <2 years; this may occur during therapy or several months after therapy; total cumulative dose should take into account previous or concomitant treatment with cardiotoxic agents or irradiation of chest; infants and children may be more susceptible to anthracycline-induced cardiotoxicity than adults; severe myelosuppression is possible when used in therapeutic doses

Precautions Reduce dosage in patients with hepatic, biliary, or renal impairment

Adverse Reactions

Cardiovascular: Cardiotoxicity, CHF (dose-related, may occur 7-8 years after treatment), arrhythmias, EKG abnormalities

Central nervous system: Fever, chills

Dermatologic: Alopecia, hyperpigmentation of skin and nail beds, urticaria, pruritus

Endocrine & metabolic: Hyperuricemia, infertility, sterility

Gastrointestinal: Stomatitis, esophagitis, nausea, vomiting, diarrhea

Genitourinary: Discoloration of urine (red-orange)

Hematologic: Myelosuppression (thrombocytopenia, leukopenia)

Hepatic: Elevated serum bilirubin, AST, and alkaline phosphatase

Local: Severe tissue necrosis with extravasation

Stability Protect from light; reconstituted solution is stable for 48 hours when refrigerated and 24 hours at room temperature; a color change from red to blue/purple indicates decomposition of the drug; unstable in solutions with a pH >8; incompatible with heparin, sodium bicarbonate, 5-FU, and dexamethasone

Mechanism of Action Inhibition of DNA and RNA synthesis by intercalating between DNA base pairs, uncoiling of the helix, and by steric obstruction; not cell cycle-specific for the S-phase of cell division; may cause free radical damage to DNA

Pharmacokinetics

Distribution: Widely distributed in tissues such as spleen, heart, kidneys, liver, and lungs; does not cross the blood-brain barrier; crosses the placenta

Metabolism: To daunorubicinol (active)

Half-life, terminal: 14-18.5 hours

Daunorubicinol, active metabolite: 26.7 hours

Elimination: 40% of dose excreted in bile; ~14% to 23% excreted in urine as metabolite and unchanged drug

Usual Dosage I.V. (refer to individual protocols):

Children <2 years or <0.5 m^2: Dosage should be calculated on the basis of body weight rather than body surface area: 1 mg/kg or per protocol with frequency dependent on regimen employed

Children:

ALL combination therapy: Remission induction: 25-45 mg/m^2 on days 1 and 8 of cycle, or 30-45 mg/m^2/day for 3 days every 3-4 weeks, or 25 mg/m^2 every week for 4 weeks

AML combination therapy: Induction: I.V. continuous infusion: 30-60 mg/m^2/day on days 1-3 of cycle, or 20 mg/m^2/day for 4 days every 14 days

Adults: 30-60 mg/m^2/day for 3-5 days, repeat dose in 3-4 weeks; total cumulative dose should not exceed 400-600 mg/m^2

AML: Single agent induction: 60 mg/m^2/day for 3 days; repeat every 3-4 weeks

AML: Combination therapy induction: 45 mg/m^2/day for 3 days of the first course of induction therapy; subsequent courses: Every day for 2 days

ALL: Combination therapy: Remission induction: 45 mg/m^2 on days 1, 2, and 3 of induction course

Dosing adjustment in hepatic or renal impairment: Reduce dose by 25% in patients with serum bilirubin of 1.2-3 mg/dL; reduce dose by 50% in patients with serum bilirubin and/or creatinine >3 mg/dL

Administration Parenteral: Drug is very irritating, do not inject I.M. or S.C.; administer IVP diluting the reconstituted dose in 10-15 mL NS and administering over 2-3 minutes into the tubing of a rapidly infusing I.V. solution of D$_5$W or NS; daunorubicin has also been diluted in 100 mL of D$_5$W or NS and infused over 30-45 minutes or as a continuous 24-hour infusion

Monitoring Parameters CBC with differential and platelet count, serum bilirubin, serum uric acid, liver function test, EKG, ventricular ejection fraction, renal function test; patency of I.V. line

Patient Information Transient red-orange discoloration of urine can occur for up to 48 hours after a dose; notify physician if fever, sore throat, bleeding, bruising, chills, signs of infection, abdominal pain, blood in stools, excessive fatigue, yellowing of eyes or skin, or difficulty breathing occurs

Nursing Implications Leukemic patients should receive prophylactic allopurinol to prevent acute urate nephropathy; avoid extravasation; if extravasation occurs, apply a cold compress immediately for 30-60 minutes, then alternate off/on every 15 minutes for 1 day; apply 1.5 mL of dimethylsulfoxide 99% (w/v) solution to the site every 6 hours for 14 days; allow to air-dry; do not cover

Additional Information Myelosuppressive effects:

WBC: Severe

Platelets: Severe

Onset (days): 7

Nadir (days): 10-14

Recovery (days): 21-28

Dosage Forms

Injection, solution, as hydrochloride: 5 mg/mL (4 mL, 10 mL) [contains mannitol]

Injection, powder for reconstitution, lyophilized, as hydrochloride: 20 mg [contains 100 mg mannitol]

References

Crom WR, Glynn-Barnhart AM, Rodman JH, et al, "Pharmacokinetics of Anticancer Drugs in Children," *Clin Pharmacokinet*, 1987, 12(3):168-213.

- **d-Biotin [OTC]** *see* Biotin *on page 173*
- **DDAVP®** *see* Desmopressin *on page 352*
- **ddC** *see* Zalcitabine *on page 1161*
- **DDI** *see* Didanosine *on page 377*
- **1-Deamino-8-D-Arginine Vasopressin** *see* Desmopressin *on page 352*
- **Debrox® [OTC]** *see* Carbamide Peroxide *on page 212*
- **Decadron®** *see* Dexamethasone *on page 354*

- ♦ **Decadron® Phosphate** *see Dexamethasone on page 354*
- ♦ **Declomycin®** *see Demeclocycline on page 348*
- ♦ **Decofed® [OTC]** *see Pseudoephedrine on page 958*

Deferoxamine (de fer OKS a meen)

U.S. Brand Names Desferal®
Canadian Brand Names PMS-Deferoxamine
Therapeutic Category Antidote, Aluminum Toxicity; Antidote, Iron Toxicity; Chelating Agent, Parenteral
Generic Available No

Use Acute iron intoxication; chronic iron overload secondary to multiple transfusions; diagnostic test for iron overload; used investigationally in the treatment of aluminum accumulation in renal failure

Pregnancy Risk Factor C

Contraindications Hypersensitivity to deferoxamine or any component; patients with severe renal disease, anuria, or primary hemochromatosis

Warnings Cataracts, decreased visual acuity, impaired peripheral and color vision, impaired night vision, and retinal pigmentary abnormalities have been reported after usage for prolonged periods at high dosages or in patients with low ferritin levels; periodic eye exams are recommended while on chronic therapy; neurotoxicity-related auditory abnormalities have been reported including high frequency sensorineural hearing loss; periodic auditory exams are recommended. ARDS has been reported following treatment of acute iron intoxication or thalassemia with high doses of deferoxamine; flushing of the skin, urticaria, hypotension, and shock have been reported after rapid I.V. administration. High doses (>60 mg/kg), especially in patients ≤3 years of age, with resulting low ferritin levels have been associated with growth retardation; a reduction in deferoxamine dosage may partially improve growth velocity; monitor growth in children receiving chronic therapy closely. In patients with aluminum-related encephalopathy, deferoxamine may exacerbate neurologic dysfunction (seizures) possibly due to an acute increase in circulating aluminum and also may decrease serum calcium aggravating hyperparathyroidism. Deferoxamine may precipitate the onset of dialysis dementia.

Patients with severe chronic iron overload treated with deferoxamine and high dose vitamin C have been reported to develop impaired cardiac function which is reversed after discontinuation of vitamin C; vitamin C increases the availability of iron for chelation with deferoxamine. To decrease the risk of impaired cardiac function, the manufacturer recommends: Avoiding vitamin C in patients with pre-existing cardiac failure; start vitamin C supplementation only after the first month of deferoxamine therapy; use vitamin C only if the patient is regularly receiving deferoxamine; do not exceed vitamin C doses of 50 mg/day in children <10 years, 100 mg/day in older children, and 200 mg/day in adults; monitor cardiac function.

Precautions Use with caution in patients with pyelonephritis; may increase susceptibility to *Yersinia enterocolitica* infections

Adverse Reactions

Cardiovascular: Flushing, hypotension with rapid I.V. injection, tachycardia, shock, edema, impaired cardiac function (see Warnings)

Central nervous system: Fever, seizures, dialysis dementia

Dermatologic: Erythema, urticaria, pruritus, rash, cutaneous wheal formation

Endocrine & Metabolic: Growth impairment (dose related; see Warnings)

Gastrointestinal: Abdominal discomfort, diarrhea, nausea, vomiting

Genitourinary: Discoloration of urine (reddish color), dysuria

Hematologic: Thrombocytopenia (rare), leukopenia (rare)

Local: Pain, induration at injection site

Neuromuscular & skeletal: Leg cramps, metaphyseal dysplasia

Ocular: Blurred vision; cataracts; impaired peripheral, color, and night vision; retinal pigmentary abnormalities

Otic: High frequency sensorineural hearing loss, tinnitus

Respiratory: ARDS (see Warnings)

Miscellaneous: Anaphylaxis, possible increased risk of infections particularly with *Y. enterocolitica*; rare cases of mucormycosis

Drug Interactions Vitamin C (see Warnings); prochlorperazine

Stability Protect from light; do not refrigerate reconstituted solutions as they will precipitate; reconstituted solutions are stable for 7 days at room temperature; due to a lack of preservatives, the manufacturer recommends immediate use after reconstitution

Mechanism of Action Complexes with trivalent ions (ferric ions) to form ferrioxamine, which is removed by the kidneys

Pharmacokinetics

Absorption: Oral: <15%

Metabolism: By plasma enzymes to ferrioxamine

Half-life:

Deferoxamine: 6.1 hours

Ferrioxamine: 5.8 hours

Elimination: Renal excretion of the metabolite iron chelate and unchanged drug

Dialysis: Dialyzable

Usual Dosage

Children:

Acute iron intoxication:

I.M.: 50 mg/kg/dose every 6 hours; maximum dose: 6 g/day

I.V.: 15 mg/kg/hour; maximum dose: 6 g/day

Alternative dosing I.M. or I.V.: 20 mg/kg or 600 mg/m^2 (not to exceed 1000 mg) initially followed by 10 mg/kg or 300 mg/m^2 (not to exceed 500 mg) at 4-hour intervals for 2 doses; subsequent doses of 10 mg/kg or 300 mg/m^2 (not to exceed 500 mg) every 4-12 hours may be repeated depending upon the clinical response; maximum dose: 6 g/day

Chronic iron overload:

I.V.: 15 mg/kg/hour; maximum dose: 12 g/day

S.C. infusion via a portable, controlled infusion device: 20-50 mg/kg/day over 8-12 hours; maximum dose: 2 g/day

Adults:

Acute iron intoxication:

I.M.: 1 g stat, then 0.5 g every 4 hours for two doses, additional doses of 0.5 g every 4-12 hours up to 6 g/day may be needed depending upon the clinical response

I.V.: 15 mg/kg/hour; maximum dose: 6 g/day

Chronic iron overload:

I.M.: 0.5-1 g/day

I.V.: 15 mg/kg/hour; maximum dose: 12 g/day

Manufacturer's recommendations: 2 g per each unit of blood transfused; maximum dose: 6 g/day if transfused or 1 g/day without transfusion

S.C. infusion via a portable, controlled infusion device: 1-2 g/day over 8-24 hours

Aluminum-induced bone disease: 20-40 mg/kg every hemodialysis treatment, frequency dependent on clinical status of the patient

Administration Parenteral: Add 2 mL SWI to 500 mg vial or 8 mL SWI to each 2 g vial, resulting in 250 mg/mL solution; for I.M. or S.C. administration, no further dilution is required; for I.V. infusion, dilute in dextrose, NS, LR: 10 mg/mL (maximum concentration: 250 mg/mL); maximum rate of infusion: 15 mg/kg/hour; the manufacturer recommends using a reduced rate of infusion (not to exceed 125 mg/hour) after the first 1000 mg has been infused; local reactions at the site of subcutaneous infusion may be minimized by diluting the deferoxamine in 5-10 mL SWI and adding 1 mg hydrocortisone to each mL of deferoxamine solution (Kirking, 1991)

Monitoring Parameters Serum ferritin, iron, total iron binding capacity; body weight, growth, ophthalmologic exam, and audiometry (with chronic use); blood pressure (with I.V. infusions)

Reference Range Effective plasma concentration: 3-15 mcg/mL

Test Interactions Gallium-67 imaging results may be distorted due to rapid urinary excretion of deferoxamine-bound gallium-67; discontinue deferoxamine at least 48 hours prior to imaging

Patient Information May cause dizziness or impairment of vision or hearing; report any hearing loss, night blindness, decreased visual acuity, impaired peripheral vision, or loss of color vision; may cause the urine to turn a reddish color

Nursing Implications Local injection site reactions may be minimized by daily rotation of subcutaneous injection sites and by applying topical corticosteroids; painful lumps formed under the skin may indicate that the rate of S.C. administration exceeds the rate of absorption from the injection site or the needle is inserted too close to the dermis

Additional Information Has been used investigationally as a single 40 mg/kg I.V. dose over 2 hours, to promote mobilization of aluminum from tissue stores as an aid in the diagnosis of aluminum-associated osteodystrophy

Dosage Forms Injection, powder for reconstitution, as mesylate: 500 mg, 2 g

References

Bentur Y, McGuigan M, and Koren G, "Deferoxamine (Desferrioxamine): New Toxicities for an Old Drug," *Drug Saf*, 1991, 6(1):37-46.

Cohen AR, Mizanin J, and Schwartz E, "Rapid Removal of Excessive Iron With Daily, High-Dose Intravenous Chelation Therapy," *J Pediatr*, 1989, 115(1):151-5.

Freedman MH, Olivieri N, Benson L, et al, "Clinical Studies on Iron Chelation in Patients With Thalassemia Major," *Haematologica*, 1990, 75(Suppl 5):74-83.

(Continued)

Deferoxamine *(Continued)*

Giardina PJ, Grady RW, Ehlers KH, et al, "Current Therapy of Cooley's Anemia: A Decade of Experience With Subcutaneous Desferrioxamine," *Ann N Y Acad Sci*, 1990, 612:275-85.

Kirking MH, "Treatment of Chronic Iron Overload," *Clin Pharm*, 1991, 10(10):775-83.

Pippard MJ, "Iron Metabolism and Iron Chelation in the Thalassemia Disorders," *Haematologica*, 1990, 75(Suppl 5):66-71.

- ◆ **Dehydral® (Can)** *see* Methenamine *on page 733*
- ◆ **Dehydrated Alcohol Injection** *see* Ethyl Alcohol *on page 465*
- ◆ **Delacort®** *see* Hydrocortisone *on page 573*
- ◆ **Del Aqua®** *see* Benzoyl Peroxide *on page 165*
- ◆ **Delatestryl®** *see* Testosterone *on page 1070*
- ◆ **Delestrogen®** *see* Estradiol *on page 456*
- ◆ **Delsym® [OTC]** *see* Dextromethorphan *on page 365*
- ◆ **Deltacortisone** *see* PredniSONE *on page 928*
- ◆ **Deltadehydrocortisone** *see* PredniSONE *on page 928*
- ◆ **Deltahydrocortisone** *see* PrednisoLONE *on page 925*
- ◆ **Deltasone®** *see* PredniSONE *on page 928*
- ◆ **Demadex®** *see* Torsemide *on page 1104*

Demeclocycline *(dem e kloe SYE kleen)*

U.S. Brand Names Declomycin®

Synonyms Demethylchlortetracycline

Therapeutic Category Antibiotic, Tetracycline Derivative

Generic Available No

Use Treatment of susceptible bacterial infections (acne, gonorrhea, pertussis, chronic bronchitis, and urinary tract infections) caused by both gram-negative and gram-positive organisms; treatment of chronic syndrome of inappropriate antidiuretic hormone (SIADH) secretion

Pregnancy Risk Factor D

Contraindications Hypersensitivity to demeclocycline, tetracyclines, or any component; pregnancy

Warnings Photosensitivity reactions occur frequently with this drug, avoid prolonged exposure to sunlight; do not use tanning equipment. Do not administer to children ≤8 years of age; use of tetracyclines during tooth development may cause permanent discoloration of the teeth and enamel hypoplasia; do not administer to pregnant women; use of tetracyclines in pregnant women may result in retardation of bone growth and skeletal development of the fetus; prolonged use may result in superinfection. Use of outdated tetracyclines have caused a Fanconi-like syndrome.

Precautions Use with caution and modify dosage in patients with impaired renal function

Adverse Reactions

Central nervous system: Elevated intracranial pressure, bulging fontanels in infants

Dermatologic: Rash, pruritus, photosensitivity, exfoliative dermatitis, discoloration of nails, Stevens-Johnson syndrome

Endocrine & metabolic: Diabetes insipidus syndrome

Gastrointestinal: Nausea, vomiting, diarrhea, anorexia, pancreatitis

Hematologic: Leukopenia, neutropenia, thrombocytopenia

Hepatic: Hepatotoxicity

Neuromuscular & skeletal: Paresthesia

Renal: Azotemia, acute renal failure

Miscellaneous: Superinfections

Drug Interactions Antacids, calcium, magnesium, zinc, bismuth salts, and iron preparations may decrease absorption of demeclocycline; decreased effect of oral contraceptives, penicillins; increased effect of warfarin

Food Interactions Food, milk, milk formulas, and dairy products decrease absorption of demeclocycline

Mechanism of Action Inhibits protein synthesis by binding with the 30S ribosomal subunits and preventing the binding of transfer RNA to those ribosomes of susceptible bacteria; may also cause alterations in the cytoplasmic membrane

Pharmacodynamics Onset of action for diuresis in SIADH: Within 5 days

Pharmacokinetics

Absorption: ~60% to 80% of dose absorbed from the GI tract; food and dairy products reduce absorption by 50% or more

Distribution: Excreted into breast milk

Protein binding: 36% to 91%

Metabolism: Small amounts metabolized in the liver to inactive metabolites; enterohepatically recycled

Half-life: 10-17 hours (prolonged with reduced renal function)

Time to peak serum concentration: Oral: Within 3-6 hours

Elimination: Excreted as unchanged drug (42% to 50%) in urine

Usual Dosage Oral:

Children >8 years: 8-12 mg/kg/day divided every 6-12 hours

Adults: 150 mg 4 times/day or 300 mg twice daily

Uncomplicated gonorrhea: 600 mg stat, 300 mg every 12 hours for 4 days (3 g total)

SIADH: Initial: 900-1200 mg/day or 13-15 mg/kg/day divided every 6-8 hours; then decrease to 600-900 mg/day

Dosing adjustment in renal impairment: Not recommended for use

Administration Oral: Administer 1 hour before or 2 hours after food or milk with plenty of fluids; do not administer with food, milk, dairy products, antacids, zinc, or iron supplements

Monitoring Parameters CBC, renal and hepatic function tests, I & O, urine output, serum sodium

Test Interactions May interfere with tests for urinary glucose (false-negative urine glucose using Clinistix®, Tes-Tape®)

Patient Information May cause photosensitivity reactions (eg, exposure to sunlight may cause severe sunburn, skin rash, redness, or itching; avoid exposure to sunlight and artificial light sources (sunlamps, tanning booth/bed); wear protective clothing, wide-brimmed hats, sunglasses, and lip sunscreen (SPF ≥15); use a sunscreen [broad-spectrum sunscreen or physical sunscreen (preferred) or sunblock with SPF ≥15]; contact physician if reaction occurs. May discolor fingernails. Avoid taking dosages at bedtime.

Dosage Forms Tablet, film coated, as hydrochloride: 150 mg, 300 mg

References

Abdi EA and Bishop S, "The Syndrome of Inappropriate Antidiuretic Hormone Secretion With Carcinoma of the Tongue," *Med Pediatr Oncol*, 1988, 16(3):210-5.

Troyer AD, "Demeclocycline. Treatment for Syndrome of Inappropriate Antidiuretic Hormone Secretion," *JAMA*, 1977, 237(25):2723-6.

♦ **Demerol®** *see* Meperidine *on page 717*

♦ **4-Demethoxydaunorubicin** *see* Idarubicin *on page 591*

♦ **Demethylchlortetracycline** *see* Demeclocycline *on page 348*

♦ **Denorex® [OTC]** *see* Coal Tar *on page 299*

♦ **Denorex® Extra Strength [OTC]** *see* Coal Tar *on page 299*

♦ **Deodorized Opium Tincture** *see* Opium Tincture *on page 836*

♦ **2'-Deoxy-3'-Thiacytidine** *see* Lamivudine *on page 650*

♦ **Depacon®** *see* Valproic Acid and Derivatives *on page 1131*

♦ **Depakene®** *see* Valproic Acid and Derivatives *on page 1131*

♦ **Depakote®** *see* Valproic Acid and Derivatives *on page 1131*

♦ **Depakote®-ER** *see* Valproic Acid and Derivatives *on page 1131*

♦ **Depakote® Sprinkle®** *see* Valproic Acid and Derivatives *on page 1131*

♦ **Depen®** *see* Penicillamine *on page 872*

♦ **Depo®-Estradiol** *see* Estradiol *on page 456*

♦ **Depo-Medrol®** *see* MethylPREDNISolone *on page 747*

♦ **Deponit® [DSC]** *see* Nitroglycerin *on page 815*

♦ **Depo-Provera®** *see* MedroxyPROGESTERone *on page 712*

♦ **Depo-Provera® Contraceptive** *see* MedroxyPROGESTERone *on page 712*

♦ **Depotest® 100 (Can)** *see* Testosterone *on page 1070*

♦ **Depo®-Testosterone** *see* Testosterone *on page 1070*

♦ **Dermarest Dri-Cort® [OTC]** *see* Hydrocortisone *on page 573*

♦ **Derma-Smoothe/FS®** *see* Fluocinolone *on page 498*

♦ **Dermazin™ (Can)** *see* Silver Sulfadiazine *on page 1019*

♦ **Dermazole (Can)** *see* Miconazole *on page 759*

♦ **Dermtex® HC [OTC]** *see* Hydrocortisone *on page 573*

♦ **Desferal®** *see* Deferoxamine *on page 346*

Desipramine (des IP ra meen)

Related Information

Comparison of Adverse Effects of Antidepressants *on page 1210*

Comparison of Usual Adult Dosage and Mechanism of Action of Antidepressants *on page 1209*

Drugs and Breast-Feeding *on page 1404*

Overdose and Toxicology *on page 1388*

U.S. Brand Names Norpramin®

(Continued)

Desipramine *(Continued)*

Canadian Brand Names Alti-Desipramine; Apo®-Desipramine; Novo-Desipramine; Nu-Desipramine; PMS-Desipramine

Therapeutic Category Antidepressant, Tricyclic

Generic Available Yes

Use Treatment of various forms of depression, often in conjunction with psychotherapy; analgesic in chronic pain, peripheral neuropathies

Pregnancy Risk Factor C

Contraindications Hypersensitivity to desipramine (cross-sensitivity with other tricyclic antidepressants may occur) or any component; use of MAO inhibitors within 14 days (potentially fatal reactions may occur, see Drug Interactions); narrow-angle glaucoma

Warnings Do not discontinue abruptly in patients receiving long-term high-dose therapy

Precautions Use with caution in patients with cardiovascular disease, conduction disturbances, urinary retention, seizure disorders, hyperthyroidism or those receiving thyroid replacement

Adverse Reactions Less sedation and anticholinergic adverse effects than amitriptyline or imipramine

Cardiovascular: Arrhythmias, hypotension; asymptomatic EKG changes and minor increases in diastolic blood pressure and heart rate have been noted in children receiving >3.5 mg/kg/day; **Note:** 4 cases of sudden death have been reported in children 5-14 years of age; an association between desipramine and sudden death was not shown to be significant in one retrospective study; further studies are needed

Central nervous system: Sedation, confusion, dizziness

Dermatologic: Photosensitivity

Endocrine & metabolic: SIADH

Gastrointestinal: Constipation, nausea, vomiting, xerostomia, weight gain

Genitourinary: Urinary retention, discoloration of urine (blue-green)

Hematologic: Blood dyscrasias

Hepatic: Hepatitis

Ocular: Blurred vision, elevated intraocular pressure

Otic: Tinnitus

Miscellaneous: Hypersensitivity reactions

Drug Interactions Cytochrome P450 isoenzyme CYP1A2 and CYP2D6 substrate; isoenzyme CYP2D6 inhibitor

May decrease effects of guanethidine and clonidine; may increase effects of CNS depressants, alcohol, adrenergic agents, anticholinergic agents; with MAO inhibitors, fever, tachycardia, hypertension, seizures, and death may occur; cimetidine may decrease desipramine clearance and increase plasma concentrations; the herbal medicine St John's wort (*Hypericum perforatum*) may increase serious side effects, its use is **not** recommended; ritonavir increases desipramine concentration by 145% (dosage reduction of desipramine is recommended); concurrent use of high dose TCAs and ritonavir may cause the serotonin syndrome; interactions similar to other TCAs may occur

Food Interactions May increase riboflavin dietary requirements

Mechanism of Action Increases the synaptic concentration of serotonin and/or norepinephrine in the CNS by inhibition of their reuptake by the presynaptic neuronal membrane

Pharmacodynamics Antidepressant effects:

Onset of action: Occasionally seen in 2-5 days

Maximum effect: After more than 2 weeks

Pharmacokinetics

Absorption: Well absorbed from the GI tract

Distribution: V_d: Adults: 21 L/kg; distributes into breast milk (concentrations approximately equal to maternal plasma)

Protein binding: 90%

Metabolism: In the liver

Half-life, adults: 12-57 hours

Elimination: 70% in urine

Usual Dosage Oral:

Children 6-12 years: 1-3 mg/kg/day in divided doses; monitor carefully with doses >3 mg/kg/day; maximum dose: 5 mg/kg/day

Adolescents: Initial: 25-50 mg/day; gradually increase to 100 mg/day in single or divided doses; maximum dose: 150 mg/day

Adults: Initial: 75 mg/day in divided doses; increase gradually to 150-200 mg/day in divided or single dose; maximum dose: 300 mg/day

Administration Oral: Administer with food to decrease GI upset

Monitoring Parameters Blood pressure, heart rate, EKG, mental status, weight
Long-term use: CBC with differential, liver enzymes, serum concentrations

Reference Range
Therapeutic: 150-300 ng/mL (SI: 560-1125 nmol/L)
Possible toxicity: >300 ng/mL (SI: >1070 nmol/L)
Toxic: >1000 ng/mL (SI: >3750 nmol/L)

Patient Information May cause drowsiness and impair ability to perform activities requiring mental alertness or physical coordination; may cause dry mouth; avoid alcohol and the herbal medicine St John's wort; limit caffeine; may discolor urine to blue-green color; do not discontinue medication abruptly; may increase appetite. May cause photosensitivity reactions (eg, exposure to sunlight may cause severe sunburn, skin rash, redness, or itching); avoid exposure to sunlight and artificial light sources (sunlamps, tanning booth/bed); wear protective clothing, wide-brimmed hats, sunglasses, and lip sunscreen (SPF ≥15); use a sunscreen [broad-spectrum sunscreen or physical sunscreen (preferred) or sunblock with SPF ≥15]; contact physician if reaction occurs.

Additional Information Place in therapy (treatment of depression): Desipramine is considered by some clinicians to be the first or second drug of choice for depressed children with excessive daytime sleepiness

Dosage Forms Tablet, as hydrochloride: 10 mg, 25 mg, 50 mg, 75 mg, 100 mg, 150 mg

References
Biederman J, Thisted RA, Greenhill LL, et al, "Estimation of the Association Between Desipramine and the Risk for Sudden Death in 5-14 Year-Old Children," *J Clin Psychiatry*, 1995, 56(3):87-93.
Levy HB, Harper CR, and Weinberg WA, "A Practical Approach to Children Failing in School," *Pediatr Clin North Am*, 1992, 39(4):895-928.

♦ **Desitin® [OTC]** *see* Zinc Oxide *on page 1167*
♦ **Desitin® Creamy [OTC]** *see* Zinc Oxide *on page 1167*

Desloratadine (des lor AT a deen)

U.S. Brand Names Clarinex®
Canadian Brand Names Aerius®
Therapeutic Category Antihistamine
Generic Available No

Use Symptomatic relief of nasal and non-nasal symptoms of allergic rhinitis; chronic idiopathic urticaria

Pregnancy Risk Factor C

Contraindications Hypersensitivity to desloratadine, loratadine, or any component

Warnings Use with caution and adjust dosage in patients with liver or renal impairment

Precautions A subset of the general population (7% in clinical trials) are slow metabolizers of desloratadine; the frequency of slow metabolism appears to be higher in African Americans; patients who are slow metabolizers may be more susceptible to dose-related side effects; use with caution in "slow metabolizers." Use cautiously in patients who are also taking ketoconazole, itraconazole, fluconazole, erythromycin, clarithromycin, or other drugs which may impair desloratadine's hepatic metabolism; although increased plasma levels of desloratadine have been observed, no adverse effects with concomitant administration have been reported, including QT interval prolongation which has occurred when similar antihistamines, terfenadine and astemizole, were combined with these agents. While less sedating than other antihistamines, desloratadine may cause drowsiness and impair ability to perform hazardous activities requiring mental alertness. Use cautiously in breast-feeding women as desloratadine passes into breast milk. RediTabs® contain aspartame which is metabolized to phenylalanine and must be used with caution in patients with phenylketonuria.

Adverse Reactions
Cardiovascular: Tachycardia, edema
Central nervous system: Somnolence, fatigue, dizziness
Dermatologic: Pruritus, urticaria
Gastrointestinal: Xerostomia, nausea, dry throat
Hepatic: Elevated liver enzymes, elevated bilirubin
Neuromuscular & skeletal: Myalgia
Respiratory: Pharyngitis, dyspnea
Miscellaneous: Hypersensitivity reactions, flu-like symptoms

Drug Interactions Increased plasma concentrations and AUC of desloratadine and its active metabolite with ketoconazole and erythromycin; no change in QT_c interval or cardiac arrhythmias have been seen (see Warnings); additive CNS depression with other CNS depressants and alcohol
(Continued)

Desloratadine *(Continued)*

Food Interactions Administration with food has no effect on desloratadine's bioavailability

Stability Store at room temperature; avoid excessive heat and moisture; RediTabs® must be used immediately after removal from blister pack

Mechanism of Action Long-acting tricyclic antihistamine with selective peripheral histamine H_1-receptor antagonistic properties; active metabolite of loratadine

Pharmacodynamics
Onset of action: 1 hour
Duration: 24 hours

Pharmacokinetics
Distribution: Distributes into breast milk
Protein binding: 82% to 87% (desloratadine), 85% to 89% (metabolite)
Metabolism: Metabolized to an active metabolite (3-hydroxydesloratadine); subset of population are slow metabolizers of desloratadine (7% of patients in clinical trials were slow-metabolizers; see Precautions)
Half-life: 27 hours (both desloratadine and active metabolite)
Time to peak serum concentration: 3 hours
Elimination: 87% eliminated via urine and feces as metabolic products

Usual Dosage Oral: Children ≥12 years and Adults: 5 mg once daily
Dosage adjustment in renal/hepatic impairment: Administer dosage every other day

Administration Oral: May administer without regard to food. Place RediTabs® directly on the tongue; tablet will disintegrate immediately; may be taken with or without water

Monitoring Parameters Improvement in signs and symptoms of allergic rhinitis

Reference Range Therapeutic serum levels (not used clinically): Desloratadine: 2.5-4 ng/mL

Test Interactions Antigen skin testing

Patient Information Drink plenty of water; may cause dry mouth; may cause drowsiness and impair ability to perform activities requiring mental alertness or physical coordination; avoid alcohol

Dosage Forms
Tablet: 5 mg
Tablet, orally-disintegrating (RediTabs®): 5 mg [contains 1.75 mg phenylalanine (as aspartame); tutti-frutti flavor]

Desmopressin *(des moe PRES in)*

U.S. Brand Names DDAVP®; Stimate®

Canadian Brand Names Apo®-Desmopressin; Minirin®; Octostim®

Synonyms 1-Deamino-8-D-Arginine Vasopressin

Therapeutic Category Antihemophilic Agent; Hemostatic Agent; Vasopressin Analog, Synthetic

Generic Available Yes (injection)

Use Treatment of diabetes insipidus, control of bleeding in hemophilia A (with factor VIII levels >5%), mild to moderate type I von Willebrand disease, and thrombocytopenia; primary nocturnal enuresis

Pregnancy Risk Factor B

Contraindications Hypersensitivity to desmopressin or any component; avoid using in patients with severe type I, type IIB or platelet-type (pseudo) von Willebrand disease, hemophilia A with factor VIII levels ≤5% or hemophilia B

Warnings Avoid intranasal use in patients with nasal mucosa changes (scarring, edema, discharge, obstruction, or severe atopic rhinitis)

Precautions Use with caution in patients with predisposition to thrombus formation, conditions associated with fluid and electrolyte imbalance (eg, cystic fibrosis), and in patients with coronary artery disease and/or hypertensive cardiovascular disease

Adverse Reactions
Cardiovascular: Facial flushing, elevated blood pressure, chest pain, palpitations, tachycardia
Central nervous system: Headache, somnolence, dizziness, insomnia, agitation
Endocrine & metabolic: Hyponatremia, water intoxication
Gastrointestinal: Nausea, abdominal cramps, dyspepsia, vomiting
Genitourinary: Vulval pain, balanitis
Local: Pain at the injection site
Ocular: Itchy or light-sensitive eyes
Respiratory: Rhinitis, upper respiratory infections, epistaxis, nasal congestion

Drug Interactions Decreased antidiuretic response with lithium, large doses of epinephrine, demeclocycline, and heparin; increased antidiuretic response with carbamazepine, chlorpropamide, fludrocortisone, and clofibrate

Stability Refrigerate injection, nasal solution and Stimate® nasal spray; nasal solution and Stimate® nasal spray are stable for 3 weeks when stored at room temperature if unopened; injection is stable for 2 weeks at room temperature; DDAVP® nasal spray is stable at room temperature

Mechanism of Action Enhances reabsorption of water in the kidneys by increasing cellular permeability of the collecting ducts; possibly causes smooth muscle constriction with resultant vasoconstriction; dose-dependent increase in plasma factor VIII and plasminogen activator

Pharmacodynamics

Oral administration:
Onset of ADH action: 1 hour
Maximum effect: 2-7 hours
Duration: 6-8 hours

Intranasal administration:
Onset of ADH action: Within 1 hour
Maximum effect: Within 1.5 hours
Duration: 5-21 hours

I.V. infusion:
Onset of increased factor VIII activity: Within 15-30 minutes
Maximum effect: 90 minutes to 3 hours

Pharmacokinetics

Absorption:
Oral tablets: 5% to 15%
Nasal solution: 10% to 20%
Nasal spray (1.5 mg/mL concentration): 3.3% to 4.1%

Metabolism: Unknown

Half-life:
Oral: 1.5-2.5 hours
I.V.:
Initial: 7.8 minutes
Terminal: 75.5 minutes (range: 0.4-4 hours)
Intranasal: 3.3-3.5 hours

Time to peak serum concentration:
Oral: 0.9 hours
Intranasal: 1.5 hours

Usual Dosage

Diabetes insipidus:

Oral:
Children ≤12 years: Initial: 0.05 mg 2 times daily; titrate to desired response (range: 0.1-0.8 mg daily)
Children >12 years and Adults: 0.05 mg 2 times daily; titrate to desired response (range: 0.1-1.2 mg divided 2-3 times/day)

Intranasal:
Children 3 months to ≤12 years: Initial (using 100 mcg/mL nasal solution): 5 mcg/day (0.05 mL/day) divided 1-2 times/day; range: 5-30 mcg/day (0.05-0.3 mL/day); adjust morning and evening doses separately for an adequate diurnal rhythm of water turnover

Children >12 years and Adults: Initial (using 100 mcg/mL nasal solution): 5-40 mcg (0.05-0.4 mL) divided 1-3 times/day; adjust morning and evening doses separately for an adequate diurnal rhythm of water turnover. **Note:** The nasal spray pump can only deliver doses of 10 mcg (0.1 mL) or multiples of 10 mcg (0.1 mL), if doses other than this are needed, the rhinal tube delivery system is preferred

I.V., S.C.: Children >12 years and Adults: 2-4 mcg/day in 2 divided doses or $^1/_{10}$ of the maintenance intranasal dose

Hemophilia:

I.V.: Children ≥3 months and Adults: 0.3 mcg/kg beginning 30 minutes before procedure; may repeat dose if needed

Intranasal: Children >12 years and Adults: Using high concentration Stimate® nasal spray:
≤50 kg: 150 mcg (1 spray)
>50 kg: 300 mcg (1 spray each nostril)
Repeat use is determined by the patient's clinical condition and laboratory work; if using preoperatively, administer 2 hours before surgery

Nocturnal enuresis:

Intranasal: Children ≥6 years: (Using 100 mcg/mL nasal solution): Initial: 20 mcg (0.2 mL) at bedtime; range: 10-40 mcg; it is recommended that $^1/_2$ of the dose be given in each nostril

Oral: Children ≥6 years: 0.2-0.6 mg once before bedtime
(Continued)

Desmopressin *(Continued)*

Administration
Intranasal: Using rhinal tube delivery system, draw solution into flexible, calibrated rhinal tube; insert one end into nostril; blow on the other end to deposit the solution deep into the nasal cavity. The Stimate® spray pump must be primed prior to first use; to prime pump, press down 4 times. Avoid spray use in children <6 years of age due to difficulty in titrating dosage; discard any solution remaining after 25 or 50 doses (2.5 or 5 mL vials, respectively) because the amount delivered may be substantially less than prescribed

Parenteral: I.V.: Dilute to a maximum concentration of 0.5 mcg/mL in NS and infuse over 15-30 minutes; if desmopressin I.V. is given preoperatively, administer 30 minutes prior to surgery

Monitoring Parameters I.V. infusion: Blood pressure and pulse should be monitored
Diabetes insipidus: Fluid intake, urine volume, specific gravity, plasma and urine osmolality, serum electrolytes
Hemophilia: Factor VIII antigen levels, APTT, Factor VIII activity level

Patient Information Avoid overhydration; blow nose before using nasal solution or spray; notify physician if headache, shortness of breath, heartburn, nausea, abdominal cramps, or vulval pain occur

Dosage Forms
Injection, solution, as acetate (DDAVP®): 4 mcg/mL (1 mL, 10 mL)
Solution, intranasal, as acetate, (DDAVP®): 100 mcg/mL (2.5 mL) [with rhinal tube]
Solution, intranasal spray, as acetate:
DDAVP®: 100 mcg/mL (5 mL) [delivers 10 mcg/spray]
Stimate®: 1.5 mg/mL (2.5 mL) [delivers 150 mcg/spray]
Tablet, as acetate (DDAVP®): 0.1 mg, 0.2 mg

References
Stenberg A and Läckgren G, "Desmopressin Tablets in the Treatment of Severe Nocturnal Enuresis in Adolescents," *Pediatrics*, 1994, 94(6 Pt 1):841-46.

+ **Desquam-E®** *see* Benzoyl Peroxide *on page 165*
+ **Desquam-X®** *see* Benzoyl Peroxide *on page 165*
+ **Desyrel®** *see* Trazodone *on page 1110*
+ **Detane® [OTC]** *see* Benzocaine *on page 163*
+ **Devrom®** *see* Bismuth *on page 174*
+ **Dex4 Glucose [OTC]** *see* Dextrose *on page 366*
+ **Dexacidin®** *see* Dexamethasone, Neomycin, and Polymyxin B *on page 357*
+ **Dexacine™** *see* Dexamethasone, Neomycin, and Polymyxin B *on page 357*
+ **Dexalone® [OTC]** *see* Dextromethorphan *on page 365*

Dexamethasone *(deks a METH a sone)*

Related Information
Carbohydrate and Alcohol Content of Liquid Medications for Use in Patients Receiving Ketogenic Diets *on page 1431*
Corticosteroids Comparison, Systemic *on page 1211*

U.S. Brand Names Decadron®; Decadron® Phosphate; Dexamethasone Intensol®; Dexasone®; Dexasone® L.A.; DexPak® TaperPak®; Maxidex®; Solurex®; Solurex L.A.®

Canadian Brand Names Diodex®; PMS-Dexamethasone

Therapeutic Category Adrenal Corticosteroid; Antiasthmatic; Antiemetic; Anti-inflammatory Agent; Anti-inflammatory Agent, Ophthalmic; Corticosteroid, Ophthalmic; Corticosteroid, Systemic; Glucocorticoid

Generic Available Yes

Use Treatment of chronic inflammation, allergic, hematologic, neoplastic, and autoimmune diseases; may be used in management of cerebral edema, septic shock, and as a diagnostic agent; adjunctive antiemetic agent in the treatment of chemotherapy-induced emesis; treatment of airway edema prior to extubation; used in neonates with bronchopulmonary dysplasia to facilitate ventilator weaning

Pregnancy Risk Factor C

Contraindications Hypersensitivity to dexamethasone or any component (see Warnings); active untreated infections; viral, fungal, or tuberculous diseases of the eye

Warnings Hypothalamic - pituitary - adrenal (HPA) suppression may occur; withdrawal and discontinuation of corticosteroids should be done carefully; acute adrenal insufficiency may occur with abrupt withdrawal after long term therapy or with stress. Immunosuppression may occur.

Injection may contain sulfites and 0.5 mg tablet may contain tartrazine, either may cause allergic reactions in susceptible individuals. Elixir contains benzoic acid; benzoic acid (benzoate) is a metabolite of benzyl alcohol; large amounts of benzyl alcohol (≥99 mg/kg/day) have been associated with a potentially fatal toxicity ("gasping syndrome") in neonates; the "gasping syndrome" consists of metabolic acidosis, respiratory distress, gasping respirations, CNS dysfunction (including convulsions, intracranial hemorrhage), hypotension and cardiovascular collapse; use dexamethasone products containing benzoic acid with caution in neonates; *in vitro* and animal studies have shown that benzoate displaces bilirubin from protein binding sites

Precautions Suppression of HPA function, suppression of linear growth, or hypercorticism (Cushing's syndrome) may occur; use with extreme caution in patients with respiratory tuberculosis, untreated systemic infections, or ocular herpes simplex; use with caution in patients with hyperthyroidism, cirrhosis, ulcerative colitis, hypertension, osteoporosis, thromboembolic tendencies, CHF, convulsive disorders, myasthenia gravis, thrombophlebitis, peptic ulcer, diabetes; prolonged use may result in cataracts or glaucoma

Adverse Reactions

Cardiovascular: Edema, hypertension

Central nervous system: Headache, vertigo, seizures, psychosis, pseudotumor cerebri, insomnia, nervousness

Dermatologic: Acne, skin atrophy

Endocrine & metabolic: Pituitary-adrenal axis suppression, growth suppression, glucose intolerance, hypokalemia, alkalosis, Cushing's syndrome

Gastrointestinal: Peptic ulcer, nausea, vomiting

Neuromuscular & skeletal: Muscle weakness, osteoporosis, fractures

Ocular: Cataracts, glaucoma

Miscellaneous: Immunosuppression

Drug Interactions Cytochrome P450 isoenzyme CYP3A3/4 substrate; isoenzyme CYP3A3/4 inducer; isoenzyme CYP3A3/4 inhibitor

Barbiturates, phenytoin, rifampin, ritonavir, saquinavir, salicylates, NSAIDs, toxoids; alcohol and caffeine may increase adverse GI effects; live virus vaccines (increase risk of viral infection); vaccines may have decreased effects

Food Interactions Systemic use of corticosteroids may require a diet with increased potassium, vitamins A, B_6, C, D, folate, calcium, zinc, and phosphorus and decreased sodium

Stability Dilution of dexamethasone sodium phosphate injection with D_5W or NS is stable for at least 24 hours

Mechanism of Action Decreases inflammation by suppression of migration of polymorphonuclear leukocytes and reversal of increased capillary permeability; suppresses normal immune response

Pharmacodynamics Duration: Metabolic effects can last for 72 hours

Pharmacokinetics

Metabolism: In the liver

Half-life: Terminal:

Extremely low birth weight infants with BPD: 9.3 hours

Children 3 months to 16 years: 4.3 hours

Healthy adults: 3 hours

Time to peak serum concentration:

Oral: Within 1-2 hours

I.M.: Within 8 hours

Elimination: In urine and bile

Usual Dosage

Neonates:

Airway edema or extubation: I.V.: Usual: 0.25 mg/kg/dose given ~4 hours prior to scheduled extubation and then every 8 hours for 3 doses total; range: 0.25-1 mg/kg/dose for 1-3 doses; maximum dose: 1 mg/kg/day. **Note:** A longer duration of therapy may be needed with more severe cases.

Bronchopulmonary dysplasia (to facilitate ventilator weaning): Oral, I.V.: Numerous dosing schedules have been proposed; range: 0.5-0.6 mg/kg/day given in divided doses every 12 hours for 3-7 days, then taper over 1-6 weeks

Children:

Airway edema or extubation: Oral, I.M., I.V.: 0.5-2 mg/kg/day in divided doses every 6 hours; begin 24 hours prior to extubation and continue for 4-6 doses after extubation

Antiemetic (chemotherapy induced): I.V.: Initial: 10 mg/m²/dose (maximum dose: 20 mg) then 5 mg/m²/dose every 6 hours

Anti-inflammatory: Oral, I.M., I.V.: 0.08-0.3 mg/kg/day or 2.5-10 mg/m²/day in divided doses every 6-12 hours

Bacterial meningitis: Infants and Children >2 months: I.V.: 0.6 mg/kg/day divided every 6 hours for the first 4 days of antibiotic treatment; start dexamethasone at the time of the first dose of antibiotic

(Continued)

Dexamethasone *(Continued)*

Cerebral edema: Oral, I.M., I.V.: Loading dose: 1-2 mg/kg/dose as a single dose; maintenance: 1-1.5 mg/kg/day (maximum dose: 16 mg/day) in divided doses every 4-6 hours

Physiologic replacement: Oral, I.M., I.V.: 0.03-0.15 mg/kg/day or 0.6-0.75 mg/m²/day in divided doses every 6-12 hours

Children and Adults: Ophthalmic:

Ointment: Apply thin coating to conjunctival sac 3-4 times/day, gradually taper dose to discontinue

Suspension: Instill 2 drops every hour during the day and every other hour during the night; gradually reduce dose to every 3-4 hours, then to 3-4 times/day

Adults:

Acute nonlymphoblastic leukemia (ANLL) protocol: I.V.: 2 mg/m²/dose every 8 hours for 12 doses

Anti-inflammatory: Oral, I.M., I.V.: 0.75-9 mg/day in divided doses every 6-12 hours

Cerebral edema: I.V.: Initial: 10 mg then 4 mg I.M./I.V. every 6 hours

Diagnosis for Cushing's syndrome: Oral: 1 mg at 11 PM, draw blood at 8 AM

Administration

Ophthalmic: Avoid contact of container tip with skin or eye

Solution: Apply finger pressure to lacrimal sac during and for 1-2 minutes after instillation to decrease risk of absorption and systemic effects

Oral: May administer with food or milk to decrease GI adverse effects

Parenteral: **Acetate injection is not for I.V. use;** I.V. (as sodium phosphate): Administer undiluted solution (4 mg/mL) I.V. push over 1-4 minutes if dose is <10 mg; high-dose therapy must be diluted in D_5W or NS and administered by I.V. intermittent infusion over 15-30 minutes

Monitoring Parameters Hemoglobin, occult blood loss, blood pressure, serum potassium and glucose

Reference Range Dexamethasone suppression test: 8 AM cortisol <6 µg/100 mL in adults given dexamethasone 1 mg at 11 PM the previous night

Test Interactions Skin tests

Patient Information Avoid alcohol; limit caffeine; do not decrease dose or discontinue drug without physician's approval; inform physician you are taking corticosteroid prior to any surgery or with any injury

Additional Information Due to long duration of effect, not suitable for every other day dosing

Dosage Forms

Elixir, as **base**: 0.5 mg/5 mL (100 mL, 240 mL) [contains 5% alcohol and 0.1% benzoic acid; raspberry flavor]

Injection, suspension, as **acetate** (Dexasone® LA, Solurex LA®): 8 mg/mL (5 mL)

Injection, solution, as **sodium phosphate**: 4 mg/mL (1 mL, 5 mL, 10 mL, 25 mL, 30 mL); 10 mg/mL (1 mL, 10 mL)

Decadron® Phosphate: 4 mg/mL (5 mL, 25 mL); 24 mg/mL (5 mL) [contains sodium bisulfite]

Dexasone®: 4 mg/mL (5 mL)

Solurex®: 4 mg/mL (5 mL, 10 mL, 30 mL)

Ointment, ophthalmic, as **sodium phosphate**: 0.05% (3.5 g)

Solution, oral, as **base**: 0.5 mg/5 mL (5 mL, 500 mL) [cherry flavor]

Solution, oral **concentrate**, as base (Dexamethasone Intensol®): 1 mg/mL (30 mL) [contains 30% alcohol]

Suspension, ophthalmic, as **base** (Maxidex®): 0.1% (5 mL, 15 mL)

Tablet, as **base**: 0.25 mg, 0.5 mg, 0.75 mg, 1 mg, 1.5 mg, 2 mg, 4 mg, 6 mg [0.5 mg tablets may contain tartrazine]

Decadron®: 0.5 mg, 0.75 mg, 4 mg

DexPak® TaperPack®: 1.5 mg [51 tablets on a 13-day taper dose card]

References

American Academy of Pediatrics Committee on Infectious Diseases, "Dexamethasone Therapy for Bacterial Meningitis in Infants and Children," *Pediatrics*, 1990, 86(1):130-3.

Bahal N and Nahata MC, "The Role of Corticosteroids in Infants and Children With Bacterial Meningitis," *DICP*, 1991, 25(5):542-5.

Couser RJ, Ferrara TB, Falde B, et al, "Effectiveness of Dexamethasone in Preventing Extubation Failure in Preterm Infants at Increased Risk for Airway Edema," *J Pediatr*, 1992, 121(4):591-6.

Durand M, Sardesai S, and McEvoy C, "Effects of Early Dexamethasone Therapy on Pulmonary Mechanics and Chronic Lung Disease in Very Low Birth Weight Infants: A Randomized, Controlled Trial," *Pediatrics*, 1995, 95(4):584-90.

Ng PC, "The Effectiveness and Side Effects of Dexamethasone in Preterm Infants With Bronchopulmonary Dysplasia," *Arch Dis Child*, 1993, 68(3 Spec No):330-6.

♦ **Dexamethasone Intensol®** *see* Dexamethasone *on page 354*

Dexamethasone, Neomycin, and Polymyxin B

(deks a METH a sone, nee oh MYE sin, & pol i MIKS in bee)

U.S. Brand Names AK-Trol®; Dexacidin®; Dexacine™; Dexasporin®; Maxitrol®; Ocu-Trol®

Canadian Brand Names Dioptrol®

Synonyms Neomycin, Dexamethasone, and Polymyxin B Polymyxin B, Dexamethasone, and Neomycin

Therapeutic Category Antibiotic, Ophthalmic; Corticosteroid, Ophthalmic

Generic Available Yes

Use Steroid-responsive inflammatory ocular conditions in which a corticosteroid is indicated and where bacterial infection or a risk of bacterial infection exists

Pregnancy Risk Factor C

Contraindications Hypersensitivity to dexamethasone, polymyxin, neomycin, or any component; viral diseases of the cornea and conjunctiva; mycobacterial infection of the eye; fungal disease of ocular structures; dendritic keratitis; use after uncomplicated removal of a corneal foreign body

Warnings Prolonged use may result in glaucoma, defects in visual acuity, posterior subcapsular cataract formation, and secondary ocular infections

Adverse Reactions

Dermatologic: Contact dermatitis, cutaneous sensitization (sensitivity to topical neomycin has been reported to occur in 5% to 15% of patients)

Local: Pain, stinging

Ocular: Development of glaucoma, cataract, elevated intraocular pressure, optic nerve damage, visual defects, blurred vision

Miscellaneous: Delayed wound healing, secondary infections

Usual Dosage Children and Adults: Ophthalmic:

Ointment: Apply a small amount (~½") in the affected eye 3-4 times/day or apply at bedtime as an adjunct with drops

Suspension: Instill 1-2 drops into affected eye(s) every 4-6 hours; in severe disease, drops may be used hourly and tapered to discontinuation

Administration Ophthalmic: Shake suspension well before using; instill drop into affected eye; avoid contacting bottle tip with skin or eye; apply finger pressure to lacrimal sac during and for 1-2 minutes after instillation to decrease risk of absorption and systemic effects

Monitoring Parameters Intraocular pressure with use >10 days

Patient Information May cause temporary blurring of vision or stinging following administration

Dosage Forms

Ointment, ophthalmic (Dexacine™, Maxitrol®, Ocu-Trol®): Dexamethasone 0.1%, neomycin sulfate 3.5 mg, and polymyxin B sulfate 10,000 units per g (3.5 g)

Suspension, ophthalmic (AK-Trol®, Dexacidin®, Dexasporin®, Maxitrol®, Ocu-Trol®): Dexamethasone 0.1%, neomycin sulfate 3.5 mg, and polymyxin B sulfate 10,000 units per mL (5 mL)

♦ **Dexasone®** see Dexamethasone on page 354

♦ **Dexasone® L.A.** see Dexamethasone on page 354

♦ **Dexasporin®** see Dexamethasone, Neomycin, and Polymyxin B on page 357

♦ **Dexedrine®** see Dextroamphetamine on page 360

♦ **Dexedrine® Spansule®** see Dextroamphetamine on page 360

♦ **Dexferrum®** see Iron Supplements (Parenteral) on page 626

♦ **DexPak® TaperPak®** see Dexamethasone on page 354

Dexrazoxane (deks ray ZOKS ane)

U.S. Brand Names Zinecard®

Therapeutic Category Antineoplastic Agent; Chelating Agent; Chemoprotectant Agent

Generic Available No

Use Reduction of anthracycline-induced (doxorubicin, daunorubicin) cardiotoxicity. Not generally recommended for use with the initiation of anthracycline therapy. Most dexrazoxane studies have been done in women with metastatic breast cancer who had received a cumulative doxorubicin dose of 300 mg/m^2.

Pregnancy Risk Factor C

Contraindications Hypersensitivity to dexrazoxane or any component; should only be used with chemotherapy regimens containing an anthracycline

Warnings Due to limited experience, the possibility of dexrazoxane interference with antineoplastic efficacy may exist; dose-limiting toxicity is myelosuppression; dexrazoxane may add to the myelosuppression caused by chemotherapeutic agents; dexrazoxane should be handled, prepared, and disposed as an antineoplastic agent (Continued)

Dexrazoxane *(Continued)*

Precautions Do not give doxorubicin prior to dexrazoxane administration. Doxorubicin should be given within 30 minutes after the beginning of a dexrazoxane infusion.

Adverse Reactions

Central nervous system: Low grade fever

Dermatologic: Alopecia (possibly dose-related)

Endocrine/metabolic: Elevated serum iron and serum triglyceride levels, decreased serum zinc and calcium levels

Gastrointestinal: Mild nausea and vomiting, diarrhea, elevated serum amylase levels

Hepatic: Transient elevation of serum transaminase level

Hematologic: **Dose-limiting, additive myelosuppression** (leukopenia and thrombocytopenia at high doses >1000 mg/m^2)

Local: Pain at injection site (13%)

Drug Interactions Dexrazoxane can have either a synergistic or inhibitory activity with different anthracyclines

Stability Reconstituted solution is stable for 6 hours at room temperature or under refrigeration. Dexrazoxane degrades rapidly at pH >7.

Mechanism of Action Dexrazoxane is a piperazine EDTA derivative that rapidly penetrates the myocardial cell membrane. It binds intracellular iron and prevents generation of oxygen free radicals by anthracyclines. Dexrazoxane is hydrolyzed intracellularly to an open-ring chelating agent which is responsible for chelating heavy metals and preventing formation of superhydroxide free radicals believed to be responsible for anthracycline-induced cardiomyopathy. Dexrazoxane may also have antitumor activity and have synergistic activity with certain cytotoxic agents.

Pharmacokinetics Minimal data in the pediatric population

Distribution: V_d:

Children: 0.67 L/kg

Adults: 1.3 L/kg

Protein binding: Insignificant

Half-life: Biphasic

Distribution half-life: 8-21 minutes

Terminal half-life: 2-3 hours

Elimination: 40% to 60% of dose excreted renally within 24 hours; removed by peritoneal or hemodialysis

Usual Dosage I.V. (refer to individual protocols):

Children: 10:1 dose ratio with doxorubicin (example: 250 mg/m^2 dexrazoxane: 25 mg/m^2 doxorubicin) is currently recommended; 20:1 ratio with doxorubicin has been studied, but due to higher incidence of adverse reactions is no longer recommended

Adults: 10:1 ratio with doxorubicin (example: 500 mg/m^2 dexrazoxane: 50 mg/m^2 doxorubicin); administer 30 minutes before doxorubicin

Administration Parenteral: Reconstitute with 0.167 Molar sodium lactate injection to a concentration of 10 mg/mL. Administer slow I.V. push or further dilute in NS or D_5W to a final concentration of 1.3-5 mg/mL and give as a rapid I.V. infusion over 15-30 minutes

Monitoring Parameters CBC with differential and platelet count; cardiac function tests; serum triglycerides, iron, calcium, and zinc levels; liver function tests

Nursing Implications To ensure optimal chemoprotectant effect, do not allow chemotherapy to be delayed following completion of dexrazoxane

Dosage Forms Injection, powder for reconstitution, as hydrochloride: 250 mg, 500 mg [contains 0.167 M sodium lactate injection diluent]

References

Sehested M, et al, "Dexrazoxane for Protection Against Cardiotoxic Effects of Anthracyclines," *J Clin Oncol*, 1996, 14:2884.

Swain SM, et al, "Cardioprotection With Dexrazoxane for Doxorubicin-Containing Therapy in Advanced Breast Cancer," *J Clin Oncol*, 1997, 15:1318-32.

Swain SM, et al, "Delayed Administration of Dexrazoxane Provides Cardioprotection for Patients With Advanced Breast Cancer Treated With Doxorubicin-Containing Therapy," *J Clin Oncol*, 1997, 15:1333-40.

Wexler LH, et al, "Randomized Trial of the Cardioprotective Agent ICRF-187 in Pediatric Sarcoma Patients Treated With Doxorubicin," *J Clin Oncol*, 1996, 14:362-72.

Dextran *(DEKS tran)*

U.S. Brand Names Gentran®; LMD®

Synonyms Dextran 40; Dextran 70; Dextran, High Molecular Weight; Dextran, Low Molecular Weight

Therapeutic Category Plasma Volume Expander

Generic Available Yes

Use Fluid replacement and blood volume expander used in the treatment of hypovolemia, shock, or near shock states; dextran 40 is also indicated for use as a priming fluid in pump oxygenators during extracorporeal circulation and for venous thrombosis and pulmonary embolism prophylaxis in patients undergoing surgery associated with a high incidence of thromboembolic complications (eg, hip surgery)

Pregnancy Risk Factor C

Contraindications Hypersensitivity to dextrans or any component; severe CHF, renal failure, severe thrombocytopenia; hypervolemia; hypofibrinogenemia; severe bleeding disorders

Warnings Use with caution in patients with CHF, pulmonary edema, renal insufficiency, thrombocytopenia, or active hemorrhage; watch for anaphylactoid reactions, have epinephrine and diphenhydramine at bedside

Precautions Use with caution in patients with extreme dehydration (renal failure may occur) and in patients with chronic liver disease

Adverse Reactions
Cardiovascular: Hypotension
Central nervous system: Fever
Dermatologic: Urticaria
Gastrointestinal: Nausea, vomiting
Hematologic: Prolongation of bleeding time with higher doses (may interfere with platelet function)
Neuromuscular & skeletal: Arthralgia
Respiratory: Wheezing, pulmonary edema with high doses, tightness of chest, dyspnea, nasal congestion
Miscellaneous: Anaphylaxis

Stability Store at room temperature; do not freeze; do not use if crystallization has occurred; discard partially used containers

Mechanism of Action Produces plasma volume expansion due to high colloidal osmotic effect (similar to albumin); draws interstitial fluid into the intravascular space; dextran 40 may also increase blood flow in microcirculation

Pharmacodynamics
Maximum effect on plasma volume:
Dextran 40: Within several minutes
Dextran 70 and dextran 75: ~1 hour

Pharmacokinetics
Metabolism: Molecules with molecular weight $\geq$50,000 are metabolized to glucose
Elimination:
Molecules with molecular weight $\leq$15,000: Rapidly eliminated in the kidney
Dextran 40: ~70% excreted in urine (unchanged) within 24 hours
Dextran 70 & 75: ~50% excreted in urine within 24 hours

Usual Dosage I.V. (dose and infusion rate are dependent upon the patient's fluid status and must be individualized):

Volume expansion/shock:
Children: Total dose should not be >20 mL/kg during first 24 hours and not >10 mL/kg/day thereafter; do not treat for >5 days
Adults: 500-1000 mL at rate of 20-40 mL/minute
Maximum daily dose: First 24 hours: 20 mL/kg and 10 mL/kg/day thereafter; therapy should not continue beyond 5 days

Administration Parenteral: I.V. infusion only; usual maximum infusion rate (adults): 4 mL/minute; maximum infusion rate in emergency situations (adults): 20-40 mL/minute

Monitoring Parameters Vital signs, signs of allergic/anaphylactoid reaction especially for 30 minutes after starting infusions; signs of circulatory overload (ie, heart rate, blood pressure, central venous pressure, hematocrit), urine output; urine specific gravity; platelets

Test Interactions Falsely elevated serum glucose when determined by methods that use high concentrations of acid (eg, sulfuric acid, acetic acid); may interfere with bilirubin assays that use alcohol and total protein assays using biuret reagents; dextran 70 may produce erythrocyte aggregation and interfere with blood typing and cross matching of blood

Nursing Implications Be prepared to treat anaphylaxis with epinephrine, antihistamines, supportive therapy, and alternative agents to dextran to maintain circulation; do not administer if cloudy or if solution contains dextran flakes; discontinue dextran if urine specific gravity is low, if oliguria or anuria occur, or if there is a rapid acute rise in central venous pressure or other signs of circulatory overload

Additional Information Dextran in sodium chloride 0.9% contains sodium chloride 154 mEq/L

Dosage Forms
Injection, solution, high molecular weight (Gentran®): 6% dextran 70 in sodium chloride 0.9% (500 mL)
(Continued)

Dextran *(Continued)*

Injection, solution, low molecular weight (Gentran®, LMD®): 10% dextran 40 in D_5W (500 mL); 10% dextran 40 in sodium chloride 0.9% (500 mL)

- ◆ **Dextran 40** *see Dextran on page 358*
- ◆ **Dextran 70** *see Dextran on page 358*
- ◆ **Dextran, High Molecular Weight** *see Dextran on page 358*
- ◆ **Dextran, Low Molecular Weight** *see Dextran on page 358*

Dextroamphetamine (deks troe am FET a meen)

Related Information

Drugs and Breast-Feeding *on page 1404*
Laboratory Detection of Drugs in Urine *on page 1400*

U.S. Brand Names Dexedrine®; Dexedrine® Spansule®; Dextrostat®

Therapeutic Category Amphetamine; Anorexiant; Central Nervous System Stimulant, Amphetamine

Generic Available Yes

Use Adjunct in treatment of attention-deficit/hyperactivity disorder (ADHD) in children, narcolepsy, exogenous obesity

Restrictions C-II

Pregnancy Risk Factor C

Contraindications Hypersensitivity to dextroamphetamine or any component (see Warnings); advanced arteriosclerosis, hypertension, hyperthyroidism, glaucoma; concurrent use or use within 14 days of MAO inhibitors (hypertensive crisis may occur)

Warnings High potential for abuse; use in weight reduction programs only when alternative therapy has been ineffective; prolonged administration may lead to drug dependence; use in psychotic children may exacerbate symptoms of thought disorder and behavior disturbance; may potentially be associated with growth inhibition (monitor growth); may exacerbate motor and phonic tics and Tourette's syndrome; Dexedrine® and Dextrostat® tablets contain tartrazine which may cause allergic reactions in susceptible individuals

Precautions Use with caution in patients with psychopathic personalities

Adverse Reactions

Cardiovascular: Hypertension, tachycardia, palpitations, cardiac arrhythmias

Central nervous system: Insomnia, headache, nervousness, dizziness, irritability, depression; exacerbation of phonic and motor tics

Endocrine & metabolic: Growth suppression, weight loss

Gastrointestinal: Anorexia, nausea, vomiting, diarrhea, abdominal cramps, metallic taste, xerostomia

Neuromuscular & skeletal: Movement disorders, tremor

Ocular: Mydriasis

Miscellaneous: Physical and psychologic dependence with long-term use

Drug Interactions Amphetamines may decrease hypotensive effects of antihypertensives and sedative effect of antihistamines; may increase effects of tricyclic antidepressants or sympathomimetics; may delay oral absorption of ethosuximide, phenobarbital, and phenytoin; may precipitate hypertensive crisis in patients receiving MAO inhibitors (avoid use within 14 days); the herbal medicine St John's wort (*Hypericum perforatum*) may increase serious side effects, its use is **not** recommended; amphetamine may precipitate arrhythmias in patients receiving general anesthetics. With propoxyphene overdose, CNS stimulation from amphetamines is potentiated (fatal convulsions may occur); tricyclic antidepressants may enhance the effects of amphetamines (avoid use or monitor for cardiovascular effects); chlorpromazine and haloperidol may inhibit the CNS stimulant effects of amphetamines. Antacids may increase the oral absorption of amphetamines; urinary alkalinizers or large doses of antacids may decrease urinary excretion of amphetamines and increase their half-life and duration of action (dosage decrease may be needed). Acids or acidifiers may decrease the oral absorption of amphetamines; urinary acidifiers may increase urinary excretion of amphetamines and decrease their half-life and duration of action (dosage adjustment may be needed).

Food Interactions Acidic foods, juices, or vitamin C may decrease GI absorption

Mechanism of Action Blocks reuptake of dopamine and norepinephrine from the synapse, thus increases the amounts of circulating dopamine and norepinephrine in cerebral cortex to reticular activating system; inhibits the action of monoamine oxidase and causes catecholamines to be released; peripherally increases blood pressure and acts as a respiratory stimulant and weak bronchodilator

Pharmacodynamics Onset of action: Oral: 60-90 minutes

Pharmacokinetics
Metabolism: In the liver
Half-life, adults: 34 hours (pH dependent)
Time to peak serum concentration: Oral: Within 3 hours
Elimination: In urine as unchanged drug and inactive metabolites; urinary excretion is pH dependent and is increased with acid urine (low pH)

Usual Dosage Oral: **Note:** Use lowest effective individualized dose; administer first dose as soon as awake
ADHD: Children:
<3 years: Not recommended
3-5 years: Initial: 2.5 mg/day given every morning; increase by 2.5 mg/day at weekly intervals until optimal response is obtained, usual range is 0.1-0.5 mg/kg/dose every morning with maximum of 40 mg/day given in 1-3 divided doses per day
≥6 years: 5 mg once or twice daily; increase in increments of 5 mg/day at weekly intervals until optimal response is reached, usual range is 0.1-0.5 mg/kg/dose every morning (5-20 mg/day) with maximum of 40 mg/day given in 1-3 divided doses per day
Note: Tablets are usually dosed 2-3 times/day and sustained release capsules are usually given 1-2 times/day
Narcolepsy:
Children 6-12 years: Initial: 5 mg/day, may increase at 5 mg increments at weekly intervals until optimal response is obtained; maximum dose: 60 mg/day
Children >12 years and Adults: Initial: 10 mg/day, may increase at 10 mg increments at weekly intervals until optimal response is obtained; maximum dose: 60 mg/day
Exogenous obesity: Children >12 years and Adults: 5-30 mg/day in divided doses of 5-10 mg given 30-60 minutes before meals

Administration Oral: Sustained release preparations should be used for once daily dosing; do not crush or chew sustained release preparations; to avoid insomnia, last daily dose should be administered no less than 6 hours before retiring

Monitoring Parameters CNS activity, blood pressure, height, weight

Test Interactions Amphetamines may interfere with urinary steroid measurements; may cause significant increase in plasma corticosteroid levels

Patient Information May impair ability to perform activities requiring mental alertness or physical coordination; may be habit-forming; avoid abrupt discontinuation after prolonged use; limit caffeine; avoid alcohol and the herbal medicine St. John's wort; may cause dry mouth

Additional Information Treatment for ADHD should include "drug holiday" or periodic discontinuation in order to assess the patient's requirements, decrease tolerance, and limit suppression of linear growth and weight

Dosage Forms
Capsule, sustained release, as sulfate (Dexedrine® Spansule®): 5 mg, 10 mg, 15 mg
Tablet, as sulfate: 5 mg, 10 mg
Dexedrine®: 5 mg [contains tartrazine]
Dextrostat®: 5 mg, 10 mg [contains tartrazine]

References
American Academy of Pediatrics, "Clinical Practice Guideline: Treatment of the School-Aged Child With Attention-Deficit/Hyperactivity Disorder," *Pediatrics*, 2001, 108(4):1033-44.
Greenhill LL, Pliszka S, Dulcan MK, et al, "Practice Parameter for the Use of Stimulant Medications in the Treatment of Children, Adolescents, and Adults," *J Am Acad Child Adolesc Psychiatry*, 2002, 41(2 Suppl):26S-49S.

Dextroamphetamine and Amphetamine
(deks troe am FET a meen & am FET a meen)

Related Information
Dextroamphetamine *on page 360*
Drugs and Breast-Feeding *on page 1404*
Laboratory Detection of Drugs in Urine *on page 1400*

U.S. Brand Names Adderall®; Adderall XR™

Synonyms Amphetamine and Dextroamphetamine

Therapeutic Category Amphetamine; Anorexiant; Central Nervous System Stimulant, Amphetamine

Generic Available Yes (tablets)

Use Attention-deficit/hyperactivity disorder (ADHD); narcolepsy

Restrictions C-II

Pregnancy Risk Factor C

Contraindications Hypersensitivity or idiosyncrasy to dextroamphetamine, amphetamine, sympathomimetic amines, or any component; advanced arteriosclerosis, (Continued)

Dextroamphetamine and Amphetamine *(Continued)*

moderate to severe hypertension, symptomatic cardiovascular disease, hyperthyroidism, glaucoma, agitated states, history of drug abuse; concurrent use or use within 14 days of MAO inhibitors (hypertensive crisis may occur)

Warnings High potential for abuse; prolonged administration may lead to drug dependence; use in psychotic children may exacerbate symptoms of thought disorder and behavior disturbance; may potentially be associated with growth inhibition (monitor growth); may exacerbate motor and phonic tics and Tourette's syndrome

Precautions Use with caution in patients with mild hypertension; prescribe or dispense least amount feasible to minimize chance of overdose

Adverse Reactions

Cardiovascular system: Hypertension: tachycardia, palpitations; cardiomyopathy (chronic use)

Central nervous system: Insomnia, headache, nervousness, overstimulation, dizziness, euphoria, dysphoria, dyskinesia, exacerbation of phonic and motor tics; psychotic episodes (rare at recommended doses); emotional lability, depression

Dermatologic: Rash, urticaria

Endocrine and metabolic: Growth suppression, weight loss

Gastrointestinal: Anorexia, diarrhea, constipation, xerostomia, unpleasant taste

Neuromuscular and skeletal: Tremor

Miscellaneous: Physical and psychological dependence with long-term use

Drug Interactions Amphetamines may decrease hypotensive effects of antihypertensives and sedative effect of antihistamines; may increase effects of tricyclic antidepressants or sympathomimetics; may delay oral absorption of ethosuximide, phenobarbital, and phenytoin; may precipitate hypertensive crisis in patients receiving MAO inhibitors (avoid use within 14 days); the herbal medicine St John's wort (*Hypericum perforatum*) may increase serious side effects, its use is **not** recommended; amphetamines may precipitate arrhythmias in patients receiving general anesthetics. With propoxyphene overdose, CNS stimulation from amphetamines is potentiated (fatal convulsions may occur); tricyclic antidepressants may enhance the effects of amphetamines (avoid use or monitor for cardiovascular effects); chlorpromazine and haloperidol may inhibit the CNS stimulant effects of amphetamines. Antacids may increase the oral absorption of amphetamines; urinary alkalinizers or large doses of antacids may decrease urinary excretion of amphetamines and increase their half-life and duration of action (dosage decrease may be needed). Acids or acidifiers may decrease the oral absorption of amphetamines; urinary acidifiers may increase urinary excretion of amphetamines and decrease their half-life and duration of action (dosage adjustment may be needed).

Food Interactions Acidic foods, juices, or vitamin C may decrease oral absorption; extended release capsules: Food does not affect the extent of absorption; a high-fat meal delays the time to peak concentrations by 2.5 hours; similar absorption occurs if capsule is opened and contents sprinkled on applesauce versus swallowing intact capsule on an empty stomach

Stability Store at controlled room temperature; dispense in tight, light-resistant container

Mechanism of Action Blocks reuptake of dopamine and norepinephrine from the synapse, thus increases the amounts of circulating dopamine and norepinephrine in cerebral cortex to reticular activating system; inhibits the action of monoamine oxidase and causes catecholamines to be released; peripherally increases blood pressure and acts as a respiratory stimulant and weak bronchodilator

Pharmacodynamics Oral:

Onset of action: Tablet: 30-60 minutes

Duration: Tablet: 4-6 hours

Pharmacokinetics

Absorption: Oral: Well-absorbed

Distribution: V_d: Adults: 3.5-4.6 L/kg; concentrates in breast milk (avoid breastfeeding); distributes into CNS, mean CSF concentrations are 80% of plasma

Metabolism: In the liver by cytochrome P450 mono-oxygenase and glucuronidation

Half-life:

d-amphetamine:

Children 6-12 years: 9 hours

Adults: 10 hours

l-amphetamine:

Children 6-12 years: 11 hours

Adults: 13 hours

Time to peak serum concentration:

Tablet (immediate release): 3 hours

Capsule (extended release): 7 hours

Elimination: 70% of a single dose is eliminated within 24 hours; excreted as unchanged amphetamine (30%), benzoic acid, hydroxy-amphetamine, hippuric acid, norephedrine and p-hydroxynorephedrine

Usual Dosage Oral: **Note:** Use lowest effective individualized dose; administer first dose as soon as awake

Tablet: **Note:** Use intervals of 4-6 hours between additional doses; tablets are usually doses 1-2 times/day

ADHD:

Children <3 years: Not recommended

Children 3-5 years: Initial 2.5 mg/day given every morning; increase daily dose by 2.5 mg at weekly intervals until optimal response is obtained; maximum dose: 40 mg/day given in 1-3 divided doses per day

Children ≥6 years: Initial: 5 mg once or twice daily; increase daily dose by 5 mg at weekly intervals until optimal response is obtained; usual maximum dose: 40 mg/day given in 1-3 divided doses per day

Narcolepsy:

Children 6-12 years: Initial: 5 mg/day; increase daily dose by 5 mg at weekly intervals until optimal response is obtained; maximum dose: 60 mg/day given in 1-3 divided doses per day

Children >12 years and Adults: Initial: 10 mg/day; increase daily dose by 10 mg at weekly intervals until optimal response is obtained; maximum dose: 60 mg/day given in 1-3 divided doses per day

Extended release capsule (Adderall XR®):

ADHD:

Children <3 years: Not recommended

Children 3-5 years: Has not been studied

Children ≥6 years: Initial: 10 mg/day given every morning (may initiate with 5 mg/day given every morning if lower dose is clinically needed); increase daily dose by 5 mg or 10 mg at weekly intervals until optimal response is obtained; maximum dose: 30 mg once daily; doses >30 mg/day have not been studied; **Note:** Patients taking divided doses of immediate release tablets may be switched to extended release capsule using the same total daily dose (taken once daily); titrate dose at weekly intervals to achieve optimal response

Administration Oral:

Tablet: To avoid insomnia, last daily dose should be administered no less than 6 hours before retiring

Extended release capsule: Avoid afternoon doses to prevent insomnia. Swallow capsule whole; do not chew or divide. May open capsule and sprinkle contents on applesauce; consume applesauce/medication mixture immediately; do not store; do not chew sprinkled beads from capsule

Monitoring Parameters CNS activity, blood pressure, height, weight

Test Interactions Amphetamines may interfere with urinary steroid measurements; may cause significant increase in plasma corticosteroid levels

Patient Information May impair ability to perform activities requiring mental alertness or physical coordination; may be habit-forming; avoid abrupt discontinuation after prolonged use; limit caffeine; avoid alcohol and the herbal medicine St John's wort; may cause dry mouth

Additional Information Treatment of ADHD should include "drug holidays" or periodic discontinuation of medication in order to assess the patient's requirments, decrease tolerance, and limit suppression of linear growth and weight; the combination of equal parts of d, l-amphetamine aspartate, d, l-amphetamine sulfate, dextroamphetamine saccharate and dextroamphetamine sulfate results in a 3:1 ratio of the dextro- and levo isomers of amphetamine.

The duration of action of Adderall® is longer than methylphenidate; behavioral effects of a single morning dose of Adderall® may last throughout the school day; a single morning dose of Adderall® has been shown in several studies to be as effective as twice daily dosing of methylphenidate for the treatment of ADHD (see Pelham, 1999a; Manos 1999; Pliszka 2000).

A recent randomized, double-blind, placebo-controlled crossover trial of Adderall® in children with ADHD demonstrated efficacy rates of 82% based on parent response, 77% based on teacher response, and 59% based on concurrence between parent and teacher response; reported side effects included decreased appetite, stomach aches, insomnia, and headaches; decreased appetite and insomnia were more problematic on the high dose (0.3 mg/kg/dose twice daily) versus the low dose (0.15 mg/kg/dose twice daily); headaches occurred more frequently on the high dose, suggesting a dose-dependency (Ahmann, 2001).

Long term use of Adderall XR® (ie, >3 weeks) has not been studied; long term usefulness should be periodically re-evaluated for the individual patient
(Continued)

Dextroamphetamine and Amphetamine *(Continued)*

Dosage Forms

Capsule, extended release (Adderall XR™):

5 mg [amphetamine aspartate monohydrate 1.25 mg, amphetamine sulfate 1.25 mg, dextroamphetamine saccharate 1.25 mg, dextroamphetamine sulfate 1.25 mg; total amphetamine base equivalence: 3.1 mg]

10 mg [amphetamine aspartate monohydrate 2.5 mg, amphetamine sulfate 2.5 mg, dextroamphetamine saccharate 2.5 mg, dextroamphetamine sulfate 2.5 mg; total amphetamine base equivalence: 6.3 mg]

15 mg [amphetamine aspartate monohydrate 3.75 mg, amphetamine sulfate 3.75 mg, dextroamphetamine saccharate 3.75 mg, dextroamphetamine sulfate 3.75 mg; total amphetamine base equivalence: 9.4 mg]

20 mg [amphetamine aspartate monohydrate 5 mg, amphetamine sulfate 5 mg, dextroamphetamine saccharate 5 mg, dextroamphetamine sulfate 5 mg; total amphetamine base equivalence: 12.5 mg]

25 mg [amphetamine aspartate monohydrate 6.25 mg, amphetamine sulfate 6.25 mg, dextroamphetamine saccharate 6.25 mg, dextroamphetamine sulfate 6.25 mg; total amphetamine base equivalence: 15.6 mg]

30 mg [amphetamine aspartate monohydrate 7.5 mg, amphetamine sulfate 7.5 mg, dextroamphetamine saccharate 7.5 mg, dextroamphetamine sulfate 7.5 mg; total amphetamine base equivalence: 18.8 mg]

Tablet: **5 mg** [amphetamine aspartate 1.25 mg, amphetamine sulfate 1.25 mg, dextroamphetamine saccharate 1.25 mg, dextroamphetamine sulfate 1.25 mg; total amphetamine base equivalence: 3.13 mg]; **10 mg** [amphetamine aspartate 2.5 mg, amphetamine sulfate 2.5 mg, dextroamphetamine saccharate 2.5 mg, dextroamphetamine sulfate 2.5 mg; total amphetamine base equivalence: 6.3 mg]; **20 mg** [amphetamine aspartate 5 mg, amphetamine sulfate 5 mg, dextroamphetamine saccharate 5 mg, dextroamphetamine sulfate 5 mg; total amphetamine base equivalence: 12.6 mg]; **30 mg** [amphetamine aspartate 7.5 mg, amphetamine sulfate 7.5 mg, dextroamphetamine saccharate 7.5 mg, dextroamphetamine sulfate 7.5 mg; total amphetamine base equivalence: 18.8 mg]

Adderall®:

5 mg [amphetamine aspartate 1.25 mg, amphetamine sulfate 1.25 mg, dextroamphetamine saccharate 1.25 mg, dextroamphetamine sulfate 1.25 mg; total amphetamine base equivalence: 3.13 mg]

7.5 mg [amphetamine aspartate 1.875 mg, amphetamine sulfate 1.875 mg, dextroamphetamine saccharate 1.875 mg, dextroamphetamine sulfate 1.875 mg; total amphetamine base equivalence: 4.7 mg]

10 mg [amphetamine aspartate 2.5 mg, amphetamine sulfate 2.5 mg, dextroamphetamine saccharate 2.5 mg, dextroamphetamine sulfate 2.5 mg; total amphetamine base equivalence: 6.3 mg]

12.5 mg [amphetamine aspartate 3.125 mg, amphetamine sulfate 3.125 mg, dextroamphetamine saccharate 3.125 mg, dextroamphetamine sulfate 3.125 mg; total amphetamine base equivalence: 7.8 mg]

15 mg [amphetamine aspartate 3.75 mg, amphetamine sulfate 3.75 mg, dextroamphetamine saccharate 3.75 mg, dextroamphetamine sulfate 3.75 mg; total amphetamine base equivalence: 9.4 mg]

20 mg [amphetamine aspartate 5 mg, amphetamine sulfate 5 mg, dextroamphetamine saccharate 5 mg, dextroamphetamine sulfate 5 mg; total amphetamine base equivalence: 12.6 mg]

30 mg [amphetamine aspartate 7.5 mg, amphetamine sulfate 7.5 mg, dextroamphetamine saccharate 7.5 mg, dextroamphetamine sulfate 7.5 mg; total amphetamine base equivalence: 18.8 mg]

Extemporaneous Preparations A 1 mg/mL oral formulation of Adderall® in 3 different vehicles (Ora-Sweet®, Ora-Plus®, and a 1:1 mixture of Ora-Sweet® and Ora-Plus®) was found to be stable for 30 days when stored in glass bottles in the dark at 25°C and 60% relative humidity; ten 10 mg Adderall® tablets were crushed in a mortar into a fine powder; approximately 20 mL of vehicle was added to the mortar and triturated well; the contents were transferred to a 4 ounce glass prescription bottle; the mortar was rinsed with approximately 20 mL of vehicle and transferred to the bottle (this was repeated until the final volume was qsad to 100 mL); label "shake well" and "protect from light"

Justice J, Kupiec TC, Matthews P, et al, "Stability of Adderall® in Extemporaneously Compounded Oral Liquids," *Am J Health Syst Pharm*, 2001, 58(15):1418-21.

References

Ahmann PA, Theye FW, Berg R, et al, "Placebo-Controlled Evaluation of Amphetamine Mixture - Dextroamphetamine Salts and Amphetamine Salts (Adderall): Efficacy Rate and Side Effects," *Pediatrics*, 2001, 107(1), http://www.pediatrics.org/cgi/content/full/107/1/e10.

American Academy of Pediatrics, "Clinical Practice Guideline: Treatment of the School-Aged Child With Attention-Deficit/Hyperactivity Disorder," *Pediatrics*, 2001, 108(4):1033-44.

Greenhill LL, Pliszka S, Dulcan MK, et al, "Practice Parameter for the Use of Stimulant Medications in the Treatment of Children, Adolescents, and Adults," *J Am Acad Child Adolesc Psychiatry*, 2002, 41(2 Suppl):26S-49S.

Manos MJ, Short EJ, and Findling RL, "Differential Effectiveness of Methylphenidate and Adderall® in School-Age Youths With Attention-Deficit/Hyperactivity Disorder," *J Am Acad Child Adolesc Psychiatry*, 1999, 38(7):813-9.

Pelham WE, Aronoff HR, Midlam JK, et al, "A Comparison of Ritalin® and Adderall®: Efficacy and Time-Course in Children With Attention-Deficit/Hyperactivity Disorder," *Pediatrics*, 1999, 103(4):e43. URL: http://www.pediatrics.org/cgi/content/full/103/4/e43

Pelham WE, Gnagy EM, Chronis AM, et al, "A Comparison of Morning-Only and Morning/Late Afternoon Adderall® to Morning-Only, Twice-Daily, and Three Times-Daily Methylphenidate in Children With Attention-Deficit/Hyperactivity Disorder," *Pediatrics*, 1999a, 104(6):1300-11.

Pliszka SR, Browne RG, Olvera RL, et al, "A Double-Blind, Placebo-Controlled Study of Adderall® and Methylphenidate in the Treatment of Attention-Deficit/Hyperactivity Disorder," *J Am Acad Child Adolesc Psychiatry*, 2000, 39(5):619-26.

Swanson JM, Wigal S, Greenhill LL, et al, "Analog Classroom Assessment of Adderall® in Children With ADHD," *J Am Acad Child Adolesc Psychiatry*, 1998, 37(5):519-26.

Dextromethorphan (deks troe meth OR fan)

U.S. Brand Names Babee Cof Syrup [OTC]; Benylin® Adult [OTC]; Benylin® Pediatric [OTC]; Creomulsion® Cough [OTC]; Creomulsion® for Children [OTC]; Creo-Terpin® [OTC]; Delsym® [OTC]; Dexalone® [OTC]; Diabe-Tuss DM [OTC]; Hold® DM [OTC]; Pertussin® DM [OTC]; Robitussin® Maximuim Strength Cough [OTC]; Robitussin® Pediatric Cough [OTC]; Scot-Tussin DM® Cough Chasers [OTC]; Silphen DM® [OTC]; Simply Cough™ [OTC]; Vicks® 44 Cough Relief [OTC]

Synonyms DM

Therapeutic Category Antitussive; Cough Preparation

Generic Available Yes

Use Symptomatic relief of coughs caused by minor viral upper respiratory tract infections or inhaled irritants

Pregnancy Risk Factor C

Contraindications Hypersensitivity to dextromethorphan or any component (see Warnings); concomitant use or use within 14 days of MAO inhibitors

Warnings Do not use for persistent or chronic cough, or for cough accompanied by excessive secretions; Creo-Terpin® contains tartrazine which may cause allergic reactions in susceptible individuals; some products may contain sodium benzoate which may cause allergic reactions in susceptible individuals; sodium benzoate has been associated with a potentially fatal toxicity ("gasping syndrome") in neonates; *in vitro* and animal studies have shown that benzoate, a metabolite of benzyl alcohol, displaces bilirubin from protein binding sites; avoid use of products containing sodium benzoate in neonates

Precautions Anecdotal reports of abuse of dextromethorphan-containing cough/cold products have increased, especially among teenagers

Adverse Reactions
Central nervous system: Drowsiness, dizziness
Gastrointestinal: Nausea

Drug Interactions Cytochrome P450 isoenzyme CYP2D6, CYP2E1, and CYP3A3/4 substrate
MAO inhibitors (increased risk of serotonin syndrome); haloperidol and fluoxetine decrease dextromethorphan metabolism; dextromethorphan decreases fluoxetine metabolism

Mechanism of Action Non-narcotic chemical relative of morphine; controls cough by depressing the medullary cough center

Pharmacodynamics
Onset of antitussive action: Within 15-30 minutes
Duration: Up to 6 hours

Pharmacokinetics
Metabolism: In the liver
Half-Life: 1.4-3.9 hours
Time to peak serum concentration: 2-2.5 hours
Elimination: Principally in urine

Usual Dosage Dosage in children <2 years of age is not well established; the following dosage recommendations in children <2 years are consistent with the dosages received when using combination products containing dextromethorphan.
Oral:
Children:
1-3 months: 0.5-1 mg every 6-8 hours
3-6 months: 1-2 mg every 6-8 hours
7 months to 1 year: 2-4 mg every 6-8 hours
≥2-6 years : 2.5-7.5 mg every 4-8 hours; extended release formulation: 15 mg twice daily (maximum: 30 mg/24 hours)
(Continued)

365

Dextromethorphan *(Continued)*

7-12 years: 5-10 mg every 4 hours or 15 mg every 6-8 hours; extended release formulation: 30 mg twice daily (maximum: 60 mg/24 hours)

Children >12 years and Adults: 10-30 mg every 4-8 hours or extended release formulation: 60 mg twice daily (maximum: 120 mg/24 hours)

Administration Oral: May administer without regard to meals

Monitoring Parameters Cough, mental status

Test Interactions Can give a false-positive on phencyclidine qualitative immunoassay screen

Patient Information If cough lasts more than 1 week or is accompanied by fever or headache, notify physician

Additional Information Dextromethorphan 15-30 mg equals 8-15 mg codeine as an antitussive

Dosage Forms

Capsule, as hydrobromide (Dexalone®): 30 mg

Liquid, as hydrobromide:

Creo-Terpin®: 10 mg/15 mL (120 mL) [contains 25% alcohol and tartrazine]

Simply Cough™: 5 mg/mL (120 mL) [contains sodium benzoate; cherry berry flavor]

Vicks 44® Cough Relief: 10 mg/5 mL (120 mL) [contains 5% alcohol, 10 mg/5 mL sodium, and sodium benzoate]

Liquid, sustained release, as polistirex, as hydrobromide (Delsym®): 30 mg/5 mL (89 mL) [contains 0.26% alcohol; orange flavor]

Lozenges, as hydrobromide:

Hold® DM: 5 mg (10s) [cherry and original flavors]

Scot-Tussin DM® Cough Chasers: 5 mg (20s)

Syrup, as hydrobromide:

Babee Cof Syrup: 7.5 mg/5 mL (120 mL) [alcohol free; dye free; cherry flavor]

Benylin® Adult: 15 mg/5 mL (120 mL) [alcohol and sugar free; raspberry flavor]

Benylin® Pediatric: 7.5 mg/mL (120 mL) [alcohol and sugar free; grape flavor]

Creomulsion® Cough: 20 mg/15 mL (120 mL) [alcohol free]

Creomulsion® for Children: 5 mg/mL (120 mL) [alcohol free; cherry flavor]

Diabe-Tuss DM: 15 mg/5 mL (120 mL)

Pertussin® DM: 15 mg/15 mL (120 mL)

Robitussin® Maximum Strength Cough: 15 mg/5 mL (120 mL, 240 mL) [contains 1.4% alcohol and sodium benzoate]

Robitussin® Pediatric Cough: 7.5 mg/mL (120 mL) [alcohol free; fruit punch flavor]

Silphen DM®: 10 mg/5 mL (120 mL)

- ◆ **Dextromethorphan and Glycerol Guaiacolate** *see* Guaifenesin and Dextromethorphan *on page 553*

- ◆ **Dextromethorphan and Guaifenesin** *see* Guaifenesin and Dextromethorphan *on page 553*

- ◆ **Dextropropoxyphene** *see* Propoxyphene *on page 950*

Dextrose *(DEKS trose)*

Related Information

Fluid and Electrolyte Requirements in Children *on page 1258*

Parenteral Nutrition (PN) *on page 1262*

U.S. Brand Names B-D™ Glucose [OTC]; Dex4 Glucose [OTC]; Enfamil® Glucose; Glutol™ [OTC]; Glutose™ [OTC]; Insta-Glucose® [OTC]

Synonyms Anhydrous Glucose; D_5W; $D_{10}W$; $D_{25}W$; $D_{30}W$; $D_{40}W$; $D_{50}W$; $D_{60}W$; $D_{70}W$; Dextrose Monohydrate; Glucose; Glucose Monohydrate; Glycosum

Therapeutic Category Antidote, Insulin; Antidote, Oral Hypoglycemic; Fluid Replacement, Enteral; Fluid Replacement, Parenteral; Hyperglycemic Agent; Hyperkalemia, Adjunctive Treatment Agent; Intravenous Nutritional Therapy

Generic Available Yes

Use

5% and 10% solutions: Peripheral infusion to provide calories and fluid replacement

10% solution: Treatment of hypoglycemia in premature neonates

25% (hypertonic) solution: Treatment of acute symptomatic episodes of hypoglycemia in infants and children to restore depressed blood glucose levels; adjunctive treatment of hyperkalemia when combined with insulin

50% (hypertonic) solution: Treatment of insulin-induced hypoglycemia (hyperinsulinemia or insulin shock) and adjunctive treatment of hyperkalemia in adolescents and adults

≥10% solutions: Infusion after admixture with amino acids for nutritional support

Pregnancy Risk Factor C

Contraindications Hypersensitivity to corn or corn products; diabetic coma with hyperglycemia; hypertonic solutions in patients with intracranial or intraspinal hemorrhage; patients with delirium tremens and dehydration; patients with anuria, hepatic coma, or glucose-galactose malabsorption syndrome

Warnings Hypertonic solutions (>10%) may cause thrombosis if infused via peripheral veins; administer hypertonic solutions via a central venous catheter; rapid administration of hypertonic solutions may produce significant hyperglycemia, glycosuria, and shifts in electrolytes; this may result in dehydration, hyperosmolar syndrome, coma, and death especially in patients with chronic uremia or carbohydrate intolerance; excessive or rapid dextrose administration in very low birth weight infants has been associated with increased serum osmolality and possible intracerebral hemorrhage; hyperglycemia and glycosuria may be functions of the rate of administration of dextrose; to minimize these effects, reduce the rate of infusion; addition of insulin may be necessary; administration of potassium free I.V. dextrose solutions may result in significant hypokalemia, particularly if highly concentrated dextrose solutions are used; add potassium to dextrose solutions for patients with adequate renal function; abrupt withdrawal of dextrose solution may be associated with rebound hypoglycemia; an unexpected rise in blood glucose level in an otherwise stable patient may be an early symptom of infection; glucose is not absorbed from the buccal cavity; it must be swallowed to be effective; do not use oral forms in unconscious patients

Parenteral dextrose solutions contain aluminum which may accumulate to toxic levels with prolonged administration particularly in patients with impaired renal function. Patients with impaired renal function including premature neonates who receive aluminum at >4-5 mcg/kg/day accumulate aluminum at levels associated with CNS and bone toxicity.

Precautions Use with caution in premature infants, especially very low birth weight infants, as rapid changes in osmolality may produce profound effects on the brain, including intraventricular hemorrhage; small incremental changes in infusion rates are necessary in these patients; use with caution also in patients with diabetes mellitus

Adverse Reactions Note: Most adverse effects are associated with excessive dosage or rate of infusion

Cardiovascular: Venous thrombosis, phlebitis, hypovolemia, hypervolemia, dehydration, edema

Central nervous system: Fever, mental confusion, unconsciousness, hyperosmolar syndrome

Endocrine & metabolic: Hyperglycemia, hypokalemia, acidosis, hypophosphatemia, hypomagnesemia

Local: Pain, vein irritation, tissue necrosis

Genitourinary: Polyuria, glycosuria, ketonuria

Gastrointestinal: Polydipsia, nausea

Respiratory: Tachypnea, pulmonary edema

Drug Interactions Corticosteroids

Stability Stable at room temperature; protect from freezing and extreme heat; store oral dextrose in airtight containers

Mechanism of Action Dextrose, a monosaccharide, is a source of calories and fluid for patients unable to obtain an adequate oral intake; may decrease body protein and nitrogen losses; promotes glycogen deposition in the liver; for the treatment of hyperkalemia, when combined with insulin, dextrose stimulates the uptake of potassium by cells, especially in muscle tissue

Pharmacodynamics

Onset of action: Treatment of hypoglycemia: Oral: 10 minutes

Maximum effect: Treatment of hyperkalemia: I.V.: 30 minutes

Pharmacokinetics

Absorption: Rapidly from the small intestine by an active mechanism

Metabolism: Metabolized to carbon dioxide and water

Time to peak serum concentration: Oral: 40 minutes

Usual Dosage

Hypoglycemia: Doses may be repeated in severe cases

I.V.:

Premature neonates: 0.1-0.2 g/kg/dose (1-2 mL/kg/dose of 10% solution); followed by continuous infusion at a rate of 4-6 mg/kg/minute

Infants ≤6 months: 0.25-0.5 g/kg/dose (1-2 mL/kg/dose of 25% solution); maximum: 25 g/dose

Infants >6 months and Children: 0.5-1 g/kg/dose (2-4 mL/kg/dose of 25% solution); maximum: 25 g/dose

Adolescents and Adults: 10-25 g (40-100 mL of 25% solution or 20-50 mL of 50% solution)

(Continued)

Dextrose *(Continued)*

Oral:

Children >2 years and Adults: 10-20 g as single dose; repeat in 10 minutes if necessary

Treatment of Hyperkalemia: I.V. (in combination with insulin):

Infants and Children: 0.5-1 g/kg (using 25% or 50% solution) combined with regular insulin 1 unit for every 4-5 g dextrose given; infuse over 2 hours (infusions as short as 30 minutes have been recommended); repeat as needed

Adolescents and Adults: 25-50 g dextrose (250-500 mL D$_{10}$W) combined with 10 units regular insulin administered over 30-60 minutes; repeat as needed or as an alternative 25 g dextrose (50 mL D$_{50}$W) combined with 5-10 units regular insulin infused over 5 minutes; repeat as needed

Note: More rapid infusions (<30 minutes) may be associated with hyperglycemia and hyperosmolality and will exacerbate hyperkalemia; avoid use in patients who are already hyperglycemic

Fluid therapy: See Fluid and Electrolyte Requirements in Children *on page 1258*

Nutrition: See Parenteral Nutrition (PN) *on page 1262*

Administration

Oral: Must be swallowed to be absorbed (see Warnings)

Parenteral: Not for S.C. or I.M. administration; dilute concentrated dextrose solutions for peripheral venous administration to a maximum concentration of 12.5%; in emergency situations, 25% dextrose has been used peripherally; for direct I.V. infusion, infuse at a maximum rate of 200 mg/kg over 1 minute; continuous infusion rates very with tolerance (see Parenteral Nutrition (PN) *on page 1262*) and range from 4.5-15 mg/kg/minute; hyperinsulinemic neonates may require up to 15-25 mg/kg/minute infusion rates

Monitoring Parameters Blood and urine sugar, serum electrolytes, I & O, caloric intake

Reference Range Normal blood sugar:

Neonates: 110-270 mg/dL

0-2 years: 60-105 mg/dL

Children >2 years and Adults: 70-110 mg/dL

Additional Information Each g of I.V. dextrose contains 3.4 kcal; glucose monohydrate 1 g is equal to 1 g anhydrous dextrose; osmolarity of 10% dextrose is 505 mOsm/L and 25% dextrose is 1330 mOsm/L. Normal body fluid osmolarity is 310 mOsm/L.

Dosage Forms

Gel, as 40% dextrose:

Glutose™: 40% (15 g, 45 g)

Insta-Glucose®: 40% (30 g)

Infusion, as 2.5% dextrose: 1000 mL

Infusion, as 5% dextrose: 25 mL, 50 mL, 100 mL, 150 mL, 250 mL, 500 mL, 1000 mL

Infusion, as 10% dextrose: 3 mL, 5 mL, 250 mL, 500 mL, 1000 mL

Infusion, as 20% dextrose: 500 mL, 1000 mL

Infusion, as 25% dextrose: 10 mL

Infusion, as 30% dextrose: 500 mL, 1000 mL

Infusion, as 40% dextrose: 500 mL, 1000 mL

Infusion, as 50% dextrose: 50 mL, 500 mL, 1000 mL, 2000 mL

Infusion, as 60% dextrose: 500 mL, 1000 mL

Infusion, as 70% dextrose: 70 mL, 500 mL, 1000 mL, 2000 mL

Solution, oral:

Enfamil® Glucose: 5% (90 mL) [5 g dextrose/100 mL]; 10% (90 mL) [10 g dextrose/100 mL]

Gluto™: 55% (180 mL) [100 g dextrose/180 mL]

Tablet, chewable:

B-D™ Glucose: 5 g

Dex4 Glucose: 4 g

- ◆ **Dextrose Monohydrate** *see* Dextrose *on page 366*
- ◆ **Dextrostat®** *see* Dextroamphetamine *on page 360*
- ◆ **DHAD** *see* Mitoxantrone *on page 771*
- ◆ **DHE** *see* Dihydroergotamine *on page 385*
- ◆ **D.H.E. 45®** *see* Dihydroergotamine *on page 385*
- ◆ **DHPG** *see* Ganciclovir *on page 530*
- ◆ **DHS™ Sal [OTC]** *see* Salicylic Acid *on page 1002*
- ◆ **DHS™ Tar [OTC]** *see* Coal Tar *on page 299*
- ◆ **DHS™ Targel [OTC]** *see* Coal Tar *on page 299*
- ◆ **DHT™** *see* Dihydrotachysterol *on page 387*

♦ **DHT™ Intensol™** see Dihydrotachysterol *on page 387*
♦ **Diaβeta®** see GlyBURIDE *on page 540*
♦ **Diabetic Tussin DM® [OTC]** see Guaifenesin and Dextromethorphan *on page 553*
♦ **Diabetic Tussin® DM Maximum Strength [OTC]** see Guaifenesin and Dextromethorphan *on page 553*
♦ **Diabetic Tussin EX® [OTC]** see Guaifenesin *on page 550*
♦ **Diabe-Tuss DM [OTC]** see Dextromethorphan *on page 365*
♦ **Diaminodiphenylsulfone** see Dapsone *on page 339*
♦ **Diamox®** see AcetaZOLAMIDE *on page 40*
♦ **Diamox Sequels®** see AcetaZOLAMIDE *on page 40*
♦ **Diarr-Eze (Can)** see Loperamide *on page 687*
♦ **Diasorb® [OTC]** see Attapulgite *on page 146*
♦ **Diastat® Rectal Delivery System** see Diazepam *on page 369*
♦ **Diazemuls® (Can)** see Diazepam *on page 369*

Diazepam (dye AZ e pam)

Related Information
Adult ACLS Algorithm, Synchronized Cardioversion *on page 1192*
Carbohydrate and Alcohol Content of Liquid Medications for Use in Patients Receiving Ketogenic Diets *on page 1431*
Drugs and Breast-Feeding *on page 1404*
Laboratory Detection of Drugs in Urine *on page 1400*
Overdose and Toxicology *on page 1388*
Preprocedure Sedatives in Children *on page 1367*

U.S. Brand Names Diastat® Rectal Delivery System; Diazepam Intensol®; Valium®
Canadian Brand Names Apo®-Diazepam; Diazemuls®
Therapeutic Category Antianxiety Agent; Anticonvulsant, Benzodiazepine; Benzodiazepine; Hypnotic; Sedative

Generic Available
Yes (injection, tablets, and solution)

Use Management of general anxiety disorders, panic disorders; to provide preoperative sedation, light anesthesia, and amnesia; treatment of status epilepticus, alcohol withdrawal symptoms; used as a skeletal muscle relaxant; rectal gel is indicated for intermittent episodes of markedly increased seizure activity in epilepsy patients on stable anticonvulsant regimens

Restrictions C-IV

Pregnancy Risk Factor D

Contraindications Hypersensitivity to diazepam or any component (see Warnings); possible cross-sensitivity with other benzodiazepines; do not use in a comatose patient, in those with pre-existing CNS depression, respiratory depression, narrow-angle glaucoma, or severe uncontrolled pain

Warnings Abrupt discontinuation may cause withdrawal symptoms or seizures. Rapid I.V. push may cause sudden respiratory depression, apnea, or hypotension. Injection and rectal gel contain benzoic acid, benzyl alcohol, and sodium benzoate; benzyl alcohol may cause allergic reactions in susceptible individuals; benzoic acid (benzoate) is a metabolite of benzyl alcohol; large amounts of benzyl alcohol (≥ 99 mg/kg/day) have been associated with a potentially fatal toxicity ("gasping syndrome") in neonates; the "gasping syndrome" consists of metabolic acidosis, respiratory distress, gasping respirations, CNS dysfunction (including convulsions, intracranial hemorrhage), hypotension and cardiovascular collapse; use diazepam products containing benzoic acid, benzyl alcohol, or sodium benzoate with caution in neonates; *in vitro* and animal studies have shown that benzoate displaces bilirubin from protein binding sites

Precautions Use with caution in patients receiving other CNS depressants, patients with low albumin, renal or hepatic dysfunction, and in neonates and young infants; neonates have decreased metabolism of diazepam and desmethyldiazepam (active metabolite), both can accumulate with repeated use and cause increased toxicity; modify dosage in patients with hepatic impairment

Adverse Reactions
Cardiovascular: Cardiac arrest, hypotension, bradycardia, cardiovascular collapse
Central nervous system: Drowsiness, somnolence, confusion, dizziness, fatigue, amnesia, slurred speech, ataxia, impaired coordination, paradoxical excitement or rage (rare)
Dermatologic: Rash, dermatitis
Local: Thrombophlebitis; pain with injection; tissue necrosis may occur following extravasation
Ocular: Blurred vision, diplopia
Respiratory: Decrease in respiratory rate, apnea, laryngospasm
(Continued)

Diazepam *(Continued)*

Miscellaneous: Physical and psychological dependence with prolonged use

Drug Interactions Cytochrome P450 isoenzyme CYP2B6, CYP2C8, CYP2C9, CYP2C19 (minor), CYP3A3/4 (minor) and CYP3A5-7 substrate; isoenzyme CYP2C19 and CYP3A3/4 inhibitor; nordiazepam is a CYP1A2 isoenzyme substrate; desmethyldiazepam is a CYP2C19 isoenzyme substrate

CNS depressants (alcohol, barbiturates, opioids) may enhance sedation and respiratory depression of diazepam; enzyme inducers may increase the hepatic metabolism of diazepam; cimetidine and erythromycin may decrease the metabolism of diazepam; valproic acid may displace diazepam from binding sites which may result in an increase in sedative effects; concurrent use of diazepam with ritonavir is not recommended

Food Interactions Grapefruit juice significantly increases oral bioavailability of diazepam

Stability Injection: Do not mix with other medications; protect from light

Mechanism of Action Depresses all levels of the CNS, including the limbic and reticular formation by binding to the benzodiazepine site on the gamma-aminobutyric acid (GABA) receptor complex and modulating GABA, which is a major inhibitory neurotransmitter in the brain

Pharmacodynamics Status epilepticus:

Onset of action:
I.V.: 1-3 minutes
Rectal: 2-10 minutes
Duration: 15-30 minutes

Pharmacokinetics

Absorption:
Oral: 85% to 100%
I.M.: Poor
Rectal (gel): Well absorbed

Distribution: Widely distributed; crosses blood-brain barrier and placenta; distributes into breast milk

Protein binding:
Neonates: 84% to 86%
Adults: 98%

Metabolism: In the liver to desmethyldiazepam (active metabolite) and N-methyloxazepam (active metabolite); these are metabolized to oxazepam (active) which undergoes glucuronide conjugation before being excreted

Bioavailability: Rectal (gel): 90%

Half-life:
Diazepam:
Neonates: 50-95 hours
Infants 1 month to 2 years: 40-50 hours
Children 2-12 years: 15-21 hours
Children 12-16 years: 18-20 hours
Adults: 20-50 hours
Increased half-life in those with severe hepatic disorders
Desmethyldiazepam (active metabolite): 50-100 hours; may be further prolonged in neonates

Time to peak serum concentration: Rectal (gel): 1.5 hours

Elimination: In urine, primarily as conjugated oxazepam (75%), desmethyldiazepam, and N-methyloxazepam

Usual Dosage

Children:
Conscious sedation for procedures: Oral: 0.2-0.3 mg/kg (maximum dose: 10 mg) 45-60 minutes prior to procedure

Febrile seizure prophylaxis: Oral: 1 mg/kg/day divided every 8 hours; initiate therapy at first sign of fever and continue for 24 hours after fever is gone

Sedation or muscle relaxation or anxiety:
Oral: 0.12-0.8 mg/kg/day in divided doses every 6-8 hours
I.M., I.V.: 0.04-0.3 mg/kg/dose every 2-4 hours to a maximum of 0.6 mg/kg within an 8-hour period if needed

Status epilepticus: I.V.:
Neonates: (Not recommended as a first-line agent; injection contains benzoic acid, benzyl alcohol, and sodium benzoate; see Warnings) 0.1-0.3 mg/kg/dose given over 3-5 minutes, every 15-30 minutes to a maximum total dose of 2 mg

Infants >30 days and Children <5 years: 0.05-0.3 mg/kg/dose given over 3-5 minutes, every 15-30 minutes to a maximum total dose of 5 mg **or** 0.2-0.5 mg/dose every 2-5 minutes to a maximum total dose of 5 mg; repeat in 2-4 hours as needed

Children ≥5 years: 0.05-0.3 mg/kg/dose given over 3-5 minutes, every 15-30 minutes to a maximum total dose of 10 mg **or** 1 mg/dose every 2-5 minutes to a maximum of 10 mg; repeat in 2-4 hours as needed

Muscle spasm associated with tetanus: I.V., I.M.:
Infants >30 days: 1-2 mg/dose every 3-4 hours as needed
Children ≥5 years: 5-10 mg/dose every 3-4 hours as needed

Anticonvulsant: Acute treatment:
Rectal gel formulation:
Infants <6 months: Not recommended
Children <2 years: Safety and efficacy have not been studied
Children 2-5 years: 0.5 mg/kg
Children 6-11 years: 0.3 mg/kg
Children ≥12 years and Adults: 0.2 mg/kg
Note: Round dose to 2.5, 5, 10, 15, and 20 mg/dose; dose may be repeated in 4-12 hours if needed; do not use more than 5 times per month or more than once every 5 days

Rectal: Undiluted 5 mg/mL parenteral formulation (filter if using ampul): 0.5 mg/kg/dose then 0.25 mg/kg/dose in 10 minutes if needed

Adolescents: Conscious sedation for procedures:
Oral: 10 mg
I.V.: 5 mg; may repeat with 2.5 mg if needed

Adults:
Anxiety:
Oral: 2-10 mg 2-4 times/day
I.M., I.V.: 2-10 mg, may repeat in 3-4 hours if needed
Skeletal muscle relaxation:
Oral: 2-10 mg 2-4 times/day
I.M., I.V.: 5-10 mg, may repeat in 2-4 hours
Status epilepticus: I.V.: 5-10 mg every 10-15 minutes up to 30 mg in an 8-hour period; may repeat in 2-4 hours
Preoperative medication: I.M.: 10 mg before surgery

Administration

Oral: Administer with food or water; do not administer with grapefruit juice; oral concentrate solution (5 mg/mL) should be diluted or mixed with water, juice, soda, applesauce, or pudding before use

Parenteral: I.V.: Rapid injection may cause respiratory depression or hypotension; infants and children: Do not exceed 1-2 mg/minute I.V. push; adults: Maximum infusion rate: 5 mg/minute; maximum concentration for administration: 5 mg/mL

Rectal: Diastat®: Place patient on side; remove protective cap and seal pin from syringe; lubricate rectal tip with lubricating jelly (provided in twin pack); turn patient on side facing you; bend upper leg forward and separate buttocks to expose rectum; insert syringe tip gently into rectum until rim fits snug against rectal opening; administer dose while slowly counting to 3 while gently pushing on plunger; slowly count to 3 again before removing syringe; hold buttocks together while slowing counting to 3 to prevent leakage; keep patient on side, facing towards you and continue to observe patient; discard syringe and all used materials safely away from children; do not reuse

Monitoring Parameters Heart rate, respiratory rate, blood pressure

Reference Range Effective therapeutic range not well established
Proposed therapeutic:
Diazepam: 0.2-1.5 µg/mL (SI: 0.7-5.3 µmol/L)
N-desmethyldiazepam (nordiazepam): 0.1-0.5 µg/mL (SI: 0.35-1.8 µmol/L)

Test Interactions False-negative urinary glucose determinations with Clinistix® or Diastix®

Patient Information Avoid alcohol and grapefruit juice; limit caffeine; may cause drowsiness and impair ability to perform activities requiring mental alertness or physical coordination; may be habit-forming; avoid abrupt discontinuation after prolonged use

Nursing Implications Avoid extravasation (tissue necrosis may occur); infuse I.V. into secure line using larger veins

Additional Information Diazepam does not have any analgesic effects. Diarrhea in a 9 month old infant receiving high-dose oral diazepam was attributed to the diazepam oral solution that contained polyethylene glycol and propylene glycol (both are osmotically active); diarrhea resolved when crushed tablets were substituted for the oral solution (see Marshall, 1995). In addition to additives listed in the Dosage Forms field, the injection contains 40% propylene glycol.

Dosage Forms

Gel, rectal delivery system (Diastat®):
Adult rectal tip [6 cm]: 5 mg/mL (15 mg, 20 mg) [contains 10% ethyl alcohol, benzoic acid, benzyl alcohol, and sodium benzoate; twin pack]

(Continued)

Diazepam *(Continued)*

Pediatric rectal tip [4.4 cm]: 5 mg/mL (2.5 mg, 5 mg) [contains 10% ethyl alcohol, benzoic acid, benzyl alcohol, and sodium benzoate; twin pack]

Universal rectal tip [for pediatric and adult use; 4.4 cm]: 5 mg/mL (10 mg) [contains 10% ethyl alcohol, benzoic acid, benzyl alcohol, and sodium benzoate; twin pack]

Injection, solution: 5 mg/mL (2 mL, 10 mL) [contains 10% alcohol, benzoic acid, 1.5% benzyl alcohol, and sodium benzoate]

Valium®: 5 mg/mL (10 mL) [contains benzoic acid, 1.5% benzyl alcohol, 10% ethyl alcohol, and 5% sodium benzoate] [DSC]

Solution, oral: 5 mg/5 mL (5 mL, 10 mL, 500 mL) [wintergreen-spice flavor]

Solution, oral **concentrate** (Diazepam Intensol®): 5 mg/mL (30 mL)

Tablet (Valium®): 2 mg, 5 mg, 10 mg

References

Dreifuss FE, Rosman NP, Cloyd JC, et al, "A Comparison of Rectal Diazepam Gel and Placebo for Acute Repetitive Seizures," *N Engl J Med*, 1998, 338(26):1869-75.

Marshall JD, Farrar HC, and Kearns GL, "Diarrhea Associated With Enteral Benzodiazepine Solutions," *J Pediatr*, 1995, 126(4):657-9.

Rosman NP, Colton T, Labazzo J, et al, "A Controlled Trial of Diazepam Administered During Febrile Illnesses to Prevent Recurrence of Febrile Seizures," *N Engl J Med*, 1993, 329(2):79-84.

Zeltzer LK, Altman A, Cohen D, et al, "Report of the Subcommittee on the Management of Pain Associated With Procedures in Children With Cancer," *Pediatrics*, 1990, 86(5 Pt 2):826-31.

♦ **Diazepam Intensol®** *see* Diazepam *on page 369*

Diazoxide *(dye az OKS ide)*

U.S. Brand Names Hyperstat®; Proglycem®

Therapeutic Category Antihypertensive Agent; Antihypoglycemic Agent; Vasodilator

Generic Available No

Use

I.V.: Emergency lowering of blood pressure

Oral: Management of hypoglycemia related to hyperinsulinism secondary to: Islet cell adenoma, carcinoma, or hyperplasia; adenomatosis; nesidioblastosis (persistent hyperinsulinemic hypoglycemia of infancy); leucine sensitivity, or extrapancreatic malignancy

Pregnancy Risk Factor C

Contraindications Hypersensitivity to diazoxide, any component, thiazides, or other sulfonamide derivatives; I.V. diazoxide is contraindicated in patients with aortic coarctation, arteriovenous shunts, dissecting aortic aneurysm

Precautions Use with caution in patients with diabetes mellitus, renal or liver disease, coronary artery disease, or cerebral vascular insufficiency

Adverse Reactions

Cardiovascular: Hypotension, tachycardia, flushing, edema (more common in young infants and adults), arrhythmias, angina, MI; CHF (due to sodium retention)

Central nervous system: Dizziness, seizure, headache; cerebral ischemia

Dermatologic: Rash, hirsutism

Endocrine & metabolic: Hyperglycemia, ketoacidosis, hyperuricemia, sodium and water retention

Gastrointestinal: Nausea, vomiting, anorexia, constipation

Hematologic: Leukopenia, thrombocytopenia

Local: Pain, burning, cellulitis/phlebitis upon extravasation

Neuromuscular & skeletal: Weakness

Miscellaneous: Extrapyramidal symptoms and development of abnormal facies with chronic oral use

Drug Interactions Diuretics and hypotensive agents may potentiate diazoxide adverse effects; use of I.V. diazoxide within 6 hours of the administration of beta-blockers, hydralazine, methyldopa, minoxidal, nitrates, papaverine-like drugs, prazosin, or reserpine is not recommended; diazoxide may increase phenytoin metabolism or free fraction; diazoxide may decrease warfarin protein binding

Stability Protect from light, heat, and freezing; avoid using darkened solutions

Mechanism of Action Inhibits insulin release from the pancreas; produces direct smooth muscle relaxation of the peripheral arterioles which results in decrease in blood pressure and reflex increase in heart rate and cardiac output

Pharmacodynamics

Hyperglycemic effects (oral):

Onset of action: Within 1 hour

Duration (normal renal function): 8 hours

Hypotensive effects (I.V.):

Maximum effect: Within 5 minutes

Duration: Usually 3-12 hours

Pharmacokinetics
Protein binding: >90%
Half-life:
Children: 9-24 hours
Adults: 20-36 hours
Elimination: 50% excreted unchanged in urine

Usual Dosage
Hyperinsulinemic hypoglycemia: Oral (**Note:** Use lower dose listed as initial dose):
Newborns and Infants: 8-15 mg/kg/day in divided doses every 8-12 hours
Children and Adults: 3-8 mg/kg/day in divided doses every 8-12 hours
Hypertension: I.V.: Children and Adults: 1-3 mg/kg (maximum dose: 150 mg in a single injection); repeat dose in 5-15 minutes until blood pressure adequately reduced; repeat administration every 4-24 hours; monitor blood pressure closely

Administration
Oral: Administer on an empty stomach 1 hour before or 1 hour after meals; shake suspension well before use
Parenteral: Do not administer I.M. or S.C.; administer I.V. (undiluted) by rapid I.V. injection over a period of 30 seconds or less

Monitoring Parameters Blood pressure, heart rate, blood glucose, serum uric acid; CBC, platelets

Nursing Implications Avoid extravasation (injection is alkaline and irritating to tissues); patient should remain supine during and for at least 1 hour after I.V. injection

Additional Information Patients may require a diuretic with repeated I.V. doses (due to sodium retention); usual duration of I.V. therapy is <4-5 days; use of injection >10 days is not recommended

Dosage Forms
Injection, solution (Hyperstat®): 15 mg/mL (20 mL)
Suspension, oral (Proglycem®): 50 mg/mL (30 mL) [contains 7.25% alcohol; chocolate-mint flavor]

♦ **Dibenzyline®** see Phenoxybenzamine on page 890

Dibucaine (DYE byoo kane)

U.S. Brand Names Nupercainal® [OTC]
Therapeutic Category Analgesic, Topical; Local Anesthetic, Topical
Generic Available Yes
Use Fast, temporary relief of pain and itching due to hemorrhoids, minor burns, other minor skin conditions
Pregnancy Risk Factor C
Contraindications Hypersensitivity to dibucaine, other amide-type anesthetics, or any component (see Warnings)
Warnings Some products may contain sulfites which may cause allergic reactions in susceptible individuals

Adverse Reactions
Cardiovascular: Edema
Dermatologic: Urticaria, cutaneous lesions, contact dermatitis
Local: Burning, tenderness, irritation, inflammation

Mechanism of Action Blocks both the initiation and conduction of nerve impulses by decreasing the neuronal membrane's permeability to sodium ions, which results in inhibition of depolarization with resultant blockade of conduction

Pharmacodynamics
Onset of action: Within 15 minutes
Duration: 2-4 hours

Pharmacokinetics Absorption: Poor through intact skin, but well absorbed through mucous membranes and excoriated skin

Usual Dosage Children and Adults:
Rectal: Hemorrhoids: Administer each morning, evening, and after each bowel movement
Topical: Apply gently to the affected areas; no more than 30 g for adults or 7.5 g for children should be used in any 24-hour period

Administration
Rectal: Insert ointment into rectum using a rectal applicator
Topical: Apply gently to affected areas; do not use near the eyes or over denuded surfaces or blistered areas

Dosage Forms
Ointment, topical: 1% (30 g, 60 g, 454 g)
Nupercainal®: 1% (30 g, 60 g) [contains sodium bisulfite]

♦ **DIC** see Dacarbazine on page 332

♦ **Dichysterol** see Dihydrotachysterol on page 387

♦ **Dickinson's® Witch Hazel™ [OTC]** *see* Hemorrhoidal Preparations *on page 556*

Diclofenac (dye KLOE fen ak)

U.S. Brand Names Cataflam®; Solaraze™; Voltaren®; Voltaren Ophthalmic®; Voltaren®-XR

Canadian Brand Names Apo®-Diclo; Apo®-Diclo Rapide; Apo®-Diclo SR; Diclotec; Novo-Difenac®; Novo-Difenac K; Novo-Difenac-SR®; Nu-Diclo; Nu-Diclo-SR; PMS-Diclofenac; PMS-Diclofenac SR; Riva-Diclofenac; Riva-Diclofenac-K; Voltaren Rapide®

Therapeutic Category Analgesic, Non-narcotic; Anti-inflammatory Agent; Nonsteroidal Anti-inflammatory Drug (NSAID), Ophthalmic; Nonsteroidal Anti-inflammatory Drug (NSAID), Oral

Generic Available Yes

Use

Oral: Acute treatment of mild to moderate pain; acute and chronic treatment of rheumatoid arthritis, ankylosing spondylitis, and osteoarthritis; used for juvenile rheumatoid arthritis, gout, dysmenorrhea

Ophthalmic solution: Treatment of postoperative inflammation after cataract extraction; temporary relief of pain and photophobia in patients undergoing corneal refractive surgery

Topical: Treatment of actinic keratosis in adults

Pregnancy Risk Factor Oral: B (D in 3rd trimester); Ophthalmic: C; Topical: B

Contraindications Hypersensitivity to diclofenac, any component (see Warnings), aspirin, or NSAIDs; active GI bleeding; ulcer disease; patients with the "aspirin triad" [asthma, rhinitis (with or without nasal polyps) and aspirin intolerance] (fatal asthmatic and anaphylactoid reactions may occur in these patients); porphyria

Warnings Oral use: Serious GI toxicities may occur including inflammation, ulceration, bleeding, or perforation; patients with a history of PUD or GI bleeding who use NSAIDs have a >10-fold higher risk for GI bleed; other factors which may increase risk for GI bleed include: Longer duration of NSAID treatment, use of oral corticosteroids or anticoagulants, alcoholism, smoking, overall poor health, and older age. Diclofenac is not recommended for use in patients with severe renal dysfunction (if therapy is needed, close monitoring of renal function is highly recommended).

Topical gel contains benzyl alcohol which may cause allergic reactions in susceptible individuals; large amounts of benzyl alcohol (≥99 mg/kg/day) have been associated with a potentially fatal toxicity ("gasping syndrome") in neonates; avoid use of diclofenac products containing benzyl alcohol in neonates; *in vitro* and animal studies have shown that benzoate, a metabolite of benzyl alcohol, displaces bilirubin from protein binding sites

Precautions Use with caution in patients with CHF, asthma, hypertension, fluid retention, dehydration (rehydrate patient before starting therapy), mild to moderate renal dysfunction, decreased hepatic function (dosage reduction may be required), history of GI disease, or those receiving anticoagulants, ACE inhibitors, or diuretics; patients should not wear soft contact lenses while using ophthalmic solution; do not apply topical gel to open skin wounds, infections, or exfoliative dermatitis; do not allow gel to come in contact with eyes; do not use topical gel in neonates, infants, or children

Adverse Reactions

Central nervous system: Dizziness, headache

Dermatologic: Rash, pruritus; topical use: Contact dermatitis, dry skin, rash, skin exfoliation (scaling), skin irritation

Endocrine & metabolic: Fluid retention

Gastrointestinal: Abdominal pain, indigestion, peptic ulcer, GI bleeding, GI perforation, constipation, diarrhea

Hematologic: Agranulocytosis, aplastic anemia (rare), inhibition of platelet aggregation

Hepatic: Elevated ALT or AST, hepatitis, jaundice

Ocular: With ophthalmic use, itching, tearing (allergic reaction); irritation, redness, burning; ocular irritation with use of hydrogel soft contact lenses

Otic: Tinnitus

Renal: Renal impairment, nephrotic-like syndrome

Drug Interactions Cytochrome P450 isoenzyme CYP2C8 and CYP2C9 substrate; CYP2C9 isoenzyme inhibitor

Diclofenac may increase serum concentrations of digoxin, methotrexate and lithium; may increase nephrotoxicity of cyclosporine; may decrease diuretic and antihypertensive effects of thiazides and furosemide; may decrease antihypertensive effects of ACE inhibitors and angiotensin II antagonists; diclofenac plus potassium-sparing diuretics may increase serum potassium; concomitant insulin or oral hypoglycemic agents may increase or decrease serum glucose; aspirin may decrease serum concentration of diclofenac (combination not recommended); gastric irritants (eg, aspirin, other NSAIDs, potassium supplements) may increase risk of GI irritation; **Note:** Concurrent use of oral NSAIDs or aspirin with diclofenac topical gel should be minimized

Food Interactions Delayed oral absorption has been reported with food for single doses but not with chronic multiple-dose administration

Stability

Ophthalmic solution: Store at room temperature; protect from light

Tablets: Store at ≤30°C (86°F); protect from moisture; dispense in tight container

Topical gel: Store at room temperature; protect from heat; do not freeze

Mechanism of Action Inhibits prostaglandin synthesis by decreasing the activity of the enzyme, cyclooxygenase, which results in decreased formation of prostaglandin precursors

Pharmacokinetics

Absorption: Topical gel: 10%

Distribution: V_d: Adults: 1.4 L/kg

Protein binding: >99%

Metabolism: In the liver; undergoes hydroxylation then glucuronide and sulfate conjugation

Bioavailability: Oral: 50%

Half-life: Adults: 2.3 hours

Time to peak serum concentration: Adults:

Cataflam®: 1 hour

Voltaren®: 2.22 hours

Voltaren®-XR: 5.25 hours

Elimination: About 65% of the dose is eliminated in the urine and ~35% in the bile (primarily as conjugated forms); little or no unchanged drug is excreted in urine or bile

Usual Dosage Note: Cataflam® tablets are immediate release and is the formulation which should be used when prompt onset of pain relief is desired; Voltaren®-XR should not be used for acute pain relief due to its extended release

Oral:

Children: 2-3 mg/kg/day divided 2-4 times/day

Adults:

Rheumatoid arthritis:

Cataflam® or Voltaren®: 100-200 mg/day in 2-4 divided doses; maximum dose: 225 mg/day

Voltaren®-XR: 100 mg/day; dose may be increased to 100 mg twice daily; maximum dose: 200 mg/day

Osteoarthritis:

Cataflam® or Voltaren®: 100-150 mg/day in 2-3 divided doses

Voltaren®-XR: 100 mg/day

Ankylosing spondylitis: Voltaren®: 100-125 mg/day in 4-5 divided doses

Analgesia and primary dysmenorrhea: Cataflam®: 50 mg given 3 times/day; some patients may have better relief with an initial dose of 100 mg

Ophthalmic:

Cataract surgery: Instill 1 drop into affected eye 4 times/day beginning 24 hours after cataract surgery and continuing for 2 weeks

Corneal refractive surgery: Instill 1-2 drops into operative eye within the hour prior to surgery, within 15 minutes after surgery, and continuing 4 times/day for up to 3 days

Topical: Adults: Apply to affected area twice daily; recommended duration of therapy: 60-90 days

Administration

Ophthalmic: Avoid contact of bottle tip with skin or eye; apply finger pressure to lacrimal sac during and for 1-2 minutes after instillation to decrease risk of absorption and systemic effects

Oral: Administer with milk or food to decrease GI upset; do not chew or crush delayed release or extended release tablets, swallow whole

Topical: Apply a small amount of gel to affected area; smooth gently over lesion; usually 0.5 g of gel is used per 5 x 5 cm lesion site

Monitoring Parameters CBC, liver enzymes; monitor urine output, BUN, serum creatinine in patients receiving diuretics

Patient Information

Oral use: Avoid alcohol; report any signs of blood in stool, GI bleeding, weight gain, edema, skin rash, yellow skin

Ophthalmic use : Do not use hydrogel soft contact lenses during ophthalmic diclofenac therapy

Topical use: Avoid exposure to sunlight or sunlamps; notify physician if rash occurs

(Continued)

Diclofenac *(Continued)*

Additional Information Vomiting, drowsiness, and acute renal failure have been reported with overdoses; the safety of concurrent use of cosmetics, sunscreens, or other topical agents with diclofenac gel is not known

Dosage Forms

Gel, topical, as **sodium** (Solaraze™): 3% (50 g) [contains benzyl alcohol]

Solution, ophthalmic, as **sodium** (Voltaren Ophthalmic®): 0.1% (2.5 mL, 5 mL)

Tablet, as **potassium** (Cataflam®): 50 mg

Tablet, enteric coated, as **sodium** (Voltaren®): 25 mg, 50 mg, 75 mg

Tablet, extended release, as **sodium** (Voltaren®-XR): 100 mg

References

Brogden RN, Heel RC, Pakes GE, et al, "Diclofenac Sodium: A Review of Its Pharmacological Properties and Therapeutic Use in Rheumatic Diseases and Pain of Varying Origin," *Drugs*, 1980, 20(1):24-48.

Haapasaari J, Wuolijoki E, and Ylijoki H, "Treatment of Juvenile Rheumatoid Arthritis With Diclofenac Sodium" *Scand J Rheumatol*, 1983, 12(4):325-30.

♦ **Diclotec (Can)** *see* Diclofenac *on page 374*

Dicloxacillin *(dye kloks a SIL in)*

Canadian Brand Names Dycill®; Pathocil®

Therapeutic Category Antibiotic, Penicillin (Antistaphylococcal)

Generic Available Yes

Use Treatment of skin and soft tissue infections, pneumonia and follow-up therapy of osteomyelitis caused by susceptible penicillinase-producing staphylococci

Pregnancy Risk Factor B

Contraindications Hypersensitivity to dicloxacillin, penicillin, or any component

Warnings Elimination is prolonged in neonates

Adverse Reactions

Central nervous system: Fever

Dermatologic: Rash

Gastrointestinal: Nausea, vomiting, diarrhea, *C. difficile* colitis

Hematologic: Eosinophilia, neutropenia, leukopenia, thrombocytopenia

Hepatic: Elevated liver enzymes

Miscellaneous: Serum sickness-like reaction

Drug Interactions Oral contraceptives (decreased effectiveness), probenecid (increase serum concentration of dicloxacillin)

Food Interactions Food decreases the rate and extent of absorption

Mechanism of Action Inhibits bacterial cell wall synthesis by binding to one or more of the penicillin-binding proteins and interfering with the final transpeptidation step of peptidoglycan synthesis

Pharmacokinetics

Absorption: 35% to 76% absorbed from the GI tract

Distribution: Into bone, bile, pleural fluid, synovial fluid, and amniotic fluid; appears in breast milk

Protein binding: 96% to 98%

Half-life: Adults: 0.6-0.8 hours; slightly prolonged in patients with renal impairment

Time to peak serum concentration: Within 0.5-2 hours

Elimination: Partially eliminated by the liver and excreted in bile; 31% to 65% eliminated in urine as unchanged drug and active metabolite

Neonates: Prolonged

CF patients: More rapid elimination than healthy patients

Dialysis: Not dialyzable (0% to 5%)

Usual Dosage Oral:

Children <40 kg: 25-50 mg/kg/day divided every 6 hours; doses of 50-100 mg/kg/day in divided doses every 6 hours have been used for follow-up therapy of osteomyelitis; maximum dose: 2 g/day

Children >40 kg and Adults: 125-500 mg every 6 hours; maximum dose: 2 g/day

Administration Oral: Administer with water 1 hour before or 2 hours after meals on an empty stomach

Monitoring Parameters Periodic monitoring of CBC, platelet count, BUN, serum creatinine, urinalysis, and liver enzymes during prolonged therapy

Additional Information Sodium content of 250 mg capsule: 0.6 mEq

Dosage Forms Capsule, as sodium: 250 mg, 500 mg

Dicyclomine *(dye SYE kloe meen)*

Related Information

Carbohydrate and Alcohol Content of Liquid Medications for Use in Patients Receiving Ketogenic Diets *on page 1431*

Overdose and Toxicology *on page 1388*

U.S. Brand Names Bentyl®
Canadian Brand Names Bentylol®; Formulex®; Lomine
Synonyms Dicycloverine
Therapeutic Category Anticholinergic Agent; Antispasmodic Agent, Gastrointestinal
Generic Available Yes
Use Treatment of functional disturbances of GI motility such as irritable bowel syndrome
Pregnancy Risk Factor B
Contraindications Hypersensitivity to dicyclomine or any component; narrow-angle glaucoma, tachycardia, GI obstruction, obstruction of the urinary tract, myasthenia gravis; should not be used in infants <6 months of age due to reports of respiratory distress, seizures, syncope, asphyxia, pulse rate fluctuations, muscular hypotonia, and coma
Precautions Use with caution in patients with hepatic or renal disease, ulcerative colitis, hyperthyroidism, cardiovascular disease, hypertension, hiatal hernia, autonomic neuropathy
Adverse Reactions Children with Down's syndrome, spastic paralysis, or brain damage are more sensitive to toxic effects than adults

Cardiovascular: Tachycardia, palpitations, orthostatic hypotension
Central nervous system: Seizures, coma, nervousness, excitement, confusion, insomnia, headache
Dermatologic: Urticaria, pruritus, dry skin
Gastrointestinal: Nausea, vomiting, constipation, xerostomia, dry throat, dysphagia
Genitourinary: Urinary retention
Local: Injection site reactions
Neuromuscular & skeletal: Muscular hypotonia, weakness
Ocular: Blurred vision, photophobia
Respiratory: Respiratory distress, asphyxia, dry nose
Miscellaneous: Decreased diaphoresis

Drug Interactions Additive adverse effects when given with medications with anticholinergic activity; may alter GI absorption of various drugs due to prolonged GI transit time; antacids; antagonizes effects of antiglaucoma agents
Stability Protect from light
Mechanism of Action Blocks the action of acetylcholine at parasympathetic sites in smooth muscle, secretory glands and the CNS
Pharmacodynamics
Onset of action: 1-2 hours
Duration: Up to 4 hours
Pharmacokinetics
Absorption: Oral: Well absorbed
Distribution: V_d: 3.65 L/kg
Bioavailability: 67%
Half-life:
Initial phase: 1.8 hours
Terminal phase: 9-10 hours
Time to peak serum concentration: Oral: 1-1.5 hours
Elimination: 80% in urine; 10% in feces
Usual Dosage
Infants >6 months: Oral: 5 mg/dose 3-4 times/day
Children: Oral: 10 mg/dose 3-4 times/day
Adults:
Oral: Initial: 20 mg 4 times/day, then increase up to 40 mg 4 times/day
I.M.: 20 mg/dose 4 times/day; oral therapy should replace I.M. therapy as soon as possible
Administration
Oral: Administer 30 minutes before eating
Parenteral: I.M. only; not for I.V. use
Patient Information Limit alcohol; may cause dry mouth
Dosage Forms
Capsule, as hydrochloride: 10 mg
Injection, solution, as hydrochloride: 10 mg/mL (2 mL)
Syrup, as hydrochloride: 10 mg/5 mL (480 mL)
Tablet, as hydrochloride: 20 mg

♦ **Dicycloverine** *see* Dicyclomine *on page 376*

Didanosine (dye DAN oh seen)
Related Information
Adult and Adolescent HIV *on page 1327*
(Continued)

Didanosine *(Continued)*

U.S. Brand Names Videx®; Videx® EC

Synonyms DDI; Dideoxyinosine

Therapeutic Category Antiretroviral Agent; HIV Agents (Anti-HIV Agents); Nucleoside Reverse Transcriptase Inhibitor (NRTI)

Generic Available No

Use Treatment of HIV infection in combination with other antiretroviral agents; **(Note:** HIV regimens consisting of **three** antiretroviral agents are strongly recommended)

Pregnancy Risk Factor B (Fatal lactic acidosis/severe hepatomegaly with steatosis has been reported in pregnant women who received the combination of didanosine and stavudine with other antiretroviral agents)

Contraindications Hypersensitivity to didanosine or any component

Warnings Major clinical toxicities of didanosine include pancreatitis and peripheral neuropathy; fatal and nonfatal pancreatitis has been reported during therapy; risk factors for developing pancreatitis include a previous history of the condition, didanosine dosage >10 mg/kg/day, concurrent cytomegalovirus or *Mycobacterium avium-intracellulare* infection, and concomitant use of stavudine with or without hydroxyurea, pentamidine, or sulfamethoxazole and trimethoprim. Dose-related (treatment-limiting) peripheral neuropathy occurs most often after 2-6 months of continuous didanosine administration; may cause retinal depigmentation in children receiving doses >300 mg/m^2/day. Fatal cases of lactic acidosis and severe hepatomegaly with steatosis have been reported with use of didanosine and other NRTIs; obesity and prolonged nucleoside exposure may be risk factors

Precautions Fat redistribution and accumulation [ie, central obesity, peripheral wasting, facial wasting, breast enlargement, dorsocervical fat enlargement (buffalo hump), and cushingoid appearance] have been observed in patients receiving antiretroviral agents (causal relationship not established). Use with caution in patients on sodium-restricted diets, patients with history of pancreatitis, and patients with renal or hepatic impairment; adjust dosage in patients with renal impairment or peripheral neuropathy; discontinue didanosine if clinical signs of pancreatitis occur; only after pancreatitis has been ruled out should dosing be resumed; chewable, dispersible tablets contain aspartame which is metabolized to phenylalanine and must be used with caution in patients with phenylketonuria.

Adverse Reactions

Central nervous system: Headache (32% to 36%), insomnia, malaise, CNS depression, fever

Dermatologic: Rash, pruritus, alopecia

Endocrine & metabolic: Hypokalemia, hyperuricemia, elevated triglycerides, hyperglycemia, lactic acidosis; central redistribution of body fat: Central obesity, buffalo hump, facial atrophy, and breast enlargement

Gastrointestinal: Diarrhea (18%), nausea, vomiting, anorexia, stomatitis, pancreatitis (9%, dose-related, less common in children than adults), abdominal pain

Hepatic: Elevated liver enzymes, hepatic failure, elevated amylase

Neuromuscular & skeletal: Peripheral neuropathy (dose-related), myalgia, arthritis, weakness

Ocular: Retinal depigmentation, optic neuritis

Respiratory: Cough, dyspnea

Drug Interactions Antacids, allopurinol, omeprazole, ganciclovir, cimetidine, and ranitidine may increase absorption of didanosine; methadone decreases didanosine concentration; decreases absorption of ketoconazole, itraconazole, indinavir, ganciclovir, dapsone, ciprofloxacin, tetracyclines (administer at least 2 hours before or 2 hours after didanosine); drugs associated with peripheral neuropathy (cisplatin, isoniazid, metronidazole, phenytoin, vincristine, stavudine, zalcitabine, dapsone, ethambutol, ethionamide, hydralazine, and nitrofurantoin) may increase the risk for didanosine peripheral neuropathy; drugs associated with pancreatitis (alcohol, I.V. pentamidine) may increase the risk of pancreatitis; concomitant administration of didanosine and delavirdine may decrease absorption of both drugs (separate dosing by at least 2 hours); concomitant administration of didanosine and ritonavir may decrease AUC of didanosine

Food Interactions Food decreases oral bioavailability by as much as 50%; do not mix with fruit juice or other acid-containing liquid since didanosine is unstable in acidic solutions

Stability Undergoes rapid degradation when exposed to an acidic environment; tablets dispersed in water are stable for 1 hour at room temperature; reconstituted buffered solution is stable for 4 hours at room temperature; reconstituted unbuffered solution is stable for 30 days if refrigerated; unbuffered powder for oral solution must be reconstituted with water and mixed with an equal volume of double strength antacid at time of preparation; when unbuffered powder for oral solution is reconstituted and admixed with a double-strength antacid to make a 20 mg/mL solution for adult once-daily

378

dosing, the admixture is stable for 24 hours at room temperature and for 30 days if refrigerated

Mechanism of Action A purine dideoxynucleoside analog converted within the cell to an active metabolite, dideoxyadenosine triphosphate which serves as a substrate and inhibitor of viral RNA-directed DNA polymerase resulting in premature termination of viral DNA synthesis

Pharmacokinetics

Distribution: Extensive intracellular distribution; low penetration into CNS; crosses the placenta

V_d:

Children: 35.6 L/m^2; range: 18.4-61 L/m^2

Adults: 18.4-60.7 L/m^2

Protein binding: <5%

Metabolism: Converted intracellularly to active triphosphate form

Bioavailability: Variable and affected by the presence of food in the GI tract, gastric pH, and the dosage form administered

Children and Adolescents: 32% to 42% (ranges from 13% to 78%)

Adults:

Tablet: 40%

Powder: 30%

Half-life:

Plasma:

Children and Adolescents: 0.8 hour

Adults: 1.3-1.6 hours

Intracellular: Adults: 25-40 hours

Elimination: Unchanged drug excreted in urine

Children: 6% to 30%

Adults: 20% to 55%

Usual Dosage Oral: (Use in combination with other antiretroviral agents):

Neonates <90 days: Based on clinical study data from PACTG 239: 50 mg/m^2/dose every 12 hours

Children <13 years: Dosing is based on body surface area (m^2): 180-300 mg/m^2/day divided every 12 hours. **Note:** Use lower dosage range for patients on combination therapy with other antiretrovirals; may need higher dose in patients with CNS disease.

Children ≥13 years and Adults: **Note:** Although once-daily dosing is available, it should only be considered for adult patients whose management requires once-daily administration (eg, in renal impairment); the preferred dosing frequency of didanosine is twice daily because there is more evidence to support the effectiveness of this dosing frequency (BMS study AI454-148)

<60 kg: 125 mg every 12 hours using 2 tablets/dose **or** 250 mg once daily using 2 tablets/dose

Buffered powder for oral solution: 167 mg every 12 hours

Delayed-release capsule: 250 mg once daily

≥60 kg: 200 mg every 12 hours using 2 tablets/dose **or** 400 mg once daily using 2 tablets/dose or a special Videx® solution in double-strength antacid which provides 400 mg/20 mL for once-daily dosing

Buffered powder for oral solution: 250 mg every 12 hours

Delayed-release capsule: 400 mg once daily

Dosing adjustment in renal impairment: Adults: Dosing based on patient weight, creatinine clearance, and dosage form:

Dosing for patients <60 kg:

Cl_{cr} 30-59 mL/minute:

Tablet: 75 mg (using 2 tablets) twice daily

Buffered powder for oral solution: 100 mg twice daily

Delayed-release capsule: 125 mg once daily

Cl_{cr} 10-29 mL/minute:

Tablet: 100 mg (using 2 tablets) once daily

Buffered powder for oral solution: 100 mg once daily

Delayed-release capsule: 125 mg once daily

Cl_{cr} <10 mL/minute:

Tablet: 75 mg (using 2 tablets) once daily

Buffered powder for oral solution: 100 mg once daily

Delayed-release capsule: Use alternate formulation

Dosing for patients ≥60 kg:

Cl_{cr} 30-59 mL/minute:

Tablet: 100 mg (using 2 tablets) twice daily

Buffered powder for oral solution: 100 mg twice daily

Delayed-release capsule: 200 mg once daily

(Continued)

Didanosine *(Continued)*

Cl_{cr} 10-29 mL/minute:
Cl_{cr} 10-29 mL/minute:
   Tablet: 150 mg (using 2 tablets) once daily
   Buffered powder for oral solution: 167 mg once daily
   Delayed-release capsule: 125 mg once daily
Cl_{cr} <10 mL/minute:
   Tablet: 100 mg (using 2 tablets) once daily
   Buffered powder for oral solution: 100 mg once daily
   Delayed-release capsule: 125 mg once daily

Administration Oral: Administer on an empty stomach 30 minutes before or at least 2 hours after a meal; tablets should be chewed, crushed, or dispersed in water for oral administration; tablets dispersed in water must be administered within 1 hour; unbuffered pediatric powder should be reconstituted with water and admixed in equal parts with a double-strength antacid to provide a final concentration of 10 mg/mL; unbuffered pediatric powder has also been reconstituted and admixed with a double-strength antacid to provide a final concentration of 20 mg/mL to be used for once-daily dosing in adults; shake oral solution well before use; administer at least 1 hour apart from indinavir or 2 hours apart from ritonavir; didanosine should be given at least 1 hour before or 2 hours after lopinavir/ritonavir; when administering chewable tablets, at least 2 tablets should be taken per dose to ensure adequate buffering capacity

Monitoring Parameters Serum potassium, glucose, uric acid, lactic acid, creatinine; hemoglobin, CBC with neutrophil and platelet count, CD4 cells; HIV RNA plasma level; liver function tests, serum amylase and triglyceride levels; weight gain; perform dilated retinal exam every 6 months; signs and symptoms of peripheral neuropathy

Patient Information Didanosine is not a cure for HIV. Avoid alcohol; the buffered powder vehicle may contribute to the development of diarrhea; inform physician if numbness, tingling, persistent severe abdominal pain, nausea, or vomiting occurs; shake oral solution well before use and keep refrigerated; discard solution after 30 days and obtain new supply

HIV medications may cause changes in body fat, including an increase in fat in the upper back and neck, breasts, and trunk; a loss of fat from the face, arms, and legs may also occur.

Additional Information
   Contents of each tablet: 11.5 mEq of sodium, 15.7 mEq of magnesium; tablets are buffered with dihydroxyaluminum sodium carbonate, magnesium hydroxide, and sodium citrate
   Sodium content of each packet of buffered powder for oral solution: 60 mEq

Dosage Forms
   Capsule, delayed-release (Videx® EC): 125 mg, 200 mg, 250 mg, 400 mg
   Powder for oral solution, buffered [single-dose packet] (Videx®): 100 mg, 167 mg, 250 mg [contains 1380 mg sodium/packet] [DSC]
   Powder for oral solution, pediatric [for 10 mg/mL solution] (Videx®): 2 g, 4 g
   Tablet, chewable/dispersible, buffered (Videx®): 25 mg, 50 mg, 100 mg, 150 mg, 200 mg [contains 36.5 mg phenylalanine (as aspartame)/tablet (all strengths); buffered with calcium carbonate and magnesium hydroxide; orange flavor]

References
Balis FM, Pizzo PA, Butler KM, et al, "Clinical Pharmacology of 2', 3'-Dideoxyinosine in Human Immuno-deficiency Virus-Infected Children," *J Infect Dis*, 1992, 165(1):99-104.
Butler KM, Husson RN, Balis FM, et al, "Dideoxyinosine in Children With Symptomatic Human Immunode-ficiency Virus Infection," *N Engl J Med*, 1991, 324(3):137-44.
Panel on Clinical Practices for Treatment of HIV Infection, "Guidelines for the Use of Antiretroviral Agents in HIV-Infected Adults and Adolescents," February 4, 2002, http://www.aidsinfo.nih.gov.
Working Group on Antiretroviral Therapy and Medical Management of HIV-Infected Children, "Guidelines for the Use of Antiretroviral Agents in Pediatric HIV Infection," December 14, 2001, http://www.aidsinfo.nih.gov.

♦ **2',3'-didehydro-3'-deoxythymidine** *see* Stavudine *on page 1039*
♦ **Dideoxycytidine** *see* Zalcitabine *on page 1161*
♦ **Dideoxyinosine** *see* Didanosine *on page 377*
♦ **Didronel®** *see* Etidronate Disodium *on page 467*
♦ **Diflucan®** *see* Fluconazole *on page 488*
♦ **Digibind®** *see* Digoxin Immune Fab *on page 383*
♦ **DigiFab™** *see* Digoxin Immune Fab *on page 383*
♦ **Digitek®** *see* Digoxin *on page 380*

Digoxin *(di JOKS in)*

Related Information
   Adult ACLS Algorithm, Narrow-Complex Supraventricular Tachycardia *on page 1190*

Blood Level Sampling Time Guidelines *on page 1386*
Carbohydrate and Alcohol Content of Liquid Medications for Use in Patients Receiving Ketogenic Diets *on page 1431*
Overdose and Toxicology *on page 1388*

U.S. Brand Names Digitek®; Lanoxicaps®; Lanoxin®

Canadian Brand Names Digoxin CSD; Novo-Digoxin

Therapeutic Category Antiarrhythmic Agent, Miscellaneous; Cardiac Glycoside

Generic Available Yes (except capsule and pediatric injection)

Use Treatment of CHF; slows the ventricular rate in tachyarrhythmias such as atrial fibrillation, atrial flutter, supraventricular tachycardia

Pregnancy Risk Factor C

Contraindications Hypersensitivity to digoxin, other digitalis preparations, or any component; ventricular fibrillation, A-V block, idiopathic hypertrophic subaortic stenosis, or constrictive pericarditis

Warnings Use with extreme caution in patients with hypoxia, hypothyroidism, acute myocarditis, electrolyte disorders, acute MI

Precautions Use with caution and reduce dosage in patients with renal impairment

Adverse Reactions

Cardiovascular: Sinus bradycardia, A-V block, S-A block, atrial or nodal ectopic beats, ventricular arrhythmias, bigeminy, trigeminy, atrial tachycardia with A-V block

Central nervous system: Drowsiness, fatigue, headache, lethargy, vertigo, disorientation

Endocrine & metabolic: Hyperkalemia with acute toxicity

Gastrointestinal: Vomiting, nausea, feeding intolerance, abdominal pain, diarrhea

Neuromuscular & skeletal: Neuralgia

Ocular: Blurred vision, halos, yellow or green vision, diplopia, photophobia, flashing lights

Drug Interactions Antacids, kaolin-pectin, cholestyramine, cisapride, colestipol, sucralfate, and metoclopramide may decrease absorption of digoxin; quinidine, nifedipine, itraconazole, indomethacin, verapamil, diltiazem, flecainide, amiodarone, erythromycin, propafenone, tetracycline, and spironolactone may increase digoxin serum concentration; the herbal medicine St John's wort (*Hypericum perforatum*) may significantly decrease digoxin serum concentrations; penicillamine may decrease digoxin's pharmacologic effects; calcium (especially rapid I.V. use) may cause severe arrhythmias; paroxetine may decrease the AUC of digoxin by 15%; ritonavir may increase or decrease digoxin levels (close monitoring of digoxin levels is recommended); suspected interaction with nevirapine (careful monitoring is recommended)

Food Interactions Meals containing increased fiber (bran) or foods high in pectin, may decrease oral absorption of digoxin; avoid natural licorice (causes sodium and water retention and increases potassium loss); maintain adequate amounts of potassium in diet to decrease risk of hypokalemia (hypokalemia may increase risk of digoxin toxicity)

Stability I.V. solution compatibility: D_5W, $D_{10}W$, NS, SWI (when diluted fourfold or greater); do not mix with other drugs; store at room temperature; protect from light

Mechanism of Action Increases the influx of calcium ions, from extracellular to intracellular cytoplasm by inhibition of sodium and potassium ion movement across the myocardial membranes; this increase in calcium ions results in a potentiation of the activity of the contractile heart muscle fibers and an increase in the force of myocardial contraction (positive inotropic effect); inhibits adenosine triphosphatase (ATPase); decreases conduction through the S-A and A-V nodes

Pharmacodynamics

Onset of action:

Oral: 0.5-2 hours

I.V.: 5-30 minutes

Maximum effect:

Oral: 2-8 hours

I.V.: 1-4 hours

Duration (adults): 3-4 days

Pharmacokinetics

Distribution: Distribution phase: 6-8 hours

V_d:

Neonates, full-term: 7.5-10 L/kg

Children: 16 L/kg

Adults: 7 L/kg

Renal disease: Decreased V_d

Protein binding: 20% to 25%

Bioavailability (dependent upon formulation):

Capsules: 90% to 100%

(Continued)

Digoxin *(Continued)*

Elixir: 70% to 85%
Tablets: 60% to 80%
Half-life, elimination (dependent upon age, renal and cardiac function):
Premature: 61-170 hours
Neonates, full-term: 35-45 hours
Infants: 18-25 hours
Children: 35 hours
Adults: 38-48 hours
Anephric adults: >4.5 days
Anuric adults: 3.5-5 days
Elimination: 50% to 70% excreted unchanged in urine
Dialysis: Nondialyzable (0% to 5%)

Usual Dosage Dosage must be individualized due to substantial individual variation; table lists dosage recommendations based on average patient response.

Dosage Recommendations for Digoxin*

Age	Total Digitalizing Dose† (mcg/kg)		Daily Maintenance Dose‡ (mcg/kg)	
	P.O.	I.V. or I.M.	P.O.	I.V. or I.M.
Neonates				
Preterm	20-30	15-25	5-7.5	4-6
Full-term	25-35	20-30	6-10	5-8
Infants and Children				
1 mo - 2 y	35-60	30-50	10-15	7.5-12
2-5 y	30-40	25-35	7.5-10	6-9
5-10 y	20-35	15-30	5-10	4-8
>10 y	10-15	8-12	2.5-5	2-3
Adults	0.75-1.5 mg	0.5-1 mg	0.125-0.5 mg	0.1-0.4 mg

*Based on lean body weight and normal renal function for age. Decrease maintenance dose in patients with decreased renal function and decrease total digitalizing dose by 50% in end-stage renal disease.

†Give one-half of the total digitalizing dose (TDD) in the initial dose, then give one-quarter of the TDD in each of two subsequent doses at 6- to 12-hour intervals. Obtain EKG 6 hours after each dose to assess potential toxicity.

‡Divided every 12 hours in infants and children <10 years of age. Given once daily to children >10 years of age and adults.

Dosing adjustment in renal impairment: (Monitor patient closely):
Total digitalizing dose: Reduce by 50% in end stage renal disease
Maintenance dose:
Cl_{cr} 10-50 mL/minute: Administer 25% to 75% of normal daily dose (divided and given at normal intervals) or administer normal dose every 36 hours
Cl_{cr} <10 mL/minute: Administer 10% to 25% of normal daily dose (divided and given at normal intervals) or give normal dose every 48 hours

Administration
Oral: Administer consistently with relationship to meals; avoid concurrent administration (ie, administer digoxin 1 hour before or 2 hours after) with meals high in fiber or pectin and with drugs that decrease oral absorption of digoxin
Parenteral: Administer I.V. doses (undiluted or diluted at least fourfold) slowly over 5-10 minutes; avoid rapid I.V. infusion since this may result in systemic and coronary arteriolar vasoconstriction; I.M. route not usually recommended due to local irritation, pain, and tissue damage

Monitoring Parameters Heart rate and rhythm, periodic EKG; follow serum potassium, magnesium, and calcium closely (especially in patients receiving diuretics or amphotericin); decreased serum potassium and magnesium, or increased serum magnesium and calcium may increase digoxin toxicity; assess renal function (serum BUN, S_{cr}) in order to adjust dose; obtain serum drug concentrations at least 8-12 hours after a dose, preferably prior to next scheduled dose

Reference Range Therapeutic: 0.8-2 ng/mL (SI: 1.0-2.6 nmol/L); Adults: <0.5 ng/mL (SI: <0.6 nmol/L) probably indicates underdigitalization unless there are special circumstances. Toxicity usually associated with levels >2 ng/mL (SI: >2.6 nmol/L).
Note: Serum concentration must be used in conjunction with clinical symptoms and EKG to confirm diagnosis of digoxin intoxication.

Test Interactions Spironolactone may interfere with digoxin radioimmunoassay

Patient Information Notify physician if decreased appetite, nausea, vomiting, diarrhea, or visual changes occur; avoid the herbal medicine St John's wort

Additional Information Digoxin-like immunoreactive substance (DLIS) may cross-react with digoxin immunoassay and falsely increase serum concentrations; DLIS has been found in patients with renal dysfunction, liver disease, CHF, neonates, and pregnant women (third trimester)

Dosage Forms

Capsule (Lanoxicaps®): 50 mcg, 100 mcg, 200 mcg [contains ethyl alcohol]

Elixir, pediatric: 50 mcg/mL (2.5 mL, 5 mL, 60 mL) [contains 10% alcohol; lime flavor]

Lanoxin®: 50 mcg/mL (60 mL) [contains 10% alcohol; lime flavor]

Injection: 250 mcg/mL (1 mL, 2 mL) [contains 10% alcohol]

Lanoxin®: 250 mcg/mL (2 mL) [contains 10% alcohol]

Injection, pediatric (Lanoxin®): 100 mcg/mL (1 mL) [contains 10% alcohol]

Tablet: 125 mcg, 250 mcg, 500 mcg

Digitek®, Lanoxin®: 125 mcg, 250 mcg

References

Bakir M and Bilgic A, "Single Daily Dose of Digoxin for Maintenance Therapy of Infants and Children With Cardiac Disease: Is It Reliable?" *Pediatr Cardiol*, 1994, 15(5):229-32.

Bendayan R and McKenzie MW, "Digoxin Pharmacokinetics and Dosage Requirements in Pediatric Patients," *Clin Pharm*, 1983, 2(3):224-35.

Johne A, Brockmoller J, Bauer S, et al, "Pharmacokinetic Interaction of Digoxin With an Herbal Extract From St John's Wort (*Hypericum perforatum*)," *Clin Pharmacol Ther*, 1999, 66(4):338-45.

Park MK, "Use of Digoxin in Infants and Children With Specific Emphasis on Dosage," *J Pediatr*, 1986, 108(6):871-7.

♦ **Digoxin CSD (Can)** *see* Digoxin *on page 380*

Digoxin Immune Fab (di JOKS in i MYUN fab)

U.S. Brand Names Digibind®; DigiFab™

Synonyms Antidigoxin Fab Fragments

Therapeutic Category Antidote, Digoxin

Generic Available No

Use Treatment of potentially life-threatening digoxin or digitoxin intoxication in carefully selected patients; use in life-threatening ventricular arrhythmias secondary to digoxin, acute digoxin ingestion (ie, >10 mg in adults or >4 mg in children), hyperkalemia (serum potassium >5 mEq/L) in the setting of digoxin toxicity

Pregnancy Risk Factor C

Contraindications Hypersensitivity to digoxin immune fab, ovine (sheep) proteins, or (DigiFab™ only) papain, chymopapain, other papaya extracts, or the pineapple enzyme bromelain

Warnings Hypokalemia has been reported to occur following reversal of digitalis intoxication; monitor serum potassium levels closely; Fab fragments may be eliminated more slowly in patients with renal failure; heart failure may be exacerbated as digoxin level is reduced; total serum digoxin concentration may rise precipitously following administration of digoxin immune Fab, but this will be almost entirely bound to the Fab fragment and not able to react with receptors in the body; digoxin immune Fab will interfere with digitalis immunoassay measurements - this will result in clinically misleading serum digoxin concentrations until the Fab fragment is eliminated from the body (several days to >1 week after digoxin immune Fab administration); serum digoxin levels drawn prior to therapy may be difficult to evaluate if 6-8 hours have not elapsed after the last dose of digoxin (time to equilibration between serum and tissue); redigitalization should not be initiated until Fab fragments have been eliminated from the body, which may occur over several days or greater than a week in patients with impaired renal function

Precautions Use with caution in renal or cardiac failure; allergic reactions possible; epinephrine should be immediately available; patients may deteriorate due to withdrawal of digoxin and may require I.V. inotropic support (eg, dobutamine) or vasodilators

Adverse Reactions

Cardiovascular: Worsening of low cardiac output or CHF, rapid ventricular response in patients with atrial fibrillation as digoxin is withdrawn

Dermatologic: Urticarial rash

Endocrine & metabolic: Hypokalemia

Miscellaneous: Facial edema and redness, allergic reactions

Stability Store in refrigerator; reconstituted solutions are stable 4 hours at 2°C to 8°C

Mechanism of Action Binds with molecules of free (unbound) digoxin or digitoxin and then is removed from the body by renal excretion

Pharmacodynamics Onset of action: Improvement in signs and symptoms occurs within 2-30 minutes following I.V. infusion

Pharmacokinetics

Distribution: V_d:

Digibind®: 0.3 L/kg

DigiFab™: 0.4 L/kg

(Continued)

Digoxin Immune Fab *(Continued)*

Half-life: Renal impairment prolongs the half-life of both agents:

Digibind®: 15-20 hours

DigiFab™: 15 hours

Elimination: Renal with levels declining to undetectable amounts within 5-7 days

Usual Dosage To determine the dose of digoxin immune Fab, first determine the total body load of digoxin (TBL) or digitoxin (depending upon which product was ingested) as follows (using either an approximation of the amount ingested or a postdistribution serum digoxin/digitoxin concentration (C)):

TBL of **digoxin** (in mg) = C (in ng/mL) x 5.6 x body weight (in kg)/1000

or

TBL = mg of **digoxin** ingested (as tablets or elixir) x 0.8

TBL of **digitoxin** (mg) = C (in ng/mL) x 0.56 x body weight (in kg)/1000

or

TBL of **digitoxin** (in mg) = mg digitoxin ingested

Dose of Digibind® **(in mg)** I.V. = TBL x 76

Dose of DigiFab™ **(in mg)** I.V. = TBL x 80

Dose of digoxin immune Fab (Digibind® or DigiFab™) **(# vials)** I.V. = TBL/0.5

See tables.

Infants and Children Dose Estimates of Digoxin Immune Fab (in mg)* From Serum Digoxin Concentration

Patient Weight (kg)	Serum Digoxin Concentration (ng/mL)						
	1	**2**	**4**	**8**	**12**	**16**	**20**
1	0.4 mg#	1 mg#	1.5 mg#	3 mg	5 mg	6-6.5 mg	8 mg
3	1 mg#	2-2.5 mg#	5 mg	9-10 mg	14 mg	18-19 mg	23-24 mg
5	2 mg#	4 mg	8 mg	15-16 mg	23-24 mg	30-32 mg	38-40 mg
10	4 mg	8 mg	15-16 mg	30-32 mg	46-48 mg	61-64 mg	76-80 mg
20	8 mg	15-16 mg	30-32 mg	61-64 mg	91-96 mg	122-128 mg	152-160 mg

*When a range in dose is listed, the lower number represents the Digibind® dose and the higher number represents the DigiFab® dose. A single dose is the same for both products.

#Dilution of reconstituted vial to 1 mg/mL may be desirable.

Adult Dose Estimate of Digoxin Immune Fab (in # of Vials) From Serum Digoxin Concentration

Patient Weight (kg)	Serum Digoxin Concentration (ng/mL)						
	1	**2**	**4**	**8**	**12**	**16**	**20**
40	0.5 v*	1 v	2 v	3 v	5 v	7 v	8 v
60	0.5 v	1 v	3 v	5 v	7 v	10 v	12 v
70	1 v	2 v	3 v	6 v	9 v	11 v	14 v
80	1 v	2 v	3 v	7 v	10 v	13 v	16 v
100	1 v	2 v	4 v	8 v	12 v	16 v	20 v

* v = vials

Administration Parenteral: I.V.: Digibind® is reconstituted by adding 4 mL SWI, resulting in a 9.5 mg/mL concentration for I.V. infusion; DigiFab™ is reconstituted with 4 mL SWI, resulting in an 10 mg/mL concentration for I.V. infusion; both formulations may be further diluted with NS to a convenient volume (eg, 1 mg/mL); infuse over 15-30 minutes; to remove protein aggregates, 0.22 micron in-line filter is needed (Digibind® only)

Monitoring Parameters Serum potassium; serum digoxin/digitoxin level prior to first dose of digoxin immune Fab; (digoxin levels will greatly increase with digoxin immune Fab use and are not an accurate determination of body stores); continuous EKG monitoring

Additional Information Each 38 mg vial (Digibind®) or 40 mg vial (DigiFab™) will bind approximately 0.5 mg digoxin or digitoxin; for individuals at increased risk of sensitivity (see Contraindications) an intradermal or scratch technique skin test using a 1:100 dilution of reconstituted digoxin immune Fab diluted in NS has been used. Skin test volume is 0.1 mL of 1:100 dilution; evaluate after 20 minutes.

Dosage Forms
Injection, powder for reconstitution, lyophilized:
Digibind®: 38 mg
DigiFab™: 40 mg

References
Hickey AR, Wenger TL, Carpenter VP, et al, "Digoxin Immune Fab Therapy in the Management of Digitalis Intoxication: Safety and Efficacy Results of an Observational Surveillance Study," *J Am Coll Cardiol*, 1991, 17(3):590-8.

Dihydroergotamine (dye hye droe er GOT a meen)

U.S. Brand Names D.H.E. 45®; Migranal®

Synonyms DHE

Therapeutic Category Alpha-Adrenergic Blocking Agent, Intranasal; Alpha-Adrenergic Blocking Agent, Parenteral; Antimigraine Agent; Ergot Alkaloid and Derivative

Generic Available No

Use Treatment of migraine headache with or without aura; injection also indicated for treatment of cluster headaches

Pregnancy Risk Factor X

Contraindications Hypersensitivity to dihydroergotamine, other ergot alkaloids, caffeine (nasal spray only), or any component; pregnancy; patients with uncontrolled hypertension, ischemic heart disease, angina pectoris, history of MI, silent ischemia, or coronary artery vasospasm including Prinzmetal's angina; patients with hemiplegic or basilar migraine; patients with peripheral vascular disease, sepsis, severe hepatic or renal dysfunction, and following vascular surgery; do not use within 24 hours of sumatriptan, zolmitriptan, other serotonin agonists, or ergot-like agents; do not use during or within 2 weeks of discontinuing MAO inhibitors; do not coadminister with potent cytochrome P450 isoenzyme CYP3A4 inhibitors (clarithromycin, erythromycin, itraconazole, and ketoconazole), protease inhibitors (indinavir, ritonavir, saquinavir, nelfinavir, amprenavir, lopinavir, or ritonavir), efavirenz, or delavirdine (see Drug Interactions)]

Warnings May cause vasospastic reactions; persistent vasospasm may lead to gangrene or death in patients with compromised circulation; discontinue if signs of vasoconstriction develop; rare reports of increased blood pressure in patients without history of hypertension; rare reports of adverse cardiac events (acute MI, life-threatening arrhythmias, death) have been reported following use of the injection; cerebral hemorrhage, subarachnoid hemorrhage, and stroke have also occurred following use of the injection; serious and/or life-threatening cerebral and peripheral ischemia have been associated with concomitant use of dihydroergotamine with potent cytochrome P450 isoenzyme CYP3A4 inhibitors, including macrolide antibiotics (erythromycin, clarithromycin) and protease inhibitors due to increased serum levels of dihydroergotamine (see Contraindications and Drug Interactions)

Precautions Prolonged use has been associated with fibrotic changes to heart and pulmonary valves (see Adverse Reactions); use with caution and only after a satisfactory cardiovascular evaluation has been performed in patients with risk factors for CAD; it is also recommended in these patients that the healthcare provider should administer the first dose; cardiovascular status should be periodically evaluated

Adverse Reactions
Cardiovascular: Cerebral hemorrhage, coronary artery vasospasm, edema, flushing, hypertension, MI, myocardial ischemia, palpitations, subarachnoid hemorrhage, transient ventricular tachycardia, ventricular fibrillation, tachycardia, bradycardia; fibrotic thickening of the aortic, mitral, tricuspid, and/or pulmonary valves (rare)
Central nervous system: Dizziness, somnolence, anxiety, headache, stroke
Dermatologic: Rash, pruritus
Endocrine & metabolic: Hot flashes
Gastrointestinal: Nausea, taste disturbance, vomiting, diarrhea, abdominal pain, cramps, diarrhea, xerostomia
Local: Application site reaction
Neuromuscular & skeletal: Asthenia, stiffness, hyperkinesis, muscular weakness, myalgia, paresthesia, tremor
Respiratory:
Nasal spray: Pharyngitis, rhinitis, nasal congestion, rhinorrhea, sneezing, nasal edema
Injection: Pleuropulmonary fibrosis
Miscellaneous: Retroperitoneal fibrosis (injection), increased sweating

Drug Interactions Cytochrome P450 isoenzyme CYP3A inhibitor
May increase serum levels of cyclosporine and tacrolimus; increased serum levels of dihydroergotamine with macrolide antibiotics (eg, erythromycin, clarithromycin, and (Continued)

Dihydroergotamine *(Continued)*

troleandomycin) and protease inhibitors may result in serious and/or life-threatening cerebral or peripheral ischemia (see Contraindications); MAO inhibitors; propranolol may potentiate the vasoconstrictive action of ergotamine; nicotine may increase ischemic response by provoking vasoconstriction; nitroglycerin may increase bioavailability of dihydroergotamine; dihydroergotamine decreases antianginal effects of nitrates; sumatriptan and other serotonin 5-HT$_1$ receptor agonists may prolong vasospastic reactions (see Contraindications); concomitant use with peripheral vasoconstrictors may cause synergistic elevation of blood pressure; use with a selective serotonin reuptake inhibitor (SSRI) (eg, dexfenfluramine, fluoxetine, paroxetine), may result in a condition known as serotonin syndrome (confusion, mental status change, diaphoresis, tremor, myoclonus, shivering, hyper-reflexia, weakness, incoordination, hypertension); delavirdine and efavirenz also increase ergotamine plasma concentrations which may result in life-threatening toxicities

Stability Store below 25°C (77°F); do not refrigerate or freeze; protect from heat and light; once the nasal spray applicator has been prepared, use within 8 hours; discard any unused nasal solution

Mechanism of Action Ergot alkaloid alpha-adrenergic blocker which aborts vascular headaches by direct vasoconstriction of vascular smooth muscle, particularly of the carotid artery bed but also peripheral and cerebral vessels, which reduces the amplitude of pulsation in the cranial arteries; it also has partial agonist or antagonist activity against tryptaminergic and dopaminergic receptors; it is less active than ergotamine

Pharmacodynamics
Onset of action:
I.M.: 15-30 minutes
Intranasal: 30 minutes
I.V.: Immediate
Duration: I.M.: 3-4 hours

Pharmacokinetics
Distribution: V_d: 14.5 L/kg (~800 L)
Bioavailability: Intranasal: 32%
Protein binding: 93%
Metabolism: Extensively in the liver; one active metabolite
Half-life: Distribution phase: 0.9-2.1 hours; terminal elimination phase: 7-32 hours
Time to peak serum concentration: I.M.: Within 15-30 minutes; intranasal: 0.5-1 hour; I.V.: 15 minutes; S.C.: 15-45 minutes
Elimination: Predominantly into bile and feces and 10% excreted in urine, mostly as metabolites
Clearance: 1.5 L/minute

Usual Dosage Adolescents and Adults: Treatment should be initiated at the first symptom or sign of an attack; nasal spray may be used at any stage of a migraine attack:
I.M., S.C.: 1 mg at first sign of headache; repeat hourly to a maximum total dose of 3 mg/day; do not exceed 6 mg/week
I.V.: 1 mg at first sign of headache; repeat hourly up to a maximum total dose of 2 mg/day; do not exceed 6 mg/week
Intranasal: 1 spray (0.5 mg) of nasal spray into each nostril (total: 1 mg); repeat if needed within 15 minutes; maximum: 4 sprays (2 mg/day); do not exceed 8 sprays (4 mg)/week
Dosing adjustment in renal impairment: Contraindicated in severe renal impairment
Dosing adjustment in hepatic impairment: Dosage reductions are probably necessary but specific guidelines are not available; contraindicated in severe hepatic dysfunction

Administration
Intranasal (For complete directions, see patient instruction booklet): Prior to administration, the nasal spray applicator must be primed (pumped 4 times); spray once into each nostril; avoid deep inhalation through the nose while spraying or immediately after spraying; do not tilt head back
I.M., S.C.: Administer without dilution
I.V.: Administer without dilution slowly over 2-3 minutes

Patient Information Take this drug as rapidly as possible when first symptoms occur; may cause dry mouth; may cause drowsiness and impair ability to perform activities requiring mental alertness or physical coordination; report heart palpitations, severe nausea or vomiting, or severe numbness of fingers or toes; do not assemble nasal spray until needed for use

Dosage Forms
Injection, solution, as mesylate (D.H.E. 45®): 1 mg/mL (1 mL) [contains ethanol]

Solution, intranasal spray, as mesylate (Migranol®): 4 mg/mL (1 mL) [0.5 mg/spray; contains 10 mg/mL caffeine]

Dihydrotachysterol (dye hye droe tak IS ter ole)

U.S. Brand Names DHT™; DHT™ Intensol™; Hytakerol®

Synonyms Dichysterol

Therapeutic Category Nutritional Supplement; Vitamin D Analog; Vitamin, Fat Soluble

Generic Available Yes

Use Treatment of hypocalcemia associated with hypoparathyroidism; prophylaxis of hypocalcemic tetany following thyroid surgery; suppression of hyperparathyroidism and treatment of renal osteodystrophy in patients with chronic renal failure

Pregnancy Risk Factor C

Contraindications Hypersensitivity to dihydrotachysterol or any component; hypercalcemia

Warnings Use cautiously in patients with renal stones, renal failure, and heart disease; calcium phosphate may precipitate if the product of serum calcium multiplied by phosphate (Ca x P) >70; adequate dietary calcium is necessary for a clinical response to therapy

Adverse Reactions Related to accompanying hypercalcemia

Central nervous system: Convulsions

Endocrine & metabolic: Hypercalcemia, metastatic calcification, polydipsia

Gastrointestinal: Nausea, vomiting, anorexia, weight loss

Hematologic: Anemia

Neuromuscular & skeletal: Weakness

Renal: Renal damage, polyuria

Drug Interactions Cholestyramine may reduce absorption; clofibrate, thiazides, phenobarbital, and phenytoin decrease the half-life of dihydrotachysterol; potential dihydrotachysterol-induced hypercalcemia may precipitate arrhythmias with cardiac glycosides

Mechanism of Action A synthetic reduction product of tachysterol, a close isomer of vitamin D; stimulates calcium and phosphate absorption from the small intestine, promotes secretion of calcium from bone to blood

Pharmacodynamics

Maximum hypercalcemic effect: Within 2 weeks

Duration: As long as 9 weeks

Pharmacokinetics

Absorption: Well absorbed from the GI tract

Metabolism: Hydroxylated in liver to 25-hydroxy-dihydrotachysterol

Usual Dosage Oral:

Hypoparathyroidism:

Neonates: 0.05-0.1 mg/day

Infants and young Children: Initial: 1-5 mg/day for 4 days, then 0.5-1.5 mg/day

Older Children and Adults: Initial: 0.75-2.5 mg/day for 4 days, then 0.2-1 mg/day; maximum dose: 1.5 mg/day

Nutritional rickets: 0.5 mg as a single dose or 13-50 mcg/day until healing occurs

Renal osteodystrophy:

Children and Adolescents: 0.1-0.5 mg/day

Adults: 0.1-0.6 mg/day

Administration Oral: May administer without regard to meals

Monitoring Parameters Serum calcium and phosphate, renal function, alkaline phosphatase, 24-hour urinary calcium

Additional Information 1 mg is approximately equivalent to 120,000 international units vitamin D_2

Dosage Forms

Capsule (Hytakerol®): 0.125 mg

Solution, oral **concentrate** (DHT™ Intensol™): 0.2 mg/mL (30 mL)

Tablet (DHT™): 0.125 mg, 0.2 mg, 0.4 mg

♦ **1,25 dihydroxycholecalciferol** see Calcitriol on page 199

♦ **Diiodohydroxyquin** see Iodoquinol on page 618

♦ **Dilacor® XR** see Diltiazem on page 388

♦ **Dilantin®** see Phenytoin on page 894

♦ **Dilaudid®** see Hydromorphone on page 577

♦ **Dilaudid-HP®** see Hydromorphone on page 577

♦ **Dilaudid-HP-Plus® (Can)** see Hydromorphone on page 577

♦ **Dilaudid® Sterile Powder (Can)** see Hydromorphone on page 577

♦ **Dilaudid-XP® (Can)** see Hydromorphone on page 577

♦ **Diltia® XT** *see* Diltiazem *on page 388*

Diltiazem (dil TYE a zem)

Related Information
Adult ACLS Algorithm, Narrow-Complex Supraventricular Tachycardia *on page 1190*

U.S. Brand Names Cardizem®; Cardizem® CD; Cardizem® LA; Cardizem® SR; Cartia XT™; Dilacor® XR; Diltia® XT; Tiazac®

Canadian Brand Names Alti-Diltiazem CD; Apo®-Diltiaz; Apo®-Diltiaz CD; Apo®-Diltiaz SR; Gen-Diltiazem; Gen-Diltiazem SR; Med-Diltiazem; Novo-Diltiazem; Novo-Diltiazem-CD; Novo-Diltiazem SR; Nu-Diltiaz; Nu-Diltiaz-CD; ratio-Diltiazem CD; Rhoxal-diltiazem CD; Rhoxal-diltiazem SR; Syn-Diltiazem®

Therapeutic Category Antianginal Agent; Antihypertensive Agent; Calcium Channel Blocker

Generic Available Yes (except extended release tablet)

Use
Oral: Treatment of chronic stable angina or angina from coronary artery spasm; hypertension (**Note:** Only extended and sustained release products are FDA approved for the treatment of hypertension)

Injection: Management of atrial fibrillation or atrial flutter; paroxysmal supraventricular tachycardias (PSVT)

Pregnancy Risk Factor C

Contraindications Hypersensitivity to diltiazem or any component; severe hypotension; second or third degree heart block; sick-sinus syndrome; acute MI with pulmonary congestion

Warnings May cause bradycardia, second or third degree heart block, hypotension, hepatic injury; may worsen CHF; use with certain medications may result in additive effects on cardiac condition (see Drug Interactions)

Precautions Use with caution in patients with CHF or impaired renal or hepatic function. Dermatologic reactions may occur; these may be transient or disappear with continued therapy; however, erythema multiforme or exfoliative dermatitis have been reported; discontinue diltiazem if skin rash persists or is severe.

Adverse Reactions
Cardiovascular: Arrhythmia, bradycardia, hypotension, A-V block, tachycardia (rare), flushing, peripheral edema, CHF

Central nervous system: Headache, dizziness, insomnia, nervousness

Dermatologic: Urticaria, rash; erythema multiforme, exfoliative dermatitis (rare); photosensitivity (<1%)

Gastrointestinal: Nausea, vomiting, constipation, dyspepsia, dysgeusia

Hematologic: Leukopenia (rare), thrombocytopenia (rare)

Hepatic: Mild to marked elevations in liver enzyme tests (rare)

Neuromuscular & skeletal: Gait abnormality, tremor, paresthesia, weakness, asthenia

Drug Interactions Cytochrome P450 isoenzyme CYP3A3/4 substrate; isoenzyme CYP1A2, CYP2D6, and CYP3A3/4 inhibitor

Cimetidine may increase diltiazem serum concentration; digoxin, beta-adrenergic blocking agents may increase risk of bradycardia or heart block; diltiazem may decrease metabolism and increase concentrations of cyclosporine, carbamazepine, digoxin, lovastatin, midazolam; diltiazem may increase the effect/toxicity of digitalis glycosides, encainide, fentanyl; rifampin may decrease diltiazem serum concentrations; cardiac effects of anesthetics may be potentiated by diltiazem (titrate doses of both carefully)

Food Interactions Food may increase absorption of diltiazem from sustained-release preparation; high fat meal does not effect extent of absorption of Cardizem® CD, Cardizem® LA, Cartia XT™, or Tiazac®; avoid natural licorice (causes sodium and water retention and increases potassium loss)

Stability
Capsule, tablet: Store at controlled room temperature; avoid excessive humidity; dispense in a tight, light resistant container

Injection: Refrigerate vials; do not freeze; may store at room temperature for up to 1 month; compatible in D_5W, NS, and $D_5\frac{1}{2}NS$ at a maximum concentration of 1 mg/mL for 24 hours when stored at room temperature or under refrigeration; not compatible with furosemide

Mechanism of Action Inhibits calcium ions from entering the "slow channels" or select voltage-sensitive areas of vascular smooth muscle and myocardium during depolarization; produces a relaxation of coronary vascular smooth muscle and coronary vasodilation; increases myocardial oxygen delivery in patients with vasospastic angina

Pharmacodynamics

Onset of action:
  Oral: Tablet: Immediate release: 30-60 minutes
  Parenteral: I.V. (bolus): Within 3 minutes
Maximum effect:
  Antiarrhythmic (I.V. bolus): 2-7 minutes
  Antihypertensive (Oral): Within 2 weeks

Pharmacokinetics

Absorption: 80%
Distribution: V_d: 1.7 L/kg; appears in breast milk
Protein binding: 70% to 80%
Metabolism: Extensive first-pass effect; metabolized in the liver; desacetyldiltiazem is an active metabolite (25% to 50% as potent as diltiazem based on coronary vasodilation effects); desacetyldiltiazem may accumulate with plasma concentrations 10% to 20% of diltiazem levels
Bioavailability: Oral: ~40%
Half-life: 3-4.5 hours, up to 8 hours with chronic high dosing
Time to peak serum concentration:
  Tablet: Immediate release: 2-4 hours
  Cardizem® CD: 10-14 hours
  Cardizem® LA: 11-18 hours
  Cardizem® SR: 6-11 hours
Elimination: In urine and bile mostly as metabolites; 2% to 4% excreted as unchanged drug in urine
Dialysis: Not dialyzable

Usual Dosage

Children: Minimal information available; some centers use the following:
  Hypertension: Oral: Initial: 1.5-2 mg/kg/day in 3-4 divided doses (extended release formulations may be dosed once or twice daily); maximum dose: 3.5 mg/kg/day; some centers use a maximum dose of 6 mg/kg/day up to 360 mg/day (see Flynn, 2000)
  Note: Doses up to 8 mg/kg/day given in 4 divided doses have been used for investigational therapy of Duchenne muscular dystrophy
Adolescents and Adults:
  Oral: Hypertension:
    Capsule, extended release:
      Cardizem® CD: 180-300 mg once daily; maximum: 480 mg once daily
      Cartia XT™: Initial: 180-240 mg once daily; usual: 240-360 mg once daily; maximum: 480 mg once daily
      Dilacor® XR: 180-240 mg once daily
      Diltia XT®: Initial: 180-240 mg once daily; usual: 180-480 mg once daily; maximum: 540 mg once daily
      Tiazac®: 120-240 mg once daily; maximum: 540 mg once daily
    Capsule, sustained release: Cardizem® SR: 60-120 mg twice daily
    Tablet, extended release: Cardizem® LA: Initial: 180-240 mg once daily; may increase dose after 14 days; limited clinical experience with doses >360 mg/day; maximum dose: 540 mg once daily
    Tablet, immediate release: 30-120 mg 3-4 times/day; dosage should be increased gradually, at 1- to 2-day intervals until optimum response is obtained; usual maintenance dose: 180-360 mg/day (see Use)
  I.V. (antiarrhythmic): Initial: 0.25 mg/kg as a bolus over 2 minutes, if response is inadequate a second bolus dose (0.35 mg/kg) may be administered after 15 minutes; further bolus doses should be individualized
  I.V. continuous infusion (start after I.V. bolus doses): 5-15 mg/hour for up to 24 hours
  Conversion from I.V. diltiazem to oral diltiazem: Start first oral dose approximately 3 hours after bolus dose
  Oral dose (mg/day) is approximately equal to [(rate in mg/hour x 3) + 3] x 10;
    Note: Dose per day may need to be divided depending on formulation used (see Usual Dosage above)
    3 mg/hour = 120 mg/day
    5 mg/hour = 180 mg/day
    7 mg/hour = 240 mg/day
    11 mg/hour = 360 mg/day (maximum recommended dose)

Administration

Oral: May be administered with or without food, but should be administered consistently with relation to meals; administer with a full glass of water; swallow extended and sustained release preparations (CD, LA, SR, XR, XT, Tiazac®) whole, do not chew, break, or crush
(Continued)

Diltiazem *(Continued)*

Tiazac® capsules (extended release) may be opened and sprinkled on applesauce; swallow applesauce immediately, do not chew; follow with some cool water (adults: 1 glass) to ensure complete swallowing; do not divide capsule contents (ie, do not administer partial doses); do not store mixture of applesauce and capsule contents, use immediately

Parenteral:

I.V. bolus: Adults: Infuse over 2 minutes

I.V. continuous infusion: May dilute with NS, D_5W, or $D_5\frac{1}{2}NS$; maximum final concentration: 1 mg/mL

Monitoring Parameters Blood pressure, renal function, liver enzymes; EKG with I.V. therapy

Patient Information Do not discontinue abruptly; report any dizziness, shortness of breath, palpitations, or edema; avoid alcohol. May cause photosensitivity reactions (eg, exposure to sunlight may cause severe sunburn, skin rash, redness, or itching); avoid exposure to sunlight and artificial light sources (sunlamps, tanning booth/bed); wear protective clothing, wide-brimmed hats, sunglasses, and lip sunscreen (SPF ≥15); use a sunscreen [broad-spectrum sunscreen or physical sunscreen (preferred) or sunblock with SPF ≥15]; contact physician if reaction occurs.

Nursing Implications Do not crush extended or sustained release preparations (CD, LA, SR, XR, XT, Tiazac®)

Additional Information Cartia XT™ is the generic version of Cardizem® CD; Diltia XT® is the generic version of Dilacor XR®

Dosage Forms

Capsule, extended release, as hydrochloride: 60 mg, 90 mg, 120 mg, 180 mg, 240 mg, 300 mg

Cardizem® CD: 120 mg, 180 mg, 240 mg, 300 mg, 360 mg

Cartia XT™: 120 mg, 180 mg, 240 mg, 300 mg

Dilacor® XR: 120 mg, 180 mg, 240 mg

Diltia® XT: 120 mg, 180 mg, 240 mg

Tiazac®: 120 mg, 180 mg, 240 mg, 300 mg, 360 mg, 420 mg

Capsule, sustained release (Cardizem® SR): 60 mg, 90 mg, 120 mg

Injection, powder for reconstitution, as hydrochloride (Cardizem®): 25 mg, 100 mg

Injection, solution, as hydrochloride: 5 mg/mL (5 mL, 10 mL, 25 mL)

Cardizem®: 5 mg/mL (5 mL, 10 mL) [DSC]

Tablet, as hydrochloride (Cardizem®): 30 mg, 60 mg, 90 mg, 120 mg

Tablet, extended release, as hydrochloride (Cardizem® LA): 120 mg, 180 mg, 240 mg, 300 mg, 360 mg, 420 mg

Extemporaneous Preparations A 12 mg/mL oral liquid preparation made from tablets (regular, not sustained release) and 3 different vehicles (cherry syrup, a 1:1 mixture of Ora-Sweet® and Ora-Plus®, or a 1:1 mixture of Ora-Sweet® SF and Ora-Plus®) was stable for 60 days when stored in amber plastic prescription bottles in the dark at room temperature (25°C) or under refrigeration (5°C); grind sixteen 90 mg tablets in a mortar into a fine powder; add 10 mL of the vehicle and mix well to form a uniform paste; mix while adding the vehicle in geometric proportions to **almost** 120 mL; transfer to a calibrated bottle and qsad with vehicle to 120 mL; label "shake well" and "protect from light"

Allen LV and Erickson MA, "Stability of Baclofen, Captopril, Diltiazem Hydrochloride, Dipyridamole, and Flecainide Acetate in Extemporaneously Compounded Oral Liquids," *Am J Health Sys Pharm*, 1996, 53(18):2179-84.

References

Bertorini TE, Palmieri GMA, Griffin JW, et al, "Effect of Chronic Treatment With the Calcium Antagonist Diltiazem in Duchenne Muscular Dystrophy," *Neurology*, 1988, 38(4):609-13.

Flynn JT and Pasko DA, "Calcium Channel Blockers: Pharmacology and Place in Therapy of Pediatric Hypertension," *Pediatr Nephrol*, 2000, 15(3-4):302-16.

♦ **Dilusol® (Can)** *see* Ethyl Alcohol *on page 465*

DimenhyDRINATE *(dye men HYE dri nate)*

Related Information

Overdose and Toxicology *on page 1388*

U.S. Brand Names Dramamine®; Hydrate® [DSC]

Canadian Brand Names Apo®-Dimenhydrinate; Gravol®

Therapeutic Category Antiemetic; Antihistamine

Generic Available Yes

Use Treatment and prevention of nausea, vertigo, and vomiting associated with motion sickness

Pregnancy Risk Factor B

Contraindications Hypersensitivity to dimenhydrinate or any component (see Warnings)

Warnings Chewable tablets contain tartrazine which may cause allergic reactions in susceptible individuals

Precautions Use with caution in patients with a history of seizure disorder; may produce excitation in the young child; use with caution in any condition which may be aggravated by anticholinergic symptoms such as prostatic hypertrophy, asthma, bladder neck obstruction, narrow-angle glaucoma, etc; chewable tablets contain aspartame which is metabolized to phenylalanine and must be used with caution in patients with phenylketonuria

Adverse Reactions

Cardiovascular: Hypotension, palpitations, tachycardia

Central nervous system: Drowsiness, headache, paradoxical CNS stimulation, dizziness

Dermatologic: Photosensitivity, urticaria, rash

Gastrointestinal: Anorexia, xerostomia, dry mucous membranes, constipation

Genitourinary: Urinary frequency, dysuria

Hematologic: Hemolytic anemia

Ocular: Blurred vision, diplopia

Otic: Tinnitus

Respiratory: Chest tightness, wheezing, thickened secretions

Drug Interactions Enhances sedative effects of other CNS depressants, may potentiate anticholinergic effects; may mask early signs and symptoms of ototoxicity in patients on aminoglycosides, furosemide, etc

Mechanism of Action Competes with histamine for H_1-receptor sites on effector cells in the GI tract, blood vessels, and respiratory tract; diminishes vestibular stimulation and depresses labyrinthine function through its central anticholinergic activity; consists of equimolar proportions of diphenhydramine and chlorotheophylline

Pharmacodynamics

Onset of action: Oral: Within 15-30 minutes

Duration: ~3-6 hours

Pharmacokinetics

Absorption: Well absorbed from the GI tract

Metabolism: Extensive in the liver

Usual Dosage Oral:

Children:

2-5 years: 12.5-25 mg every 6-8 hours, maximum dose: 75 mg/day

6-12 years: 25-50 mg every 6-8 hours, maximum dose: 150 mg/day

or

Alternately: 5 mg/kg/day or 150 mg/m²/day in 4 divided doses, not to exceed 300 mg/day

Children ≥12 years and Adults: 50-100 mg every 4-6 hours, not to exceed 400 mg/day

Administration Oral: Administer with food or water

Patient Information May cause drowsiness and impair ability to perform activities requiring mental alertness or physical coordination; may cause dry mouth. May rarely cause photosensitivity reactions (eg, exposure to sunlight may cause severe sunburn, skin rash, redness, or itching); avoid direct exposure to sunlight.

Dosage Forms

Tablet (Dramamine®): 50 mg

Tablet, chewable (Dramamine®): 50 mg [contains 1.5 mg phenylalanine (as aspartame)/tablet and tartrazine; orange flavor]

Dimercaprol (dye mer KAP role)

U.S. Brand Names BAL in Oil®

Therapeutic Category Antidote, Arsenic Toxicity; Antidote, Gold Toxicity; Antidote, Lead Toxicity; Antidote, Mercury Toxicity; Chelating Agent, Parenteral

Generic Available No

Use Antidote to gold, arsenic, and mercury poisoning; adjunct to edetate calcium disodium in lead poisoning

Pregnancy Risk Factor C

Contraindications Hypersensitivity to dimercaprol, peanuts (injection in peanut oil), or any component; hepatic insufficiency; do not use in iron, cadmium, or selenium poisoning; do not use iron supplements during therapy

Precautions Use with caution in patients with renal impairment or hypertension; produces hemolysis in persons with G-6-PD deficiency, especially in the presence of infection or other stressful situations; due to increased frequency of histamine-release related side effects, pretreatment with antihistamines is recommended; urine should be kept alkaline to prevent dissociation of chelate

Adverse Reactions

Cardiovascular: Hypertension, tachycardia

(Continued)

Dimercaprol *(Continued)*

Central nervous system: Nervousness, seizures, fever (30% of children), headache, anxiety

Gastrointestinal: Vomiting, nausea, salivation

Hematologic: Transient neutropenia

Local: Pain at the injection site, sterile abscesses

Neuromuscular & skeletal: Paresthesia of hands

Ocular: Blepharospasm, conjunctivitis, lacrimation, burning eyes

Renal: Nephrotoxicity

Respiratory: Rhinorrhea

Miscellaneous: Burning sensation of the lips, mouth, throat, and penis

Drug Interactions Iron (chelation product toxic to kidneys)

Stability Do not mix in the same syringe with edetate calcium disodium

Mechanism of Action Sulfhydryl group combines with ions of various heavy metals (arsenic, gold, mercury, lead) to form relatively stable, nontoxic, soluble chelates which are excreted in the urine

Pharmacokinetics

Distribution: To all tissues including the brain

Metabolism: Rapid to inactive products

Time to peak serum concentration: 30-60 minutes

Elimination: In urine and feces via bile

Usual Dosage Children and Adults: I.M.:

Mild arsenic and gold poisoning: 2.5 mg/kg/dose every 6 hours for 2 days, then every 12 hours on the third day, and once daily thereafter for 10 days

Severe arsenic and gold poisoning: 3 mg/kg/dose every 4 hours for 2 days then every 6 hours on the third day, then every 12 hours thereafter for 10 days

Mercury poisoning: 5 mg/kg initially followed by 2.5 mg/kg/dose 1-2 times/day for 10 days

Lead poisoning: (use with edetate calcium disodium):

Mild: 4 mg/kg/dose for one dose then 3 mg/kg/dose every 4 hours for 2-7 days

Severe and acute encephalopathy: (**blood lead levels >70 mcg/dL**): 4 mg/kg/dose every 4 hours in combination with edetate calcium disodium for at least 72 hours; may use for up to 5 days; if additional days of therapy (>5 days) are indicated, a minimum of 2 days without treatment should elapse before considering another treatment course

Administration Parenteral: Administer undiluted, deep I.M.

Monitoring Parameters Specific heavy metal levels, urine pH

Dosage Forms Injection, oil: 100 mg/mL (3 mL) [contains benzyl benzoate and peanut oil]

References

"Treatment Guidelines for Lead Exposure in Children. American Academy of Pediatrics Committee on Drugs," *Pediatrics,* 1995, 96(1 Pt 1):155-60.

♦ **Dipalmitoylphosphatidylcholine** *see* Colfosceril [DSC] *on page 304*
♦ **Dipentum®** *see* Olsalazine *on page 832*
♦ **Diphen® [OTC]** *see* DiphenhydrAMINE *on page 393*
♦ **Diphen® AF [OTC]** *see* DiphenhydrAMINE *on page 393*
♦ **Diphen® Cough [OTC]** *see* DiphenhydrAMINE *on page 393*
♦ **Diphenhist [OTC]** *see* DiphenhydrAMINE *on page 393*

DiphenhydrAMINE (dye fen HYE dra meen)

Related Information
Carbohydrate and Alcohol Content of Liquid Medications for Use in Patients Receiving Ketogenic Diets *on page 1431*
Compatibility of Medications Mixed in a Syringe *on page 1412*
OTC Cough & Cold Preparations, Pediatric *on page 1225*
Overdose and Toxicology *on page 1388*

U.S. Brand Names Aler-Dryl [OTC]; AllerMax® [OTC]; Banophen® [OTC]; Benadryl® Allergy [OTC]; Benadryl® Cream [OTC]; Benadryl® Dye-Free Allergy [OTC]; Benadryl® Extra Strength Cream [OTC]; Benadryl® Extra Strength Spray [OTC]; Benadryl® Gel [OTC]; Benadryl® Gel Extra Strength [OTC]; Benadryl® Injection; Benadryl® Itch Relief [OTC]; Benadryl® Spray [OTC]; Compoz® Nighttime Sleep Aid [OTC]; Diphen® [OTC]; Diphen® AF [OTC]; Diphen® Cough [OTC]; Diphenhist [OTC]; Genahist® [OTC]; Hydramine® [OTC]; Hydramine® Cough [OTC]; Hyrexin-50® Injection; Nytol® [OTC]; Nytol® Maximum Strength [OTC]; Scot-Tussin® Allergy Relief [OTC]; Siladryl® Allergy [OTC]; Simply Allergy® [OTC]; Simply Sleep® [OTC]; Sleepinal® [OTC]; Sominex® [OTC]; Sominex® Maximum Strength [OTC]; Tusstat®; Unisom® Maximum Strength SleepGels® [OTC]

Canadian Brand Names Allerdryl®; Allernix; PMS-Diphenhydramine

Therapeutic Category Antidote, Drug-induced Dystonic Reactions; Antidote, Hypersensitivity Reactions; Antihistamine; Sedative

Generic Available Yes

Use Symptomatic relief of allergic symptoms caused by histamine release which include nasal allergies and allergic dermatosis; mild nighttime sedation, prevention of motion sickness, as an antitussive; treatment of phenothiazine-induced dystonic reactions

Pregnancy Risk Factor B

Contraindications Hypersensitivity to diphenhydramine or any component; should not be used in acute attacks of asthma

Warnings Topical diphenhydramine should not be used to treat chickenpox, poison ivy, or sunburn, on large areas of the body, or on blistered or oozing skin, due to potential for causing toxic psychosis, particularly in children

Precautions Use with caution in patients with angle-closure glaucoma, peptic ulcer, urinary tract obstruction, hyperthyroidism; may cause paradoxical excitation in young children; chewable tablets contain phenylalanine and must be used with caution in patients with phenylketonuria

Adverse Reactions
Cardiovascular: Hypotension, palpitations, tachycardia
Central nervous system: Sedation, dizziness, paradoxical excitement, fatigue, insomnia
Dermatologic: Photosensitivity, rash, urticaria
Gastrointestinal: Nausea, vomiting, xerostomia, dry mucous membranes, anorexia, constipation, epigastric distress
Genitourinary: Urinary retention, dysuria
Hematologic: Rare: Hemolytic anemia, aplastic anemia, thrombocytopenia
Neuromuscular & skeletal: Paresthesia of hands, tremor
Ocular: Blurred vision
Respiratory: Chest tightness, thickened bronchial secretions, wheezing

Drug Interactions Cytochrome P450 isoenzyme CYP2D6 substrate
Additive sedation when given with drugs which depress the CNS; may impair absorption of aminosalicylic acid

Stability Compatible when mixed in the same syringe: atropine, chlorpromazine, cimetidine, droperidol, fentanyl, glycopyrrolate, hydromorphone, meperidine, metoclopramide, midazolam, morphine, promethazine, and ranitidine

Mechanism of Action Competes with histamine for H_1-receptor sites on effector cells in the GI tract, blood vessels, and respiratory tract

Pharmacodynamics
Maximum sedative effect: 1-3 hours after administration
Duration: 4-7 hours
(Continued)

DiphenhydrAMINE *(Continued)*

Pharmacokinetics

Absorption: Oral: Well absorbed but 40% to 60% of an oral dose reaches the systemic circulation due to first-pass metabolism

Protein-binding: 78%

Metabolism: Extensive in the liver

Half-life: 2-8 hours

Time to peak serum concentration: 2-4 hours

Usual Dosage

Oral, I.M., I.V.:

Treatment of phenothiazine dystonic reactions and moderate to severe allergic reactions:

Children: 5 mg/kg/day or 150 mg/m^2/day in divided doses every 6-8 hours, not to exceed 300 mg/day

Adults: 25-50 mg every 4 hours, not to exceed 400 mg/day

Minor allergic rhinitis or motion sickness:

Children 2 to <6 years: 6.25 mg every 4-6 hours; maximum: 37.5 mg/day

Children 6 to <12 years: 12.5-25 mg every 4-6 hours; maximum: 150 mg/day

Children ≥12 years and Adults: 25-50 mg every 4-6 hours; maximum: 300 mg/day

Antitussive: Oral:

Children 2 to <6 years: 6.25 mg every 4 hours; maximum 37.5 mg/day

Children 6 to <12 years: 12.5 mg every 4 hours; maximum 75 mg/day

Children ≥12 years and Adults: 25 mg every 4 hours; maximum 150 mg/day

Night-time sleep aid: 30 minutes before bedtime:

Children 2 to <12 years: 1 mg/kg/dose; maximum: 50 mg/dose

Children ≥12 years and Adults: 50 mg

Topical cream, gel, spray, or stick:

Children ≥2 to 12 years: Apply 1% concentration not more than 3-4 times/day

Children ≥12 years and Adults: Apply 1% or 2% concentration not more than 3-4 times/day

Administration

Oral: Administer with food to avoid GI distress

Parenteral:

I.V.: Dilute with compatible I.V. fluid to a maximum concentration of 25 mg/mL and infuse over 10-15 minutes (maximum rate of infusion: 25 mg/minute)

I.M.: 50 mg/mL concentration by deep I.M. injection

Topical: Shake well (gel); apply thin coat to affected area (see Warnings)

Test Interactions May suppress the wheal and flare reactions to skin test antigens; discontinue 4 days prior to skin testing procedures

Patient Information May cause drowsiness and impair ability to perform activities requiring mental alertness or physical coordination; may cause dry mouth. May rarely cause photosensitivity reactions (eg, exposure to sunlight may cause severe sunburn, skin rash, redness, or itching); avoid direct exposure to sunlight.

Dosage Forms

Capsule, as hydrochloride: 25 mg, 50 mg

Banophen®, Diphen®, Diphenhist®, Genahist®: 25 mg

Nytol® Maximum Strength, Sleepinal®: 50 mg

Cream, topical:

Benadryl®: Diphenhydramine hydrochloride 1% and zinc acetate 0.1% (30 g)

Benadryl® Extra Strength: Diphenhydramine hydrochloride 2% and zinc acetate 0.1% (30 g)

Elixir, as hydrochloride: 12.5 mg/5 mL (5 mL, 10 mL, 20 mL, 120 mL, 480 mL, 3780 mL)

Banophen®: 12.5 mg/5 mL (120 mL, 480 mL, 3840 mL)

Diphen AF: 12.5 mg/5 mL (120 mL, 240 mL, 480 mL, 3840 mL) [alcohol free; cherry flavor]

Genahist®: 12.5 mg/5 mL (120 mL)

Hydramine®: 12.5 mg/5 mL (120 mL) [alcohol free; cherry flavor]

Gel, topical, as hydrochloride:

Benadryl®: 1% (120 mL)

Benadryl® Extra Strength: 2% (120 mL)

Injection, solution, as hydrochloride: 10 mg/mL (30 mL); 50 mg/mL (1 mL, 10 mL)

Benadryl®: 50 mg/mL (1 mL, 10 mL)

Hyrexin®: 50 mg/mL (10 mL)

Liquid, as hydrochloride:

Benadryl® Allergy: 12.5 mg/5 mL (120 mL, 240 mL) [alcohol free; cherry flavor]

Benadryl® Dye-Free Allergy: 12.5 mg/5 mL (120 mL) [alcohol, dye, and sugar free; bubblegum flavor]

Liquid, topical (Benadryl® Itch Relief): Diphenhydramine hydrochloride 2% and zinc acetate 0.1% (14 mL)

Softgel, as hydrochloride:
Benadryl® Dye-Free Allergy: 25 mg [dye free]
Unisom® Maximum Strength SleepGels®: 50 mg

Solution, oral, as hydrochloride:
AllerMax®: 12.5 mg/5 mL (120 mL)
Diphenhist®: 12.5 mg/5 mL (120 mL, 480 mL)
Scot-Tussin® Allergy Relief: 12.5 mg/mL (120 mL, 480 mL, 3780 mL)

Spray, topical:
Benadryl®: Diphenhydramine hydrochloride 1% and zinc acetate 0.1% (60 mL)
Benadryl® Extra Strength: Diphenhydramine hydrochloride 2% and zinc acetate 0.1% (60 mL)

Syrup, as hydrochloride: 12.5 mg/5 mL (120 mL, 240 mL, 480 mL)
Diphen® Cough: 12.5 mg/5 mL (120 mL, 240 mL, 480 mL) [contains 5.1% alcohol; raspberry flavor]
Diphenhist®: 12.5 mg/5 mL (120 mL)
Hydramine® Cough: 12.5 mg/5 mL (120 mL, 480 mL) [contains 5% alcohol; fruit flavor]
Siladryl® Allergy: 12.5 mg/5 mL (120 mL, 240 mL, 480 mL)
Tusstat®: 12.5 mg/5 mL (120 mL, 240 mL, 3840 mL)

Tablet, as hydrochloride: 25 mg, 50 mg
Aler-Dryl, AllerMax®, Compoz® Nighttime Sleep Aid, Sominex® Maximum Strength: 50 mg
Banophen®, Benadryl® Allergy, Diphenhist®, Genahist®, Nytol®, Simply Allergy®, Simply Sleep®, Sominex®: 25 mg

Tablet, chewable, as hydrochloride (Benadryl® Allergy): 12.5 mg [contains 4.2 mg phenylalanine/tablet; grape flavor]

Diphenoxylate and Atropine (dye fen OKS i late & A troe peen)

U.S. Brand Names Lomotil®; Lonox®

Synonyms Atropine and Diphenoxylate

Therapeutic Category Antidiarrheal

Generic Available Yes

Use Treatment of diarrhea

Restrictions C-V

Pregnancy Risk Factor C

Contraindications Hypersensitivity to diphenoxylate, atropine, or any component; severe liver disease, jaundice, dehydration, and narrow-angle glaucoma; do not use in children <2 years of age

Warnings Reduction of intestinal motility may be deleterious in diarrhea resulting from *Shigella*, *Salmonella*, toxigenic strains of *E. coli* and from pseudomembranous enterocolitis associated with broad spectrum antibiotics; children (especially those with Down syndrome) may develop signs of atropinism (dry skin and mucous membranes, thirst, hyperthermia, tachycardia, urinary retention, flushing) even at the recommended dosages. Prolonged use may result in tolerance to antidiarrheal effects and physical dependence; abrupt discontinuation may cause withdrawal symptoms.

Precautions Use with extreme caution in patients with dehydration, cirrhosis, hepato-renal disease, renal dysfunction, and acute ulcerative colitis

Adverse Reactions
Cardiovascular: Tachycardia
Central nervous system: Sedation, dizziness, euphoria, headache, hyperthermia
Dermatologic: Pruritus, urticaria
Gastrointestinal: Nausea, vomiting, abdominal discomfort, paralytic ileus, pancreatitis, xerostomia
Genitourinary: Urinary retention
Neuromuscular & skeletal: Weakness
Ocular: Blurred vision
Respiratory: Respiratory depression (young children may be at greater risk)
Miscellaneous: Physical and psychological dependence with prolonged use

Drug Interactions MAO inhibitors (hypertensive crisis), CNS depressants, alcohol, anticholinergic agents, naltrexone; the herbal medicine St John's wort (*Hypericum perforatum*) may increase serious side effects, its use is **not** recommended

Stability Protect from light

Mechanism of Action Diphenoxylate inhibits excessive GI motility and GI propulsion; commercial preparations contain a subtherapeutic amount of atropine to discourage abuse

Pharmacodynamics
Onset of action: Within 45-60 minutes
(Continued)

Diphenoxylate and Atropine *(Continued)*

Maximum effect: Within 2 hours

Duration: 3-4 hours

Tolerance to antidiarrheal effects may occur with prolonged use

Pharmacokinetics

Absorption: Oral: Well absorbed

Metabolism: Extensive in the liver to diphenoxylic acid (active)

Half-life:

Diphenoxylate: 2.5 hours

Diphenoxylic acid: 12-24 hours

Time to peak serum concentration: ~2 hours

Elimination: Primarily in feces (via bile); ~14% is excreted in urine as metabolites; <1% excreted unchanged in urine

Usual Dosage Oral (as diphenoxylate):

Children: **Liquid: Note:** Only the liquid product is recommended for children under 13 years of age; do not exceed recommended doses; reduce dose as soon as symptoms are initially controlled; maintenance doses may be as low as 25% of initial dose; if no improvement within 48 hours of therapy, diphenoxylate is not likely to be effective

Initial: 0.3-0.4 mg/kg/day in 4 divided doses **or**

Manufacturer's recommendations: Initial:

<2 years: Not recommended

2 years (11-14 kg): 1.5-3 mL 4 times/day

3 years (12-16 kg): 2-3 mL 4 times/day

4 years (14-20 kg): 2-4 mL 4 times/day

5 years (16-23 kg): 2.5-4.5 mL 4 times/day

6-8 years (17-32 kg): 2.5-5 mL 4 times/day

9-12 years (23-55 kg): 3.5-5 mL 4 times/day

13-16 years: 5 mg (either 2 tablets or 10 mL) 3 times/day

Alternative pediatric dosing: Initial:

<2 years: Not recommended

2-5 years: 2 mg 3 times/day

5-8 years: 2 mg 4 times/day

8-12 years: 2 mg 5 times/day

Adults: Initial: 15-20 mg/day in 3-4 divided doses; maintenance: 5-15 mg/day in 2-3 divided doses

Note: Do not exceed recommended doses; reduce dose once symptoms are initially controlled; acute diarrhea usually improves within 48 hours; if chronic diarrhea dose not improve within 10 days at maximum daily doses of 20 mg, diphenoxylate is not likely to be effective.

Administration Oral: May be administered with food to decrease GI upset; **Note:** Dropper has a 2 mL (1 mg) capacity and is calibrated in increments of ½ mL (0.25 mg)

Monitoring Parameters Bowel frequency, signs and symptoms of atropinism, fluid and electrolytes

Patient Information Avoid alcohol and the herbal medicine St John's wort; may cause dizziness or drowsiness and impair ability to perform activities requiring mental alertness or physical coordination; may cause dry mouth; may be habit-forming; avoid abrupt discontinuation after prolonged use

Additional Information Naloxone reverses toxicity due to diphenoxylate; Lomotil® solution also contains sorbitol

Dosage Forms

Solution, oral: Diphenoxylate hydrochloride 2.5 mg and atropine sulfate 0.025 mg per 5 mL (5 mL, 10 mL, 60 mL)

Lomotil®: Diphenoxylate hydrochloride 2.5 mg and atropine sulfate 0.025 mg per 5 mL (60 mL) [contains 15% alcohol; cherry flavor]

Tablet (Lomotil®, Lonox®): Diphenoxylate hydrochloride 2.5 mg and atropine sulfate 0.025 mg

- ♦ **Diphenylhydantoin** *see Phenytoin on page 894*
- ♦ **Diphtheria and Tetanus Toxoids** *see page 1333*
- ♦ **Diphtheria, Tetanus, and Acellular Pertussis Vaccine** *see page 1333*
- ♦ **Diphtheria, Tetanus Toxoids, and Whole-Cell Pertussis Vaccine** *see page 1333*
- ♦ **Dipivalyl Epinephrine** *see Dipivefrin on page 396*

Dipivefrin *(dye PI ve frin)*

U.S. Brand Names Propine®

Canadian Brand Names Apo®-Dipivefrin; Ophtho-Dipivefrin™; PMS-Dipivefrin

Synonyms Dipivalyl Epinephrine; DPE

Therapeutic Category Adrenergic Agonist Agent, Ophthalmic; Ophthalmic Agent, Vasoconstrictor

Generic Available Yes

Use Reduces elevated IOP in chronic open-angle glaucoma; treatment of ocular hypertension

Pregnancy Risk Factor B

Contraindications Hypersensitivity to dipivefrin, any component (see Warnings), or epinephrine; contraindicated in patients with angle-closure glaucoma

Warnings Commercial preparation contains sodium metabisulfate which may cause allergic reactions in susceptible individuals

Precautions Use with caution in patients with vascular hypertension or cardiac disorders and in aphakic patients (dipivefrin may cause cystoid macular edema in aphakic patients)

Adverse Reactions
Central nervous system: Headache
Local: Burning, stinging
Ocular: Ocular congestion, photophobia, mydriasis, blurred vision, ocular pain, bulbar conjunctival follicles, blepharoconjunctivitis, cystoid macular edema

Drug Interactions Effects of lowering IOP may be additive when used with topical miotics, timolol, betaxolol, or carbonic anhydrase inhibitors

Stability Protect from light and avoid exposure to air; discolored or darkened solutions indicate loss of potency

Mechanism of Action Dipivefrin is a prodrug of epinephrine which is the active agent that stimulates alpha- and/or beta-adrenergic receptors increasing aqueous humor outflow

Pharmacodynamics
Onset of action:
Ocular pressure effects: Within 30 minutes
Mydriasis: Within 30 minutes
Maximum effect: Ocular pressure effects: Within 1 hour
Duration:
Ocular pressure effects: 12 hours or longer
Mydriasis: Several hours

Pharmacokinetics Absorption: Rapid into the aqueous humor; converted to epinephrine

Usual Dosage Children and Adults: Ophthalmic: Initial: Instill 1 drop every 12 hours

Administration Ophthalmic: Instill drop into eye; apply finger pressure to lacrimal sac during and for 1-2 minutes after instillation to decrease risk of absorption and systemic effects; avoid contacting bottle tip with skin or eye

Monitoring Parameters IOP

Patient Information Discolored solutions should be discarded; may cause burning or stinging, blurred vision, and sensitivity to light

Dosage Forms Solution, ophthalmic, as hydrochloride: 0.1% (5 mL, 10 mL, 15 mL)

♦ **Diprivan**® *see* Propofol *on page 947*
♦ **Diprolene**® *see* Betamethasone *on page 169*
♦ **Diprolene**® **AF** *see* Betamethasone *on page 169*
♦ **Diprolene**® **Glycol (Can)** *see* Betamethasone *on page 169*
♦ **Dipropylacetic Acid** *see* Valproic Acid and Derivatives *on page 1131*
♦ **Diprosone**® **[DSC]** *see* Betamethasone *on page 169*

Dipyridamole (dye peer ID a mole)

Related Information
Antithrombotic Therapy in Children *on page 1316*

U.S. Brand Names Persantine®

Canadian Brand Names Apo®-Dipyridamole FC; Novo-Dipiradol

Therapeutic Category Antiplatelet Agent; Vasodilator, Coronary

Generic Available Yes

Use Maintain patency after surgical grafting procedures including coronary artery bypass; with warfarin to decrease thrombosis in patients after artificial heart valve replacement; for chronic management of angina pectoris; with aspirin to prevent coronary artery thrombosis; in combination with aspirin or warfarin to prevent other thromboembolic disorders; dipyridamole may also be given 2 days prior to open heart surgery to prevent platelet activation by extracorporeal bypass pump; diagnostic agent I.V. (dipyridamole stress test) for coronary artery disease

Pregnancy Risk Factor B

Contraindications Hypersensitivity to dipyridamole or any component

(Continued)

Dipyridamole *(Continued)*

Precautions May further decrease blood pressure in patients with hypotension due to peripheral vasodilation

Adverse Reactions
Cardiovascular: Vasodilatation, flushing, syncope
Central nervous system: Dizziness, headache (dose-related)
Dermatologic: Rash, pruritus
Gastrointestinal: Abdominal distress, nausea, vomiting, diarrhea
Neuromuscular & skeletal: Weakness

Drug Interactions Heparin, warfarin, streptokinase, urokinase, alteplase, aspirin, NSAIDs, cefamandole, cefoperazone, cefotetan, and valproic acid may increase risk of bleeding; decreased coronary artery vasodilation from I.V. dipyridamole may occur in patients receiving theophylline or caffeine

Stability Do not freeze; protect I.V. preparation from light

Mechanism of Action Inhibits the activity of adenosine deaminase and phosphodiesterase, which causes an accumulation of adenosine, adenine nucleotides, and cyclic AMP; these mediators then inhibit platelet aggregation and may cause vasodilation; may also stimulate release of prostacyclin or PGD_2; causes coronary vasodilation

Pharmacokinetics Oral:
Absorption: Slow and variable
Distribution: V_d: Adults: 2-3 L/kg
Protein binding: 91% to 99%
Metabolism: In the liver to glucuronide conjugate
Bioavailability: 27% to 66%
Half-life, terminal: 10-12 hours
Time to peak serum concentration: Within 2-2.5 hours
Elimination: In feces via bile as glucuronide conjugates and unchanged drug

Usual Dosage
Children:
Oral: 3-6 mg/kg/day in 3 divided doses
Doses of 4-10 mg/kg/day have been used investigationally to treat proteinuria in pediatric renal disease
Mechanical prosthetic heart valves: 2-5 mg/kg/day [used in combination with an oral anticoagulant in children who have systemic embolism despite adequate oral anticoagulant therapy (INR 2.5-3.5), and used in combination with low-dose oral anticoagulation (INR 2-3) plus aspirin in children in whom full-dose oral anticoagulation is contraindicated]
Adults:
Oral: 75-400 mg/day in 3-4 divided doses
Dipyridamole stress test (for evaluation of myocardial perfusion): I.V.: 0.142 mg/kg/minute for a total of 4 minutes (0.57 mg/kg total); maximum dose: 60 mg; inject thallium 201 within 5 minutes after end of injection of dipyridamole
Platelet aggregation inhibitor: I.V. infusion: 250 mg/day at a rate of 10 mg/hour; maximum dose: 400 mg/day (use lower doses with aspirin)

Administration
Oral: Administer with water on an empty stomach 1 hour before or 2 hours after meals; may take with milk or food to decrease GI upset
Parenteral: I.V.: Dilute in at least a 1:2 ratio with NS, ½NS, or D_5W; infusion of undiluted dipyridamole may cause local irritation; see Usual Dosage for infusion rates

Monitoring Parameters Blood pressure, heart rate

Test Interactions Patients on theophylline may show false-negative thallium scan result on dipyridamole stress test

Patient Information Notify physician or pharmacist if taking other medications that affect bleeding, such as warfarin or NSAIDs; avoid alcohol

Dosage Forms
Injection, solution: 5 mg/mL (2 mL, 10 mL)
Tablet: 25 mg, 50 mg, 75 mg

Extemporaneous Preparations A 10 mg/mL oral liquid preparation made from tablets and 3 different vehicles (cherry syrup, a 1:1 mixture of Ora-Sweet® and Ora-Plus®, or a 1:1 mixture of Ora-Sweet® SF and Ora-Plus®) was stable for 60 days when stored in amber plastic prescription bottles in the dark, at room temperature (25°C) or under refrigeration (5°C); grind twenty-four 50 mg tablets in a mortar into a fine powder; add 20 mL of the vehicle and mix well to form a uniform paste; mix while adding the vehicle in geometric proportions to **almost** 120 mL; transfer to a calibrated bottle and qsad with vehicle to 120 mL; label "shake well" and "protect from light"
Allen LV and Erickson MA, "Stability of Baclofen, Captopril, Diltiazem Hydrochloride, Dipyridamole, and Flecainide Acetate in Extemporaneously Compounded Oral Liquids," *Am J Health Sys Pharm,* 1996, 53(18):2179-84.

References

Monagle P, Michelson AD, Bovill E, et al, "Antithrombotic Therapy in Children," *Chest*, 2001, 119(1 Suppl):344S-370S.

Rao PS, Solymar L, Mardini MK, et al, "Anticoagulant Therapy in Children With Prosthetic Valves," *Ann Thorac Surg*, 1989, 47(4):589-92.

Ueda N, Kawaguchi S, Niinomi Y, et al, "Effect of Dipyridamole Treatment on Proteinuria in Pediatric Renal Disease," *Nephron*, 1986, 44(3):174-9.

♦ **Disodium Cromoglycate** *see* Cromolyn *on page 311*

♦ **Disodium Thiosulfate Pentahydrate** *see* Sodium Thiosulfate *on page 1030*

♦ **d-Isoephedrine** *see* Pseudoephedrine *on page 958*

Disopyramide (dye soe PEER a mide)

U.S. Brand Names Norpace®; Norpace® CR

Canadian Brand Names Rythmodan®; Rythmodan®-LA

Therapeutic Category Antiarrhythmic Agent, Class I-A

Generic Available Yes

Use Treatment of life-threatening ventricular arrhythmias; suppression and prevention of unifocal and multifocal ventricular premature complexes, coupled ventricular premature complexes, and/or paroxysmal ventricular tachycardia; also effective in the conversion and prevention of recurrence of atrial fibrillation, atrial flutter, and paroxysmal atrial tachycardia

Pregnancy Risk Factor C

Contraindications Hypersensitivity to disopyramide or any component; pre-existing second or third degree A-V block; congenital QT prolongation; cardiogenic shock; do not administer with clarithromycin or erythromycin (see Drug Interactions)

Precautions Use with caution in patients with pre-existing urinary retention, existing or family history of angle-closure glaucoma, myasthenia gravis, hypotension during initiation of therapy, CHF unless caused by an arrhythmia, widening of QRS complex during therapy or lengthening of QT interval (>25% to 50% of baseline QRS complex or QT interval), sick sinus syndrome, Wolf Parkinson White syndrome (WPW) or bundle-branch block; may increase ventricular rate in patients with atrial flutter who have not received digoxin; use with caution and decrease dose in patients with renal or hepatic impairment; not recommended for use 48 hours before or 24 hours after verapamil

Adverse Reactions

Cardiovascular: CHF, edema, chest pain, syncope and hypotension, conduction disturbances including A-V block, widening QRS complex and lengthening of QT interval

Central nervous system: Fatigue, headache, malaise, nervousness, acute psychosis, depression, dizziness

Dermatologic: Generalized rashes

Endocrine & metabolic: Hypoglycemia, elevated cholesterol and triglycerides; may initiate contractions of pregnant uterus; hyperkalemia may enhance toxicities

Gastrointestinal: Xerostomia, dry throat, constipation, nausea, vomiting, diarrhea, pain, gas, anorexia, weight gain

Genitourinary: Urinary retention/hesitancy

Hepatic: Elevated liver enzymes, hepatic cholestasis

Neuromuscular & skeletal: Weakness

Ocular: Blurred vision, dry eyes

Respiratory: Dyspnea (<1%), dry nasal membranes

Drug Interactions Cytochrome P450 isoenzyme CYP3A4 substrate

Hepatic microsomal enzyme inducing agents (ie, phenytoin, phenobarbital, rifampin) may increase metabolism of disopyramide and lower serum concentrations; clarithromycin and erythromycin may increase disopyramide serum concentrations which can be life-threatening (do not use with disopyramide); other antiarrhythmic agents (quinidine, procainamide, lidocaine, propranolol) may increase adverse conduction effects (widening QRS complex, lengthening QT interval); adverse effects of disopyramide may be additive with amitriptyline, imipramine, haloperidol, thioridazine, cisapride, and other drugs that prolong the QT interval; verapamil (disopyramide is not recommended for use 48 hours before or 24 hours after verapamil)

Mechanism of Action Class IA antiarrhythmic: Decreases myocardial excitability and conduction velocity; reduces disparity in refractory period between normal and infarcted myocardium; possesses anticholinergic, peripheral vasoconstrictive, and negative inotropic effects

Pharmacodynamics

Capsules, regular:

Onset of action: 30-210 minutes

Duration: 1.5-8.5 hours

(Continued)

Disopyramide *(Continued)*

Pharmacokinetics

Protein binding: Concentration dependent, stereoselective, and ranges from 20% to 60%

Distribution: V_d: Children: 1 L/kg

Metabolism: In the liver; major metabolite has anticholinergic and antiarrhythmic effects

Bioavailability: 60% to 83%

Half-life:
  Children: 3.15 hours
  Adults: 4-10 hours (mean: 6.7 hours), increased half-life with hepatic or renal disease

Elimination: 40% to 60% excreted unchanged in urine and 10% to 15% in feces
  Clearance is greater and half-life shorter in children vs adults; clearance (children): 3.76 mL/minute/kg

Usual Dosage Oral:

Children (start with lower dose listed):
  <1 year: 10-30 mg/kg/day in 4 divided doses
  1-4 years: 10-20 mg/kg/day in 4 divided doses
  4-12 years: 10-15 mg/kg/day in 4 divided doses
  12-18 years: 6-15 mg/kg/day in 4 divided doses

Adults: **Note:** Some patients may require initial loading dose; see product information for details
  <50 kg: 100 mg every 6 hours **or** 200 mg every 12 hours (controlled release)
  >50 kg: 150 mg every 6 hours **or** 300 mg every 12 hours (controlled release); if no response, may increase to 200 mg every 6 hours; maximum dose required for patients with severe refractory ventricular tachycardia is 400 mg every 6 hours.
  Note: Use lower doses (100 mg of nonsustained release every 6-8 hours) in adults with cardiomyopathy or cardiac decompensation.

Adult dosing adjustment in renal impairment: 100 mg (nonsustained release) given at the following intervals: See table

Creatinine Clearance (mL/min)	Dosage Interval
30-40	Every 8 hours
15-30	Every 12 hours
<15	Every 24 hours

Administration Oral: Administer on an empty stomach; do not crush, break, or chew controlled release capsules, swallow whole

Monitoring Parameters Blood pressure, EKG, drug level; serum potassium, glucose, cholesterol, triglycerides, and liver enzymes; especially important to monitor EKG in patients with hepatic or renal disease, heart disease, or others with increased risk of adverse effects

Reference Range Therapeutic:
Atrial arrhythmias: 2.8-3.2 μg/mL (SI: 8.3-9.4 μmol/L)
Ventricular arrhythmias: 3.3-7.5 μg/mL (SI: 9.7-22 μmol/L)
Toxic: >7 μg/mL (SI: >20.7 μmol/L)

Patient Information Avoid alcohol; notify physician if urinary retention or worsening of CHF occurs; may cause dry mouth

Dosage Forms
Capsule, as phosphate (Norpace®): 100 mg, 150 mg
Capsule, extended release, as phosphate (Norpace® CR): 100 mg, 150 mg

Extemporaneous Preparations Extemporaneous suspensions in cherry syrup (1 mg/mL and 10 mg/mL) are stable for 4 weeks in amber glass bottles stored at 5°C, 30°C, or at room temperature; shake well before use; do not use extended release capsules for this suspension
  Mathur LK, Lai PK, and Shively CD, "Stability of Disopyramide Phosphate in Cherry Syrup," *J Hosp Pharm*, 1982, 39(2):309-10.

References

Chiba K, Koike K, Nakamoto M, et al, "Steady-State Pharmacokinetics and Bioavailability of Total and Unbound Disopyramide in Children With Cardiac Arrhythmias," *Ther Drug Monit*, 1992, 14(2):112-8.
Echizen H, Takahashi H, Nakamura H, et al, "Stereoselective Disposition and Metabolism of Disopyramide in Pediatric Patients," *J Pharmacol Exp Ther*, 1991, 259(3):953-60.

♦ **Ditropan®** *see* Oxybutynin *on page 843*
♦ **Ditropan® XL** *see* Oxybutynin *on page 843*
♦ **Diuril®** *see* Chlorothiazide *on page 261*
♦ **Dixarit® (Can)** *see* Clonidine *on page 294*

- *dl*-Alpha Tocopherol *see* Vitamin E *on page 1152*
- **DM** *see* Dextromethorphan *on page 365*
- ***D*-Mannitol** *see* Mannitol *on page 706*
- **4-DMDR** *see* Idarubicin *on page 591*
- **DMSA** *see* Succimer *on page 1043*
- **DNase** *see* Dornase Alfa *on page 406*
- **DNR** *see* DAUNOrubicin *on page 344*

DOBUTamine (doe BYOO ta meen)

Related Information
Emergency Pediatric Drip Calculations *on page 1177*
Extravasation Treatment *on page 1240*

U.S. Brand Names Dobutrex®

Therapeutic Category Adrenergic Agonist Agent; Sympathomimetic

Generic Available Yes

Use Short-term management of patients with cardiac decompensation

Pregnancy Risk Factor B

Contraindications Hypersensitivity to dobutamine or any component (see Warnings); patients with idiopathic hypertrophic subaortic stenosis (IHSS)

Warnings Potent drug; must be diluted prior to use; patient's hemodynamic status should be monitored; contains sulfites which may cause allergic reactions in susceptible individuals

Precautions Hypovolemia should be corrected prior to use; infiltration causes local inflammatory changes, extravasation may cause dermal necrosis

Adverse Reactions
Cardiovascular: Ectopic heartbeats, elevated heart rate, chest pain, palpitations, elevation in blood pressure; in higher doses ventricular tachycardia or arrhythmias may be seen; patients with atrial fibrillation or flutter are at risk of developing a rapid ventricular response
Central nervous system: Headache
Gastrointestinal: Nausea, vomiting
Local: Phlebitis
Neuromuscular & skeletal: Mild leg cramps, paresthesia
Respiratory: Dyspnea

Drug Interactions Beta-adrenergic blocking agents, general anesthetics

Stability Stable in various parenteral solutions for 24 hours; incompatible with alkaline solutions, do not give through same I.V. line as heparin, sodium bicarbonate, ethacrynic acid, cefazolin, or penicillin; compatible when coadministered with dopamine, nitroprusside, potassium chloride, protamine sulfate, tobramycin, epinephrine, atracurium, vecuronium, isoproterenol, and lidocaine; pink discoloration of dobutamine hydrochloride indicates slight oxidation, but no significant loss of potency if administered within the recommended time period

Mechanism of Action Stimulates beta$_1$-adrenergic receptors, causing increased contractility and heart rate, with little effect on beta$_2$- or alpha-receptors

Pharmacodynamics
Onset of action: I.V.: 1-10 minutes
Maximum effect: Within 10-20 minutes

Pharmacokinetics
Metabolism: In tissues and the liver to inactive metabolites
Half-life: 2 minutes

Usual Dosage I.V. continuous infusion:
Neonates: 2-15 mcg/kg/minute, titrate to desired response
Children and Adults: 2.5-15 mcg/kg/minute, titrate to desired response; maximum dose: 40 mcg/kg/minute

Administration Parenteral: Dilute in dextrose or NS; maximum recommended concentration: 5000 mcg/mL (5 mg/mL); rate of infusion (mL/hour) = dose (mcg/kg/minute) x weight (kg) x 60 minutes/hour divided by the concentration (mcg/mL); administer into large vein; use infusion device to control rate of flow

Monitoring Parameters EKG, heart rate, CVP, MAP, urine output; if pulmonary artery catheter is in place, monitor CI, PCWP, RAP, and SVR. Dobutamine lowers central venous pressure and wedge pressure but has little effect on pulmonary vascular resistance.

Dosage Forms
Infusion, as hydrochloride [premixed in dextrose]: 1 mg/mL (250 mL, 500 mL); 2 mg/mL (250 mL); 4 mg/mL (250 mL)
Injection, solution, as hydrochloride: 12.5 mg/mL (20 mL, 40 mL, 100 mL) [contains sodium bisulfite]

- **Dobutrex®** *see* DOBUTamine *on page 401*

Docusate (DOK yoo sate)

U.S. Brand Names Colace® [OTC]; Diocto® [OTC]; Dioeze® [OTC]; Docusoft-S™ [OTC]; DOK® [OTC]; DOS® [OTC]; D-S-S® [OTC]; ex-lax® Stool Softener [OTC]; Fleet® Sof-Lax® [OTC]; Genasoft® [OTC]; Phillips'® Stool Softener Laxative [OTC]; Sulfalax® [OTC]; Surfak® [OTC]

Canadian Brand Names Albert® Docusate; Colax-C®; PMS-Docusate Calcium; PMS-Docusate Sodium; Regulex®; Selax®; Soflax™

Synonyms DOSS; DSS

Therapeutic Category Laxative, Surfactant; Stool Softener

Generic Available Yes

Use Stool softener in patients who should avoid straining during defecation; constipation associated with hard, dry stools; ceruminolytic

Pregnancy Risk Factor C

Contraindications Hypersensitivity to docusate or any component; concomitant use of mineral oil; intestinal obstruction, acute abdominal pain, nausea, vomiting

Adverse Reactions
Dermatologic: Rash
Gastrointestinal: Intestinal obstruction, diarrhea, abdominal cramping
Local: Throat irritation

Drug Interactions Docusate may increase absorption of mineral oil; docusate may increase the GI toxicity of aspirin

Mechanism of Action Reduces surface tension of the oil-water interface of the stool resulting in enhanced incorporation of water and fat allowing for stool softening

Pharmacodynamics Onset of action: 12-72 hours

Usual Dosage
Infants and Children: Oral: 5 mg/kg/day in 1-4 divided doses **or** dose by age:
<3 years: 10-40 mg/day in 1-4 divided doses
3-6 years: 20-60 mg/day in 1-4 divided doses
6-12 years: 40-150 mg/day in 1-4 divided doses
Adolescents and Adults: Oral: 50-400 mg/day in 1-4 divided doses
Older Children and Adults: Rectal: Add 50-100 mg of docusate liquid (not syrup) to enema fluid (NS or water)

Administration
Oral: Administer docusate liquid (not syrup) with milk, fruit juice, or infant formula to mask the bitter taste; ensure adequate fluid intake
Rectal: Administer as a retention or flushing enema

Additional Information Docusate sodium 5-10 mg/mL **liquid** instilled in the ear as a ceruminolytic produces substantial ear wax disintegration within 15 minutes and complete disintegration after 24 hours

Dosage Forms
Capsule, as **calcium** (Sulfalax®, Surfak®): 240 mg
Capsule, as **sodium**: 100 mg, 250 mg
Colace®: 50 mg, 100 mg
Dioeze®: 250 mg
Docusoft-S™, Fleet® Sof-Lax®, Genasoft®, Phillips'® Stool Softener Laxative: 100 mg
DOK®, DOS®, D-S-S®: 100 mg, 250 mg
Liquid, as **sodium**: 150 mg/15 mL (480 mL)
Colace®: 150 mg/15 mL (30 mL)
Diocto®: 150 mg/15 mL (480 mL) [vanilla flavor]
Syrup, as **sodium**: 50 mg/15 mL (30 mL); 60 mg/15 mL (480 mL)
Colace®, Diocto®: 60 mg/15 mL (480 mL) [contains alcohol]
Tablet, as **sodium** (Ex-Lax® Stool Softener): 100 mg

References
Chen DA and Caparosa RJ, "A Nonprescription Cerumenolytic," *Am J Otol*, 1991, 12(6):475-6.

Docusate and Casanthranol (DOK yoo sate & ka SAN thra nole)

U.S. Brand Names Diocto C® [OTC]; Docusoft Plus™ [OTC]; D-S-S Plus® [OTC]; Fleet® Sof-Lax® Overnight [OTC]; Genasoft® Plus [OTC]; Peri-Colace® [OTC]

Synonyms Casanthranol and Docusate; DSS With Casanthranol

Therapeutic Category Laxative, Stimulant; Laxative, Surfactant; Stool Softener

Generic Available Yes

Use Treatment of constipation generally associated with dry, hard stools and decreased intestinal motility

Pregnancy Risk Factor C

Contraindications Hypersensitivity to docusate, casanthranol, or any component; concomitant use of mineral oil; intestinal obstruction; acute abdominal pain; nausea, vomiting

Warnings Do not use when abdominal pain, nausea, or vomiting are present

Precautions Casanthranol is habit-forming; may result in laxative dependence and loss of normal bowel function with prolonged use

Adverse Reactions
Dermatologic: Rash
Gastrointestinal: Intestinal obstruction, diarrhea, abdominal cramping
Local: Throat irritation

Drug Interactions Docusate may increase absorption of mineral oil; docusate may increase the GI toxicity of aspirin

Mechanism of Action Combination stool softener (docusate) which lowers surface tension of the stool allowing water and lipids to penetrate and a stimulant laxative (casanthranol) which produces a net intestinal fluid accumulation and laxation

Pharmacodynamics Onset of action: 8-12 hours after administration but may require up to 24 hours

Usual Dosage Oral:
Children: 5-15 mL of syrup at bedtime or 1 capsule at bedtime
Adults: 1-2 capsules or 15-30 mL syrup at bedtime, may be increased to 2 capsules or 30 mL twice daily or 3 capsules at bedtime

Administration Oral: Administer with plenty of fluids

Monitoring Parameters Bowel frequency

Dosage Forms
Capsule (Docusoft Plus™, Doxidan®, D-S-S Plus®, Fleet® Sof-Lax® Overnight, Genasoft® Plus, Peri-Colace®): Docusate sodium 100 mg and casanthranol 30 mg
Syrup (Diocto C®, Peri-Colace®): Docusate sodium 60 mg and casanthranol 30 mg per 15 mL (480 mL) [contains alcohol]

♦ **Docusoft Plus™ [OTC]** *see* Docusate and Casanthranol *on page 402*

♦ **Docusoft-S™ [OTC]** *see* Docusate *on page 402*

♦ **DOK® [OTC]** *see* Docusate *on page 402*

Dolasetron (dol A se tron)

U.S. Brand Names Anzemet®

Synonyms Hydrodolasetron

Therapeutic Category Antiemetic; 5-HT$_3$ Receptor Antagonist

Generic Available No

Use Prevention of chemotherapy-induced nausea and vomiting; prevention and treatment of postoperative nausea and vomiting

Pregnancy Risk Factor B

Contraindications Hypersensitivity to dolasetron or any component

Warnings Dolasetron may cause EKG interval changes (PR, QT$_c$, JT prolongation and QRS widening) related in magnitude and frequency to blood levels of the active metabolite, hydrodolasetron; interval prolongation could lead to cardiovascular consequences such as heart block or cardiac arrhythmias

Precautions Use with caution in patients with, or who may develop, prolongation of cardiac conduction intervals, particularly QT$_c$; conditions include hypokalemia, hypomagnesemia, or congenital QT syndrome; use with caution in patients receiving antiarrhythmic or other medications known to prolong the QT interval (eg, class I or III antiarrhythmic agents) or medications known to reduce potassium or magnesium levels (eg, diuretics)

Adverse Reactions
Cardiovascular: Prolonged QT interval and other EKG changes (see Warnings), hypertension, hypotension, edema, diaphoresis
Central nervous system: Headache, fatigue, dizziness, fever, chills, shivering, agitation, sleep disorder, confusion, anxiety, abnormal dreams
Dermatologic: Rash, urticaria
Gastrointestinal: Diarrhea, abdominal pain, constipation, dyspepsia, anorexia, pancreatitis (rarely), taste perversion
Genitourinary: Urinary retention, acute renal failure (rarely), polyuria (rarely), dysuria (rarely)
Hepatic: Transient elevations in liver enzymes
Local: Venous irritation
Neuromuscular & skeletal: Myalgia, arthralgia
Ocular: Photophobia (rarely), abnormal vision
Otic: Tinnitus (rarely)
Miscellaneous: Hypersensitivity reactions

Drug Interactions Cytochrome P450 isoenzyme CYP2D6 and CYP3A3/4 substrate
Increased hydrodolasetron (active metabolite) serum levels with cimetidine; decreased hydrodolasetron serum levels with rifampin; decreased clearance of hydrodolasetron with atenolol; (see Warnings and Precautions)
(Continued)

403

Dolasetron *(Continued)*

Stability Injection is stable after dilution in NS, D$_5$W, D$_5$1/2NS, D$_5$LR, LR, and 10% mannitol injection for 24 hours at room temperature and 48 hours under refrigeration

Mechanism of Action Dolasetron and its major metabolite, hydrodolasetron, are selective 5-HT$_3$ receptor antagonists, blocking serotonin, both peripherally on vagal nerve terminals and centrally in the chemoreceptor trigger zone

Pharmacokinetics Due to the rapid metabolism of dolasetron to hydrodolasetron (primary active metabolite), the majority of the following pharmacokinetic parameters relate to hydrodolasetron:

Distribution:
  Children: 5.9-7.4 L/kg
  Adults: 4.15-5.5 L/kg

Metabolism: Rapidly converted by carbonyl reductase to active major metabolite, hydrodolasetron; hydrodolasetron is metabolized by the cytochrome P450 CYP2D6 and CYP3A enzyme systems and flavin mono-oxygenase

Bioavailability: Oral: Children: 59% (formulation not specified), adults: 70% to 80%

Half-life, elimination:
  Dolasetron: <10 minutes
  Hydrodolasetron:
    Oral: Children: 5.7 hours, adults: 8.1 hours (range: 5-10 hours)
    I.V.: Children: 4.8 hours, adults: 7.3 hours (range: 4-8 hours)

Time to peak serum concentration:
  Oral: 1-1.5 hours
  I.V.: 0.6 hours

Elimination: Dolasetron: <1% excreted unchanged in urine; hydrodolasetron: 53% to 61% excreted unchanged in urine within 36 hours

Usual Dosage

Prevention of chemotherapy-induced nausea and vomiting: **Oral:** Administered within 1 hour before chemotherapy; or **I.V.:** Administered 30 minutes before chemotherapy:

Children ≥2 to 16 years:
  Oral, I.V.: 1.8 mg/kg as a single dose (maximum: 100 mg)

Adults:
  Oral: 100 mg as a single dose
  I.V.: 1.8 mg/kg or alternatively 100 mg as a single dose

Prevention or treatment of postoperative nausea and vomiting: **Oral:** Administered 2 hours before surgery and; **I.V.:** Administered 15 minutes prior to cessation of anaesthesia or as soon as symptoms present

Children ≥2 to 16 years:
  Oral: 1.2 mg/kg as a single dose (maximum: 100 mg)
  I.V.: 0.35 mg/kg as a single dose (maximum: 12.5 mg)

Adults:
  Oral: 100 mg as a single dose
  I.V.: 12.5 mg as a single dose

Dosage adjustment in hepatic or renal impairment: No dosage adjustment is indicated

Administration

Oral: May be administered with or without food; injection may be used orally, dilute injection in apple or apple-grape juice; stable for 2 hours at room temperature

Parenteral: I.V.: Infuse undiluted over 30 seconds or dilute in 50 mL compatible I.V. fluid and infuse over ≤15 minutes; do not mix with other medications

Monitoring Parameters Baseline EKG in high-risk patients (see Warnings and Precautions), emesis episodes

Dosage Forms

Injection, solution, as mesylate: 20 mg/mL (0.625 mL, 5 mL)
Tablet, as mesylate: 50 mg, 100 mg

References

"ASHP Therapeutic Guidelines on the Pharmacologic Management of Nausea and Vomiting in Adult and Pediatric Patients Receiving Chemotherapy or Radiation Therapy or Undergoing Surgery," *Am J Health Syst Pharm*, 1999, 56(8):729-64.

Coppes MJ, Lau R, Ingram LC, et al, "Open-Label Comparison of the Antiemetic Efficacy of Single Intravenous Doses of Dolasetron Mesylate in Pediatric Cancer Patients Receiving Moderately to Highly Emetogenic Chemotherapy," *Med Pediatr Oncol*, 1999, 33(2):99-105.

DOPamine (DOE pa meen)

Related Information
- Adult ACLS Algorithm, Bradycardia *on page 1188*
- Emergency Pediatric Drip Calculations *on page 1177*
- Extravasation Treatment *on page 1240*

Canadian Brand Names Intropin®

Therapeutic Category Adrenergic Agonist Agent; Sympathomimetic

Generic Available Yes

Use Increase cardiac output, blood pressure, and urine flow as an adjunct in the treatment of shock or hypotension which persists after adequate fluid volume replacement; in low dosage to increase renal perfusion

Pregnancy Risk Factor C

Contraindications Hypersensitivity to dopamine or any component; pheochromocytoma, or ventricular fibrillation

Warnings Potent drug; must be diluted prior to use; patient's hemodynamic status should be monitored

Precautions Blood volume depletion should be corrected, if possible, before starting dopamine therapy. Dopamine must not be used as sole therapy in hypovolemic patients. Extravasation may cause tissue necrosis (treat extravasation with phentolamine; see Extravasation Treatment *on page 1240*); due to potential gangrene of extremities, use with caution in patients with occlusive vascular disease.

Adverse Reactions
Cardiovascular: Ectopic heartbeats, tachycardia, vasoconstriction, cardiac conduction abnormalities, widened QRS complex, hypertension, ventricular arrhythmias, gangrene of the extremities (with high doses for prolonged periods or even with low doses in patients with occlusive vascular disease), anginal pain, palpitations
Central nervous system: Anxiety, headache
Gastrointestinal: Nausea, vomiting
Genitourinary: Decreased urine output (high dose)
Neuromuscular & skeletal: Piloerection
Ocular: Dilated pupils
Renal: Azotemia
Respiratory: Dyspnea

Drug Interactions Dopamine's cardiac and pressor response are prolonged and intensified by MAO inhibitors, alpha- and beta-adrenergic agonists, and oxytocic drugs; tricyclic antidepressants may decrease effects; use with phenytoin has resulted in seizures, severe hypotension, and bradycardia; use with halogenated hydrocarbon anesthetics may lead to serious arrhythmias; dopamine's cardiac effects are antagonized by beta-adrenergic blocking agents; vasoconstrictive effects are antagonized by alpha-adrenergic blocking agents

Stability Protect from light; solutions that are darker than slightly yellow should not be used; incompatible with alkaline solutions or iron salts; compatible when coadministered with dobutamine, epinephrine, isoproterenol, lidocaine, atracurium, vecuronium

Mechanism of Action Stimulates both adrenergic and dopaminergic receptors; low doses are mainly dopaminergic which stimulate and produce renal and mesenteric vasodilation; intermediate doses stimulate both dopaminergic and beta$_1$-adrenergic receptors and produce cardiac stimulation (increased heart rate and cardiac index) and increased renal blood flow; high doses stimulate alpha-adrenergic receptors primarily (vasoconstriction and increased blood pressure)

Pharmacodynamics
Onset of action: Adults: 5 minutes
Duration: Due to its short duration of action (<10 minutes) a continuous infusion must be used

Pharmacokinetics
Metabolism: In plasma, kidneys, and liver; 75% to inactive metabolites by monoamine oxidase and catechol-o-methyltransferase and 25% to norepinephrine (active)
Half-life: 2 minutes
Clearance: Neonatal clearance varies and appears to be age related. Clearance is more prolonged with combined hepatic and renal dysfunction. Dopamine has exhibited nonlinear kinetics in children; dose changes in children may not achieve steady-state for approximately 1 hour rather than 20 minutes seen in adults.

Usual Dosage I.V. infusion:
The hemodynamic effects of dopamine are dose-dependent:
Low dosage: 1-5 mcg/kg/minute, increased renal blood flow and urine output
Intermediate dosage: 5-15 mcg/kg/minute, increased renal blood flow, heart rate, cardiac contractility, cardiac output, and blood pressure
High dosage: >15 mcg/kg/minute, alpha-adrenergic effects begin to predominate, vasoconstriction, increased blood pressure
Neonates: 1-20 mcg/kg/minute continuous infusion, titrate to desired response
(Continued)

DOPamine *(Continued)*

Infants and Children: 1-20 mcg/kg/minute, maximum dose: 50 mcg/kg/minute continuous infusion, titrate to desired response

Adults: 1 mcg/kg/minute up to 50 mcg/kg/minute, titrate to desired response

If dosages >20-30 mcg/kg/minute are needed, a more direct-acting pressor may be beneficial (ie, epinephrine, norepinephrine)

Administration Parenteral: Must be diluted prior to administration; maximum concentration: 3200 mcg/mL (3.2 mg/mL); (concentrations as high as 6000 mcg/mL have been infused into large veins, safely and with efficacy, in cases of extreme fluid restriction); rate of infusion (mL/hour) = dose (mcg/kg/minute) x weight (kg) x 60 minutes/hour divided by concentration (mcg/mL); administer into large vein to prevent the possibility of extravasation; use infusion device to control rate of flow; administration into an umbilical arterial catheter is **not** recommended

Monitoring Parameters EKG, heart rate, CVP, MAP, urine output; if pulmonary artery catheter is in place, monitor CI, PWCP, SVR, RAP, and PVR

Dosage Forms

Infusion, as hydrochloride [premixed in D_5W]: 0.8 mg/mL (250 mL, 500 mL); 1.6 mg/mL (250 mL, 500 mL); 3.2 mg/mL (250 mL)

Injection, solution, as hydrochloride: 40 mg/mL (5 mL, 10 mL); 80 mg/mL (5 mL, 10 mL); 160 mg/mL (5 mL)

References

Banner W, Jr, Vernon DD, Dean JM, et al, "Nonlinear Dopamine Pharmacokinetics in Pediatric Patients," *J Pharmacol Exp Ther*, 1989, 249(1):131-3.

♦ **Dopar**® *see* Levodopa *on page 665*
♦ **Dopram**® *see* Doxapram *on page 409*

Dornase Alfa *(DOOR nase AL fa)*

U.S. Brand Names Pulmozyme®

Synonyms DNase; Recombinant Human Deoxyribonuclease

Therapeutic Category Enzyme, Inhalant; Mucolytic Agent

Generic Available No

Use Management of cystic fibrosis patients to reduce the frequency of respiratory infections and to improve pulmonary function

Pregnancy Risk Factor B

Contraindications Hypersensitivity to dornase alfa, Chinese hamster ovary cell products (eg, epoetin alfa), or any component

Warnings Safety and efficacy has not been established in children <5 years of age or in patients with forced vital capacity <40% of normal; no data exists regarding safety during lactation

Adverse Reactions

Cardiovascular: Chest pain

Dermatologic: Skin rash

Gastrointestinal: Sore throat

Hepatic: Liver disease

Ocular: Conjunctivitis

Respiratory: Increased cough, dyspnea, hemoptysis, wheezing, laryngitis, rhinitis, pharyngitis

Miscellaneous: Voice alteration, hoarseness

Drug Interactions None known at this time

Stability Must be stored in the refrigerator at 2°C to 8°C (36°F to 46°F) and protected from strong light; unopened vials left at room temperature for a total time of 24 hours should be discarded; discard solution if cloudy or discolored

Mechanism of Action Dornase alfa is a deoxyribonuclease (DNA) enzyme produced by recombinant gene technology. Dornase selectively cleaves DNA, thus reducing mucous viscosity seen in the pulmonary secretions of cystic fibrosis patients. As a result, airflow in the lung is improved and the risk of bacterial infection may be decreased.

Pharmacodynamics Onset of improved pulmonary function tests (PFTs): 3-8 days; PFTs will return to baseline 2-3 weeks after discontinuation of therapy

Pharmacokinetics Following nebulization, enzyme levels are measurable in the sputum within 15 minutes and decline rapidly thereafter

Usual Dosage

Infants and Children ≤5 years: Not approved for use, however studies using this therapy in small numbers of children as young as 3 months of age have reported efficacy and similar side effects. See References.

Children >5 years and Adults: Inhalation: 2.5 mg/day through selected nebulizers in conjunction with a Pulmo-Aide® or a Pari-Proneb® compressor; some patients, especially older than 21 years of age or with forced vital capacity (FVC) >85%, may benefit from twice daily administration

Administration Nebulization: Should not be diluted or mixed with any other drugs in the nebulizer, this may inactivate the drug

Dosage Forms Solution for inhalation: 1 mg/mL (2.5 mL)

References

Fuchs HJ, Borowitz DS, Christiansen DH, et al, "Effect of Aerosolized Recombinant Human DNase on Exacerbations of Respiratory Symptoms and on Pulmonary Function in Patients With Cystic Fibrosis," *N Engl J Med*, 1994, 331(10):637-42.

Mueller GA, Rubins G, Wessel D, et al, "Effects of Dornase Alfa on Pulmonary Function Tests in Infants with Cystic Fibrosis," *Am J Respir Crit Care Med*, 1996, 153:A70.

Rock M, Kirchner K, McCubbin M, et al, "Aerosol Delivery and Safety of rhDNASE in Young Children With Cystic Fibrosis: A Bronchoscopic Study," *Pediatr Pulmonol*, 1996, 13(Suppl):A268.

♦ **Doryx**® *see* Doxycycline *on page 415*

Dorzolamide (dor ZOLE a mide)

U.S. Brand Names Trusopt®

Therapeutic Category Carbonic Anhydrase Inhibitor, Ophthalmic

Generic Available No

Use Treatment of elevated intraocular pressure in patients with ocular hypertension or open-angle glaucoma

Pregnancy Risk Factor C

Contraindications Hypersensitivity to dorzolamide, sulfonamides, or any component

Warnings Dorzolamide, a sulfonamide, is absorbed systemically and may produce the same adverse effects seen with other sulfonamides; avoid use in patients with severe renal dysfunction (Cl_{cr} <30 mL/minute); contains the preservative benzalkonium chloride which may be absorbed by soft contact lenses; contact lenses should be removed prior to administration of the solution and may be reinserted 15 minutes following administration; concomitant use with other carbonic anhydrase inhibitors is not recommended

Precautions Use with caution in patients with hepatic impairment

Adverse Reactions

Central nervous system: Headache, fatigue, dizziness, vertigo

Dermatologic: Rash, pruritus, urticaria

Gastrointestinal: Bitter taste, nausea, throat irritation

Genitourinary: Urolithiasis

Neuromuscular & skeletal: Paresthesia

Ocular: Burning, stinging, discomfort, and pain, punctate keratitis, conjunctivitis, blurred vision, eye redness, tearing, dryness, photophobia, transient myopia, eyelid crusting, increased corneal thickness

Respiratory: Dyspnea

Drug Interactions Increased risk of nephrolithiasis when used with topiramate; additive intraocular pressure lowering with topical β-adrenergic blocking agents

Stability Store at room temperature.

Mechanism of Action Competitive, reversible inhibition of the enzyme carbonic anhydrase in the ciliary processes of the eye resulting in decreased secretion of aqueous humor

Pharmacodynamics

Peak effect: 2 hours

Duration: 8-12 hours

Average lowering of intraoptic pressure: 3-5 mm Hg or at least 15% decrease from unmedicated baseline value

Pharmacokinetics

Absorption: Topical: Reaches systemic circulation

Distribution: Accumulates in RBCs during chronic administration

Protein binding: 33%

Metabolism: In liver to active but less potent metabolite, N-desethyl dorzolamide

Half-life: Terminal RBC half-life: 147 days

Elimination: Primarily unchanged in the urine

Usual Dosage Glaucoma: Adults: 1 drop into the affected eye(s) 3 times/day

Administration Ophthalmic: Apply gentle pressure to lacrimal sac during and immediately following instillation (1 minute) or instruct patient to gently close eyelid after administration to decrease systemic absorption of ophthalmic drops; avoid contact of bottle tip with skin or eye; remove contact lenses prior to administration (see Warnings); lenses may be inserted 15 minutes after instillation; if more than one topical ophthalmic drug is being used, separate administration by at least 10 minutes

Monitoring Parameters Intraoptic pressure

Patient Information Avoid contact of bottle tip with skin or eye to prevent contamination by bacteria which may cause ocular infections; report any ocular reactions, particularly conjunctivitis and lid reactions to your physician promptly

(Continued)

Dorzolamide *(Continued)*

Additional Information Dorzolamide was used successfully in 11 pediatric patients <18 years of age (mean: 7.4 years), who were previously treated with acetazolamide (Portellos, 1998)

Dosage Forms Solution, ophthalmic, as hydrochloride: 2% (5 mL, 10 mL)

References

Portellos M, Buckley EG, and Freedman SF, "Topical Versus Oral Carbonic Anhydrase Inhibitor Therapy for Pediatric Glaucoma," *J AAPOS*, 1998, 2(1):43-7.

♦ **DOS® [OTC]** *see* Docusate *on page 402*

♦ **DOSS** *see* Docusate *on page 402*

Doxacurium *(doks a KYOO ri um)*

U.S. Brand Names Nuromax®

Therapeutic Category Neuromuscular Blocker Agent, Nondepolarizing; Skeletal Muscle Relaxant, Paralytic

Generic Available No

Use Doxacurium is indicated for use as an adjunct to general anesthesia. It provides skeletal muscle relaxation during surgery or endotracheal intubation; increases pulmonary compliance during mechanical ventilation

Pregnancy Risk Factor C

Contraindications Hypersensitivity to doxacurium or any component

Warnings Use with caution in patients with neuromuscular disease such as myasthenia gravis, cardiovascular disease; use with caution and reduce dosage in patients with renal or hepatic impairment; certain clinical conditions may result in potentiation or antagonism of neuromuscular blockade, see table on next page.

Adverse Reactions The most frequent adverse reactions appear as an extension of the agent's neuromuscular blocking actions

Cardiovascular: Hypotension (rare), bradycardia (rare)
Central nervous system: Fever
Dermatologic: Cutaneous flushing, urticaria
Neuromuscular & skeletal: Muscle weakness
Ocular: Diplopia
Respiratory: Respiratory insufficiency and apnea, bronchospasm, wheezing

Drug Interactions See table below.

Potential Drug Interactions

Potentiation	Antagonism
Inhalation anesthetics	Calcium
Desflurane, sevoflurane, enflurane and	Carbamazepine
isoflurane > halothane > nitrous	Phenytoin
oxide	Steroids (chronic administration)
Antibiotics	Theophylline
Aminoglycosides, polymyxins,	Anticholinesterases*
clindamycin, vancomycin, tetracycline	Neostigmine, pyridostigmine,
Magnesium	edrophonium, echothiophate
Antiarrhythmics	ophthalmic solution
Quinidine, procainamide, bretylium, and	Caffeine
possibly lidocaine	Azathioprine
Diuretics	
Furosemide, mannitol, thiazides	
Amphotericin B (secondary to hypokalemia)	
Local anesthetics	
Dantrolene (directly depresses skeletal muscle)	
Beta blockers	
Calcium channel blockers	
Ketamine	
Lithium	
Succinylcholine (when administered prior to nondepolarizing neuromuscular-blocking agent)	
Cyclosporine	

*Can prolong the effects of acetylcholine

Clinical Conditions Affecting Neuromuscular Blockade

Potentiation	Antagonism
Electrolyte abnormalities	Alkalosis
Severe hyponatremia	Hypercalcemia
Severe hypocalcemia	Demyelinating lesions
Severe hypokalemia	Peripheral neuropathies
Hypermagnesemia	Diabetes mellitus
Neuromuscular diseases	
Acidosis	
Acute intermittent porphyria	
Renal failure	
Hepatic failure	

Stability Stable for 24 hours at room temperature when diluted in concentrations up to 0.1 mg/mL in D_5W or NS; compatible with sufentanil, alfentanil, and fentanyl; incompatible with alkaline solutions

Mechanism of Action Doxacurium is a long-acting nondepolarizing skeletal muscle relaxant. The drug is a bis-quaternary benzylisoquinolinium diester, with a chemical structure similar to that of atracurium. Similar to other nondepolarizing neuromuscular blocking agents, doxacurium produces muscle relaxation by competing with acetylcholine for cholinergic receptor sites on the postjunctional membrane; significant presynaptic depressant activity is also observed.

Pharmacodynamics
Onset of action: 5-11 minutes
Duration: 30 minutes (range: 12-54 minutes)

Pharmacokinetics
Distribution: V_d: Adults: 0.22 L/kg
Protein binding: 30%
Half-life:
Normal: 1.5 hours
Renal dysfunction: 3.7 hours
Liver dysfunction: 1.9 hours
Elimination: Primarily as unchanged drug via the kidneys (80%) and biliary tract (20%)

Usual Dosage I.V. (in obese patients, use ideal body weight):
Children 2-12 years: Initial: 0.03-0.05 mg/kg/dose (30-50 mcg/kg/dose); maintenance: 0.005-0.01 mg/kg (5-10 mcg/kg/dose) every 30-45 minutes, or as needed depending upon individual patient response
Continuous infusion: 0.1-0.2 mcg/kg/minute or 6-12 mcg/kg/hour
Children >12 years and Adults: Initial: 0.025-0.05 mg/kg/dose (25-50 mcg/kg/dose); maintenance: 0.005-0.01 mg/kg/dose (5-10 mcg/kg/dose) every 60-100 minutes
Continuous infusion: 0.1-0.2 mcg/kg/minute or 6-12 mcg/kg/hour
Dosing adjustment in renal or hepatic impairment: Reduce initial dose and titrate carefully as duration may be prolonged

Administration Parenteral: I.V.: May be administered by rapid I.V. injection undiluted

Monitoring Parameters Peripheral nerve stimulation testing (measures twitch response), heart rate, blood pressure, assisted ventilation status

Additional Information Doxacurium is a long-acting nondepolarizing neuromuscular blocker with virtually no cardiovascular side effects. The characteristics of this agent make it especially useful in procedures requiring careful maintenance of hemodynamic stability for prolonged periods

Dosage Forms Injection, solution, as chloride: 1 mg/mL (5 mL)

References
Martin LD, Bratton SL, and O'Rourke PP, "Clinical Uses and Controversies of Neuromuscular Blocking Agents in Infants and Children," *Crit Care Med*, 1999, 27(7):1358-68.

Doxapram (DOKS a pram)

U.S. Brand Names Dopram®

Therapeutic Category Central Nervous System Stimulant, Nonamphetamine; Respiratory Stimulant

Generic Available No

Use Respiratory and CNS stimulant; idiopathic apnea of prematurity refractory to xanthines; aid in the prevention of elevation of arterial CO_2 tension during the administration of oxygen to patients with acute respiratory insufficiency superimposed on COPD

Pregnancy Risk Factor B
(Continued)

Doxapram *(Continued)*

Contraindications Hypersensitivity to doxapram or any component (see Warnings); epilepsy, cerebral edema, head injury, asthma or restrictive pulmonary disease, pheochromocytoma, cardiovascular or coronary artery disease, hypertension, hyperthyroidism, cardiac arrhythmias; concomitant use with mechanical ventilation in COPD patients

Warnings Doxapram contains benzyl alcohol which may cause allergic reactions in susceptible individuals; large amounts of benzyl alcohol ($\geq$99 mg/kg/day) have been associated with a potentially fatal toxicity ("gasping syndrome") in neonates; the "gasping syndrome" consists of metabolic acidosis, respiratory distress, gasping respirations, CNS dysfunction (including convulsions, intracranial hemorrhage), hypotension and cardiovascular collapse. Recommended doses of doxapram for treatment of neonatal apnea will deliver 5.4-27 mg/kg/day of benzyl alcohol; the use of doxapram should be reserved for neonates who are unresponsive to the treatment of apnea with therapeutic serum concentrations of theophylline or caffeine. *In vitro* and animal studies have shown that benzoate, a metabolite of benzyl alcohol, displaces bilirubin from protein-binding sites. Doxapram is not an antagonist to muscle relaxant drugs nor a specific narcotic antagonist; doxapram alone may not stimulate adequate spontaneous breathing or provide sufficient arousal in patients who are severely depressed; use as an adjunct to establish supportive measures; to reduce the potential for arrhythmias, including VT and VF, in patients who have received general anesthesia with a volatile agent known to sensitize the myocardium to catecholamines, administration of doxapram should be delayed until the complete excretion of anesthetic has occurred.

Precautions Oxygen, resuscitative equipment, and anticonvulsants should be readily available to manage excessive CNS stimulation. Frequent arterial blood gas measurements are recommended to identify and prevent the development of CO_2 retention and acidosis in COPD patients with acute hypercapnia; infusion of doxapram in premature infants has been associated with a statistically significant but moderate lengthening of QT_c interval; cardiac monitoring during treatment is suggested (Maillard, 2001)

Adverse Reactions

Cardiovascular: Hypertension (dose-related), tachycardia, arrhythmias, hypotension, flushing, chest pain

Central nervous system: CNS stimulation, restlessness, lightheadedness, jitters, hallucinations, irritability, seizures, headache, fever, hypothermia

Hematologic: Hemolysis

Gastrointestinal: Abdominal distension, nausea, vomiting, retching, increased gastric residuals

Genitourinary: Urinary retention

Local: Phlebitis

Metabolic: Hyperglycemia

Neuromuscular & skeletal: Tremor, hyper-reflexia

Ocular: Lacrimation, mydriasis

Renal: Glucosuria, albuminuria, elevated BUN

Respiratory: Coughing, laryngospasm, dyspnea

Miscellaneous: Diaphoresis

Drug Interactions Sympathomimetic drugs and MAO inhibitors may cause significant increase in blood pressure; general anesthetics (see Warnings)

Stability Stable at room temperature; incompatible with aminophylline, sodium bicarbonate, thiopental sodium, and other alkaline solutions

Mechanism of Action Stimulates respiration through action on respiratory center in medulla or through reflex stimulation of carotid, aortic, or other peripheral chemoreceptors; antagonizes opiate-induced respiratory depression, but does not affect analgesia

Pharmacodynamics Following I.V. injection:

Onset of respiratory stimulation: Within 20-40 seconds

Maximum effect: Within 1-2 minutes

Duration: 5-12 minutes

Pharmacokinetics

Metabolism: Extensive in the liver to active metabolite (keto-doxapram)

Distribution: V_d: Neonates: 4-7.3 L/kg

Half-life:

Neonates, premature: 6.6-12 hours

Adults: Mean: 3.4 hours (range: 2.4-4.1 hours)

Clearance: Neonates, premature: 0.44-0.7 L/hour/kg

Usual Dosage I.V.:

Neonatal apnea (apnea of prematurity): Initial loading dose: 2.5-3 mg/kg followed by a continuous infusion of 1 mg/kg/hour; titrate to the lowest rate at which apnea is controlled (maximum dose: 2.5 mg/kg/hour)

Adults: Respiratory depression following anesthesia:

Initial: 0.5-1 mg/kg; may repeat at 5-minute intervals; maximum total dose: 2 mg/kg

I.V. infusion: Initial: 5 mg/minute until adequate response or adverse effects seen; decrease to 1-3 mg/minute; usual total dose: 0.5-4 mg/kg or 300 mg

Administration Parenteral: I.V. use only: Dilute loading dose to a maximum concentration of 2 mg/mL and infuse over 15-30 minutes; for infusion, dilute in NS or dextrose (D_5W or $D_{10}W$) to 1 mg/mL (maximum concentration: 2 mg/mL); irritating to tissues; avoid extravasation

Monitoring Parameters Pulse oximetry, blood pressure, heart rate, deep tendon reflexes; for apnea: number, duration, and severity of apneic episodes

Reference Range Initial studies suggest a therapeutic serum level of at least 1.5 mg/L; toxicity becomes frequent at serum levels >5 mg/L

Dosage Forms Injection, solution, as hydrochloride: 20 mg/mL (20 mL) [contains benzyl alcohol]

References

Barrington KJ, Finer NN, Torok-Both G, et al, "Dose-Response Relationship of Doxapram in the Therapy for Refractory Idiopathic Apnea of Prematurity," *Pediatrics*, 1987, 80(1):22-7.

Bhatt-Mehta V and Schumacher RE, "Treatment of Apnea of Prematurity," *Paediatr Drugs*, 2003, 5(3):195-210.

Maillard C, Boutroy MJ, Fresson J, et al, "QT Interval Lengthening in Premature Infants Treated With Doxapram," *Clin Pharmacol Ther*, 2001, 70(6):540-5.

Doxepin (DOKS e pin)

Related Information

Comparison of Adverse Effects of Antidepressants *on page 1210*

Comparison of Usual Adult Dosage and Mechanism of Action of Antidepressants *on page 1209*

Drugs and Breast-Feeding *on page 1404*

Overdose and Toxicology *on page 1388*

U.S. Brand Names Prudoxin™; Sinequan®; Zonalon®

Canadian Brand Names Apo®-Doxepin; Novo-Doxepin

Therapeutic Category Antianxiety Agent; Antidepressant, Tricyclic

Generic Available Yes (capsule, solution)

Use

Oral: Treatment of various forms of depression, usually in conjunction with psychotherapy; treatment of anxiety disorders; analgesic for certain chronic and neuropathic pain

Topical: Adults: Short-term (<8 days) therapy of moderate pruritus due to atopic dermatitis or lichen simplex chronicus

Pregnancy Risk Factor C (Topical: B)

Contraindications Hypersensitivity to doxepin or any component (see Warnings); cross-sensitivity with other tricyclic antidepressants may occur; narrow-angle glaucoma; patients with urinary retention

Warnings Causes a high degree of sedation (relative to other antidepressants); may cause orthostatic hypotension and anticholinergic side effects; may worsen psychosis or precipitate mania or hypomania in patients with bipolar disease; may increase the risks associated with electroconvulsive therapy. Discontinue therapy, when possible, prior to elective surgery. Do not discontinue abruptly in patients receiving chronic high dose therapy; cream contains benzyl alcohol which may cause allergic reactions in susceptible individuals; large amounts of benzyl alcohol (≥99 mg/kg/day) have been associated with a potentially fatal toxicity ("gasping syndrome") in neonates; avoid use of doxepin products containing benzyl alcohol in neonates; *in vitro* and animal studies have shown that benzoate, a metabolite of benzyl alcohol, displaces bilirubin from protein binding sites

Precautions Use with caution in patients with cardiovascular disease, conduction disturbances, seizure disorders, urinary retention, hyperthyroidism or those receiving thyroid replacement; avoid use during lactation; use with caution in pregnancy

Drowsiness and other systemic effects may occur with topical use; occlusive dressings may increase absorption of doxepin; allergic contact dermatitis may occur with topical use, risk may be increased with use >8 days. **Note:** Cream is not recommended for use in pediatric patients; overdoses from topical administration in children have been reported.

Adverse Reactions Pronounced sedation and anticholinergic adverse effects may occur

Cardiovascular: Hypotension, arrhythmias

(Continued)

Doxepin (Continued)

Central nervous system: Sedation, confusion, dizziness, headache; drowsiness occurs in 22% of patients receiving topical cream especially if applied to >10% of body surface area; reduction in area treated, number of applications per day, amount of cream used, or discontinuation of cream may be needed if excessive drowsiness occurs

Dermatologic: Photosensitivity

Endocrine & metabolic: SIADH (rare)

Gastrointestinal: Constipation, nausea, vomiting, xerostomia, increased appetite, weight gain

Genitourinary: Urinary retention

Hematologic: Blood dyscrasias (rare)

Hepatic: Hepatitis

Local: Stinging and burning at application site; exacerbation of pruritus or eczema; allergic contact dermatitis

Neuromuscular & skeletal: Fine tremor

Ocular: Blurred vision

Otic: Tinnitus

Miscellaneous: Hypersensitivity reactions

Drug Interactions Cytochrome P450 isoenzyme CYP2D6 substrate

CNS depressants, alcohol, or antihistamines may potentiate sedative effects; use with MAO inhibitors may cause serious side effects including death (use within 14 days is not recommended); carbamazepine, guanethidine, clonidine, antithyroid agents; cimetidine (serious anticholinergic symptoms may occur); tolazamide (severe hypoglycemia may occur); the herbal medicine St John's wort (*Hypericum perforatum*) may increase serious side effects, its use is **not** recommended; use with cytochrome P450 CYP2D6 inhibitors may increase doxepin serum concentrations or effects (monitor patient and serum concentrations); concurrent use of high-dose TCAs and ritonavir may cause the serotonin syndrome

Food Interactions Oral solution is physically incompatible with carbonated beverages and grape juice; diets rich in fiber may decrease drug effects

Stability Protect from light; store cream at ≤80°F (27°C)

Mechanism of Action Increases the synaptic concentration of serotonin and/or norepinephrine in the CNS by inhibition of their reuptake by the presynaptic neuronal membrane

Pharmacodynamics Maximum antidepressant effects: Usually occur after >2 weeks; anxiolytic effects may occur sooner

Pharmacokinetics

Distribution: Crosses the placenta; appears in breast milk

Protein binding: 80% to 85%

Metabolism: Hepatic to metabolites, including desmethyldoxepin (active)

Half-life, adults: 6-8 hours

Elimination: Renal

Usual Dosage

Oral:

Children: 1-3 mg/kg/day in single or divided doses

Adolescents: Initial: 25-50 mg/day in single or divided doses; gradually increase to 100 mg/day

Adults: Initial: 30-150 mg/day at bedtime or in 2-3 divided doses; may increase up to 300 mg/day; single dose should not exceed 150 mg; select patients may respond to 25-50 mg/day

Topical: Adults: Apply to affected area 4 times/day

Administration

Oral: Administer with food to decrease GI upset; oral concentrate should be diluted in water, milk, or juice (but not grape juice) prior to administration (use 120 mL for adults); do not mix with carbonated beverages

Topical: Apply thin film of cream to affected area with at least 3-4 hours between applications; do not use occlusive dressings; do not use for >8 days; avoid contact with eyes

Monitoring Parameters Blood pressure, heart rate, mental status, weight, liver enzymes, CBC with differential

Reference Range Utility of serum level monitoring controversial

Doxepin plus desmethyldoxepin:

Proposed therapeutic concentration: 110-250 ng/mL (394-895 nmol/L)

Toxic concentration: >500 ng/mL (>1790 nmol/L) (toxicities may be seen at lower concentrations in some patients)

Patient Information May cause drowsiness and impair ability to perform activities requiring mental alertness or physical coordination; may cause dry mouth; avoid alcohol and the herbal medicine St John's wort; limit caffeine; may increase appetite;

do not discontinue abruptly. May cause photosensitivity reactions (eg, exposure to sunlight may cause severe sunburn, skin rash, redness, or itching); avoid exposure to sunlight and artificial light sources (sunlamps, tanning booth/bed); wear protective clothing, wide-brimmed hats, sunglasses, and lip sunscreen (SPF ≥15); use a sunscreen [broad-spectrum sunscreen or physical sunscreen (preferred) or sunblock with SPF ≥15]; contact physician if reaction occurs.

Nursing Implications Do not use occlusive dressings with cream (increases dermal absorption)

Additional Information Safety and effectiveness of topical cream when used for >8 days has not been established; use >8 days may result in an increase in serum concentrations and systemic effects

Dosage Forms

Capsule, as hydrochloride (Sinequan®): 10 mg, 25 mg, 50 mg, 75 mg, 100 mg, 150 mg

Cream, as hydrochloride:

Prudoxin™: 5% (45 g) [contains benzyl alcohol]

Zonalon®: 5% (30 g, 45 g) [contains benzyl alcohol]

Solution, oral **concentrate**, as hydrochloride (Sinequan®): 10 mg/mL (120 mL)

References

Levy HB, Harper CR, and Weinberg WA, " A Practical Approach to Children Failing in School," *Pediatr Clin North Am*, 1992, 39(4):895-928.

DOXOrubicin (doks oh ROO bi sin)

Related Information

Drugs and Breast-Feeding *on page 1404*

Emetogenic Potential of Single Chemotherapeutic Agents *on page 1286*

Extravasation Treatment *on page 1240*

U.S. Brand Names Adriamycin PFS®; Adriamycin RDF®; Rubex®

Synonyms ADR; Hydroxydaunomycin

Therapeutic Category Antineoplastic Agent, Anthracycline; Antineoplastic Agent, Antibiotic

Generic Available Yes

Use Treatment of various solid tumors including ovarian, breast, and bladder tumors; various lymphomas and leukemias (AML, ALL), soft tissue sarcomas, neuroblastoma, osteosarcoma

Pregnancy Risk Factor D

Contraindications Hypersensitivity to doxorubicin or any component; severe CHF, cardiomyopathy, pre-existing myelosuppression; patients who have received a total dose of 550 mg/m² of doxorubicin or 400 mg/m² in patients with previous or concomitant treatment with daunorubicin, idarubicin, mitoxantrone, cyclophosphamide, or irradiation of the cardiac region; patients who have received previous treatment with complete cumulative doses of daunorubicin, idarubicin, or other anthracycline derivatives; pregnancy

Warnings The FDA currently recommends that procedures for proper handling and disposal of antineoplastic agents be considered. **I.V. use only,** severe local tissue necrosis will result if extravasation occurs; irreversible myocardial toxicity, including potentially fatal CHF, may occur during therapy or months to years after therapy termination. The probability of developing myocardial toxicity is estimated to be 1% to 2% at a total cumulative dose of 300 mg/m² of doxorubicin, 3% to 5% at a total cumulative dose of 400 mg/m², 5% to 8% at a total cumulative dose of 450 mg/m², and 6% to 20% at 500 mg/m². Myocardial toxicity may occur at lower cumulative doses in patients with prior mediastinal irradiation, concurrent cyclophosphamide therapy, or pre-existing heart disease. Pediatric patients are at increased risk for developing delayed cardiac toxicity and CHF during early adulthood due to an increasing census of long-term survivors; periodic long-term monitoring of cardiac function is recommended. Doxorubicin may contribute to prepubertal growth failure in pediatric patients. Pediatric patients are at risk of developing secondary acute myeloid leukemia. Severe myelosuppression is also possible.

Precautions Use with caution and modify dosage in patients with impaired hepatic function

Adverse Reactions

Cardiovascular: CHF, cardiomyopathy, cardiotoxicity (transient type with abnormal EKG and arrhythmias, or a chronic, cumulative, dose-dependent type which progresses to CHF), cardiorespiratory decompensation, facial flushing

Central nervous system: Fever, chills

Dermatologic: Alopecia, hyperpigmentation of nail beds, urticaria, photosensitivity, radiation recall, urticaria

Endocrine & metabolic: Hyperuricemia, infertility, prepubertal growth failure

(Continued)

DOXOrubicin (Continued)

Gastrointestinal: Stomatitis, esophagitis, nausea, vomiting, mucositis, anorexia, diarrhea, ulceration and necrosis of the colon

Genitourinary: Discoloration of urine (red/orange), cystitis, hematuria, urinary frequency

Hematologic: Leukopenia (nadir: 10-14 days), thrombocytopenia, anemia

Hepatic: Transient elevation of liver enzymes

Local: Tissue necrosis upon extravasation, erythematous streaking along the vein if administered too rapidly, phlebitis

Ocular: Lacrimation

Miscellaneous: Anaphylaxis

Drug Interactions Cytochrome P450 isoenzyme CYP3A3/4 substrate; isoenzyme CYP2D6 inhibitor

May potentiate the toxicity of cyclophosphamide, mercaptopurine; ritonavir and cyclosporine decrease doxorubicin metabolism; doxorubicin decreases carbamazepine, digoxin, and phenytoin levels; paclitaxel decreases doxorubicin clearance resulting in increased toxicity if administered prior to doxorubicin; phenobarbital increases elimination of doxorubicin

Stability Protect from light; store vials containing powder at room temperature, refrigerate vials containing liquid; reconstituted vials stable for 7 days at room temperature and 15 days if refrigerated and protected from light. Discard unused portion of preservative free injection vial. Incompatible with hydrocortisone, fluorouracil, furosemide, sodium bicarbonate, aminophylline, heparin, cephalothin, dexamethasone; unstable in solutions with a pH <3 or >7. Color change from red to purple indicates decomposition of drug.

Mechanism of Action Inhibits DNA and RNA synthesis by intercalating between DNA base pairs and by steric obstruction inducing DNA breaks; produces oxygen-free radicals which cause DNA denaturation

Pharmacokinetics

Distribution: Into breast milk; does not penetrate into CSF; distributes into cells rapidly with high concentrations in lung, kidney, muscle, spleen, and liver

Protein binding: 75%

Metabolism: In both the liver and in plasma to both active and inactive metabolites

Half-life, triphasic:

Primary: 30 minutes

Secondary: 3-3.5 hours for its metabolites

Terminal: 17-30 hours for doxorubicin and its metabolites

Elimination: Undergoes triphasic elimination; 40% to 60% eventually excreted in bile and feces; <5% excreted in urine, primarily as unchanged drug and metabolites

Clearance:

Infants <2 years: 813 mL/minute/m^2

Children >2 years: 1540 mL/minute/m^2

Usual Dosage Patient's ideal weight should be used to calculate body surface area. Lower dose regimens should be given to patients with decreased bone marrow reserve, prior radiation therapy, or marrow infiltration with malignant cells.

I.V. (refer to individual protocols):

Children: 35-75 mg/m^2 as a single dose, repeat every 21 days; or 20-30 mg/m^2 once weekly; or 60-90 mg/m^2 given as a continuous infusion over 96 hours every 3-4 weeks

Adults: 60-75 mg/m^2 as a single dose, repeat every 21 days; or 20-30 mg/m^2/day for 2-3 days, repeat in 4 weeks or 20 mg/m^2 once weekly

Dosing adjustment in hepatic impairment:

Bilirubin 1.2-3 mg/dL: Reduce dose by 50%

Bilirubin >3 mg/dL: Reduce dose by 75%

Administration Parenteral: I.V. use only; reconstitute IVP doses with D$_5$W or NS to ensure isotonicity of the final solution; administer slow IVP at a rate no faster than over 3-5 minutes or by I.V. infusion over 1-4 hours at a concentration not to exceed 2 mg/mL, or by I.V. continuous infusion

Monitoring Parameters CBC with differential, erythrocyte and platelet count; serum uric acid, echocardiogram, radionuclide left ventricular ejection fraction, liver enzymes, and bilirubin; observe I.V. injection site for infiltration and vein irritation

Patient Information Transient red-orange discoloration of urine can occur for up to 48 hours after a dose; notify physician if fever, sore throat, bleeding, or bruising occurs; report any stinging sensation at the injection site during infusion. May cause photosensitivity reactions (eg, exposure to sunlight may cause severe sunburn, skin rash, redness, or itching); avoid exposure to sunlight and artificial light sources (sunlamps, tanning booth/bed); wear protective clothing, wide-brimmed hats, sunglasses, and lip sunscreen (SPF ≥15); use a sunscreen [broad-spectrum sunscreen or physical sunscreen (preferred) or sunblock with SPF ≥15]; contact physician if reaction occurs.

Nursing Implications Local erythematous streaking along the vein and/or facial flushing may indicate too rapid a rate of administration; drug is very irritating; avoid extravasation; if extravasation occurs, apply cold packs immediately for 30-60 minutes, then alternate off/on every 15 minutes for 1 day; apply 1.5 mL of dimethyl-sulfoxide 99% (w/v) solution to the site every 6 hours for 14 days; allow to air-dry; do not cover. Take precautions to prevent contact with the patient's urine and other body fluids for at least 5 days after each treatment.

Additional Information Myelosuppressive effects:
WBC: Moderate
Platelets: Moderate
Onset (days): 7
Nadir (days): 10-14
Recovery (days): 21-28

Dosage Forms
Injection, powder for reconstitution, lyophilized, as hydrochloride: 10 mg, 20 mg, 50 mg
Adriamycin RDF®: 10 mg, 20 mg, 50 mg, 150 mg [rapid dissolution formula]
Rubex®: 50 mg, 100 mg
Injection, solution, as hydrochloride [preservative free]: 2 mg/mL (5 mL, 10 mL, 25 mL, 100 mL)
Adriamycin PFS® [preservative free]: 2 mg/mL (5 mL, 10 mL, 25 mL, 37.5 mL, 100 mL)

References
Berg SL, Grissell DL, DeLaney TF, et al, "Principles of Treatment of Pediatric Solid Tumors," *Pediatr Clin North Am*, 1991, 38(2):249-67.
Ishii E, Hara T, Ohkubo K, et al, "Treatment of Childhood Acute Lymphoblastic Leukemia With Intermediate Dose Cytosine Arabinoside and Adriamycin," *Med Pediatr Oncol*, 1986, 14(2):73-7.
Legha SS, Benjamin RS, Mackay B, et al, "Reduction of Doxorubicin Cardiotoxicity by Prolonged Continuous Intravenous Infusion," *Ann Intern Med*, 1982, 96(2):133-9.

♦ **Doxy-100®** *see Doxycycline on page 415*

♦ **Doxycin (Can)** *see Doxycycline on page 415*

Doxycycline (doks i SYE kleen)

U.S. Brand Names Adoxa™; Doryx®; Doxy-100®; Monodox®; Vibramycin®; Vibra-Tabs®

Canadian Brand Names Apo®-Doxy; Apo®-Doxy Tabs; Doxycin; Doxytec; Novo-Doxylin; Nu-Doxycycline

Therapeutic Category Antibiotic, Tetracycline Derivative

Generic Available Yes

Use
Children, Adolescents, Adults: Treatment of Rocky Mountain spotted fever caused by susceptible *Rickettsia*; treatment of ehrlichiosis
Older Children, Adolescents, Adults: Treatment of Lyme disease, *Mycoplasma* infection, anthrax, or *Legionella*; management of malignant pleural effusions when intrapleural therapy is indicated
Adolescents and Adults: Treatment of nongonococcal pelvic inflammatory disease and urethritis due to *Chlamydia*; treatment for victims of sexual assault

Pregnancy Risk Factor D

Contraindications Hypersensitivity to doxycycline, tetracycline, or any component (see Warnings); children <8 years; severe hepatic dysfunction

Warnings Syrup contains sodium metabisulfite which may cause allergic reactions in susceptible individuals. Photosensitivity reaction may occur with this drug; avoid prolonged exposure to sunlight or tanning equipment. Do not administer to children <8 years of age due to associated retardation in skeletal development; use of tetracyclines during tooth development may cause permanent discoloration of the teeth and enamel hypoplasia; staining of teeth is dose-related so that duration of therapy should be minimized; doxycycline may be less likely to stain developing teeth than tetracycline since it binds less strongly to calcium; prolonged use may result in superinfection.

Adverse Reactions
Central nervous system: Elevated intracranial pressure, bulging fontanels in infants
Dermatologic: Rash, photosensitivity, discoloration of nails
Gastrointestinal: Nausea, diarrhea, esophagitis and esophageal ulceration with the hyclate salt formulation; anorexia, pseudomembranous colitis, oral candidiasis
Hematologic: Neutropenia, eosinophilia
Hepatic: Hepatotoxicity
Local: Phlebitis, pain at the injection site
Neuromuscular & skeletal: Retardation of skeletal development in infants
(Continued)

Doxycycline *(Continued)*

Miscellaneous: May cause discoloration of teeth in children <8 years of age

Drug Interactions Cytochrome P450 isoenzyme CYP3A3/4 substrate

Antacids containing aluminum, calcium, or magnesium, zinc, kaolin, pectin, iron, and bismuth subsalicylate may decrease doxycycline bioavailability; rifampin, barbiturates, phenytoin, and carbamazepine decrease doxycycline's half-life; doxycycline enhances the hypoprothrombinemic effect of warfarin; decreased effect of oral contraceptives

Food Interactions Administration with iron, calcium, milk or dairy products may decrease doxycycline absorption; may decrease absorption of calcium, iron, magnesium, zinc and amino acids

Stability Reconstituted oral doxycycline suspension is stable for 2 weeks at room temperature; I.V. doxycycline solutions must be protected from direct sunlight

Mechanism of Action Inhibits protein synthesis by binding to the 30S and possibly the 50S ribosomal subunit(s) of susceptible bacteria preventing additions of amino acids to the growing peptide chain; may also cause alterations in the cytoplasmic membrane

Pharmacokinetics

Absorption: Almost completely from the GI tract; absorption can be reduced by food or milk by 20%

Distribution: Widely distributed into body tissues and fluids including synovial and pleural fluid, bile, bronchial secretions; poor penetration into the CSF; appears in breast milk

Protein binding: 80% to 85%

Metabolism: Not metabolized in the liver; partially inactivated in the GI tract by chelate formation

Bioavailability: 90% to 100%

Half-life: 12-15 hours (usually increases to 22-24 hours with multiple dosing)

Time to peak serum concentration: Oral: Within 1.5-4 hours

Elimination: In the urine (23%) and feces (30%)

Dialysis: Not dialyzable (0% to 5%)

Usual Dosage

Children ≥8 years: Oral, I.V.: 2-4 mg/kg/day divided every 12-24 hours, not to exceed 200 mg/day

Lyme disease: Oral: 100 mg/dose twice daily for 14-21 days

Chlamydial infections: Oral: 100 mg/dose twice daily for 7-10 days

Anthrax (if strain is proven susceptible): **Note:** In the presence of systemic involvement, extensive edema, and/or lesions on head/neck, doxycycline should initially be administered I.V. Initial treatment should include two or more agents per CDC recommendations. Agents suggested for use in conjunction with doxycycline include rifampin, vancomycin, penicillin, ampicillin, chloramphenicol, imipenem, clindamycin, or clarithromycin. Continue combined therapy for 60 days.

Treatment: I.V.: 5 mg/kg/day divided every 12 hours for 60 days (switch to oral therapy when clinically appropriate); maximum dose: 200 mg/day

Inhalation (postexposure prophylaxis): Oral: 5 mg/kg/day divided every 12 hours for 60 days; maximum dose: 200 mg/day

Adolescents and Adults: Oral, I.V.: 100-200 mg/day in 1-2 divided doses

Anthrax (if strain is proven susceptible): Refer to Children's dosing for "Note" on route, combined therapy, and duration

Treatment: I.V.: 100 mg every 12 hours for 60 days (substitute oral antibiotics for I.V. antibiotics as soon as clinical condition improves)

Inhalation (postexposure prophylaxis): Oral: 100 mg every 12 hours for 60 days

Lyme disease: Oral: 100 mg/dose twice daily for 14-21 days

Pelvic inflammatory disease:

Hospitalized regimen: Oral, I.V.: 100 mg every 12 hours for 14 days administered with cefoxitin or cefotetan

Outpatient regimen: Oral: 100 mg every 12 hours for 14 days plus single dose ceftriaxone

Sclerosing agent for pleural effusion: 500 mg in 25-30 mL of NS instilled into the pleural space to control pleural effusions associated with metastatic tumors; or for recurrent malignant pleural effusions: 500 mg in 250 mL NS

Administration

Oral: Administer capsules or tablets with adequate amounts of fluid; avoid antacids, infant formula, milk, dairy products, and iron for 1 hour before or 2 hours after administration of doxycycline; may be administered with food to decrease GI upset; shake suspension well before use

Parenteral: For I.V. use only; administer by slow I.V. intermittent infusion over a minimum of 1-2 hours at a concentration not to exceed 1 mg/mL (may be infused over 1-4 hours); concentrations <0.1 mg/mL are not recommended

Sclerosing agent:

To control pleural effusions associated with metastatic tumors: Instill into the pleural space through a thoracostomy tube following drainage of the accumulated pleural fluid; clamp the tube then remove the fluid

For recurrent malignant pleural effusions: Administer via chest tube lavage, clamp tube for 24 hours then drain

Monitoring Parameters Periodic monitoring of renal, hematologic, and hepatic function tests; observe for changes in bowel frequency

Test Interactions False-negative urine glucose using Clinistix®, Tes-Tape®; false-positive urine glucose using Clinitest®

Patient Information May discolor teeth if <8 years of age; may discolor fingernails. May cause photosensitivity reactions (eg, exposure to sunlight may cause severe sunburn, skin rash, redness, or itching); avoid exposure to sunlight and artificial light sources (sunlamps, tanning booth/bed); wear protective clothing, wide-brimmed hats, sunglasses, and lip sunscreen (SPF ≥15); use a sunscreen [broad-spectrum sunscreen or physical sunscreen (preferred) or sunblock with SPF ≥15]; contact physician if reaction occurs.

Nursing Implications Check for signs of phlebitis; I.V. doxycycline should not be given I.M. or S.C.; avoid extravasation

Additional Information Injection contains ascorbic acid

Dosage Forms

Capsule, as **hyclate** (Vibramycin®): 50 mg, 100 mg

Capsule, as **monohydrate** (Monodox®): 50 mg, 100 mg

Capsule, coated pellets, as **hyclate** (Doryx®): 100 mg

Injection, powder for reconstitution, as **hyclate** (Doxy-100™): 100 mg

Powder for oral suspension, as **monohydrate** (Vibramycin®): 25 mg/5 mL (60 mL) [raspberry flavor]

Syrup, as **calcium** (Vibramycin®): 50 mg/5 mL (480 mL) [contains sodium metabisulfite; raspberry-apple flavor]

Tablet, film coated, as **hyclate** (Vibra-Tabs®): 100 mg

Tablet, as **monohydrate** (Adoxa™): 50 mg, 100 mg

References

Centers for Disease Control and Prevention, "2002 Guidelines for Treatment of Sexually Transmitted Diseases," *MMWR Morb Mortal Wkly Rep*, 2002, 51(RR-6):1-80.

Centers for Disease Control and Prevention, "Update: Investigation of Anthrax Associated with Intentional Exposure and Interim Public Health Guidelines, October 2001," *MMWR Morb Mortal Wkly Rep*, 2001, 50(41):889-93.

Inglesby TV, Henderson DA, Bartlett JG, et al, "Anthrax as a Biological Weapon: Medical and Public Health Management. Working Group on Civilian Biodefense," *JAMA*, 1999, 281(18):1735-45.

Dronabinol (droe NAB i nol)

U.S. Brand Names Marinol®

Synonyms Tetrahydrocannabinol; THC

Therapeutic Category Antiemetic

Generic Available No

Use Treatment of nausea and vomiting secondary to cancer chemotherapy in patients who have not responded to conventional antiemetics; treatment of anorexia associated with weight loss in AIDS patients

Restrictions C-III

Pregnancy Risk Factor C

Contraindications Hypersensitivity to dronabinol, any component, marijuana, or sesame oil; should not be used in patients with a history of schizophrenia

Warnings Dronabinol has a high potential for abuse; limit antiemetic therapy availability to current cycle of chemotherapy

Precautions Use with caution in patients with heart disease, hepatic disease, or seizure disorders; reduce dosage in patients with severe hepatic impairment

(Continued)

Dronabinol *(Continued)*

Adverse Reactions

Cardiovascular: Orthostatic hypotension, tachycardia, palpitations, vasodilation, hypotension

Central nervous system: Drowsiness, dizziness, vertigo, difficulty in concentrating, mood change, euphoria, detachment, depression, anxiety, paranoia, hallucinations, nervousness, ataxia, headache, memory lapse

Gastrointestinal: Xerostomia, diarrhea

Hepatic: Elevated liver enzymes

Neuromuscular & skeletal: Myalgia, tremor, paresthesia, weakness

Ocular: Vision difficulties

Respiratory: Sinusitis, cough, rhinitis

Miscellaneous: Diaphoresis

Drug Interactions
Cytochrome P450 isoenzyme CYP2C18 and CYP3A3/4 substrate

Additive tachycardia, hypertension with amphetamines, cocaine, sympathomimetics, tricyclic antidepressants; additive CNS effects with sedatives, antihistamines, hypnotics, psychomimetics, tricyclic antidepressants, alcohol; hypomanic state with disulfiram, fluoxetine; increases theophylline metabolism; decreases barbiturate clearance

Stability
Store in a cool place

Mechanism of Action
Dronabinol is the principal psychoactive substance found in *Cannabis sativa* (marijuana); its mechanism of action as an antiemetic is not well defined, it probably inhibits the vomiting center in the medulla oblongata

Pharmacodynamics

Onset of action: 30 minutes to 1 hour

Maximum effect: 2-4 hours

Duration: 4-6 hours

Pharmacokinetics

Absorption: Oral: 90% to 95%; first-pass metabolism results in low systemic bioavailability

Distribution: V_d: ~10L/kg

Protein binding: 97% to 99%

Metabolism: Extensive first-pass; metabolized in the liver to several metabolites some of which are active

Bioavailability: 10% to 20%

Half-life:

Biphasic: Alpha: 4 hours

Terminal: 25-36 hours

Time to peak serum concentration: Within 2-3 hours

Elimination: Biliary excretion is the major route of elimination

Usual Dosage
Oral:

Antiemetic: Children and Adults: 5 mg/m^2 1-3 hours before chemotherapy, then give 5 mg/m^2/dose every 2-4 hours after chemotherapy for a total of 4-6 doses/day; dose may be increased up to a maximum of 15 mg/m^2 per dose if needed (dosage may be increased in 2.5 mg/m^2 increments)

Appetite stimulant: Adults: 2.5 mg twice daily before lunch and dinner; if intolerant, a dosage of 2.5 mg once daily at night may be tried; maximum dosage (escalating): 5 mg 4 times/day (20 mg/day)

Administration
May be administered without regard to meals; take before meals if used to stimulate appetite

Monitoring Parameters
Heart rate, blood pressure

Patient Information
May cause drowsiness and impair ability to perform activities requiring mental alertness or physical coordination; may cause dry mouth; avoid alcohol

Dosage Forms
Capsule, gelatin: 2.5 mg, 5 mg, 10 mg

References

Lane M, Smith FE, Sullivan RA, et al, "Dronabinol and Prochlorperazine Alone and in Combination as Antiemetic Agents for Cancer Chemotherapy," *Am J Clin Oncol*, 1990, 13(6):480-4.

Droperidol *(droe PER i dole)*

Related Information

Compatibility of Medications Mixed in a Syringe *on page 1412*

U.S. Brand Names
Inapsine®

Therapeutic Category
Antiemetic; Antipsychotic Agent

Generic Available
Yes

Use
Treatment of nausea and vomiting associated with surgical and diagnostic procedures in patients for whom other treatments are ineffective or inappropriate

Pregnancy Risk Factor
C

Contraindications Hypersensitivity to droperidol or any component; known or suspected QT prolongation; congenital long QT syndrome

Warnings Cases of QT prolongation and torsade de pointes in patients treated with droperidol in doses within or even below the approved dosage range have been reported. Some cases occurred in patients with no underlying risk factors for QT prolongation; fatalities have occurred.

Droperidol should be reserved for patients who fail other treatments. Prior to its use, all patients should undergo a 12-lead EKG. If the QT interval is prolonged, droperidol should not be used. Droperidol should be used with extreme caution in patients with risk factors for prolonged QT syndrome (ie, CHF; bradycardia; cardiac hypertrophy; any clinically significant cardiac disease; diuretic use; hypokalemia; hypomagnesemia; concomitant use of Class I or Class III antiarrhythmics, MAO inhibitors, or medications known to prolong the QT interval; age >65 years; alcohol abuse; and use of medications such as benzodiazepines, volatile anesthetics and I.V. opiates).

The dosage of droperidol should be individualized; dosages should be started low and titrated upward. Continuous EKG monitoring should be done prior to treatment and for 2-3 hours after treatment to monitor for arrhythmias. I.V. fluids and other therapy to treat hypotension should be readily available; monitor patients carefully. Use reduced initial doses of opioids, if needed. Neuromalignant syndrome may rarely occur.

Precautions Use with caution in patients with impaired hepatic or renal function; severe hypertension and tachycardia may occur in patients with pheochromocytoma

Adverse Reactions

Cardiovascular: Hypotension (especially in hypovolemic patients), tachycardia; QT prolongation, torsade de pointes, cardiac arrest, ventricular tachycardia (see Warnings)

Central nervous system: Extrapyramidal reactions such as dystonic reactions, akathisia, and oculogyric crisis; anxiety, hyperactivity, drowsiness, dizziness, hallucinations, chills, dysphoria, restlessness

Respiratory: Laryngospasm, bronchospasm

Miscellaneous: Anaphylaxis; neuromalignant syndrome (rare)

Drug Interactions Concomitant use with any drug that prolongs the QT interval is **not** recommended (see Warnings); diuretics, laxatives, and mineralocorticoids may cause hypokalemia or hypomagnesemia and increase the risk of droperidol-induced QT prolongation. Use with other CNS depressants may have additive effects (CNS, respiratory depression, etc); droperidol plus fentanyl or other analgesics may increase blood pressure; conduction anesthesia may increase hypotension; droperidol plus epinephrine may decrease blood pressure due to alpha-adrenergic blockade effects of droperidol; droperidol plus atropine may cause tachycardia

Stability Store at room temperature; protect from light. Physically compatible and chemically stable with D_5W, LR, NS at a concentration of 20 mg/L

Mechanism of Action Alters the action of dopamine in the CNS, at subcortical levels, to produce sedation and a dissociative state; also possesses alpha-adrenergic blockade effects

Pharmacodynamics

Onset of action: 3-10 minutes

Maximum effect: Within 30 minutes

Duration: 2-4 hours (up to 12 hours)

Pharmacokinetics

Metabolism: In the liver

Half-life, adults: 2.3 hours

Elimination: In urine (75%) and feces (22%)

Usual Dosage Dosage must be individualized, based on age, body weight, underlying medical conditions, physical status, concomitant medications, type of anesthesia, and surgical procedure

Children 2-12 years:

Postoperative nausea and vomiting prophylaxis for high risk surgery: I.M., I.V.: Doses as low as 0.015 mg/kg/dose may be effective; usual: 0.05-0.06 mg/kg/dose administered once; maximum initial dose: 0.1 mg/kg; administer additional doses with caution and only if potential benefit outweighs risks (see Warnings); **Note:** A recent meta-analysis of 74 randomised controlled trials (29 pediatric trials) assessed droperidol use for the prevention of postoperative nausea and vomiting; the analysis suggested that 0.075 mg/kg/dose was likely to be the most effective prophylactic dose; it was also the most frequently used dose in the trials that were assessed; however, due to side effects associated with this dose, the study considered 0.05 mg/kg/dose to be the best prophylactic dose for children in cases where sedation and drowsiness should be prevented (eg, day surgery) (see Henzi, 2000)

(Continued)

Droperidol *(Continued)*

Postoperative nausea and vomiting (treatment): I.V.: Doses as low as 0.01-0.03 mg/kg/dose may be effective for breakthrough nausea and vomiting; maximum initial dose: 0.1 mg/kg; administer additional doses with caution and only if potential benefit outweighs risks (see Warnings)

Adults: Nausea and vomiting: I.M., I.V.: Maximum initial dose: 2.5 mg; additional doses of 1.25 mg may be administered to achieve desired effect; administer additional doses with caution and only if potential benefit outweighs risks (see Warnings)

Administration Parenteral: Administer by slow I.V. injection over 2-5 minutes; maximum concentration: 2.5 mg/mL (I.M. or I.V.)

Monitoring Parameters Prior to use: 12-lead EKG to identify patients with QT prolongation (use is contraindicated); continuous EKG during and for 2-3 hours after dosage administration is recommended. Blood pressure, heart rate, respiratory rate; serum potassium and magnesium; observe for dystonias, extrapyramidal side effects; temperature

Additional Information Does not possess analgesic effects; has little or no amnesic properties. A dose-dependent prolongation of the QT interval has been observed in adults; significant QT prolongation was noted at doses of 0.1 mg/kg, 0.175 mg/kg, and 0.25 mg/kg with prolongation of median QT_c interval by 37, 44, and 59 msec, respectively (see package insert)

Dosage Forms Injection, solution: 2.5 mg/mL (1 mL, 2 mL)

References

Henzi I, Sonderegger J, and Tramer MR, "Efficacy, Dose-Response, and Adverse Effects of Droperidol for Prevention of Postoperative Nausea and Vomiting," *Can J Anaesth*, 2000, 47(6):537-51.

Yaster M, Sola JE, Pegoli W Jr, et al, "The Night After Surgery: Postoperative Management of the Pediatric Outpatient - Surgical and Anesthetic Aspects," *Pediatr Clin North Am*, 1994, 41(1):199-220.

Drotrecogin Alfa (Activated) (dro TRE coe jin AL fa ak ti VAY ted)

U.S. Brand Names Xigris™

Synonyms Activated Protein C, Human Recombinant; Protein C (Activated), Human Recombinant; Recombinant Human Activated Protein C

Therapeutic Category Biological Response Modulator

Generic Available No

Use Reduction of mortality in adult patients with severe sepsis (sepsis associated with acute organ dysfunction) who have a high risk of death (ie, as determined by APACHE II score ≥25); purpura fulminans (compassionate use protocol)

Pregnancy Risk Factor C

Contraindications Hypersensitivity to drotrecogin alfa or any component; patients with active internal bleeding; recent (within 3 months) hemorrhagic stroke, recent (within 2 months) intracranial or intraspinal surgery, or severe head trauma; trauma with an increased risk of life-threatening bleeding; presence of an epidural catheter; intracranial neoplasm or mass lesion or evidence of cerebral herniation

Warnings Serious bleeding was observed in 3.5% of drotrecogin alfa-treated patients and is the most common adverse effect associated with this agent. Conditions which may increase the risk of bleeding with drotrecogin alfa include concurrent heparin administration (≥15 units/kg/hour); platelet count <30,000 x 10^6/L, INR >3, recent (within 6 weeks) gastrointestinal bleeding, recent administration (within 3 days) of thrombolytic therapy, recent administration (within 7 days) of oral anticoagulants or glycoprotein IIb/IIIa inhibitors, recent administration (within 7 days) of aspirin >650 mg/day, NSAIDs, clopidogrel, dipyridamole, or other platelet inhibitors, intracranial arteriovenous malformation or aneurysm, and chronic severe hepatic disease. If bleeding occurs, immediately stop the infusion. Once hemostasis has been achieved, restarting drotrecogin alfa may be considered. Stop drotrecogin alfa 2 hours prior to undergoing an invasive surgical procedure or procedure with an inherent risk of bleeding. Once hemostasis has been achieved, drotrecogin alfa may be restarted 12 hours after major invasive procedures or surgery or immediately after less invasive procedures.

Precautions Use with caution in patients at risk of bleeding, patients with chronic renal failure requiring dialysis, patients with hypercoagulable conditions (ie, hereditary deficiencies of protein C, protein S, or antithrombin III, suspected thromboembolism), or resistance to activated protein C

Adverse Reactions

Central nervous system: Intracranial hemorrhage

Gastrointestinal: GI hemorrhage

Genitourinary: GU hemorrhage

Hematologic: Bleeding, bruising

Drug Interactions Drugs affecting the coagulation system or platelet function may increase risk of bleeding (aspirin, glycoprotein IIb/IIIa antagonists, cilostazol, clopidogrel, dipyridamole, heparin, danaparoid, LMWHs, NSAIDs, thrombolytic agents, antithrombin III, warfarin)

Stability Refrigerate and protect unreconstituted vials from light. Drotrecogin alfa for injection contains no preservatives. Reconstituted vial is stable for 3 hours at room temperature. Once reconstituted and further diluted with NS, infusion must be completed within 12 hours. Additional studies (data on file, Lilly Research Laboratories) show that the final solution is stable for 14 hours at room temperature. If not used immediately, a prepared solution may be stored in the refrigerator for up to 12 hours. The expiration time (refrigeration and administration) should be ≤24 hours from preparation. The only compatible solutions which can be administered through the same line as drotrecogin alfa are NS, LR, dextrose, or dextrose and saline mixtures. Avoid exposing drotrecogin alfa infusion solution to heat and/or direct sunlight.

Mechanism of Action Drotrecogin alfa, a serine protease with the same amino acid sequence as human plasma-derived activated protein C, possesses profibrinolytic, antithrombotic, and anti-inflammatory activities. Activated protein C inactivates factors Va and VIIIa decreasing generation of thrombin and ultimately decreasing fibrin/clot formation; binds to plasminogen activator type 1 enhancing the action of tissue plasminogen activator and stimulates fibrinolysis; inhibits cytokine production

Pharmacodynamics Maximum effect on decreasing D-dimer levels: At the end of a 96-hour 24 mcg/kg/hour infusion

Pharmacokinetics A phase 2 pharmacokinetic study has been performed in pediatric patients, but results from this trial are not yet available (communication with Lilly Research Laboratories, Jan 2002)

　Metabolism: Plasma protease inhibitors inactivate drotrecogin alfa and endogenous activated protein C

　Half-life: 1.2 hours

Usual Dosage I.V.: Continuous infusion:

　Infants, Children, and Adults: Purpura fulminans: In a compassionate use program, 42 patients (range: >3 kg to 135 kg; >1 year of age) received a dose of 24 mcg/kg/hour for 96 hours. If the patient had improved after 96 hours, but had laboratory evidence of an ongoing coagulopathy, or had tissue still deemed to be at risk for necrosis, the drotrecogin alfa infusion could be continued. The maximum allowed infusion time was 168 hours.

　Adults: Severe sepsis: 24 mcg/kg/hour for 4 days. Infusion should be started within 24 hours of the onset of at least three signs of systemic inflammation and evidence of at least one organ/system dysfunction

Administration Parenteral: I.V.: May administer via a dedicated I.V. line or a dedicated lumen of a central venous catheter at a final concentration from 100-1000 mcg/mL in NS. When using low concentrations <200 mcg/mL at low flow rates <5 mL/hour, the infusion set must be primed for approximately 15 minutes at a flow rate of approximately 5 mL/hour.

Monitoring Parameters Hemoglobin, hematocrit, coagulation panel, CBC with differential, platelet count, signs and symptoms of bleeding; for select patients: Plasma D-dimer levels, plasma interleukin-6 level, protein C and protein S activity; for purpura fulminans: Evaluate tissue for necrosis risk

Test Interactions Drotrecogin alfa may prolong the one-stage coagulation assay based on the APTT (such as factor VIII, IX, and XI assays) so that an apparent factor concentration appears lower than the true concentration.

Additional Information Human plasma derived protein C concentrate (an alternative, investigational product) has been used in infants and children with severe meningococcemia associated with purpura fulminans (see Ettingshausen, 1999).

Dosage Forms Injection, powder for reconstitution, lyophilized: 5 mg, 20 mg

References

Alberio L, Lammle B, and Esmon CT, "Protein C Replacement in Severe Meningococcemia: Rationale and Clinical Experience," *Clin Infect Dis*, 2001, 32(9):1338-46.

Bernard GR, Vincent JL, Laterre PF, et al, "Efficacy and Safety of Recombinant Human Activated Protein C for Severe Sepsis," *N Engl J Med*, 2001, 344(10):699-709.

Ettingshausen CE, Veldmann A, Beeg T, et al, "Replacement Therapy With Protein C Concentrate in Infants and Adolescents With Meningococcal Sepsis and Purpura Fulminans," *Semin Thromb Hemost*, 1999, 25(6):537-41.

Faust SN, Levin M, Harrison OB, et al, "Dysfunction of Endothelial Protein C Activation in Severe Meningococcal Sepsis," *N Engl J Med*, 2001, 345(6):408-16.

Smith SN, Neal J, Winton EF, et al, "Purpura Fulminans and *S. pneumoniae* Sepsis With Severe Acquired Protein C Deficiency Successfully Treated With Recombinant Human Activated Protein C," *Thromb Haemost*, 1999, 82(Suppl 1):738.

- ◆ **D-S-S® [OTC]** *see Docusate on page 402*
- ◆ **D-S-S Plus® [OTC]** *see Docusate and Casanthranol on page 402*
- ◆ **DSS With Casanthranol** *see Docusate and Casanthranol on page 402*
- ◆ **DTIC-Dome®** *see Dacarbazine on page 332*
- ◆ **DTO** *see Opium Tincture on page 836*
- ◆ **Dulcolax® [OTC]** *see Bisacodyl on page 173*
- ◆ **Dull-C® [OTC]** *see Ascorbic Acid on page 131*
- ◆ **Duofilm® [OTC]** *see Salicylic Acid on page 1002*
- ◆ **Duoforte® 27 (Can)** *see Salicylic Acid on page 1002*
- ◆ **Duonalc® (Can)** *see Ethyl Alcohol on page 465*
- ◆ **Duonalc-E® Mild (Can)** *see Ethyl Alcohol on page 465*
- ◆ **Duoplant® [OTC] [DSC]** *see Salicylic Acid on page 1002*
- ◆ **Duraclon™** *see Clonidine on page 294*
- ◆ **Duragesic®** *see Fentanyl on page 479*
- ◆ **Duralith® (Can)** *see Lithium on page 684*
- ◆ **Duramist Plus® [OTC]** *see Oxymetazoline on page 849*
- ◆ **Duramorph®** *see Morphine Sulfate on page 778*
- ◆ **Duration® [OTC]** *see Oxymetazoline on page 849*
- ◆ **Duratuss® DM** *see Guaifenesin and Dextromethorphan on page 553*
- ◆ **Duratuss-G®** *see Guaifenesin on page 550*
- ◆ **Duricef®** *see Cefadroxil on page 224*
- ◆ **Duvoid® (Can)** *see Bethanechol on page 171*
- ◆ **Dycill® (Can)** *see Dicloxacillin on page 376*

Dyclonine *(DYE kloe neen)*

U.S. Brand Names Cepacol® Maximum Strength [OTC]; Sucrets® [OTC]

Therapeutic Category Local Anesthetic, Oral

Generic Available No

Use As a local anesthetic prior to laryngoscopy, bronchoscopy, or endotracheal intubation; used topically for temporary relief of pain associated with oral mucosa, skin, episiotomy, or anogenital lesions; the 0.5% topical solution may be used to block the gag reflex, and to relieve the pain of oral ulcers or stomatitis; the lozenge is used for temporary relief of sore throat pain and gum irritation

Pregnancy Risk Factor C

Contraindications Hypersensitivity to chlorobutanol (preservative used in dyclonine), dyclonine, or any component

Warnings Resuscitative equipment, oxygen and resuscitative drugs should be immediately available when dyclonine topical solution is administered to mucous membranes; may impair swallowing and enhance the danger of aspiration

Precautions Use with caution in patients with infection present in the area of application or traumatized mucosa in the area of application to avoid rapid systemic absorption; use with caution in patients with shock or heart block

Adverse Reactions Excessive dosage and rapid absorption may result in adverse CNS and cardiovascular effects

Cardiovascular: Hypotension, bradycardia, cardiac arrest, edema
Central nervous system: Excitation, drowsiness, nervousness, dizziness, seizures
Dermatologic: Rash, urticaria
Local: Slight irritation and stinging may occur when applied
Ocular: Blurred vision
Respiratory: Respiratory arrest
Miscellaneous: Allergic reactions

Stability Store in tight, light-resistant container; avoid freezing

Mechanism of Action Blocks impulses at peripheral nerve endings in skin and mucous membranes by altering cell membrane permeability to ionic transfer

Pharmacodynamics

Onset of action: Local anesthesia: 2-10 minutes
Duration: 30-60 minutes

Usual Dosage

Children and Adults:

Topical solution: Mouth sores: 5-10 mL of 0.5% or 1% to oral mucosa (swab or swish and then spit) 3-4 times/day as needed; maximum single dose: 200 mg (40 mL of 0.5% solution or 20 mL of 1% solution); solution may be diluted 1:1 with water

Bronchoscopy: Use 2 mL of the 1% solution or 4 mL of the 0.5% solution sprayed onto the larynx and trachea every 5 minutes for 2-3 applications until the reflex has been abolished

Children >3 years: Topical: Slowly dissolve 1 lozenge (1.2 mg) in mouth every 2 hours, if necessary

Children >12 years and Adults: Topical: Slowly dissolve 1 lozenge (3 mg) in mouth every 2 hours, if necessary

Administration Topical: Apply to mucous membranes of the mouth or throat area: food should not be ingested for 60 minutes following application in the mouth or throat area

Patient Information Do not chew lozenge; numbness of the tongue and buccal mucosa may result in increased risk of biting trauma; may impair swallowing

Nursing Implications Use the lowest dose needed to provide effective anesthesia; not for injection; do not apply nasally or to the eye

Dosage Forms

Lozenges, as hydrochloride (Sucrets®): 1.2 mg, 2 mg, 3 mg

Spray, oral, as hydrochloride (Cepacol® Maximum Strength): 0.1% (120 mL) [cherry and menthol flavors]

References

Carnel SB, Blakeslee DB, Oswald SG, et al, "Treatment of Radiation- and Chemotherapy-Induced Stomatitis," *Otolaryngol Head Neck Surg*, 1990, 102(4):326-30.

- ◆ **Dyna-Hex® [OTC]** *see* Chlorhexidine Gluconate *on page 257*
- ◆ **Dyrenium®** *see* Triamterene *on page 1115*
- ◆ **EarSol® HC** *see* Hydrocortisone *on page 573*
- ◆ **Easprin®** *see* Aspirin *on page 134*
- ◆ **EC-Naprosyn®** *see* Naproxen *on page 796*

Econazole (e KONE a zole)

U.S. Brand Names Spectazole®

Canadian Brand Names Ecostatin®

Therapeutic Category Antifungal Agent, Topical

Generic Available No

Use Topical treatment of tinea pedis, tinea cruris, tinea corporis, tinea versicolor, and cutaneous candidiasis

Pregnancy Risk Factor C

Contraindications Hypersensitivity to econazole or any component

Warnings Not for ophthalmic or intravaginal use

Precautions Discontinue the drug if sensitivity or chemical irritation occurs; cross-sensitization may occur with other imidazole derivatives (ie, clotrimazole, miconazole)

Adverse Reactions

Dermatologic: Pruritus, erythema, contact dermatitis

Local: Burning, stinging

Mechanism of Action Alters fungal cell wall membrane permeability; may interfere with RNA and protein synthesis, and lipid metabolism

Pharmacokinetics

Absorption: Following topical administration, <10% is percutaneously absorbed

Metabolism: In the liver to >20 metabolites

Elimination: <1% of an applied dose recovered in urine or feces

Usual Dosage Children and Adults: Topical:

Tinea cruris, corporis, pedis, and tinea versicolor: Apply once daily

Cutaneous candidiasis: Apply twice daily

Administration Topical: Apply a sufficient amount of cream to cover affected areas; do not apply to the eye or intravaginally

Patient Information For external use only. Notify physician if condition worsens or persists, or if irritation occurs.

Additional Information Candidal infections and tinea cruris, versicolor, and corporis should be treated for 2 weeks and tinea pedis for 1 month; occasionally, longer treatment periods may be required

Dosage Forms Cream, topical, as nitrate: 1% (15 g, 30 g, 85 g)

- ◆ **Econopred®** *see* PrednisoLONE *on page 925*
- ◆ **Econopred® Plus** *see* PrednisoLONE *on page 925*
- ◆ **Ecostatin® (Can)** *see* Econazole *on page 423*
- ◆ **Ecotrin® [OTC]** *see* Aspirin *on page 134*
- ◆ **Ecotrin® Adult Low Strength [OTC]** *see* Aspirin *on page 134*
- ◆ **Ecotrin® Maximum Strength [OTC]** *see* Aspirin *on page 134*
- ◆ **Ectosone (Can)** *see* Betamethasone *on page 169*
- ◆ **Edathamil Disodium** *see* Edetate Disodium *on page 425*

Edetate Calcium Disodium (ED e tate KAL see um dye SOW dee um)

U.S. Brand Names Calcium Disodium Versenate®

Synonyms Calcium Disodium Edathamil; Calcium Disodium Edetate; Calcium Edetate; Calcium EDTA

Therapeutic Category Antidote, Lead Toxicity; Chelating Agent, Parenteral

Generic Available No

Use Treatment of acute and chronic lead poisoning; also used as an aid in the diagnosis of lead poisoning

Pregnancy Risk Factor B

Contraindications Hypersensitivity to edetate calcium disodium or any component; severe renal disease, anuria

Warnings Do not exceed recommended daily dose; avoid rapid I.V. infusion in the management of lead encephalopathy, intracranial pressure may be increased to lethal levels; I.M. administration is the preferred route in these patients; if anuria, increasing proteinuria, or hematuria occurs during therapy, discontinue calcium EDTA

Precautions Renal tubular necrosis and fatal nephrosis may occur, especially with high doses; establish urine flow prior to administration

Adverse Reactions

Cardiovascular: Hypotension, arrhythmias, EKG changes

Central nervous system: Fever, headache, chills

Dermatologic: Skin lesions, cheilosis

Endocrine & metabolic: Hypercalcemia, zinc deficiency

Gastrointestinal: GI upset, anorexia, nausea, vomiting

Hematologic: Transient marrow suppression, anemia

Hepatic: Mild elevation in liver function tests

Local: Pain at injection site following I.M. injection, thrombophlebitis following I.V. infusion (when concentration >5 mg/mL)

Neuromuscular & skeletal: Arthralgia, tremor, numbness, paresthesia

Ocular: Lacrimation

Renal: Renal tubular necrosis, proteinuria, microscopic hematuria

Respiratory: Sneezing, nasal congestion

Drug Interactions Do not use simultaneously with zinc insulin preparations

Stability Dilute with NS or D_5W; physically incompatible with $D_{10}W$, LR; do not mix in the same syringe with dimercaprol

Mechanism of Action Calcium is displaced by divalent and trivalent heavy metals, forming a nonionizing soluble complex that is excreted in the urine

Pharmacodynamics

Onset of chelation with I.V. administration: 1 hour

Maximum excretion of chelated lead with I.V. administration: 24-48 hours

Pharmacokinetics

Absorption: I.M., S.C.: Well absorbed

Distribution: Into extracellular fluid; minimal CSF penetration

Half-life, plasma:

I.M.: 1.5 hours

I.V.: 20 minutes

Elimination: Rapid in urine as metal chelates or unchanged drug

Usual Dosage Several regimens have been recommended:

Diagnosis of lead poisoning: Mobilization test (not recommended by AAP guidelines): I.M., I.V.:

Children: 500 mg/m²/dose, (maximum dose: 1 g) as a single dose or divided into 2 doses

Adults: 500 mg/m²/dose

Note: Urine is collected for 24 hours after first EDTA dose and analyzed for lead content; if the ratio of mcg of lead in urine to mg calcium EDTA given is >1, then test is considered positive; for convenience, an 8-hour urine collection may be done after a single 50 mg/kg I.M. (maximum dose: 1 g) or 500 mg/m² I.V. dose; a positive test occurs if the ratio of lead excretion to mg calcium EDTA >0.5-0.6.

Treatment of lead poisoning: Children and Adults (each regimen is specific for route):

Symptoms of lead encephalopathy and/or blood lead level >70 mcg/dL: Treat 5 days; give in conjunction with dimercaprol; wait a minimum of 2 days with no treatment before considering a repeat course:

I.M.: 250 mg/m²/dose every 4 hours

I.V.: 50 mg/kg/day as 24-hour continuous I.V. infusion **or** 1-1.5 g/m² I.V. as either an 8- to 24-hour infusion or divided into 2 doses every 12 hours

Symptomatic lead poisoning **without** encephalopathy **or** asymptomatic with blood lead level >70 mcg/dL: Treat 3-5 days; treatment with dimercaprol is recommended until the blood lead level concentration <50 mcg/dL:

I.M.: 167 mg/m² every 4 hours

I.V.: 1 g/m^2 as an 8- to 24-hour infusion or divided every 12 hours

Asymptomatic **children** with blood lead level 45-69 mcg/dL: I.V.: 25 mg/kg/day for 5 days as an 8- to 24-hour infusion or divided into 2 doses every 12 hours

Depending upon the blood lead level, additional courses may be necessary; repeat at least 2-4 days and preferably 2-4 weeks apart

Adults with lead nephropathy: An alternative dosing regimen reflecting the reduction in renal clearance is based upon the serum creatinine (see table):

Alternative Dosing Regimen for Adults With Lead Nephropathy

Serum Creatinine (mg/dL)	Ca EDTA dosage
≤2	1 g/m^2/day for 5 days
>2-3	500 mg/m^2/day for 5 days
>3-4	500 mg/m^2/dose every 48 hours for 3 doses
>4	500 mg/m^2/week

Repeat these regimens monthly until lead excretion is reduced toward normal.

Administration Parenteral:

Intermittent I.V. infusion: Administer the dose I.V. over at least 1 hour in asymptomatic patients, 2 hours in symptomatic patients

Single daily I.V. continuous infusion: Dilute to 2-4 mg/mL in D$_5$W or NS and infuse over at least 8 hours, usually over 12-24 hours

I.M. injection: To minimize pain at the injection site, 1.67 mL of 2% procaine may be added to 5 mL calcium EDTA, resulting in 150 mg/mL concentration with 0.5% procaine (stable 3 months; see Nahata, 1997)

Monitoring Parameters BUN, serum creatinine, urinalysis, fluid balance, EKG, blood and urine lead concentrations

Test Interactions If calcium EDTA is given as a continuous I.V. infusion, stop the infusion for at least 1 hour before blood is drawn for lead concentration to avoid a falsely elevated value

Dosage Forms Injection, solution: 200 mg/mL (5 mL)

References

American Academy of Pediatrics Committee on Drugs, "Treatment Guidelines for Lead Exposure in Children," *Pediatrics*, 1995, 96(1 Pt 1):155-60.

Nahata MC and Hipple TF, *Pediatric Drug Formulations*, 3rd ed, Cincinnati, OH: Harvey Whitney Books Co, 1997.

Edetate Disodium (ED e tate dye SOW dee um)

U.S. Brand Names Endrate®

Synonyms Edathamil Disodium; EDTA; Sodium Edetate

Therapeutic Category Antidote, Hypercalcemia; Chelating Agent, Parenteral

Generic Available Yes

Use Emergency treatment of hypercalcemia; control digitalis-induced cardiac dysrhythmias (ventricular arrhythmias)

Pregnancy Risk Factor C

Contraindications Hypersensitivity to edetate disodium or any component; severe renal failure or anuria, hypocalcemia, patients with active tuberculosis or healed calcified tubercular lesions

Warnings Use of this drug is recommended only when the severity of the clinical condition justifies the aggressive measures associated with this type of therapy. Use with caution in patients with intracranial lesions, seizure disorders, coronary or peripheral vascular disease; cardiac function should be evaluated prior to therapy

Precautions Sudden, precipitous decreases of serum calcium may occur, a source of I.V. calcium replacement should be readily available; blood sugar and insulin requirements may be lower when used in insulin-dependent diabetics

Adverse Reactions

Cardiovascular: Arrhythmias, hypotension

Central nervous system: Seizures, headache, chills, fever

Dermatologic: Skin eruptions

Endocrine/metabolic: Hypomagnesemia, hypokalemia, hypocalcemia, hyperuricemia

Gastrointestinal: Vomiting, diarrhea, abdominal cramps

Genitourinary: Urinary urgency, dysuria

Hematologic: Anemia

Local: Thrombophlebitis, pain at injection site

Neuromuscular & skeletal: Back pain, muscle cramps, paresthesia, tetany

Renal: Nephrotoxicity, acute tubular necrosis, polyuria, oliguria, glucosuria

Respiratory: Respiratory arrest

(Continued)

Edetate Disodium *(Continued)*

Drug Interactions May reduce insulin requirements in diabetic patients treated with insulin

Stability Physically compatible with dextrose and saline I.V. solutions

Mechanism of Action Chelates with divalent or trivalent metals to form a soluble complex that is then eliminated in urine

Pharmacokinetics
Metabolism: Not metabolized
Half-life: 20-60 minutes
Elimination: Following chelation, 95% excreted in urine as chelates within 24-48 hours

Usual Dosage I.V.:
Hypercalcemia:
Children: 40-70 mg/kg/day slow infusion over 3-4 hours or more to a maximum of 3 g/24 hours; administer for 5 days and allow 5 days between courses of therapy or 50 mg/kg or 1.5 g/m^2 as a single dose
Adults: 50 mg/kg/day over 3 or more hours to a maximum of 3 g/24 hours; administer for 5 days followed by 2 days without drug and repeat course up to 15 total doses
Digitalis-induced arrhythmias: Children and Adults: 15 mg/kg/hour (maximum dose: 60 mg/kg/day) as continuous infusion

Administration Parenteral: I.V.: Must be diluted before I.V. use in D$_5$W or NS to a maximum concentration of 30 mg/mL (3%) and infused over at least 3 hours; avoid extravasation; **not for I.M. use**

Monitoring Parameters Serum and urine electrolytes (including calcium and magnesium), blood pressure (during infusion), renal function (before and during therapy), liver function, EKG

Test Interactions Colorimetric, oxalate, or other precipitation methods for measuring serum calcium

Nursing Implications Patient should remain supine for a short period after infusion

Additional Information Sodium content of 1 g: 5.4 mEq

Dosage Forms Injection, solution: 150 mg/mL (20 mL)

Edrophonium *(ed roe FOE nee um)*

Related Information
Overdose and Toxicology *on page 1388*

U.S. Brand Names Enlon®; Reversol®

Therapeutic Category Antidote, Neuromuscular Blocking Agent; Cholinergic Agent; Diagnostic Agent, Myasthenia Gravis

Generic Available Yes

Use Diagnosis of myasthenia gravis; differentiation of cholinergic crises from myasthenia crises; reversal of nondepolarizing neuromuscular blockers; treatment of paroxysmal atrial tachycardia

Pregnancy Risk Factor C

Contraindications Hypersensitivity to edrophonium or any component; GI or GU mechanical obstruction

Warnings Overdosage can cause cholinergic crisis which may be fatal; I.V. atropine should be readily available for treatment of cholinergic reactions

Precautions Use with caution in asthmatic patients, patients with cardiac dysrhythmias, and those receiving a cardiac glycoside

Adverse Reactions
Cardiovascular: Arrhythmias (especially bradycardia), hypotension, A-V block
Central nervous system: Seizures, drowsiness, headache, dysphoria
Gastrointestinal: Nausea, vomiting, diarrhea, excessive salivation, stomach cramps
Genitourinary: Urinary frequency
Local: Thrombophlebitis
Neuromuscular & skeletal: Weakness, muscle cramps, muscle spasms
Ocular: Diplopia, miosis, lacrimation, conjunctival hyperemia
Respiratory: Laryngospasm, bronchospasm, respiratory paralysis, increased bronchial secretions
Miscellaneous: Diaphoresis, hypersensitivity reactions

Drug Interactions Digoxin may enhance bradycardia potential of edrophonium; succinylcholine and decamethonium effects are prolonged by edrophonium; quinidine may antagonize effects of edrophonium; antagonizes effects of nondepolarizing muscle relaxants (eg, pancuronium, vecuronium)

Mechanism of Action Inhibits destruction of acetylcholine by acetylcholinesterase. This facilitates transmission of impulses across myoneural junction and results in increased cholinergic responses such as miosis, increased tonus of intestinal and skeletal muscles, bronchial and ureteral constriction, bradycardia, and increased salivary and sweat gland secretions

Pharmacodynamics

Onset of action:
  I.M.: 2-10 minutes
  I.V.: 30-60 seconds
Duration:
  I.M.: 5-30 minutes
  I.V.: 5-10 minutes

Pharmacokinetics

Distribution: V_d:
  Infants: 1.18 ± 0.2 L/kg
  Children: 1.22 ± 0.74 L/kg
  Adults: 0.9 ± 0.13 L/kg
Half-life:
  Infants: 73 ± 30 minutes
  Children: 99 ± 31 minutes
  Adults: 126 ± 59 minutes
Elimination: Clearance:
  Infants: 17.8 mL/kg/minute
  Children: 14.2 mL/kg/minute
  Adults: 8.3 ± 2.9 mL/kg/minute

Usual Dosage Usually administered I.V., however, if not possible, I.M. or S.C. may be used

Infants: Diagnosis of myasthenia gravis: Initial:
  I.M., S.C.: 0.5-1 mg
  I.V.: Initial: 0.1 mg, followed by 0.4 mg (if no response); total dose = 0.5 mg
Children:
  Diagnosis of myasthenia gravis: Initial:
    I.M., S.C.: ≤34 kg: 2 mg; >34 kg: 5 mg
    I.V.: 0.04 mg/kg given over 1 minute followed by 0.16 mg/kg given within 45 seconds (if no response) (maximum dose: 10 mg total)
    or
    Alternative (manufacturer's recommendations):
      ≤34 kg: 1 mg; if no response after 45 seconds, it may be repeated in 1 mg increments every 30-45 seconds to a total of 5 mg
      >34 kg: 2 mg; if no response after 45 seconds, it may be repeated in 1 mg increments every 30-45 seconds to a total of 10 mg
  Titration of oral anticholinesterase therapy: I.V.: 0.04 mg/kg once given 1 hour after oral intake of the drug being used in treatment; if strength improves, an increase in neostigmine or pyridostigmine dose is indicated
Adults:
  Diagnosis of myasthenia gravis: Initial:
    I.M., S.C.: Initial: 10 mg; if no cholinergic reaction occurs, administer 2 mg 30 minutes later to rule out false-negative reaction
    I.V.: 2 mg test dose administered over 15-30 seconds; 8 mg given 45 seconds later (if no response is seen); test dose may be repeated after 30 minutes.
  Titration of oral anticholinesterase therapy: I.V.: 1-2 mg given 1 hour after oral dose of anticholinesterase; if strength improves, an increase in neostigmine or pyridostigmine dose is indicated
  Differentiation of cholinergic from myasthenic crisis: I.V.: 1 mg, may repeat after 1 minute (**Note:** Intubation and controlled ventilation may be required if patient has cholinergic crises.)
  Reversal of nondepolarizing neuromuscular blocking agents (neostigmine with atropine usually preferred): I.V.: 10 mg over 30-45 seconds, may repeat every 5-10 minutes up to 40 mg total dose
  Termination of paroxysmal atrial tachycardia: I.V.: 5-10 mg
  Dosing adjustment in renal impairment: Dose may need to be reduced in patients with chronic renal failure

Administration Parenteral: Edrophonium is administered by direct I.V. or I.M. injection; see Usual Dosage

Monitoring Parameters Pre- and postinjection strength (cranial musculature is most useful); heart rate, respiratory rate, blood pressure, changes in fasciculations

Dosage Forms Injection, solution, as chloride: 10 mg/mL (15 mL)

♦ **EDTA** see Edetate Disodium on page 425
♦ **E.E.S.®** see Erythromycin on page 448

Efavirenz (eh FAH vih rehnz)

Related Information
Adult and Adolescent HIV *on page 1327*
Pediatric HIV *on page 1323*

U.S. Brand Names Sustiva®

Therapeutic Category Antiretroviral Agent; HIV Agents (Anti-HIV Agents); Non-nucleoside Reverse Transcriptase Inhibitor (NNRTI)

Generic Available No

Use Treatment of HIV-1 infection in combination with other antiretroviral agents. (**Note:** HIV regimens consisting of **three** antiretroviral agents are strongly recommended)

Pregnancy Risk Factor C

Contraindications Hypersensitivity to efavirenz or any component; concurrent therapy with astemizole, cisapride, midazolam, triazolam, or ergot derivatives

Warnings Efavirenz is a mixed inducer/inhibitor of CYP450 enzymes and numerous drug interactions occur. Due to potential serious and/or life-threatening drug interactions, certain drugs are contraindicated (see Contraindications and Drug Interactions). Resistance emerges rapidly if administered as monotherapy; always use efavirenz in combination with at least two other antiretroviral agents; do not add efavirenz as a single agent to antiretroviral regimens that are failing; initiate in combination with at least one other antiretroviral agent to which the patient is naive.

Precautions Use with caution in patients with a history of mental illness or substance abuse (delusions, inappropriate behavior, and severe acute depression may occur); serious CNS and psychiatric symptoms may occur (see Adverse Effects); discontinue if severe rash (involving blistering, desquamation, mucosal involvement, or fever) occurs; rash is more common and more severe in children versus adults, **consider prophylaxis with antihistamines in children**; use with caution in patients with known or suspected hepatitis B or C, those receiving other hepatotoxic medications, and those with hepatic impairment; weigh risk versus benefit in patients with persistent elevations of serum transaminases (ie, >5 times normal); cross resistance with other non-nucleoside reverse transcriptase inhibitors may occur; fat redistribution and accumulation [ie, central obesity, peripheral wasting, facial wasting, breast enlargement, dorsocervical fat enlargement (buffalo hump), and cushingoid appearance] have been observed in patients receiving antiretroviral agents (causal relationship not established)

Adverse Reactions

Central nervous system: (Note: Overall incidence of CNS adverse effects was 53% versus 25% in controls; nervous system symptoms in children have been reported to be 18%) somnolence, dizziness, drowsiness, abnormal dreams, insomnia, confusion, headache (children 11%), hypoesthesia, impaired concentration, abnormal thinking, agitation, amnesia, depersonalization, euphoria, hallucinations, delusions, inappropriate behavior; fever (children 21%); anxiety, nervousness; serious psychiatric adverse effects (patients with history of psychiatric disorders may be at greater risk): Suicidal ideation/attempts, severe acute depression, aggressive behavior, paranoid reactions, manic reactions

Dermatologic: Rash, usually pruritic maculopapular skin eruptions (incidence: children 46%, adults 26%; median onset, adults: 11 days, children: 9 days [range 6-205 days], **Note:** Most rashes in children appeared within 14 days after starting therapy; median duration, adults: 16 days, children: 6 days [range 2-37 days], **Note:** Median duration of rash in children who continued therapy was 9 days; rash may be treated with antihistamines and corticosteroids and usually resolves within one month while continuing therapy; **Note:** Blistering, desquamation, fever, mucosal involvement, or ulceration may occur and requires discontinuation of drug, see Precautions); pruritus, increased sweating

Endocrine & metabolic: Hypercholesterolemia, hypertriglyceridemia, fat redistribution and accumulation (see Precautions)

Gastrointestinal: Nausea or vomiting (children 12%), diarrhea/loose stools (children 39%), abdominal pain, asymptomatic elevations in serum amylase, pancreatitis (several cases)

Hepatic: Elevated liver enzymes (patients with hepatitis B or C may be at greater risk)

Respiratory: Cough (children 16%)

Miscellaneous: Alcohol intolerance

Drug Interactions Cytochrome P450 isoenzyme CYP3A4 and CYP2B6 substrate; mixed inducer/inhibitor of CYP450 enzymes: Induces CYP3A4 and inhibits isoenzymes CYP2C9, 2C19, and 3A4

Concurrent use of efavirenz with astemizole, cisapride, midazolam, triazolam, or ergot derivatives is contraindicated (efavirenz may inhibit the metabolism of these drugs and result in serious or life-threatening effects); efavirenz decreases serum concentrations of indinavir (indinavir dosage increase is recommended), saquinavir (use of saquinavir as sole protease inhibitor with efavirenz is not recommended), amprenavir, clarithromycin, rifabutin (a 50% increase in the daily dose of rifabutin is recommended; a doubling of rifabutin dosage in rifabutin twice weekly or 3 times weekly regimens should be considered), and methadone (monitor patients for withdrawal, increase methadone dose as required); efavirenz may potentially decrease serum concentrations of phenobarbital, phenytoin, or carbamazepine (monitor anticonvulsant levels) or antifungals such as itraconazole or ketoconazole; efavirenz increases serum concentrations of nelfinavir, ritonavir, lorazepam, ethinyl estradiol, and 14-hydroxy metabolite of clarithromycin; efavirenz may increase or decrease the effects of warfarin

Saquinavir, rifampin, phenobarbital, phenytoin, carbamazepine, and other enzyme inducing agents may decrease efavirenz serum concentrations; the herbal medicine St John's wort (*Hypericum perforatum*) may significantly decrease concentrations of efavirenz and is not recommended for concurrent use; ritonavir may increase efavirenz AUC by 20%; fluconazole may increase efavirenz AUC by 16% (but no dosage adjustment is recommended); alcohol or other CNS depressants may increase adverse effects; rash may be more common when efavirenz is used with clarithromycin (consider azithromycin use); interaction with oral contraceptives is not fully characterized (use reliable barrier method)

Food Interactions
    Capsules: Compared to fasting conditions, high fat/high caloric meals increase efavirenz AUC by 22% and peak concentrations by 39%; reduced fat/normal caloric meals increase efavirenz AUC by 17% and peak concentrations by 51%
    Tablets: Compared to fasting conditions, high fat/high caloric meals increase efavirenz AUC by 28% and peak concentrations by 79%

Stability Store at room temperature

Mechanism of Action A non-nucleoside reverse transcriptase inhibitor which specifically binds to HIV-1 reverse transcriptase and blocks RNA-dependent and DNA-dependent DNA polymerase activity including HIV-1 replication; does not require intracellular phosphorylation for antiviral activity

Pharmacokinetics Note: Pharmacokinetics in children ≥3 years of age are thought to be similar to adults
    Distribution: CSF concentrations are 0.69% of plasma (range 0.26% to 1.2%); however, CSF:plasma concentration ratio is 3 times higher than free fraction in plasma
    Protein binding: 99.5% to 99.8%, primarily to albumin
    Metabolism: In the liver, primarily by cytochrome P450 enzymes (mainly isoenzymes CYP3A4 and CYP2B6) to hydroxylated metabolites which then undergo glucuronidation; induces P450 enzymes and it's own metabolism
    Bioavailability: 42% (increased with fatty meal)
    Half-life: Adults:
        Single dose: 52-76 hours
        Multiple dose: 40-55 hours
    Time to peak serum concentration: 3-5 hours
    Elimination: <1% excreted unchanged in the urine; 14% to 34% excreted as metabolites in the urine and 16% to 61% in feces (primarily as unchanged drug)

Usual Dosage Oral: (use in combination with other antiretroviral agents)
    Neonates, Infants, and Children <3 years: Not approved for use (no information available)
    Children ≥3 years: Dose according to body weight:
        10 kg to <15 kg: 200 mg once daily
        15 kg to <20 kg: 250 mg once daily
        20 kg to <25 kg: 300 mg once daily
        25 kg to <32.5 kg: 350 mg once daily
        32.5 kg to <40 kg: 400 mg once daily
        ≥40 kg: 600 mg once daily
    Adults: 600 mg once daily

Administration Administer dose at bedtime to decrease CNS adverse effects; administer with water on an empty stomach (administration with food may increase efavirenz concentrations and adverse effects; see Food Interactions); capsules may be opened and added to small amount of food or liquid, but efavirenz tastes peppery (grape jelly may be used to improve taste)

Monitoring Parameters Signs and symptoms of rash; viral load; CD4 counts; serum amylase; liver enzymes in patients with known or suspected hepatitis B or C, those receiving concomitant ritonavir, and those receiving other hepatotoxic medications; serum cholesterol, triglycerides

Test Interactions False positive test for cannabinoids using the CEDIA DAU Multilevel THC assay

Patient Information May cause drowsiness and impair ability to perform activities requiring mental alertness or physical coordination; avoid alcohol; efavirenz is not a
(Continued)

Efavirenz *(Continued)*

cure for HIV; notify physician immediately if rash develops; report the use of other medications, nonprescription medications and herbal or natural products to your physician and pharmacist; avoid the herbal medicine St John's wort; take efavirenz everyday as prescribed; do not change dose or discontinue without physician's advice; if a dose is missed, take it as soon as possible, then return to normal dosing schedule; if a dose is skipped, do **not** double the next dose

HIV medications may cause changes in body fat, including an increase in fat in the upper back and neck, breasts, and trunk; a loss of fat from the face, arms, and legs may also occur.

Additional Information An oral liquid formulation of efavirenz (strawberry/mint-flavored solution) is available on an investigational basis from Bristol-Myers Squibb Company as part of an expanded access program for HIV-infected children and adolescents 3-16 years of age. For further details call 877-372-7097.

Dosage Forms
Capsule: 50 mg, 100 mg, 200 mg
Tablet: 600 mg

References
Adkins JC and Noble S, "Efavirenz," *Drugs*, 1998, 56(6):1055-64.

Center for Disease Control and Prevention, "Guidelines for Using Antiretroviral Agents Among HIV-Infected Adults and Adolescents. Recommendations of the Panel on Clinical Practices for Treatment of HIV," *MMWR*, 2002, 51(RR-7):1-55.

Collura JM and Kraus DM, "New Pediatric Antiretroviral Agents," *J Pediatr Health Care*, 2000, 14(4):183-90.

Maddocks S and Dwyer D, "The Role of Non-Nucleoside Reverse Transcriptase Inhibitors in Children With HIV-1 Infection," *Paediatr Drugs*, 2001, 3(9):681-702.

Panel on Clinical Practices for Treatment of HIV Infection, "Guidelines for the Use of Antiretroviral Agents in HIV-Infected Adults and Adolescents," February 4, 2002, http://www.aidsinfo.nih.gov.

Piscitelli SC, Burstein AH, Chaitt D, et al, "Indinavir Concentrations and St John's Wort," *Lancet*, 2000, 355(9203):547-8.

Starr SE, Fletcher CV, Spector SA, et al, "Combination Therapy With Efavirenz, Nelfinavir, and Nucleo-side Reverse-transcriptase Inhibitors in Children Infected with Human Immunodeficiency Virus Type 1. Pediatric AIDS Clinical Trials Group 382 Team," *N Engl J Med* 1999, 341(25):1874-81.

Working Group on Antiretroviral Therapy and Medical Management of HIV-Infected Children, "Guidelines for the Use of Antiretroviral Agents in Pediatric HIV Infection," December 14, 2001, http://www.aidsinfo.nih.gov.

Working Group on Antiretroviral Therapy and Medical Management of HIV-Infected Children, "Guidelines for the Use of Antiretroviral Agents in Pediatric HIV Infection. Hyperlink Supplement I: Pediatric Antiretroviral Drug Information," December 14, 2001, http://www.aidsinfo.nih.gov.

Enalapril/Enalaprilat (e NAL a pril/e NAL a pril at)

U.S. Brand Names Vasotec®; Vasotec® I.V.

Therapeutic Category Angiotensin-Converting Enzyme (ACE) Inhibitor; Antihypertensive Agent

Generic Available Yes

Use Management of mild to severe hypertension, CHF, and asymptomatic left ventricular dysfunction; has also been used to treat proteinuria in steroid-resistant nephrotic syndrome patients (see Additional Information)

Pregnancy Risk Factor C (1st trimester); D (may cause injury and death to the developing fetus when used during the 2nd and 3rd trimesters of pregnancy)

Contraindications Hypersensitivity to enalapril, enalaprilat, any component (see Warnings), or other ACE inhibitors; patients with idiopathic or hereditary angioedema or a history of angioedema with ACE inhibitors

Warnings Serious adverse effects including angioedema, anaphylactoid reactions, neutropenia, agranulocytosis, hypotension, and hepatic failure may occur (see Adverse Reactions); risk of neutropenia may be increased in patients with renal dysfunction and especially in patients with both collagen vascular disease and renal dysfunction

Injectable product contains benzyl alcohol (9 mg/mL) which may cause allergic reactions in susceptible individuals; large amounts of benzyl alcohol (≥99 mg/kg/day) have been associated with a potentially fatal toxicity ("gasping syndrome") in neonates; the "gasping syndrome" consists of metabolic acidosis, respiratory distress, gasping respirations, CNS dysfunction (including convulsions, intracranial hemorrhage), hypotension and cardiovascular collapse; use enalaprilat products containing benzyl alcohol with caution in neonates; *in vitro* and animal studies have shown that benzoate, a metabolite of benzyl alcohol, displaces bilirubin from protein binding sites

Precautions Use with caution and modify dosage in patients with renal impairment, especially renal artery stenosis; elevated BUN and S_{cr} may occur in these patients; dosage reduction or discontinuation of enalapril or discontinuation of concomitant diuretic may be needed; use with caution and modify dosage in patients with hyponatremia, hypovolemia, severe CHF, left ventricular outflow tract obstruction, or with coadministered diuretic therapy; experience in children is limited; severe hypotension may occur in patients who are sodium and/or volume depleted, initiate lower doses and monitor closely when starting therapy in these patients

Adverse Reactions

Cardiovascular: Hypotension, syncope

Central nervous system: Fatigue, vertigo, insomnia, dizziness, headache

Dermatologic: Rash, angioedema. **Note:** The relative risk of angioedema with ACE inhibitors is higher within the first 30 days of use (compared to >1 year of use), for Black Americans (compared to Whites), for lisinopril or enalapril (compared to captopril), and for patients previously hospitalized within 30 days (Brown, 1996).

Endocrine & metabolic: Hypoglycemia, hyperkalemia

Gastrointestinal: Nausea, diarrhea, ageusia

Genitourinary: Impotence

Hematologic: Agranulocytosis, neutropenia, anemia

Hepatic: Cholestatic jaundice, fulminant hepatic necrosis (rare, but potentially fatal)

Neuromuscular & skeletal: Muscle cramps

Renal: Deterioration in renal function

Respiratory: Cough, dyspnea, eosinophilic pneumonitis; **Note:** An isolated dry cough lasting >3 weeks was reported in 7 of 42 pediatric patients (17%) receiving ACE inhibitors (see von Vigier, 2000)

Drug Interactions Cytochrome P450 isoenzyme CYP3A3/4 substrate

Use with potassium-sparing diuretics may result in an additive hyperkalemic effect; diuretics or other antihypertensive agents may increase hypotensive effect; indomethacin or NSAIDs may decrease hypotensive effect; enalapril may increase lithium levels; use with NSAIDs in patients with compromised renal function may increase renal dysfunction (usually reversible)

Food Interactions Food does not affect absorption; limit salt substitutes or potassium-rich diet; avoid natural licorice (causes sodium and water retention and increases potassium loss)

Stability Store vials below 86°F (30°C); solutions for I.V. infusion mixed in NS, D_5W, D_5NS, or D_5LR are stable for 24 hours at room temperature

Mechanism of Action Competitive inhibitor of angiotensin-converting enzyme (ACE); prevents conversion of angiotensin I to angiotensin II, a potent vasoconstrictor; results in lower levels of angiotensin II which causes an increase in plasma renin activity and a reduction in aldosterone secretion

(Continued)

431

Enalapril/Enalaprilat *(Continued)*

Pharmacodynamics (Antihypertensive effect)
Onset of action:
Oral: Within 1 hour
I.V.: Within 15 minutes
Maximum effect:
Oral: Within 4-8 hours
I.V.: Within 1-4 hour
Duration:
Oral: 12-24 hours
I.V.: Dose dependent, usually 4-6 hours

Pharmacokinetics
Absorption: Oral: 55% to 75% (enalapril)
Protein binding: 50% to 60%
Metabolism: Enalapril is a prodrug (inactive) and undergoes biotransformation to enalaprilat (active) in the liver
Half-life:
Enalapril:
CHF neonates 10-19 days of age (n=3): 10.3 hours (range: 4.2-13.4 hours)
CHF: Infants >27 days and Children ≤6.5 years of age (n=11): 2.7 hours (range: 1.3-6.3 hours)
Healthy adults: 2 hours
CHF adults: 3.4-5.8 hours
Enalaprilat:
CHF neonates 10-19 days of age (n=3): 11.9 hours (range 5.9-15.6 hours)
CHF: Infants >27 days and Children ≤6.5 years of age (n=11): 11.1 hours (range: 5.1-20.8 hours)
Infants 6 weeks to 8 months: 6-10 hours
Adults: 35-38 hours
Time to peak serum concentration: Oral:
Enalapril: Within 0.5-1.5 hours
Enalaprilat (active): Within 3-4.5 hours
Elimination: Principally in urine (60% to 80%) with some fecal excretion

Usual Dosage Use lower listed initial dose in patients with hyponatremia, hypovolemia, severe CHF, decreased renal function, or in those receiving diuretics
Manufacturer's recommendations: Pediatric hypertensive patients: Oral: **Enalapril:** Initial: 0.08 mg/kg once daily (maximum dose: 5 mg); adjust dose according to blood pressure readings; doses >0.58 mg/kg (or >40 mg) have not been studied
Alternative pediatric dosing:
Neonates:
Oral: **Enalapril:** Initial: 0.1 mg/kg/day given every 24 hours; increase dose and interval as required every few days (see Additional Information)
I.V.: **Enalaprilat:** 5-10 mcg/kg/dose administered every 8-24 hours (as determined by blood pressure readings) has been used for the treatment of neonatal hypertension; monitor patients carefully; select patients may require higher doses
Infants and Children:
Oral: **Enalapril:** Initial: 0.1 mg/kg/day in 1-2 divided doses; increase as required over 2 weeks to maximum of 0.5 mg/kg/day; mean dose required for CHF improvement in 39 children (9 days to 17 years of age) was 0.36 mg/kg/day; investigationally, select individuals have been treated with doses up to 0.94 mg/kg/day (Leversha, 1994)
I.V.: **Enalaprilat:** 5-10 mcg/kg/dose administered every 8-24 hours (as determined by blood pressure readings); monitor patients carefully; select patients may require higher doses
Adolescents and Adults:
Oral: **Enalapril:** Initial: 2.5-5 mg/day then increase as required; usual dose for hypertension: 10-40 mg/day in 1-2 divided doses; usual dose for CHF: 5-20 mg/day in 2 divided doses; maximum dose: 40 mg/day
Asymptomatic left ventricular dysfunction: Initial: 2.5 mg twice daily; increase as tolerated; usual dose: 20 mg/day in 2 divided doses
I.V.: **Enalaprilat:** 0.625-1.25 mg/dose every 6 hours; doses as high as 5 mg/dose every 6 hours have been tolerated for up to 36 hours; little experience with doses >20 mg/day
Dosing adjustment in renal impairment: Note: Use in neonates and children ≤16 years of age with GFR <30 mL/min/1.73 m^2 is not recommended (no dosing data exists)
Cl$_{cr}$ 10-50 mL/minute: Administer 75% to 100% of dose
Cl$_{cr}$ <10 mL/minute: Administer 50% of dose

Administration

Oral: May administer without regard to food

Parenteral: I.V.: Administer as I.V. infusion (undiluted solution or further diluted) over 5 minutes; to deliver small I.V. doses, a dilution with NS to a final concentration of 25 mcg/mL can be made

Monitoring Parameters Blood pressure, renal function, WBC, serum potassium, serum glucose

Patient Information Limit alcohol; notify physician if vomiting, diarrhea, excessive perspiration, or dehydration occurs, or if swelling of face, lips, tongue, or difficulty in breathing occurs; do not use a salt substitute (potassium-containing) without physician advice

Nursing Implications Discontinue if angioedema occurs; observe closely for hypotension within 1-3 hours of first dose or with new higher dose

Additional Information Severe hypotension was reported in a **preterm** neonate (birth weight 835 g, gestational age 26 weeks, postnatal age 9 days) who was treated with enalapril 0.1 mg/kg orally; hypotension responded to I.V. plasma and dopamine; the authors suggest starting enalapril in preterm infants at 0.01 mg/kg and increasing upwards in a stepwise fashion with very close monitoring of blood pressure and urine output. However, in this case report, oral enalapril at doses of 0.01 mg/kg to 0.04 mg/kg did not adequately control blood pressure. Further studies are needed. (Schilder, 1995)

Over the years, several pediatric studies have examined the effects of ACE inhibitors on proteinuria. In a more recent retrospective study, enalapril (in doses of 2.5-5 mg/day) administered either as monotherapy (n=17; mean age: 13.7 years; range 8-17 years) or with prednisone (n=11; mean age: 12.6 years; range: 7-16 years), significantly decreased proteinuria in normotensive proteinuric children (with or without nephrotic syndrome); no significant change in blood pressure was observed (Sasinka, 1999). In a smaller study of children with persistent proteinuria (n=7; 6 with steroid resistant nephrotic syndrome; mean age: 13.5 years; range: 7-18 years), enalapril (at mean oral doses of 0.3 mg/kg/day) significantly reduced proteinuria in 5 of the 7 patients (Lama, 2000). Another recent study assessed the effects of enalapril on urinary protein electrophoretic patterns in 13 children (mean age: 8 years; range: 1.8-12 years) with steroid resistant nephrotic syndrome; oral enalapril was initially dosed at 0.2 mg/kg/day (with a maximum dose of 30 mg/day); doses were increased each month by 0.1 mg/kg/day until the patients' urinary protein decreased by 50% from baseline; prednisone was added after 2 months in 11 of the 13 children at doses of 30 mg/m^2 given every other day; four patients had a complete remission of proteinuria after 4-12 months; an 80% decrease in urinary total protein and a 70% decrease in urinary albumin was observed in the other patients; the pattern of urinary protein shifted from a nonselective to an albumin-selective urinary protein loss in all patients; significant increases in plasma total protein and albumin occurred; it is important to note that 3 of the 13 patients (23%) required interruption of enalapril during transient acute renal failure due to an infectious disease (Delucchi, 2000). Further pediatric studies are needed to identify optimal enalapril oral doses and to establish safety and efficacy for this use.

Dosage Forms

Injection, solution, as **enalaprilat** (Vasotec® I.V.): 1.25 mg/mL (1 mL, 2 mL) [contains benzyl alcohol]

Tablet, as **maleate** (Vasotec®): 2.5 mg, 5 mg, 10 mg, 20 mg

Extemporaneous Preparations

A 1 mg/mL oral suspension made from tablets, Bicitra®, and Ora-Sweet® SF is stable for 30 days when stored in a polyethylene terephthalate bottle under refrigeration (2°C to 8°C); place ten 20 mg tablets in a 200 mL polyethylene terephthalate bottle; add 50 mL of Bicitra®; shake well for at least 2 minutes; let stand for 1 hour then shake for one additional minute; add 150 mL of Ora-Sweet® SF and shake well; label "shake well" [Vasotec® tablets (package insert), 2001].

A 1 mg/mL oral liquid preparation made from tablets and 3 different vehicles (cherry syrup, a 1:1 mixture of Ora-Sweet® and Ora-Plus®, or a 1:1 mixture of Ora-Sweet® SF and Ora-Plus®) was stable for 60 days when stored in amber plastic prescription bottles in the dark at room temperature (25°C) or under refrigeration (5°C); grind six 20 mg tablets in a mortar into a fine powder; add 15 mL of the vehicle and mix well to form a uniform paste; mix while adding the vehicle in geometric proportions to **almost** 120 mL; transfer to a calibrated bottle and qsad with vehicle to 120 mL; label "shake well" and "protect from light" (Allen, 1998).

A 1 mg/mL oral liquid preparation made from tablets and 3 different vehicles (deionized water, citrate buffer solution at pH 5.0, or a 1:1 mixture of Ora-Sweet® and Ora-Plus®) was stable for 91 days when stored in plastic prescription bottles in the dark under refrigeration (4°C). When stored at room temperature (25°C), the preparations made in citrate buffer solution at pH 5.0 and the 1:1 mixture of Ora-Sweet®

(Continued)

Enalapril/Enalaprilat *(Continued)*

and Ora-Plus® were also stable for 91 days, but the preparation made in deionized water was stable for only 56 days. Grind twenty 10 mg tablets in a mortar; add a small amount of vehicle and mix well to form a smooth paste; mix while adding increasing amounts of the vehicle to make the mixture pourable; transfer to a graduated cylinder and qsad to 200 mL; **Note:** To prepare the isotonic citrate buffer solution (pH 5.0), see reference; label "shake well" and "protect from light" (Nahata, 1998).

A more dilute oral liquid preparation of 0.1 mg/mL made from tablets and an isotonic buffer solution at pH 5.0 was stable for 90 days when stored in amber, high density polyethylene bottles under refrigeration (5°C); grind one 20 mg tablet in a glass mortar into a fine powder; triturate with isotonic citrate buffer (pH 5.0) and filter; qsad to 200 mL with buffer solution; label "shake well" and "protect from light" (Boulton, 1994).

Allen LV and Erickson MA, "Stability of Alprazolam, Chloroquine Phosphate, Cisapride, Enalapril Maleate, and Hydralazine Hydrochloride in Extemporaneously Compounded Oral Liquids," *Am J Health Syst Pharm*, 1998, 55(18):1915-20.

Boulton DW, Woods DJ, Fawcett JP, et al, "The Stability of an Enalapril Maleate Oral Solution Prepared From Tablets," *Aust J Hosp Pharm*, 1994, 24(2):151-6.

Nahata MC, Morosco RS, and Hipple TF, "Stability of Enalapril Maleate in Three Extemporaneously Prepared Oral Liquids," *Am J Health Syst Pharm*, 1998, 55(11):1155-7.

Vasotec® (package insert), West Point, PA: Merck & Co., Inc; 2001.

References

Brown NJ, Ray WA, Snowden M, et al, "Black Americans Have an Increased Rate of Angiotensin-Converting Enzyme Inhibitor-Associated Angioedema," *Clin Pharmacol Ther*, 1996, 60(1):8-13.

Bult Y and van den Anker J, "Hypertension in a Preterm Infant Treated With Enalapril," *J Pediatr Pharm Pract*, 1997, 2(4):229-31.

Delucchi A, Cano F, Rodriguez E, et al, "Enalapril and Prednisone in Children With Nephrotic-Range Proteinuria," *Pediatr Nephrol*, 2000, 14(12):1088-91.

Frenneaux M, Stewart RA, Newman CM, et al, "Enalapril for Severe Heart Failure in Infancy," *Arch Dis Child*, 1989, 64(2):219-23.

Lama G, Luongo I, Piscitelli A, et al, "Enalapril: Antiproteinuric Effect in Children With Nephrotic Syndrome," *Clin Nephrol*, 2000, 53(6):432-6.

Leversha AM, Wilson NJ, Clarkson PM, et al, "Efficacy and Dosage of Enalapril in Congenital and Acquired Heart Disease," *Arch Dis Child*, 1994, 70(1):35-9.

Lloyd TR, Mahoney LT, Knoedel D, et al, "Orally Administered Enalapril for Infants With Congestive Heart Failure: A Dose Finding Study," *J Pediatr*, 1989, 114(4 Pt 1):650-4.

Marcadis ML, Kraus DM, Hatzopoulos FK, et al, "Use of Enalaprilat for Neonatal Hypertension," *J Pediatr*, 1991, 119(3):505-6.

Nakamura H, Ishii M, Sugimura T, et al, "The Kinetic Profiles of Enalapril and Enalaprilat and Their Possible Developmental Changes in Pediatric Patients With Congestive Heart Failure," *Clin Pharmacol Ther*, 1994, 56(2):160-8.

Sasinka MA, Podracka L, Boor A, et al, "Enalapril Treatment of Proteinuria in Normotensive Children," *Bratisl Lek Listy*, 1999, 100(9):476-80.

Schilder JL and Van den Anker JN, "Use of Enalapril in Neonatal Hypertension," *Acta Paediatr*, 1995, 84(12):1426-8.

von Vigier RO, Mozzettini S, Truttmann AC, et al, "Cough is Common in Children Prescribed Converting Enzyme Inhibitors," *Nephron*, 2000, 83(1):98.

Wells TG, Bunchman TE, Kearns GL, "Treatment of Neonatal Hypertension With Enalaprilat," *J Pediatr*, 1990, 117(4):664-7.

- ◆ **Enbrel®** *see* Etanercept *on page 461*
- ◆ **Endantadine® (Can)** *see* Amantadine *on page 73*
- ◆ **Endocarditis Prophylaxis** *see page 1321*
- ◆ **Endocet®** *see* Oxycodone and Acetaminophen *on page 847*
- ◆ **Endodan®** *see* Oxycodone and Aspirin *on page 848*
- ◆ **Endrate®** *see* Edetate Disodium *on page 425*
- ◆ **Enfamil® Glucose** *see* Dextrose *on page 366*
- ◆ **Enlon®** *see* Edrophonium *on page 426*

Enoxaparin (e noks ah PAIR in)

Related Information

Antithrombotic Therapy in Children *on page 1316*

U.S. Brand Names Lovenox®

Therapeutic Category Anticoagulant; Low Molecular Weight Heparin (LMWH)

Generic Available No

Use Prophylaxis and treatment of thromboembolic disorders, specifically: (in adults) prevention of DVT following hip or knee replacement surgery, abdominal surgery in patients at thromboembolic risk (ie, >40 years of age, obese, general anesthesia >30 minutes, malignancy, history of DVT or pulmonary embolism) and in medical patients at thromboembolic risk due to severely restricted mobility during acute illness; administered with warfarin: For inpatient treatment of acute DVT (with or without pulmonary embolism) and outpatient treatment of acute DVT (without pulmonary embolism); administered with aspirin: For prevention of ischemic complications of non-Q-wave MI and unstable angina

Pregnancy Risk Factor B

Contraindications Hypersensitivity to enoxaparin, heparin, any component (see Warnings), or pork products (enoxaparin is derived from porcine intestinal mucosa); active major bleeding; acute heparin-induced or low molecular weight heparin-induced thrombocytopenia

Warnings Bleeding or thrombocytopenia may occur; major hemorrhages (eg, intracranial and retroperitoneal bleeding) may be fatal; thrombocytopenia with thrombosis may occur and may be complicated by limb ischemia, organ infarction, or death. Use with extreme caution in patients with an increased risk of hemorrhage (eg, active GI ulceration or bleeding, angiodysplastic GI disease, bacterial endocarditis, bleeding disorders, hemorrhagic stroke); recent brain, spinal, or ophthalmological surgery; concomitant platelet inhibitor therapy (see Drug Interactions); or a history of heparin-induced thrombocytopenia. Do not use unit-for-unit in place of heparin or other low molecular weight heparins (units are not equivalent). Enoxaparin is not recommended for prophylaxis of thromboembolic disorders in patients with prosthetic heart valves (prosthetic heart valve thrombosis may occur; several cases occurred in pregnant women and resulted in maternal and fetal deaths; pregnant women with prosthetic heart valves may be at a higher risk for thromboembolism).

Epidural or spinal hematoma resulting in long-term or permanent paralysis may occur in patients receiving low molecular weight heparins or heparinoids during epidural/spinal anesthesia or spinal puncture; these patients must be monitored frequently for neurological impairment and treated immediately if compromised; the use of indwelling spinal catheters for analgesia, concomitant use of platelet inhibitors, NSAIDs, or other anticoagulants, and repeated or traumatic epidural/spinal puncture increase the risk for epidural/spinal hematoma; potential benefits must be weighed against the risks. Enoxaparin should be withheld (at least 2 doses) and antifactor Xa activity should be determined (if possible), prior to lumbar or epidural procedures.

Enoxaparin multidose vial contains benzyl alcohol which may cause allergic reactions in susceptible individuals; large amounts of benzyl alcohol (≥ 99 mg/kg/day) have been associated with a potentially fatal toxicity ("gasping syndrome") in neonates; the "gasping syndrome" consists of metabolic acidosis, respiratory distress, gasping respirations, CNS dysfunction (including convulsions, intracranial hemorrhage), hypotension and cardiovascular collapse; avoid use of enoxaparin products containing benzyl alcohol in neonates; use the preservative free injection; *in vitro* and animal studies have shown that benzoate, a metabolite of benzyl alcohol, displaces bilirubin from protein binding sites. Use multidose vial with caution in pregnant women and only if clearly needed (benzyl alcohol may cross the placenta).

Precautions Use with caution in patients with uncontrolled arterial hypertension, bleeding diathesis, history of recent GI ulceration, diabetic retinopathy, and hemorrhage; use with caution and consider dosage decrease in patients with severe renal dysfunction (Cl_{cr} <30 mL/minute); institute appropriate therapy if thromboembolism occurs despite enoxaparin prophylaxis

Adverse Reactions
Cardiovascular: Edema
Central nervous system: Fever
Endocrine & metabolic: Hyperlipidemia (very rare)
Gastrointestinal: Nausea
Hematologic: Hemorrhage, thrombocytopenia (incidence of heparin-induced thrombocytopenia is less than with heparin therapy)
Hepatic: Elevated SGOT and SGPT (asymptomatic, fully reversible, rarely associated with elevated bilirubin levels)
Local: Irritation, pain, hematoma, ecchymosis, erythema at S.C. injection site; epidural or spinal hematoma (see Warnings)

Drug Interactions Anticoagulants, thrombolytic agents (alteplase, streptokinase, urokinase), platelet inhibitors (aspirin, salicylates, NSAIDs including ketorolac, dipyridamole, and sulfinpyrazone) may increase the risk of bleeding

Stability Store at room temperature; does not contain preservatives, discard unused portions; do not mix with other injections or infusions

Mechanism of Action Potentiates the action of antithrombin III and inactivates coagulation factor Xa; also inactivates factor IIa (thrombin), but to a much lesser degree; ratio of antifactor Xa to antifactor IIa activity is ~4:1 (ratio for unfractionated heparin is 1:1)

Pharmacodynamics Antifactor Xa and antithrombin (antifactor IIa) activities:
Maximum effect: S.C.: 3-5 hours
Duration: ~12 hours following a 40 mg daily dose given S.C.

Pharmacokinetics Based on antifactor Xa activity
(Continued)

Enoxaparin *(Continued)*

Distribution: Does not cross the placental barrier

Mean V_d: Adults: 6 L

Protein binding: Does not bind to most heparin binding proteins

Bioavailability: S.C.: 92%

Half-life: S.C.: Adults: 4.5 hours (range 2.2-6 hours)

Elimination: 40% of I.V. dose is excreted in urine as active and inactive fragments; 8% to 20% of antifactor Xa activity is recovered within 24 hours in the urine

Clearance: Decreased by 30% in patients with Cl_{cr} <30 mL/minute

Usual Dosage S.C.:

Neonates, Infants, and Children: *Chest*, 2001 Recommendations:

Initial:

Infants <2 months:

Prophylaxis: 0.75 mg/kg every 12 hours

Treatment: 1.5 mg/kg every 12 hours

Infants >2 months and Children ≤18 years:

Prophylaxis: 0.5 mg/kg every 12 hours

Treatment: 1 mg/kg every 12 hours

Maintenance: See **Dosage Titration** table: **Note:** In a recent prospective study of 177 courses of enoxaparin in pediatric patients (146 treatment courses; 31 prophylactic courses) considerable variation in maintenance dosage requirements was observed (see Dix, 2000)

Enoxaparin Dosage Titration

Antifactor Xa	Dose Titration	Time to Repeat Antifactor Xa Level
<0.35 units/mL	Increase dose by 25%	4 h after next dose
0.35-0.49 units/mL	Increase dose by 10%	4 h after next dose
0.5-1 unit/mL	Keep same dosage	Next day, then 1 wk later, then monthly (4 h after dose)
1.1-1.5 units/mL	Decrease dose by 20%	Before next dose
1.6-2 units/mL	Hold dose for 3 h and decrease dose by 30%	Before next dose, then 4 h after next dose
>2 units/mL	Hold all doses until antifactor Xa is 0.5 units/mL, then decrease dose by 40%	Before next dose and every 12 h until antifactor Xa <0.5 units/mL

Modified from Monagle P, Michelson AD, Bovill E, et al, "Antithrombotic Therapy in Children," *Chest*, 2001, 119:344S-70S.

Adults: **Note:** Consider lower doses for patients <45 kg

Prevention of DVT:

Knee replacement surgery: 30 mg every 12 hours; give first dose 12-24 hours after surgery (provided hemostasis has been established); average duration 7-10 days, up to 14 days

Hip replacement surgery: Initial phase: 30 mg every 12 hours with first dose 12-24 hours after surgery (provided hemostasis has been established) or consider 40 mg once daily with first dose given 12 ± 3 hours prior to surgery; average duration of initial phase: 7-10 days, up to 14 days; after initial phase, give 40 mg once daily for 3 weeks

Abdominal surgery in patients at risk: 40 mg once daily; give first dose 2 hours prior to surgery; average duration: 7-10 days, up to 12 days

Medical patients at risk due to severely restricted mobility during acute illness: 40 mg once daily; average duration: 6-11 days, up to 14 days

Treatment of acute DVT and pulmonary embolism: **Note:** Initiate warfarin therapy when appropriate (usually within 72 hours of starting enoxaparin), continue enoxaparin for a minimum of 5 days (average 7 days) until INR is therapeutic

Inpatient treatment of acute DVT with or without pulmonary embolism: 1 mg/kg every 12 hours or 1.5 mg/kg once daily

Outpatient treatment of acute DVT without pulmonary embolism: 1 mg/kg every 12 hours

Dosage adjustment in renal impairment: No specific guidelines are available, but clearance is decreased when Cl_{cr} <30 mL/minute; monitor antifactor Xa activity to adjust dosage

on

Administration Parenteral: For S.C. use only; do not administer I.M. or I.V.; administer by deep S.C. injection; do not rub injection site after S.C. administration as bruising may occur

Monitoring Parameters CBC with platelets, stool occult blood tests; antifactor Xa activity in select patients (eg, neonates, infants, and children, and patients with significant renal impairment, active bleeding, or abnormal coagulation parameters); **Note**: Routine monitoring of PT and APTT is not warranted since PT and APTT are relatively insensitive measures of low molecular weight heparin activity; consider monitoring bone density in infants and children with long-term use

Reference Range Antifactor Xa level of 0.5-1 unit/mL measured 4-6 hours after S.C. administration

Nursing Implications Instruct patients on proper S.C. injection technique if patient will self-inject.

Additional Information Discontinue therapy if platelets fall <100,000/mm^3; each 10 mg of enoxaparin sodium equals ~1000 international units of antifactor Xa activity.

Enoxaparin contains fragments of unfractionated heparin produced by alkaline degradation (depolymerization) of heparin benzyl ester; enoxaparin has mean molecular weights of 3500-5600 daltons, which are much lower than mean molecular weights of unfractionated heparin (12,000-15,000 daltons). Low molecular weight heparins (LMWH) have several advantages over unfractionated heparin: better S.C. bioavailability, more convenient administration (S.C. versus I.V.), longer half-life (longer dosing interval), more predictable pharmacokinetics and pharmacodynamic (anticoagulant) effect, less intensive laboratory monitoring, reduced risk of heparin-induced thrombocytopenia, potential for outpatient use, and probable reduced risk of osteoporosis (further studies are needed).

Accidental overdosage may be treated with protamine sulfate; 1 mg protamine sulfate neutralizes 1 mg enoxaparin; first dose of protamine sulfate should equal the dose of enoxaparin injected, a second dose of 0.5 mg protamine sulfate per 1 mg enoxaparin may be given if APTT remains prolonged 2-4 hours after first dose (see Protamine *on page 955*)

Dosage Forms Note: Enoxaparin injection is available in 2 concentrations: 100 mg/mL and 150 mg/mL

Injection, solution, as sodium [ampul; preservative free]: 30 mg/0.3 mL (0.3 mL)

Injection, solution, as sodium [graduated prefilled syringe; preservative free]: 60 mg/0.6 mL (0.6 mL); 80 mg/0.8 mL (0.8 mL); 100 mg/1 mL (1 mL); 120 mg/0.8 mL (0.8 mL); 150 mg/1 mL (1 mL)

Injection, solution, as sodium [multidose vial]: 100 mg/mL (3 mL) [contains 15 mg/mL benzyl alcohol]

Injection, solution, as sodium [prefilled syringe; preservative free]: 30 mg/0.3 mL (0.3 mL); 40 mg/0.4 mL (0.4 mL)

References

deVeber G, Chan A, Monagle P, et al, "Anticoagulation Therapy in Pediatric Patients With Sinovenous Thrombosis: A Cohort Study," *Arch Neurol*, 1998, 55(12):1533-7.

Dix D, Andrew M, Marzinotto V, et al, "The Use of Low Molecular Weight Heparin in Pediatric Patients: A Prospective Cohort Study," *J Pediatr*, 2000, 136(4):439-45.

Hirsh J, Warkentin TE, Shaughnessy SG, et al, "Heparin and Low-Molecular-Weight Heparin: Mechanisms of Action, Pharmacokinetics, Dosing, Monitoring, Efficacy, and Safety," *Chest*, 2001, 119:64S-94S.

Martineau P and Tawil N, "Low-Molecular-Weight Heparins in the Treatment of Deep-Vein Thrombosis," *Ann Pharmacother*, 1998, 32(5):588-98, 601.

Massicotte P, Adams M, Marzinotto V, et al, "Low-Molecular-Weight Heparin in Pediatric Patients With Thrombotic Disease: A Dose Finding Study," *J Pediatr*, 1996, 128(3):313-8.

Monagle P, Michelson AD, Bovill E, et al, "Antithrombotic Therapy in Children," *Chest*, 2001, 119:344S-70S.

♦ **Entacyl® (Can)** *see* Piperazine [DSC] *on page 909*

♦ **Entocort™ EC** *see* Budesonide *on page 183*

♦ **Entrophen® (Can)** *see* Aspirin *on page 134*

♦ **Entsol® [OTC]** *see* Sodium Chloride *on page 1027*

♦ **Enulose®** *see* Lactulose *on page 649*

♦ **Ephedra** *see* Ephedrine *on page 437*

Ephedrine (e FED rin)

U.S. Brand Names Pretz-D® [OTC]

Synonyms Ephedra; Ephedrinum; Ma Huang

Therapeutic Category Adrenergic Agonist Agent; Antiasthmatic; Bronchodilator; Sympathomimetic

Generic Available Yes

Use Treatment of mild asthma, nasal congestion, acute bronchospasm, idiopathic orthostatic hypotension; adjunctive agent for treatment of shock

Pregnancy Risk Factor C

(Continued)

Ephedrine *(Continued)*

Contraindications Hypersensitivity to ephedrine or any component; patients with hypertension, cardiac arrhythmias, angle-closure glaucoma, and psychoneurosis; use during halothane or cyclopropane anesthesia (see Drug Interactions)

Warnings Use of ephedrine as a pressor is not a substitute for replacement of blood, plasma, fluids, and electrolytes; blood volume should be corrected as fully as possible before ephedrine therapy; must not be used as sole therapy in hypovolemic patients; hypoxia, hypercapnia, and acidosis may reduce the effectiveness and increase the incidence of side effects of ephedrine; may cause hypertension which may result in intracranial hemorrhage; long-term use may cause anxiety and symptoms of paranoid schizophrenia; the FDA has issued warnings concerning ephedrine-containing nonprescription products with claims of producing such effects as euphoria, increased sexual sensation, increased energy, and weight loss; healthcare professionals are urged to be aware of these products and counsel patients, when appropriate, about the potential adverse effects of ephedrine such as headache, dizziness, heart irregularities, seizures, and possibly death

Precautions Use with caution in patients with hyperthyroidism, diabetes mellitus, prostatic hypertrophy, coronary insufficiency, and angina

Adverse Reactions

Cardiovascular: Hypertension, precordial pain, edema, palpitations, tachycardia, arrhythmias

Central nervous system: Nervousness, anxiety, apprehension, fear, tension, agitation, excitation, restlessness, irritability, insomnia, dizziness, vertigo, confusion, delirium, hallucinations, euphoria, paranoid psychosis, headache

Dermatologic: Rash

Gastrointestinal: Nausea, vomiting, xerostomia, mild epigastric distress, anorexia

Genitourinary: Urinary retention

Neuromuscular & skeletal: Tremors, hyperactive reflexes, weakness

Drug Interactions Increased effects with other sympathomimetic agents; reduced pressor response to ephedrine with alpha-adrenergic blocking agents and methyldopa; increased cardiac irritability and arrhythmias with halothane and cyclopropane anesthesia; increased pressor effects with MAO inhibitors; cardiac glycosides may increase cardiac stimulation; medications which alkalinize or acidify the urine may result in increased or decreased ephedrine effects (see Pharmacokinetics); increased CNS and GI effects when used with theophylline

Stability Protect from light

Mechanism of Action Stimulates both alpha- and beta-adrenergic receptors and also stimulates the release of norepinephrine from storage sites resulting in bronchodilation, cardiac stimulation, and increased systolic and diastolic blood pressure; tachyphylaxis may occur

Pharmacodynamics

Bronchodilation:

Onset of action: Oral: 15-60 minutes

Duration: Oral: 2-4 hours

Pressor/cardiac effects: Duration:

Oral: 4 hours

I.M., S.C.: 1 hour

Pharmacokinetics

Absorption: Oral: Complete

Metabolism: Liver by oxidative deamination, demethylation, aromatic hydroxylation, and conjugation

Bioavailability: Oral: 85%

Half-life: 4.9-6.5 hours

Elimination: Dependent upon urinary pH with greatest excretion in acid pH; urine pH 5: 74% to 99% excreted unchanged; urine pH 8: 22% to 25% excreted unchanged

Usual Dosage

Bronchodilation and nasal decongestion:

Oral:

Children >2-6 years: 2-3 mg/kg/day or 100 mg/m^2/day in 4-6 divided doses

Children 7-11 years: 6.25-12.5 mg every 4 hours; not to exceed 75 mg/day

Children ≥12 years and Adults: 12.5-50 mg every 3-4 hours; not to exceed 150 mg/day

Spray:

Children 6-12 years: 1-2 sprays in each nostril not more than every 4 hours; do not exceed 3 days of therapy

Children >12 years and Adults: 2-3 sprays in each nostril not more than every 4 hours; do not exceed 3 days of therapy

Orthostatic hypotension: Oral: Adults: 25 mg 1-4 times/day

Adjunctive agent in the treatment of shock: Use the smallest effective dose for the shortest time:
  Children <12 years: I.M., I.V., S.C.: 3 mg/kg/day in 4-6 divided doses
  Children ≥12 years and Adults:
    I.M., S.C.: 25-50 mg (range: 10-50 mg); may repeat with a second dose of 50 mg; not to exceed 150 mg/24 hours
    I.V.: 10-25 mg; may repeat with a second dose in 5-10 minutes of 25 mg; not to exceed 150 mg/24 hours

Administration
  Oral: May be administered without regard to food
  Parenteral:
    I.M., S.C.: May be administered undiluted
    I.V.: May be administered by slow I.V. push
  Spray: Spray into each nostril while gently occluding the other

Monitoring Parameters Vital signs, pulmonary function tests, respiratory rate (when applicable)

Test Interactions May cause a false-positive test for amphetamine (by EMIT assay)

Patient Information Use for self-medication for asthma only under physician's direction; see Warnings; contact your physician if nervousness, tremor, insomnia, nausea, or loss of appetite occur; may cause dry mouth

Additional Information Because ephedrine has been used to synthesize methamphetamine, restrictions are in place to reduce the potential for misuse (diversion) and abuse; 24 g of ephedrine (in terms of base) is the limit for a single transaction for drug products containing ephedrine regardless of the form in which these drugs are packaged

Dosage Forms
  Capsule, as sulfate: 25 mg
  Injection, solution, as sulfate: 50 mg/mL (1 mL)
  Solution, intranasal spray, as sulfate (Pretz-D®): 0.25% (50 mL)

♦ **Ephedrinum** see Ephedrine on page 437

♦ **Epidermal Thymocyte Activating Factor** see Aldesleukin on page 56

♦ **Epifrin®** see Epinephrine on page 439

Epinephrine (ep i NEF rin)

Related Information
  Adult ACLS Algorithm, Asystole on page 1187
  Adult ACLS Algorithm, Bradycardia on page 1188
  Adult ACLS Algorithm, Cardiac Arrest on page 1183
  Adult ACLS Algorithm, Comprehensive ECC on page 1184
  Adult ACLS Algorithm, Pulseless Electrical Activity on page 1186
  Adult ACLS Algorithm, V. Fib and Pulseless VT on page 1185
  Asthma Guidelines on page 1376
  CPR Pediatric Drug Dosages on page 1175
  Emergency Pediatric Drip Calculations on page 1177
  Extravasation Treatment on page 1240
  Neonatal Resuscitation Algorithm on page 1178
  Pediatric ALS Algorithm, Bradycardia on page 1179
  Pediatric ALS Algorithm, Pulseless Arrest on page 1180

U.S. Brand Names Adrenalin®; Epifrin®; EpiPen®; EpiPen® Jr; Primatene® Mist [OTC]; S₂® [OTC]

Canadian Brand Names Vaponefrin®

Synonyms Adrenaline; Racemic Epinephrine

Therapeutic Category Adrenergic Agonist Agent; Antiasthmatic; Antidote, Hypersensitivity Reactions; Bronchodilator; Decongestant, Nasal; Sympathomimetic

Generic Available Yes

Use Treatment of bronchospasm, anaphylactic reactions, cardiac arrest, and management of open-angle (chronic simple) glaucoma; nasal decongestant (topical nasal formulation); upper airway obstruction and croup (racemic epinephrine)

Pregnancy Risk Factor C

Contraindications Hypersensitivity to epinephrine or any component (see Warnings); cardiac arrhythmias, angle-closure glaucoma

Warnings Some products contain sulfites which may cause allergic reactions in susceptible individuals

Precautions Use with caution in patients with diabetes mellitus, cardiovascular disease (angina, tachycardia, MI), thyroid disease, or cerebral arteriosclerosis; rebound nasal congestion may occur after frequent nasal use
(Continued)

Epinephrine *(Continued)*

Adverse Reactions

Cardiovascular: Pallor, tachycardia, hypertension, increased myocardial oxygen consumption, cardiac arrhythmias, sudden death

Central nervous system: Anxiety, headache

Gastrointestinal: Nausea

Genitourinary: Acute urinary retention in patients with bladder outflow obstruction

Neuromuscular & skeletal: Weakness, tremor

Ocular: Precipitation of or exacerbation of narrow-angle glaucoma

Renal: Decreased renal and splanchnic blood flow

Drug Interactions Increased cardiac irritability if administered concurrently with halogenated inhalational anesthetics; beta-blocking agents (ie, propranolol); alpha-blocking agents (eg, phentolamine); alpha- and beta-blocking agents (labetalol); phenothiazines with alpha-blocking activity; tricyclic antidepressants enhance pressor response to epinephrine

Stability Protect from light; incompatible with alkaline solutions (sodium bicarbonate); compatible when coadministered with dopamine, dobutamine, inamrinone (amrinone), atracurium, pancuronium, and vecuronium

Mechanism of Action Stimulates alpha-, beta$_1$- and beta$_2$-adrenergic receptors resulting in relaxation of smooth muscle of the bronchial tree, cardiac stimulation, and dilation of skeletal muscle vasculature; small doses can cause vasodilation via beta$_2$-vascular receptors; large doses may produce constriction of skeletal and vascular smooth muscle; decreases production of aqueous humor and increases aqueous outflow; dilates the pupil by contracting the dilator muscle

Pharmacodynamics

Local vasoconstriction (topical):
   Onset of action: 5 minutes
   Duration: <1 hour

Onset of bronchodilation:
   Inhalation: Within 1 minute
   S.C.: Within 5-10 minutes

Maximum ocular effect: Following conjunctival instillation intraocular pressures fall within 1 hour with a maximal response occurring within 4-8 hours

Duration: Ocular effects persist for 12-24 hours

Pharmacokinetics

Absorption: Orally ingested doses are rapidly metabolized in GI tract and liver; pharmacologically active concentrations are **not** achieved

Distribution: Crosses placenta but not blood-brain barrier

Metabolism: Extensive in the liver and other tissues by the enzymes catechol-o-methyltransferase and monoamine oxidase

Usual Dosage

Neonates: I.V., Intratracheal: 0.01-0.03 mg/kg (0.1-0.3 mL/kg of **1:10,000** solution) every 3-5 minutes as needed

Infants and Children:

   I.M.: EpiPen® and EpiPen® Jr: 0.01 mg/kg
      or as alternative
      <30 kg: 0.15 mg; >30 kg: 0.3 mg

   S.C.: 0.01 mg/kg (0.01 mL/kg/dose of **1:1000** solution) not to exceed 0.5 mg **or**
   Suspension: 0.005 mL/kg/dose (1:200); not to exceed 0.15 mL every 8-12 hours

   Bradycardia:
      I.V.: 0.01 mg/kg (0.1 mL/kg) of **1:10,000** solution (maximum dose: 1 mg or 10 mL); may repeat every 3-5 minutes as needed
      Intratracheal: 0.1 mg/kg (0.1 mL/kg) of **1:1000** solution; doses as high as 0.2 mg/kg may be effective; may repeat every 3-5 minutes as needed

   Asystole or pulseless arrest:
      I.V. or I.O.: 0.01 mg/kg (0.1 mL/kg) of **1:10,000** solution; may repeat every 3-5 minutes as needed; if ineffective, may increase dosage to 0.1 mg/kg (0.1 mL/kg of **1:1000** solution; doses as high as 0.2 mg/kg may be effective); repeat every 3-5 minutes as needed [increased dosage no longer routinely recommended by the American Heart Association (see References)]
      Intratracheal: 0.1 mg/kg (0.1 mL/kg) of **1:1000** solution (doses as high as 0.2 mg/kg may be effective)

   Continuous I.V. infusion rate: 0.1-1 mcg/kg/minute; titrate dosage to desired effect

   Nebulization: 0.25-0.5 mL of 2.25% **racemic epinephrine** solution diluted in 3 mL NS, or L-epinephrine at an equivalent dose; racemic epinephrine 10 mg = 5 mg L-epinephrine; use lower end of dosing range for younger infants

   Ophthalmic: Instill 1-2 drops in eye(s) once or twice daily

   Nasal: Children ≥6 years and Adults: Apply drops locally as needed; do not exceed 1 mL every 15 minutes

Adults:
Asystole: I.V.: 1 mg every 3-5 minutes; if this approach fails, alternative regimens include:
Intermediate: 2-5 mg every 3-5 minutes
Escalating: 1 mg, 3 mg, 5 mg at 3-minute intervals
High: 0.1 mg/kg every 3-5 minutes
Intratracheal: 1 mg (although the optimal dose is unknown, doses of 2-2.5 times the I.V. dose may be needed)
I.M., S.C.: 0.1-0.5 mg every 10-15 minutes
Continuous I.V. infusion rate: Initial: 1 mcg/minute (range: 1-10 mcg/minute); titrate dosage to desired effect
Ophthalmic: Instill 1-2 drops in eye(s) once or twice daily; when treating open-angle glaucoma, the concentration and dosage must be adjusted to the response of the patient

Administration
Inhalation: Nebulization: Dilute in 3 mL NS
Intratracheal: Dilute with NS to a total volume of 3-5 mL and follow with several positive pressure ventilations
Nasal: Apply as drops or with sterile swab
Ophthalmic: Instill drops into affected eye(s); avoid contacting bottle tip with skin or eye; apply finger pressure to lacrimal sac during and for 1-2 minutes after instillation to decrease risk of absorption and systemic effects
Oral inhalation: Shake well before use; use spacer in children <8 years of age
Parenteral:
Direct I.V. or I.O. administration: Dilute to a maximum concentration of 100 mcg/mL (if using 1:10,000 concentration, no dilution is necessary)
Continuous I.V. infusion: Rate of infusion (mL/hour) = dose (mcg/kg/minute) x weight (kg) x 60 minutes/hour divided by the concentration (mcg/mL); maximum concentration: 64 mcg/mL
I.M. (EpiPen® and EpiPen® Jr): Intramuscularly into anterolateral aspect of thigh
S.C.: Use only 1:1000 solution or 1:200 suspension

Monitoring Parameters EKG, heart rate, blood pressure, site of infusion for excessive blanching/extravasation

Nursing Implications Tissue irritant; extravasation may be treated by local small injections of a diluted phentolamine solution (mix 5 mg with 9 mL NS)

Dosage Forms
Aerosol for oral inhalation (Primatene® Mist): 0.2 mg/inhalation (15 mL, 22.5 mL)
Injection, solution [in prefilled auto injector]:
EpiPen®: 0.3 mg/0.3 mL [1:1000] (2 mL) [contains sodium metabisulfite; available as single unit or in double unit pack with training unit]
EpiPen® Jr.: 0.15 mg/0.3 mL [1:2000] (2 mL) [contains sodium metabisulfite; available as single unit or in double unit pack with training unit]
Injection, solution, as hydrochloride: 0.1 mg/mL [1:10,000] (10 mL); 1 mg/mL [1:1000] (1 mL)
Adrenalin®: 1 mg/mL [1:1000] (1 mL, 30 mL)
Solution for oral inhalation (S₂®): Racepinephrine 2.25% (0.5 mL, 15 mL) [contains d-epinephrine 1.125%, l-epinephrine 1.125%, and sodium metabisulfite]
Solution for oral inhalation, as hydrochloride (Adrenalin®): 1% [10 mg/mL - 1:100] (7.5 mL) [contains sodium bisulfite]
Solution, ophthalmic, as hydrochloride (Epifrin®): 0.5% (15 mL); 1% (15 mL); 2% (15 mL) [contains sodium metabisulfite]

References
American College of Cardiology, American Heart Association Task Force, "Adult Advanced Cardiac Life Support" and "Pediatric Advanced Life Support Guidelines," *JAMA*, 1992, 268(16):2199-241 and 2262-75.
"Guidelines 2000 for Cardiopulmonary Resuscitation and Emergency Cardiovascular Care. Part 10: Pediatric Advanced Life Support. The American Heart Association in Collaboration With the International Liaison Committee on Resuscitation," *Circulation*, 2000, 102(8 Suppl):I291-342.
"Guidelines 2000 for Cardiopulmonary Resuscitation and Emergency Cardiovascular Care. Part 11: Neonatal Resuscitation. The American Heart Association in Collaboration With the International Liaison Committee on Resuscitation," *Circulation*, 2000, 102(8 Suppl):I343-57.
Waisman Y, Klein BL, Boenning DA, et al, "Prospective Randomized Double-Blind Study Comparing L-Epinephrine and Racemic Epinephrine Aerosols in the Treatment of Laryngotracheitis (Croup)," *Pediatrics*, 1992, 89(2):302-6.

♦ **Epivir®** *see* Lamivudine *on page 650*

♦ **Epivir-HBV®** *see* Lamivudine *on page 650*

♦ **EPO** *see* Epoetin Alfa *on page 442*

Epoetin Alfa (e POE e tin AL fa)

U.S. Brand Names Epogen®; Procrit®

Canadian Brand Names Eprex®

Synonyms EPO; Erythropoietin; rHuEPO; *r*HuEPO-α

Therapeutic Category Colony-Stimulating Factor; Recombinant Human Erythropoietin

Generic Available No

Use Treatment of anemia associated with end-stage renal disease; anemia in cancer patients with nonmyeloid malignancies on chemotherapy; anemia related to AIDS and therapy with zidovudine-treated, HIV-infected patients; endogenous serum erythropoietin (EPO) levels which are inappropriately low for hemoglobin level (eg, anemia of neoplasia); anemia of prematurity; patients undergoing autologous blood donation prior to surgery (EPO may accelerate recovery of hemoglobin level and, in some cases, permit more units of blood to be donated)

Pregnancy Risk Factor C

Contraindications Hypersensitivity to epoetin alfa, albumin (human) or mammalian cell-derived products, or any component of epoetin alfa (see Warnings); uncontrolled hypertension; neutropenia in newborns

Warnings The multidose formulation contains benzyl alcohol which may cause allergic reactions in susceptible individuals; large amounts of benzyl alcohol (≥99 mg/kg/day) have been associated with a potentially fatal toxicity ("gasping syndrome") in neonates; the "gasping syndrome" consists of metabolic acidosis, respiratory distress, gasping respirations, CNS dysfunction (including convulsions, intracranial hemorrhage), hypotension and cardiovascular collapse; avoid use of multidose formulation in neonates; *in vitro* and animal studies have shown that benzoate, a metabolite of benzyl alcohol, displaces bilirubin from protein-binding sites. Pooled use of unused portions of preservative-free EPO has resulted in microbial contamination, bacteremia, and pyrogenic reactions. Preservative-free formulations are intended for single use only.

Precautions Use with caution in patients with porphyria or a history of seizures. Decrease the EPO dose if an increase in hematocrit exceeds 4 points in any 2-week period. EPO is not intended for patients who require acute corrections of anemia and is not a substitute for emergency blood transfusion.

Factors Limiting Response to Epoetin Alfa

Factor	Mechanism
Iron deficiency	Limits hemoglobin synthesis
Blood loss/hemolysis	Counteracts epoetin alfa-stimulated erythropoiesis
Infection/inflammation	Inhibits iron transfer from storage to bone marrow
	Suppresses erythropoiesis through activated macrophages
Aluminum overload	Inhibits iron incorporation into heme protein
Bone marrow replacement Hyperparathyroidism Metastatic, neoplastic disease	Limits bone marrow volume
Folic acid/vitamin B$_{12}$ deficiency	Limits hemoglobin synthesis
Patient compliance	Self-administered epoetin alfa or iron therapy

Assessment of iron stores and therapeutic iron supplementation is essential to optimal EPO therapy. Iron supplementation is necessary to provide for increased requirements during expansion of the red cell mass secondary to marrow stimulation by EPO, unless iron stores are already in excess.

Adverse Reactions

Cardiovascular: Hypertension, edema, chest pain, MI, CVA/TIA

Central nervous system: Fatigue, dizziness, headache, seizure, fever

Dermatologic: Rash, urticaria

Gastrointestinal: Nausea, diarrhea, vomiting

Hematologic: Neutropenia

Local: Pain, irritation at injection site (S.C. injection)

Neuromuscular & skeletal: Arthralgias, weakness

Respiratory: Cough

Miscellaneous: Hypersensitivity reactions

Stability Refrigerate; single-dose vials contain no preservatives; discard after entry (see Warnings). Multiple-dose vials contain benzyl alcohol preservative and are stable 2 weeks at room temperature and when refrigerated, may be used up to 21 days after initial entry. Prefilled syringes containing the preservative formulation are stable for 6 weeks refrigerated (2°C to 8°C) (Naughton, 2003). EPO is stable for 24 hours when diluted in dextrose I.V. fluid which contains at least 0.05% human albumin or parenteral nutrition solutions containing at least 0.5% amino acids. EPO may be diluted with NS or bacteriostatic NS in a 1:1 ratio at the time of S.C. administration.

Mechanism of Action Epoetin alfa, a glycoprotein manufactured by recombinant DNA technology, has the same effects as endogenous erythropoietin. EPO induces erythropoiesis by stimulating the division and differentiation of committed erythroid progenitor cells. It induces the release of reticulocytes from the bone marrow into the bloodstream, where they mature to erythrocytes (dose response relationship) resulting in an increase in reticulocyte counts followed by a rise in hematocrit and hemoglobin levels. There is normally an inverse correlation between the plasma EPO level and the hemoglobin concentration (only when the hemoglobin concentration is <10.5 g/dL).

Pharmacodynamics

Onset of action: Several days

Maximum effect: 2-6 weeks

Pharmacokinetics

Absorption: S.C.: 31.9%

Distribution: Adults: V_d: 9 L; rapid in the plasma compartment; majority of drug is taken up by the liver, kidneys, and bone marrow

Bioavailability: S.C.: ~21% to 31%

Half-life:

Neonates: S.C.: 17.6 hours on day 3 of therapy, 11.2 hours on day 10 of therapy

Adults: 4-13 hours in patients with chronic renal failure (CRF); half-life is 20% shorter in patients with normal renal function

Time to peak serum concentration: S.C.: 5-24 hours

Elimination: Some metabolic degradation does occur with small amounts recovered in the urine

Clearance: Neonates: S.C. or continuous I.V. infusion: 26-35 mL/hour/kg on day 3 of therapy and 65-87 mL/hour/kg on day 10 of therapy

Note: While a much higher peak plasma concentration is achieved after I.V. bolus administration, it declines at a more rapid rate (over 2-3 days) than after subcutaneous administration (plasma concentrations greater than endogenous are maintained for at least 4 days). Subcutaneous administration is associated with a 30% to 50% lower EPO dose requirement.

Usual Dosage Dosing schedules need to be individualized and careful monitoring of patients receiving the drug is recommended. EPO may be ineffective if other factors such as iron or B_{12}/folate deficiency limit marrow response. Dosage based upon S.C. administration; use of I.V. administration may result in the need to increase doses by as much as 30% to 50% to achieve the same outcome: I.V., S.C.:

Neonates: Anemia of prematurity: Variable regimens: 25-100 units/kg/dose 3 times/week **or** 100 units/kg/dose 5 times/week **or** 200 units/kg/dose every other day for 10 doses

Children and Adults:

Anemia in cancer patients: 150 units/kg/dose 3 times/week; maximum 1200 units/kg/week

Anemia in chronic renal failure: 50-150 units/kg/dose 3 times/week

Note: Once weekly dosage has been studied in chronic renal failure patients. When transitioning from multiple doses/week to once weekly, begin with a

Epoetin Alfa Dosage Adjustments

Target hematocrit range	30% to 33% (maximum 36%)
Reduce dose when	Target range is reached **or** hematocrit increases >4 points in any 2-week period
Increase dose when	Hematocrit does not increase by 5-6 points after 8 weeks of therapy **and** hematocrit is below target range
Stop therapy when	Hematocrit ≥40%; reinstate therapy at a lower dose after the hematocrit decreases to 36%
Maintenance dose (chronic renal failure)	Individualize: General dosage range: 25 units/kg 3 times/week

(Continued)

Epoetin Alfa (Continued)

weekly dosage equal to the current total dose per week. Allow at least 4 weeks to determine full effects of the new regimen.

Zidovudine-treated, HIV-infected patients: Initial: 100 units/kg/dose 3 times/week for 8 weeks; after 8 weeks of therapy the dose may be adjusted by 50-100 units/kg increments 3 times/week to a maximum dose of 300 units/kg 3 times/week

Presurgery, autologous blood donation: Adults: 300 units/kg/day for 10 days before surgery, the day of surgery, and 4 days after **or as an alternative**, 600 units/kg/week at 21-, 14-, and 7 days before surgery and on the day of surgery

Administration Parenteral: Do not shake as this may denature the glycoprotein rendering the drug biologically inactive

S.C. is the preferred route of administration; 1:1 dilution with bacteriostatic NS (containing benzyl alcohol) acts as a local anesthetic to reduce pain at the injection site. Multiple-dose vials already contain benzyl alcohol.

I.V.: Dilute with an equal volume of NS and infuse over 1-3 minutes; it may be administered into the venous line at the end of the dialysis procedure

Monitoring Parameters

Careful monitoring of blood pressure is indicated; problems with hypertension have been noted especially in renal failure patients treated with EPO. Other patients are less likely to develop this complication. See table.

Test	Initial Phase Frequency	Maintenance Phase Frequency
Hematocrit/hemoglobin	2 times/week	2-4 times/month
Blood pressure	3 times/week	3 times/week
Serum ferritin	Monthly	Quarterly
Transferrin saturation	Monthly	Quarterly
Serum chemistries including CBC with differential, creatinine, BUN, potassium, phosphorous	Regularly per routine	Regularly per routine
Reticulocyte count	Baseline prior to starting therapy	After 10 days of therapy

Hematocrit should be determined twice weekly until stabilization within the target range (30% to 36%), and twice weekly for at least 2-6 weeks after a dose increase.

Reference Range The decision to initiate EPO therapy may be made by utilizing an endogenous erythropoietin serum level measurement. Endogenous erythropoietin levels are inversely related to the hemoglobin (and hematocrit) level in anemias that are not attributed to impaired erythropoietin production (eg, iron deficiency anemia). A normal erythropoietin level, for subjects with normal hemoglobin and hematocrit, is 4.1-22.2 mIU/mL. Baseline erythropoietin levels in anemic patients may increase up to 100-1000 fold in untreated patients with a normal release of erythropoietin. The following table illustrates the "normal" response to anemia. EPO is indicated in patients who do not exhibit a normal response to anemia (eg, the measurement of endogenous erythropoietin is low relative to a normal response). If the patient has exhibited a normal response, addition of exogenous EPO may not be beneficial. Clinical studies involving the following disease states have established criteria for assessment of endogenous erythropoietin levels prior to initiating EPO therapy:

Zidovudine-treated HIV patients: Available evidence indicates patients with endogenous serum erythropoietin levels >500 mIU/mL are unlikely to respond

Cancer chemotherapy patients: Treatment of patients with endogenous serum erythropoietin levels >200 mIU/mL is not recommended.

Patient Information Frequent blood tests are needed to determine the correct dose; notify physician if any severe headache develops; due to increased risk of seizure activity in CRF patients during the first 90 days of therapy, avoid potentially hazardous activities (eg, driving during this period)

Additional Information Optimal response is achieved when iron stores are maintained with supplemental iron if necessary; evaluate iron stores prior to and during therapy

Reimbursement Hotline (Epogen®): 1-800-272-9376
Professional Services [Amgen]: 1-800-77-AMGEN
Reimbursement Hotline (Procrit®): 1-800-553-3851
Professional Services [Ortho Biotech]: 1-800-325-7504

Dosage Forms

Injection, solution [preservative free]: 2000 units/mL (1 mL); 3000 units/mL (1 mL); 4000 units/mL (1 mL); 10,000 units/mL (1 mL); 40,000 units/mL (1 mL) [contains human albumin]

Injection, solution [with preservative]: 10,000 units/mL (2 mL); 20,000 units/mL (1 mL) [contains benzyl alcohol and human albumin]

Inverse Relationship of Endogenous Erythropoietin to Hemoglobin

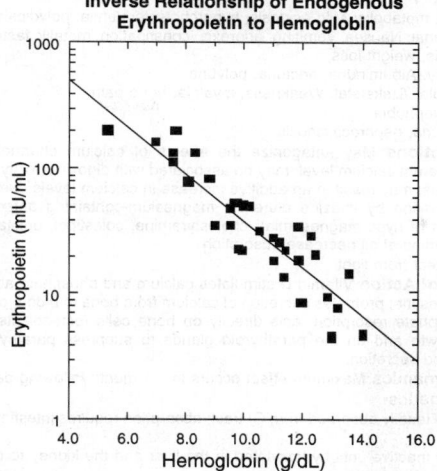

References

Blanche S, Caniglia M, Fischer A, et al, "Zidovudine Therapy in Children With Acquired Immunodeficiency Syndrome," *Am J Med*, 1988, 85(2A):203-7.

Halperin DS, Wacker P, Lacourt G, et al, "Effects of Recombinant Human Erythropoietin in Infants With the Anemia of Prematurity: A Pilot Study," *J Pediatr*, 1990, 116(5):779-86.

Naughton CA, Duppong LM, Forbes KD, et al, "Stability of Multidose, Preserved Formulation Epoetin Alfa in Syringes for Three and Six Weeks," *Am J Health Syst Pharm*, 2003, 60(5):464-8.

Ohls RK and Christensen, RD, "Stability of Human Recombinant Epoetin Alfa in Commonly Used Neonatal Intravenous Solutions," *Ann Pharmacother*, 1996, 30(5):466-468.

Ohls RK, Veerman MW, and Christensen RD, "Pharmacokinetics and Effectiveness of Recombinant Erythropoietin Administered to Preterm Infants by Continuous Infusion in Total Parenteral Nutrition Solution," *J Pediatr*, 1996, 128(4):518-23.

Rhondeau SM, Christensen RD, Ross MP, et al, "Responsiveness to Recombinant Human Erythropoietin of Marrow Erythroid Progenitors From Infants With the Anemia of Prematurity," *J Pediatr*, 1988, 112(6):935-40.

Shannon KM, Keith JF 3rd, Mentzer WC, et al, "Recombinant Human Erythropoietin Stimulates Erythropoiesis and Reduces Erythrocyte Transfusions in Very Low Birth Weight Preterm Infants," *Pediatrics*, 1995, 95(1):1-8.

Sinai-Trieman L, Salusky IB, and Fine RN, "Use of Subcutaneous Recombinant Human Erythropoietin in Children Undergoing Continuous Cycling Peritoneal Dialysis," *J Pediatr*, 1989, 114(4 Pt 1):550-4.

♦ **Epogen®** *see* Epoetin Alfa *on page 442*

♦ **Eprex® (Can)** *see* Epoetin Alfa *on page 442*

♦ **Epsom Salts (Magnesium Sulfate)** *see* Magnesium Supplements *on page 701*

Ergocalciferol (er goe kal SIF e role)

U.S. Brand Names Calciferol™; Drisdol®

Canadian Brand Names Ostoforte®

Synonyms Activated Ergosterol; Viosterol; Vitamin D_2

Therapeutic Category Nutritional Supplement; Vitamin D Analog; Vitamin, Fat Soluble

Generic Available Yes

Use Refractory rickets; hypophosphatemia; hypoparathyroidism

Pregnancy Risk Factor A (C if dose exceeds RDA recommendation)

Contraindications Hypersensitivity to ergocalciferol or any component (see Warnings); hypercalcemia; malabsorption syndrome; evidence of vitamin D toxicity

Warnings Some products contain tartrazine which may cause allergic reactions in susceptible individuals

Precautions Use with caution in patients with coronary artery disease, renal stones, and impaired renal function; adequate calcium intake is necessary for clinical response to ergocalciferol therapy; maintain adequate fluid intake; avoid hypercalcemia

Adverse Reactions

Cardiovascular: Hypertension, arrhythmias, hypotension
(Continued)

Ergocalciferol *(Continued)*

Central nervous system: Drowsiness, irritability, headache, psychosis

Dermatologic: Pruritus

Endocrine & metabolic: Mild acidosis, hypercholesterolemia, polydipsia

Gastrointestinal: Nausea, vomiting, anorexia, constipation, metallic taste, xerostomia, pancreatitis, weight loss

Genitourinary: Albuminuria, nocturia, polyuria

Neuromuscular & skeletal: Weakness, myalgia, bone pain

Ocular: Photophobia

Renal: Polyuria, nephrocalcinosis

Drug Interactions May antagonize the effects of calcium channel blockers by increasing serum calcium level; may be associated with digoxin toxicity by increasing calcium levels; may result in an additive increase in calcium levels due to decreased calcium excretion by thiazide diuretics; magnesium-containing antacids (potential development of hypermagnesemia); cholestyramine, colestipol, orlistat, and excessive use of mineral oil decrease absorption

Stability Protect from light

Mechanism of Action Vitamin D stimulates calcium and phosphate absorption from the small intestine; promotes secretion of calcium from bone to blood; promotes renal tubule phosphate resorption; acts directly on bone cells (osteoblasts) to stimulate skeletal growth and on the parathyroid glands to suppress parathyroid hormone synthesis and secretion

Pharmacodynamics Maximum effect occurs in ~1 month following daily doses

Pharmacokinetics

Absorption: Readily absorbed from GI tract; absorption requires intestinal presence of bile

Metabolism: Inactive until hydroxylated in the liver and the kidney to calcifediol and then to calcitriol (most active form)

Usual Dosage Oral dosing is preferred; use I.M. only in patients with GI, liver, or biliary disease associated with malabsorption of vitamin D:

Adequate Intake (AI) (1997 National Academy of Science Recommendations):
Neonates, Children and Adults: 200 international units/day

Dietary supplementation (each mcg = 40 USP units):
Premature infants: 10-20 mcg/day (400-800 units), up to 750 mcg/day (30,000 units)
Infants and healthy Children: 10 mcg/day (400 units)
Adults: 10 mcg/day (400 units)

Renal failure:
Children: 100-1000 mcg/day (4000-40,000 units)
Adults: 500 mcg/day (20,000 units)

Hypoparathyroidism:
Children: 1.25-5 mg/day (50,000-200,000 units) with calcium supplements
Adults: 625 mcg to 5 mg/day (25,000-200,000 units) with calcium supplements

Vitamin D-dependent rickets:
Children: 75-125 mcg/day (3000-5000 units); maximum dose: 1500 mcg/day
Adults: 250 mcg to 1.5 mg/day (10,000-60,000 units)

Nutritional rickets and osteomalacia:
Children and Adults (with normal absorption): 25-125 mcg/day (1000-5000 units) for 6-12 weeks
Children with malabsorption: 250-625 mcg/day (10,000-25,000 units)
Adults with malabsorption: 250-7500 mcg/day (10,000-300,000 units)

Vitamin D-resistant rickets:
Children: Initial: 1000-2000 mcg/day (40,000-80,000 units) with phosphate supplements; daily dosage is increased at 3- to 4-month intervals in 250-500 mcg (10,000-20,000 units) increments
Adults: 250-1500 mcg/day (10,000-60,000 units) with phosphate supplements

Administration

Oral: May be administered without regard to meals; for oral liquid, use accompanying dropper for dosage measurements

Parenteral: Injection for I.M. use only

Monitoring Parameters Serum calcium and phosphorus levels; alkaline phosphatase, BUN; bone x-ray (hypophosphatemia or hypoparathyroidism)

Reference Range Serum calcium times serum phosphorus should not exceed 70 mg/dL to avoid ectopic calcification; ergocalciferol levels: 10-60 ng/mL

Patient Information May cause dry mouth

Additional Information 1.25 mg ergocalciferol provides 50,000 units of vitamin D activity; 1 drop of 8000 units/mL = 200 units (40 drops = 1 mL)

Dosage Forms
Capsule (Drisdol®): 50,000 units [1.25 mg; contains soybean oil and tartrazine]

Injection, solution (Calciferol™): 500,000 units/mL [12.5 mg/mL] (1 mL) [contains sesame oil]

Liquid, **drops** (Calciferol™, Drisdol®): 8000 units/mL [200 mcg/mL] (60 mL) [OTC]

References
"Dietary Reference Intakes for Calcium, Phosphorus, Magnesium, Vitamin D, and Fluoride. Standing Committee on the Scientific Evaluation of Dietary Reference Intakes, Food and Nutrition Board, Institute of Medicine," National Academy of Sciences, Washington, DC: National Academy Press, 1997.

♦ **Ergomar®** *see* Ergotamine *on page 447*

Ergotamine (er GOT a meen)
Related Information
Drugs and Breast-Feeding *on page 1404*
Overdose and Toxicology *on page 1388*
U.S. Brand Names Cafergot®; Ergomar®; Wigraine®
Canadian Brand Names Cafergot®
Synonyms Ergotamine and Caffeine
Therapeutic Category Alpha-Adrenergic Blocking Agent, Oral; Antimigraine Agent; Ergot Alkaloid and Derivative
Generic Available Yes
Use Prevent or abort vascular headaches, such as migraine or cluster
Pregnancy Risk Factor X
Contraindications Hypersensitivity to ergotamine, caffeine, or any component; pregnancy; peripheral vascular disease, hepatic or renal disease, hypertension, peptic ulcer disease, sepsis, coronary heart disease; concurrent therapy with protease inhibitors (indinavir, ritonavir, saquinavir, nelfinavir, amprenavir, lopinavir/ritonavir), efavirenz, or delavirdine (see Drug Interactions)
Warnings Patients who take ergotamine for extended periods of time may become dependent on it; long-term use is also associated with fibrotic changes to heart and pulmonary valves; chronic usage may be harmful due to reduction in cerebral blood flow; concomitant use with protease inhibitors and macrolide antibiotics has been associated with serious and/or life-threatening cerebral and peripheral ischemia; some cases have resulted in amputation (see Contraindications); may precipitate angina, MI, or aggravate intermittent claudication
Precautions Avoid prolonged administration or excessive dosage because of the danger of ergotism and gangrene
Adverse Reactions
Cardiovascular: Angina-like precordial pain, transient tachycardia or bradycardia, vasospasm, vasoconstriction, claudication; fibrotic thickening of the aortic, pulmonary, mitral, and/or tricupsid valves (rare after long-term use)

Central nervous system: Rebound headaches (with abrupt withdrawal), drowsiness, dizziness

Dermatologic: Pruritus

Gastrointestinal: Nausea, vomiting, diarrhea, xerostomia, retroperitoneal fibrosis (rare)

Local: Edema

Neuromuscular & skeletal: Leg cramps, myalgia, weakness, paresthesia of the extremities

Respiratory: Pleuropulmonary fibrosis (rare)
Drug Interactions Cytochrome P450 isoenzyme CYP3A4 substrate
Serious and/or life-threatening peripheral ischemia with potent CYP3A4 inhibitors, including protease inhibitors and macrolide antibiotics (see Contraindications) due to increased blood levels of ergotamine; delavirdine and efavirenz also increase ergotamine plasma concentrations resulting in life-threatening toxicities; enhanced vasoconstriction with beta-blocking agents; increased vasoconstrictor effects with methysergide
Food Interactions Caffeine may increase GI absorption of ergotamine
Mechanism of Action Ergot alkaloid alpha-adrenergic blocker directly stimulates vascular smooth muscle to vasoconstrict peripheral and cerebral vessels; may also have antagonist effects on serotonin
Pharmacokinetics
Absorption: Oral, rectal: Erratic; absorption is enhanced by caffeine coadministration

Metabolism: Extensive in the liver

Bioavailability: Poor overall (<5%)

Time to peak serum concentration: Oral: Within 0.5-3 hours

Elimination: In bile as metabolites (90%)

(Continued)

Ergotamine *(Continued)*

Usual Dosage Note: Not for chronic daily administration

Older Children and Adolescents: Oral, S.L.: 1 mg at onset of attack; then 1 mg every 30 minutes as needed, up to a maximum of 3 mg per attack

Adults:

Oral:

Cafergot®: 2 mg at onset of attack; then 1-2 mg every 30 minutes as needed; maximum dose: 6 mg per attack; do not exceed 10 mg/week

Ergomar®: 1 tablet under tongue at first sign, then 1 tablet every 30 minutes; maximum: 3 tablets/24 hours, 5 tablets/week

Rectal, suppositories (Cafergot®, Wigraine®, Cafatine®): 1 suppository at first sign of an attack; follow with second dose after 1 hour, if needed; maximum dose: 2 per attack; do not exceed 5/week

Administration Place sublingual tablets under tongue; oral tablets may be taken without regard to meals

Patient Information Any symptoms such as nausea, vomiting, numbness or tingling, and chest, muscle, or abdominal pain should be reported to the physician at the first sign of an attack; do **not** exceed recommended dosage; avoid coffee, tea, and cola; may cause dry mouth

Dosage Forms

Suppository, rectal (Cafergot®): Ergotamine tartrate 2 mg and caffeine 100 mg (12s)

Tablet (Cafergot®, Wigraine®): Ergotamine tartrate 1 mg and caffeine 100 mg

Tablet, sublingual (Ergomar®): Ergotamine tartrate 2 mg

♦ **Ergotamine and Caffeine** *see* Ergotamine *on page 447*

♦ **E•R•O [OTC]** *see* Carbamide Peroxide *on page 212*

♦ **Erybid™ (Can)** *see* Erythromycin *on page 448*

♦ **Eryc®** *see* Erythromycin *on page 448*

♦ **Erycette®** *see* Erythromycin *on page 448*

♦ **EryDerm®** *see* Erythromycin *on page 448*

♦ **Erygel®** *see* Erythromycin *on page 448*

♦ **Ery-Ped®** *see* Erythromycin *on page 448*

♦ **Ery-Tab®** *see* Erythromycin *on page 448*

♦ **Erythra-Derm™** *see* Erythromycin *on page 448*

♦ **Erythrocin®** *see* Erythromycin *on page 448*

♦ **Erythromid® (Can)** *see* Erythromycin *on page 448*

Erythromycin *(er ith roe MYE sin)*

Related Information

Carbohydrate and Alcohol Content of Liquid Medications for Use in Patients Receiving Ketogenic Diets *on page 1431*

U.S. Brand Names Akne-Mycin®; A/T/S®; E.E.S.®; Emgel®; Eryc®; Erycette®; EryDerm®; Erygel®; Ery-Ped®; Ery-Tab®; Erythra-Derm™; Erythrocin®; PCE®; Staticin™; Theramycin™ Z; T-Stat®

Canadian Brand Names Apo®-Erythro Base; Apo®-Erythro E-C; Apo®-Erythro-ES; Apo®-Erythro-S; Diomycin®; Erybid™; Erythromid®; Nu-Erythromycin-S; PMS-Erythromycin

Synonyms Erythromycin Base

Therapeutic Category Antibiotic, Macrolide; Antibiotic, Ophthalmic

Generic Available Yes

Use Treatment of mild to moderately severe infections of the upper and lower respiratory tract, pharyngitis and skin infections due to susceptible streptococci and staphylococci; other susceptible bacterial infections including *Mycoplasma pneumoniae*, *Legionella* pneumonia, Lyme disease, diphtheria, pertussis, chancroid, *Chlamydia*, and *Campylobacter* gastroenteritis; used in conjunction with neomycin for decontaminating the bowel for surgery; ophthalmic ointment used to prevent gonococcal ophthalmia neonatorum

Pregnancy Risk Factor B

Contraindications Hypersensitivity to erythromycin or any component (see Warnings); hepatic impairment; concomitant administration with astemizole, terfenadine, or cisapride

Warnings Hepatic impairment with or without jaundice has occurred primarily in older children and adults; it may be accompanied by malaise, nausea, vomiting, abdominal colic, and fever; discontinue use if these occur; risk of serious cardiac arrhythmias exist in patients receiving erythromycin and astemizole, terfenadine, or cisapride (do not use concurrently with erythromycin)

Erythromycin lactobionate injection contains benzyl alcohol which may cause allergic reactions in susceptible individuals; large amounts of benzyl alcohol (≥99 mg/kg/day) have been associated with a potentially fatal toxicity ("gasping syndrome") in neonates; the "gasping syndrome" consists of metabolic acidosis, respiratory distress, gasping respirations, CNS dysfunction (including convulsions, intracranial hemorrhage), hypotension and cardiovascular collapse; use erythromycin lactobionate injection products containing benzyl alcohol with caution in neonates; *in vitro* and animal studies have shown that benzoate, a metabolite of benzyl alcohol, displaces bilirubin from protein binding sites

Adverse Reactions

Cardiovascular: Ventricular arrhythmias, prolongation of the QT interval; bradycardia, hypotension with I.V. administration

Central nervous system: Fever, dizziness

Dermatologic: Skin rash, pruritus

Gastrointestinal: Abdominal pain, cramping, nausea, vomiting, diarrhea, stomatitis

Hematologic: Eosinophilia

Hepatic: Cholestatic hepatitis, jaundice; (incidence of erythromycin-associated hepatotoxicity is ~0.1% in children and 0.25% in adults)

Local: Thrombophlebitis (I.V. form)

Otic: Ototoxicity (after I.V. use)

Miscellaneous: Allergic reactions, anaphylaxis

Drug Interactions
Cytochrome P450 isoenzyme CYP3A3/4 substrate; isoenzyme CYP1A2 and CYP3A3/4 inhibitor

Erythromycin decreases clearance of astemizole, terfenadine, carbamazepine, cisapride, cyclosporine, protease inhibitors, lovastatin, simvastatin, midazolam, phenytoin, alfentanil, and triazolam; erythromycin may decrease theophylline clearance, increase theophylline's half-life by up to 60%, and result in theophylline toxicity (patients on high dose theophylline and erythromycin or who have received erythromycin for >5 days may be at higher risk); may potentiate anticoagulant effect of warfarin; may increase toxicity of ergotamine; may increase serum levels of digoxin, disopyramide, and quinidine

Stability
Erythromycin lactobionate should be reconstituted with SWI without preservatives to avoid gel formation; the reconstituted solution is stable for 2 weeks when refrigerated or 24 hours at room temperature. Erythromycin I.V. infusion solution is stable at pH 6-8.

Mechanism of Action
Inhibits bacterial RNA-dependent protein synthesis at the chain elongation step; binds to the 50S ribosomal subunit resulting in blockage of transpeptidation

Pharmacokinetics

Absorption: Variable but better with salt forms like the estolate than with base form; 18% to 45% absorbed orally; ethylsuccinate may be better absorbed with food

Distribution: Crosses the placenta; distributes into body tissues, fluids, and breast milk with poor penetration into the CSF

V_d: 0.64 L/kg

Protein binding: 75% to 90%

Metabolism: In the liver by demethylation

Half-life:

Neonates (≤15 days of age): 2.1 hours

Adults: 1.5-2 hours

Time to peak serum concentration: Oral:

Base: 4 hours

Stearate: 3 hours

Ethylsuccinate: 0.5-2.5 hours

Estolate: 2-4 hours (time to peak is delayed in the presence of food except when using estolate)

Elimination: 2% to 5% unchanged drug excreted in urine, major excretion in feces (via bile)

Dialysis: Not removed by peritoneal dialysis or hemodialysis

Usual Dosage

Neonates:

Oral: Ethylsuccinate: Postnatal age:

≤7 days: 20 mg/kg/day in divided doses every 12 hours

>7 days, <1200 g: 20 mg/kg/day in divided doses every 12 hours

>7 days, 1200-2000 g: 30 mg/kg/day in divided doses every 8 hours

>7 days, >2000 g: 30-40 mg/kg/day in divided doses every 6-8 hours

Ophthalmic: Prophylaxis of neonatal gonococcal ophthalmia: 0.5-1 cm ribbon of ointment should be instilled into each conjunctival sac once

I.V.: One study (n=14, ≤15 days of age, birth weight ≤1500 g) used erythromycin lactobionate in doses of 25 or 40 mg/kg/day divided every 6 hours for treatment of *Ureaplasma urealyticum* infection

(Continued)

Erythromycin *(Continued)*

Chlamydial conjunctivitis and pneumonia: Oral: Ethylsuccinate: 50 mg/kg/day divided every 6 hours for 14 days

Infants and Children:

Oral:

Base and ethylsuccinate: 30-50 mg/kg/day divided every 6-8 hours; do not exceed 2 g/day (as base) or 3.2 g/day (as ethylsuccinate); (**Note:** Due to differences in absorption, 200 mg erythromycin ethylsuccinate produces the same serum levels as 125 mg erythromycin base or estolate)

Estolate: 30-50 mg/kg/day divided every 6-12 hours; do not exceed 2 g/day

Stearate: 30-50 mg/kg/day divided every 6 hours; do not exceed 2 g/day

Chlamydia trachomatis: Oral: 50 mg/kg/day divided every 6 hours for 10-14 days

Pertussis: Oral: 40-50 mg/kg/day divided every 6 hours for 14 days (some experts recommend using the estolate salt)

Preop bowel preparation: Oral: 20 mg/kg erythromycin base at 1, 2, and 11 PM on the day before surgery combined with mechanical cleansing of the large intestine and oral neomycin

I.V.:

Lactobionate: 15-50 mg/kg/day divided every 6 hours, not to exceed 4 g/day

Gluceptate: 15-50 mg/kg/day divided every 6 hours, not to exceed 4 g/day

Children and Adults:

Ophthalmic: Instill ointment one or more times daily depending on the severity of the infection

Topical: Apply 2% solution over the affected area twice daily after the skin has been thoroughly washed and patted dry

Adults:

Oral:

Base, delayed release: 333 mg every 8 hours

Estolate, stearate or base: 250-500 mg every 6-12 hours

Ethylsuccinate: 400-800 mg every 6-12 hours

Chancroid: Oral: Base: 500 mg 4 times/day for 7 days

Chlamydia trachomatis: Oral:

Base: 500 mg 4 times/day for 7 days **or**

Ethylsuccinate: 800 mg 4 times/day for 7 days

Preop bowel preparation: Oral: 1 g erythromycin base at 1, 2, and 11 PM on the day before surgery combined with mechanical cleansing of the large intestine and oral neomycin

I.V.: Lactobionate or gluceptate: 15-20 mg/kg/day divided every 6 hours or given as a continuous infusion over 24 hours, not to exceed 4 g/day

Prokinetic agent (to improve gastric emptying time and intestinal motility):

Children: Lactobionate or gluceptate: Initial: 3 mg/kg I.V. infused over 60 minutes followed by 20 mg/kg/day orally in 3-4 divided doses before meals, or before meals and at bedtime

Adults: Lactobionate or gluceptate: Initial: 200 mg I.V. followed by 250 mg orally 3 times/day 30 minutes before meals

Administration

Ophthalmic ointment for prevention of neonatal ophthalmia: Wipe each eyelid gently with sterile cotton; instill 0.5-1 cm ribbon of ointment in each lower conjunctival sac; massage eyelids gently to spread the ointment; after 1 minute, excess ointment can be wiped away with sterile cotton

Oral: Avoid milk and acidic beverages 1 hour before or after a dose; administer after food to decrease GI discomfort; ethylsuccinate chewable tablets should not be swallowed whole; do not chew or break delayed release capsule or enteric coated tablets, swallow whole

Parenteral: Administer by I.V. intermittent or continuous infusion diluted in either dextrose or saline solutions to a concentration of 1-2.5 mg/mL; maximum concentration: 5 mg/mL; I.V. intermittent infusions may be administered over 20-60 minutes; to decrease vein irritation, administer as a continuous infusion at a concentration ≤1 mg/mL; prolonging the infusion duration over 60 minutes or longer has been recommended to decrease the cardiotoxic effects of erythromycin

Monitoring Parameters Liver function tests; with I.V. use: Blood pressure, heart rate

Test Interactions False-positive urinary catecholamines, 17-hydroxycorticosteroids and 17-ketosteroids

Nursing Implications Do not crush enteric coated or delayed release drug products

Additional Information Treatment of erythromycin-associated cardiac toxicity with prolongation of the QT interval and ventricular tachydysrhythmias includes discontinuing erythromycin and administering magnesium.

Dosage Forms

Capsule, delayed release, enteric coated pellets, as **base** (Eryc®): 250 mg

Gel, topical, as **base**: 2% (30 g, 60 g)
  A/T/S®: 2% (30 g)
  Emgel®: 2% (27 g, 50 g)
  Erygel®: 2% (30 g, 60 g)
Granules for oral suspension, as **ethylsuccinate** (E.E.S.®): 200 mg/5 mL (100 mL, 200 mL) [cherry flavor]
Injection, powder for reconstitution, as **lactobionate** (Erythrocin®): 500 mg, 1 g [may contain benzyl alcohol]
Ointment, ophthalmic, as **base**: 5 mg/g (1 g, 3.5 g)
Ointment, topical, as **base** (Akne-Mycin®): 2% (25 g)
Powder for oral drops suspension, as **ethylsuccinate** (Ery-Ped®): 100 mg/2.5 mL (50 mL) [fruit flavor]
Powder for oral suspension, as **ethylsuccinate** (Ery-Ped®): 200 mg/5 mL (5 mL, 100 mL, 200 mL) [fruit flavor]; 400 mg/5 mL (5 mL, 60 mL, 100 mL, 200 mL) [banana flavor]
Solution, topical, as **base**: 1.5% (60 mL); 2% (60 mL)
  A/T/S®, EryDerm®, Erythra-Derm™, Theramycin™ Z, T-Stat®: 2% (60 mL)
  Staticin®: 1.5% (60 mL)
Suspension, oral, as **estolate**: 125 mg/5 mL (480 mL); 250 mg/5 mL (480 mL) [orange flavor]
Suspension, oral, as **ethylsuccinate**: 200 mg/5 mL (480 mL); 400 mg/5 mL (480 mL)
  E.E.S.®: 200 mg/5 mL (100 mL, 480 mL) [fruit flavor]; 400 mg/5 mL (100 mL, 480 mL) [orange flavor]
Swab, topical, as **base** (Erycette®, T-Stat®): 2% (60s)
Tablet, chewable, as **ethylsuccinate** (Ery-Ped®): 200 mg [fruit flavor]
Tablet, delayed release, enteric coated, as **base** (Ery-Tab®): 250 mg, 333 mg, 500 mg
Tablet, film coated, as **base**: 250 mg, 500 mg
Tablet, film coated, as **ethylsuccinate** (E.E.S.®): 400 mg
Tablet, film coated, as **stearate** (Erythrocin®): 250 mg, 500 mg
Tablet, polymer coated particles, as **base** (PCE®): 333 mg, 500 mg

References
Di Lorenzo C, Lachman R, and Hyman PE, "Intravenous Erythromycin for Postpyloric Intubation," *J Pediatr Gastroenterol Nutr*, 1990, 11(1):45-7.
Janssens J, Peeters TL, Vantrappen G, et al, "Improvement of Gastric Emptying in Diabetic Gastroparesis by Erythromycin," *N Engl J Med*, 1990, 322(15):1028-31.
Reid B, DiLorenzo C, Travis L, et al, "Diabetic Gastroparesis Due to Postprandial Antral Hypomotility in Childhood," *Pediatrics*, 1992, 90(1 Pt 1):43-6.
Thoene DE and Johnson CE, "Pharmacotherapy of Otitis Media," *Pharmacotherapy*, 1991, 11(3):212-21.
Waites KB, Sims PJ, Crouse DT, et al, "Serum Concentrations of Erythromycin After Intravenous Infusion in Preterm Neonates Treated for *Ureaplasma urealyticum* Infection," *Pediatr Infect Dis J*, 1994, 13(4):287-93.

Erythromycin and Sulfisoxazole
  (er ith roe MYE sin & sul fi SOKS a zole)

Related Information
  Carbohydrate and Alcohol Content of Liquid Medications for Use in Patients Receiving Ketogenic Diets *on page 1431*

U.S. Brand Names Eryzole®; Pediazole®

Synonyms Sulfisoxazole and Erythromycin

Therapeutic Category Antibiotic, Macrolide; Antibiotic, Sulfonamide Derivative

Generic Available Yes

Use Treatment of susceptible bacterial infections of the upper and lower respiratory tract; otitis media in children caused by susceptible strains of *Haemophilus influenzae*; other infections in patients allergic to penicillin

Pregnancy Risk Factor C

Contraindications Hypersensitivity to erythromycin, any component, or sulfonamides; hepatic dysfunction; infants <2 months of age (sulfas compete with bilirubin for binding sites which may result in kernicterus in newborns); patients with porphyria; pregnant women at term; mothers nursing infants <2 months of age; concomitant administration of astemizole, terfenadine, or cisapride

Warnings Risk of serious cardiac arrhythmias exist in patients receiving erythromycin, astemizole, terfenadine, or cisapride (do not use concurrently); fatalities due to Stevens-Johnson syndrome, toxic epidermal necrolysis, fulminant hepatic necrosis, agranulocytosis, and aplastic anemia have occurred with the administration of sulfonamides; prolonged use may result in superinfection or pseudomembranous colitis

Precautions Use with caution in patients with impaired renal or hepatic function, G-6-PD deficiency (hemolysis may occur)

Adverse Reactions
  Cardiovascular: Tachycardia, palpitations, syncope
  Central nervous system: Headache, disorientation, fever, dizziness
  (Continued)

Erythromycin and Sulfisoxazole *(Continued)*

Dermatologic: Rash, photosensitivity, Stevens-Johnson syndrome, toxic epidermal necrolysis, pruritus, urticaria

Gastrointestinal: Abdominal cramping, nausea, vomiting, diarrhea, pseudomembranous colitis, anorexia, stomatitis, pancreatitis

Genitourinary: Crystalluria, hematuria

Hematologic: Agranulocytosis, aplastic anemia, leukopenia, eosinophilia, thrombocytopenia

Hepatic: Hepatic necrosis, jaundice

Renal: Toxic nephrosis, elevated BUN and serum creatinine, acute renal failure

Respiratory: Cough, shortness of breath, pulmonary infiltrates

Miscellaneous: Anaphylaxis

Drug Interactions Erythromycin is a cytochrome P450 isoenzyme CYP3A3/4 substrate; isoenzyme CYP1A2 and CYP3A3/4 inhibitor

Erythromycin decreases clearance of astemizole, terfenadine, carbamazepine, cisapride, cyclosporine, protease inhibitors, lovastatin, simvastatin, midazolam, phenytoin, alfentanil, and triazolam; erythromycin may decrease theophylline clearance, increase theophylline's half-life by up to 60%, and result in theophylline toxicity (patients on high dose theophylline and erythromycin or who have received erythromycin for >5 days may be at higher risk); may potentiate anticoagulant effect of warfarin; may increase toxicity of ergotamine; may increase serum levels of digoxin, disopyramide, and quinidine

Sulfisoxazole may decrease the amount of thiopental needed for anesthesia; sulfisoxazole may displace methotrexate from plasma protein-binding sites increasing free methotrexate concentrations; displaces tolbutamide, chlorpropamide, oral anticoagulants from protein binding sites; PABA (antagonizes the antibacterial activity of sulfas)

Stability Reconstituted suspension is stable for 14 days when refrigerated

Mechanism of Action Erythromycin inhibits bacterial protein synthesis by binding to the 50S ribosomal subunit; sulfisoxazole competitively inhibits bacterial synthesis of folic acid from para-aminobenzoic acid

Pharmacokinetics

Erythromycin ethylsuccinate:

Absorption: Well absorbed from the GI tract

Distribution: Widely distributed into most body tissues and fluids; poor penetration into CSF; crosses the placenta; excreted in breast milk

Protein binding: 75% to 90%

Metabolism: In the liver by demethylation

Half-life: 1-1.5 hours

Elimination: Unchanged drug is excreted and concentrated in bile; <5% of dose eliminated in urine

Dialysis: Not removed by peritoneal dialysis or hemodialysis

Sulfisoxazole acetyl:

Absorption: Hydrolyzed in the GI tract to sulfisoxazole which is rapidly and completely absorbed; the small intestine is the major site of absorption

Distribution: Into extracellular space; CSF concentration ranges from 8% to 57% of blood concentration in patients with normal meninges; crosses the placenta; excreted in breast milk

Protein binding: 85%

Metabolism: Undergoes N-acetylation and N-glucuronide conjugation in the liver

Half-life: 4.6-7.8 hours, prolonged in renal impairment

Elimination: 50% in urine as unchanged drug

Dialysis: >50% removed by hemodialysis

Usual Dosage Oral (dosage recommendation is based on the product's erythromycin content):

Children ≥2 months: 40-50 mg/kg/day in divided doses every 6-8 hours; not to exceed 2 g erythromycin or 6 g sulfisoxazole/day

Adults: 400 mg erythromycin and 1200 mg sulfisoxazole every 6 hours

Administration Oral: Administer with or without food; shake suspension well before use; maintain adequate fluid intake to prevent crystalluria and kidney stone formation

Monitoring Parameters CBC with differential and platelet count, urinalysis; periodic liver function and renal function tests; observe patient for diarrhea

Test Interactions False-positive urinary protein; false-positive urinary catecholamines, 17-hydroxycorticosteroids and 17-ketosteroids

Patient Information May cause photosensitivity reactions (eg, exposure to sunlight may cause severe sunburn, skin rash, redness, or itching); avoid exposure to sunlight and artificial light sources (sunlamps, tanning booth/bed); wear protective clothing, wide-brimmed hats, sunglasses, and lip sunscreen (SPF ≥15); use a sunscreen [broad-spectrum sunscreen or physical sunscreen (preferred) or sunblock with SPF ≥15]; contact physician if reaction occurs.

Dosage Forms Suspension, oral: Erythromycin ethylsuccinate 200 mg and sulfisoxazole acetyl 600 mg per 5 mL (100 mL, 150 mL, 200 mL) [strawberry-banana flavor]

References
Rodriguez WJ, Schwartz RH, Sait T, et al, "Erythromycin-Sulfisoxazole vs Amoxicillin in the Treatment of Acute Otitis Media in Children," *Am J Dis Child*, 1985, 139(8):766-70.

♦ **Erythromycin Base** *see* Erythromycin *on page 448*

♦ **Erythropoietin** *see* Epoetin Alfa *on page 442*

♦ **Eryzole®** *see* Erythromycin and Sulfisoxazole *on page 451*

♦ **Esclim®** *see* Estradiol *on page 456*

♦ **Eserine** *see* Physostigmine *on page 901*

♦ **Eskalith®** *see* Lithium *on page 684*

♦ **Eskalith CR®** *see* Lithium *on page 684*

Esmolol (ES moe lol)

Related Information
Overdose and Toxicology *on page 1388*

U.S. Brand Names Brevibloc®

Therapeutic Category Antiarrhythmic Agent, Class II; Antihypertensive Agent; Beta-Adrenergic Blocker

Generic Available No

Use Supraventricular tachycardia (primarily to control ventricular rate) and hypertension (especially perioperatively)

Pregnancy Risk Factor C

Contraindications Hypersensitivity to esmolol, any component, or other beta-blockers; sinus bradycardia or heart block, uncompensated CHF, cardiogenic shock

Warnings Caution should be exercised when discontinuing esmolol infusions to avoid withdrawal effects

Precautions Use with extreme caution in patients with hyper-reactive airway disease; use lowest dose possible and discontinue infusion if bronchospasm occurs; use with caution in diabetes mellitus, hypoglycemia, renal failure; avoid extravasation; patients receiving beta blockers who have a history of anaphylactic reactions, may be more reactive to a repeated allergen challenge and may not be responsive to the usual epinephrine doses used to treat an allergic reaction

Adverse Reactions
Cardiovascular: Hypotension (especially with doses >200 mcg/kg/minute), bradycardia, Raynaud's phenomena
Central nervous system: Dizziness, somnolence, confusion, lethargy, depression, headache
Gastrointestinal: Nausea, vomiting
Local: Phlebitis, skin necrosis after extravasation
Respiratory: Bronchoconstriction (less than propranolol, but more likely with higher doses)
Miscellaneous: Diaphoresis, adverse reactions similar to other beta-blockers may occur

Drug Interactions Esmolol may increase digoxin or theophylline serum concentrations; morphine may increase esmolol blood concentrations; xanthines (eg, theophylline, caffeine) may decrease effects of esmolol

Food Interactions Avoid xanthine-containing foods or beverages

Mechanism of Action Class II antiarrhythmic: Competitively blocks response to $beta_1$-adrenergic stimulation with little or no effect on $beta_2$-receptors except at high doses (ie, cardioselective at lower doses); no intrinsic sympathomimetic activity; no membrane-stabilizing activity; ultrashort-acting

Pharmacodynamics
Onset of action: I.V.: Beta blockade occurs within 2-10 minutes (onset of effects is quickest when loading doses are administered)
Duration: Short (10-30 minutes)

Pharmacokinetics
Protein binding: 55%
Distribution: V_d:
Children: 2 L/kg
Adults: 3.5 L/kg (range: 2-5 L/kg)
Metabolism: In blood by esterases
Half-life, elimination:
Children:
18 months to 14 years (n=12): 2.88 ± 2.67 minutes
2.5-16 years (n=20): 4.5 ± 2.1 minutes
(Continued)

Esmolol (Continued)

Adults: 9 minutes

Elimination: ~69% of dose excreted in urine as metabolites and 2% as unchanged drug

Usual Dosage Must be adjusted to individual response and tolerance

Children: I.V.: Limited information available

Supraventricular tachycardia (SVT): Some centers have utilized initial doses of 100-500 mcg/kg given over 1 minute followed by a continuous infusion for control of SVT. One electrophysiologic study assessing esmolol-induced beta-blockade (n=20, 2-16 years of age) used an initial dose of 600 mcg/kg over 2 minutes followed by an infusion of 200 mcg/kg/minute; the infusion was titrated upward by 50-100 mcg/kg/minute every 5-10 minutes until a reduction >10% in heart rate or mean blood pressure occurred. Mean dose required: 550 mcg/kg/minute with a range of 300-1000 mcg/kg/minute (Trippel, 1991).

Postoperative hypertension: Loading doses of 500 mcg/kg/minute over 1 minute followed by a continuous infusion with doses of 50-250 mcg/kg/minute (mean 173) have been used in addition to nitroprusside in a small number of patients (7 patients, 7-19 years of age, median age 13 years) after coarctation of aorta repair (Vincent, 1990).

An open-label trial of 20 infants and children (1 month to 12 years of age; median age: 25.6 months) used the following dosing guidelines to treat postoperative hypertension following cardiac surgery: Age 0-7 days: Initial: 50 mcg/kg/minute; titrate dose by 25-50 mcg/kg/minute every 20 minutes; age 8 days to 1 month: Initial: 75 mcg/kg/minute; titrate dose by 50 mcg/kg/minute every 20 minutes; age >1 month to 1 year: Initial: 100 mcg/kg/minute; titrate dose by 50 mcg/kg/minute every 10 minutes; age >1 year to 12 years: Initial: 150 mcg/kg/minute; titrate dose by 50-100 mcg/kg/minute every 10 minutes; dose was titrated until blood pressure was ≤90th percentile for age or until maximum dose of 1000 mcg/kg/minute was reached; mean required dose: 700 mcg/kg/minute (range: 300-1000 mcg/kg/minute); final dose required was significantly higher in patients with aortic coarctation repair (mean ± SD: 830 ± 153 mcg/kg/minute) than in patients with repair of other congenital heart defects (mean ± SD: 570 ± 230 mcg/kg/minute) (Wiest, 1998)

Adults: I.V.: Loading dose: 500 mcg/kg over 1 minute; follow with a 50 mcg/kg/minute infusion for 4 minutes; if response is inadequate, rebolus with another 500 mcg/kg loading dose over 1 minute, and increase the maintenance infusion to 100 mcg/kg/minute. Repeat this process until a therapeutic effect has been achieved or to a maximum recommended maintenance dose of 200 mcg/kg/minute. Usual dosage range: 50-200 mcg/kg/minute with average dose = 100 mcg/kg/minute.

Administration Parenteral: I.V.: The 250 mg/mL ampul is **not** for direct I.V. injection, but must first be diluted to a final concentration not to exceed 10 mg/mL (ie, 2.5 g in 250 mL or 5 g in 500 mL); infuse I.V. loading dose over 1-2 minutes

Monitoring Parameters Blood pressure, EKG, heart rate, respiratory rate, I.V. site

Nursing Implications Decrease infusion rate or discontinue if hypotension, CHF, etc occur

Dosage Forms

Infusion [preservative free; premixed in sodium chloride]: 10 mg/mL (250 mL)

Injection, solution, as hydrochloride: 10 mg/mL (10 mL) [alcohol free; preservative free]; 250 mg/mL (10 mL) [contains 25% alcohol]

References

Cuneo BF, Zales VR, Blahunka PC, et al, "Pharmacodynamics and Pharmacokinetics of Esmolol, A Short-Acting Beta-Blocking Agent in Children," *Pediatr Cardiol*, 1994, 15(6):296-301.

Trippel DL, Wiest DB, and Gillette PC, "Cardiovascular and Antiarrhythmic Effects of Esmolol in Children," *J Pediatr*, 1991, 119(1):142-7.

Vincent RN, Click LA, Williams HM, et al, "Esmolol As an Adjunct in the Treatment of Systemic Hypertension After Operative Repair of Coarctation of the Aorta," *Am J Cardiol*, 1990, 65(13):941-3.

Wiest DB, Garner SS, Uber WE, et al, "Esmolol for the Management of Pediatric Hypertension After Cardiac Operations," *J Thorac Cardiovasc Surg*, 1998, 115(4):890-7.

Wiest DB, Trippel DL, Gillette PC, et al, "Pharmacokinetics of Esmolol in Children," *Clin Pharmacol Ther*, 1991, 49(6):618-23.

Esomeprazole (es oh ME pray zol)

U.S. Brand Names Nexium®

Therapeutic Category Gastric Acid Secretion Inhibitor; Gastrointestinal Agent; Gastric or Duodenal Ulcer Treatment; Proton Pump Inhibitor

Generic Available No

Use Treatment and maintenance of healing of severe erosive esophagitis; treatment of symptomatic gastroesophageal reflux disease (GERD); adjunctive treatment of duodenal ulcers associated with *Helicobacter pylori*

Pregnancy Risk Factor B

Contraindications Hypersensitivity to esomeprazole, omeprazole, lansoprazole, pantoprazole, or any component

Warnings Esomeprazole is an enantiomer of omeprazole and may share the same potential long-term side effects as omeprazole; atrophic gastritis has been noted occasionally in gastric corpus biopsies from patients treated long-term with omeprazole; in long-term (2-year) studies in rats, omeprazole produced a dose-related increase in gastric carcinoid tumors. While available endoscopic evaluations and histologic examinations of biopsy specimens from human stomachs have not detected a risk from short-term exposure to omeprazole, further human data on the effect of sustained hypochlorhydria and hypergastrinemia are needed to rule out the possibility of an increased risk for the development of tumors in humans receiving long-term therapy.

Precautions Modify dosage in patients with liver impairment.

Adverse Reactions

Cardiovascular: Chest pain, tachycardia, bradycardia, flushing, hypertension

Central nervous system: Headache, dizziness, vertigo, insomnia, anxiety, nervousness, fever, anorexia, confusion, somnolence

Dermatologic: Rash, acne, angioedema, dermatitis, pruritus, urticaria

Endocrine & metabolic: Goiter, glycosuria, hyperuricemia, hyponatremia

Gastrointestinal: Diarrhea, nausea, abdominal pain, vomiting, constipation, flatulence, dyspepsia, dysphagia, epigastric pain, eructation, gastroenteritis, GI hemorrhage, hiccup, melena, irritable colon, xerostomia, anorexia, dysgeusia, abdominal pain, taste loss, taste perversion

Genitourinary: Dysmenorrhea, vaginitis, urinary frequency, dysuria, hematuria

Hematologic: Leukopenia, pancytopenia, thrombocytopenia, anemia, leukocytosis

Hepatic: Elevated liver function tests

Neuromuscular & skeletal: Myalgia, arthralgia, back pain, arthropathy, cramps, fibromyalgia syndrome, polymyalgia rheumatica, paresthesia

Ocular: Conjunctivitis, abnormal vision

Otic: Tinnitus, earache

Renal: Hematuria, pyuria, proteinuria

Respiratory: Cough, dyspnea, larynx edema, pharyngitis, rhinitis, sinusitis

Drug Interactions Cytochrome P450 isoenzyme CYP2C19 and CYP3A4 substrate May decrease absorption of ketoconazole, itraconazole, dapsone, and iron salts; increases half-life (decreased clearance) of diazepam; may increase absorption of digoxin

Food Interactions Absorption is decreased by 33% to 53% when taken with food.

Stability Esomeprazole stability is a function of pH; it is rapidly degraded in acidic media, but has acceptable stability under alkaline conditions. Each capsule of esomeprazole contains enteric coated granules to prevent esomeprazole degradation by gastric acidity.

Mechanism of Action Esomeprazole is the S-isomer of omeprazole. Esomeprazole suppresses gastric acid secretion by inhibiting the parietal cell membrane enzyme (H^+/K^+)-ATPase or proton pump; demonstrates antimicrobial activity against *Helicobacter pylori*.

Pharmacokinetics

Distribution: Adults: V_d: 16 L

Protein binding: 97%

Metabolism: Hepatic via CYP2C19 and 3A3/4 isoenzymes to hydroxy, desmethyl, and sulfone metabolites (all inactive)

Bioavailability: 64% after a single dose; 90% with repeated administration

Half-life: Adults: 1-1.5 hours

Time to peak serum concentration: 1.5 hours

Elimination: <1% excreted unchanged in urine

Usual Dosage Oral: Adults:

Erosive esophagitis: 20-40 mg once daily for 4-8 weeks; maintenance: 20 mg once daily

Symptomatic GERD: 20 mg once daily for 4 weeks

Adjunctive therapy of duodenal ulcers associated with *Helicobacter pylori* (in combination with antibiotic therapy): 40 mg once daily for 10 days

Dosage adjustment in hepatic impairment:

Mild to moderate liver impairment (Child-Pugh Class A or B): No dosage adjustment needed

Severe liver impairment (Child-Pugh Class C): Not to exceed 20 mg daily

Administration Oral: Administer at least 1 hour before food or meals; capsule should be swallowed whole, do not chew or crush; capsules may be opened and the enteric coated pellets may be mixed with applesauce (applesauce should not be hot) and swallowed immediately; do not store mixture for future use; esomeprazole pellets also remain intact when mixed with tap water, orange juice, apple juice, and yogurt; due to

(Continued)

Esomeprazole *(Continued)*

small pellet size, the entire contents of an opened capsule may be completely delivered via small caliber and standard NG tubes when mixed with water (White, 2002)

Patient Information May cause dry mouth; do not chew or crush granules

Dosage Forms Capsule, delayed release, as esomeprazole magnesium: 20 mg, 40 mg

References

Gibbons TE and Gold BD, "The Use of Proton Pump Inhibitors in Children: A Comprehensive Review," *Paediatr Drugs*, 2003, 5(1):25-40.

White CM, Kalus JS, Quercia R, et al, "Delivery of Esomeprazole Magnesium Enteric-Coated Pellets Through Small Caliber and Standard Nasogastric Tubes and Gastrostomy Tubes *In Vitro*," *Am J Health Syst Pharm*, 2002, 59(21):2085-8.

◆ **Estar®** [OTC] *see Coal Tar on page 299*

◆ **Estimated Comparative Daily Dosages for Inhaled Corticosteroids** *see page 1382*

◆ **Estrace®** *see Estradiol on page 456*

◆ **Estraderm®** *see Estradiol on page 456*

Estradiol *(es tra DYE ole)*

U.S. Brand Names Alora®; Climara®; Delestrogen®; Depo®-Estradiol; Esclim®; Estrace®; Estraderm®; Estring®; Femring™; Gynodiol®; Vagifem®; Vivelle®; Vivelle Dot®

Canadian Brand Names Estradot®; Estrogel®; Oesclim®

Therapeutic Category Estrogen Derivative; Estrogen Derivative, Vaginal

Generic Available Yes

Use Treatment of hypoestrogenism (due to hypogonadism, castration, or primary ovarian failure), moderate to severe vasomotor symptoms of menopause, moderate to severe symptoms of vulvar and vaginal atrophy due to menopause; palliative treatment of breast cancer in select patients; palliative treatment of androgen-dependent prostate cancer; prevention of osteoporosis in postmenopausal women

Pregnancy Risk Factor X

Contraindications Hypersensitivity to estradiol or any component (see Warnings); history of or current DVT or PE; recent (eg, within past year) or current arterial thromboembolic disease (eg, MI, stroke); undiagnosed vaginal bleeding; pregnancy; known, suspected, or history of breast cancer (except in select patients being treated for metastatic disease); estrogen-dependent neoplasia

Warnings Estrogens have been reported to increase the risk of endometrial carcinoma (the addition of a progestin has been shown to decrease the risk of estrogen-induced endometrial hyperplasia, a condition thought to be a precursor to endometrial cancer). Do not use estrogens (with or without progestins) for the prevention of cardiovascular disease; a significantly increased risk of MI, stroke, PE, DVT, and invasive breast cancer was reported in postmenopausal women receiving conjugated equine estrogens combined with medroxyprogesterone acetate (see Rossouw, 2002); due to these risks, use estrogens (with or without progestins) at the lowest effective doses and for the shortest duration possible that is consistent with an individual's treatment goals and risks; periodic risk:benefit assessments should be conducted; consider topical vaginal products when estrogen is used solely for the treatment of vulvar and vaginal atrophy; if used solely for the prevention of osteoporosis in postmenopausal women, estrogens should only be considered for those at significant risk of osteoporosis and nonestrogen treatment options should be carefully considered. Do not use estrogens during pregnancy.

Since estrogens may increase the risk of venous thromboembolism, discontinue therapy, if possible, at least 4-6 weeks before surgery that is associated with an increased risk of thromboembolism, or during times of prolonged immobilization. Estrogens may increase the risk of breast cancer, gallbladder disease, hypercalcemia, and retinal vascular thrombosis (discontinue estrogen therapy in patients with sudden partial or complete loss of vision, sudden onset of diplopia, proptosis, or migraine, or if eye exam reveals retinal vascular lesions or papilledema)

Injection may contain benzyl alcohol and oral tablet may contain tartrazine, both of which may cause allergic reactions in susceptible individuals; large amounts of benzyl alcohol (≥99 mg/kg/day) have been associated with a potentially fatal toxicity ("gasping syndrome") in neonates; avoid use of estradiol products containing benzyl alcohol in neonates; *in vitro* and animal studies have shown that benzoate, a metabolite of benzyl alcohol, displaces bilirubin from protein binding sites

Precautions Use with caution in patients with asthma, epilepsy, migraines, diabetes, hypothyroidism, hypocalcemia, hypercalcemia, endometriosis, porphyria, history of cholestatic jaundice due to past estrogen use or pregnancy, cardiac, liver, or renal dysfunction; estrogens may cause premature closure of the epiphyses in young individuals; may increase blood pressure; may cause fluid retention; may greatly increase triglycerides and lead to pancreatitis and other problems in patients with familial defects of lipoprotein metabolism; Femring™ may not be suitable for women that have conditions which make the vagina more susceptible to vaginal ulceration or irritation, or make expulsion of the ring more likely (eg, vaginal stenosis, cervical prolapse, etc)

Adverse Reactions

Cardiovascular: Hypertension, edema, thromboembolic disorders

Central nervous system: Depression, headache, dizziness

Dermatologic: Chloasma, melasma

Endocrine & metabolic: Breast enlargement, breast tenderness, changes in libido, impaired glucose tolerance, hypercalcemia, folate deficiency; increased risk of endometrial hyperplasia

Gastrointestinal: Nausea, vomiting, bloating, abdominal cramps, pancreatitis, weight gain or weight loss, gall bladder disease

Genitourinary: Changes in menstrual flow

Hepatic: Cholestatic jaundice

Local: Pain at injection site; topical may cause burning or irritation

Neuromuscular & skeletal: Premature closure of epiphyses in young patients (large and repeated doses over an extended period of time)

Drug Interactions Cytochrome P450 isoenzyme CYP1A2 and CYP3A3/4 substrate; isoenzyme CYP1A2 inhibitor

Rifampin, phenobarbital, carbamazepine, and the herbal medicine St John's wort (*Hypericum perforatum*) may decrease plasma concentrations and effects of estrogens; cytochrome P450 CYP3A4 inhibitors (eg, erythromycin, clarithromycin, ketoconazole, itraconazole, ritonavir) may increase estrogen plasma concentrations and effects; anticoagulants, bromocriptine, dantrolene (increased risk of hepatotoxicity); estrogens may decrease the clearance and increase the serum concentrations and toxic effects of corticosteroids and cyclosporine

Food Interactions Larger doses of vitamin C (eg, 1 g/day in adults) may increase the serum concentrations and adverse effects of estradiol; vitamin C supplements are not recommended, but this effect may be decreased if vitamin C supplement is given 2-3 hours after estrogen; dietary intake of folate and pyridoxine may need to be increased; grapefruit juice may possibly increase estrogen plasma concentrations and effects

Mechanism of Action Increases the synthesis of DNA, RNA, and various proteins in target tissues; reduces the release of gonadotropin-releasing hormone from the hypothalamus; reduces FSH and LH release from the pituitary

Usual Dosage Adolescents and Adults: All dosage needs to be adjusted based upon the patient's response

Female hypogonadism:

I.M.:

Cypionate: 1.5-2 mg given once each month

Valerate: 10-20 mg given once each month

Oral: 0.5-2 mg/day in a cyclic regimen (3 weeks on drug, 1 week off)

Transdermal:

Once-weekly patch (Climara®): Initial: 0.025-0.05 mg/day patch applied once weekly (titrate dosage to response)

Twice-weekly patch: Alora®, Esclim®, Estraderm®: Initial: 0.05 mg patch; Vivelle®, Vivelle Dot®: Initial: 0.0375 mg patch; titrate dosage to response; apply patch twice weekly in a cyclic regimen (3 weeks on drug, 1 week off) in patients with intact uterus and continuously in patients without a uterus

Vaginal and vulval atrophy: Intravaginal: Initial: 200-400 mcg of estradiol once daily for 1-2 weeks; taper dose gradually to 100-200 mcg of estradiol once daily for 1-2 weeks; maintenance, cyclic regimen (after vaginal mucosa restored): 100 mcg of estradiol 1-3 times/week for 3 weeks, then no drug for the 4th week per cycle

Vaginal ring:

Postmenopausal vaginal atrophy, urogenital symptoms: Estring®: 2 mg intravaginally; following insertion, ring should remain in place for 90 days

Moderate to severe vasomotor symptoms associated with menopause; vulvar/vaginal atrophy: Femring™: 0.05 mg intravaginally; following insertion, ring should remain in place for 3 months; dose may be increased to 0.1 mg if needed

Administration

Oral: Administer with food or after a meal to reduce GI upset

Parenteral: Injection for I.M. use only

Transdermal: Apply to clean dry area; do not apply to breasts; do not apply to waistline (may loosen patch); rotate application sites

Vaginal ring: Exact positioning is not critical for efficacy, however, patient should not feel ring or discomfort once inserted. In case of discomfort, ring should be gently

(Continued)

Estradiol *(Continued)*

pushed further into vagina. If ring is expelled prior to 90 days, it may be rinsed off and reinserted.

Monitoring Parameters Blood pressure, weight, serum calcium, glucose, liver enzymes; bone maturation and epiphyseal effects in young patients in whom bone growth is not complete

Test Interactions Thyroid function tests: Estrogens may increase thyroid binding globulin and circulating total thyroid hormone (when measured by T_4 RIA, T_4 by column, or by PBI); decreases free T_3 resin uptake; concentration of free T_4 is not altered

Patient Information Limit alcohol, caffeine, and grapefruit juice; notify physician if sudden severe headache or vomiting, disturbance of vision or speech, numbness or weakness of extremity, sharp or crushing chest pain, calf pain, shortness of breath, severe abdominal pain or mass, mental depression, or unusual bleeding occurs

Additional Information Femring™ can remain in place during local treatment of vaginal infections.

Dosage Forms

Cream, vaginal, as **base** (Estrace®): 0.1 mg/g (12 g) [refill tube]; 0.1 mg/g (42.5 g) [tube with applicator]

Injection, oil, as **cyplonate** (Depo®-Estradiol): 5 mg/mL (5 mL) [contains chlorobu-tanol]

Injection, oil, as **valerate** (Delestrogen®): 10 mg/mL (5 mL) [contains chlorobutanol]; 20 mg/mL (5 mL) [contains benzyl alcohol and castor oil]; 40 mg/mL (5 mL) [contains benzyl alcohol and castor oil]

Tablet, micronized, as **base**: 0.5 mg, 1 mg, 2 mg

Estrace®: 0.5 mg, 1 mg, 2 mg [2 mg tablets contain tartrazine]

Gynodiol®: 0.5 mg, 1 mg, 1.5 mg, 2 mg

Tablet, vaginal, as **base** (Vagifem®): 25 mcg

Transdermal system, as **base**: 0.05 mg/24 hours (4s); 0.1 mg/24 hours (4s)

Alora® [twice weekly patch]:
0.05 mg/24 hours (8s, 24s) [18 cm²; contains 1.5 mg estradiol/patch]
0.075 mg/24 hours (8s) [27 cm²; contains 2.3 mg/patch]
0.1 mg/24 hours (8s) [36 cm²; contains 3 mg estradiol/patch]

Climara® [once weekly patch]:
0.025 mg/24 hours (4s) [6.5 cm²; contains 2 mg estradiol/patch]
0.05 mg/24 hours (4s) [12.5 cm²; contains 3.8 mg estradiol/patch]
0.075 mg/24 hours (4s) [18.75 cm²; contains 5.7 mg estradiol/patch]
0.1 mg/24 hours (4s) [25 cm²; contains 7.6 mg estradiol/patch]

Esclim® [twice weekly patch]:
0.025 mg/24 hours (8s) [11 cm²; contains 5 mg estradiol/patch]
0.0375 mg/24 hours (8s) [16.5 cm²; contains 7.5 mg estradiol/patch]
0.05 mg/24 hours (8s) [22 cm²; contains 10 mg estradiol/patch]
0.075 mg/24 hours (8s) [33 cm²; contains 15 mg estradiol/patch]
0.1 mg/24 hours (8s) [44 cm²; contains 20 mg estradiol/patch]

Estraderm® [twice weekly patch]:
0.05 mg/24 hours (8s, 24s) [10 cm²; contains 4 mg estradiol/patch]
0.1 mg/24 hours (8s, 24 s) [20 cm²; contains 8 mg estradiol/patch]

Vivelle® [twice weekly patch]:
0.025 mg/24 hours (8s) [7.25 cm²; contains 2.17 mg estradiol/patch]
0.0375 mg/24 hours (8s) [11 cm²; contains 3.28 mg estradiol/patch]
0.05 mg/24 hours (8s) [14.5 cm²; contains 4.33 mg estradiol/patch]
0.075 mg/24 hours (8s) [22 cm²; contains 6.57 mg estradiol/patch]
0.1 mg/24 hours (8s) [29 cm²; contains 8.66 mg estradiol/patch]

Vivelle Dot® [twice weekly patch]:
0.0375 mg/24 hours (8s) [3.75 cm² ; contains 0.585 mg estradiol/patch]
0.05 mg/24 hours (8s) [5 cm²; contains 0.78 mg estradiol/patch]
0.075 mg/24 hours (8s) [7.5 cm²; contains 1.17 mg estradiol/patch]
0.1 mg/24 hours (8s) [10 cm²; contains 1.56 mg estradiol/patch]

Vaginal ring, as **acetate** (Femring™): 0.05 mg [contains 12.4 mg; releases 0.05 mg/day over 3 months] (1s); 0.1 mg [contains 24.8 mg; releases 0.1 mg/day over 3 months] (1s)

Vaginal ring, as **base** (Estring®): 2 mg (1s) [gradually released over 90 days]

References

Rossouw JE, Anderson GL, Prentice RL, et al, "Risks and Benefits of Estrogen Plus Progestin in Healthy Postmenopausal Women: Principal Results From the Women's Health Initiative Randomized Controlled Trial," *JAMA*, 2002, 288(3):321-33.

♦ **Estradot®** **(Can)** *see* Estradiol *on page 456*

♦ **Estring®** *see* Estradiol *on page 456*

♦ **Estrogel®** **(Can)** *see* Estradiol *on page 456*

♦ **Estrogenic Substances, Conjugated** *see* Estrogens (Conjugated/Equine) *on page 459*

Estrogens (Conjugated/Equine) (ES troe jenz KON joo gate ed)

U.S. Brand Names Premarin®
Canadian Brand Names Cenestin; C.E.S.®; Congest
Synonyms C.E.S.; Conjugated Estrogens; Estrogenic Substances, Conjugated
Therapeutic Category Estrogen Derivative; Estrogen Derivative, Vaginal
Generic Available No
Use Treatment of dysfunctional uterine bleeding, hypoestrogenism (due to hypogonadism, castration, or primary ovarian failure), moderate to severe vasomotor symptoms of menopause; moderate to severe symptoms of vulvar and vaginal atrophy due to menopause; palliative treatment of breast cancer in select patients; palliative treatment of androgen-dependent prostate cancer; prevention of osteoporosis in postmenopausal women
Pregnancy Risk Factor X
Contraindications Hypersensitivity to estrogens or any component (see Warnings); history of or current DVT or PE; recent (eg, within past year) or current arterial thromboembolic disease (eg, MI, stroke); undiagnosed vaginal bleeding; pregnancy; known, suspected, or history of breast cancer (except in select patients being treated for metastatic disease); estrogen-dependent neoplasia
Warnings Estrogens have been reported to increase the risk of endometrial carcinoma (the addition of a progestin has been shown to decrease the risk of estrogen-induced endometrial hyperplasia, a condition thought to be a precursor to endometrial cancer). Do not use estrogens (with or without progestins) for the prevention of cardiovascular disease; a significantly increased risk of MI, stroke, PE, DVT, and invasive breast cancer was reported in postmenopausal women receiving conjugated equine estrogens combined with medroxyprogesterone acetate (see Rossouw, 2002); due to these risks, use estrogens (with or without progestins) at the lowest effective doses and for the shortest duration possible that is consistent with an individual's treatment goals and risks; periodic risk:benefit assessments should be conducted; consider topical vaginal products when estrogen is used solely for the treatment of vulvar and vaginal atrophy; if used solely for the prevention of osteoporosis in postmenopausal women, estrogens should only be considered for those at significant risk of osteoporosis and nonestrogen treatment options should be carefully considered. Do not use estrogens during pregnancy.

Since estrogens may increase the risk of venous thromboembolism, discontinue therapy, if possible, at least 4-6 weeks before surgery that is associated with an increased risk of thromboembolism, or during times of prolonged immobilization. Estrogens may increase the risk of breast cancer, gallbladder disease, hypercalcemia, and retinal vascular thrombosis (discontinue estrogen therapy in patients with sudden partial or complete loss of vision, sudden onset of diplopia, proptosis, or migraine, or if eye exam reveals retinal vascular lesions or papilledema)

Diluent for injection contains benzyl alcohol which may cause allergic reactions in susceptible individuals; large amounts of benzyl alcohol (≥99 mg/kg/day) have been associated with a potentially fatal toxicity ("gasping syndrome") in neonates; avoid use of estrogen products containing benzyl alcohol in neonates; *in vitro* and animal studies have shown that benzoate, a metabolite of benzyl alcohol, displaces bilirubin from protein binding sites

Precautions Use with caution in patients with asthma, epilepsy, migraines, diabetes, hypothyroidism, hypocalcemia, hypercalcemia, endometriosis, porphyria, history of cholestatic jaundice due to past estrogen use or pregnancy; cardiac, liver, or renal dysfunction; estrogens may cause premature closure of the epiphyses in young individuals; may increase blood pressure; may cause fluid retention; may greatly increase triglycerides and lead to pancreatitis and other problems in patients with familial defects of lipoprotein metabolism

Adverse Reactions
Cardiovascular: Hypertension, edema, thromboembolic disorder
Central nervous system: Depression, headache, dizziness
Dermatologic: Chloasma, melasma
Endocrine & metabolic: Breast enlargement, breast tenderness, changes in libido, impaired glucose tolerance, hypercalcemia, folate deficiency; increased risk of endometrial hyperplasia
Gastrointestinal: Nausea, vomiting, bloating, abdominal cramps, pancreatitis, weight gain or weight loss, gall bladder disease
Genitourinary: Changes in menstrual flow
Hepatic: Cholestatic jaundice
Local: Pain at injection site
Neuromuscular & skeletal: Premature closure of epiphyses in young patients
(Continued)

Estrogens (Conjugated/Equine) *(Continued)*

Drug Interactions Cytochrome P450 isoenzyme CYP3A4 substrate

Rifampin, phenobarbital, carbamazepine, and the herbal medicine St John's wort (*Hypericum perforatum*) may decrease plasma concentrations and effects of estrogens; cytochrome P450 CYP3A4 inhibitors (eg, erythromycin, clarithromycin, ketoconazole, itraconazole, ritonavir) may increase estrogen plasma concentrations and effects; anticoagulants, bromocriptine, dantrolene (increased risk of hepatotoxicity); estrogens may decrease the clearance and increase the serum concentrations and toxic effects of corticosteroids and cyclosporine

Food Interactions Larger doses of vitamin C (eg, 1 g/day in adults) may increase the serum concentrations and adverse effects of estrogens; vitamin C supplements are not recommended, but this effect may be decreased if vitamin C supplement is given 2-3 hours after estrogen; dietary intake of folate and pyridoxine may need to be increased; grapefruit juice may possibly increase estrogen plasma concentrations and effects

Stability Injection: Store in the refrigerator; compatible with NS, dextrose, and invert sugar solutions; not compatible with ascorbic acid, protein hydrolysate, or acidic pH

Mechanism of Action Increases the synthesis of DNA, RNA, and various proteins in target tissues; reduces the release of gonadotropin-releasing hormone from the hypothalamus; reduces FSH and LH release from the pituitary

Usual Dosage Adolescents and Adults:

Female castration or primary ovarian failure: Oral: Cyclic regimen: 1.25 mg/day for 3 weeks, then no drug for the 4th week per cycle; repeat; titrate dose to response; use lowest effective dose

Female hypogonadism: Oral:

Manufacturer's recommendation: Cyclic regimen: 0.3-0.625 mg/day for 3 weeks, then no drug for the 4th week per cycle; titrate dose to response; use lowest effective dose

Alternative dosing: 2.5-7.5 mg/day in divided doses for 20 days, off 10 days and repeat until menses occur

Dysfunctional uterine bleeding:

Stable hematocrit: Oral: 1.25 mg twice daily for 21 days; if bleeding persists after 48 hours, increase to 2.5 mg twice daily; if bleeding persists after 48 more hours, increase to 2.5 mg 4 times/day; some recommend starting at 2.5 mg 4 times/day (**Note:** Medroxyprogesterone acetate 10 mg/day is also given on days 17-21; see Neistein, 1991)

Alternatively: Oral: 2.5-5 mg/day for 7-10 days; then decrease to 1.25 mg/day for 2 weeks

Unstable hematocrit: Oral, I.V.: 5 mg 2-4 times/day; if bleeding is profuse, 20-40 mg every 4 hours up to 24 hours may be used; **Note:** A progestational-weighted contraception pill should also be given (eg, Ovral® 2 tablets stat and 1 tablet 4 times/day or medroxyprogesterone acetate 5-10 mg 4 times/day; see Neistein, 1991)

Alternatively: I.M., I.V.: 25 mg every 6-12 hours until bleeding stops

Vaginal and vulval atrophy: Intravaginal or topical: Cyclic regimen: 1.25-2.5 mg/day of conjugated estrogens for 3 weeks, then no drug for the 4th week per cycle; repeat as clinically needed

Administration

Oral: Administer with food or after eating to reduce GI upset; administration of dose at bedtime may decrease adverse effects

Parenteral: Add sterile diluent provided by manufacturer and shake gently; I.V.: Administer slow I.V. avoid vascular flushing; I.M.: may be administered I.M. for dysfunctional uterine bleeding, but I.V. use is preferred (more rapid response)

Monitoring Parameters Blood pressure, serum calcium, glucose, liver enzymes; dysfunctional uterine bleeding: Hematocrit, hemoglobin, PT; bone maturation and epiphyseal effects in young patients in whom bone growth is not complete

Test Interactions Thyroid function tests: Estrogens may increase thyroid binding globulin and circulating total thyroid hormone (when measured by T_4 RIA, T_4 by column, or by PBI); decreases free T_3 resin uptake; concentration of free T_4 is not altered

Patient Information Limit caffeine and grapefruit juice; notify physician if sudden severe headache, vomiting, disturbance of vision or speech, numbness or weakness of extremity, sharp or crushing chest pain, calf pain, shortness of breath, severe abdominal pain or mass, mental depression, or unusual bleeding occurs

Dosage Forms

Cream, vaginal: 0.625 mg/g (42.5 g)

Injection, powder for reconstitution: 25 mg [diluent contains 2% benzyl alcohol]

Tablet: 0.3 mg, 0.625 mg, 0.9 mg, 1.25 mg, 2.5 mg

References

Minjarez DA and Bradshaw KD, "Abnormal Uterine Bleeding in Adolescents," *Obstet Gynecol Clin North Am*, 2000, 27(1):63-78.

Mitan LA and Slap GB, "Adolescent Menstrual Disorders. Update," *Med Clin North Am*, 2000, 84(4):851-68.

Neistein LS, *Adolescent Health Care - A Practical Guide*, 2nd ed, Baltimore: Urban & Schwarzenberg, 1991, 661-6.

Rossouw JE, Anderson GL, Prentice RL, et al, "Risks and Benefits of Estrogen Plus Progestin in Healthy Postmenopausal Women: Principal Results From the Women's Health Initiative Randomized Controlled Trial," *JAMA*, 2002, 288(3):321-33.

♦ **ETAF** *see* Aldesleukin *on page 56*

Etanercept (et a NER cept)

U.S. Brand Names Enbrel®

Therapeutic Category Antirheumatic, Disease Modifying

Generic Available No

Use Treatment of polyarticular-course juvenile rheumatoid arthritis in patients who have had an inadequate response to one or more disease-modifying antirheumatic drugs; treatment of signs and symptoms of moderately to severely active rheumatoid arthritis in patients who have had an inadequate response to one or more disease-modifying antirheumatic drugs or in combination with methotrexate in patients who do not respond adequately to methotrexate alone; psoriatic arthritis

Pregnancy Risk Factor B

Contraindications Hypersensitivity to etanercept or any component (ie, mannitol, sucrose, tromethamine, and benzyl alcohol) (see Warnings); patients with any serious active infection or sepsis

Warnings Some patients have developed serious infections and several have died from their infections while taking etanercept; patients who develop a new infection while being treated with etanercept should be monitored closely. Etanercept should be discontinued if a patient develops a serious infection or sepsis. Rare cases of CNS demyelinating disorders, such as multiple sclerosis, myelitis, and optic neuritis, have been reported in patients undergoing etanercept therapy.

Diluent for etanercept injection contains benzyl alcohol which may cause allergic reactions in susceptible individuals; large amounts of benzyl alcohol (≥99 mg/kg/day) have been associated with a potentially fatal toxicity ("gasping syndrome") in neonates; avoid use of etanercept products containing benzyl alcohol in neonates; *in vitro* and animal studies have shown that benzoate, a metabolite of benzyl alcohol, displaces bilirubin from protein binding sites; patients with latex allergy should not handle the needle cover of the diluent syringe since it contains latex

Precautions Use with caution in patients with a history of recurrent infections or illnesses such as poorly controlled diabetes which predisposes the patient to infection; discontinue etanercept in a child who develops varicella infection or who has a significant exposure to varicella virus and consider prophylactic treatment with varicella-zoster immune globulin; anti-TNF therapies such as etanercept may affect host defenses against infections and malignancies

Adverse Reactions

Central nervous system: Headache (19%), depression, personality disorder, dizziness, seizures

Dermatologic: Rash

Gastrointestinal: Nausea (9%), abdominal pain (19%), vomiting (13%), esophagitis/gastritis, GI bleeding

Hematologic: Pancytopenia, aplastic anemia

Local: Injection site reactions (erythema, discomfort, itching, swelling)

Respiratory: Respiratory tract infection, rhinitis

Miscellaneous: Allergic reaction (hives, difficulty breathing), positive antinuclear antibodies, positive antidouble-stranded DNA antibodies

Drug Interactions Live vaccines (unknown whether secondary transmission of infection in live vaccines can occur)

Stability Store vial in the refrigerator; do not freeze; etanercept solution should be used within 6 hours of reconstitution; do not shake or agitate vigorously; do not use if discolored or cloudy; do not filter reconstituted solution; do not add or mix with other medications

Mechanism of Action Binds to tumor necrosis factor (TNF) and blocks its interaction with cell surface TNF receptors rendering TNF biologically inactive; modulates biological responses that are induced or regulated by TNF

Pharmacodynamics

Onset of action: One week of treatment

Maximum effect: Full effect is usually seen within 3 months

Pharmacokinetics

Absorption: Absorbed slowly after S.C. injection

(Continued)

Etanercept *(Continued)*

Distribution: V_d: 1.78-3.39 L/m^2
Bioavailability: S.C.: 60%
Half-life: Adults: 115 hours (range: 98-300 hours)
Time to peak serum concentration: S.C.: 72 hours (range: 48-96 hours)
Elimination: Clearance:
Children 4-17 years: 46 mL/hour/m^2
Adults: 52 mL/hour/m^2

Usual Dosage S.C.:
Children 4-17 years: 0.4 mg/kg/dose twice weekly given 72-96 hours apart; maximum dose: 25 mg
Adult: 25 mg twice weekly given 72-96 hours apart

Administration Parenteral: Administer by S.C. injection into thigh, abdomen, or upper arm; injection sites should be rotated with subsequent doses given at least 1 inch from an old site; do not inject into areas where the skin is tender, bruised, red, or hard

Monitoring Parameters Assess for joint swelling, pain, and tenderness; ESR or C-reactive protein level; CBC with differential and platelet count

Patient Information Notify physician if persistent fever, bruising, bleeding, or pallor occurs.

Dosage Forms Injection, powder for reconstitution: 25 mg [diluent contains benzyl alcohol]

References

Ilowite NT, "Current Treatment of Juvenile Rheumatoid Arthritis," *Pediatrics*, 2002, 109(1):109-15.
Lovell DJ, Giannini EH, Whitmore JB, et al, "Safety and Efficacy of Tumor Necrosis Factor Receptor P75Fc Fusion Protein (TNFR:Fc, ENBREL) in Polyarticular Course Juvenile Rheumatoid Arthritis," Presented at American College of Rheumatology National Meeting, San Diego, CA, 1998.
Moreland LW, Baumgartner SW, Schiff MH, et al, "Treatment of Rheumatoid Arthritis With a Recombinant Human Tumor Necrosis Factor Receptor (p75)-Fc Fusion Protein," *N Engl J Med*, 1997, 337(3):141-7.

Ethambutol *(e THAM byoo tole)*

U.S. Brand Names Myambutol®
Canadian Brand Names Etibi®
Therapeutic Category Antitubercular Agent
Generic Available Yes
Use Treatment of tuberculosis and other mycobacterial diseases in conjunction with other antimycobacterial agents
Pregnancy Risk Factor C
Contraindications Hypersensitivity to ethambutol or any component; optic neuritis
Warnings Optic neuropathy including optic neuritis or retrobulbar neuritis characterized by decreased visual acuity, scotoma, color blindness, and/or visual defect has been reported with ethambutol therapy and may be related to dose and treatment duration; irreversible blindness has also been reported. Loss of visual acuity is generally reversible when ethambutol is discontinued promptly. Some patients have received ethambutol again after such recovery without recurrence of visual acuity loss. Use only in children whose visual acuity can accurately be determined and monitored; fatal hepatotoxicity has been reported; not recommended for use in children <13 years of age unless benefit outweighs risk of therapy
Precautions Use with caution in patients with ocular defects or impaired renal function; modify dose in patients with renal impairment

Adverse Reactions
Central nervous system: Malaise, mental confusion, fever, headache, dizziness
Dermatologic: Rash, pruritus
Endocrine & metabolic: Elevated uric acid levels
Gastrointestinal: Nausea, vomiting, anorexia, abdominal pain
Hematologic: Thrombocytopenia, leukopenia, eosinophilia
Hepatic: Abnormal liver function tests, hepatotoxicity
Neuromuscular & skeletal: Peripheral neuropathy, arthralgia, joint pain
Ocular: Optic neuritis, decreased visual acuity, decreased red-green color discrimination, irreversible blindness
Miscellaneous: Anaphylaxis

Stability Store tablets at controlled room temperature 20°C to 25°C (68°F to 77°F)
Mechanism of Action Suppresses mycobacterial multiplication by interfering with RNA synthesis

Pharmacokinetics
Absorption: Oral: ~80%
Distribution: Well distributed throughout the body with high concentrations in kidneys, lungs, saliva, CSF, and red blood cells; crosses the placenta; excreted into breast milk
Protein binding: 20% to 30%

Metabolism: 20% by the liver to inactive metabolite

Half-life: 2.5-3.6 hours (up to 7 hours or longer with renal impairment)

Time to peak serum concentration: Within 2-4 hours

Elimination: ~50% in urine and 20% excreted in feces as unchanged drug

Dialysis: Slightly dialyzable (5% to 20%)

Usual Dosage Oral:

Tuberculosis: Infants, Children, Adolescents, and Adults: 15-25 mg/kg/day once daily **or** 50 mg/kg/dose twice weekly, not to exceed 2.5 g/dose

Nontuberculous mycobacterial infection: Children, Adolescents, and Adults: 15 mg/kg/day, not to exceed 1 g/day

Dosing interval in renal impairment:

Cl_{cr} 10-50 mL/minute: Administer every 24-36 hours

Cl_{cr} <10 mL/minute: Administer every 48 hours and/or reduce usual dose

Administration Oral: Administer with or without food; if GI upset occurs, administer with food

Monitoring Parameters Monthly examination of visual acuity and color discrimination in patients receiving >15 mg/kg/day; periodic renal, hepatic, and hematologic function tests

Patient Information Report to physician any visual changes, numbness or tingling in hands or feet, rash, fever, and chills

Dosage Forms

Tablet, film coated, as hydrochloride: 100 mg, 400 mg

Myambutol®: 100 mg, 400 mg [scored]

References

American Academy of Pediatrics, Committee on Infectious Diseases, "Chemotherapy for Tuberculosis in Infants and Children," *Pediatrics*, 1992, 89(1):161-5.

Starke JR and Correa AG, "Management of Mycobacterial Infection and Disease in Children," *Pediatr Infect Dis J*, 1995, 14:455-70.

♦ **Ethanol** *see* Ethyl Alcohol *on page 465*

Ethionamide (e thye on AM ide)

U.S. Brand Names Trecator®-SC

Therapeutic Category Antitubercular Agent

Generic Available No

Use In conjunction with other antituberculosis agents in the treatment of tuberculosis and other mycobacterial diseases

Pregnancy Risk Factor C

Contraindications Hypersensitivity to ethionamide or any component; severe hepatic impairment

Precautions Use with caution in patients receiving cycloserine or isoniazid or in diabetic patients

Adverse Reactions

Cardiovascular: Postural hypotension

Central nervous system: Drowsiness, dizziness, seizures, headache, encephalopathy, depression

Dermatologic: Rash

Endocrine & metabolic: Hypoglycemia, goiter, gynecomastia

Gastrointestinal: Nausea, vomiting, abdominal pain, diarrhea, anorexia, stomatitis, metallic taste, weight loss

Hematologic: Thrombocytopenia

Hepatic: Hepatitis; jaundice; elevated AST, ALT, and serum bilirubin

Neuromuscular & skeletal: Peripheral neuropathy, tremor

Ocular: Optic neuritis

Miscellaneous: Excessive salivation

Drug Interactions Cycloserine and isoniazid may increase nervous system adverse effects; alcohol (associated with psychotic reaction)

Food Interactions Increase dietary intake of pyridoxine to prevent neurotoxic effects of ethionamide

Mechanism of Action Inhibits peptide synthesis in susceptible organisms

Pharmacokinetics

Absorption: ~80% is rapidly absorbed from the GI tract

Distribution: Crosses the placenta; widely distributed into body tissues and fluids including liver, kidneys, and CSF

Protein binding: 10%

Metabolism: In the liver to active and inactive metabolites

Bioavailability: 80%

Half-life: 2-3 hours

Time to peak serum concentration: Oral: Within 3 hours

Elimination: As metabolites (active and inactive) and parent drug in the urine

(Continued)

Ethionamide *(Continued)*

Usual Dosage Oral:
Children: 15-20 mg/kg/day in 2-3 divided doses, not to exceed 1 g/day
Adults: 500-1000 mg/day in 1-3 divided doses

Administration Oral: Administer with meals to decrease GI distress

Monitoring Parameters Initial and periodic serum AST and ALT, blood glucose, thyroid function tests, periodic ophthalmologic exams

Nursing Implications Neurotoxic effects may be relieved by the administration of pyridoxine

Dosage Forms Tablet: 250 mg

References

Donald PR and Seifart HI,"Cerebrospinal Fluid Concentrations of Ethionamide in Children With Tuberculous Meningitis," *J Pediatr*, 1989, 115(3):483-6.

Starke JR and Correa AG, "Management of Mycobacterial Infection and Disease in Children," *Pediatr Infect Dis J*, 1995, 14(6):455-69.

Ethosuximide *(eth oh SUKS i mide)*

Related Information

Antiepileptic Drugs *on page 1374*
Blood Level Sampling Time Guidelines *on page 1386*
Carbohydrate and Alcohol Content of Liquid Medications for Use in Patients Receiving Ketogenic Diets *on page 1431*

U.S. Brand Names Zarontin®

Therapeutic Category Anticonvulsant, Succinimide

Generic Available Yes

Use Management of absence (petit mal) seizures, myoclonic seizures, and akinetic epilepsy

Pregnancy Risk Factor C

Contraindications Hypersensitivity to ethosuximide or any component

Warnings Ethosuximide may increase tonic-clonic seizures in patients with mixed seizure disorders; ethosuximide must be used in combination with other anticonvulsants in patients with both absence and tonic-clonic seizures; may cause blood dyscrasias (periodic hematology tests should be performed)

Syrup contains sodium benzoate; benzoic acid (benzoate) is a metabolite of benzyl alcohol; large amounts of benzyl alcohol (≥99 mg/kg/day) have been associated with a potentially fatal toxicity ("gasping syndrome") in neonates; the "gasping syndrome" consists of metabolic acidosis, respiratory distress, gasping respirations, CNS dysfunction (including convulsions, intracranial hemorrhage), hypotension and cardiovascular collapse; use ethosuximide products containing sodium benzoate with caution in neonates; *in vitro* and animal studies have shown that benzoate displaces bilirubin from protein binding sites

Precautions Use with caution in patients with hepatic or renal disease; abrupt withdrawal of the drug may precipitate absence status

Adverse Reactions

Central nervous system: Sedation, dizziness, lethargy, euphoria, hallucinations, insomnia, agitation, behavioral changes, headache; increase in tonic-clonic seizures (see Warnings)

Dermatologic: Rashes, urticaria

Gastrointestinal: Nausea, vomiting, anorexia, abdominal pain

Genitourinary: Vaginal bleeding

Hematologic: Rare: Leukopenia, aplastic anemia, thrombocytopenia

Ocular: Myopia

Renal: Microscopic hematuria

Miscellaneous: Hiccups, rarely systemic lupus erythematosus

Drug Interactions Cytochrome P450 isoenzyme CYP3A3/4 substrate

Phenytoin, carbamazepine, primidone, phenobarbital may increase the hepatic metabolism of ethosuximide; ethosuximide may increase phenytoin serum concentrations; isoniazid may inhibit hepatic metabolism with a resultant increase in ethosuximide serum concentrations; CNS depressants, alcohol may increase adverse effects; haloperidol may change the frequency or pattern of seizure activity; valproic acid (increases or decreases ethosuximide serum concentrations)

Food Interactions Folate requirements may be increased

Mechanism of Action Increases the seizure threshold and suppresses paroxysmal spike-and-wave pattern in absence seizures; depresses nerve transmission in the motor cortex

Pharmacokinetics

Distribution: V_d: Adults: 0.62-0.72 L/kg

Protein binding: <10%

Metabolism: ~80% metabolized in the liver to three inactive metabolites

Half-life:

Children: 30 hours

Adults: 50-60 hours

Time to peak serum concentration:

Capsule: Within 2-4 hours

Syrup: <2-4 hours

Elimination: Slow in urine as metabolites (50%) and as unchanged drug (10% to 20%); small amounts excreted in feces

Dialysis: Removed by hemodialysis and peritoneal dialysis

Usual Dosage Oral:

Children <6 years: Initial: 15 mg/kg/day in 2 divided doses (maximum dose: 250 mg/dose); increase every 4-7 days; usual maintenance dose: 15-40 mg/kg/day in 2 divided doses; maximum dose: 1.5 g/day

Children >6 years and Adults: Initial: 250 mg twice daily; increase by 250 mg/day as needed every 4-7 days up to 1.5 g/day in 2 divided doses; usual maintenance dose: 20-40 mg/kg/day in 2 divided doses

Administration Oral: Administer with food or milk to decrease GI upset

Monitoring Parameters Seizure frequency, trough serum concentrations; CBC with differential, platelets, liver enzymes, urinalysis, renal function

Reference Range

Therapeutic: 40-100 µg/mL (SI: 280-710 µmol/L)

Toxic: >150 µg/mL (SI: >1062 µmol/L)

Patient Information Avoid alcohol; may cause drowsiness and impair ability to perform activities requiring mental alertness or physical coordination; do not discontinue abruptly; notify physician if sore throat or fever occurs

Additional Information Considered to be drug of choice for simple absence seizures

Dosage Forms

Capsule: 250 mg

Syrup: 250 mg/5 mL (473 mL) [contains sodium benzoate; raspberry flavor]

References

Marquardt ED, Ishisaka DY, Batra KK, et al, "Removal of Ethosuximide and Phenobarbital by Peritoneal Dialysis in a Child," *Clin Pharm*, 1992, 11(12):1030-1.

♦ **Ethoxynaphthamido Penicillin** *see* Nafcillin *on page 789*

Ethyl Alcohol (ETH il AL koe hol)

U.S. Brand Names Lavaco® [OTC]

Canadian Brand Names Biobase™; Biobase-G™; Dilusol®; Duonalc®; Duonalc-E® Mild

Synonyms Alcohol; Dehydrated Alcohol Injection; Ethanol; EtOH

Therapeutic Category Antidote, Ethylene Glycol Toxicity; Antidote, Methanol Toxicity; Anti-infective Agent, Topical; Fat Occlusion (Central Venous Catheter), Treatment Agent; Neurolytic

Generic Available Yes

Use Antidote for the treatment of methanol and ethylene glycol intoxication; neurolysis of nerves or ganglia for the relief of intractable, chronic pain in such conditions as inoperable cancer and trigeminal neuralgia (dehydrated alcohol injection); topical anti-infective; treatment of occluded central venous catheters due to lipid deposition from fat emulsion infusion (particularly 3-in-1 admixture)

Pregnancy Risk Factor D (X if used for prolonged periods or in high doses at term)

Contraindications Hypersensitivity to ethyl alcohol; seizure disorder and diabetic coma; subarachnoid injection of dehydrated alcohol in patients receiving anticoagulants

Warnings Ethanol is a flammable liquid and should be kept cool and away from any heat source; proper positioning of the patient for neurolytic administration is essential to control localization of the injection of dehydrated alcohol (which is hypobaric) into the subarachnoid space; avoid extravasation; not for S.C. administration; do not administer simultaneously with blood due to the possibility of pseudoagglutination or hemolysis; may potentiate severe hypoprothrombic bleeding; clinical evaluation and periodic lab determinations, including serum ethanol levels, are necessary to monitor effectiveness, changes in electrolyte concentrations, and acid-base balance (when used as an antidote)

Precautions Use with caution in diabetics (alcohol decreases blood sugar), patients with gout, shock, following cranial surgery, and in anticipated postpartum hemorrhage; monitor blood glucose closely, particularly in children as treatment of ingestions is associated with hypoglycemia; avoid extravasation during I.V. administration; ethanol passes freely into breast milk at a level approximately equivalent to maternal serum level; effects on the infant are insignificant until maternal blood level reaches (Continued)

Ethyl Alcohol *(Continued)*

300 mg/dL; minimize dermal exposure of ethanol in infants as significant systemic absorption and toxicity can occur

Adverse Reactions

Cardiovascular: Tachycardia, hypertension, hypotension, arrhythmias, cardiomegaly, angina, CHF, vasodilation, flushing, hypothermia

Central nervous system: Ataxia, dementia, Wernicke-Korsakoff syndrome, amnesia, paranoia, hyperthermia, vertigo, lethargy, sedation, coma, seizures, hallucinations

Endocrine & metabolic: Hypoglycemia, acidosis, hypokalemia, hypomagnesemia, increased serum osmolality

Dermatologic: Dry skin, irritation

Gastrointestinal: Nausea, diarrhea, abdominal pain, dyspepsia, vomiting, GI hemorrhage, anorexia, pancreatitis, hiccups

Hematologic: Porphyria, megaloblastic anemia

Hepatic: Hepatic cirrhosis, fatty degeneration of liver, hepatic steatosis

Local: Phlebitis

Neuromuscular & skeletal: Hypotonia, dysarthria, myopathy, neuropathy (peripheral); postinjection neuritis with persistent pain, hyperesthesia, and paresthesia (after neurolytic use)

Ocular: Eye stinging (from vapors)

Respiratory: Respiratory depression, tachypnea, bronchial irritation

Drug Interactions Increased CNS depressant effects with sedative hypnotic agents, antihistamines, antidepressants, narcotic analgesics, dronabinol, phenothiazines, benzodiazepines, and metoclopramide; disulfiram-like reaction with cephalosporins, chlorpropamide, disulfiram, furazolidone, metronidazole, and procarbazine; increased GI blood loss and bleeding time with aspirin and salicylates; altered glucose metabolism resulting in either hypoglycemic or hyperglycemic effects with insulin, phenformin, and sulfonylureas; increases phenytoin serum levels; increased oral bioavailability of ethyl alcohol with aspirin, ranitidine, cimetidine, and nizatidine; increases theophylline levels

Stability Store at room temperature (see Warnings); do not use unless solution is clear and container is intact

Mechanism of Action Competitively inhibits the oxidation of methanol and ethylene oxide by alcohol dehydrogenase to their more toxic metabolites; as a neurolytic, ethyl alcohol produces injury to tissue cells by producing dehydration and precipitation of protoplasm; when injected in close proximity to nerve cells, it produces neuritis and nerve degeneration

Pharmacokinetics

Distribution: V_d: 0.6 L/kg

Metabolism: Hepatic to acetaldehyde or acetate by alcohol dehydrogenase

Clearance: 10-20 mL/hour

Dialysis: Hemodialysis clearance: 300-400 mL/minute with an ethanol removal rate of 280 mg/minute

Usual Dosage

Absolute ethanol/ethyl alcohol (EtOH):

Treatment of methanol or ethylene glycol ingestion: Children, Adolescents, and Adults:

Loading dose (LD):

Oral: 0.8-1 mL/kg of 95% EtOH or 2 mL/kg of 40% EtOH

I.V.: 8-10 mL/kg of 10% EtOH solution (see Administration), not to exceed 200 mL

Modified loading dose (if ingestion consists of both EtOH **and** methanol or ethylene glycol): The loading dose is reduced in a proportional manner related to the measured EtOH blood level by multiplying the calculated loading dose described above by the following factor:

$$\text{LD} \times \left[\frac{100 - (\text{patient's serum ethanol level in mg/dL})}{100} \right]$$

Maintenance dose:

	Non-Drinker	Average Drinker	Chronic Drinker
EtOH dosage by weight	66 mg/kg/h	110 mg/kg/h	154 mg/kg/h
Oral: 40% EtOH	0.2 mL/kg/h	0.3 mL/kg/h	0.4 mL/kg/h
Oral: 95% EtOH	0.1 mL/kg/h	0.15 mL/kg/h	0.2 mL/kg/h
I.V.: 10% EtOH	0.8 mL/kg/h	1.4 mL/kg/h	2 mL/kg/h

Note: Continue therapy until methanol or ethylene glycol blood level <10 mg/dL

Dosage adjustment for hemodialysis: Increase maintenance dosage by 150 mg/kg/h during hemodialysis

Treatment of fat occlusion of central venous catheters: Children and Adults: I.V. (see institutional-based protocol for catheter clearance assessment, the following assessment is a general methodology): Up to 3 mL of 70% ethanol (maximum 0.55 mL/kg); instill a volume equal to the internal volume of the catheter; may repeat if patency not restored after 30- minute dwell time; if dose repeated, reassess after 4-hour dwell time

Dehydrated alcohol injection: Therapeutic neurolysis (nerve or ganglion block): Adults: Intraneural: Dosage variable depending upon the site of injection, eg, trigeminal neuralgia: 0.05-0.5 mL as a single injection per interspace vs subarachnoid injection: 0.5-1 mL as a single injection per interspace; single doses >1.5 mL are seldom required

Liquid denatured alcohol: Topical: Children and Adults: Apply as needed

Administration

Oral: Dilute ethanol in 6 ounces orange juice and give over 30 minutes

Parenteral: Not for S.C. administration; I.V.: Dilute absolute alcohol for I.V. administration to a final concentration of 5% to 10% v/v in D_5W or $D_{10}W$ (I.V. ethanol is also available commercially in both 5% and 10% solutions; see Dosage Forms); infuse loading dose plus 1 hour of maintenance dosage over 60 minutes; for treatment of occluded central venous catheter, a 70% dilution of ethanol may be made by adding 0.8 mL SWI to 2 mL 98% ethanol; instill with a volume equal to the internal volume of the catheter; assess patency at 30 minutes (or per institutional protocol); may repeat (see Usual Dosage)

Intraneural: Separate needles should be used for each of multiple injections or sites to prevent residual alcohol deposition at sites not intended for tissue destruction; inject slowly after determining proper placement of needle; since dehydrated alcohol is hypobaric when compared with spinal fluid, proper positioning of the patient is essential to control localization of injections into the subarachnoid space

Monitoring Parameters Antidotal therapy: Blood ethanol levels (at the end of the loading dose, every hour until stabilized, and then every 8-12 hours thereafter); blood glucose, electrolytes (including serum magnesium), arterial pH, blood gases, methanol or ethylene glycol blood levels, heart rate, blood pressure

Reference Range

Symptoms associated with serum ethanol levels:

Nausea and vomiting: Serum level >100 mg/dL

Coma: Serum level >300 mg/dL

Antidote for methanol/ethylene glycol: Goal range: Blood ethanol level: 100-130 mg/dL (22-28 mmol/liter)

Patient Information May cause drowsiness and impair ability to perform activities requiring mental alertness or physical coordination

Additional Information Eighty-proof spirits contain 40% ethanol

Dosage Forms

Infusion [in D_5W]: 5% alcohol (1000 mL); 10% alcohol (1000 mL)

Injection, absolute: 98% (1 mL, 5 mL)

Injection, dehydrated: 98% (1 mL, 5 mL)

Liquid, topical, denatured (Lavacol®): 70% (473 mL)

References

Chernow B, ed, "Poisoning", *Essentials of Critical Care Pharmacology*, 2nd ed, Baltimore: Williams & Wilkins, 1994, 501-29.

Pennington CR and Pithie AD, "Ethanol Lock in the Management of Catheter Occlusion", *JPEN J Parenter Enteral Nutr*, 1987, 11(5):507-8.

Poisoning and Drug Overdose, 2nd ed, Olson KR, ed, Norwalk, Connecticut: Appleton and Lange, 1994, 339-40.

Werlin SL, Lausten T, Jessens, et al, "Treatment of Central Venous Catheter Occlusions With Ethanol and Hydrochloric Acid", *JPEN J Parenter Enteral Nutr*, 1995, 19(5):416-8.

♦ **Ethyl Aminobenzoate** *see Benzocaine on page 163*

♦ **Ethyol®** *see Amifostine on page 75*

♦ **Etibi® (Can)** *see Ethambutol on page 462*

Etidronate Disodium (e ti DROE nate dye SOW dee um)

U.S. Brand Names Didronel®

Synonyms EHDP; Sodium Etidronate

Therapeutic Category Antidote, Hypercalcemia; Bisphosphonate Derivative

(Continued)

Etidronate Disodium *(Continued)*

Generic Available No

Use Symptomatic treatment of Paget's disease of bone and prevention and treatment of heterotopic ossification following spinal cord injury or total hip replacement; hypercalcemia associated with malignancy

Pregnancy Risk Factor C

Contraindications Hypersensitivity to biphosphonates or any component; clinically overt osteomalacia

Precautions Use with caution in patients with restricted calcium and vitamin D intake; I.V. form may be nephrotoxic and should be used with caution, if at all, in patients with impaired renal function; dosage modification required in renal impairment; hyperphosphatemia may occur at doses of 10-20 mg/kg/day; monitor serum phosphate closely

Adverse Reactions Generally dose-related and most significant when taking oral doses >5 mg/kg/day

Central nervous system: Fever, convulsions, pain

Dermatologic: Angioedema, rash

Endocrine & metabolic: Hyperphosphatemia, hypocalcemia, hypomagnesemia, fluid overload

Gastrointestinal: Diarrhea, nausea, vomiting, occult blood in stools, dysgeusia

Neuromuscular & skeletal: Bone pain, increased risk of fractures, rachitic syndrome (found in children taking dosage >10 mg/kg/day over 1 year or longer)

Renal: Nephrotoxicity

Miscellaneous: Hypersensitivity reactions

Drug Interactions May increase warfarin effects

Stability When diluted in 250 mL NS, solutions are stable 48 hours at room temperature

Mechanism of Action Decreases bone resorption by inhibiting osteocystic osteolysis; decreases mineral release and matrix or collagen breakdown in bone

Pharmacodynamics

Onset of therapeutic effects: Within 1-3 months of therapy

Duration: Persists for 12 months without continuous therapy

Pharmacokinetics

Absorption: Dependent upon dose administered

Half-life: 8.7 hours (range: 6.9-10 hours)

Elimination: Primarily as unchanged drug in urine with unabsorbed drug eliminated in feces

Usual Dosage

Children and Adults: Heterotopic ossification with spinal cord injury: Oral: 20 mg/kg once daily (or in divided doses if GI discomfort occurs) for 2 weeks, then 10 mg/kg/day for 10 weeks (**Note:** This dosage has been used in children, however, treatment >1 year has been associated with a rachitic syndrome)

Adults:

Paget's disease: Oral: 5-10 mg/kg once daily for no more than 6 months; may give 11-20 mg/kg/day for up to 3 months. Daily dose may be divided if adverse GI effects occur; courses of therapy should be separated by drug-free periods of at least 3 months.

Hypercalcemia associated with malignancy:

I.V.: 7.5 mg/kg once daily for 3 days, may be continued up to 7 days if necessary; courses of therapy should be separated by at least 7 drug-free days

Oral: Start 20 mg/kg once daily (or in divided doses if GI discomfort occurs) on the last day of infusion and continue for 30-90 days

Dosing adjustment in renal impairment:

S_{cr} 2.5-4.9 mg/dL: Use with caution

S_{cr} ≥5 mg/dL: **Not recommended**

Administration

Oral: Administer on an empty stomach, 2 hours before meals; avoid giving foods/supplements with calcium, iron, or magnesium within 2 hours of drug

Parenteral: I.V.: Dilute in a minimum volume of 250 mL NS; infuse over at least 2 hours

Monitoring Parameters Serum calcium, phosphate, creatinine, BUN

Patient Information Maintain adequate intake of calcium and vitamin D

Dosage Forms

Injection, solution: 50 mg/mL (6 mL)

Tablet: 200 mg, 400 mg

♦ **EtOH** *see* Ethyl Alcohol *on page 465*

Etoposide (e toe POE side)

Related Information

Emetogenic Potential of Single Chemotherapeutic Agents *on page 1286*

U.S. Brand Names Toposar®; VePesid®

Synonyms Epipodophyllotoxin; VP-16; VP-16-213

Therapeutic Category Antineoplastic Agent, Mitotic Inhibitor

Generic Available Yes

Use Treatment of testicular and lung carcinomas, malignant lymphoma, Hodgkin's disease, leukemias (ALL, ANLL, AML), neuroblastoma; treatment of Ewing's sarcoma, rhabdomyosarcoma, osteosarcoma, Wilms' tumor, brain tumors; conditioning regimen with hematopoietic stem cell support

Pregnancy Risk Factor D

Contraindications Hypersensitivity to etoposide or any component (see Warnings); pregnancy

Warnings The FDA currently recommends that procedures for proper handling and disposal of antineoplastic agents be considered. Etoposide is mutagenic, potentially carcinogenic, teratogenic, and embryotoxic. Severe myelosuppression with resulting infection or bleeding may occur; injectable etoposide contains polysorbate 80 (polysorbate 80 has caused thrombocytopenia, ascites, and renal, pulmonary, and hepatic failure in premature infants who received an injectable vitamin E product containing polysorbate 80). Higher rates of anaphylactoid reactions have been reported in children who received I.V. infusions of etoposide at higher than recommended concentrations

Etoposide injection contains benzyl alcohol which may cause allergic reactions in susceptible individuals; large amounts of benzyl alcohol (≥99 mg/kg/day) have been associated with a potentially fatal toxicity ("gasping syndrome") in neonates; the "gasping syndrome" consists of metabolic acidosis, respiratory distress, gasping respirations, CNS dysfunction (including convulsions, intracranial hemorrhage), hypotension and cardiovascular collapse; use etoposide injection containing benzyl alcohol with caution in neonates; *in vitro* and animal studies have shown that benzoate, a metabolite of benzyl alcohol, displaces bilirubin from protein binding sites

Precautions Use with caution and consider dosage reduction in patients with hepatic impairment, bone marrow suppression, and renal impairment

Adverse Reactions

Cardiovascular: Hypotension, tachycardia, facial flushing

Central nervous system: Somnolence, fatigue, fever, headache, chills

Dermatologic: Alopecia, rash, urticaria, angioedema

Gastrointestinal: Nausea, vomiting, diarrhea, mucositis, anorexia, constipation

Hematologic: Myelosuppression, anemia (granulocyte nadir: ~7-14 days, platelet nadir: ~9-16 days)

Hepatic: Hepatotoxicity

Local: Thrombophlebitis

Neuromuscular & skeletal: Peripheral neuropathy, weakness

Respiratory: Bronchospasm

Miscellaneous: Anaphylactoid reactions

Drug Interactions Cytochrome P450 isoenzyme CYP3A3/4 substrate

Cyclosporine may increase the plasma levels of etoposide

Food Interactions Administration of food does not affect GI absorption with doses ≤200 mg

Stability Stability of diluted injection is concentration dependent (ie, 0.2 mg/mL: 96 hours; 0.4 mg/mL: 48 hours; 1 mg/mL: 2 hours; 2 mg/mL: 1 hour); at a concentration of 1 mg/mL in NS or D_5W, crystallization has occurred within 30 minutes; **incidence of precipitation increases when final infusion concentration is >0.4 mg/mL;** intact vials remain stable for 2 years at room temperature; refrigerate capsules

Mechanism of Action Inhibits mitotic activity; inhibits DNA type II topoisomerase producing single- and double-strand DNA breaks

Pharmacokinetics

Absorption: Oral: Large variability

Distribution: CSF concentration is <5% of plasma concentration

Children V_{dss}: 10 L/m^2

Adults: V_{dss}: 7-17 L/m^2

Protein binding: 94% to 97%

Metabolism: In the liver (with a biphasic decay)

Bioavailability: Averages 50% (range: 10% to 80%, dose-dependent)

Half-life, terminal:

Children: 6-8 hours

Adults: 4-15 hours with normal renal and hepatic function

Time to peak serum concentration: Oral: Within 1-1.5 hours

(Continued)

Etoposide *(Continued)*

Elimination: Both unchanged drug and metabolites are excreted in urine and a small amount (2% to 16%) in feces; up to 55% of an I.V. dose is excreted unchanged in urine in children

Usual Dosage Refer to individual protocols

Children: I.V.: 60-150 mg/m^2/day for 2-5 days every 3-6 weeks

AML:

Remission induction: 150 mg/m^2/day for 2-3 days for 2-3 cycles

Intensification or consolidation: 250 mg/m^2/day for 3 days, on courses 2-5

Brain tumor: 150 mg/m^2/day on days 2 and 3 of treatment course

Neuroblastoma: 100 mg/m^2/day over 1 hour on days 1-5 of cycle; repeat cycle every 4 weeks

High-dose conditioning regimen for allogeneic BMT: 60 mg/kg/dose as a single dose

BMT conditioning regimen used in patients with rhabdomyosarcoma or neuroblastoma: I.V. continuous infusion: 160 mg/m^2/day for 4 days

Adults:

Testicular cancer: I.V.: 50-100 mg/m^2/day on days 1-5 or 100 mg/m^2/day on days 1, 3 and 5 every 3-4 weeks for 3-4 courses

Small cell lung cancer:

Oral: Twice the I.V. dose rounded to the nearest 50 mg given once daily if total dose ≤400 mg/day or in divided doses if >400 mg/day

I.V.: 35 mg/m^2/day for 4 days or 50 mg/m^2/day for 5 days every 3-4 weeks

Dosing adjustment in renal impairment:

Cl$_{cr}$ 10-50 mL/minute: Administer 75% of normal dose

Cl$_{cr}$ <10 mL/minute: Administer 50% of normal dose

Dosing adjustment in patients with elevated serum bilirubin: Reduce dose by 50% for bilirubin 1.5-3 mg/dL; reduce dose by 75% for bilirubin >3 mg/dL

Administration

Oral: If necessary, the injection may be used for oral administration. Mix with orange juice, apple juice, or lemonade at a final concentration not to exceed 0.4 mg/mL to prevent precipitation. Etoposide has been found to be stable with no loss of potency over 3 hours when administered in apple juice or lemonade at concentrations of 1 mg/mL.

Parenteral: I.V.: Do not administer by rapid I.V. injection or by intrathecal, intraperitoneal, or intrapleural routes due to possible severe toxicity. Administer by continuous I.V. infusion or I.V. intermittent infusion via an in-line 0.22 micron filter over at least 60 minutes at a rate not to exceed 100 mg/m^2/hour (or 3.3 mg/kg/hour) to minimize the risk of hypotensive reactions at a final concentration for administration of 0.2-0.4 mg/mL in NS or D$_5$W. More concentrated I.V. solutions (0.6-1 mg/mL) can be infused but have shorter stability times (see Stability). For high-dose etoposide infusions, undiluted etoposide (20 mg/mL) has been infused as a single dose from a glass syringe via syringe pump through a central venous catheter over 1-4 hours. Problems associated with higher than recommended concentrations of etoposide infusions include cracking of hard plastic in chemo venting pins and infusion lines; inspect infusion solution for particulate matter and plastic devices for cracks and leaks.

Monitoring Parameters CBC with differential and platelet count, hemoglobin, vital signs (blood pressure), bilirubin, liver and renal function tests; inspect solution and tubing for precipitation before and during infusion

Patient Information Notify physician if fever, sore throat, painful/burning urination, extreme fatigue, pain or numbness in extremities, yellowing of eyes or skin, bruising, bleeding or shortness of breath occurs

Nursing Implications Adequate airway and other supportive measures and agents for treating hypotension or anaphylactoid reactions should be present when I.V. etoposide is given

Dosage Forms

Capsule (VePesid®): 50 mg

Injection, solution: 20 mg/mL (5 mL, 25 mL, 50 mL) [contains benzyl alcohol]

Toposar®: 20 mg/mL (5 mL, 10 mL, 25 mL) [contains benzyl alcohol]

VePesid®: 20 mg/mL (5 mL, 7.5 mL, 25 mL, 50 mL) [contains benzyl alcohol]

References

Berg SL, Grisell DL, DeLaney TF, et al, "Principles of Treatment of Pediatric Solid Tumors," *Pediatr Clin North Am*, 1991, 38(2):249-67.

Boos J, Krümpelmann S, Schulze-Westhoff P, et al, "Steady-State Levels and Bone Marrow Toxicity of Etoposide in Children and Infants: Does Etoposide Require Age-Dependent Dose Calculation?" *J Clin Oncol*, 1995, 13(12):2954-60.

Clark PL and Slevin ML, "The Clinical Pharmacology of Etoposide and Teniposide," *Clin Pharmacokinet*, 1987, 12(4):223-52.

Lazarus HM, Creger RJ, and Diaz D, "Simple Method for the Administration of High-Dose Etoposide During Autologous Bone Marrow Transplantation," *Cancer Treat Rep*, 1985, 70(6):819-20.

Nishikawa A, Nakamura Y, Nobori U, et al, "Acute Monocytic Leukemia in Children. Response to VP-16-213 as a Single Agent," Cancer, 1987, 60(9):2146-9.

O'Dwyer PJ, Leyland-Jones B, Alonso MT, et al, "Etoposide (VP-16-213): Current Status of an Active Anticancer Drug," N Engl J Med, 1985, 312(11):692-700.

♦ **Euglucon® (Can)** see GlyBURIDE on page 540

♦ **Eurax®** see Crotamiton on page 316

♦ **Eutectic Mixture of Lidocaine and Prilocaine** see Lidocaine and Prilocaine on page 675

♦ **Eutectic Mixture of Local Anesthetics** see Lidocaine and Prilocaine on page 675

♦ **Evac-u-gen [OTC]** see Senna on page 1014

♦ **Everone® 200 (Can)** see Testosterone on page 1070

♦ **Exact® Acne Medication [OTC]** see Benzoyl Peroxide on page 165

♦ **ex-lax® [OTC]** see Senna on page 1014

♦ **ex-lax® Maximum Strength [OTC]** see Senna on page 1014

♦ **ex-lax® Stool Softener [OTC]** see Docusate on page 402

♦ **Exosurf® Neonatal [DSC]** see Colfosceril [DSC] on page 304

♦ **Exsel® [DSC]** see Selenium Sulfide on page 1013

♦ **Extravasation Treatment** see page 1240

♦ **EZ-Char™ [OTC]** see Charcoal on page 250

♦ **F₃T** see Trifluridine on page 1118

Factor IX Complex (Human) (FAK ter nyne KOM pleks HYU man)

U.S. Brand Names Bebulin® VH; Profilnine® SD; Proplex® T

Therapeutic Category Antihemophilic Agent; Blood Product Derivative

Generic Available No

Use To control bleeding in patients with factor IX deficiency (hemophilia B or Christmas disease); prevention/control of bleeding in hemophilia A patients with inhibitors to factor VIII; Proplex® T is indicated to prevent or control bleeding due to factor VII deficiency

Pregnancy Risk Factor C

Contraindications Liver disease, intravascular coagulation or fibrinolysis

Precautions Use with caution in patients with liver dysfunction; risk of viral transmission is not totally eradicated, prepared from pooled human plasma

Adverse Reactions
Cardiovascular: Flushing
Central nervous system: Somnolence, fever, headache, chills
Dermatologic: Urticaria
Gastrointestinal: Nausea, vomiting
Hematologic: Disseminated intravascular coagulation, thrombosis following high dosages in hemophilia B patients
Neuromuscular & skeletal: Paresthesia
Miscellaneous: Tightness in chest and neck

Drug Interactions Increased risk of thrombosis with aminocaproic acid (some recommend to delay the administration of aminocaproic acid 8 hours after factor IX complex administration)

Stability Store unopened vials in refrigerator; do not freeze; administer within 3 hours after reconstitution; **do not refrigerate after reconstitution**; Profilnine® SD: May store unopened vials at room temperature (<30°C) for up to 3 months

Mechanism of Action Replaces deficient clotting factors including factors II, VII, IX, and X

Pharmacokinetics Cleared rapidly from the serum in two phases
Half-life:
First phase: 4-6 hours
Terminal: 22.5 hours

Usual Dosage Dose is expressed in terms of factor IX units; dose must be individualized; **Note:** 1 unit/kg raises factor IX levels 1%

Children and Adults: I.V.:
Factor IX deficiency: Hospitalized patients: 20-50 international units/kg/dose; may be higher in special cases; may be given every 24 hours or more often in special cases
Factor VIII inhibitor patients: 75-100 international units/kg/dose; may be given every 6-12 hours

Administration Parenteral: I.V. administration only; rate of administration should be individualized for patient's comfort; maximum rates of administration: Bebulin® VH: 2 mL/minute; Profilnine® SD: 10 mL/minute; Proplex® T: 3 mL/minute; use filter needle

(Continued)

Factor IX Complex (Human) *(Continued)*

to draw product into syringe; visually inspect for particulate matter and discoloration prior to administration whenever permitted by solution or container

Monitoring Parameters Levels of factors II, IX, and X; signs/symptoms of bleeding; hemoglobin, hematocrit

Reference Range Patients with severe hemophilia will have factor IX levels <1%, often undetectable. Moderate forms of the disease have levels of 1% to 10% while some mild cases may have 11% to 49% of normal factor IX. Plasma concentration is about 4 mg/L.

Additional Information AlphaNine® SD and Mononine® contain only factor IX and should not be confused with factor IX **complex**

Dosage Forms Note: Exact potency labeled on each vial

Injection, powder for reconstitution, lyophilized:
Bebulin® VH: [Single dose vial; vapor heated]
Profilnine® SD: [Single dose vial; solvent detergent treated]
Proplex® T: [Single dose vial]

References
Lusher JM, "Thrombogenicity Associated With Factor IX Complex Concentrates," *Semin Hematol*, 1991, 28(3 Suppl 6):3-5.
Shord SS and Lindley CM, "Coagulation Products and Their Uses," *Am J Health Syst Pharm*, 2000, 57(15):1403-20.

* **Factor VIII** *see* Antihemophilic Factor (Human) *on page 116*
* **Factor VIII (Recombinant)** *see* Antihemophilic Factor (Recombinant) *on page 119*
* **Factrel®** *see* Gonadorelin *on page 547*

Famciclovir *(fam SYE kloe veer)*

U.S. Brand Names Famvir®

Therapeutic Category Antiviral Agent, Oral

Generic Available No

Use Management of acute herpes zoster (shingles); treatment or suppression of recurrent genital herpes in the immunocompetent; treatment of recurrent mucocutaneous herpes simplex infections in HIV patients

Pregnancy Risk Factor B

Contraindications Hypersensitivity to famciclovir, penciclovir, or any component

Precautions Use with caution and decrease dose in patients with renal dysfunction; dosage adjustment may be needed in patients with poorly compensated hepatic impairment

Adverse Reactions
Central nervous system: Headache, fatigue, dizziness, fever, somnolence
Dermatologic: Pruritus, rash
Gastrointestinal: Nausea, diarrhea, vomiting, constipation, anorexia, abdominal pain
Neuromuscular & skeletal: Rigors, paresthesia

Drug Interactions Probenecid may increase penciclovir serum concentrations

Food Interactions Rate of absorption and/or conversion to penciclovir and peak concentration are reduced with food, but bioavailability is not affected

Mechanism of Action Synthetic guanine derivative, prodrug for penciclovir; penciclovir has inhibitory activity against varicella zoster virus (VZV) and herpes simplex virus type 1 and 2 (HSV 1 and HSV 2); penciclovir is converted to penciclovir monophosphate (by viral thymidine kinase in VZV-, HSV 1-, and HSV 2-infected cells), then to penciclovir triphosphate which competes with deoxyguanosine triphosphate for viral DNA polymerase and incorporation into viral DNA; therefore, inhibits DNA synthesis and viral replication

Pharmacokinetics Penciclovir:
Absorption: Rapid
Distribution: V_{dss}: Healthy adults: 73-85 L
Protein binding: <20%
Metabolism: Famciclovir is a prodrug which is metabolized via deacetylation and oxidation in the intestinal wall and liver to penciclovir (active) during extensive first-pass metabolism
Bioavailability: 72% to 83%
Half-life:
Serum: 2-3 hours; increased with renal dysfunction
Mean half-life, terminal:
Cl_{cr} >80 mL/minute: 2.15 hours
Cl_{cr} 60-80 mL/minute: 2.47 hours
Cl_{cr} 30-59 mL/minute: 3.87 hours
Cl_{cr} <29 mL/minute: 9.85 hours

Intracellular penciclovir triphosphate: HSV 1: 10 hours; HSV 2: 20 hours; VZV: 7 hours

Time to peak serum concentration: ~1 hour

Elimination: Primary route is the kidney with 73% excreted in urine (predominantly as penciclovir) and 27% in feces; penciclovir undergoes tubular secretion; requires dosage adjustment with renal impairment

Usual Dosage Oral:

Adolescents (AAP, 2000):

Genital herpes infection: 750 mg/day in 3 divided doses for 7-10 days

Episodic recurrent genital herpes infection: 250 mg/day in 2 divided doses for 5 days

Daily suppressive therapy: 250-500 mg/day in 2 divided doses for 1 year; then reassess for recurrence of herpes infection

Adults:

Herpes zoster: 500 mg every 8 hours for 7 days; initiate as soon as diagnosed; initiation of therapy within 48 hours of rash onset may be more beneficial; no efficacy data available for treatment initiated >72 hours after onset of rash

Recurrent genital herpes: 125 mg twice daily for 5 days; initiate at first sign or symptom; efficacy is not established if treatment is started >6 hours after onset of lesions or symptoms

Suppression of recurrent genital herpes: 250 mg twice daily for up to 1 year

HIV patients with recurrent orolabial or genital herpes: 500 mg twice daily for 7 days

Dosing interval in renal impairment: Adults:

Herpes zoster:

Cl_{cr} ≥60 mL/minute: Administer 500 mg every 8 hours

Cl_{cr} 40-59 mL/minute: Administer 500 mg every 12 hours

Cl_{cr} 20-39 mL/minute: Administer 500 mg every 24 hours

Cl_{cr} <20 mL/minute: Administer 250 mg every 24 hours

Patients on hemodialysis: Administer 250 mg after each dialysis

Recurrent genital herpes:

Cl_{cr} ≥40 mL/minute: Administer 125 mg every 12 hours

Cl_{cr} 20-39 mL/minute: Administer 125 mg every 24 hours

Cl_{cr} <20 mL/minute: Administer 125 mg every 24 hours

Patients on hemodialysis: Administer 125 mg after each dialysis

Suppression of recurrent genital herpes:

Cl_{cr} ≥40 mL/minute: Administer 250 mg every 12 hours

Cl_{cr} 20-39 mL/minute: Administer 125 mg every 12 hours

Cl_{cr} <20 mL/minute: Administer 125 mg every 24 hours

Patients on hemodialysis: Administer 125 mg after each dialysis

Recurrent orolabial or genital herpes in HIV infected patients:

Cl_{cr} ≥40 mL/minute: Administer 500 mg every 12 hours

Cl_{cr} 20-39 mL/minute: Administer 500 mg every 24 hours

Cl_{cr} <20 mL/minute: Administer 250 mg every 24 hours

Patients on hemodialysis: Administer 250 mg after each dialysis

Administration Oral: May be administered without regard to meals; may be administered with food to decrease GI upset

Monitoring Parameters Resolution of rash

Patient Information Famciclovir is not a cure for genital herpes

Dosage Forms Tablet: 125 mg, 250 mg, 500 mg

References

Boike SC, Pue MA, and Freed MI, "Pharmacokinetics of Famciclovir in Subjects With Varying Degrees of Renal Impairment," *Clin Pharmacol Ther*, 1994, 55(4):418-26.

Pickering LK, ed, *2000 Red Book, Report of the Committee on Infectious Diseases*, 25th ed, Elk Grove Village IL: American Academy of Pediatrics, 2000, 676.

Famotidine (fa MOE ti deen)

Related Information

Carbohydrate and Alcohol Content of Liquid Medications for Use in Patients Receiving Ketogenic Diets *on page 1431*

U.S. Brand Names Pepcid®; Pepcid® AC [OTC]

Canadian Brand Names Apo®-Famotidine; Gen-Famotidine; Novo-Famotidine; Nu-Famotidine; ratio-Famotidine; Rhoxal-famotidine; Riva-Famotidine

Therapeutic Category Gastrointestinal Agent, Gastric or Duodenal Ulcer Treatment; Histamine H_2 Antagonist

Generic Available Yes (tablets, injection)

Use Short-term therapy and treatment of duodenal ulcer, gastric ulcer, control gastric pH in critically ill patients, symptomatic relief in gastritis, gastroesophageal reflux disease (GERD), active benign ulcer, and pathological hypersecretory conditions; over-the-counter (OTC) formulation for use in the relief of heartburn, acid indigestion, and sour stomach

(Continued)

Famotidine *(Continued)*

Pregnancy Risk Factor B

Contraindications Hypersensitivity to famotidine, any component (see Warnings), or other H_2 antagonists

Warnings Use with caution and modify dose in patients with renal impairment. Multidose injection contains benzyl alcohol which may cause allergic reactions in susceptible individuals; large amounts of benzyl alcohol (≥99 mg/kg/day) have been associated with a potentially fatal toxicity ("gasping syndrome") in neonates; the "gasping syndrome" consists of metabolic acidosis, respiratory distress, gasping respirations, CNS dysfunction (including convulsions, intracranial hemorrhage), hypotension and cardiovascular collapse; avoid use of the multidose injection in neonates. The oral suspension contains sodium benzoate; *in vitro* and animal studies have shown that benzoate, a metabolite of benzyl alcohol, displaces bilirubin from protein binding sites; avoid use in neonates.

Precautions Pepcid® chewable tablets contain phenylalanine which should be used with caution in patients with phenylketonuria.

Adverse Reactions

Cardiovascular: Bradycardia, tachycardia, palpitations, hypertension

Central nervous system: Headache, vertigo, anxiety, dizziness, seizures, depression, insomnia, drowsiness, confusion, fever

Dermatologic: Acne, pruritus, urticaria, dry skin, alopecia

Gastrointestinal: Constipation, nausea, vomiting, diarrhea, abdominal discomfort, flatulence, belching, dysgeusia, dry mouth, anorexia

Genitourinary: Impotence

Hematologic: Thrombocytopenia, pancytopenia, leukopenia (rare)

Hepatic: Elevated liver enzymes, hepatomegaly, cholestatic jaundice

Neuromuscular & skeletal: Weakness, arthralgias, paresthesia, muscle cramps

Ocular: Orbital edema

Otic: Ototoxicity, tinnitus

Renal: Elevated BUN and serum creatinine, proteinuria

Respiratory: Bronchospasm

Drug Interactions Decreased absorption of ketoconazole, triamterene, delavirdine, itraconazole, cefpodoxime, cyanocobalamin, indomethacin, melphalan; decreased effect of tolazoline

Food Interactions Limit xanthine-containing foods and beverages

Stability Concentrate for injection must be refrigerated but is stable for 48 hours at room temperature; if concentrated injection is diluted in D_5W or NS it is stable 48 hours at room temperature; commercially available diluted solution in NS is stable at room temperature for 15 months; injection is also compatible with $D_{10}W$, LR injection, 5% bicarbonate injection, and standard parenteral nutrition solutions with electrolytes, multivitamins, and trace minerals; reconstituted oral solution is stable for 30 days at room temperature

Mechanism of Action Competitive inhibition of histamine at H_2-receptors of the gastric parietal cells, which results in inhibition of gastric acid secretion

Pharmacodynamics

Onset of GI effect: Oral, I.V.: Within 1 hour

Maximum effect:

Oral: 1-4 hours

I.V.: 30 minutes to 3 hours

Duration: 10-12 hours

Pharmacokinetics

Distribution: V_d:

Infants:

0-3 months: 1.4-1.8 ± 0.3-0.4 L/kg

>3 to 12 months: 2.3 ± 0.7 L/kg

Children: 2 ± 1.5 L/kg

Adults: 0.94-1.33 L/kg

Protein binding: 15% to 20%

Metabolism: 30% to 35% liver metabolism

Bioavailability: Oral: 40% to 45%

Half-life:

Infants:

0-3 months: 8.1-10.5 ± 3.5-5.4 hours

>3 to 12 months: 4.5 ± 1.1 hours

Children: 3.3 ± 2.5 hours

Adults: 2.5-3.5 hours; increases with renal impairment; if Cl_{cr} <10 mL/minute, half-life ≥20 hours

Anuria: 24 hours

Elimination: 65% to 70% unchanged drug in urine

Clearance:
Infants:
0-3 months: 0.13-0.21 ± 0.06 L/hour/kg
>3-12 months: 0.49 ± 0.17 L/hour/kg
Children 1 to 11 years: 0.54 ± 0.34 L/hour/kg
Adults: 0.39 ± 0.14 L/hour/kg

Usual Dosage
Neonates and Infants <3 months: Oral: GERD: 0.5 mg/kg/dose once daily
Infants ≥3 months to 1 year: Oral: GERD: 0.5 mg/kg/dose twice daily
Children 1-16 years: Oral, I.V.:
Peptic ulcer: 0.5 mg/kg/day at bedtime or divided twice daily (maximum: 40 mg/day)
GERD: 1 mg/kg/day divided twice daily (maximum: 80 mg/day)
Adults:
Oral:
Duodenal ulcer, gastric ulcer: 20 mg/day at bedtime for 4-8 weeks (a regimen of 10 mg twice daily is also effective); maximum: 40 mg/day
Hypersecretory conditions: Initial: 20 mg every 6 hours, may increase up to 160 mg every 6 hours
Esophagitis: 20-40 mg twice daily for up to 12 weeks
GERD: 20 mg twice daily for 6 weeks
Acid indigestion, heartburn, or sour stomach (OTC use): 10 mg 15-60 minutes before eating; not more than 2 tablets per day
I.V.: 20 mg every 12 hours

Dosing adjustment in renal impairment:
Cl_{cr} 10-50 mL/minute: Administer normal dose every 24 hours or 50% of dose at normal dosing interval
Cl_{cr} <10 mL/minute: Administer normal dose every 36-48 hours

Administration
Oral: May administer with food and antacids; shake suspension vigorously for 10-15 seconds prior to each use
Parenteral: I.V.: Dilute to a maximum concentration of 4 mg/mL; may be administered I.V. push at 10 mg/minute over 2 minutes or as an infusion over 15-30 minutes

Patient Information Avoid excessive amounts of coffee and aspirin; when self medicating, if the symptoms of heartburn, acid indigestion, or sour stomach persist after 2 weeks of continuous use of the drug, consult a clinician.

Dosage Forms
Capsule, gelatin (Pepcid® AC): 10 mg
Infusion [premixed in NS] (Pepcid®): 20 mg (50 mL)
Injection, solution (Pepcid®): 10 mg/2 mL (4 mL, 20 mL) [contains benzyl alcohol]
Injection, solution [preservative free] (Pepcid®): 10 mg/2 mL (2 mL)
Powder for oral suspension (Pepcid®): 40 mg/5 mL (50 mL) [contains sodium benzoate; cherry-banana-mint flavor]
Tablet, chewable (Pepcid® AC): 10 mg [contains 1.4 mg phenylalanine (as aspartame); mint flavor]
Tablet, film coated: 10 mg [OTC], 20 mg, 40 mg
Pepcid®: 20 mg, 40 mg
Pepcid® AC: 10 mg

Extemporaneous Preparations An 8 mg/mL suspension may be made by crushing seventy 40 mg tablets; work into a paste with a small amount of sterile water; add a 1:1 mixture of Ora-Plus® and Ora-Sweet® to a total volume of 350 mL; stable 95 days at 23°C to 35°C
Dentinger PJ, Swenson CF, and Anaizi NH, "Stability of Famotidine in an Extemporaneously Compounded Oral Liquid," *Am J Health Syst Pharm*, 2000, 57(14):1340-2.

References
James LP and Kearns GL, "Pharmacokinetics and Pharmacodynamics of Famotidine in Paediatric Patients," *Clin Pharmacokinet*, 1996, 31(2):103-10.
Treem WR, Davis PM, and Hyams JS, "Suppression of Gastric Acid Secretion by Intravenous Administration of Famotidine in Children," *J Pediatr*, 1991, 118(5):812-6.

♦ **FAMP** *see* Fludarabine *on page 492*

♦ **Famvir®** *see* Famciclovir *on page 472*

♦ **Fansidar®** *see* Sulfadoxine and Pyrimethamine *on page 1051*

♦ **F-ara-AMP** *see* Fludarabine *on page 492*

Fat Emulsion (fat e MUL shun)
Related Information
Parenteral Nutrition (PN) *on page 1262*
U.S. Brand Names Intralipid®; Liposyn® III
(Continued)

Fat Emulsion *(Continued)*

Synonyms Intravenous Fat Emulsion; Lipid Emulsion

Therapeutic Category Caloric Agent; Intravenous Nutritional Therapy

Generic Available No

Use Source of calories and essential fatty acids for patients requiring parenteral nutrition of extended duration

Pregnancy Risk Factor C

Contraindications Hypersensitivity to fat emulsion and severe egg or legume (soybean) allergies; pathologic hyperlipidemia; lipoid nephrosis; pancreatitis with hyperlipemia; 30% fat emulsions are not intended for direct I.V. infusion and dilution with another I.V. fluid (eg, NS does not produce a dilution equivalent to 10% or 20% I.V. fat emulsion); such dilutions should not be administered by direct I.V. infusion (see Additional Information)

Warnings Deaths in preterm neonates after infusion of I.V. fat emulsions have been reported. Autopsy findings included intravascular fat accumulation in the lungs. Use of I.V. fat emulsion in preterm neonates should be done carefully adhering to maximum daily dosages and infusing as slowly as possible (see Usual Dosage). Preterm infants have a decreased ability to eliminate infused fat and must be monitored closely using triglyceride or plasma free fatty acid levels.

Precautions Use with caution in patients with severe liver damage, pulmonary disease, anemia, or blood coagulation disorder, and in jaundiced patients

Adverse Reactions
Cardiovascular: Cyanosis, flushing, chest pain
Central nervous system: Headache, fever, sleepiness, dizziness
Gastrointestinal: Nausea, vomiting
Hematologic: Hypercoagulability, thrombocytopenia, leukopenia
Hepatic: Hyperlipemia, hepatomegaly, jaundice, cholestasis, transient increases in liver enzymes
Local: Thrombophlebitis
Respiratory: Dyspnea
Miscellaneous: Sepsis, hypersensitivity reactions, diaphoresis, splenomegaly, deposition of brown pigment in the reticuloendothelial system (clinical significance is unknown)

Stability May be stored at room temperature; do not use if emulsion appears to be layering out; exposure to light, particularly phototherapy light, used in treatment or prevention of hyperbilirubinemia has been associated with increased lipid oxidation; the clinical significance remains to be established; do not mix other drugs with fat emulsion; only heparin at a concentration of 1-2 units/mL may be added to fat emulsion

Mechanism of Action Fatty acids are essential for normal structure and function of cell membranes; I.V. fat emulsion provides a source of calories and essential fatty acids normally obtained in the enteral diet

Usual Dosage I.V. infusion: Fat emulsion should not exceed 60% of the total daily calories

Note: At the onset of therapy, the patient should be observed for any immediate allergic reactions such as dyspnea, cyanosis, and fever. Slower initial rates of infusion may be used for the first 10-15 minutes of the infusion (eg, 0.1 mL/minute of 10% or 0.05 mL/minute of 20% solution).

Premature infants: Initial dose: 0.25-0.5 g/kg/day, increase by 0.25-0.5 g/kg/day to a maximum of 3-4 g/kg/day; maximum rate of infusion: 0.15 g/kg/hour (0.75 mL/kg/hour of 20% solution) (see Warnings)

Infants and Children: Initial dose: 0.5-1 g/kg/day, increase by 0.5 g/kg/day to a maximum of 3-4 g/kg/day; maximum rate of infusion: 0.25 g/kg/hour (1.25 mL/kg/hour of 20% solution)

Adolescents and Adults: Initial dose: 1 g/kg/day, increase by 0.5-1 g/kg/day to a maximum of 2.5 g/kg/day; maximum rate of infusion: 0.25 g/kg/hour (1.25 mL/kg/hour of 20% solution); do not exceed 50 mL/hour (20%) or 100 mL/hour (10%)

Children and Adults: Fatty acid deficiency: 8% to 10% of total caloric intake; infuse once or twice weekly

Administration Parenteral: 10% and 20% emulsions may be simultaneously infused with amino acid, dextrose mixtures by means of Y-connector located near infusion site into either central or peripheral line; 30% emulsions must not be infused directly (see Contraindications and Additional Information)

Monitoring Parameters Serum triglycerides, free fatty acids, platelets, liver enzymes

Additional Information 10% = 1.1 Kcal/mL, 20% = 2 Kcal/mL, 30% = 3 Kcal/mL; 10% and 20% solutions are isotonic and may be administered peripherally; 30% solution is not intended for direct infusion; it must be diluted to a final concentration not to exceed 20% when added to 3-in-1 or total nutrient admixture; avoid use of 10%

fat emulsion in preterm infants; a greater accumulation of plasma lipids occurs due to the greater phospholipid load of the 10% fat emulsion

Dosage Forms

Injection, emulsion:

Intralipid®: 10% [100 mg/mL] (100 mL, 250 mL, 500 mL); 20% [200 mg/mL] (50 mL, 100 mL, 250 mL, 500 mL, 1000 mL); 30% [300 mg/mL] (500 mL)

Liposyn® III: 10% [100 mg/mL] (200 mL, 500 mL); 20% [200 mg/mL] (200 mL, 500 mL); 30% [300 mg/mL] (500 mL)

References

Haumont D, Richelle M, Deckelbaum RJ, et al, "Effect of Liposomal Content of Lipid Emulsions of Plasma Lipid Concentrations in Low Birth Weight Infants Receiving Parenteral Nutrition," *J Pediatr*, 1992, 121(5 Pt 1):759-63.

Neuzil J, Darlow BA, Inder TE, et al, "Oxidation of Parenteral Lipid Emulsion by Ambient and Photo-therapy Lights: Potential Toxicity of Routine Parenteral Feeding," *J Pediatr*, 1995, 126(5 Pt 1):785-90.

♦ **5-FC** *see Flucytosine on page 491*

Felbamate (FEL ba mate)

Related Information

Antiepileptic Drugs *on page 1374*

Carbohydrate and Alcohol Content of Liquid Medications for Use in Patients Receiving Ketogenic Diets *on page 1431*

U.S. Brand Names Felbatol®

Therapeutic Category Anticonvulsant, Miscellaneous

Generic Available No

Use Not a first-line agent, see Warnings; reserved for patients who do not adequately respond to alternative agents and whose epilepsy is so severe that the benefit outweighs the risk of liver failure or aplastic anemia; used as monotherapy and adjunctive therapy in patients ≥14 years of age with partial seizures with and without secondary generalization; adjunctive therapy in children ≥2 years of age who have partial and generalized seizures associated with Lennox-Gastaut syndrome

Pregnancy Risk Factor C

Contraindications Hypersensitivity to felbamate, any component, or other carbamates (eg, meprobamate); history of or current blood dyscrasia or hepatic dysfunction

Warnings Thirty-three cases of aplastic anemia (with 8 deaths) and 14 cases of hepatic failure (with 8 deaths) have been reported in patients who received felbamate. The manufacturer (Carter Wallace) and the FDA recommend the use of this agent be suspended unless withdrawal of the product would place a patient at greater risk.

Aplastic anemia: Of the 27 cases analyzed by the manufacturer, 26 occurred in adult patients (mean age: 42 years) exposed to felbamate for a mean of 170 days at a mean dose of 3168 mg/day. One case occurred in a 13-year old exposed to felbamate for 276 days at a dose of ~69 mg/kg/day. Twenty-three of 27 patients received other antiepileptic drugs (AEDs) and 9 received drugs associated with blood dyscrasias. The 8 deaths occurred in adults (mean age: 47 years). Six of the 8 patients had a history of blood dyscrasias and 6 had allergies to medications (3 to AEDs). The onset of aplastic anemia ranged from 5-30 weeks.

Hepatic failure: Of the 14 cases, 6 cases occurred in children 3-12 years of age (mean: 6 years) exposed to felbamate for 30-218 days (mean: 115 days) at a mean dose of 1520 mg/day. The overall postmarketing reported rate of hepatic failure leading to transplant or death is 6 cases per 75,000 patient years of use; this rate is underestimated due to under reporting (eg, the true rate could be as high as 1 case per 1250 patient years of use if the reporting rate is only 10%). Approximately 67% of the reported cases of hepatic failure led to liver transplantation or death, usually within 5 weeks of the onset of signs and symptoms of hepatic failure; the earliest onset of severe liver dysfunction was 3 weeks after starting felbamate; in some cases, dark urine and nonspecific prodromal symptoms (eg, malaise, anorexia, GI symptoms) preceded the onset of jaundice.

All patients receiving felbamate **must** be monitored closely; in addition, a CBC with differential and platelet count should be taken before, during, and for a significant time after discontinuing felbamate therapy; liver enzyme tests and bilirubin should be obtained before initiation and periodically during therapy. Felbamate should be immediately withdrawn if abnormal liver function tests or bone marrow suppression occur.

The FDA and the manufacturer strongly recommend that physicians discuss the risks of felbamate with each patient and a written informed consent be obtained from the patient prior to starting therapy or before continuing therapy. A patient information consent form is included as part of the package insert and is available from the local Wallace representative or by calling 609-655-6147.

(Continued)

Felbamate *(Continued)*

Precautions Use with caution in patients concurrently receiving other antiepileptic drugs due to the potential for drug interactions; decrease dosage of phenytoin, carbamazepine, or valproic acid by 20% to 30% when felbamate is added to the regimen and when felbamate doses are titrated upwards; monitor serum levels of concomitant antiepileptic drug therapy. Use with caution and reduce dose in patients with renal dysfunction.

Adverse Reactions

Central nervous system: Headache, insomnia, somnolence, fatigue, dizziness, anxiety, drowsiness, depression, behavior changes, ataxia

Dermatologic: Acne, rash, pruritus

Gastrointestinal: Anorexia, vomiting, nausea, diarrhea, constipation, dyspepsia, gum bleeding or hyperplasia, weight loss

Hematologic: Thrombocytopenia, granulocytopenia, agranulocytosis, purpura, leukopenia, aplastic anemia (100-fold increase in risk; see Warnings)

Hepatic: Elevated liver enzymes, hepatitis, acute liver failure, may be associated with death (see Warnings)

Drug Interactions Cytochrome P450 isoenzyme CYP2C19 inhibitor

Phenytoin, carbamazepine may increase and valproic acid may decrease the clearance of felbamate; felbamate increases the concentrations of phenytoin and valproic acid; felbamate decreases carbamazepine concentrations but increases the concentration of carbamazepine epoxide (active metabolite)

Food Interactions Food does **not** affect absorption

Stability Store in tightly closed container at room temperature away from excessive heat, moisture, or direct sunlight

Mechanism of Action Mechanism of action is unknown but may be similar to other anticonvulsants; has weak inhibitory effects on GABA and benzodiazepine receptor binding; does not have activity at the MK-801 receptor binding site of the NMDA receptor-ionophore complex.

Pharmacokinetics

Absorption: Oral: Rapid and almost complete

Distribution: V_d: Adults: Mean: 0.75 L/kg; range: 0.7-1.1 L/kg

Protein binding: 20% to 25%, primarily to albumin

Metabolism: In the liver via hydroxylation and conjugation

Bioavailability: >90%

Half-life: Adults: Mean: 20-30 hours; shorter (ie, 14 hours) with concomitant enzyme-inducing drugs; half-life is prolonged (by 9-15 hours) in patients with renal dysfunction

Time to peak serum concentration: 1-4 hours

Elimination: 40% to 50% excreted as unchanged drug and 40% as inactive metabolites in urine

Clearance, apparent:

Children 2-9 years: 61.3 ± 8.2 mL/kg/hour

Children 10-12 years: 34.3 ± 4.3 mL/kg/hour

Usual Dosage See Precautions regarding concomitant antiepileptic drugs

Children 2-14 years with Lennox-Gastaut: Adjunctive therapy: Initial: 15 mg/kg/day in 3-4 divided doses; increase dose by 15 mg/kg/day increments at weekly intervals; maximum dose: 45 mg/kg/day or 3600 mg/day (whichever is less)

Children ≥14 years and Adults:

Adjunctive therapy: Initial: 1200 mg/day in 3-4 divided doses; increase daily dose by 1200 mg increments every week to a maximum dose of 3600 mg/day

Conversion to monotherapy: Initial: 1200 mg/day in 3 or 4 divided doses; at week 2, increase daily dose by 1200 mg increments every week up to a maximum dose of 3600 mg/day. Decrease dose of other anticonvulsants by $\frac{1}{3}$ their original dose at initiation of felbamate, and when felbamate dose is increased at week 2; continue to reduce other anticonvulsants as clinically needed.

Monotherapy: Initial: 1200 mg/day in 3 or 4 divided doses; titrate dosage upward according to clinical response and monitor patients closely; increase daily dose in 600 mg increments every 2 weeks to 2400 mg/day; maximum dose: 3600 mg/day

Dosage adjustment in renal impairment: Reduce initial and maintenance doses by 50%

Administration Oral: May be administered without regard to meals; shake suspension well before use

Monitoring Parameters Serum concentrations of concomitant anticonvulsant therapy; liver enzymes, bilirubin, CBC with differential, platelet count prior to therapy and periodically during therapy

Reference Range Not necessary to routinely monitor serum drug levels; dose should be titrated to clinical response; therapeutic range not fully determined; proposed 30-100 µg/mL

Patient Information Do not abruptly discontinue, an increase in seizure activity may result; report any unusual symptoms, such as a rash, bruises, bleeding, sore throat, fever, yellow skin, GI complaints, loss of appetite, tiredness, and/or dark urine to physician immediately

Additional Information Monotherapy has not been associated with gingival hyperplasia, impaired concentration, weight gain, or abnormal thinking; felbamate has also been used in a small number of patients with infantile spasms (see Pellock, 1999); an open-label study in children with refractory partial seizures (n=30; mean age: 9 years; range: 2-17 years) found that children >10 years of age had a more favorable response; this was thought to be related to the higher felbamate serum concentrations (and lower apparent clearance) in children >10 years of age compared to those <10 years; the faster apparent clearance in children <10 years of age should be considered when using this agent (Carmant, 1994)

Dosage Forms

Suspension, oral: 600 mg/5 mL (240 mL, 960 mL)

Tablet: 400 mg, 600 mg

References

Carmant L, Holmes GL, Sawyer S, et al, "Efficacy of Felbamate in Therapy for Partial Epilepsy in Children," *J Pediatr*, 1994, 125(3):481-6.

Dodson WE, "Felbamate in the Treatment of Lennox-Gastaut Syndrome: Results of a 12-Month Open-Label Study Following a Randomized Clinical Trial," *Epilepsia*, 1993, 34(Suppl 7):S18-24.

Leppik IE, "Felbamate," *Epilepsia*, 1995, 36(Suppl 2):S66-72.

Pellock JM, "Managing Pediatric Epilepsy Syndromes With New Antiepileptic Drugs," *Pediatrics*, 1999, 104(5 Pt 1):1106-16.

The Felbamate Study Group in Lennox-Gastaut Syndrome, "Efficacy of Felbamate in Childhood Epileptic Encephalopathy (Lennox-Gastaut Syndrome)," *N Engl J Med*, 1993, 328(1):29-33.

Written Communication, Elisabeth Neumann, Director Medical Services, Wallace Laboratories, June 13, 1995.

- ◆ **Felbatol®** *see* Felbamate *on page 477*
- ◆ **Feldene®** *see* Piroxicam *on page 910*
- ◆ **Femilax™ [OTC]** *see* Bisacodyl *on page 173*
- ◆ **Femizol-M™ [OTC]** *see* Miconazole *on page 759*
- ◆ **Femring™** *see* Estradiol *on page 456*
- ◆ **Fenesin™ [OTC] [DSC]** *see* Guaifenesin *on page 550*
- ◆ **Fenesin™ DM** *see* Guaifenesin and Dextromethorphan *on page 553*

Fentanyl (FEN ta nil)

Related Information

Adult ACLS Algorithm, Synchronized Cardioversion *on page 1192*
Compatibility of Medications Mixed in a Syringe *on page 1412*
Narcotic Analgesics Comparison *on page 1223*
Overdose and Toxicology *on page 1388*
Preprocedure Sedatives in Children *on page 1367*
Serotonin Syndrome *on page 1420*

U.S. Brand Names Actiq®; Duragesic®; Sublimaze®

Therapeutic Category Analgesic, Narcotic; General Anesthetic

Generic Available Yes (injection)

Use Sedation; relief of pain; preoperative medication; adjunct to general or regional anesthesia; management of chronic pain (transdermal product)

Oral transmucosal: Actiq®: Breakthrough cancer pain in adult patients tolerant to opioid therapy and who are currently receiving opiates for persistent cancer pain. Patients are considered opioid tolerant if they are receiving at least 60 mg/day of morphine, 50 mcg/hour of transdermal fentanyl, or an equivalent dose of another opioid for 1 week or longer.

Restrictions C-II

Pregnancy Risk Factor C (D if used for prolonged periods or in high doses at term)

Contraindications Hypersensitivity or intolerance to fentanyl or any component; transdermal system is contraindicated in patients with hypersensitivity to contact adhesives; increased intracranial pressure; severe respiratory depression; severe liver or renal insufficiency; Actiq® is contraindicated in patients who are not opioid tolerant and in the treatment of acute or postoperative pain.

Warnings Physical and psychological dependence may occur with prolonged use; abrupt discontinuation may result in withdrawal or seizures. Symptoms of opioid withdrawal may occur in patients after conversion of one dosage form to another or after dosage adjustment.

I.V. use: Rapid I.V. infusion may result in skeletal muscle and chest wall rigidity, impaired ventilation, respiratory distress, apnea, bronchoconstriction, laryngospasm; inject slowly over 3-5 minutes; nondepolarizing skeletal muscle relaxant may be required

(Continued)

Fentanyl *(Continued)*

Actiq®: Use only for the care of cancer patients; should be used only by specialists who are knowledgeable in treating cancer pain; keep out of the reach of children and discard any open units properly; contains an amount of medication that can be fatal to children

Precautions Use with caution in patients with bradycardia, hepatic, renal, or respiratory disease or those with increased ICP, head injuries, or impaired consciousness; patients must be monitored until fully recovered; decrease dose in patients with hepatic and/or renal disease; not recommended if patient received MAO inhibitors within 14 days; use of transdermal system is not recommended in children <12 years or those <18 years who weigh <50 kg; frequent use of Actiq® may increase risk of dental caries; Actiq® contains 2 g of sugar/unit; inform diabetic patients of sugar content

Adverse Reactions

Cardiovascular: Hypotension, bradycardia, flushing

Central nervous system: CNS depression, drowsiness, dizziness, sedation, euphoria

Dermatologic: Erythema, pruritus, facial pruritus with oral transmucosal product

Endocrine & metabolic: ADH release

Gastrointestinal: Nausea, vomiting, constipation, biliary tract spasm

Genitourinary: Urinary tract spasm

Local: Transdermal system: Edema, erythema, pruritus

Neuromuscular & skeletal: Skeletal muscle and chest wall rigidity especially following rapid I.V. administration

Ocular: Miosis

Respiratory: Respiratory depression, apnea

Miscellaneous: Physical and psychological dependence with prolonged use. **Note:** Neonates who receive a total fentanyl dose >1.6 mg/kg or continuous infusion duration >5 days are more likely to develop narcotic withdrawal symptoms; children 1 week to 22 months: those who receive a total dose of 1.5 mg/kg or duration >5 days have a 50% chance of developing narcotic withdrawal and those receiving a total dose >2.5 mg/kg or duration of infusion >9 days have a 100% chance of developing withdrawal. Doses should be tapered to prevent withdrawal symptoms.

Drug Interactions Cytochrome P450 isoenzyme CYP3A3/4 substrate

CNS depressants, alcohol, phenothiazines, MAO inhibitors, tricyclic antidepressants may potentiate fentanyl's adverse effects. Cytochrome P450 inhibitors (eg, erythromycin, ketoconazole, protease inhibitors) may increase or prolong the clinical or adverse effects of fentanyl; cytochrome P450 inducers (eg, carbamazepine, phenytoin, rifampin) may decrease the effect of fentanyl; close monitoring and dosage adjustment may be needed. The herbal medicine St John's wort (*Hypericum perforatum*) may increase serious side effects, its use is **not** recommended

Stability Protect from light

Mechanism of Action Binds with stereospecific opioid mu receptors at many sites within the CNS, increases pain threshold, alters pain reception, inhibits ascending pain pathways

Pharmacodynamics Respiratory depressant effect may last longer than analgesic effect

Onset of action: Analgesia:

I.M.: 7-15 minutes

I.V.: Almost immediate

Transdermal: 6-8 hours

Transmucosal: 5-15 minutes

Maximum effect:

Transdermal: 24 hours

Transmucosal: 20-30 minutes

Duration:

I.M.: 1-2 hours

I.V.: 30-60 minutes

Transdermal: 72 hours

Transmucosal: 1-2 hours

Pharmacokinetics

Absorption: Transmucosal: Rapid; ~25% absorbed from buccal mucosa; 75% swallowed with saliva and slowly absorbed from GI tract

Distribution: Highly lipophilic, redistributes into muscle and fat

V_d: Adults: 4 L/kg

V_{dss}: Children: 0.05-14 years of age (after long-term continuous infusion): ~15 L/kg (range: 5-30 L/kg)

Protein binding: 80% to 85%, primarily to alpha-1-acid glycoprotein

Metabolism: >90% metabolized in the liver via N-dealkylation (to norfentanyl) and hydroxylation to other inactive metabolites

Bioavailability: Transmucosal: ~50% (range: 36% to 71%)

Half-life:

  Children 5 months to 4.5 years: Mean: 2.4 hours

  Children 0.5-14 years (after long-term continuous infusion): ~21 hours (range: 11-36 hours)

  Adults: I.V.: 2-4 hours

    Transdermal: 17 hours (range: 13-22); apparent half-life increased with transdermal due to continued absorption

    Transmucosal: 6.6 hours (range: 5-15 hours)

Elimination: In urine primarily as metabolites and <10% as unchanged drug

  Clearance: Newborn infants: Clearance may be significantly correlated to gestational age and birth weight (see Saarenmaa, 2000)

Usual Dosage Doses should be titrated to appropriate effects; wide range of doses, dependent upon desired degree of analgesia/anesthesia, clinical environment, and patient's status

Neonates: Analgesia: International Evidence-Based Group for Neonatal Pain recommendations (Anand, 2001):

  Intermittent doses: Slow I.V. push: 0.5-3 mcg/kg/dose

  Continuous infusion: 0.5-2 mcg/kg/hour

Neonates and younger Infants:

  Sedation/analgesia: Slow I.V. push: 1-4 mcg/kg/dose; may repeat every 2-4 hours

  Continuous sedation/analgesia: Initial I.V. bolus: 1-2 mcg/kg, then 0.5-1 mcg/kg/hour; titrate upward

    Mean required dose: Neonates with gestational age <34 weeks: 0.64 mcg/kg/hour; neonates with gestational age ≥34 weeks: 0.75 mcg/kg/hour

  Continuous sedation/analgesia during ECMO: Initial I.V. bolus: 5-10 mcg/kg slow I.V. push over 10 minutes, then 1-5 mcg/kg/hour; titrate upward; tolerance may develop; higher doses (up to 20 mcg/kg/hour) may be needed by day 6 of ECMO

Older Infants and Children 1-12 years:

  Sedation for minor procedures/analgesia: I.M., I.V.: 1-2 mcg/kg/dose; may repeat at 30- to 60-minute intervals. **Note:** Children 18-36 months of age may require 2-3 mcg/kg/dose.

  Continuous sedation/analgesia: Initial I.V. bolus: 1-2 mcg/kg then 1 mcg/kg/hour; titrate upward; usual: 1-3 mcg/kg/hour; some require 5 mcg/kg/hour

  Transdermal: Not recommended

Children >12 years and Adults:

  Sedation for minor procedures/analgesia: I.V.: 0.5-1 mcg/kg/dose; may repeat after 30-60 minutes; **or** 25-50 mcg, repeat full dose in 5 minutes if needed, may repeat 4-5 times with 25 mcg at 5-minute intervals if needed. **Note:** Higher doses are used for major procedures.

  Preoperative sedation, adjunct to regional anesthesia, postoperative pain: I.M., I.V.: 50-100 mcg/dose

  Adjunct to general anesthesia: I.M., I.V.: 2-50 mcg/kg

  General anesthesia without additional anesthetic agents: I.V. 50-100 mcg/kg with O$_2$ and skeletal muscle relaxant

  Transdermal: Initial: 25 mcg/hour system; use short-acting analgesics for first 24 hours with supplemental PRN doses thereafter; dose may be increased after 3 days; if currently receiving opiates, convert to fentanyl equivalent and administer equianalgesic dosage; (see package insert for further information); transdermal patch is usually administered every 72 hours but select patients may require every 48-hour administration; dosage increase should be tried before 48-hour schedule is used

Actiq®: Breakthrough cancer pain: Transmucosal: Adults: Titrate dose to provide adequate analgesia: Initial: 200 mcg; may repeat dose 15 minutes after completion of first dose if needed; no more than 2 units are recommended for each breakthrough cancer pain episode; titrate dose up to next higher strength if treatment of several consecutive breakthrough episodes requires >1 Actiq® per episode; evaluate each new dose over several breakthrough cancer pain episodes (generally 1-2 days) to determine proper dose of analgesia with acceptable side effects. Once dose has been determined, consumption should be limited to ≤4 units per day. Re-evaluate long-acting opioid dose if patient requires >4 units/day. If signs of excessive opioid effects occur before a dose is complete, the unit should be removed from the mouth immediately, and subsequent doses decreased.

Dosing adjustment in renal impairment:

  Cl$_{cr}$ 10-50 mL/minute: Administer 75% of dose

  Cl$_{cr}$ <10 mL/minute: Administer 50% of dose

Administration

Transdermal: Apply to nonhairy, dry, nonirritated flat area of front or back of upper torso; do **not** shave area; do not apply new patch to same place as old patch; **Note:** Transdermal patch is a membrane-controlled system; do **not** cut the patch to

(Continued)

Fentanyl (Continued)

deliver partial doses; rate of drug delivery, reservoir contents, and adhesion may be affected if cut; if partial dose is needed, surface area of patch can be blocked proportionally using adhesive bandage (see Lee, 1997); do **not** use soap, alcohol, or other solvents to remove transdermal gel if it accidentally touches skin as they may increase transdermal absorption, use copious amounts of water

Transmucosal: Foil overwrap should be removed just prior to administration; once removed, patient should place the lozenge in mouth and suck it; do not chew lozenge

Actiq®: Place in mouth between cheek and lower gum; occasionally move lozenge from one side of the mouth to the other; consume lozenge over 15 minutes; remove lozenge from mouth if signs of excessive opioid effects appear before lozenge is totally consumed

Parenteral: I.V.: Administer by slow I.V. push over 3-5 minutes or by continuous infusion; larger bolus doses (>5 mcg/kg) should be given slow I.V. push over 5-10 minutes

Monitoring Parameters Respiratory rate, blood pressure, heart rate, oxygen saturation, bowel sounds, abdominal distention

Patient Information Avoid alcohol and the herbal medicine St John's wort; may cause drowsiness and impair ability to perform activities requiring mental alertness or physical coordination; may be habit-forming; avoid abrupt discontinuation after prolonged use; an Actiq® Welcome Kit, containing educational materials and safe storage containers (to keep medication away from children), as well as a patient safety video, is available from the manufacturer; these can be obtained by healthcare professionals who call 1-800-896-5855; dispose of transmucosal and transdermal products properly; keep all products (even if used) out of the reach of children; see Actiq® Patient Leaflet for details on proper storage, administration, and disposal of Actiq®, as well as, instructions about overdose management. Frequent use of Actiq® may increase risk of dental caries; consult dentist for appropriate oral hygiene. Diabetic patients should note that Actiq® contains 2 grams of sugar/unit (about ½ teaspoon of sugar).

Nursing Implications An opioid antagonist, resuscitative and intubation equipment, and oxygen should be available; rapid I.V. injection may result in apnea. Patients with elevated temperature may have increased fentanyl absorption transdermally, observe for adverse effects, dosage adjustment may be needed; pharmacologic and adverse effects can be seen after discontinuation of transdermal system, observe patients for at least 12 hours after transdermal product removed; destroy unused portion of Actiq® according to hospital policy on controlled substances; partial unused doses of Actiq® can be dissolved under hot running tap water; dispose of handle properly

Additional Information Fentanyl is 50-100 times as potent as morphine; morphine 10 mg I.M. = fentanyl 0.1-0.2 mg I.M.; fentanyl has less hypotensive effects than morphine or meperidine due to minimal or no histamine release; keep transmucosal and transdermal products (both used and unused) out of the reach of children; special child-resistant containers are available to temporarily store partially-consumed units that cannot be disposed of immediately

Dosage Forms

Injection, solution, as citrate [preservative free]: 0.05 mg/mL (2 mL, 5 mL, 10 mL, 20 mL, 30 mL, 50 mL)

Sublimaze®: 0.05 mg/mL (2 mL, 5 mL, 10 mL, 20 mL)

Lozenge oral transmucosal, as citrate [mounted on a plastic radiopaque handle] (Actiq®): 200 mcg, 400 mcg, 600 mcg, 800 mcg, 1200 mcg, 1600 mcg [raspberry flavor]

Transdermal system (Duragesic®): 25 mcg/hour [10 cm^2] (5s); 50 mcg/hour [20 cm^2] (5s); 75 mcg/hour [30 cm^2] (5s); 100 mcg/hour [40 cm^2] (5s)

References

Anand KJ and International Evidence-Based Group for Neonatal Pain, "Consensus Statement for the Prevention and Management of Pain in the Newborn," *Arch Pediatr Adolesc Med*, 2001, 155(2):173-80.

Billmire DA, Neale HW, and Gregory RO, "Use of I.V. Fentanyl in the Outpatient Treatment of Pediatric Facial Trauma," *J Trauma*, 1985, 25(11):1079-80.

Katz R, Kelly HW, and Hsi A, "Prospective Study on the Occurrence of Withdrawal in Critically Ill Children Who Receive Fentanyl by Continuous Infusion," *Crit Care Med*, 1994, 22(5):763-7.

Lee NA and Anderson PO, "Giving Partial Doses of Transdermal Patches," *Am J Health Syst Pharm*, 1997, 54(15):1759-60.

Leuschen MP, Willett LD, Hoie EB, et al, "Plasma Fentanyl Levels in Infants Undergoing Extracorporeal Membrane Oxygenation," *J Thorac Cardiovasc Surg*, 1993, 105(5):885-91.

Roth B, Schlunder C, Houben F, et al, "Analgesia and Sedation in Neonatal Intensive Care Using Fentanyl by Continuous Infusion," *Dev Pharmacol Ther*, 1991, 17(3-4):121-7.

Saarenmaa E, Neuvonen PJ, and Fellman V, "Gestational Age and Birth Weight Effects on Plasma Clearance of Fentanyl in Newborn Infants," *J Pediatr*, 2000, 136(6):767-70.

Schechter NL, Weisman SJ, Rosenblum M, et al, "The Use of Oral Transmucosal Fentanyl Citrate for Painful Procedures in Children," *Pediatrics*, 1995, 95(3):335-9.

Zeltzer LK, Altman A, Cohen D, et al, "Report of the Subcommittee on the Management of Pain Associated With Procedures in Children With Cancer," *Pediatrics*, 1990, 86(5 Pt 2):826-31.

- ◆ **Feosol®** [OTC] *see* Iron Supplements (Oral/Enteral) *on page 623*
- ◆ **Feostat®** [OTC] *see* Iron Supplements (Oral/Enteral) *on page 623*
- ◆ **Feratab®** [OTC] *see* Iron Supplements (Oral/Enteral) *on page 623*
- ◆ **Fer-Gen-Sol®** [OTC] *see* Iron Supplements (Oral/Enteral) *on page 623*
- ◆ **Fergon®** [OTC] *see* Iron Supplements (Oral/Enteral) *on page 623*
- ◆ **Fer-In-Sol®** [OTC] *see* Iron Supplements (Oral/Enteral) *on page 623*
- ◆ **Fermalac (Can)** *see* Lactobacillus acidophilus and *Lactobacillus bulgaricus on page 648*
- ◆ **Ferretts** [OTC] *see* Iron Supplements (Oral/Enteral) *on page 623*
- ◆ **Ferrex 150®** [OTC] *see* Iron Supplements (Oral/Enteral) *on page 623*
- ◆ **Ferrlecit®** *see* Iron Supplements (Parenteral) *on page 626*
- ◆ **Ferro-Sequels®** [OTC] *see* Iron Supplements (Oral/Enteral) *on page 623*
- ◆ **Ferrous Fumarate** *see* Iron Supplements (Oral/Enteral) *on page 623*
- ◆ **Ferrous Gluconate** *see* Iron Supplements (Oral/Enteral) *on page 623*
- ◆ **Ferrous Sulfate** *see* Iron Supplements (Oral/Enteral) *on page 623*
- ◆ **FeSO₄ (Ferrous Sulfate)** *see* Iron Supplements (Oral/Enteral) *on page 623*
- ◆ **Fe-Tinic™ 150** [OTC] *see* Iron Supplements (Oral/Enteral) *on page 623*
- ◆ **Feverall®** [OTC] *see* Acetaminophen *on page 36*

Fexofenadine (feks oh FEN a deen)

U.S. Brand Names Allegra®

Therapeutic Category Antihistamine

Generic Available No

Use Symptomatic relief of seasonal allergic rhinitis and chronic idiopathic urticaria

Pregnancy Risk Factor C

Contraindications Hypersensitivity to fexofenadine, terfenadine, or any component

Warnings Adjust dosage in patients with decreased renal function

Precautions Use cautiously in patients who are also taking ketoconazole and erythromycin (see Drug Interactions); although increased plasma levels of fexofenadine have been observed, no adverse effects with concomitant administration have been reported including QT prolongation which occurred when terfenadine was combined with these agents; while less sedating than other antihistamines, fexofenadine may cause drowsiness and impair ability to perform hazardous activities requiring mental alertness

Adverse Reactions

Central nervous system: Headache, fever, drowsiness, fatigue, dizziness

Endocrine & metabolic: Dysmenorrhea

Gastrointestinal: Nausea, dyspepsia

Neuromuscular & skeletal: Back pain

Otic: Otitis media

Respiratory: Upper respiratory tract infection, cough, sinusitis

Miscellaneous: Hypersensitivity reactions, viral infections

Drug Interactions Cytochrome P450 isoenzyme CYP2D6 inhibitor (weak) and CYP3A3/4 substrate

Ketoconazole and erythromycin increase fexofenadine plasma levels; aluminum- and magnesium-containing antacids decrease fexofenadine absorption; the herbal medicine St John's wort (*Hypericum perforatum*) may decrease absorption; avoid alcohol (may increase sedative effects)

Stability Store at controlled room temperature; protect from excessive moisture

Mechanism of Action Fexofenadine is an active metabolite of terfenadine; it competes with histamine for H_1 receptor sites on effector cells in the GI tract, blood vessels, and respiratory tract; it appears that fexofenadine does not cross the blood brain barrier to any appreciable degree, resulting in a reduced potential for sedation

Pharmacodynamics

Onset of action: 1 hour

Maximum effect: 2-3 hours

Duration: ≥12 hours

Pharmacokinetics

Absorption: Rapid

Distribution: V_d: Children: 5.4-5.8 L/kg

Protein binding: 60% to 70%

Metabolism: 5% in liver; 3.5% transformed into methylester metabolite found only in feces (possibly transformed by gut microflora)

Half-life: 14-18 hours

Time to peak serum concentration: 2.6 hours

(Continued)

Fexofenadine *(Continued)*

Elimination: 11% excreted unchanged in urine; 80% excreted unchanged in feces
  Clearance: Children: 14-18 mL/minute/kg
Dialysis: Not effectively removed by hemodialysis

Usual Dosage Oral:

Children 6-11 years: 30 mg twice daily
Children ≥12 years and Adults: 60 mg twice daily or 180 mg once daily
  Dosing adjustment in renal impairment:
  Children 6-11 years: 30 mg once daily
  Children ≥12 years and Adults: 60 mg once daily

Administration May administer without respect to food

Monitoring Parameters Improvement in signs and symptoms of allergic rhinitis and chronic idiopathic urticaria

Test Interactions Antigen skin testing

Patient Information May cause drowsiness and impair ability to perform activities requiring mental alertness or physical coordination; avoid alcohol

Dosage Forms Tablet, as hydrochloride: 30 mg, 60 mg, 180 mg

♦ Fiberall® *see Psyllium on page 959*

Filgrastim *(fil GRA stim)*

U.S. Brand Names Neupogen®

Synonyms G-CSF; Granulocyte Colony Stimulating Factor

Therapeutic Category Colony-Stimulating Factor

Generic Available No

Use Reduction of the duration of neutropenia and the associated risk of infection in patients with malignancies receiving myelosuppressive chemotherapeutic regimens associated with a significant incidence of severe neutropenia with fever; cancer patients receiving bone marrow transplant; severe chronic neutropenia which includes patients with congenital neutropenia, cyclic neutropenia, or idiopathic neutropenia; mobilization of peripheral blood progenitor cells into the peripheral blood for collection by leukapheresis; AIDS patients receiving zidovudine; neonatal neutropenia

Pregnancy Risk Factor C

Contraindications Hypersensitivity to *E. coli*-derived proteins, G-CSF, or any component; use in patients receiving concomitant chemotherapy and radiation therapy

Warnings Leukocytosis (white blood cell counts ≥100,000/mm^3) has been observed in approximately 2% of patients receiving G-CSF at doses >5 mcg/kg/day

Precautions Do not administer 24 hours prior to or within 24 hours following the administration of chemotherapy; use with caution in any malignancy with myeloid characteristics due to G-CSF's potential to act as a growth factor; use with caution in patients with gout, psoriasis; monitor patients with pre-existing cardiac conditions as cardiac events (MIs, arrhythmias) have been reported in premarketing clinical studies. Be alert to the possibility of ARDS in septic patients.

Premature discontinuation of G-CSF therapy prior to the time of recovery from the expected neutrophil nadir is generally not recommended. A transient increase in neutrophil counts is typically seen 1-2 days after initiation of therapy. For a sustained therapeutic response, G-CSF should be continued until the post nadir absolute neutrophil count (ANC) reaches:

10,000/mm^3 in chemotherapy treated patients, or
>1000/mm^3 for 3 consecutive days in bone marrow transplant patients

Most patients experience a 30% to 50% decrease in circulating leukocytes within 1-2 days following discontinuation of G-CSF

Adverse Reactions

Cardiovascular: Transient decrease in blood pressure, vasculitis, chest pain
Central nervous system: Fever, headache
Dermatologic: Exacerbation of pre-existing skin disorders, alopecia, rash, pruritus
Endocrine & metabolic: Reversible increase in uric acid
Gastrointestinal: Splenomegaly, nausea, vomiting, diarrhea, mucositis
Hematologic: Thrombocytopenia, leukocytosis
Hepatic: Elevated alkaline phosphatase, lactate dehydrogenase
Neuromuscular & skeletal: Medullary bone pain (24% incidence) is generally dose-related, localized to the lower back, posterior iliac crests, and sternum; osteoporosis
Renal: Hematuria, proteinuria
Miscellaneous: Anaphylactoid reaction (rare)

Stability Store in refrigerator; do not freeze; stable for 24 hours at room temperature; solutions with concentration ≥15 mcg/mL in D_5W are stable for 24 hours; incompatible with salt solutions

Mechanism of Action Stimulates the production, maturation, and activation of neutrophils; G-CSF activates neutrophils to increase both their migration and cytotoxicity

Pharmacodynamics
Onset of action: Immediate transient leukopenia with the nadir occurring 5-15 minutes after an I.V. dose or 30-60 minutes after a S.C. dose followed by a sustained elevation in neutrophil levels within the first 24 hours reaching a plateau in 3-5 days
Duration: Upon discontinuation of G-CSF, ANC decreases by 50% within 2 days and returns to pretreatment levels within 1 week; WBC counts return to normal range in 4-7 days

Pharmacokinetics
Distribution: V_d: 150 mL/kg
Bioavailability: Not bioavailable after oral administration
Half-life: Neonates: 4.4 hours; Adults: 1.8-3.5 hours
Time to peak serum concentration: S.C.: Within 2-6 hours
Elimination: No evidence of drug accumulation over a 11- to 20-day period

Usual Dosage I.V., S.C. (refer to individual protocols):
Neonates: 5-10 mcg/kg/day once daily for 3-5 days has been administered to neutropenic neonates with sepsis. There was a rapid and significant increase in peripheral neutrophil counts and the neutrophil storage pool.
Children and Adults: 5-10 mcg/kg/day ($\sim$150-300 mcg/m²/day) once daily for up to 14 days until ANC = 10,000/mm³; dose escalations at 5 mcg/kg/day may be required in some individuals when response at 5 mcg/kg/day is not adequate; in phase 3 trials, efficacy was observed at dosages of 4-8 mcg/kg/day with myelosuppressive chemotherapy
Peripheral blood progenitor cell (PBPC) mobilization: S.C.: 10 mcg/kg/day given for 4 days before the first leukapheresis procedure and continued until the last leukapheresis
Patients with congenital neutropenia: S.C.: Initial: 6 mcg/kg/dose twice daily; dosages of 2-60 mcg/kg/day individualized according to neutrophil count have been administered to children and adults
Patients with idiopathic or cyclic neutropenia: S.C.: 5 mcg/kg/day once daily
Cancer patients receiving bone marrow transplant: I.V. infusion, S.C.: 5-10 mcg/kg/day administered ≥24 hours after cytotoxic chemotherapy and ≥24 hours after bone marrow infusion
Dosage adjustment during neutrophil recovery period: see table

Filgrastim Dose Based on Neutrophil Response

Absolute Neutrophil Count (ANC)	Filgrastim Dose Adjustment
When ANC >1000/mm³ for 3 consecutive days	Reduce to 5 mcg/kg/day
If ANC remains >1000/mm³ for 3 more consecutive days	Discontinue filgrastim
If ANC decreases to <1000/mm³	Resume at 5 mcg/kg/day

If ANC decreases <1000/mm³ during the 5 mcg/kg/day dose, increase dose to 10 mcg/kg/day and follow the above steps in the table.

Administration Parenteral:
S.C.: Administer undiluted solution
S.C. continuous infusion: Dilute dose in 10 mL D_5W and infuse at a rate of 10 mL/24 hours
I.V. continuous infusion; Administer over 15-60 minutes or as a continuous I.V. infusion at a final concentration of at least 15 mcg/mL in D_5W. If the final concentration of G-CSF in D_5W is <15 mcg/mL, then add 2 mg albumin/mL to I.V. fluid; the solution is stable for 24 hours; albumin acts as a carrier molecule to prevent drug adsorption to the I.V. tubing. Albumin should be added to the D_5W prior to addition of G-CSF; final concentration of G-CSF for administration <5 mcg/mL is not recommended; do not shake solution to avoid foaming.

Monitoring Parameters Temperature, CBC with differential and platelet count, hematocrit, uric acid, urinalysis, liver function tests

Reference Range Blood samples for monitoring the hematologic effects of G-CSF should be drawn just before the next dose at least twice weekly

Patient Information Possible bone pain; notify physician of unusual fever or chills, severe bone pain, or chest pain and palpitations

Nursing Implications Bone pain management is usually successful with non-narcotic analgesic therapy
(Continued)

Filgrastim *(Continued)*

Additional Information Reimbursement hotline: 1-800-272-9376

Dosage Forms

Injection, solution [preservative free; prefilled Singleject® syringe]: 600 mcg/mL (0.5 mL, 0.8 mL)

Injection, solution [preservative free; vial]: 300 mcg/mL (1 mL, 1.6 mL)

References

"Update of Recommendations for the Use of Hematopoietic Colony-Stimulating Factors: Evidence-based Clinical Practice Guidelines. American Society of Clinical Oncology," *J Clin Oncol*, 1996, 14(6):1957-60.

Bonilla MA, Gillio AP, Ruggeiro M, et al, "Effects of Recombinant Human Granulocyte Colony-Stimulating Factor on Neutropenia in Patients With Congenital Agranulocytosis," *N Engl J Med*, 1989, 320(24):1574-80.

Gilmore MM, Stroncek DF, and Korones DN, "Treatment of Alloimmune Neonatal Neutropenia With Granulocyte Colony-Stimulating Factor," *J Pediatr*, 1994, 125(6 Pt 1):948-51.

Hollingshead LM, Goa KL, "Recombinant Granulocyte Colony-Stimulating Factor (rG-CSF). A Review of Its Pharmacological Properties and Prospective Role in Neutropenic Conditions," *Drugs*, 1991, 42(2):300-30.

Morstyn G, Campbell L, Lieschke G, et al, "Treatment of Chemotherapy-Induced Neutropenia by Subcutaneously Administered Granulocyte Colony-Stimulating Factor With Optimization of Dose and Duration of Therapy," *J Clin Oncol*, 1989, 7(10):1554-62.

Wolach B, "Neonatal Sepsis: Pathogenesis and Supportive Therapy," *Semin Perinatol*, 1997, 21(1):28-38.

♦ **Fisalamine** *see* Mesalamine *on page 723*

♦ **FK506** *see* Tacrolimus *on page 1062*

♦ **Flagyl®** *see* Metronidazole *on page 754*

♦ **Flagyl® ER** *see* Metronidazole *on page 754*

♦ **Flamazine® (Can)** *see* Silver Sulfadiazine *on page 1019*

♦ **Flarex®** *see* Fluorometholone *on page 502*

♦ **Flatulex® [OTC]** *see* Simethicone *on page 1020*

Flecainide *(fle KAY nide)*

U.S. Brand Names Tambocor™

Therapeutic Category Antiarrhythmic Agent, Class I-C

Generic Available No

Use Prevention and suppression of documented life-threatening ventricular arrhythmias (ie, sustained ventricular tachycardia); prevention of symptomatic, disabling supraventricular tachycardias in patients without structural heart disease

Pregnancy Risk Factor C

Contraindications Hypersensitivity to flecainide or any component; pre-existing second or third degree A-V block; right bundle-branch block associated with left hemiblock (bifascicular block) or trifascicular block; cardiogenic shock, myocardial depression

Warnings The manufacturer and FDA recommend that this drug be reserved for life-threatening ventricular arrhythmias unresponsive to conventional therapy. Its use for symptomatic nonsustained ventricular tachycardia, frequent premature ventricular complexes (PVCs), uniform and multiform PVCs and/or coupled PVCs is no longer recommended. Flecainide can worsen or cause arrhythmias with an associated risk of death. Proarrhythmic effects range from an increased number of PVCs to more severe ventricular tachycardias (ie, tachycardias that are more sustained or more resistant to conversion to sinus rhythm).

Precautions Use with caution in patients with pacemakers, sick sinus syndrome, CHF, myocardial dysfunction, and renal and/or hepatic impairment; use decreased doses and cautiously titrate dose according to serum concentrations and clinical effects in patients with CHF, or myocardial, liver or renal dysfunction. Flecainide may cause increases in PR, QRS, and QT intervals and new first degree or bundle branch block; use with caution and consider dosing reduction when increases in such intervals occur.

Adverse Reactions

Cardiovascular: Bradycardia, heart block, worsening ventricular arrhythmias, CHF, palpitations, chest pain, edema; increased P-R interval and QRS duration

Central nervous system: Dizziness, fatigue, nervousness, hypoesthesia, headache

Dermatologic: Rash

Gastrointestinal: Nausea

Hematologic: Blood dyscrasias

Hepatic: Hepatic dysfunction

Neuromuscular & skeletal: Paresthesia, tremor

Ocular: Blurred vision

Respiratory: Dyspnea

Drug Interactions Cytochrome P450 isoenzyme CYP2D6 substrate

Other antiarrhythmic agents may increase adverse cardiac effects; flecainide may increase plasma digoxin concentrations; use with beta-blockers, disopyramide, or verapamil may result in possible additive negative inotropic effects; alkalinizing agents (high-dose antacids, carbonic anhydrase inhibitors or sodium bicarbonate) may decrease flecainide's clearance; urinary acidifiers may increase flecainide's clearance; amiodarone and cimetidine increase flecainide serum concentrations; concurrent use of flecainide with ritonavir or lopinavir is not recommended

Food Interactions Dairy products (milk, infant formula, yogurt) may interfere with the absorption of flecainide in infants; there is one case report of a neonate (GA 34 weeks PNA >6 days) who required extremely large doses of oral flecainide when administered every 8 hours with feedings ("milk feeds"); changing the feedings from "milk feeds" to 5% glucose feeds alone resulted in a doubling of the flecainide serum concentration and toxicity (see Russell, 1989); clearance of flecainide may be decreased in patients with strict vegetarian diets due to urinary pH ≥8

Mechanism of Action Class IC antiarrhythmic; slows conduction in cardiac tissue by altering transport of ions across cell membranes; causes slight prolongation of refractory periods; decreases the rate of rise of the action potential without affecting its duration; increases electrical stimulation threshold of ventricle, HIS-Purkinje system; possesses local anesthetic and moderate negative inotropic effects

Pharmacokinetics

Absorption: Oral: Rapid and nearly complete

Distribution: V_d: Adults: 5-13.4 L/kg

Protein binding: 40% to 50% (alpha$_1$ glycoprotein)

Metabolism: In the liver

Bioavailability: 85% to 90%

Half-life, elimination: Increased half-life with CHF or renal dysfunction

Newborns: ~29 hours

Infants: 11-12 hours

Children: 8 hours

Adults: ~20 hours (range: 12-27 hours)

Time to peak serum concentration: ~3 hours (range 1-6 hours)

Elimination: In urine as unchanged drug (10% to 50%) and metabolites

Dialysis: Not dialyzable

Usual Dosage Oral:

Children: Initial: 1-3 mg/kg/day or 50-100 mg/m^2/day in 3 divided doses; usual: 3-6 mg/kg/day or 100-150 mg/m^2/day in 3 divided doses; up to 8 mg/kg/day or 200 mg/m^2/day for uncontrolled patients with subtherapeutic levels; higher doses have been reported, however they may be associated with an increased risk of proarrhythmias; a review of world literature reports the average effective dose to be 4 mg/kg/day or 140 mg/m^2/day

Adults: Life-threatening ventricular arrhythmias: Initial: 100 mg every 12 hours, increase by 100 mg/day (given in 2 doses/day) every 4 days; usual: ≤300 mg/day; maximum: 400 mg/day; for patients receiving 400 mg/day who are not controlled and have trough concentrations <0.6 mcg/mL, dosage may be increased to 600 mg/day

Prevention of paroxysmal supraventricular arrhythmias in patients with disabling symptoms but no structural heart disease: Initial: 50 mg every 12 hours; maximum dose: 300 mg/day

Dosing adjustment in renal failure:

Manufacturer recommendations: Adults: Cl$_{cr}$ ≤35 mL/minute/1.73 m^2: Initial: 50 mg every 12 hours or 100 mg once daily; increase dose slowly at intervals >4 days; monitor plasma levels closely

Alternative adjustment: Children and Adults Cl$_{cr}$ ≤20 mL/minute: Decrease the usual dose by 25% to 50%

Administration Oral: May be administered in children and adults without regard to food; in infants receiving milk or milk based formulas, avoid concurrent administration with feedings; monitor serum concentrations and decrease the dose when the diet changes to a decreased consumption of milk

Monitoring Parameters EKG, serum concentrations [Note: Obtain serum trough concentrations at steady state (after at least 3 days when doses are started or changed) or when dietary changes due to maturation or concurrent illness occur], liver enzymes, CBC with differential

Reference Range Therapeutic: 0.2-1 µg/mL (SI: 0.4-2 µmol/L). Note: Pediatric patients may respond at the lower end of the recommended therapeutic range (0.2-0.5 µg/mL) but up to 0.8 µg/mL may be required.

Patient Information May cause dizziness; notify physician if chest pain, faintness, palpitations, dizziness or visual disturbances occur

(Continued)

Flecainide *(Continued)*

Additional Information Single oral dose flecainide for termination of PSVT in children and young adults (n=25) and combination therapy of flecainide with amiodarone for refractory tachyarrhythmias in infancy (n=9) have been reported (See References)

Dosage Forms Tablet, as acetate: 50 mg, 100 mg, 150 mg

Extemporaneous Preparations

A 5 mg/mL suspension compounded from tablets and an oral flavored commercially available diluent (Roxane®) was stable for up to 45 days when stored at 5°C or 25°C in amber glass bottles (Wiest, 1992)

A 20 mg/mL oral liquid preparation made from tablets and 3 different vehicles (cherry syrup, a 1:1 mixture of Ora-Sweet® and Ora-Plus®, or a 1:1 mixture of Ora-Sweet® SF and Ora-Plus®) was stable for 60 days when stored in amber plastic prescription bottles in the dark at room temperature (25°C) or under refrigeration (5°C); grind twenty-four 100 mg tablets in a mortar into a fine powder; add 20 mL of the vehicle and mix well to form a uniform paste; mix while adding the vehicle in geometric proportions to **almost** 120 mL; transfer to a calibrated bottle and qsad with vehicle to 120 mL; label "shake well" and "protect from light" (Allen, 1996).

Allen LV and Erickson MA, "Stability of Baclofen, Captopril, Diltiazem Hydrochloride, Dipyridamole, and Flecainide Acetate in Extemporaneously Compounded Oral Liquids," *Am J Health Syst Pharm*, 1996, 53(18):2179-84.

Wiest DB, Garner SS, and Pagacz LR, "Stability of Flecainide Acetate in an Extemporaneously Compounded Oral Suspension," *Am J Hosp Pharm*, 1992, 49(6):1467-70.

References

Fenrich AL Jr, Perry JC, and Friedman RA, "Flecainide and Amiodarone: Combined Therapy for Refractory Tachyarrhythmias in Infants," *J Am Coll Cardiol*, 1995, 25(5):1195-8.

Musto B, Cavallaro C, Musto A, et al, "Flecainide Single Oral Dose for Management of Paroxysmal Supraventricular Tachycardia in Children and Young Adults," *Am Heart J*, 1992, 124(1):110-5.

Perry JC and Garson A Jr, "Flecainide Acetate for Treatment of Tachyarrhythmias in Children: Review of World Literature on Efficacy, Safety, and Dosing," *Am Heart J*, 1992, 124(6):1614-21.

Perry JC, McQuinn RL, Smith RT Jr, et al, "Flecainide Acetate for Resistant Arrhythmias in the Young: Efficacy and Pharmacokinetics," *J Am Coll Cardiol*, 1989, 14(1):185-91.

Priestley KA, Ladusans EJ, Rosenthal E, et al, "Experience With Flecainide for the Treatment of Cardiac Arrhythmias in Children," *Eur Heart J*, 1988, 9(12):1284-90.

Russell GA and Martin RP, "Flecainide Toxicity," *Arch Dis Child*, 1989, 64(6):860-2.

Zeigler V, Gillette PC, Ross BA, et al, "Flecainide for Supraventricular and Ventricular Arrhythmias in Children and Young Adults," *Am J Cardiol*, 1988, 62(10 Pt 1):818-20.

♦ **Fleet® Babylax® [OTC]** *see* Glycerin *on page 543*

♦ **Fleet® Bisacodyl Enema [OTC]** *see* Bisacodyl *on page 173*

♦ **Fleet® Enema [OTC]** *see* Phosphate Supplements *on page 898*

♦ **Fleet® Glycerin Suppositories [OTC]** *see* Glycerin *on page 543*

♦ **Fleet® Glycerin Suppositories Maximum Strength [OTC]** *see* Glycerin *on page 543*

♦ **Fleet® Liquid Glycerin Suppositories [OTC]** *see* Glycerin *on page 543*

♦ **Fleet® Mineral Oil [OTC]** *see* Mineral Oil *on page 767*

♦ **Fleet® Mineral Oil Enema [OTC]** *see* Mineral Oil *on page 767*

♦ **Fleet® Phospho®-Soda [OTC]** *see* Phosphate Supplements *on page 898*

♦ **Fleet® Sof-Lax® [OTC]** *see* Docusate *on page 402*

♦ **Fleet® Sof-Lax® Overnight [OTC]** *see* Docusate and Casanthranol *on page 402*

♦ **Fleet® Stimulant Laxative [OTC]** *see* Bisacodyl *on page 173*

♦ **Fletcher's® Castoria® [OTC]** *see* Senna *on page 1014*

♦ **Flexeril®** *see* Cyclobenzaprine *on page 318*

♦ **Flexitec (Can)** *see* Cyclobenzaprine *on page 318*

♦ **Flonase®** *see* Fluticasone *on page 511*

♦ **Florazole® ER (Can)** *see* Metronidazole *on page 754*

♦ **Florical® [OTC]** *see* Calcium Supplements *on page 200*

♦ **Florinef® Acetate** *see* Fludrocortisone *on page 494*

♦ **Flovent®** *see* Fluticasone *on page 511*

♦ **Flovent® Diskus®** *see* Fluticasone *on page 511*

♦ **Flovent® Rotadisk®** *see* Fluticasone *on page 511*

♦ **Flubenisolone** *see* Betamethasone *on page 169*

Fluconazole *(floo KOE na zole)*

Related Information

Carbohydrate and Alcohol Content of Liquid Medications for Use in Patients Receiving Ketogenic Diets *on page 1431*

U.S. Brand Names Diflucan®

Canadian Brand Names Apo®-Fluconazole

Therapeutic Category Antifungal Agent, Systemic

Generic Available No

Use Treatment of susceptible fungal infections including oropharyngeal, esophageal, and vaginal candidiasis; treatment of systemic candidal infections including urinary tract infection, peritonitis, cystitis, and pneumonia; strains of *Candida* with decreased *in vitro* susceptibility to fluconazole are being isolated with increasing frequency; fluconazole is more active against *C. albicans* than other candidal strains like *C. parapsilosis*, *C. glabrata*, and *C. tropicalis*; treatment and suppression of cryptococcal meningitis; prophylaxis of candidiasis in patients undergoing bone marrow transplantation; alternative to amphotericin B in patients with pre-existing renal impairment or when requiring concomitant therapy with other potentially nephrotoxic drugs

Pregnancy Risk Factor C

Contraindications Hypersensitivity to fluconazole, other azoles, or any component; concurrent use with astemizole, cisapride, and terfenadine

Warnings Patients who develop abnormal liver function tests during fluconazole therapy should be monitored closely for the development of more severe hepatic injury; if clinical signs and symptoms consistent with liver disease develop that may be attributable to fluconazole, fluconazole should be discontinued

Fluconazole oral suspension contains sodium benzoate; benzoic acid (benzoate) is a metabolite of benzyl alcohol; large amounts of benzyl alcohol ($\geq$99 mg/kg/day) have been associated with a potentially fatal toxicity ("gasping syndrome") in neonates; the "gasping syndrome" consists of metabolic acidosis, respiratory distress, gasping respirations, CNS dysfunction (including convulsions, intracranial hemorrhage), hypotension and cardiovascular collapse; use fluconazole oral suspension containing sodium benzoate with caution in neonates; *in vitro* and animal studies have shown that benzoate displaces bilirubin from protein binding sites

Precautions Use with caution and modify dosage in patients with impaired renal function

Adverse Reactions
Cardiovascular: Pallor
Central nervous system: Dizziness, headache (1.9%), seizures
Dermatologic: Skin rash (1.8%), exfoliative skin disorders, Stevens-Johnson syndrome
Endocrine & metabolic: Hypokalemia, hypercholesterolemia, hypertriglyceridemia
Gastrointestinal: Nausea (2%), abdominal pain (3%), vomiting (5%), diarrhea (2%), dysgeusia
Hematologic: Eosinophilia, leukopenia, thrombocytopenia
Hepatic: Elevated AST, ALT, or alkaline phosphatase; hepatitis; cholestasis
Miscellaneous: Anaphylaxis

Drug Interactions Cytochrome P450 isoenzyme CYP2C9 inducer; CYP2C9, CYP2C18, CYP2C19 and CYP3A3/4 (weak) isoenzyme inhibitor
Oral antidiabetic agents (fluconazole reduces the metabolism and increases the concentration of tolbutamide, glyburide, and glipizide); hydrochlorothiazide (increases fluconazole AUC); warfarin (increased prothrombin time); fluconazole increases plasma cyclosporine, tacrolimus, theophylline, zidovudine, cisapride, (fatal arrhythmias including ventricular tachycardia, ventricular fibrillation, torsade de pointes, and QT prolongation have been reported in patients taking cisapride concurrently with fluconazole), astemizole, terfenadine, rifabutin, and phenytoin concentrations; rifampin increases fluconazole metabolism; antagonism may occur if amphotericin B and fluconazole are used concomitantly

Food Interactions Food decreases the rate but not the extent of absorption

Stability Incompatible with ampicillin, calcium gluconate, ceftazidime, cefotaxime, cefuroxime, ceftriaxone, clindamycin, furosemide, imipenem, ticarcillin, and piperacillin; reconstituted oral suspension is stable for 14 days at room temperature or if refrigerated

Mechanism of Action Interferes with fungal cytochrome P450 sterol C-14 alpha-demethylation activity, decreasing ergosterol synthesis (principal sterol in fungal cell membrane) and inhibiting cell membrane formation

Pharmacokinetics
Absorption: Oral: Well absorbed; food does not affect extent of absorption
Distribution: Distributes widely into body tissues and fluids including the CSF, saliva, sputum, vaginal fluid, skin, eye; excreted in breast milk
Protein binding: 11% to 12%
Bioavailability: Oral: >90%
Half-life:
Premature newborns: 73.6 hours; 6 days PNA: 53.2 hours; 12 days PNA: 46.6 hours
Children:
9 months to 13 years: 19.5-25 hours (with oral dose)
(Continued)

Fluconazole *(Continued)*

5-15 years: 15.2-17.6 hours (with multiple I.V. dosing)

Adults: 25-30 hours with normal renal function

Time to peak serum concentration: Oral: Within 2-4 hours (1-2 hours in fasted patients)

Elimination: 80% of dose excreted unchanged in urine; 11% of dose excreted in urine as metabolites

Dialysis: Hemodialysis: 3-hour session decreases plasma concentration 50%

Usual Dosage Daily dose of fluconazole is the same for oral and I.V. administration:

Oral, I.V.:

Premature neonates:

≤29 weeks gestation:

Postnatal age 0-14 days: 5-6 mg/kg/dose every 72 hours

Postnatal age >14 days: 5-6 mg/kg/dose every 48 hours

30-36 weeks gestation: Postnatal age 0-14 days: 3-6 mg/kg/dose every 48 hours

Neonates >14 days, Infants, Children: Once daily: See table

Safety profile of fluconazole has been studied in 577 children ages 1 day to 17 years. Doses as high as 12 mg/kg/day once daily (equivalent to adult doses of 400 mg/day) have been used to treat candidiasis in immunocompromised children; 10-12 mg/kg/day doses once daily have been used prophylactically against fungal infections in pediatric bone marrow transplantation patients. Do not exceed 600 mg/day.

Adults: Oral, I.V.: Once daily: See table

Indication	Day 1	Daily Therapy	Minimum Duration of Therapy
Neonates 0-14 days: Same dosage as older children but administered every 24-72 h			
Neonates >14 days, infants, and children			
Oropharyngeal candidiasis	6 mg/kg	3 mg/kg	14 d
Esophageal candidiasis	6 mg/kg	3 mg/kg up to 12 mg/kg/d	21 d
Systemic candidiasis		6-12 mg/kg/d	28 d
Cryptococcal meningitis			
acute	12 mg/kg	6 mg/kg up to 12 mg/kg/d	10-12 wk after CSF culture becomes negative
relapse		6 mg/kg	
Adults			
Oropharyngeal candidiasis	200 mg	100 mg	14 d
Esophageal candidiasis	200 mg	100-400 mg	21 d
Systemic candidiasis	400 mg	200-800 mg	28 d
Cryptococcal meningitis			
acute	400 mg	200-800 mg	10-12 wk after CSF culture becomes negative
relapse	200 mg	200 mg	

Vaginal candidiasis: Oral: 150 mg single dose

Prophylaxis against fungal infections in bone marrow transplantation patients: Oral, I.V.: 400 mg/day once daily

Dosing adjustment in renal impairment:

Cl_{cr} 21-50 mL/minute: Administer 50% of recommended dose

Cl_{cr} <20 mL/minute: Administer 25% of recommended dose

Patients receiving hemodialysis: One recommended dose after each dialysis

Administration

Oral: Administer with or without food; shake suspension well before use

Parenteral: Fluconazole must be administered by I.V. infusion over approximately 1-2 hours at a rate not to exceed 200 mg/hour and a final concentration for administration of 2 mg/mL; for pediatric patients receiving doses ≥6 mg/kg/day, administer I.V. infusion over 2 hours

Monitoring Parameters Periodic liver function and renal function tests, serum potassium, CBC with differential, and platelet count

Patient Information Notify physician of unusual bleeding or bruising, yellowing of skin and eyes, or severe skin rash

Dosage Forms

Infusion [premixed in sodium chloride or dextrose]: 2 mg/mL (100 mL, 200 mL)

Powder for oral suspension: 10 mg/mL (35 mL); 40 mg/mL (35 mL) [contains sodium benzoate; orange flavor]

Tablet: 50 mg, 100 mg, 150 mg, 200 mg

References

Como JA and Dismukes WE, "Oral Azole Drugs as Systemic Antifungal Therapy," *N Engl J Med*, 1993, 330(4):263-72.

Goodman JL, Winston DJ, Greenfield RA, et al, "A Controlled Trial of Fluconazole to Prevent Fungal Infections in Patients Undergoing Bone Marrow Transplantation," *N Engl J Med*, 1992, 326(13):845-51.

Lee JW, Seibel NL, Amantea M, et al, "Safety and Pharmacokinetics of Fluconazole in Children With Neoplastic Diseases," *J Pediatr*, 1992, 120(6):987-93.

Moncino MD and Gutman LT, "Severe Systemic Cryptococcal Disease in a Child: Review of Prognostic Indicators Predicting Treatment Failure and an Approach to Maintenance Therapy With Oral Fluconazole," *Pediatr Infect Dis J*, 1990, 9(5):363-8.

Viscoli C, Castagnola E, Fioredda F, et al, "Fluconazole in the Treatment of Candidiasis in Immunocompromised Children," *Antimicrob Agents Chemother*, 1991, 35(2):365-7.

Flucytosine (floo SYE toe seen)

Related Information
Blood Level Sampling Time Guidelines *on page 1386*

U.S. Brand Names Ancobon®

Synonyms 5-FC; 5-Flurocytosine

Therapeutic Category Antifungal Agent, Systemic

Generic Available No

Use In combination with amphotericin B in the treatment of serious *Candida, Aspergillus, Cryptococcus,* and *Torulopsis* infections (resistance emerges if flucytosine is used as a single agent)

Pregnancy Risk Factor C

Contraindications Hypersensitivity to flucytosine or any component

Precautions Use with extreme caution in patients with renal impairment, bone marrow suppression, patients with AIDS; dosage modification required in patients with impaired renal function; monitor serum flucytosine concentration

Adverse Reactions
Central nervous system: Confusion, headache, sedation, hallucinations, seizures, vertigo, ataxia

Dermatologic: Rash, pruritus, urticaria, photosensitivity

Endocrine & metabolic: Temporary growth failure

Gastrointestinal: Nausea, vomiting, diarrhea, enterocolitis, anorexia, GI hemorrhage

Hematologic: Bone marrow suppression (often observed after 10-26 days of therapy and occurs more frequently with sustained concentrations >100 mcg/mL), anemia, leukopenia, thrombocytopenia

Hepatic: Elevated liver enzymes, hepatitis

Neuromuscular & skeletal: Neuropathy, paresthesia

Renal: Elevated BUN and serum creatinine

Miscellaneous: Anaphylaxis

Drug Interactions Increased efficacy as well as toxicity (enterocolitis, myelosuppression) with concurrent amphotericin administration; antacids and aluminum or magnesium salts delay the rate of absorption

Food Interactions Food decreases the rate, but not the extent of absorption

Mechanism of Action Penetrates fungal cells and is converted to fluorouracil which competes with uracil interfering with fungal RNA and protein synthesis

Pharmacokinetics
Absorption: Oral: 75% to 90%; rate of absorption is delayed in patients with renal impairment

Distribution: Widely distributed into body tissues and fluids including CSF, aqueous humor, peritoneal fluid, bronchial secretions, liver, kidney, heart, and joints

Protein binding: 2% to 4%

Metabolism: Minimal

Bioavailability: Decreased in neonates

Half-life:
Neonates: 4-34 hours
Adults: 3-8 hours (prolonged as high as 200 hours in anuria)

Time to peak serum concentration: Oral: Within 2-6 hours

Elimination: 75% to 90% excreted unchanged in urine by glomerular filtration

Dialysis: Dialyzable (50% to 100%)

Usual Dosage Oral:
Neonates: Initial: 50-100 mg/kg/day in divided doses every 12-24 hours

Infants, Children, Adults: 100-150 mg/kg/day in divided doses every 6 hours

Dosing adjustment in renal impairment:
Cl_{cr} 20-40 mL/minute: Administer every 12 hours
Cl_{cr} 10-20 mL/minute: Administer every 24 hours
Cl_{cr} <10 mL/minute: Administer every 24-48 hours

Patients receiving hemodialysis: Administer dose postdialysis

Administration Oral: Administer with food over a 15-minute period to decrease nausea and vomiting

(Continued)

Flucytosine *(Continued)*

Monitoring Parameters Serum creatinine, BUN, alkaline phosphatase, AST, ALT, CBC, platelet count; serum flucytosine concentrations

Reference Range Therapeutic levels: 25-100 µg/mL; with invasive candidiasis, maintain peak plasma concentration between 40-60 mcg/mL; increased bone marrow suppression with sustained serum flucytosine concentration >100 µg/mL; obtain flucytosine concentration 60 minutes after an oral dose; obtain trough level immediately before the next dose; maintain trough ≥25 mcg/mL to prevent emergence of resistant strains

Test Interactions Flucytosine causes markedly false elevations in serum creatinine values when the Ektachem® analyzer is used

Patient Information May cause photosensitivity reactions (eg, exposure to sunlight may cause severe sunburn, skin rash, redness, or itching); avoid exposure to sunlight and artificial light sources (sunlamps, tanning booth/bed); wear protective clothing, wide-brimmed hats, sunglasses, and lip sunscreen (SPF ≥15); use a sunscreen [broad-spectrum sunscreen or physical sunscreen (preferred) or sunblock with SPF ≥15]; contact physician if reaction occurs.

Additional Information Resistance develops rapidly if used alone; more rapid emergence of fungal resistance may occur when lower doses are used

Dosage Forms Capsule: 250 mg, 500 mg

Extemporaneous Preparations Flucytosine oral liquid has been prepared by using the contents of ten 500 mg capsules triturated in a mortar and pestle with a small amount of distilled water; the mixture was transferred to a 500 mL volumetric flask; the mortar was rinsed several times with a small amount of distilled water and the fluid added to the flask; sufficient distilled water was added to make a total volume of 500 mL of a 10 mg/mL liquid; oral liquid was stable for 70 days when stored in glass or plastic prescription bottles at 4°C or for up to 14 days at room temperature.

Wintermeyer SM and Nahata MC, "Stability of Flucytosine in an Extemporaneously Compounded Oral Liquid," *Am J Health-Syst Pharm*, 1996, 53:407-9.

References

Baley JE, Meyers C, Kliegman RM, et al, "Pharmacokinetics, Outcome of Treatment, and Toxic Effects of Amphotericin B and 5-Fluorocytosine in Neonates," *J Pediatr*, 1990, 116(5):791-7.

♦ **Fludara®** *see Fludarabine on page 492*

Fludarabine *(floo DARE a been)*

Related Information

Emetogenic Potential of Single Chemotherapeutic Agents *on page 1286*

U.S. Brand Names Fludara®

Synonyms FAMP; F-ara-AMP

Therapeutic Category Antineoplastic Agent, Antimetabolite

Generic Available No

Use Treatment of B-cell chronic lymphocytic leukemia unresponsive to previous therapy with an alkylating agent containing regimen; non-Hodgkin's lymphoma. Fludarabine has been tested in patients with refractory acute lymphocytic leukemia and acute nonlymphocytic leukemia, but required a highly toxic dose to achieve response.

Pregnancy Risk Factor D

Contraindications Hypersensitivity to fludarabine or any component; concomitant administration with pentostatin; pregnancy

Warnings The FDA currently recommends that procedures for proper handling and disposal of antineoplastic agents be considered; doses ≥77 mg/m²/day for 5-7 days were associated with severe neurotoxicity. Neurotoxicity can occur 21-60 days after completing a course of fludarabine and appears to be dose related. Severe bone marrow suppression has been observed at therapeutic doses; bone marrow hypoplasia or aplasia resulting in death has been reported; life-threatening and sometimes fatal autoimmune hemolytic anemia has been reported after one or more cycles of treatment. Hematologic function must be frequently monitored. Concomitant therapy with pentostatin may be associated with severe pulmonary toxicity.

Precautions Use with caution in patients with pre-existing neurologic problems and in patients with renal insufficiency; dosage adjustment may be needed in patients with impaired renal function or bone marrow suppression

Adverse Reactions

Cardiovascular: Edema

Central nervous system: Neurotoxicity (primarily progressive demyelinating encephalopathy with mental status deterioration), somnolence, seizures, fever, agitation, confusion, depression, chills, fatigue, headache, coma

Dermatologic: Pruritus, rash, alopecia

Endocrine & metabolic: Metabolic acidosis, tumor lysis syndrome, (hyperuricemia, hyperphosphatemia, hypocalcemia, hyperkalemia), hyperglycemia

Gastrointestinal: Nausea, vomiting, diarrhea, stomatitis, metallic taste, GI bleeding, anorexia

Genitourinary: Hemorrhagic cystitis (rare)

Hematologic: Leukopenia, neutropenia, thrombocytopenia, lymphocytopenia, autoimmune hemolytic anemia, anemia

Hepatic: Elevated transaminase levels

Neuromuscular & skeletal: Myalgia, peripheral neuropathy, weakness

Ocular: Blindness, blurred vision, photophobia

Renal: Hematuria, renal failure

Respiratory: Interstitial pneumonitis, dyspnea, cough

Drug Interactions Cytarabine when administered with or prior to a fludarabine dose competes for deoxycytidine kinase decreasing the phosphorylation of fludarabine to the active F-ara-ATP (inhibits the antineoplastic effect of fludarabine); however, administering fludarabine prior to cytarabine may stimulate activation of cytarabine; pentostatin (increased pulmonary toxicity)

Stability Store vial in refrigerator; reconstituted 25 mg/mL fludarabine solution should be used within 8 hours after preparation since it contains no preservatives. When fludarabine is diluted in D_5W or NS to a final concentration of 1 mg/mL, the solution is stable for 24 hours at room temperature. Discard solution if a slight haze develops.

Mechanism of Action F-ara-AMP is dephosphorylated to 2-fluoro-ara-A which enters the cell by a carrier mediated transport process; it is phosphorylated intracellularly to the active metabolite F-ara-ATP. F-ara-ATP competes with deoxyadenosine triphosphate for incorporation into the A-sites of the DNA strand inhibiting DNA synthesis in the S-phase via inhibition of DNA polymerases and RNA reductase.

Pharmacokinetics

Distribution: Widely distributed with extensive tissue binding

Protein binding: 19% to 29%

Half-life: Terminal (2-fluoro-ara-A):

Children: 12.4-19 hours

Adults: 7-20 hours

Elimination: Fludarabine clearance appears to be inversely correlated with serum creatinine; at a dose of 25 mg/m²/day for 5 days, 24% of dose excreted in urine; at higher doses, 41% to 60% of dose renally excreted

Usual Dosage Not currently FDA approved for use in children (refer to individual protocols): I.V.:

Children:

Acute leukemia: 10 mg/m² bolus over 15 minutes followed by a continuous infusion of 30.5 mg/m²/day over 5 days; or 10.5 mg/m² bolus over 15 minutes followed by a continuous infusion of 30.5 mg/m²/day over 48 hours followed by cytarabine has been used in clinical trials

Solid tumors: 9 mg/m² bolus followed by 27 mg/m²/day continuous infusion over 5 days

Adults: Chronic lymphocytic leukemia: 20-25 mg/m²/day over 30 minutes for 5 days; doses up to 30 mg/m²/day as single daily doses for 5 days have also been used; courses are usually repeated every 28 days

Dosing adjustment in renal impairment:

Cl_{cr} 30-70 mL/minute/1.73 m²: Reduce dose by 20% and monitor closely for toxicity

Cl_{cr} <30 mL/minute/1.73 m²: Not recommended

Administration Parenteral: Fludarabine phosphate has been administered by intermittent I.V. infusion over 15-30 minutes and by continuous infusion; in clinical trials the loading dose has been diluted in 20 mL D_5W and administered over 15 minutes and the continuous infusion diluted to 240 mL in D_5W and administered at a constant rate of 10 mL/hour; in other clinical studies fludarabine has been diluted to a concentration of 0.25-1 mg/mL in D_5W or NS

Monitoring Parameters CBC with differential, platelet count, AST, ALT, creatinine, serum electrolytes, albumin, uric acid, and examination for visual changes

Patient Information Notify physician if fever, sore throat, bleeding, bruising, tachypnea, respiratory distress, or neurologic changes occur

Nursing Implications Prophylactic allopurinol, adequate hydration, and urinary alkalinization should be considered for patients with large initial tumor burdens

Additional Information Myelosuppressive effects:

Granulocyte nadir: 13 days (3-25)

Platelet nadir: 16 days (2-32)

Recovery: 5-7 weeks

Dosage Forms Injection, powder for reconstitution, lyophilized, as phosphate: 50 mg

(Continued)

Fludarabine *(Continued)*

References

Avramis VI, Champagne J, Sato J, et al, "Pharmacology of Fludarabine Phosphate After a Phase I/II Trial by a Loading Bolus and Continuous Infusion in Pediatric Patients," *Cancer Res*, 1990, 50(22):7226-31.
Von Hoff DD, "Phase I Clinical Trials With Fludarabine Phosphate," *Semin Oncol*, 1990, 17(5 Suppl 8):33-8.

Fludrocortisone *(floo droe KOR ti sone)*

Related Information

Corticosteroids Comparison, Systemic *on page 1211*

U.S. Brand Names Florinef® Acetate

Synonyms Fluohydrisone; Fluohydrocortisone; 9α-Fluorohydrocortisone

Therapeutic Category Adrenal Corticosteroid; Corticosteroid, Systemic; Glucocorticoid; Mineralocorticoid

Generic Available No

Use Treatment of Addison's disease; partial replacement therapy for adrenal insufficiency; treatment of salt-losing forms of congenital adrenogenital syndrome; has been used in conjunction with an increased sodium intake for the treatment of idiopathic orthostatic hypotension

Pregnancy Risk Factor C

Contraindications Hypersensitivity to fludrocortisone or any component; CHF, systemic fungal infections

Precautions Dosage should be tapered gradually if therapy is discontinued; use with caution in patients with hypertension, edema, or renal dysfunction

Adverse Reactions

Cardiovascular: Hypertension, edema, CHF

Central nervous system: Convulsions, headache

Dermatologic: Acne, rash, bruising

Endocrine & metabolic: Hypokalemic alkalosis, suppression of growth, hyperglycemia, hypothalamic-pituitary-adrenal suppression

Gastrointestinal: Peptic ulcer

Neuromuscular & skeletal: Muscle weakness

Ocular: Cataracts

Drug Interactions Digoxin (fludrocortisone-induced hypokalemia may increase digoxin toxicity); phenytoin and rifampin may increase metabolism of fludrocortisone; hypokalemia-causing medications may increase risk of hypokalemia

Food Interactions Systemic use of mineralocorticoids/corticosteroids may require a diet with increased potassium, vitamins A, B$_6$, C, D, folate, calcium, zinc, and phosphorus, and decreased sodium; with fludrocortisone a decrease in dietary sodium is often not required as the increased retention of sodium is usually the desired therapeutic effect

Mechanism of Action Potent mineralocorticoid with glucocorticoid activity; promotes increased reabsorption of sodium and loss of potassium from distal tubules

Pharmacodynamics Duration: 1-2 days

Pharmacokinetics

Absorption: Rapid and complete from GI tract

Protein binding: 42%

Metabolism: In the liver

Half-life:

Plasma: ~3.5 hours

Biological: 18-36 hours

Usual Dosage Oral:

Infants and Children: 0.05-0.1 mg/day

Congenital adrenal hyperplasia (salt losers): Maintenance: Range: 0.05-0.3 mg/day (AAP, 2000)

Adults: 0.05-0.2 mg/day

Administration Oral: May administer with food to decrease GI upset

Monitoring Parameters Serum electrolytes and glucose, blood pressure, serum renin

Patient Information Notify physician if dizziness, severe or continuing headache, swelling of feet or lower legs, or unusual weight gain occurs

Additional Information In patients with salt-losing forms of congenital adrenogenital syndrome, use along with cortisone or hydrocortisone; fludrocortisone 0.1 mg has sodium retention activity equal to DOCA® 1 mg

Dosage Forms Tablet, as acetate: 0.1 mg

References

American Academy of Pediatrics, Section on Endocrinology and Committee on Genetics, "Technical Report: Congenital Adrenal Hyperplasia," *Pediatrics*, 2000, 106(6):1511-8.

♦ Fluid and Electrolyte Requirements in Children *see page 1258*

♦ **Flumadine®** *see* Rimantadine *on page 987*

Flumazenil (FLO may ze nil)
U.S. Brand Names Romazicon®
Canadian Brand Names Anexate®
Therapeutic Category Antidote, Benzodiazepine
Generic Available No
Use Benzodiazepine antagonist; reverses sedative effects of benzodiazepines used in general anesthesia or conscious sedation; management of benzodiazepine overdose; **not indicated** for ethanol, barbiturate, general anesthetic or narcotic overdose
Pregnancy Risk Factor C
Contraindications Hypersensitivity to flumazenil, any component, or benzodiazepines; patients given benzodiazepines for control of potentially life-threatening conditions (eg, control of intracranial pressure or status epilepticus); patients with signs of serious cyclic-antidepressant overdosage
Warnings Flumazenil may precipitate seizures in patients physically dependent on benzodiazepines, in patients treated with benzodiazepines for seizure disorders or other reasons, in overdose patients with seizure activity prior to flumazenil, or in patients with serious cyclic antidepressant overdoses; higher than normal doses of benzodiazepines may be required to treat these seizures; mixed drug overdose patients who have ingested drugs that increase the likelihood of seizures (eg, cocaine, lithium, cyclosporine, cyclic antidepressants, bupropion, methylxanthines, MAO inhibitors, isoniazid, or propoxyphene) are at extremely high risk for seizures (flumazenil may be contraindicated in these patients)
Precautions Resedation may occur with flumazenil use (due to its short half-life in comparison to some benzodiazepines); pediatric patients (especially 1-5 years of age) may experience resedation; these patients may require repeat bolus doses or continuous infusion; monitor patients for return of sedation and respiratory depression. Flumazenil should be used with caution in the intensive care unit because of increased risk of unrecognized benzodiazepine dependence in such settings. Flumazenil may provoke panic attacks in patients with panic disorder. Do not use flumazenil until effects of neuromuscular blockers have been fully reversed.
Adverse Reactions
Cardiovascular: Arrhythmias, bradycardia, tachycardia, chest pain, hypertension, hypotension
Central nervous system: Seizures (more common in patients physically dependent on benzodiazepines or with cyclic antidepressant overdoses, see Warnings), fatigue, dizziness, headache, agitation, emotional lability, anxiety, euphoria, depression, abnormal crying
Endocrine & metabolic: Hot flashes
Gastrointestinal: Nausea, vomiting, xerostomia
Local: Pain at injection site
Ocular: Blurred vision
Miscellaneous: Increased diaphoresis, shivering, hiccups, sensation of coldness; can precipitate acute withdrawal symptoms in patients physically dependent on benzodiazepines
Drug Interactions Use with caution in mixed drug overdose; toxic effects of other drugs (especially with cyclic antidepressants) may occur with reversal of benzodiazepine effects
Stability Compatible with D_5W, LR, or NS for 24 hours; discard any unused solution after 24 hours
Mechanism of Action Antagonizes the effect of benzodiazepines on the GABA/benzodiazepine receptor complex. Flumazenil is benzodiazepine specific and does not antagonize other nonbenzodiazepine GABA agonists (including ethanol, barbiturates, general anesthetics); does not reverse the effects of opiates.
Pharmacodynamics
Onset of action: Benzodiazepine reversal: Within 1-3 minutes
Maximum effect: 6-10 minutes
Duration: Usually <1 hour; duration is related to dose given and benzodiazepine plasma concentrations; reversal effects of flumazenil may wear off before effects of benzodiazepine and resedation may occur
Pharmacokinetics Follows a two compartment open model; **Note:** Clearance and V_d per kg are similar for children and adults, but children display more variability
Distribution: Adults:
Initial V_d: 0.5 L/kg
V_{dss} 0.77-1.6 L/kg
Protein binding: ~50%
Metabolism: In the liver to the de-ethylated free acid and its glucuronide conjugate
(Continued)

Flumazenil *(Continued)*

Half-life:
  Children: Terminal: 20-75 minutes (mean: 40 minutes)
  Adults:
    Alpha: 7-15 minutes
    Terminal: 41-79 minutes

Elimination: Clearance dependent upon hepatic blood flow, hepatically eliminated; <1% excreted unchanged in urine

Usual Dosage I.V.:

Children:

Reversal of benzodiazepine when used in conscious sedation or general anesthesia: Initial dose: 0.01 mg/kg (maximum dose: 0.2 mg) given over 15 seconds; may repeat 0.01 mg/kg (maximum dose: 0.2 mg) after 45 seconds, and then every minute to a maximum total cumulative dose of 0.05 mg/kg or 1 mg, whichever is lower; usual total dose: 0.08-1 mg (mean: 0.65 mg)

Management of benzodiazepine overdose: Minimal information available; initial dose: 0.01 mg/kg (maximum dose: 0.2 mg) with repeat doses of 0.01 mg/kg (maximum dose: 0.2 mg) given every minute to a maximum total cumulative dose of 1 mg; as an alternative to repeat bolus doses, follow up continuous infusions of 0.005-0.01 mg/kg/hour have been used; further studies are needed

Adults:

Reversal of benzodiazepine when used in conscious sedation or general anesthesia: 0.2 mg given over 15 seconds; may repeat 0.2 mg after 45 seconds and then every 60 seconds up to a total of 1 mg, usual total dose: 0.6-1 mg. In event of resedation, may repeat doses at 20-minute intervals with maximum of 1 mg/dose (given at 0.2 mg/minute); maximum dose: 3 mg in 1 hour.

Management of benzodiazepine overdose: 0.2 mg over 30 seconds; may give 0.3 mg dose after 30 seconds if desired level of consciousness is not obtained; additional doses of 0.5 mg can be given over 30 seconds at 1-minute intervals up to a cumulative dose of 3 mg; usual cumulative dose: 1-3 mg; rarely, patients with partial response at 3 mg may require additional titration up to total dose of 5 mg; if patient has not responded 5 minutes after cumulative dose of 5 mg, the major cause of sedation is not likely due to benzodiazepines. In the event of resedation, may repeat doses at 20-minute intervals with maximum of 1 mg/dose (given at 0.5 mg/minute); maximum dose: 3 mg in 1 hour.

Dosing adjustment in hepatic impairment: Initial dose: Use normal dose; repeat doses should be decreased in size or frequency

Administration Parenteral: For I.V. use only; administer by rapid I.V. injection over 15-30 seconds via a freely running I.V. infusion into larger vein (to decrease chance of pain, phlebitis). Children: Do not exceed 0.2 mg/minute. Adults: Repeat doses: Do not exceed 0.2 mg/minute for reversal of general anesthesia and do not exceed 0.5 mg/minute for reversal of benzodiazepine overdose.

Monitoring Parameters Level of consciousness and resedation, blood pressure, heart rate, respiratory rate, continuous pulse oximetry; monitor for resedation for 1-2 hours after reversal of sedation in patients who receive benzodiazepine sedation

Patient Information Flumazenil does not consistently reverse amnesia; do not engage in activities requiring alertness for 18-24 hours after discharge; resedation may occur in patients on long-acting benzodiazepines (such as diazepam); avoid alcohol or OTC medications for 18-24 hours after flumazenil is used or if benzodiazepine effects persist; may cause dry mouth

Nursing Implications Flumazenil does not effectively reverse hypoventilation, even in alert patients

Additional Information In one study of conscious sedation reversal in 107 pediatric patients (1-17 years of age), resedation occurred between 19-50 minutes after the start of flumazenil. Flumazenil has been used to successfully treat paradoxical reactions in children associated with midazolam use (eg, agitation, restlessness, combativeness) (see Massanari, 1997).

Dosage Forms Injection, solution: 0.1 mg/mL (5 mL, 10 mL)

References

Baktai G, Szekely E, Marialigeti T, et al, "Use of Midazolam (Dormicum) and Flumazenil (Anexate) in Paediatric Bronchology," *Curr Med Res Opin*, 1992, 12(9):552-9.

Clark RF, Sage TA, Tunget C, et al, "Delayed Onset Lorazepam Poisoning Successfully Reversed By Flumazenil in a Child: Case Report and Review of the Literature," *Pediatr Emerg Care*, 1995, 11(1):32-4.

Jones RD, Lawson AD, Andrew LJ, et al, "Antagonism of the Hypnotic Effect of Midazolam in Children: A Randomized, Double Blind Study of Placebo and Flumazenil Administered After Midazolam-Induced Anaesthesia," *Br J Anaesth*, 1991, 66(6):660-6.

Massanari M, Novitsky J, and Reinstein LJ, "Paradoxical Reactions in Children Associated With Midazolam Use During Endoscopy," *Clin Pediatr*, 1997, 36(12):681-4.

Richard P, Autret E, Bardol J, et al, "The Use of Flumazenil in a Neonate," *J Toxicol Clin Toxicol*, 1991, 29(1):137-40.

Roald OK and Dahl V, "Flunitrazepam Intoxication in a Child Successfully Treated With the Benzodiazepine Antagonist Flumazenil," *Crit Care Med*, 1989, 17(12):1355-6.

Shannon M, Albers G, Burkhart K, et al, "Safety and Efficacy of Flumazenil in the Reversal of Benzodiazepine-Induced Conscious Sedation. The Flumazenil Pediatric Study Group," *J Pediatr*, 1997, 131(4):582-6.

Sugarman JM and Paul RI, "Flumazenil: A Review," *Pediatr Emerg Care*, 1994, 10(1):37-43.

Flunisolide (floo NIS oh lide)

Related Information
Asthma Guidelines *on page 1376*
Estimated Comparative Daily Dosages for Inhaled Corticosteroids *on page 1382*

U.S. Brand Names AeroBid®; AeroBid®-M; Nasalide®; Nasarel®

Canadian Brand Names Alti-Flunisolide; Apo®-Flunisolide; Rhinalar®

Therapeutic Category Adrenal Corticosteroid; Antiasthmatic; Anti-inflammatory Agent; Corticosteroid, Inhalant (Oral); Corticosteroid, Intranasal; Glucocorticoid

Generic Available No

Use
Oral inhalation: Long-term (chronic) control of persistent bronchial asthma; **NOT** indicated for the relief of acute bronchospasm. Also used to help reduce or discontinue oral corticosteroid therapy for asthma.

Intranasal: Management of seasonal or perennial rhinitis

Pregnancy Risk Factor C

Contraindications Hypersensitivity to flunisolide or any component; primary treatment of status asthmaticus; untreated nasal mucosa infection

Warnings Fatalities have occurred due to adrenal insufficiency in asthmatic patients during and after switching from systemic corticosteroids to aerosol steroids; several months may be required for full recovery of the adrenal glands; during this period, aerosol steroids do **not** provide the systemic corticosteroid needed to treat patients requiring stress doses (ie, patients with major stress such as trauma, surgery, or infections); when used at high doses, hypothalamic-pituitary-adrenal (HPA) suppression may occur; use with inhaled or systemic corticosteroids (even alternate-day dosing) may increase risk of HPA suppression; withdrawal and discontinuation of corticosteroids should be done carefully. Immunosuppression may occur.

Precautions Avoid using higher than recommended doses; suppression of HPA function, suppression of linear growth, or hypercorticism (Cushing's syndrome) may occur; use with extreme caution in patients with respiratory tuberculosis, untreated systemic infections, or ocular herpes simplex

Adverse Reactions
Cardiovascular: Palpitations (oral inhalation), hypertension (oral inhalation)

Central nervous system: Dizziness, headache, nervousness

Dermatologic: Rash, itching, eczema

Endocrine & metabolic: Adrenal suppression, potential growth suppression

Gastrointestinal: Nausea, vomiting, diarrhea, upset stomach, sore throat, bitter taste, aftertaste

Genitourinary: Menstrual disturbances (oral inhalation)

Local: Nasal burning

Respiratory: Sneezing, nasal congestion, nasal dryness, pharyngitis, epistaxis, *Candida* infections of the nose or pharynx, atrophic rhinitis, upper respiratory infections

Drug Interactions Expected interactions similar to other corticosteroids

Stability Store intranasal solutions at 59°F to 86°F

Mechanism of Action Controls the rate of protein synthesis, depresses the migration of polymorphonuclear leukocytes and fibroblasts, reverses capillary permeability, and stabilizes lysosomal membranes at the cellular level to prevent or control inflammation

Pharmacodynamics Clinical effects are due to a direct local effect rather than systemic absorption

Onset of action: Intranasal: Within a few days
Maximum effect: Intranasal: 1-2 weeks

Pharmacokinetics
Absorption: Nasal inhalation: ~50%; oral inhalation: ~40%

Metabolism: Rapid in the liver to a less active metabolite, followed by glucuronide and sulfate conjugation

Half-life: 1.8 hours

Elimination: Excreted in urine and feces

(Continued)

Flunisolide *(Continued)*

Usual Dosage Manufacturer recommendation:

Intranasal:

Children 6-14 years: Initial: 1 spray to each nostril 3 times/day or 2 sprays to each nostril 2 times/day; maximum dose: 4 sprays to each nostril per day; after symptoms are controlled, dose should be reduced to lowest effective amount; maintenance: 1 spray each nostril once daily

Adults: Initial: 2 sprays to each nostril twice daily; may increase in 4-7 days if needed to 2 sprays to each nostril 3 times/day; maximum dose: 8 sprays to each nostril per day; after symptoms are controlled, dose should be reduced to lowest effective amount; maintenance: 1 spray to each nostril once daily

Oral inhalation: Doses should be titrated to the lowest dose once asthma is controlled:

Children: 6-15 years: 2 inhalations twice daily

Adults: 2 inhalations twice daily; maximum dose: 8 inhalations/day

NIH Asthma Guidelines (NAEPP, 2002; NIH, 1997) [give in divided doses twice daily]

Children ≤12 years:

"Low" dose: 500-750 mcg/day (2-3 puffs/day)

"Medium" dose: 1000-1250 mcg/day (4-5 puffs/day)

"High" dose: >1250 mcg/day (>5 puffs/day)

Children >12 years and Adults:

"Low" dose: 500-1000 mcg/day (2-4 puffs/day)

"Medium" dose: 1000-2000 mcg/day (4-8 puffs/day)

"High" dose: >2000 mcg/day (>8 puffs/day)

Administration Shake well before use; do not spray in eyes

Oral inhalant: Use a spacer for children <8 years of age; rinse mouth after inhalation to decrease chance of oral candidiasis

Intranasal: Clear nasal passages by blowing nose prior to use

Monitoring Parameters Check mucus membranes for signs of fungal infection; monitor growth in pediatric patients; monitor blood pressure with oral inhalation

Patient Information Notify physician if condition being treated persists or worsens; do not decrease dose or discontinue without physician approval

Oral inhalant: Report sore mouth or mouth lesions to physician

Additional Information Nasalide® and Nasarel® do not contain fluorocarbons. AeroBid® and AeroBid-M® contain fluorocarbon propellants. The efficacy of Nasalide® and Nasarel® are similar; however, more nasal burning and stinging were reported with Nasalide®, and more taste problems (eg, aftertaste) were reported with Nasarel®. These differences are due to the different vehicles of the two products. If bronchospasm with wheezing occurs after use of oral inhalation, a fast-acting bronchodilator may be used.

Dosage Forms

Aerosol for oral inhalation:

AeroBid®: 250 mcg/actuation (7 g) [100 metered doses]

AeroBid-M®: 250 mcg/actuation (7 g) [100 metered doses; menthol flavor]

Solution, intranasal spray (Nasalide®, Nasarel®): 25 mcg/actuation (25 mL) [200 sprays]

References

Expert Panel Report 2, "Guidelines for the Diagnosis and Management of Asthma," *Clinical Practice Guidelines*, National Institutes of Health, National Heart, Lung, and Blood Institute, NIH Publication No. 94-4051, April, 1997.

"National Asthma Education and Prevention Program. Expert Panel Report: Guidelines for the Diagnosis and Management of Asthma Update on Selected Topics--2002," *J Allergy Clin Immunol*, 2002, 110(5 Suppl):S141-219.

Fluocinolone *(floo oh SIN oh lone)*

Related Information

Corticosteroids Comparison, Topical *on page 1212*

U.S. Brand Names Capex™; Derma-Smoothe/FS®; Synalar®

Canadian Brand Names Fluoderm

Therapeutic Category Adrenal Corticosteroid; Anti-inflammatory Agent; Corticosteroid, Topical; Glucocorticoid

Generic Available Yes

Use Relief of susceptible inflammatory dermatosis

Capex™ shampoo: Adults: Treatment of seborrheic dermatitis of the scalp

Derma-Smoothe/FS®: Children ≥2 years: Moderate to severe atopic dermatitis (for use ≤4 weeks); Adults: Atopic dermatitis or psoriasis of the scalp

Pregnancy Risk Factor C

Contraindications Hypersensitivity to fluocinolone or any component (see Warnings); fungal infection; TB of skin; herpes (including varicella)

Warnings Infants and small children may be more susceptible to adrenal axis suppression from topical corticosteroid therapy; systemic effects may occur when used on large areas of the body, denuded areas, for prolonged periods of time, or with an occlusive dressing; Derma-Smoothe/FS® contains refined peanut oil, use with caution in patients with peanut hypersensitivity (see Additional Information)

Adverse Reactions
Dermatologic: Acne, hypopigmentation, allergic dermatitis, maceration of the skin, skin atrophy, folliculitis, hypertrichosis, striae, miliaria
Endocrine & metabolic: Hypothalamic-pituitary-adrenal suppression, Cushing's syndrome, growth retardation
Local: Burning, itching, irritation, dryness
Miscellaneous: Secondary infection

Mechanism of Action Not well defined topically; possesses anti-inflammatory, antiproliferative, and immunosuppressive properties

Usual Dosage
Children and Adults: Topical: Apply thin layer 2-4 times/day
Capex™ shampoo: Adults: Thoroughly wet hair and scalp; apply ≤1 ounce to scalp area; massage well; work into lather; allow to remain on scalp for 5 minutes; then rinse hair and scalp thoroughly; repeat daily until symptoms subside; **Note:** Once patient is symptom free, once weekly use usually keeps itching and flaking of dandruff from returning
Derma-Smoothe/FS®:
Children ≥2 years: Atopic dermatitis: Apply in a thin layer to moistened skin of affected area twice daily for ≤4 weeks
Adults:
Atopic dermatitis: Apply a thin layer to affected area 3 times/day
Scalp psoriasis: Thoroughly wet or dampen hair and scalp; apply to scalp in a thin layer, massage well, cover scalp with shower cap (supplied); leave for a minimum of 4 hours or overnight, then wash hair and rinse thoroughly

Administration Topical: Apply sparingly in a thin film; rub in lightly
Capex™ shampoo: Shake well before use; do not bandage, wrap, or cover treated scalp area unless directed by physician; discard shampoo after 3 months (**Note:** Pharmacist must empty the contents of the 12 mg fluocinolone acetonide capsule into the shampoo base before dispensing to patient)
Derma-Smoothe/FS®: Do not apply to face or diaper area; avoid application to intertriginous areas (may increase local adverse effects)

Patient Information Avoid contact with eyes; do not use for longer than directed; do not overuse; notify physician if condition being treated persists or worsens

Nursing Implications Do not use tight fitting diapers or plastic pants on a child being treated in diaper area; Derma-Smoothe/FS® is not recommended for diaper dermatitis

Additional Information Considered a moderate-potency steroid (Derma-Smoothe/FS® and Capex™ shampoo are considered to be low to medium potency); Derma-Smoothe/FS® is made with 48% refined peanut oil, NF (peanut protein is not detectable at 2.5 ppm)

Dosage Forms
Cream, topical, as acetonide: 0.01% (15 g, 60 g); 0.025% (15 g, 60 g)
Synalar®: 0.025% (15 g, 60 g)
Oil, topical, as acetonide (Derma-Smoothe/FS®): 0.01% (120 mL) [contains refined peanut oil; also available in an Atopic pak containing a moisturizer]
Ointment, topical, as acetonide (Synalar®): 0.025% (15 g, 60 g)
Shampoo, topical, as acetonide (Capex™): 0.01% (120 mL)
Solution, topical, as acetonide: 0.01% (60 mL)
Synalar®: 0.01% (20 mL, 60 mL)

Fluocinonide (floo oh SIN oh nide)
Related Information
Corticosteroids Comparison, Topical on page 1212
U.S. Brand Names Lidex®; Lidex-E®
Canadian Brand Names Lidemol®; Lyderm®; Lyodnide; Tiamol®; Topsyn®
Therapeutic Category Adrenal Corticosteroid; Anti-inflammatory Agent; Corticosteroid, Topical; Glucocorticoid
Generic Available Yes
Use Inflammation of corticosteroid-responsive dermatoses
Pregnancy Risk Factor C
Contraindications Hypersensitivity to fluocinonide or any component; viral, fungal, or tubercular skin lesions; herpes (including varicella)
Warnings Infants and small children may be more susceptible to adrenal axis suppression from topical corticosteroid therapy; systemic effects may occur when used on
(Continued)

Fluocinonide *(Continued)*

large areas of the body, denuded areas, for prolonged periods of time, or with occlusive dressings

Adverse Reactions

Dermatologic: Acne, hypopigmentation, allergic dermatitis, maceration of the skin, skin atrophy, folliculitis, hypertrichosis

Endocrine & metabolic: Hypothalamic-pituitary-adrenal suppression, Cushing's syndrome, growth retardation

Local: Burning, itching, irritation, dryness

Miscellaneous: Secondary infection

Mechanism of Action Not well defined topically; possesses anti-inflammatory, antiproliferative, and immunosuppressive properties

Usual Dosage Children and Adults: Topical: Apply thin layer to affected area 2-4 times/day depending on the severity of the condition

Administration Topical: Apply sparingly in a thin film; rub in lightly

Patient Information Do not overuse; avoid contact with eyes; do not use for longer than directed; avoid use on face; notify physician if condition being treated persists or worsens

Nursing Implications Do not use tight fitting diapers or plastic pants on a child being treated in the diaper area

Additional Information Considered to be a high potency steroid

Dosage Forms

Cream, anhydrous, emollient (Lidex®): 0.05% (15 g, 30 g, 60 g, 120 g)

Cream, aqueous, emollient (Lidex-E®): 0.05% (15 g, 30 g, 60 g)

Gel, topical (Lidex®): 0.05% (15 g, 30 g, 60 g)

Ointment, topical (Lidex®): 0.05% (15 g, 30 g, 60 g)

Solution, topical (Lidex®): 0.05% (20 mL, 60 mL)

♦ **Fluoderm (Can)** *see Fluocinolone on page 498*

♦ **Fluohydrisone** *see Fludrocortisone on page 494*

♦ **Fluohydrocortisone** *see Fludrocortisone on page 494*

♦ **Fluor-A-Day [OTC]** *see Fluoride on page 500*

Fluoride *(FLOR ide)*

U.S. Brand Names ACT® [OTC]; Fluor-A-Day [OTC]; Fluorigard® [OTC]; Fluorinse®; Flura-Drops®; Flura-Loz®; Gel-Kam® [OTC]; Gel-Kam® Rinse; Lozi-Flur™; Luride®; Luride® Lozi-Tab®; NeutraCare®; NeutraGard® [OTC]; Pediaflor®; Pharmaflur®; Pharmaflur® 1.1; Phos-Flur®; Phos-Flur® Rinse [OTC]; PreviDent®; PreviDent® 5000 Plus™; Stan-gard®; Stop®; Thera-Flur-N®

Canadian Brand Names Fluotic®

Therapeutic Category Mineral, Oral; Mineral, Oral Topical

Generic Available Yes

Use Prevention of dental caries

Pregnancy Risk Factor C

Contraindications Hypersensitivity to fluoride or any component (see Warnings); when fluoride content of drinking water exceeds 0.7 ppm; low sodium or sodium-free diets; do not use 1 mg tablets in children <3 years of age or when drinking water fluoride content is ≥0.3 ppm; do not use 1 mg/5 mL rinse (as supplement) in children <6 years of age

Warnings Some products may contain tartrazine which may cause allergic reactions in susceptible individuals

Precautions Prolonged ingestion with excessive doses may result in dental fluorosis and osseous changes; dosage should be adjusted in proportion to the amount of fluoride in the drinking water; do **not** exceed recommended dosage

Adverse Reactions

Central nervous system: Headache

Dermatologic: Rash, eczema, atopic dermatitis, urticaria

Gastrointestinal: GI upset, nausea, vomiting

Miscellaneous: Products containing stannous fluoride may stain the teeth

Drug Interactions Magnesium-, aluminum-, and calcium-containing products may decrease absorption of fluoride

Food Interactions Do not administer with milk

Stability Sodium fluoride solutions decompose in glass containers; store only in tightly closed plastic containers; aqueous solutions of stannous fluoride decompose within hours of preparation; prepare solutions immediately before use

Mechanism of Action Promotes remineralization of decalcified enamel; inhibits the cariogenic microbial process in dental plaque; increases tooth resistance to acid dissolution

Pharmacokinetics

Absorption: Via GI tract, lungs, and skin

Distribution: 50% of fluoride is deposited in teeth and bone after ingestion; crosses placenta; appears in breast milk; topical application works superficially on enamel and plaque

Elimination: In urine and feces

Usual Dosage Oral:

Adequate Intake (AI) (1997 National Academy of Science Recommendations):

Children:

0-6 months: 0.01 mg/day
7-12 months: 0.5 mg/day
1-3 years: 0.7 mg/day
4-8 years: 1 mg/day
9-13 years: 2 mg/day
14-18 years: 3 mg/day

Children >19 and Adults:

Males: 4 mg/day
Females: 3 mg/day

The recommended daily fluoride intake is adjusted in proportion to the fluoride content of available drinking water; see **Recommended Daily Fluoride Dose** table

Recommended Daily Fluoride Dose

Fluoride Content of Drinking Water	Daily Dose, Oral Fluoride (mg)
<0.3 ppm	
Birth - 6 mo	0
6 mo to 3 y	0.25
3-6 y	0.5
6-16 y	1
0.3-0.6 ppm	
Birth - 3 y	0
3-6 y	0.25
6-16 y	0.5
>0.6 ppm	
All ages	0

Adapted from *AAP News*, 1995, 11(2):18.

Dental rinse: See **Sodium Fluoride Dental Rinse Dosing** table

Sodium fluoride (dosage based upon concentration of solution):

Note: 2% concentrations are administered by dental personnel only

Sodium Fluoride Dental Rinse Dosing

Age	% Solution	Dosage
6 y	0.05%	10 mL daily
6-12 y	0.02%	10 mL twice daily
	0.2%	5 mL once weekly
>12 y	0.02%	10 mL twice daily
	0.2%	10 mL once weekly

Acidulated phosphate fluoride rinse: Children 6 years and Adults: 5-10 mL of 0.02% daily at bedtime

Gel:

Acidulated phosphate fluoride: Adults: 4-8 drops of 0.5% gel daily or for desensitizing exposed root surfaces, use a few drops of 0.5% to 1.2% gel applied and brushed onto affected area each night

Stannous fluoride: Children >6 years and Adults: Apply 0.4% gel to teeth once daily

Administration Oral:

Dental gel: Do **not** swallow; gel drops are placed in trough of applicator; applicator is applied over upper and lower teeth at same time; bite down for 6 minutes

Dental rinse: Swish or rinse in mouth then expectorate; do not swallow

Tablet: Dissolve in mouth, chew, swallow whole, or add to drinking water or fruit juice; administer with food (but not milk) to eliminate GI upset

Reference Range Total plasma fluoride: 0.14-0.19 µg/mL

(Continued)

Fluoride *(Continued)*

Dosage Forms

Cream, topical, as **sodium fluoride** (PreviDent® 5000 Plus™): 1.1% (51 g) [2.5 mg fluoride/dose; fruit and spearmint flavors]

Gel-drops, as **sodium fluoride** (Thera-Flur®-N): 1.1% (24 mL) [0.5% fluoride; neutral pH, no artificial color or flavor]

Gel, topical, as **acidulated phosphate fluoride** (Phos-Flur®): 1.1% (60 g) [0.5% fluoride; cherry and mint flavors]

Gel, topical, as **sodium fluoride**:
   NeutraCare®: 1.1% (60 g) [neutral pH; grape and mint flavors]
   PreviDent®: 1.1% (60 g) [fluoride 2 mg/dose; berry, cherry, and mint flavors]

Gel, topical, as **stannous fluoride**:
   Gel-Kam®: 0.4% (129 g) [bubblegum, cinnamon, fruit/berry, and mint flavors]
   Stan-Gard®: 0.4% (122 g) [bubblegum, cherry, cinnamon, grape, mint, and raspberry flavors]
   Stop®: 0.4% (120 g) [bubblegum, cinnamon, grape, and mint flavors]

Lozenge, as **sodium**:
   Flura-Loz®: 2.2 mg [1 mg fluoride; sugar free; raspberry flavor]
   Fluor-A-Day: 2.2 mg [1 mg fluoride; mint flavor]
   Lozi-Flur™: 2.21 mg [1 mg fluoride; cherry flavor]

Solution, oral **drops**, as **sodium**:
   Flura-Drops®: 0.55 mg/drop (24 mL) [0.25 mg fluoride/drop]
   Luride®: 1.1 mg/mL (50 mL) [0.5 mg/mL fluoride; sugar free]
   Pediaflor®: 1.1 mg/mL (50 mL) [0.5 mg/mL fluoride; sugar free; contains <0.5% alcohol; cherry flavor]

Solution, oral rinse, as **sodium**:
   ACT®: 0.05% (530 mL) [0.0226% fluoride; cinnamon flavor (contains tartrazine) or bubblegum flavor]
   Fluorigard®: 0.05% (480 mL) [contains alcohol, sodium benzoate and tartrazine; mint flavor]
   Fluorinse®: 0.2% (480 mL) [alcohol free; cinnamon and mint flavors]
   NeutraGard®: 0.05% (480 mL) [neutral pH; mint and tropical blast flavors]
   Phos-Flur®: 0.44% (500 mL) [bubblegum, cherry, grape, and mint flavors]
   PreviDent®: 0.2% (250 mL) [contains alcohol; mint flavor]

Solution, oral rinse **concentrate**, as **stannous fluoride** (Gel-Kam®): 0.63% (300 mL) [7.1 mg fluoride/dose; cinnamon and mint flavors]

Tablet, chewable, as **sodium**:
   Fluor-A-Day: 0.56 mg [0.25 mg fluoride; raspberry flavor], 1.1 mg [0.5 mg fluoride; raspberry flavor], 2.21 mg [1 mg fluoride; raspberry flavor]
   Luride® Lozi-Tab®: 0.55 mg [0.25 mg fluoride; sugar free; vanilla flavor], 1.1 mg [0.5 mg fluoride; sugar free; grape flavor], 2.2 mg [1 mg fluoride; sugar free; cherry flavor]
   Pharmaflur®: 2.2 mg [1 mg fluoride; dye and sugar free; cherry flavor]
   Pharmaflur® 1.1: 1.1 mg [0.5 mg fluoride; dye and sugar free; grape flavor]

References

"Dietary Reference Intakes for Calcium, Phosphorus, Magnesium, Vitamin D, and Fluoride. Standing Committee on the Scientific Evaluation of Dietary Reference Intakes, Food and Nutrition Board, Institute of Medicine," National Academy of Sciences, Washington, DC: National Academy Press, 1997.

♦ **Fluorigard® [OTC]** *see* Fluoride *on page 500*

♦ **Fluorinse®** *see* Fluoride *on page 500*

♦ **9α-Fluorohydrocortisone** *see* Fludrocortisone *on page 494*

Fluorometholone *(flure oh METH oh lone)*

U.S. Brand Names Eflone®; Flarex®; Fluor-Op®; FML®; FML® Forte

Canadian Brand Names PMS-Fluorometholone

Therapeutic Category Adrenal Corticosteroid; Anti-inflammatory Agent, Ophthalmic; Corticosteroid, Ophthalmic; Glucocorticoid

Generic Available Yes (suspension, as base)

Use Inflammatory conditions of the eye, including keratitis, iritis, cyclitis, and conjunctivitis

Pregnancy Risk Factor C

Contraindications Hypersensitivity to fluorometholone, other corticosteroids, or any component; herpes simplex keratitis, fungal diseases of ocular structures, mycobacterial infections of the eye, and most viral diseases of cornea and conjunctiva

Warnings Not recommended for children <2 years of age

Precautions Prolonged use may result in glaucoma, increased intraocular pressure, or other ocular damage

Adverse Reactions
Local: Stinging, burning

Ocular: Elevated intraocular pressure, open-angle glaucoma, defect in visual acuity and field of vision, cataracts, photosensitivity

Mechanism of Action Decreases inflammation by suppression of migration of polymorphonuclear leukocytes and reversal of increased capillary permeability

Pharmacokinetics Absorption: Into aqueous humor with slight systemic absorption

Usual Dosage Children >2 years and Adults: Ophthalmic:

Ointment: May be applied every 4 hours in severe cases or 1-3 times/day in mild to moderate cases.

Drops: Instill 1-2 drops into conjunctival sac every hour during day, every 2 hours at night until favorable response is obtained, then use 1 drop every 4 hours; in mild or moderate inflammation: 1-2 drops into conjunctival sac 2-4 times/day.

Administration Ophthalmic: Avoid contact of medication tube or bottle tip with skin or eye; suspension: Shake well before use; apply finger pressure to lacrimal sac during and for 1-2 minutes after instillation to decrease risk of absorption and systemic effects; the preservative (benzalkonium chloride) may be absorbed by soft contact lenses; wait at least 15 minutes after administration of suspension before inserting soft contact lenses

Monitoring Parameters Intraocular pressure (if used ≥10 days)

Patient Information May cause blurring of vision; do not discontinue without consulting physician; notify physician if improvement does not occur after 2 days

Dosage Forms
Ointment, ophthalmic (FML®): 0.1% (3.5 g) [contains phenylmercuric acetate]

Suspension, ophthalmic: 0.1% (5 mL, 10 mL, 15 mL)

Fluor-Op®: 0.1% (5 mL, 10 mL, 15 mL) [contains polyvinyl alcohol]

FML®: 0.1% (1 mL, 5 mL, 10 mL, 15 mL) [contains polyvinyl alcohol]

FML® Forte: 0.25% (2 mL, 5 mL, 10 mL, 15 mL) [contains polyvinyl alcohol]

Suspension, ophthalmic, as acetate:

Eflone®: 0.1% (5 mL, 10 mL)

Flarex®: 0.1% (5 mL, 10 mL)

♦ **Fluor-Op®** see Fluorometholone on page 502

♦ **Fluoroplex®** see Fluorouracil on page 503

Fluorouracil (flure oh YOOR a sil)

Related Information
Emetogenic Potential of Single Chemotherapeutic Agents on page 1286

U.S. Brand Names Adrucil®; Carac™; Efudex®; Fluoroplex®

Synonyms 5-Fluorouracil; 5-FU

Therapeutic Category Antineoplastic Agent, Antimetabolite

Generic Available Yes (injection)

Use Treatment of carcinoma of stomach, colon, rectum, breast, and pancreas; topically for management of multiple actinic keratoses and superficial basal cell carcinomas

Pregnancy Risk Factor D

Contraindications Hypersensitivity to fluorouracil or any component; patients with poor nutritional status, bone marrow suppression, thrombocytopenia; pregnancy

Warnings The FDA currently recommends that procedures for proper handling and disposal of antineoplastic agents be considered; if intractable vomiting, diarrhea, or hemorrhage occurs, discontinue fluorouracil immediately

Precautions Use with caution and modify dosage in patients with renal or hepatic impairment

Adverse Reactions
Cardiovascular: Cardiac arrhythmias, heart failure, hypotension

Central nervous system: Headache, cerebellar ataxia (gait and speech abnormalities), somnolence, dizziness

Dermatologic: Alopecia, skin pigmentation, pruritic maculopapular rash, partial loss of nails or hyperpigmentation of nail bed, photosensitivity

Gastrointestinal: Nausea, vomiting, diarrhea, anorexia, GI hemorrhage, stomatitis, esophagitis

Hematologic: Myelosuppression, granulocytopenia, thrombocytopenia

Hepatic: Hepatotoxicity

Ocular: Visual disturbances, nystagmus, conjunctivitis

Miscellaneous: Palmar-plantar erythrodysesthesias (erythematous, desquamative rash involving hands and feet accompanied by pain, tingling, and swollen palms; this adverse effect may be treated with oral pyridoxine)

Drug Interactions Cimetidine (increases 5-FU concentration); leucovorin may potentiate the antitumor activity of 5-FU

(Continued)

Fluorouracil *(Continued)*

Food Interactions Use of acidic solutions such as orange juice or other fruit juices to dilute 5-FU for oral administration may result in precipitation of the drug and decreased absorption; increase dietary intake of thiamine

Stability Store at room temperature; protect from light; slight discoloration of injection during storage does not affect potency; if precipitate forms, redissolve drug by heating to 140°F, shake well; allow to cool to body temperature before administration; incompatible with cytarabine, diazepam, doxorubicin, methotrexate

Mechanism of Action A pyrimidine antimetabolite that inhibits thymidylate synthase leading to depletion of the DNA precursor thymidine; incorporated into RNA, DNA

Pharmacokinetics

Absorption: Oral: Erratic

Distribution: Into tumors, intestinal mucosa, liver, bone marrow, and CSF

Protein binding: <10%

Metabolism: Inactive metabolites are formed following metabolism in the liver

Bioavailability: 50% to 80%; variable due to saturable first-pass elimination process

Half-life, biphasic:

Alpha: 10-20 minutes

Terminal: 15-19 hours

Elimination: Biphasic elimination with <10% of dose excreted unchanged in the urine

Usual Dosage Children and Adults (refer to individual protocols with dose based on lean body weight):

I.V.:

Initial: 400-500 mg/m^2/day (12 mg/kg/day; maximum dose: 800 mg/day) for 4-5 days

Maintenance: 200-250 mg/m^2/dose (6 mg/kg) every other day for 4 doses; repeat in 4 weeks

Single weekly bolus dose of 15 mg/kg or 500 mg/m^2 can be administered depending on the patient's reaction to the previous course of treatment; maintenance dose of 5-15 mg/kg/week as a single dose not to exceed 1 g/week

I.V. infusion: 15 mg/kg/day or 500 mg/m^2/day (maximum daily dose: 1 g) has been given by I.V. infusion over 4 hours for 5 days; **or** 800-1200 mg/m^2 for continuous infusion over 24-120 hours

Oral: 15-20 mg/kg/day for 5-8 days has been used for colorectal carcinoma; 15 mg/kg/week for hepatoma

Dosing adjustment in hepatic impairment: Bilirubin >5 mg/dL: Not recommended for use

Topical: Cream or solution: Apply twice daily

Administration

Oral: Administer in early morning on an empty stomach; do not eat for 2 hours before and after dosage administration; dilute injectable fluorouracil solution dose in 4 oz of water or a diluted bicarbonate buffer solution to increase absorption; do not mix with orange juice or other fruit juices

Parenteral: Administer by direct I.V. injection (50 mg/mL solution needs no further dilution) over several minutes or by I.V. intermittent or continuous infusion diluted in saline or dextrose solutions; toxicity (eg, myelosuppression) may be reduced by giving the drug as a continuous infusion. Doses >750-800 mg/m^2 should be administered as a continuous infusion, **not** by bolus injection; dose-limiting toxicity with continuous infusion is mucous membrane toxicity (ie, stomatitis, diarrhea)

Topical: Apply with a nonmetallic applicator or gloved fingers in a sufficient amount to cover affected area. Avoid contact with eyes, nostrils, and mouth. Do not cover area with an occlusive dressing

1% or 2%: Apply to lesions on the head and neck for the treatment of multiple actinic keratoses

5%: Use on lesions in areas other than the head and neck for multiple actinic keratoses; only 5% preparations are used for the treatment of superficial basal cell carcinoma

Monitoring Parameters CBC with differential and platelet count, renal function tests, liver function tests; observe for changes in bowel frequency

Patient Information Maintain adequate hydration; report signs and symptoms of infection, bleeding, bruising, vision changes, unremitting nausea, vomiting, or diarrhea, chest pain or palpitations, or CNS changes. May cause photosensitivity reactions (eg, exposure to sunlight may cause severe sunburn, skin rash, redness, or itching); avoid exposure to sunlight and artificial light sources (sunlamps, tanning booth/bed); wear protective clothing, wide-brimmed hats, sunglasses, and lip sunscreen (SPF ≥15); use a sunscreen [broad-spectrum sunscreen or physical sunscreen (preferred) or sunblock with SPF ≥15]; contact physician if reaction occurs.

Nursing Implications Wash hands immediately after topical application of the cream or solution

Additional Information Myelosuppressive effects:
WBC: Mild
Platelets: Mild
Onset (days): 7-10
Nadir (days): 9-14
Recovery (days): 21

Dosage Forms
Cream, topical:
  Carac™: 0.5% (30 g)
  Efudex®: 5% (25 g) [contains propylene glycol]
  Fluoroplex®: 1% (30 g) [contains benzyl alcohol]
Injection, solution: 50 mg/mL (10 mL, 20 mL, 50 mL, 100 mL)
  Adrucil®: 50 mg/mL (10 mL, 50 mL, 100 mL)
Solution, topical:
  Efudex®: 2% (10 mL); 5% (10 mL) [contains propylene glycol]
  Fluoroplex®: 1% (30 mL) [contains propylene glycol]

References
Balis FM, Holcenberg JS and Bleyer WA, "Clinical Pharmacokinetics of Commonly Used Anticancer Drugs," *Clin Pharmacokinet*, 1983, 8(3):202-32.

♦ **5-Fluorouracil** *see* Fluorouracil *on page 503*

♦ **Fluotic® (Can)** *see* Fluoride *on page 500*

Fluoxetine (floo OKS e teen)

Related Information
Carbohydrate and Alcohol Content of Liquid Medications for Use in Patients Receiving Ketogenic Diets *on page 1431*
Comparison of Adverse Effects of Antidepressants *on page 1210*
Comparison of Usual Adult Dosage and Mechanism of Action of Antidepressants *on page 1209*
Drugs and Breast-Feeding *on page 1404*
Serotonin Syndrome *on page 1420*

U.S. Brand Names Prozac®; Prozac® Weekly™; Sarafem™

Canadian Brand Names Alti-Fluoxetine; Apo®-Fluoxetine; CO Fluoxetine; Gen-Fluoxetine; Novo-Fluoxetine; Nu-Fluoxetine; PMS-Fluoxetine; Rhoxal-fluoxetine

Therapeutic Category Antidepressant, Selective Serotonin Reuptake Inhibitor (SSRI)

Generic Available Yes (except delayed release capsule)

Use Treatment of major depressive disorder, obsessive-compulsive disorder, bulimia nervosa, premenstrual dysphoric disorder (PMDD), panic disorder with or without agoraphobia

Pregnancy Risk Factor C

Contraindications Hypersensitivity to fluoxetine or any component; use of MAO inhibitors within 14 days (potentially fatal reactions may occur, see Drug Interactions); do not use MAO inhibitors for at least 5 weeks after fluoxetine is discontinued); concurrent use of thioridazine or use within 5 weeks after fluoxetine is discontinued (see Drug Interactions)

Warnings Rash or urticaria may occur along with leukocytosis, fever, edema, arthralgia, lymphadenopathy, respiratory distress, and other symptoms; rare cases of vasculitis and lupus-like syndrome have been reported; anaphylactoid reactions including laryngospasm, bronchospasm, angioedema, and urticaria may occur; discontinue use if rash or other allergic reaction occurs

Oral solution contains benzoic acid; benzoic acid (benzoate) is a metabolite of benzyl alcohol; large amounts of benzyl alcohol (≥99 mg/kg/day) have been associated with a potentially fatal toxicity ("gasping syndrome") in neonates; avoid use of fluoxetine products containing benzoic acid in neonates; *in vitro* and animal studies have shown that benzoate displaces bilirubin from protein binding sites

Precautions May precipitate mania or hypomania in patients with bipolar disease. May cause insomnia, anxiety, nervousness, anorexia, or weight loss. Use with caution in patients where weight loss is undesirable. May impair cognitive or motor performance. Use with caution in patients with renal or hepatic impairment, seizure disorders, cardiac dysfunction, diabetes mellitus; decrease dose in liver dysfunction; use with caution in patients at high risk for suicide; add or initiate other antidepressants with caution after 5 weeks or longer after stopping fluoxetine

Fluoxetine may cause decreased growth (smaller increases in weight and height) in children and adolescent patients; currently, no studies directly evaluate fluoxetine's long term effects on growth, development, and maturation of pediatric patients; periodic monitoring of height and weight in pediatric patients is recommended **Note:** Case reports of decreased growth in children receiving fluoxetine or fluvoxamine
(Continued)

Fluoxetine *(Continued)*

(n=4; age: 11.6-13.7 years) for 6 months to 5 years suggest a suppression of growth hormone secretion during SSRI therapy (see Weintrob, 2002). Further studies are needed.

Adverse Reactions Predominant adverse effects are CNS and GI:

Cardiovascular: Vasodilation

Central nervous system: Headache, nervousness, insomnia, drowsiness, anxiety, dizziness, fatigue, sedation, somnolence, mania, hypomania, irritability, suicidal ideation, extrapyramidal reactions (rare); difficulty concentrating, abnormal dreams

Dermatologic: Rash, urticaria, pruritus

Endocrine & metabolic: Hypoglycemia; hyponatremia, SIADH (usually in volume-depleted patients); sexual dysfunction, decreased libido

Gastrointestinal: Nausea, diarrhea, xerostomia, anorexia, dyspepsia, constipation, weight loss; decreased growth in pediatric patients

Hematologic: Altered platelet function (rare)

Neuromuscular & skeletal: Tremor, asthenia, weakness

Ocular: Visual disturbances

Respiratory: Rhinitis, pharyngitis, yawn

Miscellaneous: Anaphylactoid reactions, allergies, diaphoresis, flu-like syndrome

Drug Interactions Cytochrome P450 isoenzyme CYP2D6 substrate (minor pathway), CYP3A3/4 substrate; CYP2C9 isoenzyme inducer; CYP1A2 (at higher doses), CYP2C9, CYP2C19, CYP2D6, CYP3A3/4 isoenzyme inhibitor (extent of CYP3A4 inhibition may not be clinically significant; however, the metabolite norfluoxetine is a more potent CYP3A inhibitor)

With MAO inhibitors, fever, tremors, seizures, delirium, coma may occur [use of MAO inhibitors within 14 days of fluoxetine use is contraindicated; do not use MAO inhibitors for at least 5 weeks after fluoxetine is discontinued (due to long elimination half-life of fluoxetine and its active metabolite)]; tryptophan (which can be metabolized to serotonin) may increase CNS and GI toxic effects and the herbal medicine St John's wort (*Hypericum perforatum*) may increase serious side effects (the use of these agents is **not** recommended). Fluoxetine may inhibit metabolism and increase effects of tricyclic antidepressants (dosage reduction of TCA and monitoring of TCA plasma concentrations may be needed when fluoxetine is coadministered or has been recently discontinued), trazodone, phenytoin, carbamazepine, haloperidol, clozapine, alprazolam, and diazepam; fluoxetine may inhibit the metabolism of thioridazine and increase the risk of serious adverse effects, such as QT_c prolongation, serious ventricular arrhythmias (eg, torsade de pointes) and sudden death (concurrent use of thioridazine or use within 5 weeks of discontinuation of fluoxetine is contraindicated); may antagonize buspirone effects; may displace highly protein bound drugs and cause adverse effects; may increase prothrombin time in patients receiving warfarin; use with sumatriptan may cause weakness, incoordination, and hyper-reflexia; may increase or decrease serum lithium levels (monitor levels closely); concurrent use of fluoxetine with ritonavir may cause the serotonin syndrome (monitor closely)

Food Interactions Tryptophan supplements may increase CNS and GI adverse effects (eg, restlessness, agitation, GI problems); food does not affect bioavailability, but may delay absorption by 1-2 hours

Stability Store at room temperature; protect tablets, immediate release capsules, and solution from light

Mechanism of Action Inhibits CNS neuron serotonin uptake; minimal or no effect on reuptake of norepinephrine or dopamine; does not significantly bind to alpha-adrenergic, histamine or cholinergic receptors; may therefore be useful in patients at risk from sedation, hypotension and anticholinergic effects of tricyclic antidepressants

Pharmacodynamics Maximum effect: Maximum antidepressant effects usually occur after >4 weeks; due to long half-life, resolution of adverse reactions after discontinuation may be slow

Pharmacokinetics Note: Average steady-state fluoxetine serum concentrations in children (n=10; 6 to <13 years of age) were 2-fold higher than in adolescents (n=11; 13 to <18 years of age); all patients received 20 mg/day; average steady-state norfluoxetine serum concentrations were 1.5-fold higher in the children compared with adolescents; differences in weight almost entirely explained the differences in serum concentrations

Absorption: Oral: Well absorbed; enteric-coated pellets contained in Prozac® Weekly™ resist dissolution until GI pH >5.5 and therefore delay onset of absorption 1-2 hours compared to immediate release formulations

Distribution: Adults: V_d: 20-45 L/kg; widely distributed

Protein binding: ~95% (albumin and alpha$_1$-glycoprotein)

Metabolism: In the liver to norfluoxetine (active) and other metabolites

Bioavailability: Capsules, tablets, solution, and weekly capsules are bioequivalent

Half-life: Adults:
Fluoxetine: Acute dosing: 1-3 days; chronic dosing: 4-6 days; cirrhosis: 7.6 days
Norfluoxetine: Acute and chronic dosing: 4-16 days; cirrhosis: 12 days
Time to peak serum concentration: Immediate release formulation: After 6-8 hours
Elimination: In urine as fluoxetine (2.5% to 5%) and norfluoxetine (10%)

Usual Dosage Oral:
Children and Adolescents:
Depression: 8-18 years of age: Initial: 10-20 mg/day; in patients started at 10 mg/day, may increase dose to 20 mg/day after 1 week. Lower weight children: Initial: 10 mg/day; usual: 10 mg/day; if needed, may increase dose to 20 mg/day after several weeks.
Obsessive-compulsive disorder: 7-18 years of age:
Lower weight children: Initial: 10 mg/day; if needed, may increase dose after several weeks; usual range: 20-30 mg/day; minimal experience with doses >20 mg/day; no experience with doses >60 mg/day
Higher weight children and Adolescents: Initial: 10 mg/day; may increase dose to 20 mg/day after 2 weeks; may increase dose after several more weeks, if needed; usual range: 20-60 mg/day
Elective mutism: 6 children 6-12 years of age with elective mutism were treated with initial doses of 0.2 mg/kg/day for 1 week, then 0.4 mg/kg/day for 1 week, then 0.6 mg/kg/day for 10 weeks (Black,1994); further studies are needed

Adults:
Depression or obsessive-compulsive disorder: Initial dose: 20 mg/day administered in the morning; may increase after several weeks by 20 mg/day increments; maximum dose: 80 mg/day; doses >20 mg/day can be given either once daily (in the morning) or divided into morning or noon doses
Depression: Weekly dosing: Patients maintained on 20 mg/day may be changed to Prozac® Weekly™ 90 mg/week, starting 7 days after the last 20 mg/day dose
Bulimia nervosa: 60 mg/day administered in the morning; may need to titrate up to this dose over several days in some patients; higher doses have not been well studied
Premenstrual dysphoric disorder: 20 mg/day; given continuously (every day), **or** 20 mg/day given intermittently (starting the daily dose 14 days prior to the expected onset of menstruation with administration of daily dose through the first full day of menses); repeat with each menstrual cycle; doses >60 mg/day have not been studied; maximum dose: 80 mg/day
Panic disorder: Initial: 10 mg/day; increase dose to 20 mg/day after 1 week; if needed, may increase dose further after several weeks; doses >60 mg/day have not been evaluated

Dosage adjustment in renal impairment: Adjustment not routinely needed

Dosage adjustment in hepatic impairment: Lower doses or less frequent administration are recommended

Administration Oral: May be administered without regard to food

Monitoring Parameters Liver function, weight, serum glucose; serum sodium (in volume depleted patients); monitor for rash and signs or symptoms of anaphylactoid reactions; monitor height and weight in pediatric patients periodically

Reference Range
Therapeutic: Fluoxetine 100-800 ng/mL (SI: 289-2314 nmol/L); norfluoxetine 100-600 ng/mL (SI: 289-1735 nmol/L)
Toxic: (Fluoxetine plus norfluoxetine): >2000 ng/mL (SI: >5784 nmol/L)

Patient Information Avoid alcohol, tryptophan supplements, and the herbal medicine St John's wort; may cause dizziness or drowsiness and impair ability to perform activities requiring mental alertness or physical coordination; may cause dry mouth; inform physician immediately if hives or rash develops. Some medicines should not be taken with fluoxetine or should not be taken for a while after fluoxetine has been discontinued; report the use of other medications, nonprescription medications, and herbal or natural products to your physician and pharmacist.

Nursing Implications Last dose of the day should be given before 4 PM (to avoid insomnia)

Additional Information If used for an extended period of time, long-term usefulness of fluoxetine should be periodically re-evaluated for the individual patient. A recent report describes 5 children (age: 8-15 years) who developed epistaxis (n=4) or bruising (n=1) while receiving SSRI therapy (sertraline) (Lake, 2000).

Dosage Forms Available as fluoxetine hydrochloride; mg strength refers to fluoxetine
Capsule: 10 mg, 20 mg, 40 mg
Prozac®: 10 mg, 20 mg, 40 mg
Sarafem™: 10 mg, 20 mg
Capsule, delayed release (Prozac® Weekly™): 90 mg
Solution, oral (Prozac®): 20 mg/5 mL (120 mL) [contains alcohol and benzoic acid; mint flavor]
(Continued)

Fluoxetine *(Continued)*

Tablet: 10 mg, 20 mg
Prozac®: 10 mg

Extemporaneous Preparations Dilutions of the commercially available oral solution may be made; 1 mg/mL and 2 mg/mL dilutions in Simple Syrup USP, Simple Syrup - British Pharmacopoeia, Aromatic Elixir USP, grape-cranberry drink (Ocean Spray® Cran-Grape), and deionized water were stable for 8 weeks when stored in amber glass bottles at 5°C and 30°C (Peterson, 1994).

Peterson JA, Risley DS, Anderson PN, et al, "Stability of Fluoxetine Hydrochloride in Fluoxetine Solution Diluted With Common Pharmaceutical Diluents," *Am J Hosp Pharm*, 1994, 51(10):1342-5.

References

Black B and Uhde TW, "Treatment of Elective Mutism With Fluoxetine: A Double Blind, Placebo-Controlled Study," *J Am Acad Child Adolesc Psychiatry*, 1994, 33(7):1000-6.

Como PG and Kurlan R, "An Open-Label Trial of Fluoxetine for Obsessive-Compulsive Disorder in Gilles de la Tourette's Syndrome," *Neurology*, 1991, 41(6):872-4.

DeSilva KE, Le Flore DB, Marston BJ, et al, "Serotonin Syndrome in HIV-Infected Individuals Receiving Antiretroviral Therapy and Fluoxetine," *AIDS*, 2001, 15(10):1281-5.

Emslie GJ, Rush AJ, Weinberg WA, et al, "A Double-Blind, Randomized, Placebo-Controlled Trial of Fluoxetine in Children and Adolescents With Depression," *Arch Gen Psychiatry*, 1997, 54(11):1031-7.

Findling RL, Reed MD, and Blumer JL, "Pharmacological Treatment of Depression in Children and Adolescents," *Paediatr Drugs*, 1999, 1(3):161-82.

Kurlan R, Como PG, Deeley C, et al, "A Pilot Controlled Study of Fluoxetine for Obsessive-Compulsive Symptoms in Children With Tourette's Syndrome," *Clin Neuropharmacol*, 1993, 16(2):167-72.

Lake MB, Birmaher B, Wassick S, et al, "Bleeding and Selective Serotonin Reuptake Inhibitors in Childhood and Adolescence," *J Child Adolesc Psychopharmacol*, 2000, 10(1):35-8.

Riddle MA, Hardin MT, King R, et al, "Fluoxetine Treatment of Children and Adolescents With Tourette's and Obsessive-Compulsive Disorders: Preliminary Clinical Experience," *J Am Acad Child Adolesc Psychiatry*, 1990, 29(1):45-8.

Riddle MA, Scahill L, King RA, et al, "Double-Blind, Crossover Trial of Fluoxetine and Placebo in Children and Adolescents With Obsessive-Compulsive Disorder," *J Am Acad Child Adolesc Psychiatry*, 1992, 31(6):1062-9.

Thomsen PH, "Obsessive-Compulsive Disorder: Pharmacological Treatment," *Eur Child Adolesc Psychiatry*, 2000, 9 Suppl 1:I76-84.

Weintrob N, Cohen D, Klipper-Aurbach Y, et al, "Decreased Growth During Therapy With Selective Serotonin Reuptake Inhibitors," *Arch Pediatr Adolesc Med*, 2002, 156(7):696-701.

Fluoxymesterone *(floo oks i MES te rone)*

U.S. Brand Names Halotestin®

Therapeutic Category Androgen

Generic Available Yes

Use Replacement of endogenous testicular hormone; in females used as palliative treatment of breast cancer, postpartum breast engorgement

Restrictions C-III

Pregnancy Risk Factor X

Contraindications Hypersensitivity to fluoxymesterone or any component (see Warnings); serious cardiac disease, liver or kidney disease

Warnings Some tablets (brand name) contain tartrazine which may cause allergic reactions in susceptible individuals

Precautions May accelerate bone maturation without producing compensatory gain in linear growth; in prepubertal children perform radiographic examination of the hand and wrist every 6 months to determine the rate of bone maturation and to assess the effect of treatment on the epiphyseal centers

Adverse Reactions

Cardiovascular: Edema

Central nervous system: Anxiety, mental depression, headache

Dermatologic: Acne, hirsutism

Endocrine & metabolic: Gynecomastia, amenorrhea, hypercalcemia, female virilization

Gastrointestinal: Nausea

Genitourinary: Priapism

Hematologic: Polycythemia, suppression of clotting factors II, VII, IX, X

Hepatic: Cholestatic hepatitis

Neuromuscular & skeletal: Paresthesia

Miscellaneous: Hypersensitivity reactions

Drug Interactions May potentiate the action of oral anticoagulants; may decrease blood glucose concentrations and insulin requirements in patients with diabetes; may elevate cyclosporin levels; may increase extrapyramidal side effects and other CNS effects when coadministered with lithium; may potentiate respiratory depressant effects of narcotics

Mechanism of Action Synthetic androgenic anabolic steroid hormone responsible for the normal growth and development of male sex organs and maintenance of secondary sex characteristics; synthetic testosterone derivative with significant androgen activity; stimulates RNA polymerase activity resulting in an increase in protein production; increases bone development

Pharmacokinetics
Absorption: Oral: Rapid
Protein binding: 98%
Metabolism: In the liver
Half-life: 10-100 minutes
Elimination: Enterohepatic circulation and urinary excretion (90%)
Halogenated derivative of testosterone with up to 5 times the activity of methyltestosterone

Usual Dosage Adults: Oral:
Male:
Hypogonadism: 5-20 mg/day
Delayed puberty: 2.5-20 mg/day for 4-6 months
Female:
Inoperable breast carcinoma: 10-40 mg/day in divided doses for 1-3 months
Breast engorgement: 2.5 mg after delivery, 5-10 mg/day in divided doses for 4-5 days

Monitoring Parameters Periodic radiographic exams of hand and wrist (when used in children); hemoglobin, hematocrit (if receiving high dosages or long-term therapy)

Dosage Forms
Tablet: 10 mg
Halotestin®: 2 mg, 5 mg, 10 mg [contains tartrazine]

♦ **Flura-Drops®** see Fluoride on page 500
♦ **Flura-Loz®** see Fluoride on page 500

Flurazepam (flure AZ e pam)

Related Information
Overdose and Toxicology on page 1388
U.S. Brand Names Dalmane®
Canadian Brand Names Apo®-Flurazepam
Therapeutic Category Benzodiazepine; Hypnotic; Sedative
Generic Available Yes
Use Short-term treatment of insomnia
Restrictions C-IV
Pregnancy Risk Factor X
Contraindications Hypersensitivity to flurazepam or any component (there may be cross-sensitivity with other benzodiazepines), pregnancy, pre-existing CNS depression, respiratory depression, narrow-angle glaucoma
Precautions Use with caution in patients receiving other CNS depressants and in patients with low albumin or hepatic dysfunction
Adverse Reactions
Central nervous system: Drowsiness, dizziness, confusion; residual daytime sedation; paradoxical reactions, hyperactivity, and excitement (rare), ataxia
Miscellaneous: Physical and psychological dependence with prolonged use
Drug Interactions Cytochrome P450 isoenzyme CYP3A3/4 substrate
Additive CNS depression with other CNS depressants, alcohol; cimetidine may decrease and enzyme inducers may increase metabolism of flurazepam; concurrent use of flurazepam with ritonavir is not recommended
Mechanism of Action Depresses all levels of the CNS, including the limbic and reticular formation, by binding to the benzodiazepine site on the gamma-aminobutyric acid (GABA) receptor complex and modulating GABA, which is a major inhibitory neurotransmitter in the brain
Pharmacodynamics Hypnotic effects:
Onset of action: 15-20 minutes
Maximum effect: 3-6 hours
Duration: 7-8 hours
Pharmacokinetics
Metabolism: In the liver to N-desalkylflurazepam (active)
Half-life, metabolite (adults): 40-114 hours
Usual Dosage Oral:
Children:
<15 years: Dose not established
≥15 years: 15 mg at bedtime
Adults: 15-30 mg at bedtime
Administration May be administered without regard to meals; administer dose at bedtime
(Continued)

Flurazepam (Continued)

Patient Information Avoid alcohol and other CNS depressants; may be habit-forming; avoid abrupt discontinuation after prolonged use

Dosage Forms Capsule, as hydrochloride: 15 mg, 30 mg

Flurbiprofen (flure BI proe fen)

U.S. Brand Names Ansaid®; Ocufen®

Canadian Brand Names Alti-Flurbiprofen; Apo®-Flurbiprofen; Froben®; Froben-SR®; Novo-Flurprofen; Nu-Flurprofen

Therapeutic Category Analgesic, Non-narcotic; Anti-inflammatory Agent; Anti-inflammatory Agent, Ophthalmic; Nonsteroidal Anti-inflammatory Drug (NSAID), Ophthalmic; Nonsteroidal Anti-inflammatory Drug (NSAID), Oral

Generic Available Yes

Use

Ophthalmic: For inhibition of intraoperative trauma-induced miosis; the value of flurbiprofen for the prevention and management of postoperative ocular inflammation and postoperative cystoid macular edema remains to be determined

Systemic: Management of inflammatory disease and rheumatoid disorders; dysmenorrhea; pain

Pregnancy Risk Factor B (D in 3rd trimester)

Contraindications Hypersensitivity to flurbiprofen, any component, aspirin, or other NSAIDs; active GI bleeding, ulcer disease; patients with the "aspirin triad" [asthma, rhinitis (with or without nasal polyps), and aspirin intolerance] (fatal asthmatic and anaphylactoid reactions may occur in these patients); dendritic keratitis

Warnings Use with caution in patients with history of herpes simplex, keratitis, and patients who might be affected by inhibition of platelet aggregation; with ophthalmic use, an increased bleeding of ocular tissues may occur in conjunction with ocular surgery

Precautions Use oral form with caution in renal or hepatic impairment, GI disease, cardiac disease, and patients receiving anticoagulants

Adverse Reactions

Cardiovascular: Edema

Central nervous system: Headache, fatigue, drowsiness, vertigo

Dermatologic: Pruritus, rash

Gastrointestinal: Abdominal discomfort, nausea, heartburn, constipation, vomiting, GI bleeding, ulcers, perforation

Hematologic: Thrombocytopenia, inhibits platelet aggregation; prolongs bleeding time; agranulocytosis; increased bleeding of ocular tissues with ocular surgery (ophthalmic use)

Hepatic: Hepatitis

Ocular: Slowing of corneal wound healing, mild ocular stinging, itching, burning, ocular irritation

Otic: Tinnitus

Renal: Renal dysfunction

Drug Interactions Cytochrome P450 isoenzyme CYP2C9 substrate and inhibitor

Oral: May decrease antihypertensive effects of ACE inhibitors or angiotensin II antagonists; drug interactions similar to other NSAIDs may occur

Ophthalmic: Carbachol and acetylcholine chloride may not be effective when used concurrently with flurbiprofen

Food Interactions Food may decrease the rate but not the extent of absorption

Mechanism of Action Inhibits prostaglandin synthesis by decreasing the activity of the enzyme, cyclooxygenase, which results in decreased formation of prostaglandin precursors

Pharmacokinetics Oral:

Time to peak serum concentration: Within 1.5-2 hours

Elimination: 95% in urine

Usual Dosage

Children and Adults: Ophthalmic: Instill 1 drop every 30 minutes starting 2 hours prior to surgery (total of 4 drops to each affected eye)

Adults: Oral:

Arthritis: 200-300 mg/day in 2-4 divided doses; maximum dose: 100 mg/dose; maximum: 300 mg/day

Dysmenorrhea: 50 mg 4 times/day

Administration

Oral: Administer with food, milk, or antacid to decrease GI effects

Ophthalmic: Instill drops into affected eye(s); avoid contact of container tip with skin or eye; apply finger pressure to lacrimal sac during and for 1-2 minutes after instillation to decrease risk of absorption and systemic effects

Monitoring Parameters Systemic use: CBC, platelets, BUN, serum creatinine, liver enzymes, occult blood loss; ocular use: Periodic eye exams

Patient Information Ophthalmic solution may cause mild burning or stinging, notify physician if this becomes severe or is persistent

Dosage Forms

Solution, ophthalmic, as sodium (Ocufen®): 0.03% (2.5 mL) [contains polyvinyl alcohol and thimerosal]

Tablet (Ansaid®): 50 mg, 100 mg

♦ **5-Flurocytosine** *see* Flucytosine *on page 491*

Fluticasone (floo TIK a sone)

Related Information

Asthma Guidelines *on page 1376*
Estimated Comparative Daily Dosages for Inhaled Corticosteroids *on page 1382*

U.S. Brand Names Cutivate®; Flonase®; Flovent®; Flovent® Diskus®; Flovent® Rotadisk®

Therapeutic Category Adrenal Corticosteroid; Antiasthmatic; Anti-inflammatory Agent; Corticosteroid, Inhalant (Oral); Corticosteroid, Intranasal; Corticosteroid, Topical; Glucocorticoid

Generic Available No

Use

Oral inhalation: Long-term (chronic) control of persistent bronchial asthma; NOT indicated for the relief of acute bronchospasm. Also used to help reduce or discontinue oral corticosteroid therapy for asthma (see Additional Information)

Intranasal: Management of seasonal and perennial allergic and nonallergic rhinitis

Topical: Relief of inflammation and pruritus associated with corticosteroid-responsive dermatoses [medium potency topical corticosteroid]

Pregnancy Risk Factor C

Contraindications Hypersensitivity to fluticasone or any component; primary treatment of status asthmaticus

Warnings Fatalities have occurred due to adrenal insufficiency in asthmatic patients during and after switching from systemic corticosteroids to aerosol steroids (see Additional Information); several months may be required for full recovery of the adrenal glands; patients receiving higher doses of systemic corticosteroids (eg, adults receiving ≥20 mg of prednisone per day) may be at greater risk; during this period of adrenal suppression, aerosol steroids do **not** provide the systemic corticosteroid needed to treat patients requiring stress doses (ie, patients with major stress such as trauma, surgery, or infections); when used at high doses, hypothalamic-pituitary-adrenal (HPA) suppression may occur; use with inhaled or systemic corticosteroids (even alternate-day dosing) may increase risk of HPA suppression; withdrawal and discontinuation of corticosteroids should be done carefully. Immunosuppression may occur.

Topical use: Adverse systemic effects may occur when topical steroids are used on large areas of the body, denuded areas, for prolonged periods of time, with an occlusive dressing, and/or in infants or small children; infants and small children may be more susceptible to adrenal axis suppression or other systemic toxicities due to a larger skin surface area to body mass ratio; use with caution in pediatric patients; do not use for the treatment of rosacea, perioral dermatitis, or in the presence of skin atrophy or infection at treatment site

Precautions Avoid using higher than recommended doses; suppression of HPA function, suppression of linear growth, or hypercorticism (Cushing's syndrome) may occur; these adverse effects (as well as intracranial hypertension) may occur with topical use and have been reported in pediatric patients (see also Additional Information); use with extreme caution in patients with respiratory tuberculosis, untreated systemic infections, or ocular herpes simplex; use with caution and monitor patients closely with hepatic dysfunction. Eosinophilic conditions (eosinophilia, vasculitic rash, cardiac complications, worsening pulmonary symptoms, and/or neuropathy) may occur and are usually associated with withdrawal or decrease of oral corticosteroids after the initiation of fluticasone (oral inhalation); a causal relationship by fluticasone has not been established

Adverse Reactions

Central nervous system: Headache, dizziness, malaise, fatigue, insomnia

Dermatologic:

Inhalational use: Dermatitis, rash

Topical use: Pruritus, dry skin, numbness of fingers, acne, hypopigmentation, allergic dermatitis, maceration of the skin, skin atrophy, folliculitis, hypertrichosis, itching

Endocrine & metabolic: HPA suppression, Cushing's syndrome, growth suppression

(Continued)

Fluticasone *(Continued)*

Gastrointestinal: Oral candidiasis, nausea, vomiting, diarrhea, dyspepsia

Local: Burning, irritation

Neuromuscular & skeletal: Muscular soreness

Ocular: Eye pain

Respiratory: Respiratory infection, pharyngitis, nasal congestion, sinusitis, nasal discharge, rhinitis, epistaxis (intranasal), dysphonia (oral inhalation)

Miscellaneous: Secondary infection, eosinophilic conditions (see Precautions)

Drug Interactions Cytochrome P450 isoenzyme CYP3A3/4 substrate

Ketoconazole, ritonavir, and other strong P450 3A4 isoenzyme inhibitors may increase fluticasone serum concentrations

Stability

Oral inhalation: Aerosol canister: Store between 36°F to 86°F with nozzle end down; do not store at >120°F; protect from freezing and direct sunlight; Rotadisk®: Store at controlled room temperature; keep dry; discard Rotadisk® blisters 2 months after opening moisture-proof foil overwrap (or before expiration date); Diskus®: Store at controlled room temperature; keep dry; protect from direct heat or sunlight; discard Diskus® 6 weeks (for 50 mcg strength) or 2 months (for 100 mcg and 250 mcg strengths) after opening moisture-proof foil overwrap or when dose indicator reads "0" (whichever comes first); **Note:** Diskus® device is not reusable

Intranasal: Store nasal spray between 39°F to 86°F

Mechanism of Action Controls the rate of protein synthesis, depresses the migration of polymorphonuclear leukocytes and fibroblasts, reverses capillary permeability, and stabilizes lysosomal membranes at the cellular level to prevent or control inflammation

Pharmacodynamics

Oral inhalation: Clinical effects are due to direct local effect rather than systemic absorption

Onset of action: Within 24 hours

Maximum effect: 1-2 weeks or more

Duration after discontinuation: Several days or more

Pharmacokinetics

Distribution: V_d: Adults: 4.2 L/kg

Protein binding: 91%

Metabolism: Via cytochrome P450 3A4 pathway

Bioavailability: Oral inhalation: 30% of dose delivered from activator; Diskus®: 18%

Half-life: 7.8 hours

Usual Dosage

Intranasal: Note: For optimal effects, nasal spray should be used at regular intervals (eg, once or twice daily); however, some adolescent patients ≥12 years of age and adults with seasonal allergic rhinitis may have effective control of symptoms with prn (as needed) use of 200 mcg (2 sprays to each nostril) once daily.

Children <4 years: Not recommended

Children ≥4 years and Adolescents: Initial: 1 spray (50 mcg/spray) to each nostril daily (100 mcg/day); if response is inadequate, give 2 sprays to each nostril daily (200 mcg/day); once symptoms are controlled, reduce dose to 100 mcg/day (1 spray to each nostril daily); maximum dose: 200 mcg/day (4 sprays/day)

Adults: Initial: 200 mcg/day given as 2 sprays (50 mcg/spray) to each nostril daily or 1 spray to each nostril twice daily; dosage may be reduced to 100 mcg/day (1 spray to each nostril daily) after the first few days if symptoms are controlled; maximum dose: 200 mcg/day (4 sprays/day)

Oral inhalation: If adequate response is not seen after 2 weeks of initial dosage, increase dosage; doses should be titrated to the lowest effective dose once asthma is controlled; Manufacturer recommendations:

Inhalation aerosol (Flovent®): Children ≥12 years and Adults:

Patients previously treated with bronchodilators only: Initial: 88 mcg twice daily; maximum dose: 440 mcg twice daily

Patients treated with an inhaled corticosteroid: Initial: 88-220 mcg twice daily; maximum dose: 440 mcg twice daily; may start doses above 88 mcg twice daily in poorly controlled patients or in those who previously required higher doses of inhaled corticosteroids

Patients previously treated with oral corticosteroids: Initial: 880 mcg twice daily; maximum dose: 880 mcg twice daily

NIH Asthma Guidelines (NAEPP, 2002; NIH, 1997) [give in divided doses twice daily]:

Children ≤12 years:

"Low" dose: 88-176 mcg/day (44 mcg/puff: 2-4 puffs/day)

"Medium" dose: 176-440 mcg/day (44 mcg/puff: 4-10 puffs/day or 110 mcg/puff: 2-4 puffs/day)

"High" dose: >440 mcg/day (110 mcg/puff: >4 puffs/day or 220 mcg/puff: >2 puffs/day)

Children >12 years and Adults:

"Low" dose: 88-264 mcg/day (44 mcg/puff: 2-6 puffs/day or 110 mcg/puff: 2 puffs/day)

"Medium" dose: 264-660 mcg/day (110 mcg/puff: 2-6 puffs/day)

"High" dose: >660 mcg/day (110 mcg/puff: >6 puffs/day or 220 mcg/puff: >3 puffs/day)

Inhalation powder (Flovent® Diskus® and Flovent® Rotadisk®): **Note:** Children maintained on Flovent® Rotadisk® who are switched to Flovent® Diskus® may require dosage adjustment

Children 4-11 years: Patients previously treated with bronchodilators alone or inhaled corticosteroids: Initial: 50 mcg twice daily; maximum dose: 100 mcg twice daily; may start higher initial dose in poorly controlled patients or in those who previously required higher doses of inhaled corticosteroids

Adolescents and Adults:

Patients previously treated with bronchodilators alone: Initial: 100 mcg twice daily; maximum dose: 500 mcg twice daily

Patients previously treated with inhaled corticosteroids: Initial: 100-250 mcg twice daily; maximum dose: 500 mcg twice daily; may start doses above 100 mcg twice daily in poorly controlled patients or in those who previously required higher doses of inhaled corticosteroids

Patients previously treated with oral corticosteroids: Initial: Diskus®: 500-1000 mcg twice daily (select dose based on assessment of individual patient); Rotadisk®: 1000 mcg twice daily (this dose is based on clinical data using Flovent® inhalation aerosol); maximum dose: 1000 mcg twice daily; **Note:** Inability to reduce oral corticosteroid therapy (see Additional Information) may indicate need for maximum fluticasone dose

NIH Asthma Guidelines (NAEPP, 2002) [give in divided doses twice daily]:

Children ≤12 years:

"Low" dose: 100-200 mcg/day (50 mcg/puff: 2-4 puffs/day or 100 mcg/puff: 1-2 puffs/day)

"Medium" dose: 200-400 mcg/day (50 mcg/puff: 4-8 puffs/day or 100 mcg/puff: 2-4 puffs/day)

"High" dose: >400 mcg/day (50 mcg/puff: >8 puffs/day or 100 mcg/puff: >4 puffs/day)

Children >12 years and Adults:

"Low" dose: 100-300 mcg/day (50 mcg/puff: 2-6 puffs/day or 100 mcg/puff: 1-3 puffs/day)

"Medium" dose: 300-600 mcg/day (50 mcg/puff: 6-12 puffs/day or 100 mcg/puff: 3-6 puffs/day)

"High" dose: >600 mcg/day (50 mcg/puff: >12 puffs/day or 100 mcg/puff: >6 puffs/day)

Topical:

Cream:

Infants <3 months: Not approved for use

Infants ≥3 months, Children, and Adults: **Note:** Safety and efficacy of use >4 weeks in pediatric patients have not been established:

Atopic dermatitis: Apply a thin film to affected area once or twice daily

Other dermatoses: Apply a thin film to affected area twice daily

Ointment:

Pediatric patients: Not approved for use (due to potential for adrenal suppression)

Adults: Apply sparingly in a thin film twice daily

Administration

Intranasal spray: Shake bottle gently before use; clear nasal passages by blowing nose prior to use; nasal spray pump must be primed (6 actuations) before first use or after ≥1 week of non-use; discard unit after 120 metered sprays are used

Oral inhalation: Rinse mouth after inhalation to decrease chance of oral candidiasis

Aerosol inhalation: Shake canister well before use; use a spacer device for children <8 years of age

Powder for oral inhalation:

Diskus®: Do not use with spacer device; do not exhale into Diskus®; do not wash or take apart; activate and use Diskus® in horizontal position

Rotadisk®: Do not puncture blister until taking dose with Diskhaler®; do not use with a spacer device

Topical: Apply sparingly to affected area, gently rub in until disappears; do not use on open skin; avoid application on face, underarms, or groin area unless directed by physician; avoid contact with eyes; do not occlude area unless directed; do not apply to diaper area

(Continued)

Fluticasone *(Continued)*

Monitoring Parameters Oral inhalation: Check mucus membranes for signs of fungal infection; monitor growth in pediatric patients; assess HPA suppression in patients using potent topical steroids applied to a large surface area or to areas under occlusion

Patient Information Notify physician if condition being treated persists or worsens; do not decrease dose or discontinue without physician approval; avoid exposure to chicken pox or measles; if exposed, seek medical advice without delay

Oral inhalation: Report sore mouth or mouth lesions to physician

Additional Information When using fluticasone oral inhalation to help reduce or discontinue oral corticosteroid therapy, begin prednisone taper after at least 1 week of fluticasone inhalation therapy; do not decrease prednisone faster than 2.5 mg/day on a weekly basis; monitor patients for signs of asthma instability and adrenal insufficiency (see Warnings); decrease fluticasone to lowest effective dose **after** prednisone reduction is complete. If bronchospasm with wheezing occurs after oral inhalation use, a fast-acting bronchodilator may be used.

Topical: HPA axis suppression occurred in 2 children (2 and 5 years old) of 43 pediatric patients treated topically for 4 weeks; application covered at least 35% of body surface area

Dosage Forms

Aerosol for oral inhalation, as propionate (Flovent®):
  44 mcg/inhalation (7.9 g) [60 metered doses], (13 g) [120 metered doses]
  110 mcg/inhalation (7.9 g) [60 metered doses] (13 g) [120 metered doses]
  220 mcg/inhalation (7.9 g) [60 metered doses] (13 g) [120 metered doses]

Cream, topical, as propionate (Cutivate®): 0.05% (15 g, 30 g, 60 g)

Ointment, topical, as propionate (Cutivate®): 0.005% (15 g, 30 g, 60 g)

Powder for oral inhalation, as propionate:
  Flovent® Diskus® [approved by FDA October, 2000]
    50 mcg [delivers 47 mcg/inhalation] (28 doses, 60 doses)
    100 mcg [delivers 94 mcg/inhalation] (28 doses, 60 doses)
    250 mcg [delivers 235 mcg/inhalation] (28 doses, 60 doses)
  Flovent® Rotadisk® (4 blisters of the drug per Rotadisk®, 15 Rotadisks® per pack):
    50 mcg (60s) [delivers 44 mcg/inhalation]
    100 mcg (60s) [delivers 88 mcg/inhalation]
    250 mcg (60s) [delivers 220 mcg/inhalation]

Suspension, intranasal spray, as propionate (Flonase®): 50 mcg/inhalation (16 g) [120 metered doses]

References

Expert Panel Report 2, "Guidelines for the Diagnosis and Management of Asthma," *Clinical Practice Guidelines*, National Institutes of Health, National Heart, Lung, and Blood Institute, NIH Publication No. 94-4051, April, 1997.

"National Asthma Education and Prevention Program. Expert Panel Report: Guidelines for the Diagnosis and Management of Asthma Update on Selected Topics--2002," *J Allergy Clin Immunol*, 2002, 110(5 Suppl):S141-219.

Fluticasone and Salmeterol *(floo TIK a sone & sal ME te role)*

Related Information

Asthma Guidelines *on page 1376*

U.S. Brand Names Advair™ Diskus®

Therapeutic Category Adrenal Corticosteroid; Adrenergic Agonist Agent; Antiasthmatic; Anti-inflammatory Agent; Beta$_2$-Adrenergic Agonist Agent; Bronchodilator; Corticosteroid, Inhalant; Glucocorticoid

Generic Available No

Use Maintenance treatment of asthma

Pregnancy Risk Factor C

Contraindications Hypersensitivity to salmeterol, adrenergic amines, fluticasone, or any component; primary treatment of status asthmaticus; use with other long-acting beta$_2$-adrenergic agonists; transferring patients from systemic corticosteroid therapy (see Warnings)

Warnings Fatalities have occurred due to adrenal insufficiency in asthmatic patients during and after switching from systemic corticosteroids to aerosol steroids; several months may be required for full recovery of the adrenal glands; patients receiving higher doses of systemic corticosteroids (eg, adults receiving ≥20 mg of prednisone per day) may be at greater risk; during this period of adrenal suppression, aerosol steroids do not provide the systemic corticosteroid needed to treat patients requiring stress doses (ie, patients with major stress such as trauma, surgery, or infections); when used at high doses, hypothalamic-pituitary-adrenal (HPA) suppression may occur; withdrawal and discontinuation of corticosteroid therapy should be done carefully. Immunosuppression may occur.

Cardiovascular effects are not common with salmeterol when used in recommended doses. Salmeterol/fluticasone is not meant to relieve acute asthmatic symptoms. Acute episodes should be treated with short-acting beta$_2$ agonist. Do not increase the frequency of salmeterol/fluticasone use. Paroxysmal bronchospasm (which can be fatal) has been reported with this and other inhaled beta$_2$-agonist agents. If this occurs, discontinue treatment; symptoms of laryngeal spasm, irritation, or swelling, such as stridor and choking have been reported in patients receiving fluticasone/ salmeterol; if this occurs, discontinue treatment.

Precautions Use with caution in patients with cardiovascular disorders, convulsive disorders, liver dysfunction, thyrotoxicosis, or others who are sensitive to the effects of sympathomimetic amines; avoid using higher than recommended doses; suppression of HPA function, suppression of linear growth, or hypercorticism (Cushing's syndrome) may occur; use with extreme caution in patients with respiratory tuberculosis, untreated systemic infections, or ocular herpes simplex; use with caution and monitor patients closely with hepatic dysfunction; eosinophilic conditions (eosinophilia, vasculitic rash, cardiac complications, worsening pulmonary symptoms, and/or neuropathy) may occur and are usually associated with withdrawal or decrease of oral corticosteroids after the initiation of fluticasone oral inhalation; a causal relationship by fluticasone has not been established.

Adverse Reactions See Fluticasone *on page 511* and Salmeterol *on page 1004*

Drug Interactions See Fluticasone *on page 511* and Salmeterol *on page 1004*

Stability Store at controlled room temperature; avoid direct heat or sunlight; discard device 1 month after removal from the moisture-protective foil overwrap pouch or after every blister has been used (when the dose indicator reads "0") whichever comes first.

Mechanism of Action

Fluticasone: Controls the rate of protein synthesis, depresses the migration of polymorphonuclear leukocytes and fibroblasts, reverses capillary permeability, and stabilizes lysosomal membranes at the cellular level to prevent or control inflammation.

Salmeterol: Relaxes bronchial smooth muscle by selective action on beta$_2$-receptors with little effect on heart rate

Pharmacodynamics See Fluticasone *on page 511* and Salmeterol *on page 1004*

Pharmacokinetics See Fluticasone *on page 511* and Salmeterol *on page 1004*

Usual Dosage Oral Inhalation:

Children 4-11 years without prior inhaled corticosteroid (limited data in 257 patients, per manufacturer, 2002): Fluticasone 100 mcg/salmeterol 50 mcg (Advair™ Diskus® 100/50) 1 inhalation twice daily

Children ≥12 years and Adults without prior inhaled corticosteroid: Fluticasone 100 mcg/salmeterol 50 mcg (Advair™ Diskus® 100/50) 1 inhalation twice daily

Recommended Starting Dose of Fluticasone/Salmeterol (Advair™ Diskus®) for Patients Currently Taking Inhaled Corticosteroids

Current Daily Dose of Inhaled Corticosteroid*		Recommended Strength and Dosing Schedule of Advair™ Diskus®†
Beclomethasone dipropionate (Beclovent®, Vanceril®) (40, 42, 80, or 84 mcg/spray)	≤420 mcg	100/50 twice daily
	462-840 mcg	250/50 twice daily
Budesonide (Pulmicort®) (200 mcg/spray)	≤420 mcg	100/50 twice daily
	800-1200 mcg	250/50 twice daily
	1600 mcg	500/50 twice daily
Flunisolide (AeroBid®) (250 mcg/spray)	≤1000 mcg	100/50 twice daily
	1250-2000 mcg	250/50 twice daily
Fluticasone propionate inhalation aerosol (Flovent® Diskus®) (50, 100, or 250 mcg/spray)	≤176 mcg	100/50 twice daily
	440 mcg	250/50 twice daily
	660-880 mcg	500/50 twice daily
Fluticasone proprionate inhalation powder (Flovent® Rotadisk®) (50, 100, or 250 mcg/spray)	≤200 mcg	100/50 twice daily
	500 mcg	250/50 twice daily
	1000 mcg	500/50 twice daily
Triamcinolone acetate (100 mcg/spray)	≤1000 mcg	100/50 twice daily
	1100-1600 mcg	250/50 twice daily

*Not for use in patients transferring from systemic corticosteroid therapy

†Doses are a single inhalation of listed strengths of fluticasone/salmeterol twice daily

(Continued)

Fluticasone and Salmeterol (Continued)

Children ≥12 years and Adults currently receiving an inhaled corticosteroid: The starting dose is dependent upon the current steroid therapy, see previous table

Administration Oral inhalation: The Diskus® is a device containing a double-foil blister of a powder formulation for oral inhalation; each blister contains 1 complete dose of both medications; after the medication is opened by activating the device, the medication is dispersed into the airstream created by the patient inhaling through the mouthpiece; it may not be used with a spacer. Follow the patient directions for use which are provided with each device; do not exhale into the Diskus® or attempt to take it apart. Always activate and use the Diskus® in a level, horizontal position. Do not wash the mouthpiece or any part of the Diskus®; it must be kept dry.

Monitoring Parameters Pulmonary function tests, check mucous membranes for signs of fungal infection; monitor growth in pediatric patients

Patient Information Do not use to treat acute symptoms; do not exceed the prescribed dose of fluticasone/salmeterol; report sore mouth or mouth lesions to physician; avoid exposure to chickenpox or measles; if exposed, seek medical advice without delay; do not use with spacer (see Administration)

Additional Information When fluticasone/salmeterol is initiated in patients previously receiving a short-acting beta agonist, instruct the patient to discontinue regular use of the short-acting beta agonist and to utilize the shorter-acting agent for symptomatic acute episodes only.

Dosage Forms Note: mcg strength refers to salmeterol base
Powder for oral inhalation:
    100/50: Fluticasone propionate 100 mcg and salmeterol xinafoate 50 mcg (28s, 60s)
    250/50: Fluticasone propionate 250 mcg and salmeterol xinafoate 50 mcg (28s, 60s)
    500/50: Fluticasone propionate 500 mcg and salmeterol xinafoate 50 mcg (28s, 60s)

References
"National Asthma Education and Prevention Program. Expert Panel Report: Guidelines for the Diagnosis and Management of Asthma Update on Selected Topics--2002," *J Allergy Clin Immunol*, 2002, 110(5 Suppl):S141-219.

♦ **FML®** *see* Fluorometholone *on page 502*

♦ **FML® Forte** *see* Fluorometholone *on page 502*

♦ **Foille® [OTC]** *see* Benzocaine *on page 163*

♦ **Foille® Medicated First Aid [OTC]** *see* Benzocaine *on page 163*

♦ **Foille® Plus [OTC]** *see* Benzocaine *on page 163*

♦ **Folacin** *see* Folic Acid *on page 516*

♦ **Folate** *see* Folic Acid *on page 516*

Folic Acid (FOE lik AS id)

Canadian Brand Names Apo®-Folic

Synonyms Folacin; Folate; Pteroylglutamic Acid

Therapeutic Category Nutritional Supplement; Vitamin, Water Soluble

Generic Available Yes

Use Treatment of megaloblastic and macrocytic anemias due to folate deficiency; dietary supplement to prevent neural tube defects

Pregnancy Risk Factor A (C if dose exceeds RDA recommendation)

Contraindications Hypersensitivity to folic acid or any component (see Warnings); pernicious, aplastic, or normocytic anemias

Warnings Large doses may mask the hematologic effects of B_{12} deficiency, thus obscuring the diagnosis of pernicious anemia while allowing the neurologic complications due to B_{12} deficiency to progress. Folic acid injection contains benzyl alcohol (1.5%) as preservative, which may cause allergic reactions in susceptible individuals; large amounts of benzyl alcohol (≥99 mg/kg/day) have been associated with a potentially fatal toxicity ("gasping syndrome") in neonates; the "gasping syndrome" consists of metabolic acidosis, respiratory distress, gasping respirations, CNS dysfunction (including convulsions, intracranial hemorrhage), hypotension and cardiovascular collapse; avoid use of injection in neonates; *in vitro* and animal studies have shown that benzoate, a metabolite of benzyl alcohol, displaces bilirubin from protein-binding sites

Adverse Reactions
Cardiovascular: Slight flushing
Central nervous system: Irritability, difficulty sleeping, confusion, malaise
Dermatologic: Pruritus, rash
Gastrointestinal: GI upset
Miscellaneous: Hypersensitivity reactions

Drug Interactions May decrease phenytoin serum concentration; hematologic response antagonized by chloramphenicol; folic acid antagonists (ie, methotrexate, pyrimethamine, trimethoprim) prevent the formation of tetrahydrofolic acid (active metabolite), therefore, folic acid is not effective for the treatment of overdosage of these drugs (leucovorin must be used); decreased folic acid absorption with sulfasalazine and aminosalicylic acid; decreased folic acid concentration with phenytoin, primidone, para-aminosalicylic acid

Mechanism of Action Folic acid is necessary for formation of a number of coenzymes in many metabolic systems, particularly for purine and pyrimidine synthesis; required for nucleoprotein synthesis and maintenance in erythropoiesis; stimulates WBC and platelet production in folate deficiency anemia

Pharmacodynamics Maximum effect: Oral: Within 30-60 minutes

Pharmacokinetics

Absorption: In the proximal part of the small intestine

Time to peak serum concentration: Oral: 1 hour

Elimination: Primarily via liver metabolism

Usual Dosage

Recommended daily allowance (RDA): Oral:

Premature neonates: 50 mcg (~15 mcg/kg/day)

Neonates to 6 months: 25-35 mcg

Children:

6 months to 3 years: 50 mcg

4-6 years: 75 mcg

7-10 years: 100 mcg

11-14 years: 150 mcg

Children >15 years and Adults: 200 mcg

Pregnant women: 400 mcg

Folic acid deficiency: Oral, I.M., I.V., S.C.:

Infants: 15 mcg/kg/dose daily or 50 mcg/day

Children: 1 mg/day initial dosage; maintenance dose: 1-10 years: 0.1-0.4 mg/day

Children >11 years and Adults: 1 mg/day initial dosage; maintenance dose: 0.5 mg/day

Administration

Oral: May be administered without regard to meals

Parenteral: I.V.: Dilute with SWI, dextrose or saline solution to 0.1 mg/mL; if I.M. route used, administer deep I.M.; may also administer S.C.

Monitoring Parameters CBC with differential

Reference Range Total folate: Normal: 5-15 ng/mL; folate deficiency: <5 ng/mL; megaloblastic anemia: <2 ng/mL

Additional Information Oral liquid vitamin drops (eg, Vi-Daylin®) do not contain folic acid due to the instability of folic acid in the pH of these formulations.

Dosage Forms

Injection, solution, as sodium folate: 5 mg/mL (10 mL) [contains benzyl alcohol]

Tablet: 0.4 mg, 0.8 mg, 1 mg

Extemporaneous Preparations A 50 mcg/mL oral solution may be made by mixing 1 mL (5 mg) folic acid injection in 90 mL purified water; adjust pH to 9 with sodium hydroxide 0.1 N (approximately 2.8 mL), then add purified water to make a total volume of 100 mL; stable 30 days at room temperature

Smith SG, "A Folic Acid Solution for Oral Use," *Pharm J*, 1976, 216:108.

♦ **Folinic Acid** *see* Leucovorin *on page 660*

Fomepizole (foe ME pi zole)

U.S. Brand Names Antizol®

Synonyms 4-Methylpyrazole; 4-MP

Therapeutic Category Antidote, Ethylene Glycol Toxicity; Antidote, Methanol Toxicity

Generic Available No

Use Antidote for ethylene glycol (antifreeze) or methanol toxicity; may be useful in propylene glycol toxicity

Pregnancy Risk Factor C

Contraindications Hypersensitivity to fomepizole, other pyrazoles, or any component

Warnings By inhibiting the action of alcohol dehydrogenase, fomepizole reduces the elimination of alcohol; this must be considered when using fomepizole, as alcohol is often ingested concomitantly by patients with ethylene glycol intoxication; likewise, alcohol may reduce the elimination of fomepizole by the same mechanism; safety and efficacy in pediatric patients has not been established

(Continued)

Fomepizole *(Continued)*

Precautions Management of ethylene glycol ingestion may require treatment of metabolic acidosis, acute renal failure, adult respiratory distress syndrome, and hypocalcemia; dialysis should be considered, in addition to fomepizole therapy, in patients with acute renal failure, severe metabolic acidosis, or a serum ethylene glycol concentration >50 mg/dL; adjust dosage for renal dysfunction (see Usual Dosage)

Adverse Reactions
Cardiovascular: Bradycardia, tachycardia, hypotension
Central nervous system: Headache, dizziness, seizure, slurred speech, fever, somnolence
Dermatologic: Rash
Gastrointestinal: Nausea, vomiting, diarrhea, anorexia, heartburn, metallic taste, abdominal pain
Hematologic: Eosinophilia, anemia
Hepatic: Transient elevations in transaminase levels
Local: Phlebosclerosis, vein irritation
Ocular: Nystagmus, blurred vision
Respiratory: Pharyngitis, hiccups
Miscellaneous: Hypersensitivity reactions

Drug Interactions Alcohol (see Warnings)

Stability Store at room temperature; fomepizole solidifies at temperatures <25°C (77°F); if solidification occurs, liquefy by running the vial under warm water or by holding in the hand; solidification does not affect the efficacy, safety, or stability of fomepizole; stabile diluted in NS or D_5W for 48 hours; does not contain a preservative; use within 24 hours of dilution

Mechanism of Action A competitive alcohol dehydrogenase inhibitor, fomepizole complexes and inactivates alcohol dehydrogenase thus preventing formation of the toxic metabolites of the alcohols

Pharmacokinetics
Distribution: V_d: 0.6-1.02 L/kg; rapidly distributes into total body water
Protein binding: Negligible
Metabolism: Liver; primarily to 4-carboxypyrazole; after single doses, exhibits saturable, Michaelis-Menton kinetics; with multiple dosing, fomepizole induces its own metabolism via the cytochrome P450 system; after enzyme induction elimination follows first order kinetics
Elimination: 1% to 3.5% excreted unchanged in the urine
Dialysis: Dialyzable

Usual Dosage I.V.:
Children: Has not been studied
Adults **not requiring** hemodialysis: Initial: 15 mg/kg loading dose; followed by 10 mg/kg every 12 hours for 4 doses; then 15 mg/kg every 12 hours until ethylene glycol or methanol levels have been reduced to <20 mg/dL
Adults **requiring** hemodialysis: Since fomepizole is dialyzable, follow the above dose recommendations at intervals related to institution of hemodialysis and its duration:
Dose at the beginning of hemodialysis:
If <6 hours since last fomepizole dose: Do **not** administer dose
If ≥6 hours since last fomepizole dose: Administer next scheduled dose
Dose during hemodialysis: Administer every 4 hours or as continuous infusion 1-1.5 mg/kg/hour
Dose at the time hemodialysis is completed (dependent upon the time between the last dose and the end of hemodialysis):
<1 hour: Do **not** administer at the end of hemodialysis
1-3 hours: Administer ½ of the next scheduled dose
>3 hours: Administer the next scheduled dose
Maintenance dose off hemodialysis: Give next scheduled dose 12 hours from last dose administered

Dosage adjustment in renal impairment: Fomepizole is substantially excreted by the kidney and the risk of toxic reactions to this drug may be increased in patients with impaired renal function; no dosage recommendations for patients with impaired renal function have been established

Administration Parenteral: I.V. Dilute in at least 100 mL NS or D_5W (<25 mg/mL); infuse over 30 minutes; rapid infusion of concentrations ≥25 mg/mL has been associated with vein irritation and phlebosclerosis

Monitoring Parameters Vital signs, arterial blood gases, acid-base status, urinary oxalate, anion and osmolar gaps, clinical signs and symptoms of toxicity (arrhythmias, seizures, coma); serum and urinary ethylene glycol or serum methanol level depending upon the agent ingested; formic acid level (methanol ingestion)

Reference Range Ethylene glycol or methanol serum concentration: Goal: <20 mg/dL; therapeutic plasma fomepizole level: 0.8 mcg/mL

Additional Information If ethylene glycol poisoning is left untreated, the natural progression of the poisoning leads to accumulation of toxic metabolites, including glycolic and oxalic acids; these metabolites can induce metabolic acidosis, seizures, stupor, coma, calcium oxaluria, acute tubular necrosis and death; as ethylene glycol levels diminish in the blood when metabolized to glycolate, the diagnosis of this poisoning may be difficult

Dosage Forms Injection, solution **concentrate** [preservative free]: 1 g/mL (1.5 mL)

References

Druteika DP, Zed PJ, and Ensom MH, "Role of Fomepizole in the Management of Ethylene Glycol Toxicity," *Pharmacotherapy*, 2002, 22(3):365-72.

♦ **Foradil®** *see* Formoterol *on page 519*

Formoterol (for MOH te rol)

Related Information
Asthma Guidelines *on page 1376*

U.S. Brand Names Foradil®

Canadian Brand Names Oxeze® Turbuhaler®

Therapeutic Category Adrenergic Agonist Agent; Antiasthmatic; Beta$_2$-Adrenergic Agonist Agent; Bronchodilator; Sympathomimetic

Generic Available No

Use Maintenance treatment of asthma; maintenance treatment of bronchoconstriction in COPD; prevention of bronchospasm in patients >5 years of age with reversible obstructive airway disease; prevention of exercise-induced bronchospasm in children >12 years of age and adults

Pregnancy Risk Factor C

Contraindications Hypersensitivity to formoterol, adrenergic amines, or any component

Warnings Cardiovascular effects are not common with formoterol when used in recommended doses. Do not increase the frequency of formoterol use. Paroxysmal bronchospasm (which can be fatal) has been reported with this and other inhaled agents. If this occurs, discontinue treatment. Formoterol capsules should **only** be used with the Aerolizer™ inhaler and should **not** be taken orally.

Precautions Use with caution in patients with cardiovascular disorders, convulsive disorders, thyrotoxicosis, or others who are sensitive to the effects of sympathomimetic amines

Adverse Reactions
Cardiovascular: Tachycardia, palpitations, arrhythmias, angina, hypertension, hypotension
Central nervous system: Dizziness, headache, nervousness, hyperactivity, insomnia, malaise, fatigue
Dermatologic: Rash, pruritus
Endocrine & metabolic: Hypokalemia, hyperglycemia, metabolic acidosis
Gastrointestinal: GI upset, nausea, xerostomia, tonsillitis, dysphonia
Neuromuscular & skeletal: Tremors, muscle cramps
Respiratory: Respiratory arrest, cough, pharyngitis, bronchitis, paradoxical bronchospasm (see Warnings), sinusitis, upper respiratory tract infections, rhinitis
Miscellaneous: Hypersensitivity reactions, tachyphylaxis

Drug Interactions Cytochrome P450 isoenzyme CYP2A6, CYP2C9, CYP2C19, and CYP2D6 substrate
Additive effects with beta-adrenergic agents; MAO inhibitors and tricyclic antidepressants potentiate cardiovascular effects; beta-blocking agents antagonize effects; increased potassium losses with diuretics

Stability Store in refrigerator or at controlled room temperature; capsules should always be stored in the blister pack and only removed immediately before use

Mechanism of Action Formoterol is a long-acting selective beta$_2$-adrenergic receptor agonist. It relaxes bronchial smooth muscle by selective action on beta$_2$-receptors with little effect on heart rate

Pharmacodynamics
Onset of action: 1-3 minutes
Peak effect: 30 minutes to 1 hour
Duration: Up to 12 hours

Pharmacokinetics
Protein binding: 61% to 64%
Metabolism: Extensive via glucuronidation
Half-life: 10 hours
Time to peak serum concentration: 5 minutes
Elimination: 6% to 10% eliminated unchanged in urine
(Continued)

Formoterol *(Continued)*

Usual Dosage

Bronchodilation (asthma or COPD): Children ≥5 years and Adults: Inhalation, oral: 12 mcg (contents of 1 capsule aerosolized) twice daily, 12 hours apart

Prevention of exercise-induced asthma: Children ≥12 years and Adults: Inhalation: 12 mcg (contents of 1 capsule aerosolized) 15 minutes prior to exercise; additional doses should not be used for 12 hours; patients who are using formoterol twice daily should **not** use an additional formoterol dose prior to exercise; if twice daily use is not effective during exercise, consider other appropriate therapy

Administration Inhalation: The contents of a capsule are aerosolized via a device called an Aerolizer™. Place the capsule into the Aerolizer™. The capsule is pierced by pressing and releasing the buttons on the side of the Aerolizer™. The formoterol formulation is dispersed into the air stream when the patient inhales rapidly and deeply through the mouthpiece. May not be used with spacer device.

Monitoring Parameters Pulmonary function tests

Patient Information Do not use to treat acute symptoms; do not exceed the prescribed dose of formoterol; do not stop using inhaled or oral corticosteroids without medical advice even if feeling better; may cause dry mouth; the capsule is not to be taken by mouth

Additional Information When formoterol is initiated in patients previously receiving a short-acting beta agonist, instruct the patient to discontinue the regular use of the short-acting beta agonist and to utilize the shorter-acting agent for symptomatic or acute episodes only.

Dosage Forms Capsule for oral inhalation, as fumarate: 12 mcg

References

Bisgaard H, "Long-acting Beta₂-Agonists in Management of Childhood Asthma: A Critical Review of the Literature," *Pediatr Pulmonol*, 2000, 29(3):221-34

"National Asthma Education and Prevention Program. Expert Panel Report: Guidelines for the Diagnosis and Management of Asthma Update on Selected Topics--2002," *J Allergy Clin Immunol*, 2002, 110(5 Suppl):S141-219.

♦ **Formulation R™ [OTC]** *see* Phenylephrine *on page 892*

♦ **Formulex® (Can)** *see* Dicyclomine *on page 376*

♦ **5-Formyl Tetrahydrofolate** *see* Leucovorin *on page 660*

♦ **Fortaz®** *see* Ceftazidime *on page 238*

♦ **Fortovase®** *see* Saquinavir *on page 1006*

Foscarnet *(fos KAR net)*

U.S. Brand Names Foscavir®

Synonyms PFA; Phosphonoformate; Phosphonoformic Acid

Therapeutic Category Antiviral Agent, Parenteral

Generic Available No

Use Alternative to ganciclovir for treatment of CMV infections; treatment of CMV retinitis in patients with acquired immunodeficiency syndrome; treatment of acyclovir-resistant mucocutaneous herpes simplex virus infections in immunocompromised patients and acyclovir-resistant herpes zoster infections

Pregnancy Risk Factor C

Contraindications Hypersensitivity to foscarnet or any component; Cl_{cr} <0.4 mL/minute/kg

Warnings Renal impairment occurs to some degree in the majority of patients treated with foscarnet; renal impairment may occur at any time and is usually reversible within 1 week following dose adjustment or discontinuation of therapy; however, several patients have died with renal failure within 4 weeks of stopping foscarnet; foscarnet is deposited in teeth and bone of young, growing animals; it has adversely affected tooth enamel development in rats; safety and effectiveness in children has not been studied

Serum electrolyte imbalance occurs in 6% to 30% of patients (hypocalcemia, low ionized calcium, hypo- or hyperphosphatemia, hypokalemia, or hypomagnesemia). Patients with a low ionized calcium may experience perioral tingling, numbness, parasthesia, tetany, and seizures. Risk factor for seizures include a low baseline ANC, impaired renal function, and low total serum calcium.

Precautions Use with caution in patients with renal impairment, patients with altered electrolyte levels, and patients with neurologic or cardiac abnormalities; adjust dose for patients with impaired renal function; discontinue treatment in adults if serum creatinine ≥2.9 mg/dL; therapy can be restarted if serum creatinine ≤2 mg/dL

Adverse Reactions

Cardiovascular: Hypertension, palpitations, chest pain, EKG abnormalities, hypotension, flushing, arrhythmias

Central nervous system: Fatigue, fever, headache, seizures, hallucinations, dizziness, agitation, amnesia, depression

Dermatologic: Rash, pruritus

Endocrine & metabolic: Hypocalcemia, hypomagnesemia, hypokalemia, hypo- or hyperphosphatemia

Gastrointestinal: Nausea, diarrhea, vomiting, weight loss, pancreatitis, anorexia, constipation, dyspepsia, stomatitis

Genitourinary: Vulvovaginal ulceration, penile epithelium ulceration, dysuria, urethral disorder

Hematologic: Decreases in hemoglobin and hematocrit, leukopenia

Hepatic: Elevated liver enzymes, cholecystitis, hepatitis

Local: Thrombophlebitis

Neuromuscular & skeletal: Peripheral neuropathy, paresthesia, tremor

Ocular: Ocular pain, conjunctivitis

Renal: Elevated BUN and serum creatinine, polyuria, oliguria, renal failure, proteinuria

Respiratory: Coughing, dyspnea, bronchospasm

Drug Interactions Pentamidine (additive hypocalcemia); cyclosporine, aminoglycosides, amphotericin B (additive nephrotoxicity); ciprofloxacin (increases seizure potential)

Stability Store at room temperature; refrigeration may result in crystallization of the drug; incompatible with dextrose ≥30%, I.V. solutions containing calcium, magnesium, vancomycin, TPN

Mechanism of Action Pyrophosphate analog which inhibits DNA synthesis by interfering with viral DNA polymerase and reverse transcriptase

Pharmacokinetics

Distribution: V_d: Adults: 0.6 L/kg; up to 20% of cumulative I.V. dose may be deposited in bone

Protein binding: 14% to 17%

Half-life, plasma: Adults: 2-4.5 hours

Elimination: 80% to 90% excreted unchanged in urine

Usual Dosage Children and Adults: I.V.:

CMV retinitis: Induction treatment: 180 mg/kg/day divided every 8 hours for 14-21 days

Maintenance therapy: 90-120 mg/kg/day as a single infusion once daily

Acyclovir-resistant herpes simplex virus infection: 40 mg/kg/dose every 8 hours or 40-60 mg/kg/dose every 12 hours for up to 3 weeks or until lesions heal; repeat treatment may lead to the development of resistance

Induction Treatment

Cl_{cr} (mL/min/kg)	mg/kg/8h
≥1.6	60
1.5	56.5
1.4	53
1.3	49.4
1.2	45.9
1.1	42.4
1	38.9
0.9	35.3
0.8	31.8
0.7	28.3
0.6	24.8
0.5	21.2
0.4	17.7

Maintenance Therapy

Cl_{cr} (mL/min/kg)	mg/kg
≥1.4	90-120 q24h
1-1.4	70-90 q24h
0.8-1	50-65 q24h
0.6-0.8	80-105 q48h
0.5-0.6	60-80 q48h
0.4-0.5	50-65 q48h
<0.4	not recommended

(Continued)

Foscarnet (Continued)

Dosing interval in renal impairment: See tables on previous page.

Administration Parenteral: 24 mg/mL solution may be administered without further dilution when using a central venous catheter for infusion; for peripheral vein administration, the solution **must** be diluted to a final concentration **not to exceed** 12 mg/mL with either NS or D_5W; administer by I.V. infusion at a rate **not to exceed** 60 mg/kg/dose over 1 hour or 120 mg/kg/dose over 2 hours

Monitoring Parameters Serum creatinine, calcium, phosphorus, potassium, magnesium; hemoglobin, hematocrit, ophthalmologic exams

Reference Range Therapeutic for CMV: 150 µg/mL

Patient Information Report any numbness in the extremities, paresthesias, perioral tingling, or seizures

Nursing Implications Provide adequate hydration with I.V. NS or D_5W prior to and during treatment to minimize nephrotoxicity

Dosage Forms Injection, solution, as sodium: 24 mg/mL (250 mL, 500 mL)

References

Aweeka FT, Jacobson MA, Martin-Munley S, et al, "Effect of Renal Disease and Hemodialysis on Foscarnet Pharmacokinetics and Dosing Recommendations," *J Acquir Immune Defic Syndr Hum Retrovirol*, 1999, 20(4):350-7.

Butler KM, DeSmet MD, Husson RN, et al, "Treatment of Aggressive Cytomegalovirus Retinitis With Ganciclovir in Combination With Foscarnet in a Child Infected With Human Immunodeficiency Virus," *J Pediatr*, 1992, 120(3):483-6.

Kaplan JE, Masur H, and Holmes KK, "Guidelines for Preventing Opportunistic Infections Among HIV-Infected Persons - 2002. Recommendations of the USPHS and IDSA," *MMWR*, 2002, 51(RR-8):1-27, 29-46.

♦ **Foscavir®** *see* Foscarnet *on page 520*

Fosphenytoin (FOS fen i toyn)

Related Information
Blood Level Sampling Time Guidelines *on page 1386*

U.S. Brand Names Cerebyx®

Synonyms 3-Phosphoryloxymethyl Phenytoin Disodium

Therapeutic Category Anticonvulsant, Hydantoin

Generic Available No

Use Management of generalized convulsive status epilepticus; used for short-term parenteral administration of phenytoin; prevention and management of seizures responsive to phenytoin

Pregnancy Risk Factor D

Contraindications Hypersensitivity to fosphenytoin, phenytoin, other hydantoins, or any other component; second and third degree heart block, sino-atrial block, sinus bradycardia, Adams-Stokes syndrome

Warnings Abrupt withdrawal may precipitate status epilepticus; monitor blood pressure and EKG with I.V. loading doses; use with caution in patients with severe myocardial insufficiency and hypotension; discontinue if skin rash develops, do not resume drug if rash is exfoliative, purpuric, bullous, or if SLE, Stevens-Johnson syndrome, or toxic epidermal necrolysis is suspected; discontinue if acute hepatotoxicity occurs; hematologic toxicities and lymphadenopathy have been reported with phenytoin use

Precautions Use with caution in patients with porphyria; consider the amount of phosphate delivered by fosphenytoin in patients who require phosphate restriction; sensory disturbances (burning, pruritus, tingling, paresthesia) may occur especially at higher doses (≥15 mg **PE**/kg) and at maximum I.V. infusion rates (see Adverse Reactions); use with caution and modify dosage in patients with hepatic or renal dysfunction

Adverse Reactions

Cardiovascular: Hypotension (with rapid I.V. administration), vasodilation, tachycardia, bradycardia

Central nervous system: Slurred speech, dizziness, drowsiness, headache, somnolence, ataxia, fever

Dermatologic: Rash, exfoliative dermatitis, facial edema

Endocrine & metabolic: Folic acid depletion, hyperglycemia

Gastrointestinal: Nausea, vomiting, taste perversion

Genitourinary: Pelvic pain

Hematologic: Neutropenia, thrombocytopenia, anemia (megaloblastic)

Local: Pain on injection; since fosphenytoin is water soluble and has a lower pH (8.8) than phenytoin (12), irritation at injection site or phlebitis is reduced; I.M.: Local itching

Neuromuscular & skeletal: Osteomalacia

Ocular: Nystagmus, blurred vision, diplopia

Otic: Tinnitus

Miscellaneous: Lymphadenopathy; sensory disturbances (burning, pruritus, tingling, paresthesia) occur predominately in the groin area, but may occur in the lower back, abdomen, head or neck (these effects may be related to the phosphate load); paresthesia and pruritus are more common with I.V. vs I.M. administration and are dose and infusion rate related

Drug Interactions No drugs are known to interfere with the conversion of fosphenytoin to phenytoin; see Phenytoin *on page 894* for phenytoin interactions

Stability Store unopened vials in the refrigerator; do not store unopened vials at room temperature for >48 hours; do not use vials containing particulate matter. Fosphenytoin at concentrations of 1, 8, and 20 mg phenytoin sodium equivalents **(PE)**/mL in D$_5$W or NS is stable for 30 days when stored at 25°C or 4°C in glass bottles or polyvinyl chloride infusion bags, and when frozen at -20°C in polyvinyl chloride infusion bags. After removal from the freezer, these solutions are stable for 7 days at 25°C or 4°C.

Undiluted fosphenytoin injection (50 mg **PE**/mL) is stable in polypropylene syringes for 30 days at 25°C, 4°C, or frozen at -20°C.

Fosphenytoin at concentrations of 1, 8, and 20 mg **PE**/mL prepared in D$_5$/^{1}/$_2$NS, D$_5$/^{1}/$_2$NS with KCl 20 mEq/L, D$_5$/^{1}/$_2$NS with 40 mEq/L, LR, D$_5$/LR, D$_{10}$W, amino acid 10%, mannitol 20%, hetastarch 6% in NS or Plasma-Lyte® A injection is stable in polyvinyl chloride bags for 7 days when stored at 25°C (room temperature).

Mechanism of Action Diphosphate ester salt of phenytoin which acts as a water soluble prodrug of phenytoin; after administration, plasma and tissue esterases convert fosphenytoin to phosphate, formaldehyde and phenytoin (as the active moiety); phenytoin works by stabilizing neuronal membranes and decreasing seizure activity by increasing efflux or decreasing influx of sodium ions across cell membranes in the motor cortex during generation of nerve impulses

Pharmacokinetics The pharmacokinetics of fosphenytoin-derived phenytoin are the same as those for phenytoin (see Phenytoin *on page 894*). Parameters listed below are for fosphenytoin (the prodrug) unless otherwise noted. **Note:** The pharmacokinetics of fosphenytoin have been studied in a limited number of children 5-18 years of age and have been found to be similar to the pharmacokinetics observed in young adults (see Pellock, 1996).

Bioavailability: I.M., I.V.: 100%

Distribution: Adults: V$_d$: 4.3-10.8 L; V$_d$ of fosphenytoin increases with dose and rate of administration

Protein binding: 95% to 99% primarily to albumin; binding of fosphenytoin to protein is saturable (the percent bound decreases as total concentration increases); fosphenytoin displaces phenytoin from protein binding sites; during the time fosphenytoin is being converted to phenytoin, fosphenytoin may temporarily increase the free fraction of phenytoin up to 30% unbound

Metabolism: Each millimole of fosphenytoin is metabolized to 1 millimole of phenytoin, phosphate, and formaldehyde; formaldehyde is converted to formate, which is then metabolized by a folate-dependent mechanism; conversion of fosphenytoin to phenytoin increases with increasing dose and infusion rate, most likely due to a decrease in fosphenytoin protein binding

Conversion of fosphenytoin to phenytoin: Half-life: 15 minutes

Time for complete conversion to phenytoin:

I.M.: 4 hours after injection

I.V.: 2 hours after the end of infusion

Elimination: 0% fosphenytoin excreted in urine

Usual Dosage

The dose, concentration in solutions, and infusion rates for fosphenytoin are expressed as PHENYTOIN SODIUM EQUIVALENTS (PE)

Fosphenytoin should ALWAYS be prescribed and dispensed in mg of PE; otherwise significant medication errors may occur

Children 5-18 years: I.V.: A limited number of children have been studied. Seven children received a single I.V. loading dose of fosphenytoin 10-20 mg **PE**/kg for the treatment of acute generalized convulsive status epilepticus (Pellock, 1996). Some centers are using the phenytoin dosing guidelines in children and dosing fosphenytoin using **PE** doses equal to the phenytoin doses (ie, phenytoin 1 mg = fosphenytoin 1 mg **PE**). Further pediatric studies are needed.

(Continued)

Fosphenytoin *(Continued)*

Adults:

Loading dose:

Status epilepticus: I.V.: 15-20 mg **PE**/kg

Nonemergent loading: I.M., I.V.: 10-20 mg **PE**/kg

Initial daily maintenance dose: I.M., I.V.: 4-6 mg **PE**/kg; I.M. dose may be administered as a single daily dose using 1 or 2 injection sites; some patients may require more frequent dosing

I.M. or I.V. substitution for oral phenytoin: Initial: Use the same total daily dose in **PE** of fosphenytoin (ie, phenytoin 1 mg = fosphenytoin 1 mg **PE**); plasma concentrations may increase slightly with this method because oral phenytoin sodium is 90% bioavailable and phenytoin derived from I.M. or I.V. fosphenytoin is 100% bioavailable. Monitor clinical response and phenytoin concentrations to further guide dosage adjustments after 3-4 days

Dosing adjustments in renal/hepatic impairment:

Cirrhosis: Phenytoin clearance may be substantially reduced and monitoring of plasma concentrations with dosage adjustments is advisable

Renal or hepatic disease and patients with hypoalbuminemia: Fosphenytoin conversion to phenytoin may be increased (due to lower protein binding) without a similar increase in phenytoin clearance, leading to a potential increase in the frequency and severity of adverse effects

Administration Dilute with D_5W or NS to 1.5-25 mg **PE**/mL

Children 5-18 years: An administration rate of 3 mg **PE**/kg/minute with a maximum of 150 mg **PE**/minute was used in 7 patients (see Pellock, 1996)

Adults: Administer at a rate of 100-150 mg **PE**/minute with a maximum infusion rate of 150 mg **PE**/minute

Monitoring Parameters Serum phenytoin concentrations, CBC with differential, platelets, serum glucose, liver enzymes; blood pressure, continuous EKG, respiratory function with I.V. loading doses; free (unbound) and total serum phenytoin concentrations in patients with hyperbilirubinemia, hypoalbuminemia, renal dysfunction, uremia, or hepatic disease

Reference Range Monitor **phenytoin** serum concentrations; obtain phenytoin concentrations 2 hours after the end of an I.V. infusion or 4 hours after an I.M. injection of fosphenytoin; see Phenytoin *on page 894* for phenytoin reference range

Test Interactions Falsely high plasma phenytoin concentrations (due to cross-reactivity with fosphenytoin) when measured by immunoanalytical techniques (eg, TD_x®, TD_xFL_x™, Emit® 2000) prior to complete conversion of fosphenytoin to phenytoin; see Reference Range for proper times to measure phenytoin concentrations. Phenytoin may produce falsely low results for dexamethasone or metyrapone tests.

Additional Information Dosing equivalency: Fosphenytoin sodium 1.5 mg is equivalent to phenytoin sodium 1 mg which is equivalent to fosphenytoin 1 mg **PE**

Phosphate load: Each mg **PE** of fosphenytoin delivers 0.0037 mmol of phosphate

Formaldehyde production from fosphenytoin is not expected to be clinically significant in adults with short-term use (eg, 1 week); potentially harmful amounts of phosphate and formaldehyde could occur with an overdose of fosphenytoin; fosphenytoin is more water soluble than phenytoin and, therefore, the injection does not contain propylene glycol; antiarrhythmic effects should be similar to phenytoin

Overdose may result in: Lethargy, nausea, vomiting, hypotension, syncope, tachycardia, bradycardia, asystole, cardiac arrest, hypocalcemia, and metabolic acidosis; fatalities have also been reported

Dosage Forms Injection, solution, as sodium: 75 mg/mL [equivalent to 50 mg/mL phenytoin sodium (ie, 50 mg **PE**/mL)] (2 mL, 10 mL)

References

Boucher BA, Feler CA, Dean JC, et al, "The Safety, Tolerability, and Pharmacokinetics of Fosphenytoin After Intramuscular and Intravenous Administration in Neurosurgery Patients," *Pharmacotherapy*, 1996, 16(4):638-45.

Boucher BA, "Fosphenytoin: A Novel Phenytoin Prodrug," *Pharmacotherapy*, 1996, 16(5):777-91.

Fischer JH, Cwik MS, Luer MS, et al, "Stability of Fosphenytoin Sodium With Intravenous Solutions in Glass Bottles, Polyvinyl Chloride Bags, and Polypropylene Syringes," *Ann Pharmacother*, 1997, 31(5):553-9.

Pellock JM, "Fosphenytoin Use in Children," *Neurology*, 1996, 46(6 Suppl 1):S14-6.

Wilder BJ, Campbell K, Ramsay RE, et al, "Safety and Tolerance of Multiple Doses of Intramuscular Fosphenytoin Substituted for Oral Phenytoin in Epilepsy or Neurosurgery," *Arch Neurol*, 1996, 53(8):764-8.

- **Fostex® BPO [OTC]** *see* Benzoyl Peroxide *on page 165*
- **Freezone® [OTC]** *see* Salicylic Acid *on page 1002*
- **Froben® (Can)** *see* Flurbiprofen *on page 510*
- **Froben-SR® (Can)** *see* Flurbiprofen *on page 510*

- **5-FU** *see* Fluorouracil *on page 503*
- **Fulvicin® P/G** *see* Griseofulvin *on page 549*
- **Fulvicin-U/F®** *see* Griseofulvin *on page 549*
- **Fungi-Guard® [OTC]** *see* Tolnaftate *on page 1102*
- **Fungi-Nail® [OTC]** *see* Undecylenic Acid and Derivatives *on page 1126*
- **Fungizone®** *see* Amphotericin B (Conventional) *on page 98*
- **Fung-O® [OTC]** *see* Salicylic Acid *on page 1002*
- **Fungoid® Tincture [OTC]** *see* Miconazole *on page 759*
- **Furadantin®** *see* Nitrofurantoin *on page 814*

Furazolidone [DSC] (fyoor a ZOE li done)

U.S. Brand Names Furoxone® [DSC]

Therapeutic Category Antibiotic, Miscellaneous; Antiprotozoal

Generic Available No

Use Treatment of bacterial or protozoal diarrhea and enteritis caused by susceptible organisms: *Giardia lamblia* and *Vibrio cholerae*

Pregnancy Risk Factor C

Contraindications Hypersensitivity to furazolidone or any component; concurrent use of alcohol; infants <1 month of age because of the possibility of producing hemolytic anemia; MAO inhibitors, tyramine-containing foods

Precautions Use with caution in patients with G-6-PD deficiency

Adverse Reactions
Cardiovascular: Hypotension
Central nervous system: Dizziness, drowsiness, malaise, fever, headache, polyneuritis
Dermatologic: Rash, urticaria
Endocrine & metabolic: Hypoglycemia, disulfiram-like reaction after alcohol ingestion
Gastrointestinal: Nausea, vomiting, diarrhea
Genitourinary: Discoloration of urine (brown)
Hematologic: Agranulocytosis, hemolysis in patients with G-6-PD deficiency and neonates, leukopenia
Respiratory: Pulmonary infiltration
Miscellaneous: Hypersensitivity reactions including angioedema, hypotension, fever, urticaria, arthralgia

Drug Interactions Adrenergic agents, tricyclic antidepressants, MAO inhibitors (may increase hypertensive effect); alcohol (may cause disulfiram-like reactions)

Food Interactions Avoid tyramine-containing foods (cheese, broad beans, dry or aged sausage, nonfresh meat, liver, salami, mortadella, concentrated yeast extracts, liquid and powdered protein supplements, fermented bean curd and soya bean, meat extract and hydrolyzed protein extracts, raspberries, Chianti wine, Kimchee, or sauerkraut)

Stability Protect from light

Mechanism of Action Inhibits several vital enzymatic reactions causing antibacterial and antiprotozoal action; acts as a monoamine oxidase inhibitor and may prevent acetylation of coenzyme A

Pharmacokinetics
Absorption: Oral: Poor
Metabolism: Inactivated in the intestine
Elimination: 5% of oral dose excreted in urine as active drug and metabolites

Usual Dosage Oral:
Children >1 month: 5-8.8 mg/kg/day divided every 6 hours, not to exceed 400 mg/day
Adults: 100 mg 4 times/day

Administration Oral: May be administered without regard to food

Monitoring Parameters CBC with differential

Test Interactions False-positive results for urine glucose with Clinitest®

Patient Information May discolor urine to a brown tint; avoid alcohol during treatment and for 4 days after discontinuing furazolidone; avoid tyramine-containing foods (see Food Interactions)

Dosage Forms
Suspension: 50 mg/15 mL (60 mL, 473 mL) [DSC]
Tablet, scored: 100 mg [DSC]

References
Murphy TV and Nelson JD, "Five vs Ten Days' Therapy With Furazolidone for Giardiasis," *Am J Dis Child*, 1983, 137(3):267-70.
Turner JA, "Giardiasis and Infections With Dientamoeba Fragilis," *Pediatr Clin North Am*, 1985, 32(4):865-80.

- **Furazosin** *see* Prazosin *on page 924*

Furosemide (fyoor OH se mide)

Related Information

Carbohydrate and Alcohol Content of Liquid Medications for Use in Patients Receiving Ketogenic Diets *on page 1431*

U.S. Brand Names Lasix®

Canadian Brand Names Apo®-Furosemide; Lasix® Special

Therapeutic Category Antihypertensive Agent; Diuretic, Loop

Generic Available Yes

Use Management of edema associated with CHF and hepatic or renal disease; used alone or in combination with antihypertensives in treatment of hypertension

Pregnancy Risk Factor C

Contraindications Hypersensitivity to furosemide or any component; anuria

Warnings Loop diuretics are potent diuretics; excess amounts can lead to profound diuresis with fluid and electrolyte loss

Precautions Hepatic cirrhosis (rapid alterations in fluid/electrolytes may precipitate coma)

Adverse Reactions

Cardiovascular: Orthostatic hypotension

Central nervous system: Dizziness, vertigo, headache

Dermatologic: Urticaria, photosensitivity

Endocrine & metabolic: Hypokalemia, hyponatremia, hypomagnesemia, hypocalcemia, hyperglycemia, hypochloremia, alkalosis, dehydration, hyperuricemia

Gastrointestinal: Pancreatitis, nausea; oral solutions may cause diarrhea due to sorbitol content; anorexia, vomiting, constipation, abdominal cramping

Hematologic: Agranulocytosis, anemia, thrombocytopenia

Hepatic: Ischemic hepatitis, jaundice

Otic: Potential ototoxicity

Renal: Nephrocalcinosis, prerenal azotemia, interstitial nephritis, hypercalciuria

Drug Interactions Indomethacin decreases the effect of furosemide; decreased lithium excretion; decreased glucose tolerance with antidiabetic agents; increased ototoxicity with aminoglycosides and ethacrynic acid; drugs affected by potassium depletion (ie, digoxin); increased anticoagulant activity of warfarin; increased salicylate toxicity due to decreased excretion; decreased furosemide effects when administered at the same time as sucralfate

Food Interactions Do not mix with acidic solutions; limit intake of natural licorice (causes sodium and water retention and increases potassium loss)

Stability Furosemide injection should be stored at controlled room temperature and protected from light; exposure to light may cause discoloration; do not use furosemide solutions if they have a yellow color; refrigeration may result in precipitation or crystallization, however, resolubilization at room temperature or warming may be performed without affecting the stability; furosemide solutions are unstable in acidic media but very stable in basic media; I.V. infusion solution mixed in NS or D_5W solution is stable for 24 hours at room temperature

Mechanism of Action Inhibits reabsorption of sodium and chloride in the ascending loop of Henle and distal renal tubule, interfering with the chloride-binding cotransport system, thus causing increased excretion of water, potassium, sodium, chloride, magnesium, and calcium

Pharmacodynamics

Onset of action:

Oral: Within 30-60 minutes

I.M.: 30 minutes

I.V.: 5 minutes

Maximum effect: Oral: Within 1-2 hours

Duration:

Oral: 6-8 hours

I.V.: 2 hours

Pharmacokinetics

Absorption: 65% in patients with normal renal function, decreases to 45% in patients with renal failure

Protein binding: 98%

Half-life: Adults:

Normal renal function: 30 minutes

Renal failure: 9 hours

Elimination: 50% of oral dose and 80% of I.V. dose excreted unchanged in the urine within 24 hours; the remainder is eliminated by other nonrenal pathways including liver metabolism and excretion of unchanged drug in feces

Usual Dosage

Neonates, premature (see Additional Information):

Oral: Bioavailability is poor by this route; doses of 1-4 mg/kg/dose 1-2 times/day have been used

I.M., I.V.: 1-2 mg/kg/dose given every 12-24 hours

Infants and Children:

Oral: 1-6 mg/kg/day divided every 6-12 hours

I.M., I.V.: 1-2 mg/kg/dose every 6-12 hours

Continuous infusion: 0.05 mg/kg/hour; titrate dosage to clinical effect

Adults:

Oral: Initial: 20-80 mg/dose; increase in increments of 20-40 mg/dose at intervals of 6-8 hours; usual maintenance dose interval is twice daily or every day; may be titrated up to 600 mg/day with severe edematous states

I.M., I.V.: 20-40 mg/dose; repeat in 1-2 hours as needed and increase by 20 mg/dose until the desired effect has been obtained; usual dosing interval: 6-12 hours; for acute pulmonary edema, the usual dose is 40 mg I.V.; if not adequate, may increase dose to 80 mg

Continuous I.V. infusion: Initial I.V. bolus dose of 0.1 mg/kg followed by continuous I.V. infusion doses of 0.1 mg/kg/hour doubled every 2 hours to a maximum of 0.4 mg/kg/hour

Dosing adjustment in renal impairment: Adults: Acute renal failure: High doses (up to 1-3 g/day - oral/I.V.) have been used to initiate desired response; avoid use in oliguric states

Dialysis: Not removed by hemo- or peritoneal dialysis; supplemental dose is not necessary

Dosing adjustment in hepatic disease: Diminished natriuretic effect with increased sensitivity to hypokalemia and volume depletion in cirrhosis; monitor effects, particularly with high doses

Administration

Oral: May administer with food or milk to decrease GI distress

Parenteral: I.V.: May be administered undiluted direct I.V. at a maximum rate of 0.5 mg/kg/minute for doses <120 mg and 4 mg/minute for doses >120 mg; may also be diluted for infusion 1-2 mg/mL (maximum concentration: 10 mg/mL) over 10-15 minutes (following maximum rate as above)

Monitoring Parameters Serum electrolytes, renal function, blood pressure, hearing (if high dosages used)

Patient Information May cause photosensitivity reactions (eg, exposure to sunlight may cause severe sunburn, skin rash, redness, or itching); avoid exposure to sunlight and artificial light sources (sunlamps, tanning booth/bed); wear protective clothing, wide-brimmed hats, sunglasses, and lip sunscreen (SPF ≥15); use a sunscreen [broad-spectrum sunscreen or physical sunscreen (preferred) or sunblock with SPF ≥15]; contact physician if reaction occurs.

Additional Information Single dose studies utilizing nebulized furosemide at 1-2 mg/kg/dose (diluted to a final volume of 2 mL with NS) have been shown to be effective in improving pulmonary function in preterm infants with bronchopulmonary dysplasia undergoing mechanical ventilation; no diuresis or systemic side effects were noted

Dosage Forms

Injection, solution: 10 mg/mL (2 mL, 4 mL, 8 mL, 10 mL)

Solution, oral: 10 mg/mL (60 mL, 120 mL) [orange flavor]; 40 mg/5 mL (5 mL, 500 mL) [pineapple-peach flavor]

Tablet (Lasix®): 20 mg, 40 mg, 80 mg

References

Copeland JG, Campbell DW, Plachetka JR, et al, "Diuresis With Continuous Infusion of Furosemide After Cardiac Surgery," *Am J Surg*, 1983, 146(6):796-9.

Pai VB and Nahata MC, "Aerosolized Furosemide in the Treatment of Acute Respiratory Distress and Possible Bronchopulmonary Dysplasia in Preterm Neonates," *Ann Pharmacother*, 2000, 34(3):386-92.

Rastogi A, Luayon M, Ajayi OA, et al, "Nebulized Furosemide in Infants With Bronchopulmonary Dysplasia," *J Pediatr*, 1994, 125(6 Pt 1):976-9.

Rudy DW, Voelker JR, Greene PK, et al, "Loop Diuretics for Chronic Renal Insufficiency: A Continuous Infusion Is More Efficacious Than Bolus Therapy," *Ann Intern Med*, 1991, 115(5):360-6.

♦ **Furoxone® [DSC]** *see* Furazolidone [DSC] *on page 525*

Gabapentin (GA ba pen tin)

Related Information

Antiepileptic Drugs *on page 1374*

U.S. Brand Names Neurontin®

Canadian Brand Names Apo®-Gabapentin; Novo-Gabapentin; PMS-Gabapentin

Therapeutic Category Anticonvulsant, Miscellaneous

Generic Available No

Use Adjunct for treatment of partial seizures in children >12 years and adults (with or without secondary generalized seizures); adjunct for treatment of partial seizures in (Continued)

Gabapentin *(Continued)*

children 3-12 years of age; adjunct in the treatment of neuropathic pain; management of post-herpetic neuralgia in adults

Pregnancy Risk Factor C

Contraindications Hypersensitivity to gabapentin or any component

Warnings Neuropsychiatric adverse events, such as emotional lability (eg, behavioral problems), hostility, aggressive behaviors, thought disorder (eg, problems with concentration and school performance) and hyperkinesia (eg, hyperactivity and restlessness), have been reported in pediatric patients (see Adverse Reactions); abrupt withdrawal may precipitate status epilepticus or increase in seizures; decrease dose gradually over at least 1 week

Precautions Use with caution and decrease the dose in patients with renal dysfunction; in male (but not female) rats receiving gabapentin, a high incidence of pancreatic acinar adenocarcinoma was noted, the clinical significance in humans is unknown; effectiveness in children <3 years is not established

Adverse Reactions

Cardiovascular: Peripheral edema

Central nervous system: Somnolence, dizziness, ataxia, fatigue, depression, nervousness, fever; neuropsychiatric adverse events in children 3-12 years of age: Emotional lability (behavioral problems): 6% incidence; hostility (including aggressive behaviors): 5.2%; hyperkinesia (hyperactivity, restlessness): 4.7%; thought disorder (problems with concentration and school performance): 1.7%; **Note:** Most of these pediatric neuropsychiatric adverse events are mild to moderate in terms of intensity but discontinuation of gabapentin may be required; children with mental retardation and attention deficit disorders may be at increased risk for behavioral side effects

Dermatologic: Pruritus

Gastrointestinal: Dyspepsia, constipation, nausea, vomiting, weight gain

Genitourinary: Impotence

Hematologic: Leukopenia

Neuromuscular & skeletal: Back pain, dysarthria, tremor, myalgia

Ocular: Nystagmus, diplopia

Drug Interactions Antacids reduce the bioavailability of gabapentin by 20% (separate administration times by at least 2 hours); morphine may increase gabapentin serum concentrations (monitor patients for CNS depression; reduce morphine or gabapentin dose as appropriate); hydrocodone may increase gabapentin serum concentrations; gabapentin may decrease hydrocodone serum concentrations in a dose-dependent manner; naproxen may increase the absorption of gabapentin by 12% to 15%; cimetidine may decrease the clearance of gabapentin (minor effect); gabapentin may increase levels of norethindrone (minor effect); gabapentin does not alter the pharmacokinetics of other antiepileptic drugs

Food Interactions Food slightly increases rate and extent of absorption (AUC and peak increase by 14%)

Stability Refrigerate oral solution; store capsules and tablets at room temperature

Mechanism of Action Not fully elucidated, most likely binds to an undefined neuroreceptor in the brain that is possibly linked with, or identical to a site resembling the L-system amino acid carrier protein; although structurally similar to the inhibitory neurotransmitter, gamma-aminobutyric acid (GABA), gabapentin does not significantly affect the GABA system; it does **not** bind to GABA receptors, affect GABA neuronal uptake nor mimic GABA effects

Pharmacokinetics

Absorption: Very rapid; via an active (ie, facilitated transport) saturable process; dose-dependent

Distribution: V_d: Adults: 50-60 L or 0.65-1.04 L/kg; CSF concentrations are ~20% of plasma concentrations; distributes to breast milk

Protein binding: <3% (not clinically significant)

Metabolism: Not metabolized

Bioavailability: ~60% (300 mg dose given 3 times/day); bioavailability decreases with increasing doses; bioavailability is 27% with 1600 mg dose given 3 times/day

Time to peak serum concentration: Infants 1 month to Children 12 years and Adults: 2-3 hours

Half-life, elimination:

Infants 1 month to Children 12 years: 4.7 hours

Adults, normal: 5.3 hours (range: 5-9); increased half-life with decreased renal function; anuric adult patients: 132 hours; adults during hemodialysis: 3.8 hours

Elimination: Excreted unchanged in the urine (75% to 80%) and feces (10% to 20%)

Clearance: (**Note:** Apparent oral clearance is directly proportional to Cl_{cr}): Clearance in infants is highly variable; oral clearance (per kg) in children <5 years of age is higher than in children ≥5 years of age

Usual Dosage Oral: **Note:** Do not exceed 12 hours between doses with 3 times/day dosing:

Anticonvulsant:

Children 3-12 years: Initial: 10-15 mg/kg/day divided into 3 doses/day; titrate dose upward over ~3 days; usual dose: Children 3-4 years: 40 mg/kg/day divided into 3 doses/day; children ≥5 to 12 years: 25-35 mg/kg/day divided into 3 doses/day; doses up to 50 mg/kg/day were well tolerated in one long-term study

Children >12 years and Adults: Initial: 300 mg 3 times/day; titrate dose upward if needed; usual dose: 900-1800 mg/day divided into 3 doses/day; doses up to 2400 mg/day divided in 3 doses/day are well tolerated long-term; maximum dose: 3600 mg/day

Neuropathic pain:

Children: Limited information is available; some centers use the following doses: Initial: 5 mg/kg/dose at bedtime; day 2: Increase to 5 mg/kg/dose twice daily; day 3: Increase to 5 mg/kg/dose 3 times/day; titrate to effect; usual dosage range: 8-35 mg/kg/day divided into 3 doses/day (Galloway, 2000)

Adults: Initial: 100 mg 3 times/day; titrate to effect; doses can be increased by 300 mg/day at weekly intervals; doses of at least 900 mg/day appear to be more effective; usual dosage range: 1800-2400 mg/day divided in 3 doses/day; maximum dose: 3600 mg/day (see Laird, 2000)

Post-herpetic neuralgia: Adults: Initial: Day 1: 300 mg/day; day 2: 300 mg twice daily; day 3: 300 mg 3 times/day; titrate dose as needed for relief of pain to 600 mg 3 times/day; doses of 1800-3600 mg/day have been studied; doses >1800 mg/day did not show additional benefit

Dosing adjustment in renal impairment:

Children <12 years: Dosing in renal impairment has not been studied

Children ≥12 years and Adults: See table

Gabapentin Dosing Adjustments in Renal Impairment

Creatinine Clearance (mL/min)	Total Daily Dose Range (mg/day)	Dosage Regimens (Maintenance doses) (mg)				
≥60	900-3600	300 tid	400 tid	600 tid	800 tid	1200 tid
>30-59	400-1400	200 bid	300 bid	400 bid	500 bid	700 bid
>15-29	200-700	200 qd	300 qd	400 qd	500 qd	700 qd
15[1]	100-300	100 qd	125 qd	150 qd	200 qd	300 qd
Hemodialysis[2]		Post-Hemodialysis Supplemental Dose				
		125 mg	150 mg	200 mg	250 mg	350 mg

[1]Cl$_{cr}$ <15 mL/minute: Reduce daily dose in proportion to creatinine clearance.

[2]Supplemental dose should be administered after each 4 hours of hemodialysis (patients on hemodialysis should also receive maintenance doses based on renal function as listed in the upper portion of the table)

Administration Oral: May be administered without regard to meals; administration with meals may decrease adverse GI effects; dose may be administered as combination of dosage forms; do not administer within 2 hours of magnesium- or aluminum-containing antacids

One pediatric study (Khurana, 1996) mixed the contents of the capsule in drinks (eg, orange juice) or food (eg, applesauce) for patients who could not swallow the capsule; oral solution is now available

Monitoring Parameters Seizure frequency and duration; renal function; weight; behavior in children

Reference Range Minimum effective serum concentration may be 2 μg/mL; **routine monitoring of drug levels is not required**

Test Interactions False positive urinary protein with N-Multistix SG® test

Patient Information Take only as prescribed; may cause dizziness or drowsiness and impair ability to perform activities requiring mental alertness or physical coordination; may cause somnolence, and other symptoms and signs of CNS depression; do not operate machinery or drive a car until you have experience with the drug

Nursing Implications Doses should be titrated based on clinical response; content of capsule is bitter tasting

Additional Information Gabapentin is not effective for absence seizures; gabapentin does not induce liver enzymes

Dosage Forms

Capsule: 100 mg, 300 mg, 400 mg

Solution, oral: 250 mg/5 mL (480 mL) [cool strawberry anise flavor]

Tablet, film-coated: 600 mg, 800 mg

References

Andrews CO and Fischer JH, "Gabapentin: A New Agent for the Management of Epilepsy," *Ann Pharmacother*, 1994, 28(10):1188-96.

Bourgeois BF, "Antiepileptic Drugs in Pediatric Practice," *Epilepsia*, 1995, 36(Suppl 2):S34-45.

(Continued)

Gabapentin *(Continued)*

Galloway KS and Yaster M, "Pain and Symptom Control in Terminally Ill Children," *Pediatr Clin North Am,* 2000, 47(3):711-46.

Khurana DS, Riviello J, Helmers S, et al, "Efficacy of Gabapentin Therapy in Children With Refractory Partial Seizures," *J Pediatr,* 1996, 128(6):829-33.

Laird MA and Gidal BE, "Use of Gabapentin in the Treatment of Neuropathic Pain," *Ann Pharmacother,* 2000, 34(6):802-7.

Lee DO, Steingard RJ, Cesena M, et al, "Behavioral Side Effects of Gabapentin in Children," *Epilepsia,* 1996, 37(1):87-90.

Leiderman D, Garofalo E, and LaMoreaux L, "Gabapentin Patients With Absence Seizures: Two Double-Blind, Placebo Controlled Studies," *Epilepsia,* 1993, 34(Suppl 6):45 (abstract).

Pellock JM, "Managing Pediatric Epilepsy Syndromes With New Antiepileptic Drugs," *Pediatrics,* 1999, 104(5 Pt 1):1106-16.

Pressler KL, Jabbour JT, Rose DF, et al, "Gabapentin and Aggression in Pediatric Patients: A Review of the Literature," *Journal of Pediatric Pharmacy Practice,* 1998, 3(2):100-5.

◆ **Gabitril**® *see* Tiagabine *on page 1090*

◆ **Galzin**™ *see* Zinc Supplements *on page 1167*

◆ **Gamimune**® **N** *see* Immune Globulin (Intravenous) *on page 598*

◆ **Gamma Benzene Hexachloride** *see* Lindane *on page 677*

◆ **Gammagard**® **S/D** *see* Immune Globulin (Intravenous) *on page 598*

◆ **Gammar**®**-P I.V.** *see* Immune Globulin (Intravenous) *on page 598*

Ganciclovir *(gan SYE kloe veer)*

U.S. Brand Names Cytovene®; Vitrasert®

Synonyms DHPG; GCV; Nordeoxyguanosine

Therapeutic Category Antiviral Agent, Oral; Antiviral Agent, Parenteral

Generic Available No

Use Treatment of cytomegalovirus (CMV) retinitis in immunocompromised patients, as well as CMV GI infections and pneumonitis; prevention of CMV disease in transplant patients who have been diagnosed with latent or active CMV; ganciclovir also has antiviral activity against herpes simplex virus types 1 and 2

Pregnancy Risk Factor C

Contraindications Hypersensitivity to ganciclovir, acyclovir, or any component; absolute neutrophil count <500/mm^3; platelet count <25,000/mm^3

Warnings Ganciclovir may adversely affect spermatogenesis and fertility; due to its mutagenic potential, contraceptive precautions for female and male patients need to be followed during and for at least 90 days after therapy with the drug; ganciclovir is potentially carcinogenic

Precautions Dosage adjustment or interruption of ganciclovir therapy may be necessary in patients with neutropenia and/or thrombocytopenia and patients with impaired renal function; use with extreme caution in children since long-term safety has not been determined and due to ganciclovir's potential for long-term carcinogenic and adverse reproductive effects

Adverse Reactions

Cardiovascular: Edema, arrhythmias, hypertension

Central nervous system: Headaches, seizure, confusion, nervousness, dizziness, hallucinations, coma, fever, encephalopathy, malaise

Dermatologic: Rash, pruritus, urticaria, acne

Gastrointestinal: Nausea, vomiting, diarrhea, pancreatitis

Hematologic: Neutropenia (oral ganciclovir is associated with less neutropenia and fewer bacterial infections than I.V. ganciclovir), thrombocytopenia, leukopenia, anemia, eosinophilia

Hepatic: Elevated liver enzymes

Local: Phlebitis

Ocular: Retinal detachment, photophobia, abnormal vision, loss of vision

Renal: Hematuria, elevated BUN and serum creatinine

Respiratory: Dyspnea

Drug Interactions Zidovudine (pancytopenia), imipenem/cilastatin (seizures), immunosuppressive agents increase suppression of bone marrow; amphotericin B, tacrolimus, cyclosporine increase nephrotoxicity; probenecid decreases renal clearance of ganciclovir; increases didanosine AUC (increases risk of peripheral neuropathy, pancreatitis)

Food Interactions High fat meal may increase AUC by 22%

Stability Reconstituted solution is stable for 12 hours at room temperature; **do not refrigerate**; reconstitute with SWI **not** bacteriostatic water because parabens may cause precipitation; diluted I.V. ganciclovir solutions in D$_5$W or NS with a concentration <10 mg/mL are stable for 24 hours

Mechanism of Action Ganciclovir is phosphorylated to a substrate which competitively inhibits the binding of deoxyguanosine triphosphate to DNA polymerase; ganciclovir triphosphate competes with deoxyguanosine triphosphate for incorporation into viral DNA and interferes with viral DNA chain elongation resulting in inhibition of viral replication

Pharmacokinetics

Absorption: Oral: Poor

Distribution: Distributes to most body fluids, tissues, and organs including the eyes and brain

Protein binding: 1% to 2%

Bioavailability: Fasting: 5%; following food: 6% to 9%

Half-life (prolonged with impaired renal function):

Neonates 2-49 days of age: 2.4 hours

Adults: Mean: 2.5-3.6 hours (range: 1.7-5.8 hours)

Time to peak serum concentration: Oral: 2-2.5 hours

Elimination: Majority (80% to 99%) excreted as unchanged drug in the urine

Dialysis: 40% to 50% removed by a 4-hour hemodialysis

Usual Dosage

Slow I.V. infusion:

Congenital CMV infection: Neonates and Infants: Preliminary data indicates that a higher initial dose of 15 mg/kg/day divided every 12 hours and more prolonged treatment may be more effective

Retinitis: Children >3 months and Adults:

Induction therapy: 10 mg/kg/day divided every 12 hours as a 1- to 2-hour infusion for 14-21 days

Maintenance therapy: 5 mg/kg/day as a single daily dose for 7 days/week or 6 mg/kg/day for 5 days/week

Prevention of CMV disease in transplant recipients: Children and Adults:

Initial: 10 mg/kg/day divided every 12 hours for 7-14 days, followed by 5 mg/kg/day once daily 7 days/week or 6 mg/kg/day once daily 5 days/week for 100 days

Lung/heart-lung transplant patients (CMV-positive donor with CMV-positive recipient): 6 mg/kg/day once daily for 28 days

Other CMV infections: Children and Adults: Initial: 10 mg/kg/day divided every 12 hours for 14-21 days or 7.5 mg/kg/day divided every 8 hours; maintenance therapy: 5 mg/kg/day as a single daily dose for 7 days/week or 6 mg/kg/day for 5 days/week

Oral (following induction treatment with I.V. ganciclovir):

Children: Maintenance dose, prophylaxis of CMV disease: In a study of 36 children 6 months to 16 years of age, 30 mg/kg/dose every 8 hours with food produced serum levels similar to the 1000 mg 3 times/day regimen that is effective for maintenance treatment of CMV retinitis in adults (see Frenkel, 2000).

Adults: Maintenance: 1000 mg 3 times/day **or** 500 mg 6 times/day every 3 hours during waking hours

Sustained release intravitreal implant: CMV retinitis:

Children ≥9 years: One implant every 6-9 months plus ganciclovir 30 mg/kg/dose orally 3 times/day

Adults: One implant every 6-9 months plus ganciclovir 1-1.5 g orally 3 times/day

Dosing interval in renal impairment:

Oral: Adults:

Cl$_{cr}$ 50-69 mL/minute: Administer 1500 mg/day or 500 mg 3 times/day

Cl$_{cr}$ 25-49 mL/minute: Administer 1000 mg/day or 500 mg twice daily

Cl$_{cr}$ 10-24 mL/minute: Administer 500 mg/day

Cl$_{cr}$ <10 mL/minute: Administer 500 mg 3 times/week following hemodialysis

I.V. induction:

Cl$_{cr}$ 50-69 mL/minute: Administer 2.5 mg/kg every 12 hours

Cl$_{cr}$ 25-49 mL/minute: Administer 2.5 mg/kg every 24 hours

Cl$_{cr}$ 10-24 mL/minute: Administer 1.25 mg/kg every 24 hours

Cl$_{cr}$ <10 mL/minute: Administer 1.25 mg/kg/dose 3 times/week following hemodialysis

I.V. maintenance:

Cl$_{cr}$ 50-69 mL/minute: Administer 2.5 mg/kg/dose every 24 hours

Cl$_{cr}$ 25-49 mL/minute: Administer 1.25 mg/kg/dose every 24 hours

Cl$_{cr}$ 10-24 mL/minute: Administer 0.625 mg/kg/dose every 24 hours

Cl$_{cr}$ <10 mL/minute: Administer 0.625 mg/kg/dose 3 times/week following hemodialysis

Administration

Follow same precautions utilized with antineoplastic agents when preparing and administering ganciclovir

Oral: Do not open or crush ganciclovir capsules; administer with food

Parenteral: Do not administer I.M. or S.C. since the reconstituted ganciclovir injection may cause severe tissue irritation due to its high pH; administer by slow I.V. infusion over at least 1 hour at a final concentration for administration not to exceed 10 mg/mL

(Continued)

Ganciclovir *(Continued)*

Monitoring Parameters CBC with differential and platelet count, urine output, serum creatinine, ophthalmologic exams, liver enzyme tests, blood pressure, urinalysis

Nursing Implications Handle and dispose according to guidelines issued for cytotoxic drugs; avoid direct contact of skin or mucous membranes with the powder contained in capsules or the I.V. solution; to minimize the risk of phlebitis, infuse through a large vein with adequate blood flow; maintain adequate patient hydration

Additional Information Sodium content of 1 g: 4 mEq

Dosage Forms

Capsule (Cytovene®): 250 mg, 500 mg

Implant, intravitreal (Vitrasert®): 4.5 mg [released gradually over 5-8 months]

Injection, powder for reconstitution, lyophilized, as sodium (Cytovene®): 500 mg

Extemporaneous Preparations A 100 mg/mL oral suspension can be prepared in a vertical flow hood by emptying eighty 250 mg capsules of ganciclovir into a glass mortar wetted and triturated with Ora-Sweet® to a smooth paste. Add 50 mL of Ora-Sweet® to the paste, mix, and transfer contents to an amber polyethylene terephthate bottle. Rinse the mortar with 50 mL of Ora-Sweet® and transfer contents to the bottle. Rinse the mortar with the last third of the vehicle and transfer contents to the bottle. Add enough vehicle to make a final volume of 200 mL. The suspension is stable for 123 days when stored at 23°C to 25°C.

Anaizi NH, Swenson CF, and Dentinger PJ, "Stability of Ganciclovir in Extemporaneously Compounded Oral Liquids," *Am J Health Syst Pharm*, 1999, 56(17):1738-41.

References

Fletcher C, Sawchuk R, Chinnock B, et al, "Human Pharmacokinetics of the Antiviral Drug DHPG," *Clin Pharmacol Ther*, 1986, 40(3):281-6.

Frenkel LM, Capparelli EV, Dankner WM, et al, "Oral Ganciclovir in Children: Pharmacokinetics, Safety, Tolerance, and Antiviral Effects," *J Infect Dis*, 2000, 182(6):1616-24.

Goodrich JM, Bowden RA, Fisher L, et al, "Ganciclovir Prophylaxis to Prevent Cytomegalovirus Disease After Allogeneic Marrow Transplant," *Ann Intern Med*, 1993, 118(3):173-8.

Gudnason T, Belani KK, and Balfour HH Jr, "Ganciclovir Treatment of Cytomegalovirus Disease in Immunocompromised Children," *Pediatr Infect Dis J*, 1989, 8(7):436-40.

Kaplan JE, Masur H, and Holmes KK, "Guidelines for Preventing Opportunistic Infections Among HIV-Infected Persons - 2002 Recommendations of the USPHS and IDSA," *MMWR*, 2002, 51(RR-8):1-46.

Merigan TC, Renlund DG, Keay S, et al, "A Controlled Trial of Ganciclovir to Prevent Cytomegalovirus Disease After Heart Transplantation," *N Engl J Med*, 1992, 326(18):1182-6.

♦ **Gani-Tuss® NR** *see* Guaifenesin and Codeine *on page 551*

♦ **Gantrisin®** *see* SulfiSOXAZOLE *on page 1056*

♦ **Garamycin®** *see* Gentamicin *on page 533*

♦ **Gastrocrom®** *see* Cromolyn *on page 311*

♦ **Gas-X® [OTC]** *see* Simethicone *on page 1020*

♦ **Gas-X® Extra Strength [OTC]** *see* Simethicone *on page 1020*

♦ **Gaviscon® [OTC]** *see* Antacid Preparations *on page 112*

♦ **G-CSF** *see* Filgrastim *on page 484*

♦ **GCV** *see* Ganciclovir *on page 530*

♦ **Gel-Kam® [OTC]** *see* Fluoride *on page 500*

♦ **Gel-Kam® Rinse** *see* Fluoride *on page 500*

♦ **Genac® [OTC]** *see* Triprolidine and Pseudoephedrine *on page 1122*

♦ **Gen-Acyclovir (Can)** *see* Acyclovir *on page 45*

♦ **Genahist® [OTC]** *see* DiphenhydrAMINE *on page 393*

♦ **Gen-Alprazolam (Can)** *see* Alprazolam *on page 64*

♦ **Gen-Amiodarone (Can)** *see* Amiodarone *on page 83*

♦ **Gen-Amoxicillin (Can)** *see* Amoxicillin *on page 94*

♦ **Genapap® [OTC]** *see* Acetaminophen *on page 36*

♦ **Genapap®, Children [OTC]** *see* Acetaminophen *on page 36*

♦ **Genapap® Extra Strength [OTC]** *see* Acetaminophen *on page 36*

♦ **Genapap®, Infant [OTC]** *see* Acetaminophen *on page 36*

♦ **Genaphed® [OTC]** *see* Pseudoephedrine *on page 958*

♦ **Genasal® [OTC]** *see* Oxymetazoline *on page 849*

♦ **Genasoft® [OTC]** *see* Docusate *on page 402*

♦ **Genasoft® Plus [OTC]** *see* Docusate and Casanthranol *on page 402*

♦ **Genasyme® [OTC]** *see* Simethicone *on page 1020*

♦ **Gen-Atenolol (Can)** *see* Atenolol *on page 137*

♦ **Genatuss DM® [OTC]** *see* Guaifenesin and Dextromethorphan *on page 553*

♦ **Gen-Azathioprine (Can)** *see* Azathioprine *on page 149*

♦ **Gen-Baclofen (Can)** *see* Baclofen *on page 158*

♦ **Gen-Beclo (Can)** *see* Beclomethasone *on page 160*

- **Gen-Budesonide AQ (Can)** *see* Budesonide *on page 183*
- **Gen-Buspirone (Can)** *see* BusPIRone *on page 191*
- **Gen-Captopril (Can)** *see* Captopril *on page 207*
- **Gen-Carbamazepine CR (Can)** *see* Carbamazepine *on page 209*
- **Gen-Cimetidine (Can)** *see* Cimetidine *on page 272*
- **Gen-Clonazepam (Can)** *see* Clonazepam *on page 292*
- **Gen-Cyclobenzaprine (Can)** *see* Cyclobenzaprine *on page 318*
- **Gen-Diltiazem (Can)** *see* Diltiazem *on page 388*
- **Gen-Diltiazem SR (Can)** *see* Diltiazem *on page 388*
- **Gen-Divalproex (Can)** *see* Valproic Acid and Derivatives *on page 1131*
- **Genebs® [OTC]** *see* Acetaminophen *on page 36*
- **Genebs® Extra Strength [OTC]** *see* Acetaminophen *on page 36*
- **Generlac** *see* Lactulose *on page 649*
- **Gen-Famotidine (Can)** *see* Famotidine *on page 473*
- **Genfiber® [OTC]** *see* Psyllium *on page 959*
- **Gen-Fluoxetine (Can)** *see* Fluoxetine *on page 505*
- **Gen-Glybe (Can)** *see* GlyBURIDE *on page 540*
- **Gengraf™** *see* CycloSPORINE *on page 324*
- **Gen-Hydroxyurea (Can)** *see* Hydroxyurea *on page 582*
- **Gen-Ipratropium (Can)** *see* Ipratropium *on page 620*
- **Gen-Lovastatin (Can)** *see* Lovastatin *on page 697*
- **Gen-Medroxy (Can)** *see* MedroxyPROGESTERone *on page 712*
- **Gen-Metformin (Can)** *see* Metformin *on page 729*
- **Gen-Naproxen EC (Can)** *see* Naproxen *on page 796*
- **Gen-Nitro (Can)** *see* Nitroglycerin *on page 815*
- **Gen-Nortriptyline (Can)** *see* Nortriptyline *on page 822*
- **Genoptic®** *see* Gentamicin *on page 533*
- **Genotropin®** *see* Human Growth Hormone *on page 564*
- **Genotropin Miniquick®** *see* Human Growth Hormone *on page 564*
- **Gen-Oxybutynin (Can)** *see* Oxybutynin *on page 843*
- **Gen-Piroxicam (Can)** *see* Piroxicam *on page 910*
- **Genpril® [OTC]** *see* Ibuprofen *on page 588*
- **Gen-Ranidine (Can)** *see* Ranitidine *on page 972*
- **Gen-Salbutamol (Can)** *see* Albuterol *on page 54*
- **Gen-Sertraline (Can)** *see* Sertraline *on page 1016*
- **Gen-Sotalol (Can)** *see* Sotalol *on page 1032*
- **Gentacidin®** *see* Gentamicin *on page 533*
- **Gentak®** *see* Gentamicin *on page 533*

Gentamicin (jen ta MYE sin)

Related Information
Blood Level Sampling Time Guidelines *on page 1386*
Endocarditis Prophylaxis *on page 1321*
Overdose and Toxicology *on page 1388*

U.S. Brand Names Garamycin®; Genoptic®; Gentacidin®; Gentak®

Canadian Brand Names Alcomicin®; Diogent®; Minim's Gentamicin 0.3%; SAB-Gentamicin

Therapeutic Category Antibiotic, Aminoglycoside; Antibiotic, Ophthalmic; Antibiotic, Topical

Generic Available Yes

Use Treatment of susceptible bacterial infections, normally gram-negative organisms including *Pseudomonas*, *E. coli*, *Proteus*, *Serratia*, and gram-positive *Staphylococcus*; treatment of bone infections, CNS infections, respiratory tract infections, skin and soft tissue infections, as well as abdominal and urinary tract infections, endocarditis, and septicemia; used in combination with ampicillin as empiric therapy for sepsis in newborns; prevention of bacterial endocarditis prior to surgical procedures in high risk patients; used topically to treat superficial infections of the skin or ophthalmic infections caused by susceptible bacteria

Pregnancy Risk Factor D

Contraindications Hypersensitivity to gentamicin, any component (see Warnings), or other aminoglycosides

Warnings Parenteral aminoglycosides are associated with significant nephrotoxicity or ototoxicity; the ototoxicity is directly proportional to the amount of drug given and the duration of treatment; tinnitus or vertigo are indications of vestibular injury and (Continued)

533

Gentamicin *(Continued)*

impending irreversible bilateral deafness; renal damage is usually reversible and is associated with decreased creatinine clearance and urine specific gravity, elevated BUN and serum creatinine, casts in the urine, oliguria, and proteinuria; once-daily gentamicin administration has been associated with a pyrogenic endotoxin-like reaction (fever, chills, hypotension, tachycardia); some products contain sulfites which may cause allergic reactions in susceptible individuals. Aminoglycosides can cause fetal harm when administered to a pregnant woman; aminoglycosides have been associated with several reports of total irreversible bilateral congenital deafness in pediatric patients exposed *in utero.*

Precautions Use with caution in neonates due to renal immaturity that results in a prolonged gentamicin half-life and in patients with pre-existing renal impairment, auditory or vestibular impairment, hypocalcemia, myasthenia gravis, and in conditions which depress neuromuscular transmission; modify dosage in patients with renal impairment and in neonates on extracorporeal membrane oxygenation (ECMO)

Adverse Reactions

Central nervous system: Vertigo, ataxia, gait instability, dizziness, headache, fever

Dermatologic: Rash, pruritus, erythema

Endocrine & metabolic: Hypomagnesemia

Gastrointestinal: Nausea, vomiting, anorexia

Genitourinary: Decrease in urine specific gravity, casts in urine, possible electrolyte wasting

Hematologic: Granulocytopenia, thrombocytopenia, eosinophilia

Hepatic: Elevated AST and ALT

Local: Thrombophlebitis

Neuromuscular & skeletal: Neuromuscular blockade, muscle cramps, tremor, weakness

Ocular: Optic neuritis; ophthalmic use: burning, stinging, redness, lacrimation

Otic: Ototoxicity (may be associated with high serum aminoglycoside concentrations persisting for prolonged periods) with tinnitus, hearing loss; early toxicity usually affects high-pitched sound

Renal: Nephrotoxicity (high trough levels) with proteinuria, reduction in glomerular filtration rate, elevated serum creatinine

Drug Interactions Increased toxicity: Concurrent use of amphotericin B, magnesium, cephalosporins, penicillins, loop diuretics, vancomycin, cisplatin, indomethacin; potentiates effect of neuromuscular blocking agents and botulinum toxin

Stability Incompatible with penicillins, cephalosporins, heparin

Mechanism of Action Inhibits cellular initiation of bacterial protein synthesis by binding to 30S and 50S ribosomal subunits resulting in a defective bacterial cell membrane

Pharmacokinetics

Absorption: Oral: Poorly absorbed (<2%)

Distribution: Crosses the placenta; distributes primarily in the extracellular fluid volume and in most tissues; poor penetration into CSF; drug accumulates in the renal cortex; small amounts distribute into bile, sputum, saliva, tears, and breast milk

V_d: Increased in neonates and with fever, edema, ascites, fluid overload; V_d is decreased in patients with dehydration

Neonates: 0.45 ± 0.1 L/kg

Infants: 0.4 ± 0.1 L/kg

Children: 0.35 ± 0.15 L/kg

Adolescents: 0.3 ± 0.1 L/kg

Adults: 0.2-0.3 L/kg

Protein binding: <30%

Half-life:

Neonates:

<1 week: 3-11.5 hours

1 week to 1 month: 3-6 hours

Infants: 4 ± 1 hour

Children: 2 ± 1 hour

Adolescents: 1.5 ± 1 hour

Adults with normal renal function: 1.5-3 hours

Anuria: 36-70 hours

Time to peak serum concentration:

I.M.: Within 30-90 minutes

I.V.: 30 minutes after 30-minute infusion

Elimination: Clearance is directly related to renal function; eliminated almost completely by glomerular filtration of unchanged drug with excretion into urine

Clearance:
  Neonates: 0.045 ± 0.01 L/hour/kg
  Infants: 0.1 ± 0.05 L/hour/kg
  Children: 0.1 ± 0.03 L/hour/kg
  Adolescents: 0.09 ± 0.03 L/hour/kg
Dialysis: Dialyzable (50% to 100%)

Usual Dosage Dosage should be based on an estimate of ideal body weight, except in neonates (neonatal dosage should be based on actual weight unless the patient has hydrocephalus or hydrops fetalis):

Neonates: I.M., I.V.:
  Premature neonate, <1000 g: 3.5 mg/kg/dose every 24 hours
  0-4 weeks, <1200 g: 2.5 mg/kg/dose every 18-24 hours
  Postnatal age ≤7 days: 2.5 mg/kg/dose every 12 hours
  Postnatal age >7 days:
    1200-2000 g: 2.5 mg/kg/dose every 8-12 hours
    >2000 g: 2.5 mg/kg/dose every 8 hours

Initial dose for term neonates receiving ECMO: I.V.: 2.5 mg/kg/dose every 18 hours; subsequent doses should be individualized by monitoring serum drug concentrations; when ECMO is discontinued, dosage may require readjustment due to large shifts in body water

Once daily dosing:
  Premature neonates with normal renal function: 3.5-4 mg/kg/dose every 24 hours
  Term neonates with normal renal function: 3.5-5 mg/kg/dose every 24 hours

Infants and Children <5 years: I.M., I.V.: 2.5 mg/kg/dose every 8 hours*
  Once daily dosing in patients with normal renal function: 5-7.5 mg/kg/dose every 24 hours
  Endocarditis prophylaxis (high-risk patients): 1.5 mg/kg (maximum: 120 mg) within 30 minutes of starting the procedure plus ampicillin or vancomycin (in patients allergic to ampicillin)
  Pulmonary infection in cystic fibrosis: 2.5-3.3 mg/kg/dose every 6-8 hours
  Patients on hemodialysis: 1.25-1.75 mg/kg/dose postdialysis

Children ≥5 years: I.M., I.V.: 2-2.5 mg/kg/dose every 8 hours*
  Once daily dosing in children with normal renal function: 5-7.5 mg/kg/dose every 24 hours
  Endocarditis prophylaxis (high-risk patients): 1.5 mg/kg (maximum: 120 mg) within 30 minutes of starting the procedure plus ampicillin or vancomycin (in patients allergic to ampicillin)
  Pulmonary infection in cystic fibrosis: 2.5-3.3 mg/kg/dose every 6-8 hours
  Patients on hemodialysis: 1.25-1.75 mg/kg/dose postdialysis

*Some patients may require larger or more frequent doses (eg, every 6 hours) if serum levels document the need (ie, cystic fibrosis, patients with major burns, or febrile granulocytopenic patients); modify dose based on individual patient requirements as determined by renal function, serum drug concentrations, and patient-specific clinical parameters

Intraventricular/intrathecal **(use a preservative free preparation)**:
  Newborns: 1 mg/day
  Infants >3 months and Children: 1-2 mg/day
  Adults: 4-8 mg/day

Infants, Children, and Adults:
  Topical: Apply 3-4 times/day
  Ophthalmic:
    Ointment: Apply 2-3 times/day
    Solution: Instill 1-2 drops every 2-4 hours, up to 2 drops every hour for severe infections

Adults: I.M., I.V.: 3-6 mg/kg/day in divided doses every 8 hours; studies of once daily dosing have used I.V. doses of 4-6.6 mg/kg once daily
  Endocarditis prophylaxis (high-risk patients): 1.5 mg/kg (maximum: 120 mg) within 30 minutes of starting the procedure plus ampicillin or vancomycin (in patients allergic to ampicillin)
  Patients on hemodialysis: 0.5-0.7 mg/kg/dose postdialysis

Dosing adjustment in renal impairment: I.M., I.V.: 2.5 mg/kg** (Cl_{cr} <60 mL/minute/1.73 m²) **or**
  Cl_{cr} 40-60 mL/minute: Administer every 12 hours
  Cl_{cr} 20-40 mL/minute: Administer every 24 hours
  Cl_{cr} <20 mL/minute: Administer normal dose, then monitor levels

**2-3 serum level measurements should be obtained after the initial dose to measure the patient's pharmacokinetic parameters (eg, half-life, V_d) in order to determine the frequency and amount of subsequent doses

(Continued)

Gentamicin *(Continued)*

Administration

Ophthalmic: Gentamicin solution is not for subconjunctival injection. Solution may be instilled into the affected eye or a small amount of ointment may be placed into the conjunctival sac. Avoid contaminating tip of the solution bottle or ointment tube. Solution: Apply finger pressure to lacrimal sac during and for 1-2 minutes after instillation to decrease risk of absorption and systemic effects.

Parenteral: Administer by I.M., I.V. slow intermittent infusion over 30-60 minutes or by direct injection over 15 minutes; final concentration for I.V. administration should not exceed 10 mg/mL; administer other antibiotics, such as penicillins and cephalosporins, at least 1 hour before or after gentamicin

Topical: Apply a small amount gently to the cleansed affected area

Monitoring Parameters Urinalysis, urine output, BUN, serum creatinine, peak and trough serum gentamicin concentrations, hearing test, CBC with differential

Not all infants and children who receive aminoglycosides require monitoring of serum aminoglycoside concentrations. Indications for use of aminoglycoside serum concentration monitoring include:

Treatment course >5 days

Patients with decreased or changing renal function

Patients with poor therapeutic response

Infants <3 months of age

Atypical body constituency (obesity, expanded extracellular fluid volume)

Clinical need for higher doses or shorter intervals (eg, cystic fibrosis, burns, endo-carditis, meningitis, critically ill patients, relatively resistant organism)

Patients on hemodialysis or chronic ambulatory peritoneal dialysis

Signs of nephrotoxicity or ototoxicity

Concomitant use of other nephrotoxic agents

Reference Range

Peak: 4-12 µg/mL; peak values are 2-3 times greater with once daily dosing regimens

Trough: 0.5-2 µg/mL

Test Interactions Aminoglycoside levels measured in blood taken from Silastic® central line catheters can sometimes give falsely high readings

Patient Information Report any dizziness or sensations of ringing or fullness in ears to the physician

Nursing Implications Obtain drug levels after the third or fourth dose except in neonates and patients with rapidly changing renal function in whom levels need to be measured sooner; peak gentamicin serum concentrations are drawn 30 minutes after the end of a 30-minute I.V. infusion, immediately on completion of a 1-hour I.V. infusion, or 1 hour after an intramuscular injection; trough levels are drawn within 30 minutes before the next dose; provide adequate patient hydration and perfusion

Dosage Forms

Cream, topical, as sulfate (Garamycin®): 0.1% (15 g)

Infusion, as sulfate [premixed in NS]: 40 mg (50 mL), 60 mg (50 mL, 100 mL), 70 mg (50 mL), 80 mg (50 mL, 100 mL), 90 mg (100 mL), 100 mg (50 mL, 100 mL), 120 mg (100 mL)

Injection, solution, as sulfate: 40 mg/mL (2 mL, 20 mL) [may contain sodium metabi-sulfite]

Garamycin®: 40 mg/mL (2 mL) [contains sodium bisulfite]

Injection, solution, as sulfate [ADD-Vantage® vial]: 10 mg/mL (6 mL, 8 mL, 10 mL)

Injection, solution, pediatric, as sulfate: 10 mg/mL (2 mL) [may contain sodium meta-bisulfite]

Injection, solution, pediatric, as sulfate [preservative free]: 10 mg/mL (2 mL)

Ointment, ophthalmic, as sulfate: 0.3% (3.5 g)

Ointment, topical, as sulfate (Garamycin®): 0.1% (15 g)

Solution, ophthalmic, as sulfate: 0.3% (5 mL, 15 mL)

Garamycin®, Gentacidin®: 0.3% (5 mL)

Genoptic®: 0.3% (1 mL, 5 mL)

Gentak®: 0.3% (5 mL, 15 mL)

References

Bhatt-Mehta V, Johnson CE and Schumacher RE, "Gentamicin Pharmacokinetics in Term Neonates Receiving Extracorporeal Membrane Oxygenation," *Pharmacotherapy*, 1992, 12(1):28-32.

Gilbert DN, "Once-Daily Aminoglycoside Therapy," *Antimicrob Agents Chemother*, 1991, 35(3):399-405.

Kraus DM, Pai MP, and Rodvold KA, "Efficacy and Tolerability of Extended-Interval Aminoglycoside Administration in Pediatric Patients," *Paediatr Drugs*, 2002, 4(7):469-84.

Reimche LD, Rooney, ME, Hindmarsh KW, et al, "An Evaluation of Gentamicin Dosing According to Renal Function in Neonates With Suspected Sepsis," *Am J Perinatol*, 1987, 4(3):262-5.

Shevchuk YM and Taylor DM, "Aminoglycoside Volume of Distribution in Pediatric Patients," *DICP*, 1990, 24(3):273-6.

♦ **Gentamicin and Prednisolone** *see* Prednisolone and Gentamicin *on page 927*

Gentian Violet (JEN shun VYE oh let)

Synonyms Crystal Violet; Methylrosaniline Chloride

Therapeutic Category Antibacterial, Topical; Antifungal Agent, Topical

Generic Available Yes

Use Treatment of cutaneous or mucocutaneous infections caused by *Candida albicans* and other superficial skin infections refractory to topical nystatin, clotrimazole, miconazole, or econazole

Pregnancy Risk Factor C

Contraindications Hypersensitivity to gentian violet; ulcerated areas; patients with porphyria

Warnings May result in tattooing of the skin when applied to granulation tissue

Adverse Reactions

Dermatological: Staining of skin (purple), vesicle formation

Gastrointestinal: Esophagitis

Local: Burning, irritation, vesicle formation, sensitivity reactions, ulceration of mucous membranes

Respiratory: Laryngitis, tracheitis may result from swallowing gentian violet solution, laryngeal obstruction following frequent or prolonged use

Mechanism of Action Topical antiseptic/germicide effective against some vegetative gram-positive bacteria, particularly *Staphylococcus* species, and some yeast; it is much less effective against gram-negative bacteria and is ineffective against acid-fast bacteria

Usual Dosage Topical:

Infants: Apply 3-4 drops of a 0.5% solution under the tongue or on lesion after feedings

Children and Adults: Apply 1% to 2% solution to lesion 2-3 times/day for 3 days, do not swallow

Administration Topical: Apply to lesions with cotton; do not apply to ulcerative lesions on the face

Patient Information Drug stains skin and clothing purple; proper hygiene and skin care need to be used to prevent spread of infection and reinfection

Nursing Implications Keep affected area dry and exposed to air

Additional Information 0.25% or 0.5% solution is less irritating than a 1% to 2% solution and is reported to be as effective

Dosage Forms Solution, topical: 1% (30 mL); 2% (30 mL)

♦ **Gen-Timolol (Can)** *see* Timolol *on page 1095*

♦ **Gentran®** *see* Dextran *on page 358*

♦ **Gen-Trazodone (Can)** *see* Trazodone *on page 1110*

♦ **Gen-Triazolam (Can)** *see* Triazolam *on page 1116*

♦ **Gen-Verapamil (Can)** *see* Verapamil *on page 1144*

♦ **Gen-Verapamil SR (Can)** *see* Verapamil *on page 1144*

♦ **Gen-Warfarin (Can)** *see* Warfarin *on page 1156*

♦ **Gen-XENE®** *see* Clorazepate *on page 296*

♦ **Geocillin®** *see* Carbenicillin *on page 213*

♦ **GG** *see* Guaifenesin *on page 550*

♦ **Glibenclamide** *see* GlyBURIDE *on page 540*

GlipiZIDE (GLIP i zide)

U.S. Brand Names Glucotrol®; Glucotrol® XL

Synonyms Glydiazinamide

Therapeutic Category Antidiabetic Agent, Oral; Antidiabetic Agent, Sulfonylurea; Hypoglycemic Agent, Oral

Generic Available Yes (except extended release tablet)

Use Management of type II diabetes mellitus (noninsulin-dependent, NIDDM) when hyperglycemia cannot be managed by diet alone; may be used concomitantly with metformin or insulin to improve glycemic control

Pregnancy Risk Factor C

Contraindications Hypersensitivity to glipizide, any component, or other sulfonamides; type 1 diabetes mellitus (insulin-dependent, IDDM), diabetic ketoacidosis with or without coma

Warnings Chemical similarities are present among sulfonamides, sulfonylureas, carbonic anhydrase inhibitors, thiazides, and loop diuretics (except ethacrynic acid), and although only glipizide use in patients with sulfonamide allergy is specifically contraindicated in product labeling, there is a risk of cross-reaction in patients with allergies to any of these compounds; avoid use when the previous reaction has been severe; product labeling states oral hypoglycemic drugs may be associated with an
(Continued)

GlipiZIDE *(Continued)*

increased cardiovascular mortality as compared to treatment with diet alone or diet plus insulin; data to support this association are limited, and several studies, including a large prospective trial (UKPDS) have not supported an association

Precautions Use with caution in patients with adrenal or pituitary insufficiency; hypoglycemic reactions are more prevalent in debilitated, malnourished patients, patients with mild disease or impaired hepatic or renal function; hypoglycemia may also occur with inadequate caloric intake, strenuous exercise, or concurrent use with other hypoglycemic drugs

Adverse Reactions

Cardiovascular: Edema, flushing, hypertension, arrhythmias

Central nervous system: Headache, dizziness, drowsiness, insomnia, anxiety, depression, migraine

Dermatologic: Rash, urticaria, photosensitivity

Endocrine & metabolic: Hypoglycemia, hyponatremia, weight gain

Gastrointestinal: Anorexia, nausea, vomiting, diarrhea, epigastric fullness, flatulence, constipation, heartburn

Genitourinary: Dysuria

Hematologic: Blood dyscrasias, aplastic anemia, hemolytic anemia, bone marrow suppression, thrombocytopenia, agranulocytosis

Hepatic: Cholestatic jaundice, elevated liver enzymes

Neuromuscular & skeletal: Arthralgia, leg cramps, myalgia

Ocular: Blurred vision, ocular pain, conjunctivitis

Renal: Diuretic effect (mild), SIADH, urolithiasis

Respiratory: Rhinitis, dyspnea

Drug Interactions Drugs which tend to produce hyperglycemia (eg, diuretics, corticosteroids, phenothiazines, thyroid products, estrogens, oral contraceptives, phenytoin, nicotinic acid, sympathomimetics, calcium channel-blocking drugs, rifampin, and isoniazid) may lead to a loss of glycemic control; disulfiram-like reactions with alcohol; drugs which produce an increase in glipizide's hypoglycemic effects: ACE inhibitors, cimetidine, chloramphenicol, anabolic steroids, monoamine oxidase inhibitors, fluoroquinolone antibiotics, and probenecid; since this agent is highly protein bound, use of other protein-bound drugs may result in adverse effects when glipizide therapy is initiated or discontinued; beta-adrenergic blocking agents may impair glucose tolerance, increase the frequency or severity of hypoglycemia, block hypoglycemia-induced tachycardia, delay the rate of recovery of blood glucose concentration following drug-induced hypoglycemia, and may alter the hemodynamic response to hypoglycemia; glipizide may increase cyclosporine and tacrolimus serum concentrations; cholestyramine decreases glipizide absorption

Food Interactions Food delays absorption but does not affect the extent of absorption or peak levels achieved

Stability Store at room temperature; protect from light

Mechanism of Action Stimulates insulin release from the pancreatic beta cells, reduces glucose output from the liver, and increases insulin sensitivity at peripheral target sites

Pharmacodynamics

Onset of action: Immediate release formulation: 15-30 minutes; extended release formulation: 2-3 hours

Maximum effect: Immediate release formulation: Within 2-3 hours; extended release formulation: 6-12 hours

Duration: Immediate release formulation: 12-24 hours; extended release formulation: 24 hours

Average decrease in fasting blood glucose (when used as monotherapy): 60-70 mg/dL

Pharmacokinetics

Absorption: Rapid and complete

Distribution: V_d: Adults: 11-25 L

Protein binding: 92% to 99%

Metabolism: Extensive liver metabolism to inactive metabolites

Bioavailability: 80% to 100%

Half-life: 2-4 hours

Time to peak serum concentration: Immediate release formulation: 1-3 hours

Elimination: 60% to 90% of drug excreted into urine within 24-72 hours as unchanged drug and metabolites; 5% to 20% excreted in feces within 24-96 hours

Usual Dosage Adults: Oral:

Management of noninsulin-dependent diabetes mellitus in patients **previously untreated:** Initial: 5 mg/day immediate release or extended release tablets; adjust dosage in 2.5-5 mg daily increments in intervals of 3-7 days for immediate release tablets or 5 mg daily increments in intervals of at least 7 days for extended release tablets; if total daily dose for immediate release tablets is >15 mg, divide into twice daily dosage; maximum daily dose for immediate release tablets: 40 mg; maximum daily dose for extended release tablets: 20 mg

Note: patients may be converted from immediate release tablets to extended release tablets by giving the nearest equivalent total daily dose once daily

Management of noninsulin-dependent diabetes mellitus in patients **previously maintained on insulin:**

Insulin dosage ≤20 units/day: Use recommended initial dose and abruptly discontinue insulin

Insulin dosage >20 units/day: Use recommended initial dose and reduce daily insulin dosage by 50%; continue to withdraw daily insulin dosage gradually over several days as tolerated with incremental increases of glipizide

Dosing adjustment/comments in renal impairment: Cl_{cr} <10 mL/minute: Some investigators recommend not using

Dosing adjustment in hepatic impairment: Reduce initial dosage to 2.5 mg/day

Administration Oral: Administer immediate release tablets 30 minutes before a meal; extended release tablets should be swallowed whole and administered with breakfast; do not cut, crush, or chew

Monitoring Parameters Signs and symptoms of hypoglycemia, fasting blood glucose, glycosylated hemoglobin (hemoglobin A_{1c})

Reference Range Target range:

Blood glucose: Fasting and preprandial: 80-120 mg/dL; bedtime: 100-140 mg/dL

Glycosylated hemoglobin (hemoglobin A_{1c}): <7%

Patient Information Do not change dose or discontinue without consulting prescriber; avoid alcohol while taking this medication, may cause severe reaction; maintain regular dietary intake and exercise routine; always carry quick source of sugar; if experiencing a hypoglycemic reaction, contact prescriber immediately; report severe or persistent side effects, extended vomiting or flu-like symptoms, skin rash, easy bruising or bleeding, or change in color of urine or stool; when taking extended release tablets, it is not unusual to observe a tablet in the stool; this is the nonabsorbable shell containing the active drug which has been released. May rarely cause photosensitivity reactions (eg, exposure to sunlight may cause severe sunburn, skin rash, redness, or itching); avoid direct exposure to sunlight

Additional Information When transferring from other sulfonylurea antidiabetic agents to glyburide, with the exception of chlorpropamide, the administration of the other agent may be abruptly discontinued; due to the prolonged elimination half-life of chlorpropamide, a 2- to 3-day drug-free interval may be advisable before glipizide therapy is begun

Dosage Forms

Tablet (Glucotrol®): 5 mg, 10 mg

Tablet, extended release (Glucotrol® XL): 2.5 mg, 5 mg, 10 mg

References

DeFronzo RA, "Pharmacologic Therapy for Type 2 Diabetes Mellitus," *Ann Intern Med*, 1999, 131(4):281-303.

"Intensive Blood-Glucose Control With Sulphonylureas or Insulin Compared With Conventional Treatment and Risk of Complications in Patients With Type 2 Diabetes (UKPDS 33) UK Prospective Diabetes Study (UKPDS) Group," *Lancet*, 1998, 352(9131):837-53.

♦ **GlucaGen®** *see* Glucagon (rDNA Origin) *on page 539*

♦ **GlucaGen® Diagnostic Kit** *see* Glucagon (rDNA Origin) *on page 539*

♦ **Glucagon** *see* Glucagon (rDNA Origin) *on page 539*

♦ **Glucagon Diagnostic Kit** *see* Glucagon (rDNA Origin) *on page 539*

♦ **Glucagon Emergency Kit** *see* Glucagon (rDNA Origin) *on page 539*

Glucagon (rDNA Origin) (GLOO ka gon)

U.S. Brand Names GlucaGen®; GlucaGen® Diagnostic Kit; Glucagon; Glucagon Diagnostic Kit; Glucagon Emergency Kit

Therapeutic Category Antihypoglycemic Agent

Generic Available No

Use Management of hypoglycemia; diagnostic aid in the radiologic examination of GI tract when a hypotonic state is needed; used with some success as a cardiac stimulant in management of severe cases of beta-adrenergic blocking agent overdosage

Pregnancy Risk Factor B

Contraindications Hypersensitivity to glucagon or any component

Warnings Use with caution in patients with a history of insulinoma and/or pheochromocytoma; because glucagon depletes glycogen stores, the patient should be given supplemental carbohydrates as soon as physically possible

Adverse Reactions

Cardiovascular: Hypotension

(Continued)

Glucagon (rDNA Origin) (Continued)

Dermatologic: Urticaria
Gastrointestinal: Nausea, vomiting
Respiratory: Respiratory distress
Miscellaneous: Hypersensitivity reactions

Drug Interactions Enhances anticoagulant effect of warfarin; phenytoin inhibits the stimulant effect of glucagon on insulin release by the islet cells; propranolol partially inhibits the hyperglycemic effect of glucagon

Stability Glucagon (rDNA origin) for injection (Lilly) should be stored at controlled room temperature; glucagon (rDNA origin) for injection (GlucaGen®) should be refrigerated; both injections should be used immediately after reconstitution

Mechanism of Action Glucagon (rDNA origin) is genetically engineered and identical to human glucagon. It stimulates adenylate cyclase to produce increased cyclic AMP. It promotes hepatic glycogenolysis and gluconeogenesis, causing an increase in blood glucose levels; produces both positive inotropic and chronotropic effects.

Pharmacodynamics

Blood glucose effect (after 1 mg dosage):
  Onset of action: I.M.: 8-10 minutes; I.V.: 1 minute
  Duration: I.M.: 12-27 minutes; I.V.: 9-17 minutes

GI tract effect:
  Onset of action: Within 1-10 minutes
  Duration: 12-30 minutes

Pharmacokinetics

Distribution: V_d: 0.25 L/kg
Metabolism: Extensively degraded in liver and kidneys
Half-life, plasma: 8-18 minutes
Clearance: 13.5 mL/minute/kg

Usual Dosage

Hypoglycemia or insulin shock therapy: I.M., I.V., S.C. (may repeat in 20 minutes as needed):
  Neonates, Infants and Children ≤20 kg: 0.02-0.03 mg/kg or 0.5 mg
  Children >20 kg and Adults: 1 mg
Diagnostic aid: Adults: I.M., I.V.: 0.25-2 mg 10 minutes prior to procedure

Administration Parenteral: Dilute with manufacturer provided diluent resulting in 1 mg/mL; if doses exceeding 2 mg are used, dilute with SWI instead of diluent; administer by direct I.V. injection, I.M., or S.C.

Monitoring Parameters Blood glucose, blood pressure

Additional Information 1 unit = 1 mg

Dosage Forms

Injection, powder for reconstitution, lyophilized, as hydrochloride:
  GlucaGen®, Glucagon: 1 mg [1 unit]
  GlucaGen® Diagnostic Kit: 1 mg [1 unit] [packaged with sterile water]
  Glucagon Diagnostic Kit, Glucagon Emergency Kit: 1 mg [1 unit] [packaged with diluent syringe containing 12 mg/mL glycerin and SWI]

♦ **Glucocerebrosidase** see Alglucerase on page 61
♦ **Glucophage®** see Metformin on page 729
♦ **Glucophage® XR** see Metformin on page 729
♦ **Glucose** see Dextrose on page 366
♦ **Glucose Monohydrate** see Dextrose on page 366
♦ **Glucotrol®** see GlipiZIDE on page 537
♦ **Glucotrol® XL** see GlipiZIDE on page 537
♦ **Glutol™ [OTC]** see Dextrose on page 366
♦ **Glutose™ [OTC]** see Dextrose on page 366
♦ **Glybenclamide** see GlyBURIDE on page 540
♦ **Glybenzcyclamide** see GlyBURIDE on page 540

GlyBURIDE (GLYE byoor ide)

U.S. Brand Names Diaβeta®; Glynase® PresTab®; Micronase®
Canadian Brand Names Albert® Glyburide; Apo®-Glyburide; Euglucon®; Gen-Glybe; Novo-Glyburide; Nu-Glyburide; PMS-Glyburide; ratio-Glyburide
Synonyms Diabeta; Glibenclamide; Glybenclamide; Glybenzcyclamide
Therapeutic Category Antidiabetic Agent, Oral; Antidiabetic Agent, Sulfonylurea; Hypoglycemic Agent, Oral
Generic Available Yes

Use Management of type II diabetes mellitus (noninsulin-dependent, NIDDM) when hyperglycemia cannot be managed by diet alone; may be used concomitantly with metformin or insulin to improve glycemic control

Pregnancy Risk Factor C

Contraindications Hypersensitivity to glyburide, any component, or other sulfonamides; type 1 diabetes mellitus (insulin-dependent, IDDM), diabetic ketoacidosis with or without coma

Warnings Chemical similarities are present among sulfonamides, sulfonylureas, carbonic anhydrase inhibitors, thiazides, and loop diuretics (except ethacrynic acid), and although only glyburide use in patients with sulfonamide allergy is specifically contraindicated in product labeling, there is a risk of cross-reaction in patients with allergies to any of these compounds; avoid use when the previous reaction has been severe; product labeling states oral hypoglycemic drugs may be associated with an increased cardiovascular mortality as compared to treatment with diet alone or diet plus insulin; data to support this association are limited, and several studies, including a large prospective trial (UKPDS) have not supported an association.

Precautions Use with caution in patients with adrenal or pituitary insufficiency; hypoglycemic reactions are more prevalent in debilitated, malnourished patients, patients with mild disease or impaired hepatic or renal function; hypoglycemia may also occur with inadequate caloric intake, strenuous exercise, or concurrent use with other hypoglycemic drugs

Adverse Reactions

Central nervous system: Headache, dizziness

Dermatologic: Pruritus, rash, urticaria, photosensitivity

Endocrine & metabolic: Hypoglycemia, weight gain

Gastrointestinal: Nausea, epigastric fullness, heartburn, constipation, diarrhea, anorexia

Genitourinary: Nocturia

Hematologic: Leukopenia, thrombocytopenia, hemolytic anemia, aplastic anemia, bone marrow suppression, agranulocytosis

Hepatic: Cholestatic jaundice, elevated liver enzymes

Neuromuscular & skeletal: Arthralgia, paresthesia

Ocular: Blurred vision

Renal: Diuretic effect (minor), urolithiasis

Drug Interactions Cytochrome P450 isoenzyme CYP3A3/4 enzyme substrate

Drugs which tend to produce hyperglycemia (eg, diuretics, corticosteroids, phenothiazines, thyroid products, estrogens, oral contraceptives, phenytoin, nicotinic acid, sympathomimetics, calcium channel-blocking drugs, rifampin, and isoniazid) may lead to a loss of glycemic control; disulfiram-like reactions with alcohol; drugs which produce an increase in glyburide's hypoglycemic effects: chloramphenicol, monoamine oxidase inhibitors, fluoroquinolone antibiotics, and probenecid; since this agent is highly protein bound, use of other protein-bound drugs may result in adverse effects when glyburide therapy is initiated or discontinued; beta-adrenergic blocking agents may impair glucose tolerance, increase the frequency or severity of hypoglycemia, block hypoglycemia-induced tachycardia, delay the rate of recovery of blood glucose concentration following drug-induced hypoglycemia, and may alter the hemodynamic response to hypoglycemia

Food Interactions Food does not affect absorption.

Mechanism of Action Stimulates insulin release from the pancreatic beta cells, reduces glucose output from the liver, and increases insulin sensitivity at peripheral target sites

Pharmacodynamics

Onset of action: 45-60 minutes

Maximum effect: 1.5-3 hours

Duration: Conventional formulations: 16-24 hours; micronized formulations: 12-24 hours

Average decrease in fasting blood glucose (when used as monotherapy): 60-70 mg/dL

Pharmacokinetics

Absorption: Reliably and almost completely absorbed

Distribution: V_d: 0.125 L/kg

Metabolism: Completely metabolized to one moderately active and several inactive metabolites

Protein binding: High (>99%)

Half-life: Biphasic: Terminal elimination half-life: Average: 1.4-1.8 hours (range: 0.7-3 hours); may be prolonged with renal or hepatic insufficiency

Time to peak serum concentration: Conventional formulation: 4 hours; micronized formulation: 2-3 hours

(Continued)

GlyBURIDE *(Continued)*

Elimination: 30% to 50% of dose excreted in the urine as metabolites in first 24 hours; the remainder of the metabolite via biliary excretion

Dialysis: Not dialyzable

Usual Dosage Adults: Oral: Formulations of micronized glyburide (Glynase™ PresTab™) are **not** bioequivalent with conventional formulations (Diaβeta®, Micronase®) and dosage should be retitrated when transferring patients from one formulation to the other

Management of noninsulin-dependent diabetes mellitus in patients **previously untreated**:

Tablet (Diaβeta®, Micronase®):

Initial: 2.5-5 mg/day; in patients who are more sensitive to hypoglycemic drugs (see Precautions), start at 1.25 mg/day; increase in increments of no more than 2.5 mg/day at weekly intervals

Maintenance: 1.25-20 mg/day given as single or divided doses; maximum: 20 mg/day; doses >10 mg should be divided into twice daily doses

Micronized tablets (Glynase™ PresTab™):

Initial: 1.5-3 mg/day; in patients who are more sensitive to hypoglycemic drugs (see Precautions), start at 0.75 mg/day; increase in increments of no more than 1.5 mg/day at weekly intervals

Maintenance: 0.75-12 mg/day given as a single dose or in divided doses; doses >6 mg should be divided into twice daily doses

Management of noninsulin-dependent diabetes mellitus in patients **previously maintained on insulin**: Initial dosage dependent upon previous insulin dosage, see table

Previous Daily Insulin Dosage (units)	Initial Glyburide Dosage (mg conventional formulation)	Initial Glyburide Dosage (mg micronized formulation)	Insulin Dosage Change (after glyburide started)
<20	2.5-5	1.5-3	Discontinue
20-40	5	3	Discontinue
>40	5 (increase in increments of 1.25-2.5 mg every 2-10 days)	3 (increase in increments of 0.75-1.5 mg every 2-10 days)	Reduce insulin dosage by 50% (gradually taper off insulin as glyburide dosage increased)

Dosing adjustment in renal impairment: Cl_{cr} <50 mL/minute: Not recommended

Dosing adjustment in hepatic impairment: Use conservative initial and maintenance doses and avoid use in severe disease

Administration Oral: May administer with food every morning 30 minutes before breakfast or the first main meal

Monitoring Parameters Signs and symptoms of hypoglycemia, fasting blood glucose, hemoglobin A_{1c}

Reference Range Target range:

Blood glucose: Fasting and preprandial: 80-120 mg/dL; bedtime: 100-140 mg/dL

Glycosylated hemoglobin (hemoglobin A_{1c}): <7%

Patient Information Do not change dose or discontinue without consulting prescriber; avoid alcohol while taking this medication, may cause severe reaction; maintain regular dietary intake and exercise routine; always carry quick source of sugar; if experiencing a hypoglycemic reaction, contact prescriber immediately; report severe or persistent side effects, extended vomiting or flu-like symptoms, skin rash, easy bruising or bleeding, or change in color of urine or stool. May rarely cause photosensitivity reactions (eg, exposure to sunlight may cause severe sunburn, skin rash, redness, or itching); avoid direct exposure to sunlight

Additional Information When transferring from other sulfonylurea antidiabetic agents to glyburide, with the exception of chlorpropamide, the administration of the other agent may be abruptly discontinued; due to the prolonged elimination half-life of chlorpropamide, a 2- to 3-day drug-free interval may be advisable before glyburide therapy is begun

Dosage Forms

Tablet (Diaβeta®, Micronase®): 1.25 mg, 2.5 mg, 5 mg

Tablet, micronized (Glynase® PresTab®): 1.5 mg, 3 mg, 6 mg

References

DeFronzo RA, "Pharmacologic Therapy for Type 2 Diabetes Mellitus," *Ann Intern Med*, 1999, 131(4):281-303.

"Intensive Blood-Glucose Control With Sulphonylureas or Insulin Compared With Conventional Treatment and Risk of Complications in Patients With Type 2 Diabetes (UKPDS 33) UK Prospective Diabetes Study (UKPDS) Group," *Lancet*, 1998, 352(9131):837-53.

Glycerin (GLIS er in)

U.S. Brand Names Bausch & Lomb® Computer Eye Drops [OTC]; Fleet® Babylax® [OTC]; Fleet® Glycerin Suppositories [OTC]; Fleet® Glycerin Suppositories Maximum Strength [OTC]; Fleet® Liquid Glycerin Suppositories [OTC]; Osmoglyn®; Sani-Supp® [OTC]

Synonyms Glycerol

Therapeutic Category Laxative, Osmotic

Generic Available Yes

Use Treatment of constipation; reduction of intraocular pressure; reduction of corneal edema; glycerin has been administered orally to reduce intracranial pressure; laxative used in newborns to promote bilirubin excretion by reducing enterohepatic circulation, decreasing GI transit time, and stimulating passage of meconium

Pregnancy Risk Factor C

Contraindications Hypersensitivity to glycerin or any component; severe dehydration, anuria

Precautions Use oral glycerin with caution in patients with cardiac, renal or hepatic disease and in diabetics

Adverse Reactions

Central nervous system: Dizziness, headache, confusion, disorientation

Endocrine & metabolic: Hyperglycemia, dehydration

Gastrointestinal: Diarrhea, nausea, tenesmus, thirst, cramping pain, vomiting, rectal irritation

Local: Pain/irritation with ophthalmic solution (may need to apply a topical ophthalmic anesthetic before glycerin administration)

Stability Protect from heat; freezing should be avoided

Mechanism of Action

Rectal: Osmotic dehydrating agent which increases osmotic pressure; draws fluid into colon and thus stimulates evacuation

Ophthalmic: Osmotic action reduces edema and causes clearing of corneal haze

Oral: Glycerin increases osmotic pressure of the plasma drawing water from the extravascular spaces into the blood producing a decrease in intraocular and intracranial pressure

Pharmacodynamics

Onset of action for glycerin suppository or enema: 15-30 minutes

Onset of action in decreasing intraocular pressure: Within 10-30 minutes

Duration: 4-8 hours

Increased intracranial pressure decreases within 10-60 minutes following an oral dose

Duration: ~2-3 hours

Pharmacokinetics

Absorption:

Oral: Well absorbed

Rectal: Poorly absorbed

Metabolism: Primarily in the liver with 20% metabolized in the kidney

Half-life: 30-45 minutes

Time to peak serum concentration: Oral: Within 60-90 minutes

Elimination: Only a small percentage of drug is excreted unchanged in urine

Usual Dosage

Constipation: Rectal: Administered in single doses only at infrequent intervals

Neonates: 0.5 mL/kg/dose of rectal solution as an enema

Children <6 years: 1 infant suppository as needed or 2-5 mL of rectal solution as an enema

Children ≥6 years and Adults: 1 adult suppository as needed or 5-15 mL of rectal solution as an enema

Children and Adults:

Reduction of intraocular pressure: Oral: 1-1.8 g/kg administered 1-1½ hours preoperatively; additional doses may be administered at 5-hour intervals

Reduction of intracranial pressure: Oral: 1.5 g/kg/day divided every 4 hours; 1 g/kg/dose every 6 hours has also been used

Reduction of corneal edema: Ophthalmic: Instill 1-2 drops in eye(s) every 3-4 hours

Administration

Oral: Orange or lemon juice may be added to unflavored 50% oral solution; pour solution over crushed ice and drink through a straw to improve palatability

Ophthalmic: Instill drops onto the eye; avoid contaminating tip of the solution bottle

Rectal: Insert suppository in the rectum and retain 15 minutes

Monitoring Parameters Blood glucose, intraocular pressure, evacuation of stool

(Continued)

Glycerin *(Continued)*

Patient Information Do not use if experiencing abdominal pain, nausea, or vomiting

Nursing Implications Use caution during insertion of suppository to avoid intestinal perforation, especially in neonates; instruct patient to lie down after oral glycerin administration to prevent or relieve headaches

Dosage Forms

Solution, ophthalmic, sterile (Bausch & Lomb® Computer Eye Drops): 1% (15 mL)

Solution, oral (Osmoglyn®): 50% (220 mL) [lime flavor]

Solution, rectal:
Fleet® Babylax®: 2.3 g/2.3 mL (4 mL) [6 units/box]
Fleet® Liquid Glycerin Suppositories: 5.6 g/5.5 mL (7.5 mL) [4 units/box]

Suppository, rectal: (12s, 24s, 25s, 50s) [pediatric and adult sizes]
Fleet® Glycerin Suppositories: 1 g (12s) [pediatric size], 2 g (12s, 24s, 50s) [adult size]
Fleet® Glycerin Suppositories Maximum Strength: 3 g (18s) [adult size]
Sani-Supp®: 82.5% (10s, 25s) [pediatric size]; 82.5% (10s, 25s, 50s) [adult size]

References

Heinemeyer G, "Clinical Pharmacokinetic Considerations in the Treatment of Increased Intracranial Pressure," *Clin Pharmacokinet*, 1987, 13(1):1-25.

Rottenberg DA, Hurwitz BJ, and Posner JB, "The Effect of Oral Glycerol on Intraventricular Pressure in Man," *Neurology*, 1977, 27(7):600-8.

Zenk KE, Koeppel RM, and Liem LA, "Comparative Efficacy of Glycerin Enemas and Suppository Chips in Neonates," *Clin Pharm*, 1993, 12(11):846-8.

♦ **Glycerol** *see* Glycerin *on page 543*

♦ **Glycerol Guaiacolate** *see* Guaifenesin *on page 550*

♦ **Glycerol Guaiacolate and Codeine** *see* Guaifenesin and Codeine *on page 551*

♦ **Glyceryl Trinitrate** *see* Nitroglycerin *on page 815*

♦ **Glycon (Can)** *see* Metformin *on page 729*

Glycopyrrolate *(glye koe PYE roe late)*

Related Information

Compatibility of Medications Mixed in a Syringe *on page 1412*
Overdose and Toxicology *on page 1388*

U.S. Brand Names Robinul®; Robinul® Forte

Synonyms Glycopyrronium

Therapeutic Category Anticholinergic Agent; Antispasmodic Agent, Gastrointestinal

Generic Available Yes (injection)

Use Adjunct in treatment of peptic ulcer disease; inhibition of salivation and excessive secretions of the respiratory tract; reversal of the muscarinic effects of cholinergic agents such as neostigmine and pyridostigmine during reversal of neuromuscular blockade

Pregnancy Risk Factor B

Contraindications Hypersensitivity to glycopyrrolate or any component (see Warnings); narrow-angle glaucoma; acute hemorrhage; tachycardia; ulcerative colitis; obstructive uropathy; paralytic ileus; myasthenia gravis

Warnings Infants, patients with Down syndrome, and children with spastic paralysis or brain damage may be hypersensitive to antimuscarinic effects. Injection contains benzyl alcohol which may cause allergic reactions in susceptible individuals; large amounts of benzyl alcohol (≥99 mg/kg/day) have been associated with a potentially fatal toxicity ("gasping syndrome") in neonates; the "gasping syndrome" consists of metabolic acidosis, respiratory distress, gasping respirations, CNS dysfunction (including convulsions, intracranial hemorrhage), hypotension and cardiovascular collapse; avoid use of injections containing benzyl alcohol in neonates; *in vitro* and animal studies have shown that benzoate, a metabolite of benzyl alcohol, displaces bilirubin from protein binding sites.

Precautions Use with caution in patients with fever, hyperthyroidism, hepatic or renal disease, hypertension, CHF, GI infections, diarrhea, reflux esophagitis

Adverse Reactions

Cardiovascular: Tachycardia, orthostatic hypotension, ventricular fibrillation, palpitations

Central nervous system: Drowsiness, nervousness, headache, insomnia, confusion, loss of memory, fatigue, ataxia

Dermatologic: Rash, dry skin

Gastrointestinal: Xerostomia, constipation, nausea, vomiting, dry throat, dysphagia

Genitourinary: Urinary retention, dysuria

Local: Irritation at injection site

Neuromuscular & skeletal: Weakness

Ocular: Blurred vision

Respiratory: Dry nose

Miscellaneous: Decreased diaphoresis

Drug Interactions Phenothiazines, meperidine, amantadine, tricyclic antidepressants, and quinidine (additive anticholinergic effect); wax-matrix potassium chloride (increased severity of potassium-induced GI mucosal lesions); antacids (decreased absorption); decreased effect of levodopa

Stability Unstable at pH >6; compatible in the same syringe with atropine, benzquinamide, chlorpromazine, codeine, diphenhydramine, droperidol, fentanyl, hydromorphone, hydroxyzine, lidocaine, meperidine, promethazine, morphine, neostigmine, oxymorphone, procaine, prochlorperazine, promazine, pyridostigmine, scopolamine, triflupromazine, and trimethobenzamide

Mechanism of Action Inhibits the muscarinic action of acetylcholine at postganglionic parasympathetic neuroeffector sites in smooth muscle, secretory glands, and CNS

Pharmacodynamics
Onset of action:
Oral: Within 1 hour
I.M., S.C.: 15-30 minutes
I.V.: 1-10 minutes
Maximum effect: I.M., S.C.: 30-45 minutes
Duration (anticholinergic effects):
Oral: 8-12 hours
Parenteral: 7 hours

Pharmacokinetics
Absorption: Oral: Poor and erratic; 10% absorption
Distribution: Does not adequately penetrate into CNS
Elimination: Primarily unchanged via biliary elimination (70% to 90%)

Usual Dosage
Children:
Control of secretions:
Oral: 40-100 mcg/kg/dose 3-4 times/day
I.M., I.V.: 4-10 mcg/kg/dose every 3-4 hours
Preoperative: I.M.:
<2 years: 4.4-8.8 mcg/kg 30-60 minutes before procedure
>2 years: 4.4 mcg/kg 30-60 minutes before procedure
Children and Adults: Reversal of muscarinic effects of cholinergic agents: I.V.: 0.2 mg for each 1 mg of neostigmine or 5 mg of pyridostigmine administered
Adults:
Peptic ulcer:
Oral: 1-2 mg 2-3 times/day
I.M., I.V.: 0.1-0.2 mg 3-4 times/day
Preoperative: I.M.: 4.4 mcg/kg 30-60 minutes before procedure

Administration
Oral: May be administered without regard to meals
Parenteral: Dilute to a concentration of 2 mcg/mL (maximum concentration: 200 mcg/mL); infuse over 15-20 minutes; may be administered direct I.V. at a maximum rate of 20 mcg/minute; may be administered I.M.

Monitoring Parameters Heart rate

Patient Information May cause dry mouth

Dosage Forms
Injection, solution (Robinul®): 0.2 mg/mL (1 mL, 2 mL, 5 mL, 20 mL) [contains benzyl alcohol]
Tablet:
Robinul®: 1 mg
Robinul® Forte: 2 mg

- ◆ **Glycopyrronium** see Glycopyrrolate on page 544
- ◆ **Glycosum** see Dextrose on page 366
- ◆ **Glydiazinamide** see GlipiZIDE on page 537
- ◆ **Glynase® PresTab®** see GlyBURIDE on page 540
- ◆ **Gly-Oxide® [OTC]** see Carbamide Peroxide on page 212
- ◆ **Glytuss® [OTC]** see Guaifenesin on page 550
- ◆ **GM-CSF** see Sargramostim on page 1007

Gold Sodium Thiomalate (gold SOW dee um thye oh MAL ate)

U.S. Brand Names Aurolate®
Canadian Brand Names Myochrysine®
Therapeutic Category Gold Compound
Generic Available Yes
Use Treatment of progressive rheumatoid arthritis
(Continued)

Gold Sodium Thiomalate *(Continued)*

Pregnancy Risk Factor C

Contraindications Hypersensitivity to gold compounds, any component (see Warnings), or other heavy metals; severe hepatic or renal dysfunction; systemic lupus erythematosus; history of blood dyscrasias; CHF, exfoliative dermatitis, or colitis; avoid concomitant use of antimalarials, immunosuppressive agents, penicillamine, or phenylbutazone

Warnings Explain the possibility of adverse reactions before initiating therapy; signs of gold toxicity include: decrease in hemoglobin, leukocytes, granulocytes and platelets, proteinuria, hematuria, pigmentation, pruritus, stomatitis or persistent diarrhea, rash, metallic taste; advise patient to report any symptoms of toxicity

Injection contains benzyl alcohol which may cause allergic reactions in susceptible individuals; large amounts of benzyl alcohol (≥99 mg/kg/day) have been associated with a potentially fatal toxicity ("gasping syndrome") in neonates; the "gasping syndrome" consists of metabolic acidosis, respiratory distress, gasping respirations, CNS dysfunction (including convulsions, intracranial hemorrhage), hypotension and cardiovascular collapse; *in vitro* and animal studies have shown that benzoate displaces bilirubin from protein binding sites; avoid use of gold sodium thiomalate in neonates

Precautions Frequent monitoring of patients for signs and symptoms of toxicity will prevent serious adverse reactions; NSAIDs and corticosteroids may be discontinued after initiating gold therapy; must not be injected I.V.

Adverse Reactions
Cardiovascular: Flushing
Central nervous system: Seizures, headache
Dermatologic: Exfoliative urticaria, dermatitis, erythema nodosum, alopecia, shedding of nails, pruritus, gray-to-blue pigmentation of skin and mucous membranes
Gastrointestinal: Stomatitis, nausea, diarrhea, abdominal cramps, metallic taste, gingivitis, glossitis, ulcerative enterocolitis, GI hemorrhage, dysphagia
Genitourinary: Vaginitis
Hematologic: Eosinophilia, leukopenia, agranulocytosis, thrombocytopenia
Hepatic: Hepatitis
Neuromuscular & skeletal: Arthralgias, peripheral neuropathy
Ocular: Blurred vision, conjunctivitis, corneal ulcers, iritis
Renal: Hematuria, proteinuria, nephrotic syndrome
Respiratory: Interstitial pneumonitis and fibrosis
Miscellaneous: Hypersensitivity reactions including anaphylaxis (rare)

Drug Interactions Decreased effect with penicillamine, acetylcysteine

Mechanism of Action Unknown, may decrease prostaglandin synthesis or may alter cellular mechanisms by inhibiting sulfhydryl systems

Pharmacokinetics
Distribution: Breast milk to plasma ratio: 0.02-0.3
Half-life: 3-27 days (may lengthen with multiple doses)
Time to peak serum concentration: I.M.: Within 3-6 hours
Elimination: Majority (50% to 90%) excreted in urine with smaller amounts (10% to 50%) excreted in feces (via bile)

Usual Dosage I.M.:
Children: Initial: Test dose of 10 mg I.M. is recommended, followed by 1 mg/kg I.M. weekly for 20 weeks (maximum dose: 50 mg); maintenance: 1 mg/kg/dose at 2- to 4-week intervals thereafter for as long as therapy is clinically beneficial and toxicity does not develop. Administration for 2-4 months is usually required before clinical improvement is observed.
Adults: 10 mg first week; 25 mg second week; then 25-50 mg/week until clinical improvement or a 1 g cumulative dose has been given. If improvement occurs without adverse reactions, give 25-50 mg every 2 weeks for 2-20 weeks; if continues stable, give 25-50 mg every 3-4 weeks indefinitely.

Dosage adjustment in renal impairment:
Cl_{cr} 50-80 mL/minute: Administer 50% of dose
Cl_{cr} <50 mL/minute: Avoid use

Administration Parenteral: Administer I.M. only, preferably intragluteally; addition of 0.1 mL of 1% lidocaine to each injection may reduce the discomfort associated with I.M. administration; patients should be recumbent during injection and for 10 minutes afterwards; observe closely for 15 minutes after injection

Monitoring Parameters CBC, platelets, hemoglobin, urinalysis, renal and liver function tests

Reference Range Gold: Normal: 0-0.1 µg/mL (SI: 0-0.0064 µmol/L); Therapeutic: 1-3 µg/mL (SI: 0.06-0.18 µmol/L); Urine <0.1 µg/24 hours

Dosage Forms Injection, solution: 50 mg/mL (1 mL, 10 mL) [contains benzyl alcohol]

♦ **GoLYTELY®** *see* Polyethylene Glycol-Electrolyte Solution *on page 914*

Gonadorelin (goe nad oh REL in)

U.S. Brand Names Factrel®
Canadian Brand Names Lutrepulse™
Synonyms LH-RH; LRH
Therapeutic Category Diagnostic Agent, Gonadotrophic Hormone; Gonadotropin
Generic Available No
Use Evaluation of hypothalamic-pituitary gonadotropic function; used to evaluate abnormal gonadotropin regulation as in precocious puberty and delayed puberty; treatment of primary hypothalamic amenorrhea
Pregnancy Risk Factor B
Contraindications Hypersensitivity to gonadorelin or any component (see Warnings)
Warnings Anaphylactic reactions have occurred following multiple-dose administration; multiple pregnancy is a possibility with Lutrepulse®

Diluent for injection contains benzyl alcohol which may cause allergic reactions in susceptible individuals; large amounts of benzyl alcohol (≥99 mg/kg/day) have been associated with a potentially fatal toxicity ("gasping syndrome") in neonates; avoid use of gonadorelin products containing benzyl alcohol in neonates; *in vitro* and animal studies have shown that benzoate, a metabolite of benzyl alcohol, displaces bilirubin from protein binding sites

Adverse Reactions
Cardiovascular: Flushing
Central nervous system: Lightheadedness, headache
Dermatologic: Skin rash
Gastrointestinal: Nausea, abdominal discomfort
Local: Pain, pruritus, edema
Miscellaneous: Hypersensitivity reactions

Drug Interactions Androgens, estrogens, progestins, glucocorticoids affect pituitary secretion of gonadotropins; spironolactone, levodopa may increase gonadotropin levels; oral contraceptives, digoxin may suppress gonadotropin levels; phenothiazines, dopamine antagonists may blunt response to gonadorelin
Stability Prepare immediately prior to use; after reconstitution, store at room temperature and use within 1 day; discard unused portion
Mechanism of Action Stimulates the release of luteinizing hormone (LH) from the anterior pituitary gland
Pharmacodynamics
Onset of action: Following administration, maximal LH release occurs within 20 minutes
Duration: 3-5 hours
Pharmacokinetics Half-life: 4 minutes
Usual Dosage
Children: I.V. **(as hydrochloride salt)**: 100 mcg to evaluate abnormal gonadotropin regulation
Children >12 years and Adults: I.V., S.C. **(as hydrochloride salt)**: 100 mcg; administer to women during early phase of menstrual cycle (day 1-7)
Adults: I.V. **(as acetate salt)**: 5 mcg (range: 1-20 mcg) every 90 minutes for 7 days via the Lutrepulse® pump; recommended treatment interval: 21 days
Administration Parenteral:
Hydrochloride salt: Dilute in 3 mL of NS; administer I.V. push over 30 seconds
Acetate salt (Lutrepulse®): Fill presterilized reservoir bag with reconstituted solution; administer I.V. using the Lutrepulse® pump
Monitoring Parameters Plasma LH and FSH
Hypothalamic/pituitary function evaluation: Draw blood samples for LH 15 minutes before and immediately before gonadorelin dose, then at 15, 30, 45, 60, and 120 minutes after dose
Dosage Forms
Injection, powder for reconstitution, lyophilized, as hydrochloride: 100 mcg [diluent contains benzyl alcohol]

References
Pescovitz OH, Comite F, Hench K, et al, "The NIH Experience With Precocious Puberty: Diagnostic Subgroups and Response to Short-Term Luteinizing Hormone-Releasing Hormone Analogue Therapy," *J Pediatr*, 1986, 108(1):47-54.

♦ **Gordofilm®** [OTC] *see* Salicylic Acid *on page 1002*

Granisetron (gra NI se tron)

U.S. Brand Names Kytril®
Therapeutic Category Antiemetic; 5-HT₃ Receptor Antagonist
(Continued)

Granisetron *(Continued)*

Generic Available No

Use Prophylaxis and treatment of chemotherapy and radiation-related nausea and emesis; prophylaxis and treatment of postoperative nausea and vomiting

Pregnancy Risk Factor B

Contraindications Hypersensitivity to granisetron or any component (see Warnings)

Warnings Some injectable products contain benzyl alcohol which may cause allergic reactions in susceptible individuals; large amounts of benzyl alcohol ($\geq$99 mg/kg/day) have been associated with a potentially fatal toxicity ("gasping syndrome") in neonates; the "gasping syndrome" consists of metabolic acidosis, respiratory distress, gasping respirations, CNS dysfunction (including convulsions, intracranial hemorrhage), hypotension and cardiovascular collapse; avoid use of products containing benzyl alcohol in neonates. *In vitro* and animal studies have shown that benzoate, a metabolite of benzyl alcohol, displaces bilirubin from protein-binding sites; granisetron oral solution contains sodium benzoate; avoid use of oral solution in neonates

Precautions Use with caution in patients with liver disease or in pregnant patients. Use with caution in patients following abdominal surgery; may mask progressive ileus or gastric distension.

Adverse Reactions
Cardiovascular: Hypertension, hypotension, arrhythmias such as bradycardia, atrial fibrillation, A-V block, angina, syncope
Central nervous system: Agitation, anxiety, CNS stimulation, headache, insomnia, somnolence, fever, dizziness
Dermatologic: Skin rashes
Gastrointestinal: Constipation, diarrhea, dysgeusia, abdominal pain
Hepatic: Elevated liver enzymes
Neuromuscular & skeletal: Weakness
Miscellaneous: Allergic reactions

Drug Interactions Cytochrome P450 isoenzyme CYP3A3/4 substrate
Because granisetron is metabolized by hepatic cytochrome P450 drug metabolizing enzymes, inducers or inhibitors of this system may change the clearance and half-life

Stability Tablets and injections: Store at room temperature, protect from light; injection stable when mixed in NS, D_5W for at least 24 hours

Mechanism of Action Selective 5-HT$_3$ receptor antagonist, blocking serotonin, both peripherally on vagal nerve terminals and centrally in the chemoreceptor trigger zone

Pharmacodynamics
Onset of action: I.V.: 1-3 minutes
Duration: I.V.: $\leq$24 hours

Pharmacokinetics
Distribution: V_d: 2-3 L/kg; widely distributed throughout the body
Protein binding: 65%
Metabolism: Hepatic via N-demethylation, oxidation, and conjugation; some metabolites may have 5-HT$_3$ antagonist activity
Half-life:
Cancer patients: 10-12 hours
Healthy volunteers: 3-4 hours
Elimination: Primarily nonrenal, 8% to 15% of dose excreted unchanged in urine

Usual Dosage
Treatment of chemotherapy-induced emesis: Initial dose given just prior to chemotherapy (15-60 minutes before)
Children $\geq$2 years and Adults: I.V.: Manufacturer's recommendation: 10 mcg/kg; or as an alternative based on clinical research: 20-40 mcg/kg/day divided once or twice daily; maximum: 3 mg/dose or 9 mg/day
As intervention therapy for breakthrough nausea and vomiting, during the first 24 hours following chemotherapy, 2 or 3 repeat infusions (same dose) have been administered
Adults: Oral: 2 mg once daily or 1 mg twice daily
Prevention and treatment of postoperative nausea and vomiting, before induction of surgery, immediately before reversal of anesthesia, or postoperatively: I.V.:
Children $\geq$4 years: 20-40 mcg/kg given as a single dose; not to exceed 1 mg
Adults: 1 mg given as a single dose

Administration
Oral: Given at least 1 hour prior to chemotherapy and then 12 hours later; shake oral suspension well before use
Parenteral: I.V.: Infuse over 30 seconds undiluted **or** dilute in small volume NS or D_5W and administer over 5 minutes **or** dilute in 20-50 mL of NS or D_5W and infuse over 30 minutes to 1 hour

Dosage Forms

Injection, solution, as hydrochloride: 1 mg/mL (4 mL) [contains benzyl alcohol]

Injection, solution, as hydrochloride [preservative free]: 1 mg/mL (1 mL)

Solution, oral, as hydrochloride: 2 mg/10 mL (30 mL) [contains sodium benzoate; orange flavor]

Tablet, as hydrochloride: 1 mg

Extemporaneous Preparations

A 0.2 mg/mL suspension may be made by crushing twelve 1 mg tablets. Add 30 mL distilled water, mix well, and transfer to a bottle. Rinse the mortar with 10 mL cherry syrup and add to bottle. Add enough cherry syrup to make a final volume of 60 mL. Label "shake well"; stable 14 days at room temperature or refrigerated (Quercia, 1997).

A 50 mcg/mL suspension may be made by crushing one 1 mg tablet. Add 1% methylcellulose and syrup NF to a total volume of 20 mL (may also use Ora-Sweet® or Ora-Plus® instead of methylcellulose and syrup); shake well; stable 91 days refrigerated (Nahata, 1998).

Nahata MC, Morosco RS, and Hipple TF, "Stability of Granisetron Hydrochloride in Two Oral Suspensions," *Am J Health Syst Pharm*, 1998, 55(23):2511-3.

Quercia RA, Zhang J, Fan C, et al, "Stability of Granisetron Hydrochloride in an Extemporaneously Prepared Oral Liquid," *Am J Health-Syst Pharm*, 1997, 54(12):1404-6.

References

"ASHP Therapeutic Guidelines on the Pharmacologic Management of Nausea and Vomiting in Adult and Pediatric Patients Receiving Chemotherapy or Radiation Therapy or Undergoing Surgery," *Am J Health Syst Pharm*, 1999, 56(8):729-64.

Hahlen K, Quintana E, Pinkerton CR, et al, "A Randomized Comparison of Intravenously Administered Granisetron Versus Chlorpromazine Plus Dexamethasone in the Prevention of Ifosfamide-Induced Emesis in Children," *J Pediatr*, 1995, 126(2):309-13.

Lemerle J, Amaral D, Southall DP, et al, "Efficacy and Safety of Granisetron in the Prevention of Chemotherapy-Induced Emesis in Paediatric Patients," *Eur J Cancer*, 1991, 27(9):1081-3.

♦ **Granulocyte Colony Stimulating Factor** *see* Filgrastim *on page 484*

♦ **Granulocyte Macrophage Colony Stimulating Factor** *see* Sargramostim *on page 1007*

♦ **Gravol® (Can)** *see* DimenhyDRINATE *on page 390*

♦ **Grifulvin® V** *see* Griseofulvin *on page 549*

Griseofulvin (gri see oh FUL vin)

Related Information

Carbohydrate and Alcohol Content of Liquid Medications for Use in Patients Receiving Ketogenic Diets *on page 1431*

U.S. Brand Names Fulvicin® P/G; Fulvicin-U/F®; Grifulvin® V; Gris-PEG®

Synonyms Griseofulvin Microsize; Griseofulvin Ultramicrosize

Therapeutic Category Antifungal Agent, Systemic

Generic Available Yes

Use Treatment of tinea infections of the skin, hair, and nails caused by susceptible species of *Microsporum*, *Epidermophyton*, or *Trichophyton*

Pregnancy Risk Factor C

Contraindications Hypersensitivity to griseofulvin or any component; severe liver disease, porphyria (interferes with porphyrin metabolism); pregnant women (may cause fetal harm)

Precautions Avoid exposure to intense sunlight to prevent photosensitivity reactions; use with caution in patients with penicillin hypersensitivity since cross-reactivity with griseofulvin is possible

Adverse Reactions

Central nervous system: Fatigue, confusion, impaired judgment, insomnia, headache, incoordination, dizziness

Dermatologic: Rash, urticaria, photosensitivity

Endocrine & metabolic: Estrogen-like effects in children

Gastrointestinal: Nausea, vomiting, diarrhea, oral thrush

Hematologic: Leukopenia, granulocytopenia

Hepatic: Hepatotoxicity

Neuromuscular & skeletal: Paresthesia

Renal: Proteinuria

Miscellaneous: Lupus-like syndrome

Drug Interactions Cytochrome P450 isoenzyme CYP1A2 inducer

Phenobarbital decreases griseofulvin concentrations; griseofulvin decreases warfarin effectiveness; griseofulvin decreases oral contraceptive efficacy; griseofulvin potentiates the effects of alcohol and causes flushing and tachycardia

Food Interactions Fatty meal will increase griseofulvin absorption

(Continued)

Griseofulvin *(Continued)*

Mechanism of Action Inhibits fungal cell mitosis at metaphase by disrupting the cell's mitotic spindle structure; binds to human keratin making it resistant to fungal invasion

Pharmacokinetics

Absorption: Ultramicrosize griseofulvin absorption is almost complete; absorption of microsize griseofulvin is variable (25% to 70% of an oral dose); absorbed from the duodenum

Distribution: Deposited in the keratin layer of skin, hair, and nails; concentrates in liver, fat, and skeletal muscles; crosses the placenta

Metabolism: Extensive in the liver

Half-life: 9-22 hours

Elimination: <1% excreted unchanged in urine; also excreted in feces and perspiration

Usual Dosage Oral:

Children:

Microsize: 10-20 mg/kg/day in single or 2 divided doses

Ultramicrosize: >2 years: 5-10 mg/kg/day in single or 2 divided doses

Adults:

Microsize: 500-1000 mg/day in single or divided doses

Ultramicrosize: 330-375 mg/day in single or divided doses; doses up to 750 mg/day have been used for infections more difficult to eradicate such as tinea unguium

Duration of therapy depends on the site of infection:

Tinea corporis: 2-4 weeks

Tinea capitis: 4-6 weeks or longer

Tinea pedis: 4-8 weeks

Tinea unguium: 3-6 months or longer

Administration Oral: Administer with a fatty meal (peanuts or ice cream to increase absorption), or with food or milk to avoid GI upset; shake suspension well before use

Monitoring Parameters Periodic renal, hepatic, and hematopoietic function tests

Test Interactions False-positive urinary VMA levels

Patient Information Avoid alcohol. May cause photosensitivity reactions (eg, exposure to sunlight may cause severe sunburn, skin rash, redness, or itching); avoid exposure to sunlight and artificial light sources (sunlamps, tanning booth/bed); wear protective clothing, wide-brimmed hats, sunglasses, and lip sunscreen (SPF ≥15); use a sunscreen [broad-spectrum sunscreen or physical sunscreen (preferred) or sunblock with SPF ≥15]; contact physician if reaction occurs.

Dosage Forms

Suspension, oral, microsize (Grifulvin® V): 125 mg/5 mL (120 mL) [contains 0.2% alcohol and propylene glycol]

Tablet, microsize, scored (Fulvicin-U/F®): 250 mg, 500 mg

Tablet, ultramicrosize: 125 mg, 250 mg, 330 mg

Fulvicin® P/G: 125 mg, 165 mg, 250 mg, 330 mg [scored]

Tablet, ultramicrosize, film coated, scored (Gris-PEG®): 125 mg, 250 mg

References

Ginsburg CM, McCracken GH Jr, Petruska M, et al, "Effect of Feeding on Bioavailability of Griseofulvin in Children," *J Pediatr*, 1983, 102(2):309-11.

- ◆ **Griseofulvin Microsize** *see* Griseofulvin *on page 549*
- ◆ **Griseofulvin Ultramicrosize** *see* Griseofulvin *on page 549*
- ◆ **Gris-PEG®** *see* Griseofulvin *on page 549*
- ◆ **Growth Hormone** *see* Human Growth Hormone *on page 564*

Guaifenesin *(gwye FEN e sin)*

Related Information

OTC Cough & Cold Preparations, Pediatric *on page 1225*

U.S. Brand Names Amibid LA; Breonesin® [OTC] [DSC]; Diabetic Tussin EX® [OTC]; Duratuss-G®; Fenesin™ [OTC] [DSC]; Glytuss® [OTC]; Guaifenex® G; Guaifenex LA®; Guiatuss® [OTC]; Humibid® L.A.; Humibid® Pediatric; Hytuss® [OTC]; Hytuss-2X® [OTC]; Liquibid®; Liquibid® 1200; Mucinex™ [OTC]; Organidin NR®; Phanasin [OTC]; Respa-GF; Robitussin® [OTC]; Scot-Tussin® Sugar Free Expectorant [OTC]; Touro Ex®

Canadian Brand Names Balminil Expectorant; Benylin® E Extra Strength; Koffex Expectorant

Synonyms GG; Glycerol Guaiacolate

Therapeutic Category Expectorant

Generic Available Yes

Use Temporary control of cough due to minor throat and bronchial irritation

Pregnancy Risk Factor C

Contraindications Hypersensitivity to guaifenesin or any component (see Warnings)

Warnings Some products contain tartrazine which may cause allergic reactions in susceptible individuals. Some products contain sodium benzoate; benzoic acid (benzoate) is a metabolite of benzyl alcohol; large amounts of benzyl alcohol (≥99 mg/kg/day) have been associated with a potentially fatal toxicity ("gasping syndrome") in neonates; *in vitro* and animal studies have shown that benzoate displaces bilirubin from protein binding sites; avoid use of products containing sodium benzoate in neonates

Precautions Some products contain phenylalanine which must be used with caution in patients with phenylketonuria.

Adverse Reactions
Central nervous system: Drowsiness, headache
Dermatologic: Rash
Gastrointestinal: Nausea, vomiting

Mechanism of Action Thought to act as an expectorant by irritating the gastric mucosa and stimulating respiratory tract secretions, thereby increasing respiratory fluid volumes and decreasing phlegm viscosity

Usual Dosage Oral:
Children:
<2 years: 12 mg/kg/day in 6 divided doses
2-5 years: 50-100 mg every 4 hours, not to exceed 600 mg/day
6-11 years: 100-200 mg every 4 hours, not to exceed 1.2 g/day or as extended release product 600 mg every 12 hours
Children >12 years and Adults: 200-400 mg every 4 hours or as extended release product 1200 mg every 12 hours; not to exceed 2.4 g/day

Administration Oral: Administer with a large quantity of fluid to ensure proper action

Test Interactions May cause a colorimetric interference with certain laboratory determinations of 5-hydroxyindoleacetic acid (5-HIAA) and vanillylmandelic acid (VMA)

Dosage Forms
Caplet, sustained release (Touro Ex®): 575 mg
Capsule (Breonesin® [DSC], Hytuss-2X®): 200 mg
Capsule, sustained release (Humibid® Pediatric): 300 mg
Liquid: 100 mg/5 mL (120 mL, 240 mL, 480 mL)
Diabetic Tussin EX®: 100 mg/5 mL (120 mL) [alcohol, dye, and sugar free; contains 8.4 mg phenylalanine (as aspartame)/5 mL]
Organidin NR®: 100 mg/5 mL (480 mL) [contains sodium benzoate; raspberry flavor]
Syrup: 100 mg/5 mL (120 mL, 240 mL, 480 mL)
Guiatuss®: 100 mg/5 mL (120 mL, 240 mL, 480 mL, 3840 mL) [alcohol free; fruit mint flavor]
Phanasin: 100 mg/5 mL (120 mL, 240 mL) [alcohol, sodium, and sugar free]
Robitussin®: 100 mg/5 mL (5 mL, 10 mL, 15 mL, 30 mL, 120 mL, 240 mL, 480 mL) [alcohol free]
Scot-Tussin® Sugar Free Expectorant: 100 mg/5 mL (120 mL) [alcohol and dye free; contains benzoic acid; grape flavor]
Tablet: 200 mg
Tablet:
Glytuss®, Organidin NR®: 200 mg
Hytuss®: 100 mg
Tablet, extended release (Mucinex™): 600 mg
Tablet, sustained release: 600 mg, 1200 mg
Amibid LA, Fenesin™ [DSC], Guafenex® LA, Humibid® LA, Liquibid®, Respa-GF®: 600 mg
Duratuss-G®, Liquibid® 1200: 1200 mg
Tablet, film coated (Guaifenex® G): 1200 mg [dye free]

Guaifenesin and Codeine (gwye FEN e sin & KOE deen)
Related Information
OTC Cough & Cold Preparations, Pediatric *on page 1225*

U.S. Brand Names Brontex®; Cheracol®; Gani-Tuss® NR; Guaituss AC®; Mytussin® AC; Robafen® AC; Robitussin® A-C [DSC]; Romilar® AC; Tussi-Organidin® NR; Tussi-Organidin® S-NR

Synonyms Codeine and Glycerol Guaiacolate; Codeine and Guaifenesin; Glycerol Guaiacolate and Codeine

Therapeutic Category Antitussive; Cough Preparation; Expectorant

Generic Available Yes

Use Temporary control of cough due to minor throat and bronchial irritation

Restrictions C-V

Pregnancy Risk Factor C
(Continued)

Guaifenesin and Codeine *(Continued)*

Contraindications Hypersensitivity to guaifenesin, codeine, or any component

Warnings Some products contain sodium benzoate; benzoic acid (benzoate) is a metabolite of benzyl alcohol; large amounts of benzyl alcohol (≥99 mg/kg/day) have been associated with a potentially fatal toxicity ("gasping syndrome") in neonates; *in vitro* and animal studies have shown that benzoate displaces bilirubin from protein binding sites; avoid use of sodium benzoate products in neonates

Precautions Use with caution in patients with hypersensitivity reactions to other phenanthrene derivative opioid agonists (morphine, hydrocodone, hydromorphone, levorphanol, oxycodone, oxymorphone). Some products contain phenylalanine which must be used with caution in patients with phenylketonuria.

Adverse Reactions

Codeine:

Cardiovascular: Palpitations, bradycardia, peripheral vasodilation

Central nervous system: CNS depression, dizziness, drowsiness, sedation, elevated intracranial pressure

Dermatologic: Pruritus from histamine release

Endocrine & metabolic: Antidiuretic hormone release

Gastrointestinal: Nausea, vomiting, constipation, biliary tract spasm

Genitourinary: Urinary tract spasm

Ocular: Miosis

Respiratory: Respiratory depression

Miscellaneous: Histamine release, physical and psychological dependence with prolonged use

Guaifenesin:

Central nervous system: Drowsiness, headache

Dermatologic: Rash

Gastrointestinal: Nausea, vomiting

Drug Interactions CNS depressant medications produce additive sedative properties

Mechanism of Action See individual monographs for Guaifenesin *on page 550* and Codeine *on page 301*

Usual Dosage Oral:

Children:

2-6 years: 1-1.5 mg/kg codeine/day divided into 4 doses administered every 4-6 hours (maximum dose: 30 mg/24 hours)

6-12 years: 5 mL every 4 hours, not to exceed 30 mL/24 hours

>12 years: 10 mL every 4 hours, up to 60 mL/24 hours

Adults: 5-10 mL or 1 tablet every 4-6 hours; not to exceed 120 mg (60 mL) codeine/day or 6 tablets/day

Administration Oral: Administer with a large quantity of fluid to ensure proper action; may administer with food to decrease nausea and GI upset from codeine

Test Interactions May cause a colorimetric interference with certain laboratory determinations of 5-hydroxy indoleacetic acid (5-HIAA) and vanillylmandelic acid (VMA)

Patient Information May be habit-forming; do not discontinue abruptly

Dosage Forms

Liquid: Guaifenesin 100 mg and codeine phosphate 10 mg per 5 mL (120 mL, 480 mL)

Brontex®: Guaifenesin 75 mg and codeine phosphate 2.5 mg per 5 mL (480 mL) [alcohol free; mint flavor]

Gani-Tuss® NR: Guaifenesin 100 mg and codeine phosphate 10 mg per 5 mL (480 mL) [alcohol and sugar free; raspberry flavor]

Tussi-Organidin® S-NR: Guaifenesin 100 mg and codeine phosphate 10 mg per 5 mL (120 mL) [contains sodium benzoate; raspberry flavor]

Syrup: Guaifenesin 100 mg and codeine phosphate 10 mg per 5 mL (120 mL, 480 mL)

Cheracol®: Guaifenesin 100 mg and codeine phosphate 10 mg per 5 mL (120 mL) [contains 4.75% alcohol and benzoic acid]

Guaituss AC®: Guaifenesin 100 mg and codeine phosphate 10 mg per 5 mL (120 mL, 480 mL, 3840 mL) [sugar free; contains alcohol; fruit-mint flavor]

Mytussin® AC: Guaifenesin 100 mg and codeine phosphate 10 mg per 5 mL (120 mL, 480 mL, 3840 mL) [sugar free; contains alcohol; fruit flavor]

Robafen® A-C: Guaifenesin 100 mg and codeine phosphate 10 mg per 5 mL (120 mL, 480 mL, 3840 mL)

Robitussin® AC: Guaifenesin 100 mg and codeine phosphate 10 mg per 5 mL (120 mL, 240 mL) [contains 3.5% alcohol and sodium benzoate] [DSC]

Romilar® AC: Guaifenesin 100 mg and codeine phosphate 10 mg per 5 mL (480 mL) [alcohol, dye, and sugar free; contains phenylalanine]

Tablet (Brontex®): Guaifenesin 300 mg and codeine phosphate 10 mg

Guaifenesin and Dextromethorphan
(gwye FEN e sin & deks troe meth OR fan)

Related Information

OTC Cough & Cold Preparations, Pediatric *on page 1225*

U.S. Brand Names Aquatab® DM; Benylin® Expectorant [OTC]; Cheracol D® [OTC]; Cheracol® Plus [OTC]; Diabetic Tussin DM® [OTC]; Diabetic Tussin® DM Maximum Strength [OTC]; Duratuss® DM; Fenesin™ DM; Genatuss DM® [OTC]; Guaifenex® DM; Guiatuss® DM [OTC]; Humibid® DM [OTC]; Hydro-Tussin™ DM [OTC]; Kolephrin® GG/DM [OTC]; Mytussin® DM [OTC]; Respa-DM®; Robitussin® DM [OTC]; Robitussin® Sugar Free Cough [OTC]; Safe Tussin® 30 [OTC]; Silexin® [OTC]; Tolu-Sed® DM [OTC]; Touro® DM; Tussi-Organidin® DM NR; Vicks® 44E [OTC]; Vicks® Pediatric Formula 44E [OTC]

Canadian Brand Names Balminil DM E; Benylin® DM-E; Koffex DM-Expectorant

Synonyms Dextromethorphan and Glycerol Guaiacolate; Dextromethorphan and Guaifenesin

Therapeutic Category Antitussive; Cough Preparation; Expectorant

Generic Available Yes

Use Temporary control of cough due to minor throat and bronchial irritation

Pregnancy Risk Factor C

Contraindications Hypersensitivity to guaifenesin, dextromethorphan, or any component

Warnings Some products contain sodium benzoate; benzoic acid (benzoate) is a metabolite of benzyl alcohol; large amounts of benzyl alcohol (≥99 mg/kg/day) have been associated with a potentially fatal toxicity ("gasping syndrome") in neonates; *in vitro* and animal studies have shown that benzoate displaces bilirubin from protein binding sites; avoid use of sodium benzoate products in neonates

Precautions Some products contain phenylalanine which must be used with caution in patients with phenylketonuria.

Adverse Reactions

Central nervous system: Drowsiness, dizziness, headache

Dermatologic: Rash

Gastrointestinal: Nausea

Mechanism of Action See individual monographs for Guaifenesin *on page 550* and Dextromethorphan *on page 365*

Pharmacodynamics Onset of action: Antitussive effect: Oral: 15-30 minutes

Pharmacokinetics Absorption: Dextromethorphan is rapidly absorbed from the GI tract

Usual Dosage Oral (dose expressed in mg of **dextromethorphan**):

Children: 1-2 mg/kg/day every 6-8 hours

Adults: 60-120 mg/day divided every 6-8 hours or as extended release product 30-60 mg every 12 hours; not to exceed 120 mg/day

Administration Oral: Administer with a large quantity of fluid to ensure proper effect

Test Interactions May cause a colorimetric interference with certain laboratory determinations of 5-hydroxy indoleacetic acid (5-HIAA) and vanillylmandelic acid (VMA)

Dosage Forms

Liquid: Guaifenesin 100 mg and dextromethorphan hydrobromide 10 mg per 5 mL (120 mL, 240 mL)

Diabetic Tussin® DM: Guaifenesin 100 mg and dextromethorphan hydrobromide 10 mg per 5 mL (120 mL) [alcohol, dye, and sugar free; contains 8.4 mg phenylalanine (as aspartame)/5 mL]

Diabetic Tussin® DM Maximum Strength: Guaifenesin 200 mg and dextromethorphan hydrobromide 10 mg per 5 mL (120 mL) [alcohol, dye, and sugar free; contains 8.4 mg phenylalanine (as aspartame)/5 mL]

Duratuss® DM: Guaifenesin 200 mg and dextromethorphan hydrobromide 20 mg per 5 mL (480 mL, 3840 mL) [contains 5% alcohol and sodium benzoate; fruit flavor]

Hydro-Tussin™ DM: Guaifenesin 200 mg and dextromethorphan hydrobromide 20 mg per 5 mL (480 mL) [alcohol and sugar free]

Robitussin® Sugar Free Cough: Guaifenesin 100 mg and dextromethorphan hydrobromide 10 mg per 5 mL (120 mL) [alcohol and sugar free]

Safe Tussin® 30: Guaifenesin 100 mg and dextromethorphan hydrobromide 15 mg per 5 mL (120 mL) [alcohol, dye, and sugar free; mint flavor]

Tussi-Organidin® DM NR: Guaifenesin 100 mg and dextromethorphan hydrobromide 10 mg per 5 mL (120 mL, 480 mL) [contains sodium benzoate; raspberry flavor]

Vicks® 44E: Guaifenesin 200 mg and dextromethorphan hydrobromide 20 mg per 15 mL (120 mL, 235 mL) [contains 31 mg/15 mL sodium, alcohol, and sodium benzoate]

(Continued)

Guaifenesin and Dextromethorphan *(Continued)*

Vicks® Pediatric Formula 44E: Guaifenesin 100 mg and dextromethorphan hydrobromide 10 mg per 15 mL (120 mL) [alcohol free; contains 30 mg/15 mL sodium and sodium benzoate; cherry flavor]

Syrup: Guaifenesin 100 mg and dextromethorphan hydrobromide 10 mg per 5 mL (120 mL, 240 mL, 480 mL)

Benylin® Expectorant: Guaifenesin 100 mg and dextromethorphan hydrobromide 5 mg per 5 mL (120 mL) [alcohol and sugar free; contains sodium benzoate; raspberry flavor]

Cheracol® D: Guaifenesin 100 mg and dextromethorphan hydrobromide 10 mg per 5 mL (120 mL, 180 mL) [contains alcohol and benzoic acid]

Cheracol® Plus: Guaifenesin 100 mg and dextromethorphan hydrobromide 10 mg per 5 mL (120 mL)

Genatuss DM®: Guaifenesin 100 mg and dextromethorphan hydrobromide 10 mg per 5 mL (120 mL) [cherry flavor]

Guiatuss® DM: Guaifenesin 100 mg and dextromethorphan hydrobromide 10 mg per 5 mL (120 mL, 240 mL, 480 mL, 3840 mL) [alcohol free; fruit mint flavor]

Kolephrin® GG/DM: Guaifenesin 150 mg and dextromethorphan hydrobromide 10 mg per 5 mL (120 mL) [alcohol free; cherry flavor]

Mytussin® DM: Guaifenesin 100 mg and dextromethorphan hydrobromide 10 mg per 5 mL (120 mL, 480 mL) [alcohol free; cherry flavor]

Robitussin® DM: Guaifenesin 100 mg and dextromethorphan hydrobromide 10 mg per 5 mL (5 mL, 120 mL, 240 mL, 360 mL, 480 mL) [alcohol free]

Silexin: Guaifenesin 100 mg and dextromethorphan hydrobromide 10 mg per 5 mL (45 mL, 480 mL)

Tolu-Sed® DM: Guaifenesin 100 mg and dextromethorphan hydrobromide 10 mg per 5 mL (120 mL)

Tablet (Silexin®): Guaifenesin 100 mg and dextromethorphan hydrobromide 10 mg

Tablet, extended release: Guaifenesin 600 mg and dextromethorphan hydrobromide 30 mg

Aquatab® DM: Guaifenesin 1200 mg and dextromethorphan hydrobromide 60 mg

Fenesin™ DM, Guaifenex® DM, Humibid® DM, Respa-DM®: Guaifenesin 600 mg and dextromethorphan hydrobromide 30 mg

Touro® DM: Guaifenesin 575 mg and dexiromethorphan hydrobromide 30 mg

- **Guaifenex® DM** *see Guaifenesin and Dextromethorphan on page 553*
- **Guaifenex® G** *see Guaifenesin on page 550*
- **Guaifenex LA®** *see Guaifenesin on page 550*
- **Guaituss AC®** *see Guaifenesin and Codeine on page 551*
- **Guiatuss® [OTC]** *see Guaifenesin on page 550*
- **Guiatuss® DM [OTC]** *see Guaifenesin and Dextromethorphan on page 553*
- **Gyne-Lotrimin® [OTC]** *see Clotrimazole on page 297*
- **Gyne-Lotrimin® 3 [OTC]** *see Clotrimazole on page 297*
- **Gynodiol®** *see Estradiol on page 456*
- **H₂O₂** *see Hydrogen Peroxide on page 577*
- ***Haemophilus* b Oligosaccharide Conjugate Vaccine** *see page 1333*
- **Halcion®** *see Triazolam on page 1116*
- **Haldol®** *see Haloperidol on page 554*
- **Haldol® Decanoate** *see Haloperidol on page 554*
- **Halfprin® [OTC]** *see Aspirin on page 134*

Haloperidol *(ha loe PER i dole)*

Related Information

Carbohydrate and Alcohol Content of Liquid Medications for Use in Patients Receiving Ketogenic Diets *on page 1431*

Drugs and Breast-Feeding *on page 1404*

U.S. Brand Names Haldol®; Haldol® Decanoate

Canadian Brand Names Apo®-Haloperidol; Apo®-Haloperidol LA; Haloperidol-LA Omega; Haloperidol Long Acting; Novo-Peridol; Peridol; PMS-Haloperidol LA

Therapeutic Category Antipsychotic Agent; Phenothiazine Derivative

Generic Available Yes

Use Management of schizophrenia; treatment of psychoses, Tourette's disorder, and severe behavioral problems in children; emergency sedation of severely agitated or delirious patients

Pregnancy Risk Factor C

Contraindications Hypersensitivity to haloperidol or any component (see Warnings); narrow-angle glaucoma, bone marrow suppression, CNS depression, coma, severe liver or cardiac disease, parkinsonism

Warnings May cause extrapyramidal symptoms, including pseudoparkinsonism, acute dystonic reactions, akathisia, and tardive dyskinesia (risk of these reactions is high relative to other neuroleptics). Use may be associated with neuroleptic malignant syndrome. Safety and efficacy have not been established in children <3 years of age.

Injection as deconate contains benzyl alcohol which may cause allergic reactions in susceptible individuals; large amounts of benzyl alcohol (≥99 mg/kg/day) have been associated with a potentially fatal toxicity ("gasping syndrome") in neonates; avoid use of haloperidol products containing benzyl alcohol in neonates; *in vitro* and animal studies have shown that benzoate, a metabolite of benzyl alcohol, displaces bilirubin from protein binding sites

Precautions Use with caution in patients with renal or hepatic dysfunction, thyrotoxicosis, cardiovascular disease, history of seizures, or EEG abnormalities; haloperidol may cause hypotension, precipitation of anginal pain, anticholinergic effects (low incidence relative to other neuroleptics), elevation of prolactin levels

Adverse Reactions
Cardiovascular: Tachycardia, hypotension, hypertension, EKG changes (eg, prolongation of QT interval, torsade de pointes)

Central nervous system: Extrapyramidal reactions, neuroleptic malignant syndrome, tardive dyskinesia, drowsiness, restlessness, anxiety, agitation, euphoria, insomnia, confusion, headache, lethargy, vertigo, seizures, depression, hyperpyrexia, heat stroke; exacerbation of psychotic symptoms

Dermatologic: Rash, contact dermatitis; photosensitivity (rare)

Endocrine & metabolic: Galactorrhea, gynecomastia, hyperglycemia, hypoglycemia, hyponatremia, hypomagnesemia, elevated prolactin levels, menstrual irregularities, sexual dysfunction

Gastrointestinal: Xerostomia, constipation, nausea, vomiting, diarrhea, dyspepsia, hypersalivation

Genitourinary: Urinary retention, priapism

Hematologic: Leukopenia, leukocytosis, anemia, lymphomonocytosis; agranulocytosis (rare)

Hepatic: Hepatotoxicity (rare)

Ocular: Blurred vision, retinopathy, visual disturbances

Respiratory: Bronchospasm, laryngospasm, increased depth of respiration

Miscellaneous: Diaphoresis

Drug Interactions Cytochrome P450 isoenzyme CYP1A2 (minor), CYP2D6 (minor), and CYP3A3/4 substrate; CYP2D6 isoenzyme inhibitor

CNS depressants may increase adverse effects; epinephrine may cause hypotension; fluoxetine may inhibit metabolism and increase effect of haloperidol; chlorpromazine may increase haloperidol concentrations; carbamazepine, phenobarbital, and rifampin may increase metabolism and decrease effectiveness of haloperidol; use of haloperidol with anticholinergic agents may increase intraocular pressure; concurrent use with lithium has occasionally caused acute encephalopathy-like syndrome

Food Interactions Drug may precipitate if oral concentrate is mixed with coffee or tea

Stability All dosage forms: Store at controlled room temperature; protect from light
Oral concentrate and injection, as lactate: Do not freeze
Injection, as deconate: Do not refrigerate or freeze

Mechanism of Action Competitive blockade of postsynaptic dopamine receptors in the mesolimbic dopaminergic system; depresses cerebral cortex and hypothalamus; exhibits a strong alpha-adrenergic and anticholinergic blocking activity

Pharmacokinetics
Absorption: Oral: Well absorbed, undergoes first-pass metabolism in the liver
Distribution: Crosses the placenta; appears in breast milk
Protein binding: 92%
Metabolism: In the liver, hydroxy-metabolite is active
Bioavailability: Oral: 60%
Half-life: Adults: 20 hours; range: 13-35 hours
Elimination: Excreted in urine and feces as drug and metabolites

Usual Dosage
Children:
3-12 years (15-40 kg): Oral: Initial: 0.25-0.5 mg/day given in 2-3 divided doses; increase by 0.25-0.5 mg every 5-7 days; maximum dose: 0.15 mg/kg/day; usual maintenance:
Agitation or hyperkinesia: 0.01-0.03 mg/kg/day once daily
Tourette's disorder: 0.05-0.075 mg/kg/day in 2-3 divided doses
Psychotic disorders: 0.05-0.15 mg/kg/day in 2-3 divided doses
Note: Preliminary findings of a double-blind, placebo controlled study reported the mean optimal dose in 12 schizophrenic children 5-12 years to be ~2 mg/day (range: 0.5-3.5 mg/day or 0.02-0.12 mg/kg/day) given in 3 divided doses

(Continued)

Haloperidol *(Continued)*

6-12 years: I.M. **(as lactate):** 1-3 mg/dose every 4-8 hours to a maximum of 0.15 mg/kg/day; switch to oral therapy as soon as able

Adults:

Oral: 0.5-5 mg 2-3 times/day; usual maximum dose: 30 mg/day; some patients may require 100 mg/day

I.M.:

As **lactate:** 2-5 mg every 4-8 hours as needed

As **decanoate:** Initial: 10-15 times the individual patients' stabilized oral dose, given at 3- to 4-week intervals

Administration

Oral: Administer with food or milk to decrease GI distress; prior to administration, dilute oral concentrate with ≥2 ounces of water or acidic beverage; do not mix oral concentrate with coffee or tea

Parenteral: **Decanoate** product is for I.M. use only, do not give I.V.; although not FDA-approved, haloperidol **lactate** has been administered I.V.

Monitoring Parameters Blood pressure, heart rate, CBC with differential, liver enzymes with long-term use; serum glucose, sodium, magnesium

Patient Information Avoid alcohol; may cause drowsiness and impair ability to perform activities requiring mental alertness or physical coordination; may cause dry mouth. May rarely cause photosensitivity reactions; avoid exposure to sunlight and artificial light sources (sunlamps, tanning booth/bed); use a sunscreen; contact physician if reaction occurs

Nursing Implications Observe for extrapyramidal effects

Dosage Forms

Injection, oil, as **decanoate** (Haldol® Decanoate): 50 mg/mL (1 mL, 5 mL); 100 mg/mL (1 mL, 5 mL) [contains 1.2% benzyl alcohol and sesame oil]

Injection, solution, as **lactate** (Haldol®): 5 mg/mL (1 mL, 10 mL)

Solution, oral **concentrate**, as **lactate:** 2 mg/mL (15 mL, 120 mL)

Tablet: 0.5 mg, 1 mg, 2 mg, 5 mg, 10 mg, 20 mg

References

Serrano AC, "Haloperidol - Its Use in Children," *J Clin Psychiatry*, 1981, 42(4):154-6.

Spencer EK, Kafantaris V, Padron-Gayol MV, et al, "Haloperidol in Schizophrenic Children: Early Findings From a Study in Progress," *Psychopharmacol Bull*, 1992, 28(2):183-6.

* **Haloperidol-LA Omega (Can)** *see* Haloperidol *on page 554*
* **Haloperidol Long Acting (Can)** *see* Haloperidol *on page 554*
* **Halotestin®** *see* Fluoxymesterone *on page 508*
* **Haltran® [OTC]** *see* Ibuprofen *on page 588*
* **HAT Antibody** *see* Daclizumab *on page 334*
* **hCG** *see* Chorionic Gonadotropin *on page 269*
* **HCTZ** *see* Hydrochlorothiazide *on page 569*
* **HDA Toothache® [OTC]** *see* Benzocaine *on page 163*
* **Head & Shoulders® Intensive Treatment [OTC]** *see* Selenium Sulfide *on page 1013*
* **Heavy Mineral Oil** *see* Mineral Oil *on page 767*
* **Helixate® FS** *see* Antihemophilic Factor (Recombinant) *on page 119*
* **Hemocyte™ [OTC]** *see* Iron Supplements (Oral/Enteral) *on page 623*
* **Hemofil® M** *see* Antihemophilic Factor (Human) *on page 116*
* **Hemorid® [OTC]** *see* Hemorrhoidal Preparations *on page 556*

Hemorrhoidal Preparations *(HEM or oyd al prep a RAY shuns)*

U.S. Brand Names Anusol® [OTC]; Anusol® HC-1™ [OTC]; Dickinson's® Witch Hazel™ [OTC]; Hemorid® [OTC]; Medicone® [OTC]; Nupercainal® Hemorrhoidal and Anesthetic Ointment [OTC]; Nupercainal® Hydrocortisone Cream [OTC]; Prax® [OTC]; Preparation H® [OTC]; Preparation H® Hydrocortisone [OTC]; ProcotFoam® NS [OTC]; Tronolane® [OTC]; Tucks® [OTC]

Therapeutic Category Hemorrhoidal Treatment Agent; Topical Skin Product

Generic Available Yes

Use Symptomatic relief of pain and discomfort in external and internal hemorrhoids, proctitis, papillitis, cryptitis, anal fissures, incomplete fistulas and relief of local pain following anorectal surgery

Contraindications Hypersensitivity to any component (see Warnings)

Warnings Some preparations contain sulfites which may cause allergic reactions in susceptible individuals

Adverse Reactions

Dermatologic: Rash

Local: Irritation, burning, itching

Mechanism of Action

Dibucaine, benzocaine, pramoxine: Temporarily relieves pain, itching, and irritation by blocking nerve impulses at the sensory nerve endings in the skin and mucous membranes

Emollient/protectant (glycerin, lanolin, mineral oil, petrolatum, zinc oxide, cocoa butter, shark liver oil): Form a physical barrier and lubricate tissues preventing irritation of the anorectal area and water loss

Pharmacodynamics Onset of action: Topical:

Pramoxine: 3-5 minutes

Dibucaine: <15 minutes

Benzocaine: 1 minute

Usual Dosage

Children and Adults: Topical: Apply ointment as a thin layer to the perianal area and the anal canal 3-6 times/day

Benzocaine-containing preparations: Apply up to 6 times/day

Dibucaine-containing preparations: Apply ointment into the rectum each morning and evening and after each bowel movement; ointment may be applied topically to anal tissues; apply up to 3-4 times/day

Children: No more than 7.5 g in a 24-hour period

Adults: No more than 30 g in a 24-hour period

Pramoxine-containing preparations: Apply up to 5 times/day (2-3 times/day and after bowel movements)

Adults: Rectal: Insert 1 suppository in the morning and at bedtime and after each bowel movement

Administration

Rectal: Foam, ointment, and cream for rectal use are instilled using a rectal applicator. The aerosol should not be inserted into the anus.

Topical: Apply cream or ointment to affected areas and rub in gently. A small amount of foam may be applied to the affected area using a cleansing tissue or pad.

Patient Information If anorectal symptoms do not improve in 7 days, or if bleeding, protrusion or seepage occurs, consult physician; avoid contact of topical preparations to the eyes

Dosage Forms

Cream:

Hemorid®: White petrolatum 30%, mineral oil 20%, pramoxine hydrochloride 1%, and phenylephrine hydrochloride 0.25% (30 g)

Nupercainal® Hydrocortisone Cream: Hydrocortisone 1% (30 g)

Preparation H®: Petrolatum 18%, glycerin 12%, shark liver oil 3%, and phenylephrine hydrochloride 0.25% (26 g, 52 g)

Preparation H® Hydrocortisone: Hydrocortisone 1% (26 g)

Tronolane®: Pramoxine hydrochloride 1% (30 g, 60 g)

Foam (ProcotFoam® NS): Pramoxine hydrochloride 1% (30 g)

Gel (Preparation H®): Witch hazel 50% and phenylephrine hydrochloride 0.25% (26 g, 52 g)

Lotion (Prax®): Pramoxine hydrochloride 1% (120 mL, 240 mL)

Ointment:

Anusol®: Pramoxine hydrochloride 1% and zinc oxide 12.5% (30 g)

Anusol® HC-1™: Hydrocortisone 1% (20 g)

Hemorid®: White petrolatum 82%, light mineral oil 12.5%, pramoxine hydrochloride 1%, and phenylephrine hydrochloride 0.25% (30 g)

Medicone®: Benzocaine 20% (30 g)

Nupercainal® Hemorrhoidal and Anesthetic Ointment: Dibucaine 1% (30 g, 60 g) [contains sodium bisulfite]

Preparation H®: Petrolatum 72%, mineral oil 14%, shark liver oil 3%, and phenylephrine hydrochloride 0.25% (30 g, 60 g)

Pads:

Dickinson's® Witch Hazel™: Witch hazel 50% (20s, 50s)

Preparation H®: Witch hazel 50% (48s)

Tucks®: Witch hazel 50% (12s, 40s, 100s)

Suppositories:

Anusol®: Topical starch 51% and benzyl alcohol (12s, 24s)

Medicone®: Hard fat 89% and phenylephrine hydrochloride 0.25% (18s, 24s)

Preparation H®: Cocoa butter 85%, shark liver oil 3%, and phenylephrine hydrochloride 0.25% (12s, 24s, 48s)

Tronolane®: Pramoxine hydrochloride 1% (10s, 20s)

◆ **Hemril®-HC** see Hydrocortisone on page 573

◆ **Hepalean® (Can)** see Heparin on page 558

◆ **Hepalean® Leo (Can)** see Heparin on page 558

◆ **Hepalean®-LOK (Can)** see Heparin on page 558

Heparin (HEP a rin)

Related Information
Antithrombotic Therapy in Children *on page 1316*
Overdose and Toxicology *on page 1388*

U.S. Brand Names Hep-Lock®

Canadian Brand Names Hepalean®; Hepalean® Leo; Hepalean®-LOK

Synonyms Heparin Lock Flush

Therapeutic Category Anticoagulant

Generic Available Yes

Use Prophylaxis and treatment of thromboembolic disorders

Pregnancy Risk Factor C

Contraindications Hypersensitivity to heparin or any component (see Warnings); severe thrombocytopenia, subacute bacterial endocarditis, suspected intracranial hemorrhage, shock, severe hypotension, uncontrollable bleeding (unless secondary to disseminated intravascular coagulation)

Warnings Some preparations contain sulfites or benzyl alcohol both of which may cause allergic reactions in susceptible individuals; large amounts of benzyl alcohol (≥99 mg/kg/day) have been associated with a potentially fatal toxicity ("gasping syndrome") in neonates; the "gasping syndrome" consists of metabolic acidosis, respiratory distress, gasping respirations, CNS dysfunction (including convulsions, intracranial hemorrhage), hypotension and cardiovascular collapse; avoid use of heparin products containing benzyl alcohol in neonates (use preservative free heparin); *in vitro* and animal studies have shown that benzoate, a metabolite of benzyl alcohol, displaces bilirubin from protein binding sites

Precautions Use with caution as hemorrhage may occur; risk factors for hemorrhage include: I.M. injections; peptic ulcer disease; intermittent I.V. injections (vs continuous I.V. infusion); increased capillary permeability; menstruation; recent surgery or invasive procedures; severe renal, hepatic, or biliary disease; and indwelling catheters

Heparin does not possess fibrinolytic activity and, therefore, cannot lyse established thrombi; discontinue heparin if hemorrhage occurs; severe hemorrhage or overdosage may require protamine

Adverse Reactions
Central nervous system: Fever, headache, chills

Dermatologic: Urticaria, alopecia

Gastrointestinal: Nausea, vomiting

Hematologic: Hemorrhage, thrombocytopenia (may be more common with beef lung heparin vs porcine mucosa heparin; however, if a patient receiving beef lung heparin experiences severe thrombocytopenia it is **not** recommended to switch to porcine mucosa heparin because a similar reaction may occur)

Hepatic: Elevated liver enzymes

Local: Irritation, ulceration, cutaneous necrosis has been rarely reported with deep S.C. injections

Neuromuscular & skeletal: Osteoporosis (with long-term use)

Drug Interactions Thrombolytic agents (urokinase, streptokinase, alteplase) and drugs which affect platelet function (eg, aspirin, NSAIDs, dipyridamole) may potentiate the risk of hemorrhage; digoxin, tetracycline, nicotine, antihistamines, and I.V. nitroglycerin may decrease heparin's anticoagulant effect.

Mechanism of Action Potentiates the action of antithrombin III and thereby inactivates thrombin (as well as activated coagulation factors IX, X, XI, XII, and plasmin) and prevents the conversion of fibrinogen to fibrin; heparin also stimulates release of lipoprotein lipase (lipoprotein lipase hydrolyzes triglycerides to glycerol and free fatty acids)

Pharmacodynamics Anticoagulation effect: Onset of action:
S.C.: 20-60 minutes
I.V.: Immediate

Pharmacokinetics
Absorption: S.C., I.M.: Erratic

Distribution: Does not cross the placenta; does not appear in breast milk

Metabolism: Believed to be partially metabolized in the reticuloendothelial system

Half-life: Mean: 90 minutes (range: 1-2 hours); affected by obesity, renal function, hepatic function, malignancy, presence of pulmonary embolism, and infections

Elimination: Renal; small amount excreted unchanged in urine

Usual Dosage
Line flushing: When using daily flushes of heparin to maintain patency of single and double lumen central catheters, 10 units/mL is commonly used for younger infants (eg, <10 kg) while 100 units/mL is used for older infants, children, and adults. Capped polyvinyl chloride catheters and peripheral heparin locks require flushing more frequently (eg, every 6-8 hours). Volume of heparin flush is usually similar to

volume of catheter (or slightly greater) or may be standardized according to specific hospital's policy (eg, 2-5 mL/flush). Dose of heparin flush used should not approach therapeutic unit per kg dose. Additional flushes should be given when stagnant blood is observed in catheter, after catheter is used for drug or blood administration, and after blood withdrawal from catheter.

TPN: Heparin 1 unit/mL (final concentration) may be added to TPN solutions, both central and peripheral. (Addition of heparin to peripheral TPN has been shown to increase duration of line patency.) The final concentration of heparin used for TPN solutions may need to be decreased to 0.5 units/mL in small infants receiving larger TPN volumes in order to avoid approaching therapeutic amounts.

Arterial lines: Heparinize with a usual final concentration of 1 unit/mL; range: 0.5-2 units/mL; in order to avoid large total doses and systemic effects, use 0.5 unit/mL in low birth weight/premature newborns and in other patients receiving multiple lines containing heparin

Prophylaxis for cardiac catheterization via an artery: Newborns and Children: I.V.: Bolus: 100-150 units/kg (see Monagle, 2001)

Systemic heparinization:

Neonates and Infants <1 year: I.V. infusion: Initial loading dose: 75 units/kg given over 10 minutes; then initial maintenance dose: 28 units/kg/hour; adjust dose to maintain APTT of 60-85 seconds (assuming this reflects an antifactor Xa level of 0.3-0.7); see table.

Children >1 year:

Intermittent I.V.: Initial: 50-100 units/kg, then 50-100 units/kg every 4 hours (**Note:** Continuous I.V. infusion is preferred):

I.V. infusion: Initial loading dose: 75 units/kg given over 10 minutes, then initial maintenance dose: 20 units/kg/hour; adjust dose to maintain APTT of 60-85 seconds (assuming this reflects an antifactor Xa level of 0.3-0.7); see table.

PEDIATRIC PROTOCOL FOR SYSTEMIC HEPARIN ADJUSTMENT

To be used after initial loading dose and maintenance I.V. infusion dose (see Usual Dosage listed above) to maintain APTT of 60-85 seconds (assuming this reflects antifactor Xa level of 0.3-0.7)

Obtain blood for APTT 4 hours after heparin loading dose and 4 hours after every infusion rate change

Obtain daily CBC and APTT after APTT is therapeutic

APTT (seconds)	Dosage Adjustment	Time to Repeat APTT
<50	Give 50 units/kg bolus and increase infusion rate by 10%	4 h after rate change
50-59	Increase infusion rate by 10%	4 h after rate change
60-85	Keep rate the same	Next day
86-95	Decrease infusion rate by 10%	4 h after rate change
96-120	Hold infusion for 30 minutes and decrease infusion rate by 10%	4 h after rate change
>120	Hold infusion for 60 minutes and decrease infusion rate by 15%	4 h after rate change

Modified from Monagle P, Michelson AD, Bovill E, et al, "Antithrombotic Therapy in Children," *Chest*, 2001, 119:344S-70S.

Adults:

Prophylaxis (low dose heparin): S.C.: 5000 units every 8-12 hours

Intermittent I.V.: Initial: 10,000 units, then 50-70 units/kg (5000-10,000 units) every 4-6 hours

I.V. infusion: Initial loading dose: 80 units/kg; initial maintenance dose: 18 units/kg/hour with dose adjusted according to APTT; usual range: 10-30 units/kg/hour

Adults: *Chest* 2001 Recommendations (see Hirsh, 2001):

Prophylaxis of DVT and PE: S.C.: 5000 units every 8 or 12 hours or adjusted low-dose heparin

Treatment of DVT: Initial loading dose: I.V. bolus: 5000 units, then initial maintenance dose: I.V. infusion: 32,000 units/day (1333 units/hour); adjust dose to maintain therapeutic APTT; recommendations also list S.C. 35,000-40,000 units/day (**Note:** S.C. dose which was divided into 2 daily doses, is no longer used clinically)

Unstable angina or acute MI without thrombolytic therapy: Initial loading dose: I.V. bolus: 5000 units, then initial maintenance dose: I.V. infusion: 32,000 units/day (1333 units/hour); adjust dose to maintain therapeutic APTT

(Continued)

Heparin (Continued)

Acute MI after thrombolytic therapy (role of heparin unproven): Initial loading dose: I.V. bolus: 5000 units, then initial maintenance dose: I.V. infusion: 24,000 units/day (1000 units/hour); adjust dose to maintain therapeutic APTT

Administration Parenteral: Continuous I.V. infusion is preferred vs I.V. intermittent injections; heparin lock flush solutions are intended only to maintain patency of I.V. devices and are **not** for systemic anticoagulation

Monitoring Parameters Platelet counts, signs of bleeding, hemoglobin, hematocrit, APTT; for full-dose heparin (ie, nonlow dose), the dose should be titrated according to APTT (see table). For intermittent I.V. injections, APTT is measured 3.5-4 hours after I.V. injection.

Reference Range Treatment of venous thrombotic disease: Recommended APTT should reflect a heparin level by protamine titration of 0.2-0.4 units/mL or an antifactor Xa level of 0.3-0.7 units/mL; this usually reflects an APTT of 60-85 seconds or a ratio (patient/control APTT) of 1.5-2.5; a lower therapeutic range (corresponding to antifactor Xa level of 0.14-0.34 units/mL) is recommended for patients with acute MI who received thrombolytic therapy

Test Interactions ↑ thyroxine (S) (competitive protein binding methods)

Patient Information Limit alcohol

Nursing Implications Do not administer I.M. due to pain, irritation, and hematoma formation

Additional Information To reverse the effects of heparin, use protamine (see Protamine *on page 955* for specifics); heparin is available from beef lung and from porcine intestinal mucosa sources

Duration of heparin therapy (pediatric):

DVT: At least 5 days

Extensive DVT or pulmonary embolism (PE): 7-10 days

Note: Oral anticoagulation can be started on day 1 of heparin, except for extensive DVT or PE, when it should be delayed; oral anticoagulation should be overlapped with heparin for 5 days

Dosage Forms

Infusion, as sodium [premixed in D$_5$W; porcine intestinal mucosa source]:
10,000 units [100 units/mL] (100 mL) [contains sodium bisulfite]
12,500 units [50 units/mL] (250 mL) [contains sodium bisulfite]
20,000 units [40 units/mL] (500 mL) [contains sodium bisulfite]
25,000 units [100 units/mL] (250 mL); [50 units/mL] (500 mL) [contains sodium bisulfite]

Infusion, as sodium [premixed in NaCl 0.9%; porcine intestinal mucosa source; preservative free]: 1000 units [2 unit/mL] (500 mL); 2000 units [2 units/mL] (1000 mL)

Infusion, as sodium [premixed in NaCl 0.45%]:
12,500 units [50 units/mL] (250 mL)
25,000 units [100 units/mL] (250 mL); [50 units/mL] (500 mL)

Injection, solution, as sodium [lock flush preparation; porcine intestinal mucosa source; multiple dose vial]: 10 units/mL (1 mL, 10 mL, 30 mL); 100 units/mL (1 mL, 5 mL) [contains parabens]

Injection, solution, as sodium [lock flush preparation; porcine intestinal mucosa source; multiple dose vial]: 10 units/mL (10 mL, 30 mL); 100 units/mL (10 mL, 30 mL) [contains benzyl alcohol]

Injection, solution, as sodium [lock flush preparation; porcine intestinal mucosa source; preservative free; prefilled syringe]: 10 units/mL (1 mL, 2 mL, 3 mL, 5 mL, 10 mL); 100 units/mL (1 mL, 2 mL, 3 mL, 5 mL, 10 mL)

Injection, solution, as sodium [lock flush preparation; porcine intestinal mucosa source; prefilled syringe]: 10 units/mL (1 mL, 2 mL, 2.5 mL, 3 mL, 5 mL); 100 units/mL (1 mL, 2 mL, 2.5 mL, 3 mL, 5 mL) [contains benzyl alcohol]

Injection, solution, as sodium [beef lung source; multiple dose vial]: 1000 units/mL (10 mL, 30 mL); 5000 units/mL (10 mL); 10,000 units/mL (1 mL, 4 mL) [contains benzyl alcohol]

Injection, solution, as sodium [porcine intestinal mucosa source; preservative free; vial]: 1000 units/mL (2 mL); 2000 units/mL (5 mL, 10 mL); 2500 units/mL (5 mL, 10 mL)

Injection, solution, as sodium [porcine intestinal mucosa source; multiple dose vial]: 10,000 units/mL (5 mL) [contains benzyl alcohol]

Injection, solution, as sodium [porcine intestinal mucosa source; preservative free; prefilled syringe]: 10,000 units/mL (0.25 mL, 0.5 mL, 0.75 mL, 1 mL)

Injection, solution, as sodium [porcine intestinal mucosa source; prefilled syringe]: 1000 units/mL (1 mL); 2500 units/mL (1 mL); 5000 units/mL (0.5 mL, 1 mL); 7500 units/mL (1 mL); 10,000 units/mL (1 mL); 20,000 units/mL (1 mL) [contains benzyl alcohol]

References
Andrew M, Marzinotto V, Massicotte P, et al, "Heparin Therapy in Pediatric Patients: A Prospective Cohort Study," *Pediatr Res*, 1994, 35(1):78-83.

Hirsh J, Warkentin TE, Shaughnessy SG, et al, "Heparin and Low-Molecular Weight-Heparin: Mechanisms of Action, Pharmacokinetics, Dosing, Monitoring, Efficacy and Safety," *Chest*, 2001, 119:64S-94S.

Monagle P, Michelson AD, Bovill E, et al, "Antithrombotic Therapy in Children," *Chest*, 2001, 119:344S-70S.

♦ **Heparin Lock Flush** *see* Heparin *on page 558*

♦ **Hepatitis A Vaccine** *see page 1333*

♦ **Hepatitis B Immune Globulin** *see page 1333*

♦ **Hepatitis B Vaccine** *see page 1333*

♦ **Hep-Lock®** *see* Heparin *on page 558*

♦ **Heptovir® (Can)** *See* Lamivudine *on page 650*

♦ **HES** *see* Hetastarch *on page 561*

♦ **Hespan®** *see* Hetastarch *on page 561*

Hetastarch (HET a starch)

U.S. Brand Names Hespan®; Hextend®

Synonyms HES; Hydroxyethyl Starch

Therapeutic Category Plasma Volume Expander

Generic Available Yes

Use Blood volume expander used in treatment of shock or impending shock when blood or blood products are not available; does not have oxygen-carrying capacity and is not a substitute for blood or plasma

Pregnancy Risk Factor C

Contraindications Hypersensitivity to hetastarch or any component; severe bleeding disorders, renal failure with oliguria or anuria, or severe CHF; management of cerebral vasospasm associated with subarachnoid hemorrhage or for conditions other than leukapheresis which necessitate repeated use of the drug over several days; per manufacturer, Hextend® is contraindicated in the treatment of lactic acidosis and in leukapheresis

Warnings Anaphylactoid reactions have occurred; use with caution in patients with thrombocytopenia (may interfere with platelet function); large volume may cause drops in hemoglobin concentrations; use with caution in patients at risk from overexpansion of blood volume, including the very young or aged patients, those with CHF or pulmonary edema; large volumes (>1500 mL) may interfere with platelet function and prolong PT and PTT times; use with caution in patients with a history of liver disease

Precautions Use with caution in patients allergic to corn (may have cross allergy to hetastarch). Note electrolyte content of Hextend® including calcium, lactate, and potassium (see Additional Information); use with caution in situations where electrolyte and/or acid-base disturbances may be exacerbated (renal impairment, respiratory alkalosis).

Adverse Reactions
Cardiovascular: Heart failure, circulatory overload, peripheral edema
Central nervous system: Headache, fever, chills, intracranial bleeding
Dermatologic: Urticaria, pruritus, rash
Endocrine & metabolic: Parotid gland enlargement, hyperchloremic metabolic acidosis, hypernatremia
Gastrointestinal: Vomiting, elevated amylase levels
Hematologic: Thrombocytopenia, transient prolongation of PT, PTT, clotting time, and bleeding time, anemia, DIC (rare), hemolysis (rare)
Hepatic: Elevated indirect bilirubin
Neuromuscular & skeletal: Myalgia
Ocular: Periorbital edema
Respiratory: Wheezing
Miscellaneous: Anaphylactoid reactions, flu-like symptoms

Stability Store at room temperature; do not freeze; do not use if crystalline precipitate forms or is turbid deep brown

Mechanism of Action Hetastarch. a synthetic polymer, produces plasma volume expansion by virtue of its highly colloidal starch structure

Pharmacodynamics
Onset of volume expansion: I.V.: Within 30 minutes
Duration: 24-36 hours

Pharmacokinetics
Metabolism: Molecules >50,000 daltons require enzymatic degradation by the reticuloendothelial system or amylases in the blood prior to urinary and fecal excretion
(Continued)

Hetastarch *(Continued)*

Elimination: Smaller molecular weight molecules are readily excreted in urine; approximately 40% of dose excreted in first 24 hours in patients with normal renal function

Usual Dosage I.V. infusion:

Children: 10 mL/kg/dose; the total daily dose should not exceed 20 mL/kg

Adults: 500-1000 mL (30-60 g) per dose; the total daily dose should not exceed 1.2 g/kg or 90 g (1500 mL)

Dosing adjustment in renal impairment: Cl_{cr} <10 mL/minute: Initial dose is the same but subsequent doses should be reduced by 20% to 50% of normal

Administration Parenteral: I.V.: Maximum rate of infusion: 1.2 g/kg/hour (20 mL/kg/hour)

Monitoring Parameters Volume expansion: capillary refill time, CVP, RAP, MAP, urine output, heart rate, if pulmonary artery catheter in place, monitor PWCP, SVR, and PVR; hemoglobin, hematocrit; for leukapheresis, monitor CBC, total leukocyte and platelet counts, leukocyte differential count, hemoglobin, hematocrit, prothrombin time, and partial thromboplastin time

Additional Information Hetastarch is a synthetic polymer derived from a waxy starch composed of amylopectin, average molecular weight = 450,000; each liter of Hespan® provides 154 mEq sodium chloride; each liter of Hextend® contains the following electrolytes: Sodium 143 mEq, chloride 124 mEq, lactate 28 mEq, calcium 5 mEq, magnesium 0.9 mEq, potassium 3 mEq, and dextrose 0.99 g

Dosage Forms

Infusion, solution [premixed in lactated electrolyte injection] (Hextend®): 6% (500 mL, 1000 mL) [contains calcium, chloride, magnesium, potassium, and sodium (see Additional Information)]

Infusion, solution [premixed in sodium chloride 0.9%] (Hespan®): 6% (500 mL)

References

Brutocao D, Bratton SL, Thomas JR, et al, "Comparison of Hetastarch With Albumin for Postoperative Volume Expansion in Children After Cardiopulmonary Bypass," *J Cardiothoracic Vasc Anesth,* 1996, 10(3):348-51.

♦ **Hexachlorocyclohexane** *see Lindane* *on page 677*

Hexachlorophene (heks a KLOR oh feen)

U.S. Brand Names pHisoHex®

Therapeutic Category Antibacterial, Topical; Soap

Generic Available No

Use Surgical scrub and as a bacteriostatic skin cleanser; to control an outbreak of gram-positive staphylococcal infection when other infection control procedures have been unsuccessful

Pregnancy Risk Factor C

Contraindications Hypersensitivity to halogenated phenol derivatives or hexachlorophene; use in premature infants; use on burned or denuded skin; use with an occlusive dressing; application to mucous membranes

Warnings Do not use for bathing infants; do not apply to mucous membranes; premature and low birth weight infants are particularly susceptible to hexachlorophene topical absorption; irritability, generalized clonic muscular contractions, decerebrate rigidity, and brain lesions in the white matter have occurred in infants following topical use of 6% hexachlorophene; exposure of preterm infants or patients with extensive burns has been associated with apnea, convulsions, agitation, and coma

Adverse Reactions

Central nervous system: CNS injury, seizures, irritability

Dermatologic: Dermatitis, erythema, dry skin, photosensitivity

Drug Interactions Polysorbate 80, nonionic detergents with concentration >8% may decrease antibacterial activity of hexachlorophene

Stability Store in nonmetallic container (incompatible with many metals); protect from light

Mechanism of Action Bacteriostatic polychlorinated biphenol which inhibits membrane-bound enzymes and disrupts the cell membrane

Pharmacokinetics

Absorption: Percutaneously through inflamed, excoriated and intact skin

Distribution: Crosses the placenta

Half-life, infants: 6.1-44.2 hours

Usual Dosage Children and Adults: Topical: Apply 5 mL cleanser and water to area to be cleansed; lather and rinse thoroughly under running water; for use as a surgical scrub, a second application of 5 mL cleanser should be made and the hands and forearms scrubbed for an additional 3 minutes, rinsed thoroughly with running water and dried

Administration Topical: For external use only; rinse thoroughly after each use

Patient Information Avoid prolonged contact with skin. May cause photosensitivity reactions (eg, exposure to sunlight may cause severe sunburn, skin rash, redness, or itching); avoid exposure to sunlight and artificial light sources (sunlamps, tanning booth/bed); wear protective clothing, wide-brimmed hats, sunglasses, and lip sunscreen (SPF ≥15); use a sunscreen [broad-spectrum sunscreen or physical sunscreen (preferred) or sunblock with SPF ≥15]; contact physician if reaction occurs.

Dosage Forms Liquid, topical (pHisoHex®): 3% (150 mL, 500 mL, 3840 mL)

References
Lester RS, "Topical Formulary for the Pediatrician," *Pediatr Clin North Am*, 1983, 30(4):749-65.

♦ **Hexamethylenetetramine** *see* Methenamine *on page 733*

♦ **Hexit™ (Can)** *see* Lindane *on page 677*

♦ **Hextend®** *see* Hetastarch *on page 561*

♦ **Hibiclens® [OTC]** *see* Chlorhexidine Gluconate *on page 257*

♦ **Hibidil® 1:2000 (Can)** *see* Chlorhexidine Gluconate *on page 257*

♦ **Hiprex®** *see* Methenamine *on page 733*

♦ **Hi-Vegi-Lip® [OTC]** *see* Pancreatin *on page 855*

♦ **Hivid®** *see* Zalcitabine *on page 1161*

♦ **HMS Liquifilm®** *see* Medrysone *on page 713*

♦ **HN₂** *see* Mechlorethamine *on page 708*

♦ **Hold® DM [OTC]** *see* Dextromethorphan *on page 365*

Homatropine *(hoe MA troe peen)*

U.S. Brand Names Isopto® Homatropine

Therapeutic Category Anticholinergic Agent, Ophthalmic; Ophthalmic Agent, Mydriatic

Generic Available No

Use Producing cycloplegia and mydriasis for refraction; treatment of acute inflammatory conditions of the uveal tract

Pregnancy Risk Factor C

Contraindications Hypersensitivity to homatropine or any component; narrow-angle glaucoma, acute hemorrhage

Precautions Use with caution in patients with hypertension, cardiac disease, increased intraocular pressure, obstructive uropathy, paralytic ileus, or ulcerative colitis

Adverse Reactions
Cardiovascular: Vascular congestion, edema
Central nervous system: Drowsiness
Dermatologic: Eczematoid dermatitis
Ocular: Follicular conjunctivitis, blurred vision, elevated intraocular pressure, stinging, exudate

Mechanism of Action Blocks response of iris sphincter muscle and the accommodative muscle of the ciliary body to cholinergic stimulation resulting in dilation and loss of accommodation

Pharmacodynamics Ophthalmic:
Onset of accommodation and pupil action:
Maximum mydriatic effect: Within 10-30 minutes
Maximum cycloplegic effect: Within 30-90 minutes
Duration:
Mydriasis: Persists for 6 hours to 4 days
Cycloplegia: 10-48 hours

Usual Dosage Ophthalmic:
Children:
Mydriasis and cycloplegia for refraction: Instill 1 drop of 2% solution immediately before the procedure; repeat at 10-minute intervals as needed
Uveitis: Instill 1 drop of 2% solution 2-3 times/day
Adults:
Mydriasis and cycloplegia for refraction: Instill 1-2 drops of 2% solution or 1 drop of 5% solution before the procedure; repeat at 5- to 10-minute intervals as needed
Uveitis: Instill 1-2 drops of either 2% or 5% solution 2-3 times/day up to every 3-4 hours as needed

Administration Ophthalmic: Finger pressure should be applied to lacrimal sac for 1-2 minutes after instillation to decrease risk of absorption and systemic effects

Dosage Forms Solution, ophthalmic, as hydrobromide: 2% (5 mL); 5% (5 mL, 15 mL)

♦ **Horse Antihuman Thymocyte Gamma Globulin** *see* Antithymocyte Globulin (Equine) *on page 123*

♦ **H.P. Acthar® Gel** *see* Corticotropin *on page 307*

- **HPMPC** *see* Cidofovir *on page 270*
- **Humalog®** *see* Insulin Preparations *on page 609*
- **Humalog® Mix 25™ (Can)** *see* Insulin Preparations *on page 609*
- **Humalog® Mix 75/25®** *see* Insulin Preparations *on page 609*

Human Growth Hormone (HYU man grothe HOR mone)

U.S. Brand Names Genotropin®; Genotropin Miniquick®; Humatrope®; Norditropin®; Nutropin®; Nutropin® AQ; Nutropin Depot®; Protropin®; Saizen®; Serostim®

Canadian Brand Names Nutropine®

Synonyms Growth Hormone; Somatrem; Somatropin

Therapeutic Category Growth Hormone

Generic Available No

Use Long-term treatment of growth failure in children as a result of lack or inadequate endogenous growth hormone secretion, Prader-Willi syndrome, birth at small for gestational age (SGA) with failure to catch-up growth by 2 years of age; chronic renal insufficiency (up until the time of renal transplantation); short stature associated with Turner syndrome (in patients whose epiphyses are not closed); growth hormone deficiency as a result of pituitary disease, hypothalamic disease, surgery, radiation, or trauma; Serostim®: Treatment of AIDS-related wasting or cachexia

Pregnancy Risk Factor C; Serostim® (only): B

Contraindications Hypersensitivity to human growth hormone or any component (see Warnings); do not use for growth promotion in pediatric patients with closed epiphyses; evidence of active malignancy; progression of any underlying intracranial lesion or actively growing intracranial tumor; patients with acute critical illness due to complications following open heart or abdominal surgery, multiple accidental trauma, or acute respiratory failure

Warnings Diluents for Nutropin®, Protropin®, and Saizen® contain benzyl alcohol which may cause allergic reactions in susceptible individuals; large amounts of benzyl alcohol (≥99 mg/kg/day) have been associated with a potentially fatal toxicity ("gasping syndrome") in neonates; the "gasping syndrome" consists of metabolic acidosis, respiratory distress, gasping respirations, CNS dysfunction (including convulsions, intracranial hemorrhage), hypotension and cardiovascular collapse; *in vitro* and animal studies have shown that benzoate, a metabolite of benzyl alcohol, displaces bilirubin from protein-binding sites; avoid use of benzyl alcohol containing diluents in neonates. Intracranial hypertension with papilledema, visual changes, headache, nausea, and/or vomiting has been reported; this has occurred during the first 8 weeks of therapy; all reported cases were reversible upon discontinuation of therapy; baseline and regular fundoscopic exams are recommended for assistance in recognizing this potential adverse effect.

Precautions Use with caution in patients with diabetes or family history of diabetes; insulin dosage may require adjustment when growth hormone therapy is instituted; patients with hypopituitarism may develop hypothyroidism during growth hormone therapy; children may develop slipped capital epiphyses during therapy; progression of scoliosis may occur in patients with a history of scoliosis

Adverse Reactions
Cardiovascular: Mild transient edema
Central nervous system: Headache, intracranial hypertension
Dermatologic: Increased growth of pre-existing nevi; local lipoatrophy or lipodystrophy (S.C. administration)
Endocrine & metabolic: Reversible hypothyroidism (reported in pituitary-derived growth hormone), mild hyperglycemia; gynecomastia (rare)
Gastrointestinal: Pancreatitis (rare)
Hematologic: Small risk for developing leukemia
Local: Pain at injection site
Neuromuscular & skeletal: Carpal tunnel syndrome (rare), pain in hip/knee
Renal: Glucosuria

Drug Interactions Corticosteroids may inhibit growth hormone activity

Stability For long term storage, refrigerate all products, do not freeze; once reconstituted with diluents containing preservatives and refrigerated, Humotrope® and Protropin® are stable for 14 days, Genotropin® is stable for 21 days, and Humotrope® cartridges are stable for 28 days; Nutropin® AQ (aqueous form) is stable for 28 days after initial entry; Nutropin Depot® must be used immediately after reconstitution. Genotropin MiniQuick® is stable prior to reconstitution for up to 3 months at room temperature. If diluents without preservatives are used, stability is 24 hours refrigerated. After a Norditropen® cartridge has been inserted into the NordiPen® injector, it is stable (in the pen) refrigerated for 4 weeks.

Mechanism of Action Somatropin and somatrem are purified polypeptide hormones of recombinant DNA origin; somatropin contains the identical sequence of amino acids found in human growth hormone while somatrem's amino acid sequence is identical plus an additional amino acid, methionine; human growth hormone stimulates growth of linear bone, skeletal muscle, and organs; stimulates erythropoietin which increases red blood cell mass; exerts both insulin-like and diabetogenic effects

Pharmacokinetics Somatrem and somatropin have equivalent pharmacokinetic profiles

Absorption: I.M.: Well absorbed

Distribution: V_d: 50 mL/kg

Metabolism: ~90% of dose metabolized in the liver and kidney cells

Bioavailability: S.C.: 81 ± 20%

Half-life: S.C.: 2.3 ± 0.42 hours

Elimination: 0.1% of dose excreted in urine unchanged

Usual Dosage

Children: I.M., S.C. (preferred route); not for I.V. injection:

Growth hormone inadequacy: Children:

Somatrem (Protropin®): 0.3 mg/kg (0.9 international units/kg) **weekly** divided into daily doses

Somatropin:

Genotropin®: 0.16-0.24 mg/kg **weekly** divided into daily doses (6-7 doses)

Humatrope®: 0.18 mg/kg (0.54 international units/kg) **weekly** divided into equal doses given either on alternate days or 6 times per week; maximum **weekly** dosage: 0.3 mg/kg (0.9 international units/kg)

Norditropin®: 0.024-0.034 mg/kg/dose (0.07-0.1 international units/kg/dose) 6-7 times per week

Nutropin®: 0.3 mg/kg (0.9 international units/kg) **weekly** divided into daily doses; in pubertal patients, dosage may be increased to 0.7 mg/kg (2.1 international units/kg) **weekly** divided into daily doses

Saizen®: 0.06 mg/kg (0.18 international units/kg) 3 times per week

Nutropin® Depot™: S.C. only:

Once-monthly injection: 1.5 mg/kg body weight administered on the same day of each month; patients >15 kg will require more than one injection per dose

Twice-monthly injection: 0.75 mg/kg body weight administered twice each month on the same days of each month (eg, days 1 and 15 of each month); patients >30 kg will require more than one injection per dose; twice monthly dosing is recommended in patients >45 kg

Note: Human growth hormone therapy should be individualized; discontinue therapy when the patient has reached satisfactory adult height, when epiphyses have fused, or when the patient ceases to respond. Growth of ≥5 cm/year is expected, if growth rate does not exceed 2.5 cm in a 6-month period, double the dose for the next 6 months, if there is still no satisfactory response, discontinue therapy

Chronic renal insufficiency: Nutropin®: 0.35 mg/kg (approximately 1.05 international units/kg) **weekly**; may be continued until time of transplantation

Prader-Willi syndrome: Genotropin®: 0.24 mg/kg **weekly** divided daily into 6-7 doses per week

Children SGA at birth: Genotropin®: 0.48 mg/kg **weekly** divided daily into 6-7 doses per week

Turner syndrome: Humatrope®: Weekly dosage ≤0.375 mg/kg (1.125 international units/kg) divided into equal doses daily or on 3 alternate days

Adults: Growth hormone deficiency: 0.006 mg/kg/day (0.018 international units/kg/day) once daily; may be increased to a maximum of 0.025 mg/kg/day (0.075 international units/kg) in patients <35 years of age and to a maximum of 0.0125 mg/kg/day (0.0375 international units/kg/day) in patients >35 years of age

AIDS-related wasting or cachexia: Serostim®:

Children (limited information): 0.04-0.07 mg/kg/day for 4 weeks

Adults: Administered once daily at bedtime:

<35 kg: 0.1 mg/kg

35-44 kg: 4 mg

45-55 kg: 5 mg

>55 kg: 6 mg

Administration Parenteral: Administer S.C. (preferred route) or I.M.; not for I.V. injection; do not shake; rotate injection site; administer into the thigh, buttock, or abdomen; limit S.C. injection volume to 1 mL per site

Somatrem: Protropin®: Reconstitute each 5 mg vial with 1-5 mL and each 10 mg vial with 1-10 mL bacteriostatic SWI containing benzyl alcohol; when using in neonates, reconstitute with preservative free SWI

Somatropin:

Genotropin® cartridges: Reconstitute with provided diluent resulting in the following concentrations: 1.5 mg cartridge - 1.3 mg/mL (4 international units/mL), 5.8 mg

(Continued)

Human Growth Hormone *(Continued)*

cartridge - 5 mg/mL (15 international units/mL), and 13.8 mg cartridge - 12 mg/mL (36 international units/mL)

Nutropin®: Reconstitute each 5 mg vial with 1.5-5 mL diluent; when using in neonates, reconstitute with preservative free SWI

Norditropin® Cartridges: Must be used with the NordiPen® injection pen (each cartridge has a color-coded injection pen which is graduated to deliver the appropriate dose); do not interchange

Nutropin® Depot™: Reconstitute vials with provided diluent only, resulting in 19 mg/mL concentration; swirl vigorously for 2 minutes until all the powder is fully dispersed; withdraw measured dose, change to a new needle, and administer immediately to avoid settling of the suspension in the syringe; inject S.C. at a continuous rate over no more than 5 seconds

Note: When treating chronic renal insufficiency patients, growth hormone should be administered as follows: in hemodialysis patients, administer injection at night just prior to sleeping and at least 3-4 hours after dialysis; in chronic cycling peritoneal dialysis patients, administer injection in the morning after dialysis; in chronic ambulatory peritoneal dialysis patients administer injection in the evening at the time of the overnight exchange.

Monitoring Parameters Growth curve, periodic thyroid function tests, bone age (annually), periodical urine testing for glucose, somatomedin C levels; fundoscopic exams (see Warnings); progression of scoliosis and clinical evidence of slipped capital femoral epiphysis such as a limp or hip or knee pain

Patient Information Report the development of a severe headache, acute visual changes, a limp or complaints of hip or knee pain to your physician

Additional Information S.C. administration can cause local lipoatrophy or lipodystrophy and may enhance the development of neutralizing antibodies

Dosage Forms

Injection, powder for reconstitution [rDNA origin]:

Somatrem: Protropin®: 5 mg [~15 international units]; 10 mg [~30 international units] [diluent contains benzyl alcohol]

Somatropin:

Genotropin® [preservative free]: 1.5 mg [4 international units/mL] [delivers 1.3 mg/mL]

Genotropin® [with preservative]: 5.8 mg [15 international units/mL] [delivers 5 mg/mL]; 13.8 mg [36 international units/mL] [delivers 12 mg/mL]

Genotropin Miniquick® [preservative free]: 0.2 mg, 0.4 mg, 0.6 mg, 0.8 mg, 1 mg, 1.2 mg, 1.4 mg, 1.6 mg, 1.8 mg, 2 mg [following reconstitution, each strength delivers 0.25 mL]

Humatrope®: 5 mg [~15 international units], 6 mg [18 international units], 12 mg [36 international units], 24 mg [72 international units]

Norditropin®: 4 mg [~12 international units; 8 mg [~24 international units] [diluent contains benzyl alcohol] [DSC]

Nutropin®: 5 mg [~15 international units]; 10 mg [~30 international units] [diluent contains benzyl alcohol]

Nutropin Depot® [preservative free]: 13.5 mg, 18 mg, 22.5 mg

Saizen®: 5 mg [~15 international units]; 8.8 mg [~26.4 international units] [diluent contains benzyl alcohol]

Serostim®: 4 mg [12 international units]; 5 mg [15 international units]; 6 mg [18 international units]

Injection, solution [rDNA origin]: Somatropin:

Norditropin® Cartridges: 5 mg/1.5 mL (1.5 mL); 10 mg/1.5 mL (1.5 mL); 15 mg/1.5 mL (1.5 mL)

Nutropin AQ®: 5 mg/mL [~30 international units/2 mL] (2 mL)

References

Howrie DL, "Growth Hormone for the Treatment of Growth Failure in Children," *Clin Pharm*, 1987, 6(4):283-91.

+ **Humulin® 70/30** *see* Insulin Preparations *on page 609*
+ **Humulin® L** *see* Insulin Preparations *on page 609*
+ **Humulin® N** *see* Insulin Preparations *on page 609*
+ **Humulin® R** *see* Insulin Preparations *on page 609*
+ **Humulin® R (Concentrated) U-500** *see* Insulin Preparations *on page 609*
+ **Humulin® U** *see* Insulin Preparations *on page 609*
+ **Hurricaine®** *see* Benzocaine *on page 163*

Hyaluronidase [DSC] (hye al yoor ON i dase)
Related Information
Extravasation Treatment *on page 1240*
U.S. Brand Names Wydase® [DSC]
Therapeutic Category Antidote, Extravasation
Generic Available No
Use Increase the dispersion and absorption of other drugs; increase rate of absorption of parenteral fluids given by hypodermoclysis; management of I.V. extravasations
Pregnancy Risk Factor C
Contraindications Hypersensitivity to hyaluronidase or any component; do not inject in or around infected, inflamed, or cancerous areas
Warnings Drug infiltrates in which hyaluronidase is **not** the extravasation management of choice include dopamine and alpha agonists
Precautions Hypersensitivity reactions may occur; a preliminary intradermal skin test should be performed utilizing 0.02 mL of a 150 units/mL solution
Adverse Reactions
Cardiovascular: Tachycardia, hypotension
Central nervous system: Dizziness, chills
Dermatologic: Urticaria, erythema
Gastrointestinal: Nausea, vomiting
Drug Interactions Salicylates, cortisone, ACTH, estrogens, antihistamines (decrease effectiveness of hyaluronidase)
Stability Reconstituted hyaluronidase solution prepared from a 150 unit vial of lyophilized powder for injection is stable for 24 hours; refrigerate the stabilized hyaluronidase solution for injection
Mechanism of Action Modifies the permeability of connective tissue through hydrolysis of hyaluronic acid, one of the chief ingredients of tissue cement which offers resistance to diffusion of liquids through tissues; hyaluronidase increases both the distribution and absorption of locally injected substances
Pharmacodynamics
Onset of action by the S.C. or intradermal routes for the treatment of extravasation: Immediate
Duration: 24-48 hours
Usual Dosage
Infants and Children: Management of I.V. extravasation: S.C., intradermal: Reconstitute the 150 unit vial of lyophilized powder with 1 mL NS; take 0.1 mL of this solution and dilute with 0.9 mL NS to yield 15 units/mL; using a 25- or 26-gauge needle, five 0.2 mL injections are made subcutaneously or intradermally into the extravasation site at the leading edge, changing the needle after each injection; **Note:** Some centers utilize a 150 units/mL hyaluronidase solution and, without further dilution, administer 0.2 mL injections subcutaneously or intradermally into the extravasation site at the leading edge
Adults: Absorption and dispersion of drugs: I.M., S.C.: 150 units is added to the vehicle containing the drug
Hypodermoclysis: S.C.: 15 units is added to each 100 mL of I.V. fluid to be administered
Premature Infants and Neonates: Volume of a single clysis should not exceed 25 mL/kg and the rate of administration should not exceed 2 mL/minute
Children <3 years: Volume of a single clysis should not exceed 200 mL
Children ≥3 years and Adults: Rate and volume of a single clysis should not exceed those used for infusion of I.V. fluids
Administration Management of intravenous extravasations: Do not administer I.V.; stop the infusion and remove needle; elevate extremity; administer hyaluronidase within the first few minutes to 1 hour after the extravasation is recognized
Monitoring Parameters Observe appearance of lesion for induration, swelling, discoloration, blanching, and blister formation every 15 minutes for ~2 hours
Dosage Forms Injection, stabilized solution: 150 units/mL (1 mL, 10 mL) [DSC]
References
Raszka WV, Keuser TK, Smith FR, et al, "The Use of Hyaluronidase in the Treatment of Intravenous Extravasation Injuries," *J Perinatol*, 1990, 10(2):146-9.
Zenk KE, "Hyaluronidase: An Antidote for Intravenous Extravasations," *CSHP Voice*, 1981, 66-8.
(Continued)

Hyaluronidase [DSC] (Continued)

Zenk KE, Dungy CI, and Greene GR, "Nafcillin Extravasation Injury: Use of Hyaluronidase as an Antidote," *Am J Dis Child,* 1981, 135(12):1113-4.

♦ **Hycort™ (Can)** *see* Hydrocortisone *on page 573*
♦ **Hydeltra T.B.A.® (Can)** *see* PrednisoLONE *on page 925*
♦ **Hyderm (Can)** *see* Hydrocortisone *on page 573*

HydrALAZINE (hye DRAL a zeen)

Canadian Brand Names Apo®-Hydralazine; Apresoline®; Novo-Hylazin; Nu-Hydral
Therapeutic Category Antihypertensive Agent; Vasodilator
Generic Available Yes
Use Management of moderate to severe hypertension, CHF, hypertension secondary to pre-eclampsia/eclampsia, primary pulmonary hypertension
Pregnancy Risk Factor C
Contraindications Hypersensitivity to hydralazine or any component; dissecting aortic aneurysm, mitral valve rheumatic heart disease, coronary artery disease
Warnings Monitor blood pressure closely with I.V. use; modify dosage in patients with severe renal impairment
Precautions Discontinue hydralazine in patients who develop SLE-like syndrome or positive ANA; use with caution in patients with severe renal disease or cerebral vascular accidents
Adverse Reactions
Cardiovascular: Palpitations, flushing, tachycardia, edema, orthostatic hypotension (rare)
Central nervous system: Malaise, fever, headache, dizziness
Dermatologic: Rash
Gastrointestinal: Anorexia, nausea, vomiting, diarrhea
Neuromuscular & skeletal: Arthralgias, weakness, pyridoxine deficiency-induced peripheral neuropathy (paresthesia, numbness)
Miscellaneous: Positive ANA, positive LE cells, SLE-like syndrome
Drug Interactions MAO inhibitors may cause a significant decrease in blood pressure; indomethacin may decrease hypotensive effects
Food Interactions Avoid natural licorice (causes sodium and water retention and increases potassium loss); long-term use of hydralazine may cause pyridoxine deficiency resulting in numbness, tingling, and paresthesias; if symptoms develop, pyridoxine supplements may be needed
Stability Changes color after contact with a metal filter; do not store intact ampuls in refrigerator
Mechanism of Action Direct vasodilation of arterioles (with little effect on veins) which results in decreased systemic resistance
Pharmacodynamics
Onset of action:
Oral: 20-30 minutes
I.V.: 5-20 minutes
Duration:
Oral: 2-4 hours
I.V.: 2-6 hours
Pharmacokinetics
Distribution: Crosses placenta; appears in breast milk
Protein-binding: 85% to 90%
Metabolism: Acetylated in the liver
Bioavailability: 30% to 50%; large first-pass effect orally
Half-life, adults: 2-8 hours; half-life varies with genetically determined acetylation rates
Elimination: 14% excreted unchanged in urine
Usual Dosage
Infants and Children:
Oral: Initial: 0.75-1 mg/kg/day in 2-4 divided doses, not to exceed 25 mg/dose; increase over 3-4 weeks to maximum of 5 mg/kg/day in infants and 7.5 mg/kg/day in children, given in 2-4 divided doses; maximum daily dose: 200 mg/day
I.M., I.V.: Initial: 0.1-0.2 mg/kg/dose (not to exceed 20 mg) every 4-6 hours as needed; up to 1.7-3.5 mg/kg/day divided in 4-6 doses
Adults:
Oral: Initial: 10 mg 4 times/day, increase by 10-25 mg/dose every 2-5 days to maximum of 300 mg/day
I.M., I.V.: Hypertension: Initial: 10-20 mg/dose every 4-6 hours as needed, may increase to 40 mg/dose

I.M., I.V.: Pre-eclampsia/eclampsia: 5 mg/dose then 5-10 mg every 20-30 minutes as needed

Dosing interval in renal impairment:
Cl$_{cr}$ 10-50 mL/minute: Administer every 8 hours
Cl$_{cr}$ <10 mL/minute: Administer every 8-16 hours in fast acetylators and every 12-24 hours in slow acetylators

Administration
Oral: Administer with food
Parenteral: I.V.: Do not exceed rate of 0.2 mg/kg/minute; maximum concentration for I.V. use: 20 mg/mL

Monitoring Parameters Heart rate, blood pressure, ANA titer

Patient Information Limit alcohol; notify physician if flu-like symptoms occur

Nursing Implications I.V. use: Monitor blood pressure closely

Additional Information Slow acetylators, patients with decreased renal function and patients receiving >200 mg/day (chronically) are at higher risk for SLE. Titrate dosage to patient's response. Usually administered with diuretic and a beta-blocker to counteract hydralazine's side effects of sodium and water retention and reflex tachycardia.

Dosage Forms
Injection, solution, as hydrochloride: 20 mg/mL (1 mL)
Tablet, as hydrochloride: 10 mg, 25 mg, 50 mg, 100 mg

Extemporaneous Preparations
A flavored syrup (1.25 mg/mL) has been made using seventy-five hydralazine hydrochloride 50 mg tablets, dissolved in 250 mL of distilled water with 2250 g of Lycasin® (75% w/w maltitol syrup vehicle); edetate disodium 3 g and sodium saccharin 3 g dissolved in 50 mL distilled water was added; solution was preserved with 30 mL of a solution containing methylparaben 10% (w/v) and propylparaben 2% (w/v) in propylene glycol; flavored with 3 mL orange flavoring; qsad to 3 L with distilled water and then pH adjusted to pH of 3.7 using glacial acetic acid; measured stability was 5 days at room temperature (25°C); less than 2% loss of hydralazine occurred at 2 weeks when syrup was stored at 5°C (Alexander, 1993)
A 4 mg/mL oral liquid preparation made from tablets was **not** stable for very long; preparation made in cherry syrup was not even stable for 1 day; preparation made in a 1:1 mixture of Ora-Sweet® and Ora-Plus® was stable for only 1 day under refrigeration (5°C) and not even 1 day at room temperature (25°C); preparation made in a 1:1 mixture of Ora-Sweet® SF and Ora-Plus® was stable for only 2 days under refrigeration (5°C), but not even 1 day at room temperature (25°C) (Allen, 1998).

Alexander KS, Pudipeddi M, and Parker GA, "Stability of Hydralazine Hydrochloride Syrup Compounded From Tablets," *Am J Hosp Pharm*, 1993, 50(4):683-6.
Allen LV and Erickson MA, "Stability of Alprazolam, Chloroquine Phosphate, Cisapride, Enalapril Maleate, and Hydralazine Hydrochloride in Extemporaneously Compounded Oral Liquids," *Am J Health Syst Pharm*, 1998, 55(18):1915-20.

♦ **Hydramine®** [OTC] *see* DiphenhydrAMINE *on page 393*
♦ **Hydramine® Cough** [OTC] *see* DiphenhydrAMINE *on page 393*
♦ **Hydrate®** [DSC] *see* DimenhyDRINATE *on page 390*
♦ **Hydrated Chloral** *see* Chloral Hydrate *on page 252*
♦ **Hydrea®** *see* Hydroxyurea *on page 582*
♦ **Hydrisalic™** [OTC] *see* Salicylic Acid *on page 1002*
♦ **Hydrocet®** *see* Hydrocodone and Acetaminophen *on page 571*

Hydrochlorothiazide (hye droe klor oh THYE a zide)

Related Information
Carbohydrate and Alcohol Content of Liquid Medications for Use in Patients Receiving Ketogenic Diets *on page 1431*

U.S. Brand Names Aquazide® H; Microzide™; Oretic®

Canadian Brand Names Apo®-Hydro; Novo-Hydrazide

Synonyms HCTZ

Therapeutic Category Antihypertensive Agent; Diuretic, Thiazide

Generic Available Yes

Use Management of mild to moderate hypertension; treatment of edema in CHF and nephrotic syndrome

Pregnancy Risk Factor B

Contraindications Hypersensitivity to hydrochlorothiazide or any component; cross-sensitivity with other thiazides or sulfonamides; anuria

Warnings Oral solution contains sodium benzoate; benzoic acid (benzoate) is a metabolite of benzyl alcohol; large amounts of benzyl alcohol (≥99 mg/kg/day) have (Continued)

Hydrochlorothiazide *(Continued)*

been associated with a potentially fatal toxicity ("gasping syndrome") in neonates; *in vitro* and animal studies have shown that benzoate displaces bilirubin from protein binding sites; avoid use in neonates

Precautions Use with caution in patients with severe renal disease (Cl_{cr} <10 mL/minute), impaired hepatic function, hepatic disease, gout, lupus erythematosus, diabetes mellitus

Adverse Reactions

Cardiovascular: Hypotension

Central nervous system: Drowsiness, vertigo, headache

Dermatologic: Photosensitivity

Endocrine & metabolic: Hypokalemia, hyperglycemia, hypochloremic metabolic alkalosis, hyperlipidemia, hyperuricemia

Gastrointestinal: Nausea, vomiting, anorexia, diarrhea, cramping, pancreatitis

Hematologic: Aplastic anemia, hemolytic anemia, leukopenia, agranulocytosis, thrombocytopenia

Hepatic: Hepatitis, intrahepatic cholestasis

Neuromuscular & skeletal: Muscle weakness, paresthesia

Renal: Polyuria, prerenal azotemia

Drug Interactions NSAIDs decrease antihypertensive effect; steroids, amphotericin B increase potassium losses; hydrochlorothiazide increases hypersensitivity reactions to allopurinol; decreased clearance of lithium; increased hyperglycemia with diazoxide; hydrochlorothiazide decreases effectiveness of antidiabetic agents in blood sugar control; cholestyramine decreases hydrochlorothiazide absorption

Food Interactions Avoid natural licorice (causes sodium and water retention and increases potassium loss); may need to decrease sodium and calcium and increase potassium, zinc, magnesium, and riboflavin in diet

Mechanism of Action Inhibits sodium reabsorption in the distal tubules causing increased excretion of sodium and water as well as potassium, hydrogen, magnesium, phosphate, calcium, and bicarbonate ions

Pharmacodynamics

Onset of diuretic action: Oral: Within 2 hours

Maximum effect: Within 3-6 hours

Duration: 6-12 hours

Pharmacokinetics

Absorption: Oral: ~60% to 80%

Distribution: Breast milk to plasma ratio: 0.25

Half-life: 5.6-14.8 hours

Elimination: Unchanged in urine

Usual Dosage Oral: (daily dosages should be decreased if used with other antihypertensives):

Neonates and Infants <6 months: 2-4 mg/kg/day in 2 divided doses; maximum daily dosage: 37.5 mg

Infants >6 months and Children: 2 mg/kg/day in 2 divided doses; maximum daily dosage: 200 mg

Adults: 12.5-100 mg/day in 1-2 doses; maximum dose: 200 mg/day

Dosage adjustment in renal impairment: Cl_{cr} <25-50 mL/minute: May not be effective

Administration Oral: Administer with food or milk

Monitoring Parameters Serum electrolytes, BUN, creatinine, blood pressure, fluid balance, body weight

Patient Information May cause photosensitivity reactions (eg, exposure to sunlight may cause severe sunburn, skin rash, redness, or itching); avoid exposure to sunlight and artificial light sources (sunlamps, tanning booth/bed); wear protective clothing, wide-brimmed hats, sunglasses, and lip sunscreen (SPF ≥15); use a sunscreen [broad-spectrum sunscreen or physical sunscreen (preferred) or sunblock with SPF ≥15]; contact physician if reaction occurs.

Dosage Forms

Capsule (Microzide™): 12.5 mg

Solution, oral: 50 mg/5 mL (500 mL) [contains sodium benzoate; mint flavor] [DSC]

Tablet: 25 mg, 50 mg

Aquazide® H: 50 mg

Oretic®: 50 mg

Hydrochlorothiazide and Spironolactone

(hye droe klor oh THYE a zide & speer on oh LAK tone)

U.S. Brand Names Aldactazide®

Canadian Brand Names Novo-Spirozine

Synonyms Spironolactone and Hydrochlorothiazide

Therapeutic Category Antihypertensive Agent, Combination; Diuretic, Combination

Generic Available Yes (only combination with 25 mg hydrochlorothiazide and spironolactone)

Use Management of mild to moderate hypertension; treatment of edema in CHF and nephrotic syndrome

Pregnancy Risk Factor C

Contraindications Hypersensitivity to hydrochlorothiazide, spironolactone, or any component; anuria, hyperkalemia, renal or hepatic failure; cross-sensitivity with other thiazides or sulfonamides; patients receiving triamterene or amiloride

Warnings This fixed combination is not indicated for initial therapy of hypertension; therapy requires titration to the individual patient; if dosage so determined represents this fixed combination, its use may be more convenient

Adverse Reactions See individual components, Hydrochlorothiazide *on page 569* and Spironolactone *on page 1037*, for full adverse drug reaction information

Drug Interactions Drugs that increase serum potassium (amiloride, triamterene, indomethacin, ACE inhibitors); digoxin decreases renal clearance; see individual components, Hydrochlorothiazide *on page 569* and Spironolactone *on page 1037*, for complete drug interaction information

Food Interactions Avoid food with high potassium content, natural licorice (causes sodium and water retention and increases potassium loss), and salt substitutes

Usual Dosage Oral: As the product is in a fixed combination of equal mg doses, the following dosages represent mg of either spironolactone **or** hydrochlorothiazide

Children: 1.5-3 mg/kg/day in 2-4 divided doses; maximum daily dosage: 200 mg
Adults: 12.5-200 mg in 1-2 divided doses

Administration Oral: Administer in the morning; administer the last dose of multiple doses before 6 PM unless instructed otherwise; administer with food or milk

Monitoring Parameters Blood pressure, serum electrolytes, renal function

Test Interactions Spironolactone may interfere with plasma and urinary cortisol levels and the radioimmunoassay for digoxin

Dosage Forms
Tablet: Hydrochlorothiazide 25 mg and spironolactone 25 mg
Aldactazide®: Hydrochlorothiazide 25 mg and spironolactone 25 mg; Hydrochlorothiazide 50 mg and spironolactone 50 mg

Extemporaneous Preparations A 5 mg/mL oral suspension may be compounded by crushing twenty-four 25 mg (spironolactone/HCTZ) Aldactazide® tablets; add geometric amounts of a 1:1 mixture of Ora-Sweet® and Ora-Plus®, or Ora-Sweet® SF and Ora-Plus®, or cherry syrup alone to a final volume of 120 mL; shake well, refrigerate; stable 60 days
Allen LV and Erickson MA, "Stability of Labetalol Hydrochloride, Metoprolol Tartrate, Verapamil Hydrochloride, and Spironolactone With Hydrochlorothiazide in Extemporaneously Compounded Oral Liquids," *Am J Health Syst Pharm*, 1996, 53(19):2304-9.

♦ **Hydrocil® [OTC]** *see* Psyllium *on page 959*

Hydrocodone and Acetaminophen
(hye droe KOE done & a seet a MIN oh fen)

Related Information
Narcotic Analgesics Comparison *on page 1223*
Overdose and Toxicology *on page 1388*

U.S. Brand Names Anexsia®; Bancap HC®; Ceta-Plus®; Co-Gesic®; Hydrocet®; Hydrogesic® [DSC]; Lorcet® 10/650; Lorcet®-HD; Lorcet® Plus; Lortab®; Margesic® H; Maxidone™; Norco®; Stagesic®; Vicodin®; Vicodin® ES; Vicodin® HP; Zydone®

Synonyms Acetaminophen and Hydrocodone

Therapeutic Category Analgesic, Narcotic; Antitussive; Cough Preparation

Generic Available Yes

Use Relief of moderate to severe pain; antitussive (hydrocodone)

Restrictions C-III

Pregnancy Risk Factor C

Contraindications Hypersensitivity to hydrocodone, acetaminophen, or any component; CNS depression; severe respiratory depression

Warnings Abrupt discontinuation after prolonged use may result in withdrawal symptoms or seizures

Precautions Use with caution in patients with hypersensitivity reactions to other phenanthrene derivative opioid agonists (morphine, codeine, hydromorphone, oxycodone, oxymorphone, levorphanol)
(Continued)

Hydrocodone and Acetaminophen (Continued)

Adverse Reactions
Cardiovascular: Hypotension, bradycardia, peripheral vasodilation

Central nervous system: CNS depression, drowsiness, dizziness, sedation, elevated intracranial pressure

Endocrine & metabolic: Antidiuretic hormone release

Gastrointestinal: Nausea, vomiting, constipation, biliary tract spasm

Genitourinary: Urinary tract spasm

Ocular: Miosis

Respiratory: Respiratory depression

Miscellaneous: Histamine release, physical and psychological dependence with prolonged use

Drug Interactions
Hydrocodone is a cytochrome P450 isoenzyme CYP2D6 substrate; acetaminophen is a cytochrome P450 isoenzyme CYP1A2 substrate (minor), CYP2A6, CYP2C9, CYP2D6, CYP2E1, and CYP3A3/4 isoenzyme substrate

CNS depressants, alcohol, phenothiazines, tricyclic antidepressants may potentiate the adverse effects of hydrocodone; see also Acetaminophen *on page 36*

Food Interactions
Rate of absorption of acetaminophen may be decreased when given with food high in carbohydrates

Mechanism of Action
Inhibits the synthesis of prostaglandins in the CNS and peripherally blocks pain impulse generation; produces antipyresis from inhibition of hypothalamic heat-regulating center

Pharmacodynamics
Narcotic analgesia: Oral:

Onset of action: Within 10-20 minutes

Duration: 3-6 hours

Usual Dosage
Oral:

Antitussive (doses based on hydrocodone):

Children: 0.6 mg/kg/day or 20 mg/m^2/day divided in 3-4 doses/day

<2 years: Do not exceed 1.25 mg/single dose

2-12 years: Do not exceed 5 mg/single dose

>12 years: Do not exceed 10 mg/single dose

Analgesic: **Doses should be titrated to appropriate analgesic effect**

Children: Dose has not been well established

Adults: 1-2 tablets or capsules every 4-6 hours as needed

AHCPR dosing guidelines (doses based on hydrocodone): Opioid naive patients: (See Carr, 1992 and Jacox, 1994)

Children and Adults <50 kg: Moderate to severe pain: Usual initial dose: 0.2 mg/kg every 3-4 hours

Children and Adults ≥50 kg: Moderate to severe pain: Usual initial dose: 10 mg every 3-4 hours

Administration
Oral: May administer with food or milk to decrease GI distress

Monitoring Parameters
Pain relief, respiratory rate, blood pressure

Patient Information
Avoid alcohol; may cause drowsiness and impair ability to perform activities requiring mental alertness or physical coordination; may be habit-forming; avoid abrupt discontinuation after prolonged use

Dosage Forms
Capsule (Bancap HC®, Ceta-Plus®, Hydrocet®, Hydrogesic®, Lorcet®-HD, Margesic® H, Stagesic®): Hydrocodone bitartrate 5 mg and acetaminophen 500 mg

Elixir, oral (Lortab®): Hydrocodone bitartrate 2.5 mg and acetaminophen 167 mg per 5 mL (480 mL) [contains 7% alcohol; tropical fruit punch flavor]

Tablet: Hydrocodone bitartrate 2.5 mg and acetaminophen 500 mg; hydrocodone bitartrate 5 mg and acetaminophen 500 mg; hydrocodone bitartrate 7.5 mg and acetaminophen 500 mg; hydrocodone bitartrate 7.5 mg and acetaminophen 650 mg; hydrocodone bitartrate 7.5 mg and acetaminophen 750 mg; hydrocodone bitartrate 10 mg and acetaminophen 325 mg; hydrocodone bitartrate 10 mg and acetaminophen 650 mg

Anexsia®:

5/325: Hydrocodone bitartrate 5 mg and acetaminophen 325 mg

5/500: Hydrocodone bitartrate 5 mg and acetaminophen 500 mg

7.5/325: Hydrocodone bitartrate 7.5 mg and acetaminophen 325 mg

7.5/650: Hydrocodone bitartrate 7.5 mg and acetaminophen 650 mg

10/660: Hydrocodone bitartrate 10 mg and acetaminophen 660 mg

Co-Gesic®: 5/500: Hydrocodone bitartrate 5 mg and acetaminophen 500 mg

Lorcet® 10/650: Hydrocodone bitartrate 10 mg and acetaminophen 650 mg

Lorcet® Plus: Hydrocodone bitartrate 7.5 mg and acetaminophen 650 mg

Lortab®:

2.5/500: Hydrocodone bitartrate 2.5 mg and acetaminophen 500 mg

5/500: Hydrocodone bitartrate 5 mg and acetaminophen 500 mg

7.5/500: Hydrocodone bitartrate 7.5 mg and acetaminophen 500 mg

10/500: Hydrocodone bitartrate 10 mg and acetaminophen 500 mg

Maxidone™: Hydrocodone bitartrate 10 mg and acetaminophen 750 mg

Norco®: Hydrocodone bitartrate 5 mg and acetaminophen 325 mg; hydrocodone bitartrate 7.5 mg and acetaminophen 325 mg; hydrocodone bitartrate 10 mg and acetaminophen 325 mg

Vicodin®: Hydrocodone bitartrate 5 mg and acetaminophen 500 mg

Vicodin® ES: Hydrocodone bitartrate 7.5 mg and acetaminophen 750 mg

Vicodin® HP: Hydrocodone bitartrate 10 mg and acetaminophen 660 mg

Zydone®: Hydrocodone bitartrate 5 mg and acetaminophen 400 mg; hydrocodone bitartrate 7.5 mg and acetaminophen 400 mg; hydrocodone bitartrate 10 mg and acetaminophen 400 mg

References

Carr D, Jacox A, Chapman CR, et al, "Clinical Practice Guideline Number 1: Acute Pain Management: Operative or Medical Procedures and Trauma," Rockville, Maryland: U.S. Department of Health and Human Services, Public Health Service, Agency for Health Care Policy and Research, AHCPR Publication No 92-0032, 1992.

Jacox A, Carr D, Payne R, et al, "Clinical Practice Guideline Number 9: Management of Cancer Pain," Rockville, Maryland: U.S. Department of Health and Human Services, Public Health Service, Agency for Health Care Policy and Research, AHCPR Publication No. 94-0592, 1994.

Hydrocortisone (hye droe KOR ti sone)

Related Information

Carbohydrate and Alcohol Content of Liquid Medications for Use in Patients Receiving Ketogenic Diets on page 1431

Corticosteroids Comparison, Systemic on page 1211

Corticosteroids Comparison, Topical on page 1212

U.S. Brand Names A-hydroCort®; Anucort™ HC; Anusol-HC®; Anusol® HC-1 [OTC]; Caldecort® [OTC]; Cetacort®; Colocort™; CortaGel® Maximum Strength [OTC]; Cortaid® Intensive Therapy [OTC]; Cortaid® Maximum Strength [OTC]; Cortaid® Sensitive Skin With Aloe [OTC]; Cortef®; Corticool® [OTC]; Cortifoam® [OTC]; Cortizone®-5 [OTC]; Cortizone®-10 [OTC]; Cortizone®-10 Plus [OTC]; Cortizone®-10 Quick Shot [OTC]; Cortizone® for Kids [OTC]; Delacort®; Dermarest Dri-Cort® [OTC]; Dermtex® HC [OTC]; EarSol® HC; Hemril®-HC; Hydrocortone®; Hydrocortone® Phosphate; Hytone®; LactiCare-HC®; Locoid®; Locoid Lipocream®; Nupercainal® Hydrocortisone Cream [OTC]; Nutracort®; Pandel®; Post Peel Healing Balm [OTC]; Preparation H® Hydrocortisone [OTC]; Proctocort®; ProctoCream® HC; Proctosol-HC®; Sarnol®-HC [OTC]; Solu-Cortef®; Summer's Eve® SpecialCare™ Medicated Anti-Itch Cream [OTC]; Texacort®; Theracort® [OTC]; Westcort®

Canadian Brand Names Aquacort®; Cortamed®; Cortate®; Cortenema®; Cortoderm; Emo-Cort®; Hycort™; Hyderm; HydroVal®; Prevex® HC; Sarna® HC

Synonyms Compound F; Cortisol

Therapeutic Category Adrenal Corticosteroid; Antiasthmatic; Anti-inflammatory Agent; Anti-inflammatory Agent, Rectal; Corticosteroid, Rectal; Corticosteroid, Systemic; Corticosteroid, Topical; Glucocorticoid

Generic Available Yes

Use Management of adrenocortical insufficiency; relief of inflammation and pruritus associated with corticosteroid-responsive dermatoses; adjunctive treatment of ulcerative colitis

Pregnancy Risk Factor C

Contraindications Hypersensitivity to hydrocortisone or any component (see Warnings); serious infections, except septic shock or tuberculous meningitis; viral, fungal, or tubercular skin lesions

Warnings Acute adrenal insufficiency may occur with abrupt withdrawal after long-term therapy or with stress

Topical: Adverse systemic effects may occur when topical steroids are used in large areas of the body, denuded areas, for prolonged periods of time, with an occlusive dressing, and/or in infants and small children; infants and small children may be more susceptible to HPA axis suppression or other systemic toxicities due to larger skin surface area to body mass ratio; use with caution in pediatric patients.

Solution for injection (as sodium phosphate) contains sodium bisulfite which may cause allergic reactions in susceptible individuals; manufacturer supplied diluents for injection (eg, A-hydroCort®, Solu-Cortef®) contain benzyl alcohol and topical aerosol spray and topical cream may contain benzyl alcohol which may cause allergic reactions in susceptible individuals; otic solution contains benzyl benzoate and oral suspension (see Additional Information) contains benzoic acid; benzoic acid (benzoate) is a metabolite of benzyl alcohol; large amounts of benzyl alcohol (≥99 mg/kg/day) have been associated with a potentially fatal toxicity ("gasping syndrome") in neonates; the "gasping syndrome" consists of metabolic acidosis, respiratory distress, gasping respirations, CNS dysfunction (including convulsions, intracranial hemorrhage), hypotension and cardiovascular collapse; avoid use of (Continued)

Hydrocortisone (Continued)

hydrocortisone products containing benzoic acid, benzyl alcohol, or benzyl benzoate in neonates; *in vitro* and animal studies have shown that benzoate displaces bilirubin from protein binding sites

Precautions Use with caution in patients with hyperthyroidism, cirrhosis, nonspecific ulcerative colitis, hypertension, osteoporosis, thromboembolic tendencies, CHF, convulsive disorders, myasthenia gravis, thrombophlebitis, peptic ulcer, diabetes, glaucoma, cataracts, tuberculosis, or hepatic impairment; avoid using higher than recommended doses; suppression of HPA function, suppression of linear growth, hypercorticism (Cushing's syndrome), hyperglycemia, or glucosuria may occur; titrate to lowest effective dose; these adverse effects (as well as intracranial hypertension) may also occur with topical use and have been reported in pediatric patients

Adverse Reactions

Cardiovascular: Hypertension, edema

Central nervous system: Euphoria, insomnia, headache

Dermatologic: Acne, dermatitis, skin atrophy; topical use: eczema, pruritus, stinging, dry skin, irritation, redness

Endocrine & metabolic: Hypokalemia, hyperglycemia, Cushing's syndrome, growth suppression; suppression of HPA function

Gastrointestinal: Peptic ulcer

Ocular: Cataracts

Miscellaneous: Immunosuppression

Drug Interactions Cytochrome P450 isoenzyme CYP2D6 and CYP3A3/4 substrate Barbiturates, phenytoin, rifampin, salicylates, NSAIDs, diuretics (potassium depleting), warfarin; caffeine and alcohol may increase risk for GI ulcer; live virus vaccines (increase risk of viral infection); vaccines may have decreased effects

Food Interactions Systemic use of corticosteroids may require a diet with increased potassium, vitamins A, B_6, C, D, folate, calcium, zinc, phosphorus, and decreased sodium

Mechanism of Action Decreases inflammation by suppression of migration of polymorphonuclear leukocytes and reversal of increased capillary permeability

Pharmacodynamics Anti-inflammatory effects:

Maximum effect:

Oral: 12-24 hours

I.V.: 4-6 hours

Duration: 8-12 hours

Pharmacokinetics

Absorption: Rapid by all routes, except rectally

Metabolism: In the liver

Half-life, biologic: 8-12 hours

Elimination: Renally, mainly as 17-hydroxysteroids and 17-ketosteroids

Usual Dosage Dose should be based on severity of disease and patient response; **Note:** A variety of salt forms are available and can lead to confusion in prescribing, dispensing, and administration; use the appropriate salt/dosage form for the following indications:

Acetate: For intra-articular, intrasynovial, intrabursal, intralesional, or soft tissue injection only

Cypionate: Oral suspension (see Additional Information)

Sodium phosphate: For general I.V. use

Sodium succinate: For general I.V. use, I.V. use in patients allergic to sodium phosphate salt, I.V. for shock and for intrathecal use (must reconstitute with a preservative free diluent or use a preservative free product)

Acute adrenal insufficiency: I.M., I.V.:

Infants and young Children: 1-2 mg/kg/dose I.V. bolus, then 25-150 mg/day in divided doses every 6-8 hours

Older Children: 1-2 mg/kg I.V. bolus, then 150-250 mg/day in divided doses every 6-8 hours

Adults: 100 mg I.V. bolus, then 300 mg/day in divided doses every 8 hours or as a continuous infusion for 48 hours; once patient is stable change to oral, 50 mg every 8 hours for 6 doses, then taper to 30-50 mg/day in divided doses

Anti-inflammatory or immunosuppressive:

Infants and Children:

Oral: 2.5-10 mg/kg/day or 75-300 mg/m²/day divided every 6-8 hours

I.M., I.V.: 1-5 mg/kg/day or 30-150 mg/m²/day divided every 12-24 hours

Adolescents and Adults: Oral, I.M., I.V., S.C.: 15-240 mg every 12 hours

Congenital adrenal hyperplasia: AAP Recommendations: Oral: Initial: 10-20 mg/m²/day in 3 divided doses; usual requirement: Infants: 2.5-5 mg 3 times/day; Children: 5-10 mg 3 times/day; **Note:** Administer morning dose as early as possible; tablets may result in more reliable serum concentrations than oral liquid formulation (see Additional Information); individualize dose by monitoring growth, hormone levels, and bone age; mineralocorticoid (eg, fludrocortisone) and sodium supplement may be required in salt losers

Physiologic replacement: Children:
Oral: 0.5-0.75 mg/kg/day or 20-25 mg/m²/day divided every 8 hours
I.M.: 0.25-0.35 mg/kg/day or 12-15 mg/m²/day once daily

Shock: I.V.: **Sodium succinate:**
Children: Initial: 50 mg/kg then repeated in 4 hours and/or every 24 hours if needed
Adolescents and Adults: 500 mg to 2 g every 2-6 hours

Status asthmaticus:
Children: I.V.: Optional loading dose: 4-8 mg/kg; maximum: 250 mg; then maintenance: 2 mg/kg/dose every 6 hours
Adults: 100-500 mg every 6 hours

Adolescents and Adults: Rectal: Insert 1 application 1-2 times/day for 2-3 weeks
Ulcerative colitis: One enema nightly for 21 days, or until remission occurs; clinical symptoms should subside within 3-5 days; discontinue use if no improvement within 2-3 weeks; some patients may require 2-3 months of therapy; if therapy lasts >21 days, discontinue slowly by decreasing use to every other night for 2-3 weeks

Children and Adults: Topical: Apply 3-4 times/day

Administration
Oral: Administer with food or milk to decrease GI upset (see Additional Information)
Parenteral:
I.V. bolus: Dilute to 50 mg/mL and administer over 3-5 minutes
I.V. intermittent infusion: Dilute to 1 mg/mL and administer over 20-30 minutes; maximum concentration: 5 mg/mL
Rectal: Patient should lie on left side during administration and for 30 minutes after; retain enema for at least 1 hour, preferably all night
Topical: Apply a thin film to clean, dry skin and rub in gently; avoid contact with eyes. Do not apply to face, underarms, or groin unless directed by physician. Do not wrap or bandage affected area unless directed by physician. Do not apply to diaper areas because diapers or plastic pants may be occlusive.

Monitoring Parameters Blood pressure, weight, serum glucose, electrolytes; growth in pediatric patients

Reference Range Hydrocortisone (normal endogenous morning levels) 4-30 μg/mL

Test Interactions Skin tests

Patient Information Limit caffeine; avoid alcohol; do not decrease dose or discontinue without physician's approval; avoid exposure to measles or chicken pox, advise physician immediately if exposed; notify physician if condition being treated persists or worsens. Topical: Avoid contact with eyes; do not use for longer than directed; contact physician if no improvement is seen in 2 weeks

Additional Information Cortef® oral suspension was reformulated in July 1998; the suspending agent was changed from tragacanth to xanthan gum; this suspension was found **not** to be bioequivalent to hydrocortisone tablets in the treatment of children with congenital adrenal hyperplasia; children required higher doses of the suspension (19.6 mg/m²/day) compared to the tablets (15.2 mg/m²/day); based on these findings, Cortef® suspension was voluntarily recalled from the market on July 18, 2000 (see Merke, 2001).

To facilitate retention of enema, prior antidiarrheal medication or sedation may be required (especially when beginning therapy)

Dosage Forms
Aerosol, rectal, as **acetate** (Cortifoam®): 10% (15 g) [90 mg/applicator]
Aerosol, topical spray, as **base:**
Cortizone®-10 Quick Shot: 1% (44 mL) [contains benzyl alcohol]
Dermtex® HC: 1% (52 mL)
Cream, rectal, as **acetate** (Nupercainal® Hydrocortisone Cream): 1% (30 g)
Cream, rectal, as **base:**
Cortizone®-10: 1% (30 g)
Preparation H® Hydrocortisone: 1% (27 g)
Cream, topical, as **acetate:** 0.5% (30 g); 1% (30 g)
Cortaid® Maximum Strength: 1% (15 g, 30 g, 40 g)
Cortaid® Sensitive Skin With Aloe: 0.5% (15 g)
Cream, topical, as **base:** 0.5% (15 g, 30 g, 454 g); 1% (1.5 g, 15 g, 20 g, 30 g, 120 g, 454 g); 2.5% (20 g, 30 g, 454 g)
Anusol-HC®: 2.5% (30 g) [contains benzyl alcohol]
Caldecort®: 1% (15 g, 30 g) [contains benzyl alcohol]
Cortaid® Intensive Therapy: 1% (60 g)
Cortaid® Maximum Strength: 1% (15 g, 30 g, 40 g, 60 g) [contains benzyl alcohol]
(Continued)

Hydrocortisone *(Continued)*

    Cortizone®-5: 0.5% (30 g, 60 g)
    Cortizone®-10: 1% (15 g, 30 g, 60 g)
    Cortizone®-10 Plus: 1% (30 g, 60 g) [contains vitamins A, D, E]
    Cortizone® for Kids: 0.5% (30 g)
    Dermarest Dri-Cort®: 1% (15 g, 30 g)
    Hytone®: 2.5% (30 g, 60 g)
    Post Peel Healing Balm: 1% (23 g)
    ProctoCream® HC: 2.5% (30 g) [contains benzyl alcohol]
    Proctocort®: 1% (30 g)
    Proctosol-HC®: 2.5% (30 g)
    Summer's Eve® SpecialCare™ Medicated Anti-Itch Cream: 1% (30 g)
Cream, topical, as **butyrate** (Locoid®, Locoid Lipocream®): 0.1% (15 g, 45 g)
Cream, topical, as **probutate** (Pandel®): 0.1% (15 g, 45 g, 80 g)
Cream, topical as **valerate** (Westcort®): 0.2% (15 g, 45 g, 60 g)
Gel, as **base**:
    Corticool®: 1% (45 g)
    CortaGel® Maximum Strength: 1% (15 g, 30 g)
Injection, powder for reconstitution, as **sodium succinate**: 100 mg, 250 mg, 500 mg, 1 g
    A-hydroCort®: 100 mg, 250 mg [diluent contains benzyl alcohol]
    Solu-Cortef®: 100 mg, 250 mg, 500 mg, 1 g [diluent contains benzyl alcohol]
Injection, solution, as **sodium phosphate** (Hydrocortone® Phosphate): 50 mg/mL (2 mL) [contains sodium bisulfite]
Lotion, as **base**: 0.5% (60 mL); 1% (120 mL); 2.5% (60 mL)
    Cetacort®, Sarnol®-HC: 1% (60 mL)
    Delacort®, Theracort®: 1% (120 mL)
    Hytone®: 1% (30 mL, 120 mL); 2.5% (60 mL)
    LactiCare-HC®: 1% (120 mL); 2.5% (60 mL, 120 mL)
    Nutracort®: 1% (60 mL, 120 mL); 2.5% (60 mL, 120 mL)
Ointment, topical, as **acetate**: 1% (30 g)
    Anusol® HC-1: 1% (21 g)
    Cortaid® Maximum Strength: 1% (15 g, 30 g)
Ointment, topical, as **base**: 0.5% (30 g); 1% (15 g, 20 g, 30 g, 454 g); 2.5% (20 g, 30 g, 454 g)
    Cortizone®-5: 0.5% (30 g)
    Cortizone®-10: 1% (30 g, 60 g)
    Hytone®: 2.5% (30 g)
Ointment, topical, as **butyrate** (Locoid®): 0.1% (15 g, 45 g)
Ointment, topical, as **valerate** (Westcort®): 0.2% (15 g, 45 g, 60 g)
Solution, otic, as **base** (EarSol® HC): 1% (30 mL) [contains 44% alcohol and benzyl benzoate]
Solution, rectal, as **base** (Colocort™): 100 mg/60 mL (7s) [packaged as single dose enemas]
Solution, topical, as **base** (Texacort®): 2.5% (30 mL) [contains 48% alcohol]
Solution, topical, as **butyrate** (Locoid®): 0.1% (20 mL, 60 mL) [contains 50% alcohol]
Stick, roll-on, as **base** (Cortaid® Maximum Strength): 1% (7 g)
Suppository, rectal, as **acetate**: 25 mg (12s, 24s)
    Anucort™ HC: 25 mg (12s, 24s, 100s)
    Anusol-HC®: 25 mg (12s, 24s)
    Hemril®-HC: 25 mg (12s)
    Proctocort®: 30 mg (12s, 24s)
    Proctosol-HC®: 25 mg (12s, 24s)
Suspension, oral, as **cypionate** (Cortef®): 10 mg/5 mL (120 mL) [contains benzoic acid] [DSC]
Tablet, as **base**: 20 mg
    Cortef®: 5 mg, 10 mg, 20 mg
    Hydrocortone®: 10 mg

Extemporaneous Preparations A 2.5 mg/mL oral suspension prepared from tablets (with a vehicle containing sodium carboxymethylcellulose, syrup, hydroxybenzoate 0.1% preservatives, polysorbate 80, and citric acid) and stored in the dark in amber high density polyethylene bottles was stable for 90 days when stored at 5°C or 25°C and stable for 30 days when stored at 40°C; a 2.5 mg/mL oral suspension prepared from powder and the same vehicle was stable for 90 days when stored in the dark in amber polyethylene bottles at 40°C (Fawcett, 1995).

    Fawcett JP, Boulton DW, Jiang R, et al, "Stability of Hydrocortisone Oral Suspensions Prepared From Tablets and Powder," *Ann Pharmacother*, 1995, 29(10):987-90.

References
American Academy of Pediatrics, Section on Endocrinology and Committee on Genetics, "Technical Report: Congenital Adrenal Hyperplasia," *Pediatrics*, 2000, 106(6):1511-8.

Merke DP, Cho D, Calis KA, et al, "Hydrocortisone Suspension and Hydrocortisone Tablets are not Bioequivalent in the Treatment of Children With Congenital Adrenal Hyperplasia," *J Clin Endocrinol Metab*, 2001, 86(1):441-5.

♦ **Hydrocortisone, Neomycin, (Bacitracin), and Polymyxin B** *see* Neomycin, (Bacitracin) Polymyxin B, and Hydrocortisone *on page 802*

♦ **Hydrocortone®** *see* Hydrocortisone *on page 573*

♦ **Hydrocortone® Phosphate** *see* Hydrocortisone *on page 573*

♦ **Hydrodolasetron** *see* Dolasetron *on page 403*

♦ **Hydrogen Dioxide** *see* Hydrogen Peroxide *on page 577*

Hydrogen Peroxide (HYE droe jen per OKS ide)

U.S. Brand Names Orajel® Perioseptic® Super Cleaning Rinse [OTC]; Peroxyl® [OTC]

Synonyms H_2O_2; Hydrogen Dioxide; Peroxide

Therapeutic Category Antibacterial, Otic; Antibacterial, Topical; Antibiotic, Oral Rinse

Generic Available Yes

Use Cleanse wounds, suppurating ulcers, and local infections; used in the treatment of inflammatory conditions of the external auditory canal and as a mouthwash or gargle; hydrogen peroxide concentrate (30%) has been used as a hair bleach and as a tooth bleaching agent

Contraindications Should not be used in abscesses

Warnings Hydrogen peroxide concentrate (30%) is a caustic liquid; it should not be tasted since it is strongly irritating to skin or mucous membranes

Precautions Repeat use as a mouthwash or gargle may produce irritation of the buccal mucous membrane or "hairy tongue"; bandages should not be applied too quickly after its use

Adverse Reactions
Dermatologic: Bleaching effect on hair, irritating burn
Gastrointestinal: Rupture of the colon, proctitis, ulcerative colitis, gas embolism, hairy tongue
Local: Irritation of the buccal mucous membrane

Stability Protect from light and heat; decomposes upon standing, upon repeated agitation, or when in contact with oxidizing or reducing substances

Mechanism of Action Antiseptic oxidant that slowly releases oxygen and water upon contact with serum or tissue catalase

Pharmacodynamics Duration: Only while bubbling action occurs

Usual Dosage Children and Adults:
Mouthwash or gargle: Dilute the 3% solution with an equal volume of water; swish around in the mouth over the affected area for at least 1 minute and then expel; use up to 4 times/day (after meals and at bedtime)
Topical:
1.5% to 3% solution for cleansing wounds
1.5% gel for cleansing wounds or mouth/gum irritations: Apply a small amount to the affected area for at least 1 minute, then expectorate; use up to 4 times/day (after meals and at bedtime)

Administration Topical: Do not inject or instill into closed body cavities from which released oxygen cannot escape; strong solutions (30.5%) of hydrogen peroxide should not be applied undiluted to tissues

Dosage Forms
Gel, oral (Peroxyl®): 1.5% (15 g)
Liquid, oral rinse:
Orajel® Perioseptic® Super Cleaning Rinse: 1.5% (240 mL) [contains 4% alcohol]
Peroxyl®: 1.5% (10 mL, 240 mL, 480 mL) [contains 6% alcohol; mint and cool mint flavors]
Solution, **concentrate**: 30% (100 mL, 500 mL, 4000 mL); 35% (500 mL, 4000 mL); 50% (100 mL, 500 mL, 4000 mL)
Solution, topical: 3% (120 mL, 240 mL, 480 mL, 960 mL, 3840 mL)

♦ **Hydrogesic® [DSC]** *see* Hydrocodone and Acetaminophen *on page 571*

♦ **Hydromorph Contin® (Can)** *see* Hydromorphone *on page 577*

Hydromorphone (hye droe MOR fone)

Related Information
Laboratory Detection of Drugs in Urine *on page 1400*
Narcotic Analgesics Comparison *on page 1223*
(Continued)

Hydromorphone *(Continued)*

Overdose and Toxicology *on page 1388*

U.S. Brand Names Dilaudid®; Dilaudid-HP®

Canadian Brand Names Dilaudid-HP-Plus®; Dilaudid® Sterile Powder; Dilaudid-XP®; Hydromorph Contin®; Hydromorphone HP; PMS-Hydromorphone

Therapeutic Category Analgesic, Narcotic; Antitussive

Generic Available Yes

Use Management of moderate to severe pain; antitussive at lower doses

Restrictions C-II

Pregnancy Risk Factor C

Contraindications Hypersensitivity to hydromorphone or any component (see Warnings)

Warnings Oral liquid and 8 mg tablets may contain trace amounts of sodium bisulfite which may cause allergic reactions in susceptible individuals; rubber stopper of multiple dose vials contains latex which may cause allergic reactions in susceptible individuals; abrupt discontinuation after prolonged use may result in withdrawal symptoms or seizures

Precautions Use with caution in patients with hypersensitivity reactions to other phenanthrene derivative opioid agonists (morphine, hydrocodone, levorphanol, oxycodone, oxymorphone, codeine). Use with caution and reduce the initial dose in patients with significant liver, respiratory, or renal disease; hypothyroidism or myxedema; CNS depression or coma; adrenocortical insufficiency; toxic psychoses; gall bladder disease; prostatic hypertrophy or urethral stricture; acute alcoholism; delirium tremens; or kyphoscoliosis. Seizures and myoclonus have been reported in severely compromised patients receiving high doses of parenteral hydromorphone. Use with caution in patients undergoing biliary tract surgery (narcotics may cause spasm of the sphincter of Oddi).

Adverse Reactions

Cardiovascular: Palpitations, hypotension, bradycardia, peripheral vasodilation

Central nervous system: CNS depression, elevated intracranial pressure, drowsiness, dizziness, sedation

Dermatologic: Pruritus

Endocrine & metabolic: Antidiuretic hormone release

Gastrointestinal: Nausea, vomiting, constipation, biliary tract spasm

Genitourinary: Urinary tract spasm

Ocular: Miosis

Respiratory: Respiratory depression

Miscellaneous: Histamine release, physical and psychological dependence with prolonged use

Drug Interactions CNS depressants, alcohol, phenothiazines, tricyclic antidepressants may potentiate the adverse effects of hydromorphone

Stability Protect from light; store suppositories in refrigerator; store other dosage forms at room temperature; a slight yellow discoloration of injection has not been associated with a loss of potency

Mechanism of Action Binds to opiate receptors in the CNS, causing inhibition of ascending pain pathways, altering the perception of and response to pain; causes cough suppression by direct central action in the medulla; produces generalized CNS depression

Pharmacodynamics Analgesic effects: Oral:

Onset of action: Within 15-30 minutes

Maximum effect: Within 30-90 minutes

Duration: 4-5 hours; suppository may provide longer duration of effect

Pharmacokinetics

Metabolism: Primarily in the liver

Bioavailability: Oral: 62%

Half-life: 1-3 hours

Elimination: In urine, principally as glucuronide conjugates

Usual Dosage

Antitussive: Oral:

Children 6-12 years: 0.5 mg every 3-4 hours as needed

Children >12 years and Adults: 1 mg every 3-4 hours as needed

Pain: Doses should be titrated to appropriate analgesic effects, while minimizing adverse effects; when changing routes of administration, note that oral doses are less than one-half as effective as parenteral doses (may be only $1/_5$ as effective):

Young children:

Oral: 0.03-0.08 mg/kg/dose every 3-4 hours as needed; usual maximum dose: 5 mg/dose

I.V.: 0.015 mg/kg/dose every 3-6 hours as needed

Older Children and Adults:

Oral: Initial: Opiate-naive: 1-2 mg/dose every 3-4 hours as needed; patients with prior opiate exposure may tolerate higher initial doses; usual adult dose: 2-4 mg/dose; doses up to 8 mg have been used in adults

I.M., I.V., S.C.: Initial: Opiate-naive: 0.2-0.6 mg every 2-4 hours as needed; patients with prior opiate exposure may tolerate higher initial doses

Adults: Rectal: 3 mg (1 suppository) every 6-8 hours as needed

AHCPR dosing guidelines: Opioid naive patients: (See Carr, 1992 and Jacox, 1994)

Children and Adults <50 kg: Moderate to severe pain: Usual initial dose:
Oral: 0.06 mg/kg every 3-4 hours
I.V.: 0.015 mg/kg every 3-4 hours

Children and Adults ≥50 kg: Moderate to severe pain: Usual initial dose:
Oral: 6 mg every 3-4 hours
I.M., I.V., S.C.: 1.5 mg every 3-4 hours

Administration

Oral: Administer with food or milk to decrease GI upset

Parenteral: I.V.: Administer via slow I.V. injection over at least 2-3 minutes

Rectal: Insert suppository rectally and retain

Monitoring Parameters Pain relief, respiratory rate, heart rate, blood pressure

Patient Information Avoid alcohol; may cause drowsiness and impair ability to perform activities requiring mental alertness or physical coordination; may be habit-forming; avoid abrupt discontinuation after prolonged use; if oral liquid spills on skin, remove contaminated clothing and rinse area with cool water

Additional Information Equianalgesic doses: Morphine 10 mg I.M. = hydromorphone 1.5 mg I.M.

Dosage Forms

Injection, powder for reconstitution, as hydrochloride (Dilaudid-HP®): 250 mg

Injection, solution, as hydrochloride: 1 mg/mL (1 mL); 2 mg/mL (1 mL, 20 mL); 4 mg/mL (1 mL)

Dilaudid®: 1 mg/mL (1 mL); 2 mg/mL (1 mL, 20 mL); 4 mg/mL (1 mL)

Dilaudid-HP®: 10 mg/mL (1 mL, 5 mL, 50 mL)

Liquid, oral, as hydrochloride (Dilaudid®): 1 mg/mL (480 mL) [may contain trace amounts of sodium bisulfite]

Suppository, rectal, as hydrochloride (Dilaudid®): 3 mg (6s)

Tablet, as hydrochloride (Dilaudid®): 2 mg, 4 mg, 8 mg [8 mg tablets may contain trace amounts of sodium bisulfite]

References

Berde CB and Sethna NF, "Analgesics for the Treatment of Pain in Children," *N Engl J Med*, 2002, 347(14):1094-103.

Carr D, Jacox A, Chapman CR, et al, "Clinical Practice Guideline Number 1: Acute Pain Management: Operative or Medical Procedures and Trauma," Rockville, Maryland: U.S. Department of Health and Human Services, Public Health Service, Agency for Health Care Policy and Research, AHCPR Publication No 92-0032, 1992.

Jacox A, Carr D, Payne R, et al, "Clinical Practice Guideline Number 9: Management of Cancer Pain," Rockville, Maryland: U.S. Department of Health and Human Services, Public Health Service, Agency for Health Care Policy and Research, AHCPR Publication No. 94-0592, 1994.

◆ **Hydromorphone HP (Can)** *see* Hydromorphone *on page 577*
on page 577

◆ **Hydro-Tussin™ DM** *see* Guaifenesin and Dextromethorphan *on page 553*

◆ **HydroVal® (Can)** *see* Hydrocortisone *on page 573*

◆ **Hydroxide and Magnesium Carbonate** *see* Antacid Preparations *on page 112*

Hydroxocobalamin (hye droks oh koe BAL a min)

Synonyms Vitamin B$_{12}$

Therapeutic Category Nutritional Supplement; Vitamin, Water Soluble

Generic Available Yes

Use Treatment of pernicious anemia and other vitamin B$_{12}$ deficiency states; dietary supplement particularly in conditions of increased requirements (eg, pregnancy, thyrotoxicosis, hemorrhage, malignancy, liver or kidney disease)

Pregnancy Risk Factor C

Contraindications Hypersensitivity to cyanocobalamin or any component, cobalt

Warnings Anaphylactic shock has occurred after parenteral vitamin B$_{12}$ administration; intradermal skin testing may be used prior to administration in individuals sensitive to cobalt

Precautions Serum potassium concentrations should be monitored early as severe hypokalemia has occurred after the conversion of megaloblastic anemia to normal erythropoiesis; the increase in nucleic acid degradation produced by administration of hydroxocobalamin to deficient patients may result in gout in susceptible individuals; use of hydroxocobalamin in folic acid deficient individuals may improve folate-deficient megaloblastic anemia and obscure the true diagnosis

(Continued)

Hydroxocobalamin *(Continued)*

Adverse Reactions
Cardiovascular: Peripheral vascular thrombosis
Dermatologic: Itching, exanthema, urticaria
Endocrine & metabolic: Hypokalemia
Gastrointestinal: Diarrhea
Local: Pain at injection site
Miscellaneous: Hypersensitivity reactions

Drug Interactions Decreased absorption of hydroxocobalamin from GI tract by aminoglycoside antibiotics, colchicine, extended release potassium products, aminosalicylic acid, excessive alcohol use, phenytoin, and phenobarbital; antagonism of hematopoietic response to hydroxocobalamin when administered with chloramphenicol

Stability Protect from light

Mechanism of Action Coenzyme for various metabolic functions, including fat and carbohydrate metabolism and protein synthesis, used in cell replication and hematopoiesis

Pharmacodynamics
Onset of action: I.M.:
Megaloblastic anemia:
Conversion of megaloblastic to normoblastic erythroid hyperplasia within bone marrow: 8 hours
Increased reticulocytes: 2-5 days
Complicated vitamin B$_{12}$ deficiency:
Psychiatric sequelae: 24 hours
Thrombocytopenia: 10 days
Granulocytopenia: 2 weeks

Pharmacokinetics
Distribution: Principally stored in the liver; also stored in the kidneys and adrenals
Protein binding: Bound to transcobalamin II
Metabolism: Converted in the tissues to active coenzymes methylcobalamin and deoxyadenosylcobalamin
Time to peak serum concentration: 2 hours
Elimination: 50% to 98% unchanged in the urine

Usual Dosage I.M.:
Schilling test (diagnostic for vitamin B$_{12}$ deficiency): Children and Adults: 1000 mcg once
Congenital transcobalamin deficiency: Neonates: 1000 mcg twice weekly
Vitamin B$_{12}$ deficiency or pernicious anemia: Varying regimens:
Uncomplicated disease:
Children: Initial: 100 mcg/day for 10-15 days (total dose: 1-5 mg); maintenance: 60 mcg/month
or as an alternative: 30-50 mcg/day for at least 2 weeks (total dose: 1-5 mg); maintenance: 100 mcg/month
Adults: Initial: 30 mcg/day for 5-10 days; maintenance: 100-200 mcg/monthly
or as an alternative: 1000 mcg/day for 5-10 days, followed by 100-200 mcg/month
or as an alternative: 100 mcg/day for 1 week, followed by 100 mcg every other day for 2 weeks; maintenance: 100 mcg/month
Complicated disease (eg, severe anemia with heart failure, thrombocytopenia with bleeding, granulocytopenia with infection, severe neurologic damage): Adults: 1000 mcg plus folic acid 15 mg once, followed by 100 mcg/day plus oral folic acid 5 mg/day for 1 week; maintenance dosing as above

Dosage interval in hepatic or renal impairment: A decrease in the interval between injections may be required

Administration Parenteral: I.M. injection only; do not administer S.C.

Monitoring Parameters Serum potassium, erythrocyte and reticulocyte counts, hemoglobin, hematocrit

Reference Range Normal: 200-900 pg/mL; vitamin B$_{12}$ deficiency: <200 pg/mL; megaloblastic anemia: <100 pg/mL

Patient Information Life-long therapy is required in patients with pernicious anemia or other absorption defects; do not discontinue therapy without consulting your physician; avoid alcohol

Additional Information Cyanocobalamin is preferred over hydroxocobalamin due to reports of antibody formation to the hydroxocobalamin-transcobalamin complex

Dosage Forms Injection, solution: 1000 mcg/mL (30 mL)

♦ **Hydroxy-1,4-naphthoquinone** *see* Atovaquone *on page 141*

Hydroxychloroquine (hye droks ee KLOR oh kwin)

U.S. Brand Names Plaquenil®

Therapeutic Category Antimalarial Agent; Antirheumatic, Disease Modifying

Generic Available Yes

Use Suppression or chemoprophylaxis of malaria caused by susceptible *P. vivax, P. ovale, P. malariae,* and some strains of *P. falciparum* (not active against pre-erythrocytic or exoerythrocytic tissue stages of *Plasmodium*); treatment of systemic lupus erythematosus (SLE) and rheumatoid arthritis

Pregnancy Risk Factor C

Contraindications Hypersensitivity to hydroxychloroquine, 4-aminoquinoline derivatives, or any component; retinal or visual field changes; patients with porphyria or psoriasis

Warnings Long-term use in children is **not** recommended; daily dose >6-6.5 mg/kg/day in patients with abnormal hepatic or renal function may be associated with an increased risk of retinal toxicity

Precautions Use with caution in patients with hepatic disease and G-6-PD deficiency

Adverse Reactions

Cardiovascular: Cardiomyopathy (rare)

Central nervous system: Insomnia, nervousness, nightmares, dizziness, psychosis, headache, confusion, agitation, ataxia

Dermatologic: Lichenoid dermatitis, bleaching of the hair, pruritus, alopecia, hyperpigmentation, photosensitivity, Stevens-Johnson syndrome, exfoliative dermatitis

Gastrointestinal: GI irritation, abdominal cramps, anorexia, nausea, vomiting, diarrhea

Hematologic: Bone marrow suppression, thrombocytopenia, aplastic anemia, agranulocytosis

Hepatic: Hepatic failure

Neuromuscular & skeletal: Muscle weakness, skeletal muscle palsies, neuromyopathy, depression of tendon reflexes, peripheral neuropathy

Ocular: Visual field defects, blindness, retinitis, macular degeneration, decreased night vision

Drug Interactions Increases digoxin serum levels

Food Interactions Food increases bioavailability

Stability Protect from light

Mechanism of Action Interferes with digestive vacuole function within sensitive malarial parasites by increasing the pH and interfering with lysosomal degradation of hemoglobin; inhibits locomotion of neutrophils and chemotaxis of eosinophils; impairs complement-dependent antigen-antibody reactions

Pharmacodynamics Onset of action for JRA: 2-4 months, up to 6 months

Pharmacokinetics

Absorption: Highly variable (31% to 100%)

Distribution: Extensive distribution to most body fluids and tissues; excreted into breast milk; crosses the placenta

Metabolism: In the liver

Bioavailability: Increased when administered with food

Elimination: Metabolites and unchanged drug slowly excreted in the urine

Usual Dosage Oral:

Children:

Chemoprophylaxis of malaria: 5 mg/kg **(base)** once weekly; do not exceed the recommended adult dose; begin 1-2 weeks before exposure; continue for 4 weeks after leaving endemic area

Uncomplicated acute attack of malaria: 10 mg/kg **(base)** initial dose; followed by 5 mg/kg **(base)** in 6-8 hours on day 1; 5 mg/kg **(base)** as a single dose on day 2 and on day 3

JRA or SLE: 3-5 mg/kg/day **(as sulfate)** divided 1-2 times/day to a maximum of 400 mg/day **(as sulfate)**; not to exceed 7 mg/kg/day

Adults:

Chemoprophylaxis of malaria: 310 mg **(base)** once weekly on same day each week; begin 1-2 weeks before exposure; continue for 4 weeks after leaving endemic area

Uncomplicated acute attack of malaria: 620 mg **(base)** first dose day one; 310 mg **(base)** in 6-8 hours day one; 310 mg **(base)** as a single dose day 2; and 310 mg **(base)** as a single dose on day 3

Rheumatoid arthritis: 400-600 mg/day **(as sulfate)** once daily to start; increase dose until optimum response level is reached; usually after 4-12 weeks dose should be reduced by 50% and a maintenance dose given of 200-400 mg/day **(as sulfate)** divided 1-2 times/day

(Continued)

Hydroxychloroquine *(Continued)*

Lupus erythematosus: 400 mg **(as sulfate)** every day or twice daily for several weeks depending on response; 200-400 mg/day **(as sulfate)** for prolonged maintenance therapy

Administration Oral: Administer with food or milk to decrease GI distress

Monitoring Parameters Ophthalmologic examination, CBC with differential and platelet count; check for muscular weakness with prolonged therapy

Patient Information May cause photosensitivity reactions (eg, exposure to sunlight may cause severe sunburn, skin rash, redness, or itching); avoid exposure to sunlight and artificial light sources (sunlamps, tanning booth/bed); wear protective clothing, wide-brimmed hats, sunglasses, and lip sunscreen (SPF ≥15); use a sunscreen [broad-spectrum sunscreen or physical sunscreen (preferred) or sunblock with SPF ≥15]; contact physician if reaction occurs. Notify physician if blurring of vision, vision change, or emotional change occur; may cause dizziness and vision changes, so exercise caution when driving; avoid alcohol; contraindicated during breast-feeding

Dosage Forms Tablet, film coated, as sulfate: 200 mg [equivalent to base 155 mg]

Extemporaneous Preparations A 25 mg/mL hydroxychloroquine sulfate suspension is made by removing the coating off of fifteen 200 mg hydroxychloroquine sulfate tablets with a towel moistened with alcohol; tablets are ground to a fine powder and levigated to a paste with 15 mL of Ora-Plus® suspending agent; add an additional 45 mL of suspending agent and levigate until a uniform mixture is obtained; qs ad to 120 mL with sterile water for irrigation; a 30 day expiration date is recommended, although stability testing has not been performed

Pesko LJ, "Compounding: Hydroxychloroquine," *Am Druggist*, 1993, 207:57.

References
Emery H, "Clinical Aspects of Systemic Lupus Erythematosus in Childhood," *Pediatr Clin North Am*, 1986, 33(5):1177-90.

Giannini EH and Cawkwell GD, "Drug Treatment in Children With Juvenile Rheumatoid Arthritis. Past, Present, and Future," *Pediatr Clin North Am*, 1995, 42(5):1099-125.

"Guidelines for the Management of Rheumatoid Arthritis. American College of Rheumatology Ad Hoc Committee on Clinical Guidelines," *Arthritis Rheum*, 1996, 39(5):713-22.

♦ **Hydroxydaunomycin** *see* DOXOrubicin *on page 413*
♦ **Hydroxyethyl Starch** *see* Hetastarch *on page 561*
♦ **Hydroxynorephedrine** *see* Metaraminol *on page 728*

Hydroxyurea *(hye droks ee yoor EE a)*

Related Information

Adult and Adolescent HIV *on page 1327*
Emetogenic Potential of Single Chemotherapeutic Agents *on page 1286*

U.S. Brand Names Droxia™; Hydrea®; Mylocel™

Canadian Brand Names Gen-Hydroxyurea

Therapeutic Category Antineoplastic Agent, Miscellaneous

Generic Available Yes

Use Treatment of chronic myelocytic leukemia (CML), melanoma, and ovarian carcinoma; used with radiation in treatment of tumors of the head and neck; adjunct in the management of sickle cell patients who have had at least three painful crises in the previous 12 months; combination therapy with didanosine for treatment of HIV infection

Pregnancy Risk Factor D

Contraindications Hypersensitivity to hydroxyurea or any component; severe anemia, severe bone marrow suppression; WBC <2500/mm^3 or platelet count <100,000/mm^3

Warnings The FDA currently recommends that procedures for proper handling and disposal of antineoplastic agents be considered; hydroxyurea is presumed to be a human carcinogen; secondary leukemia and skin cancer have been reported in patients receiving long-term hydroxyurea therapy. Hydroxyurea is embryotoxic and causes fetal malformations.

Precautions Use with caution and modify dose in patients with renal impairment

Adverse Reactions

Central nervous system: Dizziness, disorientation, hallucinations, drowsiness, seizures, headache, fever, chills

Dermatologic: Maculopapular rash, facial erythema, thinning of the skin, pruritus, hyperpigmentation

Endocrine & metabolic: Hyperuricemia

Gastrointestinal: Nausea, vomiting, diarrhea, constipation, anorexia, stomatitis, pancreatitis

Genitourinary: Dysuria

Hematologic: Myelosuppression (leukopenia, thrombocytopenia), megaloblastic anemia

Hepatic: Elevated hepatic enzymes

Renal: Renal tubular function impairment, elevated BUN, elevated serum creatinine

Drug Interactions Fluorouracil, cytarabine (increases cytarabine activity); didanosine (may potentiate intracellular toxicity of didanosine and precipitate didanosine-induced pancreatitis)

Stability Store in a tightly sealed container since the drug is degraded by moisture; store at room temperature

Mechanism of Action Interferes with synthesis of DNA during the S-phase of cell division without interfering with RNA synthesis; inhibits ribonucleoside diphosphate reductase preventing conversion of ribonucleotides to deoxyribonucleotides; hydroxyurea also inhibits the incorporation of thymidine into DNA; in sickle cell patients, hydroxyurea increases the production of fetal hemoglobin

Pharmacodynamics Maximum effect for sickle cell disease: 6-18 months

Pharmacokinetics

Absorption: Readily from the GI tract

Distribution: Readily crosses the blood-brain barrier and the placenta; distributes into peritoneal or pleural effusions; excreted in breast milk

Metabolism: In the liver

Half-life: 3-4 hours

Time to peak serum concentration: Within 2 hours

Elimination: 50% of drug excreted unchanged in urine; renal excretion of urea (metabolite) and respiratory excretion of CO_2 (metabolic end product)

Usual Dosage Oral (refer to individual protocols): Base dosage on ideal body weight:

Children:

Treatment of pediatric astrocytoma, medulloblastoma, and primitive neuroectodermal tumors: No FDA approved dosage regimens have been established. Dosages of 1500-3000 mg/m² as a single dose in combination with other agents, followed by a second course 2 weeks later with subsequent courses every 4-6 weeks have been used (eight-in-one regimen).

CML: Initial: 10-20 mg/kg/day once daily; adjust dose according to hematologic response

Children and Adults: Sickle cell anemia: Initial dose: 15 mg/kg/day (range: 10-20 mg/kg/day) once daily; increase dose in increments of 5 mg/kg/day every 12 weeks to a maximum dose of 35 mg/kg/day; reduced dosage of hydroxyurea alternating with erythropoietin may decrease myelotoxicity and increase levels of fetal hemoglobin in patients who have not been helped by hydroxyurea alone

Adults:

Solid tumors:

Intermittent therapy: 80 mg/kg as a single dose every third day

Continuous therapy: 20-30 mg/kg/day given as a single dose/day

Concomitant therapy with irradiation: 80 mg/kg as a single dose every third day starting at least 7 days before initiation of irradiation

Resistant chronic myelocytic leukemia: 20-30 mg/kg/day once daily

HIV infection: 500 mg twice daily (15 mg/kg/day divided twice daily) in combination with didanosine 200 mg twice daily (**Note:** HIV Adult and Adolescent guidelines state that there is insufficient data to make a recommendation for or against its use; see February 4, 2002, http://www.aidsinfo.nih.gov)

Dosing adjustment in renal impairment: Dose should be reduced 50% in patients with a GFR <10 mL/minute

Administration Oral: Administer with water on an empty stomach; for patients unable to swallow capsules, contents of capsule may be emptied into a glass of water if administered immediately

Monitoring Parameters CBC with differential and platelet count, hemoglobin, renal function and liver function tests, serum uric acid

Test Interactions False-negative triglyceride measurement by a glycerol oxidase method

Patient Information Inform physician if fever, sore throat, bruising, or bleeding develops; advise women of childbearing potential to avoid becoming pregnant while taking hydroxyurea

Additional Information Myelosuppressive effects:

WBC: Moderate

Platelets: Moderate

Onset (days): 7

Nadir (days): 10

Recovery (days): 21

Dosage Forms

Capsule: 500 mg

Droxia™: 200 mg, 300 mg, 400 mg

Hydrea®: 500 mg

(Continued)

Hydroxyurea *(Continued)*

Tablet, scored (Mylocel™): 1000 mg

References

Geyer JR, Finlay JL, Boyett JM, et al, "Survival of Infants With Malignant Astrocytomas. A Report From the Childrens Cancer Group," *Cancer*, 1995, 75(4):1045-50.

Geyer JR, Pendergrass TW, Milstein JM, et al, "Eight Drugs in One Day Chemotherapy in Children With Brain Tumors: A Critical Toxicity Appraisal," *J Clin Oncol*, 1988, 6(6):996-1000.

Maier-Redelsperger M, de Montalembert M, Flahault A, et al, "Fetal Hemoglobin and F-Cell Responses to Long-Term Hydroxyurea Treatment in Young Sickle Cell Patients. The French Study Group on Sickle Cell Disease," *Blood*, 1998, 91(12):4472-9.

Montaner JS, Zala C, Conway B, et al, "A Pilot Study of Hydroxyurea Among Patients With Advanced Human Immunodeficiency Virus (HIV) Disease Receiving Chronic Didanosine Therapy: Canadian HIV Trials Network Protocol 080," *J Infect Dis*, 1997, 175(4):801-6.

Panel on Clinical Practices for the Treatment of HIV Infection, "Guidelines for the Use of Antiretroviral Agents in HIV-Infected Adults and Adolescents," February 4, 2002, http://www.aidsinfo.nih.gov.

Rodgers GP, Dover GJ, Noguchi CT, et al, "Hematologic Responses of Patients With Sickle Cell Disease to Treatment With Hydroxyurea," *N Engl J Med*, 1990, 322(15):1037-45.

Rodgers GP, Dover GJ, Uyesaka N, et al, "Augmentation by Erythropoietin of the Fetal-Hemoglobin Response to Hydroxyurea in Sickle Cell Disease," *N Engl J Med*, 1993, 328(2):73-80.

HydrOXYzine *(hye DROKS i zeen)*

Related Information

Carbohydrate and Alcohol Content of Liquid Medications for Use in Patients Receiving Ketogenic Diets *on page 1431*

Compatibility of Medications Mixed in a Syringe *on page 1412*

U.S. Brand Names Atarax®; Vistaril®

Canadian Brand Names Apo®-Hydroxyzine; Novo-Hydroxyzin; PMS-Hydroxyzine

Therapeutic Category Antianxiety Agent; Antiemetic; Antihistamine; Sedative

Generic Available Yes

Use Treatment of anxiety; preoperative sedative; antipruritic; antiemetic

Pregnancy Risk Factor C

Contraindications Hypersensitivity to hydroxyzine or any component (see Warnings)

Warnings Subcutaneous, intra-arterial and I.V. administration **not** recommended since thrombosis and digital gangrene can occur; extravasation can result in sterile abscess and marked tissue induration

Injection may contain benzyl alcohol which may cause allergic reactions in susceptible individuals; syrup may contain sodium benzoate; benzoic acid (benzoate) is a metabolite of benzyl alcohol; large amounts of benzyl alcohol ($\geq$99 mg/kg/day) have been associated with a potentially fatal toxicity ("gasping syndrome") in neonates; the "gasping syndrome" consists of metabolic acidosis, respiratory distress, gasping respirations, CNS dysfunction (including convulsions, intracranial hemorrhage), hypotension and cardiovascular collapse; avoid use of hydroxyzine products containing benzyl alcohol or sodium benzoate in neonates; *in vitro* and animal studies have shown that benzoate displaces bilirubin from protein binding sites

Precautions Use with caution in patients with narrow-angle glaucoma, prostatic hypertrophy, bladder neck obstruction, asthma, or COPD

Adverse Reactions

Cardiovascular: Hypotension

Central nervous system: Drowsiness, dizziness, headache, ataxia

Gastrointestinal: Xerostomia

Genitourinary: Urinary retention

Local: Pain at injection site

Neuromuscular & skeletal: Weakness

Miscellaneous: Anticholinergic effects

Drug Interactions Hydroxyzine may potentiate other CNS depressants, alcohol, or anticholinergics, and can antagonize the vasopressor effects of epinephrine

Stability Protect from light

Mechanism of Action Competes with histamine for H_1-receptor sites on effector cells in the GI tract, blood vessels, and respiratory tract

Pharmacodynamics

Onset of action: Within 15-30 minutes

Duration: 4-6 hours

Usual Dosage

Children:

Oral: 2 mg/kg/day divided every 6-8 hours

I.M.: 0.5-1 mg/kg/dose every 4-6 hours as needed

Adults:

Antiemetic: I.M.: 25-100 mg/dose every 4-6 hours as needed

Anxiety: Oral: 25-100 mg 4 times/day; maximum dose: 600 mg/day

Preoperative sedation:

Oral: 50-100 mg

I.M.: 25-100 mg

Management of pruritus: Oral: 25 mg 3-4 times/day

Administration
Oral: May be administered without regard to food; shake suspension well before use
Parenteral: For I.M. administration in children, injections should be made into the midlateral muscles of the thigh; hydroxyzine has been administered slow I.V. to oncology patients via central venous lines without problems

Monitoring Parameters Relief of symptoms, mental status, blood pressure

Patient Information May cause drowsiness and impair ability to perform activities requiring mental alertness or physical coordination; may cause dry mouth; avoid alcohol

Dosage Forms
Capsule, as pamoate (Vistaril®): 25 mg, 50 mg, 100 mg
Injection, solution, as **hydrochloride**: 25 mg/mL (1 mL); 50 mg/mL (1 mL, 2 mL, 10 mL)
Vistaril®: 50 mg/mL (10 mL) [contains 0.9% benzyl alcohol]
Suspension, oral, as **pamoate** (Vistaril®): 25 mg/5 mL (120 mL, 480 mL) [lemon flavor]
Syrup, as **hydrochloride**: 10 mg/5 mL (120 mL, 480 mL, 4000 mL)
Atarax®: 10 mg/5 mL [contains 0.5% alcohol and sodium benzoate; mint flavor]
Tablet, as **hydrochloride**: 10 mg, 25 mg, 50 mg
Atarax®: 10 mg, 25 mg, 50 mg, 100 mg

References
Berde C, Ablin A, Glazer J, et al, "American Academy of Pediatrics Report of the Subcommittee on Disease-Related Pain in Childhood Cancer," Pediatrics, 1990, 86(5 Pt 2):818-25.

♦ **Hyoscine** see Scopolamine on page 1009

Hyoscyamine (hye oh SYE a meen)

U.S. Brand Names Anaspaz®; Cystospaz®; Cystospaz-M®; Hyosine; Levbid®; Levsin®; Levsinex®; Levsin/SL®; NuLev™; Spacol; Spacol T/S; Symax SL; Symax SR

Therapeutic Category Anticholinergic Agent; Antispasmodic Agent, Gastrointestinal

Generic Available Yes

Use Treatment of GI tract disorders caused by spasm; adjunctive therapy for peptic ulcers and hypermotility disorders of lower urinary tract; infant colic

Pregnancy Risk Factor C

Contraindications Hypersensitivity to hyoscyamine or any component; narrow-angle glaucoma, GI and GU obstruction, paralytic ileus, severe ulcerative colitis, myasthenia gravis

Warnings Low doses may cause a paradoxical decrease in heart rate; heat prostration may occur in hot weather. Some oral liquids contain sodium benzoate; benzoic acid (benzoate) is a metabolite of benzyl alcohol; large amounts of benzyl alcohol (≥99 mg/kg/day) have been associated with a potentially fatal toxicity ("gasping syndrome") in neonates; in vitro and animal studies have shown that benzoate displaces bilirubin from protein binding sites; avoid using products containing sodium benzoate in neonates

Precautions Use with caution in patients with hyperthyroidism, CHF, cardiac arrhythmias, prostatic hypertrophy, autonomic neuropathy, chronic lung disease, biliary tract disease, children with spastic paralysis. Disintegrating tablet (NuLev™) contains aspartame which is metabolized to phenylalanine and must be used with caution in patients with phenylketonuria.

Adverse Reactions
Cardiovascular: Tachycardia or palpitations, bradycardia (with very low doses), orthostatic hypotension
Central nervous system: Headache, lightheadedness, short-term memory loss, fatigue, delirium, restlessness, ataxia, dizziness, insomnia, psychosis, euphoria, nervousness, confusion, insomnia, fever
Dermatologic: Dry skin, photosensitivity, rash, urticaria
Gastrointestinal: Xerostomia, nausea, vomiting, constipation, dysphagia, dysgeusia, dry throat
Genitourinary: Difficult urination, urinary retention
Local: Irritation at injection site
Neuromuscular & skeletal: Weakness, tremor
Ocular: Blurred vision, photophobia, mydriasis, anisocoria, cycloplegia, elevated intraocular pressure
Respiratory: Dry nose
Miscellaneous: Decreased diaphoresis

Drug Interactions Decreased absorption when given with antacids; increased anticholinergic activity with amantadine, antimuscarinics, haloperidol, phenothiazines, tricyclic antidepressants, antihistamines; MAO inhibitors
(Continued)

Hyoscyamine *(Continued)*

Mechanism of Action Blocks the action of acetylcholine at parasympathetic sites in smooth muscle, secretory glands, and the CNS; specific anticholinergic responses are dose-related; increases cardiac output, dries secretions, antagonizes histamine and serotonin

Pharmacodynamics
Onset of action:
Oral: 20-30 minutes
Sublingual: 5-20 minutes
I.V.: 2-3 minutes
Duration: 4-6 hours

Pharmacokinetics
Absorption: Well absorbed from the GI tract
Distribution: Crosses the placenta; small amounts appear in breast milk
Protein binding: 50%
Metabolism: In the liver
Half-life: 3.5 hours
Elimination: 30% to 50% eliminated unchanged in urine within 12 hours

Usual Dosage
GI tract disorders:
Infants <2 years: Oral: The following table lists the hyoscyamine dosage using the drop formulation; hyoscyamine drops are dosed every 4 hours as needed

Hyoscyamine Drops Dosage

Weight (kg)	Dose (drops)	Maximum Daily Dose (drops)
2.3	3	18
3.4	4	24
5	5	30
7	6	36
10	8	48
15	11	66

Oral, S.L.:
Children 2-12 years: 0.0625-0.125 mg every 4 hours as needed; maximum daily dosage 0.75 mg **or** timed release 0.375 mg every 12 hours; maximum daily dosage 0.75 mg
Children >12 years to Adults: 0.125-0.25 mg every 4 hours as needed; maximum daily dosage 1.5 mg **or** timed release 0.375-0.75 mg every 12 hours; maximum daily dosage 1.5 mg
I.V., I.M., S.C.: Children >12 years to Adults: 0.25-0.5 mg at 4-hour intervals for 1-4 doses
Adjunct to anesthesia: I.M., I.V., S.C.: Children >2 years to Adults: 5 mcg/kg given 30-60 minutes prior to induction of anesthesia
Hypermotility of lower urinary tract: Oral, S.L.: Adults: 0.15-0.3 mg four times daily; timed release: 0.375 mg every 12 hours
Reversal of neuromuscular blockage: I.V., I.M., S.C.: 0.2 mg for every 1 mg neostigmine or equivalent dose of physostigmine

Administration
Oral: Administer before meals; timed release tablets are scored and may be cut for easier dosage titration; S.L.: Place under the tongue
Parenteral: May be administered I.M., I.V., and S.C.; no information is available for I.V. administration rate or dilution

Monitoring Parameters Pulse, anticholinergic effects, urine output, GI symptoms

Patient Information May cause dry mouth; maintain good oral hygiene habits, because lack of saliva may increase chance of cavities; notify physician if skin rash, flushing or eye pain occurs, or if difficulty in urinating, constipation, or sensitivity to light becomes severe or persists; may cause dizziness or blurred vision; may cause drowsiness and impair ability to perform activities requiring mental alertness or physical coordination. May rarely cause photosensitivity reactions (eg, exposure to sunlight may cause severe sunburn, skin rash, redness, or itching); avoid direct exposure to sunlight

Dosage Forms
Capsule, timed release, as sulfate (Cystospaz-M®, Levsinex®): 0.375 mg
Elixir, as sulfate: 0.125 mg/5 mL (480 mL)

Hyosine: 0.125 mg/5 mL (480 mL) [contains 20% alcohol and sodium benzoate; orange flavor]

Levsin®: 0.125 mg/5 mL (480 mL) [contains 20% alcohol; orange flavor]

Injection, solution, as sulfate (Levsin®): 0.5 mg/mL (1 mL)

Liquid, as sulfate (Spacol): 0.125 mg/5 mL (120 mL) [alcohol and sugar free; simethicone-based; bubblegum flavor]

Solution, oral drops, as sulfate: 0.125 mg/mL (15 mL)

Hyosine: 0.125 mg/5 mL (15 mL) [contains 5% alcohol and sodium benzoate; orange flavor]

Levsin®: 0.125 mg/5 mL (15 mL) [contains 5% alcohol; orange flavor]

Tablet (Cystospaz®): 0.15 mg

Tablet, as sulfate: (Anaspaz®, Levsin®, Spacol) 0.125 mg

Tablet, extended release, as sulfate (Levbid®, Spacol T/S, Symax SR): 0.375 mg

Tablet, orally disintegrating, as sulfate (NuLev™): 0.125 mg [contains 1.7 mg phenylalanine (as aspartame)/tablet; mint flavor]

Tablet, sublingual, as sulfate: 0.125 mg

Levsin/SL®: 0.125 mg [peppermint flavor]

Symax SL: 0.125 mg

Hyoscyamine, Atropine, Scopolamine, and Phenobarbital

(hye oh SYE a meen, A troe peen, skoe POL a meen & fee noe BAR bi tal)

U.S. Brand Names Donnatal®; Donnatal Extentabs®

Synonyms Atropine, Hyoscyamine, Scopolamine, and Phenobarbital; Phenobarbital, Hyoscyamine, Atropine, and Scopolamine; Scopolamine, Hyoscyamine, Atropine, and Phenobarbital

Therapeutic Category Anticholinergic Agent; Antispasmodic Agent, Gastrointestinal

Generic Available No

Use Adjunct in treatment of peptic ulcer disease, irritable bowel, spastic colitis, spastic bladder, and renal colic

Pregnancy Risk Factor C

Contraindications Hypersensitivity to hyoscyamine, atropine, scopolamine, phenobarbital, or any component of the formulation; narrow-angle glaucoma; tachycardia; GI and GU obstruction; myasthenia gravis; paralytic ileus; intestinal atony; unstable cardiovascular status in acute hemorrhage; severe ulcerative colitis; hiatal hernia associated with reflux esophagitis; acute intermittent porphyria

Warnings Heat prostration can occur in the presence of high environmental temperature

Precautions Use with caution in patients with hepatic or renal disease, hyperthyroidism, CAD, CHF, cardiac arrhythmias, tachycardia, hypertension, autonomic neuropathy

Adverse Reactions

Cardiovascular: Tachycardia, palpitations, bradycardia (with very low doses of atropine)

Central nervous system: Headache, drowsiness, nervousness, confusion, insomnia, fever, dizziness

Gastrointestinal: Xerostomia, nausea, vomiting, constipation, dysphagia, paralytic ileus, dysgeusia

Genitourinary: Impotence, urinary retention

Neuromuscular & skeletal: Weakness, musculoskeletal pain

Ocular: Blurred vision, photophobia, mydriasis, cycloplegia, elevated intraocular pressure

Respiratory: Nasal congestion

Miscellaneous: Hypersensitivity reactions, decreased diaphoresis

Drug Interactions Phenobarbital: Cytochrome P450 isoenzyme substrate CYP2C8/9, CYP2C19, CYP2E1; inducer CYP1A2, CYP2A6, CYP2B6, CYP2C8/9, CYP3A4 (see Phenobarbital monograph for complete drug interaction profile)

Additive CNS depression with CNS depressants, antihistamines, phenothiazines, tricyclic antidepressants; additive anticholinergic activity with antihistamines, phenothiazines, amantadine

Mechanism of Action Anticholinergic agents (hyoscyamine, atropine, and scopolamine) inhibit the muscarinic actions of acetylcholine at the postganglionic parasympathetic neuroeffector sites including smooth muscle, secretory glands, and CNS sites; specific anticholinergic responses are dose-related

Pharmacokinetics Absorption: Well absorbed from the GI tract

Usual Dosage Oral:

Children: Donnatal®: 0.1 mL/kg/dose every 4 hours; maximum dose: 5 mL **or** see table on next page for alternative.

Adults: Donnatal®: 1-2 tablets or capsules 3-4 times/day **or** 5-10 mL 3-4 times/day or 1 extended release tablet every 12 hours (may increase to every 8 hours if needed)

(Continued)

Hyoscyamine, Atropine, Scopolamine, and Phenobarbital
(Continued)

Donnatal® Dosage

Weight (kg)	Dose (mL)	
	Every 4 Hours	Every 6 Hours
4.5	0.5	0.75
10	1	1.5
14	1.5	2
23	2.5	3.8
34	3.8	5
≥45	5	7.5

Administration Oral: Administer 30-60 minutes before meals; do not crush or chew extended release tablets

Patient Information Maintain good oral hygiene habits because lack of saliva may increase chance of cavities; may cause dry mouth; notify physician if skin rash, flushing or eye pain occurs, or if difficulty in urinating, constipation, or sensitivity to light becomes severe or persists; observe caution while driving or performing other tasks requiring alertness, as may cause drowsiness, dizziness, or blurred vision

Dosage Forms

Elixir (Donnatal®): Hyoscyamine sulfate 0.1037 mg, atropine sulfate 0.0194 mg, scopolamine hydrobromide 0.0065 mg, and phenobarbital 16.2 mg per 5 mL (120 mL, 480 mL, 4000 mL) [contains 23% alcohol; citrus flavor]

Tablet (Donnatal®): Hyoscyamine sulfate 0.1037 mg, atropine sulfate 0.0194 mg, scopolamine hydrobromide 0.0065 mg, and phenobarbital 16.2 mg

Tablet, extended release (Donnatal Extentabs®): Hyoscyamine sulfate 0.3111 mg, atropine sulfate 0.0582 mg, scopolamine hydrobromide 0.0195 mg, and phenobarbital 48.6 mg

- ♦ **Hyosine** *see* Hyoscyamine *on page 585*
- ♦ **Hyperstat®** *see* Diazoxide *on page 372*
- ♦ **Hypotears® [OTC]** *see* Ocular Lubricant *on page 831*
- ♦ **Hyrexin-50® Injection** *see* DiphenhydrAMINE *on page 393*
- ♦ **Hytakerol®** *see* Dihydrotachysterol *on page 387*
- ♦ **Hytinic® [OTC]** *see* Iron Supplements (Oral/Enteral) *on page 623*
- ♦ **Hytone®** *see* Hydrocortisone *on page 573*
- ♦ **Hytuss® [OTC]** *see* Guaifenesin *on page 550*
- ♦ **Hytuss-2X® [OTC]** *see* Guaifenesin *on page 550*
- ♦ **Ibenzmethyzin** *see* Procarbazine *on page 937*
- ♦ **Ibidomide** *see* Labetalol *on page 645*

Ibuprofen (eye byoo PROE fen)

Related Information

Carbohydrate and Alcohol Content of Liquid Medications for Use in Patients Receiving Ketogenic Diets *on page 1431*

Overdose and Toxicology *on page 1388*

U.S. Brand Names Advil® [OTC]; Advil®, Children's [OTC]; Advil®, Infants' Concentrated Drops [OTC]; Advil®, Junior [OTC]; Advil® Migraine [OTC]; Genpril® [OTC]; Haltran® [OTC]; Ibu-Tab®; I-Prin [OTC]; Menadol® [OTC]; Midol® Maximum Strength Cramp Formula [OTC]; Motrin®; Motrin®, Children's [OTC]; Motrin® IB [OTC]; Motrin®, Infants' [OTC]; Motrin®, Junior Strength [OTC]; Motrin® Migraine Pain [OTC]

Canadian Brand Names Apo®-Ibuprofen; Novo-Profen®; Nu-Ibuprofen

Synonyms *p*-Isobutylhydratropic Acid

Therapeutic Category Analgesic, Non-narcotic; Anti-inflammatory Agent; Antipyretic; Nonsteroidal Anti-inflammatory Drug (NSAID), Oral

Generic Available Yes

Use Treatment of inflammatory diseases and rheumatoid disorders including juvenile rheumatoid arthritis (JRA); mild to moderate pain; migraine pain; fever; dysmenorrhea; gout

Pregnancy Risk Factor B (D if used in the 3rd trimester)

Contraindications Hypersensitivity to ibuprofen, any component (see Warnings); aspirin, or other NSAIDs; active GI bleeding, ulcer disease; patients with the "aspirin triad" [asthma, rhinitis (with or without nasal polyps), and aspirin intolerance] (fatal asthmatic and anaphylactoid reactions may occur in these patients)

Warnings Junior Strength Motrin® caplets contain tartrazine and Motrin® IB gelcaps contain benzyl alcohol, both of which may cause allergic reactions in susceptible individuals. Some products contain sodium benzoate (see Dosage Forms); benzoate is a metabolite of benzyl alcohol; large amounts of benzyl alcohol (≥99 mg/kg/day) have been associated with a potentially fatal toxicity ("gasping syndrome") in neonates; the "gasping syndrome" consists of metabolic acidosis, respiratory distress, gasping respirations, CNS dysfunction (including convulsions, intracranial hemorrhage), hypotension and cardiovascular collapse; avoid use of ibuprofen products containing benzyl alcohol or sodium benzoate in neonates; *in vitro* and animal studies have shown that benzoate displaces bilirubin from protein binding sites

Precautions Use with caution in patients with CHF, hypertension, decreased renal or hepatic function, dehydration, history of GI disease (bleeding or ulcers), or those receiving anticoagulants; chewable tablets contain phenylalanine which must be avoided (or used with caution) in patients with phenylketonuria.

Adverse Reactions
Cardiovascular: Edema
Central nervous system: Dizziness, drowsiness, fatigue, headache
Dermatologic: Rash, urticaria
Gastrointestinal: Dyspepsia, heartburn, nausea, vomiting, abdominal pain, peptic ulcer, GI bleed, GI perforation
Hematologic: Neutropenia, anemia, agranulocytosis, inhibition of platelet aggregation
Hepatic: Hepatitis
Ocular: Vision changes
Otic: Tinnitus
Renal: Acute renal failure

Drug Interactions Cytochrome P450 isoenzyme CYP2C8 and CYP2C9 substrate

May increase digoxin, methotrexate and lithium serum concentrations; may decrease antihypertensive effects of ACE inhibitors or angiotensin II antagonists (monitor blood pressure); may decrease effects of other antihypertensive agents, furosemide, and thiazides; aspirin may decrease ibuprofen serum concentrations; other GI irritants (eg, NSAIDs, oral potassium) may increase adverse GI effects

Food Interactions Food may decrease the rate but not the extent of oral absorption

Mechanism of Action Inhibits prostaglandin synthesis by decreasing the activity of the enzyme, cyclooxygenase, which results in decreased formation of prostaglandin precursors

Pharmacodynamics
Fever reduction:
Onset of action (single dose 8 mg/kg):
Infants ≤1 year: Mean ± SD: 69 ± 22 minutes
Children ≥6 years: 109 ± 64 minutes
Maximum effect: 2-4 hours
Duration: 6-8 hours (dose-related)

Pharmacokinetics
Absorption: Oral: Rapid (80%)
Protein binding: 90% to 99%
Metabolism: Oxidized in the liver; **Note:** Ibuprofen is a racemic mixture of R and S isomers; the R isomer (thought to be inactive) is slowly and incompletely (~60%) converted to the S isomer (active) in adults; the amount of conversion in children is not known, but it is thought to be similar to adults
Half-life:
Children: 1-2 hours; children 3 months to 10 years: Mean: 1.6 hours
Adults: 2-4 hours
Time to peak serum concentration: Tablets: 2 hours; suspension: 1 hour
Children with cystic fibrosis:
Suspension (n=22): 0.74 ± 0.43 hours (median: 30 minutes)
Chewable tablet (n=4): 1.5 ± 0.58 hours (median: 1.5 hours)
Tablet (n=12): 1.33 ± 0.95 hours (median: 1 hour)
Elimination: ~1% excreted as unchanged drug and 14% as conjugated ibuprofen in urine; 45% to 80% eliminated in urine as metabolites; some biliary excretion

Usual Dosage Oral:
Infants and Children:
Analgesic: 4-10 mg/kg/dose every 6-8 hours
Antipyretic: 6 months to 12 years: Temperature <102.5°F (39°C): 5 mg/kg/dose; temperature ≥102.5°F: 10 mg/kg/dose; give every 6-8 hours; maximum daily dose: 40 mg/kg/day
Juvenile rheumatoid arthritis: 6 months to 12 years: 30-50 mg/kg/day in 4 divided doses; start at lower end of dosing range and titrate; maximum dose: 2.4 g/day
OTC pediatric labeling (analgesic, antipyretic): 6 months to 11 years: 7.5 mg/kg/dose every 6-8 hours; maximum daily dose: 30 mg/kg
(Continued)

Ibuprofen *(Continued)*

Manufacturer's recommendations: See table; use of weight to select dose is preferred; if weight is not available, then use age; doses may be repeated every 6-8 hours; maximum: 4 doses/day

Ibuprofen Dosing

Weight (lbs)	Age	Dosage (mg)
12-17	6-11 mo	50
18-23	12-23 mo	75
24-35	2-3 y	100
35-47	4-5 y	150
48-59	6-8 y	200
60-71	9-10 y	250
72-95	11 y	300

Cystic fibrosis: Ibuprofen when taken chronically (for 4 years) in doses to achieve peak plasma concentrations of 50-100 mcg/mL has been shown to slow the progression of lung disease in mild cystic fibrosis patients >5 years of age, and especially in patients who started therapy when <13 years of age. Doses administered twice daily ranged from 16.2-31.6 mg/kg/dose with 90% of patients requiring 20-30 mg/kg/dose (mean dose: ~25 mg/kg/dose), but individual patient's dose requirements were not predictable. Patients did not take pancreatic enzymes nor eat for 2 hours after the dose (Konstan, 1995). In children with cystic fibrosis, an initial ibuprofen pharmacokinetic analyses is recommended using tablet doses of 20-30 mg/kg to optimize concentrations in the therapeutic range; blood sampling is recommended at 1, 2, and 3 hours postdose. A recent pharmacokinetic study in children with cystic fibrosis demonstrated that ibuprofen oral suspension also delivers therapeutic plasma concentrations; this study recommends using a 20 mg/kg dose of ibuprofen suspension for the initial pharmacokinetic analyses and obtaining blood samples at 30, 45, and 60 minutes postdose (Scott, 1999); further studies are needed

Adolescents and Adults:

Inflammatory disease: 400-800 mg/dose 3-4 times/day; maximum dose: 3.2 g/day

Pain/fever/dysmenorrhea: 200-400 mg/dose every 4-6 hours; maximum daily dose: 1.2 g

Administration Oral: Administer with food or milk to decrease GI upset; shake suspension well before use

Monitoring Parameters CBC, occult blood loss, liver enzymes; urine output, serum BUN, and creatinine in patients receiving diuretics, those with decreased renal function, or in patients on chronic therapy; patients receiving long-term therapy for JRA should receive periodic ophthalmological exams

Reference Range Plasma concentrations >200 µg/mL may be associated with severe toxicity; cystic fibrosis: therapeutic peak plasma concentration: 50-100 mcg/mL

Patient Information Avoid alcohol; may cause dizziness or drowsiness and impair ability to perform activities requiring mental alertness or physical coordination; notify physician if changes in vision occur

OTC (pediatrics): Do not administer to children for >3 days unless recommended by physician or other health care professional; notify physician if child's condition does not improve or if worsens within 24 hours

Additional Information Nystagmus, dizziness, hypotension, apnea and coma have been reported with overdose.

Note: A study comparing the short-term use of acetaminophen and ibuprofen in 84,192 children (6 months to 12 years of age) found no significant difference in the rates of hospitalization for acute GI bleeding, acute renal failure, anaphylaxis or Reye's syndrome. (Four of 55,785 children in the ibuprofen group and zero of 28,130 children in the acetaminophen group were hospitalized with acute GI bleeding). A low WBC occurred more frequently in the ibuprofen group (8 vs 0) (see Lesko, 1995). A subanalysis of 27,065 children <2 years of age also found no significant difference in the rates of hospitalization. (Three of 17,938 children in the ibuprofen group and zero of 9,127 children in the acetaminophen group were hospitalized with GI bleeding) (see Lesko, 1999).

There is currently no scientific evidence to support alternating acetaminophen with ibuprofen in the treatment of fever (see Mayoral, 2000)

I.V. ibuprofen was shown to be as effective as I.V. indomethacin for the treatment of PDA in preterm infants with RDS; in addition, ibuprofen was significantly less likely to cause oliguria (Van Overmeire, 2000); further studies are needed; **Note:** I.V. ibuprofen is not commercially available in the USA, but has FDA orphan drug status and may be obtained (as ibuprofen lysine) only through a compassionate-use program (sponsored by Farmacon-IL, L.L.C. of Westport, Connecticut)

Dosage Forms

Caplet: 200 mg
   Advil®: 200 mg [contains sodium benzoate]
   Junior Strength Motrin®: 100 mg [contains tartrazine]
   Menadol®, Motrin® IB, Motrin® Migraine Pain: 200 mg

Capsule, liqui-gel:
   Advil®: 200 mg
   Advil® Migraine: 200 mg [solubilized ibuprofen (present as the free acid and potassium salt) equal to 200 mg ibuprofen]

Drops: See Suspension, oral **drops**

Gelcap:
   Advil®: 200 mg
   Motrin® IB: 200 mg [contains benzyl alcohol]

Suspension, oral: 100 mg/5 mL (5 mL, 120 mL, 480 mL)
   Children's Advil®: 100 mg/5 mL (60 mL, 120 mL) [contains sodium benzoate; blue raspberry, fruit, and grape flavors]
   Children's Motrin®: 100 mg/5 mL (60 mL, 120 mL) [contains sodium benzoate; berry, dye-free berry, bubblegum, and grape flavors]

Suspension, oral **drops**:
   Infants' Advil® Concentrated Drops: 40 mg/mL (15 mL) [droppers are marked at 0.625 mL (25 mg), 1.25 mL (50 mg), and 1.875 mL (75 mg); contains sodium benzoate; fruit and grape flavors]
   Infants' Motrin®: 40 mg/mL (15 mL) [droppers are marked at 0.625 mL (25 mg) and 1.25 mL (50 mg); alcohol free; contains sodium benzoate; berry and dye-free berry flavors]

Tablet: 200 mg [OTC], 400 mg, 600 mg, 800 mg
   Advil®: 200 mg [contains sodium benzoate]
   Genpril®, Haltran®, I-Prin, Midol® Maximum Strength Cramp Formula, Motrin® IB: 200 mg
   Ibu-Tab®, Motrin®: 400 mg, 600 mg, 800 mg

Tablet, chewable:
   Children's Advil®: 50 mg [contains 2.1 mg phenylalanine (as aspartame); fruit and grape flavors]
   Junior Advil®: 100 mg [contains 2.1 mg phenylalanine (as aspartame); fruit and grape flavors]
   Children's Motrin®: 50 mg [contains 1.4 mg phenylalanine (as aspartame); orange flavor]
   Junior Strength Motrin®: 100 mg [contains 2.8 mg phenylalanine (as aspartame); grape and orange flavors]

Tablet, coated (Junior Strength Advil®): 100 mg [contains sodium benzoate]

References
Berde C, Ablin A, Glazer J, et al, "American Academy of Pediatrics Report of the Subcommittee on Disease-Related Pain in Childhood Cancer," *Pediatrics*, 1990, 86(5 Pt 2):818-25.
Brewer EJ, "Nonsteroidal Anti-inflammatory Agents," *Arthritis Rheum*, 1977, 20(2):513-25.
Kauffman RE and Nelson MV, "Effect of Age on Ibuprofen Pharmacokinetics and Antipyretic Response," *J Pediatr*, 1992, 121(6):969-73.
Konstan MW, Byard PJ, Hoppel CL, et al, "Effect of High-Dose Ibuprofen in Patients With Cystic Fibrosis," *N Engl J Med*, 1995, 332(13):848-54.
Lesko SM and Mitchell AA, "An Assessment of the Safety of Pediatric Ibuprofen. A Practitioner-Based Randomized Clinical Trial," *JAMA*, 1995, 273(12):929-33.
Lesko SM and Mitchell A, "The Safety of Acetaminophen and Ibuprofen Among Children Younger Than Two Years Old," *Pediatrics*, 1999, 104(4), http://www.pediatrics.org/cgi/content/full/104/4/e39.
Mayoral CE, Marino RV, Rosenfeld, W, et al, "Alternating Antipyretics: Is This an Alternative?" *Pediatrics*, 2000, 105(5):1009-12.
Scott CS, Retsch-Bogart GZ, Kustra RP, et al, "The Pharmacokinetics of Ibuprofen Suspension, Chewable Tablets, and Tablets in Children With Cystic Fibrosis," *J Pediatr*, 1999, 134(1):58-63.
Van Overmeire B, Smets K, Lecoutere D, et al, "A Comparison of Ibuprofen and Indomethacin for Closure of Patent Ductus Arteriosus," *N Engl J Med*, 2000, 343(10):674-81.

♦ **Ibu-Tab®** *see* Ibuprofen *on page 588*
♦ **ICN-1299** *see* Ribavirin *on page 981*
♦ **IDA** *see* Idarubicin *on page 591*
♦ **Idamycin PFS®** *see* Idarubicin *on page 591*

Idarubicin (eye da ROO bi sin)

Related Information
   Emetogenic Potential of Single Chemotherapeutic Agents *on page 1286*
U.S. Brand Names Idamycin PFS®
Synonyms 4-Demethoxydaunorubicin; 4-DMDR; IDA
   (Continued)

Idarubicin *(Continued)*

Therapeutic Category Antineoplastic Agent, Anthracycline; Antineoplastic Agent, Antibiotic

Generic Available Yes

Use Used in combination with other antineoplastic agents for treatment of acute leukemias (AML, ANLL, ALL)

Pregnancy Risk Factor D

Contraindications Hypersensitivity to idarubicin or any component; patients with pre-existing bone marrow suppression unless the benefit warrants the risk; severe CHF, cardiomyopathy, or arrhythmias; pregnancy

Warnings The FDA currently recommends that procedures for proper handling and disposal of antineoplastic agents be considered; I.V. use only, severe local tissue necrosis will result if extravasation occurs; pre-existing heart disease, chest radiation, and previous therapy with anthracyclines at high cumulative doses increase risk of idarubicin-induced cardiac toxicity (manifested by potentially fatal CHF, life-threatening arrhythmias, or cardiomyopathies); the maximum lifetime anthracycline dose for idarubicin is approximately 137.5 mg/m^2; severe myelosuppression occurs in all patients given a therapeutic dose and is the dose-limiting adverse effect associated with idarubicin

Precautions Use with caution and reduce dose in patients with impaired hepatic or renal function and patients receiving concurrent radiation therapy

Adverse Reactions
Cardiovascular: Arrhythmias, EKG changes, cardiomyopathy, CHF
Dermatologic: Alopecia, rash, urticaria
Endocrine & metabolic: Hyperuricemia
Gastrointestinal: Nausea, vomiting, diarrhea, stomatitis, anorexia, mucositis
Genitourinary: Discoloration of urine (pink or red)
Hematologic: Leukopenia (nadir: 8-29 days), thrombocytopenia (nadir: 10-15 days), anemia
Hepatic: Elevated liver enzymes or bilirubin
Local: Tissue necrosis upon extravasation, erythematous streaking
Miscellaneous: Anaphylaxis

Stability Store vials under refrigeration and protect from light; incompatible with acyclovir, ceftazidime, furosemide, hydrocortisone, sodium bicarbonate and heparin; inactivated by alkaline solutions

Mechanism of Action Intercalates with DNA causing strand breakage and affects topoisomerase II activity resulting in inhibition of chain elongation and inhibition of DNA and RNA synthesis

Pharmacokinetics
Distribution:
V_d: Large volume of distribution due to extensive tissue binding; distributes into CSF
V_{dss}: 1700 L/m^2
Protein binding:
Idarubicin: 97%
Idarubicinol: 94%
Metabolism: In the liver to idarubicinol (active metabolite)
Half-life:
Children: 18.7 hours (range: 2.5-22.4 hours)
Adults: 19 hours (range: 10.5-34.7 hours)
Idarubicinol: 45-56.8 hours
Elimination: Primarily by biliary excretion; 2.3% to 6.5% of a dose is eliminated renally

Usual Dosage I.V. (refer to individual protocols):
Children:
Leukemia: 10-12 mg/m^2 once daily for 3 days of treatment course
Solid tumors: 5 mg/m^2 once daily for 3 days of treatment course
Adults: 8-12 mg/m^2 once daily for 3 days of treatment course in combination with Ara-C; reduce dose by 25% if severe mucositis is present
Dosing adjustment in hepatic and/or renal impairment:
Serum creatinine ≥2 mg/dL: Reduce dose by 25%
Bilirubin >2.5 mg/dL: Reduce dose by 50%
Bilirubin >5 mg/dL: **Do not administer**

Administration Do not administer I.M. or S.C.
Parenteral: I.V.: Administer by I.V. intermittent infusion over 10-30 minutes into a free flowing I.V. solution of NS or D$_5$W; administer at a final concentration of 1 mg/mL

Monitoring Parameters CBC with differential, platelet count, ECHO, EKG, serum electrolytes, creatinine, uric acid, ALT, AST, bilirubin, signs of extravasation

Patient Information Notify physician if fever, sore throat, bleeding, bruising, or pain at infusion site occurs. Urine may turn pink or red. Contraceptive measures are recommended during therapy.

Nursing Implications Maintain adequate patient hydration; local erythematous streaking along the vein may indicate too rapid a rate of administration; care should be taken to avoid extravasation; if extravasation occurs, the manufacturer recommends that the affected extremity be elevated and that topical ice packs be placed over the affected area immediately for 30 minutes, then apply for 30 minutes 4 times/day for 3 days; alternative therapy includes topical application of dimethylsulfoxide

Dosage Forms Injection, solution, as hydrochloride [preservative free] (Idamycin PFS®): 1 mg/mL (5 mL, 10 mL, 20 mL)

References

Dinndorf PA, Avramis VI, Wiersma S, et al, "Phase I/II Study of Idarubicin Given With Continuous Infusion Fludarabine Followed by Continuous Infusion Cytarabine in Children With Acute Leukemia: A Report From the Children's Cancer Group," *J Clin Oncol*, 1997, 15(8):2780-5.

Leahey A, Kelly K, Rorke LB, et al, "A Phase I/II Study of Idarubicin (Ida) With Continuous Infusion Fludarabine (F-ara-A) and Cytarabine (ara-C) for Refractory or Recurrent Pediatric Acute Myeloid Leukemia (AML)," *J Pediatr Hematol Oncol*, 1997, 19(4):304-8.

Reid JM, Pendergrass TW, Krailo MD, et al, "Plasma Pharmacokinetics and Cerebrospinal Fluid Concentrations of Idarubicin and Idarubicinol in Pediatric Leukemia Patients: A Children's Cancer Study Group Report," *Cancer Res*, 1990, 50(20):6525-8.

- **Ifex®** *see* Ifosfamide *on page 593*
- **IFLrA** *see* Interferon Alfa-2a *on page 614*
- **IFN** *see* Interferon Alfa-2a *on page 614*
- **IFN-α-2** *see* Interferon Alfa-2b *on page 616*

Ifosfamide (eye FOSS fa mide)

Related Information

Emetogenic Potential of Single Chemotherapeutic Agents *on page 1286*

U.S. Brand Names Ifex®

Therapeutic Category Antineoplastic Agent, Alkylating Agent

Generic Available Yes

Use In combination with other antineoplastics in treatment of lung cancer, Hodgkin's and non-Hodgkin's lymphoma, breast cancer, acute and chronic lymphocytic leukemia, ovarian cancer, testicular cancer, and sarcomas

Pregnancy Risk Factor D

Contraindications Hypersensitivity to ifosfamide or any component; patients with severely depressed bone marrow function; pregnancy

Warnings The FDA currently recommends that procedures for proper handling and disposal of antineoplastic agents be considered. May require therapy cessation if confusion or coma occurs; monitor for hemorrhagic cystitis and severe myelosuppression; risk factors for ifosfamide-induced nephrotoxicity include previous or concurrent cisplatin therapy, pre-existing renal impairment, prior nephrectomy, children ≤5 years, or patients who have received high cumulative ifosfamide doses of 50 g/m^2

Precautions Use with caution in patients with impaired renal function or those with compromised bone marrow reserve

Adverse Reactions

Cardiovascular: Cardiotoxicity

Central nervous system: Somnolence, lethargy, confusion, depressive psychoses, hallucinations, dizziness, seizures, fever, ataxia, coma

Dermatologic: Alopecia, hyperpigmentation

Endocrine & metabolic: Metabolic acidosis

Gastrointestinal: Nausea, vomiting, stomatitis, diarrhea

Genitourinary: Dysuria, hemorrhagic cystitis

Hematologic: Myelosuppression (leukocyte nadir: 7-14 days), thrombocytopenia

Hepatic: Elevated liver enzymes and/or bilirubin

Local: Phlebitis

Neuromuscular & skeletal: Polyneuropathy

Renal: Renal tubular acidosis, hematuria, elevated BUN and serum creatinine

Drug Interactions Cytochrome P450 isoenzyme CYP2B6 and CYP3A3/4 substrate

Phenobarbital, phenytoin, chloral hydrate may increase the conversion of ifosfamide to active metabolites and increase toxicity; cisplatin may increase ifosfamide renal damage

Stability Reconstituted solution is stable for 7 days at room temperature and 21 days when refrigerated

Mechanism of Action Causes cross-linking of DNA strands by binding with nucleic acids and other intracellular structures; inhibits protein synthesis and DNA synthesis

Pharmacokinetics Dose-dependent pharmacokinetics:

Distribution: Unchanged ifosfamide penetrates the blood-brain barrier; excreted into breast milk

(Continued)

Ifosfamide *(Continued)*

Metabolism: Requires biotransformation by the cytochrome P450 enzyme system in the liver before it can act as an alkylating agent; following hydroxylation, the metabolite breaks down to acrolein (bladder irritant) and ifosfamide mustard (active drug)

Half-life: Terminal:

Low dose (1800 mg/m^2): 4-7 hours

High dose (3800-5000 mg/m^2): 11-15 hours

Elimination: 60% to 80% of a dose is excreted in urine as unchanged drug and metabolites

Usual Dosage I.V. (refer to individual protocols):

Children: 1200-1800 mg/m^2/day for 5 days every 21-28 days or 5000 mg/m^2 as a single 24-hour infusion or 3 g/m^2/day for 2 days

Adults: 700-2000 mg/m^2/day for 5 days or 2400 mg/m^2/day for 3 days every 21-28 days; 5000 mg/m^2 as a single dose over 24 hours

Administration Parenteral: Administer as a slow I.V. intermittent infusion over at least 30 minutes at a final concentration for administration not to exceed 40 mg/mL (usual concentration for administration is between 0.6-20 mg/mL), or administer as a 24-hour infusion

Monitoring Parameters CBC with differential and platelet count, urine output, urinalysis, liver function and renal function tests, serum electrolytes

Patient Information Notify physician of pain or irritation in urination, CNS changes, fever, chills, bruising, or bleeding. Contraceptive measure are recommended during therapy.

Nursing Implications Maintain adequate patient hydration

Additional Information Usually used in combination with mesna, an agent used to prevent hemorrhagic cystitis

Dosage Forms Injection, powder for reconstitution: 1 g, 3 g [packaged with Mesnex® (mesna) 1 g]

References

Ninane J, Baurain R, and de Kraker J, "Alkylating Activity in Serum, Urine, and CSF Following High-Dose Ifosfamide in Children," *Cancer Chemother Pharmacol,* 1989, 24(Suppl 1):S2-6.

Pinkerton CR, Rogers H, James C, et al, "A Phase II Study of Ifosfamide in Children With Recurrent Solid Tumors," *Cancer Chemother Pharmacol,* 1985, 15(3):258-62.

- ◆ **IGIV** *see Immune Globulin (Intravenous) on page 598*
- ◆ **IL-2** *see Aldesleukin on page 56*
- ◆ **Iletin® II Pork (Can)** *see Insulin Preparations on page 609*
- ◆ **Imidazole Carboxamide** *see Dacarbazine on page 332*

Imiglucerase *(imi GLOO ser ase)*

U.S. Brand Names Cerezyme®

Therapeutic Category Enzyme, Glucocerebrosidase; Gaucher's Disease Treatment Agent

Generic Available No

Use Long-term enzyme replacement therapy for patients with Type 1 Gaucher's disease

Pregnancy Risk Factor C

Contraindications Hypersensitivity to imiglucerase or any component

Warnings During clinical trials, 16% of patients developed IgG antibodies reactive with imiglucerase; <1% of patients experienced anaphylactoid reactions; most patients may continue therapy after a reduction in the infusion rate and pretreatment with an antihistamine and/or corticosteroid; close observation for hypersensitivity reactions is recommended

Precautions Patients experiencing respiratory symptoms during treatment should be evaluated for potential pulmonary hypertension

Adverse Reactions

Cardiovascular: Systemic hypertension (mild), pulmonary hypertension, tachycardia, flushing, peripheral edema (transient)

Central nervous system: Headache, dizziness, fatigue, fever

Dermatologic: Rash, pruritus

Gastrointestinal: Nausea, abdominal pain, diarrhea, vomiting

Genitourinary: Decreased urinary frequency

Local: Burning, swelling, pruritus, sterile abscess at injection site

Neuromuscular & skeletal: Back pain

Respiratory: Dyspnea, cough

Miscellaneous: Anaphylactoid reactions (see Warnings)

Drug Interactions No information available at this time

Stability Store in refrigerator 2°C to 8°C (36°F to 46°F); after reconstitution, stable for 12 hours refrigerated or at room temperature; after dilution in NS, 40 units/mL solution is stable for 24 hours refrigerated; do not use if opaque particles or solution discoloration are seen

Mechanism of Action Imiglucerase, produced by recombinant DNA technology, is an analog of glucocerebrosidase; it acts by replacing the missing enzyme associated with Gaucher's disease; Gaucher's disease is an inherited metabolic disorder caused by the defective activity of beta-glucosidase and the resultant accumulation of glucosyl ceramide laden macrophages in the liver, bone, and spleen; this results in one or more of the following conditions: anemia, thrombocytopenia, bone disease, hepatomegaly, splenomegaly

Pharmacodynamics
Onset of significant improvement in symptoms:
Hepatosplenomegaly and hematologic abnormalities: Within 6 months
Improvement in bone mineralization: Noted at 80-104 weeks of therapy

Pharmacokinetics
Distribution: V_d: 0.09-0.15 L/kg
Half-life, elimination: 3.6-10.4 minutes
Clearance: 9.8-20.3 mL/minute/kg

Usual Dosage I.V.: Children and Adults:
Initial: Dosage dependent upon disease severity: Usual: 60 units/kg every 2 weeks; range in dosage: 2.5 units/kg 3 times/week to 60 units/kg once weekly to every 4 weeks
Maintenance: After patient response is well established a reduction in dosage may be attempted; progressive reductions may be made at intervals of 3-6 months

Administration Parenteral: Reconstitute 200 unit vial with 5.1 mL SWI or 400 unit vial with 10.2 mL SWI resulting in a 40 units/mL concentration; further dilute in 100-200 mL NS; infuse over 1-2 hours; may filter diluted solution through an in-line low protein-binding 0.2 micron filter during administration

Monitoring Parameters CBC, platelets, liver function tests

Dosage Forms Powder for injection, lyophilized [preservative free]: 212 units [equivalent to a withdrawal dose of 200 units]; 424 units [equivalent to a withdrawal dose of 400 units]

♦ **Imipemide** see Imipenem and Cilastatin on page 595 ♦ Imipemide see Imipenem and Cilastatin on page 595

Imipenem and Cilastatin (i mi PEN em & sye la STAT in)

U.S. Brand Names Primaxin®

Synonyms Cilastatin and Imipenem; Imipemide

Therapeutic Category Antibiotic, Carbapenem

Generic Available No

Use Treatment of documented multidrug-resistant gram-negative infection of the lower respiratory tract, urinary tract, intra-abdominal, gynecologic, bone and joint, septicemias, endocarditis, and skin and skin structure due to organisms proven or suspected to be susceptible to imipenem/cilastatin; treatment of multiple organism infection in which other agents have an insufficient spectrum of activity or are contraindicated due to toxic potential; therapeutic alternative for treatment of gram-negative sepsis in immunocompromised patients

Pregnancy Risk Factor C

Contraindications Hypersensitivity to imipenem/cilastatin or any component

Warnings Serious and occasionally fatal hypersensitivity reactions have been reported in patients receiving beta-lactam therapy; careful inquiry should be made concerning previous hypersensitivity reactions to penicillins, cephalosporins, or other beta-lactams before initiating imipenem. Seizures have been reported with imipenem therapy in children with meningitis; imipenem is not recommended in pediatric patients with CNS infections. Pseudomembranous colitis has been reported in patients receiving imipenem; prolonged use may result in superinfection.

Precautions Use with caution in patients with history of seizures or who are predisposed and in patients with a history of hypersensitivity to penicillins; use with caution and adjust dose in patients with impaired renal function

Adverse Reactions
Cardiovascular: Hypotension, tachycardia
Central nervous system: Seizures, hallucinations, altered effect, confusion, fever, dizziness
Dermatologic: Rash, pruritus, urticaria
Gastrointestinal: Nausea, vomiting, diarrhea, pseudomembranous colitis, oral candidiasis
Genitourinary: Discoloration of urine, anuria, oliguria, hematuria
Hematologic: Eosinophilia, neutropenia
Hepatic: Transient elevation in liver enzymes
(Continued)

Imipenem and Cilastatin *(Continued)*

Local: Phlebitis, irritation and pain at injection site

Miscellaneous: Emergence of resistant strains of *P. aeruginosa*

Drug Interactions Beta-lactam antibiotics, probenecid; ganciclovir (increased risk of seizures)

Stability

I.V.: When reconstituted suspension is further diluted with NS, it is stable for 10 hours at room temperature or 48 hours under refrigeration; when reconstituted suspension is further diluted with D_5W, $D_{10}W$, D_5NS, or $D_5{}^1\!/_4NS$, it is stable for 4 hours at room temperature and 24 hours under refrigeration; incompatible with TPN; inactivated at alkaline or acidic pH

I.M.: Reconstituted I.M. suspension in lidocaine HCl should be used within 1 hour after preparation

Mechanism of Action Inhibits cell wall synthesis by binding to all of the penicillin-binding proteins with greatest affinity for PBP 1 and PBP 2; cilastatin prevents renal metabolism of imipenem by competitive inhibition of dehydropeptidase along the brush border of the proximal renal tubules

Pharmacokinetics

Absorption: I.M.:

Imipenem: 75%

Cilastatin: 95%

Distribution: Imipenem appears in breast milk; crosses the placenta; only low concentrations penetrate into CSF

Protein binding:

Imipenem: 13% to 21%

Cilastatin: 40%

Metabolism: Imipenem is metabolized in the kidney by dehydropeptidase; cilastatin is partially metabolized in the kidneys

Half-life, both: Prolonged with renal insufficiency

Neonates: 1.5-3 hours

Infants and Children: 1-1.4 hours

Adults: 1 hour

Elimination: When imipenem is given with cilastatin, urinary excretion of unchanged imipenem increases to 70%; 70% to 80% of a cilastatin dose is excreted unchanged in the urine

Dialysis: Moderately dialyzable (20% to 50%)

Usual Dosage Dosage recommendation based on imipenem component for non-CNS infections: I.V. infusion: (I.M. is limited to mild-moderate infections):

Neonates:

0-4 weeks, <1200 g: 20 mg/kg/dose every 18-24 hours

Postnatal age ≤7 days, 1200-1500 g: 40 mg/kg/day divided every 12 hours

Postnatal age ≤7 days, >1500 g: 50 mg/kg/day divided every 12 hours

Postnatal age >7 days, 1200-1500 g: 40 mg/kg/day divided every 12 hours

Postnatal age >7 days, >1500 g: 75 mg/kg/day divided every 8 hours

Infants 4 weeks to 3 months: 100 mg/kg/day divided every 6 hours

Infants ≥3 months and Children: 60-100 mg/kg/day divided every 6 hours; maximum dose: 4 g/day

Adults:

Serious infections: 2-4 g/day divided every 6 hours

Mild to moderate infections: 1-2 g/day in 3-4 divided doses

Dosing adjustment in renal impairment: Imipenem doses should be reduced in patients with Cl_{cr} <41-70 mL/minute/1.73 m^2: See table.

Creatinine Clearance (mL/min/1.73 m^2)	Frequency	% Decrease in Daily Maximum Dose
41-70	Every 6 hours	50
21-40	Every 8 hours	63
6-20	Every 12 hours	75

Patients with creatinine clearance ≤5 mL/minute/1.73 m^2 should not receive imipenem unless undergoing hemodialysis

Administration

I.M.: Administer suspension by deep I.M. injection into a large muscle mass such as the gluteal muscle or lateral part of the thigh; the I.M. powder for suspension should be reconstituted with lidocaine hydrochloride 1% injection (without epinephrine). **Note:** The I.M. formulation is not for I.V. use.

I.V.: Administer by I.V. intermittent infusion; final concentration should not exceed 5 mg/mL; in fluid-restricted patients, a final concentration of 7 mg/mL has been administered; doses ≤500 mg may be infused over 15-30 minutes; doses >500 mg should be infused over 40-60 minutes

Monitoring Parameters Periodic renal, hepatic, and hematologic function tests

Test Interactions Interferes with urinary glucose determination using Clinitest®; Positive Coombs' [direct]

Nursing Implications If nausea and/or vomiting occur during administration, decrease the rate of I.V. infusion

Additional Information Sodium content of 1 g I.V. formulation: 3.2 mEq; sodium content of 500 mg I.M. formulation: 1.4 mEq

Dosage Forms

Injection, powder for I.M. suspension: Imipenem 500 mg and cilastatin 500 mg
Injection, powder for reconstitution [I.V.]:
Imipenem 250 mg and cilastatin 250 mg
Imipenem 500 mg and cilastatin 500 mg

References

Ahonkhai VI, Cyhan GM, Wilson SE, et al, "Imipenem-Cilastatin in Pediatric Patients: An Overview of Safety and Efficacy in Studies Conducted in the United States," *Pediatr Infect Dis J*, 1989, 8(11):740-4.

Overturf GD, "Use of Imipenem-Cilastatin in Pediatrics," *Pediatr Infect Dis J*, 1989, 8(11):792-4.

Wong VK, Wright HT Jr, Ross LA, et al, "Imipenem/Cilastatin Treatment of Bacterial Meningitis in Children," *Pediatr Infect Dis J*, 1991, 10(2):122-5.

Imipramine (im IP ra meen)

Related Information

Comparison of Adverse Effects of Antidepressants *on page 1210*
Comparison of Usual Adult Dosage and Mechanism of Action of Antidepressants *on page 1209*
Drugs and Breast-Feeding *on page 1404*
Overdose and Toxicology *on page 1388*

U.S. Brand Names Tofranil®; Tofranil-PM®

Canadian Brand Names Apo®-Imipramine

Therapeutic Category Antidepressant, Tricyclic

Generic Available Yes (tablet)

Use Treatment of various forms of depression, often in conjunction with psychotherapy; enuresis in children; analgesic for certain chronic and neuropathic pain

Pregnancy Risk Factor D

Contraindications Hypersensitivity to imipramine (cross-sensitivity with other tricyclics may occur) or any component; use of MAO inhibitors within 14 days (potentially fatal reactions may occur, see Drug Interactions); narrow-angle glaucoma

Warnings Do not discontinue abruptly in patients receiving long-term high-dose therapy. Some generic tablets contain sodium benzoate; benzoate is a metabolite of benzyl alcohol; large amounts of benzyl alcohol (≥99 mg/kg/day) have been associated with a potentially fatal toxicity ("gasping syndrome") in neonates; avoid use of imipramine products containing sodium benzoate in neonates; *in vitro* and animal studies have shown that benzoate displaces bilirubin from protein binding sites

Precautions Use with caution in patients with cardiovascular disease, conduction disturbances, seizure disorders, urinary retention, anorexia, hyperthyroidism or those receiving thyroid replacement

Adverse Reactions Less sedation and anticholinergic effects than amitriptyline

Cardiovascular: Arrhythmias, hypotension (especially orthostatic)
Central nervous system: Drowsiness, sedation, confusion, dizziness, fatigue, anxiety, nervousness, sleep disorders, seizures
Dermatologic: Rash, photosensitivity
Gastrointestinal: Nausea, vomiting, constipation, xerostomia, decreased appetite
Genitourinary: Urinary retention
Hematologic: Blood dyscrasias
Hepatic: Hepatitis
Ocular: Blurred vision, elevated intraocular pressure
Neuromuscular & skeletal: Weakness
Miscellaneous: Hypersensitivity reactions

Drug Interactions Cytochrome P450 isoenzyme CYP1A2 (demethylation), CYP2C9 (demethylation), CYP2C19 (demethylation), CYP2D6 (hydroxylation), and CYP3A3/4 substrate

May decrease or reverse effects of guanethidine and clonidine; may increase effects of CNS depressants, alcohol, adrenergic agents, anticholinergic agents; with MAO inhibitors, fever, tachycardia, hypertension, seizures, and death may occur (do not use MAO inhibitors within 14 days of imipramine); the herbal medicine St John's wort (*Hypericum perforatum*) may increase serious side effects, its use is **not** recommended; concurrent use of high-dose TCAs and ritonavir may cause the serotonin syndrome; similar interactions as with other tricyclics may occur
(Continued)

Imipramine *(Continued)*

Food Interactions Riboflavin dietary requirements may be increased; food does not alter bioavailability

Mechanism of Action Increases the synaptic concentration of serotonin and/or norepinephrine in the CNS by inhibition of their reuptake by the presynaptic neuronal membrane

Pharmacodynamics Maximum antidepressant effects usually occur after ≥2 weeks

Pharmacokinetics

Absorption: Oral: Well absorbed

Distribution: Crosses the placenta; distributes into breast milk

V_d: Children: 14.5 L/kg; Adults: ~17 L/kg

Protein binding: >90% (primarily to alpha$_1$ acid glycoprotein and lipoproteins; to a lesser extent albumin)

Metabolism: In the liver by microsomal enzymes to desipramine (active) and other metabolites; significant first-pass effect

Bioavailability: 20% to 80%

Half-life: Adults: Range: 6-18 hours

Mean: Children: 11 hours; Adults: 16-17 hours

Desipramine (active metabolite): Adults: 22-28 hours

Time to peak serum concentration: Within 1-2 hours

Elimination: In the urine

Usual Dosage Oral:

Children:

Depression: 1.5 mg/kg/day with dosage increments of 1 mg/kg every 3-4 days to a maximum dose of 5 mg/kg/day in 1-4 divided doses; monitor carefully especially with doses ≥3.5 mg/kg/day

Enuresis: ≥6 years: Initial: 10-25 mg at bedtime, if inadequate response still seen after 1 week of therapy, increase by 25 mg/day; dose should not exceed 2.5 mg/kg/day or 50 mg at bedtime if 6-12 years of age or 75 mg at bedtime if ≥12 years of age

Adjunct in the treatment of cancer pain: Initial: 0.2-0.4 mg/kg at bedtime; dose may be increased by 50% every 2-3 days up to 1-3 mg/kg/dose at bedtime

Adolescents: Initial: 25-50 mg/day; increase gradually; maximum dose: 200 mg/day in single or divided doses

Adults: Initial: 25 mg 3-4 times/day, increase dose gradually, total dose may be given at bedtime; maximum dose: 300 mg/day

Administration Oral: May administer with food to decrease GI distress

Monitoring Parameters Heart rate, EKG, supine and standing blood pressure (especially in children), liver enzymes, CBC, serum drug concentrations (see Reference Range)

Reference Range

Therapeutic: Imipramine and desipramine 150-250 ng/mL (SI: 530-890 nmol/L); desipramine 150-300 ng/mL (SI: 560-1125 nmol/L)

Potentially toxic: >300 ng/mL (SI: >1070 nmol/L)

Toxic: >1000 ng/mL (SI: >3570 nmol/L)

Patient Information Limit caffeine; avoid alcohol and the herbal medicine St. John's wort; may cause drowsiness and impair ability to perform activities requiring mental alertness or physical coordination; may cause dry mouth. May cause photosensitivity reactions (eg, exposure to sunlight may cause severe sunburn, skin rash, redness, or itching); avoid exposure to sunlight and artificial light sources (sunlamps, tanning booth/bed); wear protective clothing, wide-brimmed hats, sunglasses, and lip sunscreen (SPF ≥15); use a sunscreen [broad-spectrum sunscreen or physical sunscreen (preferred) or sunblock with SPF ≥15]; contact physician if reaction occurs.

Dosage Forms

Capsule, as pamoate (Tofranil-PM®): 75 mg, 100 mg, 125 mg, 150 mg

Tablet, as hydrochloride (Tofranil®): 10 mg, 25 mg, 50 mg [generic tablets may contain sodium benzoate]

References

Berde C, Ablin A, Glazer J, et al, "American Academy of Pediatrics Report of the Subcommittee on Disease-Related Pain in Childhood Cancer," *Pediatrics*, 1990, 86(5 Pt 2):818-25.

Levy HB, Harper CR, and Weinberg WA, "A Practical Approach to Children Failing in School," *Pediatr Clin North Am*, 1992, 39(4):895-928.

♦ **Imitrex®** *see* Sumatriptan *on page 1059*

♦ **Immune Globulin, Intramuscular** *see page 1333*

Immune Globulin (Intravenous)

(i MYUN GLOB yoo lin, IN tra VEE nus)

U.S. Brand Names Carimune™; Gamimune® N; Gammagard® S/D; Gammar®-P I.V.; Iveegam EN; Panglobulin®; Polygam® S/D; Venoglobulin®-S

Canadian Brand Names Iveegam Immuno®

Synonyms IGIV; IVIG

Therapeutic Category Immune Globulin

Generic Available No

Use Treatment of immunodeficiency syndrome, idiopathic thrombocytopenic purpura (ITP) and B-cell chronic lymphocytic leukemia (CLL); used in conjunction with appropriate anti-infective therapy to prevent or modify acute bacterial or viral infections in patients with iatrogenically-induced or disease-associated immunodepression; autoimmune neutropenia, bone marrow transplantation patients, Kawasaki disease, pediatric HIV infection, HIV-associated thrombocytopenia, Guillain-Barré syndrome, dermatomyositis, polymyositis, demyelinating polyneuropathies

FDA and NIH Recommendations for the use of IGIV:
Primary immunodeficiencies
Kawasaki disease
Pediatric HIV infection
Chronic B-cell lymphocytic leukemia
Recent bone marrow transplantation
Immune-mediated thrombocytopenia
Chronic inflammatory demyelinating polyneuropathy

Pregnancy Risk Factor C

Contraindications Hypersensitivity to immune globulin, blood products, or any component; IgA deficiency (except with the use of Gammagard® S/D or Polygam® S/D)

Warnings Renal dysfunction and/or acute renal failure has been reported with the administration of IVIG; 88% of the cases were associated with the administration of sucrose-containing IVIG products (Sandoglobulin®, Panglobulin™, Gammar®-P I.V.)

Precautions Use with caution in patients with a history of cardiovascular disease or thrombotic episodes. Rapid IVIG infusion may be a possible risk factor for vascular occlusive events associated with IVIG. Do not exceed manufacturer's recommended initial infusion rate, use a lower IVIG concentration, and advance slowly in patients at risk. Use with caution in patients at increased risk for developing acute renal failure (patients with pre-existing renal insufficiency, diabetes mellitus, volume depletion, sepsis, paraproteinemia, and concomitant nephrotoxic drugs). Assure that patients are not volume depleted prior to the initiation of an IVIG infusion.

Adverse Reactions
Cardiovascular: Flushing of the face, hypotension, tachycardia, pallor
Central nervous system: Dizziness, fever, headache, chills, anxiety, lightheadedness, malaise, irritability, aseptic meningitis syndrome
Dermatologic: Urticaria, pruritus
Gastrointestinal: Nausea, vomiting
Hematologic: Transient neutropenia, hemolytic anemia
Neuromuscular & skeletal: Myalgia
Renal: Acute renal failure
Respiratory: Tightness in the chest, difficulty breathing
Miscellaneous: Hypersensitivity reactions, diaphoresis, aseptic meningitis

Drug Interactions Live virus vaccines (measles, mumps, rubella)

Stability Do not mix with other drugs or I.V. infusion fluids; see table for storage

Mechanism of Action Replacement therapy for primary and secondary immunodeficiencies; interference with F_c receptors on the cells of the reticuloendothelial system for autoimmune cytopenias and ITP

Pharmacokinetics Half-life: 21-29 days

Usual Dosage Children and Adults: I.V.:
Immunodeficiency syndrome: 300-400 mg/kg/dose once a month; maintain trough IgG concentration of 500 mg/dL
Chronic lymphocytic leukemia (CLL): 400 mg/kg/dose every 3 weeks
Idiopathic thrombocytopenic purpura: 400-1000 mg/kg/day for 2-5 consecutive days; maintenance dose: 400-1000 mg/kg/dose every 3-6 weeks based on clinical response and platelet count
Pediatric HIV infection: 400 mg/kg/dose every 4 weeks in those patients with hypogammaglobulinemia (IgG concentration <250 mg/dL), those with recurrent serious bacterial infections (2 or more infections in a 1-year period), those who fail to form antibodies to common antigens such as measles vaccine, and those living in areas where measles is prevalent and have not developed an antibody response after 2 doses of MMR
HIV-associated thrombocytopenia: 500-1000 mg/kg/day for 3-5 days
Kawasaki disease: 2 g/kg as a single dose, given over 10-12 hours; if signs and symptoms persist, retreatment with a second 2 g/kg infusion should be considered
Congenital and acquired immunodeficiency syndrome: 100-400 mg/kg/dose every 3-4 weeks
(Continued)

Immune Globulin (Intravenous) *(Continued)*

Adjuvant in severe cytomegalovirus infection: 500 mg/kg/dose every other day for 7 doses

Bone marrow transplant: 400-500 mg/kg/dose every week for 3 months and then once every month

Guillain-Barré syndrome: 400 mg/kg/day for 4 days **or** 1 g/kg/day for 2 days **or** 2 g/kg as a single dose

Refractory dermatomyositis: 2 g/kg/dose every month for 3-4 doses

Refractory polymyositis: 1 g/kg/day for 2 days every month for 4 doses

Chronic inflammatory demyelinating polyneuropathy: 400 mg/kg/day for 5 days once each month **or** 1 g/kg/day for 2 days once each month

Severe systemic viral and bacterial infections:

Neonates: 500 mg/kg/day for 2 days then once weekly

Children: 500-1000 mg/kg/week

Prevention of gastroenteritis: Infants and Children: Oral: 50 mg/kg/day divided every 6 hours

Administration Do not administer I.M. or S.C.

I.V. infusion: For initial treatment, use a lower concentration and/or administer at the slowest infusion rate (see recommended initial infusion rate in tables) for the first 30 minutes. Titrate infusion rate up gradually to the maximum infusion rate. If an adverse reaction occurs, reduce I.V. infusion rate to previously tolerated rate. See tables below and on next page.

Monitoring Parameters Platelet count, blood pressure, vital signs, Quantitative Immunoglobulins (QUIGS), trough IgG concentration; periodic monitoring of renal function tests and urine output in patients with an increased risk for developing acute renal failure

Patient Information Notify physician of any sudden weight gain, fluid retention/edema, decreased urine output, and/or shortness of breath

Nursing Implications Appropriate agents for treatment of a hypersensitivity reaction (eg, epinephrine) should be readily available; patients may need to be pretreated with an antipyretic, antihistamine, and/or corticosteroid to prevent chills and fever; adverse reactions may also be alleviated by decreasing the rate or the concentration of infusion or utilizing a different IGIV preparation

Intravenous Immune Globulin Product Comparison

	Gamimune® N	Gammagard® S/D	Gammar-P® IV	Iveegam®
FDA indication	Primary immuno-deficiency, ITP, bone marrow transplantation, pediatric HIV infection	Primary immuno-deficiency, ITP, CLL prophylaxis, Kawasaki disease	Primary immuno-deficiency	Primary immuno-deficiency, Kawasaki syndrome
Contraindication	IgA deficiency	None (caution with IgA deficiency)	IgA deficiency	IgA deficiency
IgA content	270 mcg/mL	1.2 mcg/mL	<25 mcg/mL	<10 mcg/mL
g sucrose/g Ig	0	0	1	0
Adverse reactions	3.5% to 14.3%	6%	16%	1%
Plasma source	>2000 paid donors	10,000 paid donors	>1000 paid donors	>6000 paid donors
Half-life	21 d	24 d	21-24 d	26-29 d
IgG subclass (%)				
IgG$_1$ (60-70)	61.3	67 (66.8)[1]	69	64.1[2]
IgG$_2$ (19-31)	27.6	25 (25.4)	23	30.3
IgG$_3$ (5-8.4)	6.8	5 (7.4)	6	4
IgG$_4$ (0.7-4)	4.3	3 (0.3)	2	1.5
Monomers	>90%	>96.4%	>98%	93.8%
Gammaglobulin	>98%	>90%	>98%	100%
Storage	Refrigerate	Room temp	Room temp	Refrigerate
Recommended **initial** infusion rate	0.01-0.02 mL/kg/min	0.5 mL/kg/h	0.01-0.02 mL/kg/min	1 mL/min
Maximum infusion rate	0.08 mL/kg/min	4 mL/kg/h	0.06 mL/kg/min	2 mL/min
Maximum concentration for infusion	10%	10%	10%	5%

	Polygam® S/D	Immune Globulin Intravenous (Human) Carimune™ or Panglobulin™	Venoglobulin®-S
FDA indication	Primary immuno-deficiency, ITP, CLL, Kawasaki disease	Primary immuno-deficiency, ITP	Primary immuno-deficiency, ITP, Kawasaki disease
Contraindication	None (caution with IgA deficiency)	IgA deficiency	IgA deficiency
IgA content	1.2 mcg/mL	720 mcg/mL	5% (15.1 mcg/mL) 10% (20-50 mcg/mL)
g sucrose/g Ig	0	1.67	0
Adverse reactions	6%	2.9%-10%	5.8%-14.8%
Plasma source	50,000 voluntary donors	>16,000 voluntary donors	>10,000 paid donors
Half-life	24 d	23 d	33.5 d
IgG subclass (%)			
IgG₁ (60-70)	67	60.5 (55.3)[1]	65.7-67.2
IgG₂ (19-31)	25	30.2 (35.7)	23.7-25.3
IgG₃ (5-8.4)	5	6.6 (6.3)	5.7-5.9
IgG₄ (0.7-4)	3	2.8 (2.6)	3-3.4
Monomers	>96.4%	92%	>95%
Gammaglobulin	>90%	>96%	>99%
Storage	Room temp	Room temp	5% Room temp 10% Refrigerate
Recommended initial infusion rate	0.5 mL/kg/h	0.01-0.03 mL/kg/min	0.01-0.02 mL/kg/min
Maximum infusion rate	4 mL/kg/h	2.5 mL/min	0.04 mL/kg/min
Maximum concentration for infusion	10%	12%	10%

[1]Skvaril F and Gardi A, "Differences Among Available Immunoglobulin Preparations for Intravenous Use," *Pediatr Infect Dis J*, 1988, 7:543-48.

[2]Roomer J, Morgenthaler JJ, Scherz R, et al, "Characterization of Various Immunoglobulin Preparations for Intravenous Application," *Vox Sang*, 1982, 42:62-73.

Reference: ASHP Commission on Therapeutics, "ASHP Therapeutic Guidelines for Intravenous Immune Globulin," *Clin Pharm*, 1992, 11:117-36.

Dosage Forms

Injection, powder for reconstitution [preservative free]:

Carimune™: 1 g, 3 g, 6 g, 12 g

Gammar®-P I.V.: 1 g, 2.5 g, 5 g, 10 g [stabilized with human albumin and sucrose]

Iveegam EN: 0.5 g, 1 g, 2.5 g, 5 g [stabilized with glucose]

Panglobulin®: 1 g, 3 g, 6 g 12 g

Injection, powder for reconstitution [preservative free; solvent detergent-treated] (Gammagard® S/D, Polygam® S/D): 2.5 g, 5 g, 10 g [stabilized with human albumin, glycine, glucose, and polyethylene glycol]

Injection, solution [preservative free; solvent detergent-treated]:

Gamimune® N: 10% [100 mg/mL] (10 mL, 50 mL, 100 mL, 200 mL)

Venoglobulin® S: 5% [50 mg/mL] (50 mL, 100 mL, 200 mL); 10% [100 mg/mL] (50 mL, 100 mL, 200 mL) [stabilized with human albumin]

References

ASHP Commission on Therapeutics, "ASHP Therapeutic Guidelines for Intravenous Immune Globulin," *Am J Hosp Pharm*, 1992, 49(3):652-4.

Blanchette VS, Luke B, Andrew M, et al, "A Prospective Randomized Trial of High-Dose Intravenous Immune Globulin G Therapy, Oral Prednisone Therapy, and No Therapy in Childhood Acute Immune Thrombocytopenic Purpura," *J Pediatr*, 1993, 123(6):989-95.

Kaplan JE, Masur H, and Holmes KK, "Guidelines for Preventing Opportunistic Infections Among HIV-infected Persons - 2002 Recommendations of the USPHS and IDSA," *MMWR*, 2002, 51(RR-8):1-46.

NIH Consensus Conference, "Intravenous Immunoglobulin, Prevention and Treatment of Disease," *JAMA*, 1990, 264(24):3189-93.

"University Hospital Consortium Expert Panel for Off-Label Use of Polyvalent Intravenously Administered Immunoglobulin Preparations Consensus Statement," *JAMA*, 1995, 273(23):1865-70.

◆ **Immunization Guidelines** *see page 1333*

◆ **Imodium® A-D [OTC]** *see Loperamide on page 687*

◆ **Imuran®** *see Azathioprine on page 149*

Inamrinone (eye NAM ri none)

Synonyms Amrinone

Therapeutic Category Phosphodiesterase Enzyme Inhibitor

Generic Available Yes

Use Short-term treatment of low cardiac output states (sepsis, CHF); reserved for patients who have not responded adequately to therapy with digitalis, diuretics, and vasodilators; adjunctive therapy of pulmonary hypertension

Pregnancy Risk Factor C

(Continued)

Inamrinone *(Continued)*

Contraindications Hypersensitivity to inamrinone lactate or any component (see Warnings); valvular obstructive disease

Warnings Injection contains sodium metabisulfite which may cause allergic reactions in susceptible individuals

Precautions Monitor for hypotension, thrombocytopenia, hepatotoxicity, and GI effects; discontinue inamrinone if significant increase in liver enzymes with symptoms of idiosyncratic hypersensitivity reaction (ie, eosinophilia) occurs; monitor fluids and electrolytes. Diuresis may result from improvement in cardiac output and may require dosage reduction of diuretics. Inamrinone may exacerbate myocardial ischemia or worsen ventricular ectopy.

Adverse Reactions

Cardiovascular: Hypotension (1.3% incidence), ventricular and supraventricular arrhythmias (3%); may be related to infusion rate

Gastrointestinal: Nausea (1.7%), vomiting (0.9%), abdominal pain (0.4%), anorexia (0.4%); GI effects may be due to an increase in gastric acid secretion and intestinal motility, secondary to phosphodiesterase inhibition

Hematologic: Thrombocytopenia (2.4%), may be dose-related; in one study, 8 of 16 children (1.5 months to 11.2 years of age) developed thrombocytopenia (mean count 66 x 10^9 platelets/L). Inamrinone bolus doses ranged from 1.2-3 mg/kg given in 4 divided doses over 1 hour and were followed by continuous infusions of 5-10 mcg/kg/minute. Thrombocytopenia developed 19-71 hours after starting inamrinone (mean ± SD = 51 ± 25 hours). Resolution of thrombocytopenia occurred 54 ± 15 hours after therapy was discontinued; thrombocytopenia developed in patients with a higher total dose, longer duration of infusion, higher plasma concentrations of N-acetylamrinone (major metabolite of inamrinone), and higher plasma ratios of N-acetylamrinone to inamrinone.

Hepatic: Hepatotoxicity (0.2%)

Drug Interactions Disopyramide may increase hypotension (one case report; use with caution); diuretics may cause significant hypovolemia (dosage reduction of diuretic may be required)

Stability Dilute only with NS or ½NS; do not directly dilute with dextrose-containing solutions, chemical interaction occurs; may be administered I.V. (via Y-site) into running dextrose infusions. Furosemide forms a precipitate when injected in I.V. lines containing inamrinone; incompatible with sodium bicarbonate; use diluted solutions of inamrinone (1-3 mg/mL) within 24 hours.

Mechanism of Action Inhibits phosphodiesterase III (PDE III), the major PDE in cardiac and vascular tissues. Inhibition of PDE III increases cyclic adenosine monophosphate (cAMP) which potentiates the delivery of calcium to myocardial contractile systems and results in a positive inotropic effect. Inhibition of PDE III in vascular tissue results in relaxation of vascular muscle and vasodilatation.

Pharmacodynamics

Onset of action: I.V.: Within 2-5 minutes

Maximum effect: Within 10 minutes

Duration: Dose dependent with low doses lasting ~30 minutes and higher doses lasting ~2 hours

Pharmacokinetics

Distribution: V_d:

Neonates: 1.8 L/kg

Infants: 1.6 L/kg

Adults: 1.2 L/kg

Protein binding: 10% to 49%

Metabolism: In the liver to several metabolites (N-acetate, N-glycolyl, N-glucuronide, and O-glucuronide)

Half-life:

Neonates, 1-2 weeks of age: 22.2 hours

Infants 6-38 weeks of age: 6.8 hours; negative correlation of age with half-life in infants 4-38 weeks of age

Infants and Children (1 month to 15 years of age): 2.2-10.5 hours

Adults, normal volunteers: 3.6 hours

Adults with CHF: 5.8 hours

Elimination: Excreted in urine as metabolites and unchanged drug; 10% to 40% as unchanged drug in the urine within 24 hours

Usual Dosage I.V.: Note: Dose should not exceed 10 mg/kg/24 hours; doses of 18 mg/kg/day have been used in adults for a short duration; titrate infusion based on patient clinical response and adverse effects

Neonates: 0.75 mg/kg I.V. bolus over 2-3 minutes followed by maintenance infusion 3-5 mcg/kg/minute; I.V. bolus may need to be repeated in 30 minutes; see Additional Information

Infants and Children: 0.75 mg/kg I.V. bolus over 2-3 minutes followed by maintenance infusion 5-10 mcg/kg/minute; I.V. bolus may need to be repeated in 30 minutes; see Additional Information

Adults: 0.75 mg/kg I.V. bolus over 2-3 minutes followed by maintenance infusion of 5-10 mcg/kg/minute; I.V. bolus may need to be repeated in 30 minutes

PALS Guidelines 2000: I.V., I.O.: Loading dose: 0.75-1 mg/kg over 5 minutes; if tolerated, loading dose may be repeated up to 2 times; maximum total loading dose: 3 mg/kg; follow with maintenance infusion of 5-10 mcg/kg/minute; **Note:** If hypotension occurs during loading dose, administer 5-10 mL/kg of NS or other appropriate fluid and position patient flat or with head down (if patient can tolerate); if hypotension continues after fluid loading, administer a vasopressor agent and do not administer further inamrinone loading doses

ACLS Guidelines 2000: Adults: 0.75 mg/kg I.V. bolus over 2-3 minutes followed by maintenance infusion of 5-15 mcg/kg/minute; I.V. bolus may need to be repeated in 30 minutes

Administration Parenteral:

I.V. bolus: Infuse over 2-3 minutes; may be administered undiluted

Continuous infusion: Dilute with NS or ½NS to final concentration of 1-3 mg/mL; use controlled infusion device (eg, I.V. pump)

Monitoring Parameters Blood pressure, heart rate, platelet count, liver enzymes, fluid status, intake and output, body weight, serum electrolytes; if Swan-Ganz catheter is present, monitor cardiac index, stroke volume, systemic vascular resistance, pulmonary vascular resistance

Reference Range Proposed: Adults: 3 µg/mL; linear correlation with cardiac index observed from 0.5-7 µg/mL

Nursing Implications Do **not** administer furosemide I.V. push via "Y" site into inamrinone solutions as precipitate will occur; monitor patients closely (see Monitoring Parameters)

Additional Information Preliminary pharmacokinetic studies estimate that total initial bolus doses of 3-4.5 mg/kg given in divided doses to neonates and infants are required to obtain serum concentrations similar to therapeutic adult levels. The use of these higher doses has been reported in a small number of infants and children. Some centers use a total loading dose of 3 mg/kg (administered as 4 doses of 0.75 mg/kg/dose given every 15 minutes); each of the 0.75 mg/kg doses is given over 5 minutes. Further pharmacodynamic studies are needed to define pediatric inamrinone dosing guidelines.

Use of inamrinone in controlled trials did not extend beyond 48 hours; due to potential serious adverse effects and limited experience, inamrinone should only be used in patients who have not responded to other therapies (ie, digoxin, diuretics, vasodilators). Inamrinone has not been shown to be safe or effective for long-term treatment of CHF.

Effective July 1, 2000, the nonproprietary name of the drug (amrinone) was officially changed by the U.S. Pharmacopeia (USP) Nomenclature Committee and the U.S. Adopted Names (USAN) Council to inamrinone to prevent confusion with amiodarone; other countries will still use the name amrinone

Dosage Forms Injection, solution, as lactate: 5 mg/mL (20 mL) [contains sodium metabisulfite]

References

Allen-Webb EM, Ross MP, Pappas JB, et al, "Age-Related Amrinone Pharmacokinetics in a Pediatric Population," Crit Care Med, 1994, 22(6):1016-24.

"Guidelines 2000 for Cardiopulmonary Resuscitation and Emergency Cardiovascular Care, Part 6: Advanced Cardiovascular Life Support, The American Heart Association in Collaboration With the International Liaison Committee on Resuscitation," Circulation, 2000, 102(8 Suppl):I86-171.

"Guidelines 2000 for Cardiopulmonary Resuscitation and Emergency Cardiovascular Care, Part 10: Pediatric Advanced Life Support, The American Heart Association in Collaboration With the International Liaison Committee on Resuscitation," Circulation, 2000, 102(8 Suppl):I291-342.

Lawless S, Burckart G, Diven W, et al, "Amrinone in Neonates and Infants After Cardiac Surgery," Crit Care Med, 1989, 17(8):751-4.

Lawless ST, Zaritsky A, and Miles MV, "The Acute Pharmacokinetics and Pharmacodynamics of Amrinone in Pediatric Patients," J Clin Pharmacol, 1991, 31(9):800-3.

Lynn AM, Sorensen GK, and Williams GD, "Hemodynamic Effects of Amrinone and Colloid Administration in Children Following Cardiac Surgery," J Cardiothorac Vasc Anesth, 1993, 7(5):560-5.

Ross MP, Allen-Webb EM, Pappas JB, et al, "Amrinone-Associated Thrombocytopenia: Pharmacokinetic Analysis," Clin Pharmacol Ther, 1993, 53(6):661-7.

♦ **Inapsine®** see Droperidol on page 418

♦ **Inderal®** see Propranolol on page 952

♦ **Inderal® LA** see Propranolol on page 952

Indinavir (in DIN a veer)

Related Information
Adult and Adolescent HIV *on page 1327*
Pediatric HIV *on page 1323*

U.S. Brand Names Crixivan®

Synonyms L-735,524; MK-639

Therapeutic Category Antiretroviral Agent; HIV Agents (Anti-HIV Agents); Protease Inhibitor

Generic Available No

Use Treatment of HIV infection in combination with other antiretroviral agents; (**Note:** HIV regimens consisting of **three** antiretroviral agents are strongly recommended); postexposure chemoprophylaxis following occupational exposure to HIV

Pregnancy Risk Factor C

Contraindications Hypersensitivity to indinavir or any component

Warnings Cases of nephrolithiasis and nephrolithiasis associated with renal insufficiency or acute renal failure have been reported. If signs and symptoms of nephrolithiasis occur (flank pain with or without hematuria), interrupt or discontinue therapy. Due to potential serious and life-threatening drug interactions, the following drugs should not be coadministered with indinavir: terfenadine, astemizole, cisapride, pimozide, ergot alkaloid derivatives, triazolam, and midazolam. Concomitant use with rifampin is contraindicated since rifampin may markedly reduce indinavir concentrations. Spontaneous bleeding episodes have been reported in patients with hemophilia A and B. New onset diabetes mellitus, exacerbation of diabetes and hyperglycemia have been reported in HIV-infected patients receiving protease inhibitors.

Precautions Fat redistribution and accumulation [ie, central obesity, peripheral wasting, facial wasting, breast enlargement, dorsocervical fat enlargement (buffalo hump), and cushingoid appearance] have been observed in patients receiving antiretroviral agents (causal relationship not established). Use with caution in patients with hepatic impairment; modify dose in patients with impaired liver function.

Adverse Reactions

Central nervous system: Insomnia, dizziness, headache, somnolence, asthenia, depression

Dermatologic: Rash, dry skin, urticaria, pruritus, paronychia

Endocrine & metabolic: Rare: Hyperglycemia, diabetes, ketoacidosis; elevated serum cholesterol and triglycerides; redistribution of body fat to cause protease paunch, buffalo hump, facial atrophy, and breast enlargement

Gastrointestinal: Nausea (10%), vomiting, diarrhea, abdominal pain, dyspepsia, metallic taste, pancreatitis

Genitourinary: Dysuria, pyelonephritis

Hematologic: Hemolytic anemia, spontaneous bleeding episodes in hemophiliacs (rare)

Hepatic: Hyperbilirubinemia (10%), elevated liver function tests, jaundice, liver cirrhosis

Neuromuscular & skeletal: Arthralgia

Renal: Nephrolithiasis, urolithiasis (pediatric patients: 29%; adult patients: 9.3%), hematuria, proteinuria, renal failure, interstitial nephritis

Respiratory: Dry throat, pharyngitis

Drug Interactions Cytochrome P450 isoenzyme CYP3A3/4 substrate; isoenzyme CYP3A3/4 inhibitor

Coadministration with didanosine will decrease indinavir absorption; coadministration with rifampin or rifabutin will greatly reduce indinavir levels; indinavir increases rifabutin concentrations (decrease daily rifabutin dose by 50%); ketoconazole and itraconazole increase indinavir concentrations (dosage reduction of indinavir is recommended); ritonavir and nelfinavir decrease the metabolism of indinavir; coadministration with nevirapine may decrease indinavir concentrations; efavirenz decreases indinavir concentrations (indinavir dosage increase is recommended); delavirdine increases indinavir concentrations (dosage reduction of indinavir is recommended); indinavir inhibits the metabolism of HMG-CoA reductase inhibitors (atorvastatin, lovastatin, simvastatin) which increases the risk of myopathy; avoid concurrent use of astemizole or cisapride with indinavir due to potential for life-threatening cardiotoxicity; coadministration of benzodiazepines with indinavir may result in prolonged sedation and respiratory depression; indinavir increases the AUC of amprenavir; the herbal medicine St John's wort (*Hypericum perforatum*) induces CYP3A enzymes and has lead to 57% reductions in indinavir AUC's and 81% reductions in serum trough concentrations, which may lead to treatment failures; (see Warnings related to potentially serious and life-threatening drug interactions)

Food Interactions Decreased absorption when administered with high amounts of protein or fatty foods; 26% decrease in AUC when administered with grapefruit juice

Stability Store capsules at room temperature in original container with desiccant since capsules are sensitive to moisture

Mechanism of Action A protease inhibitor which acts on an enzyme late in the HIV replication process after the virus has entered into the cell's nucleus preventing cleavage of the gag-pol protein precursors resulting in the production of immature, noninfectious virions; cross-resistance with other protease inhibitors is possible

Pharmacokinetics
Absorption: Rapid; presence of food decreases the extent of absorption
Protein binding: 60%
Metabolism: In the liver by CYP3A4 system to inactive metabolites
Bioavailability: Wide interpatient variability in children: 15% to 50%
Half-life: 1.8-2 hours
Time to peak serum concentration: 0.8-1 hour
Elimination: 83% in feces as unabsorbed drug and metabolites; 10% excreted in urine as unchanged drug

Usual Dosage Oral:
Neonates: Should not be administered to neonates until further studies are performed due to side effect of hyperbilirubinemia
Children: Under study in clinical trials: 500 mg/m²/dose every 8 hours; maximum dose: 800 mg/dose every 8 hours
Adolescents and Adults: 800 mg/dose every 8 hours
Chemoprophylaxis after high-risk occupational exposure to HIV: 800 mg/dose every 8 hours in combination with zidovudine and lamivudine; start treatment as soon as possible (within a few hours following exposure) and continue for 4 weeks
Protease "boosting" by ritonavir:
Indinavir 400 mg twice daily with ritonavir 400 mg twice daily
or
Indinavir 800 mg twice daily with ritonavir 100 mg or 200 mg twice daily
Dosage adjustment in mild to moderate hepatic impairment: Reduce dose by 25%

Administration Administer with water on an empty stomach or with a light snack 1 hour before or 2 hours after a meal; may administer with other liquids (ie, skim milk, apple juice) or a light snack (ie, dry toast or cornflakes with skim milk); do not administer with grapefruit juice; if coadministered with didanosine, give at least 1 hour apart on an empty stomach. Administer around-the-clock to avoid significant fluctuation in serum levels.

Monitoring Parameters Serum bilirubin, cholesterol, triglycerides, amylase, lipase, liver function tests, urinalysis, blood glucose levels, CD4 cell count, plasma levels of HIV RNA, CBC

Patient Information Indinavir is not a cure for HIV. Avoid the herbal medicine St John's wort and grapefruit juice; if dose is missed, the dose should be omitted and the next dose taken at the usual scheduled time; do not double the next dose

HIV medications may cause changes in body fat, including an increase in fat in the upper back and neck, breasts, and trunk; a loss of fat from the face, arms, and legs may also occur.

Nursing Implications Ensure adequate patient hydration to minimize the risk of nephrolithiasis

Dosage Forms Capsule, as sulfate: 100 mg, 200 mg, 333 mg, 400 mg

Extemporaneous Preparations An indinavir 10 mg/mL oral solution is stable for 2 weeks stored at 4°C. The solution is made by first preparing an indinavir 100 mg/mL concentrate: Add contents of fifteen 400 mg capsules and 54 mL of purified distilled water into a 100 mL amber glass bottle. Place bottle in an ultrasonic water bath filled with water at 37°C for 60 minutes. Filter solution; wash bottle and filter with 6 mL purified distilled water. 50 mL of 100 mg/mL indinavir concentrate is added to 360 mL of viscous sweet base, 90 mL of simple syrup, 1.8 g citric acid, 45 mg azorubine, 0.1M sodium hydroxide solution to pH 3, and 12 drops of lemon oil to make a final volume of 500 mL. Mix solution until it is homogeneous.
Hugen PW, Burger DM, ter Hofstede HJ, et al, "Development of an Indinavir Oral Liquid for Children," *Am J Health Syst Pharm*, 2000, 57(14):1332-9.

References
CDC and the National Foundation for Infectious Disease, "Update: Provisional Public Health Service Recommendations for Chemoprophylaxis After Occupational Exposure to HIV," *MMWR Morb Mortal Wkly Rep*, 1996, 45(22):468-80.
Mueller BU, Smith S, Sleasman J, et al, "A Phase I/II Study of the Protease Inhibitor Indinavir (MK-0639) in Children With HIV Infection," *Eleventh International Conference on AIDS*, Vancouver, Canada, 1996.
Panel on Clinical Practices for Treatment of HIV Infection, "Guidelines for the Use of Antiretroviral Agents in HIV-Infected Adults and Adolescents," February 4, 2002, http://www.aidsinfo.nih.gov.
Stein DS, Fish DG, Bilello JA, et al, "A 24-Week Open-Label Phase I/II Evaluation of the HIV Protease Inhibitor MK-639 (Indinavir)," *AIDS*, 1996, 10(5):485-92.
(Continued)

Indinavir *(Continued)*

Working Group on Antiretroviral Therapy and Medical Management of HIV-Infected Children, "Guidelines for the Use of Antiretroviral Agents in Pediatric HIV Infection," December 14, 2001, http://www.aidsinfo.nih.gov.

- ♦ **Indocid® (Can)** *see* Indomethacin *on page 606*
- ♦ **Indocid® P.D.A. (Can)** *see* Indomethacin *on page 606*
- ♦ **Indocin®** *see* Indomethacin *on page 606*
- ♦ **Indocin® I.V.** *see* Indomethacin *on page 606*
- ♦ **Indocin® SR** *see* Indomethacin *on page 606*
- ♦ **Indo-Lemmon (Can)** *see* Indomethacin *on page 606*

Indomethacin (in doe METH a sin)

Related Information
Overdose and Toxicology *on page 1388*

U.S. Brand Names Indocin®; Indocin® I.V.; Indocin® SR

Canadian Brand Names Apo®-Indomethacin; Indocid®; Indocid® P.D.A.; Indo-Lemmon; Indotec; Novo-Methacin; Nu-Indo; Rhodacine®

Therapeutic Category Analgesic, Non-narcotic; Anti-inflammatory Agent; Antipyretic; Nonsteroidal Anti-inflammatory Drug (NSAID), Oral; Nonsteroidal Anti-inflammatory Drug (NSAID), Parenteral

Generic Available Yes (capsule and suspension)

Use Management of inflammatory diseases and rheumatoid disorders; moderate pain; acute gouty arthritis; I.V. form used as alternative to surgery for closure of patent ductus arteriosus (PDA) in neonates

Pregnancy Risk Factor B (D if used longer than 48 hours or after 34 weeks gestation)

Contraindications Hypersensitivity to indomethacin, any component, aspirin, or other NSAIDs; active GI bleeding, ulcer disease; patients with the "aspirin triad" [asthma, rhinitis (with or without nasal polyps), and aspirin intolerance] (fatal asthmatic and anaphylactoid reactions may occur in these patients); premature neonates with necrotizing enterocolitis, impaired renal function (eg, neonates with urine output <0.6 mL/kg/hour or serum creatinine ≥1.8 mg/dL), IVH, active bleeding, thrombocytopenia

Precautions Use with caution in patients with cardiac dysfunction, hypertension, renal or hepatic impairment, epilepsy, patients receiving anticoagulants and for treatment of JRA in children (fatal hepatitis has been reported; monitor children closely; assess liver function periodically)

Adverse Reactions
Cardiovascular: Hypertension, edema

Central nervous system: Somnolence, fatigue, depression, confusion, dizziness, headache

Dermatologic: Rash

Endocrine & metabolic: Hyperkalemia, dilutional hyponatremia (I.V.), hypoglycemia (I.V.)

Gastrointestinal: Nausea, vomiting, epigastric pain, abdominal pain, anorexia, GI bleeding, ulcers, perforation

Hematologic: Hemolytic anemia, bone marrow suppression, agranulocytosis, thrombocytopenia, inhibition of platelet aggregation

Hepatic: Hepatitis

Ocular: Corneal opacities

Otic: Tinnitus

Renal: Renal failure, oliguria

Miscellaneous: Hypersensitivity reactions

Drug Interactions Cytochrome P450 isoenzyme CYP2C9 substrate

Indomethacin may increase serum concentrations of digoxin, methotrexate, lithium, and aminoglycosides (reported with I.V. use in neonates); may increase nephrotoxicity of cyclosporine; may decrease antihypertensive and diuretic effects of furosemide and thiazides; may increase serum potassium with potassium-sparing diuretics; may decrease antihypertensive effects of beta-blockers, hydralazine, ACE inhibitors and angiotensin II antagonists; aspirin may decrease and probenecid may increase indomethacin serum concentrations; other GI irritants (eg, potassium supplements, NSAIDs) may increase GI adverse effects

Food Interactions Food may decrease the rate but not the extent of absorption

Stability

Oral suspension: Store below 86°F; do not freeze

I.V. product: Protect from light; not stable in alkaline solution; reconstitute just prior to administration; discard any unused portion; do not use preservative-containing diluents for reconstitution; will precipitate if reconstituted with solutions at pH <6 (product is not buffered)

Mechanism of Action Inhibits prostaglandin synthesis by decreasing the activity of the enzyme, cyclooxygenase, which results in decreased formation of prostaglandin precursors

Pharmacokinetics
Absorption: Oral:
  Neonates: Incomplete, nonuniform
  Adults: Rapid and well absorbed
Distribution:
  Neonates: PDA: 0.36 L/kg
    Post-PDA closure: 0.26 L/kg
  Adults: 0.34-1.57 L/kg
Protein binding: 99%
Metabolism: In the liver via glucuronide conjugation and other pathways
Bioavailability: Oral:
  Neonates, premature: 13% to 20%
  Adults: ~100%
Half-life:
  Neonates:
    Postnatal age (PNA) <2 weeks: ~20 hours
    PNA >2 weeks: ~11 hours
  Adults: 2.6-11.2 hours
Elimination: Significant enterohepatic recycling; 33% excreted in feces as demethylated metabolites with 1.5% as unchanged drug; 60% eliminated in urine as drug and metabolites

Usual Dosage
Patent ductus arteriosus:
  Neonates: I.V.: Initial: 0.2 mg/kg, followed by 2 doses depending on postnatal age (PNA):
    PNA **at time of first dose** <48 hours: 0.1 mg/kg at 12- to 24-hour intervals
    PNA **at time of first dose** 2-7 days: 0.2 mg/kg at 12- to 24-hour intervals
    PNA **at time of first dose** >7 days: 0.25 mg/kg at 12- to 24-hour intervals
  In general, may use 12-hour dosing interval if urine output >1 mL/kg/hour after prior dose; use 24-hour dosing interval if urine output is <1 mL/kg/hour but >0.6 mL/kg/hour; doses should be withheld if patient has oliguria (urine output <0.6 mL/kg/hour) or anuria
Inflammatory/rheumatoid disorders: **Note:** Use lowest effective dose: Oral:
  Children ≥2 years: 1-2 mg/kg/day in 2-4 divided doses; maximum dose: 4 mg/kg/day; do not exceed 150-200 mg/day
  Adults: 25-50 mg/dose 2-3 times/day; maximum dose: 200 mg/day; extended release capsule should be given on a 1-2 times/day schedule

Administration
Oral: Administer with food, milk, or antacids to decrease GI adverse effects; extended release capsules must be swallowed whole, do not crush or chew
Parenteral: I.V.: Administer over 20-30 minutes at a concentration of 0.5-1 mg/mL in preservative free SWI or preservative free NS
Note: Do **not** administer via I.V. bolus or I.V. infusion via an umbilical catheter into vessels near the superior mesenteric artery, as these may cause vasoconstriction and can compromise blood flow to the intestines. Do not administer intra-arterially.

Monitoring Parameters BUN, serum creatinine, potassium, liver enzymes, CBC with differential; in addition, in neonates treated for PDA: heart rate, heart murmur, blood pressure, urine output, echocardiogram, serum sodium and glucose, platelet count, and serum concentrations of concomitantly administered drugs which are renally eliminated (eg, aminoglycosides, digoxin); periodic ophthalmic exams with chronic use

Patient Information Avoid alcohol; may cause dizziness

Additional Information Indomethacin may mask signs and symptoms of infections; fatalities in children have been reported, due to unrecognized overwhelming sepsis; drowsiness, lethargy, nausea, vomiting, seizures, paresthesia, headache, dizziness, tinnitus, GI bleeding, cerebral edema, and cardiac arrest have been reported with overdoses

Dosage Forms
Capsule (Indocin®): 25 mg, 50 mg
Capsule, sustained release (Indocin® SR): 75 mg
Injection, powder for reconstitution, as sodium trihydrate (Indocin® I.V.): 1 mg
Suspension, oral (Indocin®): 25 mg/5 mL (237 mL) [contains 1% alcohol; pineapple-coconut-mint flavor]

References
Coombs RC, Morgan ME, Durbin GM, et al, "Gut Blood Flow Velocities in the Newborn: Effects of Patent Ductus Arteriosus and Parenteral Indomethacin," *Arch Dis Child*, 1990, 65(10 Spec No):1067-71.
(Continued)

Indomethacin (Continued)

Gersony WM, Peckham GJ, Ellison RC, et al, "Effects of Indomethacin in Premature Infants With Patent Ductus Arteriosus: Results of a National Collaborative Study," *J Pediatr*, 1983, 102(6):895-906.

Kraus DM and Pham JT, "Neonatal Therapy," *Applied Therapeutics: The Clinical Use of Drugs*, 7th ed, Koda-Kimble MA, Young LY, eds, Baltimore, MD: Lippincott Williams & Wilkins, 2001.

- ◆ **Indotec (Can)** *see* Indomethacin *on page 606*
- ◆ **Infantaire® [OTC]** *see* Acetaminophen *on page 36*
- ◆ **Infasurf®** *see* Calfactant *on page 205*
- ◆ **InFed®** *see* Iron Supplements (Parenteral) *on page 626*
- ◆ **Inflamase® Forte** *see* PrednisoLONE *on page 925*
- ◆ **Inflamase® Mild** *see* PrednisoLONE *on page 925*

Infliximab (in FLIKS e mab)

U.S. Brand Names Remicade®

Synonyms Antitumor Necrosis Factor-Alpha

Therapeutic Category Antirheumatic, Disease Modifying; Gastrointestinal Agent, Miscellaneous

Generic Available No

Use Reduction of signs and symptoms of Crohn's disease in patients with moderate to severely active disease who have had an inadequate response to conventional therapy; reduction in the number of draining enterocutaneous fistulas in patients with fistulizing Crohn's disease; treatment of refractory ulcerative colitis; in combination with methotrexate for the reduction in signs and symptoms of rheumatoid arthritis in patients who have had an inadequate response to methotrexate

Pregnancy Risk Factor B

Contraindications Hypersensitivity to infliximab, murine proteins, or any component; patients with any serious active infection or sepsis; patients with moderate or severe (NYHA class III/IV) congestive heart failure

Warnings Higher incidence of mortality and hospitalization for worsening heart failure have been reported in patients with CHF treated with infliximab, especially those patients treated at a higher dose of 10 mg/kg; do not initiate infliximab therapy in patients with CHF. Serious infections (some fatal) including sepsis, invasive fungal infections and opportunistic infections have been reported in patients receiving infliximab while on concomitant immunosuppressive therapy; 84 cases of tuberculosis have been reported in association with infliximab therapy; the majority of cases occurred after ≤3 infusions of infliximab; patients should be evaluated for risk of tuberculosis prior to initiating infliximab therapy; patients who develop a new infection while receiving infliximab should be monitored closely; if a patient develops a serious infection while on treatment, infliximab therapy should be discontinued. Infliximab administration has been associated with infusion-related hypersensitivity reactions which include urticaria, dyspnea, and/or hypotension that occurred during or within 2 hours of infusion; discontinue infliximab if severe reaction occurs; medications for treatment of hypersensitivity reactions must be readily available for use in case of a reaction

Precautions Use with caution in patients with a history of recurrent infections or illnesses which predispose the patient to infection; anti-TNF therapies such as infliximab may affect host defenses against infections and malignancies

Adverse Reactions

Cardiovascular: Hypotension, hypertension, chest pain, syncope, edema, tachycardia, arrhythmia, cardiac arrest

Central nervous system: Headache, dizziness, fatigue, fever, chills, seizures, anxiety, confusion, delirium, somnolence, depression, suicide attempt, multiple sclerosis

Dermatologic: Urticaria, rash, pruritus, moniliasis, furunculosis

Endocrine & metabolic: Weight decrease

Gastrointestinal: Nausea, vomiting, diarrhea, abdominal pain, pancreatitis, intestinal obstruction, GI hemorrhage, stomatitis

Genitourinary: Urinary tract infection

Hematologic: Anemia, thrombocytopenia, leukopenia

Hepatic: Cholestatic jaundice, cholecystitis, elevated AST and ALT

Neuromuscular & skeletal: Myalgia, back pain, arthropathy, septic arthritis, chronic osteomyelitis

Ophthalmologic: Endophthalmitis, optic neuritis

Renal: Renal failure

Respiratory: Dyspnea, cough, upper respiratory tract infections

Miscellaneous: Anaphylaxis, serum-sickness-like reaction (fever, rash, headache, sore throat, myalgias, polyarthralgias, hand and facial edema, dysphagia, antibodies to infliximab, loss of drug efficacy 3-12 days after reinstitution of infliximab following an extended period without treatment); lupus-like syndrome; infection

Drug Interactions Live vaccines (decreased immune response may allow live vaccine to produce infection, do not administer concurrently with infliximab); immunosuppressant agents (may reduce frequency of infusion reactions and antibodies to infliximab)

Stability Store vial in refrigerator; do not freeze; infliximab solution should be used immediately after reconstitution since the vial contains no preservative; do not shake or agitate vigorously; do not use if discolored or cloudy; the reconstituted dose must be further diluted in NS and the infusion should begin within 3 hours of preparation

Mechanism of Action Chimeric monoclonal antibody which binds specifically to human tumor necrosis factor alpha (TNFα); inhibits functional activity of TNFα by binding to its receptors

Pharmacodynamics

Onset:

Crohn's disease: 1-2 weeks

Rheumatoid arthritis: 3-7 days

Duration:

Crohn's disease: 8-48 weeks

Rheumatoid arthritis: 6-12 weeks

Pharmacokinetics

Distribution: Within the vascular compartment

V_d: Adults: 3 L

Half-life, terminal: 8-12 days

Usual Dosage I.V. infusion:

Children: Crohn's disease: 5 mg/kg/dose; in an open-label retrospective chart review (n=19; mean age: 14.4 years, range 9-19 years) patients received 1-3 infusions of infliximab for active intestinal Crohn's disease over a 12-week period for corticosteroid-resistant disease (n=7) or corticosteroid-dependence (n=12); infliximab provided rapid, short-term clinical improvement; however, additional infusion doses may be needed in some patients due to return of disease symptoms weeks to months after the initial infusion. Further studies are needed (Hyams, 2001).

Adults:

Crohn's disease: 5 mg/kg as a single dose

Patients with fistulizing disease: Initial: 5 mg/kg; repeat 5 mg/kg/dose at 2 and 6 weeks after the first infusion

Rheumatoid arthritis (in combination with methotrexate): Initial: 3 mg/kg; repeat 3 mg/kg/dose at 2 and 6 weeks after the first infusion, then every 8 weeks thereafter. If the response is incomplete, may increase dose up to 10 mg/kg or treat as often as every 4 weeks.

Administration Parenteral: Administer by I.V. infusion over 2 hours at a final concentration between 0.4-4 mg/mL in NS. Administer through an in-line, sterile, nonpyrogenic, low-protein-binding filter with pore size of ≤1.2 μm; do not infuse in the same I.V. line as other agents

Monitoring Parameters Urinalysis, blood chemistry, ESR, blood pressure, signs of infection, CBC; tuberculin skin test prior to initiation of therapy

Crohn's disease: C-reactive protein, frequency of stools, abdominal pain

Rheumatoid arthritis: C-reactive protein, rheumatoid factor, decrease in pain, swollen joints, stiffness

Additional Information A retrospective study of 57 children receiving 361 infliximab infusions reported that the rate of infusion-related reactions in children was similar to that in adults (9.7% incidence shown). Female gender, immunosuppressive use for <4 months, and prior infusion reactions were risk factors for subsequent infusion reactions in children (see Crandall, 2003)

Dosage Forms Injection, powder for reconstitution, lyophilized: 100 mg

References

Crandall WV and Mackner LM, "Infusion Reactions to Infliximab in Children and Adolescents: Frequency, Outcome and a Predictive Model," *Aliment Pharmacol Ther*, 2003, 17(1):75-84.

Hyams JS, "Use of Infliximab in the Treatment of Crohn's Disease in Children and Adolescents," *J Pediatr Gastroenterol Nutr*, 2001, 33 (Suppl 1):S36-9.

Hyams JS, Markowitz J, and Wyllie R, "Use of Infliximab in the Treatment of Crohn's Disease in Children and Adolescents," *J Pediatr*, 2000, 137(2):192-6.

Serrano MS, Schmidt-Sommerfeld E, Kilbaugh TJ, et al, "Use of Infliximab in Pediatric Patients With Inflammatory Bowel Disease," *Ann Pharmacother*, 2001, 35(7-8):823-8.

♦ **Influenza Virus Vaccine** *see page 1333*

♦ **Infumorph®** *see Morphine Sulfate on page 778*

♦ **INH** *see Isoniazid on page 629*

♦ **Insta-Glucose® [OTC]** *see Dextrose on page 366*

Insulin Preparations (IN su lin prep a RAY shuns)

U.S. Brand Names Humalog®; Humalog® Mix 75/25®; Humulin® 50/50; Humulin® 70/30; Humulin® L; Humulin® N; Humulin® R; Humulin® R (Concentrated) U-500; (Continued)

Insulin Preparations *(Continued)*

Humulin® U; Lantus®; Lente® Iletin® II; Novolin® 70/30; Novolin® L; Novolin® N; Novolin® R; NovoLog®; NovoLog® Mix 70/30; NPH Iletin® II; Pork Regular Iletin® II; Velosulin® BR Human (Buffered)

Canadian Brand Names Humalog® Mix 25™; Iletin® II Pork; Novolin® ge; NovoRapid®

Therapeutic Category Antidiabetic Agent, Parenteral

Generic Available No

Use Treatment of insulin-dependent diabetes mellitus, also noninsulin-dependent diabetes mellitus unresponsive to treatment with diet and/or oral hypoglycemics; to assure proper utilization of glucose and reduce glucosuria in nondiabetic patients receiving parenteral nutrition whose glucosuria cannot be adequately controlled with infusion rate adjustments or those who require assistance in achieving optimal caloric intakes; treatment of hyperkalemia (use with glucose to shift potassium into cells to lower serum potassium levels)

Pregnancy Risk Factor B

Contraindications Hypersensitivity to the insulin source (pork) or any components; hypoglycemia; only regular insulin may be given intravenously

Warnings Any change of insulin should be made cautiously; changing manufacturers, type, source, and/or method of manufacture, may result in the need for a change of dosage; human insulin differs from pork insulin; hypoglycemia may result from increased work or exercise without eating

Adverse Reactions Primarily symptoms of hypoglycemia

Cardiovascular: Palpitations, tachycardia, pallor

Central nervous system: Fatigue, mental confusion, loss of consciousness, headache, hypothermia

Dermatologic: Urticaria, redness

Endocrine & metabolic: Hypoglycemia, hypokalemia

Gastrointestinal: Hunger, nausea, numbness of mouth

Local: Itching, redness, edema, stinging (particularly with insulin glargine), or warmth at injection site, atrophy or hypertrophy of S.C. fat tissue

Neuromuscular & skeletal: Muscle weakness, tremors, tingling of fingers

Ocular: Transient presbyopia or blurred vision

Miscellaneous: Diaphoresis, anaphylaxis

Drug Interactions See table.

Drug Interactions With Insulin

Decrease Hypoglycemic Effects	Increase Hypoglycemic Effects
Acetazolamide	ACE inhibitors
Alcohol (chronic use)	Alcohol (acute use)
Antiretrovirals	Alpha-blockers
Asparaginase	Anabolic steroids
Calcitonin	Beta blockers, nonselective
Contraceptives, oral	Calcium
Corticosteroids	Chloroquine
Cyclophosphamide	Clofibrate
Danazol	Disopyramide
Diazoxide	Fluoxetine
Diltiazem	Guanethidine
Dobutamine	Lithium
Epinephrine	MAO inhibitors
Estrogens	Mebendazole
Ethacrynic acid	Octreotide
Isoniazid	Oral antidiabetic agents
Lithium	(oral hypoglycemic agents)
Morphine	Pentamidine
Niacin	Phenylbutazone
Nicotine	Propoxyphene
Phenothiazines	Pyridoxine
Phenytoin	Salicylates
Somatropin	Sulfinpyrazone
Terbutaline	Sulfonamides
Thiazide diuretics	Tetracyclines
Thyroid hormone	

Stability

Insulin is stable at room temperature up to 1 month and 3 months refrigerated; cold (freezing) causes more damage to insulin than room temperatures up to 100°F;

avoid direct sunlight; cold injections should be avoided; visually inspect insulin for the presence of frosting (a frosty appearance due to freezing or overheating of vials and insulin precipitation on the walls of the vial), particulates, clumping (a potential problem with suspensions), and changes in clarity or color. NPH, Lente®, Ultralente®, and premixed insulins are cloudy, white suspensions. All other insulins should be clear.

Insulin Mixture Compatibility

Insulin Preparations	Compatible Mixed With
Insulin injection (regular)	NPH, Lente®, Ultralente®
Insulin aspart (NovoLog™)	NPH
Lispro insulin solution (Humalog®)*	Ultralente®, NPH
Isophane insulin suspension (NPH)	Regular, Humalog®*, NovoLog™
Insulin zinc suspension (Lente®)	Regular, Ultralente®
Extended insulin zinc suspension (Ultralente®)	Regular, Lente®, Humalog®*
Insulin glargine (Lantus®)	Do not mix with any other insulin

*Mixtures with Humalog® should be used within 5 minutes of mixing

When mixing with NPH insulin in any proportion, the excess protamine may combine with regular insulin and may reduce or delay activity of regular insulin (does not appear to be clinically significant); Lente® insulin binds with short-acting insulins and delays the onset of action; degree of binding varies with the ratio and species of the two insulins. Binding equilibrium may not be reached for 24 hours; if mixed, standardize the interval between mixing and injection

Stability of parenteral admixture of regular insulin in NS or 1/2 NS at room temperature (25°C) and at refrigeration temperature (4°C): 24 hours; all bags should be prepared fresh; tubing should be flushed 30 minutes prior to administration to allow adsorption as time permits

Mechanism of Action The principal hormone required for proper glucose utilization in normal metabolic processes; it is obtained from pork pancreas or a biosynthetic process converting pork insulin to human insulin; insulin analogs have been made by modifying the amino acid sequence of the insulin molecule; insulins are categorized into 4 groups related to promptness, duration, and intensity of action

Pharmacodynamics Onset and duration of hypoglycemic effects depend upon the route of administration (absorption and onset of action are more rapid after deeper I.M. injections than after S.C.), site of injection (onset and duration are progressively slower with subcutaneous injection into the abdomen, arm, buttock, or thigh), volume

Pharmacodynamics of Insulin Preparations

Insulin Preparations	Onset (h)	Peak (h)	Duration (h)
Rapid-Acting			
Insulin aspart (NovoLog™)	0.17-0.33	1-3	3-5
Lispro insulin (Humalog®)	0.25-0.5	0.5-1.5	3-5
Short-Acting			
Insulin injection (regular)	0.5-1	1-5	3-10
Insulin, buffered (regular) (Velosulin® BR)	0.5	1-3	8
Intermediate-Acting			
Isophane insulin suspension (NPH)	1-4	4-14	10-24
Insulin zinc suspension (Lente®)	1-4	4-14	12-24+
Long-Acting			
Extended insulin zinc suspension (Ultralente®)	4-10	8-30	18-36
Insulin glargine (Lantus®)	1-2	2-20*	20-24+

*Has no pronounced peak

(Continued)

Insulin Preparations (Continued)

and concentration of injection, and the preparation administered; exercise, local heat, and massage also increase the rate of absorption; see table on previous page for specifics related to product.

Usual Dosage Maintaining the proper dosage requires continuous medical supervision; only regular insulin may be given I.V. or I.M.. The daily dose should be divided up depending upon the product used and the patient's response (see table).

Children and Adults: S.C.: 0.5-1 unit/kg/day in divided doses

Adolescents (during growth spurt) S.C.: 0.8-1.2 units/kg/day in divided doses

Commonly used regimens include:

Newly diagnosed patients: $^2/_3$ of total daily dose as an intermediate-acting insulin (eg, NPH) and a short-acting insulin in a 2:1 ratio before breakfast and $^1/_3$ of the total daily dose of the two insulins in a 1:1 ratio before the evening meal or $^1/_2$ the daily dose as a long-acting insulin and $^1/_2$ as a rapid- or short-acting insulin before meals with the amount used proportional to the carbohydrate intake. **Note:** Twice daily administration is only recommended during the "honeymoon" period immediately after diagnosis.

Three injections: Rapid -or short-acting insulin before each meal and an intermediate-acting insulin before breakfast and dinner.

Four injections: Rapid -or short-acting insulin before each meal and a long-acting insulin at bedtime.

When changing from once daily intermediate insulin (eg, NPH or Lente) to long-acting insulin (eg, Lantus®), the same total daily dose in units may be used. If changing from twice daily intermediate to long-acting in order to reduce the risk of hypoglycemia, the initial dose should be the sum of both doses (in units) but reduced by 20%.

Diabetic ketoacidosis: Children: I.V. loading dose: 0.1 unit/kg, then maintenance continuous infusion: 0.1 unit/kg/hour (range: 0.05-0.2 unit/kg/hour depending upon the rate of decrease of serum glucose). Decreasing the serum glucose level too rapidly may lead to cerebral edema; optimum rate of decrease (serum glucose): 80-100 mg/dL/hour

Note: Newly diagnosed patients with juvenile onset diabetes mellitus presenting in DKA and patients with blood sugars <800 mg/dL may be relatively "sensitive" to insulin and should receive loading and initial maintenance doses approximately $^1/_2$ of those indicated above.

Sliding scale: Use only for brief transitional periods of treatment; newly diagnosed patients with juvenile onset diabetes may be "sensitive" to exogenous insulin and should be treated with the lower end of these ranges; see table.

Insulin Dosing Sliding Scale

Urine Glucose	Insulin Dose (units/kg)	
	Urine Ketones (-)	Urine Ketones (+)
0-$^1/_2$%	0	0
$^3/_4$%	0.03-0.1	0.05-0.12
1%	0.07-0.2	0.1-0.25
2%	0.15-0.4	0.2-0.5

To optimize caloric intake in neonates while on parenteral nutrition:

Continuous infusion: I.V.: Neonates: 0.01-0.1 unit/kg/hour; neonates are very sensitive to insulin; start at low end of infusion rate and monitor closely

Treatment of hyperkalemia (after treatment with I.V. calcium gluconate and NaHCO₃):

Children: Dextrose 0.5-1 g/kg (using 25% or 50%) combined with insulin 1 unit for every 4-5 g dextrose; infuse over 2 hours **or** dextrose 0.5-1 g/kg infused over 15-30 minutes followed by 0.1 unit/kg insulin S.C. or I.V.

Adults: 50% dextrose at 0.5-1 mL/kg and insulin 1 unit for every 4-5 g dextrose given

Dosing adjustment in renal impairment: Children and Adults:

Cl$_{cr}$ 10-50 mL/minute: Administer 75% of recommended dose

Cl$_{cr}$ <10 mL/minute: Administer 25% to 50% of recommended dose (follow blood sugar closely)

Administration

Parenteral: S.C.: Administration is usually made into the subcutaneous fat of the thighs, arms, buttocks, or abdomen, with sites rotated; only regular insulin may be administered I.M.; when mixing regular insulin with other preparations of insulin, regular insulin should be drawn into syringe first; insulin lispro (when used as "meal-time" insulin, due to a rapid onset of effect) should be administered 15 minutes before meals or immediately after meals and insulin aspart 5-10 minutes before meals; regular insulin should be administered 30-60 minutes before meals; insulin glargine (Lantus®) should be administered once daily at bedtime; do not mix Velosulin® BR or Lantus® with other insulins; to achieve complete suspension, containers (vials, cartridges, prefilled syringes) with insulin suspensions should be gently agitated (rolled between palms 10 times and inverted 10 times) but not vigorously shaken; insulin pens should be rolled and inverted at least 20 times before injection

I.V. (**only regular insulin** may be administered I.V.; Humulin® BR contains a phosphate buffer to decrease crystal formation; it should not be administered I.V.) infusion (requires use of an infusion pump): To minimize adsorption problems to I.V. solution bag and tubing:

If new tubing is **not** needed: Wait a minimum of 30 minutes between the preparation of the solution and the initiation of the infusion

If new tubing is needed: After receiving the insulin drip solution, the administration set should be attached to the I.V. container and the line should be flushed with the insulin solution, wait 30 minutes, then flush the line again with the insulin solution prior to initiating the infusion.

Because of adsorption, the actual amount of insulin being administered could be substantially less than the apparent amount. Therefore, adjustment of the insulin drip rate should be based on effect and not solely on the apparent insulin dose. Furthermore, the apparent I.V. infusion dose should not be used as the basis for determining the subsequent insulin dose upon discontinuing the insulin drip. Dosage adjustment requires continuous medical supervision.

Monitoring Parameters Urine sugar and acetone, blood sugar, serum electrolytes, hemoglobin A_{1c}

Reference Range Target range:

Blood glucose:
Fasting and preprandial: 80-120 mg/dL
Bedtime: 100-140 mg/dL

Serum glucose:
Fasting and preprandial: 90-130 mg/dL
Bedtime: 110-150 mg/dL

Glycosolated hemoglobin (hemoglobin A_{1c}): <7%

Patient Information Do not change insulins without physician's approval; patients should be counseled by someone experienced in diabetes education regarding signs and symptoms of hyper- and hypoglycemia, exercise and diet, blood glucose monitoring, and other related topics. If injections are painful, be sure to inject insulin which is at room temperature; allow alcohol on skin surface to dry before injecting the dose; relax the muscles around the injection site, insert the needle quickly keeping the angle of the needle insertion constant and use a fresh needle.

Additional Information The term "purified" refers to insulin preparations containing no more than 10 ppm proinsulin (purified and human insulins are less immunogenic); buffering agent in Velosulin® BR may alter the activity of other insulin products

Dosage Forms

Rapid-Acting:

Injection, solution, aspart, human:
NovoLog®: 100 units/mL (10 mL vial)
NovoLog® [PenFill®]: 100 units/mL (3 mL cartridge)

Injection, solution, lispro, human (Humalog®): 100 units/mL (1.5 mL cartridge, 3 mL disposable pen, 10 mL vial)

Short-Acting:

Injection, solution, regular, human:
Humlin® R: 100 units/mL (10 mL vial)
Novolin® R: 100 units/mL (1.5 mL prefilled syringe, 10 mL vial)
Novolin® R [PenFill®]: 100 units/mL (1.5 mL cartridge, 3 mL cartridge)

Injection, solution, regular, human, buffered (Velosulin® BR): 100 units/mL (10 mL vial)

Injection, solution, regular, human, **concentrate** (Humulin® R U-500): 500 units/mL (20 mL vial)

Injection, solution, regular, purified pork (Regular Iletin® II): 100 units/mL (10 mL vial)

Intermediate-Acting:

Injection, suspension, lente, human [zinc] (Humulin® L, Novolin® L): 100 units/mL (10 mL vial)

Injection, suspension, lente, purified pork [zinc] (Lente® Iletin® II): 100 units/mL (10 mL vial)

Injection, suspension, NPH, human [isophane]:
Humulin® N: 100 units/mL (3 mL disposable pen, 10 mL vial)
Novolin® N: 100 units/mL (1.5 mL prefilled syringe, 10 mL vial)

(Continued)

Insulin Preparations (Continued)

Novolin® N [PenFill®]: 100 units/mL (1.5 mL cartridge, 3 mL cartridge)

Injection, suspension, NPH, purified pork [isophane] (NPH Iletin® II): 100 units/mL (10 mL vial)

Long-Acting:

Injection, solution, glargine, human (Lantus®): 100 unit/mL (10 mL vial)

Injection, suspension, Ultralente®, human [zinc] (Humulin® U Ultralente®): 100 units/mL (10 mL vial)

Combination, Intermediate-Acting:

Injection, aspart protamine human suspension 75% and rapid-acting aspart human solution 30% (NovoLog® Mix 70/30): 100 units/mL (3 mL cartridge, 3 mL prefilled syringe)

Injection, lispro human suspension 75% and rapid-acting lispro human solution 25% (Humalog® Mix 75/25®): 100 units/mL (3 mL disposable pen, 10 mL vial)

Injection, NPH human insulin suspension 50% and short-acting regular human insulin solution 50% (Humulin® 50/50): 100 units/mL (10 mL vial)

Injection, NPH human insulin suspension 70% and short-acting regular human insulin solution 30%:

Humulin® 70/30: 100 units/mL (3 mL disposable pen, 10 mL vial)

Novolin® 70/30: 100 units/mL (1.5 mL prefilled syringe, 10 mL vial)

Novolin® 70/30 [PenFill®]: 100 units/mL (1.5 mL cartridge, 3 mL cartridge)

References

"American Diabetes Association: Clinical Practice Recommendations 2002." *Diabetes Care*, 2002, 25(Suppl 1):S1-147.

Simeon PS, Geffner ME, Levin SR, et al, "Continuous Insulin Infusions in Neonates: Pharmacologic Availability of Insulin in Intravenous Solutions," *J Pediatr*, 1994, 124(5 Pt 1):818-20.

♦ **Intal®** *see Cromolyn on page 311*

♦ **α-2-interferon** *see Interferon Alfa-2b on page 616*

Interferon Alfa-2a (in ter FEER on AL fa too aye)

U.S. Brand Names Roferon-A®

Synonyms IFLrA; IFN; rIFN-α

Therapeutic Category Antineoplastic Agent, Miscellaneous; Biological Response Modulator; Interferon

Generic Available No

Use FDA approved in patients >18 years of age: Hairy cell leukemia, AIDS-related Kaposi's sarcoma, Philadelphia chromosome-positive chronic myelogenous leukemia, hemangiomas of infancy; multiple unlabeled uses

Pregnancy Risk Factor C

Contraindications Hypersensitivity to alpha interferon or any component (see Warnings)

Warnings The FDA currently recommends that procedures for proper handling and disposal of antineoplastic agents be considered. Interferon alfa-2a may cause life-threatening neuropsychiatric, autoimmune, and infectious disorders. Patients with persistently severe or worsening symptoms of these conditions should be withdrawn from therapy. Alpha interferons suppress bone marrow function which may result in severe cytopenias or aplastic anemia. Discontinue alpha interferon in patients who develop severe decreases in neutrophil count or platelet counts. Safety and efficacy in children <18 years of age have not been established.

Interferon alfa-2a injection contains benzyl alcohol which may cause allergic reactions in susceptible individuals; large amounts of benzyl alcohol (≥99 mg/kg/day) have been associated with a potentially fatal toxicity ("gasping syndrome") in neonates; the "gasping syndrome" consists of metabolic acidosis, respiratory distress, gasping respirations, CNS dysfunction (including convulsions, intracranial hemorrhage), hypotension and cardiovascular collapse; use interferon alfa-2a products containing benzyl alcohol with caution in neonates; *in vitro* and animal studies have shown that benzoate, a metabolite of benzyl alcohol, displaces bilirubin from protein binding sites

Precautions Use with caution in patients with seizure disorders, psychiatric disorders, brain metastases, multiple sclerosis, compromised CNS, and patients with pre-existing cardiac disease, myelosuppression, or severe renal/hepatic impairment

Adverse Reactions Flu-like symptoms (fever, fatigue/malaise, myalgia, chills, headache, arthralgia, rigors) begin about 2-6 hours after the dose is given and may persist as long as 24 hours; severity of flu-like symptoms increase with higher dosages; usually patient can build up a tolerance to side effects

Cardiovascular: Tachycardia, arrhythmias, hypotension, edema, chest pain, syncope

Central nervous system: Fatigue/malaise, dizziness, depression, confusion, sensory neuropathy, psychiatric symptoms (psychosis, mania, depression, suicidal behavior), fever, headache, EEG abnormalities, chills

Dermatologic: Partial alopecia, rash, dry skin

Endocrine & metabolic: Elevated uric acid level, thyroid dysfunction, hyperglycemia, hypertriglyceridemia

Gastrointestinal: Anorexia, xerostomia, nausea, vomiting, diarrhea, abdominal cramps, dysgeusia, weight loss, stomatitis

Hematologic: Leukopenia (mainly neutropenia); anemia; thrombocytopenia; neutralizing antibodies

Hepatic: Elevated ALT and AST

Local: Burning, pain, erythema, rash at the site of injection, pruritus

Neuromuscular & skeletal: Myalgia, arthralgia, rigors, leg cramps, spastic diplegia

Ocular: Blurred vision, retinal hemorrhage

Renal: Proteinuria, elevated BUN and serum creatinine

Respiratory: Coughing, nasal congestion

Miscellaneous: Diaphoresis

Drug Interactions

Interferon Alfa-2b: Possible competitive binding to same receptors

Acyclovir: Possible synergistic effects

Theophylline: Clearance of theophylline is reduced

Vinblastine: May increase interferon toxicity; increased neurotoxicity

Zidovudine: Possible additive myelosuppression

Stability Store in refrigerator; do not shake; after reconstitution stable at room temperature for 24 hours; do not store in syringes for prolonged periods

Mechanism of Action Inhibits cellular growth, alters the state of cellular differentiation, interferes with oncogene expression, alters cell surface antigen expression, increases phagocytic activity of macrophages and augments cytotoxicity of lymphocytes for target cells

Pharmacokinetics

Absorption: I.M., S.C.: >80%

Metabolism: In the kidney, filtered, and absorbed at the renal tubule

Half-life:

I.M., I.V.: 2 hours

S.C.: 3 hours

Time to peak serum concentration: Within 3-8 hours

Usual Dosage Refer to individual protocols

Infants and Children:

Hemangiomas of infancy, pulmonary hemangiomatosis: S.C.: 1-3 million units/m^2/day once daily

Philadelphia chromosome-positive CML: I.M., S.C.: 2.5-5 million units/m^2 daily

Chronic hepatitis B: S.C.: 5-10 million units/m^2 3 times/week

Chronic hepatitis C: S.C.: 3 million units/m^2 3 times/week

Children >18 years and Adults: I.M., S.C.:

Hairy cell leukemia: Induction dose is 3 million units/day for 16-24 weeks; maintenance: 3 million units 3 times/week

AIDS-related Kaposi's sarcoma: Induction dose: 36 million units/day for 10-12 weeks; maintenance: 36 million units 3 times/week (may begin with dose escalation from 3 to 9 to 18 million units each day over 3 consecutive days followed by 36 million units/day for the remainder of the 10-12 weeks of induction); or 20 million units/m^2 daily for 4 weeks, then if responding, 20 million units/m^2 3 times/week

CML: 9 million units daily

Hepatitis C: Initial: 6 million units 3 times/week for 3 months followed by 3 million units 3 times/week for 9 months

Melanoma: 12 million units/m^2 3 times/week for 3 months

Administration Parenteral: S.C. (rather than I.M.) administration is suggested for those patients who are at risk for bleeding or are thrombocytopenic; rotate S.C. injection site to help minimize local reactions

Monitoring Parameters Baseline EKG, CBC with differential and platelet count, hemoglobin, hematocrit, blood glucose, electrolytes, liver and renal function tests, weight, neuropsychiatric monitoring

Patient Information Do not change brands as changes in dosage may result; possible mental status changes may occur while on therapy; may cause dry mouth

Nursing Implications Patient should be well hydrated; pretreatment with NSAIDs or acetaminophen can decrease fever and its severity and alleviate headache

Additional Information Indications and dosage regimens are specific for a particular brand of interferon; other brands of interferon (ie, Intron® A) have different indications (Continued)

Interferon Alfa-2a *(Continued)*

and dosage guidelines; do not change brands of interferon as changes in dosage may result

Dosage Forms

Injection, solution [multidose vial]: 6 million units/mL (3 mL) [contains benzyl alcohol]

Injection, solution [single-dose prefilled syringe; S.C. use only]: 3 million units/0.5 mL; 6 million units/0.5 mL (0.5 mL); 9 million units/0.5 mL (0.5 mL) [contains benzyl alcohol]

Injection, solution [single-dose vial]: 36 million units/mL (1 mL) [contains benzyl alcohol]

References

Ezekowitz RAB, Mulliken JB, and Folkman J, "Interferon Alfa-2a Therapy for Life-Threatening Hemangiomas of Infancy," *N Engl J Med*, 1992, 326(22):1456-63.

Jonas MM, Ott MJ, Nelson SP, et al, "Interferon-Alpha Treatment of Chronic Hepatitis C Virus Infection in Children," *Pediatr Infect Dis J*, 1998, 17(3):241-6.

Ozen H, Kocak N, Yuce A, et al, "Retreatment With Higher Dose Interferon Alpha in Children With Chronic Hepatitis B Infection," *Pediatr Infect Dis J*, 1999, 18(8):694-7.

White CW, Sondheimer HM, Crouch EC, et al, "Treatment of Pulmonary Hemangiomatosis With Recombinant Interferon Alfa-2a," *N Engl J Med*, 1989, 320(18):1197-200.

Interferon Alfa-2b (in ter FEER on AL fa too bee)

U.S. Brand Names Intron® A

Synonyms IFN-α-2; α-2-interferon; rIFN-α2

Therapeutic Category Antineoplastic Agent, Miscellaneous; Biological Response Modulator; Interferon

Generic Available No

Use Induce hairy cell leukemia remission; treatment of AIDS-related Kaposi's sarcoma; condylomata acuminata; adjuvant therapy of melanoma following surgical excision; chronic hepatitis C; chronic hepatitis B; hemangiomas of infancy

Pregnancy Risk Factor C

Contraindications Hypersensitivity to interferon alfa-2b or any component (see Warnings)

Warnings Safety and efficacy in children <18 years of age have not been established. The FDA currently recommends that procedures for proper handling and disposal of antineoplastic agents be considered. Alpha interferons suppress bone marrow function which may result in severe cytopenias or aplastic anemia. Alpha interferons may cause or aggravate fatal or life-threatening neuropsychiatric, autoimmune, ischemic, and infectious disorders. Patients with severe or worsening signs or symptoms of these conditions should be withdrawn from therapy.

Diluent for interferon alfa-2b injection contains benzyl alcohol which may cause allergic reactions in susceptible individuals; large amounts of benzyl alcohol (≥99 mg/kg/day) have been associated with a potentially fatal toxicity ("gasping syndrome") in neonates; the "gasping syndrome" consists of metabolic acidosis, respiratory distress, gasping respirations, CNS dysfunction (including convulsions, intracranial hemorrhage), hypotension and cardiovascular collapse; avoid use of interferon alfa-2b products containing benzyl alcohol in neonates; *in vitro* and animal studies have shown that benzoate, a metabolite of benzyl alcohol, displaces bilirubin from protein binding sites

Precautions Use with caution in patients with seizure disorders, brain metastases, compromised CNS, multiple sclerosis, and patients with pre-existing cardiac disease, severe renal or hepatic impairment, or myelosuppression

Adverse Reactions Flu-like symptoms (fever, fatigue/malaise, myalgia, chills, headache, arthralgia, rigors) begin about 2-6 hours after the dose is given and may persist as long as 24 hours; usually patient can build up a tolerance to side effects

Cardiovascular: Tachycardia, arrhythmias, hypotension, edema, chest pain, syncope

Central nervous system: Fatigue/malaise, dizziness, depression, confusion, sensory neuropathy, psychiatric symptoms (psychosis, mania, depression, suicidal behavior), fever, headache, EEG abnormalities, chills

Dermatologic: Partial alopecia, rash

Endocrine & metabolic: Elevated uric acid level, thyroid dysfunction, hyperglycemia, hypertriglyceridemia

Gastrointestinal: Anorexia, xerostomia, nausea, vomiting, diarrhea, abdominal cramps, dysgeusia, weight loss

Hematologic: Leukopenia (mainly neutropenia); anemia; thrombocytopenia; neutralizing antibodies

Hepatic: Elevated ALT and AST

Local: Burning, pain, erythema, rash at the site of injection, pruritus

Neuromuscular & skeletal: Myalgia, arthralgia, rigors

Ocular: Blurred vision, retinal hemorrhage

Renal: Proteinuria, elevated BUN and serum creatinine
Respiratory: Coughing, nasal congestion
Miscellaneous: Diaphoresis

Drug Interactions
Interferon Alfa-2a: May competitively bind to same receptors
Acyclovir: Possible synergistic effect
Theophylline: Clearance of theophylline is reduced
Vinblastine: May increase interferon toxicity; increased neurotoxicity
Zidovudine: Possible additive myelosuppression

Stability Refrigerate; reconstituted solution is stable for 1 month when refrigerated

Mechanism of Action Inhibits cellular growth, alters the state of cellular differentiation, interferes with oncogene expression, alters cell surface antigen expression, increases phagocytic activity of macrophages, and augments cytotoxicity of lymphocytes for target cells

Pharmacokinetics
Metabolism: Majority of dose is thought to be metabolized in the kidney, filtered and absorbed at the renal tubule
Half-life, elimination:
I.M., I.V.: 2 hours
S.C.: 3 hours
Time to peak serum concentration: I.M., S.C.: ~6-8 hours

Usual Dosage Refer to individual protocols:
Children: S.C.:
Chronic hepatitis B: 3-10 million units/m² 3 times/week
Chronic hepatitis C: 3-5 million units/m² 3 times/week
Hemangiomas: 3 million units/m² daily
Adults:
Hairy cell leukemia: I.M., S.C.: 2 million units/m² 3 times/week
AIDS-related Kaposi's sarcoma: I.M., S.C.: 30 million units/m² 3 times/week or 50 million units/m² I.V. 5 days/week every other week
Condylomata acuminata: Intralesionally: 1 million units/lesion 3 times/week for 3 weeks; not to exceed 5 million units per treatment (maximum dose: 5 lesions at one time) (use only the 10 million units vial)
Chronic hepatitis B: I.M., S.C.: 5 million units given once daily **or** 10 million units given 3 times/week for 4 months
Chronic hepatitis C: I.M., S.C.: 3 million units 3 times/week for approximately a 6-month course; relapse of hepatitis has occurred after treatment was stopped
Melanoma adjuvant therapy:
Induction: I.V.: 20 million units/m²/day 5 days/week for 4 weeks
Maintenance: S.C.: 10 million units/m²/day 3 days/week for 48 weeks

Administration Parenteral: S.C. (rather than I.M.) administration is suggested for those patients who are at risk for bleeding or are thrombocytopenic; rotate S.C. injection site

Monitoring Parameters Baseline EKG, CBC with differential and platelet count, hemoglobin, hematocrit, blood glucose, liver function tests, electrolytes, weight, chest x-ray, neuropsychiatric monitoring

Patient Information Do not change brands of interferon as changes in dosage may result; do not operate heavy machinery while on therapy since changes in mental status may occur; may cause dry mouth

Nursing Implications Patient should be well hydrated; may pretreat with NSAID or acetaminophen to decrease fever and its severity and to alleviate headache

Additional Information Myelosuppressive effects:
WBC: Mild
Platelets: Mild
Onset (days): 7-10
Nadir (days): 14
Recovery (days): 21

Dosage Forms
Injection, powder for reconstitution: 3 million units; 5 million units; 10 million units; 18 million units; 25 million units; 50 million units [contains human albumin; diluent contains benzyl alcohol]
Injection, solution [multidose prefilled pens]:
Delivers 3 million units/0.2 mL (1.5 mL) [delivers 6 doses; 18 million units]
Delivers 5 million units/0.2 mL (1.5 mL) [delivers 6 doses; 30 million units]
Delivers 10 million units/0.2 mL (1.5 mL) [delivers 6 doses; 60 million units]
Injection, solution [multidose vial]: 6 million units/mL (3 mL); 10 million units/mL (2.5 mL)
Injection, solution [single-dose vial]: 3 million units/0.5 mL (0.5 mL); 5 million units/0.5 mL (0.5 mL); 10 million units/mL (1 mL)

(Continued)

Interferon Alfa-2b *(Continued)*

References

Davis GL, Balart LA, Schiff ER, et al, "Treatment of Chronic Hepatitis C With Recombinant Interferon Alfa. A Multicenter Randomized, Controlled Trial. Hepatitis Interventional Therapy Group," *N Engl J Med*, 1989, 321(22):1501-6.

Garmendia G, Miranda N, Borroso S, et al, "Regression of Infancy Hemangiomas With Recombinant IFN-Alpha 2b," *J Interferon Cytokine Res*, 2001, 21(1):31-8.

Gurakan F, Kocak N, Ozen H, et al, "Comparison of Standard and High Dosage Recombinant Interferon Alpha 2b for Treatment of Children With Chronic Hepatitis B Infection," *Pediatr Infect Dis J*, 2000, 19(1):52-6.

Kirkwood JM, Ibrahim JG, Sondak VK, et al, "High- and Low-Dose Interferon Alfa-2b in High-Risk Melanoma: First Analysis of Intergroup Trial E1690/S9111/C9190," *J Clin Oncol*, 2000, 18(12):2444-58.

Zwiener RJ, Fielman BA, Cochran C, et al, "Interferon-Alpha-2b Treatment of Chronic Hepatitis C in Children With Hemophilia," *Pediatr Infect Dis J*, 1996, 15(10):906-8.

- ◆ **Interleukin-2** *see* Aldesleukin *on page 56*
- ◆ **Intralipid®** *see* Fat Emulsion *on page 475*
- ◆ **Intravenous Fat Emulsion** *see* Fat Emulsion *on page 475*
- ◆ **Intron® A** *see* Interferon Alfa-2b *on page 616*
- ◆ **Intropin® (Can)** *see* DOPamine *on page 405*
- ◆ **Invirase®** *see* Saquinavir *on page 1006*
- ◆ **Iodex [OTC]** *see* Iodine *on page 618*

Iodine (EYE oh dyne)

Related Information
Drugs and Breast-Feeding *on page 1404*

U.S. Brand Names Iodex [OTC]; Iodoflex™; Iodosorb®

Therapeutic Category Topical Skin Product

Generic Available Yes

Use Used topically as an antiseptic in the management of minor, superficial skin wounds and has been used to disinfect the skin preoperatively

Pregnancy Risk Factor D

Contraindications Hypersensitivity to iodine preparations or any component; neonates

Warnings May be highly toxic if ingested

Adverse Reactions
Local: Skin irritation, discoloration, and burns
Miscellaneous: Hypersensitivity, allergic reactions

Mechanism of Action Free iodine oxidizes microbial protoplasm making it effective against bacteria, fungi, yeasts, protozoa, and viruses; complexes with amino groups in tissue compounds to form iodophors from which the iodine is slowly released causing a sustained action

Usual Dosage Apply topically as necessary to affected areas of skin

Administration Topical: Apply to affected areas; avoid tight bandages because iodine may cause burns on occluded skin

Patient Information May stain skin and clothing

Additional Information Sodium thiosulfate inactivates iodine and is an effective chemical antidote for iodine poisoning; solutions of sodium thiosulfate may be used to remove iodine stains from skin and clothing

Dosage Forms
Dressing, topical (Iodoflex™): 0.9% (5 g, 10 g) [gel pad]
Gel, topical (Iodosorb®): 0.9% (40 g)
Ointment (Iodex): 4.7% (30 g, 720 g)
Solution: 2% (500 mL, 4000 mL); 5% (100 mL, 500 mL, 4000 mL)
Tincture: 2% (30 mL, 480 mL, 500 mL, 4000 mL); 7% (30 mL, 100 mL, 480 mL, 500 mL, 4000 mL)

- ◆ **Iodine Sodium** *see* Trace Metals *on page 1106*
- ◆ **Iodoflex™** *see* Iodine *on page 618*
- ◆ **Iodopen®** *see* Trace Metals *on page 1106*

Iodoquinol (eye oh doe KWIN ole)

U.S. Brand Names Yodoxin®

Canadian Brand Names Diodoquin®

Synonyms Diiodohydroxyquin

Therapeutic Category Amebicide

Generic Available No

Use Treatment of acute and chronic intestinal amebiasis due to *Entamoeba histolytica*; asymptomatic cyst passers; *Blastocystis hominis* infections; iodoquinol alone is ineffective for amebic hepatitis or hepatic abscess

Pregnancy Risk Factor C

Contraindications Hypersensitivity to iodine, iodoquinol, or any component; hepatic or renal damage; pre-existing optic neuropathy

Precautions Use with caution in patients with thyroid disease or neurological disorders

Adverse Reactions
Central nervous system: Agitation, retrograde amnesia, fever, chills, headache, ataxia
Dermatologic: Anal pruritus, rash, acne
Endocrine & metabolic: Enlargement of the thyroid
Gastrointestinal: Nausea, vomiting, diarrhea, gastritis, anorexia, constipation
Neuromuscular & skeletal: Weakness, peripheral neuropathy, myalgia
Ocular: Optic neuritis, optic atrophy, visual impairment

Mechanism of Action Contact amebicide that works in the lumen of the intestine by an unknown mechanism

Pharmacokinetics
Absorption: Oral: Poor and irregular
Metabolism: In the liver
Elimination: In feces; metabolites appear in urine

Usual Dosage Oral:
Children: 30-40 mg/kg/day in 3 divided doses for 20 days; not to exceed 1.95 g/day
Adults: 650 mg 3 times/day after meals for 20 days; not to exceed 2 g/day

Administration Oral: Administer medication after meals; tablets may be crushed and mixed with applesauce or chocolate syrup

Monitoring Parameters Ophthalmologic exam

Test Interactions May increase protein-bound serum iodine concentrations reflecting a decrease in iodine 131 uptake; false-positive ferric chloride test for phenylketonuria

Patient Information Notify physician if rash occurs

Dosage Forms
Powder: 25 g, 100 g
Tablet: 210 mg, 650 mg

♦ **Iodosorb®** *see* Iodine *on page 618*
♦ **Ionil® [OTC]** *see* Salicylic Acid *on page 1002*
♦ **Ionil® Plus [OTC]** *see* Salicylic Acid *on page 1002*
♦ **Iostat™ [OTC]** *see* Potassium Iodide *on page 918*

Ipecac Syrup (IP e kak SIR up)

Therapeutic Category Antidote, Emetic

Generic Available Yes

Use Treatment of acute oral drug overdosage and certain poisonings; use only in alert conscious patients who have ingested potentially toxic amounts of substance

Pregnancy Risk Factor C

Contraindications Hypersensitivity to ipecac syrup or any component; do not use in unconscious patients, patients with absent gag reflex or seizures; ingestion of strong bases or acids, other corrosive substances, volatile oils, hydrocarbons with high potential for aspiration

Warnings Avoid use in patients with coagulopathy or bleeding problems (risk of gastroesophageal hemorrhage) and in patients receiving calcium channel blockers, beta-blockers, clonidine, or digitalis glycosides (risk of exaggerated vagal stimulation with gagging, resulting in severe bradycardia); do not confuse ipecac syrup with ipecac fluid extract; fluid extract is 14 times more potent than syrup

Precautions Use with caution in patients with cardiovascular disease and bulimics

Adverse Reactions
Cardiovascular: Cardiotoxicity
Central nervous system: Lethargy, drowsiness
Gastrointestinal: Protracted vomiting, diarrhea; Mallory-Weiss syndrome, gastric rupture
Neuromuscular & skeletal: Myopathy
Respiratory: Aspiration (can be fatal)

Drug Interactions Activated charcoal may decrease effectiveness

Food Interactions Milk, carbonated beverages may decrease effectiveness

Mechanism of Action Irritates the gastric mucosa and stimulates the medullary chemoreceptor trigger zone to induce vomiting

Pharmacodynamics
Onset of vomiting after oral dose: Within 15-30 minutes; usual: 20 minutes
(Continued)

Ipecac Syrup (Continued)

Duration: 20-25 minutes; can last longer, up to 1-2 hours

Usual Dosage Oral:

Children:

<6 months: Not recommended

6-12 months: 5-10 mL followed by 10-20 mL/kg or 120-240 mL of water; repeat dose one time if vomiting does not occur within 20-30 minutes

1-12 years: 15 mL followed by 10-20 mL/kg or 120-240 mL of water; repeat dose one time if vomiting does not occur within 20-30 minutes

Adolescents and Adults: 30 mL followed by 240 mL of water; repeat dose one time if vomiting does not occur within 20-30 minutes

Administration Oral: Administer within 60 minutes of ingestion; follow administration with water; do not administer with milk or carbonated beverages

Nursing Implications Do **not** administer to unconscious patients

Additional Information Patients should be kept active and moving following administration of ipecac; if vomiting does not occur after second dose, gastric lavage may be considered to remove ingested substance

The Position Statement of The American Academy of Clinical Toxicology and The European Association of Poisons Centres and Clinical Toxicologists does not recommend routine administration of ipecac syrup to poisoned patients; scientific literature does not support that ipecac improves patient outcome; this paper states that the **routine** administration of ipecac syrup in the emergency room should be abandoned. Also, scientific literature cannot support or exclude giving ipecac syrup soon after toxic ingestions; administration of ipecac syrup may delay the administration or decrease the effectiveness of activated charcoal, oral antidotes, or whole bowel irrigation; its use should be considered only if it can be given within 60 minutes after ingestion of poison.

Dosage Forms Syrup: 70 mg/mL (30 mL, 500 mL, 4000 mL) [contains alcohol]

References

"Position Statement: Ipecac Syrup. American Academy of Clinical Toxicology; European Association of Poisons Centres and Clinical Toxicologists," *J Toxicol Clin Toxicol*, 1997, 35(7):699-709.

Quang LS and Woolf AD, "Past, Present, and Future Role of Ipecac Syrup," *Curr Opin Pediatr*, 2000, 12(2):153-62.

Shannon M, "Ingestion of Toxic Substances by Children," *N Engl J Med*, 2000, 342(3):186-91.

Ipratropium (i pra TROE pee um)

Related Information

Asthma Guidelines on page 1376

U.S. Brand Names Atrovent®

Canadian Brand Names Alti-Ipratropium; Apo®-Ipravent; Gen-Ipratropium; Novo-Ipramide; Nu-Ipratropium; PMS-Ipratropium

Therapeutic Category Antiasthmatic; Anticholinergic Agent; Bronchodilator

Generic Available Yes (solution for nebulization)

Use Anticholinergic bronchodilator used in bronchospasm associated with asthma, COPD, bronchitis, and emphysema; symptomatic relief of rhinorrhea associated with allergic and nonallergic rhinitis

Pregnancy Risk Factor B

Contraindications Hypersensitivity to ipratropium, atropine, or its derivatives

Warnings Not indicated for the initial treatment of acute episodes of bronchospasm

Precautions Use with caution in patients with narrow-angle glaucoma, bladder neck obstruction, or prostatic hypertrophy

Adverse Reactions

Note: Ipratropium is poorly absorbed from the lung, so systemic effects are rare

Cardiovascular: Palpitations, tachycardia, flushing, hypotension, hypertension

Central nervous system: Nervousness, dizziness, headache, fatigue, drowsiness, insomnia

Dermatologic: Rash, pruritus, alopecia

Gastrointestinal: Nausea, xerostomia, constipation

Genitourinary: Dysuria

Ocular: Blurred vision

Respiratory: Cough, hoarseness, dry secretions, epistaxis (with nasal spray)

Drug Interactions Additive effects with anticholinergics or drugs with anticholinergic properties

Stability Compatible for 1 hour when mixed with albuterol or metaproterenol in a nebulizer

Mechanism of Action Blocks the action of acetylcholine at parasympathetic sites in bronchial smooth muscle causing bronchodilation; inhibits secretions from the serous and seromucous glands lining the nasal mucosa

Pharmacodynamics
Onset of bronchodilation: 1-3 minutes after administration
Maximal effect: Maximal effect within 1.5-2 hours
Duration: Bronchodilation persists for up to 4-6 hours

Pharmacokinetics
Absorption: Not readily absorbed into the systemic circulation from the surface of the lung or from the GI tract
Distribution: Following inhalation, 15% of dose reaches the lower airways
Half-life: 2 hours

Usual Dosage
Acute exacerbation of asthma (NIH guidelines):
Children: Nebulization: 250 mcg every 20 minutes for 3 doses then every 2-4 hours
Metered inhaler: 4-8 puffs as needed
Children >12 years and Adults: Nebulization: 500 mcg every 30 minutes for 3 doses then every 2-4 hours as needed
Metered inhaler: 4-8 puffs as needed

Maintenance treatments (nonacute):
Neonates: Nebulization: 25 mcg/kg/dose 3 times/day
Infants and Children: Nebulization: 125-250 mcg 3 times/day
Children 3-12 years: Metered inhaler: 1-2 inhalations 3 times/day, up to 6 inhalations/24 hours
Children ≥12 years and Adults:
Nebulization: 500 mcg 3-4 times/day
Metered inhaler: 2 inhalations 4 times/day, up to 12 inhalations/24 hours
Nasal spray:
Children >6 years and Adults: 0.03%: 2 sprays in each nostril 2-3 times/day
Children >5 years and Adults: 0.06%: 2 sprays in each nostril 3-4 times/day

Administration
Nasal spray: Pump must be primed before usage by 7 actuations into the air away from the face; if not used for >24 hours, pump must be reprimed with 2 actuations; if not used >7 days, reprime with 7 actuations
Nebulization: May be administered with or without dilution in NS; use of a nebulizer with a mouth piece rather than a face mask may be preferred to prevent contact with eyes
Oral Inhalation: Shake well before use; use spacer device in children <8 years

Patient Information
May cause dry mouth

Dosage Forms
Solution for nebulization, as bromide (Atrovent®): 0.02% (2.5 mL)
Solution for oral inhalation, as bromide: 18 mcg/actuation (14 g)
Solution, intranasal spray, as bromide: 0.03% (30 mL); 0.06% (15 mL)

References
"Guidelines for the Diagnosis and Management of Asthma. NAEPP Expert Panel Report 2," July 1997, www.nhlbi.nih.gov/guidelines/asthma/asthgdln.pdf.
Henry RI, Hiller EG, Milner AD, et al, "Nebulised Ipratropium Bromide and Sodium Cromoglycate in the First 2 Years of Life," Arch Dis Child, 1984, 59(1):54-7.
Mann NP and Hiller RG, "Ipratropium Bromide in Children With Asthma," Thorax, 1982, 37(1):72-4.
"National Asthma Education and Prevention Program. Expert Panel Report: Guidelines for the Diagnosis and Management of Asthma Update on Selected Topics--2002," J Allergy Clin Immunol, 2002, 110(5 Suppl):S141-219.
Schuh S, Johnson DW, Callahan S, et al, "Efficacy of Frequent Nebulized Ipratropium Added to Frequent High-Dose Albuterol Therapy in Severe Childhood Asthma," J Pediatr, 1995, 126(4):639-45.
Schuh S, Johnson D, Canny G, et al, "Efficacy of Adding Nebulized Ipratropium Bromide to Nebulized Albuterol Therapy in Acute Bronchiolitis," Pediatrics, 1992, 90(6): 920-3.
Wang EE, Milner R, Allen U, et al, "Bronchodilators for Treatment of Mild Bronchiolitis: A Factorial Randomized Trial," Arch Dis Child, 1992, 67(3):289-93.
Wilkie RA and Bryan MH, "Effect of Bronchodilators on Airway Resistance in Ventilator-dependent Neonates With Chronic Lung Disease," J Pediatr, 1987, 111(2):278-82.

♦ I-Prin [OTC] see Ibuprofen on page 588
♦ Iproveratril see Verapamil on page 1144
♦ Ircon® [OTC] see Iron Supplements (Oral/Enteral) on page 623

Irinotecan (eye rye no TEE kan)
U.S. Brand Names Camptosar®
Synonyms Camptothecin-11; CPT-11
Therapeutic Category Antineoplastic Agent, Topoisomerase Inhibitor
Generic Available No
Use Childhood refractory solid tumors including neuroblastoma, hepatocellular tumor, Wilms' tumor, osteosarcoma, and rhabdomyosarcoma; recurrent or refractory CNS tumors such as medulloblastoma, ependymoma, brain stem glioma, or astrocytoma; adult brain tumors; colorectal, breast, and prostate cancer; leukemia, lymphoma, small and nonsmall cell lung cancer, and gastric, ovarian, and cervical cancer
(Continued)

Irinotecan *(Continued)*

Pregnancy Risk Factor D

Contraindications Hypersensitivity to irinotecan or any component; pregnancy

Warnings The FDA currently recommends that procedures for proper handling and disposal of antineoplastic agents be considered. Irinotecan is potentially embryotoxic and teratogenic if administered to pregnant women.

Early and late forms of severe diarrhea have been reported with irinotecan administration. Early diarrhea has occurred during or shortly after infusion and may be accompanied by symptoms of rhinitis, increased salivation, miosis, lacrimation, diaphoresis, flushing, and abdominal cramping. Atropine 0.01 mg/kg I.V. (maximum dose: 0.4 mg) may be used to prevent or treat symptoms of early diarrhea. Late diarrhea has occurred >24 hours after irinotecan administration and can be prolonged leading to life-threatening dehydration and electrolyte imbalance. Treat late diarrhea promptly with loperamide until a normal pattern of bowel movements returns (see Additional Information for loperamide dosing recommendation); fluid and electrolyte replacement may be needed for dehydration. Interrupt or reduce subsequent irinotecan doses if National Cancer Institute (NCI) grade 3 (increase of 7-9 stools daily, or incontinence, or severe cramping) or grade 4 (increase ≥10 stools daily, grossly bloody stool, or need for parenteral support) late diarrhea occurs.

Deaths due to sepsis following severe myelosuppression have been reported with irinotecan administration. Patients with abnormal glucuronidation of bilirubin, such as Gilbert's syndrome, may also be at greater risk of myelosuppression when receiving irinotecan. Temporarily discontinue therapy if neutropenic fever occurs or if absolute neutrophil count is <1000/mm^3.

Precautions Use with caution and reduce initial irinotecan dose in patients with elevated total serum bilirubin concentration (1-2 mg/dL) who previously received pelvic/abdominal radiation therapy or in patients with baseline total serum bilirubin concentration >2 mg/dL.

Adverse Reactions

Cardiovascular: Facial flushing

Central nervous system: Fever, asthenia, tremor, headache, dizziness, confusion, insomnia

Dermatologic: Alopecia, rash

Endocrine & metabolic: Hyponatremia, hypernatremia, hypokalemia, metabolic acidosis

Gastrointestinal: Diarrhea (see Warnings), nausea, vomiting, abdominal pain, anorexia, constipation, mucositis, colitis

Genitourinary: Hematuria, proteinuria, glucosuria

Hematologic: Leukopenia, neutropenia, thrombocytopenia, thromboembolism

Hepatic: Elevated transaminases, alkaline phosphatase, bilirubin

Local: Pain at infusion site

Renal: Elevated serum creatinine, acute renal failure (rare)

Respiratory: Pulmonary infiltrates, pneumonitis, dyspnea, cough

Miscellaneous: Anaphylaxis

Drug Interactions Cytochrome P450 isoenzyme CYP2B6 and CYP3A3/4 substrate

Concurrent administration of erythromycin, cimetidine, fluconazole, or itraconazole with irinotecan may result in increased exposure to irinotecan; phenytoin, phenobarbital, and carbamazepine may decrease systemic exposure to SN-38, the active metabolite; prochlorperazine may increase incidence of akathisia

Stability Store unopened vials at room temperature; protect from light. Once injectable solution is mixed with D$_5$W, solution is stable for 24 hours if stored at room temperature or 48 hours if stored refrigerated. Injectable solution mixed with NS is stable for 24 hours if stored at room temperature. Do not refrigerate solutions mixed in NS since visible particulates may develop.

Mechanism of Action Prodrug undergoes de-esterification by cellular carboxylesterases to a potent active metabolite (SN-38) which is a topoisomerase I inhibitor. Binds to topoisomerase I-DNA complex preventing religation of single-strand DNA breaks.

Pharmacokinetics

Protein binding:

Irinotecan: 30% to 68%

SN-38 (active metabolite): 95%

Half-life, terminal: Adults:

Irinotecan: 6-12 hours

SN-38 (active metabolite): 10-20 hours

Metabolism: Irinotecan is converted to its active metabolite SN-38 by carboxylesterase-mediated cleavage of the carbamate bond. SN-38 undergoes conjugation to a glucuronide metabolite in the liver. Irinotecan also undergoes oxidation by cytochrome P450 3A4 to yield to 2 inactive metabolites.

Elimination: 11% to 20% of irinotecan and <1% SN-38 is excreted in the urine

Usual Dosage I.V. infusion (refer to individual protocols):

Children:

Refractory solid tumor (low-dose, protracted schedule): 20 mg/m^2/day for 5 days for 2 consecutive weeks followed by a week of rest; repeat cycle every 3 weeks

Refractory solid tumor or CNS tumor: 50 mg/m^2/day for 5 days; repeat cycle every 21 days

Adults:

Colorectal cancer that has recurred or progressed following fluorouracil-containing chemotherapy: 300-350 mg/m^2/dose once every 3 weeks or 125 mg/m^2/dose once weekly (maximum dose: 150 mg/m^2) for 4 weeks followed by a 2-week rest period; repeat courses every 6 weeks (4 weeks of therapy followed by 2 weeks off)

Small cell lung cancer: 100-125 mg/m^2/dose once weekly (maximum dose: 150 mg/m^2) or 350 mg/m^2/dose once every 3 weeks; or 60-70 mg/m^2 once weekly for 3 weeks in combination with other agents

Note: A new cycle of irinotecan therapy should not begin until serious treatment-induced toxicity has fully resolved, granulocyte count recovers to ≥1500/mm^3, and platelet count recovers to ≥100,000/mm^3. Treatment should be delayed 1-2 weeks to allow for recovery from treatment-related toxicities. If the patient has not recovered after a 2-week delay, consider discontinuing irinotecan.

Administration Parenteral: I.V. infusion: Irinotecan can be further diluted in D$_5$W (preferred diluent) or NS to a final concentration of 0.12-2.8 mg/mL. Infuse over 60-90 minutes depending on protocol. Higher incidence of cholinergic symptoms have been reported with more rapid infusion rates.

Monitoring Parameters Signs of diarrhea and dehydration, serum electrolytes, serum BUN and creatinine; infusion site for signs of inflammation; CBC with differential and platelet count, liver function tests, and serum bilirubin

Patient Information Advise women of childbearing potential to avoid becoming pregnant while receiving irinotecan. Avoid the use of laxatives. Notify physician if diarrhea, vomiting, fever, or symptoms of dehydration such as fainting, lightheadedness, or dizziness occur. Initiate loperamide therapy at the first episode of poorly formed or loose stools after irinotecan administration (see Additional Information).

Nursing Implications Avoid extravasation. If extravasation occurs, flush the site with sterile water and apply an ice pack. To prevent emesis, pretreat with a 5HT-3 antagonist and dexamethasone 30 minutes prior to irinotecan therapy.

Additional Information Loperamide dosing for treatment of late diarrhea: Oral:

8-10 kg: 1 mg after the first loose bowel movement followed by 0.5 mg every 3 hours until a normal pattern of bowel movement returns. Take 0.75 mg every 4 hours during the night rather than every 3 hours.

10.1-20 kg: 1 mg after the first loose bowel movement followed by 1 mg every 3 hours until a normal pattern of bowel movement returns. Take 1 mg every 4 hours during the night rather than every 3 hours.

20.1-30 kg: 2 mg after the first loose bowel movement followed by 1 mg every 3 hours until a normal pattern of bowel movement returns. Take 2 mg every 4 hours during the night rather than every 3 hours.

30.1-43 kg: 2 mg after the first loose bowel movement followed by 1 mg every 2 hours until a normal pattern of bowel movement returns. Take 2 mg every 4 hours during the night rather than every 2 hours.

>43 kg: 4 mg after the first loose bowel movement followed by 2 mg every 2 hours until the patient is diarrhea free for 12 hours. Take 4 mg every 4 hours during the night rather than every 2 hours.

Dosage Forms Injection, solution, as hydrochloride: 20 mg/mL (2 mL, 5 mL)

References

Cosetti M, Wexler LH, Calleja E, et al, "Irinotecan for Pediatric Solid Tumors: The Memorial Sloan-Kettering Experience," *J Pediatr Hematol Oncol*, 2002, 24(2):101-5.

Gajjar A, Chintagumpala MM, Bowers DC, et al, "Effect of Intrapatient Dosage Escalation of Irinotecan on Its Pharmacokinetics in Pediatric Patients Who Have High-Grade Gliomas and Receive Enzyme-Inducing Anticonvulsant Therapy," *Cancer*, 2003, 97(9 Suppl):2374-80.

♦ **Iron Dextran** *see* Iron Supplements (Parenteral) *on page 626*

♦ **Iron Sucrose** *see* Iron Supplements (Parenteral) *on page 626*

♦ **Iron Sulfate (Ferrous Sulfate)** *see* Iron Supplements (Oral/Enteral) *on page 623*

Iron Supplements (Oral/Enteral) (EYE ern SUP la ments)

Related Information

Carbohydrate and Alcohol Content of Liquid Medications for Use in Patients Receiving Ketogenic Diets *on page 1431*

Overdose and Toxicology *on page 1388*

(Continued)

Iron Supplements (Oral/Enteral) *(Continued)*

U.S. Brand Names Feosol® [OTC]; Feostat® [OTC]; Feratab® [OTC]; Fer-Gen-Sol [OTC]; Fergon® [OTC]; Fer-In-Sol® [OTC]; Ferretts [OTC]; Ferrex 150® [OTC]; Ferro-Sequels® [OTC]; Fe-Tinic™ 150 [OTC]; Hemocyte™ [OTC]; Hytinic® [OTC]; Ircon® [OTC]; Nephro-Fer® [OTC]; Niferex® [OTC]; Niferex® 150 [OTC]; Nu-Iron® 150 [OTC]; Poly-Iron 150 [OTC]; Slow FE® [OTC]

Synonyms FeSO$_4$ (Ferrous Sulfate); Iron Sulfate (Ferrous Sulfate)

Available Salts Ferrous Fumarate; Ferrous Gluconate; Ferrous Sulfate

Therapeutic Category Iron Salt; Mineral, Oral

Generic Available Yes

Use Prevention and treatment of iron deficiency anemias; supplemental therapy for patients receiving epoetin alfa

Pregnancy Risk Factor A

Contraindications Hypersensitivity to iron salts or any component (see Warnings); hemochromatosis, hemolytic anemia

Warnings Avoid use in premature infants until the vitamin E stores, deficient at birth, are replenished; some products contain sulfites and/or tartrazine which may cause allergic reactions in susceptible individuals

Precautions Avoid using for longer than 6 months, except in patients with conditions that require prolonged therapy; avoid in patients with peptic ulcer, enteritis, or ulcerative colitis; avoid in patients receiving frequent blood transfusions

Adverse Reactions

Gastrointestinal: GI irritation, epigastric pain, nausea, diarrhea, dark stools, constipation

Genitourinary: Discoloration of urine (black or dark)

Miscellaneous: Liquid preparations may temporarily stain the teeth

Drug Interactions Absorption of oral preparation of iron and tetracyclines are decreased when both of these drugs are given together; concurrent administration of antacids and cimetidine may decrease iron absorption; iron may decrease absorption of penicillamine, levothyroxine, methyldopa, and levodopa when given at the same time; response to iron therapy may be delayed in patients receiving chloramphenicol; concurrent administration of ≥200 mg vitamin C per 30 mg elemental iron increases absorption of oral iron; absorption of quinolones may be decreased due to formation of a ferric ion-quinolone complex

Food Interactions Milk, cereals, dietary fiber, tea, coffee, or eggs decrease absorption of iron

Mechanism of Action Iron is released from the plasma and eventually replenishes the depleted iron stores in the bone marrow where it is incorporated into hemoglobin

Pharmacodynamics

Onset of action: Hematologic response to either oral or parenteral iron salts is essentially the same; red blood cell form and color changes within 3-10 days

Maximum effect: Peak reticulocytosis occurs in 5-10 days, and hemoglobin values increase within 2-4 weeks

Pharmacokinetics

Absorption: Oral: Iron is absorbed in the duodenum and upper jejunum; in persons with normal iron stores 10% of an oral dose is absorbed, this is increased to 20% to 30% in persons with inadequate iron stores; food and achlorhydria will decrease absorption

Elimination: Iron is largely bound to serum transferrin and excreted in the urine, sweat, sloughing of intestinal mucosa, and by menses

Usual Dosage Note: Multiple salt forms of iron exist; close attention must be paid to the salt form when ordering and administering iron; incorrect selection

Recommended Daily Allowance of Iron
(dosage expressed as elemental iron)

Age	RDA (mg)
<5 mo	5
5 mo to 10 y	10
Male	
11-18 y	12
>18 y	10
Female	
11-50 y	15
>50 y	10

or substitution of one salt for another without proper dosage adjustment may result in serious over- or underdosing.

Oral (dose expressed in terms of **elemental** iron):
Recommended Daily Allowance, see table on previous page.
Premature neonates: 2-4 mg elemental iron/kg/day divided every 12-24 hours (maximum dose: 15 mg/day)
Infants and Children:
Severe iron deficiency anemia: 4-6 mg elemental iron/kg/day in 3 divided doses
Mild to moderate iron deficiency anemia: 3 mg elemental iron/kg/day in 1-2 divided doses
Prophylaxis: 1-2 mg elemental iron/kg/day up to a maximum of 15 mg elemental iron/day
Adults:
Iron deficiency: 2-3 mg/kg/day or 60-100 mg elemental iron twice daily up to 60 mg elemental iron 4 times/day, or 50 mg elemental iron (extended release) 1-2 times/day
Prophylaxis: 60-100 mg elemental iron/day; see table

Elemental Iron Content of Iron Salts

Iron Salt	Elemental Iron Content (% of salt form)	Approximate Equivalent Doses (mg of iron salt)
Ferrous fumarate	33	197
Ferrous gluconate	11.6	560
Ferrous sulfate	20	324
Ferrous sulfate, exsiccated	30	217

Administration Oral: Do not chew or crush sustained release preparations; administer with water or juice between meals for maximum absorption; may administer with food if GI upset occurs; do not administer with milk or milk products

Monitoring Parameters Serum iron, total iron binding capacity, reticulocyte count, hemoglobin, ferritin

Reference Range
Serum iron:
Newborns: 110-270 µg/dL
Infants: 30-70 µg/dL
Children: 55-120 µg/dL
Adults: Male: 75-175 µg/dL; Female: 65-165 µg/dL
Total iron binding capacity:
Newborns: 59-175 µg/dL
Infants: 100-400 µg/dL
Children and Adults: 230-430 µg/dL
Transferrin: 204-360 mg/dL
Percent transferrin saturation: 20% to 50%
Iron levels >300 µg/dL may be considered toxic; should be treated as an overdosage
Ferritin: 13-300 ng/mL

Test Interactions False-positive for blood in stool by the guaiac test

Patient Information May color the stools and urine black; do not take within 2 hours of tetracyclines or fluoroquinolones, do not take with milk or antacids; keep out of reach of children

Additional Information When treating iron deficiency anemias, treat for 3-4 months after hemoglobin/hematocrit return to normal in order to replenish total body stores; elemental iron dosages as high as 15 mg/kg/day have been used to supplement neonates receiving concomitant epoetin alpha in the treatment of anemia of prematurity

Dosage Forms
Ferrous fumarate:
Suspension, oral (Feostat® [DSC]): 100 mg/5 mL (240 mL) [33 mg/5 mL elemental iron]
Tablet: 325 mg [106 mg elemental iron]
Ferretts: 325 mg [106 mg elemental iron]
Hemocyte™: 324 mg [106 mg elemental iron]
Icron®: 200 mg [66 mg elemental iron]
Nephro-Fer®: 350 mg [115 mg elemental iron]
Tablet, chewable (Feostat®): 100 mg [33 mg elemental iron; chocolate flavor]
Tablet, timed release (Ferro-Sequels®): 150 mg [50 mg elemental iron; contains 100 mg docusate sodium]
(Continued)

Iron Supplements (Oral/Enteral) *(Continued)*

Ferrous gluconate:
Tablet: 240 mg [27 mg elemental iron]; 246 mg [28 mg elemental iron]; 300 mg [34 mg elemental iron]; 324 mg [37 mg elemental iron]; 325 mg [38 mg elemental iron]

Fergon®: 240 mg [27 mg elemental iron; contains tartrazine]

Ferrous sulfate:
Liquid, oral **drops**: 75 mg/0.6 mL (50 mL) [15 mg/0.6 mL elemental iron]

Fer-Gen-Sol: 75 mg/0.6 mL (50 mL) [15 mg/0.6 mL elemental iron; lemon-lime flavor]

Fer-In-Sol®: 75 mg/0.6 mL (50 mL) [15 mg/0.6 mL elemental iron; contains 0.2% alcohol and sodium bisulfite]

Tablet: 324 mg [65 mg elemental iron]; 325 mg [65 mg elemental iron]

Feratab®: 300 mg [60 mg elemental iron]

Tablet, exsiccated (Feosol®): 200 mg [65 mg elemental iron]

Tablet, exsiccated, timed release (Slow FE®): 160 mg [50 mg elemental iron]

Polysaccharide - iron complex:
Capsule, as elemental iron (Ferrex 150®, Fe-Tinic™ 150, Hytinic®, Niferex® 150, Nu-Iron® 150, Poly-Iron 150): 150 mg

Elixir, as elemental iron (Niferex®): 100 mg/5 mL (240 mL) [contains alcohol]

Tablet, as elemental iron (Niferex®): 50 mg

Iron Supplements (Parenteral) (EYE ern SUP la ments)

U.S. Brand Names Dexferrum®; Ferrlecit®; InFed®; Venofer®

Synonyms Iron Dextran; Iron Sucrose

Available Salts Sodium Ferric Gluconate

Therapeutic Category Iron Salt, Parenteral; Mineral, Parenteral

Generic Available No

Use

Iron dextran: Treatment of microcytic, hypochromic anemia resulting from iron deficiency when oral iron administration is infeasible or ineffective

Ferric gluconate and iron sucrose: Treatment of microcytic, hypochromic anemia in combination with erythropoietin in hemodialysis patients when iron administration is not feasible or ineffective

Pregnancy Risk Factor B (ferric gluconate, iron sucrose); C (iron dextran)

Contraindications Hypersensitivity to the iron formulation or any component (see Warnings); anemias that are not associated with iron deficiency; hemochromatosis; hemolytic anemia; iron overload

Warnings Deaths associated with parenteral iron administration following anaphylactic-type reactions have been reported; treatment agents for anaphylactic reactions (eg, epinephrine, steroids, diphenhydramine) should be immediately available; a test dose is recommended prior to initial therapy; rapid I.V. administration is associated with flushing, fatigue, weakness, chest, back, groin, or flank pain, and hypotension; use parenteral iron only in patients where the iron deficient state is not amenable to oral iron therapy; only iron dextran is approved for I.M. administration.

Ferric gluconate formulation contains benzyl alcohol which may cause allergic reactions in susceptible individuals; large amounts of benzyl alcohol (≥99 mg/kg/day) have been associated with a potentially fatal toxicity ("gasping syndrome") in neonates; the "gasping syndrome" consists of metabolic acidosis, respiratory distress, gasping respirations, CNS dysfunction (including convulsions, intracranial hemorrhage), hypotension and cardiovascular collapse; *in vitro* and animal studies have shown that benzoate, a metabolite of benzyl alcohol, displaces bilirubin from protein-binding sites; avoid use of ferric gluconate formulation in neonates

Precautions Use with caution in patients with histories of significant allergies, asthma, hepatic impairment, rheumatoid arthritis

Adverse Reactions Anaphylactoid reactions: Respiratory difficulties and cardiovascular collapse have been reported and occur most frequently within the first several minutes of administration

Cardiovascular: Cardiovascular collapse, hypotension, flushing, chest pain, syncope, tachycardia, MI, hypovolemia

Central nervous system: Dizziness, fever, headache, chills, shivering, malaise, insomnia, agitation, somnolence

Dermatologic: Urticaria, pruritus, rash

Gastrointestinal: Nausea, vomiting, diarrhea, metallic taste, abdominal pain, dyspepsia, flatulence, eructation, melena

Genitourinary: Discoloration of urine

Hematologic: Leukocytosis

Hepatic: Elevated liver enzymes

Local: Pain, staining of skin at the site of I.M. injection, phlebitis

Neuromuscular & skeletal: Arthralgia, arthritic reactivation in patients with quiescent arthritis, backache, paresthesia, leg cramps, weakness

Ocular: Blurred vision, conjunctivitis

Renal: Hematuria

Respiratory: Dyspnea, cough, rhinitis, upper respiratory infection, pulmonary edema, pneumonia

Miscellaneous: Lymphadenopathy, diaphoresis

Note: Sweating, urticaria, arthralgia, fever, chills, dizziness, headache, and nausea may be delayed 24-48 hours after I.V. administration or 3-4 days after I.M. administration

Stability Store at room temperature; use immediately after dilution in NS; product literature states parenteral iron formulations should not be mixed with other medications or in parenteral nutrition solutions

Mechanism of Action Replaces iron found in hemoglobin, myoglobin, and specific enzymes; allows transportation of oxygen via hemoglobin

Pharmacodynamics

Onset of action: Hematologic response to either oral or parenteral iron salts is essentially the same; red blood cell form and color changes within 3-10 days

Maximum effect: Peak reticulocytosis occurs in 5-10 days, and hemoglobin values increase within 2-4 weeks

Pharmacokinetics

Absorption: I.M.: 60% absorbed after 3 days; 90% after 1-3 weeks, the balance is slowly absorbed over months

Following I.V. doses, the uptake of iron by the reticuloendothelial system appears to be constant at about 10-20 mg/hour

Elimination: By the reticuloendothelial system and excreted in urine and feces (via bile)

Dialysis: Not dialyzable

Usual Dosage Multiple forms for parenteral iron exist; close attention must be paid to the specific product when ordering and administering; incorrect selection or substitution of one form for another without proper dosage adjustment may result in serious over or under dosing; test doses are recommended before starting therapy

Ferric gluconate: Adults: I.V.: **Dosage expressed in mg elemental iron:** Test dose: 25 mg (2 mL); repletion dose: 125 mg (10 mL) during hemodialysis; most patients will require a cumulative dose of 1 g over ~8 sequential dialysis treatments to achieve a favorable response

Iron dextran:

Iron deficiency anemia:

I.M., I.V.: Test dose (given 1 hour prior to starting iron dextran therapy):

Infants: 12.5 mg (0.25 mL)

Children, Adolescents, and Adults: 25 mg (0.5 mL)

Total replacement dosage of iron dextran for iron deficiency anemia:

(mL) = 0.0476 x LBW (kg) x (Hb_n - Hb_o) + 1 mL/per 5 kg LBW (up to maximum of 14 mL)

LBW = lean body weight

Hb_n = desired hemoglobin (g/dL) = 12 if <15 kg or 14.8 if >15 kg

Hb_o = measured hemoglobin (g/dL)

Total iron replacement dosage for acute blood loss: Assumes 1 mL of normocytic, normochromic red cells = 1 mg elemental iron: Iron dextran (mL) = 0.02 x blood loss (mL) x hematocrit (expressed as a decimal fraction)

Note: Total dose infusions have been used safely and are the preferred method of administration

I.M.: Maximum daily dose: Injected in daily or less frequent increments:

Infants <5 kg: 25 mg

Children 5-10 kg: 50 mg

Children >10 kg and Adults: 100 mg

Anemia of prematurity: I.V.: Neonates: 0.2-1 mg/kg/day or 20 mg/kg/week with epoetin alfa therapy

Anemia of chronic renal failure: I.V.: Children and Adults: 2 mg/kg three times/week with epoetin alfa therapy

Iron sucrose: Adults: I.V. **(doses expressed in mg of elemental iron):**

Test dose: 50 mg (while product labeling does not indicate need for a test dose in product-naive patients, test doses were administered in some clinical trials); 100 mg (5 mL) administered 1-3 times/week during dialysis, for a total dose of 1000 mg (10 doses); administer no more than 3 times/week; may continue to administer at lowest dose necessary to maintain target hemoglobin, hematocrit, and iron storage parameters

(Continued)

Iron Supplements (Parenteral) *(Continued)*

Administration Parenteral: Avoid dilution in dextrose due to an increased incidence of local pain and phlebitis

Iron dextran:
> I.M.: Use Z-track technique for I.M. administration (deep into the upper outer quadrant of buttock)
> I.V.: Infuse test dose over at least 5 minutes; dilute replacement dose in NS (50-100 mL), maximum concentration 50 mg/mL and infuse over 1-6 hours at a maximum rate of 50 mg/minute

Ferric gluconate:
> I.V. infusion: Dilute test dose in 50 mL NS and infuse over 1 hour; dilute repletion dose (125 mg) in 100 mL NS and infuse over at least 1 hour; do not exceed 2.1 mg/minute; **not for I.M. administration**
> Slow I.V. injection: 1 mL (12.5 mg iron) of undiluted solution per minute (5 minutes/vial)

Iron sucrose:
> Slow I.V. injection: 1 mL (20 mg iron) of undiluted solution per minute (5 minutes/vial)
> Infusion: Dilute 1 vial (5 mL) in maximum of 100 mL NS; infuse over at least 15 minutes; **not for I.M. administration**

Monitoring Parameters Vital signs and other symptoms of anaphylactoid reactions (during I.V. infusion); reticulocyte count, serum ferritin, hemoglobin, serum iron concentrations, and TIBC may not be meaningful for 3 weeks after administration, especially after large I.V. doses

Reference Range
Serum iron:
> Newborns: 110-270 µg/dL
> Infants: 30-70 µg/dL
> Children: 55-120 µg/dL
> Adults: Male: 75-175 µg/dL; female: 65-165 µg/dL

Total iron binding capacity:
> Newborns: 59-175 µg/dL
> Infants: 100-400 µg/dL
> Children and Adults: 230-430 µg/dL

Transferrin: 204-360 mg/dL
Percent transferrin saturation: 20% to 50%
Iron levels >300 µg/dL may be considered toxic; should be treated as an overdosage
Ferritin: 13-300 ng/mL

Test Interactions May cause falsely elevated values of serum bilirubin and falsely decreased values of serum calcium

Nursing Implications Only iron dextran is approved for I.M. administration

Additional Information Iron storage may lag behind the appearance of normal red blood cell morphology; use periodic hematologic determination to assess therapy; VLBW infants receiving I.V. iron sucrose 2 mg/kg/day with erythropoietin showed improved erythropoiesis when compared with oral iron supplementation and erythropoietin (Pollak, et al)

Dosage Forms Expressed as mg of **elemental iron:**
Injection, solution, as **ferric gluconate** (Ferrlecit®): 12.5 mg/mL (5 mL) [contains 9 mg benzyl alcohol/mL]
Injection, solution, as **iron dextran:**
> Dexferrum®: 50 mg/mL (1 mL, 2 mL)
> InFed®: 50 mg/mL (2 mL)

Injection, solution, as **iron sucrose** [preservative free] (Venofer®): 20 mg/mL (5 mL)

References
Auerbach M, Witt D, Toler W, et al, "Clinical Use of the Total Dose Intravenous Infusion of Iron Dextran," *J Lab Clin Med*, 1988, 111(5):566-70.
Benito RP and Guerrero TC, "Response to a Single Intravenous Dose Versus Multiple Intramuscular Administration of Iron-Dextran Complex: A Comparative Study," *Curr Ther Res Clin Exp*, 1973, 15(7):373-82.
Pollak A, Hayde M, Hayn M, et al, "Effect of Intravenous Iron Supplementation on Erythropoiesis in Erythropoietin-Treated Premature Infants," *Pediatrics*, 2001, 107(1):78-85.

♦ **Isoamyl Nitrite** *see* Amyl Nitrite *on page 111*

Isoetharine [DSC] *(eye soe ETH a reen)*
Related Information
Asthma Guidelines *on page 1376*
Canadian Brand Names Beta-2®; Bronkometer®; Bronkosol®
Therapeutic Category Adrenergic Agonist Agent; Antiasthmatic; Bronchodilator; Sympathomimetic
Generic Available Yes

Use Bronchodilator used in asthma and for the reversible bronchospasm occurring with bronchitis and emphysema

Pregnancy Risk Factor C

Contraindications Hypersensitivity to isoetharine, any component (see Warnings), or other sympathomimetics

Warnings Isoetharine hydrochloride solution contains sulfites which may cause allergic reactions in susceptible individuals

Precautions Excessive, prolonged use may lead to decreased effectiveness; use with caution in patients with hyperthyroidism, hypertension, acute coronary artery disease, cerebral arteriosclerosis

Adverse Reactions

Cardiovascular: Tachycardia, hypertension, palpitations

Central nervous system: Anxiety, dizziness, restlessness, excitement, headache, nervousness, insomnia, lightheadedness

Gastrointestinal: Nausea, vomiting, xerostomia

Neuromuscular & skeletal: Tremor, weakness

Drug Interactions Additive effects when used in combination with other sympathomimetics; decreased effect with beta-blocking agents

Mechanism of Action Relaxes bronchial smooth muscle and peripheral vasculature by action on $beta_2$-receptors with little effect on heart rate

Pharmacodynamics

Maximum effect: Following oral inhalation: Within 5-15 minutes

Duration: 1-4 hours

Pharmacokinetics

Metabolism: In many tissues including the liver and lungs

Elimination: Renal, primarily (90%) as metabolites

Usual Dosage Treatments are usually not repeated more often than every 4 hours, except in severe cases

Nebulizer:

Children: 0.01 mL/kg (0.1 mg/kg) of 1% solution; minimum dose 0.1 mL (1 mg); maximum dose: 0.5 mL (5 mg)

Adults: 0.5-1 mL (2.5-5 mg) of a 0.5% solution or equivalent dosages using 0.125%, 0.2%, 0.25%, or 1% solutions

Inhalation: Adults: 1-2 inhalations every 4 hours as needed

Administration

Nebulization: Dilute dosage of 0.5% or 1% solutions in 2-3 mL NS; 0.125%, 0.2%, and 0.25% solutions may be administered without dilution

Oral inhalation: Shake well before use; use spacer device in children <8 years of age

Monitoring Parameters Heart rate, blood pressure, respiratory rate

Patient Information May cause dry mouth

Dosage Forms Solution for oral inhalation, as hydrochloride: 1% (10 mL) [contains sodium bisulfite and sodium sulfite] [DSC]

References

"National Asthma Education and Prevention Program. Expert Panel Report: Guidelines for the Diagnosis and Management of Asthma Update on Selected Topics--2002," *J Allergy Clin Immunol*, 2002, 110(5 Suppl):S141-219.

Rachelefsky GS and Siegel SC, "Asthma in Infants and Children - Treatment of Childhood Asthma: Part 11," *J Allergy Clin Immunol*, 1985, 76(3):409-25.

Isoniazid (eye soe NYE a zid)

Related Information

Overdose and Toxicology *on page 1388*

U.S. Brand Names Nydrazid®

Canadian Brand Names Isotamine®; PMS-Isoniazid

Synonyms INH; Isonicotinic Acid Hydrazide

Therapeutic Category Antitubercular Agent

Generic Available Yes

Use Treatment of susceptible mycobacterial infection due to *M. tuberculosis* and prophylactically to those individuals exposed to tuberculosis

Pregnancy Risk Factor C

Contraindications Hypersensitivity to isoniazid or any component; acute liver disease; previous history of hepatic damage during isoniazid therapy

Warnings Severe and sometimes fatal hepatitis may occur or develop even after many months of treatment; the administration of isoniazid in combination with rifampin is associated with an increased incidence of hepatotoxicity if isoniazid dose is >10 mg/kg/day; patients must report any prodromal symptoms of hepatitis such as fatigue, weakness, malaise, anorexia, nausea, vomiting, dark urine, or yellowing of eyes

Precautions Use with caution in patients with renal impairment and chronic liver disease

(Continued)

Isoniazid *(Continued)*

Adverse Reactions

Central nervous system: Seizure, stupor, dizziness, agitation, euphoria, psychosis, fever, ataxia

Dermatologic: Skin eruptions, rash, acne

Endocrine & metabolic: Hyperglycemia, metabolic acidosis, pellagra

Gastrointestinal: Nausea, vomiting, epigastric distress; diarrhea (associated with administration of syrup formulation)

Hematologic: Agranulocytosis, hemolytic anemia, aplastic anemia, thrombocytopenia, eosinophilia, leukopenia

Hepatic: Hepatitis, 3% to 10% of children experience transient elevated liver transaminase levels

Local: Irritation at I.M. injection site

Neuromuscular & skeletal: Peripheral neuropathy

Ocular: Optic neuritis

Otic: Tinnitus

Miscellaneous: Hypersensitivity reaction

Drug Interactions Cytochrome P450 isoenzyme CYP2E1 substrate; isoenzyme CYP2E1 inducer; isoenzyme CYP1A2, CYP2C, CYP2C9, CYP2C19, and CYP3A3/4 inhibitor

May increase serum concentrations of phenytoin, carbamazepine, diazepam; aluminum salts may decrease isoniazid absorption; prednisolone may increase isoniazid metabolism; cycloserine, ethionamide (additive CNS toxicity); disulfiram (coordination difficulty, psychotic episode); meperidine (serotonin syndrome); rifampin (increased hepatotoxicity)

Food Interactions Rate and extent of isoniazid absorption may be reduced when administered with food; avoid foods with histamine or tyramine (cheese, broad beans, dry sausage, salami, nonfresh meat, liver pate, soya bean, liquid and powdered protein supplements, wine); increase dietary intake of folate, niacin, magnesium, and pyridoxine; the American Academy of Pediatrics recommends that pyridoxine supplementation (1-2 mg/kg/day) should be administered to patients with nutritional deficiencies including all symptomatic HIV-infected children, children or adolescents on meat or milk-deficient diets, breast-feeding infants and their mothers, pregnant adolescents and women, and those predisposed to neuritis to prevent peripheral neuropathy

Stability Protect from light and excessive heat; avoid freezing

Mechanism of Action Inhibits mycolic acid synthesis resulting in disruption of the bacterial cell wall

Pharmacokinetics

Absorption: Oral, I.M.: Rapid and complete

Distribution: Crosses the placenta; appears in breast milk; distributes into most body tissues and fluids including the CSF

Protein binding: 10% to 15%

Metabolism: By the liver to acetylisoniazid with decay rate determined genetically by acetylation phenotype; undergoes further hydrolysis to isonicotinic acid and acetylhydrazine

Half-life: May be prolonged in patients with impaired hepatic function or severe renal impairment

Fast acetylators: 30-100 minutes

Slow acetylators: 2-5 hours

Time to peak serum concentration: Oral: Within 1-2 hours

Elimination: 75% to 95% excreted in urine as unchanged drug and metabolites; small amounts excreted in feces and saliva

Dialysis: Dialyzable (50% to 100%)

Usual Dosage Oral, I.M.:

Infants and Children:

Treatment: 10-15 mg/kg/day in 1-2 divided doses; maximum dose: 300 mg/day

Prophylaxis: 10 mg/kg/day given once daily, not to exceed 300 mg/day

Adults:

Treatment: 5 mg/kg/day given daily (usual dose: 300 mg)

Disseminated disease: 10 mg/kg/day in 1-2 divided doses

Prophylaxis: 300 mg/day given daily

American Thoracic Society and CDC currently recommend twice weekly therapy as part of a short-course regimen which follows 1-2 months of daily treatment for uncomplicated pulmonary tuberculosis in **compliant** patients

Children: 20-30 mg/kg/dose (up to 900 mg/dose) twice weekly

Adults: 15 mg/kg/dose (up to 900 mg/dose) twice weekly

Duration of therapy:
Asymptomatic infection (positive skin test):
Isoniazid susceptible: 9 months of isoniazid
Isoniazid resistant: 9 months of rifampin
Pulmonary, hilar adenopathy, and extrapulmonary infection other than meningitis, bone/joint, or disseminated infection:
6 months which includes 2-month therapy of isoniazid, rifampin, and pyrazinamide daily followed by 4 months of isoniazid and rifampin daily **or** 2 months of isoniazid, rifampin, and pyrazinamide daily, followed by 4 months of isoniazid and rifampin twice weekly under direct observation
alternatively
9 months of isoniazid and rifampin daily **or** 1 month of isoniazid and rifampin daily followed by 8 months of isoniazid and rifampin twice weekly under direct observation; if isoniazid resistance is identified, rifampin and ethambutol should be continued for a maximum of 12 months
Note: If drug resistance is possible, ethambutol or streptomycin should be added to the initial therapy regimen until susceptibility is determined
Meningitis, bone/joint, and disseminated infection:
12 months which includes 2 months of isoniazid, rifampin, pyrazinamide, and streptomycin daily followed by 10 months of isoniazid and rifampin daily **or** 2 months of isoniazid, rifampin, pyrazinamide, and streptomycin daily followed by 10 months of isoniazid and rifampin twice weekly under direct observation

Administration
Oral: Administer 1 hour before or 2 hours after meals with water; administration of isoniazid syrup has been associated with diarrhea
Parenteral: I.M.: Administer I.M. when oral therapy is not possible

Monitoring Parameters Periodic liver function tests; monitor for prodromal signs of hepatitis; ophthalmologic exam; chest x-ray

Test Interactions False-positive urinary glucose with Clinitest®

Patient Information Report any prodromal symptoms of hepatitis (fatigue, weakness, nausea, vomiting, dark urine, or yellowing of eyes) or any burning, tingling, or numbness in the extremities; avoid alcohol

Dosage Forms
Injection, solution (Nydrazid®): 100 mg/mL (10 mL)
Syrup: 50 mg/5 mL (473 mL) [contains 70% sorbitol; orange flavor]
Tablet: 100 mg, 300 mg

References
Ad Hoc Committee of the Scientific Assembly on Microbiology, Tuberculosis, and Pulmonary Infections, "Treatment of Tuberculosis and Tuberculosis Infection in Adults and Children," *Clin Infect Dis*, 1995, 21:9-27.
American Academy of Pediatrics, Committee on Infectious Diseases, "Chemotherapy for Tuberculosis in Infants and Children," *Pediatrics*, 1992, 89(1):161-5.
Starke JR, "Modern Approach to the Diagnosis and Treatment of Tuberculosis in Children," *Pediatr Clin North Am*, 1988, 35(3):441-64.
Starke JR, "Multidrug Therapy for Tuberculosis in Children," *Pediatr Infect Dis J*, 1990, 9(11):785-93.
Van Scoy RE and Wilkowske CJ, "Antituberculous Agents: Isoniazid, Rifampin, Streptomycin, Ethambutol, and Pyrazinamide," *Mayo Clin Proc*, 1983, 58(4):233-40.

♦ **Isonicotinic Acid Hydrazide** *see* Isoniazid *on page 629*
♦ **Isonipecaine** *see* Meperidine *on page 717*
♦ **Isoprenaline** *see* Isoproterenol *on page 631*

Isoproterenol (eye soe proe TER e nole)
Related Information
Adult ACLS Algorithm, Stable Ventricular Tachycardia *on page 1191*
Asthma Guidelines *on page 1376*
Emergency Pediatric Drip Calculations *on page 1177*

U.S. Brand Names Isuprel®

Synonyms Isoprenaline

Therapeutic Category Adrenergic Agonist Agent; Antiasthmatic; Beta$_1$ & Beta$_2$-Adrenergic Agonist Agent; Bronchodilator; Sympathomimetic

Generic Available Yes

Use Treatment of asthma or COPD (reversible airway obstruction); ventricular arrhythmias due to A-V nodal block; hemodynamically compromised bradyarrhythmias or atropine-resistant bradyarrhythmias, temporary use in third degree A-V block until pacemaker insertion; low cardiac output or vasoconstrictive shock states

Pregnancy Risk Factor C

Contraindications Hypersensitivity to isoproterenol, other sympathomimetic amines, or any component (see Warnings); angina, pre-existing cardiac arrhythmias (ventricular); tachycardia or A-V block caused by cardiac glycoside intoxication; narrow-angle glaucoma
(Continued)

Isoproterenol *(Continued)*

Warnings Tolerance may occur with prolonged use; when discontinuing an isoproterenol continuous infusion used for bronchodilation, the infusion **must** be gradually tapered over a 24- to 48-hour period to prevent rebound bronchospasm; injection contains sulfites which may cause allergic reactions in susceptible individuals

Precautions Use with caution in diabetics, renal or cardiovascular disease, hyperthyroidism, prostatic hypertrophy

Adverse Reactions

Cardiovascular: Flushing of the face or skin, ventricular arrhythmias, tachycardia, hypotension, chest pain, palpitations, hypertension

Central nervous system: Nervousness, restlessness, anxiety, dizziness, headache, vertigo, insomnia

Endocrine & metabolic: Parotid glands swelling

Gastrointestinal: Heartburn, GI distress, nausea, vomiting, dry throat, xerostomia

Neuromuscular & skeletal: Tremor, weakness, trembling

Miscellaneous: Diaphoresis

Drug Interactions Additive effects and increased cardiotoxicity when administered concomitantly with other sympathomimetic amines; beta-adrenergic blocking agents may decrease effectiveness due to beta blockade; may increase theophylline elimination

Mechanism of Action Stimulates beta$_1$- and beta$_2$-receptors resulting in relaxation of bronchial, GI, and uterine smooth muscle; increases heart rate and contractility; causes vasodilation of peripheral vasculature

Pharmacodynamics

Onset of action: I.V.: Immediately

Duration: I.V. (single dose): Few minutes

Pharmacokinetics

Metabolism: By conjugation in many tissues including the liver and lungs

Half-life: 2.5-5 minutes

Elimination: In urine principally as sulfate conjugates

Usual Dosage

Neonates, Infants, and Children: I.V. infusion: 0.05-2 mcg/kg/minute; rate (mL/hour) = dose (mcg/kg/minute) x weight (kg) x 60 minutes/hour divided by concentration (mcg/mL)

Adults: I.V. infusion: 2-20 mcg/minute

Administration Parenteral: For continuous infusions, dilute in dextrose or NS to a maximum concentration of 20 mcg/mL; concentrations as high as 64 mcg/mL have been used safely and with efficacy in situations of extreme fluid restriction

Monitoring Parameters Heart rate, blood pressure, respiratory rate, arterial blood gases, central venous pressure, EKG

Patient Information May cause dry mouth

Additional Information Hypotension is more common in hypovolemic patients

Dosage Forms Injection, solution, as hydrochloride: 0.02 mg/mL (10 mL); 0.02% [0.2 mg/mL = 1:5000] (1 mL, 5 mL) [contains sodium metabisulfite]

References

"National Asthma Education and Prevention Program. Expert Panel Report: Guidelines for the Diagnosis and Management of Asthma Update on Selected Topics--2002," *J Allergy Clin Immunol*, 2002, 110(5 Suppl):S141-219.

Rachelefsky GS and Siegel SC, "Asthma in Infants and Children - Treatment of Childhood Asthma: Part 1I," *J Allergy Clin Immunol*, 1985, 76(3):409-25.

♦ **Isoptin® (Can)** *see* Verapamil *on page 1144*

♦ **Isoptin® I.V. (Can)** *see* Verapamil *on page 1144*

♦ **Isoptin® SR** *see* Verapamil *on page 1144*

♦ **Isopto® Atropine** *see* Atropine *on page 144*

♦ **Isopto® Carpine** *see* Pilocarpine *on page 903*

♦ **Isopto® Eserine (Can)** *see* Physostigmine *on page 901*

♦ **Isopto® Homatropine** *see* Homatropine *on page 563*

♦ **Isopto® Hyoscine** *see* Scopolamine *on page 1009*

♦ **Isotamine® (Can)** *see* Isoniazid *on page 629*

Isotretinoin *(eye soe TRET i noyn)*

U.S. Brand Names Accutane®

Canadian Brand Names Isotrex®

Synonyms 13-*cis*-Retinoic Acid

Therapeutic Category Acne Products; Retinoic Acid Derivative; Vitamin A Derivative

Generic Available No

Use Treatment of severe recalcitrant cystic and/or conglobate acne unresponsive to conventional therapy; used investigationally for the treatment of children with high-risk neuroblastoma that does not respond to conventional therapy

Restrictions

Prescriptions for Accutane® may not be dispensed unless they are affixed with a yellow self-adhesive Accutane® qualification sticker filled out by the prescriber. Telephone, fax, or computer-generated prescriptions are no longer valid. Prescriber should prescribe no more than a 1-month supply with no refills. Prescription must be dispensed with a patient education guide.

Prescriptions for females must be filled within 7 days of the date noted on the yellow sticker.

Prescribers will be provided with Accutane® qualification stickers after they have read the S.M.A.R.T. program booklet and have signed and mailed to the manufacturer their agreement to participate.

Pregnancy Risk Factor X

Contraindications Hypersensitivity to isotretinoin, parabens, vitamin A or other retinoids; patients who are pregnant or intend to become pregnant during treatment; nursing mothers

Warnings Major human fetal abnormalities to isotretinoin administration have been documented; during pregnancy, it can cause fetal defects in the CNS (cerebral abnormalities, hydrocephalus, microcephaly, cranial nerve deficit, cerebellar malformation), skull, ear, eye, and cardiovascular systems, cleft palate, and parathyroid hormone deficiency; not to be used in women of childbearing potential unless woman is capable of complying with effective contraceptive measures. Prescription for isotretinoin should not be issued until a female patient has had negative results from 2 urine or serum pregnancy tests, one performed in the prescriber's office when the patient is qualified for therapy, the second one performed on the second day of next normal menstrual period or 11 days after the last unprotected act of sexual intercourse, whichever is later. Effective contraception must be used for at least 1 month before beginning therapy, during therapy, and for 1 month after discontinuation of therapy. Isotretinoin may cause depression, psychosis, and suicidal ideations; concomitant use with tetracyclines has been associated with cases of pseudotumor cerebri; avoid concomitant treatment with tetracyclines

Precautions Use with caution in patients with diabetes mellitus or hypertriglyceridemia

Adverse Reactions

Cardiovascular: Palpitations, tachycardia, vascular thrombotic stroke, edema, vasculitis

Central nervous system: Fatigue, headache, dizziness, pseudotumor cerebri, psychosis, mental depression, suicidal ideation, seizures, insomnia

Dermatologic: Pruritus, alopecia, cheilitis, photosensitivity, rash

Endocrine & metabolic: Hypertriglyceridemia, hyperuricemia, hyperglycemia, hypercalcemia

Gastrointestinal: Xerostomia, anorexia, nausea, vomiting, inflammatory bowel syndrome, acute pancreatitis

Hematologic: Elevation in erythrocyte sedimentation rate, decrease in hemoglobin and hematocrit, neutropenia

Hepatic: Hepatitis; elevated AST, ALT, and alkaline phosphatase

Neuromuscular & skeletal: Bone pain, arthralgia, myalgia, skeletal hyperostosis, premature epiphyseal closure, rhabdomyolysis (rare)

Ocular: Conjunctivitis, corneal opacities, cataracts, blurred vision, decreased night vision

Otic: Hearing impairment

Renal: Hematuria, proteinuria

Respiratory: Epistaxis, bronchospasm

Miscellaneous: Hypersensitivity reactions

Drug Interactions Increased clearance of carbamazepine; vitamin A supplements increase toxic effects; alcohol may potentiate an increase in serum triglycerides; concomitant use with tetracyclines has been associated with cases of pseudotumor cerebri (avoid tetracyclines)

Food Interactions Food or milk increases isotretinoin bioavailability

Stability Protect from light

Mechanism of Action Reduces sebaceous gland size and reduces sebum production; regulates cell proliferation and differentiation

Pharmacokinetics

Absorption: Oral: Demonstrates biphasic absorption

Distribution: Crosses the placenta; appears in breast milk, bile

Protein binding: 99% to 100%

Metabolism: In the liver; major metabolite: 4-oxo-isotretinoin (active); undergoes enterohepatic circulation

(Continued)

Isotretinoin *(Continued)*

Half-life, terminal: 10-20 hours for isotretinoin, and 17-50 hours for its metabolite

Time to peak serum concentration: Within 3 hours

Elimination: Excreted in feces as unchanged drug and in urine as metabolites

Usual Dosage Oral:

Children: Maintenance therapy for neuroblastoma: 160 mg/m^2/day in 2 divided doses for 14 consecutive days in a 28-day cycle has been used investigationally

Children and Adults: Acne: 0.5-2 mg/kg/day in 2 divided doses (dosages as low as 0.05 mg/kg/day have been reported to be beneficial) for 15-20 weeks or until the total cyst count decreases by 70%, whichever is sooner

Administration Oral: Capsules can be swallowed or chewed and swallowed; the capsule may be opened with a large needle and the contents placed on apple sauce or ice cream for patients unable to swallow the capsule; administer with meals

Monitoring Parameters CBC with differential, platelet count, baseline ESR, serum triglyceride, liver enzymes, CPK, ophthalmologic exam, blood glucose; pregnancy test in female patients of childbearing potential (see Warnings)

Patient Information Do not take vitamin supplements containing vitamin A; use caution when driving at night since decreased night vision can develop suddenly; patients who wear contact lenses may experience decreased tolerance to the lenses; avoid alcohol; may cause dry mouth; notify physician of any headache, blurred vision, yellowing of skin or eyes, bone or muscle pain, vision changes, suicidal thoughts, dark urine, abdominal pain, rectal bleeding, or severe diarrhea; female patients of childbearing potential must be counseled to use 2 effective forms of contraception simultaneously, unless absolute abstinence is the chosen method; patients should not self-medicate with St John's Wort due to a possible interaction with hormonal contraceptives; provide female patients instruction to join the Accutane® survey and watch a videotape that provides information about contraceptive methods; inform patients not to donate blood during therapy and for 1 month following discontinuation of therapy

May cause photosensitivity reactions (eg, exposure to sunlight may cause severe sunburn, skin rash, redness, or itching); avoid exposure to sunlight and artificial light sources (sunlamps, tanning booth/bed); wear protective clothing, wide-brimmed hats, sunglasses, and lip sunscreen (SPF ≥15); use a sunscreen [broad-spectrum sunscreen or physical sunscreen (preferred) or sunblock with SPF ≥15]; contact physician if reaction occurs.

Dosage Forms Capsule, liquid-filled: 10 mg, 20 mg, 40 mg

References

American Academy of Pediatrics Committee on Drugs, "Retinoid Therapy for Severe Dermatological Disorders," *Pediatrics*, 1992, 90(1 Pt 1):119-20.

DiGiovanna JJ and Peck GL, "Oral Synthetic Retinoid Treatment in Children," *Pediatr Dermatol*, 1983, 1(1):77-88.

Matthay KK, Villablanca JG, Seeger RC, et al, "Treatment of High-Risk Neuroblastoma With Intensive Chemotherapy, Radiotherapy, Autologous Bone Marrow Transplantation, and 13-cis-Retinoic Acid. Children's Cancer Group," *N Engl J Med*, 1999, 341:1165-73.

Reynolds CP, Kane DJ, Einhorn PA, et al, "Response of Neuroblastoma to Retinoic Acid *In Vitro*, and *In Vivo*," *Prog Clin Biol Res*, 1991, 366:203-11

♦ **Isotrex® (Can)** *see* Isotretinoin *on page 632*

♦ **Isoxazolyl Penicillin** *see* Oxacillin *on page 840*

♦ **Isuprel®** *see* Isoproterenol *on page 631*

Itraconazole *(i tra KOE na zole)*

U.S. Brand Names Sporanox®

Therapeutic Category Antifungal Agent, Systemic

Generic Available No

Use Treatment of susceptible systemic fungal infections in immunocompromised and nonimmunocompromised patients including blastomycosis, coccidioidomycosis, paracoccidioidomycosis, histoplasmosis, and aspergillosis in patients who do not respond to or cannot tolerate amphotericin B; treatment of oropharyngeal or esophageal candidiasis (oral solution only)

Pregnancy Risk Factor C

Contraindications Hypersensitivity to itraconazole or any component; concomitant administration with terfenadine, astemizole, cisapride, pimozide, quinidine, dofetilide, alprazolam, triazolam, or HMG-CoA reductase inhibitors metabolized by CYP3A4 isoenzyme (ie, lovastatin, simvastatin)

Warnings Itraconazole has induced bone defects (decreased bone plate activity, thinning of the zona compacta of large bones, increased bone fragility) and changes in tooth appearance in rats. Severe cardiovascular effects including QT interval prolongation, ventricular tachycardia, ventricular fibrillation, cardiac arrest, palpitations, syncope, and death have occurred in patients receiving itraconazole concomitantly with terfenadine, astemizole, or cisapride; **itraconazole solution and capsules should not be used interchangeably**

Precautions Use with caution in patients with hypersensitivity to other azole antifungal agents, patients with left ventricular dysfunction or a history of CHF, and in patients with hepatic impairment; discontinue if signs and symptoms of liver disease or CHF develop

Adverse Reactions

Cardiovascular: Hypertension, ventricular fibrillation, edema, CHF

Central nervous system: Headache, dizziness, somnolence, fever, fatigue

Dermatologic: Rash, pruritus, urticaria, angioedema, toxic epidermal necrolysis

Endocrine & metabolic: Hypokalemia, adrenal insufficiency, gynecomastia

Gastrointestinal: Nausea, vomiting, diarrhea, abdominal pain, anorexia

Hematologic: Thrombocytopenia, leukopenia

Hepatic: Elevated liver enzymes, hepatitis

Otic: Tinnitus

Renal: Albuminuria

Drug Interactions Cytochrome P450 isoenzyme CYP3A3/4 substrate; isoenzyme CYP3A3/4 inhibitor

Decreased effect of itraconazole with rifampin, rifabutin, carbamazepine, isoniazid, phenytoin, and phenobarbital (increases itraconazole's metabolism); H_2 antagonists, omeprazole, antacids, didanosine (decreases absorption)

Increased effect of cyclosporine, tacrolimus (interferes with clearance); digoxin, warfarin, amlodipine, buspirone, corticosteroids, protease inhibitors (ie, indinavir), and hypoglycemic agents (decreased metabolism)

Increased toxicity of terfenadine, astemizole, alprazolam, triazolam, oral midazolam, cisapride, lovastatin, simvastatin, vinca alkaloids; see Warnings

Food Interactions Grapefruit juice decreases itraconazole AUC by 30%; avoid drinking grapefruit juice while taking oral itraconazole; absorption of capsule and oral solution are increased when taken with a cola beverage

Capsule: Food increases bioavailability

Solution: 31% increase in AUC if taken without food

Stability Store at room temperature; protect from light. Avoid freezing. A precise mixing ratio of itraconazole injection in NS diluent resulting in a 3.33 mg/mL concentration is required for a stable admixture. Following dilution of itraconazole injection in NS, the solution is stable for up to 48 hours when refrigerated and protected from light.

Mechanism of Action Inhibits ergosterol synthesis in fungal cell membranes by inhibiting fungal cytochrome P450

Pharmacokinetics

Absorption:

Capsule: Rapid and complete when capsule is given immediately after a meal (bioavailability: 100%); decreased absorption reported when administered via nasogastric tube

Oral solution: Solution better absorbed on empty stomach

Distribution: High affinity for tissues (liver, lung, kidney, adipose tissue, brain, vagina, dermis, epidermis); poor penetration into CSF, eye fluid, saliva; distributes into breast milk, bronchial exudate, and sputum

Protein binding: 99%

Metabolism: Saturable hepatic metabolism to active and inactive metabolites

Bioavailability: Capsules:

Fasted state: 40%

Fed state: Dose administered immediately after a meal: 100%

Half-life: 17-30 hours

Elimination: Metabolites are excreted in urine (35%) and bile (55%)

Dialysis: Nondialyzable

Usual Dosage

Oral:

Children: Efficacy of itraconazole has not been established; a limited number of children have been treated with itraconazole using doses of 3-5 mg/kg/day once daily; doses as high as 5-10 mg/kg/day divided every 12-24 hours have been used in 32 patients with chronic granulomatous disease for prophylaxis against *Aspergillus* infection; doses of 6-8 mg/kg/day have been used in the treatment of disseminated histoplasmosis

Prophylaxis for first episode of *Cryptococcus neoformans* or *Histoplasma capsulatum* in HIV-infected infants and children: 2-5 mg/kg/dose every 12-24 hours

Prophylaxis for recurrence of opportunistic disease in HIV-infected infants and children:

Cryptococcus neoformans: 2-5 mg/kg/dose every 12-24 hours

(Continued)

Itraconazole (Continued)

Histoplasma capsulatum: 2-5 mg/kg/dose every 12-48 hours

Adults:

Blastomycosis and nonmeningeal histoplasmosis: Initial: 200 mg once daily; if poor response, increase dose in 100 mg increments to a maximum of 400 mg/day in 2 divided doses

Life-threatening infection and aspergillosis: Initial loading dose can be administered as follows: 600 mg/day in 3 divided doses for the first 3-4 days; maintenance dose: 200-400 mg/day in 2 divided doses; maximum dose: 600 mg/day in 3 divided doses

Esophageal candidiasis: Vigorously swish 10 mL in the mouth for several seconds and then swallow daily; maximum dose: 200 mg/day

Oropharyngeal candidiasis: Vigorously swish 10 mL in the mouth for several seconds at a time once daily (20 mL total daily dose), or 10 mL twice daily in patients refractory to oral fluconazole

I.V.: Adults: Blastomycosis, aspergillosis, or histoplasmosis: 200 mg twice daily for 4 doses then decrease dose to 200 mg once daily. Safety and efficacy of I.V. itraconazole administered for longer than 14 days has not been established; therapy should be completed using oral itraconazole

Dosing adjustment in renal impairment: Cl_{cr} <30 mL/minute: Itraconazole injection is not recommended.

Administration

Oral: Avoid grapefruit juice

Capsules: Administer with food

Solution: Administer on an empty stomach

Parenteral I.V. infusion: Dilute entire contents of an ampul (250 mg) in 50 mL of NS diluent provided by the manufacturer to provide a solution with a final concentration of 3.33 mg/mL. Calculate itraconazole dosage volume needed and infuse over 60 minutes using the infusion set provided by the manufacturer and a dedicated I.V. line. Do not mix with other drugs. After completion of infusion, flush infusion set with 15-20 mL NS over 5-15 minutes via the two-way stopcock, then discard the entire I.V. line. Do not flush the infusion set with bacteriostatic NS.

Monitoring Parameters Periodic liver function tests, serum potassium; monitor for prodromal signs of hepatitis

Reference Range Therapeutic blood level: >250 ng/mL

Patient Information Report any prodromal symptoms of hepatitis (fatigue, weakness, nausea, vomiting, dark urine, or yellowing of eyes); avoid grapefruit juice

Nursing Implications Do not administer with antacids or H_2 antagonists

Dosage Forms

Capsule: 100 mg

Injection, solution: 10 mg/mL (25 mL) [contains propylene glycol and hydroxypropyl-B-cyclodextrin; packaged in a kit containing 0.9% sodium chloride (50 mL); filtered infusion set (1)]

Solution, oral: 100 mg/10 mL (150 mL) [contains propylene glycol and hydroxypropyl-B-cyclodextrin; cherry flavor]

References

Cowie F, Meller ST, Cushing P, et al, "Chemoprophylaxis for Pulmonary Aspergillosis During Intensive Chemotherapy," *Arch Dis Child*, 1994, 70(2):136-8.

Mouy R, Veber F, Blanche S, et al, "Long-Term Itraconazole Prophylaxis Against *Aspergillus* Infections in Thirty-Two Patients With Chronic Granulomatous Disease," *J Pediatr*, 1994, 125(6 Pt 1):998-1003.

Tobon AM, Franco L, Espinal D, et al, "Disseminated Histoplasmosis in Children: The Role of Itraconazole Therapy," *Pediatr Infect Dis J*, 1996; 15:1002-8.

"1999 USPHS/IDSA Guidelines for the Prevention of Opportunistic Infections in Persons Infected With Human Immunodeficiency Virus. USPHS/IDSA Prevention of Opportunistic Infections Working Group," *MMWR Morb Mortal Wkly Rep*, 1999, 48 (RR-10):1-66.

Kaolin and Pectin (KAY oh lin & PEK tin)

Related Information

Carbohydrate and Alcohol Content of Liquid Medications for Use in Patients Receiving Ketogenic Diets *on page 1431*

U.S. Brand Names Kaodene® NN [OTC]; Kao-Spen® [OTC]; Kapectolin® [OTC]

Synonyms Pectin and Kaolin

Therapeutic Category Antidiarrheal

Generic Available Yes

Use Treatment of uncomplicated diarrhea

Pregnancy Risk Factor C

Contraindications Hypersensitivity to kaolin, pectin, or any component

Warnings Not to be used for self-medication of diarrhea for >48 hours or in presence of high fever in infants and children <3 years of age; do not use for diarrhea associated with pseudomembraneous enterocolitis or in diarrhea caused by toxigenic bacteria

Precautions Some products have added bismuth subsalicylate; use these products with caution in patients with bleeding disorders, salicylate sensitivity; do not use the subsalicylate-containing products in children <16 years of age who have chickenpox or flu symptoms due to the association with Reye's syndrome

Drug Interactions Kaolin and pectin may decrease absorption of quinidine, chloroquine, lincomycin, and digoxin (tablets only)

Usual Dosage Adequate controlled clinical studies documenting the efficacy of these combination products are lacking. Their usage and dosage have been primarily empiric; the table lists the manufacturer's recommended dosage.

Kaolin and Pectin Dosage*
(*mL/dose after each bowel movement)

Product	Dosage (by age)		
	3-6 y	6-12 y	>12 y to adult
Kao-Spen®	—	—	60-120 mL
Kaolin w/pectin (Kapectolin®)	15-30 mL	30-60 mL	60-120 mL
Kaodene® NN	15 mL	22.5 mL	45 mL

Administration May be administered without regard to meals

Dosage Forms

Suspension, oral: Kaolin 967 mg and pectin 22 mg per 5 mL (30 mL, 180 mL)
Kaodene® NN: Kaolin 650 mg and pectin 32.4 mg per 5 mL (120 mL) [contains 2.8 mg/5 mL bismuth subsalicylate]
Kao-Spen®: Kaolin 866 mg and pectin 43.3 mg per 5 mL (3780 mL)
Kapectolin®: Kaolin 15 g and pectin 333 mg per 5 mL (120 mL, 240 mL, 480 mL)

♦ **Kerr Insta-Char®** [OTC] *see* Charcoal *on page 250*

♦ **Ketalar®** *see* Ketamine *on page 638*

Ketamine (KEET a meen)

Related Information

Adult ACLS Algorithm, Synchronized Cardioversion *on page 1192*

Preprocedure Sedatives in Children *on page 1367*

U.S. Brand Names Ketalar®

Therapeutic Category General Anesthetic

Generic Available Yes

Use Anesthesia, short surgical procedures, dressing changes

Restrictions C-III

Pregnancy Risk Factor D

Contraindications Hypersensitivity to ketamine or any component; elevated intracranial pressure; patients with hypertension, aneurysms, thyrotoxicosis, CHF, angina, psychotic disorders

Warnings Use only by or under the direct supervision of physicians experienced in administering general anesthetics. Resuscitative equipment should be available for use; respiratory depression may occur with rapid administration rates or with overdose. Postanesthetic emergence reactions which can manifest as vivid dreams, hallucinations and/or frank delirium occur in 12% of patients; these reactions are less common in pediatric patients; emergence reactions may occur up to 24 hours postoperatively and may be reduced by minimization of verbal, tactile, and visual patient stimulation during recovery, or by pretreatment with a benzodiazepine (using lower recommended doses of ketamine). Severe emergent reactions may require treatment with a small hypnotic dose of a short or ultra-short acting barbiturate. Prolonged use may cause physical dependence (withdrawal symptoms on discontinuation) and tolerance.

Precautions Use with caution in patients with gastroesophageal reflux; use with caution and decrease the dose in patients with hepatic dysfunction; use with caution in patients with a full stomach, patients should fast (ie, be NPO) for an appropriate time before being sedated for elective procedures; use with caution in patients with elevated CSF pressure, chronic alcoholics, and in acutely intoxicated patients; do not use as sole anesthetic in surgery or diagnostic procedures of the pharynx, larynx, or bronchial tree or in surgical procedures involving visceral pain pathways

Adverse Reactions

Cardiovascular: Hypertension, tachycardia, increased cardiac output, paradoxical direct myocardial depression, hypotension, bradycardia, increases cerebral blood flow, arrhythmias

Central nervous system: Tonic-clonic movements, elevated intracranial pressure, hallucinations

Dermatologic: Transient erythema, morbilliform rash

Endocrine & metabolic: Increased metabolic rate

Gastrointestinal: Hypersalivation, vomiting, postoperative nausea, anorexia

Local: Pain and exanthema at injection site

Neuromuscular & skeletal: Increased skeletal muscle tone, tremor, purposeless movement, fasciculations

Ocular: Diplopia, nystagmus, elevated intraocular pressure

Respiratory: Increased airway resistance, cough reflex may be depressed, decreased bronchospasm; respiratory depression or apnea with large doses or rapid infusions, laryngospasm; increased bronchial mucous gland secretion

Miscellaneous: Emergence reactions; anaphylaxis; physical and psychological dependence with prolonged use

Drug Interactions Cytochrome P450 isoenzyme CYP3A substrate

Barbiturates, narcotics, hydroxyzine prolong recovery from anesthesia

Stability Protect from light; do not mix with barbiturates or diazepam as precipitation may occur

Mechanism of Action Produces dissociative anesthesia by direct action on the cortex and limbic system; does not usually impair pharyngeal or laryngeal reflexes

Pharmacodynamics

Onset of action:

Anesthesia:

I.M.: 3-4 minutes

I.V.: Within 30 seconds

Analgesia:

Oral: Within 30 minutes

I.M.: Within 10-15 minutes

Duration: Following single dose:
Anesthesia:
   I.M.: 12-25 minutes
   I.V.: 5-10 minutes
Analgesia: I.M.: 15-30 minutes
Recovery:
   I.M.: 3-4 hours
   I.V.: 1-2 hours

Pharmacokinetics
   Metabolism: In the liver via N-dealkylation, hydroxylation of cyclohexone ring, glucu-ronide conjugation, and dehydration of hydroxylated metabolites
   Half-life:
      Alpha: 10-15 minutes
      Terminal: 2.5 hours

Usual Dosage Titrate dose to effect
   Children:
      Oral: 6-10 mg/kg for 1 dose (mixed in cola or other beverage) given 30 minutes before the procedure
      I.M.: 3-7 mg/kg
      I.V.: Range: 0.5-2 mg/kg, use smaller doses (0.5-1 mg/kg) for sedation for minor procedures; usual induction dosage: 1-2 mg/kg
      Continuous I.V. infusion: Sedation: 5-20 mcg/kg/minute; start at lower dosage listed and titrate to effect
   Adults:
      I.M.: 3-8 mg/kg
      I.V.: Range: 1-4.5 mg/kg; usual induction dosage: 1-2 mg/kg
   Children and Adults: Maintenance: Supplemental doses of $^1/_3$ to $^1/_2$ of initial dose

Administration
   Oral: Use 100 mg/mL I.V. solution and mix the appropriate dose in 0.2-0.3 mL/kg of cola or other beverage
   Parenteral: I.V.: Administer slowly, do not exceed 0.5 mg/kg/minute; do not administer faster than 60 seconds; maximum concentration for slow I.V. push: 50 mg/mL; **Note:** Do not inject 100 mg/mL concentration I.V. without proper dilution; dilute with an equal volume of SWI, NS, or D_5W to produce 50 mg/mL concentration for slow I.V. push. Maximum concentration for intermittent or continuous infusion: 2 mg/mL

Monitoring Parameters Cardiovascular effects, heart rate, blood pressure, respiratory rate, transcutaneous O_2 saturation

Patient Information May cause drowsiness and impair ability to perform activities requiring mental alertness or physical coordination; do not engage in such activities for at least 24 hours after ketamine anesthesia.

Nursing Implications Resuscitative equipment should be available for use. Ensure that outpatients have fully recovered from ketamine anesthesia before being released and that they are accompanied by a responsible adult.

Additional Information Used in combination with anticholinergic agents to decrease hypersalivation; should not be used for sedation for procedures that require a total lack of movement (eg, MRI, radiation therapy) due to association with purposeless movements

Dosage Forms Injection, solution, as hydrochloride: 10 mg/mL (20 mL); 50 mg/mL (10 mL); 100 mg/mL (5 mL)

References
Cote CJ, "Sedation for the Pediatric Patient: A Review," *Pediatr Clin North Am,* 1994, 41(1):31-58.
Gutstein HB, Johnson KL, Heard MN, et al, "Oral Ketamine Premedication in Children," *Anesthesiology,* 1992, 76(1):28-33.
Tobias JD, Phipps S, Smith B, et al, "Oral Ketamine Premedication to Alleviate the Distress of Invasive Procedures in Pediatric Oncology Patients," *Pediatrics,* 1992, 90(4):537-41.
Tobias JD and Rasmussen GE, "Pain Management and Sedation in the Pediatric Intensive Care Unit," *Pediatr Clin North Am,* 1994, 41(6):1269-92.

Ketoconazole (kee toe KOE na zole)

U.S. Brand Names Nizoral®; Nizoral® A-D [OTC]
Canadian Brand Names Apo®-Ketoconazole; Ketoderm®; Novo-Ketoconazole
Therapeutic Category Antifungal Agent, Systemic; Antifungal Agent, Topical
Generic Available Yes
Use Treatment of susceptible fungal infections, including candidiasis, oral thrush, blastomycosis, histoplasmosis, paracoccidioidomycosis, chronic mucocutaneous candidiasis, as well as certain recalcitrant cutaneous dermatophytoses; used topically for treatment of tinea corporis, tinea cruris, tinea versicolor, and cutaneous candidiasis; shampoo is used for dandruff
Pregnancy Risk Factor C
(Continued)

Ketoconazole (Continued)

Contraindications Hypersensitivity to ketoconazole or any component; single agent in the treatment of CNS fungal infections (due to poor CNS penetration); concomitant administration of astemizole, terfenadine, or cisapride

Warnings Has been associated with hepatotoxicity, including some fatalities; perform periodic liver function tests; high doses of ketoconazole may depress adrenocortical function and decrease serum testosterone concentrations; risk of serious cardiac arrhythmias in patients receiving ketoconazole and astemizole, terfenadine, or cisapride

Precautions Gastric acidity is necessary for the dissolution and absorption of ketoconazole; avoid concomitant (within 2 hours) administration of antacids, H_2-blockers, anticholinergics; use with caution in patients with impaired hepatic function

Adverse Reactions

Central nervous system: Lethargy, nervousness, headache, dizziness, somnolence, fever, chills, bulging fontanelles

Dermatologic: Pruritus, rash, dry skin

Endocrine & metabolic: Adrenocortical insufficiency, gynecomastia, decreased libido

Gastrointestinal: Nausea, vomiting, abdominal discomfort, GI bleeding, diarrhea

Genitourinary: Oligospermia

Hematologic: Leukopenia, thrombocytopenia, hemolytic anemia

Hepatic: Hepatotoxicity; elevated AST, ALT, and alkaline phosphatase; jaundice

Local: Irritation, stinging

Miscellaneous: Anaphylaxis

Drug Interactions Cytochrome P450 isoenzyme CYP3A3/4 substrate; CYP1A2, CYP2C, CYP2C9 (weak), CYP2C19 (weak), CYP3A3/4, and CYP3A5-7 isoenzyme inhibitor

Drugs that decrease ketoconazole absorption (raise gastric pH) such as antacids, didanosine, sodium bicarbonate, omeprazole, H_2-receptor blockers; sucralfate decreases absorption of ketoconazole by 20%; drugs that decrease serum concentrations of ketoconazole (rifampin, isoniazid, phenytoin); drug concentrations that are increased by ketoconazole (phenytoin, astemizole, cisapride, digoxin, cyclosporine, tacrolimus, triazolam, midazolam, HMG-CoA reductase inhibitors, corticosteroids, terfenadine, indinavir, saquinavir, warfarin); drugs that cause hepatotoxicity; alcohol may cause disulfiram-like reactions; increased trough concentrations of delavirdine if given with ketoconazole (see Warnings)

Food Interactions Food may increase ketoconazole absorption; administration with an acidic beverage (eg, Coca-Cola, Pepsi, citrus juice) increases ketoconazole absorption

Mechanism of Action Alters the permeability of the cell wall; inhibits fungal biosynthesis of triglycerides and phospholipids; inhibits several fungal enzymes that results in a build-up of toxic concentrations of hydrogen peroxide

Pharmacokinetics

Absorption: Oral: Rapid (~75%)

Distribution: Minimal penetration into the CNS; distributes to bile, saliva, urine, sweat, synovial fluid, lungs, liver, kidney and bone marrow

Protein binding: 84% to 99%

Metabolism: Partially in the liver by enzymes to inactive compounds

Bioavailability: Decreases as pH of the gastric contents increase

Half-life, biphasic:

Alpha: 2 hours

Terminal: 8 hours

Time to peak serum concentration: Oral: Within 1-2 hours

Elimination: Primarily in feces (57%) with smaller amounts excreted in urine (~13%)

Dialysis: Not dialyzable (0% to 5%)

Usual Dosage

Infants and Children: Oral: 3.3-6.6 mg/kg/day once daily

Prophylaxis for recurrence of mucocutaneous candidiasis with HIV infection: 5-10 mg/kg/day divided every 12-24 hours; maximum: 800 mg/day divided twice daily

Adults: Oral: 200-400 mg/day as a single daily dose; maximum: 800 mg/day divided twice daily

Children and Adults:

Shampoo: Shampoo twice weekly (at least 3 days should elapse between each shampoo) for 4 weeks

Topical: Apply once daily to twice daily

Administration

Oral: May administer with or without food or with juice; administer with food to decrease nausea and vomiting; administer 2 hours prior to antacids, didanosine, proton pump inhibitors, or H_2-receptor antagonists to prevent decreased ketoconazole absorption; shake suspension well before use

Shampoo: Apply to wet hair and massage over entire scalp for 1 minute; rinse hair thoroughly and reapply shampoo for 3 minutes; rinse

Topical: Apply a sufficient amount and rub gently into the affected and surrounding area

Monitoring Parameters Liver function tests, signs of adrenal dysfunction

Patient Information Cream is for topical application to the skin only; avoid contact with the eye; notify physician of unusual fatigue, weakness, vomiting, dark urine, or yellowing of eyes; avoid alcohol

Dosage Forms
Cream: 2% (15 g, 30 g, 60 g)
Shampoo (Nizoral® A-D): 1% (6 mL, 120 mL, 210 mL)
Tablet (Nizoral®): 200 mg

Extemporaneous Preparations A 20 mg/mL suspension may be made by pulverizing twelve 200 mg ketoconazole tablets to a fine powder; add 40 mL Ora-Plus® in small portions with thorough mixing; incorporate Ora-Sweet® to make a final volume of 120 mL and mix thoroughly; shake well before using; protect from light; stable for 60 days when stored without light at 5°C and 25°C

Allen LV and Erickson MA, "Stability of Ketoconazole, Metolazone, Metronidazole, Procainamide, Hydrochloride, and Spironolactone in Extemporaneously Compounded Oral Liquids," *AM J Health-Syst Pharm*, 1996, 53:2073-8.

References
Como JA and Dismukes WE, "Oral Azole Drugs as Systemic Antifungal Therapy," *N Engl J Med*, 1994, 330(4):263-72.

Ginsburg AM, McCracken GH Jr, and Olsen K, "Pharmacology of Ketoconazole Suspension in Infants and Children," *Antimicrob Agents Chemother*, 1983, 23(5):787-9.

Herrod HG, "Chronic Mucocutaneous Candidiasis in Childhood and Complications of non-*Candida* Infection: A Report of the Pediatric Immunodeficiency Collaborative Study Group," *J Pediatr*, 1990, 116(3):377-82.

♦ **Ketoderm® (Can)** *see* Ketoconazole *on page 639*

Ketorolac (KEE toe role ak)

U.S. Brand Names Acular®; Acular® P.F.; Toradol®

Canadian Brand Names Apo®-Ketorolac; Apo®-Ketorolac Injectable; Novo-Ketorolac

Therapeutic Category Analgesic, Non-narcotic; Anti-inflammatory Agent; Antipyretic; Nonsteroidal Anti-inflammatory Drug (NSAID), Ophthalmic; Nonsteroidal Anti-inflammatory Drug (NSAID), Oral; Nonsteroidal Anti-inflammatory Drug (NSAID), Parenteral

Generic Available Yes (injection and tablet)

Use
Oral, I.M., I.V.,: Short-term (≤5 days) management of moderate to severe pain, usually postoperative pain; has also been used to treat visceral pain associated with cancer, pain associated with trauma. **Note:** In adults, oral ketorolac is indicated only as continuation therapy to I.M. or I.V. ketorolac; the combined duration of oral and parenteral ketorolac should not be >5 days due to the increased risk of serious adverse effects. Only single-dose ketorolac injection is approved for use in children 2-16 years of age.

Ophthalmic:
Acular®: Treatment of ocular itch associated with seasonal allergic conjunctivitis; postoperative inflammation following cataract extraction
Acular® P.F.: Reduction of ocular pain and photophobia after incisional refractive surgery

Pregnancy Risk Factor C (D if used in 3rd trimester)

Contraindications Hypersensitivity to ketorolac, any component, aspirin, or other NSAIDs; patients with the "aspirin triad" [asthma, rhinitis (with or without nasal polyps), and aspirin intolerance] (fatal asthmatic and anaphylactoid reactions may occur in these patients); patients with active peptic ulcer disease (PUD), recent GI bleeding or perforation, or history of PUD or GI bleeding; advanced renal dysfunction; patients at risk for renal failure due to hypovolemia; women in late pregnancy; women in labor and delivery or breast-feeding; preoperative or intraoperative use; patients with cerebrovascular bleeding, incomplete hemostasis, hemorrhagic diathesis, or at high risk of bleeding; contraindicated for epidural or intrathecal use due to alcohol content; do not administer with aspirin, NSAIDs, or probenecid

Warnings Serious GI adverse effects (eg, GI bleeding, ulceration, perforation) may occur; these effects may be related to dose and duration of therapy. Ketorolac may inhibit platelet aggregation; pediatric patients may be at a greater risk for bleeding when using ketorolac following tonsillectomy (see Additional Information). Anaphylactoid reactions may occur (even in patients without previous exposure or hypersensitivity to aspirin, ketorolac, or other NSAIDs). Decreased renal function or acute renal failure may occur (patients with impaired renal function, dehydration, heart failure, (Continued)

Ketorolac *(Continued)*

liver impairment, or patients taking diuretics may be at greatest risk); correct hypovolemia before starting ketorolac. Fluid retention, edema, and sodium retention may occur; use with caution in patients with CHF, hypertension, cardiac decompensation, or similar conditions.

Precautions Use with caution and reduce dose in patients with decreased renal function; use with caution in patients with hepatic impairment and in patients in whom prolongation of bleeding time would cause adverse effects; not recommended after plastic or neurosurgery due to increased risk of bleeding.

Use ocular product with caution in patients with complicated ocular surgeries, corneal denervation or epithelial defects, ocular surface diseases (eg, dry eye syndrome), repeated ocular surgeries within a short period of time, diabetes mellitus, rheumatoid arthritis; these patients may be at risk for corneal adverse events that may be sight threatening (see Adverse Reactions)

Adverse Reactions

Cardiovascular: Edema (4%), hypertension

Central nervous system: Somnolence, drowsiness (6%), dizziness (7%), headache (17%), insomnia, euphoria, hallucinations, malaise (<1%)

Dermatologic: Rash, pruritus, purpura, urticaria

Gastrointestinal: Dyspepsia (12%), nausea (12%), diarrhea (7%), GI pain, peptic ulcer, melena, rectal bleeding, constipation, vomiting

Genitourinary: Urinary frequency

Hematologic: Inhibits platelet aggregation, may prolong bleeding time

Hepatic: Elevated liver enzymes

Local: Pain at injection site (2%)

Ocular: Blurred vision; ocular use: Transient stinging, burning, corneal edema, allergic reactions, ocular irritation or inflammation, delayed ocular healing; keratitis; epithelial breakdown, corneal thinning, erosion, ulceration, or perforation in susceptible patients (may be sight threatening; discontinue use; monitor closely); **Note:** Use >24 hours before surgery and >14 days after surgery may increase risk of corneal adverse events

Renal: Oliguria, interstitial nephritis, acute renal failure (rare)

Respiratory: Dyspnea, wheezing

Miscellaneous: Anaphylaxis, hypersensitivity reactions

Drug Interactions Warfarin, heparin, lithium, methotrexate, salicylates, NSAIDs, GI irritants (eg, potassium supplements), probenecid (significantly increases ketorolac half-life and plasma levels), furosemide, phenytoin, carbamazepine; ketorolac may decrease antihypertensive effects of ACE inhibitors and angiotensin II antagonists

Food Interactions High-fat meals may delay time to peak (by ~1 hour) and decrease peak concentrations

Stability Protect from light; Injection: Color change indicates degradation; do not administer in same syringe with narcotics; ketorolac will precipitate if mixed with morphine, meperidine, promethazine, or hydroxyzine. Discard single-use Acular® P.F. vial immediately after administration (solution does not contain preservative).

Mechanism of Action Inhibits prostaglandin synthesis by decreasing the activity of the enzyme, cyclooxygenase, which results in decreased formation of prostaglandin precursors

Pharmacodynamics Analgesia:

Onset of action:

Oral: 30-60 minutes

I.M., I.V.: ~30 minutes

Maximum effect:

Oral: 1.5-4 hours

I.M., I.V.: 1-2 hours

Duration: 4-6 hours

Pharmacokinetics

Absorption:

Oral: Well absorbed; 100%

I.M.: Rapid and complete

Distribution: Crosses placenta, crosses into breast milk, poor penetration into CSF; follows two-compartment model

V_d beta:

Children 4-8 years: 0.19-0.44 L/kg (mean: 0.26 L/kg)

Adults: 0.11-0.33 L/kg (mean: 0.18 L/kg)

Protein binding: 99%

Metabolism: In the liver; undergoes hydroxylation and glucuronide conjugation; in children 4-8 years, V_{dss} and plasma clearance were twice as high as adults, but terminal half-life was similar

Bioavailability: Oral, I.M.: 100%
Half-life, terminal:
  Children 4-8 years: ~6 hours; range: 3.5-10 (n=10)
  Adults: Mean: ~5 hours; range: 4-9 hours
    With renal impairment: S_{cr} 1.9-5 mg/dL: Mean: ~11 hours; range: 4-19 hours
    Renal dialysis patients: Mean: ~14 hours; range: 8-40 hours
Time to peak serum concentration:
  Oral: ~45 minutes
  I.M.: 30-45 minutes
  I.V.: 1-3 minutes
Elimination: Renal excretion: 60% in urine as unchanged drug with 40% as metabolites; 6% of dose excreted in feces

Usual Dosage Note: Ketorolac injection is approved for use in pediatric patients only as a single I.M. or I.V. dose in children 2-16 years of age; the use of ketorolac injection in children <2 years of age, the use of multiple doses of the injection in children <16 years of age, and the use of the tablets in children <16 years of age are outside of product labeling; ophthalmic solutions are approved for use in children ≥3 years of age

Children 2-16 years: **Do not exceed adult doses**; see Additional Information
  Single-dose treatment:
    Manufacturer's recommendations:
      I.M.: 1 mg/kg as a single dose; maximum dose: 30 mg
      I.V.: 0.5 mg/kg as a single dose; maximum dose: 15 mg
    Alternative dosing:
      I.M., I.V.: 0.4-1 mg/kg as a single dose; **Note:** Limited information exists. Single I.V. doses of 0.5 mg/kg, 0.75 mg/kg, 0.9 mg/kg and 1 mg/kg have been studied in children 2-16 years of age for postoperative analgesia. One study (Maunuksela, 1992) used a titrating dose starting with 0.2 mg/kg I.V. up to a total of 0.5 mg/kg (median dose required: 0.4 mg/kg).
      Oral: One study used 1 mg/kg as a single dose for analgesia in 30 children (mean ± SD age: 3 ± 2.5 years) undergoing bilateral myringotomy
  Multiple-dose treatment: I.M., I.V., Oral: No pediatric studies exist; one report (Buck, 1994) of the clinical experience with ketorolac in 112 children, 6 months to 19 years of age (mean: 9 years), described usual I.V. maintenance doses of 0.5 mg/kg every 6 hours (mean dose: 0.52 mg/kg; range: 0.17-1 mg/kg)
Children >16 years and >50 kg and Adults <65 years:
  Single-dose treatment:
    I.M.: 60 mg as a single dose
    I.V.: 30 mg as a single dose
  Multiple-dose treatment:
    I.M., I.V.: 30 mg every 6 hours; maximum dose: 120 mg/day
    Oral: Initial: 20 mg, then 10 mg every 4-6 hours; maximum dose: 40 mg/day
Adults ≥65 years, renally impaired, or <50 kg:
  Single-dose treatment:
    I.M.: 30 mg as a single dose
    I.V.: 15 mg as a single dose
  Multiple-dose treatment:
    I.M., I.V.: 15 mg every 6 hours; maximum dose: 60 mg/day
    Oral: 10 mg every 4-6 hours; maximum dose: 40 mg/day

Children ≥3 years and Adults: Ophthalmic:
  Seasonal allergic conjunctivitis (Acular®): Instill 1 drop in eye(s) 4 times/day
  Postoperative inflammation (Acular®): Instill 1 drop in affected eye(s) 4 times/day starting 24 hours after cataract surgery and through 14 days after surgery
  Postoperative pain and photophobia (Acular® P.F.): Instill 1 drop in affected eye(s) 4 times/day as needed for up to 3 days after incisional refractive surgery

Administration
Ophthalmic: Instill drops into affected eye(s); avoid contact of container tip with skin or eyes; apply finger pressure to lacrimal sac during and for 1-2 minutes after instillation to decrease risk of absorption and systemic effects. Acular® P.F.: Administer to one or both eyes immediately after opening single-use vial; discard vial immediately after use
Oral: May administer with food or milk to decrease GI upset
Parenteral:
  I.M.: Administer slowly and deeply into muscle; 60 mg/2 mL vial is for I.M. use only
  I.V. bolus: Administer over at least 15 seconds; maximum concentration: 30 mg/mL; **Note:** I.V. ketorolac has been infused over 1-5 minutes in children
Monitoring Parameters Signs of pain relief (eg, increased appetite and activity); BUN, serum creatinine, liver enzymes, occult blood loss, urinalysis, urine output
(Continued)

Ketorolac *(Continued)*

Reference Range Serum concentration:
Therapeutic: 0.3-5 µg/mL
Toxic: >5 µg/mL

Patient Information Avoid alcohol; may cause dizziness or drowsiness and impair ability to perform activities requiring mental alertness or physical coordination; do not exceed 5 days total use (I.M., I.V., oral). Do not use ophthalmic solution while wearing contact lenses.

Additional Information 30 mg provides analgesia comparable to 12 mg of morphine or 100 mg of meperidine; ketorolac may possess an opioid-sparing effect; diarrhea, pallor, vomiting, and labored breathing may occur with overdose

Note: A single I.V. dose of ketorolac (0.75 mg/kg) in 21 children (2.5-9 years of age) undergoing outpatient strabismus surgery was associated with less postoperative emesis than morphine plus metoclopramide (Munro, 1994). However, a single dose of I.V. ketorolac (1 mg/kg) in 25 children (2-15 years of age) undergoing tonsillectomy was associated with an increase in surgical bleeding, more patients requiring extra hemostatic measures (eg, synthetic collagen, extra Neo-Synephrine® packing), and a higher estimated blood loss compared to rectal acetaminophen (Rusy, 1995); further studies are needed.

Dosage Forms

Injection, solution, as tromethamine [single use vial] (Toradol®): 15 mg/mL (1 mL); 30 mg/mL (1 mL, 2 mL) [contains 10% alcohol]

Solution, ophthalmic, as tromethamine (Acular®): 0.5% (3 mL, 5 mL, 10 mL)

Solution, ophthalmic, as tromethamine [single use vial; preservative free] (Acular® P.F.): 0.5% (0.4 mL)

Tablet, as tromethamine (Toradol®): 10 mg

References

Buck ML, "Clinical Experience With Ketorolac in Children," *Ann Pharmacother*, 1994, 28(9):1009-13.

Maunuksela E, Kokki H, and Bullingham RES, "Comparison of Intravenous Ketorolac With Morphine for Postoperative Pain in Children," *Clin Pharmacol Ther*, 1992, 52(4):436-43.

Munro HM, Reigger LQ, Reynolds PI, et al, "Comparison of the Analgesic and Emetic Properties of Ketorolac and Morphine for Paediatric Outpatient Strabismus Surgery," *Br J Anaesth*, 1994, 72(6):624-8.

Rusy LM, Houck CS, Sullivan LJ, et al, "A Double-Blind Evaluation of Ketorolac Tromethamine Versus Acetaminophen in Pediatric Tonsillectomy: Analgesia and Bleeding," *Anesth Analg*, 1995, 80(2):226-9.

Watcha MF, Jones MB, Lagueruela RG, et al, "Comparison of Ketorolac and Morphine as Adjuvants During Pediatric Surgery," *Anesthesiology*, 1992, 76(3):368-72.

Labetalol (la BET a lole)

Related Information
Overdose and Toxicology *on page 1388*
U.S. Brand Names Normodyne®; Trandate®
Canadian Brand Names Apo®-Labetalol
Synonyms Ibidomide
Therapeutic Category Alpha-/Beta- Adrenergic Blocker; Antihypertensive Agent
Generic Available Yes
Use Treatment of mild to severe hypertension; I.V. for hypertensive emergencies
Pregnancy Risk Factor C
Contraindications Hypersensitivity to labetalol or any component; asthma, obstructive airway disease, cardiogenic shock, uncompensated CHF, bradycardia, pulmonary edema, or heart block; history of asthma or obstructive airway disease
Warnings Orthostatic hypotension may occur with I.V. administration; patient should remain supine during and for up to 3 hours after I.V. administration; use with extreme caution when reducing severely elevated blood pressure; cerebral and cardiac adverse effects (infarction/ischemia) may occur if blood pressure is decreased too rapidly; blood pressure should be lowered over as long a period of time that is compatible with the status of the patient

Tablets may contain sodium benzoate; benzoic acid (benzoate) is a metabolite of benzyl alcohol; large amounts of benzyl alcohol ($\geq$99 mg/kg/day) have been associated with a potentially fatal toxicity ("gasping syndrome") in neonates; the "gasping syndrome" consists of metabolic acidosis, respiratory distress, gasping respirations, CNS dysfunction (including convulsions, intracranial hemorrhage), hypotension and cardiovascular collapse; avoid use of labetalol products containing sodium benzoate in neonates; *in vitro* and animal studies have shown that benzoate displaces bilirubin from protein binding sites
Precautions Paradoxical increase in blood pressure has been reported with treatment of pheochromocytoma or clonidine withdrawal syndrome; use with extreme caution in patients with hyper-reactive airway disease, CHF, diabetes mellitus, hepatic dysfunction

Adverse Reactions
Cardiovascular: Orthostatic hypotension especially with I.V. administration, edema, CHF, A-V conduction disturbances (but less than with propranolol), bradycardia
Central nervous system: Drowsiness, fatigue, dizziness, behavior disorders, headache
Dermatologic: Rash, tingling in scalp or skin (transient with initiation of therapy)
Gastrointestinal: Nausea, xerostomia
Genitourinary: Sexual dysfunction, urinary problems
Neuromuscular & skeletal: Reversible myopathy has been reported in 2 children, paresthesia
Respiratory: Bronchospasm, nasal congestion
Drug Interactions Cytochrome P450 isoenzyme CYP2D6 substrate and inhibitor
Cimetidine may potentiate labetalol action; additive hypotensive effects with other hypotensive drugs; halothane may cause synergistic hypotension; tricyclic antidepressants; beta agonists; nitroglycerin; calcium antagonists
(Continued)

Labetalol *(Continued)*

Food Interactions Avoid natural licorice (causes sodium and water retention and increases potassium loss); food may increase bioavailability

Stability

Injection: Store at room temperature; do not freeze; protect from light; stable in D_5W, NS, dextrose/saline combinations, D_5/LR, $D_5/Ringer's$, LR, and Ringer's injection for 24 hours; incompatible with sodium bicarbonate, furosemide; most stable in pH of 2-4

Tablets: Store at room temperature; protect unit dose boxes from excessive moisture

Mechanism of Action Blocks alpha-, beta$_1$- and beta$_2$-adrenergic receptor sites; elevated renins are reduced

Pharmacodynamics

Onset of action:
  Oral: 20 minutes to 2 hours
  I.V.: 2-5 minutes
Maximum effect:
  Oral: 1-4 hours
  I.V.: 5-15 minutes
Duration:
  Oral: 8-24 hours (dose dependent)
  I.V.: 2-4 hours

Pharmacokinetics

Distribution: Crosses the placenta; small amounts in breast milk
  V_d: Adults: 3-16 L/kg; mean: 9.4 L/kg
Protein-binding: 50%
Metabolism: In the liver primarily via glucuronide conjugation; extensive first-pass effect
Bioavailability: Oral: 25%; increased bioavailability with liver disease, elderly
Half-life: 5-8 hours
Elimination: Possible decreased clearance in neonates/infants; <5% excreted in urine unchanged

Usual Dosage

Children: **Note**: Limited information regarding labetalol use in pediatric patients is currently available in the literature; labetalol should be initiated cautiously in pediatric patients (using the lower doses listed) with careful dosage adjustment and blood pressure monitoring

Oral: Some centers recommend initial oral doses of 4 mg/kg/day in 2 divided doses. (Reported oral doses have started at 3 mg/kg/day and 20 mg/kg/day and have increased up to 40 mg/kg/day.)

I.V., intermittent bolus doses: Initial doses of 0.2-0.5 mg/kg/dose with a range of 0.2-1 mg/kg/dose have been suggested; maximum dose: 20 mg/dose

Treatment of pediatric hypertensive emergencies: Initial continuous infusions of 0.4-1 mg/kg/hour with a maximum of 3 mg/kg/hour have been used; one study used initial bolus dose of 0.2-1 mg/kg (maximum dose: 20 mg, mean: 0.5 mg/kg) followed by a continuous infusion of 0.25-1.5 mg/kg/hour (mean: 0.78 mg/kg/hour)

Adults:

Oral: Initial: 100 mg twice daily, may increase as needed every 2-3 days by 100 mg until desired response is obtained; usual dose: 200-400 mg twice daily; not to exceed 2.4 g/day

I.V.: Initial: 20 mg; may give 40-80 mg at 10-minute intervals, up to 300 mg total dose

I.V. infusion: Initial: 2 mg/minute; titrate to response

Administration

Oral: May administer with food but should be administered in a consistent manner with regards to meals

Parenteral:

I.V. bolus: Administer over 2-3 minutes; do not administer faster than 2 mg/minute; maximum concentration: 5 mg/mL

I.V. continuous infusion: Dilute to 1 mg/mL; undiluted labetalol injection (5 mg/mL) has been administered to a very small number of adult patients who were extremely fluid restricted

Monitoring Parameters Blood pressure, heart rate, pulse, EKG

Test Interactions False-positive urine catecholamines, VMA if measured by fluorometric or photometric methods; use HPLC or specific catecholamine radioenzymatic technique

Patient Information Limit alcohol; may cause dizziness or drowsiness and impair ability to perform activities requiring mental alertness or physical coordination; do not stop medication abruptly; may cause dry mouth

Nursing Implications Instruct patient regarding compliance; do **not** abruptly withdraw medication in patients with ischemic heart disease; labetalol may mask other signs and symptoms of diabetes mellitus, but sweating can still occur

Dosage Forms

Injection, solution, as hydrochloride (Normodyne®): 5 mg/mL (20 mL, 40 mL)
Injection, solution, as hydrochloride [prefilled syringe; single dose]: 5 mg/mL (4 mL)
Normodyne®: 5 mg/mL (4 mL, 8 mL)
Tablet, as hydrochloride: 100 mg, 200 mg, 300 mg
Normodyne®: 100 mg, 200 mg, 300 mg
Trandate®: 100 mg, 200 mg [contains sodium benzoate], 300 mg

Extemporaneous Preparations

A 40 mg/mL labetalol hydrochloride oral liquid preparation made from tablets and 3 different vehicles (cherry syrup, a 1:1 mixture of Ora-Sweet® and Ora-Plus®, or a 1:1 mixture of Ora-Sweet® SF and Ora-Plus®) was stable for 60 days when stored in amber plastic prescription bottles in the dark at room temperature (25°C) or under refrigeration (5°C); grind sixteen 300 mg tablets in a mortar into a fine powder; add 20 mL of the vehicle and mix well to form a uniform paste; mix while adding the vehicle in geometric proportions to **almost** 120 mL; transfer to a calibrated bottle and qsad with vehicle to make 120 mL; label "shake well" and "protect from light" (Allen, 1996).

Extemporaneously prepared solutions of labetalol hydrochloride (approximate concentrations 7-10 mg/mL) prepared in distilled water, simple syrup, apple juice, grape juice, and orange juice were stable for 4 weeks when stored in amber glass or plastic prescription bottles at 23°C and 4°C (Nahata, 1991).

Allen LV and Erickson MA, "Stability of Labetalol Hydrochloride, Metoprolol Tartrate, Verapamil Hydrochloride, and Spironolactone With Hydrochlorothiazide in Extemporaneously Compounded Oral Liquids," *Am J Health Syst Pharm*, 1996, 53(19):2304-9.

Nahata MC, "Stability of Labetolol Hydrochloride in Distilled Water, Simple Syrup, and Three Fruit Juices," *DICP*, 1991, 25(5):465-9.

References

Bunchman TE, Lynch RE, and Wood EG, "Intravenously Administered Labetalol for Treatment of Hypertension in Children," *J Pediatr*, 1992, 120(1):140-4.

Farine M and Arbus GS, "Management of Hypertensive Emergencies in Children," *Pediatr Emerg Care*, 1989, 5(1):51-5.

Ishisaka DY, Yonan CD, Housel BF, "Labetalol for Treatment of Hypertension in a Child," *Clin Pharm*, 1991, 10(7):500-1 (case report).

Jones SE, "Coarctation in Children. Controlled Hypotension Using Labetalol and Halothane," *Anaesthesia*, 1979, 34(10):1052-5.

Jureidini KF, "Oral Labetalol in a Child With Phaeochromocytoma and Five Children With Renal Hypertension," *N Z Med J*, 1980, 10:479 (abstract).

Mueller JB and Solhaug MJ, "Labetalol in Pediatric Hypertensive Emergencies," *Pediatr Res*, 1988, 23(Pt 2):543A (abstract).

Wesley AG, Hariparsad D, Pather M, et al, "Labetalol in Tetanus. The Treatment of Sympathetic Nervous System Overactivity," *Anaesthesia*, 1983, 38(3):243-9.

♦ **Laboratory Detection of Drugs in Urine** *see page 1400*
♦ **Lac-Hydrin®** *see* Lactic Acid and Ammonium Hydroxide *on page 647*
♦ **LAClotion™** *see* Lactic Acid and Ammonium Hydroxide *on page 647*
♦ **Lacri-Lube® SOP [OTC]** *see* Ocular Lubricant *on page 831*

Lactic Acid and Ammonium Hydroxide

(LAK tik AS id with a MOE nee um hye DROKS ide)

U.S. Brand Names AmLactin® [OTC]; Lac-Hydrin®; LAClotion™

Synonyms Ammonium Hydroxide and Lactic Acid; Ammonium Lactate

Therapeutic Category Topical Skin Product

Generic Available No

Use Topical humectant used in the treatment of ichthyosis vulgaris, ichthyosis xerosis, and dry skin conditions

Pregnancy Risk Factor B

Contraindications Hypersensitivity to ammonium lactate, parabens, or any component

Warnings May cause photosensitivity reaction (see Patient Information)

Precautions Use with caution on face due to potential irritation, particularly in fair-skinned individuals

Adverse Reactions

Dermatologic: Rash, erythema, peeling, photosensitivity
Local: Burning, stinging

Drug Interactions Mixture of calcipotriene ointment with ammonium lactate lotion may result in a significant decrease in the calcipotriene concentration within 24 hours and continued decrease over the next 10 days

Stability Store at room temperature

(Continued)

Lactic Acid and Ammonium Hydroxide *(Continued)*

Mechanism of Action Ammonium lactate is a formulation of lactic acid neutralized with ammonium hydroxide. Lactic acid is an alpha-hydroxy acid which increases hydration of the skin, decreases corneocyte adhesion, reduces excessive epidermal keratinization in hyperkeratotic conditions, and induces synthesis of mucopolysaccharides and collagen in photodamaged skin.

Pharmacodynamics Onset of action: Ichthyosis xerosis: 3-7 days

Pharmacokinetics Bioavailability: 6%

Usual Dosage Infants, Children, and Adults: Topical: Apply twice daily

Administration Topical: Apply a small amount to the affected area(s) and rub in thoroughly; avoid contact with eyes, lips, or mucous membranes; shake lotion well before use

Monitoring Parameters Physical examination of skin condition

Patient Information Avoid contact with eyes, lips, or mucous membranes; may cause stinging or burning when applied to skin with fissures, erosions, or abrasions. May cause photosensitivity reactions (eg, exposure to sunlight may cause severe sunburn, skin rash, redness, or itching); avoid exposure to sunlight and artificial light sources (sunlamps, tanning booth/bed); wear protective clothing, wide-brimmed hats, sunglasses, and lip sunscreen (SPF ≥15); use a sunscreen [broad-spectrum sunscreen or physical sunscreen (preferred) or sunblock with SPF ≥15]; contact physician if reaction occurs. Do not use cosmetics or other skin care products on the treated skin area.

Dosage Forms

Cream, topical:

AmLactin®: Lactic acid 12% with ammonium hydroxide (140 g)

Lac-Hydrin®: Lactic acid 12% with ammonium hydroxide (280 g, 385 g)

Lotion, topical (AmLactin®, Lac-Hydrin®, LAClotion™): Lactic acid 12% with ammonium hydroxide (225 g, 400 g)

♦ **LactiCare-HC®** *see* Hydrocortisone *on page 573*

♦ **Lactinex® [OTC]** *see Lactobacillus acidophilus* and *Lactobacillus bulgaricus* on page 648

Lactobacillus acidophilus and *Lactobacillus bulgaricus*

(lak toe ba SIL us as i DOF fil us & lak toe ba SIL us bul GAR i cus)

U.S. Brand Names Bacid® [OTC]; Kala [OTC]; Lactinex® [OTC]; Megadophilus® [OTC]; More-Dophilus® [OTC]; Superdophilus® [OTC]

Canadian Brand Names Fermalac

Therapeutic Category Antidiarrheal

Generic Available Yes

Use Treatment of uncomplicated diarrhea particularly that caused by antibiotic therapy; re-establish normal physiologic and bacterial flora of the intestinal tract

Contraindications Allergy to milk or lactose

Warnings Discontinue if high fever present

Adverse Reactions Gastrointestinal: Intestinal flatus

Stability Store in the refrigerator

Mechanism of Action Creates an environment unfavorable to potentially pathogenic fungi or bacteria through the production of lactic acid, and favors establishment of an aciduric flora, thereby suppressing the growth of pathogenic microorganisms; helps re-establish normal intestinal flora

Pharmacokinetics

Absorption: Not orally absorbed

Distribution: Locally, primarily in the colon

Elimination: In feces

Usual Dosage Children and Adults: Oral:

Capsule: 1-2 capsules 2-4 times/day

Granules: 1 packet added to or taken with cereal, food, milk, fruit juice, or water, 3-4 times/day

Powder: 1/4-1 teaspoon 1-3 times/day with liquid

Tablet, chewable: 4 tablets 3-4 times/day; may follow each dose with a small amount of milk, fruit juice, or water

Recontamination protocol for BMT unit: 1 packet 3 times/day for 6 doses for those patients who refuse yogurt

Administration Oral: Granules, powder, or contents of capsules may be added to or administered with cereal, food, milk, fruit juice, or water

Dosage Forms

Capsule: *Lactobacillus acidophilus* 100 million units

Bacid®: *Lactobacillus acidophilus* 500 million units

Megadophilus®, Superdophilus®: *Lactobacillus acidophilus* 2 billion units [available in dairy-based or dairy-free formulation]

Granules (Lactinex®): Mixed culture *Lactobacillus acidophilus* and *Lactobacillus bulgaricus* per 1 g packet (12s)

Powder for suspension:

More-Dophilus®: *Lactobacillus acidophilus* 12.4 billion units/5 mL (30 g, 120 g) [carrot derived]

Megadophilus®, Superdophilus®: *Lactobacillus acidophilus* 2 billion units/2.5 mL (49 g) [available in dairy-based or dairy-free formulations]

Tablet (Kala): *Lactobacillus acidophilus* 200 million units [soy based]

Tablet, chewable (Lactinex®): Mixed culture *Lactobacillus acidophilus* and *Lactobacillus bulgaricus*

♦ **Lactoflavin** *see* Riboflavin *on page 983*

Lactulose (LAK tyoo lose)

Related Information

Carbohydrate and Alcohol Content of Liquid Medications for Use in Patients Receiving Ketogenic Diets *on page 1431*

U.S. Brand Names Cholac®; Constilac®; Constulose®; Enulose®; Generlac; Kristalose®

Canadian Brand Names Acilac; Apo®-Lactulose; Laxilose; PMS-Lactulose

Therapeutic Category Ammonium Detoxicant; Hyperammonemia Agent; Laxative, Miscellaneous

Generic Available Yes

Use Adjunct in the prevention and treatment of portal-systemic encephalopathy (PSE); treatment of chronic constipation

Pregnancy Risk Factor B

Contraindications Hypersensitivity to lactulose or any component; galactosemia or patients requiring low galactose diet

Warnings Accumulation of hydrogen gas in intestine could result in an explosion if the patient were to undergo electrocautery procedure

Precautions Use with caution in patients with diabetes mellitus; do not use with other laxatives especially when initiating PSE treatment as increased loose stools may falsely suggest adequate lactulose dosage

Adverse Reactions Gastrointestinal: Flatulence, abdominal discomfort, diarrhea, nausea, vomiting

Drug Interactions Oral antibiotics may interfere with desired degradation of lactulose by eliminating key GI bacteria; nonabsorbable antacids may eliminate desired lactulose-induced decreased GI tract pH

Food Interactions Contraindicated in patients on galactose-restricted diet

Stability Store at room temperature to reduce viscosity; discard solution if cloudy or very dark

Mechanism of Action The bacterial degradation of lactulose resulting in an acidic pH inhibits the diffusion of NH_3 into the blood by causing the conversion of NH_3 to NH_4+; also enhances the diffusion of NH_3 from the blood into the gut where conversion to NH_4+ occurs; produces an osmotic effect in the colon with resultant distention promoting peristalsis and elimination of NH_4+ from the body

Pharmacokinetics

Absorption: Oral: Not absorbed appreciably

Metabolism: By colonic flora to lactic acid and acetic acid

Elimination: Primarily in feces and urine (~3%)

Usual Dosage

Prevention and treatment of portal systemic encephalopathy (PSE): Oral:

Infants: 2.5-10 mL/day divided 3-4 times/day, adjust dosage to produce 2-3 soft stools per day

Children: 40-90 mL/day divided 3-4 times/day, adjust dosage to produce 2-3 soft stools per day

Adults:

Oral:

Acute episodes of PSE: 30-45 mL (20-30 g) at 1- to 2-hour intervals until laxative effect observed, then adjust dosage to produce 2-3 soft stools per day

Chronic therapy: 30-45 mL/dose (20-30 g/dose) 3-4 times/day; titrate dose every 1-2 days to produce 2-3 soft stools per day

Rectal: 300 mL diluted with 700 mL of water or NS, and given via a rectal balloon catheter and retained for 30-60 minutes; may give every 4-6 hours

Constipation: Oral:

Children: 7.5 mL/day (5 g/day) after breakfast

Adults: 15-30 mL/day (10-20 g/day); increase to a maximum of 60 mL/day (40 g/day) if needed

(Continued)

Lactulose *(Continued)*

Administration
Oral: Administer with juice, milk, or water; dissolve crystals in 4 ounces of water or juice

Rectal: See Usual Dosage

Monitoring Parameters Serum ammonia, serum potassium, fluid status, stool output

Additional Information Upon discontinuation of therapy, allow 24-48 hours for resumption of normal bowel movements

Dosage Forms
Crystals for reconstitution (Kristalose®): 10 g/packet (30s), 20 g/packet (30s)

Syrup: 10 g/15 mL (15 mL, 30 mL, 237 mL, 473 mL, 946 mL, 1000 mL, 1890 mL)

Cholac®, Constilac®: 10 g/15 mL (30 mL, 240 mL, 480 mL, 960 mL, 1920 mL, 3875 mL)

Constulose®: 10 g/15 mL (240 mL, 960 mL)

Enulose®: 10 g/15 mL (480 mL, 1900 mL)

Generlac: 10 g/15 mL (480 mL, 1920 mL)

♦ **L-AmB** *see* Amphotericin B Liposome *on page 102*

♦ **Lamictal®** *see* Lamotrigine *on page 653*

Lamivudine *(la MI vyoo deen)*

Related Information
Adult and Adolescent HIV *on page 1327*

Pediatric HIV *on page 1323*

U.S. Brand Names Epivir®; Epivir-HBV®

Canadian Brand Names Heptovir®; 3TC®

Synonyms 2'-Deoxy-3'-Thiacytidine; 3TC

Therapeutic Category Antiretroviral Agent; HIV Agents (Anti-HIV Agents); Nucleoside Reverse Transcriptase Inhibitor (NRTI)

Generic Available No

Use Treatment of HIV infection in combination with other antiretroviral agents. (**Note:** HIV regimens consisting of **three** antiretroviral agents are strongly recommended); chemoprophylaxis after occupational exposure to HIV; management of chronic hepatitis B infection associated with evidence of hepatitis B viral replication and active liver inflammation

Pregnancy Risk Factor C

Contraindications Hypersensitivity to lamivudine or any component

Warnings The major clinical toxicity of lamivudine in pediatric patients is pancreatitis which has occurred in 14% of patients in one open-label, uncontrolled study; discontinue lamivudine therapy if clinical signs, symptoms, or laboratory abnormalities suggestive of pancreatitis occur. Lactic acidosis and severe hepatomegaly with steatosis have been reported with the use of lamivudine. A majority of these cases have been in women. Obesity and prolonged nucleoside exposure may be risk factors. Discontinue lamivudine if clinical or laboratory abnormalities suggestive of lactic acidosis or pronounced hepatotoxicity occur. If treatment doses used for chronic hepatitis B are administered as monotherapy to a patient with unrecognized or untreated HIV infection, rapid emergence of HIV resistance will occur.

Precautions Fat redistribution and accumulation [ie, central obesity, peripheral wasting, facial wasting, breast enlargement, dorsocervical fat enlargement (buffalo hump), and cushingoid appearance] have been observed in patients receiving antiretroviral agents (causal relationship not established). Use with extreme caution and only if there is no satisfactory alternative therapy in pediatric patients with a history of pancreatitis or other significant risk factors for the development of pancreatitis; reduce dosage in patients with impaired renal function; mothers should not breast-feed if they are receiving lamivudine

Adverse Reactions
Central nervous system: Headache (6% to 11%), fatigue, insomnia, psychomotor disorders (11% to 15%), dizziness, depressive disorder

Dermatologic: Rash, pruritus, urticaria, alopecia

Endocrine & metabolic: Lactic acidosis, hyperglycemia; central redistribution of body fat: Central obesity, buffalo hump, facial atrophy, and breast enlargement

Gastrointestinal: Nausea, feeding problem (12% to 19%), abdominal discomfort (10% to 12%), pancreatitis (14%; primarily seen in children with advanced HIV receiving multiple medications), diarrhea, vomiting, anorexia, stomatitis

Hematologic: Neutropenia, anemia, thrombocytopenia

Hepatic: Elevated ALT, AST, bilirubin, and amylase; hepatic steatosis, severe hepatomegaly

Neuromuscular & skeletal: Paresthesias, peripheral neuropathy, musculoskeletal pain (8% to 11%), gait disorder, myalgia, muscle weakness, rhabdomyolysis, elevated CPK

Respiratory: Cough, wheezing

Drug Interactions Coadministration with trimethoprim/sulfamethoxazole increases the AUC of lamivudine (significance is unknown); when used with zidovudine, may prevent emergence of zidovudine resistance; lamivudine and zalcitabine may inhibit intracellular phosphorylation of each other (concurrent use of lamivudine and zalcitabine is **not** recommended)

Stability Store tablets and oral solution at room temperature in tightly closed bottles

Mechanism of Action A synthetic nucleoside analogue that is converted intracellularly to the active triphosphate metabolite which inhibits reverse transcription via viral DNA chain termination after incorporation of the nucleoside analogue. Lamivudine triphosphate is a weak inhibitor of DNA polymerase alpha- and beta-mitochondrial DNA polymerase.

Pharmacokinetics

Distribution: Into extravascular spaces
   Children: CSF/plasma ratio: 0.11
Protein binding: <36%
Metabolism: Converted intracellularly to the active triphosphate form
Bioavailability:
   Children: 66%
   Adolescents and Adults: 86%
Half-life:
   Intracellular: 10-15 hours
   Elimination:
      Children 4 months to 14 years: 2 ± 0.6 hours
      Adults with normal renal function: 3-6 hours
Time to peak serum concentration:
   Fasting state: 0.9 hours
   Fed state: 3.2 hours
Elimination: 70% of dose eliminated unchanged in urine; 5.2% of dose is eliminated as a trans-sulfoxide metabolite

Usual Dosage Oral:

HIV:
   Neonates <30 days: 2 mg/kg/dose twice daily is being studied in clinical trials
   Infants > 3 months and Children: 4 mg/kg/dose twice daily; maximum dose: 150 mg/dose every 12 hours
   Adolescents and Adults, body weight <50 kg: 2 mg/kg/dose twice daily
   Adolescents (in later puberty: Tanner V) and Adults, body weight ≥50 kg: 150 mg/dose twice daily or 300 mg/dose once daily
      Chemoprophylaxis after occupational exposure to HIV: 150 mg/dose twice daily in combination with zidovudine 200 mg 3 times/day or 300 mg twice daily and indinavir 800 mg 3 times/day are first-line agents after exposures for which prophylaxis is recommended.
Chronic hepatitis B infection:
   Children 2-17 years: 3 mg/kg/dose once daily; maximum dose: 100 mg/day
   Adolescents ≥16 years and Adults: 100 mg/dose once daily

Dosing adjustment in renal impairment for HIV: Adults:
   Cl_{cr} 30-49 mL/minute: 150 mg once daily
   Cl_{cr} 15-29 mL/minute: 150 mg first dose, then 100 mg once daily
   Cl_{cr} 5-14 mL/minute: 150 mg first dose, then 50 mg once daily
   Cl_{cr} <5 mL/minute: 50 mg first dose, then 25 mg once daily

Dosing adjustment in renal impairment for chronic hepatitis B: Adults:
   Cl_{cr} 30-49 mL/minute: 100 mg first dose, then 50 mg once daily
   Cl_{cr} 15-29 mL/minute: 100 mg first dose, then 25 mg once daily
   Cl_{cr} 5-14 mL/minute: 35 mg first dose, then 15 mg once daily
   Cl_{cr} <5 mL/minute: 35 mg first dose, then 10 mg once daily

Dosing adjustment in hepatic impairment: No data

Administration Oral: Administer with or without food

Monitoring Parameters CBC with differential, hemoglobin, ALT, AST, serum amylase, bilirubin, CD4 cell count, HIV RNA plasma levels; signs and symptoms of pancreatitis, lactic acidosis, and pronounced hepatotoxicity

Patient Information Lamivudine is not a cure for HIV; notify physician if persistent severe abdominal pain, nausea, vomiting, numbness, or tingling occur; avoid alcohol

HIV medications may cause changes in body fat, including an increase in fat in the upper back and neck, breasts, and trunk; a loss of fat from the face, arms, and legs may also occur.

(Continued)

Lamivudine (Continued)

Dosage Forms
Solution:

Epivir®: 10 mg/mL (240 mL) [contains 6% alcohol and propylene glycol; strawberry-banana flavor]

Epivir-HBV®: 5 mg/mL (240 mL) [contains propylene glycol; strawberry-banana flavor]

Tablet, film-coated:

Epivir®: 150 mg, 300 mg

Epivir-HBV®: 100 mg

References

"U.S. Public Health Service Guidelines for the Management of Occupational Exposures to HBV, HCV, and HIV and Recommendations for Postexposure Prophylaxis," MMWR Morb Mortal Wkly Rep, 2001, 50(RR-11):1-52.

Eron JJ, Benoit SL, Jemsek J, et al, "Treatment With Lamivudine, Zidovudine, or Both in HIV-Positive Patients With 200 to 500 CD4+ Cells Per Cubic Millimeter," N Engl J Med, 1995, 333(25):1662-9.

Lai CL, Chien RN, Leung NW, et al, "A One-Year Trial of Lamivudine for Chronic Hepatitis B," N Engl J Med, 1998, 339(2):61-8.

Lewis LL, Mueller B, Schock R, et al, "A Phase I/II Study to Evaluate the Safety, Toxicity, and Preliminary Efficacy of Combinations of Lamivudine (3TC), Zidovudine (AZT) and Didanosine (ddI) in Children With HIV Infection," Natl Conf Hum Retroviruses Relat Infect (2nd), 1995, Jan 29-Feb 2:103.

Lewis LL, Venzon D, Church J, et al, "Lamivudine in Children With Human Immunodeficiency Virus Infection: A Phase I/II Study," J Infect Dis, 1996, 174(1):16-25.

Working Group on Antiretroviral Therapy and Medical Management of HIV-Infected Children, "Guidelines for the Use of Antiretroviral Agents in Pediatric HIV Infection," December 14, 2001, http://www.aidsinfo.nih.gov.

♦ Lamivudine, Abacavir, and Zidovudine see Abacavir, Lamivudine, and Zidovudine on page 32

Lamivudine and Zidovudine (la MI vyoo deen & zye DOE vyoo deen)

U.S. Brand Names Combivir®

Synonyms AZT and 3TC; 3TC and AZT; 3TC and ZDV; Zidovudine and Lamivudine; ZVD and 3TC

Therapeutic Category Antiretroviral Agent; HIV Agents (Anti-HIV Agents); Nucleoside Reverse Transcriptase Inhibitor (NRTI)

Generic Available No

Use Treatment of HIV-1 infection in combination with at least one other antiretroviral agent; **(Note:** HIV regimens consisting of **three** antiretroviral agents are strongly recommended)

Pregnancy Risk Factor C

Contraindications Hypersensitivity to lamivudine, zidovudine, or any component

Warnings This product contains lamivudine and zidovudine as a fixed-dose combination; ordinarily, concomitant use of Combivir® with either lamivudine or zidovudine is not recommended. The major clinical toxicity of lamivudine in pediatric patients is pancreatitis; discontinue therapy if clinical signs, symptoms, or laboratory abnormalities suggestive of pancreatitis occur. Zidovudine is associated with hematologic toxicity including granulocytopenia and severe anemia requiring transfusions; use with caution in patients with ANC <1000 cells/mm³ or hemoglobin <9.5 g/dL; discontinue treatment in children with an ANC <500 cells/mm³ until marrow recovery is observed; use of erythropoietin, filgrastim, or reduced zidovudine dosage may be necessary in some patients; prolonged use of zidovudine may cause myositis and myopathy; zidovudine has been shown to be carcinogenic in rats and mice.

Cases of lactic acidosis, severe hepatomegaly with steatosis, and death have been reported with the use of lamivudine, zidovudine and other antiretroviral agents; most of these cases have been in women; prolonged nucleoside use, obesity, and prior liver disease may be risk factors; use with extreme caution in patients with other risk factors for liver disease; discontinue therapy in patients who develop laboratory or clinical evidence of lactic acidosis or pronounced hepatotoxicity.

Precautions Always use Combivir® in combination with another antiretroviral agent; use with extreme caution and only if there is no satisfactory alternative therapy in pediatric patients with a history of pancreatitis or other significant risk factors for pancreatitis; use with caution in patients with bone marrow compromise or in patients with impaired renal or hepatic function. The dose of lamivudine should be reduced in patients with renal dysfunction; the dose of zidovudine should be reduced or therapy interrupted in patients with anemia, granulocytopenia, myopathy, renal or hepatic impairment, or liver cirrhosis; use of the fixed-dose combination product (Combivir®) is **not** recommended for patients who need a dosage reduction (use individual antiretroviral agents to appropriately adjust dosages).

Fat redistribution and accumulation [ie, central obesity, peripheral wasting, facial wasting, breast enlargement, dorsocervical fat enlargement (buffalo hump), and cushingoid appearance] have been observed in patients receiving antiretroviral agents (causal relationship not established). HIV-infected patients who are coinfected with hepatitis B may experience clinical symptoms or laboratory evidence of hepatitis when lamivudine is discontinued; most cases are self-limited, but fatalities have been reported; monitor patients closely for at least several months after discontinuation of lamivudine and zidovudine.

Adverse Reactions See Lamivudine *on page 650* and Zidovudine *on page 1163*

Drug Interactions See Lamivudine *on page 650* and Zidovudine *on page 1163*

Food Interactions Food does not affect the extent of of absorption

Mechanism of Action See Lamivudine *on page 650* and Zidovudine *on page 1163*

Pharmacokinetics One Combivir® tablet is bioequivalent to one lamivudine 150 mg tablet plus one zidovudine 300 mg tablet; see Lamivudine *on page 650* and Zidovudine *on page 1163*

Usual Dosage Oral: Adolescents ≥12 years and Adults: One tablet twice daily

> **Dosage adjustment in hepatic impairment:** Mild to moderate hepatic dysfunction or liver cirrhosis: Not recommended (use individual antiretroviral agents to reduce dosage)
>
> **Dosage adjustment in renal impairment:** Cl_{cr} ≤50 mL/minute: Not recommended (use individual antiretroviral agents to reduce dosage)

Administration Oral: May be administered without regard to meals

Monitoring Parameters CBC with differential, hemoglobin, MCV, reticulocyte count, liver enzymes, serum amylase, bilirubin, CD4 cell count, HIV RNA plasma levels, renal and hepatic function tests; signs and symptoms of pancreatitis, lactic acidosis, pronounced hepatotoxicity, anemia, and bone marrow suppression

Patient Information Avoid alcohol; Combivir® is not a cure; notify physician if persistent severe abdominal pain, nausea, or vomiting occurs; take Combivir® every day as prescribed; do not change dose or discontinue without physician's advice. If a dose is missed, take it as soon as possible, then return to normal dosing schedule; if a dose is skipped, do **not** double the next dose

HIV medications may cause changes in body fat, including an increase in fat in the upper back and neck, breasts, and trunk; a loss of fat from the face, arms, and legs may also occur.

Dosage Forms Tablet: Lamivudine 150 mg and zidovudine 300 mg

♦ **Lamivudine, Zidovudine, and Abacavir** *see* Abacavir, Lamivudine, and Zidovudine *on page 32*

Lamotrigine (la MOE tri jeen)

Related Information
Antiepileptic Drugs *on page 1374*
Carbohydrate and Alcohol Content of Liquid Medications for Use in Patients Receiving Ketogenic Diets *on page 1431*

U.S. Brand Names Lamictal®

Synonyms BW-430C; LTG

Therapeutic Category Anticonvulsant, Miscellaneous

Generic Available No

Use Adjunctive treatment of partial seizures and generalized seizures of Lennox-Gastaut syndrome in children ≥2 years of age and adults; monotherapy of partial seizures in adults who are converted from a single enzyme-inducing AED

> **Note:** Preliminary investigations have shown potential efficacy as add-on therapy for absence, atypical absence, generalized tonic-clonic, atonic, tonic, and myoclonic seizures; and as monotherapy in adults and adolescents for partial seizures and idiopathic generalized tonic-clonic seizures; additional studies are underway

Pregnancy Risk Factor C

Contraindications Hypersensitivity to lamotrigine or any component

Warnings Skin rash may occur (10%) and can be serious enough to require hospitalization or discontinuation of drug; serious skin rashes (including Stevens-Johnson syndrome) occur in 0.8% of pediatric patients and in 0.3% of adults; rare cases of toxic epidermal necrolysis have been reported; rash-related deaths have occurred in pediatric and adult patients. In addition to pediatric age, the risk of rash may be increased in patients receiving valproic acid, high initial doses, or with rapid dosage increases; rash usually appears in the first 2-8 weeks of therapy, but may occur after prolonged treatment (eg, 6 months). Benign rashes may occur, but one cannot predict which rashes will become serious or life-threatening; the manufacturer recommends (ordinarily) discontinuation of lamotrigine at the first sign of rash (unless rash is clearly not drug related); discontinuation of lamotrigine may not prevent rash from becoming life-threatening or permanently disfiguring or disabling
(Continued)

Lamotrigine *(Continued)*

Potentially fatal hypersensitivity reactions may occur; these may include multiorgan failure or dysfunction; early symptoms of hypersensitivity reaction (eg, lymphadenopathy, fever) may occur without rash; discontinue lamotrigine if another cause for symptoms cannot be established. Blood dyscrasias may occur.

Precautions Use with caution and decrease the dose in patients with renal or moderate to severe hepatic dysfunction; do not abruptly discontinue; when discontinuing therapy, gradually reduce the dose by ~50% per week and taper over at least 2 weeks unless safety concerns require a more rapid withdrawal. Lamotrigine binds to melanin and may possibly accumulate in the eye and other tissues rich in melanin; long-term ophthalmologic effects are unknown.

Adverse Reactions

Cardiovascular: Edema

Central nervous system: Dizziness, sedation, somnolence, headache, agitation, ataxia, fever; exacerbation of seizures has been reported

Dermatologic: Rash (higher incidence in children and in patients receiving valproic acid, high initial lamotrigine doses, or rapid dosage increases), angioedema, Stevens-Johnson syndrome, photosensitivity; toxic epidermal necrolysis (rare)

Gastrointestinal: Nausea, vomiting, diarrhea, abdominal pain, dyspepsia, constipation

Hematologic: Leukopenia, neutropenia, anemia, thrombocytopenia, pancytopenia, aplastic anemia (rare), pure red cell aplasia (rare)

Neuromuscular & skeletal: Tremor, asthenia

Ocular: Diplopia, amblyopia, nystagmus

Miscellaneous: Hypersensitivity reactions, lymphadenopathy; acute multiorgan failure (rare)

Drug Interactions Acetaminophen may increase the clearance of lamotrigine; carbamazepine, when administered at the same time as lamotrigine, may increase adverse effects such as dizziness, diplopia, ataxia (space administration of drugs by at least 1 hour); valproic acid may increase incidence of rash and increases half-life and serum concentrations of lamotrigine; enzyme-inducing drugs (eg, carbamazepine, phenytoin) decrease lamotrigine's half-life by ~50%; lamotrigine may increase the clearance of valproic acid

Food Interactions Absorption is not affected by food

Stability Store at room temperature in a dry place away from heat and light

Mechanism of Action A triazine derivative which affects voltage-sensitive sodium channels and inhibits presynaptic release of glutamate and aspartate (excitatory amino acid CNS neurotransmitters)

Pharmacokinetics

Absorption: Oral: Rapid, 97.6% absorbed

Distribution: V_d: Adults: 1.1 L/kg; range: 0.9-1.3 L/kg; crosses into breast milk

Protein binding: 55% (primarily albumin)

Metabolism: >75% metabolized in the liver via glucuronidation; autoinduction may occur

Bioavailability: 98%

Half-life:

Children:

With enzyme-inducing AEDs (eg, phenytoin, carbamazepine): ~7-10 hours

With enzyme inducer and valproic acid (VPA): ~15-27 hours

With VPA: ~44-94 hours

Adults:

Normal: Single dose: 33 hours; multiple dose: ~25 hours

With enzyme-inducing AEDs: ~13-14 hours (range: 8-33 hours)

With enzyme inducer and VPA: ~27 hours

With VPA: 59 hours (range: 30-89 hours)

Hepatic dysfunction: Child-Pugh classification:

Grade A: 36 hours

Grade B: 60 hours

Grade C: 110 hours

Renal dysfunction (Cl_{cr} 13 mL/minute): ~43 hours

Severe renal dysfunction (Cl_{cr} <10 mL/minute): 57.4 hours

During dialysis: 13 hours

Time to peak serum concentration: Oral: ~2 hours (range: 1.4-4.8 hours); select patients may have second peak at 4-6 hours due to enterohepatic recirculation

Elimination: 75% to 90% excreted as glucuronide metabolites and 10% as unchanged drug

Dialysis: ~20% is removed during 4-hour hemodialysis period

Usual Dosage Note: Dosage depends on patient's concomitant medications, ie, valproic acid and enzyme-inducing AEDs (such as phenytoin, phenobarbital, carbamazepine, and primidone) (see Additional Information)

Adjunctive (add-on) therapy:

Children 2-12 years: **Note: Only whole tablets should be used for dosing**; children 2-6 years will likely require maintenance doses at the higher end of recommended range; patients weighing <30 kg may need as much as a 50% increase in maintenance dose, compared with patients weighing >30 kg; titrate dose to clinical effect

Patients receiving AED regimens **containing valproic acid**:

Weeks 1 and 2: 0.15 mg/kg/day in 1-2 divided doses; round dose down to the nearest whole tablet; use 2 mg every other day for patients weighing >6.7 kg and <14 kg

Weeks 3 and 4: 0.3 mg/kg/day in 1-2 divided doses; round dose down to the nearest whole tablet

Maintenance dose: Titrate dose to effect; after week 4, increase dose every 1-2 weeks by a calculated increment; calculate increment as 0.3 mg/kg/day rounded down to the nearest whole tablet; add this amount to the previously administered daily dose; usual maintenance: 1-5 mg/kg/day in 1-2 divided doses; maximum: 200 mg/day. **Note:** Usual maintenance dose in children adding lamotrigine to valproic acid **alone**: 1-3 mg/kg/day

Patients receiving **enzyme-inducing** AED regimens **without valproic acid**:

Weeks 1 and 2: 0.6 mg/kg/day in 2 divided doses; round dose down to the nearest whole tablet

Weeks 3 and 4: 1.2 mg/kg/day in 2 divided doses; round dose down to the nearest whole tablet

Maintenance dose: Titrate dose to effect; after week 4, increase dose every 1-2 weeks by a calculated increment; calculate increment as 1.2 mg/kg/day rounded down to the nearest whole tablet; add this amount to the previously administered daily dose; usual maintenance: 5-15 mg/kg/day in 2 divided doses; maximum: 400 mg/day

Children >12 years and Adults:

Patients receiving AED regimens **containing valproic acid**:

Weeks 1 and 2: 25 mg every other day

Weeks 3 and 4: 25 mg every day

Maintenance dose: Titrate dose to effect; after week 4, increase dose every 1-2 weeks by 25-50 mg/day; usual maintenance: 100-400 mg/day in 1-2 divided doses; usual maintenance in patients adding lamotrigine to valproic acid **alone**: 100-200 mg/day

Patients receiving **enzyme-inducing** AED regimens **without valproic acid**:

Weeks 1 and 2: 50 mg/day

Weeks 3 and 4: 100 mg/day in 2 divided doses

Maintenance dose: Titrate dose to effect; after week 4, increase dose every 1-2 weeks by 100 mg/day; usual maintenance: 300-500 mg/day in 2 divided doses; doses as high as 700 mg/day in 2 divided doses have been used

Conversion from single enzyme-inducing AED to lamotrigine monotherapy: **Note:** First add lamotrigine and titrate it to the recommended maintenance monotherapy dose, while maintaining the enzyme-inducing AED at a fixed level; then gradually withdraw the enzyme-inducing AED over a 4-week period

Children ≥16 years and Adults:

Weeks 1 and 2: 50 mg/day

Weeks 3 and 4: 100 mg/day in 2 divided doses

Maintenance dose: After week 4, increase dose every 1-2 weeks by 100 mg/day; recommended maintenance monotherapy dose: 500 mg/day in 2 divided doses

Dosage adjustment in hepatic impairment:

Moderate impairment, Child-Pugh Grade B: Reduce initial, escalation, and maintenance doses by ~50%

Severe impairment, Child-Pugh Grade C: Reduce initial, escalation, and maintenance doses by ~75%

Note: Adjust escalation and maintenance doses by clinical response

Administration Oral: May be administered without regard to food

Regular tablet: Do not chew, as a bitter taste may result

Chewable, dispersible tablet: Only whole tablets should be administered; may swallow whole, chew, or disperse in water or diluted fruit juice; if chewed, administer a small amount of water or diluted fruit juice to help in swallowing. To disperse, add tablets to a small amount of liquid (~1 teaspoon or enough to cover the medication); when the tablets are completely dispersed (in about 1 minute), swirl the solution and administer the entire amount immediately. Do not attempt to administer partial quantities of dispersed tablets.

Monitoring Parameters Seizure frequency, duration, and severity

Reference Range Clinical value of serum concentrations not well established; proposed therapeutic range: 1-5 µg/mL

(Continued)

Lamotrigine *(Continued)*

Patient Information Report any rash, fever, or swelling of glands to the physician immediately. May cause photosensitivity reactions (eg, exposure to sunlight may cause severe sunburn, skin rash, redness, or itching); avoid exposure to sunlight and artificial light sources (sunlamps, tanning booth/bed); wear protective clothing, wide-brimmed hats, sunglasses, and lip sunscreen (SPF ≥15); use a sunscreen [broad-spectrum sunscreen or physical sunscreen (preferred) or sunblock with SPF ≥15]; contact physician if reaction occurs.

Additional Information Low water solubility. Does **not** induce P450 microsomal enzymes. The effect of AEDs (other than enzyme-inducing AEDs and valproic acid) on the metabolism of lamotrigine is not known and no specific dosing guidelines are recommended; prudence dictates conservative initial doses and titration (as with regimens containing valproic acid); expected maintenance dosing would fall between maintenance doses with valproic acid and maintenance doses of enzyme-inducing AED regimens without valproic acid.

Dosage Forms
Tablet: 25 mg, 100 mg, 150 mg, 200 mg
Tablet, chewable, dispersible: 2 mg, 5 mg, 25 mg [black currant flavor]

Extemporaneous Preparations A 1 mg/mL oral suspension made from tablets and 2 different vehicles (a 1:1 mixture of Ora-Sweet® and Ora-Plus®, or a 1:1 mixture of Ora-Sweet® SF and Ora-Plus®) was stable for 91 days when stored in amber plastic prescription bottles at room temperature (25°C) or under refrigeration (4°C); grind one 100 mg tablet in a mortar into a fine powder; add a small amount of the vehicle and mix well to form a uniform paste; mix while adding the vehicle in geometric proportions to almost 100 mL; transfer the mixture to a graduated cylinder and qsad with vehicle to make 100 mL; label "shake well" and "protect from light" (Nahata, 1999)

Nahata MC, Morosco RS, and Hipple TF, "Stability of Lamotrigine in Two Extemporaneously Prepared Oral Suspensions at 4°C and 25°C," *Am J Health Syst Pharm*, 1999, 56(3):240-2.

References
Battino D, Estienne M, and Avanzini G, "Clinical Pharmacokinetics of Antiepileptic Drugs in Paediatric Patients: Part II. Phenytoin, Carbamazepine, Sulthiame, Lamotrigine, Vigabatrin, Oxcarbazepine, and Felbamate," *Clin Pharmacokinet*, 1995, 29(5):341-69.
Besag FM, Wallace SJ, Dulac O, et al, "Lamotrigine for the Treatment of Epilepsy in Childhood," *J Pediatr*, 1995, 127(6):991-7.
Burstein AH, "Lamotrigine," *Pharmacotherapy*, 1995, 15(2):129-43.
Dooley J, Camfield P, Gordon K, et al, "Lamotrigine-Induced Rash in Children," *Neurology*, 1996, 46(1):240-2.
Fitton A, and Goa KL, "Lamotrigine: An Update of its Pharmacology and Therapeutic Use in Epilepsy," *Drugs*, 1995, 50(4):691-713.
Messenheimer JA, "Lamotrigine," *Epilepsia*, 1995, 36(Suppl 2):S87-94.
Messenheimer JA, Giorgi L, and Risner ME, "The Tolerability of Lamotrigine in Children," *Drug Saf*, 2000, 22(4):303-12.
Nahata MC, Morosco RS, and Hipple RT, "Stability of Lamotrigine in Two Extemporaneously Prepared Oral Suspensions at 4°C and 25°C," *Am J Health Syst Pharm*, 1999, 56(93):240-2.

♦ **Lamprene®** *see* Clofazimine *on page 291*

♦ **Lanacane® [OTC]** *see* Benzocaine *on page 163*

♦ **Lanoxicaps®** *see* Digoxin *on page 380*

♦ **Lanoxin®** *see* Digoxin *on page 380*

Lansoprazole *(lan SOE pra zole)*

U.S. Brand Names Prevacid®; Prevacid® SoluTab™

Therapeutic Category Gastric Acid Secretion Inhibitor; Gastrointestinal Agent, Gastric or Duodenal Ulcer Treatment; Proton Pump Inhibitor

Generic Available No

Use Short-term treatment (up to 4 weeks) for healing and symptomatic relief of active duodenal ulcer; short-term treatment (up to 8 weeks) for healing and symptomatic relief of all grades of erosive esophagitis; maintenance of healed erosive esophagitis; treatment of pathological hypersecretory conditions, including Zollinger-Ellison syndrome; adjuvant therapy in the treatment of *Helicobacter pylori*-associated antral gastritis; short-term treatment of symptomatic gastroesophageal reflux disease (GERD); prevention and treatment of NSAID-associated gastric ulcers

Pregnancy Risk Factor B

Contraindications Hypersensitivity to lansoprazole, pantoprazole, esomeprazole, omeprazole, or any component

Warnings Long-term effects are not known; enterochromaffin (ECF)-like hyperplasia and subsequent carcinoids have developed in rats following lifetime exposure to high doses (150 mg/kg/day)

Precautions Symptomatic response to therapy does not preclude the presence of gastric malignancy; use with caution in patients with liver disease, reduce dosage with severe impairment; Prevacid® SoluTabs™ contain aspartame which is metabolized to phenylalanine and must be used with caution in patients with phenylketonuria

Adverse Reactions

Cardiovascular: Angina, hypertension, hypotension, palpitations

Central nervous system: Fatigue, dizziness, headache, insomnia

Dermatologic: Rash

Gastrointestinal: Abdominal pain, nausea, melena, anorexia, cholelithiasis, xerostomia, dyspepsia, eructation, discoloration of feces, flatulence, hypergastrinemia, increased appetite, diarrhea, constipation

Hepatic: Elevated serum transaminases

Otic: Tinnitus

Renal: Proteinuria

Drug Interactions Cytochrome P450 isoenzyme CYP2C19 and CYP3A3/4 substrate

Due to profound and long-lasting inhibition of gastric acid secretion, potential for interfering with the absorption of drugs where acid pH is important exists (such as ketoconazole, ampicillin, iron salts, and digoxin); sucralfate delays and decreases lansoprazole absorption by 30%; lansoprazole increases theophylline clearance mildly (~10%)

Food Interactions Food decreases lansoprazole's bioavailability by 50%

Stability Store at room temperature; protect from light and moisture; lansoprazole is unstable in acidic media (eg, stomach contents) and is available only as enteric coated granules

Mechanism of Action Suppresses gastric acid secretion by selectively inhibiting the parietal cell membrane enzyme (H+, K+)-ATPase or proton pump; demonstrates antimicrobial activity against *Helicobacter pylori*

Pharmacodynamics

Duration of antisecretory activity: >24 hours

Relief of symptoms:

Gastric or duodenal ulcers: 1 week

Reflux esophagitis: 1-4 weeks

Ulcer healing:

Duodenal: 2 weeks

Gastric: 4 weeks

Pharmacokinetics

Absorption: Extremely acid labile and will degrade in acid pH of stomach; enteric coated granules improve bioavailability (80%)

Distribution: V_d: Children: 0.61-0.9 L/kg

Protein binding: 97%

Metabolism: Extensive by the liver to inactive metabolites; in acid media of gastric parietal cell, lansoprazole is transformed to active sulfanilamide metabolite

Bioavailability: 80% (reduced by 50% if given 30 minutes after food)

Half-life:

Children: 1.2-1.5 hours

Adults: 1.3-1.7 hours

Time to peak serum concentration: 1.7 hours

Elimination: 14% to 25% in urine as metabolites; <1% as unchanged drug; biliary excretion is major route of elimination

Clearance: Children: 0.57-0.71 L/hour/kg

Usual Dosage Oral:

Children: Limited data in single dose studies in children 3 months to 14 years; dosing range used: 0.5-1.6 mg/kg; limited multiple dose studies in pediatric patients 1-11 years of age for GERD treatment:

<10 kg: 7.5 mg once daily

10-30 kg: 15 mg once or twice daily

≥30 kg: 30 mg once or twice daily

Children ≥12 years and Adults:

Duodenal ulcer: 15 mg once daily for 4 weeks; maintenance therapy: 15 mg once daily

Primary gastric ulcer (and also associated with NSAID use): 30 mg once daily for up to 8 weeks

Erosive esophagitis: 30 mg once daily for up to 8 weeks; additional 8 weeks may be tried in those patients who failed to respond or for a recurrence of esophagitis; maintenance: 15 mg once daily

GERD: 15 mg once daily for up to 8 weeks

Pathological hypersecretory conditions: Initial: 60 mg once daily; adjust dosage based upon patient response; doses of 90 mg twice daily have been used; administer doses >120 mg/day in divided doses

Reflux esophagitis: 30-60 mg once daily for 8 weeks

Helicobacter pylori-associated antral gastritis: 30 mg twice daily for 2 weeks (in combination with 1 g amoxicillin and 500 mg clarithromycin given twice daily for

(Continued)

Lansoprazole *(Continued)*

14 days). Alternatively, in patients allergic to or intolerant of clarithromycin or in whom resistance to clarithromycin is known or suspected, lansoprazole 30 mg every 8 hours and amoxicillin 1 g every 8 hours may be given for 2 weeks

NSAID-associated gastric ulcer:

Healing: 30 mg once daily for up to 8 weeks

Prevention: 15 mg once daily for up to 12 weeks

Dosage adjustment in hepatic impairment: Reduce dosage for severe impairment

Administration Oral: Administer before eating

Capsules: Capsules may be opened and mixed with small amount of applesauce prior to administration without affecting the bioavailability; do not chew or crush granules; for nasogastric tube administration, the capsules can be opened, the granules mixed with 40 mL of apple, cranberry, grape, orange, pineapple, prune, tomato, and V-8® vegetable juice, and then administered through the NG tube; granules remain intact when mixed and stored for up to 30 minutes

Granules for oral suspension: Mix in 2 tablespoons (30 mL) water. Do not mix with other liquids or foods; stir well and drink immediately; do not chew granules. If any material remains after drinking, add more water and drink immediately. This product is not intended to be administered through a feeding tube due to increased viscosity from xanthan gum used in formulation and resulting blockage of tube.

Tablet, orally disintegrating: Place the tablet on the tongue and allow to disintegrate with or without water until the particles can be swallowed; do not chew or crush

Monitoring Parameters Patients with Zollinger-Ellison syndrome should be monitored for gastric acid output, which should be maintained at 10 mEq/hour or less during the last hour before the next lansoprazole dose; lab monitoring should include CBC, liver function, renal function, and serum gastrin levels

Reference Range Plasma levels do not correlate with pharmacologic activity

Patient Information May cause dry mouth

Dosage Forms

Capsule, delayed release: 15 mg, 30 mg

Granules for oral suspension, delayed release: 15 mg/packet (30s), 30 mg/packet (30s)

Tablet, orally disintegrating (Prevacid® SoluTabs™): 15 mg [contains 2.5 mg phenylalanine (as aspartame)/tablet; strawberry flavor], 30 mg [contains 5.1 mg phenylalanine (as aspartame)/tablet; strawberry flavor] [expected product availability early 2003]

Extemporaneous Preparations A 3 mg/mL suspension of lansoprazole is prepared by emptying the contents of ten 30 mg capsules and adding 100 mL 8.4% sodium bicarbonate solution; stir for 30 minutes; protect from light; stable for 8 hours at room temperature and for 14 days refrigerated (DiGiacinto, 2000). **Note:** The same formulation was studied by Phillips, et al. A 2-week stability at room temperature and 4-week stability under refrigeration were reported.

DiGiacinto JL, Olsen KM, Bergman KL, et al, "Stability of Suspension Formulations of Lansoprazole and Omeprazole Stored in Amber-Colored Plastic Oral Syringes," *Ann Pharmacother*, 2000, 34(5):600-4.

Phillips JO, Metzler MH, and Olsen K, "The Stability of Simplified Lansoprazole Suspension (SLS)," *Gastroen*, 1999, 116:A89.

References

Chun AH, Eason CJ, Shi HH, et al, "Lansoprazole: An Alternative Method of Administration of a Capsule Dosage Formulation," *Clin Ther*, 1995, 17(3):441-7.

Gibbons TE and Gold BD, "The Use of Proton Pump Inhibitors in Children: A Comprehensive Review," *Paediatr Drugs*, 2003, 5(1):25-40.

Oderda G, Chiorboli E, Haitink AR, "Inhibition of Hastric ACidity in Children by Lansoprazole Granules," *Gastroent*, 1998, 114(4pt2):A295.

Scott LJ, "Lansoprazole: In the Management of Gastroesophageal Reflux Disease in Children," *Paediatr Drugs*, 2003, 5(1):57-61.

Tran A, et al, "Pharmacokinetics/Pharmacodynamics Study of Oral Lansoprazole in Children," *Fundam Clin Pharmacol*, 1996, 10:A221.

♦ **Lantus®** *see* Insulin Preparations *on page 609*

♦ **Largactil®** *(Can) see* ChlorproMAZINE *on page 263*

♦ **Larodopa®** *see* Levodopa *on page 665*

Laronidase *(lair OH ni days)*

U.S. Brand Names Aldurazyme®

Synonyms Recombinant Human α-L-Iduronidase

Therapeutic Category Enzyme; Mucopolysaccharidosis I (MPS I) Disease, Treatment Agent

Generic Available No

Use Treatment of patients with mucopolysaccharidosis I (MPS I) lysosomal storage disease who have one of the following clinical syndromes: Hurler's syndrome (severe), Hurler-Scheie syndrome (intermediate), or patients with the Scheie form who have moderate to severe symptoms

Pregnancy Risk Factor B

Contraindications Hypersensitivity to laronidase or any component

Warnings Hypersensitivity reactions can occur at any time during laronidase therapy. Resuscitation equipment, oxygen, diphenhydramine, and a corticosteroid should be readily available to treat hypersensitivity or anaphylactic reactions. Use epinephrine with caution in patients with MPS I due to an increased prevalence of coronary artery disease in these patients.

Precautions The risks and benefits of administering laronidase following a severe anaphylactic or hypersensitivity reaction should be considered. If laronidase is to be readministered, use caution and have appropriate resuscitation measures available.

Adverse Reactions
Cardiovascular: Flushing, chest pain, edema, hypotension
Central nervous system: Chills, fever, headache
Dermatologic: Rash, urticaria, pruritus, angioedema
Hematologic: Thrombocytopenia
Local: Injection site reaction
Neuromuscular & skeletal: Hyper-reflexia, paresthesia
Respiratory: Dyspnea, cough, bronchospasm
Miscellaneous: Anaphylaxis, antibodies to laronidase

Drug Interactions No information available at this time.

Stability Store vials in refrigerator at 2°C to 8°C (36°F to 46°F). Do not freeze or shake. Diluted infusion solution is stable for up to 32 hours when stored at 2°C to 8°C (36°F to 46°F). Do not mix laronidase with any other drugs.

Mechanism of Action MPS I is a mucopolysaccharide storage disorder caused by a deficiency of the lysosomal enzyme, α-L-iduronidase which is required for the catabolism of glycosaminoglycans (GAG). Laronidase catalyses the hydrolysis of terminal α-L-iduronic acid residues of dermatan sulfate and heparan sulfate decreasing the accumulation of GAG substrates.

Pharmacokinetics
Distribution: V_d: 0.24 to 0.6 L/kg
Half-life: 1.5-3.6 hours
Clearance: Plasma: 1.7 to 2.7 mL/minute/kg

Usual Dosage Children, Adolescents, and Adults: I.V. infusion:
Patients ≤20 kg: 0.58 mg/kg/dose once weekly. Dose is delivered in a total volume of 100 mL.
Patients >20 kg: 0.58 mg/kg/dose once weekly. Dose is delivered in a total volume of 250 mL.

Administration I.V. infusion:
Determine the number of vials to be diluted. Remove vials from the refrigerator and allow them to reach room temperature. Do not use if the solution is discolored or contains particulate matter. Determine the total infusion volume based on the patient's weight (dose delivered in a total volume of 100 mL or 250 mL); prepare an infusion bag of 0.1% albumin in NS; gently rotate infusion bag after addition of albumin.

Remove and discard volume of 0.1% albumin in NS equal to volume of laronidase injection solution to be added to the infusion bag. Add laronidase; do not agitate solution as it denatures the enzyme. Administer with an in-line, low protein binding 0.2 micron filter.

An initial 10 mcg/kg/hour infusion rate may be incrementally increased every 15 minutes during the first hour if tolerated; increase to a maximum infusion rate of 200 mcg/kg/hour which is maintained for the remainder of the infusion (approximately 3 hours). See the following:
Initial infusion rate: 10 mcg/kg/hour for 15 minutes: If stable, increase rate to:
20 mcg/kg/hour for 15 minutes: If stable, increase rate to:
50 mcg/kg/hour for 15 minutes: If stable, increase rate to:
100 mcg/kg/hour for 15 minutes: If stable, increase rate to:
200 mcg/kg/hour for ~3 hours (remainder of the infusion)

Monitoring Parameters Vital signs, FVC, height, weight, range of motion, serum antibodies to α-L-iduronidase, urine levels of glycosaminoglycans (GAG), change in liver size

Nursing Implications Premedication with acetaminophen and/or diphenhydramine should be administered 30-60 minutes prior to starting infusion. If an infusion reaction occurs, decrease the infusion rate, temporarily stop the infusion, and/or administer antipyretics, antihistamines, and/or steroids

Dosage Forms Injection, solution [preservative free]: 0.58 mg/mL (5 mL)
(Continued)

Laronidase *(Continued)*

References

Kakkis ED, Muenzer J, Tiller GE, et al, "Enzyme-Replacement Therapy in Mucopolysaccharidosis I," *N Engl J Med*, 2001, 344(3):182-8.

- **Lasix®** *see* Furosemide *on page 526*
- **Lasix® Special (Can)** *see* Furosemide *on page 526*
- **LASP** *see* Asparaginase *on page 132*
- **Lassar's Zinc Paste** *see* Zinc Oxide *on page 1167*
- **Lavacol® [OTC]** *see* Ethyl Alcohol *on page 465*
- **Laxilose (Can)** *see* Lactulose *on page 649*
- ***L*-Bunolol** *see* Levobunolol *on page 665*
- **L-carnitine** *see* Carnitine *on page 219*
- **LCD** *see* Coal Tar *on page 299*
- **LCR** *see* VinCRIStine *on page 1149*
- ***L*-Dopa** *see* Levodopa *on page 665*
- **LEA-103** *see* Ropivacaine *on page 998*
- **Lenoltec (Can)** *see* Acetaminophen and Codeine *on page 39*
- **Lente® Iletin® II** *see* Insulin Preparations *on page 609*

Leucovorin (loo koe VOR in)

Synonyms Citrovorum Factor; Folinic Acid; 5-Formyl Tetrahydrofolate

Therapeutic Category Antidote, Methotrexate; Folic Acid Derivative

Generic Available Yes

Use Reduce toxic effects of methotrexate ("leucovorin rescue"); antidote for folic acid antagonist overdosage; treatment of folate deficient megaloblastic anemias of infancy, sprue, or pregnancy; nutritional deficiency when oral folate therapy is not possible; adjunctive treatment with sulfadiazine and pyrimethamine to prevent hematologic toxicity

Pregnancy Risk Factor C

Contraindications Hypersensitivity to leucovorin or any component; pernicious anemia and other megaloblastic anemias secondary to the lack of vitamin B_{12}; not to be administered by intrathecal or intraventricular route

Warnings Administer promptly; when the time interval between administration of folic acid antagonists and leucovorin rescue increases, its effectiveness in treatment of toxicity diminishes

Adverse Reactions

Dermatologic: Rash, pruritus, erythema, urticaria

Hematologic: Thrombocytosis

Respiratory: Wheezing

Miscellaneous: Anaphylactoid reactions

Drug Interactions Leucovorin enhances the toxicity of fluorouracil; high doses of leucovorin may reduce the efficacy of intrathecally administered methotrexate

Stability When powder for injection is reconstituted with bacteriostatic SWI, stability is 7 days at room temperature; protect from light; when doses >10 mg/m^2 are used, prepare leucovorin with preservative free SWI to decrease the amount of benzyl alcohol intake; do not mix in the same solution with 5-fluorouracil as precipitation occurs

Mechanism of Action A derivative of tetrahydrofolic acid, a reduced form of folic acid; does not require a reduction by dihydrofolate reductase for activation; allows for purine and thymidine synthesis, a necessity for normal erythropoiesis; leucovorin supplies the necessary cofactor blocked by methotrexate, enters the cells via the same active transport system as methotrexate

Pharmacodynamics Onset of action:

Oral: Within 30 minutes

I.V.: Within 5 minutes

Pharmacokinetics

Absorption: Oral, I.M.: Rapid

Metabolism: Rapidly converted to (5MTHF) 5-methyl-tetrahydrofolate (active) in the intestinal mucosa and by the liver

Bioavailability:

Oral absorption is saturable in doses >25 mg; apparent bioavailability:

Tablet, 25 mg: 97%

Tablet, 50 mg: 75%

Tablet, 100 mg: 37%

Tablet, 200 mg: 31%

Injection solution, when administered orally, provides equivalent bioavailability

Half-life:
  Leucovorin: 15 minutes
  5MTHF: 33-35 minutes
Elimination: Primarily in urine (80% to 90%) with small losses appearing in feces (5% to 8%)

Usual Dosage Children and Adults:

  Treatment of folic acid antagonist overdosage (eg, pyrimethamine, trimethoprim): Oral: 2-15 mg/day for 3 days or until blood counts are normal or 5 mg every 3 days; doses of 6 mg/day are needed for patients with platelet counts <100,000/mm^3

  Folate deficient megaloblastic anemia: I.M.: 1 mg/day

  Megaloblastic anemia secondary to congenital deficiency of dihydrofolate reductase: I.M.: 3-6 mg/day

  Leucovorin rescue: I.V.: 10 mg/m^2 to start, then 10 mg/m^2 every 6 hours orally for 72 hours; if serum creatinine 24 hours after methotrexate administration is elevated ≥50% **or** the serum methotrexate concentration is >5 x 10^{-6} M, increase leucovorin dose to 100 mg/m^2/dose every 3 hours until serum methotrexate level is less than 1 x 10^{-8} M (see graph for further dosing recommendations as a function of plasma methotrexate level vs. time)

LEUCOVORIN RESCUE DOSE
(Determined by Plasma Methotrexate Level and Time After Start of Methotrexate Infusion)

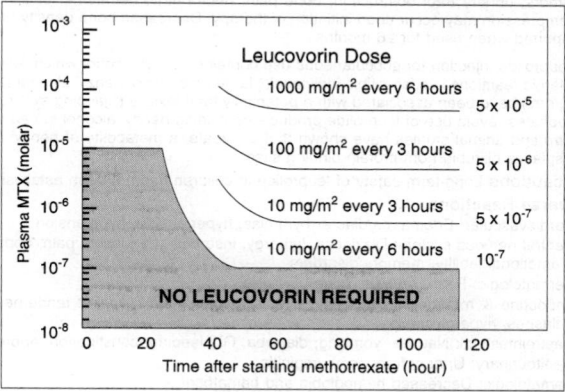

Adjunctive treatment with sulfadiazine to prevent hematologic toxicity (for toxoplasmosis): Infants, Children, and Adults: Oral, I.V.: 5-10 mg once daily; repeat every 3 days (see Sulfadiazine *on page 1050*)

Adjunctive treatment with pyrimethamine to prevent hematologic toxicity (*Pneumocystis carinii*): Adolescents and Adults: Oral, I.V.: 25 mg once weekly

Investigational: Post I.T. methotrexate: Oral, I.V.: 12 mg/m^2 as a single dose; post high-dose methotrexate: 100-1000 mg/m^2/dose until the serum methotrexate level is less than 1 x 10^{-7} molar

Administration
  Oral: **This drug should be given parenterally instead of orally in patients with GI toxicity, nausea, vomiting, and when individual doses are >25 mg.**
  Parenteral: I.M., I.V.: Reconstitute 50 mg or 100 mg powder for injection vials with 5-10 mL SWI (350 mg vial requires 17 mL diluent resulting in 20 mg/mL final concentration); for I.V. administration, infuse at a maximum rate of 160 mg/minute; not for intrathecal or intraventricular administration.

Monitoring Parameters CBC with differential; plasma methotrexate concentration as a therapeutic guide to high-dose methotrexate therapy with leucovorin rescue. Leucovorin is continued until the plasma methotrexate level is less than 1 x 10^{-7} molar. Each dose of leucovorin is increased if the plasma methotrexate concentration is excessively high. With 4- to 6-hour high-dose methotrexate infusions, plasma drug values in excess of 5 x 10^{-5} and 10^{-6} molar at 24 and 48 hours after starting the infusion, respectively, are often predictive of delayed methotrexate clearance; see leucovorin rescue dose graph.

Dosage Forms
  Injection, powder for reconstitution, as calcium: 50 mg, 100 mg, 200 mg, 350 mg
  Injection, solution, as calcium: 10 mg/mL (50 mL)
  Tablet, as calcium: 5 mg, 10 mg, 15 mg, 25 mg

♦ **Leukeran®** *see* Chlorambucil *on page 254*

♦ **Leukine®** *see* Sargramostim *on page 1007*

Leuprolide (loo PROE lide)

U.S. Brand Names Eligard™; Lupron®; Lupron Depot®; Lupron Depot-Ped®; Viadur®

Synonyms Leuprorelin

Therapeutic Category Antineoplastic Agent, Hormone (Gonadotropin Hormone-Releasing Analog); Luteinizing Hormone-Releasing Hormone Analog

Generic Available Yes (injection)

Use Treatment of precocious puberty; palliative treatment of advanced prostate carcinoma

Pregnancy Risk Factor X

Contraindications Hypersensitivity to leuprolide, gonadotropin-releasing hormone (GnRH), GnRH agonist analogs, or any component (see Warnings); pernicious anemia; pregnancy

Warnings The FDA currently recommends that procedures for proper handling and disposal of antineoplastic agents be considered; gonadotropin-releasing hormone (GnRH) analog treatment of rodents has shown an increased incidence of pituitary tumors; urinary tract obstruction, bone pain, neuropathy, hematuria, or spinal cord compression may occur upon initiation of therapy. Decreased bone density has been reported when used for ≥6 months.

Leuprolide injection for subcutaneous use contains benzyl alcohol which may cause allergic reactions in susceptible individuals; large amounts of benzyl alcohol (≥99 mg/kg/day) have been associated with a potentially fatal toxicity ("gasping syndrome") in neonates; avoid use of leuprolide products containing benzyl alcohol in neonates; *in vitro* and animal studies have shown that benzoate, a metabolite of benzyl alcohol, displaces bilirubin from protein binding sites

Precautions Long-term safety of leuprolide in children has not been established

Adverse Reactions

Cardiovascular: Edema, cardiac arrhythmias, hypertension, hypotension

Central nervous system: Dizziness, lethargy, insomnia, headache, pain, depression, emotional lability, memory disorders

Dermatologic: Rash, pruritus, acne

Endocrine & metabolic: Estrogenic effects (gynecomastia, breast tenderness), hot flashes, hyperglycemia

Gastrointestinal: Nausea, vomiting, diarrhea, GI bleeding, constipation, anorexia

Genitourinary: Urinary frequency, vaginitis

Hematologic: Decreased hemoglobin and hematocrit

Neuromuscular & skeletal: Myalgia, paresthesia, bone pain, weakness, neuropathy, arthralgia, decreased bone density

Ocular: Blurred vision

Renal: Hematuria, elevated BUN

Miscellaneous: Diaphoresis, anaphylaxis

Stability Refrigerate leuprolide acetate injection; leuprolide (Depot®) powder for suspension and its diluent may be stored at room temperature; upon reconstitution, the suspension is stable for 24 hours; protect from light and heat; do not freeze vials; leuprolide implant may be stored at room temperature

Mechanism of Action Continuous daily administration results in suppression of ovarian and testicular steroidogenesis due to decreased levels of LH and FSH so that puberty and the pubertal growth spurt are arrested; produces a "medical castration" in prostate cancer patients; inhibits pituitary gonadotropin secretion

Pharmacodynamics Onset of action: Serum testosterone levels first increase within 3 days of therapy, then decrease after 2-4 weeks with continued therapy

Pharmacokinetics

Absorption: Requires parenteral administration since it is rapidly destroyed within the GI tract

Protein binding: 43% to 49%

Bioavailability:

Oral: 0%

S.C.: 94%

Half-life: 3 hours

Elimination: Not well defined

Usual Dosage Refer to individual protocol

Children: Precocious puberty:

I.M. (Depot®) formulation: 0.15-0.3 mg/kg/dose given every 28 days; minimum dose: 7.5 mg; younger children generally require higher dosages on a mg/kg basis than older children. Consider discontinuing leuprolide therapy in girls by age 11 and boys by age 12.

Initial dose for girls <8 years or boys <9 years (titrate dose in 3.75 mg increments every 4 weeks until clinical or laboratory tests indicate no disease progression):
<25 kg: 7.5 mg every 4 weeks
25-37.5 kg: 11.25 mg every 4 weeks
>37.5 kg: 15 mg every 4 weeks

S.C.: 35-50 mcg/kg once daily; may titrate dose upward by 10 mcg/kg/day if suppression of ovarian or testicular steroidogenesis is not achieved.

Adults: Advanced prostatic carcinoma:

I.M. (Depot® formulation): 7.5 mg/dose given monthly, **or** 22.5 mg once every 3 months, **or** 30 mg once every 4 months

Implant: Insert 65 mg implant subcutaneously every 12 months

S.C.: 1 mg/day

S.C. (Eligard™ Depot): 7.5 mg/dose given monthly, **or** 22.5 mg once every 3 months, **or** 30 mg once every 4 months

Administration

Implant: Insert subcutaneously in the inner aspect of the upper arm. Keep site clean and dry for 24 hours after insertion

Parenteral: Do not administer I.V.:

I.M.: For the Depot® formulation, diluent is added to the vial to form a milky suspension

S.C.: 5 mg/mL solution is administered undiluted into areas on the arm, thigh, or abdomen

Monitoring Parameters Precocious puberty: Height, weight, bone age, Tanner staging test, GnRH testing (blood LH and FSH levels), testosterone in males and estradiol in females; closely monitor patients with prostatic carcinoma for plasma testosterone, acid phosphatase, and signs of weakness, paresthesias, and urinary tract obstruction during the first few weeks of therapy

Test Interactions Interferes with diagnostic tests of pituitary gonadotropic and gonadal function for up to 3 months after therapy

Patient Information Female patients should be informed that menstruation or spotting may occur for the first 2 months of therapy; notify physician if vaginal bleeding continues after 2 months of drug therapy

Nursing Implications Rotate S.C. and I.M. injection sites periodically

Dosage Forms

Implant, as acetate (Viadur®): 65 mg free base [released over 12 months]

Injection, solution, as acetate (Lupron®): 5 mg/mL (2.8 mL) [contains benzyl alcohol]

Injection, powder for reconstitution, as acetate [depot formulation]:

Eligard™: 7.5 mg [released over 1 month], 22.5 mg [released over 3 months], 30 mg [released over 4 months]

Lupron Depot®: 3.75 mg, 7.5 mg

Lupron Depot-3® Month: 11.25 mg, 22.5 mg

Lupron Depot-4® Month: 30 mg

Lupron Depot-Ped®: 7.5 mg, 11.25 mg, 15 mg

References

Kappy MS, Stuart T, and Perelman A, "Efficacy of Leuprolide Therapy in Children With Central Precocious Puberty," *Am J Dis Child*, 1988, 142(10):1061-4.

Lee PA and Page JG, "Effects of Leuprolide in the Treatment of Central Precocious Puberty," *J Pediatr*, 1989, 114(2):321-4.

♦ **Leuprorelin** *see* Leuprolide *on page 662*

♦ **Leurocristine** *see* VinCRIStine *on page 1149*

♦ **Leustatin®** *see* Cladribine *on page 284*

Levalbuterol (leve al BYOO ter ole)

U.S. Brand Names Xopenex™

Synonyms Levosalbutamol; R-albuterol; R-salbutamol

Therapeutic Category Adrenergic Agonist Agent; Antiasthmatic; Beta$_2$-Adrenergic Agonist Agent; Bronchodilator; Sympathomimetic

Generic Available No

Use Treatment and prevention of bronchospasm in patients with reversible obstructive airway disease

Pregnancy Risk Factor C

Contraindications Hypersensitivity to levalbuterol, any component, albuterol, or adrenergic amine

Warnings Paradoxical bronchospasm may occur, especially with the first use
(Continued)

Levalbuterol *(Continued)*

Precautions Use with caution in patients with hyperthyroidism, hypokalemia, diabetes mellitus, cardiovascular disorders including coronary insufficiency, hypertension, or history of arrhythmias; excessive or prolonged use can lead to tolerance

Adverse Reactions

Cardiovascular: Tachycardia, hypertension, hypotension, syncope, EKG abnormalities, chest pain

Central nervous system: Nervousness, dizziness, anxiety, headache, insomnia

Endocrine & metabolic: Hyperglycemia, hypokalemia

Gastrointestinal: Dyspepsia, diarrhea, xerostomia, dry throat, gastroenteritis, nausea

Neuromuscular & skeletal: Leg cramps, pain, tremor

Ocular: Eye itching

Respiratory: Cough, rhinitis, sinusitis, turbinate edema, paradoxical bronchospasm

Miscellaneous: Hypersensitivity reactions, flu-like syndrome

Drug Interactions Action of levalbuterol is antagonized by beta-adrenergic blocking agents such as propranolol; cardiovascular effects are potentiated in patients also receiving MAO inhibitors or tricyclic antidepressants; concomitant administration of sympathomimetics may result in enhanced cardiovascular effects; may decrease serum digoxin level

Food Interactions Caffeinated beverages may increase side effects of levalbuterol

Stability Store at room temperature; protect from light; after the foil covering is removed, use within 2 weeks; discard vial if solution is not colorless

Mechanism of Action R-enantiomer of racemic albuterol; relaxes bronchial smooth muscle by action on beta$_2$-receptors with little effect on heart rate

Pharmacodynamics

Onset of action: 10-17 minutes

Maximum effect: 1.5 hours

Duration: 5-6 hours

Pharmacokinetics Nebulization:

Distribution: V$_d$: Adults: 1900 L

Metabolism: In the liver to an inactive sulfate

Half-life: 3.3-4.0 hours

Time to peak serum concentration: 0.2-1.8 hours

Elimination: 3% to 6% excreted unchanged in urine

Usual Dosage Inhalation by nebulization (**dosage expressed in terms of mg levalbuterol**):

Children 2-11 years: In a randomized, double-blind, single dose, crossover study (Gawchik, 1999), doses ranging from 0.16-1.25 mg were used safely with clinically significant improvements in pulmonary function tests

Children 6-11 years: 0.31 mg 3 times/day, every 6-8 hours; not to exceed 0.63 mg 3 times/day

Children ≥12 years and Adults: 0.63 mg 3 times/day, every 6-8 hours; may be increased to 1.25 mg 3 times/day

Administration Inhalation: By nebulization only; no dilution required

Monitoring Parameters Serum potassium, heart rate, asthma symptoms, pulmonary function tests, respiratory rate; arterial or capillary blood gases (if patient's condition warrants)

Patient Information Do not exceed recommended dosage; may cause dry mouth; rinse mouth with water following each inhalation to help with dry throat and mouth; if more than one inhalation is necessary, wait at least 1 full minute between inhalations; notify physician if palpitations, tachycardia, chest pain, muscle tremors, dizziness, or headache occur, or if breathing difficulty persists; limit caffeinated beverages

Additional Information 0.63 mg levalbuterol comparable to 1.25 mg albuterol (Lotvall, 2001)

Dosage Forms Solution, for inhalation: 0.31 mg/3 mL [0.36 mg levalbuterol hydrochloride] (24s); 0.63 mg/3 mL [0.73 mg levalbuterol hydrochloride] (24s); 1.25 mg/3 mL [1.44 mg levalbuterol hydrochloride] (24s)

References

Gawchik SM, Saccar CL, Noonan M, et al, "The Safety and Efficacy of Nebulized Levalbuterol Compared With Racemic Albuterol and Placebo in the Treatment of Asthma in Pediatric Patients," *J Allergy Clin Immunol*, 1999, 103(4):615-21.

Lotvall J, Palmqvist M, Arvidsson P, et al, "The Therapeutic Ratio of R-Albuterol is Comparable With That of RS-Albuterol in Asthmatic Patients," *J Allergy Clin Immunol*, 2001, 108(5):726-31.

Milgrom H, Skoner DP, Bensch G, et al, "Low-Dose Levalbuterol in Children With Asthma: Safety and Efficacy in Comparison With Placebo and Racemic Albuterol," *J Allergy Clin Immunol*, 2001, 108(6):938-45.

"National Asthma Education and Prevention Program. Expert Panel Report: Guidelines for the Diagnosis and Management of Asthma Update on Selected Topics--2002," *J Allergy Clin Immunol*, 2002, 110(5 Suppl):S141-219.

♦ **Levaquin®** *see* Levofloxacin *on page 667*

* **Levarterenol** see Norepinephrine on page 820
* **Levate® (Can)** see Amitriptyline on page 89
* **Levbid®** see Hyoscyamine on page 585

Levobunolol (lee voe BYOO noe lole)

U.S. Brand Names Betagan® Liquifilm®
Canadian Brand Names Apo®-Levobunolol; Novo-Levobunolol; Optho-Bunolol®; PMS-Levobunolol
Synonyms L-Bunolol
Therapeutic Category Beta-Adrenergic Blocker, Ophthalmic
Generic Available Yes
Use To lower intraocular pressure in chronic open-angle glaucoma or ocular hypertension
Pregnancy Risk Factor C
Contraindications Hypersensitivity to levobunolol or any component (see Warnings); asthma, severe COPD, sinus bradycardia, second or third degree A-V block, cardiogenic shock
Warnings Contains metabisulfite which may cause allergic reactions in susceptible individuals; use only in combination with miotic for patients with angle closure glaucoma; products contain sulfites which may cause allergic reactions in susceptible individuals
Precautions Use with caution in patients with CHF, diabetes mellitus, hyperthyroidism, myasthenia gravis
Adverse Reactions
  Cardiovascular: Bradycardia, arrhythmias, hypotension, palpitations, cerebral ischemia, cerebral vascular accident, syncope, heart block, CHF
  Central nervous system: Dizziness, headache, depression, ataxia, cerebral ischemia
  Dermatologic: Rash, alopecia, itching
  Endocrine & metabolic: Masked symptoms of hypoglycemia in diabetics
  Gastrointestinal: Nausea, heartburn, diarrhea
  Ocular: Stinging, burning, erythema, itching, blepharoconjunctivitis, keratitis, ptosis, decreased visual acuity, conjunctivitis, tearing
  Respiratory: Bronchospasm
Drug Interactions May have additive toxicity with systemic beta-adrenergic blocking drugs; ophthalmic epinephrine decreases effectiveness
Mechanism of Action A nonselective beta-adrenergic blocking agent that lowers intraocular pressure by reducing aqueous humor production
Pharmacodynamics
  Onset of action: Following ophthalmic instillation, decreases in intraocular pressure can be noted within 1 hour
  Maximum effect: Within 2-6 hours
  Maximal effectiveness: 2-3 weeks
  Duration: 1-7 days
Pharmacokinetics
  Absorption: May be absorbed systemically and produce systemic side effects
  Metabolism: Extensively metabolized into several metabolites; primary metabolite (active) dihydrolevobunolol
  Elimination: Not well defined
Usual Dosage Adults: 1-2 drops of 0.5% solution in eye(s) once daily or 1-2 drops of 0.25% solution twice daily; may increase to 1 drop of 0.5% solution twice daily
Administration Intraocular: Apply drops into conjunctival sac of affected eye(s); avoid contacting bottle tip with skin; apply gentle pressure to lacrimal sac during and immediately following instillation (1-2 minutes) to decrease systemic absorption; see manufacturer's information regarding proper usage of C Cap (compliance cap)
Monitoring Parameters Intraocular pressure
Dosage Forms
  Solution, ophthalmic, as hydrochloride: 0.25% [2.5 mg/mL] (5 mL, 10 mL); 0.5% [5 mg/mL] (5 mL, 10 mL, 15 mL) [contains sodium metabisulfite]
    Betagan® Liquifilm®: 0.25% [2.5 mg/mL] (5 mL, 10 mL); 0.5% [5 mg/mL] (2 mL, 5 mL, 10 mL, 15 mL) [contains sodium metabisulfite]

* **Levocarnitine** see Carnitine on page 219

Levodopa (lee voe DOE pa)

Related Information
  Serotonin Syndrome on page 1420
U.S. Brand Names Dopar®; Larodopa®
Synonyms L-3-Hydroxytyramine; L-Dopa
(Continued)

Levodopa *(Continued)*

Therapeutic Category Anti-Parkinson's Agent; Diagnostic Agent, Growth Hormone Function

Use Diagnostic agent for growth hormone deficiency; treatment of Parkinson's disease

Pregnancy Risk Factor C

Contraindications Hypersensitivity to levodopa or any component; narrow-angle glaucoma, use of MAO inhibitors within prior 14 days (however, may be administered concomitantly with the manufacturer's recommended dose of a MAO inhibitor with selectivity for MAO type B), melanomas, or any undiagnosed skin lesions

Warnings GI hemorrhage has occurred in patients with a history of peptic ulcer disease; sudden discontinuation of levodopa may cause a worsening of Parkinson's disease

Precautions Use cautiously in patients with severe cardiovascular disease or pulmonary disease, asthma, occlusive cerebrovascular disease, renal, hepatic, or endocrine disease, affective disorders, major psychoses, cardiac arrhythmias, and chronic wide-angle glaucoma; use with caution in patients with risk of hypotension; may cause orthostatic hypotension

Adverse Reactions

Cardiovascular: Orthostatic hypotension, palpitations, cardiac arrhythmias, hypertension

Central nervous system: Memory loss, nervousness, anxiety, insomnia, fatigue, hallucinations, dystonic movements, ataxia, headache, confusion

Endocrine & metabolic: Hyperhomocysteinemia

Gastrointestinal: Nausea, vomiting, GI bleeding, constipation, anorexia, xerostomia

Hematologic: Hemolytic anemia

Neuromuscular & skeletal: Muscle twitching

Ocular: Blurred vision, eyelid spasms

Miscellaneous: Discoloration of sweat

Drug Interactions Antacids and metoclopramide increase bioavailability of levodopa; benzodiazepines, antipsychotics, clonidine, tacrine, hydantoins, methionine, papaverine, and pyridoxine decrease levodopa's effectiveness; iron salts, TCAs, and anticholinergics decrease GI absorption of levodopa; MAO inhibitors and linezolid may increase hypertensive reaction; levodopa may decrease metoclopramide's effects; methyldopa may have additive hypotensive effects

Food Interactions High protein diets may decrease the efficacy of levodopa when used for parkinsonism via competition with amino acids in crossing the blood-brain barrier; avoid foods high in pyridoxine content such as liver, fish, whole grain cereals, peas, and beans

Mechanism of Action Increases dopamine levels in the brain; stimulates dopaminergic receptors in the basal ganglia to improve the balance between cholinergic and dopaminergic activity

Pharmacokinetics

Metabolism: Majority of drug is peripherally decarboxylated to dopamine; small amounts of levodopa reach the brain where it is also decarboxylated to active dopamine

Half-life: 1.2-2.3 hours

Time to peak serum concentration: Oral: Within 1-2 hours

Elimination: Primarily in urine (80%) as dopamine, norepinephrine, and homovanillic acid

Usual Dosage Oral:

Diagnostic agent for growth hormone deficiency: Children: 0.5 g/m² as a single dose, not to exceed 500 mg **or** as an alternative

<30 lb: 125 mg

30-70 lb: 250 mg

>70 lb: 500 mg

Parkinson's disease: Adults: 500-1000 mg/day in divided doses every 6-12 hours; increase by 100-750 mg/day every 3-7 days until response or total dose of 8000 mg is reached

Administration Oral: Administer with food

Monitoring Parameters Growth hormone level

Test Interactions False-positive reaction for urinary glucose with Clinitest®; false-negative reaction using Clinistix®; false-positive urine ketones with Acetest®, Ketostix®, Labstix®; false-positive Coombs' test; false increase in uric acid with colorimetric method

Patient Information May cause dry mouth

Dosage Forms Tablet: 250 mg

References

Cara JF and Johanson HJ, "Growth Hormone for Short Stature Not Due to Classic Growth Hormone Deficiency," *Pediatr Clin North Am*, 1990, 37(6):1229-54.

Levofloxacin (lee voe FLOKS a sin)

U.S. Brand Names Levaquin®; Quixin™

Therapeutic Category Antibiotic, Ophthalmic; Antibiotic, Quinolone

Generic Available No

Use Treatment of acute maxillary sinusitis, lower respiratory tract infections, skin and skin structure infections, complicated urinary tract infections and acute pyelonephritis due to multidrug-resistant organisms susceptible to levofloxacin including *Streptococcus pneumoniae* (including penicillin-resistant strains), *S. aureus, Haemophilus influenzae, H. parainfluenzae, Moraxella catarrhalis, Klebsiella pneumoniae, Legionella pneumophila, Chlamydia pneumoniae, Mycoplasma pneumoniae, E. coli, Enterococcus fecalis, S. pyogenes, Proteus mirabilis, Enterobacter cloacae,* (less active than ciprofloxacin against *Pseudomonas aeruginosa*); infectious diarrhea due to enterotoxigenic *E. coli, Shigella, Salmonella, Campylobacter* spp, *Vibrio parahaemolyticus.* Used ophthalmically for treatment of bacterial conjunctivitis due to *S. aureus* (methicillin-susceptible strains), *S. epidermidis, S. pneumoniae, Streptococcus* (groups C/F), *Streptococcus* (group G), Viridans group *Streptococci, Corynebacterium* spp, *H. influenzae, Acinetobacter iwoffii,* or *Serratia marcescens.*

Pregnancy Risk Factor C

Contraindications Hypersensitivity to levofloxacin, any component, or other quinolones; not recommended for use in pregnant women or during breast-feeding

Warnings Not recommended in children <18 years of age; levofloxacin increased the incidence and severity of osteochondrosis in immature rats and dogs. Fluoroquinolones have caused arthropathy with erosions of the cartilage in weight-bearing joints of immature animals; Achilles tendonitis and tendon rupture have been reported with fluoroquinolones with risk increased in patients taking concomitant corticosteroids; prolonged use may result in superinfection; CNS stimulation and increased intracranial pressure may occur resulting in tremors, restlessness, confusion, and rarely hallucinations or convulsive seizures; serious and occasionally fatal hypersensitivity and/or anaphylactic reactions have been reported often following the first dose

Precautions Use with caution in patients with known or suspected CNS disorders, seizure disorders, or renal impairment; modify dosage in patients with renal impairment. Rare cases of torsade de pointes have been reported in patients taking levofloxacin so use with caution in patients on concurrent therapy with Class Ia or Class III antiarrhythmics or in patients with bradycardia, cardiomyopathy, hypokalemia, or hypomagnesemia

Adverse Reactions

Cardiovascular: Cardiac failure, hypertension, hypotension, bradycardia, tachycardia, edema, torsade de pointes (rare)

Central nervous system: Dizziness, fever, headache, insomnia, seizures, fatigue, nervousness, restlessness, confusion, hallucinations, anxiety, lightheadedness

Dermatologic: Photosensitivity, pruritus, urticaria, rash, Stevens-Johnson syndrome, toxic epidermal necrolysis

Gastrointestinal: Nausea, vomiting, diarrhea, constipation, anorexia, abdominal pain, pseudomembranous colitis

Genitourinary: Vaginitis

Hematologic: Granulocytopenia, leukopenia, thrombocytopenia

Hepatic: Elevated liver enzymes

Local: With I.V.: Phlebitis, burning, pain, erythema, swelling

Neuromuscular & skeletal: Tremor, arthralgia, tendonitis

Ocular: Ophthalmic solution: Foreign body sensation, transient decreased vision; ocular pain, burning, itching, dryness, discomfort, photophobia

Miscellaneous: Anaphylaxis

Drug Interactions Cytochrome P450 isoenzyme CYP1A2 enzyme inhibitor (minor)

Decreased absorption with antacids containing aluminum, magnesium, and/or calcium, sucralfate, metal cations (ie, zinc, iron, copper, magnesium), and didanosine; may decrease serum levels of phenytoin; cimetidine and probenecid increase serum levels and half-life of levofloxacin; concomitant use with foscarnet or NSAIDs may increase risk of seizures

Food Interactions Iron and mineral supplements decrease levofloxacin concentrations

Stability Injection is stable for 72 hours when diluted to 5 mg/mL in a compatible I.V. fluid (ie, D_5W, NS, D_5W with NaCl and KCl, D_5LR) and stored at room temperature; stable for 14 days when stored under refrigeration; incompatible with mannitol, sodium bicarbonate, multivalent cations (eg, magnesium)

Mechanism of Action L-isomer of the racemate, ofloxacin, levofloxacin inhibits DNA gyrase (bacterial topoisomerase II) thereby inhibiting relaxation of supercoiled DNA and promoting breakage of DNA strands. DNA gyrase maintains the superhelical structure of DNA and is required for DNA replication, transcription, repair, recombination and transposition.

(Continued)

Levofloxacin *(Continued)*

Pharmacokinetics

Absorption: Well absorbed

Distribution: Widely distributed in the body including blister fluid, macrophages, lung tissue; excreted in breast milk

V_d: Adults: 89-112

Protein binding: 24% to 38%

Bioavailability: Oral: 99%

Half-life: 6-8 hours

Time to peak serum concentration: Oral: Within 1-2 hours; food prolongs the time to peak by approximately 1 hour and decreases the peak concentration by 14%

Elimination: 87% excreted unchanged in urine over 48 hours by tubular secretion and glomerular filtration

Dialysis: Not removed by hemodialysis or peritoneal dialysis

Usual Dosage

Oral, I.V.:

Children: **Note:** Limited information regarding levofloxacin use in pediatric patients is currently available in the literature; some centers recommend initial doses of 5-10 mg/kg/dose every 24 hours; maximum dose: 500 mg

Adults:

Chronic bronchitis: 500 mg every 24 hours for 7 days

Community-acquired pneumonia: 500 mg every 24 hours for 7-14 days

Acute maxillary sinusitis: 500 mg every 24 hours for 10-14 days

Uncomplicated skin infections: 500 mg every 24 hours for 7-10 days

Complicated UTI or acute pyelonephritis: 250 mg every 24 hours for 10 days

Drug-resistant tuberculosis: 500-1000 mg every 24 hours (maximum dose: 1 g)

Travelers' diarrhea: 500 mg every 24 hours for up to 3 days

Children ≥1 year and Adults: Ophthalmic:

Treatment day 1 and day 2: Instill 1-2 drops into affected eye(s) every 2 hours while awake, up to 8 times/day

Treatment day 3 through 7: Instill 1-2 drops into affected eye(s) every 4 hours while awake, up to 4 times/day

Dosing interval in renal impairment:

Cl_{cr} 20-49 mL/minute: Administer 250 mg every 24 hours (initial dose: 500 mg)

Cl_{cr} 10-19 mL/minute: Administer 250 mg every 48 hours (initial dose: 500 mg for most infections; 250 mg for UTI or pyelonephritis)

Administration

Oral: May administer with or without food; avoid antacid use within 2 hours of administration; drink plenty of fluids to maintain proper hydration and urine output

Parenteral: Final concentration for administration should not exceed 5 mg/mL; administer by slow I.V. infusion over 60 minutes; avoid rapid or bolus I.V. infusion due to risk of hypotension

Ophthalmic: Not for subconjunctival injection or for use into anterior chamber of the eye. Contact lenses should not be worn during treatment; instill drops into conjunctival sac of affected eye(s); apply finger pressure to lacrimal sac during and for 1-2 minutes after instillation to decrease risk of absorption and systemic effects; avoid contacting bottle tip with skin

Monitoring Parameters Patient receiving concurrent levofloxacin and theophylline should have serum levels of theophylline monitored; monitor INR in patients receiving warfarin; monitor blood glucose in patients receiving antidiabetic agents; monitor renal, hepatic, and hematopoietic function periodically; number and type of stools/day for diarrhea

Patient Information Drink plenty of fluids; may cause dizziness or lightheadedness and impair ability to perform activities requiring mental alertness or physical coordination; notify physician if tendon pain or swelling occurs, or if palpitations or chest pain, signs of allergy, difficulty breathing, or persistent diarrhea occurs. May cause photosensitivity reactions (eg, exposure to sunlight may cause severe sunburn, skin rash, redness, or itching); avoid exposure to sunlight and artificial light sources (sunlamps, tanning booth/bed); wear protective clothing, wide-brimmed hats, sunglasses, and lip sunscreen (SPF ≥15); use a sunscreen [broad-spectrum sunscreen or physical sunscreen (preferred) or sunblock with SPF ≥15]; contact physician if reaction occurs.

Nursing Implications Do not administer antacids with or within 2 hours before or 2 hours after a levofloxacin dose; ensure adequate patient hydration

Dosage Forms

Infusion [premixed in D_5W] (Levaquin®): 5 mg/mL (50 mL, 100 mL, 150 mL)

Injection, solution [preservative free] (Levaquin®): 25 mg/mL (20 mL, 30 mL)

Solution, ophthalmic (Quixen™): 0.5% (5 mL)

Tablet, film-coated (Levaquin®): 250 mg, 500 mg, 750 mg

Extemporaneous Preparations A 50 mg/mL oral suspension made from tablets and two different vehicles (a 1:1 mixture of Ora-Plus® and strawberry syrup NF) was stable for 57 days when stored in amber plastic prescription bottles at room temperature (23°C to 25°C) or under refrigeration (3°C to 5°C); crush six 500 mg tablets in a mortar into a fine powder; add a small amount of the vehicle and mix well to form a uniform paste; mix while adding the vehicle in geometric proportions to **almost** 60 mL; transfer the mixture to a graduated cylinder and qsad with vehicle to make 60 mL; label "shake well."

VandenBussche HL, Johnson CE, Fontana EM, et al, "Stability of Levofloxacin in an Extemporaneously Compounded Oral Liquid," *Am J Health Syst Pharm*, 1999, 56(22):2316-8.

References

Ernst ME, Ernst EJ, and Klepser ME, "Levofloxacin and Trovafloxacin: The Next Generation of Fluoro-quinolones?" *Am J Health Syst Pharm*, 1997, 54(22):2569-84.

Schaad UB, "Role of the New Quinolones in Pediatric Practice," *Pediatr Infect Dis J*, 1992, 11(12):1043-6.

♦ **Levophed®** *see* Norepinephrine *on page 820*

♦ **Levosalbutamol** *see* Levalbuterol *on page 663*

♦ **Levo-T™** *see* Levothyroxine *on page 669*

♦ **Levothroid®** *see* Levothyroxine *on page 669*

Levothyroxine (lee voe thye ROKS een)

U.S. Brand Names Levo-T™; Levothroid®; Levoxyl®; Novothyrox; Synthroid®; Unithroid®

Canadian Brand Names Eltroxin®

Synonyms *L*-Thyroxine; T_4 Thyroxine

Therapeutic Category Thyroid Product

Generic Available Yes

Use Replacement or supplemental therapy in congenital or acquired hypothyroidism; treatment or prevention of euthyroid goiters (TSH suppression) including thyroid nodules and chronic lymphocytic thyroiditis; as adjunctive therapy with surgery and radioiodine in the management of thyrotropin-dependent well-differentiated thyroid cancer

Pregnancy Risk Factor A

Contraindications Hypersensitivity to levothyroxine sodium or any component; recent MI or thyrotoxicosis; uncorrected adrenal insufficiency; untreated subclinical thyrotoxicosis (suppressed TSH levels with normal T_3 and T_4 levels)

Warnings Not for use in the treatment of obesity or for weight loss; in euthyroid patients, doses within the range of daily hormonal requirements are ineffective for weight reduction; larger doses may produce serious or even life-threatening toxic effects particularly when used with some anorectic drugs (sympathomimetic amines). Overtreatment may result in craniosynostosis in infants and premature closure of epiphyses in children; monitor use closely.

Precautions Use with extreme caution in patients with cardiovascular disease, adrenal insufficiency, hypertension or coronary artery disease; patients with diabetes mellitus and insipidus may have their symptoms exaggerated or aggravated; in the first 2 weeks of therapy, neonates and infants should be monitored for cardiac overload, arrhythmias, and aspiration from avid suckling

Adverse Reactions

Cardiovascular: Palpitations, tachycardia, cardiac arrhythmias, angina, CHF, hypertension

Central nervous system: Nervousness, insomnia, fever, headache, pseudotumor cerebri

Dermatologic: Alopecia

Gastrointestinal: Diarrhea, abdominal cramps, increased appetite, weight loss

Neuromuscular & skeletal: Tremor, slipped capital femoral epiphysis

Miscellaneous: Diaphoresis

Drug Interactions Antacids (aluminum-, magnesium-, and calcium carbonate-containing), cholestyramine resin, iron salts, sodium polystyrene sulfonate, and sucralfate decrease absorption; estrogens, clofibrate, methadone, fluorouracil, mitotane, and tamoxifen increase thyroid requirements; levothyroxine increases effect of oral anticoagulants; phenytoin, carbamazepine, phenobarbital, rifampin, amiodarone, propylthiouracil, and β-adrenergic antagonists may decrease levothyroxine levels; androgens, anabolic steroids, asparaginase, glucocorticoids, and slow-release nicotinic acid decrease thyroid requirements; concurrent use with sympathomimetics, TCAs, and SSRIs may enhance the toxic effects of both drugs; use with ketamine may produce significant tachycardia and hypertension; may increase insulin and other antidiabetic agent requirements

(Continued)

Levothyroxine *(Continued)*

Food Interactions Limit intake of goitrogenic foods (asparagus, cabbage, peas, turnip greens, broccoli, spinach, brussel sprouts, lettuce, soybeans); soybean-based formulas, cottonseed meal, walnuts, and dietary fiber may decrease absorption

Stability Store at room temperature; protect from light and moisture; I.V. form must be administered immediately after preparation

Mechanism of Action Primary active compound is T_3 (triiodothyronine), which may be converted from T_4 (thyroxine) by deiodination in liver and peripheral tissues; exact mechanism of action is unknown; however, it is believed the thyroid hormone exerts its many metabolic effects through control of DNA transcription and protein synthesis; involved in normal metabolism, growth, and development; promotes gluconeogenesis, increases utilization and mobilization of glycogen stores, and stimulates protein synthesis, increases basal metabolic rate

Pharmacodynamics
Onset of action:
  Oral: 3-5 days for therapeutic effects
  I.V.: Within 6-8 hours
Maximum effect: 4-6 weeks

Pharmacokinetics
Absorption: Oral: Erratic (40% to 80%); decreases with age
Protein binding: >99%
Metabolism: In the liver and other peripheral sites by deiodination to triiodothyronine (active) T_3
Half-life: 6-7 days
Time to peak serum concentration: Within 2-4 hours
Elimination: Thyroid hormones are eliminated primarily in urine with 20% of T_4 excreted in feces

Usual Dosage
Neonates, Infants, and Children: Daily dosage:
  Oral:
    0-3 months: 10-15 mcg/kg; if the infant is at risk for development of cardiac failure use a lower starting dose ~25 mcg/day; if the initial serum T_4 is very low (<5 mcg/dL) begin treatment at a higher dosage ~50 mcg/day
    >3-6 months: 8-10 mcg/kg or 25-50 mcg
    >6-12 months: 6-8 mcg/kg or 50-75 mcg
    >1-5 years: 5-6 mcg/kg or 75-100 mcg
    6-12 years: 4-5 mcg/kg or 100-125 mcg
    >12 years: 2-3 mcg/kg or ≥150 mcg
    Growth and puberty complete: 1.7 mcg/kg
    Note: Hyperactivity in older children may be minimized by starting at one-quarter of the recommended dose and increasing each week by that amount until the full dose is achieved (4 weeks)
  I.V., I.M.: 50% to 75% of the oral dose
Adults:
  Hypothyroidism:
    Oral: 1.7 mcg/kg/day or 100-200 mcg/day; if severe hypothyroidism, use 12.5-50 mcg/day to start, then increase by 25-50 mcg/day at intervals of 2-4 weeks
    I.V., I.M.: 50% of the oral dose
  Subclinical hypothyroidism (if treated): Oral: 1 mcg/kg
  Myxedema coma or stupor: I.V.: 200-500 mcg one time, then 75-300 mcg daily; due to potential poor absorption of oral levothyroxine, avoid oral use in acute treatment
  Thyroid suppression therapy: Oral: 2-6 mcg/kg/day for 7-10 days

Administration
Oral: Administer on an empty stomach; 1-1.5 hours prior to breakfast
Parenteral: Dilute vial with 5 mL NS; use immediately after reconstitution; administer by direct I.V. infusion over 2- to 3-minute period; may administer I.M.

Monitoring Parameters T_4, TSH, heart rate, blood pressure, clinical signs of hypo- and hyperthyroidism; growth, bone development (children); TSH is the most reliable guide for evaluating adequacy of thyroid replacement dosage. TSH may be elevated during the first few months of thyroid replacement despite patients being clinically euthyroid. In cases where T_4 remains low and TSH is within normal limits, an evaluation of "free" (unbound) T_4 is needed to evaluate further increase in dosage.

In congenital hypothyroidism, adequacy of replacement should be determined using both TSH and total- or free-T_4. During the first 3 years of life, total- or free-T_4 should be maintained in the upper $1/2$ of the normal range; this should result in normalization of the TSH. In some patients, TSH may not normalize due to a resetting of the pituitary-thyroid feedback as a result of *in utero* hypothyroidism.

Suggested frequency for monitoring thyroid function tests in children: Every 1-2 months during the first year of life, every 2-3 months between ages 1-3 years, and every 3-12 months thereafter until growth is completed; repeat tests two weeks after any change in dosage.

Reference Range See normal values in Normal Laboratory Values for Children *on page 1353*

Test Interactions Many drugs may have effects on thyroid function tests: para-aminosalicylic acid, aminoglutethimide, amiodarone, barbiturates, carbamazepine, chloral hydrate, clofibrate, colestipol, corticosteroids, danazol, diazepam, estrogens, ethionamide, fluorouracil, I.V. heparin, insulin, lithium, methadone, methimazole, mitotane, nitroprusside, oxyphenbutazone, phenylbutazone, PTU, perphenazine, phenytoin, propranolol, salicylates, sulfonylureas, and thiazides

Patient Information Do not change brands without physician's knowledge; report immediately to physician any chest pain, increased pulse, palpitations, heat intolerances, excessive sweating; do not discontinue without notifying physician

Additional Information 15-37.5 mcg liothyronine = 50-60 mcg levothyroxine = 60 mg thyroid USP = 45 mg Thyroid Strong® = 60 mg thyroglobulin = 50-60 mcg liotrix

Dosage Forms

Injection, powder for reconstitution, lyophilized, as sodium (Synthroid®): 0.2 mg, 0.5 mg

Tablet, as sodium: 25 mcg, 50 mcg, 75 mcg, 88 mcg, 100 mcg, 112 mcg, 125 mcg, 150 mcg, 175 mcg, 200 mcg, 300 mcg

Levo-T™, Unithroid®: 25 mcg, 50 mcg, 75 mcg, 88 mcg, 100 mcg, 112 mcg, 125 mcg, 150 mcg, 175 mcg, 200 mcg, 300 mcg

Levothroid®, Levoxyl®, Synthroid®: 25 mcg, 50 mcg, 75 mcg, 88 mcg, 100 mcg, 112 mcg, 125 mcg, 137 mcg, 150 mcg, 175 mcg, 200 mcg, 300 mcg

Novothyrox: 25 mcg, 50 mcg, 75 mcg, 88 mcg, 100 mcg, 112 mcg, 125 mcg, 137 mcg, 150 mcg, 175 mcg, 200 mcg, 300 mcg [dye free]

Extemporaneous Preparations A 25 mcg/mL extemporaneous suspension may be compounded by crushing twenty-five 0.1 mg tablets; measure 40 mL glycerol; triturate powder into a pourable suspension with a small amount of glycerol and transfer to a calibrated 100 mL amber bottle; rinse the mortar with about 10 mL of the glycerol and pour into the bottle; repeat until the glycerol is used up; add water to bring the oral liquid to a total volume of 100 mL; label "shake well" and "refrigerate". The suspension is stable 8 days refrigerated.

Boulton DV, Fawcett JP, and Woods DJ, "Stability of an Extemporaneously Compounded Levothyroxine Sodium Oral Liquid," *Am J Health-Syst Pharm*, 1996; 53:1157-61.

♦ **Levoxyl®** *see* Levothyroxine *on page 669*

♦ **Levsin®** *see* Hyoscyamine *on page 585*

♦ **Levsinex®** *see* Hyoscyamine *on page 585*

♦ **Levsin/SL®** *see* Hyoscyamine *on page 585*

♦ **LH-RH** *see* Gonadorelin *on page 547*

♦ **LidaMantle®** *see* Lidocaine *on page 671*

♦ **Lidemol® (Can)** *see* Fluocinonide *on page 499*

♦ **Lidex®** *see* Fluocinonide *on page 499*

♦ **Lidex-E®** *see* Fluocinonide *on page 499*

Lidocaine (LYE doe kane)

Related Information

Adult ACLS Algorithm, Stable Ventricular Tachycardia *on page 1191*
Adult ACLS Algorithm, V. Fib and Pulseless VT *on page 1185*
CPR Pediatric Drug Dosages *on page 1175*
Emergency Pediatric Drip Calculations *on page 1177*
Pediatric ALS Algorithm, Pulseless Arrest *on page 1180*
Pediatric ALS Algorithm, Tachycardia - Rapid Rhythm and Adequate Perfusion *on page 1181*
Pediatric ALS Algorithm, Tachycardia - Rapid Rhythm and Evidence of Poor Perfusion *on page 1182*

U.S. Brand Names Anestacon®; Band-Aid® Hurt-Free™ Antiseptic Wash [OTC]; Burnamycin [OTC]; Burn Jel [OTC]; Burn-O-Jel [OTC]; ELA-Max® [OTC]; ELA-Max® 5 [OTC]; LidaMantle®; Lidoderm®; Premjact® [OTC]; Solarcaine® Aloe Extra Burn Relief [OTC]; Topicaine® [OTC]; Xylocaine®; Xylocaine® MPF; Xylocaine® Viscous; Zilactin®-L [OTC]

Canadian Brand Names Lidodan™; Xylocard®

Synonyms Lignocaine

Therapeutic Category Analgesic, Topical; Antiarrhythmic Agent, Class I-B; Local Anesthetic, Injectable; Local Anesthetic, Topical

(Continued)

Lidocaine *(Continued)*

Generic Available Yes (gel, injection, ointment, and solution)

Use Treatment of ventricular ectopy, ventricular tachycardia (VT), ventricular fibrillation (VF); for pulseless VT or VF **after** defibrillation and epinephrine; control of hemodynamically compromising premature ventricular contractions; stable, monomorphic VT (with normal or impaired cardiac function); stable, polymorphic VT (with normal baseline or prolonged QT interval); local anesthetic; pain relief of postherpetic neuralgia

Pregnancy Risk Factor B

Contraindications Hypersensitivity to lidocaine, amide-type local anesthetics, or any component (see Warnings); patients with Adams-Stokes syndrome or with severe degree of S-A, A-V, or intraventricular heart block (without a pacemaker)

Warnings Decrease dose in patients with decreased cardiac output or hepatic disease; do not use lidocaine solutions containing epinephrine for treatment of arrhythmias; do not use preservative-containing solution for I.V. use; do not apply patch to larger areas or for longer than recommended (toxicities may result)

Topical gel may contain tartrazine or benzyl alcohol; topical and rectal creams may contain benzyl alcohol; tartrazine and benzyl alcohol may cause allergic reactions in susceptible individuals; large amounts of benzyl alcohol (≥99 mg/kg/day) have been associated with a potentially fatal toxicity ("gasping syndrome") in neonates; the "gasping syndrome" consists of metabolic acidosis, respiratory distress, gasping respirations, CNS dysfunction (including convulsions, intracranial hemorrhage), hypotension and cardiovascular collapse; avoid use of lidocaine products containing benzyl alcohol in neonates; *in vitro* and animal studies have shown that benzoate, a metabolite of benzyl alcohol, displaces bilirubin from protein binding sites

Precautions Hepatic disease, heart failure, marked hypoxia, severe respiratory depression, hypovolemia or shock; incomplete heart block or bradycardia, atrial fibrillation

Adverse Reactions

Cardiovascular: Bradycardia, hypotension, heart block, arrhythmias, cardiovascular collapse

Central nervous system: Lethargy, coma, agitation, slurred speech, seizures, anxiety, euphoria, hallucinations

Gastrointestinal: Nausea, vomiting

Local: Thrombophlebitis; with patch: Erythema, edema, abnormal sensation

Neuromuscular & skeletal: Paresthesia, muscle twitching

Ocular: Blurred vision, diplopia

Respiratory: Respiratory depression or arrest

Miscellaneous: Allergic and anaphylactoid reactions (rare)

Drug Interactions Cytochrome P450 isoenzyme CYP1A2, CYP2B6, CYP2D6, and CYP3A3/4 substrate; isoenzyme CYP1A2 inhibitor

Cimetidine or beta-blockers may increase lidocaine serum concentration and toxicity; Class I antiarrhythmic agents (mexiletine, tocainide) may increase adverse or toxic effects

Mechanism of Action Class IB antiarrhythmic; suppresses automaticity of conduction tissue by increasing electrical stimulation threshold of ventricle, HIS-Purkinje system, and spontaneous depolarization of the ventricles during diastole by a direct action on the tissues; blocks both the initiation and conduction of nerve impulses by decreasing the neuronal membrane's permeability to sodium ions, which results in inhibition of depolarization with resultant blockade of conduction

Pharmacodynamics

Antiarrhythmic effect:

Onset of action (single I.V. bolus dose): 45-90 seconds

Duration: 10-20 minutes

Local anesthetic effect: Duration: 1-2 hours

Pharmacokinetics

Distribution: V_d alterable by many patient factors; decreased V_d in CHF and liver disease

Protein binding: 60% to 80%; binds to alpha$_1$-acid glycoprotein

Metabolism: 90% in the liver; active metabolites monoethylglycinexylidide (MEGX) and glycinexylidide (GX) can accumulate and may cause CNS toxicity

Half-life, biphasic:

Alpha: 7-30 minutes

Beta, terminal:

Infants, premature: 3.2 hours

Adults: 1.5-2 hours

CHF, liver disease, shock, severe renal disease: Prolonged half-life

Elimination: <10% excreted unchanged in urine

Dialysis: Dialyzable (0% to 5%)

Usual Dosage

Children and Adults:

Topical: Apply to affected area as needed; maximum dose: 3 mg/kg/dose; do not repeat within 2 hours

Injectable local anesthetic: Dose varies with procedure, degree of anesthesia needed, vascularity of tissue, duration of anesthesia required, and physical condition of patient; maximum dose: 4.5 mg/kg/dose; do not repeat within 2 hours

Children:

I.V., I.O.: (**Note:** For use in pulseless VT or VF, give after defibrillation and epinephrine): Loading dose: 1 mg/kg; follow with continuous infusion; may administer second bolus of 0.5-1 mg/kg if delay between bolus and start of infusion is >15 minutes; continuous infusion: 20-50 mcg/kg/minute. Use 20 mcg/kg/minute in patients with shock, hepatic disease, cardiac arrest, mild CHF; moderate to severe CHF may require ½ loading dose and lower infusion rates to avoid toxicity.

E.T.: 2-10 times the I.V. bolus dose

Adults (decrease the dose in patients with CHF, acute MI with hypotension, shock, poor peripheral perfusion states, or hepatic disease; usual bolus dose, but ½ of normal maintenance infusion should be used in these patients):

I.V.:

Antiarrhythmic: Initial bolus: 1-1.5 mg/kg; may repeat doses of 0.5-0.75 mg/kg every 5-10 minutes if needed to a total of 3 mg/kg; continuous infusion: Initial: 1-4 mg/minute

Ventricular fibrillation or pulseless VT (after defibrillation and epinephrine or vasopressin): Initial dose: 1-1.5 mg/kg IVP; may repeat 0.5-0.75 mg in 3-5 minutes; maximum total dose: 3 mg/kg; follow with continuous infusion after return of perfusion; continuous infusion: 1-4 mg/min; **Note:** Use only bolus doses for cardiac arrest caused by VF or pulseless VT

Patients with impaired cardiac function: Initial bolus: 0.5-0.75 mg/kg IVP; may repeat every 5-10 minutes; follow with continuous infusion: Initial: 1-4 mg/min; maximum total dose: 3 mg/kg (administered over 1 hour)

Prevention of ventricular fibrillation: I.V.: Initial bolus: 0.5 mg/kg; repeat every 5-10 minutes to a total dose of 2 mg/kg

Refractory ventricular fibrillation: Repeat 1.5 mg/kg bolus may be given 3-5 minutes after initial dose

E.T.: 2-2.5 times the I.V. bolus dose

I.M.: Prehospital post-MI antiarrhythmic prophylaxis: 300 mg

Lidoderm® patch: Postherpetic neuralgia: Apply patch to most painful areas; up to 3 patches may be applied per application; patch may remain in place for up to 12 hours in any 24-hour period

Administration

Endotracheal:

Children: Dilute to 5 mL with NS prior to E.T. administration; follow ET administration with 5 manual ventilations

Adults: Dilute in 10 mL NS or distilled water prior to E.T. administration (**Note:** Use of distilled water results in greater absorption, but a greater adverse effect on PaO₂)

Parenteral: I.V.: Solutions of 40-200 mg/mL must be diluted for I.V. use; final concentration not to exceed 20 mg/mL for I.V. push or 8 mg/mL for I.V. infusion; I.V. push rate of administration should not exceed 0.7 mg/kg/minute or 50 mg/minute, whichever is less; I.V. continuous infusion must be administered with a calibrated infusion device

Transdermal: Apply patch to intact skin so most painful area is covered; do not apply to broken or inflamed skin; patch may be cut to appropriate size; remove immediately if burning sensation occurs; wash hands after applying patch; avoid eye contact; keep out of the reach of children; dispose of used patch properly (see Additional Information)

Monitoring Parameters Monitor EKG continuously; serum concentrations with continuous infusion; I.V. site (local thrombophlebitis may occur with prolonged infusions)

Reference Range

Therapeutic: 1.5-5 µg/mL (SI: 6-21 µmol/L)

Potentially toxic: >6 µg/mL (SI: >26 µmol/L)

Toxic: >9 µg/mL (SI: >38 µmol/L)

Nursing Implications Multiple products and concentrations exist; use of an I.V. fluid filter is recommended where possible

Additional Information Transdermal patches (both used and unused) may cause toxicities in children; used patches still contain large amounts of lidocaine; store and dispose patches out of the reach of children

(Continued)

Lidocaine *(Continued)*

Dosage Forms

Cream, rectal (ELA-Max® 5): 5% (30 g) [contains benzyl alcohol]

Cream, topical (ELA-Max®): 4% (5 g, 30 g) [contains benzyl alcohol]

Cream, topical, as hydrochloride (LidaMantle®): 3% (30 g)

Gel, topical:

    Burn-O-Jel: 0.5% (90 g)

    Topicaine®: 4% (1 g, 10 g, 30 g, 113 g) [contains benzyl alcohol]

Gel, topical, as hydrochloride: 2% (30 g)

    Burn Jel: 2% (3.5 g, 120 g)

    Solarcaine® Aloe Extra Burn Relief: 0.5% (226 g) [contains tartrazine]

Infusion, as hydrochloride [premixed in D_5W]: 0.4% [4 mg/mL] (250 mL, 500 mL); 0.8% [8 mg/mL] (250 mL, 500 mL)

Injection, solution, as hydrochloride: 0.5% [5 mg/mL] (50 mL); 1% [10 mg/mL] (5 mL, 20 mL, 30 mL, 50 mL); 1.5% [15 mg/mL] (20 mL); 2% [20 mg/mL] (2 mL, 5 mL, 20 mL, 30 mL, 50 mL)

    Xylocaine®: 0.5% [5 mg/mL] (50 mL); 1% [10 mg/mL] (10 mL, 20 mL, 50 mL); 2% [20 mg/mL] (1.8 mL, 10 mL, 20 mL, 50 mL); 4% [40 mg/mL] (5 mL)

Injection, solution, as hydrochloride [preservative free]: 0.5% [5 mg/mL] (50 mL); 1% [10 mg/mL] (2 mL, 5 mL, 30 mL); 1.5% [15 mg/mL] (20 mL); 2% [20 mg/mL] (5 mL, 10 mL); 4% [40 mg/mL] (5 mL); 10% [100 mg/mL] (10 mL); 20% [200 mg/mL] (10 mL)

    Xylocaine® MPF: 0.5% [5 mg/mL] (50 mL); 1% [10 mg/mL] (2 mL, 5 mL, 10 mL, 20 mL, 30 mL); 1.5% [15 mg/mL] (10 mL, 20 mL); 2% [20 mg/mL] (2 mL, 5 mL, 10 mL); 4% [40 mg/mL] (5 mL)

Injection, solution, as hydrochloride [premixed in $D_{7.5}W$; preservative free]: 5% [50 mg/mL] (2 mL)

    Xylocaine® MPF: 1.5% [15 mg/mL] (2 mL)

Jelly, topical, as hydrochloride:

    Anestacon®: 2% (15 mL, 240 mL)

    Xylocaine®: 2% (5 mL, 10 mL, 20 mL, 30 mL)

Liquid, topical (Zilactin®-L): 2.5% (7.5 mL)

Ointment, topical: 5% (37 g)

    Xylocaine®: 2.5% (35 g) [OTC]; 5% (3.5 g, 35 g) [mint or unflavored]

Patch, transdermal (Lidoderm®): 5% (30s)

Solution, topical, as hydrochloride: 4% [40 mg/mL] (50 mL)

    Band-Aid® Hurt-Free™ Antiseptic Wash: 2% (180 mL)

    Xylocaine®: 4% [40 mg/mL] (50 mL)

Solution, viscous, as hydrochloride: 2% [20 mg/mL] (20 mL, 100 mL)

    Xylocaine® Viscous: 2% [20 mg/mL] (20 mL, 100 mL, 450 mL)

Spray, topical:

    Burnamycin: 0.5% (60 mL)

    Premjact®: 9.6% (13 mL)

    Solarcaine® Aloe Extra Burn Relief: 0.5% (127 g)

References

"Guidelines 2000 for Cardiopulmonary Resuscitation and Emergency Cardiovascular Care, Part 6: Advanced Cardiovascular Life Support, The American Heart Association in Collaboration With the International Liaison Committee on Resuscitation," *Circulation*, 2000, 102(8 Suppl):I86-171.

"Guidelines 2000 for Cardiopulmonary Resuscitation and Emergency Cardiovascular Care, Part 10: Pediatric Advanced Life Support, The American Heart Association in Collaboration With the International Liaison Committee on Resuscitation," *Circulation*, 2000, 102(8 Suppl): I291-342.

Lidocaine and Epinephrine *(LYE doe kane & ep i NEF rin)*

U.S. Brand Names Xylocaine® MPF With Epinephrine; Xylocaine® With Epinephrine

Synonyms Epinephrine and Lidocaine

Therapeutic Category Local Anesthetic, Injectable

Generic Available Yes

Use Local infiltration anesthesia

Pregnancy Risk Factor B

Contraindications Hypersensitivity to epinephrine, lidocaine, amide-type local anesthetics, or any component (see Warnings)

Warnings Some products contain sodium metabisulfite which may cause allergic reactions in susceptible individuals

Precautions Do not use solutions in distal portions of the body (digits, nose, ears, penis); do not use large doses in patients with conduction defects (ie, heart block)

Adverse Reactions

Cardiovascular: Hypotension, bradycardia

Central nervous system: Lightheadedness, nervousness, confusion, dizziness, drowsiness, convulsions

Dermatologic: Urticaria

Neuromuscular & skeletal: Tremor
Ocular: Blurred vision
Otic: Tinnitus

Mechanism of Action Lidocaine blocks both the initiation and conduction of nerve impulses via decreased permeability of sodium ions; epinephrine increases the duration of action of lidocaine by causing vasoconstriction (via alpha effects) which slows the vascular absorption of lidocaine

Pharmacodynamics
Maximum effect: Within 5 minutes
Duration: 2-6 hours, dependent on dose and anesthetic procedure

Usual Dosage Dosage varies with the anesthetic procedure
Children: Use lidocaine concentrations of 0.5% or 1% (or even more dilute) to decrease possibility of toxicity; lidocaine dose (when using combination product of lidocaine and epinephrine) should not exceed 7 mg/kg/dose; do not repeat within 2 hours

Administration Local injection: Before injecting, withdraw syringe plunger to make sure that injection is not into vein or artery; do not administer I.V. or intra-arterially

Additional Information Use preservative free solutions for epidural or caudal use

Dosage Forms
Injection, solution, as hydrochloride, with epinephrine 1:50,000 (Xylocaine® With Epinephrine): Lidocaine 2% [20 mg/mL] (1.8 mL) [contains sodium metabisulfite]
Injection, solution, as hydrochloride, with epinephrine 1:100,000: Lidocaine 1% [10 mg/mL] (20 mL, 30 mL, 50 mL); lidocaine 2% [20 mg/mL] (20 mL, 30 mL, 50 mL)
Xylocaine® With Epinephrine: Lidocaine 1% [10 mg/mL] (10 mL, 20 mL, 50 mL); lidocaine 2% [20 mg/mL] (1.8 mL, 10 mL, 20 mL, 50 mL) [contains sodium metabisulfite]
Injection, solution, as hydrochloride, with epinephrine 1:200,000: Lidocaine 0.5% [5 mg/mL] (50 mL)
Xylocaine® With Epinephrine: Lidocaine 0.5% [5 mg/mL] (50 mL) [contains sodium metabisulfite]
Injection, solution, as hydrochloride, with epinephrine 1:200,000 [methylparaben free]: Lidocaine 1% [10 mg/mL] (30 mL); lidocaine 1.5% [15 mg/mL] (5 mL, 30 mL); lidocaine 2% [20 mg/mL] (20 mL) [contains sodium metabisulfite]
Xylocaine® MPF With Epinephrine: Lidocaine 1% [10 mg/mL] (5 mL, 10 mL, 30 mL); 1.5% [15 mg/mL] (5 mL, 10 mL, 30 mL); lidocaine 2% [20 mg/mL] (5 mL, 10 mL, 20 mL) [contains sodium metabisulfite]

Lidocaine and Prilocaine (LYE doe kane & PRIL oh kane)

U.S. Brand Names EMLA®

Synonyms Eutectic Mixture of Lidocaine and Prilocaine; Eutectic Mixture of Local Anesthetics; Prilocaine and Lidocaine

Therapeutic Category Analgesic, Topical; Antipruritic, Topical; Local Anesthetic, Topical

Generic Available No

Use Topical anesthetic for use on normal intact skin to provide local analgesia for minor procedures such as I.V. cannulation or venipuncture; topical anesthetic for superficial minor surgery of genital mucous membranes and as an adjunct for local infiltration anesthesia in genital mucous membranes; has also been used for painful procedures such as lumbar puncture and skin graft harvesting

Pregnancy Risk Factor B

Contraindications Hypersensitivity to lidocaine, prilocaine, amide-type local anesthetics, or any component; patients with congenital or idiopathic methemoglobinemia, neonates <37 weeks gestation, infants <12 months of age who are receiving concurrent treatment with methemoglobin-inducing agents (ie, sulfas, acetaminophen, benzocaine, chloroquine, dapsone, nitrofurantoin, nitroglycerin, nitroprusside, phenobarbital, phenytoin, primaquine, quinine)

Precautions Use with caution in patients with severe hepatic disease, patients with G-6-PD deficiency, and patients taking drugs associated with drug-induced methemoglobinemia; adjust dosage by using smaller areas for application in small children (especially infants <3 months of age) or patients with impaired renal or hepatic function

Adverse Reactions
Cardiovascular: Bradycardia, hypotension, shock, angioedema
Central nervous system: Nervousness, euphoria, confusion, dizziness, drowsiness, convulsions, CNS excitation, alteration in temperature sensation
Dermatologic: Rash, urticaria
Hematologic: Methemoglobinemia
Local: Blanching, itching, erythema, edema
Neuromuscular & skeletal: Tremor
(Continued)

Lidocaine and Prilocaine *(Continued)*

Ocular: Blurred vision
Otic: Tinnitus
Respiratory: Respiratory depression, bronchospasm

Drug Interactions Class IB antiarrhythmic drugs (tocainide, mexiletine): toxic effects are additive; drugs known to induce methemoglobinemia (see Contraindications)

Stability Store at room temperature

Mechanism of Action Local anesthetic action occurs by stabilization of neuronal membranes and inhibiting the ionic fluxes required for the initiation and conduction of impulses

Pharmacodynamics

Onset of action: 1 hour for sufficient dermal analgesia
Maximum effect: 2-3 hours
Duration: 1-2 hours after removal of the cream

Pharmacokinetics

Absorption: Topical: Related to the duration of application and to the area over which it is applied
3-hour application: 3.6% lidocaine and 6.1% prilocaine were absorbed
24-hour application: 16.2% lidocaine and 33.5% prilocaine were absorbed
Distribution: Both cross the blood-brain barrier; lidocaine and probably prilocaine are excreted in breast milk; V_d:
Lidocaine: 1.1-2.1 L/kg
Prilocaine: 0.7-4.4 L/kg
Protein binding:
Lidocaine: 70%
Prilocaine: 55%
Metabolism:
Lidocaine: Metabolized by the liver to inactive and active metabolites
Prilocaine: Metabolized in both the liver and kidneys
Half-life:
Lidocaine: 65-150 minutes, prolonged with cardiac or hepatic dysfunction
Prilocaine: 10-150 minutes, prolonged in hepatic or renal dysfunction

Usual Dosage Topical:
Newborns ≥37 weeks gestation, Infants, Children, and Adults: For minor procedures, apply 2.5 g/site for at least 60 minutes; for painful procedures, apply 2 g/10 cm^2 of skin and leave on for at least 2 hours; see table.
Note: Preliminary results in a study of 30 preterm neonates (n=30) using a single 0.5 g dose of EMLA® applied to the heel for 1 hour resulted in no measurable changes in methemoglobin levels

EMLA® Cream Maximum Recommended Dose and Application Area* for Infants and Children Based on Application to Intact Skin

Age and Body Weight Requirements	Maximum Total Dose of EMLA®	Maximum Application Area	Maximum Application Time
Birth to 3 mo or <5 kg	1 g	10 cm^2	1 h
3-12 mo and >5 kg	2 g	20 cm^2	4 h
1-6 y and >10 kg	10 g	100 cm^2	4 h
7-12 y and >20 kg	20 g	200 cm^2	4 h

Adult male genital skin as an adjunct prior to local anesthetic infiltration: Apply 1 g/10 cm^2 to skin surface for 15 minutes followed immediately by local anesthetic infiltration after removal of EMLA® cream

Administration Topical: Do not use on mucous membranes or the eyes; apply a thick layer of cream to intact skin and cover with an occlusive dressing

Patient Information Not for ophthalmic use; for external use only. EMLA® may block sensation in the treated skin.

Nursing Implications In small infants and children, an occlusive bandage should be placed over the EMLA® cream to prevent the child from placing the cream in his/her mouth or smearing the cream on the eyes

Dosage Forms

Cream: Lidocaine 2.5% and prilocaine 2.5% (5 g, 30 g) [each 5 g tube is packaged with 2 Tegaderm® dressings]
Disc, topical: 1 g (2s, 10s) [contains 25 mg lidocaine and 25 mg prilocaine per 10 cm^2 disc]

References

Broadman LM, Soliman IE, Hannallah RS, et al, "Analgesic Efficacy of Eutectic Mixture of Local Anesthetics (EMLA®) vs Intradermal Infiltration Prior to Venous Cannulation in Children," *Am J Anaesth*, 1987, 34:S56.

Halperin DL, Koren G, Attias D, et al, "Topical Skin Anesthesia for Venous Subcutaneous Drug Reservoir and Lumbar Puncture in Children," *Pediatrics*, 1989, 84(2):281-4.

Robieux I, Kumar R, Radhakrishnan S, et al, "Assessing Pain and Analgesia With a Lidocaine-Prilocaine Emulsion in Infants and Toddlers During Venipuncture," *J Pediatr*, 1991, 118(6):971-3.

Taddio A, Shennan AT, Stevens B, et al, "Safety of Lidocaine-Prilocaine Cream in the Treatment of Preterm Neonates," *J Pediatr*, 1995, 127(6):1002-5.

♦ **Lidodan™ (Can)** *see* Lidocaine *on page 671*
♦ **Lidoderm®** *see* Lidocaine *on page 671*
♦ **LID-Pack® (Can)** *see* Bacitracin and Polymyxin B *on page 157*
♦ **Lignocaine** *see* Lidocaine *on page 671*
♦ **Lin-Amox (Can)** *see* Amoxicillin *on page 94*
♦ **Lin-Buspirone (Can)** *see* BusPIRone *on page 191*

Lindane (LIN dane)

Canadian Brand Names Hexit™; PMS-Lindane

Synonyms Benzene Hexachloride; Gamma Benzene Hexachloride; Hexachlorocyclohexane

Therapeutic Category Antiparasitic Agent, Topical; Pediculocide; Scabicidal Agent; Shampoos

Generic Available Yes

Use Alternative treatment of scabies (*Sarcoptes scabiei*), *Pediculus capitis* (head lice), and *Pediculus pubis* (crab lice); (the AAP and CDC consider permethrin 5% to be the scabicide of choice due to its safety and efficacy profile; many clinicians no longer recommend lindane as initial therapy for pediculosis due to reports of resistance and neurotoxicity)

Pregnancy Risk Factor B

Contraindications Hypersensitivity to lindane or any component; premature neonates; pregnant or lactating women; acutely inflamed skin or raw, weeping surfaces

Warnings Avoid contact with the face, eyes, mucous membranes, and urethral meatus

Precautions Use with caution in infants, small children and patients with pre-existing seizure disorders due to its potential for neurologic toxicity; if used in young children, cover hands to prevent accidental lindane ingestion from thumbsucking; **consider alternative therapy for the treatment of scabies in infants and young children <2 years of age (ie, permethrin)**

Adverse Reactions
Cardiovascular: Cardiac arrhythmia
Central nervous system: Dizziness, restlessness, seizures, headache, ataxia
Dermatologic: Eczematous eruptions, contact dermatitis, rash
Gastrointestinal: Nausea, vomiting
Hematologic: Aplastic anemia
Hepatic: Hepatitis
Local: Burning and stinging
Ocular: Conjunctivitis
Renal: Hematuria
Respiratory: Pulmonary edema

Mechanism of Action Directly absorbed by parasites and ova through the exoskeleton; stimulates the nervous system resulting in seizures and death of parasitic arthropods

Pharmacokinetics
Absorption: Topical: Up to 13% absorbed systemically (absorption is greater when applied to damaged skin, face, scalp, neck, or scrotum)
Distribution: Stored in body fat and accumulates in the brain; skin and adipose tissue may act as repositories
Metabolism: By the liver
Half-life, children: 17-22 hours
Time to peak serum concentration: Children: Topical: 6 hours
Elimination: In urine and feces

Usual Dosage Children and Adults: Topical:
Scabies: Apply a thin layer of lotion and massage it on skin from the neck to the toes (head to toe in infants).
Infants: Wash off 6 hours after application
Children: Wash off 6-8 hours after application
Adults: Bathe and remove drug 8-12 hours after application
Do not reapply sooner than 1 week later if live mites appear
Pediculosis: 15-30 mL of shampoo is applied and lathered for 4 minutes; rinse hair thoroughly and comb with a fine tooth comb to remove nits; repeat treatment in 7 days if lice or nits are still present
(Continued)

Lindane (Continued)

Pediculosis of the eyelashes: Do not treat with lindane; instead, apply an occlusive ophthalmic ointment like petrolatum to the eyelid margins twice daily for 10 days

Administration

For topical use only; do not apply to face; avoid getting in eyes; do **not** apply lotion immediately after a hot, soapy bath; lotion should be applied to dry, cool skin

Before applying lindane shampoo, wash hair with a plain shampoo, then dry

Patient Information Clothing and bedding should be washed in hot water or by dry cleaning to kill the scabies mite; combs and brushes may be washed with lindane shampoo then thoroughly rinsed with water

Nursing Implications

Children <6 years: ~30 mL lotion is sufficient volume for one application

Children ≥6 years and Adults: ~30-60 mL lotion is sufficient volume for one application

Pruritus associated with scabies or pediculosis may persist for longer than 1 week following treatment with drug. Oral antihistamine and/or topical corticosteroid may be used to help relieve pruritus.

Additional Information Excessive absorption may result in overdose with signs and symptoms which include nausea, vomiting, seizures, headaches, arrhythmias, apnea, pulmonary edema, hematuria, hepatitis, coma, and even death

Dosage Forms

Lotion: 1% (60 mL, 473 mL)

Shampoo: 1% (60 mL, 473 mL)

References

Eichenfield LF, Honig PJ, "Blistering Disorders in Childhood," *Pediatr Clin North Am*, 1991, 38(4):959-76.

Hogan DJ, Schachner L, Tanglertsampan C, "Diagnosis and Treatment of Childhood Scabies and Pediculosis," *Pediatr Clin North Am*, 1991, 38(4):941-57.

Pramanik AK and Hansen RC, "Transcutaneous Gamma Benzene Hexachloride Absorption and Toxicity in Infants and Children," *Arch Dermatol*, 1979, 115(10):1224-5.

Linezolid (li NE zoh lid)

U.S. Brand Names Zyvox™

Canadian Brand Names Zyvoxam®

Synonyms PNU-100766

Therapeutic Category Antibiotic, Oxazolidinone

Generic Available No

Use Treatment of community-acquired pneumonia, hospital-acquired pneumonia, skin and soft tissue infections, bacteremia caused by susceptible vancomycin-resistant *Enterococcus faecium* (VREF), *Streptococcus pneumoniae*, *Staphylococcus aureus* including MRSA, *Streptococcus pyogenes*, or *Streptococcus agalactiae*

Pregnancy Risk Factor C

Contraindications Hypersensitivity to linezolid or any component

Warnings Linezolid is a reversible, nonselective MAO inhibitor with the potential to have the same interactions as other MAO inhibitors. Avoid use with serotonergic agents such as tricyclic antidepressants, venlafaxine, trazodone, sibutramine, meperidine, dextromethorphan, and SSRIs. Thrombocytopenia, anemia, leukopenia, and pancytopenia have been reported in patients receiving linezolid and may be dependent on duration of therapy (generally >2 weeks of treatment); monitor patients' CBC weekly during linezolid therapy; discontinuation of therapy may be required; *C. difficile*-associated colitis has been reported. Peripheral and optic neuropathy have been reported primarily in patients treated for longer then 28 days with linezolid. Oral suspension contains sodium benzoate; benzoic acid (benzoate) is a metabolite of benzyl alcohol; large amounts of benzyl alcohol (≥99 mg/kg/day) have been associated with a potentially fatal toxicity ("gasping syndrome") in neonates; use caution when administering oral suspension containing sodium benzoate to neonates; *in vitro* and animal studies have shown that benzoate displaces bilirubin from protein binding sites

Precautions Use with caution in patients with uncontrolled hypertension, pheochromocytoma, carcinoid syndrome, severe renal or hepatic impairment, or untreated hyperthyroidism; linezolid suspension contains aspartame which is metabolized to phenylalanine and must be used with caution in patients with phenylketonuria.

Adverse Reactions

Cardiovascular: Hypertension

Central nervous system: Headache, insomnia, dizziness, fever

Dermatologic: Rash

Endocrine & metabolic: Lactic acidosis

Gastrointestinal: Nausea, diarrhea, vomiting, constipation, pseudomembranous colitis

Hematologic: Neutropenia, thrombocytopenia, anemia, leukopenia, pancytopenia

Hepatic: Elevated ALT

Neuromuscular & skeletal: Peripheral neuropathy

Ocular: Optic neuropathy

Drug Interactions Enhanced vasopressor effects if used with sympathomimetic agents such as dopamine, epinephrine, pseudoephedrine; serotonin syndrome (hyperpyrexia, cognitive dysfunction) if used in patients receiving concomitant serotonergic agents including tricyclic antidepressants, venlafaxine, trazodone, sibutramine, meperidine, dextromethorphan, and SSRIs (see Warnings)

Food Interactions Ingestion of tyramine-containing foods may cause hypertensive crisis; limit intake of tyramine-containing foods to less than 100 mg/meal

Stability Store at room temperature; protect from light. Store infusion bags in overwrap until ready for use. The yellow color of the injectable solution may intensify over time without adversely affecting potency. Use reconstituted suspension within 21 days. Linezolid injection is physically incompatible with amphotericin B, chlorpromazine, diazepam, erythromycin lactobionate, pentamidine, phenytoin, sulfamethoxazole and trimethoprim, and ceftriaxone. Linezolid injection is compatible with D_5W, NS, and LR.

Mechanism of Action Inhibits initiation of protein synthesis by binding to a site on the bacterial 23S ribosomal RNA of the 50S subunit preventing the formation of a functional 70S initiation complex which is an essential component of the bacterial translation process

Pharmacokinetics

Absorption: Well absorbed orally

Distribution: Well-perfused tissues

V_d: Children: 0.73 ± 0.18 L/kg

Protein binding: 31%

Metabolism: Oxidation to 2 inactive metabolites

Bioavailability: 100%

Half-life:

Preterm neonate <1 week: 5.6 hours

Full term neonate <1 week: 3 hours

Full term neonate ≥1 week to ≤28 days: 1.5 hours

Infants: 1.8 hours

Children: 3 ± 1.1 hours

Adolescents: 4.1 hours

Adults: 4-5 hours

Time to peak serum concentration: 1-2 hours

Elimination: 65% nonrenal; 30% renal; 2 metabolites of linezolid may accumulate in patients with severe renal impairment

Clearance: Children: 0.34 ± 0.15 L/hour/kg

Dialysis: Removed by hemodialysis

Usual Dosage Note: No dosage adjustment needed when switching from I.V. to oral

Neonates <7 days: Oral, I.V.: 10 mg/kg/dose every 12 hours

Neonates ≥7 days, Infants, and Children: Oral, I.V.: 10 mg/kg/dose every 8 hours

Sixty-six children 12 months to 17 years of age with community-acquired pneumonia were enrolled in a Phase II, open-label multicenter study of I.V. linezolid followed by oral linezolid with a mean total treatment duration of 12.2 ± 6.2 days (range: 6-41 days); 92.4% of patients were considered cured, one failed (methicillin-resistant *Staphylococcus aureus*) and 4 were considered indeterminate (Kaplan, 2001); pharmacokinetic data obtained in pediatric patients 0.3-16 years of age support an I.V. linezolid dose of 10 mg/kg/dose 2-3 times/day (Kearns, 2000)

Children 5-11 years: Uncomplicated skin and skin structure infections: Oral: 10 mg/kg/dose every 12 hours for 10-14 days

Children ≥12 years and Adolescents:

Uncomplicated skin and skin structure infections: Oral: 600 mg every 12 hours for 10-14 days

Complicated skin and skin structure infections, nosocomial or community-acquired pneumonia including concurrent bacteremia: Oral, I.V.: 600 mg every 12 hours for 10-14 days

VREF infections: Oral, I.V.: 600 mg every 12 hours for 14-28 days

Adults:

Uncomplicated skin and skin structure infections: Oral: 400 mg every 12 hours for 10-14 days

Complicated skin and skin structure infection, nosocomial or community-acquired pneumonia including concurrent bacteremia: Oral, I.V.: 600 mg every 12 hours for 10-14 days

VREF infections: Oral, I.V.: 600 mg every 12 hours for 14-28 days

Administration

Oral: Administer with or without food. Gently invert suspension bottle 3-5 times before use. Do not shake. Store at room temperature.

(Continued)

Linezolid *(Continued)*

Parenteral: I.V.: Infuse over 30-120 minutes. 2 mg/mL infusion should be administered without further dilution. Do not mix or infuse with other medications. Flush line before and after infusion with a linezolid-compatible I.V. solution like D₅W, NS, or LR.

Monitoring Parameters CBC and platelet counts particularly in patients at increased risk for bleeding, patients with pre-existing thrombocytopenia or myelosuppression, or concomitant medications that decrease platelet count or function or produce bone marrow suppression, and inpatients requiring >2 weeks of therapy; number and type of stools/day for diarrhea

Patient Information Avoid excessive amounts of tyramine-containing foods while taking linezolid: Red wine, aged cheese, smoked or pickled fish, beef or chicken liver, sauerkraut, dried sausage, fava or broad bean pods; notify physician of persistent or worsening symptoms of infection; complete entire course of therapy even if symptoms improve

Additional Information Sodium content of 200 mg/100 mL infusion bag (1.7 mEq), 400 mg/200 mL infusion bag (3.3 mEq), 600 mg/300 mL infusion bag (5 mEq); sodium content of tablet: 0.1 mEq per tablet regardless of strength; sodium content of suspension: 0.4 mEq/5 mL

Dosage Forms

Injection [premixed]: 200 mg (100 mL); 400 mg (200 mL); 600 mg (300 mL)
Suspension, oral: 20 mg/mL (150 mL) [contains 20 mg phenylalanine (as aspartame) per 5 mL and sodium benzoate; orange flavor]
Tablet: 400 mg, 600 mg

References

Clemett D and Markham A, "Linezolid," *Drugs,* 2000, 59(4):815-27.
Kaplan SL, Patterson L, Edwards KM, et al, "Linezolid for the Treatment of Community-Acquired Pneumonia in Hospitalized Children. Linezolid Pediatric Pneumonia Study Group," *Pediatr Infect Dis J,* 2001, 20(5):488-94.
Kearns GL, Abdel-Rahman SM, Blumer JL, et al, "Single Dose Pharmacokinetics of Linezolid in Infants and Children," *Pediatr Infect Dis J,* 2000, 19(12):1178-84.

♦ **Lin-Megestrol (Can)** *see Megestrol on page 714*
♦ **Lin-Sotalol (Can)** *see Sotalol on page 1032*
♦ **Lioresal®** *see Baclofen on page 158*
♦ **Liotec (Can)** *see Baclofen on page 158*

Liothyronine *(lye oh THYE roe neen)*

U.S. Brand Names Cytomel®; Triostat®

Synonyms *L*-Triiodothyronine; T₃

Therapeutic Category Thyroid Product

Generic Available Yes

Use Replacement or supplemental therapy in congenital or acquired hypothyroidism; treatment or prevention of euthyroid goiters including thyroid nodules and chronic lymphocytic thyroiditis; as a diagnostic aid in suppression tests to differentiate suspected mild hyperthyroidism or thyroid gland autonomy

Pregnancy Risk Factor A

Contraindications Hypersensitivity to liothyronine sodium or any component; recent MI or thyrotoxicosis; uncorrected adrenal insufficiency

Warnings Not for use in the treatment of obesity or for weight loss; in euthyroid patients, doses within the range of daily hormonal requirements are ineffective for weight reduction; larger doses may produce serious or even life-threatening toxic effects particularly when used with some anorectic drugs (sympathomimetic amines). Short duration of action permits more rapid assessment of dosage changes and rapid diminution of adverse effects upon discontinuation; transient partial loss of hair in pediatrics may be seen in the first few months of therapy.

Precautions Use with extreme caution in patients with cardiovascular disease, adrenal insufficiency, or coronary artery disease; use with extreme caution in patients receiving digoxin or vasopressors (see Drug Interactions); use with caution in patients with diabetes mellitus and diabetes insipidus as symptoms of their disease may be exaggerated or aggravated; myxedematous patients are very sensitive to thyroid supplements; initiate therapy at very low doses and increase gradually

Adverse Reactions

Cardiovascular: Palpitations, tachycardia, cardiac arrhythmias, angina, CHF, hypertension
Central nervous system: Nervousness, insomnia, fever, headache, irritability
Dermatologic: Alopecia, dermatitis herpetiformis, hair loss (transient)
Gastrointestinal: Diarrhea, abdominal cramps, increased appetite, weight loss
Local: Phlebitis with parenteral form
Neuromuscular & skeletal: Tremor
Miscellaneous: Diaphoresis

Drug Interactions Antacids (aluminum-, magnesium-, and calcium carbonate-containing), cholestyramine resin, iron salts, sodium polystyrene sulfonate, and sucralfate decrease absorption; estrogens, clofibrate, methadone, fluorouracil, mitotane, and tamoxifen increase thyroid requirements; liothyronine increases effect of oral anticoagulants; phenytoin, carbamazepine, phenobarbital, rifampin, amiodarone, propylthiouracil, and β-adrenergic antagonists may decrease thyroid levels; androgens, anabolic steroids, asparaginase, glucocorticoids, and slow-release nicotinic acid decrease thyroid requirements; concurrent use with sympathomimetics, TCAs, and SSRIs may enhance the toxic effects of both drugs; use with ketamine may produce significant tachycardia and hypertension; may increase insulin and other antidiabetic agent requirements; increases the adrenergic effect of catecholamines (epinephrine, norepinephrine); may potentiate the toxic effects of digoxin

Food Interactions Limit intake of goitrogenic foods (asparagus, cabbage, peas, turnip greens, broccoli, spinach, brussel sprouts, lettuce, soybeans)

Stability Store tablets at controlled room temperature; refrigerate parenteral solution at temperatures between 2°C and 8°C (36°F to 46°F)

Mechanism of Action Primary active compound is T_3 (triiodothyronine), which may be converted from T_4 (thyroxine) by deiodination in liver and peripheral tissues; exact mechanism of action is unknown; however, it is believed the thyroid hormone exerts its many metabolic effects through control of DNA transcription and protein synthesis; involved in normal metabolism, growth, and development; promotes gluconeogenesis, increases utilization and mobilization of glycogen stores, and stimulates protein synthesis, increases basal metabolic rate

Pharmacodynamics I.V., Oral:
Onset of action: Within a few hours
Maximum effect: Within 48 hours
Duration: Up to 72 hours

Pharmacokinetics
Absorption: Oral: Well absorbed (~85% to 90%)
Metabolism: In the liver to inactive compounds
Half-life: 25 hours (range: 16-49 hours); hypothyroid 1.4 days; hyperthyroid 0.6 days
Elimination: 76% to 83% In urine

Usual Dosage
Congenital hypothyroidism (Cretinism): Neonates, Infants, and Children <3 years:
Oral: 5 mcg/day; increase by 5 mcg every 3 days to a maximum dosage of 20 mcg/day for neonates and infants, 50 mcg/day for children 1-3 years of age
Hypothyroidism:
Children: Oral: 5 mcg/day increase in 5 mcg/day increments every 3-4 days;
Usual maintenance dose:
Infants: 20 mcg/day
Children 1-3 years: 50 mcg/day
Children >3 years: Full adult dosage may be necessary
Adults: Oral: 25 mcg/day increase in 12.5-25 mcg/day increments every 1-2 weeks to a maximum of 100 mcg/day
Goiter, nontoxic:
Children: Oral: 5 mcg/day increase in 5 mcg/day increments every 1-2 weeks; usual maintenance dose 15-20 mcg/day
Adults: Oral: 5 mcg/day; increase in 5-10 mcg/day increments every 1-2 weeks; when 25 mcg is reached, increase dosage in 12.5-25 mcg increments every 1-2 weeks; usual maintenance dosage: 75 mcg/day
T_3 suppression test: Adults: Oral: 75-100 mcg/day for 7 days
Myxedema coma: Adults:
I.V.: 25-50 mcg; reduce dosage in patients with known or suspected cardiovascular disease to 10-20 mcg
Note: Normally, at least 4 hours should be allowed between I.V. doses to adequately assess therapeutic response and no more than 12 hours should elapse between doses to avoid fluctuations in hormone levels.
Oral (**Note:** Due to potential poor oral absorption in the acute phase of myxedema, oral therapy should be avoided until the clinical situation has been stabilized): 5 mcg/day; increase in 5-10 mcg/day increments every 1-2 weeks; when 25 mcg/day is reached; increase by 5-25 mcg/day increments every 1-2 weeks; usual maintenance dose: 50-100 mcg/day

Administration
Oral: Administer on an empty stomach
Parenteral: I.V.: For I.V. use only; do not administer S.C. or I.M.; should not be admixed with other solutions

Monitoring Parameters T_3, TSH, heart rate, blood pressure, clinical signs of hypo- and hyperthyroidism; TSH is the most reliable guide for evaluating adequacy of
(Continued)

Liothyronine *(Continued)*

thyroid replacement dosage. TSH may be elevated during the first few months of thyroid replacement despite patients being clinically euthyroid.

Suggested frequency for monitoring thyroid function tests in children: Every 1-2 months during the first year of life, every 2-3 months between ages 1-3 years, and every 3-12 months thereafter until growth is completed; repeat tests two weeks after any change in dosage.

Reference Range See normal values in Normal Laboratory Values for Children *on page 1353*

Test Interactions Many drugs may have effects on thyroid function tests (ie, para-aminosalicylic acid, aminoglutethimide, amiodarone, barbiturates, carbamazepine, chloral hydrate, clofibrate, colestipol, corticosteroids, danazol, diazepam, estrogens, ethionamide, fluorouracil, I.V. heparin, insulin, lithium, methadone, methimazole, mitotane, nitroprusside, oxyphenbutazone, phenylbutazone, PTU, perphenazine, phenytoin, propranolol, salicylates, sulfonylureas, and thiazides)

Patient Information Do not change brands without physician's knowledge; report immediately to physician any chest pain, increased pulse, palpitations, heat intolerance, excessive sweating; do not discontinue without notifying physician

Additional Information 15-37.5 mcg liothyronine = 50-60 mcg levothyroxine = 60 mg thyroid USP

Dosage Forms

Injection, solution, as sodium (Triostat®): 10 mcg/mL (1 mL) [contains 6.8% alcohol]

Tablet, as sodium (Cytomel®): 5 mcg, 25 mcg, 50 mcg

- ◆ **Lipancreatin** *see Pancrelipase on page 856*
- ◆ **Lipid Emulsion** *see Fat Emulsion on page 475*
- ◆ **Liposyn® III** *see Fat Emulsion on page 475*
- ◆ **Lipram™ 4500** *see Pancrelipase on page 856*
- ◆ **Lipram™-CR** *see Pancrelipase on page 856*
- ◆ **Lipram™-PN** *see Pancrelipase on page 856*
- ◆ **Lipram™-UL** *see Pancrelipase on page 856*
- ◆ **Liquibid®** *see Guaifenesin on page 550*
- ◆ **Liquibid® 1200** *see Guaifenesin on page 550*
- ◆ **Liqui-Char® [OTC]** *see Charcoal on page 250*
- ◆ **Liquid Antidote** *see Charcoal on page 250*
- ◆ **Liquid Paraffin** *see Mineral Oil on page 767*
- ◆ **Liquiprin® for Children [OTC]** *see Acetaminophen on page 36*

Lisinopril *(lyse IN oh pril)*

Related Information

Carbohydrate and Alcohol Content of Liquid Medications for Use in Patients Receiving Ketogenic Diets *on page 1431*

U.S. Brand Names Prinivil®; Zestril®

Canadian Brand Names Apo®-Lisinopril

Therapeutic Category Angiotensin-Converting Enzyme (ACE) Inhibitor; Antihypertensive Agent

Generic Available Yes

Use Management of hypertension; adjunctive treatment of CHF; adjunctive therapy in hemodynamically stable post MI patients to improve survival

Pregnancy Risk Factor C (1st trimester); D (may cause injury and death to the developing fetus when used during the 2nd and 3rd trimesters of pregnancy)

Contraindications Hypersensitivity to lisinopril, any component, or other ACE inhibitors; patients with idiopathic or hereditary angioedema or a history of angioedema with previous ACE inhibitor use

Warnings Serious adverse effects including angioedema, anaphylactoid reactions, neutropenia, agranulocytosis, hypotension, and hepatic failure may occur (see Adverse Reactions); risk of neutropenia may be increased in patients with renal dysfunction, especially if the patients have collagen vascular diseases

Precautions Use with caution and modify dosage in patients with renal impairment, especially renal artery stenosis; elevated BUN and S_{cr} may occur in these patients; discontinuation of concomitant diuretic or lisinopril may be needed; use with caution and modify dosage in patients with hyponatremia, hypovolemia, severe CHF, left ventricular outflow tract obstruction, or with coadministered diuretic therapy. Severe hypotension may occur in patients who are sodium and/or volume depleted; initiate lower doses and monitor closely when starting therapy in these patients.

Adverse Reactions

Cardiovascular: Hypotension, chest discomfort, orthostatic hypotension

Central nervous system: Dizziness, headache, fatigue

Dermatologic: Rash, angioedema. **Note:** The relative risk of angioedema with ACE inhibitors is higher within the first 30 days of use (compared to >1 year of use), for Black Americans (compared to Whites), for lisinopril or enalapril (compared to captopril), and for patients previously hospitalized within 30 days (Brown, 1996).

Endocrine & metabolic: Hyperkalemia

Gastrointestinal: Diarrhea, nausea, vomiting, ageusia

Hematologic: Neutropenia, agranulocytosis

Hepatic: Cholestatic jaundice, fulminant hepatic necrosis (rare, but potentially fatal)

Renal: Elevated BUN, elevated serum creatinine

Respiratory: Cough, dyspnea, eosinophilic pneumonitis; **Note:** An isolated dry cough lasting >3 weeks was reported in 7 of 42 pediatric patients (17%) receiving ACE inhibitors (see von Vigier, 2000)

Neuromuscular & skeletal: Weakness

Drug Interactions Use with potassium-sparing diuretics may result in an additive hyperkalemic effect; diuretics and other antihypertensive agents may increase hypotensive effect; indomethacin or NSAIDs may decrease hypotensive effect; lisinopril may increase lithium levels; use with NSAIDs in patients with renal impairment may further decrease renal function (usually reversible)

Food Interactions Food does not effect oral absorption; limit salt substitutes or potassium-rich diet; avoid natural licorice (causes sodium and water retention and increases potassium loss)

Mechanism of Action Competitive inhibitor of angiotensin-converting enzyme (ACE); prevents conversion of angiotensin I to angiotensin II, a potent vasoconstrictor; results in lower levels of angiotensin II which causes an increase in plasma renin activity and a reduction in aldosterone secretion

Pharmacodynamics

Onset of action (decrease in blood pressure): 1 hour

Maximum effect: 6-8 hours

Duration: 24 hours

Pharmacokinetics

Absorption: Oral: 25%

Protein binding: 25%

Half-life: 11-13 hours; half-life increases with renal dysfunction

Elimination: Excreted in urine as unchanged drug

Usual Dosage Oral: Dosage must be titrated according to patient's response; use lower doses (~1/2 of those listed) for patients with hyponatremia, hypovolemia, severe CHF, decreased renal function, or in those receiving diuretics:

Children: Currently, no pediatric dosing information is available

Adults:

Hypertension (**Note:** If possible, discontinue diuretics 2-3 days prior to initiating lisinopril; restart diuretic, if needed, after blood pressure is stable): Initial: 10 mg/day given once daily: increase dose by 5-10 mg/day at 1- to 2-week intervals; usual dose: 20-40 mg/day given once daily; doses up to 80 mg/day have been used, but do not appear to have a greater effect

CHF: Initial: 5 mg once daily (with diuretics and digitalis); increase dose by ≤10 mg/day at ≥2 week intervals based on clinical response; usual dose: 5-40 mg/day given once daily; maximum dose: 40 mg/day

Dosing adjustment in renal impairment:

Cl_{cr} 10-30 mL/minute: Administer 50% of normal dose

Cl_{cr} <10 mL/minute: Administer 25% of normal dose

Administration Oral: May be administered without regard to food

Monitoring Parameters Blood pressure, BUN, serum creatinine, renal function, WBC, and serum potassium

Patient Information Limit alcohol; notify physician if vomiting, diarrhea, excessive perspiration, or dehydration occurs or if swelling of face, lips, tongue or difficulty in breathing occurs; do not use a salt substitute (potassium-containing) without physician advice

Nursing Implications Discontinue if angioedema occurs; observe closely for hypotension after the first dose or initiation of a new higher dose (keep in mind that maximum effect on blood pressure occurs at 6-8 hours)

Dosage Forms Tablet: 2.5 mg, 5 mg, 10 mg, 20 mg, 30 mg, 40 mg

Extemporaneous Preparations A 2 mg/mL lisinopril syrup made from powder (Sigma Chemical Company, St. Louis, MO) and simple syrup was stable for 30 days when stored in amber plastic prescription bottles at room temperature (23°C) or under refrigeration (5°C); dissolve 1 gram of lisinopril powder in 30 mL of distilled water; incorporate resultant solution into syrup using geometric dilution and qsad to 500 mL; label "shake well" and "refrigerate"; **Note:** Although no visual evidence of microbial (Continued)

Lisinopril *(Continued)*

growth was observed, the authors recommend storage at 5°C to inhibit microbial growth (Webster, 1997).

Webster AA, English BA, and Rose DJ, "The Stability of Lisinopril as an Extemporaneous Syrup," *Intr J Pharmaceut Compound*, 1997, 1:352-3.

References

Brown NJ, Ray WA, Snowden M, et al, "Black Americans Have an Increased Rate of Angiotensin-Converting Enzyme Inhibitor-Associated Angioedema," *Clin Pharmacol Ther*, 1996, 60(1):8-13.

Chase SL and Sutton JD, "Lisinopril: A New Angiotensin-Converting Enzyme Inhibitor," *Pharmacotherapy*, 1989, 9(3):120-30.

Raia JJ Jr, Barone JA, Byerly WG, et al, "Angiotensin-Converting Enzymes Inhibitors: A Comparative Review," *DICP*, 1990, 24(5):506-25.

von Vigier RO, Mozzettini S, Truttmann AC, et al, "Cough is Common in Children Prescribed Converting Enzyme Inhibitors," *Nephron*, 2000, 84(1):98.

♦ **Lithane™ (Can)** see Lithium *on page 684*

Lithium *(LITH ee um)*

Related Information

Carbohydrate and Alcohol Content of Liquid Medications for Use in Patients Receiving Ketogenic Diets *on page 1431*

Drugs and Breast-Feeding *on page 1404*

Serotonin Syndrome *on page 1420*

U.S. Brand Names Eskalith®; Eskalith CR®; Lithobid®

Canadian Brand Names Apo®-Lithium; Carbolith™; Duralith®; Lithane™; PMS-Lithium Carbonate; PMS-Lithium Citrate

Therapeutic Category Antidepressant, Miscellaneous; Antimanic Agent

Generic Available Yes (except controlled release tablet)

Use Management of acute manic episodes, mania in individuals with bipolar disorder (maintenance treatment diminishes or prevents intensity of subsequent manic episodes), and depression

Pregnancy Risk Factor D

Contraindications Hypersensitivity to lithium or any component (see Warnings). Generally, avoid use in patients with severe cardiovascular or renal disease, severe dehydration or debilitation, sodium depletion, and in patients receiving ACE inhibitors or diuretics (these patients are at very high risk of lithium toxicity)

Warnings Lithium toxicity is closely related to serum levels and can occur at therapeutic doses; serum lithium determinations are required to monitor therapy; chronic lithium therapy may result in diminished renal concentrating ability (eg, nephrogenic diabetes insipidus). An encephalopathic syndrome (resembling neuroleptic malignant syndrome) may occur in patients receiving lithium with haloperidol or other antipsychotic agents (see Drug Interactions).

Capsule may contain benzyl alcohol which may cause allergic reactions in susceptible individuals; large amounts of benzyl alcohol (≥99 mg/kg/day) have been associated with a potentially fatal toxicity ("gasping syndrome") in neonates; avoid use of lithium products containing benzyl alcohol in neonates; *in vitro* and animal studies have shown that benzoate, a metabolite of benzyl alcohol, displaces bilirubin from protein binding sites

Precautions Use with caution in patients with cardiovascular or thyroid disease, patients receiving medications that alter sodium excretion (eg, diuretics, ACE inhibitors, or NSAIDs; monitor lithium levels closely, lithium dosage reduction may be required); use with caution and modify dose in patients with renal dysfunction

Adverse Reactions

Cardiovascular: Arrhythmias, sinus node dysfunction, hypotension, severe bradycardia, syncope

Central nervous system: Sedation, confusion, somnolence, seizures, fatigue, headache, vertigo, dizziness, slurred speech, blackout spells, restlessness, ataxia, dystonia

Dermatologic: Rash, drying and thinning of hair, alopecia, anesthesia of skin, chronic folliculitis, exacerbation of psoriasis

Endocrine & metabolic: Nephrogenic diabetes insipidus (thirst, polyuria, polydipsia), goiter, hypothyroidism; rarely hyperthyroidism

Gastrointestinal: Nausea, diarrhea, vomiting, xerostomia, anorexia, gastritis, salivary gland swelling, excessive salivation

Genitourinary: Oliguria, polyuria, albuminuria, glycosuria

Hematologic: Leukocytosis

Neuromuscular & skeletal: Muscle hyperirritability, muscle weakness, tremor, choreoathetoid movements

Ocular: Nystagmus, blurred vision

Miscellaneous: Coldness and painful discoloration of fingers and toes

Drug Interactions Diuretics, indomethacin, NSAIDs, cyclooxygenase-2 (COX-2) inhibitors, ACE inhibitors, metronidazole may decrease lithium renal excretion and enhance lithium toxicity (monitor lithium levels closely); iodide salts (or iodine) may increase hypothyroid effects; use with haloperidol or other antipsychotic agents may result in an encephalopathic syndrome (monitor patients closely; discontinue therapy promptly if neurological toxicity occurs); lithium may prolong the effects of neuromuscular blocking agents (use with caution; monitor closely); carbamazepine, calcium channel blocking agents, methyldopa may increase neurotoxic side effects; acetazolamide, alkalinizing agents (eg, sodium bicarbonate), urea and xanthine products may increase urinary lithium excretion and decrease lithium serum concentrations; fluoxetine may increase or decrease lithium serum concentrations (monitor closely); use of lithium with SSRIs may increase GI and CNS adverse effects; phenytoin may increase lithium toxicity

Food Interactions Avoid changes in sodium content of diet (reduction in sodium intake can increase lithium toxicity); syrup may precipitate in tube feedings

Stability Store at controlled room temperature; protect slow-release tablets from moisture

Mechanism of Action Alters cation transport across cell membrane in nerve and muscle cells and influences reuptake of serotonin and/or norepinephrine

Pharmacokinetics
Distribution: Crosses the placenta; appears in breast milk at 35% to 50% of the concentrations in serum
Adults:
V_d: Initial: 0.3-0.4 L/kg
V_{dss}: 0.7-1 L/kg
Half-life, terminal: Adults: 18-24 hours, can increase to more than 36 hours in patients with renal impairment
Time to peak serum concentration (nonsustained release product): Within 0.5-2 hours
Elimination: 90% to 98% of a dose is excreted in the urine as unchanged drug; other excretory routes include feces (1%) and sweat (4% to 5%)
Dialysis: Dialyzable (50% to 100%)

Usual Dosage Oral: Monitor serum concentrations and clinical response (efficacy and toxicity) to determine proper dose

Children: 15-60 mg/kg/day in 3-4 divided doses; dose not to exceed usual adult dosage; initiate at lower dose and adjust dose weekly based on levels
Adolescents: 600-1800 mg/day in 3-4 divided doses for regular tablets or 2 divided doses for sustained release tablets
Adults: 300 mg 3-4 times/day; usual maximum maintenance dose: 2.4 g/day or 450-900 mg of sustained release tablets twice daily
Dosing adjustment in renal impairment:
Cl_{cr} 10-50 mL/minute: Administer 50% to 75% of normal dose
Cl_{cr} <10 mL/minute: Administer 25% to 50% of normal dose

Administration Oral: Administer with meals to decrease GI upset; do not crush or chew slow- or controlled-release dosage form, swallow whole

Monitoring Parameters Serum lithium every 3-4 days during initial therapy; once patient is clinically stable and serum concentrations are stable, serum lithium may be obtained every 1-2 months; obtain lithium serum concentrations 8-12 hours postdose (ie, just before next dose); renal, hepatic, thyroid and cardiovascular function; CBC with differential, urinalysis, serum sodium, calcium, potassium

Reference Range
Therapeutic: Acute mania: 0.6-1.2 mEq/L (SI: 0.6-1.2 mmol/L); protection against future episodes in most patients with bipolar disorder: 0.8-1 mEq/L (SI: 0.8-1 mmol/L). A higher rate of relapse is described in subjects who are maintained <0.4 mEq/L (SI: <0.4 mmol/L)
Toxic: >2 mEq/L (SI: >2 mmol/L)
Concentration-related adverse effects:
GI complaints/tremor: 1.5-2 mEq/L
Confusion/somnolence: 2-2.5 mEq/L
Seizures/death: >2.5 mEq/L

Patient Information Limit caffeine; limit alcohol; avoid tasks requiring psychomotor coordination until CNS effects are known; may cause dry mouth; blood level monitoring is required to determine the proper dose; maintain a steady salt and fluid intake especially during the summer months; avoid dehydration; notify physician if vomiting, diarrhea, muscle weakness, tremor, drowsiness, or ataxia occur (these may be signs of lithium toxicity)

Nursing Implications Avoid dehydration

Dosage Forms
Capsule, as **carbonate**: 150 mg, 300 mg, 600 mg
Eskalith®: 300 mg [contains benzyl alcohol]
(Continued)

Lithium (Continued)

Syrup, as **citrate**: 300 mg/5 mL (5 mL, 10 mL, 480 mL) [each 5 mL = 8 mEq lithium equivalent to 300 mg lithium carbonate; contains alcohol]

Tablet, as **carbonate**: 300 mg

Tablet, controlled release, as **carbonate** (Eskalith CR®): 450 mg

Tablet, slow release, as **carbonate** (Lithobid®): 300 mg

References

Levy HB, Harper CR, and Weinberg WA, "A Practical Approach to Children Failing in School," *Pediatr Clin North Am*, 1992, 39(4):895-928.

♦ **Lithobid®** *see* Lithium *on page 684*

♦ **LMD®** *see* Dextran *on page 358*

♦ **LoCHOLEST®** *see* Cholestyramine Resin *on page 267*

♦ **LoCHOLEST® Light** *see* Cholestyramine Resin *on page 267*

♦ **Locoid®** *see* Hydrocortisone *on page 573*

♦ **Locoid Lipocream®** *see* Hydrocortisone *on page 573*

♦ **Lomine (Can)** *see* Dicyclomine *on page 376*

♦ **Lomotil®** *see* Diphenoxylate and Atropine *on page 395*

Lomustine (loe MUS teen)

Related Information

Emetogenic Potential of Single Chemotherapeutic Agents *on page 1286*

U.S. Brand Names CeeNU®

Synonyms CCNU

Therapeutic Category Antineoplastic Agent, Alkylating Agent (Nitrosourea)

Generic Available No

Use Treatment of brain tumors, Hodgkin's disease, non-Hodgkin's lymphomas, melanoma, renal carcinoma, lung cancer, colon cancer

Pregnancy Risk Factor D

Contraindications Hypersensitivity to lomustine or any component; pregnancy

Warnings The FDA currently recommends that procedures for proper handling and disposal of antineoplastic agents be considered. Bone marrow suppression, notably thrombocytopenia and leukopenia, may lead to bleeding and overwhelming infections in an already compromised patient; nadir: ~6 weeks; do not give courses more frequently than every 6 weeks because the toxicity is cumulative; lomustine has been found to be mutagenic, teratogenic, and carcinogenic in animals.

Precautions Use with caution in patients with depressed platelet, leukocyte or erythrocyte counts; reduce dosage by 25% when platelet nadirs are 50,000-74,999/mm^3; reduce dosage by 50% when platelet nadirs are 25,000-49,999/mm^3; reduce dosage by 75% when platelet nadirs are <25,000/mm^3

Adverse Reactions

Central nervous system: Disorientation, lethargy, ataxia

Dermatologic: Alopecia

Gastrointestinal: Nausea, vomiting, stomatitis, anorexia, diarrhea

Hematologic: Anemia, thrombocytopenia, leukopenia, myelosuppression (occurs 4-6 weeks after a dose and may persist 1-2 weeks)

Hepatic: Hepatotoxicity, elevation of hepatic enzymes

Neuromuscular & skeletal: Dysarthria

Ocular: Blindness

Renal: Renal failure, interstitial nephritis

Respiratory: Pulmonary fibrosis with total cumulative dose >1 g/m^2

Drug Interactions Cytochrome P450 isoenzyme CYP2D6 inhibitor

Phenobarbital may increase metabolism and reduce activity of lomustine; cimetidine may decrease metabolism and increase myelotoxicity of lomustine

Food Interactions Avoid concurrent administration of food/drugs that cause vomiting

Stability Avoid exposure to excessive heat (>40°C) and prolonged exposure to moisture

Mechanism of Action Inhibits DNA and RNA synthesis through DNA alkylation and DNA cross-linking; carbamoylates amine groups on proteins; inhibits DNA polymerase activity, RNA and protein synthesis

Pharmacokinetics

Absorption: Rapid and complete absorption from the GI tract (30-60 minutes)

Distribution: Lomustine and/or its metabolites penetrate into the CNS; metabolites are present in breast milk

Metabolism: Rapid conversion to 4-hydroxy metabolites (active) partially by liver microsomal enzymes during first pass through the liver

Half-life, terminal (active metabolite): 1.3-2 days

Time to peak serum concentration (of active metabolite): Within 3 hours

Elimination: Excreted primarily in urine as metabolites; <5% fecal excretion

Usual Dosage Oral (refer to individual protocol):

Children: 75-150 mg/m^2 as a single dose every 6 weeks; subsequent doses are readjusted after initial treatment according to platelet and leukocyte counts (see Precautions)

Adults: 100-130 mg/m^2 as a single dose every 6 weeks; readjust after initial treatment according to platelet and leukocyte counts (see Precautions)

With compromised marrow function: Initial dose: 100 mg/m^2 as a single dose every 6 weeks

Administration Oral: Administer with fluids on an empty stomach; do not administer food or drink for 2 hours after lomustine administration to decrease incidence of nausea and vomiting

Monitoring Parameters CBC with differential and platelet count, hepatic and renal function tests, pulmonary function tests

Patient Information Notify physician if fever, sore throat, bleeding, bruising, dry cough, shortness of breath, mental confusion, or yellowing of the eyes or skin occur; avoid alcohol for short periods after taking lomustine

Dosage Forms

Capsule: 10 mg, 40 mg, 100 mg

Capsule [dose pack]: 10 mg (2s); 40 mg (2s); 100 mg (2s)

References

Berg SL, Grisell DL, DeLaney TF, et al, "Principles of Treatment of Pediatric Solid Tumors," *Pediatr Clin North Am*, 1991, 38(2):249-67.

Pendergrass TW, Milstein JM, Geyer JR, et al, "Eight Drugs in One Day Chemotherapy for Brain Tumors: Experience in 107 Children and Rationale for Preradiation Chemotherapy," *J Clin Oncol*, 1987, 5(8):1221-31.

♦ **Loniten**® *see* Minoxidil *on page 768*

♦ **Lonox**® *see* Diphenoxylate and Atropine *on page 395*

♦ **Loperacap (Can)** *see* Loperamide *on page 687*

Loperamide (loe PER a mide)

Related Information

Carbohydrate and Alcohol Content of Liquid Medications for Use in Patients Receiving Ketogenic Diets *on page 1431*

U.S. Brand Names Imodium® A-D [OTC]; Imodium® Advanced

Canadian Brand Names Apo®-Loperamide; Diarr-Eze; Loperacap; Novo-Loperamide; PMS-Loperamide; Rho®-Loperamine; Riva-Loperamine

Therapeutic Category Antidiarrheal

Generic Available Yes (except caplet)

Use Treatment of acute diarrhea and chronic diarrhea associated with inflammatory bowel disease; chronic functional diarrhea (idiopathic), chronic diarrhea caused by bowel resection or organic lesions; to decrease the volume of ileostomy discharge

Pregnancy Risk Factor B

Contraindications Hypersensitivity to loperamide or any component; patients who must avoid constipation; infectious diarrhea resulting from organisms that penetrate the intestinal mucosa (eg, *Shigella*, *Salmonella*); patients with pseudomembranous colitis; bloody diarrhea

Warnings Imodium® A-D contains benzoic acid and sodium benzoate; benzoic acid (benzoate) is a metabolite of benzyl alcohol; large amounts of benzyl alcohol (≥99 mg/kg/day) have been associated with a potentially fatal toxicity ("gasping syndrome") in neonates; *in vitro* and animal studies have shown that benzoate displaces bilirubin from protein binding sites; avoid use in neonates

Precautions If clinical improvement in acute diarrhea is not observed in 48 hours, discontinue use; monitor patients with hepatic dysfunction closely for CNS toxicity

Adverse Reactions

Central nervous system: Sedation, fatigue, dizziness

Dermatologic: Rash

Gastrointestinal: Nausea, vomiting, constipation, abdominal cramping, xerostomia

Miscellaneous: Hypersensitivity reactions

Drug Interactions Additive CNS toxicity with CNS depressants, phenothiazines, tricyclic antidepressants, alcohol

Mechanism of Action Acts directly on intestinal muscles to inhibit peristalsis and prolong transit time

Pharmacodynamics Onset of action: Within 30-60 minutes

Pharmacokinetics

Absorption: Oral: 40%

Protein binding: 97%

Metabolism: Hepatic (>50%) to inactive compounds

Half-life: 9-14 hours

(Continued)

Loperamide *(Continued)*

Time to peak serum concentration:
Capsules: 5 hours
Liquid: 2.5 hours
Elimination: Fecal and urinary (1%) excretion of metabolites and unchanged drug (30% to 40%)

Usual Dosage Oral:

Acute diarrhea:

Children: Initial doses (in first 24 hours):

2-5 years: 1 mg 3 times/day

6-8 years: 2 mg twice daily

8-12 years: 2 mg 3 times/day

After initial dosing, 0.1 mg/kg doses after each loose stool but not exceeding initial dosage

Or as an alternative (manufacturer's recommendations):

6-8 years: 2 mg after first loose stool followed by 1 mg after each subsequent stool; maximum dose: 4 mg/day

9-11 years: 2 mg after first loose stool followed by 1 mg after each subsequent stool; maximum dose: 6 mg/day

12 years to Adults: 4 mg after first loose stool followed by 2 mg after each subsequent stool; maximum dose: 8 mg/day

Adults: 4 mg initially, followed by 2 mg after each loose stool, up to 16 mg/day

Chronic diarrhea: Children: 0.08-0.24 mg/kg/day divided 2-3 times/day, maximum dose: 2 mg/dose

Administration Oral: Drink plenty of fluids to help prevent dehydration

Patient Information Do not exceed maximum daily dosage; may cause drowsiness and impair ability to perform activities requiring mental alertness or physical coordination; if acute diarrhea lasts longer than 48 hours, consult physician; may cause dry mouth; avoid alcohol

Dosage Forms

Caplet, as hydrochloride:
Imodium® A-D: 2 mg
Imodium® Advanced: 2 mg [contains 125 mg simethicone]

Capsule, as hydrochloride: 2 mg

Liquid, oral, as hydrochloride: 1 mg/5 mL (5 mL, 10 mL, 120 mL)
Imodium® A-D: 1 mg/5 mL (60 mL, 120 mL) [contains benzoic acid and sodium benzoate; cherry mint flavor]

Tablet, as hydrochloride: 2 mg

Tablet, chewable, as hydrochloride (Imodium® Advanced): 2 mg [contains 125 mg simethicone; mint flavor]

Lopinavir and Ritonavir *(lop IN uh veer & rit ON uh veer)*

U.S. Brand Names Kaletra™

Synonyms ABT-378/Ritonavir; Ritonavir and Lopinavir

Therapeutic Category Antiretroviral Agent; HIV Agents (Anti-HIV Agents); Protease Inhibitor

Generic Available No

Use Treatment of HIV infection in combination with other antiretroviral agents (**Note:** HIV regimens consisting of three antiretroviral agents are strongly recommended)

Pregnancy Risk Factor C

Contraindications Hypersensitivity to lopinavir, ritonavir, or any component; concurrent therapy with medications that largely rely on cytochrome P450 isoenzymes CYP3A or CYP2D6 for clearance and that have an association between increased plasma concentrations and serious or life-threatening effects (eg, astemizole, cisapride, dihydroergotamine, ergonovine, ergotamine, flecainide, methylergonovine, midazolam, pimozide, propafenone, terfenadine, triazolam)

Warnings Lopinavir and ritonavir are potent CYP3A isoenzyme inhibitors that interact with numerous drugs. Due to potential serious and/or life-threatening drug interactions, some drugs are contraindicated (see Contraindications and Drug Interactions) and other medications may require concentration monitoring or dosage adjustment if coadministered with lopinavir and ritonavir (see Drug Interactions). Concomitant use with certain medications may require dosage adjustment of lopinavir and ritonavir (see Drug Interactions).

Potentially fatal pancreatitis may occur; markedly elevated serum triglycerides is a risk factor for developing pancreatitis; advanced HIV disease or a history of pancreatitis may also place patients at increased risk; discontinue lopinavir and ritonavir therapy if clinical signs, symptoms, or laboratory abnormalities suggestive of pancreatitis occur. New onset diabetes mellitus, exacerbations of diabetes, and hyperglycemia have been reported in HIV-infected patients receiving protease inhibitors.

Precautions Use with caution in patients with hepatic impairment (lopinavir and ritonavir are primarily metabolized by the liver); hepatitis or markedly elevated transaminases prior to therapy may increase risk for further elevations in liver enzymes or for hepatic decompensation; hepatic dysfunction (including fatalities) have been reported; in general, these occurred in patients with advanced HIV disease who were taking multiple concomitant medications and who had underlying chronic hepatitis or cirrhosis; a causal relationship with lopinavir/ritonavir has not been established; consider more frequent monitoring of liver enzymes in these patients, especially during the first few months of lopinavir/ritonavir therapy. Spontaneous bleeding episodes have been reported in patients with hemophilia type A and B receiving protease inhibitors. Large increases in total cholesterol and triglycerides have been reported; patients should be monitored prior to therapy and periodically during treatment. Fat redistribution and accumulation [ie, central obesity, peripheral wasting, facial wasting, breast enlargement, dorsocervical fat enlargement (buffalo hump), and cushingoid appearance] have been observed in patients receiving antiretroviral agents (causal relationship not established).

Adverse Reactions

Central nervous system: Headache (2% to 7%), insomnia (1% to 2%), pain

Dermatologic: Rash (1% to 4%; children 3%)

Endocrine & metabolic: Hyperglycemia (1% to 5%), hypertriglyceridemia (9% to 32%), hypercholesterolemia (9% to 33%), hyperuricemia (up to 4%); new onset diabetes, exacerbation of diabetes mellitus; decreased serum sodium (children 3%), decreased serum phosphorus (up to 2%); fat redistribution and accumulation (see Precautions)

Gastrointestinal: Nausea (2% to 15%), vomiting (2% to 5%), diarrhea (16% to 24%), abnormal stools (up to 6%), abdominal pain (2% to 5%), elevated amylase (3% to 6%)

Hematologic: Decreased platelets (children 4%), decreased neutrophils (1% to 4%), possible spontaneous bleeding in hemophiliacs

Hepatic: Elevated liver enzymes, elevated bilirubin (children 3%)

Neuromuscular & skeletal: Asthenia (4% to 8%)

Drug Interactions Cytochrome P450 isoenzyme CYP3A substrate and inhibitor; CYP2D6 isoenzyme inhibitor (to a lesser degree than CYP3A); may induce glucuronidation; does not inhibit CYP1A2, CYP2B6, CYP2C9, CYP2C19, or CYP2E1 at clinically obtained concentrations

Lopinavir/ritonavir may inhibit the metabolism of the following drugs and cause serious or life-threatening adverse effects: Astemizole, cisapride, dihydroergotamine, ergonovine, ergotamine, flecainide, methylergonovine, midazolam, pimozide, propafenone, terfenadine, triazolam (concurrent therapy with these drugs and lopinavir/ritonavir is contraindicated). Lopinavir/ritonavir may increase the toxic effects of amiodarone, bepridil, systemic lidocaine, quinidine, warfarin, cyclosporine, tacrolimus, rapamycin (serum concentration monitoring of these drugs is necessary). Lopinavir/ritonavir may increase the concentrations of the following drugs: Clarithromycin (decrease clarithromycin dosage in patients with renal impairment), ketoconazole (high dose ketoconazole is not recommended), itraconazole (high dose itraconazole is not recommended), rifabutin and rifabutin metabolite (rifabutin dose should be decreased by at least 75% of the normal dose; further reduction in dosage may be needed, monitor closely for adverse effects). Lopinavir/ritonavir may also increase serum concentrations or toxicity of lovastatin or simvastatin (concurrent use of these agents is not recommended), atorvastatin or cerivastatin (use lowest possible dose of these agents, monitor closely; consider use of pravastatin, fluvastatin), nifedipine, felodipine, nicardipine, sildenafil. When given with reduced doses of concurrent protease inhibitors, lopinavir/ritonavir may increase the trough concentrations of amprenavir, indinavir, and saquinavir, but AUCs may be similar (appropriate doses of combination protease inhibitors have not been established).

Lopinavir/ritonavir may decrease the concentrations of atovaquone and methadone (increased doses of these agents may be needed). Lopinavir/ritonavir may decrease the efficacy of estrogen-based oral contraceptives (additional or alternative contraceptive methods should be used). Lopinavir/ritonavir may potentially decrease abacavir and zidovudine concentrations through induction of glucuronidation (clinical significance unknown).

Rifampin may significantly reduce lopinavir/ritonavir plasma concentrations and should not be used concurrently. The herbal medicine St John's wort (*Hypericum perforatum*) may significantly decrease concentrations of lopinavir/ritonavir and is not recommended for concurrent use. Efavirenz and nevirapine decrease lopinavir concentrations (an increased dose of lopinavir/ritonavir should be considered). (Continued)

Lopinavir and Ritonavir *(Continued)*

Phenobarbital, phenytoin, carbamazepine, dexamethasone may decrease lopinavir concentrations (these agents may decrease effectiveness of lopinavir/ritonavir, use with caution). Delavirdine and ritonavir may increase lopinavir concentrations.

Oral solution contains alcohol and may produce disulfiram-like reaction when coadministered with disulfiram or metronidazole. Didanosine should be given at least 1 hour before or 2 hours after lopinavir/ritonavir.

Food Interactions Compared to fasting, a moderate fat meal increased lopinavir AUC by 48% (capsules) and 80% (oral solution); a high fat meal increased lopinavir AUC by 97% (capsules) and 130% (oral solution)

Stability Capsules and oral solution: Store at 2°C to 8°C (36°F to 46°F) until dispensed; refrigerated products are stable until labeled expiration date; stability at room temperature: 2 months; avoid exposure to excessive heat

Mechanism of Action This product is a fixed-dose combination of lopinavir and ritonavir; antiretroviral effects are due to lopinavir, a protease inhibitor; lopinavir acts on an enzyme (protease) late in the HIV replication process after the virus has entered into the cell's nucleus. Lopinavir binds to the protease activity site and inhibits the activity of the enzyme, thus preventing cleavage of viral polyprotein precursors (gag-pol protein precursors) into individual functional proteins found in infectious HIV. This results in the formation of immature, noninfectious viral particles. Ritonavir inhibits the metabolism of lopinavir via the cytochrome P450 CYP3A isoenzyme pathway and significantly increases plasma concentrations of lopinavir.

Pharmacokinetics Information below refers to Lopinavir; see Ritonavir *on page 993* for additional information.

Protein binding: 98% to 99%; binds to both alpha$_1$ - acid glycoprotein and albumin; higher affinity for alpha$_1$-acid glycoprotein

Metabolism: Primarily oxidative, via cytochrome P450 CYP3A isoenzyme; 13 oxidative metabolites identified; may induce its own metabolism

Bioavailability: Absolute bioavailability not established; AUC for oral solution was 22% lower than capsule when given under fasting conditions; concentrations were similar under nonfasting conditions

Half-life: Adults: Mean: 5-6 hours

Elimination: 2.2% of dose eliminated unchanged in urine; 83% of dose eliminated in feces

Clearance: (Apparent oral): Adults: 6-7 L/hour

Dialysis: Unlikely to remove significant amounts of drug (due to high protein binding)

Usual Dosage Oral:

Patients receiving concomitant antiretroviral therapy **without** efavirenz or nevirapine:
Children 6 months to 12 years: Dosage based on weight and lopinavir component:
7 to <15 kg: Lopinavir 12 mg/kg twice daily
15-40 kg: Lopinavir 10 mg/kg twice daily
>40 kg: Lopinavir 400 mg (3 capsules or 5 mL) twice daily
Children >12 years and Adults: Lopinavir 400 mg/ritonavir 100 mg (3 capsules or 5 mL) twice daily

Treatment of experienced patients with suspected reduced susceptibility to lopinavir who are receiving concomitant antiretroviral therapy **with efavirenz or nevirapine**:
Children 6 months to 12 years: Dosage based on weight and lopinavir component:
7 to <15 kg: Lopinavir 13 mg/kg twice daily
15-45 kg: Lopinavir 11 mg/kg twice daily
>45 kg: Lopinavir 533 mg (4 capsules or 6.5 mL) twice daily
Children >12 years and Adults: Lopinavir 533 mg/ritonavir 133 mg (4 capsules or 6.5 mL) twice daily

Dosing adjustment in renal impairment: Has not been studied in patients with renal impairment; however, a decrease in clearance is not expected

Dosing adjustment in hepatic impairment: Plasma levels may be increased in patients with hepatic impairment

Administration Oral: Administer with food to enhance bioavailability and decrease kinetic variability

Monitoring Parameters Signs and symptoms of pancreatitis; serum electrolytes, glucose, triglycerides, cholesterol, liver enzymes, bilirubin, amylase, CBC with differential, platelets, CD4 cell count, viral load

Patient Information Lopinavir and ritonavir is not a cure for HIV; notify physician if symptoms of pancreatitis occur (nausea, vomiting, abdominal pain); report the use of other medications, nonprescription medications and herbal or natural products to your physician and pharmacist; avoid the herbal medicine St John's wort; take lopinavir and ritonavir everyday as prescribed; do not change dose or discontinue without physician's advice; if a dose is missed, take it as soon as possible, then return to normal dosing schedule; if a dose is skipped, do not double the next dose

HIV medications may cause changes in body fat, including an increase in fat in the upper back and neck, breasts, and trunk; a loss of fat from the face, arms, and legs may also occur.

Additional Information Oral solution contains 42.4% alcohol (v/v); overdose in a child may cause potentially lethal alcohol toxicity; treatment should be supportive and include general poisoning management; activated charcoal may help remove unabsorbed medication; dialysis unlikely to be of benefit

Preliminary studies have reported response rates (defined as viral loads <400 copies/mL) of 91%, 81%, and 33% for patients with 0-5, 6-7, and 8-10 protease mutations at baseline, respectively (see Hurst, 2000)

Dosage Forms
Capsule: Lopinavir 133.3 mg and ritonavir 33.3 mg
Solution, oral: Lopinavir 80 mg and ritonavir 20 mg per mL (160 mL) [contains 42.4% alcohol]

References
Center for Disease Control and Prevention, "Guidelines for Using Antiretroviral Agents Among HIV-Infected Adults and Adolescents. Recommendations of the Panel on Clinical Practices for Treatment of HIV," *MMWR*, 2002, 51(RR-7):1-55.

Hurst M and Faulds D, "Lopinavir," *Drugs*, 2000, 60(6):1371-9.

Mangum EM and Graham KK, "Lopinavir-Ritonavir: A New Protease Inhibitor," *Pharmacotherapy*, 2001, 21(11):1352-63.

Panel on Clinical Practices for Treatment of HIV Infection, "Guidelines for the Use of Antiretroviral Agents in HIV-Infected Adults and Adolescents," February 4, 2002, http://www.aidsinfo.nih.gov.

Piscitelli SC, Burstein AH, Chaitt D, et al, "Indinavir Concentrations and St John's Wort," *Lancet*, 2000, 355(9203):547-8.

Working Group on Antiretroviral Therapy and Medical Management of HIV-Infected Children, "Guidelines for the Use of Antiretroviral Agents in Pediatric HIV Infection," December 14, 2001, http://www.aidsinfo.nih.gov.

Working Group on Antiretroviral Therapy and Medical Management of HIV-Infected Children, "Guidelines for the Use of Antiretroviral Agents in Pediatric HIV Infection. Hyperlink Supplement I: Pediatric Antiretroviral Drug Information," December 14, 2001, http://www.aidsinfo.nih.gov.

♦ **Lopremone** *see* Protirelin *on page 956*

♦ **Lopressor®** *see* Metoprolol *on page 752*

♦ **Lorabid®** *see* Loracarbef *on page 691*

Loracarbef (lor a KAR bef)
Related Information
Carbohydrate and Alcohol Content of Liquid Medications for Use in Patients Receiving Ketogenic Diets *on page 1431*
U.S. Brand Names Lorabid®
Therapeutic Category Antibiotic, Carbacephem
Generic Available No
Use Treatment of mild to moderate community-acquired infections of the respiratory tract, skin and skin structure, and urinary tract that are caused by susceptible *S. pneumoniae*, *H. influenzae*, *M. catarrhalis*, *S. aureus*, *S. pyogenes*, and *E. coli*
Pregnancy Risk Factor B
Contraindications Hypersensitivity to loracarbef, any component, or cephalosporins
Warnings Prolonged use may result in superinfection or pseudomembranous colitis
Precautions Use with caution in patients with a previous history of hypersensitivity to other beta-lactam antibiotics (eg, penicillins); use with caution in patients with impaired renal function and patients with a history of colitis; modify dosage in patients with renal impairment
Adverse Reactions
Cardiovascular: Vasodilation
Central nervous system: Headache, somnolence, nervousness, dizziness, insomnia
Dermatologic: Skin rashes, urticaria, pruritus, erythema multiforme, Stevens-Johnson syndrome
Gastrointestinal: Diarrhea, nausea, vomiting, abdominal pain, anorexia, pseudomembranous colitis
Genitourinary: Candidal vaginitis
Hematologic: Transient thrombocytopenia, leukopenia, eosinophilia, prolongation of prothrombin time
Hepatic: Transient elevations of ALT, AST, alkaline phosphatase; cholestasis, jaundice
Renal: Transient elevation of BUN and serum creatinine
Respiratory: Rhinitis
Miscellaneous: Anaphylaxis, superinfection
Drug Interactions Probenecid inhibits renal excretion and increases the serum concentration of loracarbef
Food Interactions Administration with food decreases and delays the peak plasma concentration
(Continued)

Loracarbef *(Continued)*

Stability After reconstitution, suspension may be stored at room temperature for 14 days

Mechanism of Action Inhibits bacterial cell wall synthesis by binding to one or more of the penicillin binding proteins; inhibits the final transpeptidation step of peptidoglycan synthesis in bacterial cell walls, thus inhibiting cell wall biosynthesis. Upon exposure to beta-lactam antibiotics, bacteria eventually lyse due to ongoing activity of cell wall autolytic enzymes (autolysins and murein hydrolases) while cell wall assembly is arrested.

Pharmacokinetics

Absorption: Oral: Rapid; 90% absorbed from the GI tract

Distribution: Loracarbef middle-ear fluid concentration approximates 48% of the plasma concentration 2 hours after a dose in pediatric patients

Protein binding: 25%

Bioavailability: 90%

Half-life, elimination:

Children (suspension): ~0.78-0.85 hours

Adults, normal renal function: ~1 hour

Time to peak serum concentration: 0.5-1 hour after administration

Elimination: Primarily by the kidneys as unchanged drug in the urine

Usual Dosage Oral:

Children 6 months to 12 years:

Acute otitis media: 30 mg/kg/day divided every 12 hours for 10 days (should be treated with the **suspension** which results in higher peak plasma concentrations than the capsule)

Acute maxillary sinusitis: 30 mg/kg/day divided every 12 hours for 10 days

Pharyngitis/tonsillitis/skin and skin structure infections: 15 mg/kg/day divided every 12 hours

Adults:

Pneumonia, chronic bacterial bronchitis, sinusitis: 400 mg every 12 hours

Acute bacterial bronchitis: 200-400 mg every 12 hours

Uncomplicated urinary tract infections: 200 mg once daily for 7 days

Skin and skin structure: 200 mg every 12 hours

Uncomplicated pyelonephritis: 400 mg every 12 hours for 14 days

Dosing adjustment in renal impairment:

Cl_{cr} 10-49 mL/minute: 50% of usual dose at usual interval or usual dose given half as often

Cl_{cr} <10 mL/minute: Give usual dose every 3-5 days

Hemodialysis: Removed by hemodialysis; postdialysis dose should be administered when appropriate

Administration Oral: Administer on an empty stomach at least 1 hour before or 2 hours after meals; shake suspension well before use

Monitoring Parameters Observe patient for diarrhea; with prolonged therapy, monitor renal function periodically

Dosage Forms

Capsule: 200 mg, 400 mg

Powder for oral suspension: 100 mg/5 mL (100 mL); 200 mg/5 mL (100 mL) [strawberry-bubblegum flavor]

References

Force RW and Nahata MC, "Loracarbef: A New Orally Administered Carbacephem Antibiotic," *Ann Pharmacother*, 1993, 27(3):321-9.

Foshee WS, "Loracarbef (LY163892) Versus Amoxicillin-Clavulanate in the Treatment of Acute Otitis Media With Effusion," *J Pediatr*, 1992, 120(6):980-6.

Nelson JD, Shelton S, and Kusmiesz H, "Pharmacokinetics of LY163892 in Infants and Children," *Antimicrob Agents Chemother*, 1988, 32(11):1738-9.

Loratadine *(lor AT a deen)*

U.S. Brand Names Alavert™ [OTC]; Claritin® [OTC]; Claritin® RediTab® [OTC]

Canadian Brand Names Apo®-Loratadine

Therapeutic Category Antihistamine

Generic Available No

Use Symptomatic relief of nasal and non-nasal symptoms of allergic rhinitis; treatment of chronic idiopathic urticaria

Pregnancy Risk Factor B

Contraindications Hypersensitivity to loratadine or any component

Warnings Use with caution and adjust dosage in patients with severe liver impairment or renal impairment; Claritin® syrup contains sodium benzoate; benzoic acid (benzoate) is a metabolite of benzyl alcohol; large amounts of benzyl alcohol (≥99 mg/kg/day) have been associated with a potentially fatal toxicity ("gasping syndrome") in neonates; *in vitro* and animal studies have shown that benzoate displaces bilirubin from protein binding sites; avoid use in neonates

Precautions Use cautiously in patients who are also taking ketoconazole, itraconazole, fluconazole, erythromycin, clarithromycin, or other drugs which may impair loratadine's hepatic metabolism; although increased plasma levels of loratadine have been observed, no adverse effects with concomitant administration have been reported including QT interval prolongation which has occurred when similar antihistamines, terfenadine and astemizole, were combined with these agents; while less sedating than other antihistamines, loratadine may cause drowsiness and impair ability to perform hazardous activities requiring mental alertness. Use cautiously in breast-feeding women as breast milk levels of loratadine are equivalent to serum levels. Alavert™ contains phenylalanine which must be avoided (or used with caution) in patients with phenylketonuria.

Adverse Reactions

Cardiovascular: Hypotension, hypertension, palpitations, tachycardia, chest pain, syncope

Central nervous system: Headache, somnolence, fatigue, anxiety, depression, dizziness, fever, migraine, agitation, nervousness, hyperactivity

Dermatologic: Alopecia, dermatitis, dry skin, rash, pruritus, photosensitivity

Gastrointestinal: Xerostomia, nausea, vomiting, gastritis, abdominal pain, diarrhea

Endocrine & metabolic: Breast pain and enlargement (rare), menorrhagia, dysmenorrhea

Neuromuscular & skeletal: Hyperkinesia, arthralgias, myalgias, leg cramps

Ocular: Blurred vision, altered lacrimation, eye pain, conjunctivitis

Genitourinary: Discoloration of urine

Respiratory: Nasal dryness, pharyngitis, dyspnea, nasal congestion, wheezing, nose bleed

Miscellaneous: Diaphoresis

Drug Interactions Cytochrome P450 isoenzyme CYP2D6 and CYP3A3/4 substrate Increased plasma concentrations and AUC of loratadine and its active metabolite with ketoconazole, erythromycin, and cimetidine; no change in QT_c interval or cardiac arrhythmias have been seen (see Warnings); a prolonged QT interval was reported in one patient who was receiving quinidine and loratadine; additive CNS depression with other CNS depressants, alcohol, and procarbazine; prolonged anticholinergic effects with MAO inhibitors

Food Interactions Administration with food increases loratadine's bioavailability by 40%

Mechanism of Action Long-acting tricyclic antihistamine with selective peripheral histamine H_1 receptor antagonistic properties

Pharmacodynamics

Onset of action: Within 1-3 hours

Maximum effect: 8-12 hours

Duration: >24 hours

Pharmacokinetics

Absorption: Rapid; food increases total bioavailability (AUC) by 40%

Distribution: Binds preferentially to peripheral nervous system H_1 receptors; no appreciable entry into CNS; loratadine and metabolite pass easily into breast milk and achieve concentrations equivalent to plasma levels; breast milk to plasma ratio: 1.17

Protein binding: 97% (loratadine), 73% to 77% (metabolite)

Metabolism: Extensive first-pass metabolism by cytochrome P450 system to an active metabolite (descarboethoxyloratadine)

Half-life: 8.4 hours (loratadine), 28 hours (metabolite)

Time to peak serum concentration: 1-2 hours

Elimination: 80% eliminated via urine & feces as metabolic products

Usual Dosage Oral:

Children 2-5 years: 5 mg once daily

Children ≥6 years and Adults: 10 mg once daily

Dosing interval in renal (GFR <30 mL/minute) or hepatic impairment: Administer dosage every other day

Administration Oral: Administer on an empty stomach or before meals; place Claritin® RediTab® (rapidly disintegrating tablet) on the tongue; tablet disintegration occurs rapidly; may administer with or without water

Monitoring Parameters Improvement in signs and symptoms of allergic rhinitis or chronic idiopathic urticaria

Reference Range Therapeutic serum levels (not used clinically): Loratadine: 2.5-100 ng/mL; active metabolite: 0.5-100 ng/mL

Test Interactions Antigen skin testing

(Continued)

Loratadine *(Continued)*

Patient Information Drink plenty of water; may cause dry mouth; may color urine; may cause drowsiness and impair ability to perform activities requiring mental alertness or physical coordination; notify physician if fainting episode occurs; avoid alcohol. May rarely cause photosensitivity reactions (eg, exposure to sunlight may cause severe sunburn, skin rash, redness, or itching); avoid direct exposure to sunlight

Dosage Forms
Syrup (Claritin®): 1 mg/mL (480 mL) [contains sodium benzoate]
Tablet (Claritin®): 10 mg
Tablet, rapid-disintegrating:
Alavert™: 10 mg [contains 8.4 mg phenylalanine/tablet]
Claritin® RediTab®: 10 mg [mint flavor]

References
Lin CC, Radwanski E, Affrime M, et al, "Pharmacokinetics of Loratadine in Pediatric Subjects," *Am J Therapeut*, 1995, 2:504-8.
Luck JC and Evrard HM, "Atrial Fibrillation Associated With Loratadine Use," *J Allergy Clin Immunol*, 1995, 95(2):282.
Lutsky BN, Klose P, Melon J, et al, "A Comparative Study of the Efficacy and Safety of Loratadine Syrup and Terfenadine Suspension in the Treatment of 3 to 6 Year Old Children With Seasonal Allergic Rhinitis," *Clin Ther*, 1993, 15(5):855-65.
Salmun LM, Herron JM, Banfield C, et al, "The Pharmacokinetics, Electrocardiographic Effects, and Tolerability of Loratadine Syrup in Children Aged 2 to 5 Years," *Clin Ther*, 2000, 22(5):613-21.

Loratadine and Pseudoephedrine
(lor AT a deen & soo doe e FED rin)
U.S. Brand Names Claritin-D® 12-Hour [OTC]; Claritin-D® 24-Hour [OTC]
Therapeutic Category Antihistamine/Decongestant Combination
Generic Available No
Use Symptomatic relief of symptoms of seasonal allergic rhinitis and nasal congestion
Pregnancy Risk Factor B
Contraindications Hypersensitivity to loratadine, pseudoephedrine, or any component; MAO inhibitor therapy; severe hypertension; severe coronary artery disease; narrow-angle glaucoma
Precautions Use with caution and adjust dosage in patients with renal impairment; use with caution in patients with hyperthyroidism, diabetes mellitus, prostatic hypertrophy, mild to moderate hypertension, arrhythmias; use cautiously in patients who are also taking ketoconazole, itraconazole, fluconazole, erythromycin, clarithromycin, or other drugs which may impair loratadine's hepatic metabolism; although increased plasma levels of loratadine have been observed, no adverse effects with concomitant administration have been reported including QT interval prolongation which has occurred when similar antihistamines, terfenadine and astemizole, were combined with these agents; while less sedating than other antihistamines, loratadine may cause drowsiness and impair ability to perform hazardous activities requiring mental alertness, the CNS stimulant properties of pseudoephedrine may counteract this effect. Use cautiously in breast-feeding women as breast milk levels of loratadine are equivalent to serum levels.
Adverse Reactions See individual monographs for Loratadine *on page 692* and Pseudoephedrine *on page 958*.
Drug Interactions See individual monographs for Loratadine *on page 692* and Pseudoephedrine *on page 958*.
Food Interactions Administration with food increases loratadine's bioavailability by 40%
Mechanism of Action Loratadine is a long-acting tricyclic antihistamine with selective peripheral histamine H_1-receptor antagonistic properties. Pseudoephedrine directly stimulates alpha-adrenergic receptors of respiratory mucosa causing vasoconstriction and directly stimulates beta-adrenergic receptors causing bronchial relaxation, increased heart rate and contractility
Pharmacokinetics See individual monographs for Loratadine *on page 692* and Pseudoephedrine *on page 958*.
Usual Dosage Oral: Children ≥12 years and Adults:
Claritin-D® 12-Hour: 1 tablet every 12 hours
Claritin-D® 24-Hour: 1 tablet every 24 hours
Dosage adjustment in renal impairment: Cl_{cr} <30 mL/minute:
Claritin-D® 12-Hour: 1 tablet every 24 hours
Claritin-D® 24-Hour: 1 tablet every other day
Administration Oral: Administer on an empty stomach or before meals; swallow extended release tablets whole, do not chew or crush
Monitoring Parameters Improvement in signs and symptoms of allergic rhinitis or nasal congestion

Reference Range Therapeutic serum levels (not used clinically): Loratadine: 2.5-100 ng/mL; active metabolite: 0.5-100 ng/mL

Test Interactions Antigen skin testing; false-positive test for amphetamines by EMIT assay

Patient Information Drink plenty of water; may cause dry mouth; may color urine; notify physician if fainting episode occurs; avoid alcohol. May rarely cause photosensitivity reactions (eg, exposure to sunlight may cause severe sunburn, skin rash, redness, or itching); avoid direct exposure to sunlight

Dosage Forms
Tablet, extended release:
Claritin-D® 12-hour: Loratadine 5 mg and pseudoephedrine sulfate 120 mg
Claritin-D® 24-hour: Loratadine 10 mg and pseudoephedrine sulfate 240 mg

Lorazepam (lor A ze pam)

Related Information
Carbohydrate and Alcohol Content of Liquid Medications for Use in Patients Receiving Ketogenic Diets *on page 1431*
Drugs and Breast-Feeding *on page 1404*
Overdose and Toxicology *on page 1388*
Preprocedure Sedatives in Children *on page 1367*

U.S. Brand Names Ativan®; Lorazepam Intensol®

Canadian Brand Names Apo®-Lorazepam; Novo-Lorazepam®; Nu-Loraz; Riva-Lorazepam

Therapeutic Category Antianxiety Agent; Anticonvulsant, Benzodiazepine; Antiemetic; Benzodiazepine; Hypnotic; Sedative

Generic Available Yes

Use Management of anxiety; status epilepticus; preoperative sedation and amnesia

Restrictions C-IV

Pregnancy Risk Factor D

Contraindications Hypersensitivity to lorazepam or any component (see Warnings); there may be a cross-sensitivity with other benzodiazepines; do not use in a comatose patient, those with pre-existing CNS depression, narrow-angle glaucoma, severe uncontrolled pain, severe hypotension

Warnings Dilute injection prior to I.V. use with equal volume of compatible diluent (D_5W, NS, SWI); do not inject intra-arterially, arteriospasm and gangrene may occur; abrupt discontinuation after prolonged use may result in withdrawal symptoms or seizures

Injection contains 2% benzyl alcohol, polyethylene glycol, and propylene glycol, which may be toxic to newborns in high doses; benzyl alcohol may cause allergic reactions in susceptible individuals; large amounts of benzyl alcohol (≥99 mg/kg/day) have been associated with a potentially fatal toxicity ("gasping syndrome") in neonates; the "gasping syndrome" consists of metabolic acidosis, respiratory distress, gasping respirations, CNS dysfunction (including convulsions, intracranial hemorrhage), hypotension and cardiovascular collapse; use lorazepam products containing benzyl alcohol with caution in neonates; *in vitro* and animal studies have shown that benzoate, a metabolite of benzyl alcohol, displaces bilirubin from protein binding sites

Precautions Use with caution in neonates, especially in preterm infants (several cases of neurotoxicity and myoclonus have been reported); use with caution in patients with renal or hepatic impairment, compromised pulmonary function, or those receiving other CNS depressants

Adverse Reactions
Cardiovascular: Bradycardia, circulatory collapse, hypertension, or hypotension
Central nervous system: Confusion, CNS depression, sedation, drowsiness, lethargy, hangover effect, dizziness, transitory hallucinations, ataxia, rhythmic myoclonic jerking in preterm infants
Gastrointestinal: Constipation, xerostomia, nausea, vomiting
Genitourinary: Urinary incontinence or retention
Local: Pain with injection
Ocular: Diplopia, nystagmus
Respiratory: Respiratory depression, apnea
Miscellaneous: Physical and psychological dependence with prolonged use

Drug Interactions Other CNS or respiratory depressants may increase adverse effects

Stability Do not use if injection is discolored or contains precipitate; protect from light; refrigerate injectable form and oral solution; injection is stable at room temperature for 8 weeks
(Continued)

Lorazepam *(Continued)*

Mechanism of Action Depresses all levels of the CNS, including the limbic and reticular formation, by binding to the benzodiazepine site on the gamma-aminobutyric acid (GABA) receptor complex and modulating GABA, which is a major inhibitory neurotransmitter in the brain

Pharmacodynamics Sedation:

Onset of action:

Oral: Within 60 minutes

I.M.: 30-60 minutes

I.V.: 15-30 minutes

Duration: 8-12 hours

Pharmacokinetics

Absorption: Oral, I.M.: Rapid, complete

Distribution: Crosses into placenta; crosses into breast milk

V_d:

Neonates: 0.76 L/kg

Adults: 1.3 L/kg

Protein binding: ~85%

Metabolism: Primarily by glucuronide conjugation in the liver

Bioavailability: Oral: 90% to 93%

Half-life:

Full-term neonates: 40.2 hours; range: 18-73 hours

Older Children: 10.5 hours; range: 6-17 hours

Adults: 12.9 hours; range: 10-16 hours

Elimination: In urine primarily as the glucuronide conjugate

Usual Dosage

Adjunct to antiemetic therapy:

Children: I.V.: Limited information exists in the literature, especially for multiple doses:

Single dose: 0.04-0.08 mg/kg/dose prior to chemotherapy (maximum dose: 4 mg)

Multiple doses: Some centers use 0.02-0.05 mg/kg/dose (maximum dose: 2 mg) every 6 hours as needed

Adults: Oral, I.V.: 0.5-2 mg every 4-6 hours as needed

Anxiety/sedation:

Infants and Children: Oral, I.V.: Usual: 0.05 mg/kg/dose (maximum dose: 2 mg/dose) every 4-8 hours; range: 0.02-0.1 mg/kg

Adults: Oral: 1-10 mg/day in 2-3 divided doses; usual dose: 2-6 mg/day in divided doses

Insomnia: Adults: Oral: 2-4 mg at bedtime

Operative amnesia: Adults: I.V.: up to 0.05 mg/kg; maximum dose: 4 mg/dose

Preoperative: Adults: I.M.: 0.05 mg/kg administered 2 hours before surgery; maximum dose: 4 mg/dose; I.V.: 0.044 mg/kg 15-20 minutes before surgery; usual maximum dose: 2 mg/dose

Sedation (preprocedure): Infants and Children:

Oral, I.M., I.V.: Usual: 0.05 mg/kg; range: 0.02-0.09 mg/kg

I.V.: may use smaller doses (eg, 0.01-0.03 mg/kg) and repeat every 20 minutes, as needed to titrate to effect

Status epilepticus: I.V.:

Neonates: 0.05 mg/kg over 2-5 minutes; may repeat in 10-15 minutes (see warning regarding benzyl alcohol)

Infants and Children: 0.1 mg/kg slow I.V. over 2-5 minutes, do not exceed 4 mg/single dose; may repeat second dose of 0.05 mg/kg slow I.V. in 10-15 minutes if needed

Adolescents: 0.07 mg/kg slow I.V. over 2-5 minutes; maximum dose: 4 mg/dose; may repeat in 10-15 minutes

Adults: 4 mg/dose given slowly over 2-5 minutes; may repeat in 10-15 minutes; usual total maximum dose per 12-hour period: 8 mg

Administration

Oral: May administer with food to decrease GI distress; dilute oral solution in water, juice, soda, or semisolid food (eg, applesauce, pudding)

Parenteral: I.V.: Do not exceed 2 mg/minute or 0.05 mg/kg over 2-5 minutes; dilute I.V. dose with equal volume of compatible diluent (D_5W, NS, SWI); administer I.V. using repeated aspiration with slow I.V. injection, to make sure the injection is not intra-arterial and that perivascular extravasation has not occurred

Monitoring Parameters Respiratory rate, blood pressure, heart rate; CBC with differential and liver function with long-term use

Patient Information Avoid alcohol; limit caffeine; may be habit-forming; avoid abrupt discontinuation after prolonged use; may cause drowsiness and impair ability to perform activities requiring mental alertness or physical coordination; may cause dry mouth

Additional Information Single oral doses >0.09 mg/kg produced increased ataxia without increasing sedative benefit vs lower doses; since both strengths of injection contain 2% benzyl alcohol, Neofax® recommends using the 4 mg/mL strength for dilution with **preservative free** SWI to make a 0.4 mg/mL dilution for I.V. use in neonates (in order to decrease the amount of benzyl alcohol delivered to the neonate); however, the stability of this dilution has not been studied. Diarrhea in a 9 month old infant receiving high-dose oral lorazepam was attributed to the lorazepam oral solution that contained polyethylene glycol and propylene glycol (both are osmotically active); diarrhea resolved when crushed tablets were substituted for the oral solution (see Marshall, 1995).

Dosage Forms

Injection, solution (Ativan®): 2 mg/mL (1 mL, 10 mL); 4 mg/mL (1 mL, 10 mL) [contains 2% benzyl alcohol, polyethylene glycol, and propylene glycol]

Solution, oral **concentrate** (Lorazepam Intensol®): 2 mg/mL (30 mL) [alcohol and dye free]

Tablet (Ativan®): 0.5 mg, 1 mg, 2 mg

References

Crawford TO, Mitchell WG, and Snodgrass SR, "Lorazepam in Childhood Status Epilepticus and Serial Seizures: Effectiveness and Tachyphylaxis," *Neurology*, 1987, 37(2):190-5.

Deshmukh A, Wittert W, Schnitzler E, et al, "Lorazepam in the Treatment of Refractory Neonatal Seizures: A Pilot Study," *Am J Dis Child*, 1986, 140(10):1042-4.

Henry DW, Burwinkle JW, and Klutman NE, "Determination of Sedative and Amnestic Doses of Lorazepam in Children," *Clin Pharm*, 1991, 10(8):625-9.

Lee DS, Wong HA, and Knoppert DC, "Myoclonus Associated With Lorazepam Therapy in Very-Low-Birth-Weight Infants," *Biol Neonate*, 1994, 66(6):311-5.

Marshall JD, Farrar HC, and Kearns GL, "Diarrhea Associated With Enteral Benzodiazepine Solutions," *J Pediatr*, 1995, 126(4):657-9.

McDermott CA, Kowalczyk AL, Schnitzler ER, et al, "Pharmacokinetics of Lorazepam in Critically Ill Neonates With Seizures," *J Pediatr*, 1992, 120(3):479-83.

♦ **Lorazepam Intensol®** *see* Lorazepam *on page 695*

♦ **Lorcet® 10/650** *see* Hydrocodone and Acetaminophen *on page 571*

♦ **Lorcet®-HD** *see* Hydrocodone and Acetaminophen *on page 571*

♦ **Lorcet® Plus** *see* Hydrocodone and Acetaminophen *on page 571*

♦ **Loroxide® [OTC]** *see* Benzoyl Peroxide *on page 165*

♦ **Lortab®** *see* Hydrocodone and Acetaminophen *on page 571*

♦ **Losec® (Can)** *see* Omeprazole *on page 832*

♦ **Lotrimin®** *see* Clotrimazole *on page 297*

♦ **Lotrimin AF® [OTC]** *see* Clotrimazole *on page 297*

♦ **Lotrimin® AF Powder/Spray [OTC]** *see* Miconazole *on page 759*

Lovastatin (LOE va sta tin)

U.S. Brand Names Altocor™; Mevacor®

Canadian Brand Names Apo®-Lovastatin; Gen-Lovastatin; ratio-Lovastatin

Synonyms Mevinolin; Monacolin K

Therapeutic Category Antilipemic Agent; HMG-CoA Reductase Inhibitor

Generic Available Yes (immediate release tablet)

Use Adjunct to dietary therapy to decrease elevated serum total and low density lipoprotein cholesterol (LDL-C) concentrations in primary hypercholesterolemia and adolescent patients with heterozygous familial hypercholesterolemia; primary prevention of coronary artery disease [patients without symptomatic disease with average to moderately elevated total and LDL-C and below average high density lipoprotein cholesterol (HDL-C)]

Pregnancy Risk Factor X

Contraindications Hypersensitivity to lovastatin or any component; active liver disease; unexplained persistent elevations of serum transaminases; pregnancy; breast-feeding

Warnings Rhabdomyolysis with or without acute renal failure secondary to myoglobinuria has occurred rarely and is dose-related. Risk is increased with concurrent use of clarithromycin, danazol, diltiazem, fluvoxamine, indinavir, nefazodone, nelfinavir, ritonavir, verapamil, troleandomycin, cyclosporine, fibric acid derivatives, erythromycin, niacin, azole antifungals and large quantities of grapefruit juice (>1 quart/day). Assess the risk versus benefit before combining any of these drugs with lovastatin. Temporarily discontinue lovastatin in any patient experiencing an acute or serious condition predisposing to renal failure secondary to rhabdomyolysis.

Precautions Persistent increases in serum transaminases have occurred; liver function must be monitored by laboratory assessment at the initiation of therapy, at 6 and 12 weeks after initiation of therapy, and periodically thereafter; use with caution in patients with history of heavy alcohol use; use with caution and modify dose in (Continued)

Lovastatin *(Continued)*

patients with renal impairment or receiving concomitant amiodarone, cyclosporine, fibrates, lipid-lowering doses of niacin, or verapamil. Lovastatin is less effective in patients with rare **homozygous** familial hypercholesterolemia and may be more likely to elevate serum transaminases.

Adverse Reactions

Cardiovascular: Chest pain

Central nervous system: Headache, dizziness, insomnia, tremor, vertigo, memory loss, psychic disturbances, anxiety, depression

Dermatologic: Rash, alopecia, pruritus, dermatomyositis

Endocrine & metabolic: Gynecomastia, abnormal thyroid function tests

Gastrointestinal: Abdominal pain, constipation, diarrhea, dyspepsia, flatulence, nausea, acid regurgitation, xerostomia, vomiting, anorexia

Hepatic: Hepatitis, cholestatic jaundice, cirrhosis, hepatic necrosis, hepatoma, elevated hepatic enzymes

Neuromuscular & skeletal: Increased CPK, myalgia, weakness, muscle cramps, leg pain, arthralgia, paresthesia, rhabdomyolysis

Ocular: Blurred vision, eye irritation, cataracts, ophthalmoplegia

Miscellaneous: Hypersensitivity syndrome (including one or more of the following features: Anaphylaxis, angioedema, lupus erythematous-like syndrome, polymyalgia rheumatica, dermatomyositis, vasculitis, purpura, leukopenia, hemolytic anemia, erythema multiforme)

Drug Interactions Cytochrome P450 isoenzyme CYP3A3/4 substrate

Plasma concentrations may be decreased when given with magnesium-aluminum hydroxide containing antacids; cholestyramine reduces absorption; amiodarone, clofibrate, danazol, fenofibrate, gemfibrozil, niacin (1 g/day), and cyclosporine may increase the risk of myopathy and rhabdomyolysis (see Warnings); CYP3A3/4 inhibitors (clarithromycin, cyclosporine, danazol, diltiazem, fluconazole, fluvoxamine, erythromycin, indinavir, itraconazole, ketoconazole, miconazole, nefazodone, nelfinavir, ritonavir, saquinavir, indinavir, amprenavir, troleandomycin, and verapamil) increase lovastatin blood levels and may increase the risk of lovastatin-induced myopathy and rhabdomyolysis (see Warnings); lovastatin may increase the hypoprothrombinemic response to warfarin; the herbal medicine St John's wort (*Hypericum perforatum*) may decrease lovastatin levels

Food Interactions Food increases the absorption of lovastatin; serum concentrations of active drug under fasting conditions are approximately two-thirds of that when administered with food. Lovastatin serum concentrations may be increased if taken with grapefruit juice; the risk of myopathy/rhabdomyolysis is increased with daily intake of large quantities of grapefruit juice (>1 quart/day); avoid concurrent use.

Stability Immediate release tablets should be stored at temperatures between 5°C to 30°C (41°F to 86°F); extended release tablets should be stored at temperatures between 20°C to 25°C (68°F to 77°F); avoid excessive heat and humidity

Mechanism of Action Lovastatin acts by competitively inhibiting 3-hydroxyl-3-methylglutaryl-coenzyme A (HMG-CoA) reductase, the enzyme that catalyzes the rate-limiting step in cholesterol biosynthesis

Pharmacodynamics

Onset of action: 3 days

Maximum effect: 4-6 weeks

Average LDL-C reduction: 18% to 55%

Average HDL-C increase: 5% to 15%

Average triglyceride reduction: 7% to 30%

Pharmacokinetics

Absorption: Oral: 30% absorbed but less than 5% reaches the systemic circulation due to an extensive first-pass effect; absorption increased with extended release tablets

Protein binding: 95%

Half-life: 1.1-1.7 hours

Time to peak serum concentration: 2-4 hours

Elimination: ~80% to 85% of dose excreted in feces and 10% in urine

Usual Dosage Oral:

Treatment of heterozygous familial hypercholesterolemia: Children and Adolescents 10-17 years: Begin treatment if after adequate trial of diet the following are present: LDL-C >189 mg/dL or LDL-C remains >160 mg/dL and positive family history of premature cardiovascular disease or meets NCEP classification (see Chart):

Initial (using immediate release formulation): 10 mg once daily, increase to 20 mg once daily after 8 weeks and 40 mg once daily after 16 weeks as needed. (**Note:** Girls must be at least 1 year post-menarche)

Adults: Initial:

Immediate release tablet: 20 mg once daily; adjust dosage at 4-week intervals; maximum dose: 80 mg/day; for patients requiring LDL-C reductions <20%, a lower initial dose of 10 mg once daily may be used.

Extended release tablet: 20 mg once daily; adjust dosage at 4-week intervals; maximum dose: 60 mg/day

Dosing adjustment in patients who are concomitantly receiving amiodarone or verapamil: Dose should not exceed 40 mg/day

Dosage adjustment in patients who are concomitantly receiving cyclosporine: Initial: 10 mg once daily, not to exceed 20 mg/day

Dosage adjustment in patients who are concomitantly receiving fibrates or lipid-lowering doses of niacin (≥1 g/day): Dose should not exceed 20 mg/day

Dosing adjustment in renal impairment: Cl_{cr} <30 mL/minute: Doses exceeding 20 mg/day should be carefully considered and implemented cautiously

Administration Oral: Administer with evening meal; avoid administration with grapefruit juice; do not crush or chew extended release tablets

Monitoring Parameters Serum cholesterol (total and fractionated), creatine phosphokinase levels (CPK); liver function tests (see Precautions and Warnings)

Reference Range Hypercholesterolemia: See table below; HDL-C <40 mg/dL

Classification of Blood Cholesterol, LDL-C, and Triglyceride Concentrations*

Classification	Cholesterol (mg/dL)		LDL-C (mg/dL)		Triglycerides (mg/dL)
	Children	Adults	Children	Adults	Adults
Acceptable/optimal	<170	<200	<110	<100	<150
Above optimal	†	†	†	100-129	†
Borderline high	170-199	200-239	110-129	130-159	150-199
High	≥200	≥240	≥130	160-189	200-499
Very high	†	†	†	≥190	≥500

*Adapted from American Academy of Pediatrics Committee on Nutrition, "Cholesterol in Childhood," *Pediatrics*, 1998, 101(1 Pt 1):141-7 and "Third Report of the National Cholesterol Education Program Expert Panel on Detection, Evaluation, and Treatment of High Blood Cholesterol in Adults (Adult Treatment Panel III)," May 2001, www.nhlbi.nih.gov/guidelines/cholesterol.

†Lack of specific type of classification in either pediatric or adult recommendations.

Patient Information Avoid grapefruit juice and the herbal medicine, St John's wort. Report severe and unresolved gastric upset, any vision changes, unexplained muscle pain or weakness, changes in color of urine or stool, yellowing of skin or eyes, and any unusual bruising. Female patients of childbearing age must be counseled to use 2 effective forms of contraception simultaneously, unless absolute abstinence is the chosen method; this drug may cause severe fetal defects.

Additional Information The current recommendation for treatment of hypercholesterolemia in children is limited to children ≥10 years of age who, after a 6-month to 1-year trial of diet therapy, continue to have LDL-C concentrations ≥190 mg/dL alone, or LDL-C concentrations ≥160 mg/dL and a family history of premature coronary artery disease, or two or more other coronary artery disease risk factors (AAP Committee on Nutrition, 1998). For more specific risk assessment and treatment recommendations for adults, see the NIH Guidelines, 2001.

Dosage Forms

Tablet (Mevacor®): 10 mg, 20 mg, 40 mg

Tablet, extended release (Altocor™): 10 mg, 20 mg, 40 mg, 60 mg

References

American Academy of Pediatrics Committee on Nutrition, "Cholesterol in Childhood," *Pediatrics*, 1998, 101(1 Pt 1):141-7.

American Academy of Pediatrics, "National Cholesterol Education Program: Report of the Expert Panel on Blood Cholesterol Levels in Children and Adolescents," *Pediatrics*, 1992, 89(3 Pt 2):525-84.

Duplaga BA, "Treatment of Childhood Hypercholesterolemia With HMG-CoA Reductase Inhibitors," *Ann Pharmacother*, 1999, 33(11):1224-7.

Lambert M, Lupien PJ, Gagne C, et al, "Treatment of Familial Hypercholesterolemia in Children and Adolescents: Effect of Lovastatin. Canadian Lovastatin in Children Study Group," *Pediatrics*, 1996, 97(5):619-28.

Stein EA, Illingworth DR, Kwiterovich PO Jr, et al, "Efficacy and Safety of Lovastatin in Adolescent Males With Heterozygous Familial Hypercholesterolemia: A Randomized Controlled Trial," *JAMA*, 1999, 281(2):137-44.

"Third Report of the National Cholesterol Education Program Expert Panel on Detection, Evaluation, and Treatment of High Blood Cholesterol in Adults (Adult Treatment Panel III)," May 2001, www.nhlbi.nih.gov/guidelines/cholesterol.

♦ **Lovenox®** *see Enoxaparin on page 434*
♦ **Lozi-Flur™** *see Fluoride on page 500*
♦ **L-PAM** *see Melphalan on page 716*

- **LRH** *see* Gonadorelin *on page 547*
- **L-Sarcolysin** *see* Melphalan *on page 716*
- **LTG** *see* Lamotrigine *on page 653*
- ***L*-Thyroxine** *see* Levothyroxine *on page 669*
- ***L*-Triiodothyronine** *see* Liothyronine *on page 680*
- **Lugol's Solution** *see* Potassium Iodide *on page 918*
- **Luminal® Sodium** *see* Phenobarbital *on page 888*
- **Lupicare™ Dandruff [OTC]** *see* Salicylic Acid *on page 1002*
- **Lupicare™ II Psoriasis [OTC]** *see* Salicylic Acid *on page 1002*
- **Lupicare™ Psoriasis [OTC]** *see* Salicylic Acid *on page 1002*
- **Lupron®** *see* Leuprolide *on page 662*
- **Lupron Depot®** *see* Leuprolide *on page 662*
- **Lupron Depot-Ped®** *see* Leuprolide *on page 662*
- **Luride®** *see* Fluoride *on page 500*
- **Luride® Lozi-Tab®** *see* Fluoride *on page 500*
- **Lutrepulse™ (Can)** *see* Gonadorelin *on page 547*
- **Luxiq®** *see* Betamethasone *on page 169*
- **LY139603** *see* Atomoxetine *on page 138*
- **Lyderm® (Can)** *see* Fluocinonide *on page 499*
- **Lydonide (Can)** *see* Fluocinonide *on page 499*
- **Lymphocyte Mitogenic Factor** *see* Aldesleukin *on page 56*
- **Lyteprep™ (Can)** *see* Polyethylene Glycol-Electrolyte Solution *on page 914*
- **Maalox® Fast Release [OTC]** *see* Antacid Preparations *on page 112*
- **Maalox® Max [OTC]** *see* Antacid Preparations *on page 112*
- **Maalox® Max Quick Dissolve [OTC]** *see* Calcium Supplements *on page 200*
- **Maalox® Quick Dissolve [OTC]** *see* Antacid Preparations *on page 112*
- **Maalox® Quick Dissolve [OTC]** *see* Calcium Supplements *on page 200*
- **Maalox® TC [OTC]** *see* Antacid Preparations *on page 112*
- **Macrobid®** *see* Nitrofurantoin *on page 814*
- **Macrodantin®** *see* Nitrofurantoin *on page 814*

Mafenide (MA fe nide)

U.S. Brand Names Sulfamylon®
Therapeutic Category Antibiotic, Topical
Generic Available No
Use Adjunct in the treatment of second and third degree burns to prevent septicemia caused by susceptible organisms such as *Pseudomonas aeruginosa*
Pregnancy Risk Factor C
Contraindications Hypersensitivity to mafenide or any component (see Warnings)
Warnings Superinfection with nonsusceptible organisms has occurred in burn wounds treated with mafenide; some products contain sulfites which may cause allergic reactions in susceptible individuals
Precautions Use with caution in patients with renal impairment and in patients with G-6-PD deficiency
Adverse Reactions
    Dermatologic: Erythema, rash, pruritus, urticaria
    Endocrine & metabolic: Hyperchloremia, metabolic acidosis
    Hematologic: Bone marrow suppression, hemolytic anemia, bleeding, porphyria, eosinophilia
    Local: Burning sensation, excoriation, pain, swelling
    Respiratory: Hyperventilation, tachypnea
    Miscellaneous: Hypersensitivity reactions, facial edema
Stability Prepared topical solution is stable for 48 hours at room temperature
Mechanism of Action Interferes with bacterial cellular metabolism and bacterial folic acid synthesis through competitive inhibition of para-aminobenzoic acid
Pharmacokinetics
    Absorption: Diffuses through devascularized areas and is rapidly absorbed from burned surface
    Metabolism: To para-carboxybenzene sulfonamide which is a carbonic anhydrase inhibitor
    Time to peak serum concentration: Topical: 2-4 hours
    Elimination: In urine as metabolites
Usual Dosage Children ≥3 months and Adults: Topical
    Cream: Apply once or twice daily; apply to a thickness of approximately 16 mm; the burned area should be covered with cream at all times

Solution: Irrigate dressing every 4 hours or as needed to keep gauze moistened

Administration Topical:

Cream: Apply to cleansed, debrided, burned area with a sterile-gloved hand

Solution: Reconstitute 50 g powder by adding to 1 liter sterile water or 1 liter NS for irrigation; mix until completely dissolved; filter solution through a 0.22 micron filter before use; cover area with gauze and the dressing wetted with mafenide solution; wound dressing may be left undisturbed for up to 5 days

Monitoring Parameters Acid base balance, improvement of wound healing

Patient Information Inform physician if rash, blisters, or swelling appear

Nursing Implications For external use only

Dosage Forms

Cream, topical, as acetate: 85 mg/g (60 g, 120 g, 454 g) [contains sodium metabisulfite]

Powder for topical solution: 5% (5s) [50 g/packet]

♦ **Mag-Carb® [OTC]** *see Magnesium Supplements on page 701*

♦ **Mag G® [OTC]** *see Magnesium Supplements on page 701*

♦ **Maginex™ [OTC]** *see Magnesium Supplements on page 701*

♦ **Maginex™ DS [OTC]** *see Magnesium Supplements on page 701*

♦ **Magnesia Magma (Magnesium Hydroxide)** *see Magnesium Supplements on page 701*

♦ **Magnesium Carbonate** *see Magnesium Supplements on page 701*

♦ **Magnesium Chloride** *see Magnesium Supplements on page 701*

♦ **Magnesium Citrate** *see Magnesium Supplements on page 701*

♦ **Magnesium Gluconate** *see Magnesium Supplements on page 701*

♦ **Magnesium Hydroxide** *see Magnesium Supplements on page 701*

♦ **Magnesium Hydroxide and Mineral Oil Emulsion** *see Magnesium Supplements on page 701*

♦ **Magnesium Lactate** *see Magnesium Supplements on page 701*

♦ **Magnesium L-Aspartate Hydrochloride** *see Magnesium Supplements on page 701*

♦ **Magnesium Oxide** *see Magnesium Supplements on page 701*

♦ **Magnesium Sulfate** *see Magnesium Supplements on page 701*

Magnesium Supplements (mag NEE zee um SUP la ments)

Related Information

Adult ACLS Algorithm, Stable Ventricular Tachycardia *on page 1191*

Adult ACLS Algorithm, V. Fib and Pulseless VT *on page 1185*

CPR Pediatric Drug Dosages *on page 1175*

Pediatric ALS Algorithm, Pulseless Arrest *on page 1180*

U.S. Brand Names Almora® [OTC]; Mag-Carb® [OTC]; Mag G® [OTC]; Maginex™ [OTC]; Maginex™ DS [OTC]; Magonate® [OTC]; Mag-Ox 400® [OTC]; Mag-Tab SR® [OTC]; Magtrate® [OTC]; Phillips'® Milk of Magnesia [OTC]; Phillips'® M-O [OTC]; Slow-Mag® [OTC]; Uro-Mag® [OTC]

Synonyms Citrate of Magnesia (Magnesium Citrate); Epsom Salts (Magnesium Sulfate); Magnesia Magma (Magnesium Hydroxide); Milk of Magnesia (Magnesium Hydroxide); MOM (Magnesium Hydroxide)

Available Salts Magnesium Carbonate; Magnesium Chloride; Magnesium Citrate; Magnesium Gluconate; Magnesium Hydroxide; Magnesium Hydroxide and Mineral Oil Emulsion; Magnesium Lactate; Magnesium Oxide; Magnesium Sulfate; Magnesium L-Aspartate Hydrochloride

Therapeutic Category Antacid; Anticonvulsant, Miscellaneous; Electrolyte Supplement, Oral; Electrolyte Supplement, Parenteral; Laxative, Osmotic; Magnesium Salt

Generic Available Yes

Use

Treatment and prevention of hypomagnesemia **(magnesium chloride, magnesium lactate, magnesium carbonate, magnesium sulfate, magnesium gluconate, magnesium l-aspartate hydrochloride, and magnesium oxide)**

Treatment of hypertension **(magnesium sulfate)**

Treatment of torsade de pointes **(magnesium sulfate)**

Treatment of encephalopathy and seizures associated with acute nephritis **(magnesium sulfate)**

Short-term treatment of constipation **(magnesium citrate, magnesium hydroxide, and magnesium oxide)**

Treatment of hyperacidity symptoms **(magnesium hydroxide and magnesium oxide)**

Unlabeled use: Adjunctive treatment for bronchodilation in moderate to severe acute asthma **(magnesium sulfate)**

(Continued)

Magnesium Supplements *(Continued)*

Pregnancy Risk Factor B

Contraindications Hypersensitivity to magnesium salt(s) or any component (see Warnings); serious renal impairment, myocardial damage, heart block; patients with colostomy or ileostomy, intestinal obstruction, impaction, or perforation, appendicitis, abdominal pain

Warnings Magnesium chloride injection contains benzyl alcohol which may cause allergic reactions in susceptible individuals; large amounts of benzyl alcohol (≥99 mg/kg/day) have been associated with a potentially fatal toxicity ("gasping syndrome") in neonates; the "gasping syndrome" consists of metabolic acidosis, respiratory distress, gasping respirations, CNS dysfunction (including convulsions, intracranial hemorrhage), hypotension and cardiovascular collapse; avoid or use magnesium chloride injection with caution in neonates

Magonate® solution contains sodium benzoate; benzoic acid (benzoate) is a metabolite of benzyl alcohol; large amounts of benzyl alcohol (≥99 mg/kg/day) have been associated with a potentially fatal toxicity ("gasping syndrome") in neonates; *in vitro* and animal studies have shown that benzoate displaces bilirubin from protein binding sites; avoid use of Magonate® solution in neonates

Precautions Use with caution in patients with impaired renal function (accumulation of magnesium may lead to magnesium intoxication); use with caution in digitalized patients (may alter cardiac conduction leading to heart block)

Adverse Reactions Adverse effects with magnesium therapy are primarily related to the magnesium serum level

>3 mg/dL: Depressed CNS, blocked peripheral neuromuscular transmission leading to anticonvulsant effects

>5 mg/dL: Depressed deep tendon reflexes, flushing, somnolence

>12 mg/dL: Respiratory paralysis, complete heart block

Other effects:
Cardiovascular: Hypotension
Endocrine & metabolic: Hypermagnesemia
Gastrointestinal: Diarrhea, abdominal cramps, gas formation
Neuromuscular & skeletal: Muscle weakness

Drug Interactions Magnesium salts, when given orally, may decrease the absorption of the following: H_2 antagonists, phenytoin, iron salts, penicillamine, tetracycline, ciprofloxacin, benzodiazepines, chloroquine, steroids, and glyburide; systemic magnesium may enhance the effects of calcium channel blockers and neuromuscular blockers; may share additive CNS depressant effects with CNS depressants; if sufficient alkalinization of the urine by magnesium salts occurs, the excretion of salicylates is enhanced and the tubular reabsorption of quinidine is enhanced (increased effect)

Mechanism of Action Magnesium is important as a cofactor in many enzymatic reactions in the body. There are at least 300 enzymes which are dependent upon magnesium for normal functioning. Actions on lipoprotein lipase have been found to be important in reducing serum cholesterol. Magnesium is necessary for the maintaining of serum potassium and calcium levels due to its effect on the renal tubule. In the heart, magnesium acts as a calcium channel blocker. It also activates sodium potassium ATPase in the cell membrane to promote resting polarization and produce arrhythmias. Promotes bowel evacuation by causing osmotic retention of fluid which distends the colon and produces increased peristaltic activity when taken orally. To reduce stomach acidity, it reacts with hydrochloric acid in the stomach to form magnesium chloride.

Pharmacodynamics

Onset of action:
Anticonvulsant:
I.M.: 60 minutes
I.V.: Immediately
Laxative: Oral: 4-8 hours
Duration: Anticonvulsant:
I.M.: 3-4 hours
I.V.: 30 minutes

Pharmacokinetics

Absorption: Oral: Up to 30%
Elimination: Renal with unabsorbed drug excreted in feces

Usual Dosage Note: Multiple salt forms of magnesium exist; close attention must be paid to the salt form when ordering and administering magnesium; **incorrect selection or substitution of one salt for another without proper dosage adjustment may result in serious over- or underdosing.**

Recommended daily allowance of magnesium: Oral: See table.

Magnesium - Recommended Daily Allowance (RDA) and Estimated Average Requirement (EAR) (in terms of elemental magnesium)

Age	RDA (mg/day)	EAR (mg/day)
<6 mo	40	30
6-12 mo	60	75
1-3 y	80	65
4-8 y	130	110
Male		
9-13 y	240	200
14-18 y	410	340
19-30 y	400	330
Female		
9-13 y	240	200
14-18 y	360	300
19-30 y	310	255

HYPOMAGNESEMIA:

Neonates: I.V.:

Magnesium sulfate: 25-50 mg/kg/dose (0.2-0.4 mEq/kg/dose) every 8-12 hours for 2-3 doses

Magnesium chloride: 0.2-0.4 mEq/kg/dose every 8-12 hours for 2-3 doses

Children:

I.M., I.V.:

Magnesium sulfate: 25-50 mg/kg/dose (0.2-0.4 mEq/kg/dose) every 4-6 hours for 3-4 doses; maximum single dose: 2000 mg (16 mEq)

Magnesium chloride: 0.2-0.4 mEq/kg/dose every 4-6 hours for 3-4 doses; maximum single dose 16 mEq

Oral:

Magnesium chloride, gluconate, lactate, L-aspartate, carbonate, or oxide salts: 10-20 mg/kg **elemental magnesium** per dose 4 times/day

Adults:

Magnesium gluconate: Oral: 500-1000 mg 3 times/day

Magnesium sulfate:

I.M., I.V.: 1 g every 6 hours for 4 doses, or 250 mg/kg over a 4-hour period; for severe hypomagnesemia: 8-12 g/day in divided doses has been used

DAILY MAINTENANCE MAGNESIUM: I.V.:

Magnesium sulfate or magnesium chloride:

Neonates, Infants, and Children ≤45 kg: 0.25-0.5 mEq/kg/day

Adolescents >45 kg and Adults: 0.2-0.5 mEq/kg/day or 3-10 mEq/1000 kcal/day (maximum 8-16 mEq/day)

MANAGEMENT OF SEIZURES AND HYPERTENSION: I.M., I.V.:

Magnesium sulfate:

Children: 20-100 mg/kg/dose every 4-6 hours as needed; in severe cases doses as high as 200 mg/kg/dose have been used

Adults: 1 g every 6 hours for 4 doses as needed

TREATMENT OF TORSADE DE POINTES VT: I.V.:

Magnesium sulfate: Infants and Children: 25-50 mg/kg/dose; not to exceed 2 g/dose

BRONCHODILATION (adjunctive treatment in moderate to severe acute asthma): I.V.:

Magnesium sulfate:

Children: 25 mg/kg/dose (maximum dose 2 g) as a single dose

Adults: 2 g as a single dose

Note: Literature evaluating magnesium sulfate's efficacy in the relief of bronchospasm has utilized single dosages in patient's with acute symptomatology who have received aerosol β-agonist therapy (see References) with inconsistent results. A recent study (Ciarallo, 2000) showed significant improvement in pulmonary function in children who received a single dose of 40 mg/kg magnesium sulfate vs. placebo; pulmonary index scores after magnesium sulfate 75 mg/kg (maximum: 2.5 g) vs. placebo were not statistically different in 54 children between 1-18 years of age (Scarfone, 2000).

(Continued)

Magnesium Supplements *(Continued)*

CATHARTIC: Oral:

Magnesium citrate (Citrate of magnesia):
  <6 years: 2-4 mL/kg given once or in divided doses
  6-12 years: 100-150 mL
  ≥12 years and Adults: 150-300 mL

Magnesium hydroxide (Milk of magnesia, MOM):
  Liquid: Dosage based upon regular strength liquid (400 mg/5 mL); when using concentrated magnesium hydroxide solution, reduce recommended dose by ½:
    <2 years: 0.5 mL/kg/dose
    2-5 years: 5-15 mL/day once before bedtime or in divided doses
    6-11 years: 15-30 mL/day once before bedtime or in divided doses
    ≥12 years and adults: 30-60 mL/day once before bedtime or in divided doses
  Tablet:
    2-5 years: 311-622 mg (1-2 tablets) once before bedtime or in divided doses
    6-11 years: 933-1244 mg (3-4 tablets) once before bedtime or in divided doses
    ≥12 years and Adults: 1866-2488 mg (6-8 tablets) once before bedtime or in divided doses

Magnesium hydroxide and mineral oil (Haley's M-O®) (infant dosage to provide equivalent dosage of magnesium hydroxide listed above)
    <2 years: 0.6 mL/kg/dose
    2-5 years: 5-15 mL/day once or in divided doses
    6-11 years: 15-30 mL/day once or in divided doses
    ≥12 years and Adults: 30-60 mL once or in divided doses

Magnesium oxide: Adults: 2-4 g at bedtime with full glass of water

ANTACID Oral:

Magnesium hydroxide:
  Children:
    Liquid: 2.5-5 mL/dose, up to 4 times/day
    Tablet: 311 mg (1 tablet) up to 4 times/day
  Adults:
    Liquid: 5-15 mL/dose, up to 4 times/day
    Liquid concentrate: 2.5-7.5 mL/dose, up to 4 times/day
    Tablet: 622-1244 mg/dose (2-4 tablets) up to 4 times/day

Magnesium oxide: Adults: 140 mg 3-4 times/day or 400-840 mg/day

Elemental Magnesium Content of Magnesium Salts

Magnesium Salt	Elemental Magnesium (mg per 500 mg salt)	mEq Magnesium per 500 mg salt
Magnesium carbonate	140	11.7
Magnesium chloride	59	4.9
Magnesium gluconate	27	2.4
Magnesium lactate	50	4.2
Magnesium L-aspartate	49.6	4.1
Magnesium oxide	302	25
Magnesium sulfate	49.3	4.1

Dosing in renal impairment: Patients in severe renal failure should not receive magnesium due to toxicity from accumulation. Patients with a Cl_{cr} <25 mL/minute receiving magnesium should have serum magnesium levels monitored.

Administration

Oral:
  Solution: Mix with water and administer on an empty stomach; chill **magnesium citrate** prior to administration to improve palatability
  Tablet: Take with full glass of water; chew **magnesium hydroxide** chewable tablets thoroughly; do not chew or crush sustained release formulations
  Granules: Mix each packet in 4 ounces water or juice prior to administration

Parenteral: Intermittent infusion: Dilute to a concentration of 0.5 mEq/mL (60 mg/mL of **magnesium sulfate**) (maximum concentration: 1.6 mEq/mL, 200 mg/mL of **magnesium sulfate**) and infuse over 2-4 hours; do not exceed 1 mEq/kg/hour (125 mg/kg/hour of **magnesium sulfate**); in severe circumstances, half of the dosage to be administered may be infused over the first 15-20 minutes; for I.M. administration, dilute **magnesium sulfate** to a maximum concentration of 200 mg/mL prior to injection; rapid infusions (utilized for treatment of severe asthma or torsade de pointes VT) over 10-20 minutes may be used **(magnesium sulfate)**

Monitoring Parameters Serum magnesium, deep tendon reflexes, respiratory rate, renal function, blood pressure, stool output (laxative use)

Reference Range
Neonates and Infants: 1.5-2.3 mEq/L
Children: 1.5-2.0 mEq/L
Adults: 1.4-2.0 mEq/L

Additional Information 1 g elemental magnesium = 83.3 mEq = 41.1 mmol

Dosage Forms
Magnesium carbonate:
Capsule, gelatin (Mag-Carb®): 250 mg [5.8 mEq; equivalent to 70 mg elemental magnesium]

Magnesium chloride:
Injection, solution: 20% (50 mL) [1.97 mEq mg/mL; contains 1% benzyl alcohol]
Tablet (Slow-Mag®): 64 mg [as elemental magnesium; also contains 106 mg elemental calcium]

Magnesium citrate:
Solution: 290 mg/5 mL (300 mL) [cherry and lemon flavors]
Tablet: 100 mg [as elemental magnesium]

Magnesium gluconate:
Solution (Magonate®): 1000 mg/5 mL (480 mL) [4.8 mEq; equivalent to 54 mg elemental magnesium; contains sodium benzoate]
Tablet (Almora®, Mag G®, Magonate®, Magtrate®): 500 mg [2.4 mEq; equivalent to 27 mg elemental magnesium]

Magnesium hydroxide:
Liquid: 400 mg/5 mL (10 mL, 480 mL, 3780 mL)
Phillips'® Milk of Magnesia: 400 mg/5 mL (120 mL, 240 mL, 360 mL, 780 mL) [original, mint, and cherry flavors]
Liquid, **concentrate**: 800 mg/5 mL (100 mL, 400 mL)
Concentrated Phillips'® Milk of Magnesia: 800 mg/5 mL (240 mL) [strawberry flavor]
Tablet, chewable (Phillips'® Milk of Magnesia): 311 mg [mint flavor]

Magnesium hydroxide and mineral oil:
Suspension (Phillips'® M-O): Magnesium hydroxide 300 mg and mineral oil 1.25 mL per 5 mL (360 mL, 780 mL) [mint flavor]

Magnesium lactate:
Caplet, sustained release (Mag-Tab SR®): 835 mg [7 mEq; equivalent to 84 mg elemental magnesium]

Magnesium L-aspartate hydrochloride:
Granules (Maginex™ DS): 1230 mg [10 mEq; 122 mg] per packet [lemon flavor]
Tablet, enteric coated (Maginex™): 615 mg [5 mEq; 61 mg]

Magnesium oxide:
Capsule (Uro-Mag®): 140 mg [7 mEq; equivalent to 84 mg elemental magnesium]
Tablet (Mag-Ox 400®): 400 mg [20 mEq; equivalent to 242 mg elemental magnesium]

Magnesium sulfate:
Infusion [premixed in D_5W]: 10 mg/mL (100 mL); 20 mg/mL (500 mL, 1000 mL)
Infusion [premixed in water for injection]: 40 mg/mL (100 mL, 500 mL, 1000 mL); 80 mg/mL (50 mL)
Injection, solution: 125 mg/mL (8 mL); 500 mg/mL (2 mL, 5 mL, 10 mL, 20 mL, 50 mL)

References
Bloch H, Silverman R, Mancherje N, et al, "Intravenous Magnesium Sulfate as an Adjunct in the Treatment of Acute Asthma," *Chest*, 1995, 107(6):1576-81.
Chernow B, Smith J, Rainey TG, et al, "Hypomagnesemia: Implications for the Critical Care Specialist," *Crit Care Med*, 1982, 10(3):193-6.
Ciarallo L, Brousseau D, and Reinert S, "Higher-Dose Intravenous Magnesium Therapy for Children With Moderate to Severe Acute Asthma," *Arch Pediatr Adolesc Med*, 2000, 154(10):979-83.
Ciarallo L, Sauer AH, and Shannon MW, "Intravenous Magnesium Therapy for Moderate to Severe Pediatric Asthma: Results of a Randomized, Placebo-Controlled Trial," *J Pediatr*, 1996, 129(6):809-14.
"Dietary Reference Intakes for Calcium, Phosphorus, Magnesium, Vitamin D, and Fluoride. Standing Committee on the Scientific Evaluation of Dietary Reference Intakes, Food and Nutrition Board, Institute of Medicine," National Academy of Sciences, Washington, DC: National Academy Press, 1997.
Engel J, "Normal Laboratory Values," *Pocket Guide to Pediatric Assessment*, St Louis, MO: CV Mosby, 1989, 259.
"Guidelines 2000 for Cardiopulmonary Resuscitation and Emergency Cardiovascular Care. Part 10: Pediatric Advanced Life Support. The American Heart Association in Collaboration With the International Liaison Committee on Resuscitation," *Circulation*, 2000, 102(8 Suppl):I291-342.
Scarfone RJ, Loiselle JM, Joffe MD, et al, "A Randomized Trial of Magnesium in the Emergency Department Treatment of Children With Asthma," *Ann Emerg Med*, 2000, 36(6):572-8.

♦ **Magonate® [OTC]** *see Magnesium Supplements on page 701*

- ◆ **Mag-Ox 400® [OTC]** *see* Magnesium Supplements *on page 701*
- ◆ **Mag-Tab SR® [OTC]** *see* Magnesium Supplements *on page 701*
- ◆ **Magtrate® [OTC]** *see* Magnesium Supplements *on page 701*
- ◆ **Ma Huang** *see* Ephedrine *on page 437*
- ◆ **Mallamint® [OTC]** *see* Calcium Supplements *on page 200*

Malt Soup Extract (malt soop EKS trakt)

U.S. Brand Names Maltsupex® [OTC]
Therapeutic Category Laxative, Bulk-Producing
Generic Available No
Use Short-term treatment of constipation
Contraindications Hypersensitivity to barley malt extract or any component
Warnings Do not use when abdominal pain, nausea, or vomiting are present
Adverse Reactions Gastrointestinal: Abdominal cramps, diarrhea, rectal obstruction
Mechanism of Action Holds water in stool, reduces fecal pH
Pharmacodynamics Onset of action: Effect is usually apparent in 12-24 hours
Pharmacokinetics Hydrolyzed in the colon, metabolized by the liver
Usual Dosage Oral:

Infants >1 month:
Breast-fed:
Liquid: 1-2 teaspoonfuls in 2-4 oz of water or fruit juice 1-2 times/day for 3-4 days
Powder: 4 g in 2-4 oz of water or fruit juice daily for 3-4 days
Bottle-fed:
Liquid: ½ to 2 tablespoonfuls/day in formula for 3-4 days, then 1-2 teaspoonfuls/day
Powder: 8-16 g/day in formula for 3-4 days, then 4-8 g/day
Children:
2-6 years:
Liquid: 7.5 mL 1-2 times/day for 3-4 days
Powder: 8 g twice daily for 3-4 days
6-12 years:
Liquid: 15-30 mL 1-2 times/day for 3-4 days
Powder: Up to 16 g/day for 3-4 days
Children ≥12 years and Adults:
Liquid: 30 mL twice daily for 3-4 days, then 15-30 mL at bedtime
Powder: Up to 32 g twice daily for 3-4 days, then 16-32 g at bedtime
Tablets: 4 tablets 4 times/day (maximum dose: 64 g/day)

Administration Oral: Add to warm water and stir; then add milk, formula, water, or fruit juice until dissolved
Dosage Forms

Liquid: Nondiastatic barley malt extract 16 g/15 mL (240 mL, 480 mL)
Powder: Nondiastatic barley malt extract 8 g/tablespoonful (240 g, 480 g)
Tablet: Nondiastatic barley malt extract 750 mg

- ◆ **Maltsupex® [OTC]** *see* Malt Soup Extract *on page 706*
- ◆ **Mandelamine®** *see* Methenamine *on page 733*
- ◆ **Manganese Chloride** *see* Trace Metals *on page 1106*
- ◆ **Manganese Sulfate** *see* Trace Metals *on page 1106*

Mannitol (MAN i tole)

U.S. Brand Names Osmitrol®; Resectisol®
Synonyms *D*-Mannitol
Therapeutic Category Diuretic, Osmotic
Generic Available Yes
Use Reduction of increased intracranial pressure (ICP) associated with cerebral edema; promotion of diuresis in the prevention and/or treatment of oliguria or anuria due to acute renal failure; reduction of increased intraocular pressure; promotion of urinary excretion of toxic substances. Resectisol® is used for urologic irrigation for transurethral prostatic resection (see package insert for further information on this use).
Pregnancy Risk Factor C
Contraindications Hypersensitivity to mannitol or any component; severe renal disease, dehydration, active intracranial bleeding, severe pulmonary edema or congestion
Adverse Reactions

Cardiovascular: Circulatory overload, CHF (due to inadequate urine output and over-expansion of extracellular fluid)
Central nervous system: Convulsions, headache

Endocrine & metabolic: Fluid and electrolyte imbalance, hyponatremia or hypernatremia, hypokalemia or hyperkalemia, water intoxication, dehydration and hypovolemia secondary to rapid diuresis

Gastrointestinal: Xerostomia

Local: Tissue necrosis

Respiratory: Pulmonary edema

Miscellaneous: Allergic reactions

Drug Interactions Lithium

Stability Store at room temperature (15°C to 30°C); protect from freezing; crystallization may occur at low temperatures; do not use solutions that contain crystals; heating
in a hot water bath and vigorous shaking may be utilized for resolubilization of
crystals; cool solutions to body temperature before using; incompatible with strongly
acidic or alkaline solutions; potassium chloride or sodium chloride may cause precipitation of mannitol 20% or 25% solution

Mechanism of Action Increases the osmotic pressure of glomerular filtrate, which
inhibits tubular reabsorption of water and electrolytes and increases urinary output

Pharmacodynamics After I.V. injection:
Diuresis: Onset of action: Within 1-3 hours
Reduction in ICP:
  Onset of action: Within 15 minutes
  Duration: 3-6 hours

Pharmacokinetics
Distribution: Remains confined to extracellular space; does not penetrate blood-brain
  barrier (except in very high concentrations or with acidosis)
Metabolism: Minimal amounts in the liver to glycogen
Half-life: 1.1-1.6 hours
Elimination: Primarily unchanged in urine by glomerular filtration

Usual Dosage I.V.:
Children:
  Test dose (to assess adequate renal function): 200 mg/kg (maximum dose: 12.5 g)
    over 3-5 minutes to produce a urine flow of at least 1 mL/kg/hour for 1-3 hours
  Initial: 0.5-1 g/kg
  Maintenance: 0.25-0.5 g/kg every 4-6 hours
Adults:
  Test dose: 12.5 g (200 mg/kg) over 3-5 minutes to produce a urine flow of at least
    30-50 mL of urine per hour over the next 2-3 hours
  Initial: 0.5-1 g/kg
  Maintenance: 0.25-0.5 g/kg every 4-6 hours

Administration Parenteral: In-line filter set (≤5 micron) should always be used for
mannitol infusion with concentrations ≥20%; administer test dose (for oliguria) I.V.
push over 3-5 minutes; for cerebral edema or elevated ICP, administer over 20-30
minutes; maximum concentration for administration: 25%

Monitoring Parameters Renal function, daily fluid intake and output, serum electrolytes, serum and urine osmolality; for treatment of elevated intracranial pressure,
maintain serum osmolality 310-320 mOsm/kg

Patient Information May cause dry mouth

Nursing Implications Avoid extravasation; crenation and agglutination of red blood
cells may occur if administered with whole blood

Additional Information Approximate osmolarity: Mannitol 20%: 1100 mOsm/L;
mannitol 25%: 1375 mOsm/L

Dosage Forms
Injection, solution: 5% [50 mg/mL] (1000 mL); 10% [100 mg/mL] (500 mL, 1000 mL);
  15% [150 mg/mL] (500 mL); 20% [200 mg/mL] (150 mL, 250 mL, 500 mL); 25%
  [250 mg/mL] (50 mL)
Osmitrol®: 5% [50 mg/mL] (1000 mL); 10% [100 mg/mL] (500 mL, 1000 mL); 15%
  [150 mg/mL] (500 mL); 20% [200 mg/mL] (250 mL, 500 mL)
Solution, urologic (Resectisol®): 5% [50 mg/mL] (2000 mL, 4000 mL)

- ♦ **3M™ Avagard™ [OTC]** *see* Chlorhexidine Gluconate *on page 257*
- ♦ **Maxair™** *see* Pirbuterol *on page 910*
- ♦ **Maxair™ Autohaler™** *see* Pirbuterol *on page 910*
- ♦ **Maxidex®** *see* Dexamethasone *on page 354*
- ♦ **Maxidone™** *see* Hydrocodone and Acetaminophen *on page 571*
- ♦ **Maxipime®** *see* Cefepime *on page 228*
- ♦ **Maxitrol®** *see* Dexamethasone, Neomycin, and Polymyxin B *on page 357*
- ♦ **Maxivate®** *see* Betamethasone *on page 169*
- ♦ **MCT Oil® [OTC]** *see* Medium Chain Triglycerides *on page 711*
- ♦ **Measles and Rubella Vaccines, Combined** *see page 1333*
- ♦ **Measles, Mumps, and Rubella Vaccines, Combined** *see page 1333*
- ♦ **Measles Virus Vaccine, Live, Attenuated** *see page 1333*
- ♦ **Mebaral®** *see* Mephobarbital *on page 720*

Mebendazole (me BEN da zole)

U.S. Brand Names Vermox®
Therapeutic Category Anthelmintic
Generic Available Yes
Use Treatment of enterobiasis (pinworm infection), trichuriasis (whipworm infection), ascariasis (roundworm infection), and hookworm infections caused by *Necator americanus* or *Ancylostoma duodenale*; drug of choice in the treatment of capillariasis
Pregnancy Risk Factor C
Contraindications Hypersensitivity to mebendazole or any component
Warnings Pregnancy and children <2 years of age are relative contraindications since safety has not been established
Adverse Reactions
  Central nervous system: Dizziness, fever, headache
  Dermatologic: Rash, pruritus, alopecia
  Gastrointestinal: Diarrhea, abdominal pain, nausea, vomiting
  Hematologic: Neutropenia, anemia, leukopenia
  Hepatic: Transient abnormalities in liver function tests
  Otic: Tinnitus
  Renal: Hematuria
Drug Interactions Anticonvulsants such as carbamazepine and phenytoin may increase metabolism of mebendazole
Food Interactions Food increases mebendazole absorption
Mechanism of Action Selectively and irreversibly blocks uptake of glucose and other nutrients in susceptible intestine-dwelling helminths
Pharmacokinetics
  Absorption: Oral: 2% to 10%
  Distribution: To Liver, fat, muscle, plasma, and hepatic cysts
  Protein binding: 95%
  Metabolism: Extensive in the liver
  Half-life: 2.8-9 hours
  Time to peak serum concentration: Variable (0.5-7 hours)
  Elimination: Primarily in feces as inactive metabolites with 5% to 10% eliminated in urine
  Dialysis: Not dialyzable
Usual Dosage Children and Adults: Oral:
  Pinworms: Single chewable tablet (100 mg); may need to repeat after 2 weeks
  Whipworms, roundworms, hookworms: 100 mg twice daily, morning and evening on 3 consecutive days; if patient is not cured within 3-4 weeks, a second course of treatment may be administered
  Capillariasis: 200 mg twice daily for 20 days
Administration Oral: Administer with food; tablet can be crushed and mixed with food, swallowed whole, or chewed
Monitoring Parameters For treatment of trichuriasis, ascariasis, hookworm, or mixed infections, check for helminth ova in the feces within 3-4 weeks following the initial therapy
Dosage Forms Tablet, chewable: 100 mg
References
  Hotez PJ, "Hookworm Disease in Children," *Pediatr Infect Dis J*, 1989, 8(8):516-20.

Mechlorethamine (me klor ETH a meen)

Related Information
  Emetogenic Potential of Single Chemotherapeutic Agents *on page 1286*
  Extravasation Treatment *on page 1240*

U.S. Brand Names Mustargen®

Synonyms HN₂; Mustine; Nitrogen Mustard

Therapeutic Category Antineoplastic Agent, Alkylating Agent (Nitrogen Mustard)

Generic Available No

Use Combination therapy of Hodgkin's disease, brain tumors, non-Hodgkin's lymphoma, and malignant lymphomas; palliative treatment of lung, breast, and ovarian carcinoma; sclerosing agent in intracavitary therapy of pleural, pericardial, and other malignant effusions

Pregnancy Risk Factor D

Contraindications Hypersensitivity to mechlorethamine or any component; pre-existing profound myelosuppression; pregnancy

Warnings The FDA currently recommends that procedures for proper handling, administration, and disposal of mechlorethamine powder and solution be followed. Avoid inhalation of dust or vapors and contact with skin or mucous membranes. Mechlorethamine is potentially carcinogenic, teratogenic, and mutagenic. It may cause permanent sterility and birth defects. Extravasation of the drug into subcutaneous tissues results in painful inflammation, erythema, and induration; sloughing may occur; promptly infiltrate the area with sterile isotonic sodium thiosulfate ($\frac{1}{6}$ molar) and apply a cold compress for 6-12 hours. See Extravasation Treatment *on page 1240*

Precautions Use with caution in patients with myelosuppression; patients with lymphoma should receive adequate hydration, alkalinization of the urine and/or prophylactic allopurinol to prevent complications such as uric acid nephropathy and hyperuricemia

Adverse Reactions
Cardiovascular: Thrombosis
Central nervous system: Vertigo, fever, headache, drowsiness, lethargy, encephalopathy (high dose)
Dermatologic: Rash, alopecia
Endocrine & metabolic: Amenorrhea, impaired spermatogenesis, hyperuricemia
Gastrointestinal: Nausea, vomiting, anorexia, diarrhea, metallic taste, mucositis
Hematologic: Myelosuppression (leukopenia, thrombocytopenia), hemolytic anemia
Local: Thrombophlebitis, tissue necrosis upon extravasation
Neuromuscular & skeletal: Weakness
Ocular: Lacrimation
Otic: Tinnitus, deafness
Miscellaneous: Hypersensitivity reactions, diaphoresis, anaphylaxis

Stability Highly unstable in neutral or alkaline solutions; use immediately after reconstitution; discard any unused drug after 60 minutes (although manufacturer reports only 15 minutes of stability after reconstitution, other studies indicate it is stable longer)

Mechanism of Action Alkylating agent that inhibits DNA and RNA synthesis via formation of carbonium ions which can attach to nucleic acids at the N^7 position of guanine; cross-links strands of DNA causing miscoding, breakage, and failure of replication

Pharmacokinetics
Absorption: Incomplete after intracavitary administration secondary to rapid deactivation by body fluids
Distribution: Following I.V. administration, drug undergoes rapid hydrolysis to a highly reactive alkylating intermediate; unchanged drug is undetectable in the blood within a few minutes
Half-life: <1 minute
Elimination: <0.01% of unchanged drug is recovered in urine

Usual Dosage Refer to individual protocols
Children:
Lymphoma: MOPP regimen: Mustargen® (mechlorethamine), Oncovin® (vincristine), procarbazine, and prednisone: I.V.: 6 mg/m² on days 1 and 8 of a 28-day cycle
Brain tumors: MOPP regimen: I.V.: 3 mg/m² on days 1 and 8 of a 28-day cycle
Adults:
I.V.: 0.4 mg/kg or 12-16 mg/m² as a single monthly dose or divided into 0.1 mg/kg/day once daily for 4 days, repeated at 4- to 6-week intervals
Intracavitary: 10-30 mg or 0.2-0.4 mg/kg

Administration
Intracavitary: Dilute dose in up to 100 mL NS; paracentesis is performed to remove most of the fluid from the cavity prior to administration; inject drug slowly with frequent aspiration to ensure that a free flow of fluid is present; change patient's position every 5-10 minutes for 1 hour following injection to distribute drug uniformly throughout the cavity
(Continued)

Mechlorethamine (Continued)

Parenteral: **DO NOT ADMINISTER I.M. or S.C.** Administer I.V. push through a side port of an established I.V. line over 1-5 minutes at a concentration not to exceed 1 mg/mL

Monitoring Parameters CBC with differential and platelet count, hemoglobin; serum uric acid in lymphoma patients

Patient Information Report to physician any pain or irritation at the site of injection, fever, sore throat, bruising, bleeding, shortness of breath, itching, or wheezing

Nursing Implications Avoid extravasation, inhalation of vapors, or contact with skin, mucous membranes, and eyes since mechlorethamine is a potent vesicant. If accidental eye contact occurs, copious irrigation for at least 15 minutes with NS or a balanced salt ophthalmic irrigating solution should be instituted immediately followed by prompt ophthalmologic consultation. If accidental skin contact occurs, irrigate the affected area with copious amounts of water for at least 15 minutes while removing contaminated clothing, followed by application of a 2% sodium thiosulfate solution; contaminated clothing should be destroyed. Medical attention should be sought immediately. For mechlorethamine extravasations, infiltrate area with a 1/6 molar sodium thiosulfate solution and apply cold compresses for 6-12 hours; 1/6 molar sodium thiosulfate solution can be prepared by diluting 4 mL of 10% sodium thiosulfate injection with 6 mL of SWI; Dorr recommends to inject 2 mL of the 1/6 molar solution into site for each milligram of mechlorethamine extravasated

Additional Information Myelosuppressive effects:

WBC: Severe
Platelets: Severe
Onset (days): 4-7
Nadir (days): 14
Recovery (days): 21

Dosage Forms Injection, powder for reconstitution, as hydrochloride: 10 mg

References

Ater JL, van Eys J, Woo SY, et al, "MOPP Chemotherapy Without Irradiation as Primary Postsurgical Therapy for Brain Tumors in Infants and Young Children," *J Neurooncol*, 1997, 32(3):243-52.

Berg SL, Grisell DL, DeLaney TF, et al, "Principles of Treatment of Pediatric Solid Tumors," *Pediatr Clin North Am*, 1991, 38(2):249-67.

Dorr RT, Soble M, and Alberts DS, "Efficacy of Sodium Thiosulfate as a Local Antidote to Mechlorethamine Skin Toxicity in the Mouse," *Cancer Chemother Pharmacol*, 1988, 22(4):299-302.

Krischer JP, Ragab AH, Kun L, et al, "Nitrogen Mustard, Vincristine, Procarbazine, and Prednisone as Adjuvant Chemotherapy in the Treatment of Medulloblastoma. A Pediatric Oncology Group Study," *J Neurosurg*, 1991, 74(6):905-9.

♦ **Meclastine** see Clemastine on page 287

Meclizine (MEK li zeen)

Related Information

Overdose and Toxicology on page 1388

U.S. Brand Names Antivert®; Bonine® [OTC]; Dramamine® Less Drowsy Formula [OTC]

Canadian Brand Names Bonamine™

Synonyms Meclozine

Therapeutic Category Antiemetic; Antihistamine

Generic Available Yes

Use Prevention and treatment of motion sickness; management of vertigo

Pregnancy Risk Factor B

Contraindications Hypersensitivity to meclizine or any component

Precautions Use with caution in patients with angle-closure glaucoma or obstructive diseases of the GI or GU tract

Adverse Reactions

Cardiovascular: Hypotension, palpitations, tachycardia

Central nervous system: Drowsiness, fatigue, auditory and visual hallucinations, restlessness, excitation, insomnia, nervousness

Dermatologic: Urticaria, rash

Gastrointestinal: Xerostomia, anorexia, nausea, vomiting, diarrhea, constipation, appetite increase, weight gain

Hepatic: Cholestatic jaundice, hepatitis

Neuromuscular & skeletal: Myalgia, tremor, paresthesia

Ocular: Blurred vision, diplopia

Otic: Tinnitus

Respiratory: Bronchospasm, epistaxis

Drug Interactions Additive sedation with CNS depressants (eg, sedatives, alcohol, antihistamines)

Mechanism of Action Has central anticholinergic action and CNS depressant activity; decreases excitability of the middle ear labyrinth and blocks conduction in the middle ear vestibular-cerebellar pathways

Pharmacodynamics
Onset of action: Oral: 30-60 minutes
Duration: 12-24 hours

Pharmacokinetics
Metabolism: In the liver
Half-life: 6 hours
Elimination: As metabolites in urine and as unchanged drug in feces

Usual Dosage Children >12 years and Adults: Oral:
Motion sickness: 25-50 mg 1 hour before travel, repeat dose every 24 hours if needed
Vertigo: 25-100 mg/day in divided doses

Administration Oral: Administer with food to decrease GI distress

Patient Information May cause drowsiness and impair ability to perform activities requiring mental alertness or physical coordination; may cause dry mouth; avoid alcohol

Dosage Forms
Tablet, as hydrochloride: 12.5 mg, 25 mg
Antivert®: 12.5 mg, 25 mg, 50 mg
Dramamine® Less Drowsy Formula: 25 mg
Tablet, chewable, as hydrochloride (Bonine®): 25 mg

- **Mecloprodin** *see* Clemastine *on page 287*
- **Meclozine** *see* Meclizine *on page 710*
- **Med-Diltiazem (Can)** *see* Diltiazem *on page 388*
- **Medicinal Carbon** *see* Charcoal *on page 250*
- **Medicinal Charcoal** *see* Charcoal *on page 250*
- **Medicone® [OTC]** *see* Hemorrhoidal Preparations *on page 556*
- **Medicone® [OTC]** *see* Phenylephrine *on page 892*
- **Mediplast® [OTC]** *see* Salicylic Acid *on page 1002*

Medium Chain Triglycerides (mee DEE um chane trye GLIS er ides)

U.S. Brand Names MCT Oil® [OTC]

Synonyms Triglycerides, Medium Chain

Therapeutic Category Caloric Agent; Nutritional Supplement

Generic Available No

Use Nutritional supplement for those who cannot digest long chain fats; malabsorption associated with disorders such as pancreatic insufficiency, bile salt deficiency, and bacterial overgrowth of the small bowel; induce ketosis as a prevention for seizures (akinetic, clonic, and petit mal)

Pregnancy Risk Factor C

Contraindications Hypersensitivity to medium chain triglycerides or any component; should not be used in patients with hepatic encephalopathy due to earlier observations which report that short chain fatty acids may have a narcotic effect on the CNS and inhibit oxidative phosphorylation

Warnings Patients with cirrhosis demonstrate higher concentrations of medium chain fatty acids in the serum and CSF than normal individuals; impaired hepatic clearance of medium chain fatty acids due to parenchymal dysfunction of medium chain fatty acid oxidation, portal systemic shunt, and impaired protein binding of fatty acid enhance the passive diffusion of medium chain fatty acids into the CSF

Precautions Use with caution in patients with hepatic cirrhosis and complications such as portacaval shunts or encephalopathy

Adverse Reactions
Central nervous system: Sedation, narcosis, coma (cirrhotics)
Endocrine & metabolic: Ketosis
Gastrointestinal: Nausea, vomiting, abdominal pain, diarrhea, borborygmi

Mechanism of Action A semisynthetic class of lipids; medium chain triglycerides (MCT) are composed of fatty acids with chain length varying from 6-12 carbon atoms; preparations contain approximately 75% octanoic (caprylic), 20% to 25% decanoic (capric), 1% hexanoic (caproic), and 1% dodecanoic (lauric) acids

MCT are hydrolyzed in the stomach and in the small intestine by pancreatic lipase to form medium chain fatty acids; the medium chain fatty acids are incorporated into bile salts for more rapid solubilization and entrance into the mucosal cell and into the portal venous blood; MCT can also be absorbed unchanged as a triglycerides into the mucosal cell; medium chain fatty acids presented to the liver are minimally converted to hepatic lipid and are rapidly oxidized to carbon dioxide, ketones, and acetate; the medium chain fatty acids are also esterified to long chain triglycerides

(Continued)

Medium Chain Triglycerides *(Continued)*

Pharmacodynamics Onset of action: Octanoic acid appeared in each subject by 30 minutes following ingestion; effect on seizures in children: Within 6 weeks

Pharmacokinetics

Absorption: Up to 30% of dose can be absorbed unchanged as a triglyceride in the mucosal cell

Metabolism: Almost entirely oxidized by the liver to acetyl CoA fragments and to carbon dioxide; little deposited in adipose tissue or elsewhere

Elimination: As much as 20% of oral dose of MCT, recovered in expired CO_2 in 50 minutes; <10% elimination of medium chain fatty acids in feces

Usual Dosage Oral:

Infants: Nutritional supplement: Initial: 0.5 mL every other feeding, then advance to every feeding, then increase in increments of 0.25-0.5 mL/feeding at intervals of 2-3 days as tolerated

Children: Seizures: About 40 mL with each meal or 50% to 70% (800-1120 kcal) of total calories (1600 kcal) as the oil will induce the ketosis necessary for seizure control

Children and Adults: Cystic fibrosis: 3 tablespoons/day in divided doses

Adults: Malabsorption syndromes: 15 mL 3-4 times/day

Administration Oral:

Dilute with at least an equal volume of water or mix with some other vehicle such as fruit juice (should not be cold; flavoring may be added); mixture should be sipped slowly; administer no more than 15-20 mL at any one time (up to 100 mL may be administered in divided doses in a 24-hour period)

Possible GI side effects from medication can be prevented if therapy is initiated with small supplements at meals and gradually increased according to patient's tolerance

Monitoring Parameters

Nutritional supplement and malabsorption: Weight gain, height, stool output

Seizure treatment: Reduction in seizures, urine ketones

Patient Information GI symptoms may occur during the first few days of administration and then disappear; it is important to continue therapy with at least the smallest dose

Additional Information Does not provide any essential fatty acids; contains only saturated fats; supplementation with safflower, corn oil, or other polyunsaturated vegetable oil must be given to provide the patient with the essential fatty acids; caloric content: 8.3 calories/g; 115 calories/15 mL

Dosage Forms Oil: 14 g/15 mL (960 mL)

♦ **Medrol®** *see* MethylPREDNISolone *on page 747*

MedroxyPROGESTERone (me DROKS ee proe JES te rone)

U.S. Brand Names Depo-Provera®; Depo-Provera® Contraceptive; Provera®

Canadian Brand Names Alti-MPA; Gen-Medroxy; Novo-Medrone

Synonyms Acetoxymethylprogesterone; Methylacetoxyprogesterone

Therapeutic Category Contraceptive, Progestin Only; Progestin

Generic Available Yes (tablet)

Use Secondary amenorrhea or abnormal uterine bleeding due to hormonal imbalance; prevention of pregnancy

Pregnancy Risk Factor X

Contraindications Hypersensitivity to medroxyprogesterone or any component; thrombophlebitis; cerebral apoplexy, undiagnosed vaginal bleeding, liver dysfunction, thromboembolic disorders, breast cancer, pregnancy (known or suspected)

Warnings Discontinue if there is a sudden partial or complete loss of vision, proptosis, diplopia, migraine, if papilledema or retinal vascular lesions are present, or any other symptom of a thromboembolic event

Precautions Use with caution in patients with mental depression, diabetes, epilepsy, asthma, migraines, renal or cardiac dysfunction

Adverse Reactions

Cardiovascular: Edema, thromboembolic disorders

Central nervous system: Depression, dizziness, nervousness, fever, insomnia

Dermatologic: Melasma, chloasma, urticaria, acne, alopecia, hirsutism

Endocrine & metabolic: Menstrual irregularities, amenorrhea, breakthrough bleeding, breast tenderness

Gastrointestinal: Weight gain or loss, anorexia

Hepatic: Cholestatic jaundice

Local: Pain at injection site, thrombophlebitis

Neuromuscular & skeletal: Weakness

Drug Interactions Aminoglutethimide depresses serum concentrations of medroxy-progesterone acetate

Mechanism of Action Inhibits secretion of pituitary gonadotropins, which prevents follicular maturation and ovulation, transforms a proliferative endometrium into a secretory one

Pharmacokinetics
Absorption: I.M.: Slow
Protein binding: 90%
Metabolism: In the liver
Bioavailability: 0.6% to 10%
Half-life: 30 days
Elimination: Oral: In urine and feces

Usual Dosage Adolescents and Adults:
Amenorrhea: Oral: 5-10 mg/day for 5-10 days or 2.5 mg/day
Abnormal uterine bleeding: Oral: 5-10 mg for 5-10 days starting on day 16 or day 21 of menstrual cycle
Contraception: I.M.: 150 mg every 3 months; first dose to be given only during first 5 days of normal menstrual period; only within 5 days postpartum if not breast-feeding, or only at sixth postpartum week if exclusively breast-feeding

Administration
Oral: Administer with food
Parenteral: I.M. only; in upper arm or buttock; not for I.V. use; shake well before drawing into syringe

Test Interactions Altered thyroid and liver function tests, prothrombin time, factors VII, VIII, IX, X, metyrapone test

Patient Information Notify physician if sudden loss of vision, severe headache, sharp chest pain, coughing up blood, weakness or numbness in an arm or leg, severe pain or swelling in calf, unusual heavy vaginal bleeding or severe pain or tenderness in lower abdominal area

Additional Information I.M. dosing is recommended only for contraceptive purposes or in the treatment of endometrial or renal carcinoma

Dosage Forms
Injection, suspension, as acetate:
Depo-Provera®: 400 mg/mL (2.5 mL, 10 mL)
Depo-Provera® Contraceptive: 150 mg/mL (1 mL) [available in prefilled syringe or vial]
Tablet, as acetate (Provera®): 2.5 mg, 5 mg, 10 mg

Medrysone (ME dri sone)

U.S. Brand Names HMS Liquifilm®

Therapeutic Category Anti-inflammatory Agent, Ophthalmic; Corticosteroid, Ophthalmic

Generic Available No

Use Treatment of allergic conjunctivitis, vernal conjunctivitis, episcleritis, ophthalmic epinephrine sensitivity reaction

Pregnancy Risk Factor C

Contraindications Hypersensitivity to medrysone or any component; ocular fungal, viral, or tuberculosis infections; acute superficial herpes simplex

Warnings Medrysone is not recommended for use in uveitis or iritis (effectiveness has not been established); may delay healing after cataract surgery and increase risk of bleb formation; effectiveness and safety have not been established in children <3 years of age

Precautions Prolonged use has been associated with the development of glaucoma, corneal or scleral perforation, and posterior subcapsular cataracts; use with caution in patients with glaucoma (monitor IOP frequently); may mask or enhance the establishment of acute purulent untreated infections of the eye; dose should be tapered to avoid disease exacerbation; re-evaluate patient if symptoms do not improve after 2 days; secondary ocular infections may occur (especially with prolonged use)

Adverse Reactions
Endocrine & metabolic: Systemic hypercorticoidism (rare)
Local: Stinging, burning
Ocular: Corneal thinning, elevated intraocular pressure, glaucoma, damage to the optic nerve, defects in visual activity, cataracts, foreign body sensation, acute anterior uveitis, perforation of the globe; rarely: Keratitis, corneal ulcers, conjunctivitis, mydriasis, ptosis, conjunctival hyperemia, loss of accommodation
Miscellaneous: Hypersensitivity reactions

Stability Store at temperatures up to 25°C (77°F); do not freeze

Mechanism of Action Inhibits inflammatory response by suppression of migration of polymorphonuclear leukocytes and reversal of increased capillary permeability
(Continued)

Medrysone *(Continued)*

Pharmacokinetics
Absorption: Through aqueous humor
Metabolism: In the liver
Elimination: By the kidneys and feces

Usual Dosage Children ≥3 years and Adults: Ophthalmic: Instill 1 drop in conjunctival sac 2-4 times/day up to every 4 hours; may use every 1-2 hours during first 1-2 days

Administration Ophthalmic: Shake well before use; do not touch dropper to the eye or skin; finger pressure should be applied to lacrimal sac during and for 1-2 minutes after instillation to decrease risk of absorption and systemic reactions

Monitoring Parameters Monitor IOP if duration of therapy is >10 days; periodic examination of lens (with prolonged use)

Patient Information If eye pain or inflammation persists >48 hours or becomes worse, discontinue medrysone and contact physician.

Additional Information Medrysone is a synthetic corticosteroid; structurally related to progesterone; duration of therapy: 3-4 days to several weeks dependent on type and severity of disease

Dosage Forms Solution, ophthalmic: 1% (5 mL, 10 mL)

♦ **Mefoxin**® *see* Cefoxitin *on page 234*

♦ **Megace**® *see* Megestrol *on page 714*

♦ **Megadophilus**® **[OTC]** *see* Lactobacillus acidophilus and Lactobacillus bulgaricus *on page 648*

Megestrol *(me JES trole)*

U.S. Brand Names Megace®
Canadian Brand Names Apo®-Megestrol; Lin-Megestrol; Nu-Megestrol
Therapeutic Category Antineoplastic Agent, Miscellaneous; Progestin
Generic Available Yes

Use Appetite stimulation and promotion of weight gain in cachexia (particularly in HIV patients) which is unresponsive to nutritional supplementation; palliative treatment of breast and endometrial carcinomas

Pregnancy Risk Factor X

Contraindications Hypersensitivity to megestrol or any component; pregnancy (known or suspected); concomitant use with dofetilide

Warnings The FDA currently recommends that procedures for proper handling and disposal of antineoplastic agents be considered. May cause fetal harm when administered during pregnancy; women of childbearing age should use appropriate contraceptive measures. May suppress HPA axis during chronic administration; acute adrenal insufficiency may occur with abrupt withdrawal after long-term use or with stress; withdrawal or discontinuation of megesterol should be done carefully. Consider providing exogenous glucocorticoids during periods of stress or severe infection.

Oral suspension contains sodium benzoate; benzoic acid (benzoate) is a metabolite of benzyl alcohol; large amounts of benzyl alcohol (≥99 mg/kg/day) have been associated with a potentially fatal toxicity ("gasping syndrome") in neonates; *in vitro* and animal studies have shown that benzoate, a metabolite of benzyl alcohol, displaces bilirubin from protein-binding sites; avoid use of products containing sodium benzoate in neonates. Megesterol may inhibit the elimination of dofetilide resulting in increased dofetilide plasma concentrations and potential serious ventricular arrhythmias associated with QT interval prolongation; concomitant use with dofetilide is not recommended.

Precautions Use with caution in patients with history of thromboembolic disease and diabetes mellitus

Adverse Reactions
Cardiovascular: Cardiomyopathy, palpitations, edema, hypertension, chest pain
Central nervous system: Insomnia, depression, fever, headache, confusion, mood changes, lethargy, malaise, asthenia
Dermatologic: Rash, alopecia
Endocrine & metabolic: Breakthrough bleeding and amenorrhea, spotting, changes in menstrual flow or vaginal bleeding pattern, changes in cervical erosion and secretions, increased breast tenderness, hyperglycemia, HPA axis suppression, adrenal insufficiency, Cushing's syndrome, hypercalcemia
Gastrointestinal: Constipation, xerostomia, weight gain, nausea, vomiting, diarrhea, flatulence, abdominal pain, dyspepsia
Genitourinary: Impotence, gynecomastia, urinary incontinence
Hematologic: Leukopenia, anemia
Hepatic: Hepatomegally, cholestatic jaundice, hepatotoxicity

Local: Thrombophlebitis
Neuromuscular & skeletal: Weakness, paresthesia, carpal tunnel syndrome
Respiratory: Hyperpnea, dyspnea, pulmonary embolism, hyperventilation
Miscellaneous: Diaphoresis

Drug Interactions Megesterol may inhibit the elimination of dofetilide resulting in increased dofetilide plasma concentrations and potential serious ventricular arrhythmias associated with QT interval prolongation.

Stability Store tablets and oral suspension at room temperature; protect from heat

Mechanism of Action A synthetic progestin with antiestrogenic properties which disrupt the estrogen receptor cycle. Megesterol interferes with the normal estrogen cycle and results in a lower LH titer. It may also have a direct effect on the endometrium. As an antineoplastic progestin, it is thought to act through an antileutenizing effect mediated via the pituitary. The exact mechanism for appetite stimulation has not been determined but is postulated to be due in part to a direct effect on the hypothalamus.

Pharmacodynamics Onset of action:
Antineoplastic: 2 months of continuous therapy
Weight gain: 2-4 weeks

Pharmacokinetics
Absorption: Well absorbed
Metabolism: In the liver
Half-life: Adults: 10-120 hours
Time to peak serum concentration:
Tablet: 2-3 hours
Suspension: 3-5 hours
Elimination: In urine (57% to 78%) and feces (8% to 30%) within 10 days

Usual Dosage Oral:
Appetite stimulant in cachexia: Titrate dosage to response; decrease dose if weight gain is excessive:
Children: Limited data has been reported in cachectic children with cystic fibrosis, HIV, and solid tumors: 7.5-10 mg/kg/day in 1-4 divided doses; not to exceed 800 mg/day or 15 mg/kg/day
Adolescents & Adults: 800 mg/day in 1-4 divided doses; titrate dose to response; doses between 400-800 mg/day have been clinically effective
Breast carcinoma: Female Adults: 40 mg 4 times/day
Endometrial carcinoma: Female Adults: 40-320 mg/day in divided doses; not to exceed 800 mg/day
Uterine bleeding: Female Adults: 40 mg 2-4 times/day

Administration Oral: Shake oral suspension well before administering; administer without regard to food

Monitoring Parameters Monitor for signs of thromboembolic phenomena and adrenal axis suppression
Appetite stimulation: Weight, caloric intake, basal cortisol level
Antineoplastic: Tumor response

Patient Information Follow dosage schedule and do not take more than prescribed. May cause photosensitivity reactions (eg, exposure to sunlight may cause severe sunburn, skin rash, redness, or itching); avoid exposure to sunlight and artificial light sources (sunlamps, tanning booth/bed); wear protective clothing, wide-brimmed hats, sunglasses, and lip sunscreen (SPF ≥15); use a sunscreen [broad-spectrum sunscreen or physical sunscreen (preferred) or sunblock with SPF ≥15]; contact physician if reaction occurs. May cause dry mouth. Report absent or altered menses, abdominal pain, vaginal itching, irritation, or discharge; report warmth, redness, or swelling of extremities, sudden onset of difficulty breathing, severe headache, or change in vision. May cause fetal harm particularly in the first 4 months of pregnancy; use appropriate contraception.

Dosage Forms
Suspension, oral, as acetate: 40 mg/mL (240 mL) [contains alcohol 0.06% and sodium benzoate]
Tablet, as acetate: 20 mg, 40 mg

References
Eubanks V, Koppersmith N, Wooldridge N, et al, "Effects of Megestrol Acetate on Weight Gain, Body Composition, and Pulmonary Function in Patients With Cystic Fibrosis," *J Pediatr*, 2002, 140(4):439-44.

Nasr SZ, Hurwitz ME, Brown RW, et al, "Treatment of Anorexia and Weight Loss With Megestrol Acetate in Patients With Cystic Fibrosis," *Pediatr Pulmonol*, 1999, 28(5):380-2.

Stockheim JA, Daaboul JJ, Yogev R, et al, "Adrenal Suppression in Children With the Human Immunodeficiency Virus Treated With Megestrol Acetate," *J Pediatr*, 1999, 134(3):368-70.

Tchekmedyian NS, Hickman M, and Heber D, "Treatment of Anorexia and Weight Loss With Megestrol Acetate in Patients With Cancer or Acquired Immunodeficiency Syndrome," *Semin Oncol*, 1991, 18(1 Suppl 2):35-42.

◆ **Mellaril® [DSC]** *see* Thioridazine *on page 1085*

Melphalan (MEL fa lan)

Related Information
Emetogenic Potential of Single Chemotherapeutic Agents *on page 1286*

U.S. Brand Names Alkeran®

Synonyms L-PAM; L-Sarcolysin; Phenylalanine Mustard

Therapeutic Category Antineoplastic Agent, Alkylating Agent (Nitrogen Mustard)

Generic Available No

Use Palliative treatment of multiple myeloma and nonresectable epithelial ovarian carcinoma; neuroblastoma, rhabdomyosarcoma, breast cancer, sarcoma; I.V. formulation: Use in patients in whom oral therapy is not appropriate

Pregnancy Risk Factor D

Contraindications Hypersensitivity to melphalan or any component; severe bone marrow suppression; patients whose disease was resistant to prior therapy; pregnancy

Warnings The FDA currently recommends that procedures for proper handling and disposal of antineoplastic agents be considered; potentially mutagenic, carcinogenic, and teratogenic; long-term oral dosing can increase the chance of developing secondary leukemia; produces amenorrhea

Precautions Cross-sensitivity may exist between melphalan and chlorambucil; reduce dosage or discontinue therapy if leukocyte count is <3000/mm^3 or platelet count is <100,000/mm^3; use with caution in patients with bone marrow suppression and impaired renal function; dosage reduction may be necessary in patients with impaired renal function

Adverse Reactions
Cardiovascular: Vasculitis, chest pain; hypotension, diaphoresis, and cardiac arrest have been reported following I.V. administration

Dermatologic: Alopecia, rash, pruritus, vesiculation of skin, urticaria

Endocrine & metabolic: Amenorrhea, sterility, SIADH

Gastrointestinal: Nausea, vomiting, diarrhea, stomatitis, mucositis, anorexia

Hematologic: Leukopenia, thrombocytopenia, anemia, agranulocytosis, hemolytic anemia

Hepatic: Hepatic veno-occlusive disease, hepatitis, jaundice

Local: Burning, discomfort, skin ulceration at injection site, tissue necrosis

Respiratory: Pulmonary fibrosis, interstitial pneumonitis, dyspnea

Miscellaneous: Hypersensitivity reaction

Drug Interactions Cyclosporine (development of severe renal failure); cimetidine and other H$_2$ antagonists decrease bioavailability of oral melphalan; nalidixic acid may increase incidence of severe hemorrhagic necrotic enterocolitis

Food Interactions Food interferes with oral absorption

Stability Protect from light and store at room temperature; reconstituted 5 mg/mL solution for injection is stable 90 minutes at room temperature; do not refrigerate since it may precipitate; once reconstituted solution is further diluted for I.V. infusion with NS, administration must be completed within 1 hour

Mechanism of Action Alkylating agent that inhibits DNA and RNA synthesis via formation of carbonium ions; cross-links strands of DNA

Pharmacokinetics
Absorption: Oral: Variable and incomplete

Distribution: Distributes throughout total body water; V$_{dss}$: 0.5 L/kg

Protein binding: 60% to 90%

Metabolism: Nonenzymatic hydrolysis to mono- or dihydroxy products; some conjugation to glutathione

Bioavailability: Ranges from 49% to 95% depending on the presence of food; average: 60%

Half-life, terminal: 75-120 minutes

Time to peak serum concentration: Oral: Within 2 hours

Elimination: 10% to 15% of dose excreted unchanged in urine; after oral administration, 20% to 50% excreted in stool

Usual Dosage Refer to individual protocols
Children:

I.V.:

Pediatric rhabdomyosarcoma: 10-35 mg/m^2/dose every 21-28 days

High-dose melphalan with bone marrow transplantation for neuroblastoma: 70-100 mg/m^2/day on day 7 and 6 before BMT; or 140-220 mg/m^2 single dose before BMT; or 50 mg/m^2/day for 4 days; or 70 mg/m^2/day for 3 days

Oral: 4-20 mg/m^2/day for 1-21 days

Adults:

Multiple myeloma:

Oral: 6 mg/day once daily initially adjusted as indicated or 0.15 mg/kg/day for 7 days; or 0.25 mg/kg/day for 4 days or 8-10 mg/m^2 for 4 days, repeat at 4- to 6-week intervals

I.V.: 16 mg/m^2/dose every 2 weeks for 4 doses, then repeat monthly as per protocol for multiple myeloma

Ovarian carcinoma: Oral: 0.2 mg/kg/day for 5 days, repeat in 4-5 weeks

Dosing adjustment in renal impairment:

BUN >30 mg/dL: Reduce dose by 50%

Serum creatinine >1.5 mg/dL: Reduce dose by 50%

Administration

Oral: Administer on an empty stomach

Parenteral: I.V.: Reconstitute 50 mg vial for injection with special diluent to yield a 5 mg/mL solution; dilute the reconstituted solution with NS to a final concentration not to exceed 2 mg/mL for I.V. central line administration or 0.45 mg/mL for peripheral I.V. administration; administer by I.V. infusion over 15-30 minutes at a rate not to exceed 10 mg/minute but total infusion should be administered within 1 hour

Monitoring Parameters CBC with differential and platelet count, serum electrolytes, hemoglobin

Test Interactions Positive Coombs' [direct]

Patient Information Notify physician if fever, shortness of breath, persistent cough, sore throat, bleeding, or bruising occurs

Nursing Implications Ensure adequate patient hydration; care should be taken to avoid extravasation

Additional Information Myelosuppressive effects:

WBC: Moderate

Platelets: Moderate

Onset (days): 7

Nadir (days): 14-21

Recovery (days): 42-50

Dosage Forms

Injection, powder for reconstitution, as hydrochloride: 50 mg [diluent contains ethanol and propylene glycol]

Tablet: 2 mg

References

Berg SL, Grisell DL, DeLaney TF, et al, "Principles of Treatment of Pediatric Solid Tumors," *Pediatr Clin North Am*, 1991, 38(2):249-67.

Pole JG, Casper J, Elfenbein G, et al, "High-Dose Chemoradiotherapy Supported by Marrow Infusions for Advanced Neuroblastoma: A Pediatric Oncology Group Study," *J Clin Oncol*, 1991, 9(1):152-8.

Schroeder H, Pinkerton CR, Powles RL, et al, "High-Dose Melphalan and Total Body Irradiation With Autologous Marrow Rescue in Childhood Acute Lymphoblastic Leukemia After Relapse," *Bone Marrow Transplant*, 1991, 7(1):11-15.

♦ **Menadol® [OTC]** *see* Ibuprofen *on page 588*

♦ **Meningococcal Polysaccharide Vaccine, Groups A, C, Y, and W-135** *see page 1333*

Meperidine (me PER i deen)

Related Information

Adult ACLS Algorithm, Synchronized Cardioversion *on page 1192*

Compatibility of Medications Mixed in a Syringe *on page 1412*

Narcotic Analgesics Comparison *on page 1223*

Overdose and Toxicology *on page 1388*

Preprocedure Sedatives in Children *on page 1367*

Serotonin Syndrome *on page 1420*

U.S. Brand Names Demerol®

Synonyms Isonipecaine; Pethidine

Therapeutic Category Analgesic, Narcotic

Generic Available Yes

Use Management of moderate to severe pain; adjunct to anesthesia and preoperative sedation

Restrictions C-II

Pregnancy Risk Factor B (D if used for prolonged periods or in high doses at term)

Contraindications Hypersensitivity to meperidine or any component (see Warnings); use of MAO inhibitors within 14 days (potentially fatal reactions may occur, see Drug Interactions)

Warnings Abrupt discontinuation after prolonged use may cause withdrawal symptoms or seizures; multiple dose vial may contain sulfites which may cause allergic reactions in susceptible individuals; syrup contains benzoic acid or sodium benzoate; benzoic acid (benzoate) is a metabolite of benzyl alcohol; large amounts of benzyl (Continued)

Meperidine *(Continued)*

alcohol (≥99 mg/kg/day) have been associated with a potentially fatal toxicity ("gasping syndrome") in neonates; the "gasping syndrome" consists of metabolic acidosis, respiratory distress, gasping respirations, CNS dysfunction (including convulsions, intracranial hemorrhage), hypotension and cardiovascular collapse; use meperidine products containing benzoic acid or sodium benzoate with caution in neonates; *in vitro* and animal studies have shown that benzoate displaces bilirubin from protein binding sites

Precautions Use with caution in patients with pulmonary, hepatic, or renal disorders; use with caution in patients with tachycardias, biliary colic, increased intracranial pressure, seizure disorders or those receiving high-dose meperidine because normeperidine (an active metabolite and CNS stimulant) may accumulate and precipitate twitches, tremors, or seizures; decrease the dose in patients with renal or hepatic impairment

Adverse Reactions

Cardiovascular: Palpitations, hypotension, bradycardia, peripheral vasodilation, tachycardia

Central nervous system: CNS depression, dizziness, drowsiness, sedation, elevated intracranial pressure; active metabolite (normeperidine) may precipitate twitches, tremors, or seizures

Dermatologic: Pruritus

Endocrine & metabolic: Antidiuretic hormone release

Gastrointestinal: Nausea, vomiting, constipation, biliary tract spasm

Genitourinary: Urinary tract spasm

Local: Induration, irritation (repeated S.C. use)

Ocular: Miosis

Respiratory: Respiratory depression

Miscellaneous: Physical and psychological dependence, histamine release

Drug Interactions Cytochrome P450 isoenzyme CYP2D6 substrate

May aggravate the adverse effects of isoniazid; MAO inhibitors greatly potentiate the effects of meperidine (acute opioid overdosage symptoms can be seen, including severe toxic reactions); the herbal medicine St John's wort (*Hypericum perforatum*) may increase serious side effects, its use is **not** recommended; CNS depressants, alcohol, tricyclic antidepressants, phenothiazines may potentiate the effects of meperidine; phenytoin may decrease the analgesic effects; concurrent use of meperidine with ritonavir is not recommended

Stability Incompatible with aminophylline, heparin, phenobarbital, phenytoin, and sodium bicarbonate

Mechanism of Action Binds to opiate receptors in the CNS, causing inhibition of ascending pain pathways, altering the perception of and response to pain; produces generalized CNS depression

Pharmacodynamics Analgesia:

Onset of action:

Oral, I.M., S.C.: Within 10-15 minutes

I.V.: Within 5 minutes

Maximum effect:

Oral, I.M., S.C.: Within 1 hour

I.V.: 5-7 minutes

Duration:

Oral, I.M., S.C.: 2-4 hours

I.V.: 2-3 hours

Pharmacokinetics

Distribution: Crosses the placenta; appears in breast milk

V_{dss}:

Neonates: Preterm 1-7 days: 8.8 L/kg; term 1-7 days: 5.6 L/kg

Infants: 1 week to 2 months: 8 L/kg; 3-18 months: 5 L/kg; 5-8 years: 2.8 L/kg

Adults: 3-4 L/kg

Protein binding: (to alpha$_1$-acid glycoprotein)

Neonates: 52%

Infants: 3-18 months: 85%

Adults: ~60% to 80%

Metabolism: In the liver via hydrolysis and N-demethylation

Bioavailability: ~50% to 60%, increased bioavailability with liver disease

Half-life, terminal:

Preterm infants 3.6-65 days of age: 11.9 hours (range: 3.3-59.4 hours)

Term infants:

0.3-4 days of age: 10.7 hours (range: 4.9-16.8 hours)

26-73 days of age: 8.2 hours (range: 5.7-31.7 hours)

Neonates: 23 hours (range: 12-39 hours)

Infants 3-18 months: 2.3 hours
Children 5-8 years: 3 hours
Adults: 2.5-4 hours
Adults with liver disease: 7-11 hours
Normeperidine (active metabolite): Neonates: 30-85 hours; Adults: 8-16 hours; normeperidine half-life is dependent on renal function and can accumulate with high doses or in patients with decreased renal function; normeperidine may precipitate tremors or seizures
Elimination: ~5% meperidine eliminated unchanged in urine

Usual Dosage Doses should be titrated to appropriate analgesic effect; **when changing route of administration, note that oral doses are about half as effective as parenteral dose**

Children:
Oral, I.M., I.V., S.C.: Usual: 1-1.5 mg/kg/dose every 3-4 hours as needed; 1-2 mg/kg as a single dose preoperative medication may be used; maximum dose: 100 mg/dose
I.V. continuous infusion: Loading dose: 0.5-1 mg/kg followed by initial rate: 0.3 mg/kg/hour; titrate dose to effect; may require 0.5-0.7 mg/kg/hour
Adults: Oral, I.M., I.V.: S.C.: 50-150 mg/dose every 3-4 hours as needed
AHCPR dosing guidelines: Opioid naive patients: **Note:** Oral route not recommended (See Carr, 1992 and Jacox, 1994):
Children and Adults <50 kg: Moderate to severe pain: I.M., I.V., S.C.: Usual initial dose: 0.75 mg/kg every 2-3 hours
Children and Adults ≥50 kg: Moderate to severe pain: I.M., I.V., S.C.: Usual initial dose: 100 mg every 3 hours

Dosing adjustment in renal impairment:
Cl_{cr} 10-50 mL/minute: Administer 75% of normal dose
Cl_{cr} <10 mL/minute: Administer 50% of normal dose

Administration
Oral: Administer with water; dilute syrup in water prior to use (use 4 oz water for adults)
Parenteral:
Slow I.V. push: Do not administer rapid I.V., administer over at least 5 minutes and dilute to ≤10 mg/mL
Intermittent infusion: Dilute to 1 mg/mL and administer over 15-30 minutes

Monitoring Parameters Respiratory and cardiovascular status; relief of pain, level of sedation

Patient Information Avoid alcohol and the herbal medicine St John's wort; may be habit-forming; avoid abrupt discontinuation after prolonged use; may cause drowsiness and impair ability to perform activities requiring mental alertness or physical coordination

Additional Information Equianalgesic doses: morphine 10 mg I.M. = meperidine 75-100 mg I.M.. **Note:** Although meperidine has been used in combination with chlorpromazine and promethazine as a premedication ("Lytic Cocktail"), this combination may have a higher rate of adverse effects compared to alternative sedatives and analgesics (See American Academy of Pediatrics Committee on Drugs, 1995)

Dosage Forms
Injection, solution, as hydrochloride [ampul]: 50 mg/mL (1.5 mL, 2 mL)
Injection, solution, as hydrochloride [prefilled syringe]: 25 mg/mL (1 mL); 50 mg/mL (1 mL); 75 mg/mL (1 mL); 100 mg/mL (1 mL)
Injection, solution, as hydrochloride [prefilled syringe for PCA pump]: 10 mg/mL (50 mL)
Injection, solution, as hydrochloride [vial]: 50 mg/mL (1 mL, 30 mL); 100 mg/mL (20 mL) [may contain sodium metabisulfite]
Syrup, as hydrochloride: 50 mg/5 mL (5 mL, 500 mL) [contains sodium benzoate]
Demerol®: 50 mg/5 mL (480 mL) [contains benzoic acid; banana flavor]
Tablet, as hydrochloride (Demerol®): 50 mg, 100 mg

References
American Academy of Pediatrics Committee on Drugs, "Reappraisal of Lytic Cocktail/Demerol®, Phenergan®, and Thorazine® (DPT) for the Sedation of Children," *Pediatrics*, 1995, 95(4):598-602.
Carr D, Jacox A, Chapman CR, et al, "Clinical Practice Guideline Number 1: Acute Pain Management: Operative or Medical Procedures and Trauma," Rockville, Maryland: U.S. Department of Health and Human Services, Public Health Service, Agency for Health Care Policy and Research, AHCPR Publication No 92-0032, 1992.
Cole TB, Sprinkle RH, Smith SJ, et al, "Intravenous Narcotic Therapy for Children With Severe Sickle Cell Pain Crisis," *Am J Dis Child*, 1986, 140(12):1255-9.
Jacox A, Carr D, Payne R, et al, "Clinical Practice Guideline Number 9: Management of Cancer Pain," Rockville, Maryland: U.S. Department of Health and Human Services, Public Health Service, Agency for Health Care Policy and Research, AHCPR Publication No. 94-0592, 1994.
Olkkola KT, Hamunen K, and Maunuksela EL, "Clinical Pharmacokinetics and Pharmacodynamics of Opioid Analgesics in Infants and Children," *Clin Pharmacokinet*, 1995, 28(5):385-404.

(Continued)

Meperidine *(Continued)*

Pokela ML, Olkkola KT, Koivisto ME, et al, "Pharmacokinetics and Pharmacodynamics of Intravenous Meperidine in Neonates and Infants," *Clin Pharmacol Ther*, 1992, 52(4):342-9.

Mephobarbital *(me foe BAR bi tal)*

U.S. Brand Names Mebaral®

Synonyms Methylphenobarbital

Therapeutic Category Anticonvulsant, Barbiturate; Barbiturate; Sedative

Generic Available No

Use Treatment of generalized tonic-clonic and simple partial seizures

Restrictions C-IV

Pregnancy Risk Factor D

Contraindications Hypersensitivity to mephobarbital or any component; pre-existing CNS depression; respiratory depression; severe uncontrolled pain; history of porphyria

Precautions Use with caution in patients with hepatic or renal impairment or respiratory diseases

Adverse Reactions
Central nervous system: Drowsiness, lethargy, paradoxical excitement (especially in children)
Dermatologic: Rash, including Stevens-Johnson syndrome or erythema multiforme
Gastrointestinal: Nausea, vomiting
Hematologic: Agranulocytosis, thrombocytopenic purpura
Miscellaneous: Psychological and physical dependence

Drug Interactions Cytochrome P450 isoenzyme CYP2C, CYP2C8, and CYP2C19 substrate
Mephobarbital is expected to have similar drug interactions as phenobarbital, since mephobarbital is metabolized in the liver to phenobarbital (see Phenobarbital *on page 888*)

Food Interactions High doses of pyridoxine may decrease drug effect; barbiturates may increase the metabolism of vitamin D & K; dietary requirements of vitamin D, K, C, B_{12}, folate and calcium may be increased with long-term use

Mechanism of Action Increases seizure threshold in the motor cortex; depresses monosynaptic and polysynaptic transmission in the CNS; depresses CNS activity by binding to barbiturate site at GABA-receptor complex enhancing GABA activity; depresses reticular activating system; higher doses may be gabamimetic

Pharmacokinetics Values listed are for mephobarbital; see also Phenobarbital *on page 888*
Absorption: Oral: ~50%
Metabolism: In the liver via N-demethylation to phenobarbital

Usual Dosage Epilepsy: Oral:
Children: 4-10 mg/kg/day in 2-4 divided doses
Adults: 200-600 mg/day in 2-4 divided doses

Administration Oral: Administer with water, milk, or juice

Monitoring Parameters Phenobarbital serum concentrations; CBC with differential, platelet count, hepatic and renal function

Reference Range Phenobarbital level should be in the range of 15-40 µg/mL (SI: 65-172 µmol/L)

Patient Information May cause drowsiness and impair ability to perform activities requiring mental alertness or physical coordination; avoid alcohol; limit caffeine; may be habit-forming; avoid abrupt discontinuation after prolonged use

Additional Information Sometimes used in specific patients who have excessive sedation or hyperexcitability from phenobarbital

Dosage Forms Tablet: 32 mg, 50 mg, 100 mg

♦ **Mephyton®** *see Phytonadione on page 902*

♦ **Mepron®** *see Atovaquone on page 141*

Mercaptopurine *(mer kap toe PYOOR een)*

Related Information
Emetogenic Potential of Single Chemotherapeutic Agents *on page 1286*

U.S. Brand Names Purinethol®

Synonyms 6-Mercaptopurine; 6-MP

Therapeutic Category Antineoplastic Agent, Antimetabolite; Antineoplastic Agent, Purine

Generic Available No

Use Use in conjunction with methotrexate for maintenance therapy in childhood ALL; use in combination regimens for the treatment of AML, CML; non-Hodgkin's lymphoma

Pregnancy Risk Factor D

Contraindications Hypersensitivity to mercaptopurine or any component; severe liver disease; severe bone marrow suppression; patients whose disease showed prior resistance to mercaptopurine or thioguanine

Warnings The FDA currently recommends that procedures for proper handling and disposal of antineoplastic agents be considered; mercaptopurine may cause birth defects; potentially carcinogenic

Avoid using the terms "6-mercaptopurine" or "6-MP" which have been associated with medication errors resulting in sixfold overdosages.

Precautions Use with caution and adjust dosage in patients with renal impairment or hepatic failure; patients who receive allopurinol concurrently should have the mercaptopurine dose reduced by 66% to 75%

Adverse Reactions
Central nervous system: Drug fever
Dermatologic: Rash, hyperpigmentation, alopecia
Endocrine & metabolic: Hyperuricemia
Gastrointestinal: Mild nausea or vomiting, diarrhea, stomatitis, anorexia
Genitourinary: Oligospermia
Hematologic: Myelosuppression (leukopenia, thrombocytopenia, anemia), eosinophilia
Hepatic: Hepatotoxicity, hyperbilirubinemia, jaundice, elevation of liver enzymes
Renal: Renal toxicity (oliguria, hematuria)

Drug Interactions Allopurinol may potentiate the effect of bone marrow suppression (blocks metabolism of **orally** administered mercaptopurine by inhibiting xanthine oxidase); mercaptopurine decreases anticoagulant effect of warfarin; doxorubicin, hepatotoxic drugs (may potentiate liver toxicity)

Food Interactions Food decreases bioavailability

Stability Intact vials and tablets should be stored at room temperature and protected from light; reconstitute 500 mg vial with 49.8 mL SWI; the 10 mg/mL solution is stable for 24 hours

Mechanism of Action Prodrug incorporated into DNA and RNA; blocks purine synthesis and inhibits DNA and RNA synthesis

Pharmacokinetics
Absorption: Oral: Variable and incomplete (16% to 50%)
Distribution: Distributed throughout total body water; penetrates into CSF at low concentrations
Protein binding: 19%
Metabolism: Undergoes first-pass metabolism in the GI mucosa and liver; metabolized in the liver to sulfate conjugates, 6-thiouric acid, and other inactive compounds
Bioavailability: Oral: <20% (variable)
Half-life: Age dependent
  Children: <60 minutes
  Adults: 36-90 minutes
Time to peak serum concentration: Oral: Within 2 hours
Elimination: 20% excreted unchanged in urine

Usual Dosage Refer to individual protocols
Children:
Oral:
  Induction: 2.5-5 mg/kg/day given once daily, or 70-100 mg/m²/day once daily
  Maintenance: 1.5-2.5 mg/kg/day given once daily or 50-75 mg/m²/day once daily
I.V. continuous infusion (investigational; distributed under the auspices of the NCI for authorized studies): 50 mg/m²/hour for 24-48 hours, or 1000 mg/m²/day for 24 hours
Adults: Oral:
  Induction: 2.5-5 mg/kg/day given once daily, or 80-100 mg/m²/day given once daily
  Maintenance: 1.5-2.5 mg/kg/day given once daily
Dosing adjustment in renal impairment: Children and Adults:
  Cl_cr <50 mL/minute: Administer every 48 hours

Administration
Oral: Do not administer with meals. For pediatric patients with ALL, studies suggest that evening administration may lower the risk of relapse compared to morning administration.
Parenteral: Administer by slow I.V. push over several minutes or by slow I.V. continuous infusion to reduce the incidence of vein irritation; further dilute the 10 mg/mL
(Continued)

Mercaptopurine *(Continued)*

reconstituted solution in NS or D₅W to a final concentration for administration of 1-2 mg/mL

Monitoring Parameters CBC with differential and platelet count, liver function tests, uric acid, urinalysis

Patient Information Report to physician if fever, sore throat, bleeding, bruising, shortness of breath, or painful urination occurs; avoid alcohol

Nursing Implications Avoid extravasation

Additional Information Myelosuppressive effects:

WBC: Moderate
Platelets: Moderate
Onset (days): 7-10
Nadir (days): 14
Recovery (days): 21

Dosage Forms

Injection [investigational use only]: 500 mg vial
Tablet, scored: 50 mg

Extemporaneous Preparations A 50 mg/mL oral suspension can be prepared in a vertical flow hood using a 1:1 mixture of methylcellulose 1% and simple syrup; crush thirty 50 mg tablets into a fine powder in a mortar; add a small amount of methylcellulose and simple syrup mixture to make a uniform paste; mix while adding 1:1 mixture of methylcellulose 1% and simple syrup to a final volume of 30 mL. **Note:** May use ultrasonication dispersal. Preparation is stable for 14 days when stored at room temperature; label "shake well" and "caution chemotherapy"

Nahata MC and Hipple TF, *Pediatric Drug Formulations*, 4th ed, Cincinnati, OH: Harvey Whitney Books, 2000.

References

Zimm S, Ettinger LJ, Holcenberg JS, et al, "Phase I and Clinical Pharmacological Study of Mercaptopurine Administered as a Prolonged Intravenous Infusion," *Cancer Res*, 1988, 45(4):1869-73.

♦ **6-Mercaptopurine** *see* Mercaptopurine *on page 720*

♦ **Mercapturic Acid** *see* Acetylcysteine *on page 43*

♦ **Meribin® [OTC]** *see* Biotin *on page 173*

Meropenem *(mer oh PEN em)*

U.S. Brand Names Merrem® I.V.

Synonyms SM-7338

Therapeutic Category Antibiotic, Carbapenem

Generic Available No

Use Treatment of multidrug-resistant gram-negative and gram-positive aerobic and anaerobic pathogens documented or suspected to be susceptible to meropenem; used in treatment of meningitis, lower respiratory tract infections, urinary tract infections, intra-abdominal infections, skin and skin structure infections and sepsis caused by susceptible *S. aureus*, group A *Streptococcus*, *S. pneumoniae*, *H. influenzae*, *N. meningitidis*, *M. catarrhalis*, *E. coli*, *Klebsiella*, *Enterobacter*, *Serratia*, *P. aeruginosa*, *B. cepacia*, and *B. fragilis*

Pregnancy Risk Factor B

Contraindications Hypersensitivity to meropenem, any component, other carbapenems, or in patients who have experienced anaphylactic reactions to beta-lactams

Warnings Safety and efficacy in children <3 months of age have not been established; pseudomembranous colitis has been reported with the use of meropenem; prolonged use may result in superinfection

Precautions Use with caution in patients with a history of seizures, CNS disease, CNS infection, and/or compromised renal function; dosage adjustment required in patients with renal impairment

Adverse Reactions

Cardiovascular: Hypotension
Central nervous system: Seizures (<0.38%), headache, pain, insomnia, dizziness, agitation
Dermatologic: Rash (1.4%), pruritus
Gastrointestinal: Nausea, vomiting (1%), diarrhea (4.3%), melena, constipation, oral moniliasis
Hematologic: Leukopenia, neutropenia
Hepatic: Elevated AST, ALT, alkaline phosphatase, LDH, and bilirubin
Local: Phlebitis (1.2%), inflammation at the injection site
Renal: Elevated BUN and serum creatinine
Respiratory: Dyspnea

Drug Interactions Probenecid inhibits renal excretion of meropenem

Stability Meropenem reconstituted with SWI is stable for up to 2 hours at room temperature or for up to 12 hours when refrigerated; when reconstituted with NS to a final concentration between 2.5-50 mg/mL, the solution is stable for up to 2 hours at room temperature or 18 hours when refrigerated; when reconstituted with D_5W to a final concentration between 2.5-50 mg/mL, the solution is stable for up to 1 hour at room temperature or 8 hours when refrigerated; solutions prepared for infusion in plastic I.V. bags with NS at concentrations ranging from 2.5-20 mg/mL are stable for 4 hours at room temperature or 24 hours when refrigerated

Mechanism of Action Inhibits cell wall synthesis by binding to penicillin-binding proteins (PBPs) with its strongest affinities for PBPs 2, 3 and 4 of *E. coli* and *P. aeruginosa* and PBPs 1, 2 and 4 of *S. aureus*

Pharmacokinetics

Distribution: Penetrates into most tissues and body fluids including CSF, urinary tract, peritoneal fluid, bone, bile, lung, bronchial mucosa, muscle tissue, and heart valves

Protein binding: 2%

Metabolism: 20% is hydrolyzed in plasma to an inactive metabolite

Half-life:

Premature newborns: 3 hours

Full-term newborns: 2 hours

Infants 3 months to 2 years: 1.4 hours

Children 2-12 years and Adults: 1 hour

Elimination: Cleared by the kidney with 70% excreted unchanged in urine

Usual Dosage I.V.:

Neonates:

Postnatal age 0-7 days: 20 mg/kg/dose every 12 hours

Postnatal age >7 days:

Weight 1200-2000 g: 20 mg/kg/dose every 12 hours

Weight >2000 g: 20 mg/kg/dose every 8 hours

Children ≥3 months: 60 mg/kg/day divided every 8 hours; meningitis: 120 mg/kg/day divided every 8 hours; maximum dose: 6 g/day

Adults:

Mild to moderate infection: 1.5-3 g/day divided every 8 hours

Meningitis: 6 g/day divided every 8 hours

Dosage adjustment in renal impairment:

Cl_{cr} 26-50 mL/minute: Standard dose every 12 hours

Cl_{cr} 10-25 mL/minute: One-half dose every 12 hours

Cl_{cr} <10 mL/minute: One-half dose every 24 hours

Administration Administer by I.V. push or I.V. intermittent infusion; final concentration for administration should not exceed 50 mg/mL; infuse I.V. push injection over 3-5 minutes; intermittent infusion dose should be administered over 15-30 minutes

Monitoring Parameters Periodic renal, hepatic, and hematologic function tests

Test Interactions Positive Coombs' [direct]

Additional Information Sodium content 1 g: 3.92 mEq

Dosage Forms Injection, powder for reconstitution, as trihydrate: 500 mg, 1 g

References

Blummer JL, "Pharmacokinetic Determinants of Carbapenem Therapy in Neonates and Children," *Pediatr Infect Dis J*, 1996, 15(8):733-7.

Blummer JL, Reed MD, Kearns GL, et al, "Sequential, Single-Dose Pharmacokinetic Evaluation of Meropenem in Hospitalized Infants and Children," *Antimicrob Agents Chemother*, 1995, 39(8):1721-5.

Bradley, JS, "Meropenem: A New, Extremely Broad Spectrum Beta-lactam Antibiotic for Serious Infections in Pediatrics," *Pediatr Infect Dis J*, 1997, 16:263-8.

Odio CM, Puig JR, Feris JM, et al, "Prospective, Randomized, Investigator-Blinded Study of the Efficacy and Safety of Meropenem vs. Cefotaxime Therapy in Bacterial Meningitis in Children. Meropenem Meningitis Study Group," *Pediatr Infect Dis J*, 1999, 18(7):581-90.

Wiseman LR, Wagstaff AJ, Brogden RN, et al, "Meropenem. A Review of its Antibacterial Activity, Pharmacokinetic Properties and Clinical Efficacy," *Drugs*, 1995, 50(1):73-101.

♦ **Merrem® I.V.** *see* Meropenem on page 722

Mesalamine (me SAL a meen)

Related Information

Drugs and Breast-Feeding on page 1404

U.S. Brand Names Asacol®; Canasa™; Pentasa®; Rowasa®

Canadian Brand Names Mesasal®; Novo-5 ASA; Quintasa®; Salofalk®

Synonyms 5-Aminosalicylic Acid; 5-ASA; Fisalamine; Mesalazine

Therapeutic Category 5-Aminosalicylic Acid Derivative; Anti-inflammatory Agent; Anti-inflammatory Agent, Rectal

Generic Available No

Use Treatment of ulcerative colitis (UC), proctosigmoiditis, and proctitis

Pregnancy Risk Factor B

(Continued)

Mesalamine *(Continued)*

Contraindications Hypersensitivity to mesalamine, any component (see Warnings), or salicylates

Warnings Pericarditis should be considered in patients with chest pain (has occurred rarely with mesalamine containing products); pancreatitis should be considered in any patient with new abdominal complaints; has been implicated in the production of an acute intolerance syndrome or exacerbation of colitis (<3%), prompt discontinuation is required if this develops.

Some products may contain sulfites which may cause allergic reactions in susceptible individuals. Rowasa® suspension contains sodium benzoate; benzoic acid (benzoate) is a metabolite of benzyl alcohol; large amounts of benzyl alcohol (≥99 mg/kg/day) have been associated with a potentially fatal toxicity ("gasping syndrome") in neonates; *in vitro* and animal studies have shown that benzoate displaces bilirubin from protein binding sites; avoid use of Rowasa® suspension in neonates.

Precautions Use with caution in patients with hypersensitivity to sulfasalazines or patients with renal disease

Adverse Reactions

Cardiovascular: Pericarditis, chest pain, myocarditis, T-wave abnormalities, edema

Central nervous system: Chills, dizziness, fever, headache, insomnia, malaise, anxiety, depression

Dermatologic: Psoriasis, dry skin, urticaria, pyoderma gangrenosum, erythema nodosum, photosensitivity, lichen planus, alopecia

Endocrine & metabolic: Amenorrhea, menorrhagia, breast pain

Gastrointestinal: Abdominal pain, cramps, flatulence, bloody diarrhea, anal irritation, anorexia, pancreatitis, gastritis, dyspepsia, eructation, vomiting, hemorrhoids, constipation, dysgeusia

Genitourinary: Epididymitis, dysuria, discoloration of urine (yellow-brown)

Hematologic: Rare: Agranulocytosis, thrombocytopenia, eosinophilia, aplastic anemia

Hepatic: Elevated liver enzymes, jaundice, cholestatic jaundice, liver necrosis/failure

Neuromuscular & skeletal: Weakness

Renal: Interstitial nephritis, renal papillary necrosis, nephrotic syndrome

Respiratory: Interstitial pneumonitis, pulmonary infiltrates, sinusitis, asthma exacerbation, pleuritis, fibrosing alveolitis

Miscellaneous: Kawasaki-like syndrome, lupus-like syndrome

Drug Interactions Decreased digoxin bioavailability

Stability Unstable in presence of water or light; once foil has been removed, unopened bottles have an expiration of 1 year following the date of manufacture; store suppositories at room temperature; do not refrigerate

Mechanism of Action Mesalamine (5-aminosalicylic acid) is the active component of sulfasalazine; the specific mechanism of action of mesalamine is unknown; however, it is thought that it modulates local chemical mediators of the inflammatory response, especially leukotrienes; action appears topical rather than systemic

Pharmacokinetics

Absorption:

Capsule: 20% to 30%

Rectal: ~15%; variable and dependent upon retention time, underlying GI disease, and colonic pH

Tablet: 28%

Distribution: Breast milk to plasma ratio:

5-ASA: 0.27

Acetyl 5-ASA: 5.1

Metabolism: In the liver by acetylation to acetyl-5-aminosalicylic acid (acetyl-5-ASA, an active metabolite) and to glucuronide conjugates; intestinal metabolism may also occur

Half-life:

5-ASA: 0.5-1.5 hours

Acetyl 5-ASA: 5-10 hours

Time to peak serum concentration: Oral, Rectal: Within 4-7 hours

Elimination: Most metabolites are excreted in urine with <2% appearing in feces

Usual Dosage Oral (usual course of therapy is 3-6 weeks):

(Oral products are formulated to slowly release therapeutic quantities of drug throughout the GI tract):

Capsule (ethylcellulose-coated, controlled release):

Children: 50 mg/kg/day divided every 6-12 hours

Adults: 1 g 4 times/day for up to 8 weeks

Tablet (coated with acrylic-based resin; drug released after reaches terminal ileum):

Children: 50 mg/kg/day divided every 8-12 hours

Adults: Treatment: 800 mg 3 times/day; maintenance for remission of UC: 1.6 g daily in divided doses up to 6 months

Retention enema: Adults: 60 mL (4 g) at bedtime, retained overnight, approximately 8 hours for 3-6 weeks

Rectal suppository: Adults: Insert 1 suppository (500 mg) in rectum twice daily, for 3-6 weeks; may increase to 3 times daily if ineffective response noted after 2 weeks of therapy

Administration

Oral: Administer with food; swallow tablets whole, do not break outer coating

Rectal: Retain enema for 8 hours or as long as practical; shake rectal suspension well before use; retain suppository for 1-3 hours

Patient Information May discolor urine yellow-brown. May rarely cause photosensitivity reactions (eg, exposure to sunlight may cause severe sunburn, skin rash, redness, or itching); avoid direct exposure to sunlight. Suppositories will cause staining of direct contact surfaces including fabrics.

Dosage Forms

Capsule, controlled release (Pentasa®): 250 mg

Suppository, rectal (Canasa™): 500 mg

Suspension, rectal (Rowasa®): 4 g/60 mL (7s) [contains potassium metabisulfite and sodium benzoate]

Tablet, delayed release, enteric coated (Asacol®): 400 mg

References

Grand RJ, Ramakrishna J, and Calenda KA, "Inflammatory Bowel Disease in the Pediatric Patient," *Gastroenterol Clin North Am*, 1995, 24(3):613-32.

♦ **Mesalazine** *see* Mesalamine *on page 723*

♦ **Mesasal® (Can)** *see* Mesalamine *on page 723*

♦ **M-Eslon® (Can)** *see* Morphine Sulfate *on page 778*

Mesna (MES na)

U.S. Brand Names Mesnex®

Canadian Brand Names Uromitexan™

Synonyms Sodium 2-Mercaptoethane Sulfonate

Therapeutic Category Antidote, Cyclophosphamide-induced Hemorrhagic Cystitis; Antidote, Ifosfamide-induced Hemorrhagic Cystitis

Generic Available Yes (injection)

Use Detoxifying agent used as a protectant against hemorrhagic cystitis induced by ifosfamide and cyclophosphamide

Pregnancy Risk Factor B

Contraindications Hypersensitivity to mesna, other thiol compounds, or any component (see Warnings)

Warnings Mesna injection contains benzyl alcohol which may cause allergic reactions in susceptible individuals; large amounts of benzyl alcohol (≥99 mg/kg/day) have been associated with a potentially fatal toxicity ("gasping syndrome") in neonates; the "gasping syndrome" consists of metabolic acidosis, respiratory distress, gasping respirations, CNS dysfunction (including convulsions, intracranial hemorrhage), hypotension and cardiovascular collapse; avoid use of mesna products containing benzyl alcohol in children <2 years of age; a benzyl alcohol free (preservative free) injection is available (see Additional Information); *in vitro* and animal studies have shown that benzoate, a metabolite of benzyl alcohol, displaces bilirubin from protein binding sites

Precautions Examine morning urine specimen for hematuria prior to ifosfamide or cyclophosphamide treatment; if hematuria develops, reduce the ifosfamide/cyclophosphamide dose or discontinue the drug and consider increasing the mesna dosage

Adverse Reactions

Cardiovascular: Hypotension

Central nervous system: Malaise, headache

Dermatologic: Skin rash

Gastrointestinal: Diarrhea, nausea, vomiting, dysgeusia

Neuromuscular & skeletal: Limb pain

Stability Diluted solutions in D_5W, D_5/NS, NS, or LR are chemically and physically stable for 48 hours at room temperature; compatible with solutions containing ifosfamide or cyclophosphamide; incompatible with cisplatin

Mechanism of Action In the urinary bladder, mesna binds with and detoxifies acrolein and other urotoxic metabolites of ifosfamide and cyclophosphamide via an active sulfhydryl group on mesna

Pharmacokinetics

Distribution: No tissue penetration; following glomerular filtration, mesna disulfide is reduced in the renal tubules back to mesna and delivered to the bladder in the active form

(Continued)

Mesna (Continued)

Bioavailability: Oral: 50%

Half-life: 24 minutes (mesna); after I.V. administration, mesna is rapidly oxidized intravascularly to mesna disulfide (half-life: 72 minutes)

Elimination: Unchanged drug and metabolite are excreted primarily in the urine; time for maximum urinary mesna excretion: 1 hour after I.V. and 2-3 hours after an oral mesna dose

Usual Dosage Children and Adults (refer to individual protocols): **Mesna dose depends on dose of antineoplastic agent used:**

When used with ifosfamide: I.V.: Mesna dose is 20% w/w of ifosfamide dose 15 minutes before and 4 and 8 hours later or combined with ifosfamide administration; for high-dose ifosfamide, mesna has been administered at a dose of 20% w/w 15 minutes before and every 3 hours for 3-6 doses or combined with ifosfamide administration; **(Note:** In clinical protocols, total daily mesna dose ranged between 60% to 160% w/w of the daily ifosfamide dose)

When used with cyclophosphamide: I.V.: Mesna dose is 20% w/w of cyclophosphamide dose 15 minutes before and every 3 hours for 3-4 doses or combined with cyclophosphamide administration; **(Note:** In clinical protocols, total daily mesna dose ranged between 60% to 160% w/w of the daily cyclophosphamide dose)

I.V. continuous infusion: Mesna doses equivalent to 60% to 100% of the ifosfamide or cyclophosphamide dose have been used

Oral: Mesna dose is 40% w/w of the antineoplastic agent dose in 3 doses at 4-hour intervals or 20 mg/kg/dose every 4 hours x 3 (oral mesna is not recommended for the first dose before ifosfamide or cyclophosphamide)

Administration

Oral: Dilute mesna solution before oral administration to decrease sulfur odor; mesna can be diluted 1:1 to 1:10 in carbonated cola drinks, fruit juices (grape, apple, tomato, and orange juice) or in plain or chocolate milk (most palatable in chilled grape juice)

Parenteral: Administer by I.V. infusion over 15-30 minutes, or by continuous I.V. infusion, or per protocol; mesna may be diluted in D_5W or NS to a final concentration of 1-20 mg/mL; may be added to solutions containing ifosfamide or cyclophosphamide

Monitoring Parameters Urinalysis

Test Interactions False-positive urinary ketones with Chemstrip®, Multistix®, or Labstix®

Nursing Implications Used concurrently with and/or following high-dose ifosfamide or cyclophosphamide; ensure adequate patient hydration; report vomiting within 1 hour of an oral mesna dose to physician so that I.V. mesna can be administered

Additional Information pH of the commercial 100 mg/mL solution: 6.5-8.5. A preservative free formulation of Mesnex® injection may be obtained directly from the manufacturer. It is restricted for use in children <2 years and others who are sensitive to benzyl alcohol. Contact Bristol-Myers Squibb Company at 800-437-0994 for additional information.

Dosage Forms

Injection, solution (Mesnex®): 100 mg/mL (10 mL) [contains benzyl alcohol]

Tablet (Mesnex®): 400 mg

References

Ben Yehuda A, Heyman A and Steiner Salz D, "False Positive Reaction for Urinary Ketones With Mesna," *Drug Intell Clin Pharm*, 1987, 21(6): 547-8.

Brock N and Pohl J, "The Development of Mesna for Regional Detoxification," *Cancer Treat Rev*, 1983, 10(Suppl A):33-43.

"Cancer Chemotherapy," *Med Lett Drugs Ther*, 1989, 31(793):49-56.

Schoenike SE and Dana WJ, "Ifosfamide and Mesna," *Clin Pharm*, 1990, 9(3):179-91.

Metaproterenol (met a proe TER e nol)

Related Information

Asthma Guidelines *on page 1376*

Carbohydrate and Alcohol Content of Liquid Medications for Use in Patients Receiving Ketogenic Diets *on page 1431*

U.S. Brand Names Alupent®

Synonyms Orciprenaline

Therapeutic Category Adrenergic Agonist Agent; Antiasthmatic; Beta$_2$-Adrenergic Agonist Agent; Bronchodilator; Sympathomimetic

Generic Available Yes (except inhaler)

Use Bronchodilator in reversible airway obstruction due to asthma or COPD

Pregnancy Risk Factor C

Contraindications Hypersensitivity to metaproterenol or any component; pre-existing cardiac arrhythmias associated with tachycardia; narrow-angle glaucoma

Warnings Excessive use may result in cardiac arrest and death; do not use concurrently with other sympathomimetic bronchodilators. Some products contain sodium benzoate; benzoic acid (benzoate) is a metabolite of benzyl alcohol; large amounts of benzyl alcohol (≥99 mg/kg/day) have been associated with a potentially fatal toxicity ("gasping syndrome") in neonates; *in vitro* and animal studies have shown that benzoate displaces bilirubin from protein binding sites; avoid use of sodium benzoate containing products in neonates.

Precautions Use with caution in patients with ischemic heart disease, hypertension, hyperthyroidism, seizure disorders, CHF, cardiac arrhythmias, and diabetes mellitus

Adverse Reactions

Cardiovascular: Tachycardia, palpitations, hypertension

Central nervous system: Nervousness, dizziness, headache, fatigue, vertigo

Gastrointestinal: Nausea, vomiting, diarrhea, GI distress, xerostomia, dysgeusia, throat irritation

Neuromuscular & skeletal: Tremor, weakness, muscle cramps

Respiratory: Exacerbation of asthma, hoarseness, cough, nasal congestion

Drug Interactions Beta-adrenergic blockers (eg, propranolol) may antagonize metaproterenol's effects; sympathomimetics may increase adverse effects if administered concomitantly; MAO inhibitors may cause hypertensive crisis

Stability Protect from light

Mechanism of Action Relaxes bronchial smooth muscle and peripheral vasculature by action on beta$_2$-receptors

Pharmacodynamics

Onset of bronchodilation:

Oral: Within 30 minutes

Inhalation: Within 60 seconds

Maximum effect: Oral: Within 1 hour

Duration: (approximately 1-5 hours) regardless of route administered

Pharmacokinetics

Absorption: Oral: Well absorbed

Metabolism: Extensive first-pass in the liver (~40% of oral dose is available)

Elimination: Mainly as glucuronic acid conjugates

Usual Dosage

Oral:

Children:

<2 years: 0.4 mg/kg/dose given 3-4 times/day; in infants, the dose can be given every 8-12 hours

2-6 years: 1.3-2.6 mg/kg/day divided every 6-8 hours

6-9 years: 10 mg/dose given 3-4 times/day

Children >9 years and Adults: 20 mg/dose given 3-4 times/day

Inhalation: Children >12 years and Adults: 2-3 inhalations every 3-4 hours, up to 12 inhalations in 24 hours

Nebulizer:

Infants and Children: 0.01-0.02 mL/kg (0.5-1 mg/kg) of 5% solution; minimum dose: 0.1 mL (5 mg); maximum dose: 0.3 mL (15 mg) every 4-6 hours (may be given more frequently according to need); equivalent doses using more dilute solutions may be administered at the same frequency

Adolescents and Adults: 0.2 to 0.3 mL (10-15 mg) of 5% metaproterenol every 4-6 hours (can be given more frequently according to need); equivalent doses using more dilute solutions may be administered at the same frequency

Administration

Nebulization: Dilute 5% solution in 2-3 mL NS; more dilute solutions may be used without dilution

Oral: Administer with food to decrease GI distress

Monitoring Parameters Heart rate, respiratory rate, blood pressure, arterial or capillary blood gases if applicable, pulmonary function tests

Patient Information May cause dry mouth

(Continued)

Metaproterenol (Continued)

Dosage Forms

Aerosol for oral inhalation, as sulfate (Alupent®): 0.65 mg/inhalation (14 g) [200 doses]

Solution for oral inhalation, as sulfate [preservative free]: 0.4% [4 mg/mL] (2.5 mL); 0.6% [6 mg/mL] (2.5 mL); 5% [50 mg/mL] (10 mL, 30 mL)

Syrup, as sulfate: 10 mg/5 mL (480 mL) [may contain sodium benzoate]

Tablet, as sulfate: 10 mg, 20 mg

References

"National Asthma Education and Prevention Program. Expert Panel Report: Guidelines for the Diagnosis and Management of Asthma Update on Selected Topics--2002," *J Allergy Clin Immunol*, 2002, 110(5 Suppl):S141-219.

♦ Metaradrine *see* Metaraminol *on page 728*

Metaraminol (met a RAM i nole)

U.S. Brand Names Aramine®

Synonyms Hydroxynorephedrine; Metaradrine

Therapeutic Category Adrenergic Agonist Agent; Alpha-Adrenergic Agonist; Sympathomimetic

Generic Available No

Use Prevention and treatment of an acute hypotensive state occurring with spinal anesthesia; treatment of shock which persists after adequate fluid volume replacement

Pregnancy Risk Factor C

Contraindications Hypersensitivity to metaraminol or any component (see Warnings); use with cyclopropane or halothane anesthesia

Warnings Contains sulfites which may cause allergic reactions in susceptible individuals; extravasant; may cause tissue necrosis and sloughing of surrounding skin if I.V. infiltration occurs; see Extravasation Treatment *on page 1240*; use of MAO inhibitors may result in potentiation of its pressor effects

Precautions Blood/volume depletion should be corrected, if possible, before metaraminol therapy; use with caution in patients with heart or thyroid disease, hypertension, diabetes mellitus, and cirrhosis; because of its prolonged action, a cumulative effect is possible resulting in a prolonged elevation of blood pressure despite discontinuation of therapy; may provoke a relapse in patients with a history of malaria

Adverse Reactions

Cardiovascular: Tachycardia, bradycardia, hypertension, cardiac arrhythmias, palpitations, cardiac arrest

Central nervous system: Headache, dizziness, apprehension

Gastrointestinal: Nausea

Local: Tissue necrosis, sloughing at injection site, abscess formation

Neuromuscular & skeletal: Tremors

Miscellaneous: Diaphoresis

Drug Interactions Atropine may block the reflex bradycardia caused by metaraminol and enhance the pressor response; tricyclic antidepressants, MAO inhibitors, and ergot alkaloids may potentiate the effects of metaraminol; ectopic arrhythmias with concurrent use of digoxin; phentolamine and other alpha-adrenergic blocking agents will reduce metaraminol's effects

Stability Stable at room temperature; stable when diluted in D_5W, NS, Ringer's injection, LR injection, Normosol®-R, and Normosol®-M in D_5W; use diluted solutions within 24 hours

Mechanism of Action Predominantly stimulates alpha-adrenergic receptors resulting in vasoconstriction and increased systemic blood pressure; it also stimulates beta$_1$-adrenergic receptors causing increased contractility and heart rate; clinically the chronotropic effect (increased heart rate) is overcome by increased vagal activity occurring as a reflex to increased arterial blood pressure; bradycardia usually results; metaraminol also has an indirect effect by releasing norepinephrine from storage sites

Pharmacodynamics

Onset of action:

I.V.: 1-2 minutes

I.M.: 10 minutes

S.C.: 5-20 minutes

Duration: 20-90 minutes depending upon the route of administration

Usual Dosage Use the lowest effective dosage for the shortest possible time:

Prevention of hypotension: I.M., S.C.:

Children: 0.1 mg/kg or 3 mg/m²; repeat as needed, after at least 10 minutes

Adults: 2-10 mg; repeat as needed, after at least 10 minutes

Adjunctive treatment of shock: I.V.:
   Children: 0.01 mg/kg or 0.3 mg/m^2; may follow with infusion of 0.4 mg/kg or 12 mg/m^2 at a rate adjusted to maintain the desired blood pressure
   Adults: 0.5-5 mg; may follow with infusion of 15-100 mg at a rate adjusted to maintain the desired blood pressure

Administration Parenteral: Due to potentially severe tissue irritation, use S.C. route only if other routes are unavailable; may administer single doses without dilution by direct I.V. infusion slowly; for continuous infusion, dilute 15-100 mg in 500 mL of D$_5$W or NS; concentrations as high as 1 mg/mL have been used; administer I.V. infusions in large peripheral veins or use central venous access

Monitoring Parameters Blood pressure, heart rate, urine output, peripheral perfusion

Nursing Implications Monitor I.V. site closely for signs of infiltration/extravasation

Dosage Forms Injection, solution, as bitartrate: 10 mg/mL (10 mL) [contains sodium bisulfite]

♦ **Meted® [OTC]** *see* Sulfur and Salicylic Acid *on page 1058*

Metformin (met FOR min)

U.S. Brand Names Glucophage®; Glucophage® XR
Canadian Brand Names Alti-Metformin; Apo®-Metformin; Gen-Metformin; Glycon; Novo-Metformin; Nu-Metformin; PMS-Metformin; Rho®-Metformin; Rhoxal-metformin FC
Synonyms Metformin Hydrochloride
Therapeutic Category Antidiabetic Agent, Oral; Antidiabetic Agent, Biguanide; Hypoglycemic Agent, Oral
Generic Available Yes (except extended release)
Use Management of type II diabetes mellitus (noninsulin-dependent, NIDDM) as monotherapy when hyperglycemia cannot be managed with diet alone; may be used concomitantly with a sulfonylurea or insulin to improve glycemic control
Pregnancy Risk Factor B
Contraindications Hypersensitivity to metformin or any component; renal disease or renal dysfunction (S$_{cr}$ ≥1.5 mg/dL in males or ≥1.4 mg/dL in females); clinical conditions such as cardiovascular collapse, respiratory failure, acute MI, acute CHF, and septicemia [which may result in decreased renal function (see Warnings)]; acute or chronic metabolic acidosis with or without coma (including diabetic ketoacidosis)
Warnings Lactic acidosis is a rare, but potentially severe consequence of therapy with metformin; withhold therapy in clinical conditions which may predispose to the development of lactic acidosis (eg, hypoxemia, dehydration, hypoperfusion, sepsis) or in any patient with CHF requiring pharmacologic management; the risk of accumulation and lactic acidosis increases with the degree of impairment of renal function and age; avoid use in patients with renal function below the limit of normal for their age; therapy should be suspended for any surgical procedures (resume only after normal intake resumed and normal renal function is verified); temporarily discontinue therapy for 48 hours in patients undergoing radiologic studies involving the intravascular administration of iodinated contrast materials (potential for acute alteration in renal function); avoid use in patients with impaired liver function; avoid excessive acute or chronic ethanol use; lactic acidosis should be suspected in any diabetic patient receiving metformin who has evidence of acidosis when evidence of ketoacidosis is lacking
Precautions Use with caution in patients receiving medications that may affect renal function, particularly tubular secretion, as they may also affect metformin disposition; hypoglycemia (rare with metformin) may occur with inadequate caloric intake, strenuous exercise, or concurrent use with other hypoglycemic drugs
Adverse Reactions
   Cardiovascular: Chest discomfort, flushing, palpitation
   Central nervous system: Headache, chills, dizziness, lightheadedness
   Dermatologic: Rash, urticaria
   Endocrine & metabolic: Hypoglycemia (rare), lactic acidosis
   Gastrointestinal: Anorexia, nausea, vomiting, diarrhea, flatulence, indigestion, abdominal discomfort, abdominal distention, abnormal stools, constipation, dyspepsia, heartburn, metallic taste
   Hematologic: Megaloblastic anemia (rare)
   Neuromuscular & skeletal: Weakness, myalgia
   Respiratory: Dyspnea, upper respiratory tract infection
   Miscellaneous: Decreased vitamin B$_{12}$ levels, increased sweating, flu-like syndrome, nail disorder
Drug Interactions Drugs which tend to produce hyperglycemia (eg, diuretics, corticosteroids, phenothiazines, thyroid products, estrogens, oral contraceptives, phenytoin, nicotinic acid, sympathomimetics, calcium channel blocking drugs, isoniazid) may lead to a loss of glycemic control; alcohol potentiates the effects of metformin on
(Continued)

Metformin *(Continued)*

lactate metabolism; cationic drugs (eg, amiloride, digoxin, morphine, procainamide, quinidine, quinine, ranitidine, triamterene, trimethoprim, and vancomycin) which are eliminated by renal tubular secretion have the potential for interaction with metformin by competing for common renal tubular transport systems; cimetidine increases (by 60%) peak metformin blood concentrations; in a single dose study, furosemide increased the metformin blood concentration without altering metformin renal clearance; nifedipine may enhance the absorption of metformin

Food Interactions Food decreases the extent and slightly delays the absorption (clinical significance unknown); may decrease absorption of vitamin B_{12} and folic acid

Stability Store at 20°C to 25°C (68°F to 77°F); protect from light

Mechanism of Action Decreases hepatic glucose production, decreases intestinal absorption of glucose, and improves insulin sensitivity (increases peripheral glucose uptake and utilization)

Pharmacodynamics

Onset of action: Within days, maximum effects up to 2 weeks

Average decrease in fasting blood glucose: 60-70 mg/dL

Pharmacokinetics

Absorption: Oral: Slowly and incompletely absorbed

Distribution: Adults: V_d: 654 ± 358 L

Protein binding, plasma: Negligible

Bioavailability: Oral: 50% to 60% (under fasting conditions)

Half-life, plasma elimination: 3-6 hours

Time to peak serum concentration: 2-4 hours

Elimination: Renal: tubular secretion is major route

Dialysis: Removed by hemodialysis; clearance up to 170 mL/minute

Usual Dosage Oral: **Note:** While significant responses may not be seen at doses <1500 mg daily, a lower recommended starting dose and gradual increase in dosage is recommended to minimize GI symptoms

Treatment of type 2 diabetes mellitus (noninsulin-dependent) in previously untreated patients or patients currently receiving sulfonylurea oral antidiabetic agents:

Children 10-16 years: Initial: 500 mg twice daily; dosage increases should be made weekly, in increments of 500 mg/day in divided doses, up to a maximum of 2000 mg/day.

Children ≥17 years and Adults:

Initial: 500 mg twice daily; dosage increases should be made weekly, in increments of 500 mg/day in 2 divided doses, up to a maximum of 2500 mg/day; doses >2000 mg/day may be better tolerated divided 3 times/day

Alternative dose: Initial: 850 mg once daily; dosage increases should be made in increments of 850 mg every 2 weeks, given in divided doses, up to a maximum of 2550 mg/day

Glucophage® XR (extended release tablets): Initial: 500 mg once daily; dosage may be increased by 500 mg weekly; maximum dose: 2000 mg once daily. If glycemic control is not achieved at maximum dose, may divide dose to 1000 mg twice daily; if doses >2000 mg/day are needed, switch to regular release tablets and titrate to maximum dose of 2550 mg/day

Adjunctive agent to diabetic patient receiving insulin: Children ≥17 years and Adults: Initial: 500 mg metformin or metformin extended release once daily, continue current insulin dose; increase by 500 mg every week; maximum dose: 2500 mg metformin or 2000 mg metformin extended release; decrease insulin dose by 10% to 25% when fasting blood glucose <120 mg/dL

Dosing adjustment in renal impairment: Metformin is contraindicated in the presence of renal dysfunction (see Contraindications)

Dosing adjustment in hepatic impairment: Avoid metformin; liver disease is a risk factor for the development of lactic acidosis during metformin therapy.

Administration Oral:

Glucophage®: Administer in divided doses with meals

Glucophage® XR: Administer with evening meal; extended release tablets should be swallowed whole; do not cut, crush, or chew

Monitoring Parameters Fasting blood glucose, hemoglobin A_{1c}, initial and periodic monitoring of hemoglobin, hematocrit, and red blood cell indices; renal function (baseline and annually)

Reference Range Target range:

Blood glucose: Fasting and preprandial: 80-120 mg/dL; bedtime: 100-140 mg/dL

Glycosylated hemoglobin (hemoglobin A_{1c}): <7%

Patient Information Do not change dose or discontinue without consulting prescriber; avoid alcohol while taking this medication, could cause severe reaction; maintain regular dietary intake and exercise routine; always carry quick source of sugar with you; during the first weeks of therapy, side effects such as headache, nausea, vomiting, or diarrhea may occur; consult prescriber if these persist; report severe or persistent side effects, extended vomiting or flu-like symptoms, skin rash, easy bruising or bleeding, or change in color of urine or stool; contact your healthcare provider immediately if you feel very weak, tired, or uncomfortable, have unusual muscle pain, trouble breathing, unusual stomach discomfort, are dizzy or lightheaded, or suddenly develop a slow or irregular heartbeat; parts of the extended release tablet (which do not contain active ingredient) may be found excreted in the stool

Additional Information When transferring therapy from chlorpropamide to metformin, monitor the patient closely during the first 2 weeks due to the prolonged retention of chlorpropamide in the body, leading to overlapping drug effects and possible hypoglycemia; if the patient has not responded to 4 weeks at the maximum metformin dosage, consider a gradual addition of a sulfonylurea antidiabetic agent, even if prior primary or secondary failure to a sulfonylurea has occurred; continue metformin at the maximum dose

Dosage Forms
Tablet, as hydrochloride (Glucophage®): 500 mg, 850 mg, 1000 mg
Tablet, extended release, as hydrochloride (Glucophage® XR): 500 mg

References
DeFronzo RA, "Pharmacologic Therapy for Type 2 Diabetes Mellitus," *Ann Intern Med*, 1999, 131(4):281-303.

Jones K, Arlanian S, McVie R, et al, "Metformin Improves Glycemic Control in Children With Type 2 Diabetes," *Diabetes*, 2000, 49(Suppl 1):A75.

"Type 2 Diabetes in Children and Adolescents. American Diabetes Association," *Diabetes Care*, 2000, 23(3):381-9.

♦ **Metformin Hydrochloride** *see* Metformin *on page 729*

Methadone (METH a done)

Related Information
Narcotic Analgesics Comparison *on page 1223*
Overdose and Toxicology *on page 1388*

U.S. Brand Names Dolophine®; Methadone Intensol™; Methadose®
Canadian Brand Names Metadol™
Therapeutic Category Analgesic, Narcotic
Generic Available Yes (solution and tablets)
Use Management of severe pain, used in narcotic detoxification maintenance programs and for the treatment of iatrogenic narcotic dependency
Restrictions C-II
Pregnancy Risk Factor B (D if used for prolonged periods or in high doses at term)
Contraindications Hypersensitivity to methadone or any component
Warnings Tablets are to be used only for oral administration and **must not** be used for injection; abrupt discontinuation after prolonged use may result in withdrawal symptoms or seizures
Precautions Due to the cumulative effects of methadone, the dose and frequency of administration need to be reduced with repeated use; use with caution in patients with respiratory diseases; methadone's effect on respiration lasts longer than analgesic effects

Adverse Reactions
Cardiovascular: Hypotension, bradycardia, peripheral vasodilation
Central nervous system: CNS depression, elevated intracranial pressure, drowsiness, dizziness, sedation (marked sedation seen after repeated administration)
Endocrine & metabolic: Antidiuretic hormone release
Gastrointestinal: Nausea, vomiting, constipation, xerostomia, biliary tract spasm
Genitourinary: Urinary tract spasm
Ocular: Miosis
Respiratory: Respiratory depression
Miscellaneous: Histamine release, physical and psychological dependence with prolonged use

Drug Interactions Cytochrome P450 isoenzyme CYP1A2, CYP2D6, CYP3A3/4 substrate; CYP2D6 isoenzyme inhibitor
CNS depressants, alcohol, phenothiazines, tricyclic antidepressants may potentiate the adverse effects of methadone; barbiturates, carbamazepine, phenytoin, primidone, efavirenz, nevirapine, ritonavir, nelfinavir, amprenavir, lopinavir, and rifampin may increase the metabolism of methadone and may precipitate withdrawal (monitor patients, larger doses of methadone may be required); methadone may decrease stavudine (no dosage adjustment needed) and didanosine concentrations (consider increase in didanosine dose)

Mechanism of Action Binds to opiate receptors in the CNS, causing inhibition of ascending pain pathways, altering the perception of and response to pain; produces generalized CNS depression
(Continued)

Methadone *(Continued)*

Pharmacodynamics Analgesia:
Onset of action:
- Oral: Within 30-60 minutes
- Parenteral: Within 10-20 minutes

Maximum effect: Parenteral: 1-2 hours

Duration: Oral: 6-8 hours; after repeated doses, duration increases to 22-48 hours

Pharmacokinetics
Distribution: Crosses the placenta; appears in breast milk

V_d: (Mean ± SD)
- Children: 7.1 ± 2.5 L/kg
- Adults: 6.1 ± 2.4 L/kg

Protein binding: 80% to 85%

Metabolism: N-demethylated in the liver

Half-life: May be prolonged with alkaline pH
- Children: 19 ± 14 hours (range: 4-62 hours)
- Adults: 35 ± 22 hours (range: 9-87 hours)

Elimination: In urine (<10% as unchanged drug); increased renal excretion with urine pH <6

Usual Dosage Doses should be titrated to appropriate effects:
Neonatal abstinence syndrome: Oral, I.V.: Initial: 0.05-0.2 mg/kg/dose given every 12-24 hours or 0.5 mg/kg/day divided every 8 hours; individualize dose and tapering schedule to control symptoms of withdrawal; usually taper dose by 10% to 20% per week over 1 to 1½ months. **Note**: Due to long elimination half-life, tapering is difficult; consider alternate agent.

Children:

Analgesia:
- I.V.: Initial: 0.1 mg/kg/dose every 4 hours for 2-3 doses, then every 6-12 hours as needed; maximum dose: 10 mg/dose
- Oral, I.M., S.C.: Initial: 0.1 mg/kg/dose every 4 hours for 2-3 doses, then every 6-12 hours as needed or 0.7 mg/kg/24 hours divided every 4-6 hours as needed; maximum dose: 10 mg/dose

Iatrogenic narcotic dependency: Oral: Controlled studies have not been conducted; several clinically used dosing regimens have been reported. Methadone dose **must be individualized** and will depend upon patient's previous narcotic dose and severity of opioid withdrawal; patients who have received higher doses of narcotics will require higher methadone doses.

General guidelines: Initial: 0.05-0.1 mg/kg/dose every 6 hours; increase by 0.05 mg/kg/dose until withdrawal symptoms are controlled; after 24-48 hours, the dosing interval can be lengthened to every 12-24 hours; to taper dose, wean by 0.05 mg/kg/day; if withdrawal symptoms recur, taper at a slower rate

Adults:
- Analgesia: Oral, I.M., I.V., S.C.: 2.5-10 mg every 3-8 hours as needed, up to 5-20 mg every 6-8 hours
- Detoxification: Oral: 15-40 mg/day
- Maintenance of opiate dependence: Oral: 20-120 mg/day

Dosing adjustment in renal impairment: Children and Adults:
Cl_{cr} <10 mL/minute: Administer 50% to 75% of normal dose

Administration Oral: Administer with juice or water; dispersible tablet should be completely dissolved before administration; oral dose for detoxification and maintenance may be administered in Tang®, Kool-Aid®, apple juice, grape Crystal Light®

Monitoring Parameters Respiratory, cardiovascular, and mental status, pain relief (if used for analgesia), abstinence scoring system (if used for neonatal abstinence syndrome)

Patient Information Avoid alcohol; may be habit-forming; avoid abrupt discontinuation after prolonged use; may cause drowsiness and impair ability to perform activities requiring mental alertness or physical coordination; may cause dry mouth

Additional Information Methadone accumulates with repeated doses and dosage may need to be adjusted downward after 3-5 days to prevent toxic effects. Some patients may benefit from every 8- to 12-hour dosing interval (pain control).

Methadone 10 mg I.M. = morphine 10 mg I.M.

Dosage Forms
Injection, solution, as hydrochloride (Dolophine®): 10 mg/mL (20 mL)

Solution, oral, as hydrochloride: 5 mg/5 mL (500 mL); 10 mg/5 mL (500 mL) [contains 8% alcohol; citrus flavor]

Solution, oral **concentrate**, as hydrochloride:
- Methadone Intensol™: 10 mg/mL (30 mL)
- Methadose®: 10 mg/mL (30 mL) [cherry flavor]

Tablet, as hydrochloride (Dolophine®, Methadose®): 5 mg, 10 mg

Tablet, dispersible, as hydrochloride (Methadose®): 40 mg

References

Anand KJ and Arnold JH, "Opioid Tolerance and Dependence in Infants and Children," *Crit Care Med*, 1994, 22(2):334-42.

Berde C, Ablin A, Glazer J, et al, "American Academy of Pediatrics Report of the Subcommittee on Disease-Related Pain in Childhood Cancer," *Pediatrics*, 1990, 86(5 Pt 2):818-25.

Lauriault G, LeBelle MJ, Lodge BA, et al, "Stability of Methadone in Four Vehicles for Oral Administration," *Am J Hosp Pharm*, 1991, 48(6):1252-6.

Olkkola KT, Hamunen K, and Maunuksela EL, "Clinical Pharmacokinetics and Pharmacodynamics of Opioid Analgesics in Infants and Children," *Clin Pharmacokinet*, 1995, 28(5):385-404.

♦ **Methadone Intensol™** *see* Methadone *on page 731*

♦ **Methadose®** *see* Methadone *on page 731*

Methenamine (meth EN a meen)

U.S. Brand Names Hiprex®; Mandelamine®; Urex®

Canadian Brand Names Dehydral®; Urasal®

Synonyms Hexamethylenetetramine

Therapeutic Category Antibiotic, Miscellaneous

Generic Available Yes

Use Prophylaxis or suppression of recurrent urinary tract infections

Pregnancy Risk Factor C

Contraindications Hypersensitivity to methenamine or any component (see Warnings); severe dehydration, renal insufficiency (methenamine is ineffective in patients with renal impairment), hepatic insufficiency in patients receiving hippurate salt

Warnings Dosage of 8 g/day has been associated with bladder irritation, albuminuria, and hematuria; Hiprex® tablets contain tartrazine which may cause allergic reactions in susceptible individuals

Precautions Use with caution in patients with hepatic impairment

Adverse Reactions

Central nervous system: Headache

Dermatologic: Rash, pruritus, urticaria

Gastrointestinal: Nausea, vomiting, diarrhea, abdominal cramping, anorexia, stomatitis

Genitourinary: Bladder irritation, painful and frequent micturition, dysuria, crystalluria

Hepatic: Elevated AST and ALT (with hippurate formulation)

Otic: Tinnitus

Renal: Hematuria

Respiratory: Lipoid pneumonitis (with mandelate suspension), dyspnea

Drug Interactions Sulfamethizole (precipitates in acid urine); sodium bicarbonate, acetazolamide (decrease effect of methenamine)

Food Interactions Foods/diets which alkalinize urine pH >5.5 decrease activity of methenamine; cranberry juice can be used to acidify urine and increase activity of methenamine

Stability Protect from excessive heat

Mechanism of Action Methenamine is hydrolyzed to formaldehyde and ammonia in acidic urine; formaldehyde has nonspecific bactericidal action

Pharmacokinetics

Absorption: Readily from the GI tract; 10% to 30% of the drug will be hydrolyzed by gastric juices unless it is protected by an enteric coating

Distribution: Distributes into breast milk; crosses the placenta

Metabolism: ~10% to 25% in the liver

Half-life: 3-6 hours

Elimination: Excretion occurs via glomerular filtration and tubular secretion with ~70% to 90% of dose excreted unchanged in urine within 24 hours

Usual Dosage Oral:

Children 6-12 years: Mandelate: 75 mg/kg/day divided every 12 hours or 50-75 mg/kg/day divided every 6-8 hours; maximum dose: 4 g/day

Adults:

Hippurate: 1 g twice daily

Mandelate: 1 g 4 times/day after meals and at bedtime

Administration Oral: Administer with food to minimize GI upset; shake suspension well before use; patient should drink plenty of fluids to ensure adequate urine flow; administer with cranberry juice, ascorbic acid, or ammonium chloride to acidify urine; avoid intake of alkalinizing agents (sodium bicarbonate, antacids)

Monitoring Parameters Urinary pH, urinalysis, periodic liver function tests in patients receiving hippurate salt

Test Interactions Formaldehyde interferes with fluorometric procedures causing falsely increased results for catecholamines and VMA (U); falsely decreased urine estriol concentration with tests using acid hydrolysis

(Continued)

Methenamine (Continued)

Nursing Implications Urine should be acidic, pH <5.5 for maximum effect

Additional Information Should not be used to treat infections outside of the lower urinary tract (ie, pyelonephritis)

Dosage Forms

Tablet, scored, as **hippurate** (Hiprex®, Urex®): 1 g [Hiprex® contains tartrazine]

Tablet, enteric coated, as **mandelate** (Mandelamine®): 500 mg, 1 g

Tablet, film coated, as **mandelate**: 500 mg, 1 g

References

"Practice Parameter: The Diagnosis, Treatment, and Evaluation of the Initial Urinary Tract Infection in Febrile Infants and Young Children. American Academy of Pediatrics. Committee on Quality Improvement. Subcommittee on Urinary Tract Infection," *Pediatrics*, 1999, 103(4 Pt 1):843-52.

Methimazole (meth IM a zole)

U.S. Brand Names Tapazole®

Synonyms Thiamazole

Therapeutic Category Antithyroid Agent

Generic Available Yes

Use Palliative treatment of hyperthyroidism, to return the hyperthyroid patient to a normal metabolic state prior to thyroidectomy, and to control thyrotoxic crisis that may accompany thyroidectomy

Pregnancy Risk Factor D

Contraindications Hypersensitivity to methimazole or any component, nursing mothers per manufacturer, however, expert analysis and the American Academy of Pediatrics state this drug may be used with caution in nursing mothers (see Drugs and Breast-Feeding *on page 1404*)

Precautions Use with extreme caution in patients receiving other drugs known to cause agranulocytosis

Adverse Reactions

Cardiovascular: Edema, periarteritis

Central nervous system: Drowsiness, vertigo, headache, CNS stimulation, neuropathies, CNS depression, fever, dizziness

Endocrine & metabolic: Goiter

Dermatologic: Rash, urticaria, pruritus, alopecia, skin pigmentation, exfoliative dermatitis

Gastrointestinal: Ageusia, nausea, vomiting, epigastric distress, splenomegaly, constipation, weight gain

Hematologic: Agranulocytosis, hypoprothrombinemia

Hepatic: Cholestatic jaundice, hepatitis

Neuromuscular & skeletal: Arthralgia, myalgia, paresthesia, neuritis

Renal: Nephritis

Respiratory: Interstitial pneumonitis

Miscellaneous: Lupus-like syndrome, lymphadenopathy, insulin autoimmune syndrome

Drug Interactions Lithium and potassium iodide may potentiate hypothyroid effects; potentiates warfarin's anticoagulant effects

Mechanism of Action Inhibits the synthesis of thyroid hormones by blocking the oxidation of iodine in the thyroid gland, blocking iodine's ability to combine with tyrosine to form thyroxine (T_4) and triiodothyronine (T_3)

Pharmacodynamics Antithyroid effect:

Onset of action: 12-18 hours

Duration: 36-72 hours

Pharmacokinetics

Distribution: Found in high concentrations in breast milk; breast milk to plasma ratio: 1.0

Bioavailability: 80% to 95%

Half-life: 5-13 hours

Time to peak serum concentration: 1 hour

Elimination: <12% excreted in urine

Usual Dosage Oral:

Children:

Initial: 0.4 mg/kg/day in 3 divided doses; maintenance: 0.2 mg/kg/day in 3 divided doses

or

Initial: 0.5-0.7 mg/kg/day or 15-20 mg/m²/day in 3 divided doses

Maintenance: $1/3$ to $2/3$ of initial dose; maximum dose: 30 mg/day

Adults: Initial: 5 mg every 8 hours; 10 mg every 8 hours for moderately severe disease and up to 20 mg every 8 hours for severe hyperthyroidism; maintenance: 5-15 mg/day

Administration Oral: Administer with meals

Monitoring Parameters CBC with differential, liver function (baseline and as needed); serum thyroxine, free thyroxine index, prothrombin time

Patient Information Notify physician of fever, sore throat, unusual bleeding or bruising, headache, rash, or yellowing of skin

Dosage Forms Tablet: 5 mg, 10 mg

References

Raby C, Lagorce JF, Jambut-Absil AC, et al, "The Mechanism of Action of Synthetic Antithyroid Drugs: Iodine Complexation During Oxidation of Iodide," *Endocrinology*, 1990, 126(3):1683-91.

Methocarbamol (meth oh KAR ba mole)

U.S. Brand Names Robaxin®

Therapeutic Category Skeletal Muscle Relaxant, Nonparalytic

Generic Available Yes (tablet)

Use Treatment of muscle spasm associated with acute painful musculoskeletal conditions; supportive therapy in tetanus

Pregnancy Risk Factor C

Contraindications Hypersensitivity to methocarbamol or any component

Warnings Solution is hypertonic, avoid extravasation; avoid using injection in patients with impaired renal function because the polyethylene glycol vehicle may be irritating to the kidneys

Precautions Use injectable form cautiously in patients with suspected or known seizure disorders

Adverse Reactions

Cardiovascular: Syncope, bradycardia, hypotension

Central nervous system: Drowsiness, dizziness, lightheadedness, headache, fever, vertigo, seizures

Dermatologic: Urticaria, pruritus

Gastrointestinal: Nausea, metallic taste, GI upset, vomiting

Genitourinary: Discoloration of urine (brown, black, or green)

Hematologic: Leukopenia

Local: Pain and phlebitis at injection site, thrombophlebitis

Ocular: Blurred vision, conjunctivitis, nystagmus, diplopia

Respiratory: Nasal congestion

Miscellaneous: Hypersensitivity reactions

Stability Injection when diluted to 4 mg/mL in SWI, D_5W, or NS is stable for 6 days at room temperature; do **not** refrigerate after dilution

Mechanism of Action CNS depressant with sedative and skeletal muscle relaxant effects; exact mechanism of action is unknown

Pharmacodynamics Onset of action: 30 minutes

Pharmacokinetics Oral:

Metabolism: Extensive in the liver

Half-life: 0.9-1.8 hours

Time to peak serum concentration: Within ~1-2 hours

Usual Dosage

Tetanus: I.V.:

Children (recommended **only** for use in tetanus): 15 mg/kg/dose or 500 mg/m²/dose, may repeat every 6 hours if needed; maximum dose: 1.8 g/m²/day for 3 days only

Adults: 1-2 g by direct I.V. injection followed by additional 1-2 g (maximum dose: 3 g total); repeat with 1-2 g every 6 hours until NG tube or oral therapy possible; total daily dose of up to 24 g may be needed

Muscle spasm: Adults:

Oral: 1.5 g 3-4 times/day or 750 mg every 4 hours for 2-3 days, then decrease to 4-4.5 g/day in 3-6 divided doses

I.M., I.V.: 1 g every 8 hours if oral not possible; maximum dose: 3 g/day for 3 consecutive days (except when treating tetanus); may be reinstituted after 2 drug-free days

Dosing adjustment in renal impairment: Do not administer parenteral formulation to patients with renal dysfunction

Administration

Parenteral: I.V.: May be injected directly I.V. without dilution at a maximum rate of 180 mg/m²/minute but not >3 mL/minute; may also be diluted in NS or D_5W to a concentration of 4 mg/mL and infused more slowly; patient should be in the recumbent position during and for 10-15 minutes after I.V. administration

I.M.: Do not inject more than 3 mL per site; not recommended for S.C. administration

Test Interactions 5-hydroxyindoleacetic acid (5-HIAA) and vanillylmandelic acid (VMA)

(Continued)

Methocarbamol *(Continued)*

Patient Information May cause drowsiness and impair ability to perform activities requiring mental alertness or physical coordination; urine may darken to brown, black, or green

Nursing Implications Avoid infiltration, extremely irritating to tissues

Dosage Forms

Injection, solution (Robaxin®): 100 mg/mL (10 mL) [in polyethylene glycol]

Tablet (Robaxin®): 500 mg, 750 mg

Methohexital *(meth oh HEKS i tal)*

Related Information

Adult ACLS Algorithm, Synchronized Cardioversion *on page 1192*

Preprocedure Sedatives in Children *on page 1367*

U.S. Brand Names Brevital® Sodium

Therapeutic Category Barbiturate; General Anesthetic; Sedative

Generic Available No

Use Induction and maintenance of general anesthesia for short procedures; induction of hypnotic state

Restrictions C-IV

Pregnancy Risk Factor B

Contraindications Hypersensitivity to methohexital, barbiturates, or any component; porphyria; patients in whom general anesthesia is contraindicated

Warnings Continuously monitor respiratory function, pulse oximetry, and cardiac function. Resuscitative drugs, ventilation and intubation equipment, and trained personnel should be immediately available. For deep sedation, a designated individual (other than the person performing the procedure) should be present to continuously monitor the patient.

Precautions Use with extreme caution in patients with liver impairment, asthma, cardiovascular instability; may precipitate seizures in patients with history of convulsions, especially partial seizure disorders; prolonged administration may result in increased CNS, respiratory, and cardiovascular effects; use with caution in patients with obstructive pulmonary disease, severe hypertension or hypotension, myocardial disease, CHF, severe anemia, extreme obesity, renal impairment, or endocrine disorders

Adverse Reactions

Cardiovascular: Hypotension, peripheral vascular collapse, tachycardia (following induction)

Central nervous system: Seizures, headache, somnolence, unconsciousness

Gastrointestinal: Nausea, vomiting, abdominal pain

Local: Pain on I.M. injection, thrombophlebitis

Hepatic: Elevated liver enzymes

Neuromuscular & skeletal: Twitching, rigidity, tremor, involuntary muscle movement

Respiratory: Apnea, respiratory depression, laryngospasm, coughing

Miscellaneous: Hiccups

Drug Interactions CNS depressants may increase effects; prior chronic use of phenytoin, barbiturates, or other enzyme inducing agents may decrease effect of methohexital; methohexital may affect absorption or elimination of phenytoin, anticoagulants, corticosteroids, halothane, ethanol, propylene glycol containing solutions

Stability Do not dilute with solutions containing bacteriostatic agents; acceptable diluents: D_5W, NS, SWI, or accompanying diluent (for 500 mg vial to make a 1% solution); SWI is the preferred diluent except for making the 0.2% solution for I.V. continuous infusion (use of SWI to make the 0.2% solution will result in extreme hypotonicity; D_5W or NS should be used). Do not use I.V./I.M. solutions if not clear and colorless. Solutions are alkaline (pH 9.5-11) and incompatible with acids (eg, atropine sulfate, succinylcholine chloride); incompatible with phenol-containing solutions, silicone, and LR

Mechanism of Action Ultra short-acting I.V. barbiturate anesthetic; depresses CNS activity by binding to barbiturate site at GABA-receptor complex enhancing GABA activity; depresses reticular activating system; higher doses may be gabamimetic

Pharmacodynamics

Onset of action:

I.M. (pediatric patients): 2-10 minutes

I.V.: 1 minute

Rectal (pediatric patients): 5-15 minutes

Duration:

I.M.: 1-1.5 hours

I.V.: 7-10 minutes

Rectal: 1-1.5 hours

Pharmacokinetics

Metabolism: In the liver via demethylation and oxidation

Bioavailability: Rectal: 17%

Elimination: Through the kidney via glomerular filtration

Usual Dosage Doses must be titrated to effect

Manufacturer's recommendations:

Infants <1 month: Safety and efficacy not established

Infants ≥1 month and Children:

I.M.: Induction: 6.6-10 mg/kg of a 5% solution

Rectal: Induction: Usual: 25 mg/kg of a 1% solution

Alternative pediatric dosing:

Children 3-12 years:

I.M.: Preoperative: 5-10 mg/kg/dose

I.V.: Induction: 1-2 mg/kg/dose (additional studies are needed)

Rectal: Preoperative/induction: 20-35 mg/kg/dose; usual: 25 mg/kg/dose; maximum dose: 500 mg/dose; give as 10% aqueous solution

Adults: I.V.:

Induction: Range: 50-120 mg or 1-1.5 mg/kg; usual: 70 mg (**Note:** This provides anesthesia for 5-7 minutes)

Maintenance: Intermittent I.V. bolus injection: 20-40 mg (2-4 mL of a 1% solution) every 4-7 minutes OR Continuous infusion: Average dose: 6 mg/minute (eg, 3 mL/minute of a 0.2% solution); titrate to effect; reduce administration rate gradually for longer surgical procedures

Administration

Parenteral:

I.M.: Reconstitute with NS to a maximum concentration of 50 mg/mL (5% solution)

I.V.: Adults:

Bolus: Dilute with SWI (preferred), NS, or D_5W to a maximum concentration of 10 mg/mL (1% solution); for induction, infuse a 1% solution at a rate of 1 mL/5 seconds

Continuous infusion: Dilute with D_5W or NS to prepare a 0.2% solution (see Usual Dosage)

Rectal: Dilute with acceptable diluent (see Stability) to a recommended concentration of 10 mg/mL (1% solution)

Monitoring Parameters Blood pressure, heart rate, respiratory rate, oxygen saturation, pulse oximetry

Patient Information May cause drowsiness and impair ability to perform activities requiring mental alertness or physical coordination; do not drive a motor vehicle or operate machinery until 8-12 hours after medication was administered, or until normal functions return (whichever is longer)

Nursing Implications Check catheter placement prior to I.V. injection; avoid extravasation; avoid intra-arterial administration (thrombosis, necrosis, and gangrene may occur)

Additional Information Does not possess analgesic properties; Brevital® has FDA-approved labeling for I.V. use in adults, and for rectal and I.M. use only in pediatric patients >1 month of age; 100 pediatric patients (3 months to 5 years of age) received rectal methohexital (25 mg/kg) for sedation prior to computed tomography (CT) scan; sedation was adequate in 95% of patients; mean time for full sedation = 8.2 ± 3.9 minutes; mean duration of action = 79.3 ± 30.9 minutes; 10% of patients had transient side effects (see Pomeranz, 2000)

Dosage Forms Injection, powder for reconstitution, as sodium: 500 mg, 2.5 g, 5 g

References

Cote' CJ, "Sedation for the Pediatric Patient," Pediatr Clin North Am, 1994, 41(1):31-58.

Pomeranz ES, Chudnofsky CR, Deegan TJ, et al, "Rectal Methohexital Sedation for Computed Tomography Imaging of Stable Pediatric Emergency Department Patients," Pediatrics, 2000, 105(5):1110-4.

Methotrexate (meth oh TREKS ate)

Related Information

Drugs and Breast-Feeding on page 1404

Emetogenic Potential of Single Chemotherapeutic Agents on page 1286

U.S. Brand Names Rheumatrex®; Trexall™

Canadian Brand Names Apo®-Methotrexate; ratio-Methotrexate

Synonyms Amethopterin; MTX

Therapeutic Category Antineoplastic Agent, Antimetabolite; Antirheumatic, Disease Modifying

Generic Available Yes

(Continued)

Methotrexate *(Continued)*

Use Treatment of trophoblastic neoplasms, leukemias, histiocytoses, osteosarcoma, non-Hodgkin's lymphoma; psoriasis; children with severe polyarticular juvenile rheumatoid arthritis who have failed to respond to other agents

Pregnancy Risk Factor D

Contraindications Hypersensitivity to methotrexate or any component (see Warnings); severe renal or hepatic impairment; pre-existing profound bone marrow suppression; high-dose methotrexate (>1 g/m²) should not be administered to patients with a creatinine clearance of <50% to 75% of normal

Warnings The FDA currently recommends that procedures for proper handling and disposal of antineoplastic agents be considered. Due to the possibility of severe toxic reactions, fully inform patient of the risks involved; do not use in women of child-bearing age unless benefit outweighs risks; may cause hepatotoxicity, fibrosis and cirrhosis, along with marked bone marrow suppression; death from intestinal perforation may occur.

Some injections contain benzyl alcohol which may cause allergic reactions in susceptible individuals; large amounts of benzyl alcohol (≥99 mg/kg/day) have been associated with a potentially fatal toxicity ("gasping syndrome") in neonates; the "gasping syndrome" consists of metabolic acidosis, respiratory distress, gasping respirations, CNS dysfunction (including convulsions, intracranial hemorrhage), hypotension and cardiovascular collapse; avoid use of methotrexate products containing benzyl alcohol in neonates; *in vitro* and animal studies have shown that benzoate, a metabolite of benzyl alcohol, displaces bilirubin from protein binding sites

Precautions Use with caution in patients with peptic ulcer disease, ulcerative colitis, pre-existing bone marrow suppression; use with caution and reduce dosage in patients with renal or hepatic impairment, ascites, and pleural effusion

Adverse Reactions
  Cardiovascular: Vasculitis
  Central nervous system: Malaise, fatigue, dizziness, encephalopathy, seizures, confusion, fever, headache, chills
  Dermatitis: Alopecia, rash, depigmentation or hyperpigmentation of skin, photosensitivity, pruritus, urticaria
  Endocrine & metabolic: Hyperuricemia
  Gastrointestinal: Nausea, vomiting, diarrhea, anorexia, stomatitis, enteritis
  Genitourinary: Cystitis
  Hematologic: Myelosuppression, leukopenia, thrombocytopenia, anemia, hemorrhage
  Hepatic: Hepatotoxicity, elevated liver enzymes, hyperbilirubinemia
  Neuromuscular & skeletal: Arthralgia
  Ocular: Blurred vision
  Renal: Nephropathy (azotemia, hematuria, renal failure)
  Respiratory: Interstitial pneumonitis
  Miscellaneous: Anaphylaxis

Drug Interactions Salicylates may delay MTX's clearance; sulfonamides, phenytoin displace MTX from protein binding sites; live virus vaccines, pyrimethamine, 5-FU; NSAIDs increase toxicity of MTX by elevating serum MTX concentrations; penicillins may decrease renal clearance of MTX; probenecid decreases the renal elimination of MTX

Food Interactions Milk-rich foods may decrease MTX absorption; folate may decrease drug response

Stability Protect from light; incompatible with fluorouracil, cytarabine, prednisolone, and sodium phosphate

Mechanism of Action An antimetabolite that binds to dihydrofolate reductase blocking the reduction of dihydrofolate to tetrahydrofolic acid; depletion of tetrahydrofolic acid leads to depletion of DNA precursors and inhibition of DNA and purine synthesis

Pharmacodynamics Approximate time to benefit in treatment of rheumatoid arthritis: 1-2 months

Pharmacokinetics
  Absorption:
    Oral: Average: 30%; variable absorption at low doses (<30 mg/m²); incomplete absorption after large doses
    I.M.: Completely absorbed
  Distribution: Small amounts excreted into breast milk; crosses the placenta; does not achieve therapeutic concentrations in the CSF; sustained concentrations are retained in the kidney and liver
  Metabolism: In the liver to 7-hydroxymethotrexate
  Protein binding: 50% to 60%

Time to peak serum concentration:
Oral: 0.5-4 hours
Parenteral: 0.5-2 hours
Half-life: 8-12 hours
Elimination: Small amounts in feces; primarily excreted unchanged in urine (90%) via glomerular filtration and active secretion by the renal tubule; 1% to 11% of a dose is excreted as the 7-hydroxy metabolite

Usual Dosage Refer to individual protocols:

Children:
Dermatomyositis: Oral: 15-20 mg/m^2/week as a single dose once weekly or 0.3-1 mg/kg/dose once weekly
Juvenile rheumatoid arthritis: Oral, I.M., S.C.: 5-15 mg/m^2/week as a single dose or in 3 divided doses given 12 hours apart; folic acid 1 mg daily or folinic acid ≤5 mg weekly are often used to prevent folate depletion from methotrexate
Antineoplastic dosage range:
Oral:, I.M.: 7.5-30 mg/m^2/week or every 2 weeks
I.V.: 10 mg to 33,000 mg/m^2 bolus dosing or continuous infusion over 6-42 hours
Antineoplastic dosing schedules (adapted from Dorr RT and Von Hoff DD, *Cancer Chemotherapy Handbook*, 2nd ed, 1994): See table

Methotrexate Dosing Schedules

	Dose	Route	Frequency
Conventional dose	15-20 mg/m^2	Oral	Twice weekly
	30-50 mg/m^2	Oral, I.V.	Weekly
	15 mg/day for 5 days	Oral, I.M.	Every 2-3 weeks
Intermediate dose	50-150 mg/m^2	I.V. push	Every 2-3 weeks
	240 mg/m^2*	I.V. infusion	Every 4-7 days
	0.5-1 g/m^2*	I.V. infusion	Every 2-3 weeks
High dose	1-12 g/m^2*	I.V. infusion	Every 1-3 weeks

*Followed with leucovorin rescue

Pediatric solid tumors:
<12 years: 12 g/m^2 (dosage range: 12-18 g)
≥12 years: 8 g/m^2 (maximum dose: 18 g)
Meningeal leukemia: I.T.: 10-15 mg/m^2 (maximum: 15 mg) by protocol **or**
≤3 months: 3 mg dose
4-11 months: 6 mg dose
1 year: 8 mg dose
2 years: 10 mg dose
≥3 years: 12 mg dose
I.T. doses are administered at 2- to 5-day intervals until CSF counts return to normal followed by a dose once weekly for 2 weeks then monthly thereafter
ALL (high dose): I.V.: Loading dose: 200 mg/m^2 followed by a 24-hour infusion of 1200 mg/m^2/day
ANLL: I.V.: 7.5 mg/m^2/day on days 1-5 of treatment course
Resistant ANLL: I.V.: 100 mg/m^2/dose on day 1 of treatment course
Non-Hodgkin's lymphoma: I.V.: 200-500 mg/m^2; repeat every 28 days
Induction of remission in acute lymphoblastic leukemias: Oral: 3.3 mg/m^2/day for 4-6 weeks
Remission maintenance: Oral, I.M.: 20-30 mg/m^2 2 times/week

Adults:
Trophoblastic neoplasms: Oral, I.M.: 15-30 mg/day for 5 days, repeat in 7 days for 3-5 courses
Head and neck cancer: Oral, I.M. I.V.: 25-50 mg/m^2 once weekly
Rheumatoid arthritis: Oral: 7.5 mg once weekly or 2.5 mg every 12 hours for 3 doses/week; not to exceed 20 mg/week
Psoriasis: Oral: 2.5-5 mg/dose every 12 hours for 3 doses/week given once weekly **or**
Oral, I.M.: 10-25 mg given once weekly

Dosing adjustment in renal impairment:
Cl$_{cr}$ 61-80 mL/minute: Decrease dose by 25%
Cl$_{cr}$ 51-60 mL/minute: Decrease dose by 33%
Cl$_{cr}$ 10-50 mL/minute: Decrease dose by 50% to 70%

Administration Parenteral:
Methotrexate may be administered I.V. push, I.V. intermittent infusion, or I.V. continuous infusion at a concentration <25 mg/mL; doses >100-300 mg/m^2 are usually
(Continued)

Methotrexate *(Continued)*

administered by I.V. continuous infusion and are followed by a course of leucovorin rescue

For intrathecal use, mix methotrexate without preservatives with NS, Elliotts B solution, or LR to a concentration not greater than 2 mg/mL

Monitoring Parameters CBC with differential and platelet count, creatinine clearance, serum creatinine, BUN, hepatic function tests, serum electrolytes, urinalysis, plasma MTX concentrations (see leucovorin rescue graph *on page 661* to evaluate plasma MTX concentration versus leucovorin rescue dose)

Reference Range Serum levels >1 x 10^{-7} mol/L for more than 40 hours are toxic

Patient Information Report to physician any fever, sore throat, bleeding or bruising, shortness of breath, painful urination; avoid alcohol. May cause photosensitivity reactions (eg, exposure to sunlight may cause severe sunburn, skin rash, redness, or itching); avoid exposure to sunlight and artificial light sources (sunlamps, tanning booth/bed); wear protective clothing, wide-brimmed hats, sunglasses, and lip sunscreen (SPF ≥15); use a sunscreen [broad-spectrum sunscreen or physical sunscreen (preferred) or sunblock with SPF ≥15]; contact physician if reaction occurs.

Nursing Implications Intensive hydration should be administered and urine should be alkalinized prior to high doses to enhance methotrexate solubility

Additional Information Myelosuppressive effects:

WBC: Mild
Platelets: Moderate
Onset (days): 7
Nadir (days): 10
Recovery (days): 21

Dosage Forms

Injection, powder for reconstitution, as sodium [preservative free]: 20 mg, 1 g

Injection, solution, as sodium: 25 mg/mL (2 mL, 10 mL) [contains benzyl alcohol]

Injection, solution, as sodium [preservative free]: 25 mg/mL (2 mL, 4 mL, 8 mL, 10 mL)

Tablet, as sodium: 2.5 mg
Rheumatrex®: 2.5 mg [scored]
Trexall™: 5 mg, 7.5 mg, 10 mg, 15 mg [scored]

Tablet, dose pack, as sodium (Rheumatrex®): 2.5 mg [4 cards with 2, 3, 4, 5, or 6 tablets each; scored]

References

Berg SL, Grisell DL, DeLaney TF, et al, "Principles of Treatment of Pediatric Solid Tumors," *Pediatr Clin North Am*, 1991, 38(2):249-67.

Bleyer WA, "Clinical Pharmacology of Intrathecal Methotrexate II. An Approved Dosage Regimen Derived From Age-Related Pharmacokinetics," *Cancer Treat Rep*, 1977, 61(8):1419-25.

Crom WR, Glynn-Barnhart AM, Rodman JH, et al, "Pharmacokinetics of Anticancer Drugs in Children," *Clin Pharmacokinet*, 1987, 12(3):168-213.

Giannini EH, Brewer EJ, Kuzmina N, et al, "Methotrexate in Resistant Juvenile Rheumatoid Arthritis. Results of the USA-USSR Double-Blind, Placebo-Controlled Trial," *N Engl J Med*, 1992, 326(16):1043-9.

Greaves MW and Weinstein GD, "Treatment of Psoriasis," *N Engl J Med*, 1995, 332(9):581-8.

Rose CD, Singsen BH, and Eichenfield AH, "Safety and Efficacy of Methotrexate Therapy for Juvenile Rheumatoid Arthritis," *J Pediatr*, 1990, 117(4):653-9.

Methsuximide *(meth SUKS i mide)*

Related Information

Antiepileptic Drugs *on page 1374*

U.S. Brand Names Celontin®

Therapeutic Category Anticonvulsant, Succinimide

Generic Available No

Use Control of absence (petit mal) seizures; useful adjunct in refractory, partial complex (psychomotor) seizures

Pregnancy Risk Factor C

Contraindications Hypersensitivity to methsuximide, other succinimides, or any component

Warnings Blood dyscrasias (sometimes fatal) have been reported (monitor hematologic function periodically); SLE has been reported with the use of succinimides

Precautions Use with caution in patients with hepatic or renal disease; avoid abrupt withdrawal. Methsuximide may increase tonic clonic seizures in some patients.

Adverse Reactions

Central nervous system: Dizziness, drowsiness, lethargy, euphoria, nervousness, hallucinations, insomnia, mental confusion, headache, ataxia

Dermatologic: Rash, urticaria, Stevens-Johnson syndrome

Gastrointestinal: Nausea, vomiting, anorexia, diarrhea, abdominal pain

Genitourinary: Microscopic hematuria, proteinuria

Hematologic: Leukopenia, thrombocytopenia, eosinophilia, pancytopenia, monocytosis

Ocular: Periorbital edema

Miscellaneous: Hiccups

Drug Interactions Methsuximide may increase phenytoin and phenobarbital serum concentrations (monitor serum levels)

Stability Store at room temperature; protect from light, moisture, and heat; **Note:** Methsuximide has a relatively low melting temperature (124°F); do not store in conditions that promote high temperatures (eg, in a closed vehicle)

Mechanism of Action Increases the seizure threshold and suppresses paroxysmal spike-and-wave pattern in absence seizures; depresses nerve transmission in the motor cortex

Pharmacokinetics

Metabolism: Rapidly demethylated in the liver to N-desmethylmethsuximide (active metabolite)

Half-life: 2-4 hours

N-desmethylmethsuximide:

Children: 26 hours

Adults: 28-80 hours

Time to peak serum concentration: Within 1-3 hours

Elimination: <1% in urine as unchanged drug

Usual Dosage Oral:

Children: Initial: 10-15 mg/kg/day in 3-4 divided doses; increase weekly up to maximum of 30 mg/kg/day; mean dose required:

<30 kg: 20 mg/kg/day

>30 kg: 14 mg/kg/day

Adults: 300 mg/day for the first week; may increase by 300 mg/day at weekly intervals up to 1.2 g in 2-4 divided doses/day

Administration Oral: Administer with food

Monitoring Parameters CBC with differential, liver enzymes, urinalysis; measure trough serum levels for efficacy and 3-hour postdose concentrations for toxicity

Reference Range Measure N-desmethylmethsuximide concentrations:

Therapeutic: 10-40 μg/mL (SI: 53-212 μmol/L)

Toxic: >40 μg/mL (SI: >212 μmol/L)

Patient Information May cause drowsiness and impair ability to perform activities requiring mental alertness or physical coordination; do not discontinue abruptly; notify physician if sore throat or fever develop; do not store capsules in conditions that promote high temperatures (eg, in closed cars or other vehicles), as medication may melt

Dosage Forms Capsule: 150 mg, 300 mg

References

Miles MV, Tennison MB, and Greenwood RS, "Pharmacokinetics of N-desmethylmethsuximide in Pediatric Patients," J Pediatr, 1989, 114(4 Pt 1):647-50.

Tennison MB, Greenwood RS, Miles MV, "Methsuximide for Intractable Childhood Seizures," Pediatrics, 1991, 87(2):186-9.

♦ **Methylacetoxyprogesterone** see MedroxyPROGESTERone on page 712

Methyldopa (meth il DOE pa)

Canadian Brand Names Apo®-Methyldopa; Nu-Medopa

Therapeutic Category Alpha-Adrenergic Inhibitors, Central; Antihypertensive Agent

Generic Available Yes

Use Management of moderate to severe hypertension

Pregnancy Risk Factor B

Contraindications Hypersensitivity to methyldopa or any component (see Warnings); liver disease, pheochromocytoma

Warnings Injection contains sodium bisulfite which may cause allergic reactions in susceptible individuals

Precautions Use with caution and adjust dose in patients with renal dysfunction; active metabolite may accumulate in uremia

Adverse Reactions:

Cardiovascular: Orthostatic hypotension, bradycardia, edema

Central nervous system: Drowsiness, sedation, vertigo, headache, depression, memory lapse, fever

Dermatologic: Rash

Endocrine & metabolic: Gynecomastia, sexual dysfunction, sodium retention

Gastrointestinal: Nausea, vomiting, diarrhea, xerostomia, "black" tongue

Genitourinary: Discoloration of urine (red or brown)

Hematologic: Hemolytic anemia, positive Coombs' test, leukopenia

Hepatic: Hepatitis, elevated liver enzymes, jaundice, cirrhosis

(Continued)

Methyldopa *(Continued)*

Neuromuscular & skeletal: Weakness

Respiratory: Nasal congestion

Drug Interactions May increase lithium toxicity; concomitant oral administration of iron salts may decrease oral absorption of methyldopa and result in an increase in blood pressure, spacing drugs 2 hours apart may decrease this effect

Food Interactions Avoid natural licorice (causes sodium and water retention and increases potassium loss); dietary requirements for vitamin B_{12} and folate may be increased with high doses of methyldopa

Mechanism of Action Stimulates inhibitory alpha-adrenergic receptors via alpha-methylnorepinephrine (false transmitter); this results in a decreased sympathetic outflow to the heart, kidneys, and peripheral vasculature; may decrease plasma renin activity

Pharmacodynamics Hypotensive effects:

Maximum effect: Oral, I.V.: Single-dose: Within 3-6 hours; multiple-dose: 2-3 days

Duration:

Oral: Single-dose: 12-24 hours; multiple-dose: 1-2 days

I.V.: 10-16 hours

Pharmacokinetics

Absorption: Oral: ~50%

Distribution: Crosses placenta; appears in breast milk

Protein binding: <15%

Metabolism: In the intestine and the liver

Half-life: Elimination:

Neonates: 10-20 hours

Adults: 1-3 hours

Elimination: ~70% of systemic dose eliminated in urine as drug and metabolites

Dialysis: Slightly dialyzable (5% to 20%)

Usual Dosage

Children:

Oral: Initial: 10 mg/kg/day in 2-4 divided doses; increase every 2 days as needed to maximum dose of 65 mg/kg/day; do not exceed 3 g/day

I.V.: Initial: 2-4 mg/kg/dose; if response is not seen within 4-6 hours, may increase to 5-10 mg/kg/dose; administer doses every 6-8 hours; maximum daily dose: 65 mg/kg or 3 g, whichever is less

Adults:

Oral: Initial: 250 mg 2-3 times/day; increase every 2 days as needed; usual dose 500 mg to 2 g daily in 2-4 divided doses; maximum dose: 3 g/day

I.V.: 250-1000 mg every 6-8 hours; maximum dose: 4 g/day

Dosing interval in renal impairment: Children and Adults:

Cl_{cr} >50 mL/minute: Administer normal dose every 8 hours

Cl_{cr} 10-50 mL/minute: Administer normal dose every 8-12 hours

Cl_{cr} <10 mL/minute: Administer normal dose every 12-24 hours

Administration

Oral: May be administered without regard to food; administer new dosage increases in the evening to minimize sedation

Parenteral: I.V.: Infuse I.V. dose slowly over 30-60 minutes at a concentration ≤10 mg/mL

Monitoring Parameters Blood pressure, CBC with differential, hemoglobin, hematocrit, Coombs' test [direct], liver enzymes

Test Interactions Urinary uric acid, serum creatinine (alkaline picrate method), AST (colorimetric method), and urinary catecholamines (falsely high levels)

Patient Information Avoid alcohol; may cause drowsiness and impair ability to perform activities requiring mental alertness or physical coordination; may cause dry mouth; rise slowly from prolonged sitting or lying position; may cause urine to turn red or brown; notify physician of unexplained prolonged general tiredness, fever, or jaundice

Nursing Implications Transient sedation or depression may occur for first 72 hours of therapy, or when doses are increased

Additional Information Most effective if used with diuretic; titrate dose to optimal blood pressure control with minimal side effects

Dosage Forms

Injection, solution, as methyldopate hydrochloride: 50 mg/mL (5 mL) [contains sodium bisulfite]

Tablet: 250 mg, 500 mg

Extemporaneous Preparations A 50 mg/mL oral liquid preparation made from tablets and 2 different vehicles [unpreserved simple syrup (Syrup, USP) and a 1:1 mixture of simple syrup (containing 0.5% citric acid) and hydrochloric acid 0.2 N] was stable for 14 days when stored in glass prescription bottles in the dark, at room temperature (25°C) or under refrigeration (5°C); grind ten 250 mg tablets in a glass mortar into a fine powder. To make formulation with unpreserved simple syrup (Syrup, USP), levigate with Syrup, USP to form a uniform paste; add a small amount of Syrup, USP; mix well; transfer to a calibrated bottle; rinse the mortar and pestle several times with vehicle; transfer to calibrated bottle and qsad to 50 mL. To make formulation with second vehicle, levigate powdered tablets with 25 mL of hydrochloric acid 0.2 N (0.73% w/v); dilute this mixture to 50 mL with simple syrup containing 0.5% citric acid by the method described above. Label "shake well" and "protect from light."

Newton DW, Rogers AG, Becker CH, et al, "Extemporaneous Preparation of Meth-yldopa in Two Syrup Vehicles," *Am J Hosp Pharm*, 1975, 32(8):817-21.

Methylene Blue (METH i leen bloo)

U.S. Brand Names Urolene Blue®

Therapeutic Category Antidote, Cyanide; Antidote, Drug-induced Methemoglobi-nemia

Generic Available Yes

Use Antidote for cyanide poisoning and drug-induced methemoglobinemia, indicator dye, bacteriostatic genitourinary antiseptic

Pregnancy Risk Factor C (D if injected intra-amniotically)

Contraindications Hypersensitivity to methylene blue or any component; renal insuf-ficiency

Warnings Do not inject subcutaneously or intrathecally as necrotic abscesses (S.C.) and neural damage (I.T.) including paraplegia have occurred

Precautions Use with caution in patients with G-6-PD deficiency; continued use can cause profound anemia

Adverse Reactions
Cardiovascular: Hypertension, cyanosis, large I.V. doses have been associated with precordial pain
Central nervous system: Dizziness, mental confusion, headache, fever
Dermatologic: Stains skin
Gastrointestinal: Nausea, vomiting, abdominal pain, diarrhea, discoloration of feces (blue-green)
Genitourinary: Bladder irritation, discoloration of urine (blue-green)
Hematologic: Formation of methemoglobin
Miscellaneous: Diaphoresis

Mechanism of Action Weak germicide; in low concentrations hastens the conversion of methemoglobin to hemoglobin; has opposite effect at high concentrations by converting ferrous iron of reduced hemoglobin to ferric iron to form methemoglobin; in cyanide toxicity, it combines with cyanide to form cyanmethemoglobin preventing the interference of cyanide with the cytochrome system

Pharmacokinetics
Absorption: Well absorbed from GI tract
Elimination: In bile, feces, and urine

Usual Dosage
Methemoglobinemia: Children and Adults: I.V.: 1-2 mg/kg or 25-50 mg/m²; may be repeated after 1 hour if necessary
Chronic methemoglobinemia: Adults: Oral: 100-300 mg/day
NADPH-methemoglobin reductase deficiency: Children: Oral: 1-1.5 mg/kg/day (maximum dose: 300 mg/day) given with 5-8 mg/kg/day ascorbic acid
Genitourinary antiseptic: Adults: Oral: 65-130 mg 3 times/day; maximum dose: 390 mg/day
Chronic urolithiasis: Adults: Oral: 65 mg 3 times/day

Administration
Parenteral: Administer undiluted by direct I.V. injection over several minutes
Oral: Administer after meals with a full glass of water

Patient Information May discolor urine and feces blue-green; may discolor skin on contact

Additional Information Has been used topically (0.1% solutions) in conjunction with polychromatic light to photoinactivate viruses such as herpes simplex (this is an unlabeled indication); has been used alone or in combination with vitamin C for the management of chronic urolithiasis; skin stains may be removed using a hypochlorite solution

Dosage Forms
Injection, solution: 10 mg/mL (1 mL, 10 mL)
Tablet (Urolene Blue®): 65 mg

- ◆ **Methylin™** *see* Methylphenidate *on page 744*
- ◆ **Methylin™ ER** *see* Methylphenidate *on page 744*

♦ **Methylmorphine** *see* Codeine *on page 301*

Methylphenidate (meth il FEN i date)

U.S. Brand Names Concerta®; Metadate® CD; Metadate® ER; Methylin™; Methylin™ ER; Ritalin®; Ritalin® LA; Ritalin-SR®

Canadian Brand Names PMS-Methylphenidate; Riphenidate

Therapeutic Category Central Nervous System Stimulant, Nonamphetamine

Generic Available Yes (tablets)

Use Attention-deficit/hyperactivity disorder (ADHD); narcolepsy

Restrictions C-II

Pregnancy Risk Factor C

Contraindications Hypersensitivity to methylphenidate or any component; glaucoma; motor tics; Tourette's syndrome (diagnosis or family history); patients with marked agitation, tension, and anxiety; use of MAO inhibitors within 14 days (hypertensive crisis may occur)

Warnings Suppression of growth may occur with long-term use in children (monitor carefully); may exacerbate symptoms of thought disorder and behavior disturbance in psychotic children; do not use for severe depression or normal fatigue states; may lower seizure threshold; rare cases of visual disturbances may occur; EKG abnormalities and 4 cases of sudden cardiac death have been reported in children receiving clonidine with methylphenidate; reduce dose of methylphenidate by 40% when used concurrently with clonidine; consider EKG monitoring. A potential for GI obstruction exists with Concerta® (tablet is nondeformable); do not ordinarily use in patients with severe GI narrowing (eg, esophageal motility disorders, small bowel inflammatory disease, short gut syndrome, history of cystic fibrosis, peritonitis, chronic intestinal pseudo-obstruction, or Meckel's diverticulum)

Precautions Use with caution in patients with hypertension, seizures, acute stress reactions, emotional instability, patients with history of drug dependence; hematological monitoring is advised with long term use (see Monitoring Parameters)

Adverse Reactions

Cardiovascular: Tachycardia, hypertension, hypotension, palpitations, cardiac arrhythmias

Central nervous system: Nervousness, insomnia, dizziness, drowsiness, movement disorders, motor tics, precipitation of Tourette's syndrome; fever, headache, toxic psychosis (rare); neuroleptic malignant syndrome (very rare and usually in patients receiving medications associated with the syndrome; one case with concurrent first dose of venlafaxine has been reported)

Dermatologic: Rash

Endocrine & metabolic: Growth retardation

Gastrointestinal: Anorexia, nausea, vomiting, abdominal pain, weight loss, potential for GI obstruction with Concerta® (see Warnings)

Hematologic: Thrombocytopenia

Ocular: Visual disturbances (rare), blurred vision, problems with accommodation

Miscellaneous: Hypersensitivity reactions; physical and psychological dependence

Drug Interactions Use with clonidine may potentially increase EKG effects (see Warnings); methylphenidate increases serum concentrations of tricyclic antidepressants, selective serotonin reuptake inhibitors, phenylbutazone, warfarin, phenytoin, phenobarbital and primidone (a decrease in the dose of these agents may be required, monitor closely); use of MAO inhibitors within 14 days may result in hypertensive crisis, use of MAOI within 14 days of methylphenidate is contraindicated; the herbal medicine St John's wort (*Hypericum perforatum*) may increase serious side effects, its use is **not** recommended; effects of guanethidine, bretylium may be antagonized by methylphenidate

Food Interactions Food may increase oral absorption

Concerta®: A high fat meal does not alter pharmacokinetics or pharmacodynamics; no evidence of dose dumping occurs when administered with or without food

Metadate® CD: Food delays the early peak by ~1 hour; a high fat meal increases peak concentrations by 30% and AUC by 17%; one adult study showed no difference in bioavailability when Metadate® CD capsules were opened and contents sprinkled onto 1 tablespoon of applesauce (compared to fasting conditions; see Pentikin, 2002).

Ritalin® LA: Compared to fasting, food does not affect the first peak concentration, extent of absorption, or time to second peak concentration; however, the second peak was 25% lower. A high fat meal delays absorption. Compared to fasting, no differences in pharmacokinetics occurred when Ritalin® LA capsules were administered with applesauce. No evidence of dose dumping occurs when administered with or without food.

Stability Store at room temperature; dispense in tight, light-resistant container; **Note:** Metadate® CD should be dispensed in the original dose pack of 30 capsules

Methylin™ ER, Ritalin-SR®: Protect from moisture

Concerta®: Protect from humidity

Mechanism of Action Blocks the reuptake mechanism of dopaminergic neurons, appears to act at the cerebral cortex and subcortical structures

Pharmacodynamics Cerebral stimulation:

Maximum effect:

Immediate release tablet: Within 2 hours

Sustained release tablet: Within 4-7 hours

Duration (AAP, 2001):

Immediate release tablet (short-acting): Methylin™, Ritalin®: 3-5 hours

Sustained release, extended release (intermediate-acting): Metadate® ER, Methylin™ ER, Ritalin-SR®: 3-8 hours

Extended release (long-acting): Concerta®, Metadate® CD, Ritalin® LA: 8-12 hours

Pharmacokinetics

Absorption: From the GI tract, slow and incomplete

Protein binding: 15%

Metabolism: In the liver via hydroxylation to ritalinic acid (alpha-phenyl-2-piperidine acetic acid)

Half-life: 2-4 hours

Elimination: 90% of dose is eliminated in the urine as metabolites and unchanged drug; main urinary metabolite (ritalinic acid) accounts for 80% of the dose; drug is also excreted in feces via bile

Usual Dosage Oral: **Note:** Discontinue medication if no improvement is seen after appropriate dosage adjustment over a one-month period of time:

Immediate release tablets (Methylin™, Ritalin®):

Children ≥6 years: ADHD: Initial: 0.3 mg/kg/dose or 2.5-5 mg/dose given before breakfast and lunch; increase by 0.1 mg/kg/dose or by 5-10 mg/day at weekly intervals; usual dose: 0.3-1 mg/kg/day; maximum dose: 2 mg/kg/day or 60 mg/day; specific patients may require 3 doses/day (ie, additional dose at 4 PM)

Adults: Narcolepsy: 10 mg 2-3 times/day; maximum dose: 60 mg/day

Metadate® ER, Methylin™ ER, Ritalin-SR®: Children ≥6 years and Adults: Sustained release and extended release tablets (duration of action ~8 hours) may be given in place of regular tablets, once the daily dose is titrated using the regular tablets and the titrated 8-hour dosage corresponds to sustained release tablet size

Concerta®: Children ≥6 years and Adults:

Methylphenidate naive patients: Initial: 18 mg once daily; may increase by 18 mg/day increments at weekly intervals; maximum dose: 54 mg once daily

Switching from methylphenidate immediate release 5 mg 2-3 times/day, or sustained release 20 mg daily: Initial: 18 mg once daily; may increase by 18 mg/day increments at weekly intervals; maximum dose: 54 mg once daily

Switching from methylphenidate immediate release 10 mg 2-3 times/day, or sustained release 40 mg daily: Initial: 36 mg once daily; may increase by 18 mg/day increments at weekly intervals; maximum dose: 54 mg once daily

Switching from methylphenidate immediate release 15 mg 2-3 times/day, or sustained release 60 mg daily: Initial: 54 mg once daily; maximum dose: 54 mg once daily

Metadate® CD: Children ≥6 years and Adults: Initial: 20 mg once daily; may increase by 20 mg/day increments at weekly intervals; maximum dose: 60 mg once daily

Ritalin® LA: Children ≥6 years and Adults:

Methylphenidate naive patients: Initial: 20 mg once daily; may increase by 10 mg/day increments at weekly intervals; maximum dose: 60 mg once daily; **Note:** Patients may begin therapy with an immediate release product, if a lower initial dose is desired; patients may be switched to Ritalin® LA once immediate release dosage is titrated to 10 mg twice daily (see below)

Recommended Ritalin® LA Dose for Patients Receiving Methylphenidate

Previous Methylphenidate Dose	Recommended Ritalin® LA Dose
10 mg methylphenidate twice daily or 20 mg methylphenidate sustained release	20 mg once daily
15 mg methylphenidate twice daily	30 mg once daily
20 mg methylphenidate twice daily or 40 mg methylphenidate sustained release	40 mg once daily
30 mg methylphenidate twice daily or 60 mg methylphenidate sustained release	60 mg once daily

(Continued)

Methylphenidate *(Continued)*

Patients currently receiving methylphenidate: Initial dose: See table; may increase by 10 mg/day increments at weekly intervals; maximum dose: 60 mg once daily

Administration Oral: Immediate and sustained release tablets: Administer on an empty stomach ~30-45 minutes before meals; do not crush, chew, or break sustained or extended release dosage form, swallow whole; to avoid insomnia, last daily dose should be administered several hours before retiring.

Concerta®: May be administered without regard to food, but must be taken with water, milk, or juice; administer dose once daily in the morning.

Metadate® CD: Administer dose once daily in the morning, before breakfast, with water, milk, or juice; capsule may be swallowed whole or opened and contents sprinkled on a small amount (one tablespoonful) of applesauce; immediately consume drug/applesauce mixture; do not store for future use; drink fluids after consuming drug/applesauce mixture to ensure complete swallowing of beads; do not crush, chew, or divide capsules or its contents

Ritalin® LA: Administer dose once daily in the morning; may be administered with or without food (but some food may delay absorption); capsule may be swallowed whole or may be opened and contents sprinkled on a small amount (one spoonful) of applesauce (**Note:** Applesauce should not be warm); immediately consume drug/applesauce mixture; do not store for future use; do not crush, chew, or divide capsule or its contents

Monitoring Parameters CBC with differential, platelet count, blood pressure, height, weight, heart rate

Patient Information Avoid caffeine and the herbal medicine St John's wort; may be habit-forming; avoid abrupt discontinuation after prolonged use; may cause dizziness or drowsiness and impair ability to perform activities requiring mental alertness or physical coordination; intact Concerta® tablet shell may appear in stool (this is normal); report the use of other medications and herbal or natural products to your physician and pharmacist.

Additional Information Treatment with methylphenidate should include "drug holidays" or periodic discontinuation in order to assess the patient's requirements, decrease tolerance and limit suppression of linear growth and weight. Concerta®, Metadate® CD, and Ritalin® LA are formulated to deliver methylphenidate in a biphasic release profile; Concerta® is an osmotic controlled release formulation, with an immediate release (within 1 hour) outer coating; once daily Concerta® has been shown to be as effective as immediate release methylphenidate tablets administered 3 times/day (see Pelham, 2001). Metadate® CD capsules contain both immediate release beads (30% of the dose) and extended release beads (70% of the dose). Ritalin® LA capsules contain both immediate release beads (50% of the dose) and enteric coated, delayed release beads (50% of the dose). Methylin™, Methylin™ ER, and Ritalin-SR® tablets are color and additive free.

Dosage Forms

Capsule, extended release, as hydrochloride:
Metadate® CD: 20 mg
Ritalin® LA: 20 mg, 30 mg, 40 mg

Tablet, as hydrochloride (Methylin™, Ritalin®): 5 mg, 10 mg, 20 mg

Tablet, extended release, as hydrochloride: 20 mg
Concerta®: 18 mg, 27 mg, 36 mg, 54 mg [osmotic controlled release]
Metadate® ER, Methylin™ ER: 10 mg, 20 mg

Tablet, sustained release, as hydrochloride (Ritalin-SR®): 20 mg

References

American Academy of Pediatrics. Subcommittee on Attention-Deficit/Hyperactivity Disorder, "Clinical Practice Guideline: Treatment of the School-Aged Child With Attention-Deficit/Hyperactivity Disorder," *Pediatrics,* 2001, 108(4):1033-44.

Greenhill LL, "Pharmacologic Treatment of Attention Deficit Hyperactivity Disorder," *Psychiatr Clin North Am,* 1992, 15(1):1-27.

Greenhill LL, Pliszka S, Dulcan MK, et al, "Practice Parameter for the Use of Stimulant Medications in the Treatment of Children, Adolescents, and Adults," *J Am Acad Child Adolesc Psychiatry,* 2002, 41(2 Suppl):26S-49S.

Kelly DP and Aylward GP, "Attention Deficits in School-Aged Children and Adolescents," *Pediatr Clin North Am,* 1992, 39(3):487-512.

Pelham WE, Gnagy EM, Burrows-Maclean L, et al, "Once-a-Day Concerta Methylphenidate Versus Three-Times-Daily Methylphenidate in Laboratory and Natural Settings," *Pediatrics,* 2001, 107(6), http://www.pediatrics.org/cgi/content/full/107/6/e105.

Pentikis HS, Simmons RD, Benedict MF, et al, "Methylphenidate Bioavailability in Adults When an Extended-Release Multiparticulate Formulation is Administered Sprinkled on Food or as an Intact Capsule," *J Am Acad Child Adolesc Psychiatry,* 2002, 41(4):443-9.

Wilens TE and Biederman J, "The Stimulants," *Psychiatr Clin North Am,* 1992, 15(1):191-222.

♦ **Methylphenobarbital** *see* Mephobarbital *on page 720*
♦ **Methylphenyl** *see* Oxacillin *on page 840*
♦ **Methylphytyl Napthoquinone** *see* Phytonadione *on page 902*

MethylPREDNISolone (meth il pred NIS oh lone)

Related Information
Asthma Guidelines *on page 1376*
Corticosteroids Comparison, Systemic *on page 1211*

U.S. Brand Names A-Methapred®; Depo-Medrol®; Medrol®; Solu-Medrol®

Synonyms 6-α-Methylprednisolone

Therapeutic Category Adrenal Corticosteroid; Antiasthmatic; Anti-inflammatory Agent; Corticosteroid, Systemic; Glucocorticoid

Generic Available Yes

Use Anti-inflammatory or immunosuppressant agent in the treatment of a variety of diseases including those of hematologic, allergic, inflammatory, neoplastic, and auto-immune origin

Pregnancy Risk Factor C

Contraindications Hypersensitivity to methylprednisolone or any component (see Warnings); administration of live virus vaccines; systemic fungal infections

Warnings Hypothalamic pituitary adrenal (HPA) suppression may occur; acute adrenal insufficiency may occur with abrupt withdrawal after long-term use or with stress; withdrawal or discontinuation of corticosteroids should be done carefully. Immunosuppression may occur. Corticosteroids may mask signs of infection.

Methylprednisolone **acetate** I.M. injection (multiple-dose vial) and the diluent for methylprednisolone **sodium succinate** injection contain benzyl alcohol which may cause allergic reactions in susceptible individuals; large amounts of benzyl alcohol (≥99 mg/kg/day) have been associated with a potentially fatal toxicity ("gasping syndrome") in neonates; the "gasping syndrome" consists of metabolic acidosis, respiratory distress, gasping respirations, CNS dysfunction (including convulsions, intracranial hemorrhage), hypotension and cardiovascular collapse; avoid use of methylprednisolone products containing benzyl alcohol in neonates; *in vitro* and animal studies have shown that benzoate, a metabolite of benzyl alcohol, displaces bilirubin from protein binding sites

Precautions Avoid using higher than recommended doses; suppression of HPA axis, suppression of linear growth, or hypercorticism (Cushing's syndrome) may occur; use with caution in patients with hypothyroidism, cirrhosis, ocular herpes simplex, peptic ulcer disease, osteoporosis, myasthenia gravis, hypertension, CHF, ulcerative colitis, thromboembolic disorders

Adverse Reactions
Cardiovascular: Edema, hypertension
Central nervous system: Vertigo, seizures, psychoses, pseudotumor cerebri, head-ache
Dermatologic: Acne, skin atrophy, impaired wound healing
Endocrine & metabolic: Cushing's syndrome, HPA axis suppression, growth suppression, glucose intolerance, hypokalemia, alkalosis
Gastrointestinal: Peptic ulcer, nausea, vomiting
Hematologic: Transient leukocytosis
Neuromuscular & skeletal: Muscle weakness, osteoporosis, fractures
Ocular: Cataracts, glaucoma
Miscellaneous: Infections

Drug Interactions Cytochrome P450 isoenzyme CYP3A3/4 inducer
Barbiturates, phenytoin, rifampin may increase the clearance of methylprednisolone; salicylates; toxoids; methylprednisolone may increase cyclosporine and tacrolimus serum concentrations; live virus vaccines (increase risk of viral infection); vaccines may have decreased effects

Food Interactions Systemic use of corticosteroids may require a diet with increased potassium, vitamins A, B$_6$, C, D, folate, calcium, zinc and phosphorus and decreased sodium; grapefruit juice may significantly increase the bioavailability of oral methylprednisolone

Mechanism of Action Decreases inflammation by suppression of migration of polymorphonuclear leukocytes and reversal of increased capillary permeability

Pharmacodynamics The time of maximum effects and the duration of these effects is dependent upon the route of administration. See table.

Route	Maximum Effect	Duration
Oral	1-2 h	30-36 h
I.M. (acetate)	4-8 d	1-4 wk
Intra-articular	1 wk	1-5 wk

(Continued)

MethylPREDNISolone *(Continued)*

Usual Dosage Note: Only sodium succinate salt may be given I.V.

NIH Asthma Guidelines (NAEPP, 2002):

Children ≤12 years:

Asthma exacerbations (emergency medical care or hospital doses): Oral, I.V.: 1 mg/kg every 6 hours for 48 hours; then 1-2 mg/kg/day (maximum: 60 mg/day) in divided doses given twice daily until peak expiratory flow is 70% of predicted or personal best

Short-course "burst" (acute asthma):

Oral: 1-2 mg/kg/day in divided doses 1-2 times/day for 3-10 days; longer treatment may be required; usually given for 5 days; maximum dose: 60 mg/day

I.M. **(acetate):** 7.5 mg/kg as a one-time dose; maximum dose: 240 mg **(Note:** This may be given in place of short-course "burst" of oral steroids in patients who are vomiting or if compliance is a problem)

Long-term treatment: Oral: 0.25-2 mg/kg/day given as a single dose in the morning or every other day as needed for asthma control; maximum dose: 60 mg/day

Children >12 years and Adults:

Asthma exacerbations (emergency medical care or hospital doses): Oral, I.V.: 120-180 mg/day in divided doses 3-4 times/day for 48 hours; then 60-80 mg/day in divided doses given twice daily until peak expiratory flow is 70% of predicted or personal best

Short-course "burst" (acute asthma):

Oral: 40-60 mg/day in divided doses 1-2 times/day for 3-10 days; longer treatment may be required; usually given for 5 days

I.M. **(acetate):** 240 mg as a one time dose **(Note:** This may be given in place of short-course "burst" of oral steroids in patients who are vomiting or if compliance is a problem)

Long-term treatment: Oral: 7.5-60 mg daily given as a single dose in the morning or every other day as needed for asthma control

Children:

Anti-inflammatory or immunosuppressive: Oral, I.M., I.V.: 0.5-1.7 mg/kg/day or 5-25 mg/m^2/day in divided doses every 6-12 hours

"Pulse" therapy: 15-30 mg/kg/dose over ≥30 minutes given once daily for 3 days

Status asthmaticus: I.V.: Loading dose: 2 mg/kg/dose, then 0.5-1 mg/kg/dose every 6 hours

Lupus nephritis: I.V.: 30 mg/kg over ≥30 minutes every other day for 6 doses

Acute spinal cord injury: I.V.: 30 mg/kg over 15 minutes followed in 45 minutes by a continuous infusion of 5.4 mg/kg/hour for 23 hours

Adults:

Oral: 2-60 mg/day in 1-4 divided doses

High-dose therapy: I.V.: 30 mg/kg over ≥30 minutes; repeat as needed every 4-6 hours for 48-72 hours

I.M. **(acetate):** 10-80 mg/day once daily

I.V.: 40-250 mg every 4-6 hours

Lupus nephritis: High-dose "pulse" therapy: I.V.: 1 g/day for 3 days

Intra-articular, intralesional: 4-40 mg, up to 80 mg for large joints every 1-5 weeks

Administration

Oral: Administer after meals or with food or milk; do not administer with grapefruit juice

Parenteral: I.V.: **Succinate:** Low dose (eg, ≤1.8 mg/kg or ≤125 mg/dose): I.V. push over 3-15 minutes; moderate dose (eg, ≥2 mg/kg or 250 mg/dose): administer over 15-30 minutes; high dose (eg, 15 mg/kg or ≥500 mg/dose): administer over ≥30 minutes; doses >15 mg/kg or ≥1 g: administer over 1 hour. Do **not** administer high-dose I.V. push; hypotension, cardiac arrhythmia, and sudden death have been reported in patients given high-dose methylprednisolone I.V. push over <20 minutes; administer intermittent infusion over 15-60 minutes; maximum concentration: I.V. push: 125 mg/mL; I.V. infusion: 2.5 mg/mL. **Do not give acetate form I.V.**

Monitoring Parameters Blood pressure, serum glucose, and electrolytes

Test Interactions Interferes with skin tests

Patient Information Avoid alcohol; avoid grapefruit juice if taking oral methylprednisolone; limit caffeine; do not decrease or discontinue dose without physician's approval

Additional Information Sodium content of 1 g sodium succinate injection: 2.01 mEq; methylprednisolone sodium succinate 53 mg = methylprednisolone base 40 mg

Dosage Forms

Injection, powder for reconstitution, as **sodium succinate**: 40 mg, 125 mg, 500 mg

A-Methapred®: 40 mg, 125 mg, 500 mg, 1000 mg [diluent contains benzyl alcohol]

Solu-Medrol®: 500 mg, 1 g, 2 g [diluent contains benzyl alcohol]

Solu-Medrol® [single dose vial]: 40 mg, 125 mg, 500 mg, 1000 mg [diluent contains benzyl alcohol]

Injection, suspension, as **acetate** (Depo-Medrol®): 20 mg/mL (5 mL); 40 mg/mL (5 mL); 80 mg/mL (5 mL) [contains benzyl alcohol]

Injection, suspension, as **acetate** [single dose vial] (Depo-Medrol®): 40 mg/mL (1 mL); 80 mg/mL (1 mL)

Tablet: 4 mg

Medrol®: 2 mg, 4 mg, 8 mg, 16 mg, 32 mg

Tablet, dose pack: 4 mg (21s)

References

"National Asthma Education and Prevention Program. Expert Panel Report: Guidelines for the Diagnosis and Management of Asthma Update on Selected Topics--2002," *J Allergy Clin Immunol*, 2002, 110(5 Suppl):S141-219.

♦ **6-α-Methylprednisolone** *see* MethylPREDNISolone *on page 747*

♦ **4-Methylpyrazole** *see* Fomepizole *on page 517*

♦ **Methylrosaniline Chloride** *see* Gentian Violet *on page 537*

Metoclopramide (met oh kloe PRA mide)

Related Information

Carbohydrate and Alcohol Content of Liquid Medications for Use in Patients Receiving Ketogenic Diets *on page 1431*

Compatibility of Medications Mixed in a Syringe *on page 1412*

Drugs and Breast-Feeding *on page 1404*

U.S. Brand Names Reglan®

Canadian Brand Names Apo®-Metoclop; Nu-Metoclopramide

Therapeutic Category Antiemetic; Gastrointestinal Agent, Prokinetic

Generic Available Yes

Use Treatment of gastroesophageal reflux; prevention of nausea and vomiting associated with chemotherapy; prevention of postoperative nausea and vomiting; facilitates intubation of the small intestine and symptomatic treatment of diabetic gastric stasis

Pregnancy Risk Factor B

Contraindications Hypersensitivity to metoclopramide or any component; GI obstruction, pheochromocytoma, history of seizure disorder or patients receiving drugs likely to cause extrapyramidal reactions

Warnings Some products contain sodium benzoate; benzoic acid (benzoate) is a metabolite of benzyl alcohol; large amounts of benzyl alcohol (≥99 mg/kg/day) have been associated with a potentially fatal toxicity ("gasping syndrome") in neonates; *in vitro* and animal studies have shown that benzoate displaces bilirubin from protein binding sites; avoid use of sodium benzoate containing products in neonates.

Precautions Use with caution and reduce dosage in patients with renal impairment, hypertension, or depression; transient increases in plasma aldosterone may occur which could result in fluid retention or volume overload. Patients with CHF or cirrhosis of the liver may be at increased risk for development of fluid retention and volume overload. Use with caution in these patients and discontinue therapy if symptoms of excessive body fluids occurs.

Adverse Reactions Extrapyramidal reactions occur most frequently in children and young adults and following I.V. administration of high doses, usually within 24-48 hours after starting therapy

Cardiovascular: Hypertension, hypotension, SVT, bradycardia, A-V block

Central nervous system: Drowsiness, fatigue, restlessness, anxiety, agitation, depression, tardive dyskinesia, dystonia, seizures, hallucinations, neuroleptic malignant syndrome

Endocrine & metabolic: Gynecomastia, amenorrhea, galactorrhea, hyperprolactinemia

Gastrointestinal: Constipation, diarrhea

Genitourinary: Urinary frequency, impotence

Hematologic: Methemoglobinemia, neutropenia, leukopenia, agranulocytosis

Hepatic: Porphyria

Ocular: Visual disturbances

Miscellaneous: Hypersensitivity reactions

Drug Interactions Cytochrome P450 isoenzyme CYP1A2 and CYP2D6 substrate

Decreased cimetidine and digoxin GI absorption; increased cyclosporine GI absorption; levodopa decreases metoclopramide effects; increases hypertensive episodes with MAO inhibitors; increased neuromuscular blocking effects of succinylcholine; anticholinergics and narcotic analgesics antagonize GI motility effects of metoclopramide; metoclopramide may increase tacrolimus serum levels

(Continued)

Metoclopramide *(Continued)*

Stability Protect from light; stable for 48 hours at room temperature when admixed with ascorbic acid, cimetidine (in NS only), cytarabine, dexamethasone sodium phosphate, diphenhydramine, doxorubicin, heparin, benztropine, dexamethasone hydrochloride, hydrocortisone sodium phosphate, lidocaine, magnesium sulfate, mannitol, potassium acetate, potassium chloride, and potassium phosphate; stable for 24 hours at room temperature when admixed with clindamycin (in NS only) and cyclophosphamide; incompatible with cephalothin, chloramphenicol, and sodium bicarbonate

Mechanism of Action Potent dopamine receptor antagonist; blocks dopamine receptors in chemoreceptor trigger zone of the CNS, preventing emesis; accelerates gastric emptying and intestinal transit time without stimulating gastric, biliary, or pancreatic secretions

Pharmacodynamics

Onset of action:

Oral: Within 30-60 minutes

I.M.: Within 10-15 minutes

I.V.: Within 1-3 minutes

Duration: Therapeutic effects persist for 1-2 hours, regardless of route administered

Pharmacokinetics

Distribution: V_d: 3.5 L/kg; crosses the placenta; appears in breast milk; breast milk to plasma ratio: 0.5-4.06

Protein binding: 30%

Bioavailability: Oral: $80 \pm 15.5\%$

Half-life: 2.5-6 hours (half-life and clearance may be dose-dependent)

Elimination: Primarily as unchanged drug in the urine and feces

Usual Dosage

Intubation of small intestine to facilitate radiographic examination of upper GI tract: I.V.:

Children:

<6 years: 0.1 mg/kg

6-14 years: 2.5-5 mg

Children >14 years and Adults: 10 mg

Gastroesophageal reflux: Oral, I.M., I.V.:

Neonates, Infants and Children: 0.4-0.8 mg/kg/day in 4 divided doses

Adults: 10-15 mg 4 times/day

Postoperative nausea and vomiting: I.V.:

Children: 0.1-0.2 mg/kg/dose; repeat every 6-8 hours as needed

Children >14 years and Adults: 10 mg; repeat every 6-8 hours as needed

Antiemetic **(chemotherapy-induced emesis)**: Oral, I.V.:

Children and Adults: 1-2 mg/kg/dose every 2-4 hours; pretreatment with diphenhydramine will decrease risk of extrapyramidal reactions to this dosage

Diabetic gastroparesis: Adults: Oral, I.V.: 10 mg before each meal and at bedtime for 2-8 weeks

Dosing adjustment in renal impairment: Children and Adults:

Cl_{cr} 40-50 mL/minute: Administer 75% of recommended dose

Cl_{cr} 10-40 mL/minute: Administer 50% of recommended dose

Cl_{cr} <10 mL/minute: Administer 25% to 50% of recommended dose

Administration

Oral: Administer 30 minutes before meals and at bedtime

Parenteral: Dilute to 0.2 mg/mL (maximum concentration: 5 mg/mL) and infuse over 15-30 minutes (maximum rate of infusion: 5 mg/minute); rapid I.V. administration is associated with a transient but intense feeling of anxiety and restlessness, followed by drowsiness

Monitoring Parameters Renal function; blood pressure and heart rate (when rapid I.V. administration is used)

Patient Information May cause drowsiness and impair ability to perform activities requiring mental alertness or physical coordination

Dosage Forms

Injection, solution, as hydrochloride [preservative free] (Reglan®): 5 mg/mL (2 mL, 10 mL, 30 mL)

Solution, oral **concentrate**, as hydrochloride: 10 mg/mL (30 mL) [DSC]

Syrup, as hydrochloride: 5 mg/5 mL (10 mL, 480 mL) [sugar free; some products contain sodium benzoate]

Tablet, as hydrochloride (Reglan®): 5 mg, 10 mg

Metolazone *(me TOLE a zone)*

U.S. Brand Names Mykrox®; Zaroxolyn®

Therapeutic Category Antihypertensive Agent; Diuretic, Miscellaneous

Generic Available No

Use Management of mild to moderate hypertension (Zaroxolyn® only); treatment of edema in CHF, nephrotic syndrome, and impaired renal function

Pregnancy Risk Factor B

Contraindications Hypersensitivity to metolazone, any component, other thiazide diuretics, or sulfonamide-derived drugs; anuria; patients with hepatic coma

Warnings Mykrox® is **not** therapeutically equivalent to Zaroxolyn® and should not be interchanged for Zaroxolyn®

Precautions Use with caution in patients with severe renal disease, impaired hepatic function, gout, lupus erythematosus, diabetes mellitus, moderate-high cholesterol concentrations, and/or high triglycerides

Adverse Reactions
Cardiovascular: Palpitations, chest pain, orthostatic hypotension, precordial pain
Central nervous system: Vertigo, headache, chills, drowsiness
Dermatologic: Rash, dry skin, photosensitivity, toxic epidermal necrolysis, Stevens-Johnson syndrome, cutaneous vasculitis, urticaria
Endocrine & metabolic: Hypokalemia, hyponatremia, hypochloremia, metabolic alkalosis, hyperglycemia, hyperuricemia, hypomagnesemia
Gastrointestinal: Abdominal bloating, GI irritation, bitter taste, nausea, vomiting, anorexia, xerostomia
Hematologic: Blood dyscrasias, aplastic anemia, hemolytic anemia, leukopenia, agranulocytosis, thrombocytopenia
Hepatic: Hepatitis
Neuromuscular & skeletal: Arthralgia, back pain, paresthesias
Ocular: Eye itching, transient blurred vision
Otic: Tinnitus
Renal: Polyuria, prerenal azotemia, uremia
Respiratory: Cough, sinus congestion, epistaxis

Drug Interactions Increased digoxin toxicity (due to potassium and magnesium depletion); increased lithium toxicity; additive potassium losses with amphotericin B and steroids; salicylates and NSAIDs decrease antihypertensive effects; allopurinol increases hypersensitivity reactions; rare occurrence of hemolytic anemia with methyldopa; cholestyramine and colestipol decrease metolazone absorption

Food Interactions Avoid natural licorice (causes sodium and water retention and increases potassium loss)

Mechanism of Action Inhibits sodium reabsorption in the cortical diluting site and proximal convoluted tubules causing increased excretion of sodium and water as well as potassium and hydrogen ions

Pharmacodynamics
Onset of action: 1 hour
Maximum effect (Mykrox®): Hypertension: 2 weeks
Duration: 12-24 hours

Pharmacokinetics
Absorption: Oral: Rate and extent vary with the preparation
Protein binding: 95%
Half-life: 6-20 hours
Elimination: Enterohepatic recycling; 70% to 95% excreted unchanged in urine

Usual Dosage Oral (dosage based on Zaroxolyn®, lower dosages may be used with Mykrox®):

Children: 0.2-0.4 mg/kg/day divided every 12-24 hours
Adults:
Edema: 5-10 mg/dose every 24 hours
Edema associated with renal disease or cardiac failure: 5-20 mg/dose every 24 hours
Hypertension:
Zaroxolyn®: 2.5-5 mg/dose every 24 hours
Mykrox®: 0.5 mg/day; increase to a maximum of 1 mg/day, if needed

Administration Oral: Administer with food to decrease GI distress

Monitoring Parameters Serum electrolytes, renal function, blood pressure

Patient Information May cause dry mouth; may cause drowsiness and impair ability to perform activities requiring mental alertness or physical coordination. May cause photosensitivity reactions (eg, exposure to sunlight may cause severe sunburn, skin rash, redness, or itching); avoid exposure to sunlight and artificial light sources (sunlamps, tanning booth/bed); wear protective clothing, wide-brimmed hats, sunglasses, and lip sunscreen (SPF ≥15); use a sunscreen [broad-spectrum sunscreen or physical sunscreen (preferred) or sunblock with SPF ≥15]; contact physician if reaction occurs.

Dosage Forms
Tablet:
Mykrox®: 0.5 mg
(Continued)

Metolazone *(Continued)*

Zaroxolyn®: 2.5 mg, 5 mg, 10 mg

Extemporaneous Preparations A 1 mg/mL suspension may be made by crushing one 10 mg Zaroxolyn® tablet; add simple syrup to total volume of 10 mL. Label "shake well"; stable 3 months refrigerated

Nahata MC, Morosco RS, and Hipple TF, "Stability of Metolazone in an Extemporaneously Prepared Suspension," *Hosp Pharm*, 1997, 32:691-3.

References

Arnold WC, "Efficacy of Metolazone and Furosemide in Children With Furosemide-Resistant Edema," *Pediatrics*, 1984, 74(5):872-5.

Wells TG, "The Pharmacology and Therapeutics of Diuretics in the Pediatric Patient," *Pediatr Clin North Am*, 1990, 37(2):463-504.

♦ **Metopirone®** *see* Metyrapone *on page 756*

Metoprolol *(me toe PROE lole)*

U.S. Brand Names Lopressor®; Toprol XL®

Canadian Brand Names Apo®-Metoprolol; Betaloc®; Betaloc® Durules®; Novo-Metoprolol; Nu-Metop; PMS-Metoprolol

Therapeutic Category Antianginal Agent; Antiarrhythmic Agent, Class II; Antihypertensive Agent; Antimigraine Agent; Beta-Adrenergic Blocker

Generic Available Yes [injection and tablets (nonsustained release)]

Use Management of hypertension, angina pectoris, and arrhythmias (such as multifocal atrial tachycardia); prevention of MI and migraine headaches; extended release tablets are also indicated to reduce mortality and hospitalization in adults with CHF (stable NYHA Class II or III) who are receiving ACE inhibitors, diuretics, and/or digoxin

Pregnancy Risk Factor C (D if used in 2nd of 3rd trimester)

Contraindications Hypersensitivity to metoprolol or any component; sinus bradycardia; heart block greater then first degree (except in patients with a functioning artificial pacemaker); cardiogenic shock; uncompensated CHF

Warnings May depress myocardial activity and precipitate CHF, use with caution and monitor closely, especially in patients with compensated heart failure. In patients with coronary artery disease, exacerbation of angina and, in some cases, MI may occur following abrupt discontinuation of therapy. Beta-blockers should generally be avoided in patients with bronchospastic disease; metoprolol, with relative beta$_1$ selectivity, should be used with caution and closely monitored in patients with bronchospastic disease; beta$_2$ stimulants and the lowest possible dose of metoprolol should be used in these patients. Metoprolol may block hypoglycemia-induced tachycardia and blood pressure changes; use with caution in patients with diabetes mellitus. May mask signs of thyrotoxicosis. Use with caution with verapamil, diltiazem, or anesthetic agents that decrease myocardial function.

Precautions Use with caution in patients with hepatic dysfunction. Patients who have a history of severe anaphylactic hypersensitivity reactions to various substances may be more reactive while receiving beta-blockers; these patients may not be responsive to the normal doses of epinephrine used to treat hypersensitivity reactions

Adverse Reactions

Cardiovascular: Bradycardia, reduced peripheral circulation, palpitations, CHF, hypotension, peripheral edema, worsening of AV conduction disturbances

Central nervous system: Dizziness, tiredness, depression, mental confusion, insomnia

Dermatologic: Rash, pruritus, worsening of psoriasis

Gastrointestinal: Diarrhea, nausea, abdominal pain, xerostomia, constipation

Hematologic (potential): Agranulocytosis, thrombocytopenia

Hepatic: Hepatitis, hepatic dysfunction, jaundice; rare: elevated transaminase, alkaline phosphatase, LDH

Respiratory: Bronchospasm, wheezing, dyspnea

Drug Interactions Cytochrome P450 isoenzyme CYP2D6 substrate

Catecholamine-depleting drugs, such as reserpine, may have additive effects (hypotension, bradycardia); hypotensive agents, diuretics, cardiac glycosides, amiodarone, calcium channel blockers, agents that slow AV conduction, and myocardial depressant general anesthetics may have additive effects with beta-blockers; verapamil may significantly increase the oral bioavailability of metoprolol (avoid concomitant use or reduce metoprolol dose and monitor closely); cimetidine, ciprofloxacin, fluoxetine, hydralazine, oral contraceptives, propoxyphene, and quinidine may increase metoprolol serum concentrations and effects. Abrupt withdrawal of clonidine while receiving beta-blockers may result in an exaggerated hypertensive crisis; NSAIDs may decrease the antihypertensive effects of beta-blockers; barbiturates and rifampin may increase the metabolism of metoprolol and decrease metoprolol serum concentrations; metoprolol may increase lidocaine serum concentrations

Food Interactions

Metoprolol tartrate: Food may enhance the extent of oral absorption

Metoprolol succinate (extended release tablets): Food does not significantly affect bioavailability

Stability

Tablets and extended release tablets: Store at controlled room temperature 15°C to 30°C (59°F to 86°F)

Tablets: Protect from moisture and dispense in tight, light-resistant container

Injection: Do not store above 30°C (86°F); protect from light

Mechanism of Action

Selective inhibitor of beta$_1$-adrenergic receptors at lower doses; competitively blocks beta$_1$ adrenergic receptors with little or no effect on beta$_2$-receptors at doses in adults <100 mg/day; inhibits beta$_2$- receptors at higher doses; does not exhibit membrane stabilizing or intrinsic sympathomimetic activity

Pharmacodynamics

Beta blockade:

Onset of action: Oral: Metoprolol tartrate tablets: Within 1 hour

Maximum effect: I.V.: 20 minutes

Duration: Dose dependent

Antihypertensive effect:

Onset of action: Oral: Metoprolol tartrate tablets: Within 15 minutes

Maximum effect: Oral (multiple dosing): After 1 week

Duration: Oral: Metoprolol tartrate tablets (single dose): 6 hours; metoprolol succinate (extended release tablets): Up to 24 hours

Pharmacokinetics

Absorption: Rapid and complete, with large first-pass effect

Distribution: Crosses the blood brain barrier; CSF concentrations are 78% of plasma concentrations

Protein binding: 12% bound to albumin

Metabolism: Significant first-pass metabolism; extensive metabolism in the liver

Bioavailability: Oral: 50%

Half-Life:

Neonates: 5-10 hours

Adults: 3-7 hours

Adults with chronic renal failure: Similar to normal adults

Elimination: 10% of an I.V. dose and <5% of an oral dose is excreted unchanged in the urine

Usual Dosage (See Additional Information)

Oral: Hypertension:

Children: No pediatric studies are available

Adolescents: Limited information is available. Sixteen hypertensive adolescents (≥13 years of age) were treated with an initial dose of 50 mg twice daily; patients were seen every 4-6 weeks and doses were increased to 100 mg twice daily if blood pressure was not controlled (see Falkner, 1982)

Adults:

Tablets (nonsustained release): Initial: 100 mg/day in single or divided doses, increase at weekly intervals to desired effect; usual dosage range: 100-450 mg/day; doses >450 mg/day have not been studied

Note: Lower once-daily dosing (especially 100 mg/day) may not control blood pressure for 24 hours; larger or more frequent dosing may be needed. Patients with bronchospastic diseases should receive the lowest possible daily dose; dose should initially be divided into 3 doses per day (to avoid high plasma concentrations).

Extended release tablets: Initial: 50-100 mg/day as a single dose; increase at weekly intervals to desired effect; doses >400 mg/day have not been studied.

Oral: Congestive heart failure: Adults: Extended release tablets: Initial: NYHA Class II heart failure: 25 mg once daily; more severe heart failure: 12.5 mg once daily; may double the dose every 2 weeks as tolerated; maximum: 200 mg/day

Administration Oral:

Metoprolol tartrate tablets: Administer with food or immediately after meals

Metoprolol succinate extended release tablets: May be administered without regard to meals; do not chew, crush, or break extended release tablets

Monitoring Parameters

Blood pressure, heart rate, respirations, circulation in extremities

Additional Information

Do not abruptly discontinue therapy, taper dosage gradually over 1-2 weeks. Beta-blockers without intrinsic sympathomimetic activity (such as (Continued)

Metoprolol *(Continued)*

metoprolol) have been shown to decrease morbidity and mortality when initiated in the acute treatment of MI and continued long term; metoprolol injection is used for early treatment of definitive or suspected MI; consult adult reference for further information.

Limited pediatric dosing information is available in the literature; in one case report, oral metoprolol (2 mg/kg/day in 3 divided doses) helped control paroxysmal supraventricular tachycardia in a 6 month old infant receiving digoxin (see Hepner, 1983). Low dose oral metoprolol (initial: 0.1 mg/kg/dose given twice daily, then increased slowly as needed to a maximum of 0.9 ± 0.7 mg/kg/day) was used to treat severe CHF that failed conventional therapy in 4 children (mean age: 7.8 years) with cardiomyopathy who were under consideration for heart transplantation (see Shaddy, 1998). A follow-up report in 15 children, 2.5-15 years of age (mean: 8.6 ± 1.3 years), used low dose oral metoprolol [Initial: 0.1-0.2 mg/kg/dose given twice daily, then increased slowly as needed to a maximum of 1.1 ± 0.1 mg/kg/day (range: 0.5-2.3 mg/kg/day)] to treat dilated cardiomyopathy and CHF; all patients received ACE inhibitors, digoxin, and diuretics before starting metoprolol (see Shaddy, 1999). Two studies (Muller, 1993; O'Marcaigh, 1994) assessed metoprolol for unexplained syncope in children at I.V. doses of 0.1 to 0.2 mg/kg for tilt table testing; in both studies, oral metoprolol was given after tilt table testing to select patients; initial oral doses of 0.8-2.8 mg/kg/day were used in 15 patients (8-20 years of age), but treatment was discontinued in 3 patients receiving 1.8-2.8 mg/kg/day due to adverse effects (Muller, 1993); oral doses of 1 to 2 mg/kg/day, rounded to the nearest 25 mg/day and divided into 2 doses daily were used in 19 patients (7-18 years of age) with unexplained syncope; the mean effective dose was 1.5 mg/kg/day (O'Marcaigh, 1994). High-dose beta-blocker therapy has been recommended to treat childhood hypertrophic cardiomyopathy (see Ostman-Smith 1999). Further pediatric studies are required before these doses can be recommended.

Dosage Forms

Injection, solution, as **tartrate** (Lopressor®): 1 mg/mL (5 mL)

Tablet, as **tartrate** (Lopressor®): 50 mg, 100 mg

Tablet, extended release, as **succinate** (Toprol XL®): 25 mg, 50 mg, 100 mg, 200 mg [mg strength refers to tartrate equivalent]

Extemporaneous Preparations

A 10 mg/mL metoprolol tartrate oral liquid preparation made with twelve 100 mg tablets and qsad to 120 mL with 3 different vehicles (a 1:1 mixture of Ora-Sweet® and Ora-Plus®, a 1:1 mixture of Ora-sweet® SF and Ora-Plus®, or cherry syrup) was found to be stable for 60 days when stored in amber plastic bottles in the dark at 5°C and 25°C. Microbial growth was not determined. Label "shake well" and "protect from light".

Allen LV and Erickson MA, "Stability of Labetalol Hydrochloride, Metoprolol Tartrate, Verapamil Hydrochloride, and Spironolactone With Hydrochlorothiazide in Extemporaneously Compounded Oral Liquids," *Am J Health Syst Pharm*, 1996, 53(19):2304-9.

References

Falkner B, Lowenthal DT, and Affrime MB, "The Pharmacodynamic Effectiveness of Metoprolol in Adolescent Hypertension," *Pediatr Pharmacol (New York)*, 1982, 2(1):49-55.

Hepner SI, and Davoli E, "Successful Treatment of Supraventricular Tachycardia With Metoprolol, a Cardioselective Beta Blocker," *Clin Pediatr (Phila)*, 1983, 22(7):522-3.

Morselli PL, Boutroy MJ, Bianchetti G, et al, "Pharmacokinetics of Antihypertensive Drugs in the Neonatal Period," *Dev Pharmacol Ther*, 1989, 13(2-4):190-8.

Muller G, Deal BJ, Strasburger JF, et al, "Usefulness of Metoprolol for Unexplained Syncope and Positive Response to Tilt Testing in Young Persons," *Am J Cardiol*, 1993, 71(7):592-5.

O'Marcaigh AS, MacLellan-Tobert SG, and Porter CJ, "Tilt-Table Testing and Oral Metoprolol Therapy in Young Patients With Unexplained Syncope," *Pediatrics*, 1994, 93(2):278-83.

Ostman-Smith I, Wettrell G, and Riesenfield T, "A Cohort Study of Childhood Hypertrophic Cardiomyopathy: Improved Survival Following High-Dose Beta-Adrenoceptor Antagonist Treatment," *J Am Coll Cardiol*, 1999, 34(6):1813-22.

Shaddy RE, "Beta-Blocker Therapy in Young Children With Congestive Heart Failure Under Consideration for Heart Transplantation," *Am Heart J*, 1998, 136(1):19-21.

Shaddy RE, Tani LY, Gidding SS, et al, "Beta-Blocker Treatment of Dilated Cardiomyopathy With Congestive Heart Failure in Children: A Multi-Institutional Experience," *J Heart Lung Transplant*, 1999, 18(3):269-74.

♦ **MetroCream®** *see Metronidazole on page 754*

♦ **MetroGel®** *see Metronidazole on page 754*

♦ **MetroGel-Vaginal®** *see Metronidazole on page 754*

♦ **MetroLotion®** *see Metronidazole on page 754*

Metronidazole *(me troe NI da zole)*

Related Information

Drugs and Breast-Feeding *on page 1404*

U.S. Brand Names Flagyl®; Flagyl® ER; MetroCream®; MetroGel®; MetroGel-Vaginal®; MetroLotion®; Noritate™

Canadian Brand Names Apo®-Metronidazole; Florazole® ER; Nidagel™; Novo-Nidazol

Therapeutic Category Amebicide; Antibiotic, Anaerobic; Antibiotic, Topical; Antiprotozoal

Generic Available Yes (tablets)

Use Treatment of susceptible anaerobic bacterial and protozoal infections in the following conditions: amebiasis (liver abscess, dysentery), giardiasis, symptomatic and asymptomatic trichomoniasis; skin and skin structure infections, CNS infections, intra-abdominal infections, and systemic anaerobic bacterial infections; topically for the treatment of acne rosacea; treatment of antibiotic-associated pseudomembranous colitis (AAPC) caused by *C. difficile*; bacterial vaginosis

Pregnancy Risk Factor B

Contraindications Hypersensitivity to metronidazole or any component; 1st trimester of pregnancy

Warnings Has been shown to be carcinogenic in rodents

Precautions Use with caution in patients with liver impairment, blood dyscrasias, CNS disease; metronidazole injection should be used with caution in patients receiving corticosteroids or patients predisposed to edema (injection contains 28 mEq of sodium/g metronidazole); reduce dosage in patients with severe liver impairment; dosage adjustment is not necessary in patients with moderate to severe renal insufficiency

Adverse Reactions

Central nervous system: Dizziness, confusion, seizures, headache, insomnia, hallucinations, paresthesias

Dermatologic: Rash

Endocrine & Metabolic: Disulfiram-type reaction with alcohol

Gastrointestinal: Metallic taste, nausea, xerostomia, diarrhea, furry tongue, vomiting

Genitourinary: Urethral burning, discoloration of urine (dark or reddish brown)

Hematologic: Leukopenia, neutropenia

Local: Thrombophlebitis

Neuromuscular & skeletal: Peripheral neuropathy

Drug Interactions Disulfiram (psychotic episodes); phenobarbital and rifampin (may increase metabolism of metronidazole); increased levels/toxicity of phenytoin, lithium, warfarin; alcohol may cause disulfiram-like reactions

Food Interactions Peak concentration is decreased and delayed when administered with food

Stability Do not refrigerate neutralized solution because precipitation may occur; reconstituted vials are chemically stable for 96 hours when stored at room temperature; protect from light

Mechanism of Action Reduced to a product which interacts with DNA to cause a loss of helical DNA structure and strand breakage resulting in inhibition of protein synthesis and cell death in susceptible organisms

Pharmacokinetics

Absorption: Oral: Well absorbed

Distribution: Excreted in breast milk; widely distributed into body tissues, fluids including bile, liver, bone, pleural fluid, vaginal secretions, CSF, erythrocytes, and hepatic abscesses

Protein binding: <20%

Metabolism: 30% to 60% in the liver to hydroxylated metabolite (60% to 80% bioactive), acetic acid metabolites, glucuronide, and sulfated conjugates

Half-life (increases with hepatic impairment):

Neonates: 25-75 hours

Children and Adults:

Metronidazole: 6-12 hours

Hydroxymetronidazole: 9.5-20 hours

Time to peak serum concentration: Within 1-2 hours

Elimination: Excreted via the urine (20% as unchanged drug) and feces (6% to 15%)

Dialysis: Extensively removed by hemodialysis and peritoneal dialysis

Usual Dosage

Neonates: Anaerobic infections: Oral, I.V.:

0-4 weeks, <1200 g: 7.5 mg/kg every 48 hours

Postnatal age ≤7 days:

1200-2000 g: 7.5 mg/kg/day given every 24 hours

>2000 g: 15 mg/kg/day in divided doses every 12 hours

Postnatal age >7 days:

1200-2000 g: 15 mg/kg/day in divided doses every 12 hours

>2000 g: 30 mg/kg/day in divided doses every 12 hours

(Continued)

Metronidazole *(Continued)*

Infants and Children:

Amebiasis: Oral: 35-50 mg/kg/day in divided doses every 8 hours

Other parasitic infections: Oral: 15-30 mg/kg/day in divided doses every 8 hours

Anaerobic infections: Oral, I.V.: 30 mg/kg/day in divided doses every 6 hours; maximum dose: 4 g/day

AAPC: Oral: 30 mg/kg/day divided every 6 hours for 7-10 days

Helicobacter pylori infection (has been used in combination with amoxicillin and bismuth subsalicylate): Oral: 15-20 mg/kg/day in 2 divided doses for 4 weeks

Adults:

Amebiasis: Oral: 500-750 mg every 8 hours

Other parasitic infections: Oral: 250 mg every 8 hours or 2 g as a single dose

Anaerobic infections: Oral, I.V.: 30 mg/kg/day in divided doses every 6 hours; not to exceed 4 g/day

AAPC: Oral: 250-500 mg 3-4 times/day for 10-14 days

Helicobacter pylori infection: Oral: 250-500 mg 3 times/day in combination with at least one other agent active against *H. pylori*

STD prophylaxis for acute sexual assault: Oral: 2 g in a single dose in combination with ceftriaxone and doxycycline

Topical: Apply a thin film twice daily to affected areas

Vaginal: One applicatorful (5 g) intravaginally 2 times/day for 5 days

Dosing adjustment in hepatic impairment: 50% to 67% decrease in dosage

Administration

Intravaginal: Use only **vaginal gel** intravaginally; do not apply to the eye

Oral: Administer on an empty stomach; may administer with food if GI upset occurs

Parenteral: Administer I.V. by slow intermittent infusion over 30-60 minutes at a final concentration for administration of 5-8 mg/mL

Topical: Wash affected areas with a mild cleanser; wait 15-20 minutes, then apply a thin film of drug to the affected area and rub in. Do not apply to the eye.

Monitoring Parameters WBC count

Test Interactions May cause falsely decreased AST and ALT levels

Patient Information May discolor urine dark or reddish brown; avoid alcohol; do not take alcohol for at least 48 hours after the last dose; may cause dry mouth

Nursing Implications Avoid contact between the drug and aluminum in the infusion set

Additional Information Sodium content of 500 mg ready-to-use vial: 14 mEq

Dosage Forms

Capsule (Flagyl®): 375 mg

Cream, topical:

MetroCream®: 0.75% (45 g) [contains benzyl alcohol]

Noritate™: 1% (30 g)

Gel, topical (MetroGel®): 0.75% (30 g, 45 g)

Gel, vaginal (MetroGel-Vaginal®): 0.75% (70 g)

Infusion [premixed iso-osmotic sodium chloride solution]: 5 mg/mL (100 mL)

Injection, powder for reconstitution, as hydrochloride (Flagyl®): 500 mg [contains mannitol]

Lotion, topical (MetroLotion®): 0.75% (60 mL) [contains benzyl alcohol]

Tablet: 250 mg, 500 mg [scored]

Tablet, extended release, film coated (Flagyl® ER): 750 mg

Tablet, film coated (Flagyl®): 250 mg, 500 mg

Extemporaneous Preparations A 50 mg/mL oral suspension can be made using a 1:1 mixture of Ora-Sweet® and Ora-Plus®; crush twenty-four 250 mg tablets into a fine powder in a mortar; add a small amount of vehicle and mix to make a uniform paste; mix while adding the vehicle in geometric portions to almost 120 mL; transfer to a calibrated bottle and qsad with vehicle to 120 mL; preparation is stable for 60 days when stored at room temperature or under refrigeration; label "shake well"

Allen LV Jr and Erickson MA III, "Stability of Ketoconazole, Metolazone, Metronidazole, Procainamide Hydrochloride, and Spironolactone in Extemporaneously Compounded Oral Liquids," *Am J Health Syst Pharm*, 1996, 53(17):2073-8.

References
Committee on Adolescence, American Academy of Pediatrics, "Sexual Assault and the Adolescent," *Pediatrics*, 1994, 94(5):761-5.

Israel DM and Hassall E, "Treatment and Long-Term Follow-up of *Helicobacter pylori*-Associated Duodenal Ulcer Disease in Children," *J Pediatr*, 1993, 123(1):53-8.

Kelly CP, Pothoulakis C, and LaMont JT, "*Clostridium difficile* Colitis," *N Engl J Med*, 1994, 330(4):257-62.

Oldenburg B and Speck WT, "Metronidazole," *Pediatr Clin North Am*, 1983, 30(1):71-5.

Metyrapone *(me TEER a pone)*

U.S. Brand Names Metopirone®

Therapeutic Category Diagnostic Agent, Hypothalamic-Pituitary ACTH Function

Generic Available No

Use Diagnostic drug for testing hypothalamic-pituitary ACTH function

Pregnancy Risk Factor C

Contraindications Hypersensitivity to metyrapone or any component; adrenal cortical insufficiency

Warnings All corticosteroid therapy should be discontinued prior to and during the metyrapone test; administration of metyrapone may induce acute adrenal insufficiency in patients with reduced adrenal secretory capacity; patients with suspected adrenocortical insufficiency should be observed closely over 24 hours

Precautions The test may be abnormal in the presence of thyroid dysfunction; demonstrate the ability of the adrenals to respond to exogenous ACTH before using metyrapone

Adverse Reactions
Cardiovascular: Hypotension, tachycardia
Central nervous system: Dizziness, headache, sedation
Dermatologic: Rash
Gastrointestinal: Abdominal discomfort, nausea, vomiting
Hematologic: Bone marrow suppression (rare)

Drug Interactions Phenytoin, chlorpromazine, amitriptyline, cyproheptadine, estrogens, phenobarbital may reduce test effectiveness; metyrapone inhibits glucuronidation of acetaminophen

Stability Protect from light

Mechanism of Action Reduces cortisol and corticosterone production by inhibition of 11-beta-hydroxylation of precursors in the adrenal cortex. Continued inhibition stimulates increased ACTH production by the pituitary; increased precursor levels have a weak suppressive activity on ACTH release. Elevated levels of precursor metabolites (17-hydroxycorticosteroids [17-OHCS] or 17-ketogenic steroids [17-KGS]) appear in the urine which can easily serve as an index of pituitary ACTH responsiveness. Production of aldosterone may also be suppressed by metyrapone. The adrenal cortex must have the ability to respond to ACTH before metyrapone is employed to test the capacity of the pituitary to respond to a decreased concentration of plasma cortisol.

Pharmacodynamics Maximum effect: Peak excretion of steroid during the first 24 hours after administration

Pharmacokinetics
Absorption: Oral: Well absorbed
Half-life, elimination: 1.9 ± 0.7 hours
Time to peak serum concentration: 1 hour
Elimination: 5.3% of dose excreted in urine unchanged

Usual Dosage Oral:
Children: 15 mg/kg/dose or 300 mg/m^2/dose every 4 hours for 6 doses; minimum: 250 mg/dose **or as an alternative** 30 mg/kg as a single dose (maximum: 3 g) given at midnight the night before the test
Adults: 750 mg every 4 hours for 6 doses **or as an alternative** 3 g as a single dose given at midnight the night before the test

Administration Oral: May administer with food or milk to reduce GI irritation

Reference Range
Normal response to metyrapone:
Plasma ACTH: 44 pmol/L (200 ng/L)
Plasma II desoxycortisol: 0.2 µmol/L (70 µg/L)
24 hour urinary excretion of 17-OHCS: 2-4 time increase
24 hour urinary excretion of 17-KGS: 2 time increase
A subnormal response may be indicative of panhypopituitarism or partial hypopituitarism. An excessive response is suggestive of Cushing's syndrome associated with adrenal hyperplasia.

Patient Information Arise slowly from prolonged sitting or lying position; may cause drowsiness and impair ability to perform activities requiring mental alertness or physical coordination

Dosage Forms Capsule: 250 mg

♦ **Mevacor**® *see* Lovastatin *on page 697*
♦ **Mevinolin** *see* Lovastatin *on page 697*

Mexiletine (MEKS i le teen)

U.S. Brand Names Mexitil®
Canadian Brand Names Novo-Mexiletine
Therapeutic Category Antiarrhythmic Agent, Class I-B
Generic Available Yes
(Continued)

Mexiletine *(Continued)*

Use Management of serious ventricular arrhythmias; suppression of premature ventricular contractions; diabetic neuropathy

Pregnancy Risk Factor C

Contraindications Hypersensitivity to mexiletine or any component (see Warnings); cardiogenic shock, second or third degree heart block

Warnings Exercise extreme caution in patients with pre-existing sinus node dysfunction; mexiletine can worsen bradycardias and other arrhythmias

Capsules may contain benzyl alcohol which may cause allergic reactions in susceptible individuals; large amounts of benzyl alcohol (≥99 mg/kg/day) have been associated with a potentially fatal toxicity ("gasping syndrome") in neonates; the "gasping syndrome" consists of metabolic acidosis, respiratory distress, gasping respirations, CNS dysfunction (including convulsions, intracranial hemorrhage), hypotension and cardiovascular collapse; avoid use of mexiletine capsules containing benzyl alcohol in neonates; *in vitro* and animal studies have shown that benzoate, a metabolite of benzyl alcohol, displaces bilirubin from protein binding sites

Precautions Use with caution in patients with seizure disorders, severe CHF, hypotension

Adverse Reactions

Cardiovascular: Palpitations, bradycardia, chest pain, syncope, hypotension, atrial or ventricular arrhythmias

Central nervous system: Dizziness, confusion, ataxia

Dermatologic: Rash

Gastrointestinal: Nausea, vomiting, diarrhea

Hematologic: Rarely thrombocytopenia

Hepatic: Hepatitis

Neuromuscular & skeletal: Paresthesia, tremor

Ocular: Diplopia

Otic: Tinnitus

Respiratory: Dyspnea

Miscellaneous: Positive antinuclear antibody

Drug Interactions Cytochrome P450 isoenzyme CYP2D6 substrate; CYP1A2 isoenzyme inhibitor

Phenobarbital, phenytoin, rifampin, and other hepatic enzyme inducers may lower mexiletine plasma levels; cimetidine may increase mexiletine levels; antacids, narcotics, or anticholinergics may decrease rate of absorption; metoclopramide may increase rate of absorption; drugs which affect urine pH can increase or decrease excretion of mexiletine; mexiletine may increase the serum concentrations of theophylline and caffeine

Food Interactions Food may decrease the rate, but not the extent of oral absorption; diets which affect urine pH can increase or decrease excretion of mexiletine; avoid dietary changes that alter urine pH

Mechanism of Action Class IB antiarrhythmic; structurally related to lidocaine; may cause increase in systemic vascular resistance and decrease in cardiac output; no significant negative inotropic effect

Pharmacodynamics Onset of action: Oral: 30-120 minutes

Pharmacokinetics

Distribution: V_d: 5-7 L/kg; found in breast milk in similar concentrations as plasma

Protein-binding: 50% to 70%

Metabolism: Extensive in the liver (some minor active metabolites)

Bioavailability: Oral: 88%

Half-life, adults: 10-14 hours; increase in half-life with hepatic or heart failure

Elimination: 10% to 15% excreted unchanged in urine; urinary acidification increases excretion

Usual Dosage Oral:

Children: Range: 1.4-5 mg/kg/dose (mean: 3.3 mg/kg/dose) given every 8 hours; start with lower initial dose and increase according to effects and serum concentrations

Adults: Initial: 200 mg every 8 hours (may load with 400 mg if necessary); adjust dose every 2-3 days; usual dose: 200-300 mg every 8 hours; some patients may respond to the same daily dose divided every 12 hours; maximum dose: 1.2 g/day

Dosing adjustment in renal impairment: Children and Adults: Cl_{cr} <10 mL/minute: Administer 50% to 75% of normal dose

Dosing adjustment in hepatic disease: Children and Adults: Administer 25% to 30% of normal dose; patients with severe liver disease may require even lower doses, monitor closely

Administration Oral: Administer with food or milk to decrease GI upset

Monitoring Parameters Liver enzymes, EKG, heart rate, serum concentrations

Reference Range
Therapeutic range: 0.5-2 µg/mL
Potentially toxic: >2 µg/mL

Patient Information Limit caffeine; may cause dizziness; notify physician if persistent abdominal pain, nausea, vomiting, yellowing of the eyes or skin, pale stools, dark urine, fever, sore throat, bleeding, or bruising occurs

Additional Information I.V. form under investigation

Dosage Forms Capsule, as hydrochloride: 150 mg, 200 mg, 250 mg [may contain benzyl alcohol]

Extemporaneous Preparations A 10 mg/mL oral suspension can be made using capsules and distilled water or sorbitol USP; grind the contents of eight 150 mg capsules to a powder in a mortar and pestle; then add a small amount of distilled water or sorbitol; mix to make a uniform paste; add distilled water or sorbitol in geometric amounts (while mixing) to almost 120 mL; transfer to a graduated cylinder and qsad 120 mL while mixing; suspension made with sorbitol is stable in plastic prescription bottles for 2 weeks at room temperature (25°C) and 4 weeks if refrigerated (4°C); suspension made with distilled water is stable in plastic prescription bottles for 7 weeks at room temperature (25°C) and 13 weeks if refrigerated (4°C); extended storage at 4°C is recommended to minimize microbial contamination; shake well before use

Nahata MC, Morosco RS, and Hipple TF, "Stability of Mexiletine in Two Extemporaneous Liquid Formulations Stored Under Refrigeration and at Room Temperature," *J Am Pharm Assoc*, 2000, 40(2):257-9.

References
Moak JP, Smith RT, and Garson A Jr, "Mexiletine: An Effective Antiarrhythmic Drug for Treatment of Ventricular Arrhythmias in Congenital Heart Disease," *J Am Coll Cardiol*, 1987, 10(4):824-9.

Miconazole (mi KON a zole)

U.S. Brand Names Aloe Vesta® 2-n-1 Antifungal [OTC]; Baza® Antifungal [OTC]; Carrington Antifungal [OTC]; Femizol-M™ [OTC]; Fungoid® Tincture [OTC]; Lotrimin® AF Powder/Spray [OTC]; Micatin® [OTC]; Micro-Guard® [OTC]; Mitrazol™ [OTC]; Monistat® 1 [OTC]; Monistat® 3 [OTC]; Monistat® 7 [OTC]; Monistat-Derm®; Triple Care® Antifungal [OTC]; Zeasorb®-AF [OTC]

Canadian Brand Names Dermazole; Micozole

Therapeutic Category Antifungal Agent, Topical; Antifungal Agent, Vaginal

Generic Available Yes

Use Topical: Treatment of vulvovaginal candidiasis; topical treatment of superficial fungal infections

Pregnancy Risk Factor C

Contraindications Hypersensitivity to miconazole or any component; vaginal preparation should not be used in the first trimester of pregnancy unless the drug is essential to patient's welfare

Warnings The safety of miconazole in infants <1 year of age has not been established

Precautions Use with caution in patients allergic to other imidazole-derivative antifungals (eg, clotrimazole, econazole, ketoconazole)

Adverse Reactions
Central nervous system: Headache
Dermatologic: Maceration, urticaria, rash, pruritus
Genitourinary: Pelvic cramps
Local: Irritation, burning, itching, phlebitis

Drug Interactions Cytochrome P450 isoenzyme CYP3A3/4 substrate; isoenzyme CYP2C, CYP3A3/4 (moderate), and CYP3A5-7 inhibitor
Enhanced hypoprothrombinemia with warfarin; oral sulfonylureas (severe hypoglycemia); may be antagonistic with amphotericin B; inhibits cisapride metabolism

Stability Store at room temperature

Mechanism of Action Inhibits biosynthesis of ergosterol, damaging the fungal cell wall membrane which increases permeability and causes leaking of nutrients

Pharmacokinetics
Absorption: Vaginal: Small amount absorbed systemically
(Continued)

Miconazole *(Continued)*

Distribution: Into body tissues, joints, and fluids; poor penetration into sputum, saliva, urine, and CSF

Protein binding: 91% to 93%

Metabolism: In the liver

Half-life: Multiphasic degradation:
Alpha: 40 minutes
Beta: 126 minutes
Terminal: 24 hours

Elimination: ~50% excreted in feces and <1% in urine as unchanged drug

Usual Dosage

Infants and Children:
Topical: Apply twice daily

Adolescents and Adults:
Vaginal: Insert contents of 1 applicator of vaginal cream or 100 mg vaginal suppository at bedtime for 7 days, or 200 mg vaginal suppository at bedtime for 3 days
Topical: Apply twice daily

Administration

Topical: Apply sparingly to the cleansed, dry affected area; if intertriginous areas are involved, rub cream gently into the skin

Vaginal: Wash hands before using; gently insert tablet or full applicator of cream into vagina at bedtime. Wash applicator with soap and water following use. Remain lying down for 30 minutes following administration.

Monitoring Parameters Hematocrit, hemoglobin, serum electrolytes and lipids

Patient Information Avoid contact with the eyes; do not use vaginal cream or suppositories for self-medication if patient has abdominal pain, fever, or malodorous vaginal discharge; inform physician if vaginal pruritus or discomfort occurs; avoid intercourse during therapy if using vaginal product

Dosage Forms

Combination products: Miconazole nitrate vaginal suppository 200 mg (3s) and miconazole nitrate external cream 2%; miconazole nitrate vaginal suppository 100 mg (7s) and miconazole nitrate external cream 2%

Monistat® 1 Combination Pack: Miconazole nitrate vaginal insert 1200 mg (1) and miconazole external cream 2% (5 g) [Note: Do not confuse with 1-Day™ (formerly Monistat® 1) which contains tioconazole]

Monistat® 3 Combination Pack: Miconazole nitrate vaginal suppository 200 mg (3s) and miconazole nitrate external cream 2%

Monistat® 3 Cream Combination Pack: Miconazole nitrate vaginal cream 4% and miconazole nitrate external cream 2%

Monistat® 7 Combination Pack: Miconazole nitrate vaginal suppository 100 mg (7s) and miconazole nitrate external cream 2%

Cream, topical, as nitrate: 2% (15 g, 30 g, 45 g)
Baza® Antifungal: 2% (4 g, 57 g, 142 g) [zinc oxide based formula]
Carrington Antifungal: 2% (150 g)
Micatin®: 2% (15 g)
Micro-Guard®, Mitrazol™: 2% (60 g)
Monistat-Derm®: 2% (15 g, 30 g, 85 g)
Triple Care® Antifungal: 2% (60 g, 98 g)

Cream, vaginal, as nitrate 2% (45 g) [available in prefilled applicators or with single refillable applicator]
Femizol-M™: 2% (47 g)
Monistat® 3: 4% (15 g, 25 g)
Monistat® 7: 2% (45 g)

Liquid spray, topical, as nitrate (Micatin®): 2% (90 mL, 105 mL) [contains alcohol and dimethylether propellant]

Lotion/powder, topical, as nitrate (Zeasorb®-AF): 2% (60 g) [contains 70% alcohol]

Ointment, topical, as nitrate (Aloe Vesta® 2-n-1 Antifungal): 2% (60 g, 150 g)

Powder, topical, as nitrate:
Lotrimin® AF, Micatin®, Micro-Guard®: 2% (90 g)
Mitrazol™: 2% (30 g)
Zeasorb®-AF: 2% (70 g)

Powder spray, topical, as nitrate (Lotrimin® AF): 2% (100 g) [contains alcohol and isobutane propellant]

Suppository, vaginal, as nitrate: 100 mg (7s); 200 mg (3s)
Monistat® 3: 200 mg (3s)
Monistat® 7: 100 mg (7s)

Tincture, topical, as nitrate (Fungoid®): 2% (30 mL, 473 mL) [contains benzyl alcohol and 30% isopropyl alcohol]

♦ **Micozole (Can)** *see* Miconazole *on page 759*

- **MICRhoGAM®** *see* Rh$_o$(D) Immune Globulin *on page 978*
- **Micro-Guard® [OTC]** *see* Miconazole *on page 759*
- **Micro-K®** *see* Potassium Supplements *on page 919*
- **Micronase®** *see* GlyBURIDE *on page 540*
- **Micronor®** *see* Norethindrone *on page 821*
- **Microzide™** *see* Hydrochlorothiazide *on page 569*
- **Midamor®** *see* Amiloride *on page 78*

Midazolam (MID aye zoe lam)

Related Information
Adult ACLS Algorithm, Synchronized Cardioversion *on page 1192*
Compatibility of Medications Mixed in a Syringe *on page 1412*
Drugs and Breast-Feeding *on page 1404*
Overdose and Toxicology *on page 1388*
Preprocedure Sedatives in Children *on page 1367*

U.S. Brand Names Versed®

Canadian Brand Names Apo®-Midazolam

Therapeutic Category Anticonvulsant, Benzodiazepine; Benzodiazepine; Hypnotic; Sedative

Generic Available Yes (injection)

Use Sedation, anxiolysis, amnesia prior to procedure or before induction of anesthesia; conscious sedation prior to diagnostic or radiographic procedures; continuous I.V. sedation of intubated and mechanically ventilated patients; status epilepticus

Restrictions C-IV

Pregnancy Risk Factor D

Contraindications Hypersensitivity to midazolam, any component (see Warnings), or cherries (syrup); cross-sensitivity with other benzodiazepines may occur; uncontrolled pain; existing CNS depression; shock; narrow-angle glaucoma

Warnings Midazolam may cause respiratory depression/arrest; deaths and hypoxic encephalopathy have resulted when these were not promptly recognized and treated appropriately; dose must be individualized and patients must be appropriately monitored; serious respiratory adverse events occur most often when midazolam is used in combination with other CNS depressants; personnel and equipment needed for standard respiratory resuscitation should be immediately available during midazolam use; a dedicated individual (other than the one performing the procedure) should monitor the deeply sedated pediatric patient throughout the procedure

Syrup contains sodium benzoate and injection may contain benzyl alcohol which may cause allergic reactions in susceptible individuals; large amounts of benzyl alcohol (≥99 mg/kg/day) have been associated with a potentially fatal toxicity ("gasping syndrome") in neonates; the "gasping syndrome" consists of metabolic acidosis, respiratory distress, gasping respirations, CNS dysfunction (including convulsions, intracranial hemorrhage), hypotension and cardiovascular collapse; avoid use of midazolam products containing benzyl alcohol or sodium benzoate in neonates; a benzyl alcohol free (preservative free) injection is available; *in vitro* and animal studies have shown that benzoate, a metabolite of benzyl alcohol, displaces bilirubin from protein binding sites

Precautions Use with caution in patients with CHF, renal impairment, pulmonary disease, hepatic dysfunction and in neonates (especially premature neonates); several cases of myoclonus have been reported in premature infants; benzodiazepine withdrawal may occur if abruptly discontinued in patients receiving prolonged I.V. continuous infusions; doses should be tapered slowly with prolonged use; do not administer by rapid I.V. injection (especially in neonates where severe hypotension and seizures have occurred after rapid I.V. administration)

Adverse Reactions
Cardiovascular: Cardiac arrest, hypotension, bradycardia
Central nervous system: Drowsiness, sedation, amnesia, dizziness, paradoxical excitement, hyperactivity, combativeness, headache, ataxia, rhythmic myoclonic jerking in preterm infants (~8% incidence), nystagmus
Gastrointestinal: Nausea, vomiting
Local:
  I.M., I.V.: Pain and local reactions at injection site (severity less than diazepam)
  Nasal: Burning, irritation, discomfort
Neuromuscular & skeletal: Tonic/clonic movements, muscle tremor
Ocular: Blurred vision, diplopia, lacrimation
Respiratory: Respiratory depression, oxygen desaturation, apnea, laryngospasm, bronchospasm, cough
Miscellaneous: Physical and psychological dependence with prolonged use, hiccups

Drug Interactions Cytochrome P450 isoenzyme CYP3A3/4 substrate
(Continued)

Midazolam *(Continued)*

CNS depressants, alcohol may increase sedation and respiratory depression; narcotic agents may increase hypotension (especially in neonates); doses of anesthetic agents should be reduced when used in conjunction with midazolam; cimetidine, ranitidine, erythromycin, diltiazem, verapamil, fluconazole, ketoconazole, itraconazole may increase midazolam serum concentrations; theophylline may antagonize the sedative effects of midazolam; rifampin reduces the plasma concentration of oral midazolam by >90%; carbamazepine and phenytoin may increase hepatic metabolism of midazolam; protease inhibitors (indinavir, nelfinavir, ritonavir, saquinavir) and delavirdine may decrease midazolam's metabolism and increase midazolam serum concentrations; concurrent use of midazolam with protease inhibitors or delavirdine is not recommended. Long-term administration (≥2 weeks) of the herbal medicine St John's wort (*Hypericum perforatum*) may significantly decrease serum concentrations of oral midazolam (Wang, 2001).

Food Interactions Grapefruit juice delays the absorption and significantly increases bioavailability of oral midazolam

Stability Stable at a concentration of 0.5 mg/mL for 24 hours in D_5W or NS and for 4 hours in LR

Mechanism of Action Depresses all levels of the CNS, including the limbic and reticular formation, by binding to the benzodiazepine site on the gamma-aminobutyric acid (GABA) receptor complex and modulating GABA, which is a major inhibitory neurotransmitter in the brain

Pharmacodynamics Sedation:

Onset of action:

Oral: Children: Within 10-20 minutes

I.M.:

Children: Within 5 minutes

Adults: Within 15 minutes

I.V.: Within 1-5 minutes

Intranasal: Within 5 minutes

Maximum effect:

I.M.:

Children: 15-30 minutes

Adults: 30-60 minutes

I.V.: 5-7 minutes

Intranasal: 10 minutes

Duration:

I.M.: Mean: 2 hours, up to 6 hours

I.V.: 20-30 minutes

Intranasal: 30-60 minutes

Note: Full recovery may take more than 24 hours

Pharmacokinetics

Absorption: Oral, nasal: Rapid

Distribution: V_d:

Preterm infants (n=24; GA: 26-34 weeks; PNA: 3-11 days): Median: 1.1 L/kg (range: 0.4-4.2 L/kg)

Infants and Children 6 months to 16 years: 1.24-2.02 L/kg

Adults: 1-3.1 L/kg

Increased V_d with CHF and chronic renal failure; widely distributed in body including CSF and brain; crosses placenta; enters fetal circulation; crosses into breast milk

Protein binding: Children >1 year and Adults: 97%; primarily to albumin

Metabolism: Extensive in the liver via cytochrome P450 CYP3A4 enzyme; undergoes hydroxylation and then glucuronide conjugation; primary metabolite (alpha-hydroxy-midazolam) is active and equipotent to midazolam

Bioavailability: Oral: 15% to 45% (syrup: 36%); I.M.: >90%; intranasal: ~60%; rectal: ~40% to 50%

Half-life, elimination: Increased half-life with cirrhosis, CHF, obesity, elderly, and acute renal failure

Preterm infants (n=24; GA: 26-34 weeks; PNA: 3-11 days): Median: 6.3 hours (range: 2.6-17.7 hours)

Neonates: 4-12 hours; seriously ill neonates: 6.5-12 hours

Children: I.V.: 2.9-4.5 hours; syrup: 2.2-6.8 hours

Adults: 3 hours (range: 1.8-6.4 hours)

Elimination: 63% to 80% excreted as alpha-hydroxy-midazolam glucuronide in urine; ~2% to 10% in feces, <1% eliminated as unchanged drug in the urine

Clearance:

Preterm infants (n=24; GA: 26-34 weeks; PNA: 3-11 days): Median: 1.8 mL/minute/kg (range: 0.7-6.7 mL/minute/kg)

Neonates <39 weeks GA: 1.17 mL/minute/kg

Neonates >39 weeks GA: 1.84 mL/minute/kg
Seriously ill neonates: 1.2-2 mL/minute/kg
Infants >3 months: 9.1 mL/minute/kg
Children >1 year: 3.2-13.3 mL/minute/kg
Healthy adults: 4.2-9 mL/minute/kg
Adults with acute renal failure: 1.9 mL/minute/kg

Usual Dosage Dosage must be individualized and based on patient's age, underlying diseases, concurrent medications, and desired effect; decrease dose (by ~30%) if narcotics or other CNS depressants are administered concomitantly; use multiple small doses and titrate to desired sedative effect; allow 3-5 minutes between doses to decrease the chance of oversedation

Neonates:

Conscious sedation during mechanical ventilation: I.V. continuous infusion:
<32 weeks: Initial: 0.03 mg/kg/hour (0.5 mcg/kg/minute)
>32 weeks: Initial: 0.06 mg/kg/hour (1 mcg/kg/minute)

Note: Do not use I.V. loading doses in neonates; for faster achievement of sedation, infuse the continuous infusion at a faster rate for the first several hours; use the smallest dose possible

Infants >2 months and Children:

Status epilepticus refractory to standard therapy: I.V.: Loading dose: 0.15 mg/kg followed by a continuous infusion of 1 mcg/kg/minute; titrate dose upward every 5 minutes until clinical seizure activity is controlled; mean infusion rate required in 24 children was 2.3 mcg/kg/minute with a range of 1-18 mcg/kg/minute (Rivera, 1993)

Infants ≥6 months and Children:

Sedation, anxiolysis, and amnesia prior to procedure or before induction of anesthesia: Oral: Single dose: 0.25-0.5 mg/kg, depending on patient status and desired effect, usual: 0.5 mg/kg; maximum dose: 20 mg;
Patient-specific dosing:

Infants 6 months to <6 years, and less cooperative patients: Higher doses (up to 1 mg/kg) may be required

Children 6 to ≥16 years, or cooperative patients (especially if intensity and duration of sedation is less critical): 0.25 mg/kg may suffice

High risk pediatric patients (respiratory or cardiac compromised, concomitant CNS depressants, higher risk surgical patients): 0.25 mg/kg should be considered

Children:

Preoperative sedation or conscious sedation for procedures:
I.M.: Usual: 0.1-0.15 mg/kg 30-60 minutes before surgery or procedure; range: 0.05-0.15 mg/kg; doses up to 0.5 mg/kg have been used in more anxious patients; maximum total dose: 10 mg
I.V.:

Infants <6 months: Limited information is available in nonintubated infants; dosing recommendations are unclear; infants <6 months are at higher risk for airway obstruction and hypoventilation; titrate dose with small increments to desired clinical effect; monitor carefully

Infants 6 months to Children 5 years: Initial: 0.05-0.1 mg/kg; titrate dose carefully; total dose of 0.6 mg/kg may be required; usual total dose maximum dose: 6 mg

Children 6-12 years: Initial: 0.025-0.05 mg/kg; titrate dose carefully; total doses of 0.4 mg/kg may be required; usual total dose maximum: 10 mg

Children 12-16 years: Dose as adults; usual total dose maximum: 10 mg

Intranasal: Usual: 0.2 mg/kg; may repeat in 5-15 minutes; range: 0.2-0.3 mg/kg/dose

Conscious sedation during mechanical ventilation: I.V.: Continuous infusion: Loading dose: 0.05-0.2 mg/kg given slow I.V. over 2-3 minutes, then follow with initial continuous infusion: 0.06-0.12 mg/kg/hour (1-2 mcg/kg/minute); titrate to the desired effect; range: 0.4-6 mcg/kg/minute

Adults:

Preoperative sedation: I.M.: 0.07-0.08 mg/kg 30-60 minutes presurgery; usual dose: 5 mg

Conscious sedation: I.V.: Titrate dose slowly to desired effect; administer slowly over at least 2 minutes and wait another 2 or more minutes to evaluate effect. Some adults may respond to doses as low as 1 mg; do not give more than 2.5 mg over a period of 2 minutes. Titrate as needed, using small increments every 2-3 minutes. Usual total dose: 2.5-5 mg; total dose >5 mg is generally not needed; maintenance doses may be given by slow titration, if needed, in increments of 25% of the original dose used to reach sedative endpoint.

(Continued)

Midazolam *(Continued)*

Conscious sedation during mechanical ventilation: I.V.: Optional loading dose: 0.01-0.05 mg/kg (~0.5-4 mg/dose); may repeat at 10- to 15-minute intervals until patient is adequately sedated, then begin continuous infusion

Continuous infusion: Initial: 0.02-0.1 mg/kg/hour (1-7 mg/hour); use lowest doses listed for patients receiving other sedatives, or opioids, or having residual anesthetic effects; titrate the infusion to achieve adequate level of sedation; use lowest effective dose

Administration

Intranasal: Administer using a 1 mL needleless syringe into the nares over 15 seconds; use the 5 mg/mL injection; $\frac{1}{2}$ of the dose may be administered to each nare; **Note:** The 5 mg/mL injection has also been administered as a nasal spray using a graded pump device (see Ljungman, 2000)

Oral: Administer on empty stomach (feeding is usually contraindicated prior to sedation for procedures); do not administer with grapefruit juice

Parenteral:

I.V.: Administer by slow I.V. injection over at least 2-5 minutes at a concentration of 1-5 mg/mL (maximum concentration: 5 mg/mL) or by I.V. infusion; avoid extravasation; do not administer intra-arterially

I.M.: Maximum concentration: 1 mg/mL

Monitoring Parameters
Level of sedation, respiratory rate, heart rate, blood pressure, oxygen saturation (ie, pulse oximetry)

Patient Information
Report the use of other medications, nonprescription medications, and herbal or natural products to your physician and pharmacist; avoid alcohol; avoid grapefruit juice if taking oral midazolam

Nursing Implications
Abrupt discontinuation after prolonged use may result in withdrawal symptoms

Additional Information
Sodium content of injection: 0.14 mEq/mL. For Neonates: Since both concentrations of Versed® injection contain 1% benzyl alcohol, use the 5 mg/mL injection and dilute to 0.5 mg/mL with SWI without preservatives to decrease the amount of benzyl alcohol delivered to the neonate, or use preservative free injection. With continuous infusion, midazolam may accumulate in peripheral tissues; use lowest effective infusion rate to reduce accumulation effects. Midazolam is 3-4 times as potent as diazepam. Paradoxical reactions associated with midazolam use in children (eg, agitation, restlessness, combativeness) have been successfully treated with flumazenil (see Massanari, 1997)

Dosage Forms

Injection, solution, as hydrochloride (Versed®): 1 mg/mL (2 mL, 5 mL, 10 mL); 5 mg/mL (1 mL, 2 mL, 5 mL, 10 mL) [contains 1% benzyl alcohol]

Injection, solution, as hydrochloride [preservative free]: 1 mg/mL (2 mL, 5 mL); 5 mg/mL (1 mL, 2 mL)

Syrup, as hydrochloride (Versed®): 2 mg/mL (118 mL) [contains sodium benzoate; cherry flavor]

References
Adrian ER, "Intranasal Versed®: The Future of Pediatric Conscious Sedation," *Pediatr Nurs*, 1994, 20(3):287-92.

Booker PD, Beechey A, and Lloyd-Thomas AR, "Sedation of Children Requiring Artificial Ventilation Using an Infusion of Midazolam," *Br J Anaesth*, 1986, 58(10):1104-8.

Burtin P, Jacqz-Aigrain E, Girard P, et al, "Population Pharmacokinetics of Midazolam in Neonates," *Clin Pharmacol Ther*, 1994, 56(6 Pt 1):615-25.

de Wildt SN, Kearns GL, Hop WC, et al, "Pharmacokinetics and Metabolism of Intravenous Midazolam in Preterm Infants," *Clin Pharmacol Ther*, 2001, 70(6):525-31.

Jacqz-Aigrain E, Daoud P, Burtin P, et al, "Placebo-Controlled Trial of Midazolam Sedation in Mechanically Ventilated Newborn Babies," *Lancet*, 1994, 344(8923):646-50.

Kupietzky A and Houpt MI, "Midazolam: A Review of Its Use for Conscious Sedation of Children," *Pediatr Dent*, 1993, 15(4):237-41.

Ljungman G, Kreuger A, Andreasson S, et al, "Midazolam Nasal Spray Reduces Procedural Anxiety in Children," *Pediatrics*, 2000, 105(1 Pt 1):73-8.

Lugo RA, Fishbein M, Nahata MC, et al, "Complication of Intranasal Midazolam," *Pediatrics*, 1993, 92(4):638.

Magny JF, Zupan V, Dehan M, et al, "Midazolam and Myoclonus in Neonate," *Eur J Pediatr*, 1994, 153(5):389-90.

Malinovsky JM, Populaire C, Cozian A, et al, "Premedication With Midazolam in Children, Effect of Intranasal, Rectal and Oral Routes on Plasma Midazolam Concentrations," *Anaesthesia*, 1995, 50(4):351-4.

Massanari M, Novitsky J, and Reinstein LJ, "Paradoxical Reactions in Children Associated With Midazolam Use During Endoscopy," *Clin Pediatr*, 1997, 36(12):681-4.

Riva J, Lejbusiewicz G, Papa M, et al, "Oral Premedication With Midazolam in Paediatric Anaesthesia. Effects on Sedation and Gastric Contents," *Paediatr Anaesth*, 1997, 7(3):191-6.

Rivera R, Segnini M, Baltodano A, et al, "Midazolam in the Treatment of Status Epilepticus in Children," *Crit Care Med*, 1993, 21(7):991-4.

Silvasi DL, Rosen DA, and Rosen KR, "Continuous Intravenous Midazolam Infusion for Sedation in the Pediatric Intensive Care Unit," *Anesth Analg*, 1988, 67(3):286-8.

Wang Z, Gorski JC, Hamman MA, et al, "The Effects of St John's Wort (*Hypericum perforatum*) on Human Cytochrome P450 Activity," *Clin Pharmacol Ther*, 2001, 70(4):317-26.

◆ **Midol® Maximum Strength Cramp Formula [OTC]** *see Ibuprofen on page 588*

◆ **Migranal®** *see Dihydroergotamine on page 385*

◆ **Milk of Magnesia (Magnesium Hydroxide)** *see Magnesium Supplements on page 701*

Milrinone (MIL ri none)

U.S. Brand Names Primacor®

Therapeutic Category Phosphodiesterase Enzyme Inhibitor

Generic Available No

Use Short-term treatment of acute decompensated heart failure

Pregnancy Risk Factor C

Contraindications Hypersensitivity to milrinone, any component, or inamrinone (amrinone)

Warnings Longer treatment of heart failure (>48 hours) has not been shown to be safe and effective (there are no controlled trials using milrinone infusions for >48 hours); long-term oral use for heart failure was associated with no improvement in symptoms, increased risk of hospitalization, and increased risk of sudden death; monitor EKG continuously to promptly detect and manage ventricular arrhythmias

Precautions Avoid use in patients with severe obstructive aortic or pulmonic valvular disease; use in patients with hypertrophic subaortic stenosis may increase outflow tract obstruction; use with caution in patients with a history of ventricular arrhythmias, atrial fibrillation, or atrial flutter; use with caution and modify dosage in patients with impaired renal function

Adverse Reactions

Central nervous system: Headaches (mild to moderate, 2.9%)

Cardiovascular: Ventricular arrhythmias (12.1%) including ventricular ectopic activity (8.5%), nonsustained ventricular tachycardia (2.8%), sustained ventricular tachycardia (1%), and ventricular fibrillation (0.2%); supraventricular arrhythmias (3.8%); hypotension (2.9%); angina/chest pain (1.2%)

Endocrine & metabolic: Hypokalemia (0.6%)

Hematologic: Thrombocytopenia (0.4%)

Hepatic: Abnormal liver function tests

Neuromuscular & skeletal: Tremor (0.4%)

Respiratory: Bronchospasm (rare)

Stability Incompatible with furosemide (a precipitate forms when furosemide is injected into I.V. lines containing milrinone); compatible with ½NS, NS, and D_5W

Mechanism of Action Inhibits phosphodiesterase III (PDE III), the major PDE in cardiac and vascular tissues. Inhibition of PDE III increases cyclic adenosine monophosphate (cAMP) which potentiates the delivery of calcium to myocardial contractile systems and results in a positive inotropic effect. Inhibition of PDE III in vascular tissue results in relaxation of vascular muscle and vasodilatation.

Pharmacodynamics Onset of action (improved hemodynamic function): Within 5-15 minutes

Pharmacokinetics

Distribution: V_d beta

Infants (after cardiac surgery): 0.9 ± 0.4 L/kg

Children (after cardiac surgery): 0.7 ± 0.2 L/kg

Adults:

After cardiac surgery: 0.3 ± 0.1 L/kg

CHF (with single injection): 0.38 L/kg

CHF (with infusion): 0.45 L/kg

Protein binding: 70%

Half-life:

Infants (after cardiac surgery): 3.15 ± 2 hours

Children (after cardiac surgery): 1.86 ± 2 hours

Adults:

After cardiac surgery: 1.69 ± 0.18 hours

CHF: 2.3-2.4 hours

Renal impairment: Prolonged half-life

Elimination: Excreted in the urine as unchanged drug (83%) and glucuronide metabolite (12%)

Clearance:

Infants (after cardiac surgery): 3.8 ± 1 mL/kg/minute

Children (after cardiac surgery): 5.9 ± 2 mL/kg/minute

Children (with septic shock): 10.6 ± 5.3 mL/kg/minute

Adults:

After cardiac surgery: 2 ± 0.7 mL/kg/minute

CHF: 2.2-2.3 mL/kg/minute

Renal impairment: Decreased clearance

(Continued)

Milrinone (Continued)

Usual Dosage

Neonates, Infants, and Children: I.V.: A limited number of studies have used different dosing schemes (see Additional Information). Two recent pharmacokinetic studies propose per kg doses for pediatric patients with septic shock that are greater than those recommended for adults (Lindsay, 1998) and in infants and children after cardiac surgery (Ramamoorthy, 1998). Further pharmacodynamic studies are needed to define pediatric milrinone guidelines. Several centers are using the following guidelines:

Loading dose: 50 mcg/kg administered over 15 minutes followed by a continuous infusion of 0.5 mcg/kg/minute; range: 0.25-0.75 mcg/kg/minute; titrate dose to effect

PALS Guidelines 2000: I.V., I.O.: Loading dose: 50-75 mcg/kg administered over 15 minutes followed by a continuous infusion of 0.5-0.75 mcg/kg/minute

Adults: I.V.: Loading dose: 50 mcg/kg slow I.V. over 10 minutes, followed by a continuous infusion of 0.5 mcg/kg/minute; range: 0.375-0.75 mcg/kg/minute; titrate does to effect; maximum daily dose: 1.13 mg/kg/day

Dosing adjustment in renal impairment: For continuous infusion:

Cl_{cr} 50 mL/minute/1.73 m^2: Administer 0.43 mcg/kg/minute

Cl_{cr} 40 mL/minute/1.73 m^2: Administer 0.38 mcg/kg/minute

Cl_{cr} 30 mL/minute/1.73 m^2: Administer 0.33 mcg/kg/minute

Cl_{cr} 20 mL/minute/1.73 m^2: Administer 0.28 mcg/kg/minute

Cl_{cr} 10 mL/minute/1.73 m^2: Administer 0.23 mcg/kg/minute

Cl_{cr} 5 mL/minute/1.73 m^2: Administer 0.2 mcg/kg/minute

Administration

Loading dose: Administer slow I.V. push over 15 minutes for pediatric patients and over 10 minutes in adults; loading dose may be given as undiluted solution, but may dilute to 10-20 mL (in adults) for ease of administration.

I.V. continuous infusion: Dilute with ½NS, NS, or D_5W and administer via infusion pump or syringe pump; usual concentration: ≤200 mcg/mL; 250 mcg/mL in NS has been used (see Barton, 1996)

Monitoring Parameters Blood pressure, heart rate, cardiac output, CI, SVR, PVR, CVP, EKG, platelet count, serum potassium, renal function; clinical signs and symptoms of CHF

Nursing Implications Do not administer furosemide I.V. push via "Y" site into milrinone solutions as precipitate will occur; decrease the infusion rate if significant hypotension occurs

Additional Information Dosing schemes and proposed dosing based on pharmacokinetic data:

Neonates: A loading dose of 50 mcg/kg administered over 15 minutes, followed by a continuous infusion of 0.5 mcg/kg/minute for 30 minutes in 10 neonates (3-27 days old, median age 5 days) improved hemodynamic parameters and was well tolerated (see Chang, 1995). Further neonatal studies of longer duration are needed.

Infants and children with septic shock: Twelve patients (9 months to 15 years of age) were administered a loading dose of 50 mcg/kg, followed by a continuous infusion of 0.5 mcg/kg/minute. At 1 hour after the loading dose, if patients did not respond (defined as a ≥20% increase in CI or an improvement in peripheral perfusion), an additional loading dose of 25 mcg/kg was given and the infusion rate was increased to 0.75 mcg/kg/minute. Nine of 12 patients required the additional loading dose and increased rate of infusion (see Barton 1996). A subsequent pharmacokinetic analysis of these patients recommended larger loading doses of 75 mcg/kg and infusion rates of 0.75-1 mcg/kg/minute. However, these doses were based on a one-compartment pharmacokinetic model and are higher then the mean infusion rate of 0.69 mcg/kg/minute used in the study (see Lindsay 1998). Further studies are needed.

Infants and Children after open heart surgery: Group A: Eleven patients received a loading dose of 25 mcg/kg given over 5 minutes followed by an infusion of 0.25 mcg/kg/minute; 30 minutes later, a second 25 mcg/kg loading dose was given and the infusion was increased to 0.5 mcg/kg/minute. Group B: 8 patients received a loading dose of 25 mcg/kg given over 10 minutes followed by an infusion of 0.5 mcg/kg/minute; 30 minutes later, a second loading dose of 25 mcg/kg was given and the infusion was increased to 0.75 mcg/kg/minute. Patients in both groups received a third loading dose of 25 mcg/kg if needed. A two-compartment model and NONMEM pharmacokinetic analyses were performed. Based on the NONMEM analysis, the authors propose the following doses: Infants: Loading dose: 104 mcg/kg and continuous infusion of 0.49 mcg/kg/minute; children: loading dose: 67 mcg/kg and continuous infusion of 0.61 mcg/kg/minute. Further studies are needed before these proposed doses can routinely be used in the pediatric population.

Dosage Forms

Infusion, as lactate [premixed in D5W]: 200 mcg/mL (100 mL, 200 mL)

Injection, solution, as lactate: 1 mg/mL (5 mL, 10 mL, 20 mL)

References

Barton P, Garcia J, Kouatli A, et al, "Hemodynamic Effects of I.V. Milrinone Lactate in Pediatric Patients With Septic Shock. A Prospective Double-Blinded, Randomized, Placebo-Controlled, Interventional Study," *Chest*, 1996, 109(5):1302-12.

Chang AC, Atz AM, Wernovsky G, et al, "Milrinone: Systemic and Pulmonary Hemodynamic Effects in Neonates After Cardiac Surgery," *Crit Care Med*, 1995, 23(11):1907-14.

"Guidelines 2000 for Cardiopulmonary Resuscitation and Emergency Cardiovascular Care, Part 10: Pediatric Advanced Life Support, The American Heart Association in Collaboration With the International Liaison Committee on Resuscitation," *Circulation*, 2000, 102(8 Suppl): I291-342.

Lindsay CA, Barton P, Lawless S, et al, "Pharmacokinetics and Pharmacodynamics of Milrinone Lactate in Pediatric Patients With Septic Shock," *J Pediatr*, 1998, 132(2):329-34.

Ramamoorthy C, Anderson GD, Williams GD, et al, "Pharmacokinetics and Side Effects of Milrinone in Infants and Children After Open Heart Surgery," *Anesth Analg*, 1998, 86(2):283-9.

Mineral Oil (MIN er al oyl)

U.S. Brand Names Fleet® Mineral Oil [OTC]; Fleet® Mineral Oil Enema [OTC]; Kondremul® [OTC]

Synonyms Heavy Mineral Oil; Liquid Paraffin; White Mineral Oil

Therapeutic Category Laxative, Lubricant

Generic Available Yes

Use Temporary relief of constipation, to relieve fecal impaction, preparation for bowel studies or surgery

Pregnancy Risk Factor C

Contraindications Patients with a colostomy or an ileostomy, appendicitis, ulcerative colitis, diverticulitis, dysphagia or hiatal hernia

Warnings Oral form should be avoided in children <4 years of age because of the risk of aspiration

Adverse Reactions

Gastrointestinal: Nausea, vomiting, diarrhea, abdominal cramps, anal itching, anal seepage

Respiratory: Lipid pneumonitis with aspiration

Drug Interactions May impair absorption of fat-soluble vitamins, oral contraceptives, coumarin; increased absorption with docusate

Food Interactions May decrease absorption of fat-soluble vitamins, carotene, calcium, and phosphorus

Mechanism of Action Eases passage of stool by decreasing water absorption, softens stool, and lubricates the intestine

Pharmacodynamics Onset of action: ~6-8 hours

Pharmacokinetics

Absorption: Minimal following oral or rectal administration

Distribution: Into intestinal mucosa, liver, spleen, and mesenteric lymph nodes

Elimination: In feces

Usual Dosage

Children:

Oral: 5-11 years: 5-15 mL once daily or in divided doses; should not be used for longer than 1 week

Rectal: 2-11 years: 30-60 mL as a single dose

Children ≥12 years and Adults:

Oral: 15-45 mL/day once daily or in divided doses; should not be used for longer than 1 week

Rectal: Contents of one retention enema (range 60-150 mL)/day as a single dose

Administration

Oral: Nonemulsified mineral oil may be administered at bedtime on an empty stomach; emulsified mineral oil should be shaken before using; may be administered with meals (more palatable than nonemulsified mineral oil)

Rectal: Gently insert enema tip into rectum with a slight side-to-side movement with tip pointing toward the navel; have patient bear down

Monitoring Parameters Evacuation of stool; anal leakage indicates dose too high or need for disimpaction

Patient Information Do not take if experiencing abdominal pain, nausea, or vomiting. Rectal enema: Do not take if experiencing rectal bleeding

Dosage Forms

Liquid, oral: 480 mL

Fleet® Mineral Oil: 480 mL

Kondremul®: 55% (480 mL) [sugar free; contains benzoic acid]

Liquid, rectal (Fleet® Mineral Oil Enema): 133 mL

Liquid, topical: 10 mL, 30 mL, 120 mL, 240 mL, 500 mL

(Continued)

Mineral Oil *(Continued)*

References

Baker SS, Liptak GS, Colletti RB, et al, "A Medical Position Statement of the North American Society for Pediatric Gastroenterology and Nutrition; Constipation in Infants and Children: Evaluation and treatment," www.naspgn.org/constipation, 2000, 1-34.

♦ **Minim's Atropine Solution (Can)** *see* Atropine *on page 144*

♦ **Minim's Gentamicin 0.3% (Can)** *see* Gentamicin *on page 533*

♦ **Minipress®** *see* Prazosin *on page 924*

♦ **Minirin® (Can)** *see* Desmopressin *on page 352*

♦ **Minitran™** *see* Nitroglycerin *on page 815*

♦ **Minox (Can)** *see* Minoxidil *on page 768*

Minoxidil *(mi NOKS i dil)*

U.S. Brand Names Loniten®; Rogaine® Extra Strength for Men [OTC]; Rogaine® for Men [OTC]; Rogaine® for Women [OTC]

Canadian Brand Names Apo®-Gain; Minox

Therapeutic Category Antihypertensive Agent; Vasodilator

Generic Available Yes

Use Management of severe hypertension; topically for management of alopecia or male pattern alopecia

Pregnancy Risk Factor C

Contraindications Hypersensitivity to minoxidil or any component; pheochromocytoma

Warnings May cause pericarditis, pericardial effusion and tamponade, angina, and sodium and water retention; use of minoxidil should be reserved for treatment of hypertension in patients who have not adequately responded to maximum doses of a diuretic and 2 other antihypertensive agents; minoxidil is usually used with a beta-blocker (to treat minoxidil-induced tachycardia) and a diuretic (for treatment of water retention/edema); avoid concomitant use of minoxidil with guanethidine (see Drug Interactions); minoxidil may rapidly control blood pressure; too rapid control of blood pressure may lead to syncope, CVA, MI, or ischemia

Precautions Use with caution in patients with coronary artery disease or with recent MI, pulmonary hypertension, significant renal dysfunction, CHF; renal failure or dialysis patients may require dosage reduction

Adverse Reactions

Cardiovascular: Edema, CHF, tachycardia, angina, pericardial effusion and tamponade, EKG changes

Central nervous system: Dizziness, fatigue, headache

Dermatologic: Hypertrichosis (commonly occurs within 1-2 months of therapy), coarsening facial features, dermatologic reactions, rash, Stevens-Johnson syndrome, photosensitivity

Endocrine & metabolic: Sodium and water retention

Gastrointestinal: Weight gain

Respiratory: Pulmonary hypertension, pulmonary edema

Drug Interactions Concurrent administration with guanethidine may cause profound orthostatic hypotensive effects; additive hypotensive effects with other hypotensive agents or diuretics

Food Interactions Avoid natural licorice (causes sodium and water retention and increases potassium loss)

Stability Store at controlled room temperature 20°C to 25°C (68°F to 77°F)

Mechanism of Action Produces vasodilation by directly relaxing arteriolar smooth muscle, with little effect on veins; effects may be mediated by cyclic AMP; stimulation of hair growth is secondary to vasodilation, increased cutaneous blood flow and stimulation of resting hair follicles

Pharmacodynamics Hypotensive effects:

Onset of action: Oral: Within 30 minutes

Maximum effect: Within 2-8 hours

Duration: Up to 2-5 days

Pharmacokinetics

Metabolism: 88% primarily via glucuronidation

Protein-binding: None

Bioavailability: Oral: 90%

Half-life, adults: 3.5-4.2 hours

Elimination: 12% excreted unchanged in urine

Dialysis: Dialyzable (50% to 100%)

Usual Dosage

Children <12 years: Hypertension: Oral: Initial: 0.1-0.2 mg/kg once daily; maximum dose: 5 mg/day; increase gradually every 3 days; usual dosage: 0.25-1 mg/kg/day in 1-2 divided doses; maximum dose: 50 mg/day

Children >12 years and Adults:

Hypertension: Oral: Initial: 5 mg once daily, increase gradually every 3 days; usual dose: 10-40 mg/day in 1-2 divided doses; maximum dose: 100 mg/day

Alopecia: Apply twice daily

Administration Oral: May be administered without regard to food

Monitoring Parameters Fluids and electrolytes, body weight, blood pressure

Patient Information May cause dizziness; rise slowly from prolonged lying or sitting position. May cause photosensitivity reactions (eg, exposure to sunlight may cause severe sunburn, skin rash, redness, or itching); avoid exposure to sunlight and artificial light sources (sunlamps, tanning booth/bed); wear protective clothing, wide-brimmed hats, sunglasses, and lip sunscreen (SPF ≥15); use a sunscreen [broad-spectrum sunscreen or physical sunscreen (preferred) or sunblock with SPF ≥15]; contact physician if reaction occurs.

Additional Information May take 1-6 months for hypertrichosis to totally reverse after minoxidil therapy is discontinued

Dosage Forms

Solution, topical: 2% [20 mg/metered dose] (60 mL); 5% [50 mg/metered dose] (60 mL)

Rogaine® Extra Strength for Men: 5% [50 mg/metered dose] (60 mL)

Rogaine® for Men, Rogaine® for Women: 2% [20 mg/metered dose] (60 mL)

Tablet (Loniten®): 2.5 mg, 10 mg

- ◆ **Mintezol**® *see* Thiabendazole *on page 1080*
- ◆ **Miochol-E**® *see* Acetylcholine *on page 43*
- ◆ **MiraLax**™ *see* Polyethylene Glycol-Electrolyte Solution *on page 914*

Misoprostol (mye soe PROST ole)

U.S. Brand Names Cytotec®

Canadian Brand Names Apo®-Misoprostol; Novo-Misoprostol

Therapeutic Category Gastrointestinal Agent, Gastric Ulcer Treatment; Prostaglandin

Generic Available Yes

Use Prevention of NSAID-induced gastric ulcers; improvement in fat absorption in cystic fibrosis patients when used in conjunction with pancreatic enzyme supplements (unlabeled use)

Pregnancy Risk Factor X

Contraindications Hypersensitivity to misoprostol or any component; pregnancy

Warnings Not to be used for reducing the risk of NSAID-induced ulcers in pregnant women or women of childbearing potential unless the woman is capable of complying with effective contraceptive measures; women should have a negative serum pregnancy test within 2 weeks prior to initiating therapy with therapy begun on the second or third day of next menstrual period; may cause abortion, premature labor, or birth defects if given to pregnant women

Precautions Use with caution in patients with inflammatory bowel disease (due to potential for development of diarrhea with misoprostol) and renal impairment

Adverse Reactions

Central nervous system: Headache

Gastrointestinal: Nausea, vomiting, constipation, flatulence, diarrhea, abdominal pain, dyspepsia

Genitourinary: Uterine stimulation, vaginal bleeding, menstrual irregularities, uterine rupture (when taken after the eighth week of pregnancy)

Drug Interactions Magnesium containing antacids enhance diarrhea associated with misoprostol

Mechanism of Action Misoprostol, a gastric antisecretory agent, is a synthetic prostaglandin E₁ analog that replaces the protective prostaglandins consumed with prostaglandin-inhibiting therapies (eg, NSAIDs) resulting in reduction of acid secretion from the gastric parietal cell and stimulation of bicarbonate production from the gastric and duodenal mucosa

Pharmacodynamics Inhibition of gastric acid secretion:

Onset of action: 30 minutes

Maximum effect: 60-90 minutes

Duration: 3 hours

Pharmacokinetics

Absorption: Rapid

Protein binding (misoprostol acid): 80% to 90%

(Continued)

Misoprostol *(Continued)*

Metabolism: Extensive "first pass" de-esterification to misoprostol acid (active metabolite)

Bioavailability: 88%

Half-life (metabolite): 20-40 minutes

Time to peak serum concentration (active metabolite): Within 15-30 minutes

Elimination: In urine (64% to 73% in 24 hours) and feces (15% in 24 hours)

Usual Dosage Oral:

Prevention of NSAID-induced ulcers: Adults: 200 mcg 4 times/day; if not tolerated, may decrease dose to 100 mcg 4 times/day or 200 mcg twice daily; take for the duration of NSAID therapy

Improvement of fat malabsorption in cystic fibrosis (limited data available in children): Children 8-16 years: 100 mcg four times daily

Administration Oral: Administer after meals and at bedtime

Patient Information May cause diarrhea when first being used; avoid taking with magnesium-containing antacids; do not take if you are pregnant

Nursing Implications Incidence of diarrhea may be lessened by having patient take dose right after meals

Dosage Forms Tablet: 100 mcg, 200 mcg

References

Cleghorn GJ, Shepherd RW, and Holt TL, "The Use of a Synthetic Prostaglandin E1 Analogue (Misoprostol) as an Adjunct to Pancreatic Enzyme Replacement in Cystic Fibrosis," *Scand J Gastroenterol Suppl*, 1988, 143:142-7.

Robinson PJ, Smith AL, and Sly PD, "Duodenal pH in Cystic Fibrosis and Its Relationship to Fat Malabsorption," *Dig Dis Sci*, 1990, 35(10):1299-304.

Mitomycin *(mye toe MYE sin)*

Related Information

Emetogenic Potential of Single Chemotherapeutic Agents *on page 1286*

U.S. Brand Names Mutamycin®

Synonyms Mitomycin-C; MTC

Therapeutic Category Antineoplastic Agent, Antibiotic

Generic Available Yes

Use Therapy of disseminated adenocarcinoma of stomach, colon, or pancreas in combination with other approved chemotherapeutic agents; bladder cancer, breast cancer

Pregnancy Risk Factor D

Contraindications Hypersensitivity to mitomycin or any component; platelet counts <75,000/mm^3; leukocyte counts <3000/mm^3 or serum creatinine >1.7 mg/dL; coagulation disorders; pregnancy

Warnings The FDA currently recommends that procedures for proper handling and disposal of antineoplastic agents be considered. Bone marrow suppression, notably thrombocytopenia and leukopenia, may contribute to the development of a secondary infection; hemolytic uremic syndrome, a serious and often fatal syndrome consisting of microangiopathic hemolytic anemia, thrombocytopenia, and irreversible renal failure has occurred in patients receiving systemic therapy; the risk of hemolytic uremic syndrome increases with a total cumulative dose >50 mg/m^2; mitomycin is potentially mutagenic and teratogenic.

Precautions Use with caution in patients with myelosuppression, impaired renal or hepatic function; modify dosage in patients with myelosuppression or renal impairment

Adverse Reactions

Cardiovascular: CHF (rare)

Central nervous system: Fever, headache, confusion

Dermatologic: Alopecia, pruritus

Gastrointestinal: Nausea, vomiting, mouth ulcers, diarrhea, anorexia

Hematologic: Bone marrow suppression (leukopenia, thrombocytopenia), microangiopathic hemolytic anemia

Hepatic: Veno-occlusive disease

Local: Thrombophlebitis; necrosis and sloughing of tissue with extravasation

Neuromuscular & skeletal: Paresthesia, weakness

Renal: Hemolytic uremic syndrome, nephrotoxicity, elevated serum creatinine

Respiratory: Pulmonary toxicity, interstitial pneumonia, bronchospasm, dyspnea, cough

Drug Interactions Anthracyclines (may enhance cardiotoxicity)

Stability Store intact vials at room temperature; protect from light; reconstitute vial with SWI to a concentration of 0.5 mg/mL; the reconstituted solution must be protected from light if not used within 24 hours; stable for 7 days at room temperature and 14 days when refrigerated; I.V. infusion in D$_5$W is stable for 3 hours at room temperature;

in NS solution is stable for 12 hours at room temperature; physically compatible with ondansetron for 4 hours

Mechanism of Action Inhibits DNA and RNA synthesis by alkylating and cross-linking the strands of DNA

Pharmacokinetics

Distribution: Into bile and ascites fluid; high drug concentrations found in kidney, muscle, heart, and lung tissue

Metabolism: Primarily hepatic with metabolism also occurring in other tissues

Half-life, terminal: 50 minutes

Elimination: Primarily by hepatic metabolism followed by urinary excretion (<10% as unchanged drug) and to a small extent biliary excretion

Usual Dosage Children and Adults: I.V. (refer to individual protocols): 10-20 mg/m^2/dose every 6-8 weeks, or 3 mg/m^2/day for 5 days every 4-6 weeks; subsequent doses should be adjusted to platelet and leukocyte response; see table.

Nadir After Prior Dose/mm^3		% of Prior Dose to Be Given
Leukocytes	Platelets	
4000	>100,000	100
3000-3999	75,000-99,999	100
2000-2999	25,000-74,999	70
2000	<25,000	50

Very high doses (40-50 mg/m^2 as a single dose) have been administered by hepatic artery infusion followed by autologous bone marrow transplantation.

Dosing adjustment in renal impairment: Cl$_{cr}$ <10 mL/minute: Administer 75% of normal dose

Administration Parenteral: Administer by short I.V. infusion over 30-60 minutes or by slow I.V. push over 5-10 minutes through a Y-site of a running I.V.; short I.V. infusions are usually administered at a final concentration of 20-40 mcg/mL (in 50-250 mL of D$_5$W or NS); I.V. slow push can be administered at a concentration not to exceed 0.5 mg/mL

Monitoring Parameters Platelet count, CBC with differential, hemoglobin, prothrombin time, renal and pulmonary function tests; observe I.V. injection site for infiltration and vein irritation

Patient Information Notify physician if fever, sore throat, bruising, bleeding, shortness of breath, or painful urination occur

Nursing Implications Care should be taken to avoid extravasation since ulceration and tissue sloughing can occur; mitomycin extravasation has been treated using a 99% (w/v) solution of dimethylsulfoxide (DMSO); apply 1.5 mL to the site every 6 hours for 14 days; allow to air-dry; do not cover

Additional Information Bladder fibrosis/contraction which in rare cases required cystectomy has been reported with intravesical administration of mitomycin (non-FDA approved route of administration).

Myelosuppressive effects:

WBC: Moderate

Platelets: Severe

Onset (days): 21

Nadir (days): 36

Recovery (days): 42-56

Dosage Forms Injection, powder for reconstitution: 5 mg, 20 mg, 40 mg [contains mannitol]

References

Alberts DS and Dorr RT, "Case Report: Topical DMSO for Mitomycin C-Induced Skin Ulceration," *Oncol Nurs Forum*, 1991, 18(4):693-5.

♦ **Mitomycin-C** *see* Mitomycin *on page 770*

Mitoxantrone (mye toe ZAN trone)

Related Information

Emetogenic Potential of Single Chemotherapeutic Agents *on page 1286*

U.S. Brand Names Novantrone®

Synonyms DHAD

Therapeutic Category Antineoplastic Agent, Anthracenedione; Antineoplastic Agent, Antibiotic

Generic Available No

Use For remission-induction therapy of acute nonlymphocytic leukemia (ANLL) and acute myelogenous leukemia (AML); mitoxantrone is also active against other leukemias, lymphoma, breast cancer, and moderately active against pediatric sarcoma; treatment of patients with pain related to advanced hormone refractory prostate (Continued)

Mitoxantrone *(Continued)*

cancer; reducing neurologic disability and/or frequency of clinical relapses in patients with secondary progressive, progressive relapsing, or worsening relapsing-remitting multiple sclerosis

Pregnancy Risk Factor D (may cause fetal harm when administered to a pregnant woman)

Contraindications Hypersensitivity to mitoxantrone or any component; patients with multiple sclerosis who have hepatic impairment; patients with baseline left ventricular ejection fraction <50% or cumulative lifetime mitoxantrone dose ≥140 mg/m^2 should not be treated with mitoxantrone

Warnings Avoid in patients with pre-existing myelosuppression; mitoxantrone is less cardiotoxic than anthracyclines. The predisposing factors for mitoxantrone-induced cardiotoxicity include prior anthracycline therapy, prior cardiovascular disease, and mediastinal irradiation. The risk of developing cardiotoxicity is <3% when the cumulative mitoxantrone dose is <140 mg/m^2; interstitial pneumonitis has been reported in patients receiving combination chemotherapy that included mitoxantrone; extravasation can result in tissue necrosis with resultant need for debridement and skin grafting; the FDA currently recommends that procedures for proper handling and disposal of antineoplastic agents be considered. Secondary leukemias have been reported in patients treated with mitoxantrone; intrathecal administration is not recommended since local nerve demyelinization, seizures, coma, and paraplegia have been reported with this route.

Precautions Dosage should be reduced in patients with pre-existing bone marrow suppression, previous treatment with cardiotoxic agents, and patients with impaired hepatobiliary function

Adverse Reactions

Cardiovascular: Cardiotoxicity (arrhythmias, CHF), hypotension, tachycardia, cardiomyopathy

Central nervous system: Seizures, headache

Dermatologic: Alopecia, pruritus, skin desquamation, rash, discoloration of skin (blue-green)

Gastrointestinal: Nausea, diarrhea, vomiting, stomatitis (occurs more frequently with "daily times 3 day" regimens than once every 3 week schedules), mucositis

Genitourinary: Discoloration of urine (blue-green)

Hematologic: Myelosuppression (leukopenia, pancytopenia), mild anemia, thrombocytopenia

Hepatic: Transient elevation of liver enzymes, jaundice

Local: Phlebitis, tissue necrosis with extravasation

Respiratory: Interstitial pneumonitis

Miscellaneous: Anaphylaxis

Drug Interactions Cytochrome P450 isoenzyme CYP2E1 inducer (weak)

High-dose cytarabine (therapeutic synergy)

Stability After penetration of the stopper, undiluted mitoxantrone solution is stable for 7 days at room temperature or 14 days when refrigerated; incompatible with heparin; physically compatible with ondansetron for at least 4 hours

Mechanism of Action Inhibits DNA and RNA synthesis by intercalating with DNA and causing template disordering and steric obstruction; replication is decreased by binding to DNA topoisomerase II (enzyme responsible for DNA helix supercoiling); active throughout entire cell cycle. Mitoxantrone inhibits B cell, T cell, and macrophage proliferation; impairs antigen presentation and secretion of interferon gamma, TNF$_\alpha$, IL-2.

Pharmacokinetics

Distribution: Distributes into thyroid, liver, pancreas, spleen, heart, bone marrow, and red blood cells; prolonged retention in tissues; excreted in breast milk

Protein binding: 78%

Half-life, terminal: 23-215 hours and may be prolonged with liver impairment

Elimination: Slowly excreted in urine (6% to 11%) and bile as unchanged drug and metabolites

Usual Dosage I.V. (refer to individual protocols):

Leukemias:

Children ≤2 years: 0.4 mg/kg/day once daily for 3-5 days

Children >2 years and Adults: 12 mg/m^2/day once daily for 2-3 days; acute leukemia in relapse: 8-12 mg/m^2/day once daily for 4-5 days; ANLL: 10 mg/m^2/day once daily for 3-5 days

Solid tumors:

Children: 18-20 mg/m^2 once every 3-4 weeks

Adults: 12-14 mg/m^2 once every 3-4 weeks

Multiple sclerosis: Adults: 12 mg/m^2/dose every 3 months

Dosing adjustment in hepatic impairment: Although official dosage adjustment recommendations have not been established, dosage reduction of 50% in patients with serum bilirubin of 1.5-3 mg/dL and dosage reduction of 75% in patients with serum bilirubin >3 mg/dL have been recommended

Administration Do not administer by S.C., I.M., intrathecal, or intra-arterial injection

Parenteral: I.V.: Do **not** administer I.V. push over <3 minutes; may administer by I.V. bolus over >3 minutes, I.V. intermittent infusion over 15-60 minutes or I.V. continuous infusion at a concentration of 0.02-0.5 mg/mL in D_5W or NS

Monitoring Parameters CBC with differential, serum uric acid, liver function tests, echocardiogram with monitoring of left ventricular ejection fraction; women of child-bearing potential should have a pregnancy test prior to dose

Patient Information May discolor skin, sclera, tears, sweat, and urine to a blue-green color; contraceptive measures are recommended during therapy

Nursing Implications Mitoxantrone is a nonvesicant; if extravasation occurs, the drug should be discontinued and restarted in another vein; extravasation may result in erythema, swelling, pain, burning, and/or a blue discoloration of the skin

Additional Information Myelosuppression (leukocyte nadir: 10-14 days; recovery: 21 days); injection contains 0.14 mEq of sodium/mL

Dosage Forms Injection, solution, as hydrochloride: 2 mg of mitoxantrone base/mL (10 mL, 12.5 mL, 15 mL)

References
Koeller J and Eble M, "Mitoxantrone: A Novel Anthracycline Derivative," *Clin Pharm*, 1988, 7(8):574-81.
LeMaistre CF and Herzig R, "Mitoxantrone: Potential for Use in Intensive Therapy," *Semin Oncol*, 1990, 17(1 Suppl 3):43-8.
Pratt CB, Vietti TJ, Etcubanas E, et al, "Novantrone® for Childhood Malignant Solid Tumors. A Pediatric Oncology Group Phase II Study," *Invest New Drugs*, 1986, 4(1):43-8.
Stevens RF, Hann IM, Wheatley K, et al, "Marked Improvements in Outcome With Chemotherapy Alone in Paediatric Acute Myeloid Leukemia: Results of the United Kingdom Medical Research Council's 10th AML Trial. MRC Childhood Leukaemia Working Party," *Br J Haematol*, 1998, 101(1):130-40.

♦ Mitrazol™ [OTC] *see* Miconazole *on page 759*
♦ Mivacron® *see* Mivacurium *on page 773*

Mivacurium (mye va KYOO ree um)

U.S. Brand Names Mivacron®

Therapeutic Category Neuromuscular Blocker Agent, Nondepolarizing; Skeletal Muscle Relaxant, Paralytic

Potential Drug Interactions

Potentiation	Antagonism
Inhalation anesthetics	Calcium
Desflurane, sevoflurane, enflurane and	Carbamazepine
isoflurane > halothane > nitrous	Phenytoin
oxide	Steroids (chronic administration)
Antibiotics	Theophylline
Aminoglycosides, polymyxins,	Anticholinesterases*
clindamycin, vancomycin, tetracycline	Neostigmine, pyridostigmine,
Magnesium	edrophonium, echothiophate
Antiarrhythmics	ophthalmic solution
Quinidine, procainamide, bretylium, and	Caffeine
possibly lidocaine	Azathioprine
Diuretics	
Furosemide, mannitol, thiazides	
Amphotericin B (secondary to hypokalemia)	
Local anesthetics	
Dantrolene (directly depresses skeletal muscle)	
Beta blockers	
Calcium channel blockers	
Ketamine	
Lithium	
Succinylcholine (when administered prior to nondepolarizing neuromuscular-blocking agent)	
Cyclosporine	

*Can prolong the effects of acetylcholine
(Continued)

Mivacurium *(Continued)*

Generic Available No

Use Short-acting nondepolarizing neuromuscular blocking agent used as an adjunct to general anesthesia; facilitates endotracheal intubation; provides skeletal muscle relaxation during surgery or mechanical ventilation

Pregnancy Risk Factor C

Contraindications Hypersensitivity to mivacurium chloride, any component (see Warnings), or other benzylisoquinolinium agents

Warnings Multidose vials contain benzyl alcohol which may cause allergic reactions in susceptible individuals; large amounts of benzyl alcohol (≥99 mg/kg/day) have been associated with a potentially fatal toxicity ("gasping syndrome") in neonates; the "gasping syndrome" consists of metabolic acidosis, respiratory distress, gasping respirations, CNS dysfunction (including convulsions, intracranial hemorrhage), hypotension and cardiovascular collapse; avoid use of multidose vials in neonates. *In vitro* and animal studies have shown that benzoate, a metabolite of benzyl alcohol, displaces bilirubin from protein-binding sites.

Precautions Use cautiously in patients with reduced plasma cholinesterase activity, asthma, severe cardiovascular disease

Adverse Reactions

Cardiovascular: Hypotension, bradycardia, tachycardia, flushing, cardiac arrhythmias

Central nervous system: Dizziness

Dermatologic: Cutaneous erythema, rash

Neuromuscular & skeletal: Muscle spasms

Local: Injection site reaction

Respiratory: Bronchospasm, wheezing

Miscellaneous: Endogenous histamine release

Drug Interactions See table on previous page.

Stability Store at room temperature; stable in D_5W, D_5/LR, NS for 24 hours; avoid exposure to direct ultraviolet light; incompatible with alkaline solutions; compatible with Y-site administration with sufentanil, fentanyl, alfentanil, midazolam, droperidol

Mechanism of Action Mivacurium is a short-acting, nondepolarizing, neuromuscular-blocking agent. Like other nondepolarizing drugs, mivacurium antagonizes acetylcholine by competitively binding to cholinergic sites on motor endplates in skeletal muscle.

Pharmacodynamics

Onset of action: 1-3 minutes

Duration: Short due to rapid hydrolysis by plasma cholinesterases; recovery from muscular paralysis occurs within 9-20 minutes

Pharmacokinetics Mivacurium exists as a mixture of isomers; the most potent are the *trans-trans* and *cis-trans* isomers

Distribution: V_d: *Trans-trans* isomer: 0.15 L/kg; *cis-trans* isomer: 0.27 L/kg

Metabolism: Enzymatic hydrolysis by plasma cholinesterase

Half-life: *Trans-trans* isomer: 2.3 minutes (range: 1.4-3.6); *cis-trans* isomer: 2.1 minutes (range: 0.8-4.8)

Clearance: *Trans-trans* isomer: 53 mL/minute/kg; *cis-trans* isomer: 99 mL/minute/kg

Usual Dosage Children require higher doses mg/kg than adults and more frequent maintenance doses; I.V.:

Children 2-12 years: 0.2 mg/kg; continuous infusion: 10-14 mcg/kg/minute; doses as high as 31 mcg/kg/minute have been used

Adults: 0.15-0.2 mg/kg; for prolonged neuromuscular block, continuous infusion: 9-10 mcg/kg/minute

Administration Parenteral: Administer undiluted by rapid I.V. injection; infusions diluted in D_5W to a maximum concentration of 0.5 mg/mL

Monitoring Parameters Assisted ventilation status, heart rate, blood pressure, peripheral nerve stimulator measuring twitch response

Nursing Implications Does not alter the patient's state of consciousness; addition of sedation is recommended

Dosage Forms

Injection, solution, as chloride: 2 mg/mL (20 mL, 50 mL) [contains benzyl alcohol]

Injection, solution, as chloride [preservative free]: 2 mg/mL (5 mL, 10 mL)

References

Martin LD, Bratton SL, and O'Rourke PP, "Clinical Uses and Controversies of Neuromuscular Blocking Agents in Infants and Children," *Crit Care Med*, 1999, 27(7):1358-68.

- ◆ **MK-639** *see* Indinavir *on page 604*
- ◆ **Modane® Bulk [OTC]** *see* Psyllium *on page 959*
- ◆ **Modane® Tablets [OTC]** *see* Bisacodyl *on page 173*
- ◆ **Moisture-Eyes™ PM [OTC]** *see* Ocular Lubricant *on page 831*

♦ **Mollifene®** [OTC] *see* Carbamide Peroxide *on page 212*
♦ **Molypen®** *see* Trace Metals *on page 1106*

Mometasone Furoate (moe MET a sone FYOOR oh ate)

U.S. Brand Names Elocon®; Nasonex®

Therapeutic Category Adrenal Corticosteroid; Anti-inflammatory Agent; Corticosteroid, Intranasal; Corticosteroid, Topical; Glucocorticoid

Generic Available Yes (ointment)

Use

Intranasal: Treatment of seasonal and perennial allergic rhinitis in children ≥2 years and adults; prevention of seasonal allergic rhinitis in adolescents ≥12 years and adults

Topical: Relief of the inflammation and pruritus associated with corticosteroid-responsive dermatoses [medium potency topical corticosteroid]; **Note:** Due to lack of established safety and efficacy in specific age groups, the cream and ointment are not recommended for use in children <2 years of age and the lotion is not recommended for use in children <12 years of age (see also Additional Information)

Pregnancy Risk Factor C

Contraindications Hypersensitivity to mometasone or any component

Warnings

Nasal: Acute adrenal insufficiency or corticosteroid withdrawal may occur when replacing a systemic corticosteroid with a nasal corticosteroid; hypothalamic-pituitary-adrenal (HPA) axis suppression or hypercorticism may occur, especially in younger children or in patients receiving high doses for a prolonged period of time. Immunosuppression may occur; avoid exposure to chickenpox and measles.

Topical: Adverse systemic effects may occur when topical steroids are used on large areas of the body, denuded areas, for prolonged periods of time, with an occlusive dressing, and/or in infants or small children; infants and small children may be more susceptible to HPA axis suppression or other systemic toxicities due to a larger skin surface area to body mass ratio; use with caution in pediatric patients and for no longer than 3 weeks

Precautions Avoid using higher than recommended doses; suppression of HPA axis function, suppression of linear growth, hypercorticism (Cushing's syndrome), hyperglycemia, or glucosuria may occur; titrate to lowest effective dose; these adverse effects (as well as intracranial hypertension) may also occur with topical use and have been reported in pediatric patients (see also Additional Information). Do not use topical mometasone furoate products for the treatment of diaper dermatitis. Use with extreme caution in patients with respiratory tuberculosis, untreated systemic infections, ocular herpes simplex. Nasal corticosteroids are not recommended for patients with recent nasal trauma, nasal surgery, or nasal septum ulcers, due to inhibition of wound healing. Rarely, local fungal infections, immediate hypersensitivity reactions, nasal septum perforation, or increased intraocular pressure may occur with intranasal corticosteroid use; glaucoma and/or cataracts have also been reported.

Adverse Reactions

Intranasal use:

Cardiovascular: Chest pain

Central nervous system: Headache

Endocrine & metabolic: Dysmenorrhea

Gastrointestinal: Vomiting, nausea, diarrhea, dyspepsia; oral candidiasis (rare)

Neuromuscular & skeletal: Musculoskeletal pain, arthralgia, myalgia

Ocular: Conjunctivitis

Otic: Earache, otitis media

Respiratory: Pharyngitis, cough, epistaxis, upper respiratory tract infection, sinusitis, asthma, bronchitis, nasal irritation, rhinitis, wheezing; nasal burning and irritation; nasal ulcers (rare), nasal candidiasis (rare), nasal septum perforation (rare)

Miscellaneous: Viral infection, flu-like symptoms; cases of anaphylaxis and angioedema have been reported

Topical use: Dermatologic: Bacterial skin infection, burning, tingling, stinging, furunculosis, pruritus, skin atrophy, folliculitis, moniliasis, paresthesia, skin depigmentation, acneform reaction, itching, rosacea

Drug Interactions Cytochrome P450 isoenzyme CYP3A4 substrate
No drug interactions have been reported.

Stability

Cream: Store between 2°C to 25°C (36°F to 77°F)

Lotion: Store between 2°C to 30°C (36°F to 86°F)

Nasal spray: Store between 2°C to 25°C (36°F to 77°F); protect from light

Ointment: Store at 25°C (77°F); excursions permitted to 15°C to 30°C (59°F to 86°F)

(Continued)

Mometasone Furoate *(Continued)*

Mechanism of Action Controls the rate of protein synthesis, depresses the migration of polymorphonuclear leukocytes and fibroblasts, reverses capillary permeability, and stabilizes lysosomal membranes at the cellular level to prevent or control inflammation

Pharmacodynamics

Onset of action: Intranasal: Improvement in allergic rhinitis symptoms may be seen within 11 hours

Maximum effect: Intranasal: Within 1-2 weeks after starting therapy

Pharmacokinetics

Absorption:

Intranasal: Undetectable in plasma

Topical: 0.4% of the applied dose of the cream and 0.7% of the applied dose of the ointment enter the circulation after 8 hours of contact with normal skin (without occlusion); absorption is increased by occlusive dressings or with decreased integrity of skin (eg, inflammation or skin disease)

Protein binding: 98% to 99%

Metabolism: Extensive in the liver to multiple metabolites; no major metabolites are detectable in the plasma; *in vitro* incubation studies identified one minor metabolite, 6 Beta-hydroxymometasone furoate, formed via cytochrome P450 CYP3A4 pathway

Half-life: 5.8 hours

Elimination: Metabolites are excreted primarily via the bile with a limited amount via urine

Usual Dosage

Nasal spray: Titrate to lowest effective dose

Children 2-11 years: 1 spray (50 mcg) in each nostril once daily

Children ≥12 years and Adults: 2 sprays (100 mcg) in each nostril once daily; when used for the prevention of allergic rhinitis, treatment should begin 2-4 weeks prior to pollen season

Topical: Apply sparingly, do not use occlusive dressings. Discontinue therapy when control is achieved; reassess diagnosis if no improvement is seen in 2 weeks.

Cream, ointment: Children ≥2 years and Adults: Apply a thin film to affected area once daily; do not use in pediatric patients for >3 weeks

Lotion: Children ≥12 years and Adults: Apply a few drops to affected area once daily; massage lightly into skin

Administration

Intranasal spray: Shake well prior to each use; clear nasal passages by blowing nose prior to use; occlude one nostril while administering to the other. Nasal spray must be primed before first use (10 actuations or until a fine spray appears) or after >1 week of nonuse (2 actuations or until a fine spray appears); discard unit after 120 metered sprays are used. Spray should be administered once daily, at a regular interval. Do not spray into eyes or directly onto nasal septum. After removing nasal spray from container, avoid prolonged exposure of product to direct light; brief exposure to light (with normal use) is acceptable.

Topical: Apply sparingly; avoid contact with eyes. Do not apply to face, underarms, or groin unless directed by physician. Do not wrap or bandage affected area unless directed by physician. Do not use for treatment of diaper dermatitis or in diaper area.

Lotion: Hold nozzle of bottle close to affected area and gently squeeze bottle

Monitoring Parameters Monitor growth in pediatric patients; assess HPA axis suppression in patients using topical steroids applied to a large surface area or to areas under occlusion. Intranasal: Check mucous membranes for signs of fungal infection

Patient Information Notify physician if condition being treated persists or worsens. Avoid exposure to chickenpox or measles; if exposed, seek medical advice without delay

Topical: Avoid contact with eyes; do not use occlusive dressings or other corticosteroid-containing products unless directed by physician; do not use for longer than directed; contact physician if no improvement is seen in 2 weeks

Additional Information Several studies conducted in children 6-23 months of age with atopic dermatitis demonstrated a high incidence of adrenal suppression when topical mometasone furoate products were applied once daily for approximately 3 weeks over an average body surface area of about 40%. Of the patients with normal baseline adrenal function, adrenal suppression occurred in 16% of patients using the cream, 27% of patients using the ointment, and 29% of patients using the lotion. Follow-up testing 2-4 weeks after discontinuation of therapy demonstrated suppressed HPA axis function in 1 of 5 patients who used the cream, 3 of 8 patients who used the ointment, and 1 of 8 patients who used the lotion.

Dosage Forms
Cream, topical (Elocon®): 0.1% (15 g, 45 g) [contains propylene glycol stearate]

Lotion, topical (Elocon®): 0.1% (30 mL, 60 mL) [contains 40% isopropyl alcohol and propylene glycol]

Ointment, topical (Elocon®): 0.1% (15 g, 45 g) [contains propylene glycol stearate]

Suspension, intranasal spray, as monohydrate (Nasonex®): 50 mcg (anhydrous)/ spray (17 g) [delivers 120 sprays; contains benzalkonium chloride]

- ◆ **MOM (Magnesium Hydroxide)** see Magnesium Supplements on page 701
- ◆ **Monacolin K** see Lovastatin on page 697
- ◆ **Monarc® M** see Antihemophilic Factor (Human) on page 116
- ◆ **Monistat® 1 [OTC]** see Miconazole on page 759
- ◆ **Monistat® 3 [OTC]** see Miconazole on page 759
- ◆ **Monistat® 7 [OTC]** see Miconazole on page 759
- ◆ **Monistat-Derm®** see Miconazole on page 759
- ◆ **Monoclate-P®** see Antihemophilic Factor (Human) on page 116
- ◆ **Monoclonal Antibody** see Muromonab-CD3 on page 784
- ◆ **Monodox®** see Doxycycline on page 415

Montelukast (mon te LOO kast)

Related Information
Asthma Guidelines on page 1376

U.S. Brand Names Singulair®

Therapeutic Category Antiasthmatic; Leukotriene Receptor Antagonist

Generic Available No

Use Prophylaxis and chronic treatment of asthma; relief of symptoms of seasonal allergic rhinitis

Pregnancy Risk Factor B

Contraindications Hypersensitivity to montelukast or any component

Warnings Montelukast is not indicated for use in the reversal of bronchospasm in acute asthma attacks, including status asthmaticus; it is not indicated as monotherapy for the treatment and management of exercise-induced bronchospasm; therapy with montelukast can be continued during acute exacerbations of asthma; rare cases of systemic eosinophilia, sometimes presenting with clinical features of vasculitis have been reported; this may be associated with a reduction in corticosteroid dosage; a causal association with montelukast has not been established

Precautions Phenobarbital reduces the AUC of montelukast ~40% following a single 10 mg dosage; no dosage adjustment of montelukast is indicated, however, appropriate clinical monitoring is indicated when potent cytochrome P450 enzyme inducers, such as phenobarbital or rifampin, are coadministered with montelukast. Chewable tablets contain phenylalanine which must be avoided (or used with caution) in patients with phenylketonuria.

Adverse Reactions
Central nervous system: Headache, fever, dizziness, drowsiness, irritability, restlessness, dream abnormalities, seizure (rare)

Dermatologic: Rash

Gastrointestinal: Diarrhea, nausea, abdominal pain, dyspepsia, pancreatitis (rare)

Hepatic: Elevated liver enzymes, hepatic eosinophilic infiltration

Neuromuscular & skeletal: Myalgia, cramps

Otic: Otitis

Respiratory: Sinusitis, laryngitis, nasal congestion, cough, rhinorrhea

Miscellaneous: Viral infection, influenza, hypersensitivity reactions

Drug Interactions Cytochrome P450 isoenzyme CYP2A6, CYP2C9, and CYP3A3/4 substrate

Phenobarbital (see Precautions)

Stability Store at room temperature; protect from moisture and light; granules must be administered within 15 minutes of opening the packet

Mechanism of Action Montelukast is a selective leukotriene receptor antagonist that inhibits the cysteinyl leukotriene CysLT$_1$ receptor. This activity produces inhibition of the effects of this leukotriene on bronchial smooth muscle resulting in the attenuation of bronchoconstriction and decreased vascular permeability, mucosal edema, and mucus production.

Pharmacokinetics
Absorption: Rapid

Distribution: V$_d$: Adults: 8-11 L

Protein binding: >99%

Metabolism: Extensive by cytochrome P450 3A4 and 2C9

(Continued)

Montelukast *(Continued)*

Bioavailability: Tablet:
5 mg: 63% to 73%
10 mg: 64%
Time to peak serum concentration: Tablet:
4 mg: 2 hours
5 mg: 2-2.5 hours
10 mg: 3-4 hours
Elimination: Exclusively via bile; <0.2% excreted in urine

Usual Dosage Oral:
Children
1-5 years: 4 mg/day
6-14 years: 5 mg/day
Adolescents >14 years and Adults: 10 mg/day
Note: None of the clinical trials evaluated the safety and efficacy of therapy with morning dosing; the pharmacokinetics of montelukast are similar whether dosed in the morning or evening

Administration Oral: Administer in the evening without regard to meals. Granules may be administered directly into the mouth or mixed in cold or room temperature soft foods; based on stability studies, only applesauce, mashed carrots, rice, and ice cream should be used; granules are not intended to be dissolved in liquid and must be administered within 15 minutes of opening the packet; liquids may be taken subsequent to administration

Monitoring Parameters Pulmonary function tests (FEV-1), improvement in asthma symptoms

Patient Information Take regularly as prescribed, even during symptom-free periods. Do not use to treat acute episodes of asthma. Do not decrease the dose or stop taking any other asthma medications unless instructed by a physician.

Dosage Forms
Granules, as sodium: 4 mg/packet
Tablet, as sodium: 10 mg
Tablet, chewable, as sodium: 4 mg [contains 0.674 mg phenylalanine (as aspartame); cherry flavor], 5 mg [contains 0.842 mg phenylalanine (as aspartame); cherry flavor]

References
"National Asthma Education and Prevention Program. Expert Panel Report: Guidelines for the Diagnosis and Management of Asthma Update on Selected Topics--2002," *J Allergy Clin Immunol*, 2002, 110(5 Suppl):S141-219.

♦ **More-Dophilus® [OTC]** *see* Lactobacillus acidophilus and Lactobacillus bulgaricus on page 648

♦ **Morphine HP® (Can)** *see* Morphine Sulfate on page 778

♦ **Morphine LP® Epidural (Can)** *see* Morphine Sulfate on page 778

Morphine Sulfate (MOR feen SUL fate)

Related Information
Compatibility of Medications Mixed in a Syringe on page 1412
Laboratory Detection of Drugs in Urine on page 1400
Narcotic Analgesics Comparison on page 1223
Overdose and Toxicology on page 1388
Preprocedure Sedatives in Children on page 1367

U.S. Brand Names Astramorph/PF™; Avinza™; Duramorph®; Infumorph™; Kadian®; MS Contin®; MSIR®; Oramorph SR®; RMS®; Roxanol™; Roxanol™ 100; Roxanol™ T

Canadian Brand Names M-Eslon®; Morphine HP®; Morphine LP® Epidural; M.O.S.-Sulfate®; MS-IR®; ratio-Morphine SR; Statex®

Synonyms MS

Therapeutic Category Analgesic, Narcotic

Generic Available Yes (except capsules, controlled release tablets, and sustained release tablets)

Use Relief of moderate to severe acute and chronic pain; pain of MI; relieves dyspnea of acute left ventricular failure and pulmonary edema; preanesthetic medication

Restrictions C-II

Pregnancy Risk Factor B (D if used for prolonged periods or in high doses at term)

Contraindications Hypersensitivity to morphine sulfate or any component (see Warnings); severe respiratory depression; acute or severe asthma; severe liver or renal insufficiency; GI obstruction especially known or suspected paralytic ileus

Warnings Respiratory depression may occur; neonates and infants <3 months of age are more susceptible to respiratory depression, use with caution and in reduced doses in this age group; use only preservative free injections for epidural or intrathecal administration and in neonates; abrupt discontinuation after prolonged use may result in withdrawal symptoms; use with extreme caution in patients with COPD, cor pulmonale, hypoxia, hypercapnia, pre-existing respiratory depression, significantly decreased respiratory reserve, head injury, increased ICP, other intracranial lesions; severe hypotension may occur; use with caution in patients with circulatory shock

Injection may contain sodium metabisulfite which may cause allergic reactions in susceptible individuals; oral solution may contain sodium benzoate; benzoic acid (benzoate) is a metabolite of benzyl alcohol; large amounts of benzyl alcohol ($\geq$99 mg/kg/day) have been associated with a potentially fatal toxicity ("gasping syndrome") in neonates; the "gasping syndrome" consists of metabolic acidosis, respiratory distress, gasping respirations, CNS dysfunction (including convulsions, intracranial hemorrhage), hypotension and cardiovascular collapse; avoid use of morphine sulfate products containing sodium benzoate in neonates; *in vitro* and animal studies have shown that benzoate displaces bilirubin from protein binding sites

Precautions Use with caution in patients with hypersensitivity reactions to other phenanthrene derivative opioid agonists (codeine, hydrocodone, hydromorphone, levorphanol, oxycodone, oxymorphone). Use with caution in patients with biliary tract disease or acute pancreatitis (morphine may cause spasm of the sphincter of Oddi); use with caution and decrease the dose in patients with Addison's disease, hypothyroidism, urethral stricture, prostatic hypertrophy, or in debilitated patients; use with caution in patients with CNS depression, toxic psychosis, seizure disorders, acute alcoholism, and delirium tremens. MS Contin® 200 mg tablets are for use in opioid tolerant patients only. Kadian® should be discontinued 24 hours prior to cordotomy or other interruption of pain transmission pathways (use parenteral short-acting opioids to control pain)

Adverse Reactions

Cardiovascular: Palpitations, hypotension, bradycardia, peripheral vasodilation

Central nervous system: CNS depression, drowsiness, dizziness, sedation, elevated intracranial pressure

Dermatologic: Pruritus (more common with epidural or intrathecal administration)

Endocrine & metabolic: Antidiuretic hormone release

Gastrointestinal: Nausea, vomiting, constipation, biliary tract spasm, intestinal obstruction

Genitourinary: Urinary tract spasm (may be more common with epidural or intrathecal administration), urinary retention

Ocular: Miosis

Respiratory: Respiratory depression

Miscellaneous: Physical and psychological dependence, histamine release

Drug Interactions Cytochrome P450 isoenzyme CYP2D6 substrate

CNS depressants, alcohol, phenothiazines, tricyclic antidepressants may potentiate the adverse effects of morphine

Food Interactions

Avinza™: A high fat meal may delay absorption

Kadian®: Food may decrease the rate, but not the extent of absorption

MS Contin®: A fatty meal may slightly decrease peak plasma concentrations

Oral solution: Food may increase bioavailability

Oramorph SR®: Food has little to no effect on bioavailability

Stability Refrigerate suppositories; do not freeze; degradation depends on pH and presence of oxygen; relatively stable in pH $\leq$4; darkening of solutions indicates degradation; Avinza™ and Kadian®: Protect from light and moisture

Dosage	Analgesia	
Form/Route	Peak	Duration
Tablets	1 h	3-5 h
Oral solution	1 h	3-5 h
Epidural	1 h	12-20 h
Extended release tablets	3-4 h	8-12 h
Suppository	20-60 min	3-7 h
Subcutaneous injection	50-90 min	3-5 h
I.M. injection	30-60 min	3-5 h
I.V. injection	20 min	3-5 h

(Continued)

Morphine Sulfate (Continued)

Mechanism of Action Binds to opiate receptors in the CNS, causing inhibition of ascending pain pathways, altering the perception of and response to pain; produces generalized CNS depression

Pharmacodynamics See table on previous page.

Pharmacokinetics

Absorption: Oral: Variable

Distribution: V_d, apparent: Children 1.7-18.7 years with cancer: Median: 5.2 L/kg; a significantly higher V_d was observed in children <11 years (median: 7.1 L/kg) versus >11 years (median: 4.7 L/kg) (see Hunt, 1999)

Protein binding:

Premature Infants: <20%

Adults: ~35%

Metabolism: In the liver via glucuronide conjugation to morphine-6-glucuronide (active) and morphine-3-glucuronide (inactive)

Half-life:

Preterm: 10-20 hours

Neonates: 7.6 hours (range: 4.5-13.3 hours)

Infants 1-3 months: 6.2 hours (range: 5-10 hours)

Infants 6 months to Children 2.5 years: 2.9 hours (range: 1.4-7.8 hours)

Preschool Children: 1-2 hours

Children 6-19 years with sickle cell disease: Mean ~1.3 hours

Adults: 2-4 hours

Elimination: Excreted unchanged in urine

Neonates: 3% to 15%

Adults: 6% to 10%

Clearance: **Note:** Adult values are reached by 6 months to 2.5 years of age

Preterm: 0.5-3 mL/minute/kg

Neonates 1-7 days: Median: 5.5 mL/minute/kg (range: 3.2-8.4 mL/minute/kg)

Neonates 8-30 days: Median: 7.4 mL/minute/kg (range: 3.4-13.8 mL/minute/kg)

Infants 1-3 months: Median: 10.5 mL/minute/kg (range: 9.8-20.1 mL/minute/kg)

Infants 3-6 months: Median: 13.9 mL/minute/kg (range: 8.3-24.1 mL/minute/kg)

Infants 6 months to Children 2.5 years: Median: 21.7 mL/minute/kg (range: 5.8-28.6 mL/minute/kg)

Preschool Children: 20-40 mL/minute/kg

Children 1.7-18.7 years with cancer: Median: 23.1 mL/minute/kg; a significantly higher clearance was observed in children <11 years (median: 37.4 mL/minute/kg) versus >11 years (median: 21.9 mL/minute/kg) (see Hunt, 1999)

Children 6-19 years with sickle cell disease: Mean ~36 mL/minute/kg (range: 6-59 mL/minute/kg)

Adults: 10-20 mL/minute/kg

Usual Dosage Doses should be titrated to appropriate effect; when changing routes of administration in chronically treated patients, please note that oral doses are approximately one-half as effective as parenteral dose

Neonates (see Warnings; use preservative free formulation):

I.M., I.V., S.C.: Initial: 0.05 mg/kg every 4-8 hours; titrate carefully to effect; maximum dose: 0.1 mg/kg/dose

I.V. continuous infusion: Initial: 0.01 mg/kg/hour (10 mcg/kg/hour); do **not** exceed infusion rates of 0.015-0.02 mg/kg/hour due to decreased elimination, increased CNS sensitivity, and adverse effects; **Note:** Some centers may use slightly higher doses, especially in neonates who develop tolerance

International Evidence-Based Group for Neonatal Pain recommendations (Anand, 2001): I.V.:

Intermittent dose: 0.05-0.1 mg/kg/dose

Continuous infusion: Range: 0.01-0.03 mg/kg/hour

Infants and Children:

Oral: Tablet and solution (prompt release): 0.2-0.5 mg/kg/dose every 4-6 hours as needed

I.M., I.V., S.C.: 0.1-0.2 mg/kg/dose every 2-4 hours as needed; may initiate at 0.05 mg/kg/dose; usual maximum dose: 15 mg/dose

I.V., S.C. continuous infusion:

Sickle cell or cancer pain: Initial: Infants: 0.02 mg/kg/hour (20 mcg/kg/hour); Children: 0.03 mg/kg/hour (30 mcg/kg/hour); conversion from intermittent I.V. morphine: Administer the patient's total daily I.V. morphine dose over 24 hours as a continuous infusion; titrate dose to appropriate effect; in one study (Miser, 1980), children with severe pain from terminal cancer required a median dose of 0.04-0.07 mg/kg/hour (40-70 mcg/kg/hour); range: 0.025-2.6 mg/kg/hour

Postoperative pain: 0.01-0.04 mg/kg/hour

Sedation/analgesia for procedures: I.V.: 0.05-0.1 mg/kg 5 minutes before the procedure

Epidural (use preservative free): 0.03-0.05 mg/kg (30-50 mcg/kg); maximum dose: 0.1 mg/kg (100 mcg/kg) or 5 mg/24 hours

Children: Oral: Controlled release tablet: 0.3-0.6 mg/kg/dose every 12 hours

Conversion from prompt release tablets and solution: Administer $1/2$ of the patient's total daily oral morphine dose every 12 hours or $1/3$ of the patient's total daily oral morphine dose every 8 hours

Adolescents >12 years: Sedation/analgesia for procedures: I.V.: 3-4 mg; may repeat in 5 minutes if necessary

Adults:

Oral:

Prompt release: 10-30 mg every 4 hours as needed

Controlled release: 15-30 mg every 8-12 hours

Avinza™ extended release capsules (chronic pain): Conversion from other oral morphine products: Administer the patient's total daily oral morphine dose as Avinza™ capsules once daily; do not administer more often than every 24 hours; supplemental pain medication may be needed (up to 4 days) until response to daily Avinza™ dosage has been stabilized; see package insert for more details; maximum dose: 1600 mg/day; higher doses contain quantity of fumaric acid that may result in nephrotoxicity

Kadian® sustained release capsules (chronic pain): Conversion from other oral morphine products: Administer $1/2$ of the patient's total daily oral morphine dose as Kadian® capsules every 12 hours or administer the total daily oral morphine dose as Kadian® capsules every 24 hours; do not administer more often than every 12 hours; see package insert for more details

I.M., I.V., S.C.: 2.5-20 mg/dose every 2-6 hours as needed; usual: 10 mg/dose every 4 hours as needed

I.V., S.C. continuous infusion: 0.8-10 mg/hour; may increase depending on pain relief/adverse effects; usual range up to 80 mg/hour

Epidural (use preservative free): Initial: 5 mg in lumbar region; if inadequate pain relief within 1 hour, give 1-2 mg, maximum dose: 10 mg/24 hours

Intrathecal ($1/10$ of epidural dose, use preservative free): 0.2-1 mg/dose; repeat doses **not** recommended

Dosing adjustment in renal impairment: Children and Adults:

Cl_{cr} 10-50 mL/minute: Administer 75% of normal dose

Cl_{cr} <10 mL/minute: Administer 50% of normal dose

Administration

Oral: Administer with food; swallow extended, sustained, and controlled release products whole; do not chew, crush, break, or dissolve (this would result in rapid release and absorption of a potentially toxic dose of drug)

Avinza™ and Kadian® capsules may be administered without regard to meals. Avinza™ (extended release capsules) and Kadian® (sustained release capsules) may be opened and contents sprinkled on a small amount of applesauce immediately prior to ingestion; swallow mixture; rinse mouth with water and swallow to ensure all beads have been ingested; do not chew, crush, or dissolve beads or pellets from capsule (this would result in rapid release and absorption of a potentially toxic dose of drug). Kadian® capsules may be opened and contents sprinkled into ~10 mL of water, then flushed while swirling through a pre-wetted 16-French gastrostomy tube fitted with a funnel at the port end; flush with water to transfer all pellets and flush the tube; do not attempt to administer via NG tube.

Parenteral:

I.V. push: Administer over at least 5 minutes at a final concentration of 0.5-5 mg/mL (rapid I.V. administration may increase adverse effects)

Intermittent infusion: Administer over 15-30 minutes at a final concentration of 0.5-5 mg/mL

Continuous I.V. infusion: 0.1-1 mg/mL in D_5W, $D_{10}W$, or NS

Epidural and intrathecal: Use only preservative free injections

Monitoring Parameters Respiratory and cardiovascular status, oxygen saturation, pain relief (if used for analgesia), level of sedation

Patient Information Avoid alcohol; may cause drowsiness and impair ability to perform activities requiring mental alertness or physical coordination; may be habit-forming; avoid abrupt discontinuation after prolonged use

Nursing Implications Do not administer rapidly I.V.

Additional Information Less adverse effects are associated with epidural compared to intrathecal route of administration; equianalgesic doses: Codeine: 120 mg I.M. = morphine 10 mg I.M. = single dose oral morphine 60 mg **or** chronic dosing oral morphine 15-25 mg

(Continued)

Morphine Sulfate *(Continued)*

Avinza™ capsules contain both immediate release and extended release beads; also contains fumaric acid (as an osmotic agent and local pH modifier); this product is intended for once daily oral administration only; not for PRN or postoperative use. Kadian® capsules contain sustained release pellets that are polymer-coated; this product is intended for every 12 hour or every 24 hour dosing. The pharmacokinetics of Avinza™ and Kadian® have not been studied in patients <18 years of age; the available capsule mg strength may not be appropriate for pediatric patients who are very young; sprinkling capsule contents on applesauce is **not** a suitable alternative for these patients; other oral products should be used.

Dosage Forms

Capsule (MSIR®): 15 mg, 30 mg

Capsule, extended release (Avinza™): 30 mg, 60 mg, 90 mg, 120 mg

Capsule, sustained release (Kadian®): 20 mg, 30 mg, 50 mg, 60 mg, 100 mg

Infusion [premixed in D_5W]: 0.2 mg/mL (250 mL, 500 mL); 1 mg/mL (100 mL, 250 mL, 500 mL)

Injection, solution: 2 mg/mL (1 mL); 4 mg/mL (1 mL); 5 mg/mL (1 mL); 8 mg/mL (1 mL); 10 mg/mL (1 mL, 2 mL, 10 mL); 15 mg/mL (1 mL, 20 mL); 25 mg/mL (4 mL, 10 mL, 20 mL, 40 mL) [some preparations contain sodium metabisulfite]

Injection, solution [epidural or intrathecal infusion via microinfusion device; preservative free] (Infumorph®): 10 mg/mL (20 mL); 25 mg/mL (20 mL)

Injection, solution [epidural, intrathecal, or I.V. infusion; preservative free]:
Astramorph/PF™: 0.5 mg/mL (2 mL, 10 mL); 1 mg/mL (2 mL, 10 mL)
Duramorph®: 0.5 mg/mL (10 mL); 1 mg/mL (10 mL)

Injection, solution [I.V. infusion via PCA pump]: 1 mg/mL (50 mL); 5 mg/mL (50 mL)

Injection, solution [preservative free]: 0.5 mg/mL (10 mL); 1 mg/mL (10 mL, 30 mL); 10 mg/mL (10 mL); 15 mg/mL (20 mL); 25 mg/mL (4 mL, 10 mL, 20 mL, 40 mL); 50 mg/mL (10 mL, 20 mL, 50 mL)

Solution, oral: 10 mg/5 mL (5 mL, 10 mL, 100 mL, 500 mL); 20 mg/5 mL (100 mL, 500 mL); 20 mg/mL (30 mL, 120 mL, 240 mL)
MSIR®: 10 mg/5 mL (120 mL); 20 mg/5 mL (120 mL); 20 mg/mL (30 mL, 120 mL) [contains sodium benzoate]
Roxanol™: 20 mg/mL (30 mL, 120 mL)
Roxanol™ 100: 100 mg/5 mL (240 mL) [with calibrated spoon]
Roxanol™ T: 20 mg/mL (30 mL, 120 mL) [tinted and flavored]

Suppository, rectal (RMS®): 5 mg (12s), 10 mg (12s), 20 mg (12s), 30 mg (12s)

Tablet (MSIR®): 15 mg, 30 mg

Tablet, controlled release (MS Contin®): 15 mg, 30 mg, 60 mg, 100 mg, 200 mg

Tablet, extended release: 15 mg, 30 mg, 60 mg, 100 mg, 200 mg

Tablet, sustained release (Oramorph SR®): 15 mg, 30 mg, 60 mg, 100 mg

References

Berde C, Ablin A, Glazer J, et al, "American Academy of Pediatrics Report of the Subcommittee on Disease-Related Pain in Childhood Cancer," *Pediatrics*, 1990, 86(5 Pt 2):818-25.

Dampier CD, Setty BN, Logan J, et al, "Intravenous Morphine Pharmacokinetics in Pediatric Patients With Sickle Cell Disease," *J Pediatr*, 1995, 126(3):461-7.

Henneberg SW, Hole P, Madsen de Haas I, et al, "Epidural Morphine for Postoperative Pain Relief in Children," *Acta Anaesthesiol Scand*, 1993, 37(7):664-7.

Hunt A, Joel S, Dick G, et al, "Population Pharmacokinetics of Oral Morphine and Its Glucuronides in Children Receiving Morphine as Immediate-Release Liquid or Sustained-Release Tablets for Cancer Pain," *J Pediatr*, 1999, 135(1):47-55.

McRorie TI, Lynn AM, Nespeca MK, et al, "The Maturation of Morphine Clearance and Metabolism," *Am J Dis Child*, 1992, 147(8):972-6.

Miser AW, Davis DM, Hughes CS, et al, "Continuous Subcutaneous Infusion of Morphine in Children With Cancer," *Am J Dis Child*, 1983, 137(4):383-5.

Miser AW, Miser JS, and Clark BS, "Continuous Intravenous Infusion of Morphine Sulfate for Control of Severe Pain in Children With Terminal Malignancy," *J Pediatr*, 1980, 96(5):930-2.

Olkkola KT, Hamunen K, and Maunuksela EL, "Clinical Pharmacokinetics and Pharmacodynamics of Opioid Analgesics in Infants and Children," *Clin Pharmacokinet*, 1995, 28(5):385-404.

Mupirocin (myoo PEER oh sin)

U.S. Brand Names Bactroban®; Bactroban® Nasal

Synonyms Pseudomonic Acid A

Therapeutic Category Antibiotic, Topical

Generic Available No

Use Ointment: Topical treatment of impetigo caused by *Staphylococcus aureus* and *Streptococcus pyogenes*; topical treatment of folliculitis, furunculosis, minor wounds, burns, and ulcers caused by susceptible organisms; Cream: Treatment of secondarily-infected traumatic skin lesions due to susceptible strains of *S. aureus* and *S. pyogenes*; prophylactic agent applied to intravenous catheter exit sites; Intranasal ointment: Eradication of *S. aureus* from nasal and perineal carriage sites

Pregnancy Risk Factor B

Contraindications Hypersensitivity to mupirocin, polyethylene glycol, or any component

Warnings Potentially toxic amounts of polyethylene glycol (PEG) contained in the vehicle may be absorbed percutaneously in patients with extensive burns or open wounds; the PEG vehicle may irritate mucous membranes and increase nasal secretions if applied intranasally; prolonged use may result in overgrowth of nonsusceptible organisms

Precautions Use with caution in patients with impaired renal function and in burn patients

Adverse Reactions

Dermatologic: Pruritus, rash, erythema, dry skin

Local: Burning, stinging, pain, tenderness, local edema

Stability Do not mix with Aquaphor®, coal tar solution, or salicylic acid

Mechanism of Action Binds to bacterial isoleucyl transfer-RNA synthetase preventing isoleucine incorporation resulting in the inhibition of protein and RNA synthesis

Pharmacokinetics

Absorption: Following topical administration, penetrates the outer layers of the skin; systemic absorption is minimal through intact skin

Protein binding: 95%

Metabolism: Extensive in the liver and skin to monic acid

Half-life: 17-36 minutes

Elimination: Metabolite is excreted in urine

Usual Dosage

Intranasal: Children and Adults: Apply small amount 2-4 times/day for 5-14 days

Topical:

Cream: Infants ≥3 months, Children, and Adults: Apply small amount 3 times/day for 10 days

Ointment: Infants ≥2 months, Children, and Adults: Apply a small amount 3-5 times/day for 5-14 days

Administration Cream and ointment: For topical use only; do not apply into the eye; may cover with gauze dressing; Intranasal: Avoid contact with eyes; apply one-half of the ointment from the single-use tube into each nostril

Additional Information Contains polyethylene glycol vehicle

Dosage Forms

Cream, topical, as calcium (Bactroban®): 2% (15 g, 30 g) [contains benzyl alcohol] (Continued)

Mupirocin *(Continued)*

Ointment, intranasal, as calcium (Bactroban® Nasal): 2% (1 g) [single use tube]

Ointment, topical (Bactroban®): 2% (22 g) [contains polyethylene glycol]

References

Britton JW, Fajardo JE, and Krafte-Jacobs B, "Comparison of Mupirocin and Erythromycin in the Treatment of Impetigo," *J Pediatr*, 1990, 117(5):827-9.

Hayakawa T, Hayashidera T, Katsura S, et al, "Nasal Mupirocin Treatment of Pharynx-Colonized Methicillin Resistant *Staphylococcus aureus*: Preliminary Study With 10 Carrier Infants," *Pediatr Int*, 2000, 42(1):67-70.

Hitomi S, Kubota M, Mori N, et al, "Control of a Methicillin-Resistant *Staphylococcus aureus* Outbreak in a Neonatal Intensive Care Unit by Unselective Use of Nasal Mupirocin Ointment," *J Hosp Infect*, 2000, 46(2):123-9.

Oh J, von Baum H, Klaus G, et al, "Nasal Carriage of *Staphylococcus aureus* in Families of Children on Peritoneal Dialysis. European Pediatric Peritoneal Dialysis Study Group (EPPS)," *Adv Perit Dial*, 2000, 16:324-7.

◆ **Murine® Ear [OTC]** *see* Carbamide Peroxide *on page 212*

◆ **Muro 128® [OTC]** *see* Sodium Chloride *on page 1027*

Muromonab-CD3 *(myoo roe MOE nab see dee three)*

U.S. Brand Names Orthoclone OKT®3

Synonyms Monoclonal Antibody; OKT3

Therapeutic Category Immunosuppressant Agent

Generic Available No

Use Treatment of acute allograft rejection in renal transplant patients; effective in reversing acute hepatic, cardiac, and bone marrow transplant rejection episodes resistant to conventional treatment

Pregnancy Risk Factor C

Contraindications Hypersensitivity to OKT3 or any Murine® product; patients in fluid overload or those with >3% weight gain within 1 week prior to start of OKT3

Warnings May result in an increased susceptibility to infection; severe pulmonary edema has occurred in patients with fluid overload; first-dose effect (flu-like symptoms, anaphylactic-type reaction) may occur within 30 minutes to 6 hours, up to 24 hours after the first dose. Cardiopulmonary resuscitation may be needed. Methylprednisolone sodium succinate given prior to first OKT3 dose and I.V. hydrocortisone sodium succinate given 30 minutes after administration are strongly recommended to decrease the incidence of reactions to the first dose.

Precautions Dosage of concomitant immunosuppressants should be reduced by 50%, and cyclosporine discontinued or decreased by 50% during OKT3 therapy (see Additional Information); maintenance immunosuppression and cyclosporine should be resumed about 3 days before stopping OKT3 to protect against rebound rejection

Adverse Reactions

Cardiovascular: Tachycardia, hypertension, hypotension, perioral and peripheral cyanosis

Central nervous system: Aseptic meningitis, seizures, headache, pyrexia, confusion

Dermatologic: Pruritus, rash

Gastrointestinal: Diarrhea, nausea, vomiting

Neuromuscular & skeletal: Arthralgia, tremor, myalgia

Ocular: Photophobia

Renal: Elevated BUN, elevated serum creatinine

Respiratory: Dyspnea, chest pain, tightness, wheezing, pulmonary edema

Miscellaneous: Flu-like symptoms (ie, fever, chills), anaphylactic-type reactions

Stability Store in refrigerator; do not freeze or shake; OKT3 left out of the refrigerator for more than 4 hours must not be used

Mechanism of Action Coats the circulating T lymphocytes subjecting these cells to opsonization by the reticuloendothelial system; modulates the T lymphocyte antigen receptor CD3 complex which results in the removal of all CD3 molecules from the cell surface so that the cell lacks the ability to function as a T lymphocyte

Pharmacokinetics

Distribution: V_d is closely related to the apparent volume of distribution for albumin

Half-life: 18 hours

Elimination: Binds to T lymphocytes with resultant opsonization and removal by the reticuloendothelial system

Usual Dosage I.V. (refer to individual protocols):

Note: Children and Adults: Methylprednisolone sodium succinate 1 mg/kg I.V. given 2-6 hours prior to first OKT3 administration and I.V. hydrocortisone sodium succinate 50-100 mg given 30 minutes after administration are strongly recommended to decrease the incidence of reactions to the first dose; patient temperature should not exceed 37.8°C (100°F) at time of administration

Children <12 years: 0.1 mg/kg/day once daily for 10-14 days **or** patients ≤30 kg: 2.5 mg once daily for 10-14 days; patients >30 kg: 5 mg once daily for 10-14 days

Children ≥12 years and Adults: 5 mg/day once daily for 10-14 days

Administration Parenteral: Filter each dose through a low protein-binding 0.22 micron filter (Millex GV) before administration; administer I.V. push over 1 minute at a final concentration of 1 mg/mL

Monitoring Parameters Chest x-ray, weight gain, CBC with differential, BUN and S_{cr}, vital signs (blood pressure, temperature, pulse, respiration) and immunologic monitoring of T cells, serum levels of OKT3, CD3+ cell count

Reference Range Mean serum trough levels rise during the first 3 days, then average 0.9 µg/mL on days 3-14; if serum trough OKT3 concentrations are maintained at 1 µg/mL, then CD3 counts remain low

Nursing Implications Inform patient of expected first dose effects which may include fever, chills, chest tightness, wheezing, nausea, vomiting, and diarrhea; first-dose reaction usually starts 40-60 minutes after the injection and lasts for several hours; first-dose effects are markedly reduced with subsequent doses; monitor patient closely for 48 hours after the first dose; corticosteroids are recommended; acetaminophen and antihistamines can be given concomitantly with OKT3 to reduce early reactions

Additional Information Recommend decreasing dose of prednisone to 0.5 mg/kg, azathioprine to 0.5 mg/kg (approximate 50% decrease in dose), and discontinuing cyclosporine or decreasing cyclosporine dose by 50% while patient is receiving OKT3

Dosage Forms Injection, solution: 1 mg/mL (5 mL)

References

Ettenger RB, Marik JL, Rosenthal JT, et al, "OKT₃ for Rejection Reversal in Pediatric Renal Transplantation," *Clin Transpl*, 1988, 2:180-4.

Hooks MA, Wade CS, and Millikan WJ Jr, "Muromonab CD-3: A Review of Its Pharmacology, Pharmacokinetics, and Clinical Use in Transplantation," *Pharmacotherapy*, 1991, 11(1):26-37.

Niaudet P, Murcia I, Jean G, et al, "A Comparative Trial of OKT₃ and Antilymphocyte Serum in the Preventive Treatment of Rejection After Kidney Transplantation in Children," *Ann Pediatr Paris*, 1990, 37(2):83-5.

Todd PA and Brogden RN, "Muromonab CD3 A Review of Its Pharmacology and Therapeutic Potential," *Drugs*, 1989, 37(6):871-99.

♦ **Muse® Pellet (Can)** see Alprostadil *on page 66*

♦ **Mustargen®** see Mechlorethamine *on page 708*

♦ **Mustine** see Mechlorethamine *on page 708*

♦ **Mutamycin®** see Mitomycin *on page 770*

♦ **Myambutol®** see Ethambutol *on page 462*

♦ **Mycelex®** see Clotrimazole *on page 297*

♦ **Mycelex®-7 [OTC]** see Clotrimazole *on page 297*

♦ **Myciguent [OTC]** see Neomycin *on page 801*

♦ **Mycinettes® [OTC]** see Benzocaine *on page 163*

♦ **Mycitracin® [OTC]** see Neomycin, Polymyxin B, and Bacitracin *on page 804*

♦ **Mycobutin®** see Rifabutin *on page 983*

Mycophenolate (mye koe FEN oh late)

U.S. Brand Names CellCept®

Synonyms RS61443

Therapeutic Category Immunosuppressant Agent

Generic Available No

Use Immunosuppressant agent used in conjunction with other immunosuppressive therapies (eg, cyclosporine and corticosteroids with or without antithymocyte induction) for the prophylaxis of organ rejection in patients receiving allogeneic renal, hepatic, or cardiac transplants; add-on immunosuppressant agent that is typically used in place of azathioprine in combination regimens for the treatment of refractory acute kidney graft rejection; use of mycophenolate is also being studied in bone marrow transplant patients

Pregnancy Risk Factor C

Contraindications Hypersensitivity to mycophenolate mofetil, mycophenolic acid, polysorbate 80 (I.V. formulation), or any component

Warnings Immunosuppression with mycophenolate may result in an increased susceptibility to infection and an increased risk of developing lymphomas and other malignancies, particularly of the skin. Mycophenolate has been shown to have teratogenic effects in animals; in women of childbearing potential, effective contraception must be initiated before starting mycophenolate therapy and continued for 6 weeks after it has been discontinued.

Precautions Use with caution in patients with active serious digestive disease and in patients with renal impairment; modify dosage in patients with severe chronic renal impairment (GFR <25 mL/minute/1.73 m² outside of the immediate post-transplant period) and in patients with neutropenia. Avoid use in patients with rare hereditary deficiency of hypoxanthineguanine phosphoribosyl-transferase (HGPRT) such as (Continued)

Mycophenolate *(Continued)*

Lesch-Nyhan and Kelley-Seegmiller syndrome. The oral suspension contains aspartame which is metabolized to phenylalanine and must be used with caution in patients with phenylketonuria.

Adverse Reactions

Cardiovascular: Hypertension, chest pain, peripheral edema, tachycardia

Central nervous system: Insomnia, dizziness, fever, headache, anxiety

Dermatologic: Rash, acne

Endocrine & metabolic: Hypercholesterolemia, hypophosphatemia, hypokalemia, hyperkalemia, hyperglycemia

Gastrointestinal: Diarrhea, constipation, nausea, vomiting, oral moniliasis, abdominal pain, dyspepsia, GI tract hemorrhage, colitis, pancreatitis, anorexia

Genitourinary: Hematuria

Hematologic: Leukopenia, neutropenia, anemia, thrombocytopenia, leukocytosis

Local: Phlebitis, thrombosis

Neuromuscular & skeletal: Tremor, back pain, myalgia, weakness

Renal: Renal tubular necrosis

Respiratory: Dyspnea, cough, pharyngitis, pulmonary fibrosis

Miscellaneous: 1% incidence of lymphoproliferative disease

Drug Interactions Aluminum- and magnesium-containing antacids decrease mycophenolate absorption; cholestyramine decreases mycophenolate bioavailability by 40% (interrupts enterohepatic recirculation of mycophenolic acid); acyclovir and ganciclovir may compete with mycophenolic acid glucuronide (MPAG) for renal tubular secretion resulting in increased concentrations of both drugs and MPAG; drugs which inhibit renal tubular secretion (probenecid) increase mycophenolate and MPAG concentrations; azathioprine (potential for additive bone marrow suppression); live vaccines (vaccination may be less effective, but influenza vaccine may be of value)

Food Interactions Presence of food decreases mycophenolate peak concentration by 40% but has no effect on the extent of absorption

Stability Store at room temperature

Suspension: Store reconstituted suspension in refrigerator or at room temperature; stable for 60 days after reconstitution

Injection: Mycophenolate I.V. infusion solution is stable for 12 hours at room temperature after preparation; administration of the infusion solution should be within 4 hours from reconstitution and dilution of the drug. Do not mix mycophenolate with any other drugs.

Mechanism of Action Hydrolyzed to form mycophenolic acid (MPA), the active metabolite, which is a potent, noncompetitive reversible inhibitor of inosine monophosphate dehydrogenase (IMPDH) in the purine biosynthesis pathway; inhibition of IMPDH results in a depletion of guanosine triphosphate and deoxyguanosine triphosphate, thereby inhibiting T- and B-cell proliferation, cytotoxic T-cell generation and antibody secretion.

Pharmacokinetics

Absorption: Rapid and extensive; early post-transplant period MPA AUC values are approximately 45% to 53% lower than later post-transplant period (>3 months) MPA AUC values in pediatric patients 1-18 years.

Distribution: Mean V_d (adults): 4 L/kg

Protein binding:

Mycophenolate: 97%

Mycophenolate glucuronide: 82%

Metabolism: Mycophenolate mofetil undergoes hydrolysis to mycophenolic acid (MPA is the active metabolite); MPA is metabolized by glucuronyl transferase to mycophenolic acid glucuronide (MPAG is inactive). MPAG is converted to MPA via enterohepatic recirculation.

Bioavailability: 94% based on MPA; enterohepatic recirculation contributes to MPA concentration; two 500 mg tablets have been shown to be bioequivalent to four 250 mg capsules or 1000 mg of oral suspension

Half-life:

Oral: 17.9 hours

I.V.: 16.6 hours

Time to peak serum concentration: 0.8-1.3 hours

Elimination: 93% of dose recovered in urine, 6% in feces; 87% of mycophenolic acid dose recovered as MPAG in urine; <1% of dose excreted as MPA in urine

Dialysis: Not dialyzable

Usual Dosage

Oral:

Children: 600 mg/m^2/dose twice daily; maximum dose: 2 g/day; **Note:** Limited information regarding mycophenolate use in pediatric patients is currently available in the literature: 32 pediatric patients (14 underwent living donor and 18 receiving cadaveric donor renal transplants) received mycophenolate 8-30 mg/kg/dose orally twice daily with cyclosporine, prednisone, and Atgam® induction. However, pharmacokinetic studies suggest that doses of mycophenolate adjusted to body surface area resulted in AUCs which better approximated those of adults versus doses adjusted for body weight which resulted in lower AUCs in pediatric patients.

or

BSA 1.25 m^2 to 1.5 m^2: 750 mg twice daily

BSA >1.5 m^2: 1 g twice daily

Adults:

Renal transplant: 1 g twice daily in combination with corticosteroids and cyclosporine; dosages as high as 3-3.5 g/day were used in clinical trials, but no efficacy advantage was established

Cardiac transplant: 1.5 g twice daily

Hepatic transplant: 1.5 g twice daily

I.V. infusion (administer within 24 hours following transplantation; can be given for up to 14 days; patients should be switched to oral formulation as soon as oral medication is tolerated):

Adults:

Renal transplant: 1 g twice daily

Cardiac transplant: 1.5 g twice daily

Hepatic transplant: 1 g twice daily

Dosing adjustment in renal impairment: Renal transplant: GFR <25 mL/minute/1.73 m^2 outside the immediate post-transplant period: Avoid doses >1 g twice daily

Administration

Oral: Administer on an empty stomach; one center has mixed the contents of the capsule in chocolate syrup; mycophenolate suspension can be administered orally or via a nasogastric tube with a minimum size of 8 French; shake suspension well before use

I.V.: Reconstitute vial with D$_5$W and further dilute to a final concentration of 6 mg/mL using D$_5$W. Administer by slow I.V. infusion over a period of no less than 2 hours.

Monitoring Parameters CBC with differential, platelet count, serum electrolytes, glucose, phosphate, cholesterol, and renal function tests; blood pressure. Pregnancy test in female patients of childbearing potential within 1 week prior to beginning therapy.

Patient Information Do not take within 1 hour before or 2 hours after antacids or cholestyramine; maintain adequate hydration. You will be susceptible to infection (avoid crowds and people with infections). Report to physician any chest pain, acute headache or dizziness, respiratory infection symptoms, difficulty breathing, or unusual bleeding or bruising. You may be at increased risk for skin cancer (wear protective clothing and use sunscreen). Women of childbearing age should use 2 effective forms of contraception simultaneously unless abstinence is the chosen method before starting mycophenolate therapy, during therapy, and for 6 weeks after discontinuing mycophenolate.

Nursing Implications Mycophenolate capsules should not be opened or crushed; avoid inhalation or direct contact of the capsule contents with skin or mucous membranes; mycophenolate tablets should not be crushed

Dosage Forms

Capsule, as mofetil: 250 mg

Injection, powder for reconstitution, as mofetil hydrochloride: 500 mg

Powder for oral suspension, as mofetil: 200 mg/mL (225 mL) [contains 0.56 mg/mL phenylalanine (as aspartame); mixed fruit flavor]

Tablet, as mofetil: 500 mg [contains ethyl alcohol]

Extemporaneous Preparations A 50 mg/mL suspension can be prepared in a vertical flow hood by emptying six 250 mg mycophenolate mofetil capsules into a mortar wetted and triturated with 7.5 mL Ora-Plus® to a smooth paste. Add 15 mL of cherry syrup and triturate to make a final volume of 30 mL. The suspension is stable for 210 days when stored at 5°C, stable for 28 days when stored at 37°C or 25°C, and stable for 11 days when stored at 45°C.

Venkataramanan R, McCombs JR, Zudarnan S, et al, "Stability of Mycophenolate Mofetil as an Extemporaneous Suspension," *Ann Pharmacother*, 1998, 32:755-7.

References

Ettenger R, Warshaw B, Menster M, et al, "Mycophenolate Mofetil in Pediatric Renal Transplantation: A Report of the Ped MMF Study Group." Abstract: 1996, Annual Meeting, ASTP.

(Continued)

Mycophenolate *(Continued)*

Sollinger HW, "Mycophenolate Mofetil for the Prevention of Acute Rejection in Primary Cadaveric Renal Allograft Recipients. U.S. Renal Transplant Mycophenolate Mofetil Study Group," *Transplantation*, 1995, 60:225-32.

- ◆ **Mycostatin®** *see* Nystatin *on page 827*
- ◆ **Mydfrin®** *see* Phenylephrine *on page 892*
- ◆ **Mydriacyl®** *see* Tropicamide *on page 1125*
- ◆ **Mykrox®** *see* Metolazone *on page 750*
- ◆ **Mylanta® CalciTabs [OTC]** *see* Antacid Preparations *on page 112*
- ◆ **Mylanta® Calci Tabs Extra Strength [OTC]** *see* Calcium Supplements *on page 200*
- ◆ **Mylanta® Calci Tabs Ultra [OTC]** *see* Calcium Supplements *on page 200*
- ◆ **Mylanta®, Children's [OTC]** *see* Calcium Supplements *on page 200*
- ◆ **Mylanta® Extra Strength [OTC]** *see* Antacid Preparations *on page 112*
- ◆ **Mylanta Gas® [OTC]** *see* Simethicone *on page 1020*
- ◆ **Mylanta Gas® Maximum Strength [OTC]** *see* Simethicone *on page 1020*
- ◆ **Mylanta® Supreme [OTC]** *see* Antacid Preparations *on page 112*
- ◆ **Myleran®** *see* Busulfan *on page 193*
- ◆ **Mylicon®, Infants [OTC]** *see* Simethicone *on page 1020*
- ◆ **Mylocel™** *see* Hydroxyurea *on page 582*
- ◆ **Myochrysine® (Can)** *see* Gold Sodium Thiomalate *on page 545*
- ◆ **Myotonachol® (Can)** *see* Bethanechol *on page 171*
- ◆ **Mysoline®** *see* Primidone *on page 931*
- ◆ **Mytussin® AC** *see* Guaifenesin and Codeine *on page 551*
- ◆ **Mytussin® DM [OTC]** *see* Guaifenesin and Dextromethorphan *on page 553*
- ◆ **NAC** *see* Acetylcysteine *on page 43*
- ◆ **N-Acetylcysteine** *see* Acetylcysteine *on page 43*
- ◆ **N-Acetyl-L-Cysteine** *see* Acetylcysteine *on page 43*
- ◆ **N-Acetyl-P-Aminophenol** *see* Acetaminophen *on page 36*
- ◆ **NaCl** *see* Sodium Chloride *on page 1027*

Nadolol *(nay DOE lole)*

Related Information
Overdose and Toxicology *on page 1388*

U.S. Brand Names Corgard®

Canadian Brand Names Alti-Nadolol; Apo®-Nadol; Novo-Nadolol

Therapeutic Category Antianginal Agent; Antiarrhythmic Agent, Class II; Antihypertensive Agent; Antimigraine Agent; Beta-Adrenergic Blocker

Generic Available Yes

Use Treatment of hypertension and angina pectoris; prophylaxis of migraine headaches

Pregnancy Risk Factor C

Contraindications Hypersensitivity to nadolol or any component; uncompensated CHF, cardiogenic shock, bradycardia or heart block, bronchial asthma, bronchospasms

Precautions Therapy should not be discontinued abruptly; reduce dosage gradually over a period of 1-2 weeks; increase dosing interval in patients with renal dysfunction; use with caution in patients with diabetes mellitus

Adverse Reactions
Cardiovascular: Persistent bradycardia, orthostatic hypotension, Raynaud's syndrome, CHF, edema
Central nervous system: Fatigue, dizziness
Dermatological: Rash
Gastrointestinal: GI discomfort
Respiratory: Bronchospasm

Drug Interactions Other hypotensive agents, diuretics and phenothiazines may increase hypotensive effects of nadolol; abrupt withdrawal of clonidine while receiving beta-blockers may result in an exaggerated hypertensive crisis; nadolol may enhance neuromuscular blocking agents and will antagonize beta-sympathomimetic drugs; other drug interactions similar to propranolol may occur

Food Interactions Avoid natural licorice (causes sodium and water retention and increases potassium loss)

Mechanism of Action Competitively blocks response to beta-adrenergic stimulation; nonselective beta-blocker

Pharmacodynamics Duration: 24 hours

Pharmacokinetics

Absorption: Oral: 30% to 40%

Distribution: Concentration in human breast milk is 4.6 times higher than serum

Protein-binding: 28%

Half-life, elimination:

Increased half-life with decreased renal function

Infants 3-22 months (n=3): 3.2-4.3 hours

Children 10 years (n=1): 15.7 hours

Children ~15 years (n=1): 7.3 hours

Adults: 10-24 hours

Dialysis: Moderately dialyzable (20% to 50%)

Usual Dosage Oral:

Children: Very limited information (ie, one study) regarding pediatric dosage currently available in literature: The study used oral nadolol to control supraventricular tachycardia (SVT) in 26 children 3 months to 15 years of age. SVT was well controlled in 23 out of 26 children; recommended initial dose: 0.5-1 mg/kg once daily; monitor carefully, gradually increase dose; median dose required: 1 mg/kg/day; maximum dose: 2.5 mg/kg/day.

Adults: Initial: 40 mg once daily; increase gradually; usual dosage: 40-80 mg/day; may need up to 240-320 mg/day; doses as high as 640 mg/day have been used

Dosage adjustment in adults with renal impairment:

Cl_{cr} 10-50 mL/minute: Administer 50% of normal dose

Cl_{cr} <10 mL/minute: Administer 25% of normal dose

Administration Oral: May administer without regard to meals

Monitoring Parameters Blood pressure, heart rate, fluid intake and output, weight

Patient Information Limit alcohol; do not abruptly discontinue; may mask symptoms of hypoglycemia, but sweating may still occur

Dosage Forms Tablet: 20 mg, 40 mg, 80 mg, 120 mg, 160 mg

References

Devlin RG and Duchin KL, "Nadolol in Human Serum and Breast Milk," Br J Clin Pharmacol, 1981, 12(3):393-6.

Mehta AV and Chidambaram B, "Efficacy and Safety of Intravenous and Oral Nadolol for Supraventricular Tachycardia in Children," J Am Coll Cardiol, 1992, 19(3):630-5.

Mehta AV and Chidambaram B, and Rice PJ, "Pharmacokinetics of Nadolol in Children With Supraventricular Tachycardia," J Clin Pharmacol, 1992, 32(1):1023-7.

◆ **Nadopen-V® (Can)** see Penicillin V Potassium on page 877

Nafcillin (naf SIL in)

Related Information

Extravasation Treatment on page 1240

Canadian Brand Names Nallpen®; Unipen®

Synonyms Ethoxynaphthamido Penicillin

Therapeutic Category Antibiotic, Penicillin (Antistaphylococcal)

Generic Available Yes

Use Treatment of bacterial infections such as osteomyelitis, septicemia, endocarditis, and CNS infections due to susceptible penicillinase-producing strains of *Staphylococcus*

Pregnancy Risk Factor B

Contraindications Hypersensitivity to nafcillin, any component, or penicillins

Warnings Elimination rate will be decreased in neonates; avoid using in neonates during the first 2 weeks of life

Precautions Extravasation of I.V. infusions should be avoided; modification of dosage is necessary in patients with both severe renal and hepatic impairment; use with caution in patients with cephalosporin hypersensitivity

Adverse Reactions

Central nervous system: Fever

Dermatologic: Skin rash

Endocrine & metabolic: Hypokalemia

Gastrointestinal: Nausea, diarrhea

Hematologic: Neutropenia, anemia, eosinophilia

Hepatic: Elevated AST

Local: Pain, thrombophlebitis

Renal: Acute interstitial nephritis (rare), hematuria

Miscellaneous: Hypersensitivity reactions

Drug Interactions Probenecid (decreases rate of nafcillin elimination), oral anticoagulants (may decrease half-life of warfarin), may increase hepatic metabolism of cyclosporine

Food Interactions Food decreases GI absorption

(Continued)

Nafcillin *(Continued)*

Stability Refrigerate oral suspension after reconstitution, discard after 7 days. Reconstituted nafcillin 250 mg/mL solution for injection is stable for 3 days at room temperature and 7 days when refrigerated; when diluted for I.V. intermittent infusion in D_5W or NS, solution is stable for 24 hours at room temperature and 96 hours when refrigerated; incompatible with aminoglycosides

Mechanism of Action Interferes with bacterial cell wall synthesis during active multiplication by binding to one or more of the penicillin-binding proteins; inhibits the final transpeptidation step of peptidoglycan synthesis causing cell wall death and resultant bactericidal activity against susceptible bacteria

Pharmacokinetics

Absorption: Oral: Poor and erratic

Distribution: Distributes into bile, synovial, pleural, and pericardial fluids and into bone and liver; CSF penetration is poor unless meninges are inflamed; crosses the placenta

Protein binding: 90%

Metabolism: 70% to 90%

Half-life:

Neonates:

<3 weeks: 2.2-5.5 hours

4-9 weeks: 1.2-2.3 hours

Children 1 month to 14 years: 0.75-1.9 hours

Adults with normal renal and hepatic function: 0.5-1.5 hours

Time to peak serum concentration:

Oral: Within 2 hours

I.M.: Within 30-60 minutes

Elimination: Primarily in bile and 10% to 30% in urine as unchanged drug; undergoes enterohepatic recycling

Dialysis: Not dialyzable (0% to 5%)

Usual Dosage

Neonates: I.M., I.V.:

0-4 weeks, <1200 g: 50 mg/kg/day in divided doses every 12 hours

≤7 days:

1200-2000 g: 50 mg/kg/day in divided doses every 12 hours

>2000 g: 75 mg/kg/day in divided doses every 8 hours

>7 days:

1200-2000 g: 75 mg/kg/day in divided doses every 8 hours

>2000 g: 100 mg/kg/day in divided doses every 6 hours

Children:

I.M., I.V.:

Mild to moderate infections: 50-100 mg/kg/day in divided doses every 6 hours

Severe infections: 100-200 mg/kg/day in divided doses every 4-6 hours

Maximum dose: 12 g/day

Oral: 50-100 mg/kg/day divided every 6 hours

Adults:

Oral: 250-500 mg every 4-6 hours, up to 1 g every 4-6 hours for more severe infections

I.M.: 500 mg every 4-6 hours

I.V.: 500-2000 mg every 4-6 hours

Dosing adjustment in patients with both severe renal/hepatic impairment: Use lower range of usual dose or reduce dose 33% to 50%

Administration

Oral: Administer on an empty stomach with water 1 hour before or 2 hours after meals

Parenteral:

I.M.: Administer deep I.M. into a large muscle (ie, gluteus maximus) using a solution containing 250 mg/mL

I.V.: Nafcillin may be administered by I.V. push over 5-10 minutes or by I.V. intermittent infusion over 15-60 minutes at a final concentration not to exceed 40 mg/mL; in fluid-restricted patients, a maximum concentration of 100 mg/mL may be administered

Monitoring Parameters Periodic CBC with differential, urinalysis, BUN, serum creatinine, AST, and ALT

Test Interactions False-positive urinary and serum proteins

Nursing Implications Extravasation may cause tissue sloughing and necrosis; hyaluronidase infiltration may help avoid injury

Additional Information Sodium content of 1 g injection: 2.9 mEq

Dosage Forms

Infusion, as sodium [premixed iso-osmotic dextrose solution]: 1 g (50 mL); 2 g (100 mL)

Injection, powder for reconstitution, as sodium: 1 g, 2 g, 10 g

References

Banner W Jr, Gooch WM 3d, Burckart G, et al, "Pharmacokinetics of Nafcillin in Infants With Low Birth Weights," *Antimicrob Agents Chemother*, 1980, 17(4):691-4.

Zenk KE, Dungy CL, and Greene CR, "Nafcillin Extravasation Injury: Use of Hyaluronidase as an Antidote," *Am J Dis Child*, 1981, 135(12):1113-4.

♦ **NaHCO₃** *see* Sodium Bicarbonate *on page 1025*

Nalbuphine (NAL byoo feen)

U.S. Brand Names Nubain®

Therapeutic Category Analgesic, Narcotic; Opiate Partial Agonist

Generic Available Yes

Use Relief of moderate to severe pain

Pregnancy Risk Factor B (D if used for prolonged periods or in high doses at term)

Contraindications Hypersensitivity to nalbuphine or any component

Warnings Abrupt discontinuation after prolonged use may result in narcotic withdrawal; administration to patients receiving chronic opiates may precipitate narcotic withdrawal

Precautions Reduce dose in patients with hepatic impairment; use with caution in patients with impaired respiration, recent MI, or biliary tract surgery; may produce respiratory depression; use with caution in patients with a history of drug dependence, head trauma or increased intracranial pressure, decreased hepatic or renal function, pregnancy, or patients suspected to be opioid dependent

Adverse Reactions

Cardiovascular: Hypotension, tachycardia, bradycardia, peripheral vasodilation

Central nervous system: CNS depression, drowsiness, headache, dizziness, sedation, elevated ICP

Dermatologic: Urticaria, pruritus, rash

Gastrointestinal: Anorexia, nausea, vomiting, xerostomia, biliary tract spasm

Genitourinary: Urinary tract spasm, urinary retention

Ocular: Blurred vision, miosis

Respiratory: Respiratory depression

Miscellaneous: Histamine release, physical and psychological dependence, narcotic withdrawal in patients receiving opiate agonists chronically

Drug Interactions CNS depressants, alcohol, phenothiazine, tricyclic antidepressants may potentiate adverse effects

Mechanism of Action Binds to opiate receptors in the CNS, causing inhibition of ascending pain pathways, altering the perception of and response to pain; produces generalized CNS depression; opiate antagonistic effect may result from competitive inhibition at the opiate mu receptor

Pharmacodynamics

Onset of action:

I.M., S.C.: Within 15 minutes

I.V.: 2-3 minutes

Maximum effect:

I.M.: 30 minutes

I.V.: 1-3 minutes

Duration: 3-6 hours

Pharmacokinetics

Metabolism: In the liver; extensive first-pass metabolism

Protein binding: ~50%

Half-life, terminal:

Children 1-8 years: 0.9 hours

Adults 23-32 years: ~2 hours; range: 3.5-5 hours

Adults 65-90 years: 2.3 hours

Time to peak serum concentration:

I.M.: 30 minutes

I.V.: 1-3 minutes

Elimination: Metabolites primarily in feces (via bile) and in urine; 4% to 7% eliminated unchanged in the urine

Usual Dosage I.M., I.V., S.C.:

Children 1-14 years: Premedication: 0.2 mg/kg; maximum dose: 20 mg/dose

Children: Analgesia: 0.1-0.15 mg/kg every 3-6 hours as needed

Adults: 10 mg/70 kg every 3-6 hours as needed; maximum single-dose: 20 mg; maximum daily dose: 160 mg

Administration Parenteral: I.V.: Administer over 5-10 minutes; larger doses should be administered over 10-15 minutes

Monitoring Parameters Relief of pain, respiratory and mental status, blood pressure

(Continued)

Nalbuphine (Continued)

Patient Information Avoid alcohol; may cause drowsiness and impair ability to perform activities requiring mental alertness or physical coordination; may impair judgment; may be habit-forming; avoid abrupt discontinuation after prolonged use; will cause withdrawal in patients currently dependent on narcotics; may cause dry mouth

Nursing Implications Observe patient for excessive sedation, respiratory depression, implement safety measures, assist with ambulation; observe for narcotic withdrawal (nausea, vomiting, abdominal cramps, lacrimation, rhinorrhea, piloerection, anxiety, restlessness, increased temperature)

Additional Information Analgesic potency: 1 mg nalbuphine ~1 mg morphine

Dosage Forms Injection, solution, as hydrochloride: 10 mg/mL (1 mL, 10 mL); 20 mg/mL (1 mL, 10 mL)

References

Jaillon P, Gardin ME, Lecocq B, et al, "Pharmacokinetics of Nalbuphine in Infants, Young Healthy Volunteers, and Elderly Patients," *Clin Pharmacol Ther*, 1989, 46(2):226-33.

Nalidixic Acid (nal i DIKS ik AS id)

U.S. Brand Names NegGram®

Synonyms Nalidixinic Acid

Therapeutic Category Antibiotic, Quinolone

Generic Available No

Use Lower urinary tract infections due to susceptible gram-negative organisms including *E. coli*, *Enterobacter*, *Klebsiella*, and *Proteus* (inactive against *Pseudomonas*)

Pregnancy Risk Factor B

Contraindications Hypersensitivity to nalidixic acid or any component; history of convulsive disorders; infants <3 months of age; treatment of UTI in febrile infants and young children in whom renal involvement is likely

Warnings Use with caution in prepubertal children since nalidixic acid has been shown to cause cartilage degeneration and arthropathy in immature animals; usefulness may be limited by the emergence of bacterial resistance to nalidixic acid during treatment

Precautions Use with caution in patients with impaired hepatic or renal function, patients with G-6-PD deficiency, severe cerebral arteriosclerosis, or respiratory insufficiency

Adverse Reactions

Central nervous system: Malaise, drowsiness, vertigo, confusion, toxic psychosis, convulsions, fever, headache, elevated intracranial pressure, chills, depression, insomnia

Dermatologic: Rash, urticaria, pruritus, photosensitivity

Endocrine & metabolic: Metabolic acidosis (in premature infants)

Gastrointestinal: Nausea, vomiting, diarrhea, abdominal pain

Hematologic: Leukopenia, thrombocytopenia, eosinophilia, hemolytic anemia

Hepatic: Hepatotoxicity, cholestatic jaundice

Neuromuscular & skeletal: Myalgia, weakness, arthralgia with joint stiffness, peripheral neuritis

Ocular: Visual disturbances, nystagmus

Drug Interactions Warfarin (increases anticoagulant effect due to displacement of warfarin from albumin binding sites), antacids (decrease nalidixic acid absorption); may increase incidence of severe hemorrhagic necrotic enterocolitis in patients taking melphalan

Mechanism of Action Inhibits DNA topoisomerase in susceptible organisms resulting in inhibition of DNA polymerization at late stages of chromosomal replication and promotion of double-stranded DNA breakage

Pharmacokinetics

Absorption: Rapid and complete from the GI tract

Distribution: Crosses the placenta; appears in breast milk; negligible amounts enter CSF; achieves significant antibacterial concentrations only in the urinary tract

Protein binding: 90%

Metabolism: Partial in the liver to hydroxynalidixic acid (active metabolite)

Half-life: 6-7 hours (increases significantly with renal impairment)

Time to peak serum concentration: 1-2 hours

Elimination: In urine as unchanged drug and 80% as metabolites; small amounts appear in feces

Usual Dosage Oral:

Children >3 months: 55 mg/kg/day divided every 6 hours

Prophylaxis of UTI: 30 mg/kg/day divided every 12 hours

Adults: Initial: 1 g 4 times/day for 2 weeks; then suppressive therapy of 500 mg 4 times/day

Administration Oral: Administer 1 hour before meals; may administer with food to minimize GI upset; shake suspension well before use

Monitoring Parameters Urinalysis, urine culture; CBC, renal and hepatic function tests

Test Interactions False-positive urine glucose with Clinitest®, false increase in urinary VMA

Patient Information May cause photosensitivity reactions (eg, exposure to sunlight may cause severe sunburn, skin rash, redness, or itching); avoid exposure to sunlight and artificial light sources (sunlamps, tanning booth/bed); wear protective clothing, wide-brimmed hats, sunglasses, and lip sunscreen (SPF ≥15); use a sunscreen [broad-spectrum sunscreen or physical sunscreen (preferred) or sunblock with SPF ≥15]; contact physician if reaction occurs.

Additional Information In a study of 31 case-control pairs, short treatment periods (1-2 weeks) with nalidixic acid in children <15 years of age did not cause arthropathies or hamper growth

Dosage Forms

Suspension, oral: 250 mg/5 mL (473 mL) [raspberry flavor]

Tablet: 250 mg, 500 mg, 1 g [scored]

References

Nuutinen M, Turtinen J, and Uhari M, "Growth and Joint Symptoms in Children Treated With Nalidixic Acid," *Pediatr Infect Dis J*, 1994, 13(9):798-800.

"Practice Parameter: The Diagnosis, Treatment, and Evaluation of the Initial Urinary Tract Infection in Febrile Infants and Young Children. American Academy of Pediatrics. Committee on Quality Improvement. Subcommittee on Urinary Tract Infection," *Pediatrics*, 1999, 103(4 Pt 1):843-52.

Stutman HR and Marks MI, "Review of Pediatric Antimicrobial Therapies," *Semin Pediatr Infect Dis*, 1991, 2:3-17.

♦ **Nalidixinic Acid** *see* Nalidixic Acid *on page 792*
♦ **Nallpen® (Can)** *see* Nafcillin *on page 789*
♦ **N-allylnoroxymorphine** *see* Naloxone *on page 793*

Naloxone (nal OKS one)

Related Information

CPR Pediatric Drug Dosages *on page 1175*

U.S. Brand Names Narcan®

Synonyms N-allylnoroxymorphine

Therapeutic Category Antidote for Narcotic Agonists

Generic Available Yes

Use Reverses CNS and respiratory depression in suspected narcotic overdose; neonatal opiate depression; coma of unknown etiology; used as low dose I.V. continuous infusion for the treatment of narcotic-induced pruritus; adjunct in the treatment of septic shock (see Additional Information); used investigationally for phencyclidine and alcohol ingestion

Pregnancy Risk Factor B

Contraindications Hypersensitivity to naloxone or any component

Warnings May precipitate withdrawal symptoms (hypertension, sweating, agitation, irritability, shrill cry, failure to feed) in patients with physical dependence to opiates (including newborns of narcotic dependent mothers)

Precautions Use with caution in patients with chronic cardiac or pulmonary disease or coronary artery disease. Following the use of narcotics during surgery, naloxone may reverse analgesia and increase blood pressure; use with caution and administer in smaller increments to patients suspected to be opioid dependent and in postoperative patients (to avoid large cardiovascular changes)

Adverse Reactions

Cardiovascular: Hypertension, hypotension, tachycardia, ventricular arrhythmias, cardiac arrest

Gastrointestinal: Nausea, vomiting

Miscellaneous: Increased diaphoresis

Stability Protect from light; stable in NS and D_5W at 4 mcg/mL for 24 hours; do not mix with alkaline solutions

Mechanism of Action Competes and displaces narcotics at narcotic receptor sites

Pharmacodynamics

Onset of action:

E.T., I.M., S.C.: Within 2-5 minutes

I.V.: Within 2 minutes

Duration: (20-60 minutes) is shorter than that of most opioids; therefore, repeated doses are usually needed

(Continued)

Naloxone *(Continued)*

Pharmacokinetics

Distribution: Crosses the placenta

Metabolism: Primarily by glucuronidation in the liver

Half-life:

Neonates: 1.2-3 hours

Adults: 0.5-1.5 hours (mean: ~1 hour)

Elimination: In urine as metabolites

Usual Dosage

PALS 2000 Guidelines: I.V. (**Note:** May be administered I.M., S.C., or E.T., but onset of action may be delayed, especially if patient has poor perfusion; recommended PALS E.T. doses are 2-10 times the I.V. dose; see also Administration):

For total reversal of narcotic effect: **Note:** Doses may need to be repeated:

Infants and Children ≤ 5 years or ≤20 kg: 0.1 mg/kg

Children >5 years or >20 kg: 2 mg/dose

Alternative dosing to avoid sudden hemodynamic effects from opioid reversal: Use repeated doses of 0.01-0.03 mg/kg

Neonatal opioid-induced depression: I.V., I.M., S.C.: Manufacturer's recommendations: Initial: Usual: 0.01 mg/kg; may repeat every 2-3 minutes as needed based on response; may need to repeat every 1-2 hours

I.M., I.V. (preferred), E.T. (preferred if I.V. route not available), S.C.: **Note:** The dose for pediatric postoperative narcotic reversal is **one-tenth** of the dose used for opiate intoxication:

Opiate intoxication:

Birth (including premature infants) to 5 years or <20 kg: 0.1 mg/kg; repeat every 2-3 minutes if needed; may need to repeat doses every 20-60 minutes

>5 years or ≥20 kg: 2 mg/dose; if no response, repeat every 2-3 minutes; may need to repeat doses every 20-60 minutes

Children and Adults: I.V. continuous infusion: If continuous infusion is required, calculate the initial dosage/hour based on the effective intermittent dose used and duration of adequate response seen; titrate dose; a range of: 2.5-160 mcg/kg/hour has been reported; taper continuous infusion gradually to avoid relapse

Adults: 0.4-2 mg every 2-3 minutes as needed; may need to repeat doses every 20-60 minutes; **Note:** Use 0.1-0.2 mg increments in patients who are opioid dependent and in postoperative patients to avoid large cardiovascular changes

Postanesthesia narcotic reversal: Infants and Children: **0.01 mg/kg**; may repeat every 2-3 minutes as needed based on response

Manufacturer's recommendations (postoperative opioid depression): I.V.: Initial: 0.005-0.01 mg/dose every 2-3 minutes as needed based on response; may need to repeat every 1-2 hours

Treatment of narcotic-induced pruritus: Limited pediatric information is available; one retrospective study reported the following doses: Children and Adolescents 3-20 years (n=30): I.V.: Continuous infusion: Initial: 2 mcg/kg/hour; **Note:** Most initial nonresponders received antihistamines; may increase by 0.5 mcg/kg/hour every few hours if pruritus continues; mean (± SD) dose: 2.3 ± 0.68 mcg/kg/hour; monitor closely; doses ≥3 mcg/kg/hour may increase risk for loss of pain control and patients may require an increase in opioid dose (see Vrchoticky, 2000).

Administration

Endotracheal: Dilute to 1-2 mL with NS; PALS Guidelines 2000 recommendations: Dilute to 3-5 mL with NS; follow with several positive-pressure ventilations

Parenteral:

I.V. continuous infusion: Dilute to 4 mcg/mL in D_5W or NS

I.V. push: Administer over 30 seconds as undiluted preparation

Note: I.M. or S.C. administration in hypotensive patients or patients with peripheral vasoconstriction or hypoperfusion may result in erratic or delayed absorption

Monitoring Parameters Respiratory rate, heart rate, blood pressure

Nursing Implications Use of neonatal naloxone (0.02 mg/mL) is no longer recommended because unacceptably high fluid volumes will result, especially in small neonates; the 0.4 mg/mL preparation is available and can be accurately dosed with appropriately sized syringes (1 mL)

Additional Information Contains methyl and propylparabens. Naloxone has been used to increase blood pressure in patients with septic shock; increases in blood pressure may last several hours; however, an increase in patient survival has not been demonstrated and in some studies serious adverse effects (eg, agitation, pulmonary edema, hypotension, cardiac arrhythmias, seizures) have been reported; naloxone should be used with caution for septic shock, especially in patients with underlying pain or opioid tolerance; optimal dosage for this indication has not been established; one neonatal study (n=2) reported a positive blood pressure response, but one neonate developed intractable seizures and died.

Dosage Forms

Injection, neonatal solution, as hydrochloride: 0.02 mg/mL (2 mL)

Injection, solution, as hydrochloride: 0.4 mg/mL (1 mL, 10 mL); 1 mg/mL (2 mL, 10 mL)

References

American Academy of Pediatrics Committee on Drugs, "Naloxone Dosage and Route of Administration for Infants and Children: Addendum to Emergency Drug Doses for Infants and Children," *Pediatrics*, 1990, 86(3):484-5.

Chamberlain JM and Klein BL, "A Comprehensive Review of Naloxone for the Emergency Physician," *Am J Emerg Med*, 1994, 12(6):650-60.

"Guidelines 2000 for Cardiopulmonary Resuscitation and Emergency Cardiovascular Care, Part 10: Pediatric Advanced Life Support, The American Heart Association in Collaboration With the International Liaison Committee on Resuscitation," *Circulation*, 2000, 102(8 Suppl): I291-342.

"Guidelines 2000 for Cardiopulmonary Resuscitation and Emergency Cardiovascular Care, Part 11: Neonatal Resuscitation, The American Heart Association in Collaboration With the International Liason Committee on Resuscitation," *Circulation*, 2000, 102(8 Suppl): I343-357.

Vrchoticky T, "Naloxone for the Treatment of Narcotic Indiced Pruritus," *Journal of Pediatric Pharmacy Practice*, 2000, 5(2):92-7.

Naphazoline (naf AZ oh leen)

U.S. Brand Names AK-Con™; Albalon®; Allersol®; Clear Eyes® [OTC]; Clear Eyes® ACR [OTC]; Naphcon® [OTC]; Privine® [OTC]; VasoClear® [OTC]

Canadian Brand Names Naphcon Forte®; Vasocon®

Therapeutic Category Adrenergic Agonist Agent, Ophthalmic; Decongestant, Nasal; Nasal Agent, Vasoconstrictor; Ophthalmic Agent, Vasoconstrictor

Generic Available Yes (ophthalmic solution)

Use Topical ocular vasoconstrictor (to soothe, refresh, moisturize, and relieve redness due to minor eye irritation); temporarily relieves nasal congestion associated with rhinitis, sinusitis, hay fever, or the common cold

Pregnancy Risk Factor C

Contraindications Hypersensitivity to naphazoline or any component; narrow-angle glaucoma; prior to peripheral iridectomy (in patients susceptible to angle block)

Warnings Excessive dosage may cause marked sedation in children, particularly infants

Precautions Rebound congestion may occur with extended use (use no longer than 3-5 days); use with caution in the presence of hypertension, diabetes mellitus, hyperthyroidism, heart disease, coronary artery disease, cerebral arteriosclerosis, or long-standing asthma

Adverse Reactions

Cardiovascular: Systemic cardiovascular stimulation (rare), pallor

Central nervous system: Dizziness, headache, nervousness, anxiety, tenseness, drowsiness, hallucinations, convulsions, CNS depression, prolonged psychosis

Gastrointestinal: Nausea, vomiting

Local: Transient stinging, nasal mucosa irritation, dryness

Ocular: Mydriasis, elevated intraocular pressure, blurring of vision, blepharospasm (ophthalmic formulations)

Respiratory: Respiratory difficulty, sneezing, rebound nasal congestion (nasal formulations)

Miscellaneous: Diaphoresis

Drug Interactions Anesthetics (discontinue naphazoline prior to use of anesthetics that sensitize the myocardium to sympathomimetics, ie, cyclopropane, halothane); MAO inhibitors, methyldopa, tricyclic antidepressants increase hypertensive response

Mechanism of Action Stimulates alpha-adrenergic receptors in the arterioles of the conjunctiva and the nasal mucosa to produce vasoconstriction

Pharmacodynamics

Onset of action: Following topical administration, decongestion occurs within 10 minutes

Duration: 2-6 hours

Pharmacokinetics Elimination: Not well defined

Usual Dosage

Nasal: Intranasal not recommended for use in children <6 years of age (especially in infants) due to CNS depression; therapy should not exceed 3-5 days

Children 6-12 years: 0.05%, 1 drop or spray every 6 hours if needed

Children >12 years to Adults: 0.05%, 1-2 drops or sprays every 3-6 hours if needed

Ophthalmic: Therapy should generally not exceed 3-4 days; not recommended for use in children <6 years of age due to CNS depression (especially in infants)

Children >6 years and Adults (0.01% to 0.1%): Instill 1-2 drops every 3-4 hours

(Continued)

Naphazoline *(Continued)*

Administration

Ophthalmic: Instill drops into conjunctival sac of affected eye; finger pressure should be applied to lacrimal sac during and for 1-2 minutes after instillation to decrease risk of absorption and systemic reactions; avoid contact of bottle tip with skin or eye

Nasal: Spray or drop medication into one nostril while gently occluding the other; then reverse procedure

Patient Information Discontinue eye drops if visual changes or ocular pain occur

Dosage Forms

Solution, intranasal **drops**, as hydrochloride (Privine®): 0.05% (25 mL)

Solution, intranasal spray, as hydrochloride (Privine®): 0.05% (20 mL, 480 mL)

Solution, ophthalmic, as hydrochloride: 0.1% (15 mL)

AK-Con™, Albalon®, Allersol®: 0.1% (15 mL)

Clear Eyes®: 0.012% (6 mL, 15 mL, 30 mL) [contains 0.2% glycerin]

Clear Eyes® ACR: 0.012% (15 mL, 30 mL) 0.2% glycerin, and 0.25% zinc sulfate]

Naphcon®: 0.012% (15 mL)

VasoClear®: 0.02% (15 mL)

♦ **Naphcon**® **[OTC]** *see* Naphazoline *on page 795*

♦ **Naphcon Forte**® **(Can)** *see* Naphazoline *on page 795*

♦ **Naprelan**® *see* Naproxen *on page 796*

♦ **Naprosyn**® *see* Naproxen *on page 796*

Naproxen (na PROKS en)

Related Information

Carbohydrate and Alcohol Content of Liquid Medications for Use in Patients Receiving Ketogenic Diets *on page 1431*

Overdose and Toxicology *on page 1388*

U.S. Brand Names Aleve® [OTC]; Anaprox®; Anaprox® DS; EC-Naprosyn®; Naprelan®; Naprosyn®

Canadian Brand Names Apo®-Napro-Na; Apo®-Napro-Na DS; Apo®-Naproxen; Apo®-Naproxen SR; Gen-Naproxen EC; Naxen®; Novo-Naproc EC; Novo-Naprox; Novo-Naprox Sodium; Novo-Naprox Sodium DS; Novo-Naprox SR; Nu-Naprox; Riva-Naproxen

Therapeutic Category Analgesic, Non-narcotic; Anti-inflammatory Agent; Antipyretic; Nonsteroidal Anti-inflammatory Drug (NSAID), Oral

Generic Available Yes

Use Management of inflammatory disease and rheumatoid disorders (including juvenile rheumatoid arthritis); acute gout; mild to moderate pain; dysmenorrhea; fever

Pregnancy Risk Factor B (D in 3rd trimester)

Contraindications Hypersensitivity to naproxen, any component, aspirin, or other NSAIDs; active GI bleeding, ulcer disease; patients with the "aspirin triad" [asthma, rhinitis (with or without nasal polyps), and aspirin intolerance] (fatal asthmatic and anaphylactoid reactions may occur in these patients)

Precautions Use with caution in patients with GI disease, cardiac disease, renal or hepatic impairment, and patients receiving anticoagulants

Adverse Reactions

Cardiovascular: Edema

Central nervous system: Fatigue, drowsiness, vertigo, headache

Dermatologic: Pruritus, rash; pseudoporphyria (ie, increased skin fragility and blistering with scarring in sun-exposed skin), incidence: 12% in naproxen-treated children with JRA (discontinue therapy if this occurs)

Gastrointestinal: Abdominal discomfort, nausea, heartburn, constipation, vomiting, GI bleed, ulcers, perforation

Hematologic: Thrombocytopenia, inhibits platelet aggregation, prolongs bleeding time, agranulocytosis

Hepatic: Hepatitis

Ocular: Visual disturbances

Otic: Tinnitus

Renal: Renal dysfunction

Miscellaneous: Hypersensitivity reactions

Drug Interactions Cytochrome P450 isoenzyme CYP2C8 (5-hydroxylation), CYP2C9 (5-hydroxylation), and CYP2C18 substrate

Naproxen may increase serum concentrations of methotrexate and decrease the effects of furosemide; may decrease antihypertensive effects of ACE inhibitors or angiotensin II antagonists; aspirin may decrease and probenecid may increase naproxen serum concentrations; drug interactions similar to other NSAIDs may also occur; other GI irritants (eg, oral potassium supplements) may increase GI adverse effects

Stability Store at room temperature; avoid excessive heat and high humidity

Mechanism of Action Inhibits prostaglandin synthesis by decreasing the activity of the enzyme, cyclooxygenase, which results in decreased formation of prostaglandin precursors

Pharmacokinetics

Absorption: Oral: Almost 100%

Distribution: Crosses the placenta; ~1% distributed into breast milk

Protein binding: 99%

Metabolism: In the liver

Half-life, elimination: Children: Range: 8-17 hours

Children 8-14 years: 8-10 hours

Adults: 10-20 hours

Time to peak serum concentration: Within 1-2 hours for naproxen sodium; within 2-4 hours for naproxen

Elimination: 10% excreted unchanged in the urine

Usual Dosage Oral as naproxen:

Children >2 years:

Analgesia: 5-7 mg/kg/dose every 8-12 hours

Inflammatory disease: Usual: 10-15 mg/kg/day in 2 divided doses; range: 7-20 mg/kg/day; maximum dose: 1000 mg/day

Adults:

Rheumatoid arthritis, osteoarthritis, and ankylosing spondylitis: 500-1000 mg/day in 2 divided doses

Acute gout: 250 mg every 8 hours

Mild to moderate pain or dysmenorrhea: Initial: 500 mg, then 250 mg every 6-8 hours; maximum dose: 1250 mg/day

Administration Oral: Administer with food, milk, or antacids to decrease GI adverse effects; shake suspension well before use

Monitoring Parameters CBC with differential, platelets, BUN, serum creatinine, liver enzymes, occult blood loss, periodic ophthalmologic exams, hemoglobin

Patient Information Avoid alcohol; may cause drowsiness and impair ability to perform activities requiring mental alertness or physical coordination; children with JRA: Protect skin from sun; use sunscreen, wide-brimmed hats, etc; report weight gain or edema to physician; do not use OTC products containing naproxen with other pain relievers, or for >10 days for pain or for >3 days for fever (notify physician if pain or fever persists)

Additional Information In a multicenter, retrospective chart review, 19 children, 4-14 years of age (mean: 9.1 ± 2.9) with rheumatic fever (but without carditis, chorea, or rashes), were treated solely with naproxen (10-20 mg/kg/day divided in 2 doses) until ESR normalized (between 4-8 weeks); fever and arthritis resolved within a median of 1 day of starting therapy; no patient had side effects, or developed carditis over the following 6 months; comparative studies with aspirin that include patients with mild carditis are needed to confirm these findings (see Uziel, 2000)

Dosage Forms

Caplet, as sodium (Aleve®): 220 mg [equivalent to 200 mg naproxen and 20 mg sodium]

Gelcap, as sodium (Aleve®): 220 mg [equivalent to 200 mg naproxen and 20 mg sodium]

Suspension, oral (Naprosyn®): 125 mg/5 mL (480 mL) [contains 0.3 mEq/mL sodium; orange-pineapple flavor]

Tablet (Naprosyn®): 250 mg, 375 mg, 500 mg

Tablet, as sodium: 220 mg [equivalent to 200 mg naproxen and 20 mg sodium]; 275 mg [equivalent to 250 mg naproxen and 25 mg sodium]; 550 mg [equivalent to 500 mg naproxen and 50 mg sodium]

Aleve®: 220 mg [equivalent to 200 mg naproxen and 20 mg sodium]

Anaprox®: 275 mg [equivalent to 250 mg naproxen and 25 mg sodium]

Anaprox® DS: 550 mg [equivalent to 500 mg naproxen and 50 mg sodium]

Tablet, controlled release, as sodium: 550 mg [equivalent to 500 mg naproxen and 50 mg sodium]

Naprelan®: 421.5 mg [equivalent to 375 mg naproxen and 37.5 mg sodium]; 550 mg [equivalent to 500 mg naproxen and 50 mg sodium]

Tablet, delayed release, enteric coated (EC-Naprosyn®): 375 mg, 500 mg

References

Berde C, Ablin A, Glazer J, et al, "American Academy of Pediatrics Report of the Subcommittee on Disease-Related Pain in Childhood Cancer," *Pediatrics*, 1990, 86(5 Pt 2):818-25.

Lang BA and Finlayson LA, "Naproxen-Induced Pseudoporphyria in Patients With Juvenile Rheumatoid Arthritis," *J Pediatr*, 1994, 124(4):639-42.

Uziel Y, Hashkes PJ, Kassem E, et al, "The Use of Naproxen in the Treatment of Children With Rheumatic Fever," *J Pediatr*, 2000, 137(2):269-71.

Wells TG, Mortensen ME, Dietrich A, et al, "Comparison of the Pharmacokinetics of Naproxen Tablets and Suspension in Children," *J Clin Pharmacol*, 1994, 34(1):30-3.

NEDOCROMIL

- ♦ **Narcan®** *see* Naloxone *on page 793*
- ♦ **Narcotic Analgesics Comparison** *see page 1223*
- ♦ **Naropin™** *see* Ropivacaine *on page 998*
- ♦ **Nasacort®** *see* Triamcinolone *on page 1112*
- ♦ **Nasacort® AQ** *see* Triamcinolone *on page 1112*
- ♦ **NaSal™ [OTC]** *see* Sodium Chloride *on page 1027*
- ♦ **Nasalcrom® [OTC]** *see* Cromolyn *on page 311*
- ♦ **Nasalide®** *see* Flunisolide *on page 497*
- ♦ **Nasal Moist® [OTC]** *see* Sodium Chloride *on page 1027*
- ♦ **Nasarel®** *see* Flunisolide *on page 497*
- ♦ **Nascobal®** *see* Cyanocobalamin *on page 316*
- ♦ **Nasonex®** *see* Mometasone Furoate *on page 775*
- ♦ **Natulan® (Can)** *see* Procarbazine *on page 937*
- ♦ **Natural Lung Surfactant** *see* Beractant *on page 168*
- ♦ **Navane®** *see* Thiothixene *on page 1088*
- ♦ **Naxen® (Can)** *see* Naproxen *on page 796*
- ♦ **Na-Zone® [OTC]** *see* Sodium Chloride *on page 1027*
- ♦ **Nebcin®** *see* Tobramycin *on page 1097*
- ♦ **NebuPent®** *see* Pentamidine *on page 879*

Nedocromil (ne doe KROE mil)

Related Information
Asthma Guidelines *on page 1376*
U.S. Brand Names Alocril™; Tilade®
Therapeutic Category Antiallergic, Ophthalmic; Antiasthmatic; Inhalation, Miscellaneous
Generic Available No
Use
Aerosol: Maintenance therapy in patients with mild to moderate asthma
Ophthalmic: Treatment of itching associated with allergic conjunctivitis
Pregnancy Risk Factor B
Contraindications Hypersensitivity to nedocromil or any component
Warnings If systemic or inhaled steroid therapy is at all reduced, monitor patients carefully; nedocromil is **not** a bronchodilator and, therefore, should not be used for reversal of acute bronchospasm
Precautions Refrain from wearing contact lenses while exhibiting the signs and symptoms of allergic conjunctivitis
Adverse Reactions
Cardiovascular: Chest pain
Central nervous system: Dizziness, dysphonia, headache, fatigue
Dermatologic: Rash
Gastrointestinal: Nausea, vomiting, dyspepsia, diarrhea, abdominal pain, xerostomia, dysgeusia, unpleasant taste
Hepatic: Elevated ALT
Neuromuscular and skeletal: Arthritis, tremor
Ocular: Burning, irritation, stinging, conjunctivitis, eye redness, photophobia (ophthalmic formulation)
Respiratory: Cough, pharyngitis, rhinitis, bronchitis, upper respiratory infection, bronchospasm, increased sputum production, pneumonitis with eosinophilia (PIE syndrome) (inhalation formulation)
Stability Store at room temperature; do not freeze; the remaining contents of Alocril® unit dose solution should be discarded immediately after use
Mechanism of Action Inhibits the activation of and mediator release from a variety of inflammatory cell types associated with asthma including eosinophils, neutrophils, macrophages, mast cells, monocytes, and platelets; it inhibits the release of histamine, leukotrienes, and slow-reacting substance of anaphylaxis; it inhibits the development of early and late bronchoconstriction responses to inhaled antigen
Pharmacodynamics Inhalation: Duration: 2 hours; maximum therapeutic benefit is seen after at least 1 week of therapy
Pharmacokinetics
Absorption: Systemic: Inhalation: 7% to 9%; ophthalmic: <4%
Protein binding, plasma: 89%
Elimination: Excreted unchanged in urine 70%; feces 30%
Usual Dosage
Inhalation: Children ≥6 years and Adults: 2 inhalations 4 times/day; may reduce dosage to 2-3 times/day once desired clinical response to initial dose is observed

Ophthalmic: Children ≥3 years and Adults: 1-2 drops in each eye twice daily throughout the period of exposure to allergen

Administration

Oral inhalation: Shake well before use; must be primed by 3 actuations prior to first use; if canister remains unused for >7 days, reprime with 3 actuations; discard canister after 104 actuations

Ophthalmic: Instill drops into conjunctival sac; avoid contact of bottle tip with skin or eye

Patient Information May cause dry mouth

Additional Information Has no known therapeutic systemic activity when delivered by inhalation

Dosage Forms

Aerosol for inhalation, as sodium (Tilade®): 1.75 mg/activation (16.2 g)

Solution, ophthalmic, as sodium (Alocril™): 2% (5 mL)

♦ **NegGram®** see Nalidixic Acid on page 792

Nelfinavir (nel FIN a veer)

Related Information

Adult and Adolescent HIV on page 1327

Pediatric HIV on page 1323

U.S. Brand Names Viracept®

Therapeutic Category Antiretroviral Agent; HIV Agents (Anti-HIV Agents); Protease Inhibitor

Generic Available No

Use Treatment of HIV infection in combination with other antiretroviral agents. (**Note:** HIV regimens consisting of **three** antiretroviral agents are strongly recommended)

Pregnancy Risk Factor B

Contraindications Hypersensitivity to nelfinavir or any component

Warnings Due to potential serious and life-threatening drug interactions, the following drugs should not be coadministered with nelfinavir: terfenadine, astemizole, cisapride, triazolam, midazolam, ergot derivatives, amiodarone, or quinidine; concurrent use with some anticonvulsants may significantly limit nelfinavir's effectiveness; spontaneous bleeding episodes have been reported in patients with hemophilia A and B; new onset diabetes mellitus, exacerbations of diabetes and hyperglycemia have been reported in HIV-infected patients receiving protease inhibitors

Precautions Fat redistribution and accumulation [ie, central obesity, peripheral wasting, facial wasting, breast enlargement, dorsocervical fat enlargement (buffalo hump), and cushingoid appearance] have been observed in patients receiving antiretroviral agents (causal relationship not established). Use caution in patients with hepatic insufficiency since nelfinavir is metabolized in the liver and excreted predominantly in the feces. Powder formulation contains aspartame which is metabolized to phenylalanine and must be used with caution in patients with phenylketonuria.

Adverse Reactions

Cardiovascular: Hypertension

Central nervous system: Decreased concentration, anxiety, depression, dizziness, emotional lability, hyperkinesia, insomnia, migraine, seizures, sleep disorder, somnolence, suicide ideation, fever, headache, asthenia, malaise

Dermatologic: Rash, pruritus, urticaria, diaphoresis

Endocrine & metabolic: Hyperlipemia, hyperuricemia; rare: hyperglycemia, diabetes, ketoacidosis; central redistribution of body fat: Central obesity, buffalo hump, facial atrophy, and breast enlargement

Gastrointestinal: Diarrhea (30%), nausea, flatulence, abdominal pain, anorexia, dyspepsia, epigastric pain, mouth ulceration, GI bleeding, pancreatitis, vomiting

Genitourinary: Kidney calculus, sexual dysfunction

Hematologic: Anemia, leukopenia, thrombocytopenia; rare: spontaneous bleeding episodes in hemophiliacs

Hepatic: Hepatitis, elevated liver function tests

Neuromuscular & skeletal: Weakness, arthralgia, arthritis, cramps, myalgia, myasthenia, myopathy, paresthesia, back pain

Ocular: Acute iritis

Respiratory: Dyspnea, pharyngitis, rhinitis, sinusitis

Drug Interactions Cytochrome P450 isoenzyme CYP3A3/4 substrate, inducer and inhibitor

Nelfinavir inhibits the metabolism and increases the levels of cisapride, terfenadine, astemizole, amiodarone, quinidine, cyclosporine, tacrolimus, sildenafil, ergot derivatives, midazolam, and triazolam; nelfinavir increases rifabutin plasma AUC by 207% so reduce rifabutin dose by 50% when coadministering with nelfinavir; rifampin decreases nelfinavir plasma AUC by ~82% (concurrent use not recommended); phenobarbital, phenytoin, and carbamazepine decrease nelfinavir

(Continued)

Nelfinavir *(Continued)*

concentration; ketoconazole, indinavir, and ritonavir increase nelfinavir concentration; nelfinavir decreases hormone levels of oral contraceptives (ethinyl estradiol, norethindrone); nelfinavir increases levels of saquinavir and indinavir; coadministration with delavirdine increases nelfinavir concentrations by twofold and decreases delavirdine concentrations by 50%; if coadministered with didanosine, administer nelfinavir 2 hours before or 1 hour after didanosine

Food Interactions Administer with food to increase absorption; do not administer with acidic food or juice (ie, orange juice, apple juice, applesauce) since the combination may result in a bitter taste

Stability Store at room temperature

Mechanism of Action A protease inhibitor which acts on an enzyme late in the HIV replication process after the virus has entered into the cell's nucleus preventing cleavage of the gag-pol protein precursors resulting in the production of immature, noninfectious virions; cross-resistance with other protease inhibitors is possible

Pharmacokinetics

Absorption: AUC is two- to threefold higher under fed conditions versus fasting

Distribution: V_d: 2-7 L/kg

Protein binding: 98%

Metabolism: Via multiple cytochrome P450 isoforms including CYP3A4 to inactive and an active metabolite which has comparable activity to the parent drug

Half-life: 3.5-5 hours

Time to peak serum concentration: 2-4 hours

Elimination: 98% to 99% excreted in feces (78% as metabolites and 22% as unchanged nelfinavir); 1% to 2% excreted in urine

Usual Dosage Oral:

Neonates: Investigational, under study in PACTG 353: 40 mg/kg/dose twice daily

Children and Adolescents (early puberty, Tanner I-II): 20-30 mg/kg/dose 3 times/day (some experts administer a minimum dose of 30 mg/kg/dose 3 times/day); maximum dose: 750 mg/dose 3 times/day

Adolescents (late puberty, Tanner V) and Adults: 750 mg 3 times/day or 1250 mg/dose twice daily

Administration Administer with a meal or light snack to optimize absorption; do not mix with any acidic food or juice because of resulting bitter taste; if patient is unable to swallow tablets, consider using oral powder formulation mixed in small amount of water, milk, formula, dietary supplementation, ice cream, or pudding; do not store mixture for more than 6 hours; tablet can be readily dissolved in water to produce a dispersion that can be mixed with milk or chocolate milk or tablets can be crushed and administered with pudding; if coadministered with didanosine, nelfinavir should be administered 2 hours before or 1 hour after didanosine

Monitoring Parameters Liver function tests, blood glucose levels, CBC with diff, CD4 cell count, plasma levels of HIV RNA

Patient Information Nelfinavir is not a cure for HIV. Use an alternative method of contraception to birth control pills during nelfinavir therapy. If a nelfinavir dose is missed, take the dose as soon as possible and then return to the normal schedule. However, if a dose is skipped, the patient should not double the next dose.

HIV medications may cause changes in body fat, including an increase in fat in the upper back and neck, breasts, and trunk; a loss of fat from the face, arms, and legs may also occur.

Nursing Implications Do not add water to bottles of oral powder; a special scoop is provided with powder for measuring purposes. If diarrhea occurs, it may be treated with an antimotility agent like loperamide

Dosage Forms

Powder for oral suspension, as mesylate: 50 mg/g (144 g) [contains 11.2 mg phenylalanine (as aspartame)/g]

Tablet, film coated, as mesylate: 250 mg

References

McDonald CK and Kuritzkes DR, "Human Immunodeficiency Virus Type I Protease Inhibitors," *Arch Intern Med*, 1997, 157(9):951-9.

Working Group on Antiretroviral Therapy and Medical Management of HIV-Infected Children, "Guidelines for the Use of Antiretroviral Agents in Pediatric HIV Infection," December 14, 2001, http://www.aidsinfo.nih.gov.

♦ **Nembutal®** *see* Pentobarbital *on page 882*

♦ **NeoCeuticals™ Acne Spot Treatment [OTC]** *see* Salicylic Acid *on page 1002*

♦ **Neo-Fradin™** *see* Neomycin *on page 801*

♦ **Neoloid® [OTC]** *see* Castor Oil *on page 222*

♦ **Neomixin®** *see* Neomycin, Polymyxin B, and Bacitracin *on page 804*

Neomycin (nee oh MYE sin)

Related Information

Emetogenic Potential of Single Chemotherapeutic Agents *on page 1286*

Overdose and Toxicology *on page 1388*

U.S. Brand Names Myciguent [OTC]; Neo-Fradin™; Neo-Rx

Therapeutic Category Ammonium Detoxicant; Antibiotic, Aminoglycoside; Antibiotic, Topical; Hyperammonemia Agent

Generic Available Yes

Use Administered orally to prepare GI tract for surgery; treat minor skin infections; treat diarrhea caused by *E. coli*; adjunct in the treatment of hepatic encephalopathy

Pregnancy Risk Factor C

Contraindications Hypersensitivity to neomycin or any component; patients with intestinal obstruction

Warnings Neomycin is more toxic than other aminoglycosides when given parenterally; **do not administer parenterally**; topical neomycin is a contact sensitizer with sensitivity occurring in 5% to 15% of patients treated with the drug; systemic absorption can occur when neomycin is utilized for irrigation of wounds or surgical sites

Precautions Use with caution in patients with renal impairment, pre-existing hearing impairment, neuromuscular disorders; modify dosage in patients with renal impairment

Adverse Reactions

Dermatologic: Contact dermatitis, erythema, rash, urticaria

Gastrointestinal: Nausea, vomiting, diarrhea, colitis, malabsorption

Local: Burning

Neuromuscular & skeletal: Neuromuscular blockade

Ocular: Contact conjunctivitis

Otic: Ototoxicity

Renal: Nephrotoxicity

Miscellaneous: Candidiasis

Drug Interactions Oral neomycin may potentiate the effects of oral anticoagulants; may decrease GI absorption of digoxin and methotrexate; synergistic effects seen with penicillins; increase adverse effects with other neurotoxic, ototoxic or nephrotoxic drugs

Stability Reconstituted neomycin solution is stable for 7 days when refrigerated

Mechanism of Action Interferes with bacterial protein synthesis by binding to 30S ribosomal subunits

Pharmacokinetics

Absorption: Poor orally (3%) or percutaneously; readily absorbed through denuded or abraded skin and body cavities

Distribution: V_d: 0.36 L/kg

Half-life: 2-3 hours (age and renal function dependent)

Time to peak serum concentration:

I.M.: Within 2 hours

Oral: 1-4 hours

Elimination: In urine (30% to 50% as unchanged drug); 97% of an oral dose eliminated unchanged in feces

Dialysis: Dialyzable (50% to 100%)

Usual Dosage

Neonates: Oral: Diarrhea: 50 mg/kg/day divided every 6 hours

Children: Oral: 50-100 mg/kg/day in divided doses every 6-8 hours

Preoperative bowel antisepsis: 90 mg/kg/day divided every 4 hours for 2 days; or 25 mg/kg at 1, 2, and 11 PM on the day preceding surgery as an adjunct to mechanical cleansing of the intestine and in combination with erythromycin base

Hepatic coma: 2.5-7 g/m²/day divided every 4-6 hours for 5-6 days not to exceed 12 g/day

Diarrhea caused by enteropathogenic *E. coli*: 50 mg/kg/day divided every 6 hours for 2-3 days

Children and Adults: Topical: Apply ointment 1-3 times/day; topical solutions containing 0.1% to 1% neomycin have been used for irrigation

Adults: Oral: 500-2000 mg every 6-8 hours

Preoperative bowel antisepsis: 1 g each hour for 4 doses then 1 g every 4 hours for 5 doses; or 1 g at 1 PM, 2 PM, and 11 PM with oral erythromycin on day preceding surgery as an adjunct to mechanical cleansing of the bowel; or 6 g/day divided every 4 hours for 2-3 days

Hepatic coma: 4-12 g/day divided every 4-6 hours

Diarrhea caused by enteropathogenic *E. coli*: 3 g/day divided every 6 hours

Monitoring Parameters Renal function tests

Patient Information Notify physician if ringing in the ears, hearing impairment, or dizziness occurs

(Continued)

Neomycin *(Continued)*

Dosage Forms

Ointment, topical, as sulfate (Myciguent): 0.5% [3.5 mg neomycin base/g] (15 g, 30 g)

Powder, micronized, as sulfate [for prescription compounding] (Neo-Rx): (10 g, 100 g)

Solution, oral, as sulfate (Neo-Fradin™): 125 mg/5 mL [87.5 mg neomycin base/5 mL] (480 mL) [contains benzoic acid; cherry flavor]

Tablet, as sulfate: 500 mg [350 mg neomycin base]

References

Feigin RD and Cherry JD, *Textbook of Pediatric Infectious Diseases*, 4th ed, Philadelphia, PA: WB Saunders Co, 1997.

Neomycin and Polymyxin B (nee oh MYE sin & pol i MIKS in bee)

U.S. Brand Names Neosporin® G.U. Irrigant

Canadian Brand Names Cortimyxin®

Synonyms Polymyxin B and Neomycin

Therapeutic Category Antibiotic, Topical; Antibiotic, Urinary Irrigation; Genitourinary Irrigant

Generic Available No

Use Short-term use as a continuous irrigant or rinse in the urinary bladder to prevent bacteriuria and gram-negative rod septicemia associated with the use of indwelling catheters

Pregnancy Risk Factor D if used as GU irrigant

Contraindications Hypersensitivity to neomycin, polymyxin B, or any component; ophthalmic use; irrigation should be avoided in patients with defects in the bladder mucosa or wall

Warnings Topical neomycin is a contact sensitizer

Precautions Use with caution in patients with impaired renal function, dehydrated patients, burn patients, and patients receiving a high dose for prolonged treatment

Adverse Reactions

Dermatologic: Contact dermatitis, erythema, rash, urticaria

Genitourinary: Bladder irritation

Local: Burning

Neuromuscular & skeletal: Neuromuscular blockade

Otic: Ototoxicity

Renal: Nephrotoxicity

Stability Store irrigant solution in the refrigerator

Mechanism of Action Neomycin inhibits bacterial protein synthesis by binding to the 30S ribosomal subunits; polymyxin B interacts with phospholipid components in the cytoplasmic membranes of susceptible bacteria disrupting the osmotic integrity of the cell membrane

Pharmacokinetics Absorption: Not absorbed following topical application to intact skin; absorbed through denuded or abraded skin, peritoneum, wounds, or ulcers

Usual Dosage Children and Adults: Bladder irrigation: 1 mL is added to 1 L of NS with administration rate adjusted to patient's urine output; usually administered via a 3-way catheter (approximately 40 mL/hour); continuous irrigation or rinse of the urinary bladder should not exceed 10 days

Administration Bladder irrigant: Do not inject irrigant solution; concentrated irrigant solution must be diluted in 1 liter NS before administration; connect irrigation container to the inflow lumen of a 3-way catheter to permit continuous irrigation of the urinary bladder

Monitoring Parameters Urinalysis, renal function

Patient Information Notify physician if condition worsens or if rash/irritation develops

Additional Information GU irrigant contains methylparaben

Dosage Forms Solution, urogenital irrigant: Neomycin 40 mg and polymyxin B 200,000 units per mL (1 mL [preservative free], 20 mL)

Neomycin, (Bacitracin) Polymyxin B, and Hydrocortisone

(nee oh MYE sin, bas i TRAY sin, pol i MIKS in bee, & hye droe KOR ti sone)

U.S. Brand Names AK-Spore H.C.® [DSC]; Antibiotic® Ear; Cortisporin®; Pediotic®

Canadian Brand Names Cortimyxin®

Synonyms Bacitracin, Neomycin, Polymyxin B, and Hydrocortisone; Hydrocortisone, Neomycin, (Bacitracin), and Polymyxin B; Polymyxin B, Neomycin, (Bacitracin), and Hydrocortisone

Therapeutic Category Antibacterial, Otic; Antibiotic, Ophthalmic; Antibiotic, Otic; Antibiotic, Topical; Corticosteroid, Ophthalmic; Corticosteroid, Otic; Corticosteroid, Topical

Generic Available Yes

Use Steroid-responsive inflammatory condition for which a corticosteroid is indicated and where bacterial infection or a risk of bacterial infection exists

Pregnancy Risk Factor C

Contraindications Hypersensitivity to hydrocortisone, polymyxin B sulfate, bacitracin, neomycin sulfate, or any component (see Warnings); herpes simplex, vaccinia and varicella; otic use: perforated tympanic membrane

Warnings Neomycin may cause cutaneous and conjunctival sensitization; children are more susceptible to topical corticosteroid-induced hypothalamic pituitary-adrenal axis suppression and Cushing's syndrome; otic solution contains potassium metabisulfate which may cause allergic reactions in susceptible individuals

Precautions Use with caution in patients with chronic otitis media and when the integrity of the tympanic membrane is in question

Adverse Reactions
Dermatologic: Contact dermatitis
Local: Itching, pain, stinging, burning, local edema
Ocular: Elevated intraocular pressure, glaucoma, cataracts, conjunctival erythema; blurring of vision (ophthalmic formulation)
Otic: Ototoxicity
Miscellaneous: Sensitization to neomycin, secondary infections

Usual Dosage
Children: Otic: Solution and suspension: 3 drops into affected ear 3-4 times/day
Adults: Otic: Solution and suspension: 4 drops into affected ear 3-4 times/day
Children and Adults:
Topical ointment: Apply thin layer to affected area 2-4 times/day
Ophthalmic:
Ointment: Apply $1/2$" ribbon to inside of lower lid every 3-4 hours until improvement occurs then 1-3 times/day
Suspension: Instill 1-2 drops in the affected eye every 3-4 hours

Administration Shake ophthalmic and otic suspension well before use
Ophthalmic: Avoid contamination of the tip of the eye dropper or ointment tube; solution and suspension: Apply finger pressure to lacrimal sac during and for 1-2 minutes after instillation to decrease risk of absorption and systemic effects
Otic: Drops can be instilled directly into the affected ear, or a cotton wick may be saturated with suspension and inserted in ear canal. Keep wick moist with suspension every 4 hours; wick should be replaced every 24 hours.
Topical: Apply a thin layer to the cleansed, dry affected area; may cover with a sterile bandage

Patient Information Ophthalmic: May cause sensitivity to bright light; may cause temporary blurring of vision or stinging following administration

Additional Information Otic **suspension** is the preferred otic preparation; otic **suspension** can be used for the treatment of infections of mastoidectomy and fenestration cavities caused by susceptible organisms; otic **solution** is used **only** for superficial infections of the external auditory canal (ie, swimmer's ear)

Dosage Forms
Cream, topical (Cortisporin®): Neomycin sulfate 5 mg [equivalent to 3.5 mg base], polymyxin B sulfate 10,000 units, and hydrocortisone 5 mg per g (7.5 g)
Ointment, ophthalmic (AK-Spore H.C.® [DSC], Cortisporin®): Neomycin sulfate 5 mg [equivalent to 3.5 mg base], bacitracin 400 units, polymyxin B sulfate and hydrocortisone 10 mg per g (3.5 g)
Ointment, topical (Cortisporin®): Neomycin sulfate 5 mg [equivalent to 3.5 mg base], bacitracin 400 units, polymyxin B sulfate 5000 units and hydrocortisone 10 mg per g (15 g)
Solution, otic (Antibiotic Ear, Cortisporin®): Neomycin sulfate 5 mg [equivalent to 3.5 mg base], polymyxin B sulfate 10,000 units, and hydrocortisone 10 mg per mL (10 mL) [contains potassium metabisulfite and propylene glycol]
Suspension, ophthalmic (Cortisporin®): Neomycin sulfate 5 mg [equivalent to 3.5 mg base], polymyxin B sulfate 10,000 units and hydrocortisone 10 mg per mL (7.5 mL) [contains propylene glycol and thimerosal]
Suspension, otic: Neomycin sulfate 5 mg [equivalent to 3.5 mg base], polymyxin B sulfate 10,000 units and hydrocortisone 10 mg per mL (10 mL)
Antibiotic Ear, Cortisporin®: Neomycin sulfate 5 mg [equivalent to 3.5 mg base], polymyxin B sulfate 10,000 units, and hydrocortisone 10 mg per mL (10 mL)
Pediotic®: Neomycin sulfate 5 mg [equivalent to 3.5 mg base], polymyxin B sulfate 10,000 units, and hydrocortisone 10 mg per mL (7.5 mL)

♦ **Neomycin, Dexamethasone, and Polymyxin B** Polymyxin B, Dexamethasone, and Neomycin *see* Dexamethasone, Neomycin, and Polymyxin B *on page 357*

Neomycin, Polymyxin B, and Bacitracin
(nee oh MYE sin, pol i MIKS in bee, & bas i TRAY sin)

U.S. Brand Names Mycitracin® [OTC]; Neomixin®; Neosporin® Ophthalmic Ointment; Neosporin® Topical [OTC]; Triple Antibiotic®

Canadian Brand Names Neotopic®

Synonyms Bacitracin, Neomycin, and Polymyxin B; Polymyxin B, Neomycin, and Bacitracin

Therapeutic Category Antibiotic, Ophthalmic; Antibiotic, Topical

Generic Available Yes

Use Help prevent infection in minor cuts, scrapes and burns; short-term treatment of superficial external ocular infections caused by susceptible organisms

Pregnancy Risk Factor C

Contraindications Hypersensitivity to neomycin, polymyxin B, zinc bacitracin, or any component

Warnings Symptoms of neomycin sensitization include itching, reddening, edema, failure to heal; ophthalmic ointments may retard corneal healing

Precautions Prolonged use may result in overgrowth of nonsusceptible organisms

Adverse Reactions
Local: Rash and hypersensitivity reactions ranging from generalized itching, local edema, and erythema have been reported; contact dermatitis
Ocular: Conjunctival sensitization, blurring of vision (ophthalmic formulation)

Usual Dosage Children and Adults:
Ophthalmic ointment: Instill into the conjunctival sac 1 or more times daily every 3-4 hours for 7-10 days
Topical: Apply 1-3 times/day

Administration
Ophthalmic: Avoid contamination of the tip of the ointment tube
Topical: Apply a thin layer to the cleansed affected area; may cover with a sterile bandage

Patient Information Ophthalmic: May cause sensitivity to bright light; may cause temporary blurring of vision or stinging following administration

Dosage Forms
Ointment, ophthalmic (Neosporin®): Bacitracin 400 units, neomycin sulfate 3.5 mg, and polymyxin B sulfate 10,000 units per g (3.5 g)
Ointment, topical (Triple Antibiotic®): Bacitracin 400 units, neomycin sulfate 3.5 mg, and polymyxin B sulfate 5000 units per g (0.9 g, 15 g, 30 g, 454 g)
Mycitracin®: Bacitracin 400 units, neomycin sulfate 3.5 mg, and polymyxin B sulfate 5000 units per g (14 g)
Neosporin®: Bacitracin 400 units, neomycin sulfate 3.5 mg, and polymyxin B sulfate 5000 units per g (0.9 g, 15 g, 30 g)

Neomycin, Polymyxin B, and Prednisolone
(nee oh MYE sin, pol i MIKS in bee, & pred NIS oh lone)

U.S. Brand Names Poly-Pred® Liquifilm®

Synonyms Polymyxin B, Neomycin, and Prednisolone; Prednisolone, Neomycin, and Polymyxin B

Therapeutic Category Antibiotic, Ophthalmic; Corticosteroid, Ophthalmic

Generic Available No

Use Used for steroid-responsive inflammatory ocular condition in which bacterial infection or a risk of bacterial ocular infection exists

Pregnancy Risk Factor C

Contraindications Hypersensitivity to neomycin, polymyxin B, prednisolone, or any component; dendritic keratitis, viral disease of the cornea and conjunctiva, mycobacterial infection of the eye, fungal disease of the ocular structure, or after uncomplicated removal of a corneal foreign body

Warnings Symptoms of neomycin sensitization include itching, reddening, edema, or failure to heal

Precautions Prolonged use may result in overgrowth of nonsusceptible organisms, glaucoma, damage to the optic nerve, defects in visual acuity, and cataract formation

Adverse Reactions
Dermatologic: Cutaneous sensitization, skin rash, delayed wound healing
Ocular: Elevated intraocular pressure, glaucoma, optic nerve damage, cataracts, conjunctival sensitization

Usual Dosage Children and Adults:
Ophthalmic: Instill 1-2 drops every 3-4 hours; acute infections may require every 30-minute instillation initially with frequency of administration reduced as the infection is brought under control

To treat the eye lids: Instill 1-2 drops every 3-4 hours, close the eye and rub the excess on the lids and lid margins.

Administration Ophthalmic: Avoid contamination of the dropper tip; shake suspension well before using; apply finger pressure to lacrimal sac during and for 1-2 minutes after instillation to decrease risk of absorption and systemic effects

Patient Information Ophthalmic: May cause sensitivity to bright light; may cause temporary blurring of vision or stinging following administration

Dosage Forms Suspension, ophthalmic: Neomycin sulfate 0.35%, polymyxin B sulfate 10,000 units and prednisolone acetate 0.5% per mL (5 mL, 10 mL) [contains propylene glycol and thimerosal]

- ◆ **Neonatal Resuscitation Algorithm** *see page 1178*
- ◆ **Neonatal Trace Metals** *see Trace Metals on page 1106*
- ◆ **Neoral®** *see CycloSPORINE on page 324*
- ◆ **Neo-Rx** *see Neomycin on page 801*
- ◆ **Neosar®** *see Cyclophosphamide on page 321*
- ◆ **Neosporin® G.U. Irrigant** *see Neomycin and Polymyxin B on page 802*
- ◆ **Neosporin® Ophthalmic Ointment** *see Neomycin, Polymyxin B, and Bacitracin on page 804*
- ◆ **Neosporin® Topical [OTC]** *see Neomycin, Polymyxin B, and Bacitracin on page 804*

Neostigmine (nee oh STIG meen)

Related Information
Overdose and Toxicology *on page 1388*

U.S. Brand Names Prostigmin®

Therapeutic Category Antidote, Neuromuscular Blocking Agent; Cholinergic Agent; Diagnostic Agent, Myasthenia Gravis

Generic Available Yes (injection)

Use Treatment of myasthenia gravis; prevention and treatment of postoperative bladder distention and urinary retention; reversal of the effects of nondepolarizing neuromuscular blocking agents after surgery

Pregnancy Risk Factor C

Contraindications Hypersensitivity to neostigmine, bromides, or any component; GI or GU obstruction, peritonitis

Warnings Does **not** antagonize, and may prolong the phase I block of depolarizing muscle relaxants (eg, succinylcholine); adequate facilities should be available for cardiopulmonary resuscitation when testing and adjusting dose for myasthenia gravis; have atropine and epinephrine ready to treat hypersensitivity reactions; anticholinesterase insensitivity can develop for brief or prolonged periods

Precautions Use with caution in patients with epilepsy, asthma, bradycardia, hyperthyroidism, cardiac arrhythmias, peptic ulcer, vagotonia, or recent coronary occlusion

Adverse Reactions
Cardiovascular: Bradycardia, hypotension, asystole, A-V block, nodal rhythms, flushing, syncope
Central nervous system: Restlessness, agitation, seizures, dysphonia, dizziness, drowsiness, headache
Dermatologic: Rash, urticaria
Gastrointestinal: Hyperperistalsis, nausea, vomiting, diarrhea, dysphagia, flatulence, abdominal cramps; increased salivary, gastric, and intestinal secretions
Genitourinary: Urinary frequency and incontinence
Local: Thrombophlebitis
Neuromuscular & skeletal: Weakness, muscle cramps, arthralgia, tremor, dysarthria
Ocular: Miosis, lacrimation, diplopia, conjunctival hyperemia
Respiratory: Bronchoconstriction, increased secretions, laryngospasm, dyspnea, respiratory arrest, bronchospasm, respiratory paralysis
Miscellaneous: Allergic reactions, diaphoresis

Drug Interactions Antagonizes effects of nondepolarizing muscle relaxants (eg, pancuronium, tubocurarine); atropine and magnesium antagonize the muscarinic effects of neostigmine; corticosteroids may decrease neostigmine effects; prolongs effects of depolarizing muscle relaxants (eg, succinylcholine)

Mechanism of Action Competitively inhibits the hydrolysis of acetylcholine by acetylcholinesterase facilitating transmission of impulses across the myoneural junction and producing cholinergic activity

Pharmacodynamics
Onset of action:
Oral: 45-75 minutes
I.M.: Within 20-30 minutes
I.V.: Within 1-20 minutes
(Continued)

Neostigmine *(Continued)*

Duration:
Oral: 2-4 hours
I.M.: 2-4 hours
I.V.: 1-2 hours

Pharmacokinetics
Absorption: Oral: Poor (~1% to 2%)
Metabolism: In the liver
Half-life: 0.5-2.1 hours
Elimination: 50% excreted renally as unchanged drug

Usual Dosage
Myasthenia gravis:
Diagnosis: I.M. (all cholinesterase medications should be discontinued at least 8 hours before; atropine should be administered I.V. immediately prior to or I.M. 30 minutes before neostigmine):
Children: 0.025-0.04 mg/kg as a single dose
Adults: 0.02 mg/kg as a single dose
Treatment (dosage requirements are variable; adjust dosage so patient takes larger doses at times of greatest fatigue):
Children:
Oral: 2 mg/kg/day or 60 mg/m^2/day every 3-4 hours; not to exceed 375 mg/day
I.M., I.V., S.C.: 0.01-0.04 mg/kg every 2-4 hours
Adults:
Oral: Initial: 15 mg/dose every 3-4 hours, gradually increase every 1-2 days; usual daily range: 15-375 mg
I.M., I.V., S.C.: 0.5-2.5 mg every 1-3 hours up to 10 mg/24 hours maximum
Reversal of nondepolarizing neuromuscular blockade after surgery in conjunction with atropine or glycopyrrolate: I.V.:
Infants: 0.025-0.1 mg/kg/dose
Children: 0.025-0.08 mg/kg/dose
Adults: 0.5-2.5 mg; total dose not to exceed 5 mg
Bladder atony: Adults: I.M., S.C.:
Prevention: 0.25 mg every 4-6 hours for 2-3 days
Treatment: 0.5-1 mg every 3 hours for 5 doses after bladder has emptied

Dosing adjustment in renal impairment:
Cl_{cr} 10-50 mL/minute: Administer 50% of normal dose
Cl_{cr} <10 mL/minute: Administer 25% of normal dose

Administration
Parenteral: May be administered undiluted by slow I.V. injection over several minutes; may be administered I.M. or S.C.
Oral: Divide dosages so patient receives larger doses at times of greatest fatigue; may be administered with or without food

Monitoring Parameters Muscle strength, heart rate, respiratory rate

Patient Information The side effects are generally due to exaggerated pharmacologic effects; the most common side effects are salivation and muscle fasciculations; notify physician if nausea, vomiting, muscle weakness, severe abdominal pain, or difficulty breathing occurs

Dosage Forms
Injection, solution, as methylsulfate: 0.5 mg/mL (1 mL, 10 mL); 1 mg/mL (10 mL)
Tablet, as bromide: 15 mg

- **Neo-Synephrine® 12 Hour [OTC]** *see* Oxymetazoline *on page 849*
- **Neo-Synephrine® 12 Hour Extra Moisturizing [OTC]** *see* Oxymetazoline *on page 849*
- **Neo-Synephrine® Extra Strength [OTC]** *see* Phenylephrine *on page 892*
- **Neo-Synephrine® Mild [OTC]** *see* Phenylephrine *on page 892*
- **Neo-Synephrine® Ophthalmic** *see* Phenylephrine *on page 892*
- **Neo-Synephrine® Regular Strength [OTC]** *see* Phenylephrine *on page 892*
- **Neotopic® (Can)** *see* Neomycin, Polymyxin B, and Bacitracin *on page 804*
- **Neotrace-4®** *see* Trace Metals *on page 1106*
- **Nephro-Calci® [OTC]** *see* Calcium Supplements *on page 200*
- **Nephrocaps®** *see page 1213*
- **Nephro-Fer® [OTC]** *see* Iron Supplements (Oral/Enteral) *on page 623*
- **Nephrovite** *see page 1213*
- **NESP** *see* Darbepoetin Alfa *on page 341*
- **Neupogen®** *see* Filgrastim *on page 484*
- **Neurontin®** *see* Gabapentin *on page 527*
- **Neut®** *see* Sodium Bicarbonate *on page 1025*

♦ **NeutraCare®** *see* Fluoride *on page 500*

♦ **NeutraGard® [OTC]** *see* Fluoride *on page 500*

♦ **Neutra-Phos® [OTC]** *see* Phosphate Supplements *on page 898*

♦ **Neutra-Phos®-K [OTC]** *see* Phosphate Supplements *on page 898*

♦ **Neutrogena® Acne Mask [OTC]** *see* Benzoyl Peroxide *on page 165*

♦ **Neutrogena® Acne Wash [OTC]** *see* Salicylic Acid *on page 1002*

♦ **Neutrogena® Body Clear™ [OTC]** *see* Salicylic Acid *on page 1002*

♦ **Neutrogena® Clear Pore [OTC]** *see* Salicylic Acid *on page 1002*

♦ **Neutrogena® Clear Pore Shine Control [OTC]** *see* Salicylic Acid *on page 1002*

♦ **Neutrogena® Healthy Scalp [OTC]** *see* Salicylic Acid *on page 1002*

♦ **Neutrogena® Maximum Strength T/Sal® [OTC]** *see* Salicylic Acid *on page 1002*

♦ **Neutrogena® On The Spot® Acne Patch [OTC]** *see* Salicylic Acid *on page 1002*

♦ **Neutrogena® On The Spot® Acne Treatment [OTC]** *see* Benzoyl Peroxide *on page 165*

♦ **Neutrogena® T/Gel [OTC]** *see* Coal Tar *on page 299*

Nevirapine (ne VYE ra peen)

Related Information
Adult and Adolescent HIV *on page 1327*
Pediatric HIV *on page 1323*

U.S. Brand Names Viramune®

Therapeutic Category Antiretroviral Agent; HIV Agents (Anti-HIV Agents); Non-nucleoside Reverse Transcriptase Inhibitor (NNRTI)

Generic Available No

Use Treatment of HIV infection in combination with other antiretroviral agents. (**Note:** HIV regimens consisting of **three** antiretroviral agents are strongly recommended)

Pregnancy Risk Factor C

Contraindications Hypersensitivity to nevirapine or any component; concurrent therapy with ketoconazole (see Drug Interactions)

Warnings Severe and life-threatening skin reactions (eg, Stevens-Johnson syndrome) have occurred in patients receiving nevirapine. Discontinue nevirapine in patients who develop a severe rash or rash accompanied by fever, blistering, oral lesions, conjunctivitis, swelling, muscle or joint aches, or malaise. Majority of skin reactions occur within the first 6 weeks of therapy. Initiating therapy at a lower dose for the first 14 days of therapy has been shown to reduce the frequency of rash. Concomitant use of prednisone during the first 6 weeks of therapy was associated with an increase in incidence and severity of rash. Use of prednisone to prevent nevirapine-associated rash is not recommended. Severe, life-threatening, and fatal cases of hepatotoxicity have been reported with the use of nevirapine. Sixty-six percent of serious hepatic events occurred during the first 12 weeks of therapy. Patients with elevated AST or ALT levels, coinfection with hepatitis B or C, CD4$^+$ cell count >350 cells/mm^3, and women may be at higher risk for hepatic adverse events. Permanently discontinue nevirapine therapy if clinical hepatotoxicity occurs and do not restart after recovery. Nevirapine induces hepatic cytochrome P450 3A and has the potential for interacting with numerous drugs; drugs having suspected interactions and that should only be used with careful monitoring include rifampin, rifabutin, triazolam, midazolam, oral contraceptives, oral anticoagulants, digoxin, phenytoin, and theophylline.

Precautions Fat redistribution and accumulation [ie, central obesity, peripheral wasting, facial wasting, breast enlargement, dorsocervical fat enlargement (buffalo hump), and cushingoid appearance] have been observed in patients receiving antiretroviral agents (causal relationship not established). Use caution in patients with either renal or hepatic dysfunction; elevated AST or ALT levels and/or a history of chronic hepatitis (B or C) infection are associated with a greater risk of hepatic adverse events

Adverse Reactions
Central nervous system: Headache, fever, sedation

Dermatologic: Rash (usually maculopapular erythematous cutaneous eruptions with or without pruritus, located on the trunk, face, and extremities; 19% of pediatric patients developed rash), toxic epidermal necrolysis, Stevens-Johnson syndrome (see Warnings)

Endocrine & metabolic: Central redistribution of body fat: Central obesity, buffalo hump, facial atrophy, and breast enlargement

Gastrointestinal: Nausea, diarrhea

Hematologic: Eosinophilia, granulocytopenia

Hepatic: Elevated liver enzymes, hepatitis (rare), liver failure

Neuromuscular & skeletal: Myalgia, arthralgia, paresthesia

Miscellaneous: Anaphylaxis; redistribution of body fat to cause central obesity, buffalo hump, facial atrophy, and breast enlargement

(Continued)

Nevirapine (Continued)

Drug Interactions Cytochrome P450 isoenzyme CYP3A3/4 substrate, inducer, and inhibitor

Cimetidine, ketoconazole (not recommended for concurrent use), macrolides increase nevirapine plasma concentrations; rifabutin, rifampin decrease nevirapine plasma concentrations; nevirapine decreases indinavir and saquinavir concentrations; decreases hormonal contraceptive efficacy; decreases metabolism of triazolam, midazolam, oral anticoagulants, digoxin, phenytoin, theophylline; the herbal medicine St John's wort (*Hypericum perforatum*) may decrease serum concentration of nevirapine and is not recommended for concurrent use; increased incidence and severity of rash when nevirapine is used with prednisone; nevirapine may reduce plasma concentration of methadone (avoid concurrent use since acute withdrawal symptoms have been reported)

Stability Store at room temperature

Mechanism of Action A non-nucleoside reverse transcriptase inhibitor which specifically binds to HIV-1 reverse transcriptase blocking the RNA-dependent and DNA-dependent DNA polymerase activity and disrupting the virus' life cycle. Nevirapine does not inhibit HIV-2 reverse transcriptase or human DNA polymerase.

Pharmacokinetics

Absorption: Rapid and readily absorbed

Distribution: V_d: 1.21 L/kg; widely distributed; crosses the placenta; excreted in breast milk; 45% of the plasma concentration in CSF

Metabolism: Metabolized by cytochrome P450 isozymes from the CYP3A family to hydroxylated metabolites; autoinduction of metabolism occurs in 2-4 weeks with a 1.5-2 times increase in clearance; nevirapine is more rapidly metabolized in pediatric patients than in adults

Protein binding, plasma: 60%

Bioavailability: 91% to 93%

Half-life: Single dose (45 hours); multiple dosing (25-30 hours)

Time to peak serum concentration: 4 hours

Elimination: 81.3% in urine as metabolites, 10.1% in feces; <3% of the total dose is eliminated in urine as parent drug

Usual Dosage Oral:

Neonates to 3 months (Investigational, under study in PACTG 365): 5 mg/kg/dose once daily for 14 days, followed by 120 mg/m²/dose every 12 hours for 14 days, followed by 200 mg/m²/dose every 12 hours

Children >3 months: 120 mg/m²/dose once daily for 14 days; increase to 120-200 mg/m²/dose every 12 hours if no rash or other adverse effects occur; maximum dose: 200 mg/dose every 12 hours.

Note: In addition to the Working Group's dosage recommendation, the manufacturer recommends:

Children 2 months to 8 years: Initial: 4 mg/kg/day divided once daily for the first 14 days of therapy; increase to 7 mg/kg/dose every 12 hours if no rash or other adverse effects occur; maximum dose: 400 mg/day

Children ≥8 years: Initial: 4 mg/kg/day divided once daily for the first 14 days of therapy; increase to 4 mg/kg/dose every 12 hours; maximum dose: 400 mg/day

Adolescents and Adults: Initial: 200 mg/dose once daily for the first 14 days; increase to full dose if no rash or other adverse effects occur; maintenance dose: 200 mg every 12 hours

Administration Oral: May be administered with or without food; may be administered with an antacid or didanosine; shake suspension gently prior to administration

Monitoring Parameters Clinical chemistry tests, CD4 cell count, plasma levels of HIV RNA; liver function tests at baseline, prior to dose escalation, and at 2 weeks postdose escalation during therapy initiation followed by frequent monitoring thereafter

Patient Information Nevirapine is not a cure for HIV; avoid the herbal medicine St John's wort; inform physician immediately of any rash or symptoms of fatigue, malaise, anorexia, or nausea; use an alternative method of contraception from birth control pills during nevirapine therapy; if a dose is missed, take the next dose as soon as possible, however, if a dose is skipped, do not double the next dose

HIV medications may cause changes in body fat, including an increase in fat in the upper back and neck, breasts, and trunk; a loss of fat from the face, arms, and legs may also occur.

Dosage Forms

Suspension, oral: 10 mg/mL (240 mL)

Tablet, scored: 200 mg

References

D'Aquila RT, Hughes MD, Johnson VA, et al, "Nevirapine, Zidovudine, and Didanosine Compared With Zidovudine and Didanosine in Patients With HIV-1 Infection. A Randomized, Double-Blind, Placebo-

Controlled Trial. National Institute of Allergy and Infectious Diseases AIDS Clinical Trials Group Protocol 241 Investigators," *Ann Intern Med*, 1996, 124(12):1019-30.

Mueller BU, Sei S, Anderson B, et al, "Comparison of Virus Burden in Blood and Sequential Lymph Node Biopsy Specimens From Children Infected With Human Immunodeficiency Virus," *J Pediatr*, 1996, 129(3):410-8.

Working Group on Antiretroviral Therapy and Medical Management of HIV-Infected Children, "Guidelines for the Use of Antiretroviral Agents in Pediatric HIV Infection," December 14, 2001, http://www.aidsinfo.nih.gov.

♦ **Nexium®** *see* Esomeprazole *on page 454*

♦ **NH₄Cl** *see* Ammonium Chloride *on page 93*

Niacin (NYE a sin)

U.S. Brand Names Niacor®; Niaspan®; Nicotinex [OTC]; Slo-Niacin® [OTC]

Synonyms Nicotinic Acid; Vitamin B₃

Therapeutic Category Antilipemic Agent; Nutritional Supplement; Vitamin, Water Soluble

Generic Available Yes

Use Adjunctive treatment of hyperlipidemias; peripheral vascular disease and circulatory disorders; treatment of pellagra; dietary supplement; **Note:** Niacin may be used in combination with lovastatin or bile acid sequestrants for treatment of hyperlipidemias in patients who fail monotherapy; combination therapy is not indicated as initial therapy

Pregnancy Risk Factor A (C if used in doses greater than RDA suggested doses)

Contraindications Hypersensitivity to niacin or any component; significant liver disease, active peptic ulcer, severe hypotension, arterial hemorrhaging; GERD (relative contraindication)

Warnings Hepatotoxicity may occur and may be more common if extended release product is substituted for immediate release product at same dosage

Precautions May elevate uric acid levels, use with caution in patients predisposed to gout; large doses should be administered with caution to patients with gallbladder disease, jaundice, liver disease, diabetes, unstable angina, MI, renal dysfunction or heavy alcohol use; niacin may cause small increases in prothrombin time (use with caution in patients receiving anticoagulants; monitor closely)

Adverse Reactions

Cardiovascular: Flushing, hypotension, tachycardia, syncope, vasovagal attacks, arrhythmias, palpitations, orthostasis, edema

Central nervous system: Dizziness, headache, chills, insomnia

Dermatologic: Pruritus, increased sebaceous gland activity, tingling skin, burning, acanthosis nigricans (reversible), dry skin, rash, urticaria, hyperpigmentation

Endocrine & metabolic: Hyperuricemia, hyperglycemia, transient hypophosphatemia

Gastrointestinal: GI upset, nausea, vomiting, heartburn, diarrhea, anorexia, peptic ulcers

Hematologic: Small increases in prothrombin time

Hepatic: Abnormal liver function tests, jaundice, chronic liver damage, hepatitis

Neuromuscular & skeletal: Asthenia, myalgia

Ocular: Blurred vision

Miscellaneous: Sweating

Drug Interactions May inhibit uricosuric effects of sulfinpyrazone and probenecid; adrenergic blocking agents and other vasodilating drugs may cause additive vasodilating effect and postural hypotension; bile acid sequestrants may decrease the absorption of niacin (separate administration by at least 4-6 hours); vitamins containing large amounts of niacin, nicotinamide, and related substances may increase adverse effects; use with lipid-lowering agents will enhance antilipid effects; HMG-CoA reductase inhibitors may increase risk of rhabdomyolysis, myopathy; use with anticoagulants may have additive effect on prothrombin time (monitor closely)

Food Interactions Concurrent intake of hot drinks or alcohol may increase flushing and pruritus (avoid around the time of niacin administration)

Mechanism of Action Component of two coenzymes necessary for tissue respiration, lipid metabolism, and glycogenolysis; inhibits the synthesis of very low density lipoproteins

Pharmacodynamics Vasodilation:

Onset of action: Within 20 minutes
Extended release: Within 1 hour
Duration: 20-60 minutes
Extended release: 8-10 hours

Pharmacokinetics

Absorption: Oral: Rapid and extensive; ≥60% to 76% of dose is absorbed

Distribution: Crosses into breast milk

Metabolism: Extensive first-pass effect; niacin in smaller doses is converted to niacinamide which is metabolized in the liver; niacin undergoes conjugation with glycine

(Continued)

Niacin *(Continued)*

to form nicotinuric acid; nicotinamide and other niacin metabolites are formed via saturable pathways

Half-life: 45 minutes

Time to peak serum concentration: Immediate release: ~45 minutes; extended release: 4-5 hours

Elimination: In urine, with ~33% as unchanged drug; with larger doses, a greater percentage is excreted unchanged in urine

Usual Dosage Oral:

Children:

Recommended daily allowances (RDA):

0-0.5 years: 5 mg/day

0.5-1 year: 6 mg/day

1-3 years: 9 mg/day

4-6 years: 12 mg/day

7-10 years: 13 mg/day

Male:

11-14 years: 17 mg/day

15-18 years: 20 mg/day

19-24 years: 19 mg/day

Female: 11-24 years: 15 mg/day

Hyperlipidemia: Initial: 100-250 mg/day (maximum dose: 10 mg/kg/day) in 3 divided doses with meals; increase weekly by 100 mg/day or increase every 2-3 weeks by 250 mg/day as tolerated; evaluate efficacy and adverse effects with laboratory tests at 20 mg/kg/day or 1000 mg/day (whichever is less); continue to increase if needed and as tolerated; re-evaluate at each 500 mg increment; doses up to 2250 mg/day have been used; **Note:** Routine use in children and adolescents is not recommended due to limited safety and efficacy information

Pellagra: 50-100 mg/dose 3 times/day

Adults:

Recommended daily allowances (RDA):

Male:

25-50 years: 19 mg/day

>51 years: 15 mg/day

Female:

25-50 years: 15 mg/day

>51 years: 13 mg/day

Hyperlipidemia:

Immediate release products: Initial: 50-100 mg twice daily for 1 week; increase slowly over 1 month (by doubling daily dose every week) to 1-1.5 g/day divided in 2-3 doses; assess therapy at 4 and 8 weeks of therapy; if needed, dose may be increased slowly to 3 g/day or until desired result is attained; maximum dose: 3 g/day in 3 divided doses; **Note:** Some patients may require a slower dose titration

Extended release products: Initial: 500 mg/day divided in 2 doses for 1 week; increase to 500 mg twice daily for 3 weeks; if needed, dose may be increased to 2 g/day or until desired result is attained; maximum dose: 2 g/day

Niacin deficiency: 10-20 mg/day, maximum dose: 100 mg/day

Pellagra: 50-100 mg 3-4 times/day, maximum dose: 500 mg/day

Classification of Blood Cholesterol, LDL-C, and Triglyceride Concentrations*

Classification	Cholesterol (mg/dL)		LDL-C (mg/dL)		Triglycerides (mg/dL)
	Children	Adults	Children	Adults	Adults
Acceptable/optimal	<170	<200	<110	<100	<150
Above optimal	†	†	†	100-129	†
Borderline high	170-199	200-239	110-129	130-159	150-199
High	≥200	≥240	≥130	160-189	200-499
Very high				≥190	≥500

*Adapted from American Academy of Pediatrics Committee on Nutrition, "Cholesterol in Childhood," *Pediatrics*, 1998, 101(1 Pt 1):141-7 and "Third Report of the National Cholesterol Education Program Expert Panel on Detection, Evaluation, and Treatment of High Blood Cholesterol in Adults (Adult Treatment Panel III)," May 2001, www.nhlbi.nih.gov/guidelines/cholesterol.

†Lack of specific type of classification in either pediatric or adult recommendations.

Administration Oral: Administer with food or milk to decrease GI upset; swallow timed release tablet and capsule whole; do not chew or crush; to minimize flushing, administer dose at bedtime, take aspirin (adults: 325 mg) 30 minutes before niacin, and avoid alcohol or hot drinks around the time of administration

Monitoring Parameters Blood glucose; serum uric acid, periodic liver function tests (with large doses or prolonged therapy); Treatment of hyperlipidemias: Baseline: Liver enzymes, uric acid, fasting glucose, and minimum of 2 fasting lipid profiles; repeat 4-6 weeks after dose is stabilized; once LDL-C goal is reached, repeat every 2-3 months for first year and then every 6-12 months if no sign of toxicity develops and dose remains stable

Reference Range Hypercholesterolemia: See previous table; HDL-C <40 mg/dL

Test Interactions False elevations in some fluorometric determinations of urinary catecholamines; false-positive urine glucose (Benedict's reagent)

Patient Information Transient flushing of the skin and a sensation of warmth (especially of face and upper body), itching, tingling or headache may occur; if dizziness occurs, avoid sudden changes in posture and notify physician; notify physician if taking vitamins or other products that contain niacin or nicotinamide; do not change brands once dosage is stabilized; report signs and symptoms of hepatotoxicity (nausea, vomiting, loss of appetite, yellow skin, dark urine, general feeling of weakness) to physician

Additional Information Discontinue use if liver enzymes increase to ≥3 times the upper limit of normal

Dosage Forms

Capsule, extended release: 125 mg, 250 mg, 400 mg, 500 mg

Capsule, timed release: 250 mg

Elixir (Nicotinex®): 50 mg/5 mL (473 mL) [contains 10% alcohol]

Tablet: 50 mg, 100 mg, 250 mg, 500 mg

Niacor®: 500 mg

Tablet, controlled release (Slo-Niacin®): 250 mg, 500 mg, 750 mg

Tablet, extended release (Niaspan®): 500 mg, 750 mg, 1000 mg

Tablet, timed release: 250 mg, 500 mg, 750 mg, 1000 mg

References
American Academy of Pediatrics Committee on Nutrition, "Cholesterol in Childhood," *Pediatrics*, 1998, 101(1 Pt 1):141-7.

"ASHP Therapeutic Position Statement on the Safe Use of Niacin in the Management of Dyslipidemias. American Society of Health-System Pharmacists," *Am J Health Syst Pharm*, 1997, 54(24):2815-9.

Colletti RB, Neufeld EJ, Roff NK, et al, "Niacin Treatment of Hypercholesterolemia in Children." *Pediatrics*, 1993, 92(1):78-82.

Schuna AA, "Safe Use of Niacin," *Am J Health Syst Pharm*, 1997, 54(24):2803.

"Third Report of the National Cholesterol Education Program Expert Panel on Detection, Evaluation, and Treatment of High Blood Cholesterol in Adults (Adult Treatment Panel III)," May 2001, www.nhlbi.nih.gov/guidelines/cholesterol.

♦ **Niacor®** *see* Niacin *on page 809*

♦ **Niaspan®** *see* Niacin *on page 809*

♦ **Nicotinex [OTC]** *see* Niacin *on page 809*

♦ **Nicotinic Acid** *see* Niacin *on page 809*

♦ **Nidagel™ (Can)** *see* Metronidazole *on page 754*

♦ **Nifedical™ XL** *see* NIFEdipine *on page 811*

NIFEdipine (nye FED i peen)

U.S. Brand Names Adalat® CC; Nifedical™ XL; Procardia®; Procardia XL®

Canadian Brand Names Apo®-Nifed; Apo®-Nifed PA; Novo-Nifedin; Nu-Nifed

Therapeutic Category Antianginal Agent; Antihypertensive Agent; Calcium Channel Blocker

Generic Available Yes

Use Treatment of angina, hypertrophic cardiomyopathy; hypertension (extended release only)

Pregnancy Risk Factor C

Contraindications Hypersensitivity to nifedipine or any component; recent MI

Warnings Excessive hypotension may occur, especially during initiation of therapy or dosage increase (more common with concurrent beta-blocker therapy; monitor blood pressure closely); profound hypotension, MI, and death have been reported in adults when immediate release nifedipine has been used (orally or sublingually) for acute reduction of blood pressure (manufacturer does **not** recommended use of capsules for acute reduction of blood pressure); immediate release nifedipine is not FDA approved for long-term control of essential hypertension (appropriate studies to determine optimal dose or dosing interval have not been conducted)

Precautions May increase frequency, duration, and severity of angina or precipitate acute MI during initiation of therapy; use with caution in patients with CHF or aortic stenosis (especially with concomitant beta-blocker)

(Continued)

NIFEdipine (Continued)

Adverse Reactions

Cardiovascular: Flushing, hypotension, tachycardia, palpitations, syncope, peripheral edema

Central nervous system: Dizziness, fever, headache, chills

Dermatologic: Dermatitis, urticaria, purpura; photosensitivity (rare)

Gastrointestinal: Nausea, diarrhea, constipation, gingival hyperplasia

Hematologic: Thrombocytopenia, leukopenia, anemia

Hepatic: Elevated liver enzymes, cholestasis, jaundice; allergic hepatitis (rare)

Neuromuscular & skeletal: Joint stiffness, arthritis with elevated ANA

Ocular: Blurred vision, transient blindness

Respiratory: Shortness of breath

Miscellaneous: Diaphoresis

Drug Interactions Cytochrome P450 isoenzyme CYP3A3/4 and CYP3A5-7 substrate
Beta-blockers may increase cardiovascular adverse effects; anesthetic doses of fentanyl may cause hypotension; cimetidine may increase nifedipine serum concentration; nifedipine may increase phenytoin, cyclosporine, and possibly digoxin serum concentrations; nifedipine may decrease quinidine serum concentrations; combined use of nifedipine with cyclosporine may significantly increase gingival hyperplasia; delavirdine may decrease the metabolism of nifedipine and increase nifedipine levels; concurrent use of delavirdine and nifedipine is not recommended; saquinavir may increase nifedipine levels

Food Interactions Capsule is rapidly absorbed orally if it is administered without food but may result in vasodilator side effects; administration with low-fat meals may decrease flushing; grapefruit juice may significantly increase the oral bioavailability of nifedipine; food may decrease the rate but not the extent of absorption of Procardia XL®

Stability Store at room temperature; protect from light and moisture

Mechanism of Action Inhibits calcium ions from entering the "slow channels" or select voltage-sensitive areas of vascular smooth muscle and myocardium during depolarization; produces a relaxation of coronary vascular smooth muscle and coronary vasodilation; increases myocardial oxygen delivery in patients with vasospastic angina

Pharmacodynamics

Onset of action:

S.L. or "bite and swallow": Within 1-5 minutes

Oral:

Immediate release: Within 20-30 minutes

Extended release: 2-2.5 hours

Duration:

Immediate release: 4-8 hours

Extended release: 24 hours

Pharmacokinetics

Protein-binding: 92% to 98% (concentration-dependent)

Metabolism: In the liver to inactive metabolites

Bioavailability:

Capsules: 45% to 75%

Extended release: 65% to 86%

Half-life:

Normal adults: 2-5 hours

Cirrhosis: 7 hours

Elimination: In the urine with >90% of the dose excreted as inactive metabolites

Usual Dosage Oral, S.L. or "bite and swallow" (eg, patient bites capsule to release liquid contents and then swallows) (see Warnings):

Note: Doses are usually titrated upward over 7 to 14 days; may increase over 3 days if clinically necessary:

Children:

Hypertensive emergencies: 0.25-0.5 mg/kg/dose; maximum dose: 10 mg/dose; may repeat if needed every 4-6 hours; monitor carefully; maximum dose: 1-2 mg/kg/day

Hypertrophic cardiomyopathy: 0.6-0.9 mg/kg/24 hours in 3-4 divided doses

Hypertension (chronic treatment): Limited information is available; some centers use the following:

Extended release: Initial: 0.25-0.5 mg/kg/day given once daily or divided in 2 doses per day; titrate dose to effect; maximum dose: 3 mg/kg/day up to 180 mg/day (see Flynn, 2000)

Adolescents and Adults: Initial: 10 mg 3 times/day (capsules) or 30-60 mg once daily (extended release tablet); maintenance: 10-30 mg 3-4 times/day (capsules); maximum dose: 180 mg/24 hours (capsules) or 120 mg/day (extended release)

Administration Oral: Administer with food; do not administer with grapefruit juice; swallow sustained release tablets whole, do not crush, break, or chew; liquid-filled capsule may be punctured and drug solution administered sublingually or orally; when measuring smaller doses from the liquid-filled capsules, consider the following concentrations (for Procardia®) 10 mg capsule = 10 mg/0.34 mL; 20 mg capsule = 20 mg/0.45 mL

> **Note:** When nifedipine is administered sublingually, only a small amount is absorbed sublingually; the observed effects are actually due to swallowing of the drug with subsequent rapid oral absorption

Monitoring Parameters Blood pressure, CBC, platelets, periodic liver enzymes

Patient Information Avoid alcohol and grapefruit juice; rise slowly from prolonged sitting or lying position; insoluble shell of extended release tablet may appear in the stool (this is normal). May rarely cause photosensitivity reactions; avoid exposure to sunlight and artificial light sources (sunlamps, tanning booth/bed); use a sunscreen; contact physician if reaction occurs

Dosage Forms

Capsule, liquid-filled (Procardia®): 10 mg, 20 mg

Tablet, extended release: 30 mg, 60 mg, 90 mg

Adalat® CC, Procardia XL®: 30 mg, 60 mg, 90 mg

Nifedical™ XL: 30 mg, 60 mg

References

Adcock KG and Wilson JT, "Nifedipine Labeling Illustrates the Pediatric Dilemma for Off-Patent Drugs," *Pediatrics*, 2002, 109(2):319-21.

Dilmen U, Çağlar MK, Senses A, et al, "Nifedipine in Hypertensive Emergencies of Children," *Am J Dis Child*, 1983, 137(12):1162-5.

Flynn JT and Pasko DA, "Calcium Channel Blockers: Pharmacology and Place in Therapy of Pediatric Hypertension," *Pediatr Nephrol*, 2000, 15(3-4):302-16.

Lopez-Herce J, Albajara L, Cagigas P, et al, "Treatment of Hypertensive Crisis in Children With Nifedipine," *Intensive Care Med*, 1988, 14(5):519-21.

Rosen WJ and Johnson CE, "Evaluation of Five Procedures for Measuring Nonstandard Doses of Nifedipine Liquid," *Am J Hosp Pharm*, 1989, 46(11):2313-7.

♦ **Niferex® [OTC]** *see* Iron Supplements (Oral/Enteral) *on page 623*

♦ **Niferex® 150 [OTC]** *see* Iron Supplements (Oral/Enteral) *on page 623*

♦ **Nilstat (Can)** *see* Nystatin *on page 827*

♦ **Nimbex®** *see* Cisatracurium *on page 279*

♦ **Nipride® (Can)** *see* Nitroprusside *on page 818*

Nitisinone (ni TIS i known)

Therapeutic Category Tyrosinemia Type 1, Treatment Agent

Use Adjunct to dietary restriction of tyrosine and phenylalanine in the treatment of hereditary tyrosinemia type 1 (HT-1)

Pregnancy Risk Factor C

Contraindications Hypersensitivity to nitisinone or any component

Warnings Nitisinone therapy should be initiated by individuals experienced in the treatment of HT-1. Dietary restriction of tyrosine and phenylalanine must be used in conjunction with nitisinone; inadequate dietary restriction can result in elevations in plasma tyrosine leading to toxic ophthalmic effects (corneal ulcers, corneal opacities, keratitis, conjunctivitis, eye pain, and photophobia), skin effects (painful hyperkeratotic plaques on the soles and palms), and variable degrees of mental retardation and developmental delay. Nitisinone dosage should not be adjusted in order to lower the plasma tyrosine level. Transient thrombocytopenia has been reported; platelet and WBC counts should be monitored regularly during nitisinone therapy.

Precautions Slit-lamp examination of the eyes should be done prior to initiation of nitisinone therapy; patients who develop photophobia, eye pain or signs of inflammation such as redness, swelling, or burning of the eyes during treatment should be re-examined and a plasma tyrosine level measured; if the plasma tyrosine level is >500 µmol/L a more restrictive diet is indicated. Patients with HT-1 are at risk for developing porphyric crises, liver failure, or hepatic neoplasm; regular liver monitoring by imaging (ultrasound, CT scan, MRI), liver function tests, and measurement of serum alpha-fetoprotein concentration is recommended; an increase in serum alpha-fetoprotein or signs of nodules in the liver during treatment may be a sign of inadequate therapy or hepatic malignancy.

Adverse Reactions Many adverse reactions noted in clinical trials are consistent with symptomatology of HT-1

Cardiovascular: Cyanosis

Central nervous system: Headache, seizures, encephalopathy, brain tumor, nervousness, somnolence

Endocrine & metabolic: Dehydration, hypoglycemia, amenorrhea

Dermatologic: Pruritus, exfoliative dermatitis, dry skin, maculopapular rash, alopecia

(Continued)

Nitisinone *(Continued)*

Gastrointestinal: Abdominal pain, diarrhea, gastritis, gastroenteritis, GI hemorrhage, melena, tooth discoloration

Hematologic: Thrombocytopenia, leukopenia, porphyria

Hepatic: Liver failure, hepatic neoplasm, hepatomegaly, elevated liver enzymes

Ocular: Conjunctivitis, corneal opacity, keratitis, photophobia, blepharitis, eye pain, cataracts

Respiratory: Bronchitis, respiratory insufficiency, epistaxis

Miscellaneous: Infection, septicemia

Drug Interactions None as yet have been identified

Stability Store in refrigerator 2°C to 8°C (36°F to 46°F)

Mechanism of Action Nitisinone is a competitive inhibitor of 4-hydroxyphenyl-pyruvate dioxygenase, an enzyme of the tyrosine metabolic pathway. Hereditary tyrosinemia type 1 occurs due to a deficiency in fumarylacetoacetase (FAH) the final enzyme in the tyrosine metabolic pathway. This deficiency results in an accumulation of maleylacetoacetate and fumarylacetoacetate. These catabolic intermediates are converted to the toxic metabolites succinylacetone and succinylacetoacetate which are responsible for progressive liver failure, increased risk of hepatocellular carcinoma, coagulopathy, painful neurologic crises, and renal tubular dysfunction with rickets. Nitisinone prevents the formation of these toxic metabolites.

Pharmacokinetics

Half-life: Adults: 54 hours

Time to peak serum concentration: 3 hours

Usual Dosage Oral: Infants, Children, and Adults: 1 mg/kg/day twice daily; may increase after 1 month of treatment to 1.5 mg/kg/day if needed; not to exceed 2 mg/kg/day

Administration Oral: Administer on an empty stomach, at least one hour before a meal. Capsules may be opened and mixed with a small amount of water, formula, or applesauce immediately before use.

Monitoring Parameters Urine succinylacetone level, alpha-fetoprotein, plasma tyrosine level, liver function, CBC, platelets, ophthalmic exams (see Warnings and Precautions)

Reference Range Plasma tyrosine level <500 µmol/L

Patient Information Advise patients and caregivers of the need to maintain a diet low in tyrosine and phenylalanine; report eye symptoms (see Precautions), rash, jaundice, or excessive bleeding to a physician promptly

Dosage Forms Capsule: 2 mg, 5 mg, 10 mg

References

Holme E and Lindstedt S, "Diagnosis and Management of Tyrosinemia Type I," *Curr Opin Pediatr,* 1995, 7(6):726-32.

- ◆ **Nitrek®** *see* Nitroglycerin *on page 815*
- ◆ **Nitro-Bid®** *see* Nitroglycerin *on page 815*
- ◆ **Nitro-Dur®** *see* Nitroglycerin *on page 815*
- ◆ **Nitroferricyanide** *see* Nitroprusside *on page 818*

Nitrofurantoin *(nye troe fyoor AN toyn)*

Related Information

Carbohydrate and Alcohol Content of Liquid Medications for Use in Patients Receiving Ketogenic Diets *on page 1431*

U.S. Brand Names Furadantin®; Macrobid®; Macrodantin®

Canadian Brand Names Apo®-Nitrofurantoin; Novo-Furantoin

Therapeutic Category Antibiotic, Miscellaneous

Generic Available Yes (capsule, macrocrystal)

Use Prevention and treatment of urinary tract infections caused by susceptible gram-negative and some gram-positive organisms including *E. coli*, *Klebsiella*, *Enterobacter*, enterococci, and *S. aureus*; *Pseudomonas*, *Serratia*, and most species of *Proteus* are generally resistant to nitrofurantoin

Pregnancy Risk Factor B; contraindicated in pregnant women at term and during labor (due to possible hemolytic anemia in the neonate)

Contraindications Hypersensitivity to nitrofurantoin or any component; renal impairment; infants <1 month of age (due to the possibility of hemolytic anemia); pregnant patients at term; should not be used to treat UTI in febrile infants and young children in whom renal involvement is likely

Warnings Therapeutic concentrations of nitrofurantoin are not attained in the urine of patients with renal insufficiency (Cl_{cr} <40 mL/minute, anuria, or oliguria)

Precautions Use with caution in patients with G-6-PD deficiency, patients with anemia, vitamin B deficiency, diabetes mellitus, or electrolyte abnormalities

Adverse Reactions

Central nervous system: Dizziness, headache, chills, fever, vertigo, drowsiness

Dermatologic: Rash, exfoliative dermatitis, urticaria

Gastrointestinal: Nausea, vomiting, anorexia, pancreatitis, pseudomembranous colitis (rare)

Genitourinary: Discoloration of urine (dark yellow or brown)

Hematologic: Hemolytic anemia, eosinophilia, leukopenia, granulocytopenia, thrombocytopenia, megaloblastic anemia

Hepatic: Hepatotoxicity, cholestatic jaundice, hepatitis

Neuromuscular & skeletal: Arthralgia, peripheral neuropathy, muscle weakness, asthenia

Respiratory: Interstitial pneumonitis and/or fibrosis

Miscellaneous: Hypersensitivity reactions

Drug Interactions Probenecid decreases renal excretion of nitrofurantoin, antacids decrease extent and rate of absorption of nitrofurantoin; drugs which delay gastric emptying increase the extent of nitrofurantoin absorption

Food Interactions Food increases the total amount absorbed; cranberry juice and other urinary acidifiers may enhance the action of nitrofurantoin; ensure diet is adequate in protein and vitamin B complex

Stability Protect from light

Mechanism of Action Inhibits several bacterial enzyme systems including acetyl coenzyme A; reduced by bacterial enzymes to active intermediates that may alter ribosomal proteins resulting in inhibition of protein, DNA, RNA, and cell wall synthesis

Pharmacokinetics

Absorption: Well absorbed from the GI tract; macrocrystalline form is absorbed more slowly due to slower dissolution, but causes less GI distress than formulations containing microcrystals of the drug

Distribution: V_d: 0.8 L/kg; crosses the placenta; appears in breast milk and bile

Protein binding: ~40%

Metabolism: Partially in the liver

Bioavailability: Presence of food increases bioavailability

Half-life: 20-60 minutes and is prolonged with renal impairment

Elimination: As metabolites and unchanged drug (40%) in the urine and small amounts in the bile; renal excretion is via glomerular filtration and tubular secretion

Usual Dosage Oral:

Children: 5-7 mg/kg/day divided every 6 hours; maximum dose: 400 mg/day

Prophylaxis of UTI: 1-2 mg/kg/day as a single daily dose; maximum dose: 100 mg/day

Adults: 50-100 mg/dose every 6 hours

Prophylaxis of UTI: 50-100 mg/dose at bedtime

Administration Oral: Administer with food or milk; suspension may be mixed with water, milk, fruit juice, or infant formula

Monitoring Parameters Signs of pulmonary reaction; signs of numbness or tingling of the extremities; periodic liver and renal function tests

Test Interactions Causes false-positive urine glucose with Clinitest®

Patient Information May discolor urine to a dark yellow or brown color; avoid alcohol

Dosage Forms

Capsule, macrocrystal: 50 mg, 100 mg

Macrodantin®: 25 mg, 50 mg, 100 mg

Capsule, macrocrystal/monohydrate (Macrobid®): 100 mg

Suspension, microcrystals, oral (Furadantin®): 25 mg/5 mL (470 mL)

References

Brendstrup L, Hjelt K, Petersen KE, et al, "Nitrofurantoin Versus Trimethoprim Prophylaxis in Recurrent Urinary Tract Infections in Children," *Acta Paediatr Scand*, 1990. 79(12):1225-34.

Coraggio MJ, Gross TP, and Roscelli JD, "Nitrofurantoin Toxicity in Children," *Pediatr Infect Dis J*, 1989, 8(3):163-6.

"Practice Parameter: The Diagnosis, Treatment, and Evaluation of the Initial Urinary Tract Infection in Febrile Infants and Young Children. American Academy of Pediatrics. Committee on Quality Improvement. Subcommittee on Urinary Tract Infection," *Pediatrics*, 1999, 103(4 Pt 1):843-52.

♦ **Nitrogard®** *see* Nitroglycerin *on page 815*

♦ **Nitrogen Mustard** *see* Mechlorethamine *on page 708*

Nitroglycerin (nye troe GLI ser in)

U.S. Brand Names Deponit® [DSC]; Minitran™; Nitrek®; Nitro-Bid®; Nitro-Dur®; Nitrogard®; Nitrol®; Nitrolingual®; NitroQuick®; Nitrostat®; Nitro-Tab®; Nitro-Time®

Canadian Brand Names Gen-Nitro; Rho-Nitro; Transderm-Nitro®

Synonyms Glyceryl Trinitrate; Nitroglycerol; NTG

Therapeutic Category Antianginal Agent; Antihypertensive Agent; Nitrate; Vasodilator; Vasodilator, Coronary

Generic Available Yes (capsule, injection, patch, and tablet)

(Continued)

Nitroglycerin *(Continued)*

Use Acute treatment and prophylaxis of angina pectoris; I.V. for treatment of CHF (especially when associated with acute MI); pulmonary hypertension; hypertensive emergencies occurring perioperatively (especially during cardiovascular surgery)

Pregnancy Risk Factor C

Contraindications Hypersensitivity to nitroglycerin, organic nitrates, or any component (including adhesives in transdermal patches); glaucoma; severe anemia; increased ICP; concurrent use with sildenafil (see Drug Interactions); I.V. product is also contraindicated in hypotension, uncontrolled hypokalemia, pericardial tamponade, or constrictive pericarditis

Warnings May cause severe hypotension; use with caution in hypovolemia, hypotension, and right ventricular infarctions

Adverse Reactions

Cardiovascular: Flushing, hypotension, pallor, reflex tachycardia, cardiovascular collapse; severe hypotension, bradycardia, and acute coronary vascular insufficiency with abrupt withdrawal

Central nervous system: Dizziness, restlessness, headache

Dermatologic: Allergic contact dermatitis, exfoliative dermatitis

Endocrine & metabolic: Alcohol intoxication from one I.V. formulation

Gastrointestinal: Nausea, vomiting

Miscellaneous: Perspiration

Drug Interactions I.V. nitroglycerin may antagonize the anticoagulant effect of heparin, monitor closely, may need to decrease heparin dosage when nitroglycerin is discontinued; alcohol, beta-blockers, calcium channel blockers may enhance nitroglycerin's hypotensive effect; sildenafil may increase vasodilatory effects and result in severe hypotension

Stability Nitroglycerin adsorbs to plastics; I.V. must be prepared in glass bottles and special administration sets intended for nitroglycerin (nonpolyvinyl chloride) must be used; do not mix with other drugs; store sublingual tablets and ointment in tightly closed container; store at 15°C to 30°C

Mechanism of Action Reduces cardiac oxygen demand by decreasing left ventricular end diastolic pressure and systemic vascular resistance; dilates coronary arteries and improves collateral flow to ischemic regions; vasodilates veins more than arteries

Pharmacodynamics Onset and duration of action is dependent upon dosage form administered; see table.

Nitroglycerin*

Dosage Form	Onset (min)	Duration
I.V.	1-2	3-5 min
Sublingual	1-3	30-60 min
Translingual spray	2	30-60 min
Buccal, extended release	2-3	3-5 h
Oral, sustained release	40	4-8 h
Topical ointment	20-60	2-12 h
Transdermal	40-60	18-24 h

*Hemodynamic and antianginal tolerance often develops within 24-48 h of continuous nitrate administration.

Adapted from Corwin S and Reiffel, JA, "Nitrate Therapy for Angina Pectoris," *Arch Intern Med*, 1985, 145:538-43 and Franciosa JA, "Nitroglycerin and Nitrates in Congestive Heart Failure," *Heart and Lung*, 1980, 9(5):873-82.

Pharmacokinetics

Protein binding: 60%

Metabolism: Extensive first-pass

Half-life: 1-4 minutes

Elimination: Excretion of inactive metabolites in urine

Usual Dosage Tolerance to the hemodynamic and antianginal effects can develop within 24-48 hours of continuous use

Children: I.V. continuous infusion: Initial: 0.25-0.5 mcg/kg/minute; titrate by 0.5-1 mcg/kg/minute every 3-5 minutes as needed; usual dose: 1-3 mcg/kg/minute; usual maximum dose: 5 mcg/kg/minute; doses up to 20 mcg/kg/minute may be used

Adults:

Oral: 2.5-9 mg every 8-12 hours

I.V. continuous infusion: Initial: 5 mcg/minute, increase by 5 mcg/minute every 3-5 minutes to 20 mcg/minute, then increase as needed by 10 mcg/minute every 3-5 minutes, up to 200 mcg/minute

Sublingual: 0.2-0.6 mg every 5 minutes for maximum of 3 doses in 15 minutes

Ointment: 1" to 2" every 8 hours

Patch, transdermal: Initial: 0.2-0.4 mg/hour, titrate to 0.4-0.8 mg/hour; use a "patch-on" period of 12-14 hours per day and a "patch-off" period of 10-12 hours per day to minimize tolerance

Lingual: 1-2 sprays into mouth onto or under tongue every 3-5 minutes for maximum of 3 sprays in 15 minutes; may administer 5-10 minutes before activities that may precipitate angina

Buccal: Initial: 1 mg every 5 hours while awake (3 times/day); titrate dosage upward if angina occurs with tablet in place

Administration

Oral:

Buccal tablet: Place in buccal pouch and allow to dissolve; do not swallow, chew, or crush

Lingual spray: Do not shake container; spray onto or under tongue with container as close to mouth as possible; do not inhale spray; avoid swallowing immediately after spray; do not expectorate or rinse mouth for 5-10 minutes after use

Sublingual tablet: Place under tongue and allow to dissolve, do not swallow, chew, or crush; do not eat or drink while tablet dissolves

Regular or sustained release capsule/tablet: Administer with a full glass of water on an empty stomach; swallow sustained release capsules/tablets whole, do not crush or chew

Parenteral: I.V. continuous infusion: Dilute in D_5W or NS to 50-100 mcg/mL; maximum concentration not to exceed 400 mcg/mL; rate of infusion (mL/hour) = dose (mcg/kg/minute) x weight (kg) x 60 minutes/hour divided by the concentration (mcg/mL); administer via controlled infusion device

Transdermal: Place on hair-free area of skin; rotate patch sites; **Note:** Some products are a membrane-controlled system (eg, Transderm-Nitro®); do **not** cut these patches to deliver partial doses; rate of drug delivery, reservoir contents, and adhesion may be affected; if partial dose is needed, surface area of patch can be blocked proportionally using adhesive bandage (see Lee, 1997 and see specific product labeling)

Monitoring Parameters Blood pressure, heart rate (continuously with I.V. use)

Patient Information Avoid alcohol; may cause dizziness, headache; if no relief of chest pains after 3 sublingual doses, seek emergency care immediately

Nursing Implications Transdermal patches are now labeled as mg/hour (rates of release used to be described as mg/24 hours)

Additional Information I.V. preparations contain alcohol and/or propylene glycol; may need to use nitrate-free interval (10-12 hours/day) to avoid tolerance development; tolerance may possibly be reversed with acetylcysteine; gradually decrease dose in patients receiving NTG for prolonged period to avoid withdrawal reaction; lingual spray contains 20% alcohol, do not spray toward flames

Dosage Forms

Aerosol, translingual spray (Nitrolingual®): 0.4 mg/metered spray (12 g) [contains 20% alcohol; 200 metered sprays]

Capsule, extended release (Nitro-Time®): 2.5 mg, 6.5 mg, 9 mg

Infusion [premixed in D_5W]: 0.1 mg/mL (250 mL, 500 mL); 0.2 mg/mL (250 mL); 0.4 mg/mL (250 mL, 500 mL)

Injection, solution: 5 mg/mL (5 mL, 10 mL) [contains alcohol and propylene glycol]

Ointment, topical:

Nitro-Bid®: 2% [20 mg/g] (30 g, 60 g)

Nitrol®: 2% [20 mg/g] (3 g, 60 g)

Tablet, buccal, extended release (Nitrogard®): 2 mg, 3 mg

Tablet, sublingual (NitroQuick®, Nitrostat®, Nitro-Tab®): 0.3 mg, 0.4 mg, 0.6 mg

Transdermal system [once daily patch]: 0.1 mg/hour (30s); 0.2 mg/hour (30s); 0.4 mg/hour (30s); 0.6 mg/hour (30s)

Deponit®: 0.1 mg/hour (30s), 0.2 mg/hour (30s), 0.4 mg/hour (30s) [DSC]

Minitran™: 0.1 mg/hour (30s), 0.2 mg/hour (30s), 0.4 mg/hour (30s), 0.6 mg/hour (30s)

Nitrek®: 0.2 mg/hour (30s), 0.4 mg/hour (30s), 0.6 mg/hour (30s)

Nitro-Dur®: 0.1 mg/hour (30s), 0.2 mg/hour (30s), 0.3 mg/hour (30s), 0.4 mg/hour (30s), 0.6 mg/hour (30s), 0.8 mg/hour (30s)

References
Elkayam U, "Tolerance to Organic Nitrates: Evidence, Mechanisms, Clinical Relevance, and Strategies for Prevention," *Ann Intern Med*, 1991, 114(8):667-77.

Lee HA and Anderson PO, "Giving Partial Doses of Transdermal Patches," *Am J Health Syst Pharm*, 1997, 54(15):1759-60.

♦ **Nitroglycerol** *see* Nitroglycerin *on page 815*

♦ **Nitrol**® *see* Nitroglycerin *on page 815*

♦ **Nitrolingual**® *see* Nitroglycerin *on page 815*

♦ **Nitropress**® *see* Nitroprusside *on page 818*

Nitroprusside (nye troe PRUS ide)

U.S. Brand Names Nitropress®

Canadian Brand Names Nipride®

Synonyms Nitroferricyanide

Therapeutic Category Antihypertensive Agent; Vasodilator

Generic Available Yes (injection, solution)

Use Management of hypertensive crises; CHF; used for controlled hypotension during anesthesia

Pregnancy Risk Factor C

Contraindications Hypersensitivity to nitroprusside or any component; decreased cerebral perfusion; arteriovenous shunt or coarctation of the aorta (ie, compensatory hypertension)

Warnings Use only as an infusion with D_5W; continuously monitor patient's blood pressure; excessive amounts of nitroprusside can cause cyanide toxicity (usually in patients with decreased liver function) or thiocyanate toxicity (usually in patients with decreased renal function, or in patients with normal renal function but prolonged nitroprusside use)

Precautions Use with caution in patients with severe renal impairment, hepatic failure, hypothyroidism, hyponatremia, increased intracranial pressure

Adverse Reactions

Cardiovascular: Excessive hypotensive response, palpitations, substernal distress

Central nervous system: Restlessness, disorientation, psychosis, headache, elevated intracranial pressure

Endocrine & metabolic: Thyroid suppression

Gastrointestinal: Nausea, vomiting

Hematologic: Thiocyanate toxicity

Neuromuscular & skeletal: Weakness

Miscellaneous: Diaphoresis, cyanide toxicity

Stability Discard solution 24 hours after reconstitution and dilution; discard highly colored solutions

Mechanism of Action Causes peripheral vasodilation by direct action on venous and arteriolar smooth muscle, thus reducing peripheral resistance; will increase cardiac output by decreasing afterload; reduces aortal and left ventricular impedance

Pharmacodynamics Hypotensive effects:

Onset of action: Within 2 minutes

Duration: 1-10 minutes

Pharmacokinetics

Metabolism: Converted to cyanide by erythrocyte and tissue sulfhydryl group interactions; cyanide is converted in the liver by the enzyme rhodanase to thiocyanate

Half-life: <10 minutes

Thiocyanate: 2.7-7 days

Elimination: Thiocyanate is excreted in the urine

Usual Dosage Children and Adults: I.V. continuous infusion: Start 0.3-0.5 mcg/kg/minute, titrate to effect; usual dose: 3 mcg/kg/minute; rarely need >4 mcg/kg/minute; maximum dose: 8-10 mcg/kg/minute

Rate (mL/hour) = dose (mcg/kg/minute) x weight (kg) x 60 minutes/hour divided by concentration (mcg/mL)

Administration Parenteral: I.V. continuous infusion only via controlled infusion device; not for direct injection; dilute in plain dextrose solutions only (eg, D_5W); solution should be protected from light, but not necessary to wrap administration set or I.V. tubing. Final concentration for administration: Usual maximum: 200 mcg/mL; in fluid restricted patients a final maximum concentration of 1000 mcg/mL in D_5W has been used. Do not add other medications to nitroprusside solutions.

Monitoring Parameters Blood pressure, heart rate; monitor for cyanide and thiocyanate toxicity; monitor acid-base status as acidosis can be the earliest sign of cyanide toxicity; monitor thiocyanate levels if requiring prolonged infusion (>3 days) or dose ≥4 mcg/kg/minute or patient has renal dysfunction; monitor cyanide blood levels in patients with decreased hepatic function

Reference Range

Thiocyanate:

Toxic: 35-100 µg/mL

Fatal: >200 µg/mL

Cyanide:

Normal <0.2 µg/mL

Normal (smoker): <0.4 µg/mL

Toxic: >2 µg/mL

Potentially lethal: >3 µg/mL

Additional Information Thiocyanate toxicity includes psychoses, blurred vision, confusion, weakness, tinnitus, seizures; cyanide toxicity includes metabolic acidosis, tachycardia, pink skin, decreased pulse, decreased reflexes, altered consciousness, coma, almond smell on breath, methemoglobinemia, dilated pupils

Dosage Forms
Injection, solution, as sodium: 25 mg/mL (2 mL)
Injection, powder for reconstitution, as sodium: 50 mg

♦ **NitroQuick®** *see* Nitroglycerin *on page 815*

♦ **Nitrostat®** *see* Nitroglycerin *on page 815*

♦ **Nitro-Tab®** *see* Nitroglycerin *on page 815*

♦ **Nitro-Time®** *see* Nitroglycerin *on page 815*

♦ **Nix® [OTC]** *see* Permethrin *on page 885*

Nizatidine (ni ZA ti deen)

U.S. Brand Names Axid®; Axid® AR [OTC]

Canadian Brand Names Apo®-Nizatidine; Novo-Nizatidine; PMS-Nizatidine

Therapeutic Category Gastrointestinal Agent, Gastric or Duodenal Ulcer Treatment; Histamine H_2 Antagonist

Generic Available Yes (capsule)

Use Treatment and maintenance therapy of duodenal ulcer; treatment of active benign gastric ulcer; esophagitis; gastroesophageal reflux disease (GERD); over-the-counter (OTC) formulation for use in the relief of heartburn, acid indigestion, and sour stomach; adjunctive therapy in the treatment of *Helicobacter pylori*-associated duodenal ulcer

Pregnancy Risk Factor B

Contraindications Hypersensitivity to nizatidine, H_2 antagonists, or any component

Precautions Use with caution and modify dosage in patients with impaired renal function

Adverse Reactions
Cardiovascular: Chest pain, ventricular tachycardia (short, asymptomatic episodes)
Central nervous system: Headache, fever, dizziness, insomnia, somnolence, anxiety, nervousness
Dermatologic: Rash, pruritus
Endocrine & metabolic: Hyperuricemia
Gastrointestinal: Nausea, vomiting, diarrhea, flatulence, dyspepsia, constipation, dry mouth, anorexia, abdominal pain
Genitourinary: Impotence
Hematologic: Anemia, thrombocytopenia, eosinophilia, leukopenia
Hepatic: Elevated liver enzymes, jaundice, hepatitis
Neuromuscular & skeletal: Back pain, asthenia, myalgia
Ocular: Amblyopia
Respiratory: Rhinitis, pharyngitis, sinusitis, cough
Miscellaneous: Hypersensitivity reactions, serum sickness

Drug Interactions May increase salicylate serum concentration (high-dose salicylate therapy); decreases absorption of itraconazole, delavirdine, and ketoconazole

Food Interactions Limit xanthine-containing foods and beverages

Stability Nizatidine is stable for 48 hours at room temperature when the contents of a capsule are mixed in Gatorade® lemon-lime, Cran-Grape® grape-cranberry drink, V8®, apple juice, or aluminum- and magnesium hydroxide suspension (approximate concentration 2.5 mg/mL)

Mechanism of Action Competitive inhibition of histamine at H_2-receptors of the gastric parietal cells, which inhibits gastric acid secretion

Pharmacodynamics Maximum effect: Duodenal ulcer: 4 weeks

Pharmacokinetics
Distribution: V_d: 0.8-1.5 L/kg (adults)
Protein binding: 35%
Bioavailability: Oral: 70%
Half-life, elimination: 1-2 hours; anuric: 3.5-11 hours
Time to peak serum concentration: 0.5-3 hours
Elimination: 60% excreted unchanged in urine

Usual Dosage Oral:
Infants 6 months to Children 11 years: Limited information available: 6-10 mg/kg/day divided twice daily (see References)
Adults:
Active duodenal and gastric ulcers: 300 mg once daily at bedtime or 150 mg twice daily
Maintenance of healed duodenal ulcer: 150 mg once daily
(Continued)

Nizatidine *(Continued)*

GERD, esophagitis: 150 mg twice daily

Relief of heartburn, acid indigestion, sour stomach (OTC use): 75 mg 30-60 minutes before meals; no more than 2 tablets/day

Helicobacter pylori-associated duodenal ulcer (limited information): 150 mg twice daily for 4 weeks (combined with clarithromycin and bismuth formulation; followed by 300 mg/day)

Dosing adjustment in renal impairment: Adults:

Cl_{cr} 50-80 mL/minute: Administer 75% of normal dose

Cl_{cr} 10-50 mL/minute: Administer 50% of normal dose or 150 mg/day for active treatment and 150 mg every other day for maintenance treatment

Cl_{cr} <10 mL/minute: Administer 25% of normal dose or 150 mg every other day for treatment and 150 mg every 3 days for maintenance treatment

Administration Oral: May administer with or without food; see Stability

Test Interactions False-positive urobilinogen with Multistix®

Patient Information Avoid excessive amounts of caffeinated beverages and aspirin; with self medication, if the symptoms of heartburn, acid indigestion, or sour stomach persist after 2 weeks of continuous use of the drug, consult clinician

Dosage Forms

Capsule (Axid®): 150 mg, 300 mg

Tablet (Axid® AR): 75 mg

Extemporaneous Preparations A 2.5 mg/mL solution may be made by opening a 300 mg capsule into a mortar and grinding to a fine powder. Add incremental amounts of SW to a total volume of 120 mL; shake well; stable for 2 days at room temperature or refrigerated.

Lantz MD and Wozniak TJ, "Stability of Nizatidine in Extemporaneous Oral Liquid Preparations," *Am J Hosp Pharm*, 1990, 47(12):2716-9.

References

Mikawa K, Nishina K, Maekawa N, et al, "Effects of Oral Nizatidine on Preoperative Gastric Fluid pH and Volume in Children," *Br J Anaesth*, 1994, 73(5):600-4.

Simeone D, Caria MC, Miele E, et al, "Treatment of Childhood Peptic Esophagitis: A Double-Blind Placebo-Controlled Trial of Nizatidine," *J Pediatr Gastroenterol Nur*, 1997, 25(1):51-5.

♦ **Nizoral®** *see* Ketoconazole *on page 639*

♦ **Nizoral® A-D [OTC]** *see* Ketoconazole *on page 639*

♦ **Noradrenaline Acid Tartrate** *see* Norepinephrine *on page 820*

♦ **Norco®** *see* Hydrocodone and Acetaminophen *on page 571*

♦ **Norcuron®** *see* Vecuronium *on page 1138*

♦ **Nordeoxyguanosine** *see* Ganciclovir *on page 530*

♦ **Norditropin®** *see* Human Growth Hormone *on page 564*

Norepinephrine *(nor ep i NEF rin)*

Related Information

Extravasation Treatment *on page 1240*

U.S. Brand Names Levophed®

Synonyms Levarterenol; Noradrenaline Acid Tartrate

Therapeutic Category Adrenergic Agonist Agent; Alpha-Adrenergic Agonist; Sympathomimetic

Generic Available No

Use Treatment of shock which persists after adequate fluid volume replacement; severe hypotension; cardiogenic shock

Pregnancy Risk Factor C

Contraindications Hypersensitivity to norepinephrine or any component (see Warnings)

Warnings Potent drug; must be diluted prior to use; monitor hemodynamic status; injection contains sodium metabisulfite which may cause allergic reactions in susceptible individuals

Precautions Blood/volume depletion should be corrected, if possible, before norepinephrine therapy; extravasation may cause severe tissue necrosis; do **not** give to patients with peripheral or mesenteric vascular thrombosis because ischemia may be increased and the area of infarct extended; use with caution during cyclopropane or halothane anesthesia and in patients with occlusive vascular disease

Adverse Reactions

Cardiovascular: Cardiac arrhythmias, palpitations, bradycardia, tachycardia, hypertension, chest pain, pallor

Central nervous system: Anxiety, headache

Endocrine & metabolic: Uterine contractions

Gastrointestinal: Vomiting

Local: Organ ischemia (due to vasoconstriction of renal and mesenteric arteries), ischemic necrosis and sloughing of superficial tissue after extravasation

Ocular: Photophobia

Respiratory: Respiratory distress

Miscellaneous: Diaphoresis

Drug Interactions Atropine sulfate may block the reflex bradycardia caused by norepinephrine and enhance the pressor response; tricyclic antidepressants, MAO inhibitors, antihistamines (diphenhydramine, tripelennamine), guanethidine, ergot alkaloids, and methyldopa may potentiate the effect of norepinephrine

Stability Readily oxidized, do not use if brown coloration; dilute with D_5W or D_5W/NS; not recommended for dilution in NS; not stable with alkaline solutions

Mechanism of Action Stimulates beta$_1$-adrenergic receptors and alpha-adrenergic receptors causing increased contractility and heart rate as well as vasoconstriction, thereby increasing systemic blood pressure and coronary blood flow; clinically, alpha effects (vasoconstriction) are greater than beta effects (inotropic and chronotropic effects)

Pharmacodynamics

Onset of action: Very rapid

Duration: Limited duration following I.V. injection

Pharmacokinetics

Metabolism: By catechol-o-methyltransferase (COMT) and monoamine oxidase (MAO)

Elimination: In urine (84% to 96% as inactive metabolites)

Usual Dosage I.V. (dose stated in terms of **norepinephrine base**):

Children: Initial: 0.05-0.1 mcg/kg/minute, titrate to desired effect; maximum dose: 1-2 mcg/kg/minute

Rate (mL/hour) = dose (mcg/kg/minute) x weight (kg) x 60 minutes/hour divided by concentration (mcg/mL)

Adults: Initial: 4 mcg/minute; titrate to desired response; usual dose: 8-12 mcg/minute as an infusion

ACLS Guidelines 2000: Initial 0.5-1 mcg/minute; titrate to effect

Refractory shock: 8-30 mcg/minute may be required

Administration Parenteral: Administer into large vein to avoid potential extravasation; standard concentration: 4 mcg/mL but 16 mcg/mL has been used safely and with efficacy in situations of extreme fluid restriction

Monitoring Parameters Blood pressure, heart rate, urine output, peripheral perfusion

Additional Information Treat extravasations with local injections of phentolamine (see Extravasation Treatment *on page 1240*)

Dosage Forms Injection, solution, as bitartrate: 1 mg/mL norepinephrine base (4 mL) [contains sodium metabisulfite]

Norethindrone (nor eth IN drone)

Related Information

Oral Contraceptives *on page 1243*

U.S. Brand Names Aygestin®; Micronor®; Nor-QD®

Canadian Brand Names Norlutate®

Synonyms Norethisterone

Therapeutic Category Contraceptive, Oral; Contraceptive, Progestin Only; Progestin

Generic Available Yes (tablet, as acetate)

Use Treatment of amenorrhea, abnormal uterine bleeding, endometriosis, oral contraceptive

Pregnancy Risk Factor X

Contraindications Hypersensitivity to norethindrone or any component; thromboembolic disorders, severe hepatic disease, breast cancer, cerebral hemorrhage, undiagnosed vaginal bleeding; known or suspected pregnancy; as a diagnostic test for pregnancy

Warnings Discontinue if sudden partial or complete loss of vision, proptosis, diplopia, or migraine occur; **there is a higher rate of failure with progestin only contraceptives**; progestin-induced withdrawal bleeding occurs within 3-7 days after discontinuation of drug

Precautions Use with caution in patients with asthma, diabetes mellitus, seizure disorder, migraine, cardiac or renal dysfunction, psychic depression; may affect lipid and carbohydrate metabolism; women with diabetes mellitus or hyperlipidemias should be monitored closely

Adverse Reactions

Cardiovascular: Edema, thromboembolic disorders, hypertension

(Continued)

Norethindrone *(Continued)*

Central nervous system: Mental depression, nervousness, dizziness, fatigue, headache

Dermatologic: Hirsutism, rash, melasma or chloasma

Endocrine & metabolic: Breakthrough bleeding, spotting, changes in menstrual flow

Gastrointestinal: Weight gain or loss

Hepatic: Cholestatic jaundice

Drug Interactions Rifampin decreases pharmacologic effect of norethindrone

Food Interactions High-dose vitamin C (1 g/day) may increase adverse effects; increase dietary intake of folate and pyridoxine

Mechanism of Action Inhibits secretion of pituitary gonadotropin (LH) which prevents follicular maturation and ovulation; in the presence of adequate endogenous estrogen, transforms a proliferative endometrium to a secretory one

Pharmacokinetics

Protein binding: 80%

Metabolism: In the liver

Half-life: 5-14 hours

Time to peak serum concentration: 0.5-4 hours

Usual Dosage Adolescents and Adults: Oral:

Amenorrhea and abnormal uterine bleeding: Norethindrone acetate 2.5-10 mg/day for 5-10 days beginning during the latter half of the menstrual cycle

Endometriosis: Norethindrone acetate 5 mg/day for 14 days; increase at increments of 2.5 mg/day every 2 weeks up to 15 mg/day

Contraception: Progesterone only: Norethindrone 0.35 mg every day of the year starting on first day of menstruation

Administration Oral: Administer with food

Test Interactions Thyroid function test, metyrapone test, liver function tests, coagulation tests (prothrombin time, factors VII, VIII, IX, X)

Patient Information Progestin-induced withdrawal bleeding occurs within 3-7 days after discontinuation of the drug; when used for contraception, if one dose is missed take as soon as remembered, then take the next tablet at the regular time; if two doses are missed, take one of the missed doses, discard the other, and take daily dose at usual time; if three doses are missed, use another form of birth control until menses appear or pregnancy is ruled out; limit caffeine

Dosage Forms

Tablet (Micronor®, Nor-QD®): 0.35 mg

Tablet, as acetate (Aygestin®): 5 mg

- ◆ **Norethisterone** *see Norethindrone on page 821*
- ◆ **Noritate™** *see Metronidazole on page 754*
- ◆ **Norlutate® (Can)** *see Norethindrone on page 821*
- ◆ **Normal Human Serum Albumin** *see Albumin on page 52*
- ◆ **Normal Laboratory Values for Children** *see page 1353*
- ◆ **Normal Saline** *see Sodium Chloride on page 1027*
- ◆ **Normal Serum Albumin (Human)** *see Albumin on page 52*
- ◆ **Normodyne®** *see Labetalol on page 645*
- ◆ **Norpace®** *see Disopyramide on page 399*
- ◆ **Norpace® CR** *see Disopyramide on page 399*
- ◆ **Norpramin®** *see Desipramine on page 349*
- ◆ **Nor-QD®** *see Norethindrone on page 821*
- ◆ **North and South American Antisnake-bite Serum** *see Crotalidae Polyvalent Antivenin (Equine) on page 313*

Nortriptyline *(nor TRIP ti leen)*

Related Information

Comparison of Adverse Effects of Antidepressants *on page 1210*

Comparison of Usual Adult Dosage and Mechanism of Action of Antidepressants *on page 1209*

U.S. Brand Names Aventyl® HCl; Pamelor®

Canadian Brand Names Alti-Nortriptyline; Apo®-Nortriptyline; Gen-Nortriptyline; Novo-Nortriptyline; Nu-Nortriptyline; PMS-Nortriptyline

Therapeutic Category Antidepressant, Tricyclic

Generic Available Yes

Use Treatment of various forms of depression, often in conjunction with psychotherapy; nocturnal enuresis

Pregnancy Risk Factor D

Contraindications Hypersensitivity to nortriptyline or amitriptyline (cross-sensitivity with other tricyclics may occur) or any component (see Warnings); angle-closure glaucoma, use of MAO inhibitors within 14 days (potentially fatal reactions may occur, see Drug Interactions)

Warnings Do not discontinue abruptly in patients receiving high doses chronically; use with extreme caution with renal or hepatic impairment

Capsule may contain sodium bisulfite and/or benzyl alcohol, both of which may cause allergic reactions in susceptible individuals; solution contains benzoic acid; benzoic acid (benzoate) is a metabolite of benzyl alcohol; large amounts of benzyl alcohol (≥99 mg/kg/day) have been associated with a potentially fatal toxicity ("gasping syndrome") in neonates; avoid use of nortriptyline products containing benzoic acid or benzyl alcohol in neonates; *in vitro* and animal studies have shown that benzoate displaces bilirubin from protein binding sites

Precautions Use with caution in patients with cardiac conduction disturbances, cardiovascular disease, seizure disorder, history of urinary retention, hyperthyroidism, or those receiving thyroid hormone replacement

Adverse Reactions Nortriptyline has lower anticholinergic and sedative effects compared to amitriptyline

Cardiovascular: Postural hypotension, arrhythmias, tachycardia, sudden death

Central nervous system: Sedation, fatigue, anxiety, impaired cognitive function, seizures

Dermatologic: Photosensitivity

Endocrine & metabolic: Rarely SIADH

Gastrointestinal: Xerostomia, constipation, increased appetite, weight gain

Genitourinary: Urinary retention

Hematologic: Rarely agranulocytosis, leukopenia, eosinophilia

Hepatic: Cholestatic jaundice, elevated liver enzymes

Neuromuscular & skeletal: Tremor, weakness

Ocular: Blurred vision, elevated intraocular pressure

Miscellaneous: Allergic reactions

Drug Interactions Cytochrome P450 isoenzyme CYP1A2 and CYP2D6 (hydroxylation) substrate

Nortriptyline may decrease the effects of guanethidine and clonidine (use with clonidine may result in possible hypertensive crisis); nortriptyline may increase the effects of other CNS depressants (including alcohol), adrenergic agents (epinephrine, isoproterenol), anticholinergic agents and warfarin

With MAO inhibitors, hyperpyrexia, hypertension, tachycardia, confusion, seizures, and death have been reported (see Contraindications); concurrent use of high-dose TCAs and ritonavir may cause the serotonin syndrome; the herbal medicine St John's wort (*Hypericum perforatum*) may increase serious side effects, its use is **not** recommended

Cimetidine, fluoxetine, and methylphenidate may decrease the metabolism and phenobarbital may increase the metabolism of nortriptyline

Food Interactions Riboflavin dietary requirements may be increased

Stability Protect from light

Mechanism of Action Increases the synaptic concentration of serotonin and/or norepinephrine in the CNS by inhibition of their reuptake by the presynaptic neuronal membrane

Pharmacodynamics Onset of action: Therapeutic antidepressant effects begin in 7-21 days; maximum effects may not occur for ≥2-3 weeks

Pharmacokinetics

Absorption: Oral: Rapid; well absorbed

Distribution: V_d: 14-22 L/kg; crosses placenta; enters breast milk

Protein binding: 93% to 95%

Metabolism: Undergoes significant first-pass metabolism; primarily detoxified in the liver via hydroxylation followed by glucuronide conjugation

Half-life:

Children (mean ± SD): 18 ± 4 hours

Adults (mean ± SD): 46 ± 24 hours

Time to peak serum concentration: Oral: Within 7-8.5 hours

Elimination: Metabolites and small amounts of unchanged drug excreted in urine; small amounts of biliary elimination occur

Dialysis: Not Dialyzable

Usual Dosage Oral:

Nocturnal enuresis: Children (give dose 30 minutes before bedtime):

6-7 years (20-25 kg): 10 mg/day

8-11 years (25-35 kg): 10-20 mg/day

>11 years (35-54 kg): 25-35 mg/day

(Continued)

Nortriptyline *(Continued)*

Depression:
Children 6-12 years: 1-3 mg/kg/day or 10-20 mg/day in 3-4 divided doses
Adolescents: 1-3 mg/kg/day or 30-50 mg/day in 3-4 divided doses; usual maximum dose: 150 mg/day
Adults: 25 mg 3-4 times/day up to 150 mg/day

Dosing adjustment in hepatic impairment: Use lower doses and slower titration; individualization of dosage is recommended

Administration Oral: May administer with food to decrease GI upset; dilute oral solution in water, milk, or fruit juice immediately before use; do not dilute in grape juice or carbonated beverages

Monitoring Parameters Heart rate, blood pressure, mental status, weight, plasma concentrations

Reference Range Therapeutic: 50-150 ng/mL (SI: 190-570 nmol/L)

Patient Information Avoid alcohol and the herbal medicine St John's wort; limit caffeine; do not discontinue medication abruptly; may cause drowsiness and impair ability to perform activities requiring mental alertness or physical coordination; may cause dry mouth. May cause photosensitivity reactions (eg, exposure to sunlight may cause severe sunburn, skin rash, redness, or itching); avoid exposure to sunlight and artificial light sources (sunlamps, tanning booth/bed); wear protective clothing, wide-brimmed hats, sunglasses, and lip sunscreen (SPF ≥15); use a sunscreen [broad-spectrum sunscreen or physical sunscreen (preferred) or sunblock with SPF ≥15]; contact physician if reaction occurs.

Nursing Implications Treatment duration of nocturnal enuresis is usually ≤3 months

Dosage Forms

Capsule, as hydrochloride: 10 mg, 25 mg, 50 mg, 75 mg
Aventyl® HCl: 10 mg, 25 mg
Pamelor®: 10 mg, 25 mg, 50 mg, 75 mg [may contain benzyl alcohol; 50 mg may also contain sodium bisulfite]
Solution, as hydrochloride (Aventyl® HCl, Pamelor®): 10 mg/5 mL (473 mL) [contains 4% alcohol and benzoic acid]

References
Levy HB, Harper CR, and Weinberg WA, "A Practical Approach to Children Failing in School," *Pediatr Clin North Am,* 1992, 39(4):895-928

- **Norvasc®** *see* Amlodipine *on page 91*
- **Norvir®** *see* Ritonavir *on page 993*
- **Norvir® SEC (Can)** *see* Ritonavir *on page 993*
- **Nostril® [OTC]** *see* Phenylephrine *on page 892*
- **Nōstrilla® [OTC]** *see* Oxymetazoline *on page 849*
- **Novamoxin® (Can)** *see* Amoxicillin *on page 94*
- **Novantrone®** *see* Mitoxantrone *on page 771*
- **Novarel™** *see* Chorionic Gonadotropin *on page 269*
- **Novasen (Can)** *see* Aspirin *on page 134*
- **Novel Erythropoiesis Stimulating Protein** *see* Darbepoetin Alfa *on page 341*
- **Novo-5 ASA (Can)** *see* Mesalamine *on page 723*
- **Novo-Alprazol (Can)** *see* Alprazolam *on page 64*
- **Novo-Amiodarone (Can)** *see* Amiodarone *on page 83*
- **Novo-Ampicillin (Can)** *see* Ampicillin *on page 103*
- **Novo-Atenol (Can)** *see* Atenolol *on page 137*
- **Novo-AZT (Can)** *see* Zidovudine *on page 1163*
- **Novo-Buspirone (Can)** *see* BusPIRone *on page 191*
- **Novo-Captopril (Can)** *see* Captopril *on page 207*
- **Novo-Carbamaz (Can)** *see* Carbamazepine *on page 209*
- **Novo-Cefaclor (Can)** *see* Cefaclor *on page 223*
- **Novo-Cefadroxil (Can)** *see* Cefadroxil *on page 224*
- **Novo-Chlorpromazine (Can)** *see* ChlorproMAZINE *on page 263*
- **Novo-Cholamine (Can)** *see* Cholestyramine Resin *on page 267*
- **Novo-Cholamine Light (Can)** *see* Cholestyramine Resin *on page 267*
- **Novo-Cimetidine (Can)** *see* Cimetidine *on page 272*
- **Novo-Clonazepam (Can)** *see* Clonazepam *on page 292*
- **Novo-Clonidine® (Can)** *see* Clonidine *on page 294*
- **Novo-Clopate® (Can)** *see* Clorazepate *on page 296*
- **Novo-Cloxin® (Can)** *see* Cloxacillin *on page 298*
- **Novo-Cycloprine® (Can)** *see* Cyclobenzaprine *on page 318*
- **Novo-Desipramine® (Can)** *see* Desipramine *on page 349*

- **Novo-Difenac® (Can)** see Diclofenac on page 374
- **Novo-Difenac K (Can)** see Diclofenac on page 374
- **Novo-Difenac-SR® (Can)** see Diclofenac on page 374
- **Novo-Digoxin (Can)** see Digoxin on page 380
- **Novo-Diltazem (Can)** see Diltiazem on page 388
- **Novo-Diltazem-CD (Can)** see Diltiazem on page 388
- **Novo-Diltazem SR (Can)** see Diltiazem on page 388
- **Novo-Dipiradol (Can)** see Dipyridamole on page 397
- **Novo-Divalproex (Can)** see Valproic Acid and Derivatives on page 1131
- **Novo-Doxepin (Can)** see Doxepin on page 411
- **Novo-Doxylin (Can)** see Doxycycline on page 415
- **Novo-Famotidine (Can)** see Famotidine on page 473
- **Novo-Fluoxetine (Can)** see Fluoxetine on page 505
- **Novo-Flurprofen (Can)** see Flurbiprofen on page 510
- **Novo-Furantoin (Can)** see Nitrofurantoin on page 814
- **Novo-Gabapentin (Can)** see Gabapentin on page 527
- **Novo-Glyburide (Can)** see GlyBURIDE on page 540
- **Novo-Hydrazide (Can)** see Hydrochlorothiazide on page 569
- **Novo-Hydroxyzin (Can)** see HydrOXYzine on page 584
- **Novo-Hylazin (Can)** see HydrALAZINE on page 568
- **Novo-Ipramide (Can)** see Ipratropium on page 620
- **Novo-Ketoconazole (Can)** see Ketoconazole on page 639
- **Novo-Ketorolac (Can)** see Ketorolac on page 641
- **Novo-Levobunolol (Can)** see Levobunolol on page 665
- **Novo-Lexin® (Can)** see Cephalexin on page 244
- **Novolin® 70/30** see Insulin Preparations on page 609
- **Novolin® ge (Can)** see Insulin Preparations on page 609
- **Novolin® L** see Insulin Preparations on page 609
- **Novolin® N** see Insulin Preparations on page 609
- **Novolin® R** see Insulin Preparations on page 609
- **NovoLog®** see Insulin Preparations on page 609
- **NovoLog® Mix 70/30** see Insulin Preparations on page 609
- **Novo-Loperamide (Can)** see Loperamide on page 687
- **Novo-Lorazepam® (Can)** see Lorazepam on page 695
- **Novo-Medrone (Can)** see MedroxyPROGESTERone on page 712
- **Novo-Metformin (Can)** see Metformin on page 729
- **Novo-Methacin (Can)** see Indomethacin on page 606
- **Novo-Metoprol (Can)** see Metoprolol on page 752
- **Novo-Mexiletine (Can)** see Mexiletine on page 757
- **Novo-Misoprostol (Can)** see Misoprostol on page 769
- **Novo-Mucilax (Can)** see Psyllium on page 959
- **Novo-Nadolol (Can)** see Nadolol on page 788
- **Novo-Naproc EC (Can)** see Naproxen on page 796
- **Novo-Naprox (Can)** see Naproxen on page 796
- **Novo-Naprox Sodium (Can)** see Naproxen on page 796
- **Novo-Naprox Sodium DS (Can)** see Naproxen on page 796
- **Novo-Naprox SR (Can)** see Naproxen on page 796
- **Novo-Nidazol (Can)** see Metronidazole on page 754
- **Novo-Nifedin (Can)** see NIFEdipine on page 811
- **Novo-Nizatidine (Can)** see Nizatidine on page 819
- **Novo-Nortriptyline (Can)** see Nortriptyline on page 822
- **Novo-Oxybutynin (Can)** see Oxybutynin on page 843
- **Novo-Pen-VK® (Can)** see Penicillin V Potassium on page 877
- **Novo-Peridol (Can)** see Haloperidol on page 554
- **Novo-Pirocam® (Can)** see Piroxicam on page 910
- **Novo-Prazin (Can)** see Prazosin on page 924
- **Novo-Prednisolone® (Can)** see PrednisoLONE on page 925
- **Novo-Profen® (Can)** see Ibuprofen on page 588
- **Novo-Quinidin (Can)** see Quinidine on page 967
- **Novo-Ranidine (Can)** see Ranitidine on page 972
- **NovoRapid® (Can)** see Insulin Preparations on page 609
- **Novo-Sertraline (Can)** see Sertraline on page 1016

- Novo-Sotalol (Can) *see* Sotalol *on page 1032*
- Novo-Soxazole® (Can) *see* SulfiSOXAZOLE *on page 1056*
- Novo-Spiroton (Can) *see* Spironolactone *on page 1037*
- Novo-Spirozine (Can) *see* Hydrochlorothiazide and Spironolactone *on page 570*
- Novo-Sucralate (Can) *see* Sucralfate *on page 1046*
- Novo-Sundac (Can) *see* Sulindac *on page 1058*
- Novo-Tetra (Can) *see* Tetracycline *on page 1074*
- Novo-Theophyl SR (Can) *see* Theophylline *on page 1076*
- Novothyrox *see* Levothyroxine *on page 669*
- Novo-Trazodone (Can) *see* Trazodone *on page 1110*
- Novo-Trimel (Can) *see* Sulfamethoxazole and Trimethoprim *on page 1052*
- Novo-Trimel D.S. (Can) *see* Sulfamethoxazole and Trimethoprim *on page 1052*
- Novo-Veramil (Can) *see* Verapamil *on page 1144*
- Novo-Veramil SR (Can) *see* Verapamil *on page 1144*
- NPH Iletin® II *see* Insulin Preparations *on page 609*
- NS *see* Sodium Chloride *on page 1027*
- NSC-373364 *see* Aldesleukin *on page 56*
- NTG *see* Nitroglycerin *on page 815*
- Nu-Acyclovir (Can) *see* Acyclovir *on page 45*
- Nu-Alprax (Can) *see* Alprazolam *on page 64*
- Nu-Amoxi (Can) *see* Amoxicillin *on page 94*
- Nu-Ampi (Can) *see* Ampicillin *on page 103*
- Nu-Atenol (Can) *see* Atenolol *on page 137*
- Nu-Baclo (Can) *see* Baclofen *on page 158*
- Nubain® *see* Nalbuphine *on page 791*
- Nu-Beclomethasone (Can) *see* Beclomethasone *on page 160*
- Nu-Buspirone (Can) *see* BusPIRone *on page 191*
- Nu-Capto® (Can) *see* Captopril *on page 207*
- Nu-Carbamazepine® (Can) *see* Carbamazepine *on page 209*
- Nu-Cefaclor (Can) *see* Cefaclor *on page 223*
- Nu-Cephalex® (Can) *see* Cephalexin *on page 244*
- Nu-Cimet® (Can) *see* Cimetidine *on page 272*
- Nu-Clonazepam (Can) *see* Clonazepam *on page 292*
- Nu-Clonidine® (Can) *see* Clonidine *on page 294*
- Nu-Cloxi® (Can) *see* Cloxacillin *on page 298*
- Nu-Cotrimox® (Can) *see* Sulfamethoxazole and Trimethoprim *on page 1052*
- Nu-Cromolyn (Can) *see* Cromolyn *on page 311*
- Nu-Cyclobenzaprine (Can) *see* Cyclobenzaprine *on page 318*
- Nu-Desipramine (Can) *see* Desipramine *on page 349*
- Nu-Diclo (Can) *see* Diclofenac *on page 374*
- Nu-Diclo-SR (Can) *see* Diclofenac *on page 374*
- Nu-Diltiaz (Can) *see* Diltiazem *on page 388*
- Nu-Diltiaz-CD (Can) *see* Diltiazem *on page 388*
- Nu-Divalproex (Can) *see* Valproic Acid and Derivatives *on page 1131*
- Nu-Doxycycline (Can) *see* Doxycycline *on page 415*
- Nu-Erythromycin-S (Can) *see* Erythromycin *on page 448*
- Nu-Famotidine (Can) *see* Famotidine *on page 473*
- Nu-Fluoxetine (Can) *see* Fluoxetine *on page 505*
- Nu-Flurprofen (Can) *see* Flurbiprofen *on page 510*
- Nu-Glyburide (Can) *see* GlyBURIDE *on page 540*
- Nu-Hydral (Can) *see* HydrALAZINE *on page 568*
- Nu-Ibuprofen (Can) *see* Ibuprofen *on page 588*
- Nu-Indo (Can) *see* Indomethacin *on page 606*
- Nu-Ipratropium (Can) *see* Ipratropium *on page 620*
- Nu-Iron® 150 [OTC] *see* Iron Supplements (Oral/Enteral) *on page 623*
- NuLev™ *see* Hyoscyamine *on page 585*
- Nu-Loraz (Can) *see* Lorazepam *on page 695*
- NuLYTELY® *see* Polyethylene Glycol-Electrolyte Solution *on page 914*
- Nu-Medopa (Can) *see* Methyldopa *on page 741*
- Nu-Megestrol (Can) *see* Megestrol *on page 714*
- Nu-Metformin (Can) *see* Metformin *on page 729*
- Nu-Metoclopramide (Can) *see* Metoclopramide *on page 749*

- **Nu-Metop (Can)** *see* Metoprolol *on page 752*
- **Nu-Naprox (Can)** *see* Naproxen *on page 796*
- **Nu-Nifed (Can)** *see* NIFEdipine *on page 811*
- **Nu-Nortriptyline (Can)** *see* Nortriptyline *on page 822*
- **Nu-Oxybutyn (Can)** *see* Oxybutynin *on page 843*
- **Nu-Pentoxifylline SR (Can)** *see* Pentoxifylline *on page 884*
- **Nu-Pen-VK® (Can)** *see* Penicillin V Potassium *on page 877*
- **Nupercainal® [OTC]** *see* Dibucaine *on page 373*
- **Nupercainal® Hemorrhoidal and Anesthetic Ointment [OTC]** *see* Hemorrhoidal Preparations *on page 556*
- **Nupercainal® Hydrocortisone Cream [OTC]** *see* Hemorrhoidal Preparations *on page 556*
- **Nupercainal® Hydrocortisone Cream [OTC]** *see* Hydrocortisone *on page 573*
- **Nu-Pirox (Can)** *see* Piroxicam *on page 910*
- **Nu-Prazo (Can)** *see* Prazosin *on page 924*
- **Nu-Prochlor (Can)** *see* Prochlorperazine *on page 938*
- **Nu-Propranolol (Can)** *see* Propranolol *on page 952*
- **Nu-Ranit (Can)** *see* Ranitidine *on page 972*
- **Nuromax®** *see* Doxacurium *on page 408*
- **Nu-Sotalol (Can)** *see* Sotalol *on page 1032*
- **Nu-Sucralate (Can)** *see* Sucralfate *on page 1046*
- **Nu-Sundac (Can)** *see* Sulindac *on page 1058*
- **Nu-Tetra (Can)** *see* Tetracycline *on page 1074*
- **Nu-Timolol (Can)** *see* Timolol *on page 1095*
- **Nutracort®** *see* Hydrocortisone *on page 573*
- **Nu-Trazodone (Can)** *see* Trazodone *on page 1110*
- **Nutropin®** *see* Human Growth Hormone *on page 564*
- **Nutropin® AQ** *see* Human Growth Hormone *on page 564*
- **Nutropin Depot®** *see* Human Growth Hormone *on page 564*
- **Nutropine® (Can)** *see* Human Growth Hormone *on page 564*
- **Nu-Verap (Can)** *see* Verapamil *on page 1144*
- **Nyaderm (Can)** *see* Nystatin *on page 827*
- **Nydrazid®** *see* Isoniazid *on page 629*

Nystatin (nye STAT in)

Related Information
Carbohydrate and Alcohol Content of Liquid Medications for Use in Patients Receiving Ketogenic Diets *on page 1431*

U.S. Brand Names Bio-Statin®; Mycostatin®; Nystat-Rx®; Nystop®; Pedi-Dri®

Canadian Brand Names Candistatin®; Nilstat; Nyaderm; PMS-Nystatin

Therapeutic Category Antifungal Agent, Oral Nonabsorbed; Antifungal Agent, Topical; Antifungal Agent, Vaginal

Generic Available Yes (cream, ointment, suspension, and tablet)

Use Treatment of susceptible cutaneous, mucocutaneous, oral cavity and vaginal fungal infections normally caused by the *Candida* species

Pregnancy Risk Factor B

Contraindications Hypersensitivity to nystatin or any component

Adverse Reactions
Dermatologic: Contact dermatitis, Stevens-Johnson syndrome
Gastrointestinal: Nausea, vomiting, diarrhea
Local: Irritation

Stability Store vaginal inserts in refrigerator; protect from moisture and light

Mechanism of Action Binds to sterols in fungal cell membrane, changing the cell wall permeability allowing for leakage of cellular contents

Pharmacodynamics Onset of action: Symptomatic relief from candidiasis: Within 24-72 hours

Pharmacokinetics
Absorption: Not absorbed through mucous membranes or intact skin; poorly absorbed from the GI tract
Elimination: In feces as unchanged drug

Usual Dosage
Oral candidiasis:
Neonates: 100,000 units 4 times/day or 50,000 units to each side of mouth 4 times/day
(Continued)

Nystatin *(Continued)*

Infants: 200,000 units 4 times/day or 100,000 units to each side of mouth 4 times/day

Children and Adults: 400,000-600,000 units 4 times/day; troche: 200,000-400,000 units 4-5 times/day

Cutaneous candidal infections: Children and Adults: Topical: Apply 2-4 times/day

Intestinal infections: Adults: Oral: 500,000-1,000,000 units every 8 hours

Vaginal infections: Adolescents and Adults: Vaginal tablets: Insert 1 tablet/day at bedtime for 2 weeks

Administration

Oral: Shake suspension well before use; suspension should be swished about the mouth and retained in the mouth for as long as possible (several minutes) before swallowing. For neonates and infants, paint nystatin suspension into recesses of the mouth. Troches must be allowed to dissolve slowly and should not be chewed or swallowed whole.

Topical:

Cream or ointment: Gently massage formulation into the skin

Intravaginal: Insert vaginal tablet high in the vagina

Powder: Dust in shoes, in stockings, and on feet for treatment of candidal infection of the feet; also used on very moist lesions

Patient Information Inform physician if irritation or sensitization occur during therapy

Dosage Forms

Capsule (Bio-Statin®): 500,000 units, 1 million units

Cream: 100,000 units/g (15 g, 30 g) [contains propylene glycol]

Mycostatin®: 100,000 units/g (30 g) [contains propylene glycol]

Lozenge (Mycostatin®): 200,000 units

Ointment, topical: 100,000 units/g (15 g, 30 g)

Powder for prescription compounding: 50 million units (10 g), 150 million units (30 g), 500 million units (100 g), 2 billion units (400 g)

Nystat-Rx®: 50 million units (10 g), 150 million units (30 g), 500 million units (100 g), 1 billion units (190 g), 2 billion units (350 g)

Powder, topical:

Mycostatin®, Nystop®: 100,000 units/g (15 g) [dispersed in talc]

Pedi-Dri®: 100,000 units/g (56.7 g)

Suspension, oral: 100,000 units/mL (5 mL, 60 mL, 480 mL)

Mycostatin®: 100,000 units/mL (60 mL, 480 mL) [contains ≤1% alcohol; cherry-mint flavor]

Tablet, film coated, oral (Mycostatin®): 500,000 units

Tablet, vaginal: 100,000 units (15s) [packaged with applicator]

References
Dismukes WE, Wade JS, Lee JY, et al, "A Randomized, Double-Blind Trial of Nystatin Therapy for the Candidiasis Hypersensitivity Syndrome," *N Engl J Med*, 1990, 323(25):1717-23.

♦ **Nystat-Rx®** *see* Nystatin *on page 827*
♦ **Nystop®** *see* Nystatin *on page 827*
♦ **Nytol® [OTC]** *see* DiphenhydrAMINE *on page 393*
♦ **Nytol® Maximum Strength [OTC]** *see* DiphenhydrAMINE *on page 393*
♦ **Occlusal™ (Can)** *see* Salicylic Acid *on page 1002*
♦ **Occlusal®-HP [OTC]** *see* Salicylic Acid *on page 1002*
♦ **Ocean [OTC]** *see* Sodium Chloride *on page 1027*
♦ **OCL® [DSC]** *see* Polyethylene Glycol-Electrolyte Solution *on page 914*
♦ **Octostim® (Can)** *see* Desmopressin *on page 352*

Octreotide Acetate *(ok TREE oh tide AS e tate)*

U.S. Brand Names Sandostatin®; Sandostatin LAR®

Therapeutic Category Antidiarrheal; Antisecretory Agent; Somatostatin Analog

Generic Available No

Use Control of symptoms in patients with metastatic carcinoid, vasoactive intestinal peptide-secreting tumors (VIPomas), and secretory diarrhea; acromegaly

Unlabeled use: AIDS-associated secretory diarrhea, control of bleeding of esophageal varices, breast cancer, cryptosporidiosis, Cushing's syndrome, insulinomas, small bowel fistulas, postgastrectomy dumping syndrome, chemotherapy-induced diarrhea, GVHD-induced diarrhea, Zollinger-Ellison syndrome, persistent hyperinsulinemic hypoglycemia of infancy (nesidioblastosis), postoperative chylothorax, treatment of sulfonylurea overdosage

Pregnancy Risk Factor B

Contraindications Hypersensitivity to octreotide or any component

Warnings Dosage adjustment may be required to maintain symptomatic control; insulin requirements may be reduced as well as sulfonylurea requirements

Precautions Patients must be monitored closely for biliary tract abnormalities (including biliary obstruction, cholecystitis, and cholelithiasis), hypothyroidism, and glucose tolerance; use with caution in patients with renal impairment and consider dosage modification in patients with severe renal failure requiring dialysis; use with caution in diabetic patients with gastroparesis; chronic usage is associated with depressed vitamin B_{12} levels; monitor vitamin B_{12} levels in patients receiving long-term therapy; suppression of growth hormone (animal data) is of concern when used as long-term therapy in children

Adverse Reactions

Cardiovascular: Flushing, edema, chest pain, hypertension, palpitations, CHF, ortho-static hypotension, syncope, bradycardia, arrhythmias, conduction abnormalities

Central nervous system: Dizziness, fatigue, anxiety, headache, depression, insomnia, fever, chills, seizures, vertigo, hyperesthesia, Bell's palsy

Dermatologic: Erythema, alopecia, bruising, pruritus, rash

Endocrine & metabolic: Hypoglycemia, hyperglycemia, galactorrhea, hypothyroidism

Gastrointestinal: Nausea, diarrhea, abdominal pain, vomiting, constipation, flatulence, fat malabsorption, GI bleeding (rare), xerostomia, dyspepsia, steatorrhea, choleli-thiasis, biliary sludge, pancreatitis

Genitourinary: Prostatitis

Hepatic: Hepatitis, jaundice, elevated liver enzymes

Local: Injection site pain, thrombophlebitis

Neuromuscular & skeletal: Weakness, increased CPK, backache, muscle spasm, muscle cramps, arthralgia, tremor, numbness

Ocular: Visual disturbance, ocular burning

Renal: Oliguria, urinary hyperosmolarity

Respiratory: Shortness of breath, rhinorrhea

Drug Interactions Cytochrome P450 isoenzyme CYP2D6 (high dose) and CYP3A inhibitor

May decrease cyclosporine levels (case report of a transplant rejection) possibly due to decreased cyclosporine bioavailability; may alter insulin and oral hypoglycemic agent requirements

Food Interactions Schedule injections between meals to decrease GI effects; may decrease vitamin B_{12} levels and decrease absorption of dietary fats

Stability Store in refrigerator; Sandostatin® injection is stable 14 days at room temper-ature if protected from light; stable in D_5W or NS for 4 days at room temperature; not compatible in TPN solutions due to glycosyl octreotide conjugate which may have decreased activity; Sandostatin LAR® Depot must be used immediately after reconsti-tution

Mechanism of Action A synthetic polypeptide which mimics natural somatostatin by inhibiting serotonin release, and the secretion of gastrin, vasoactive intestinal peptide (VIP), insulin, glucagon, secretin, motilin, and pancreatic polypeptide; in animals, also a potent inhibitor of growth hormone; decreases GI motility and inhibits intestinal secretion of water and electrolytes

Pharmacodynamics Duration (immediate release formulation): S.C.: 6-12 hours

Pharmacokinetics

Absorption:

S.C.: Rapid

I.M.(Sandostatin LAR® Depot): 60% to 63% when compared with S.C. immediate release formulation

Distribution: V_d:

Adults: 13.6 L/kg

Adults with acromegaly: 21.6 ± 8.5 L

Metabolism: Extensive by the liver

Half-life: 1.7 hours

Time to peak serum concentration: S.C.: 0.4 hours

Elimination: 32% excreted unchanged in urine

Clearance:

Adults: 10 L/hour

Adults with acromegaly: 18 L/hour

Note: When using Sandostatin LAR® Depot formulation, steady state levels are achieved after 3 injections (3 months of therapy)

Usual Dosage Dosage should be individualized according to the patient's response

Sandostatin®:

Diarrhea:

Infants and Children (limited data from case reports):

I.V., S.C.: Doses of 1-10 mcg/kg every 12 hours have been used in children beginning at the low end of the range and increasing based upon the clinical response

(Continued)

Octreotide Acetate *(Continued)*

I.V. continuous infusion: An initial 1 mcg/kg bolus dose followed by a continuous infusion of 1 mcg/kg/hour has been used successfully in several cases of severe diarrhea secondary to graft vs host disease

Adults:

S.C.: Initial: 50 mcg 1-2 times/day

I.V.: Initial: 50-100 mcg every 8 hours; increase by 100 mcg/dose at 48-hour intervals; maximum dose: 500 mcg every 8 hours

The following are effective dosing ranges for specific therapies: S.C., I.V.:

Children (limited data in case reports):

Persistent hyperinsulinemic hypoglycemia of infancy (nesidioblastosis): 2-10 mcg/kg/day initially divided every 12 hours; increase dosage depending upon patient response by either using a more frequent interval (every 6-8 hours) or larger dose; doses of 40 mcg/kg/day have been used

GI bleed: 1 mcg/kg initial bolus followed by 1 mcg/kg/hour continuous infusion; titrate infusion rate to response; taper dose by 50% every 12 hours when no active bleeding occurs for 24 hours; may discontinue when dose is 25% of initial dose

Chylothorax: 1-4 mcg/kg/hour continuous infusion has been used; titrate dose to response

Treatment of sulfonylurea overdose: 1 mcg/kg/dose every 12 hours or a single 25 mcg dose; the duration of treatment is dependent upon the sulfonylurea ingested and its half-life.

Adults:

Carcinoid: 100-600 mcg/day in 2-4 divided doses

VIPomas: 200-300 mcg/day in 2-4 divided doses; tachyphylaxis may occur requiring an increase in dosage up to 1000 mcg/day

Esophageal varices bleeding: I.V. bolus: 25-50 mcg followed by continuous I.V. infusion of 25-50 mcg/hour for 48 hours

Acromegaly: 50 mcg 3 times/day; increase as needed (usual requirement: 100 mcg 3 times/day); maximum dose: 500 mcg 3 times/day; hold dose for 4 weeks per year in patients who have been irradiated, to assess disease activity; resume therapy if growth hormone or somatomedin C (IGF-I) levels increase and signs and symptoms recur

AIDS-related diarrhea: 50-250 mcg every 8 hours; doses as high as 1500 mcg/day have been used; an improved response rate is reported in patients without infection-related diarrhea

Sandostatin LAR® Depot: May be used in patients who have responded to the immediate release formulation; Adults: I.M.:

Acromegaly: Initial: 20 mg at 4-week intervals for 3 months; dosage may be adjusted based upon the following:

Maintain same dosage IF: Growth hormone level <2.5 ng/mL, IGF-I normal, and clinical symptoms controlled

Increase dosage to 30 mg IF: Growth hormone level >2.5 ng/mL, IGF-I elevated, and clinical symptoms uncontrolled

Reduce dosage to 10 mg IF: Growth hormone level ≤1 ng/mL, IGF-I normal, and clinical symptoms controlled

[May increase dosage to maximum 40 mg every 4 weeks if 30 mg dosage ineffective; it is not recommended to administer dosage at intervals >4 weeks; hold dose for 8 weeks per year in patients who have been irradiated, to assess disease activity; resume therapy if growth hormone or somatomedin C (IGF-I) levels increase and signs and symptoms recur.]

VIPomas, carcinoid: Initial: 20 mg at 4-week intervals; due to the need for serum octreotide to reach therapeutically effective levels following initial injection for Sandostatin LAR® Depot, subcutaneous Sandostatin® injection should be continued at the current dosage **at the same time** for at least the first 2 weeks of therapy (some patients may require 3 or 4 weeks of such therapy). Adjust Sandostatin LAR® Depot dosage after 2 months of therapy depending upon patient response; doses >30 mg are not recommended

Dosage adjustment in renal impairment: Clearance is decreased by 50% in patients with severe renal failure requiring dialysis; consider dosage modification in these patients

Administration Parenteral: Only Sandostatin® injection may be administered I.V., I.M., and S.C.; Sandostatin LAR® Depot may only be administered I.M.

I.V. infusion: Dilute Sandostatin® injection in 50-200 mL NS or D$_5$W and infuse over 15-30 minutes or over 24 hours as a continuous infusion; in emergency situations, may be administered undiluted by direct I.V. push over 3 minutes; see Stability for compatibility information; allow solution to come to room temperature before administration

I.M. administration: Reconstitute with provided diluent; use immediately after reconstitution; administer into gluteal area only (avoid deltoid injections due to significant pain and discomfort at injection site)

Monitoring Parameters Baseline and periodic ultrasound evaluations for cholelithiasis, blood sugar, baseline and periodic thyroid function tests, fluid and electrolyte balance, fecal fat, and serum carotene determinations; for carcinoid, monitor urinary 5-hydroxyindole acetic acid (5-HIAA), plasma serotonin, plasma substance P; for VIPoma, monitor VIP; vitamin B_{12} levels (chronic therapy); for acromegaly: growth hormone levels, IGF-I (somatomedin C)

Reference Range Vasoactive intestinal peptide (VIP): <75 ng/L; levels vary considerably between laboratories; growth hormone level: <5 ng/mL; IGF-I (somatomedin C): males: <1.9 units/mL, females: <2.2 units/mL

Patient Information May cause dry mouth

Dosage Forms

Injection, microspheres for suspension, as acetate [depot formulation] (Sandostatin LAR®): 10 mg, 20 mg, 30 mg [packaged with diluent and syringe]

Injection, solution, as acetate (Sandostatin®): 0.05 mg/mL (1 mL); 0.1 mg/mL (1 mL); 0.2 mg/mL (5 mL); 0.5 mg/mL (1 mL); 1 mg/mL (5 mL)

References

Beckman RA, Siden R, Yanik GA, et al, "Continuous Octreotide Infusion for the Treatment of Secretory Diarrhea Caused by Acute Intestinal Graft-Versus-Host Disease in a Child," *J Pediatr Hematol Oncol*, 2000, 22(4):344-50.

Cheung Y, Leung MP, and Yip M, "Octreotide for Treatment of Postoperative Chylothorax," *J Pediatr*, 2001, 139(1):157-9.

Couper RT, Berzen A, Berall G, et al, "Clinical Response to the Long-Acting Somatostatin Analogue SMS 201-995 in a Child With Congenital Microvillus Atrophy," *Gut*, 1989, 30(7):1020-4.

Jaros W, Biller J, Greer S, et al, "Successful Treatment of Idiopathic Secretory Diarrhea of Infancy With the Somatostatin Analogue SMS 201-995," *Gastroenterology*, 1988, 94(1):189-93.

Katz MD and Erstad BL, "Octreotide, A New Somatostatin Analogue," *Clin Pharm*, 1989, 8(4):255-73.

Pratap U, Slavik Z, Ofoe VD, et al, "Octreotide to Treat Postoperative Chylothorax After Cardiac Operations in Children," *Ann Thorac Surg*, 2001, 72(5):1740-2.

Siafakas C, Fox VL, and Nurko S, "Use of Octreotide for the Treatment of Severe Gastrointestinal Bleeding in Children," *J Pediatr Gastroenterol Nutr*, 1998, 26(3):356-9.

Stanley CA, "Hyperinsulinism in Infants and Children," *Pediatr Clin North Am*, 1997, 44(2):363-74.

♦ **OcuClear®** [OTC] [DSC] see Oxymetazoline *on page 849*

♦ **Ocufen®** see Flurbiprofen *on page 510*

Ocular Lubricant (OK yoo lar LOO bri kant)

U.S. Brand Names Hypotears® [OTC]; Lacri-Lube SOP [OTC]; Moisture-Eyes™ PM [OTC]; Puralube® [OTC]; Refresh PM® [OTC]; Tears Naturale® PM [OTC]; Tears Renewed® [OTC]

Therapeutic Category Lubricant, Ocular; Ophthalmic Agent, Miscellaneous

Generic Available Yes

Use Ocular lubricant

Contraindications Hypersensitivity to any component

Warnings Discontinue if eye pain, vision change, redness or eye irritation occurs or if condition worsens or persists >72 hours

Adverse Reactions Ocular: Temporary blurring of vision, irritation

Stability Store away from heat

Mechanism of Action Forms an occlusive film on the surface of the eye to lubricate and protect the eye from drying

Usual Dosage Children and Adults: Ophthalmic: Apply ¼" of ointment to the inside of the lower lid as needed

Administration Ophthalmic: Do not use with contact lenses; to avoid contamination, do not touch tip of container to any surface

Additional Information Contains petrolatum, mineral oil, chlorobutanol and lanolin alcohols

Dosage Forms

Ointment, ophthalmic: 3.5 g [mineral oil and white petrolatum]

Hypotears®, Moisture-Eyes™ PM, Puralube®, Refresh PM®, Tears Naturale® PM, Tears Renewed®: 3.5 g [mineral oil and white petrolatum]

Lacri-Lube® SOP: 3.5 g, 7 g [mineral oil and white petrolatum]

♦ **Oculinum®** see Botulinum Toxin Type A *on page 178*

♦ **Ocu-Pentolate®** see Cyclopentolate *on page 319*

♦ **Ocusert Pilo-20®** [DSC] see Pilocarpine *on page 903*

♦ **Ocusert Pilo-40®** [DSC] see Pilocarpine *on page 903*

♦ **Ocusulf-10** see Sulfacetamide *on page 1048*

♦ **Ocu-Trol®** see Dexamethasone, Neomycin, and Polymyxin B *on page 357*

♦ **Ocu-Tropine®** see Atropine *on page 144*

♦ **Oesclim® (Can)** see Estradiol *on page 456*

- ♦ **OKT3** *see* Muromonab-CD3 *on page 784*
- ♦ **Oleovitamin A** *see* Vitamin A *on page 1151*
- ♦ **Oleum Ricini** *see* Castor Oil *on page 222*

Olsalazine (ole SAL a zeen)

U.S. Brand Names Dipentum®

Therapeutic Category 5-Aminosalicylic Acid Derivative; Anti-inflammatory Agent

Generic Available No

Use Maintenance of remission of ulcerative colitis in patients intolerant to sulfasalazine

Pregnancy Risk Factor C

Contraindications Hypersensitivity to olsalazine, salicylates, or any component

Warnings Diarrhea is a common adverse effect of olsalazine

Precautions Use with caution in patients with hypersensitivity to sulfasalazine, salicylates, or mesalamine

Adverse Reactions

Cardiovascular: Pericarditis, heart block, hypertension, orthostatic hypotension, edema, chest pain, tachycardia

Central nervous system: Headache, fatigue, drowsiness, depression, insomnia, vertigo, fever

Dermatologic: Erythema nodosum, photosensitivity, rash, pruritus

Gastrointestinal: Diarrhea, cramps, nausea, dyspepsia, bloating, vomiting, pancreatitis, rectal bleeding, xerostomia

Genitourinary: Urinary frequency, dysuria

Hematologic: Leukopenia, neutropenia, lymphopenia, eosinophilia, thrombocytopenia

Hepatic: Mild cholestatic hepatitis, elevated AST and ALT

Neuromuscular & skeletal: Arthralgia, tremor, paresthesia

Ocular: Blurred vision, dry eyes

Renal: Hematuria, proteinuria

Respiratory: Bronchospasm, respiratory infection

Drug Interactions Increases effects of warfarin

Mechanism of Action Olsalazine is a sodium salt of a salicylate compound that is effectively bioconverted by colonic bacteria to 5-aminosalicylic acid (5-ASA). The exact mechanism of action appears to be topical rather than systemic. It may diminish colonic inflammation by blocking cyclooxygenase and inhibiting colon prostaglandin production in the bowel mucosa.

Pharmacokinetics

Absorption: <3%; very little intact olsalazine is systemically absorbed

Protein binding: >99%

Metabolism: Mostly by colonic bacteria to the active drug, 5-aminosalicylic acid

Bioavailability: 2.4%

Half-life, elimination: 56 minutes (in serum)

Elimination: Primarily in feces; <1% eliminated in urine

Usual Dosage Adults: Oral: 1 g/day in 2 divided doses

Administration Oral: Administer with food in evenly divided doses

Patient Information Contact physician if diarrhea occurs. May cause dry mouth. May rarely cause photosensitivity reactions (eg, exposure to sunlight may cause severe sunburn, skin rash, redness, or itching); avoid direct exposure to sunlight.

Dosage Forms Capsule, as sodium: 250 mg

Omeprazole (oh ME pray zol)

U.S. Brand Names Prilosec®

Canadian Brand Names Losec®

Therapeutic Category Gastric Acid Secretion Inhibitor; Gastrointestinal Agent, Gastric or Duodenal Ulcer Treatment; Proton Pump Inhibitor

Generic Available Yes

Use Treatment and maintenance of healing of severe erosive esophagitis (grade 2 or above); treatment of active duodenal ulcer; treatment of active benign gastric ulcers; treatment of symptomatic gastroesophageal reflux disease (GERD); treatment of pathological hypersecretory conditions; treatment of peptic ulcer disease; adjunctive treatment of duodenal ulcers associated with *Helicobacter pylori*

Pregnancy Risk Factor C

Contraindications Hypersensitivity to omeprazole, pantoprazole, esomeprazole, lansoprazole, or any component

Warnings In long-term (2-year) studies in rats, omeprazole produced a dose-related increase in gastric carcinoid tumors. While available endoscopic evaluations and histologic examinations of biopsy specimens from human stomachs have not detected a risk from short-term exposure to omeprazole, further human data on the effect of sustained hypochlorhydria and hypergastrinemia are needed to rule out the possibility of an increased risk for the development of tumors in humans receiving long-term therapy.

Adverse Reactions

Cardiovascular: Chest pain, tachycardia, bradycardia, palpitations

Central nervous system: Headache, dizziness, vertigo, insomnia, anxiety, hemifacial dysesthesia, nervousness, fever

Dermatologic: Rash, dry skin

Endocrine & metabolic: Hypoglycemia

Gastrointestinal: Diarrhea, nausea, abdominal pain, vomiting, constipation, flatulence, discoloration of feces, irritable colon, xerostomia, anorexia, dysgeusia, abdominal pain

Genitourinary: Urinary frequency

Hematologic: Agranulocytosis, pancytopenia, thrombocytopenia, anemia, leukocytosis

Hepatic: Hepatitis, elevated liver function tests, jaundice

Neuromuscular & skeletal: Muscle cramps, myalgia, arthralgia, leg pain, paresthesia, back pain

Otic: Tinnitus

Renal: Hematuria, pyuria, proteinuria, glycosuria

Respiratory: Pharyngeal pain, cough, epistaxis

Drug Interactions
Cytochrome P450 isoenzyme CYP1A2 inducer; isoenzyme CYP2C8, CYP2C18, CYP2C19, and CYP3A3/4 substrate; isoenzyme CYP2C9, CYP3A3/4, CYP2C8, and CYP2C19 inhibitor

Omeprazole inhibits oxidative metabolism; the full potential related to specific drugs remains to be determined; decreases absorption of ketoconazole, itraconazole, iron salts, ampicillin esters; increases half-life (decreased clearance) of diazepam, phenytoin, and warfarin; may increase absorption of digoxin and didanosine; may decrease elimination of methotrexate

Food Interactions
A 25% reduction in peak plasma concentration was measured when the 20 mg capsule was mixed with applesauce; there was no change in AUC; the clinical significance is unknown. There was no change in peak plasma level or AUC when the 40 mg capsule was mixed with applesauce.

Stability
Omeprazole stability is a function of pH; it is rapidly degraded in acidic media, but has acceptable stability under alkaline conditions. Each capsule of omeprazole contains enteric coated granules to prevent omeprazole degradation by gastric acidity.

Mechanism of Action
Suppresses gastric acid secretion by inhibiting the parietal cell membrane enzyme (H^+/K^+)-ATPase or proton pump; demonstrates antimicrobial activity against *Helicobacter pylori*

Pharmacodynamics
Onset of action: 1 hour

Maximum effect: 2 hours

Duration: 72 hours

Maximum secretory inhibition: 4 days

Pharmacokinetics
Protein binding: 95%

Metabolism: Extensive first-pass metabolism in the liver

Bioavailability: 30% to 40%; improves slightly with repeated administration

Half-life: 0.5-1 hour

Note: Half-life and AUC were significantly reduced for omeprazole suspension when compared with an equivalent dose via the commercially available capsule in 7 adults (Song, 2001).

Usual Dosage
Oral:

GERD, ulcers, esophagitis:

Children: 1 mg/kg/day once or twice daily; range of effective dosages in the literature: 0.2-3.5 mg/kg/day (Hassall, 2000; Zimmermann, 2001). Higher doses may be necessary in children between 1-6 years of age due to increased metabolic clearance (Andersson, 2000). In critically ill children to maintain gastric pH >5, administration every 6-8 hours may be necessary (1.5-2 mg/kg/day) (Kaufman, 2002)

Manufacturer's recommendations (as an alternative): Children ≥2 years:

≤20 kg: 10 mg once daily

>20 kg: 20 mg once daily

Adults:

Active duodenal ulcer: 20 mg/day for 4-8 weeks

Gastric ulcers: 40 mg/day for 4-8 weeks

GERD or severe erosive esophagitis: 20 mg/day for 4-8 weeks

Pathological hypersecretory conditions: 60 mg/day to start; doses up to 120 mg 3 times/day have been administered; administer daily doses >80 mg in divided doses

(Continued)

Omeprazole *(Continued)*

Adjunctive therapy of duodenal ulcers associated with *Helicobacter pylori* [in combination with antibiotic therapy]:

Children (Gottrand, 2001):

15-30 kg: 10 mg twice daily

>30 kg: 20 mg twice daily

Adults: 20 mg twice daily or 40 mg once daily

Administration Oral: Administer before food or meals; capsule should be swallowed whole, do not chew or crush; because the enteric coating of granules will dissolve in alkaline pH, administration via NG tube should be in acidic juice (eg, apple juice or cranberry juice); stable 30 minutes after mixing; may add contents of capsule to applesauce and swallow immediately; do not crush or chew granules; to administer via jejunostomy tube, crush the granules and dissolve in a mixture of water to which a crushed 650 mg sodium bicarbonate tablet has been added

Patient Information May cause dry mouth; do not chew or crush granules

Dosage Forms

Capsule, delayed release: 10 mg, 20 mg

Prilosec®: 10 mg, 20 mg, 40 mg

Extemporaneous Preparations Omeprazole 2 mg/mL suspension may be made by adding 100 mL 8.4% sodium bicarbonate solution to the contents of ten 20 mg omeprazole capsules; stir for 30 minutes; protect from light; stable 14 days at room temperature and 45 days refrigerated

DiGiacinto JL, Olsen KM, Bergman KL, et al, "Stability of Suspension Formulations of Lansoprazole and Omeprazole Stored in Amber-colored Plastic Oral Syringes," *Ann Pharmacother*, 2000, 34(5):600-4.

References

Andersson T, Hassall E, Lundborg P, et al, "Pharmacokinetics of Orally Administered Omeprazole in Children. International Pediatric Omeprazole Pharmacokinetic Group," *Am J Gastroenterol*, 2000, 95(11):3101-6.

Gibbons TE and Gold BD, "The Use of Proton Pump Inhibitors in Children: A Comprehensive Review," *Paediatr Drugs*, 2003, 5(1):25-40.

Gottrand F, Kalach N, Spyckerelle C, et al, "Omeprazole Combined With Amoxicillin and Clarithromycin in the Eradication of *Helicobacter pylori* in Children With Gastritis: A Prospective Randomized Double-Blind Trial," *J Pediatr*, 2001, 139(5):664-8.

Gunasekaran TS and Hassall EG, "Efficacy and Safety of Omeprazole for Severe Gastroesophageal Reflux in Children," *J Pediatr*, 1993, 123(1):148-54.

Hassall E, Israel D, Shepherd R, "Omeprazole for Treatment of Chronic Erosive Esophagitis in Children: A Multicenter Study of Efficacy, Safety, Tolerability and Dose Requirements. International Pediatric Omeprazole Study Group," *J Pediatr*, 2000, 137(6):800-7.

Kane DL, "Administration of Omeprazole (Prilosec™) in the Atypical Patient," *Int J Pharm Compounding*, 1997, 1(1):13.

Kato S, Ebina K, Fujii K, et al, "Effect of Omeprazole in the Treatment of Refractory Acid-Related Diseases in Childhood: Endoscopic Healing and Twenty-Four Hour Intragastric Acidity," *J Pediatr*, 1996, 128(3):415-21.

Kaufman SS, Lyden ER, Brown CR, et al, "Omeprazole Therapy in Pediatric Patients After Liver and Intestinal Transplantation," *J Pediatr Gastroenterol Nutr*, 2002, 34(2):194-8.

Song JC, Quercia RA, Fan C, et al, "Pharmacokinetic Comparison of Omeprazole Capsules and a Simplified Omeprazole Suspension," *Am J Health Syst Pharm*, 2001, 58(8):689-94.

Zimmermann AE, Walters JK, Katona BG, et al, "A Review of Omeprazole Use in the Treatment of Acid-Related Disorders in Children," *Clin Ther*, 2003, 23(5):660-79.

♦ **Omnicef®** *see Cefdinir on page 226*

♦ **Oncaspar®** *see Pegaspargase on page 869*

♦ **Oncovin® [DSC]** *see VinCRIStine on page 1149*

Ondansetron *(on DAN se tron)*

U.S. Brand Names Zofran®; Zofran® ODT

Therapeutic Category Antiemetic; 5-HT$_3$ Receptor Antagonist

Generic Available No

Use Prevention of nausea and vomiting associated with highly emetogenic cancer chemotherapy or radiotherapy and prevention of postoperative nausea and vomiting

Pregnancy Risk Factor B

Contraindications Hypersensitivity to ondansetron, other 5-HT$_3$ receptor antagonists, or any component

Warnings Zofran® solution contains sodium benzoate; benzoic acid (benzoate) is a metabolite of benzyl alcohol; large amounts of benzyl alcohol (≥99 mg/kg/day) have been associated with a potentially fatal toxicity ("gasping syndrome") in neonates; *in vitro* and animal studies have shown that benzoate displaces bilirubin from protein binding sites; avoid use of Zofran® solution in neonates.

Precautions Zofran® ODT tablets contain aspartame; use with caution in patients with phenylketonuria

Adverse Reactions

Cardiovascular: Tachycardia, bradycardia, angina, syncope

Central nervous system: Lightheadedness, seizures, headache, dizziness, drowsiness, sedation, fatigue, fever, shivers

Dermatologic: Rash, local injection site reaction

Endocrine & metabolic: Hypokalemia

Gastrointestinal: Constipation, diarrhea, abdominal pain, xerostomia

Hepatic: Transient elevations in liver enzymes

Neuromuscular & skeletal: Weakness, musculoskeletal pain, tremor, twitching, ataxia

Ocular: Blurred vision

Respiratory: Bronchospasm

Miscellaneous: Hypersensitivity reactions

Drug Interactions Cytochrome P450 isoenzyme CYP1A2, CYP2D6, CYP2E1, and CYP3A3/4 substrate

No documented drug interactions; however, ondansetron does contain the same imidazole nucleus as cimetidine and omeprazole; patients receiving concurrent theophylline, phenytoin, or warfarin should be followed closely

Stability

Compatible for 7 days at room temperature when diluted in saline or dextrose solutions; Y-site injection compatibility with bleomycin, carboplatin, carmustine, chlorpromazine, cisplatin, cyclophosphamide, cytarabine, dacarbazine, dactinomycin, daunorubicin, dexamethasone, diphenhydramine, doxorubicin, droperidol, etoposide, fludarabine, ifosfamide, mechlorethamine, methotrexate, mesna, metoclopramide, mitoxantrone, prochlorperazine, promethazine, teniposide, vinblastine, and vincristine

Incompatible with acyclovir, ampicillin, aminophylline, furosemide, ganciclovir, lorazepam, methylprednisolone, and piperacillin

Mechanism of Action Selective 5-HT$_3$ receptor antagonist, blocking serotonin, both peripherally on vagal nerve terminals and centrally in the chemoreceptor trigger zone

Pharmacokinetics

Absorption: Oral: 100%; nonlinear absorption occurs with increasing oral doses; Zofran® ODT tablets are bioequivalent to Zofran® tablets; absorption does not occur via oral mucosa

Distribution: V$_d$: Children: 1.6-1.7 L/kg; Adults: 1.9 L/kg

Protein binding, plasma: 70% to 76%

Metabolism: Extensive first-pass metabolism; primarily by hydroxylation, followed by glucuronidation and sulfate conjugation

Bioavailability: Oral: 50% to 70% due to significant first-pass metabolism; in cancer patients (adult) 85% to 87% bioavailability possibly related to changes in metabolism

Half-life:

Children: 3-7 years: 2.6 hours; 7-12 years: 3.1 hours

Adults: 4-5 hours

Elimination: In urine and feces; <5% of the parent drug is recovered unchanged in urine

Clearance:

Children: 3-7 years: 0.5 L/hour/kg; 7-12 years: 0.39 L/hour/kg

Adults: 25-50.7 L/hour (normal); 16-32 L/hour (cancer)

Usual Dosage

Prevention of chemotherapy- or radiotherapy-induced nausea and vomiting:

Oral (all doses given 30 minutes before chemotherapy or 1-2 hours prior to radiotherapy and repeated at 8-hour intervals):

Children <4 years: No FDA-approved oral dosage; however, the following dosages based upon body surface area have been used:

<0.3 m^2: 1 mg 3 times/day

0.3-0.6 m^2: 2 mg 3 times/day

0.6-1 m^2: 3 mg 3 times/day

>1 m^2: 4 mg 3 times/day

or

Children 4-11 years: 4 mg 3 times/day

Children >11 years and Adults: 8 mg 3 times/day or 24 mg once daily

Adults: Total body irradiation: 8 mg 1-2 hours before each fraction of radiotherapy administered each day

Single high-dose fraction radiotherapy to abdomen: 8 mg 1-2 hours before irradiation, then 8 mg every 8 hours after first dose for 1-2 days after completion of radiotherapy

Daily fractionated radiotherapy to abdomen: 8 mg 1-2 hours before irradiation, then 8 mg every 8 hours after first dose for each day of radiotherapy

I.V.:

Children >3 years: 0.15 mg/kg/dose infused 30 minutes before the start of emetogenic chemotherapy, with subsequent doses administered 4 and 8 hours after the first dose

(Continued)

Ondansetron *(Continued)*

Adults: A single 32 mg dose/day or 0.15 mg/kg/dose or 45-80 kg: 8 mg, >80 kg: 12 mg infused 30 minutes before the start of emetogenic chemotherapy with subsequent doses administered 4 and 8 hours after the first dose; a few studies have evaluated a single 8 mg loading dose followed by a continuous 1 mg/hour infusion

Prevention of postoperative nausea and vomiting: I.V.: Give immediately before induction of anesthesia, or postoperatively if the patient is symptomatic:

Children ≥2 years <40 kg: 0.1 mg/kg

Children >40 kg and Adults: 4 mg

Note: Repeating a second ondansetron dose in patients who did not achieve adequate control of postoperative nausea and vomiting after a single dose will not provide additional control.

Dosing adjustment in severe hepatic impairment: Adults: Once daily dosage; maximum 8 mg per dose

Administration

Oral: May administer without regard to meals; Zofran® ODT tablet: Place tablet on tongue, it will disintegrate immediately; may also swallow with fluids as whole tablet

Parenteral:

I.V.: Dilute in 50 mL I.V. fluid (maximum concentration: 1 mg/mL) and infuse over 15 minutes; single doses for prevention of postoperative nausea/vomiting may be administered I.V. undiluted over 2-5 minutes

I.M.: Administer as undiluted injection

Patient Information May cause dry mouth

Dosage Forms

Infusion, as **hydrochloride** [premixed in dextrose] (Zofran®): 32 mg (50 mL)

Injection, solution, as **hydrochloride** (Zofran®): 2 mg/mL (2 mL, 20 mL)

Solution, as **hydrochloride** (Zofran®): 4 mg/5 mL (50 mL) [contains sodium benzoate; strawberry flavor]

Tablet, as **hydrochloride** (Zofran®): 4 mg, 8 mg, 24 mg

Tablet, orally disintegrating, as **base** (Zofran® ODT): 4 mg, 8 mg [contains <0.03 mg phenylalanine (as aspartame)/tablet; strawberry flavor]

References

"ASHP Therapeutic Guidelines on the Pharmacologic Management of Nausea and Vomiting in Adult and Pediatric Patients Receiving Chemotherapy or Radiation Therapy or Undergoing Surgery," *Am J Health Syst Pharm,* 1999, 56(8):729-64.

Carden PA, Mitchell SL, Waters KD, et al, "Prevention of Cyclophosphamide/Cytarabine-Induced Emesis With Ondansetron in Children With Leukemia," *J Clin Oncol,* 1990, 8(9):1531-5.

Marty M, Pouillart P, Scholl S, et al, "Comparison of the 5-hydroxytryptamine 3 (Serotonin) Antagonist Ondansetron (GR 38032F) With High-Dose Metoclopramide in the Control of Cisplatin-Induced Emesis," *N Engl J Med,* 1990, 322(12):816-21.

Pinkerton CR, Williams D, Wootton C, et al, "5-HT$_3$ Antagonist Ondansetron - An Effective Outpatient Antiemetic in Cancer Treatment," *Arch Dis Child,* 1990, 65(8):822-5.

Roila F and Del Favero A, "Ondansetron Clinical Pharmacokinetics," *Clin Pharmacokinet,* 1995, 29(2):95-109.

Seynaeve C, Schuller J, Buser K, et al, "Comparison of the Anti-emetic Efficacy of Different Doses of Ondansetron, Given as Either a Continuous Infusion or a Single Intravenous Dose, in Acute Cisplatin-Induced Emesis," *Br J Cancer* 1992, 66(1):192-7.

Spahr-Schopfer IA, Lerman J, Sikich N, et al, "Pharmacokinetics of Intravenous Ondansetron in Healthy Children Undergoing Ear, Nose, and Throat Surgery," *Clin Pharmacol Ther,* 1995, 58(3):316-21.

Spector JI, Lester EP, Chevlen EM, et al, "A Comparison of Oral Ondansetron and Intravenous Granisetron for the Prevention of Nausea and Emesis Associated With Cisplatin-Based Chemotherapy," *Oncologist,* 1998, 3(6):432-438.

♦ **Ophthetic®** *see* Proparacaine *on page 946*

♦ **Ophtho-Dipivefrin™ (Can)** *see* Dipivefrin *on page 396*

♦ **Ophtho-Tate® (Can)** *see* PrednisoLONE *on page 925*

Opium Tincture *(OH pee um TING chur)*

Related Information

Overdose and Toxicology *on page 1388*

Synonyms Deodorized Opium Tincture; DTO; Tincture of Opium

Therapeutic Category Analgesic, Narcotic; Antidiarrheal

Generic Available Yes

Use Treatment of diarrhea or relief of pain; **a 25-fold dilution with water** (final concentration 0.4 mg/mL morphine) can be used to treat neonatal abstinence syndrome (opiate withdrawal)

Restrictions C-II

Pregnancy Risk Factor B (D if used for prolonged periods or in high doses at term)

Contraindications Hypersensitivity to opium, morphine, or any component; diarrhea caused by poisoning until the toxic material has been removed; increased intracranial pressure, severe respiratory depression, severe liver or renal insufficiency

Warnings Do not confuse opium tincture with paregoric; opium tincture is 25 times as potent as paregoric; opium shares the toxic potential of opiate agonists, usual precautions of opiate agonist therapy should be observed; opium may mask dehydration by producing fluid retention in the bowel; monitor patients with prolonged or severe diarrhea carefully; abrupt discontinuation after prolonged use may result in withdrawal symptoms

Precautions Use with caution in patients with respiratory, hepatic, or renal dysfunction, severe prostatic hypertrophy, or history of narcotic abuse; infants <3 months of age are more susceptible to respiratory depression, use with caution and in reduced doses in this age group

Adverse Reactions

Cardiovascular: Hypotension, bradycardia, peripheral vasodilation

Central nervous system: CNS depression, elevated intracranial pressure, drowsiness, dizziness, sedation

Dermatologic: Pruritus

Endocrine & metabolic: Antidiuretic hormone release

Gastrointestinal: Nausea, vomiting, constipation

Genitourinary: Urinary tract spasm, urinary retention

Hepatic: Biliary tract spasm

Ocular: Miosis

Respiratory: Respiratory depression

Miscellaneous: Physical and psychological dependence, histamine release

Drug Interactions CNS depressants (eg, alcohol, narcotics, benzodiazepines, tricyclic antidepressants, MAO inhibitors, phenothiazines) may increase effects/toxicity

Stability Protect from light and excessive heat; do not refrigerate, decreased solubility and precipitation may occur

Mechanism of Action Contains many narcotic alkaloids including morphine; gastric motility inhibition is primarily due to morphine content; decreases digestive secretions, increases GI muscle tone, and reduces GI propulsion

Pharmacodynamics Duration: 4-5 hours

Pharmacokinetics

Absorption: Variable from GI tract

Metabolism: In the liver

Elimination: In urine and bile

Usual Dosage Oral:

Neonates (full-term): Neonatal abstinence syndrome (opiate withdrawal): **Use a 25-fold dilution of opium tincture** (final concentration: 0.4 mg/mL morphine); Initial: Give 0.1 mL/kg or 2 drops/kg of the 25-fold dilution per dose with feedings every 3-4 hours; increase as needed by 0.1 mL/kg or 2 drops/kg of the 25-fold dilution every 3-4 hours until withdrawal symptoms are controlled; usual dose: 0.2-0.5 mL of the 25-fold dilution per dose given every 3-4 hours; it is rare to exceed 0.7 mL of the 25-fold dilution per dose; stabilize withdrawal symptoms for 3-5 days, then gradually decrease the dosage (keeping the same dosage interval) over a 2- to 4- week period

Children:

Diarrhea: 0.005-0.01 mL/kg/dose every 3-4 hours for a maximum of 6 doses/24 hours

Analgesia: 0.01-0.02 mL/kg/dose every 3-4 hours

Adults:

Diarrhea: Usual: 0.6 mL/dose; range: 0.3-1 mL/dose every 3-6 hours to maximum of 6 mL/24 hours

Analgesia: 0.6-1.5 mL/dose every 3-4 hours; usual maximum dose: 6 mL/24 hours

Administration Oral: May administer with food to decrease GI upset; for neonatal abstinence syndrome (opiate withdrawal), use a 25-fold dilution of opium tincture

Monitoring Parameters Respiratory rate, blood pressure, heart rate, resolution of diarrhea or pain, mental status; if using a 25-fold dilution to treat neonatal abstinence syndrome, monitor for resolution of withdrawal symptoms (such as irritability, high-pitched cry, stuffy nose, rhinorrhea, vomiting, poor feeding, diarrhea, sneezing, yawning etc) and signs of overtreatment (such as bradycardia, lethargy, hypotonia, irregular respirations, respiratory depression etc). An abstinence scoring system (eg, Finnegan abstinence scoring system) can be used to more objectively assess neonatal opiate withdrawal symptoms and the need for dosage adjustment. Monitor fluid and electrolyte balance in young children being treated for prolonged or severe diarrhea.

Patient Information Avoid alcohol; may cause drowsiness and impair ability to perform activities requiring mental alertness or physical coordination; may be habit-forming; avoid abrupt discontinuation after prolonged use

(Continued)

Opium Tincture *(Continued)*

Nursing Implications Observe patient for excessive sedation, respiratory depression; implement safety measures; assist with ambulation; do not abruptly discontinue after prolonged use

Additional Information Opium tincture contains 10 mg/mL morphine and 17% to 21% alcohol; for treatment of neonatal abstinence syndrome, a 25-fold dilution of opium tincture (final concentration: 0.4 mg/mL morphine) is preferred over paregoric; the 25-fold dilution of opium tincture contains the same morphine concentration as paregoric, but without the high amount of alcohol or additives of paregoric

Dosage Forms Liquid: 10% (120 mL, 480 mL) [0.6 mL equivalent to morphine 6 mg; contains 19% alcohol]

References

Kraus DM and Pham JT, "Neonatal Therapy," *Applied Therapeutics: The Clinical Use of Drugs*, 7th ed, Koda-Kimble MA, Young LY, eds, Baltimore, MD: Lippincott Williams & Wilkins, 2001.

Levy M and Spino M, "Neonatal Withdrawal Syndrome: Associated Drugs and Pharmacologic Management," *Pharmacotherapy*, 1993, 13(3):202-11.

"Neonatal Drug Withdrawal. American Academy of Pediatrics Committee on Drugs," *Pediatrics*, 1998, 101(6):1079-88.

- **Optho-Bunolol® (Can)** *see* Levobunolol *on page 665*
- **Opticaine®** *see* Tetracaine *on page 1073*
- **Opticrom®** *see* Cromolyn *on page 311*
- **Opticyl®** *see* Tropicamide *on page 1125*
- **Optimyxin® (Can)** *see* Bacitracin and Polymyxin B *on page 157*
- **Optimyxin Plus® (Can)** *see* Bacitracin and Polymyxin B *on page 157*
- **Optivar™** *see* Azelastine *on page 151*
- **Orabase®-B [OTC]** *see* Benzocaine *on page 163*
- **Oracit®** *see* Citrate and Citric Acid *on page 282*
- **Oracort (Can)** *see* Triamcinolone *on page 1112*
- **Orajel® [OTC]** *see* Benzocaine *on page 163*
- **Orajel® Baby [OTC]** *see* Benzocaine *on page 163*
- **Orajel® Baby Nighttime [OTC]** *see* Benzocaine *on page 163*
- **Orajel® Maximum Strength [OTC]** *see* Benzocaine *on page 163*
- **Orajel® Perioseptic Spot Treatment [OTC]** *see* Carbamide Peroxide *on page 212*
- **Orajel® Perioseptic® Super Cleaning Rinse [OTC]** *see* Hydrogen Peroxide *on page 577*
- **Oral Contraceptives** *see page 1243*
- **Oramorph SR®** *see* Morphine Sulfate *on page 778*
- **Oranyl [OTC]** *see* Pseudoephedrine *on page 958*
- **Orapred®** *see* PrednisoLONE *on page 925*
- **Orasol® [OTC]** *see* Benzocaine *on page 163*
- **Orazinc® [OTC]** *see* Zinc Supplements *on page 1167*
- **Orciprenaline** *see* Metaproterenol *on page 726*
- **Oretic®** *see* Hydrochlorothiazide *on page 569*
- **Organidin NR®** *see* Guaifenesin *on page 550*
- **ORG NC 45** *see* Vecuronium *on page 1138*
- **ORO-Clense (Can)** *see* Chlorhexidine Gluconate *on page 257*
- **Orthoclone OKT®3** *see* Muromonab-CD3 *on page 784*
- **Os-Cal® 500 [OTC]** *see* Calcium Supplements *on page 200*

Oseltamivir (o sel TAM e veer)

U.S. Brand Names Tamiflu®

Therapeutic Category Antiviral Agent, Oral; Neuraminidase Inhibitor

Generic Available No

Use Treatment of uncomplicated acute illness due to influenza A and B infection in patients who have been symptomatic for **no more than 2 days**; prophylaxis of influenza A and B (oseltamivir is not a substitute for annual flu vaccination)

Pregnancy Risk Factor C

Contraindications Hypersensitivity to oseltamivir, any component, or other sialic acid-based neuraminidase inhibitors

Warnings Oral suspension contains sodium benzoate; benzoic acid (benzoate) is a metabolite of benzyl alcohol; large amounts of benzyl alcohol (≥99 mg/kg/day) have been associated with a potentially fatal toxicity ("gasping syndrome") in neonates; use oral suspension containing sodium benzoate with caution in neonates; *in vitro* and animal studies have shown that benzoate displaces bilirubin from protein binding sites

Precautions Use with caution and modify dosage in patients with renal impairment; oseltamivir does not prevent complication of serious bacterial infection which may begin with or coexist with influenza

Adverse Reactions

Cardiovascular: Unstable angina, arrhythmia

Central nervous system: Dizziness, headache, fatigue, insomnia, vertigo, seizure, confusion

Dermatologic: Rash, toxic epidermal necrolysis

Endocrine & metabolic: Aggravation of diabetes mellitus

Gastrointestinal: Nausea, vomiting, diarrhea, abdominal pain, pseudomembranous colitis

Hematologic: Anemia

Hepatic: Hepatitis

Ocular: Conjunctivitis

Respiratory: Bronchitis, epistaxis

Miscellaneous: Swelling of face or tongue

Drug Interactions Probenecid (increases serum oseltamivir carboxylate concentration due to decreased tubular secretion in the kidney)

Food Interactions Food has no significant effect on peak oseltamivir plasma concentration or AUC

Stability Store capsule and powder for oral suspension at room temperature. Store reconstituted suspension at room temperature or under refrigeration; stable for 10 days; do not freeze.

Mechanism of Action Inhibits influenza virus neuraminidase which is responsible for detachment of virions from the infected cell's membrane and for viral penetration through respiratory secretions resulting in the inability of the virus to spread within the respiratory tract

Pharmacodynamics Reduction in the median time to improvement: 1.3 days

Pharmacokinetics

Absorption: Well absorbed from the GI tract

Distribution: Adults: V_{dss}: 23-26 L

Protein binding: 3% (oseltamivir carboxylate); 42% (oseltamivir phosphate)

Metabolism: Prodrug oseltamivir phosphate is metabolized by hepatic esterases to oseltamivir carboxylate (active); neither oseltamivir phosphate or oseltamivir carboxylate are a substrate, inducer, or inhibitor of cytochrome P450 isoenzymes

Half-life:

Oseltamivir phosphate: 1-3 hours

Oseltamivir carboxylate: 6-10 hours

Elimination: >99% of oseltamivir carboxylate is eliminated by renal excretion via glomerular filtration and tubular secretion

Usual Dosage Oral:

Treatment of influenza (treatment should begin within 2 days of onset of flu symptoms):

Children ≥1-12 years:

≤15 kg: 2 mg/kg/dose (maximum dose: 30 mg) twice daily for 5 days

>15 kg to 23 kg: 45 mg/dose twice daily for 5 days

>23 kg to 40 kg: 60 mg/dose twice daily for 5 days

>40 kg: 75 mg/dose twice daily for 5 days

Children >12 years and Adults: 75 mg/dose twice daily for 5 days

Prophylaxis of influenza: Adults: 75 mg/dose once daily for at least 7 days or for up to 6 weeks; therapy should begin within 2 days of exposure.

Dosing adjustment in renal impairment: Adults:

Cl_{cr} 10-30 mL/minute:

Treatment of influenza: 75 mg/dose once daily

Prophylaxis of influenza: 75 mg/dose every other day

Cl_{cr} <10 mL/minute: No recommended dosage regimens are available for patients with end-stage renal disease

Administration May administer with or without food; may decrease stomach upset if administered with food; shake suspension well before use

Monitoring Parameters Renal function, serum glucose in patients with diabetes mellitus

Patient Information Oseltamivir is not a substitute for the annual flu vaccination.

Dosage Forms

Capsule, as phosphate: 75 mg

Powder for oral suspension, as phosphate: 12 mg/mL (25 mL) [contains sodium benzoate; tutti-frutti flavor]

References

Hayden FG, Atmar RL, Schilling M, et al, "Use of the Selective Oral Neuraminidase Inhibitor Oseltamivir to Prevent Influenza," *N Engl J Med*, 1999, 341(18):1336-43.

(Continued)

Oseltamivir *(Continued)*

Treanor JJ, Hayden FG, Vrooman PS, et al, "Efficacy and Safety of the Oral Neuraminidase Inhibitor Oseltamivir in Treating Acute Influenza: A Randomized Controlled Trial. US Oral Neuraminidase Study Group," *JAMA*, 2000, 283(8):1016-24.

- ◆ **Osmitrol®** *see* Mannitol *on page 706*
- ◆ **Osmoglyn®** *see* Glycerin *on page 543*
- ◆ **Ostoforte® (Can)** *see* Ergocalciferol *on page 445*
- ◆ **OTC Cough & Cold Preparations, Pediatric** *see page 1225*
- ◆ **Ovace™** *see* Sulfacetamide *on page 1048*
- ◆ **Overdose and Toxicology** *see page 1388*
- ◆ **Ovol® (Can)** *see* Simethicone *on page 1020*

Oxacillin (oks a SIL in)

Synonyms Isoxazolyl Penicillin; Methylphenyl

Therapeutic Category Antibiotic, Penicillin (Antistaphylococcal)

Generic Available Yes

Use Treatment of bacterial infections such as osteomyelitis, septicemia, endocarditis, and CNS infections due to susceptible penicillinase-producing strains of *Staphylococcus*

Pregnancy Risk Factor B

Contraindications Hypersensitivity to oxacillin, other penicillins, or any component

Warnings Elimination rate will be decreased in neonates

Precautions Use with caution in patients with hypersensitivity to cephalosporins, severe renal impairment; dosage modification required in patients with renal impairment

Adverse Reactions

Central nervous system: Fever

Dermatologic: Rash

Gastrointestinal: Diarrhea, nausea, vomiting, *C. difficile* colitis

Hematologic: Mild leukopenia, agranulocytosis, thrombocytopenia, eosinophilia

Hepatic: Elevated AST, hepatotoxicity

Local: Thrombophlebitis

Renal: Acute interstitial nephritis; hematuria and azotemia have occurred in neonates and infants receiving high-dose oxacillin; albuminuria

Miscellaneous: Hypersensitivity reactions, serum sickness-like reactions

Drug Interactions Probenecid (decreases oxacillin elimination rate)

Stability Reconstituted oxacillin 250 mg/1.5 mL solution for injection is stable for 3 days at room temperature or 7 days when refrigerated; injection is incompatible with aminoglycosides and tetracyclines

Mechanism of Action Interferes with bacterial cell wall synthesis during active multiplication by binding to one or more of the penicillin-binding proteins; inhibits the final transpeptidation step of peptidoglycan synthesis causing cell death and resultant bactericidal activity against susceptible bacteria

Pharmacokinetics

Distribution: Distributes into bile, pleural, synovial, and pericardial fluids and into lungs and bone; penetrates the blood-brain barrier only when meninges are inflamed; crosses the placenta; appears in breast milk

Protein binding: 90% to 95%

Metabolism: In the liver to active and inactive metabolites

Half-life (prolonged with reduced renal function):

Neonates 8-15 days: 1.6 hours

Children 1 week to 2 years: 0.9-1.8 hours

Adults: 0.3-0.8 hours

Time to peak serum concentration: I.M.: Within 30-60 minutes

Elimination: By the kidneys and to small degree via bile as parent drug and metabolites

Dialysis: Not dialyzable (0% to 5%)

Usual Dosage

Neonates: I.M., I.V.:

Postnatal age ≤7 days:

≤2000 g: 50 mg/kg/day in divided doses every 12 hours

>2000 g: 75 mg/kg/day in divided doses every 8 hours

Postnatal age >7 days:

<1200 g: 50 mg/kg/day in divided doses every 12 hours

1200-2000 g: 75 mg/kg/day in divided doses every 8 hours

>2000 g: 100 mg/kg/day in divided doses every 6 hours

Infants and Children: I.M., I.V.:

Mild to moderate infections: 100-150 mg/kg/day in divided doses every 6 hours

Severe infections: 150-200 mg/kg/day in divided doses every 4-6 hours; maximum dose: 12 g/day

Adults: I.M., I.V.: 250 mg to 2 g/dose every 4-6 hours

Dosing interval in renal impairment: Cl_{cr} <10 mL/minute: Use lower range of the usual dosage

Administration Parenteral:

I.V. push: Administer over 10 minutes at a maximum concentration of 100 mg/mL

I.V. intermittent infusion: Administer over 15-30 minutes at a final concentration ≤40 mg/mL

Monitoring Parameters Periodic CBC with differential, urinalysis, BUN, serum creatinine, AST and ALT

Test Interactions False-positive urinary and serum proteins

Additional Information Sodium content: 1 g injection: 2.8-3.1 mEq

Dosage Forms

Infusion [premixed iso-osmotic dextrose solution]: 1 g (50 mL); 2 g (50 mL)

Injection, powder for reconstitution, as sodium: 1 g, 2 g, 10 g

References

Olans RN and Weiner LB, "Reversible Oxacillin Hepatotoxicity," *J Pediatr*, 1976, 89(5):835-8.

Prober LS, Stevenson DK, and Benitz WE, "The Use of Antibiotics in Neonates Weighing Less Than 1200 Grams," *Pediatr Infect Dis J*, 1990, 9(2):111-21.

Oxcarbazepine (ox car BAZ e peen)

U.S. Brand Names Trileptal®

Therapeutic Category Anticonvulsant, Miscellaneous

Generic Available No

Use Adjunctive treatment of partial seizures in pediatric and adult patients; monotherapy of partial seizures in adults

Pregnancy Risk Factor C

Contraindications Hypersensitivity to oxcarbazepine or any component

Warnings Significant hyponatremia may occur; a serum sodium <125 mEq/L has been reported in 2.5% of patients; consider monitoring serum sodium especially in patients who receive other drugs that may cause hyponatremia and in patients with symptoms of hyponatremia (eg, nausea, headache, malaise, confusion, lethargy, obtundation, or an increase in seizure frequency or severity). Do not abruptly discontinue therapy, withdraw gradually to lessen chance for increased seizure frequency (unless a more rapid withdrawal is required due to safety concerns). Cross-hypersensitivity reactions with carbamazepine may occur (incidence: 25% to 30%); discontinue oxcarbazepine immediately if signs or symptoms of hypersensitivity develop

Precautions CNS adverse effects may occur including somnolence, fatigue, coordination abnormalities (ataxia and gait disturbances), and cognitive symptoms (difficulty concentrating, speech or language problems, and psychomotor slowing); these effects may be more common when oxcarbazepine is used as add-on therapy versus monotherapy. Use with caution and modify dose in patients with renal impairment. Multiple drug interactions may occur (see Drug Interactions).

Adverse Reactions

Central nervous system: Headache, dizziness, somnolence, fatigue, ataxia, tremor, insomnia, cognitive symptoms (psychomotor slowing, difficulty concentrating, speech or language problems), vertigo, anxiety, nervousness, emotional lability

Dermatologic: Rash; rare: Stevens-Johnson syndrome, erythema multiforme, toxic epidermal necrolysis

Endocrine and Metabolic: Hyponatremia (incidence: 2.5%; usually occurs within the first 3 months of therapy, but has been reported in patients more than 1 year after starting medication; serum sodium returns towards normal after discontinuation, reduction of dose, or with conservative treatment such as fluid restriction); reduction in T_4 levels

Gastrointestinal: Nausea, vomiting, abdominal pain, dyspepsia

Neuromuscular & skeletal: Abnormal gait

Ocular: Diplopia, abnormal vision, nystagmus

Miscellaneous: Hypersensitivity reactions; a rare, multi-organ hypersensitivity reaction with rash, lymphadenopathy, fever, eosinophilia, abnormal liver function tests, and arthralgia has also been reported

Drug Interactions Cytochrome P450 isoenzyme CYP2C19 inhibitor; CYP3A4 and CYP3A5 inducer

Oxcarbazepine may inhibit hepatic metabolism and increase the serum concentrations of phenobarbital (by 14%) and phenytoin (by 40% with high-dose oxcarbazepine; dosage reduction of phenytoin may be needed); may induce hepatic metabolism and decrease serum concentrations of felodipine, lamotrigine, and oral contraceptives such as ethinyl estradiol and levonorgestrel (alternative methods of contraception are recommended); use with alcohol may increase sedative effects

(Continued)

Oxcarbazepine *(Continued)*

P450 enzyme inducers such as carbamazepine, phenobarbital, and phenytoin, may significantly decrease MHD concentrations by 25% to 40%; valproic acid decreases MHD concentrations by 18% and verapamil decreases MHD concentrations by 20%

Food Interactions

Tablets: Food does not affect rate or extent of absorption

Suspension: Effect of food has not been studied, but bioavailability is not likely to be affected

Stability Store at controlled room temperature (25°C); dispense in tight container; suspension is stable for 7 weeks after first opening the bottle

Mechanism of Action Active 10-monohydroxy metabolite (MHD) is primarily responsible for anticonvulsant activity; exact mechanism unknown; both MHD and oxcarbazepine are thought to decrease the spread of seizure activity by blockade of sodium channels; also increases conductance of potassium and modulates activity of high-voltage activated calcium channels

Pharmacokinetics

Absorption: Oral: Complete

Distribution: MHD: V_d (apparent): Adults: 49 L

Protein binding: Oxcarbazepine: 67%; MHD: 40%, primarily to albumin; parent drug and metabolite do not bind to alpha-1-acid glycoprotein

Metabolism: Oxcarbazepine is extensively metabolized in the liver to its active 10-monohydroxy metabolite (MHD); MHD undergoes further metabolism via glucuronide conjugation; 4% of dose is oxidized to the 10,11-dihydroxy metabolite (DHD) (inactive); 70% of serum concentration appears as MHD, 2% as unchanged oxcarbazepine, and the rest as minor metabolites; **Note:** Unlike carbamazepine, autoinduction of metabolism has not been observed and biotransformation of oxcarbazepine does not result in an epoxide metabolite

Bioavailability: Tablets and suspension have similar bioavailability (based on MDH serum concentrations)

Half-life:

Adults:

Oxcarbazepine: 2 hours

MHD: 9 hours

Adults with renal impairment (Cl_{cr} <30 mL/minute): MHD: 19 hours

Time to peak serum concentration: Adults:

Tablets: 3-13 hours (median: 4.5 hours)

Suspension: Median: 6 hours

Elimination: >95% of dose is excreted in the urine with <1% as unchanged parent drug, 27% as unchanged MHD, 49% as MHD glucuronides, 3% as DHD (inactive), and 13% as conjugate of oxcarbazepine and MHD; <4% excreted in feces

Clearance:

Children <8 years: Increased by 30% to 40% compared to children >8 years and adults

Children >8 years: Values approach adult clearance

Hepatic impairment: Mild to moderate: No effect on pharmacokinetics; Severe: Not studied

Usual Dosage Oral: **Note:** Oral suspension and tablets are interchangeable on a mg per mg basis:

Neonates, Infants, and Children <4 years: Not approved for use; controlled trials in children <2 years have not been conducted

Children 4-16 years: Adjunctive therapy: Initial: 8-10 mg/kg/day given in 2 divided doses (usual maximum: 600 mg/day); increase dose slowly over 2 weeks to weight-dependent target maintenance dose:

20-29 kg: 900 mg/day in 2 divided doses

29.1-39 kg: 1200 mg/day in 2 divided doses

>39 kg: 1800 mg/day in 2 divided doses

Note: Use of these pediatric target maintenance doses in one clinical trial resulted in doses ranging from 6-51 mg/kg/day (median dose: 31 mg/kg/day)

Adults:

Adjunctive therapy: Initial: 300 mg twice daily; increase if needed by no more than 600 mg/day at approximately weekly intervals; recommended maintenance dose: 600 mg twice daily; **Note:** Doses >1200 mg/day may have greater efficacy, but most patients are not able to tolerate 2400 mg/day (mostly due to CNS effects); monitor patient closely and measure concentrations of concomitant antiepileptic agents during dosage titration and especially with oxcarbazepine doses >1200 mg/day

Conversion to monotherapy: Initial: 300 mg twice daily with a simultaneous initial reduction of the dose of concomitant antiepileptic drugs (AEDs); withdraw concomitant AEDs completely over 3-6 weeks, while increasing oxcarbazepine dose as needed by no more than 600 mg/day at approximately weekly intervals; recommended oxcarbazepine dose (1200 mg twice daily) should be reached in about 2-4 weeks; **Note:** A lower dose (1200 mg/day) was effective in one study in patients who initiated oxcarbazepine monotherapy

Initiation of monotherapy: Initial: 300 mg twice daily; increase by 300 mg/day every third day to 1200 mg/day; a higher dose (2400 mg/day) was effective in patients who were converted from other AEDs to oxcarbazepine monotherapy.

Dosing adjustment in renal impairment: Cl_{cr} <30 mL/minute: Initial dose: Administer 50% of the normal starting dose; slowly increase the dose if needed, using a slower dosage titration than normal

Dosing adjustment in hepatic impairment:
Mild to moderate hepatic impairment: No dosage adjustment recommended
Severe hepatic impairment: Not evaluated

Administration Oral: May be taken without regard to meals

Suspension: Prior to using for the first time, firmly insert the manufacturer supplied plastic adapter into the neck of the bottle; cover the adapter with child-resistant cap when not in use; shake suspension well (for at least 10 seconds) before use; remove child-resistant cap and insert manufacturer supplied oral syringe to withdraw appropriate dose; dose may be administered directly from syringe or mixed in a small amount of water immediately prior to use; after use, rinse oral syringe with warm water and allow to dry thoroughly; discard any unused portion 7 weeks after first opening bottle

Monitoring Parameters Seizure frequency, duration and severity; symptoms of CNS depression (dizziness, headache, somnolence) and allergic reaction; consider monitoring serum sodium (particularly during first three months of therapy) especially in patients who receive other drugs that may cause hyponatremia and in patients with symptoms of hyponatremia (see Warnings)

Patient Information Inform prescriber if allergic to carbamazepine; do not abruptly discontinue, an increase in seizure activity may result; report excessive somnolence or allergic reactions to physician immediately; report unusual symptoms such as nausea, headache, malaise, confusion, lethargy, obtundation, or a worsening of seizures to physician immediately (blood test for serum sodium may be needed); avoid alcohol; may cause drowsiness and impair ability to perform activities requiring mental alertness or physical coordination; oxcarbazepine may decrease the effectiveness of oral contraceptives (use an alternative, nonhormonal, form of contraception)

Additional Information Symptoms of overdose may include CNS depression (somnolence, ataxia, obtundation); treatment is symptomatic and supportive; consider general poisoning management (eg, gastric lavage, activated charcoal); largest reported overdose is 24 g; oxcarbazepine is a keto analogue of carbamazepine; suspension also contains propylene glycol

Dosage Forms
Suspension, oral: 300 mg/5 mL (250 mL) [contains ethanol]
Tablet: 150 mg, 300 mg, 600 mg

References
Tecoma ES, "Oxcarbazepine," *Epilepsia*, 1999, 40(Suppl 5): S37-46.

♦ **Oxeze® Turbuhaler® (Can)** *see* Formoterol *on page 519*
♦ **Oxipor® VHC [OTC]** *see* Coal Tar *on page 299*
♦ **Oxpentifylline** *see* Pentoxifylline *on page 884*
♦ **Oxy 10® Balanced Medicated Face Wash [OTC]** *see* Benzoyl Peroxide *on page 165*
♦ **Oxy 10® Balance Spot Treatment [OTC]** *see* Benzoyl Peroxide *on page 165*
♦ **Oxy Balance® [OTC]** *see* Salicylic Acid *on page 1002*
♦ **Oxy Balance® Deep Pore [OTC]** *see* Salicylic Acid *on page 1002*

Oxybutynin (oks i BYOO ti nin)

Related Information
Carbohydrate and Alcohol Content of Liquid Medications for Use in Patients Receiving Ketogenic Diets *on page 1431*

U.S. Brand Names Ditropan®; Ditropan® XL; Oxytrol™

Canadian Brand Names Gen-Oxybutynin; Novo-Oxybutynin; Nu-Oxybutyn; PMS-Oxybutynin

Therapeutic Category Antispasmodic Agent, Urinary

Generic Available Yes (except extended release tablet or transdermal patch)

Use Relief of bladder spasms associated with voiding in patients with uninhibited and reflex neurogenic bladder; treatment of overactive bladder with symptoms of urge urinary incontinence, urgency, and frequency

Pregnancy Risk Factor B
(Continued)

Oxybutynin (Continued)

Contraindications Hypersensitivity to oxybutynin or any component; glaucoma (angle-closure), myasthenia gravis, partial or complete GI obstruction, GU obstruction; megacolon, toxic megacolon

Precautions Use with caution in patients with hepatic or renal disease, heart disease, hyperthyroidism, reflux esophagitis, hypertension, prostatic hypertrophy, autonomic neuropathy, ulcerative colitis, intestinal atony

Adverse Reactions

Cardiovascular: Tachycardia, palpitations, vasodilation

Central nervous system: Drowsiness, dizziness, insomnia, fever, hallucinations

Dermatologic: Rash

Endocrine & metabolic: Hot flashes

Gastrointestinal: Xerostomia, nausea, vomiting, constipation, decreased GI motility

Genitourinary: Impotence, urinary hesitancy or retention

Local: Application site reactions, such as rash, macular rash, and burning (transdermal formulation)

Neuromuscular & skeletal: Weakness

Ocular: Blurred vision, mydriasis, decreased lacrimation, amblyopia, cycloplegia

Miscellaneous: Hypersensitivity reactions, decreased diaphoresis

Drug Interactions Additive sedation with CNS depressants and alcohol; additive anticholinergic effects with antihistamines and anticholinergic agents; decreased haloperidol serum concentrations; may increase digoxin serum levels

Stability Store at controlled room temperature; protect syrup from light; keep transdermal patch in sealed pouch

Mechanism of Action Direct antispasmodic effect on smooth muscle, also inhibits the action of acetylcholine on smooth muscle; does not block effects at skeletal muscle or at autonomic ganglia

Pharmacodynamics

Immediate release formulation:

Onset of action: Oral: Within 30-60 minutes

Maximum effect: 3-6 hours

Duration: 6-10 hours

Extended release formulation: Maximum effects: 3 days

Transdermal formulation: Duration: 96 hours

Pharmacokinetics

Absorption: Oral: Rapid and well absorbed

Distribution: V_d: Adults: 193 L

Metabolism: Extensive first pass effect; metabolized in the liver to active and inactive metabolites

Half-life: Adults: 1-2.3 hours

Time to peak serum concentration:

Immediate release: Within 60 minutes

Extended release: 12-13 hours

Transdermal: 24-48 hours

Elimination: <0.1% excreted unchanged in urine

Usual Dosage

Children: Oral:

1-5 years: 0.2 mg/kg/dose 2-4 times/day

>5 years: 5 mg twice daily, up to 5 mg 4 times/day

Adults:

Oral: 5 mg 2-3 times/day up to 5 mg 4 times/day maximum **or** extended release tablet (Ditropan® XL) 5-10 mg once daily; maximum 30 mg once daily

Transdermal: 3.9 mg/day system applied twice weekly (every 3-4 days)

Note: Should be discontinued periodically to determine whether the patient can manage without the drug and to minimize tolerance to the drug

Administration

Oral: May administer with food or milk to decrease GI distress; extended release formulation may be administered with or without food; swallow extended release tablets whole; do not chew or crush.

Transdermal: Apply to dry intact skin on the abdomen, hip, or buttock. Rotate site of application with each administration and avoid application to the same site within 7 days

Patient Information May cause drowsiness and impair ability to perform activities requiring mental alertness or physical coordination; may cause heat prostration (fever and heat stroke due to decreased sweating) when used in hot climates; avoid alcohol; may cause dry mouth; nonabsorbable tablet shell may be seen in stool, but active drug has been released

Dosage Forms

Syrup, as chloride (Ditropan®): 5 mg/5 mL (473 mL)

Tablet, as chloride (Ditropan®): 5 mg

Tablet, extended release, as chloride (Ditropan® XL): 5 mg, 10 mg, 15 mg

Transdermal system (Oxytrol™): 3.9 mg/day (8s, 24s) [39 cm²; total oxybutynin 36 mg]

♦ **Oxycocet® (Can)** *see* Oxycodone and Acetaminophen *on page 847*

♦ **Oxycodan® (Can)** *see* Oxycodone and Aspirin *on page 848*

Oxycodone (oks i KOE done)

U.S. Brand Names OxyContin®; Oxydose™; OxyFast®; OxyIR®; Percolone® [DSC]; Roxicodone™; Roxicodone™ Intensol™

Canadian Brand Names Supeudol®

Therapeutic Category Analgesic, Narcotic

Generic Available Yes

Use Relief of moderate to severe pain

Controlled release tablets (OxyContin®) are indicated for around-the-clock management of moderate to severe pain when an analgesic is needed for an extended period of time; **Note:** OxyContin® is not intended for use as a PRN analgesic or for treatment of mild pain, pain that is not expected to persist for an extended period of time, or for immediate postoperative pain (within 12-24 hours after surgery); OxyContin® may be used for postoperative pain only if the patient received it prior to surgery or if moderate to severe persistent pain is anticipated.

Restrictions C-II

Pregnancy Risk Factor B (D if used for prolonged periods or in high doses at term)

Contraindications Hypersensitivity to oxycodone or any component; significant respiratory depression (in settings without resuscitative equipment or without adequate respiratory monitoring); patients with hypercarbia, severe or acute asthma, paralytic ileus (known or suspected)

Warnings Respiratory depression may occur; use with extreme caution in patients with pre-existing respiratory depression, decreased respiratory reserve, hypoxia, hypercapnia, significant COPD, or cor pulmonale. Hypotension may occur, especially in hypovolemic patients or those receiving medications that compromise vasomotor tone; use with extreme caution in patients with circulatory shock. Orthostatic hypotension may occur in ambulatory patients; physical and psychological dependence may occur; abrupt discontinuation after prolonged use may result in withdrawal symptoms; warn patient of possible impairment of alertness or physical coordination (see Patient Information); interactions with other CNS drugs may occur (see Drug Interactions). Controlled release 80 mg and 160 mg tablets should only be used in patients who are opioid tolerant and who require daily doses of ≥160 mg and ≥320 mg, respectively (administration of these tablet strengths to opioid naive patients may cause fatal respiratory depression). Healthcare provider should be alert to problems of abuse, misuse, and diversion.

Oral concentrate contains sodium benzoate; benzoic acid (benzoate) is a metabolite of benzyl alcohol; large amounts of benzyl alcohol (≥99 mg/kg/day) have been associated with a potentially fatal toxicity ("gasping syndrome") in neonates; the "gasping syndrome" consists of metabolic acidosis, respiratory distress, gasping respirations, CNS dysfunction (including convulsions, intracranial hemorrhage), hypotension and cardiovascular collapse; avoid use of oxycodone products containing sodium benzoate in neonates; *in vitro* and animal studies have shown that benzoate displaces bilirubin from protein binding sites

Precautions Use with caution in patients with hypersensitivity to other phenanthrene derivative opioid agonists (morphine, codeine, hydrocodone, hydromorphone, oxymorphone, levorphanol). Use with caution in patients with head injury; increased intracranial pressure; CNS depression; respiratory depression; coma; toxic psychosis; seizures; acute abdominal conditions; biliary tract disease, pancreatitis; severe renal, respiratory, or hepatic insufficiency; hypothyroidism; Addison's disease; urethral stricture and in debilitated patients. Use care in prescribing, dispensing, and administering the oral concentrated solution, inappropriate use may cause overdose.

Adverse Reactions

Cardiovascular system: Hypotension, bradycardia, peripheral vasodilation

Central nervous system: CNS depression, elevated intracranial pressure, dizziness, drowsiness, sedation, lightheadedness, dysphoria, headache, fatigue

Dermatologic: Pruritus, skin rash

Endocrine & metabolic: Antidiuretic hormone release

Gastrointestinal: Nausea, vomiting, constipation, biliary tract spasm, xerostomia

Genitourinary: Urinary tract spasm, urinary retention

Ocular: Miosis

Respiratory: Respiratory depression

(Continued)

Oxycodone *(Continued)*

Miscellaneous: Physical and psychological dependence, histamine release, diaphoresis

Drug Interactions Cytochrome P450 isoenzyme CYP2D6 substrate

CNS depressants, phenothiazines, tricyclic antidepressants may potentiate the CNS adverse effects of oxycodone (dosage reduction of one or both agents is recommended; some recommend starting opioid analgesics at $1/3$ to $1/2$ of the normal dose in patients receiving other CNS depressants)

Food Interactions Food does not significantly affect absorption of controlled release tablets; high fat meal may increase peak concentrations of OxyContin® 160 mg tablet by 25%

Stability Store at room temperature; protect from light and moisture

OxyFast® oral concentrate: Stable for 90 days after opening

Mechanism of Action Binds to opiate receptors in the CNS, causing inhibition of ascending pain pathways, altering the perception of and response to pain; produces generalized CNS depression

Pharmacodynamics Duration of pain relief: Oral:

Immediate release: 4-5 hours

Controlled release: 12 hours

Pharmacokinetics

Distribution: Distributes into breast milk; V_{dss}:

Children 2-10 years: Mean: 2.1 L/kg; range: 1.2-3.7 L/kg

Adults: 2.6 L/kg

Protein binding: 38% to 45%

Metabolism: In the liver primarily to noroxycodone (via demethylation) and oxymorphone (via CYP2D6); noroxycodone is the major circulating metabolite, but has much weaker activity than oxycodone; oxymorphone is active, but present in low concentrations; <15% of the dose is metabolized to oxymorphone via CYP2D6; drug and metabolites undergo glucuronide conjugation

Bioavailability: Adults: 60% to 87%

Half-life, apparent: Adults:

Immediate release: 3.2 hours

Controlled release (OxyContin®): 4.5 hours

Half-life, elimination:

Children 2-10 years: 1.8 hours; range: 1.2-3 hours

Adults: 3.7 hours

Adults with renal dysfunction (Cl$_{cr}$ <60 mL/minute): Half-life increases by 1 hour, but peak oxycodone concentrations increase by 50% and AUC increases by 60%

Adults with mild to moderate hepatic dysfunction: Half-life increases by 2.3 hours, peak oxycodone concentrations increase by 50%, and AUC increases by 95%

Elimination: In the urine as unchanged drug (≤19%) and metabolites: Conjugated oxycodone (≤50%), conjugated oxymorphone (≤14%), noroxycodone, and conjugated noroxycodone

Usual Dosage Oral: **Doses should be titrated to appropriate effect:**

Immediate release products:

Children: 0.05-0.15 mg/kg/dose every 4-6 hours as needed

Adults: Initial: 5 mg every 6 hours as needed; usual: 10-30 mg every 4 hours as needed; more severe pain: ≥30 mg every 4 hours

AHCPR dosing guidelines: Opioid naive patients: (See Carr, 1992 and Jacox, 1994)

Children and Adults <50 kg: Moderate to severe pain: Usual initial dose: 0.2 mg/kg every 3-4 hours

Children and Adults ≥50 kg: Moderate to severe pain: Usual initial dose: 10 mg every 3-4 hours

Controlled release product: Adolescents ≥18 years and Adults: Initial: 10 mg every 12 hours; use immediate-release analgesics as needed for rescue from breakthrough pain or prior to predictable pain from procedures or activities; rescue analgesic should be $1/4$ to $1/3$ of the 12-hour controlled release oxycodone dose; increase the dose of controlled release oxycodone if >2 doses of rescue analgesic are required within 24 hours; dose of controlled release oxycodone may be adjusted every 1-2 days by 25% to 50% (initial increase may be from 10 mg to 20 mg every 12 hours). Mean doses used in open-label trials: Opioid naive patients: 40 mg/day; cancer patients: 105 mg/day (range: 20-720 mg/day).

Note: To convert patients from other opioid or nonopioid analgesics to oxycodone controlled release tablets: See OxyContin® package insert

Dosing adjustment in renal impairment: Cl$_{cr}$ <60 mL/minute: Initiate doses conservatively and carefully titrate dose to appropriate effect

Dosing adjustment in hepatic impairment: Initial: $1/3$ to $1/2$ of the usual dose; carefully titrate dose to appropriate effect

Administration May administer with food to decrease GI upset; swallow controlled (sustained) release tablets whole; do not crush, chew, or break (this would result in rapid release and absorption of a potentially fatal dose of drug); avoid high fat meals when initiating controlled release 160 mg tablets

Monitoring Parameters Pain relief, respiratory rate, mental status, blood pressure

Patient Information May cause dry mouth; may cause drowsiness and impair ability to perform activities requiring mental alertness or physical coordination; avoid alcohol; report the use of other prescription and nonprescription medications to your physician and pharmacist. May be habit-forming; do not discontinue abruptly if therapy lasts more than a few weeks; dose should be tapered to prevent withdrawal. Do not crush, chew, or break controlled release tablets (OxyContin®), as risk of overdose (and possibly death) may occur. Empty controlled release tablets may appear in stool after medication is absorbed (this is normal).

Additional Information OxyContin® tablets deliver medication over 12 hours; release is pH independent. Equianalgesic doses: oral oxycodone 30 mg = morphine 10 mg I.M. = single oral dose morphine 60 mg **or** chronic dosing oral morphine 30 mg

Dosage Forms

Capsule, immediate release, as hydrochloride (OxyIR®): 5 mg

Solution, oral, as hydrochloride (Roxicodone™): 5 mg/5 mL (5 mL, 500 mL) [contains alcohol]

Solution, oral **concentrate**, as hydrochloride:
OxyFast®, Roxicodone™ Intensol™: 20 mg/mL (30 mL) [contains sodium benzoate]
Oxydose™: 20 mg/mL (30 mL) [contains sodium benzoate; berry flavor]

Tablet, controlled release, as hydrochloride (OxyContin®): 10 mg, 20 mg, 40 mg, 80 mg, 160 mg

Tablet, immediate release, as hydrochloride: 5 mg
Percolone®: 5 mg [DSC]
Roxicodone™: 5 mg, 15 mg, 30 mg

References

Carr D, Jacox A, Chapman CR, et al, "Clinical Practice Guideline Number 1: Acute Pain Management: Operative or Medical Procedures and Trauma," Rockville, Maryland: U.S. Department of Health and Human Services, Public Health Service, Agency for Health Care Policy and Research, AHCPR Publication No 92-0032, 1992.

Jacox A, Carr D, Payne R, et al, "Clinical Practice Guideline Number 9: Management of Cancer Pain," Rockville, Maryland: U.S. Department of Health and Human Services, Public Health Service, Agency for Health Care Policy and Research, AHCPR Publication No. 94-0592, 1994.

Olkkola KT, Hamunen K, and Maunuksela EL, "Clinical Pharmacokinetics and Pharmacodynamics of Opioid Analgesics in Infants and Children," Clin Pharmacokinet, 1995, 28(5):385-404.

Olkkola KT, Hamunen K, Seppala T, et al, "Pharmacokinetics and Ventilatory Effects of Intravenous Oxycodone in Postoperative Children," Br J Clin Pharmacol, 1994, 38(1):71-6.

Oxycodone and Acetaminophen
(oks i KOE done & a seet a MIN oh fen)

Related Information

Narcotic Analgesics Comparison on page 1223
Overdose and Toxicology on page 1388

U.S. Brand Names Endocet®; Percocet® 2.5/325; Percocet® 5/325; Percocet® 7.5/325; Percocet® 7.5/500; Percocet® 10/325; Percocet® 10/650; Roxicet®; Roxicet® 5/500; Tylox®

Canadian Brand Names Oxycocet®; Percocet®-Demi

Synonyms Acetaminophen and Oxycodone

Therapeutic Category Analgesic, Narcotic

Generic Available Yes

Use Relief of moderate to severe pain

Restrictions C-II

Pregnancy Risk Factor C

Contraindications Hypersensitivity to oxycodone, acetaminophen, or any component (see Warnings); severe respiratory depression, severe liver or renal insufficiency

Warnings Abrupt discontinuation after prolonged use may result in withdrawal symptoms; some preparations contain sodium metabisulfite which may cause allergic reactions in susceptible individuals; capsule may contain sodium benzoate; benzoic acid (benzoate) is a metabolite of benzyl alcohol; large amounts of benzyl alcohol (≥99 mg/kg/day) have been associated with a potentially fatal toxicity ("gasping syndrome") in neonates; the "gasping syndrome" consists of metabolic acidosis, respiratory distress, gasping respirations, CNS dysfunction (including convulsions, intracranial hemorrhage), hypotension and cardiovascular collapse; avoid use of oxycodone and acetaminophen products containing sodium benzoate in neonates; in vitro and animal studies have shown that benzoate displaces bilirubin from protein binding sites
(Continued)

Oxycodone and Acetaminophen *(Continued)*

Precautions Use with caution in patients with hypersensitivity to other phenanthrene derivative opioid agonists (morphine, codeine, hydrocodone, hydromorphone, oxymorphone, levorphanol)

Adverse Reactions
Cardiovascular: Hypotension, bradycardia, peripheral vasodilation
Central nervous system: CNS depression, elevated intracranial pressure, drowsiness, sedation
Dermatologic: Pruritus
Endocrine & metabolic: Antidiuretic hormone release
Gastrointestinal: Nausea, vomiting, constipation, biliary tract spasm
Genitourinary: Urinary tract spasm
Ocular: Miosis
Respiratory: Respiratory depression
Miscellaneous: Physical and psychological dependence, histamine release

Drug Interactions See Acetaminophen *on page 36* and Oxycodone *on page 845*

Food Interactions Rate of absorption of acetaminophen may be decreased when given with food high in carbohydrates

Mechanism of Action See Acetaminophen *on page 36* and Oxycodone *on page 845*

Pharmacodynamics
Onset of action: Within 10-15 minutes
Maximum effect: Within 1 hour
Duration: 3-6 hours

Pharmacokinetics See Acetaminophen *on page 36* and Oxycodone *on page 845*

Usual Dosage Oral (titrate dose to appropriate analgesic effects):
Children: Based on **oxycodone component**: 0.05-0.15 mg/kg/dose up to 5 mg/dose every 4-6 hours as needed
Adults: 1-2 tablets every 4-6 hours as needed for pain; maximum daily dose of acetaminophen: 4 g/day

Administration Oral: May administer with food or milk to decrease GI upset

Monitoring Parameters Pain relief, respiratory rate, mental status, blood pressure

Patient Information Avoid alcohol; may cause drowsiness and impair ability to perform activities requiring mental alertness or physical coordination. May be habit-forming; do not discontinue abruptly if therapy lasts more than a few weeks; dose should be tapered to prevent narcotic withdrawal.

Dosage Forms
Caplet (Roxicet® 5/500): Oxycodone hydrochloride 5 mg and acetaminophen 500 mg
Capsule: Oxycodone hydrochloride 5 mg and acetaminophen 500 mg
Tylox®: Oxycodone hydrochloride 5 mg and acetaminophen 500 mg [contains sodium benzoate and sodium metabisulfite]
Solution, oral (Roxicet®): Oxycodone hydrochloride 5 mg and acetaminophen 325 mg per 5 mL (5 mL, 500 mL) [contains 0.4% alcohol; mint flavor]
Tablet: Oxycodone hydrochloride 5 mg and acetaminophen 325 mg; oxycodone hydrochloride 7.5 mg and acetaminophen 500 mg; oxycodone hydrochloride 10 mg and acetaminophen 650 mg
Endocet®: Oxycodone hydrochloride 5 mg and acetaminophen 325 mg
Percocet® 2.5/325: Oxycodone hydrochloride 2.5 mg and acetaminophen 325 mg
Percocet® 5/325: Oxycodone hydrochloride 5 mg and acetaminophen 325 mg
Percocet® 7.5/325: Oxycodone hydrochloride 7.5 mg and acetaminophen 325 mg
Percocet® 7.5/500: Oxycodone hydrochloride 7.5 mg and acetaminophen 500 mg
Percocet® 10/325: Oxycodone hydrochloride 10 mg and acetaminophen 325 mg
Percocet® 10/650: Oxycodone hydrochloride 10 mg and acetaminophen 650 mg
Roxicot®: Oxycodone hydrochloride 5 mg and acetaminophen 325 mg

References
Olkkola KT, Hamunen K, and Maunuksela EL, "Clinical Pharmacokinetics and Pharmacodynamics of Opioid Analgesics in Infants and Children," *Clin Pharmacokinet,* 1995, 28(5):385-404.

Oxycodone and Aspirin *(oks i KOE done & AS pir in)*

Related Information
Overdose and Toxicology *on page 1388*

U.S. Brand Names Endodan®; Percodan®; Percodan®-Demi [DSC]

Canadian Brand Names Oxycodan®

Synonyms Aspirin and Oxycodone

Therapeutic Category Analgesic, Narcotic

Generic Available Yes

Use Relief of moderate to moderately severe pain

Restrictions C-II

Pregnancy Risk Factor D

Contraindications Hypersensitivity to oxycodone, aspirin, or any component; severe respiratory depression, severe liver, or renal insufficiency

Warnings Contains aspirin, do not use aspirin-containing products in children <16 years of age for chickenpox or flu symptoms due to the association with Reye's syndrome

Precautions Use with caution in patients with hypersensitivity to other phenanthrene derivative opioid agonists (morphine, codeine, hydrocodone, hydromorphone, oxymorphone, levorphanol); contains aspirin, use with caution in patients with impaired renal function, erosive gastritis, peptic ulcer, gout

Adverse Reactions

Cardiovascular: Hypotension, bradycardia, peripheral vasodilation

Central nervous system: CNS depression, elevated intracranial pressure, drowsiness, sedation

Dermatologic: Pruritus, rash

Endocrine & metabolic: Antidiuretic hormone release

Gastrointestinal: Nausea, vomiting, constipation, biliary tract spasm, GI distress

Genitourinary: Urinary tract spasm

Hematologic: Inhibition of platelet aggregation (due to aspirin)

Hepatic: Hepatotoxicity (due to aspirin)

Ocular: Miosis

Respiratory: Respiratory depression

Miscellaneous: Histamine release, physical and psychological dependence

Drug Interactions See Aspirin *on page 134* and Oxycodone *on page 845*

Food Interactions Aspirin may increase renal excretion of vitamin C and may decrease serum folate levels

Mechanism of Action See Aspirin *on page 134* and Oxycodone *on page 845*

Pharmacokinetics See Aspirin *on page 134* and Oxycodone *on page 845*

Usual Dosage Oral: Based on **oxycodone-combined salt component**:

Children: 0.05-0.15 mg/kg/dose every 4-6 hours as needed; maximum dose: 5 mg/dose (1 tablet Percodan® or 2 tablets Percodan®-Demi/dose)

or alternatively:

Percodan®-Demi:

6-12 years: $^1/_4$ tablet every 6 hours as needed for pain

>12 years: $^1/_2$ tablet every 6 hours as needed for pain

Adults: Percodan®: 1 tablet every 6 hours as needed for pain or Percodan®-Demi: 1-2 tablets every 6 hours as needed for pain

Administration Oral: May administer with food or milk to decrease GI upset

Monitoring Parameters Pain relief, respiratory rate, mental status, blood pressure

Patient Information Avoid alcohol; may cause drowsiness and impair ability to perform activities requiring mental alertness or physical coordination. May be habit-forming; do not discontinue abruptly if therapy lasts more than a few weeks; dose should be tapered to prevent narcotic withdrawal.

Additional Information One tablet (Percodan®) contains ~5 mg oxycodone as combined salt

Dosage Forms

Tablet: Oxycodone hydrochloride 4.5 mg, oxycodone terephthalate 0.38 mg, and aspirin 325 mg

Endodan®, Percodan®: Oxycodone hydrochloride 4.5 mg, oxycodone terephthalate 0.38 mg, and aspirin 325 mg

Percodan®-Demi: Oxycodone hydrochloride 2.25 mg, oxycodone terephthalate 0.19 mg, and aspirin 325 mg [DSC]

♦ **OxyContin®** *see Oxycodone on page 845*

♦ **Oxyderm™ (Can)** *see Benzoyl Peroxide on page 165*

♦ **Oxydose™** *see Oxycodone on page 845*

♦ **OxyFast®** *see Oxycodone on page 845*

♦ **OxyIR®** *see Oxycodone on page 845*

Oxymetazoline (oks i met AZ oh leen)

Related Information

OTC Cough & Cold Preparations, Pediatric *on page 1225*

U.S. Brand Names Afrin® [OTC]; Afrin® Extra Moisturizing [OTC]; Afrin® Original [OTC]; Afrin® Severe Congestion [OTC]; Afrin® Sinus [OTC]; Duramist Plus® [OTC]; Duration® [OTC]; Genasal® [OTC]; Neo-Synephrine® 12 Hour [OTC]; Neo-Synephrine® 12 Hour Extra Moisturizing [OTC]; Nöstrilla® [OTC]; OcuClear® [OTC] [DSC]; Twice-A-Day® [OTC]; Vicks® Sinex® 12 Hour Ultrafine Mist [OTC]; Visine® L.R. [OTC]; 4-Way® Long Acting [OTC]

(Continued)

Oxymetazoline *(Continued)*

Canadian Brand Names Claritin® Allergic Decongestant; Dristan® Long Lasting Nasal; Drixoral® Nasal

Therapeutic Category Adrenergic Agonist Agent; Decongestant, Nasal; Nasal Agent, Vasoconstrictor; Vasoconstrictor, Nasal; Vasoconstrictor, Ophthalmic

Generic Available Yes

Use Symptomatic relief of nasal mucosal congestion associated with acute or chronic rhinitis, the common cold, sinusitis, hay fever, or other allergies

Pregnancy Risk Factor C

Contraindications Hypersensitivity to oxymetazoline or any component (see Warnings); patients on MAO inhibitor therapy

Warnings Use for periods exceeding 3 days may result in severe rebound nasal congestion; excessive dosage in children may cause profound CNS depression. Some products contain benzyl alcohol which may cause allergic reactions in susceptible individuals; large amounts of benzyl alcohol (≥99 mg/kg/day) have been associated with a potentially fatal toxicity ("gasping syndrome") in neonates; the "gasping syndrome" consists of metabolic acidosis, respiratory distress, gasping respirations, CNS dysfunction (including convulsions, intracranial hemorrhage), hypotension and cardiovascular collapse; *in vitro* and animal studies have shown that benzoate, a metabolite of benzyl alcohol, displaces bilirubin from protein binding sites; avoid use of these products in neonates

Precautions Use with caution in patients with hyperthyroidism, heart disease, hypertension, diabetes mellitus, increased intraocular pressure, or prostatic hypertrophy

Adverse Reactions

Cardiovascular: Hypertension, palpitations, reflex bradycardia, pallor

Central nervous system: Nervousness, dizziness, insomnia, headache, anxiety, tenseness, drowsiness, CNS depression, convulsions, hallucinations

Gastrointestinal: Nausea, vomiting

Ocular: Stinging to eye, mydriasis, elevated intraocular pressure, blurred vision

Respiratory: Sneezing, respiratory difficulty, rebound congestion with prolonged use, dryness of nasal mucosa

Miscellaneous: Diaphoresis

Drug Interactions Anesthetics (discontinue oxymetazoline prior to use of anesthetics that sensitize the myocardium to sympathomimetics, ie, cyclopropane, halothane); MAO inhibitors, methyldopa, tricyclic antidepressants increase hypertensive response

Mechanism of Action Stimulates alpha-adrenergic receptors in the arterioles of the nasal mucosa and arterioles of the conjunctiva to produce vasoconstriction

Pharmacodynamics

Onset of action: Intranasal: Within 5-10 minutes

Duration: 5-6 hours

Pharmacokinetics Metabolic fate is unknown

Usual Dosage

Nasal: Therapy should not exceed 3-5 days; avoid use in children <6 years of age

Children ≥6 years and Adults: 2-3 drops or 2-3 sprays or 1-2 metered sprays (Nostrilla®) into each nostril twice daily

Ophthalmic: Children ≥6 years and Adults: Instill 1-2 drops into the affected eye(s) 2-4 times/day (≥6 hours apart)

Administration

Nasal: Spray or apply drops into each nostril while gently occluding the other

Ophthalmic: Instill drops into conjunctival sac of affected eye(s); avoid contact of bottle tip with skin or eye; finger pressure should be applied to lacrimal sac during and for 1-2 minutes after instillation to decrease the risk of absorption and systemic reactions

Dosage Forms

Solution, intranasal spray, as hydrochloride: 0.05% (15 mL, 30 mL)

Afrin®, Afrin® Extra Moisturizing, Afrin® Sinus: 0.05% (15 mL) [contains benzyl alcohol; no drip formula]

Afrin® Original: 0.05% (15 mL, 30 mL, 45 mL)

Afrin® Severe Congestion: 0.05% (15 mL) [contains benzyl alcohol; no drip formula]

Duramist® Plus, Neo-Synephrine® 12 Hour, Nostrilla®, Vicks Sinex® 12 Hour Ultrafine Mist, 4-Way® Long Acting Nasal: 0.05% (15 mL)

Duration®: 0.05% (30 mL)

Genasal®: 0.05% (15 mL, 30 mL)

Neo-Synephrine® 12 Hour Extra Moisturizing: 0.05% (15 mL) [contains glycerin]

Solution, ophthalmic, as hydrochloride (OcuClear® [DSC], Visine® L.R.): 0.025% (15 mL, 30 mL)

♦ **Oxytrol**™ *see* Oxybutynin *on page 843*

♦ **Oysco®** [OTC] *see* Calcium Supplements *on page 200*
♦ **Oyst-Cal 500** [OTC] *see* Calcium Supplements *on page 200*
♦ **P-071** *see* Cetirizine *on page 249*
♦ **Pacerone®** *see* Amiodarone *on page 83*

Paclitaxel (PAK li taks el)

U.S. Brand Names Taxol®
Therapeutic Category Antineoplastic Agent, Antimicrotubular
Generic Available No
Use Treatment of advanced metastatic breast cancer, metastatic ovarian cancer, and AIDS-related Kaposi's sarcoma that is refractory to conventional therapy; active in lung cancer, head and neck cancer, bladder cancer, malignant melanoma, and other refractory solid tumors, and leukemias
Pregnancy Risk Factor D
Contraindications Hypersensitivity to paclitaxel, Cremophor® EL (polyoxyethylated castor oil) or any component
Warnings The FDA currently recommends that procedures for proper handling and disposal of antineoplastic agents be considered. Anaphylaxis and severe hypersensitivity reactions have occurred in 2% of patients receiving paclitaxel in clinical trials during first or subsequent infusions. **All patients should be premedicated with a corticosteroid, diphenhydramine, and an H_2-receptor antagonist to prevent hypersensitivity reactions.** Patients who experience severe hypersensitivity reactions to paclitaxel should not be rechallenged with the drug. Be prepared to treat a severe hypersensitivity reaction with epinephrine, I.V. fluids, diphenhydramine and a corticosteroid.

CNS toxicity has been reported in pediatric patients receiving high doses of paclitaxel (350-420 mg/m^2 as a 3-hour infusion) which may have resulted from the ethanol contained in the formulation. Severe bone marrow suppression (primarily neutropenia) with resulting infection may occur. In general, do not administer paclitaxel to patients with baseline neutrophil counts <1500/mm^3.

Precautions Use with caution in patients with moderate or severe hepatic impairment; dosage adjustment may be necessary in patients with hepatic impairment, severe neutropenia, or peripheral neuropathy
Adverse Reactions
Cardiovascular: Hypotension or hypertension, bradycardia, arrhythmias, flushing, syncope, edema
Central nervous system: Seizures, ataxia, fatigue, headache, fever, confusion
Dermatologic: Alopecia, rash, changes in nail pigmentation
Endocrine & metabolic: Elevations in serum triglyceride levels
Gastrointestinal: Mild to moderate nausea/vomiting, diarrhea, mucositis
Hematologic: Severe neutropenia (dose-limiting toxicity), leukopenia, thrombocytopenia, anemia
Hepatic: Elevated AST, alkaline phosphatase, bilirubin
Local: Erythema, tenderness, swelling at the injection site
Neuromuscular & skeletal: Peripheral neuropathy (dose-dependent, characterized by paresthesia with numbness and tingling in a stocking-and-glove distribution), myalgia, muscle weakness, motor dysfunction, arthralgia
Ocular: Loss of visual acuity, diplopia
Renal: Elevated serum creatinine
Respiratory: Dyspnea
Miscellaneous: Anaphylactoid reactions (dyspnea, bronchospasm, hypotension, generalized urticaria), ethanol intoxication
Drug Interactions Cytochrome P450 isoenzyme CYP2C8 and CYP3A3/4 substrate
Paclitaxel clearance decreases approximately 33% when administered following cisplatin. Since paclitaxel is metabolized by cytochrome P450 3A4 and 2C8 isozymes, potential drug interactions can occur with agents that are isoenzyme inducers which reduce plasma paclitaxel concentration (ie, phenytoin) or inhibitors (ie, ketoconazole, verapamil, diazepam, cyclosporine, vincristine, etoposide, dexamethasone) which may increase plasma paclitaxel concentration; opiates, antihistamines, or other CNS depressants may potentiate CNS depression caused by ethanol in the paclitaxel formulation
Stability Refrigerate intact vials or store at room temperature; undiluted vials of paclitaxel may precipitate upon refrigeration, but will redissolve at room temperature with no loss in potency; dilution of paclitaxel from 0.3 mg/mL to 1.2 mg/mL in NS or D$_5$W is stable for up to 48 hours at room temperature; incompatible with amphotericin B, chlorpromazine, hydroxyzine, methylprednisolone, and mitoxantrone
Mechanism of Action An antimicrotubule agent that promotes the assembly of microtubules from tubulin dimers and stabilizes microtubules by preventing
(Continued)

Paclitaxel *(Continued)*

depolymerization; results in the inhibition of mitotic cellular functions and cell replication by blocking cells in the late G2 phase and M phase of the cell cycle

Pharmacokinetics

Distribution: Biphasic with initial rapid distribution to the peripheral compartment; later phase is a slow efflux of paclitaxel from the peripheral compartment

V_d: 227-688 L/m^2

Protein binding: 89% to 98%

Metabolism: Cytochrome P450 hepatic isoenzymes metabolize paclitaxel to 6 alpha-hydroxypaclitaxel

Half-life (varies with dose and infusion duration):

Children: 4.6-17 hours

Adults: 1.5-8.4 hours

Elimination: Urinary recovery of unchanged drug: 1.3% to 12.6%

Dialysis: No significant drug removal by hemodialysis

Usual Dosage I.V. infusion (refer to individual protocols):

Children:

Treatment for refractory leukemia is still undergoing investigation: 250-360 mg/m^2/dose infused over 24 hours every 14 days

Recurrent Wilms' tumor: 250-350 mg/m^2/dose infused over 24 hours every 3 weeks

Adults:

Ovarian carcinoma: 135-175 mg/m^2/dose infused over 1-24 hours every 3 weeks

Metastatic breast cancer: 175 mg/m^2/dose infused over 3 hours every 3 weeks (protocols have used dosages ranging between 135-250 mg/m^2/dose over 1-24 hours every 3 weeks)

Kaposi's sarcoma: 135 mg/m^2/dose infused over 3 hours every 3 weeks, or 100 mg/m^2/dose infused over 3 hours every 2 weeks

Dosage adjustment in renal impairment: None

Dosage adjustment in hepatic impairment:

Total bilirubin ≤1.5 mg/dL and AST >2x normal limits: Total dose <135 mg/m^2

Total bilirubin 1.6-3.0 mg/dL: Total dose ≤75 mg/m^2

Total bilirubin ≥3.1 mg/dL: Total dose ≤50 mg/m^2

Administration Parenteral: I.V.: Patients should be premedicated with a corticosteroid, diphenhydramine and an H$_2$-receptor antagonist 30-60 minutes prior to paclitaxel administration. To minimize patient exposure to the plasticizer diethylhexylphthalate (DEHP) from polyoxyl 35 castor oil-induced leaching of polyvinyl chloride-containing I.V. infusion bags and administration sets, prepare paclitaxel infusions in glass or in polypropylene or polyolefin bags and administer through polyethylene lined administration sets with a 0.22 micron in-line filter. Paclitaxel can be further diluted in D$_5$W, NS, D$_5$/NS or D$_5$ in Ringer's injection to a final concentration of 0.3-1.2 mg/mL. Paclitaxel has been infused over short (1-3 hours) and long periods (24, 72, and 96 hours to 14 days continuous infusion)

Monitoring Parameters CBC with differential, platelet count, vital signs, ECG, liver function test; observe I.V. injection site for extravasation

Patient Information Avoid alcohol; may cause drowsiness and impair ability to perform activities requiring mental alertness or physical coordination

Dosage Forms Injection: 30 mg/5 mL vial [vehicle contains polyoxyethylated castor oil and dehydrated alcohol]

References

Woo MH, Gregornik D, Shearer PD, et al, "Pharmacokinetics of Paclitaxel in an Anephric Patient," *Cancer Chemother Pharmacol*, 1999, 43(1):92-6.

♦ **Palgic® D** *see* Carbinoxamine and Pseudoephedrine *on page 214*

♦ **Palgic® DS** *see* Carbinoxamine and Pseudoephedrine *on page 214*

Palivizumab (pah li VIZ u mab)

U.S. Brand Names Synagis®

Therapeutic Category Monoclonal Antibody

Generic Available No

Use Prevention of serious lower respiratory tract disease caused by respiratory syncytial virus (RSV) in infants and children <2 years of age with chronic lung disease who have required medical therapy for their chronic lung disease within 6 months before the anticipated RSV season; prevention of serious RSV disease in patients with a history of prematurity (≤28 weeks gestation) up to 12 months of age or infants born at 29-32 weeks of gestation up to 6 months of age; prophylaxis of infants with severe immune deficiency exposed to RSV

Pregnancy Risk Factor C

Contraindications Hypersensitivity to palivizumab or any component; not recommended for children with cyanotic congenital heart disease

Warnings Rare cases of anaphylaxis have been reported following re-exposure to palivizumab. Severe acute hypersensitivity reactions have also been reported following administration of palivizumab. Palivizumab should be permanently discontinued if a severe hypersensitivity reaction occurs. If anaphylaxis or severe allergic reaction occurs, administer epinephrine (1:1000) and provide supportive care as required.

Precautions Use with caution in patients with thrombocytopenia or any coagulation disorder. Safety and efficacy have not been demonstrated for treatment of established RSV disease.

Adverse Reactions
Dermatologic: Rash
Gastrointestinal: Diarrhea, vomiting
Hepatic: Elevated SGOT
Local: Injection site reaction, erythema, induration
Respiratory: Upper respiratory infection, otitis media, rhinitis, pharyngitis, cough
Miscellaneous: Anaphylaxis

Drug Interactions No formal drug interaction studies have been conducted. Note: No interference with measles, mumps, and rubella vaccines (combined) and varicella vaccine occurs

Stability Store in refrigerator at a temperature between 2°C to 8°C (35.6°F to 46.4°F) in original container; do not freeze; the single-use vial does not contain a preservative

Reconstitute single-use vial with 1 mL of SWI; swirl vial gently for 30 seconds to avoid foaming. Do not shake vial. Allow solution to stand at room temperature for 20 minutes until it clears; solution should be administered within 6 hours of reconstitution.

Mechanism of Action Humanized monoclonal antibody directed to an epitope in the A antigenic site of the respiratory syncytial virus F protein resulting in neutralizing and fusion-inhibitory activity against RSV

Pharmacokinetics
Half-life:
Children <24 months: 20 days
Adults: 18 days
Time to achieve adequate serum antibody titers: 48 hours

Usual Dosage Children:
I.M.: 15 mg/kg once monthly during RSV season
I.V. (I.V. route is investigational): 15 mg/kg has been administered to patients who could not receive I.M. injections; use has been investigated in hematopoietic stem cell transplant patients with active RSV upper respiratory tract infection.

Administration Parenteral:
I.M.: Administer I.M., preferably in the anterolateral aspect of the thigh; gluteal muscle should not be used routinely as an injection site because of the risk of damage to the sciatic nerve; injection volume over 1 mL should be given as a divided dose
I.V. (I.V. route is investigational): Administer IVP or I.V. intermittent infusion at a rate not to exceed 1-2 mL/minute at a final concentration of 20 mg/mL in SWI. Filter through a 0.22 micron low protein binding filter (Millex-GV) prior to administration.

Monitoring Parameters Observe for anaphylactic or severe allergic reactions

Additional Information RSV prophylaxis should be initiated at the onset of the RSV season. In most areas of the United States, onset of RSV outbreaks is October to December, and termination is March to May, but regional differences occur.

Dosage Forms Injection, powder for reconstitution, lyophilized: 50 mg, 100 mg

References
Boeckh M, Berrey MM, Bowden RA, et al, "Phase 1 Evaluation of the Respiratory Syncytial Virus-Specific Monoclonal Antibody Palivizumab in Recipients of Hematopoietic Stem Cell Transplants," *J Infect Dis*, 2001, 184(3):350-4.

"Palivizumab, a Humanized Respiratory Syncytial Virus Monoclonal Antibody, Reduces Hospitalization From Respiratory Syncytial Virus Infection in High-Risk Infants. The Impact-RSV Study Group," *Pediatrics*, 1998, 102(3 Pt 1):531-7.

"Prevention of Respiratory Syncytial Virus Infections: Indications for the Use of Palivizumab and Update on the Use of RSV-IGIV. American Academy of Pediatrics Committee on Infectious Diseases and Committee on Fetus and Newborn," *Pediatrics*, 1998, 102(5):1211-6.

♦ **Palmer's® Skin Success Acne [OTC]** *see* Benzoyl Peroxide *on page 165*
♦ **Palmer's® Skin Success Acne Cleanser [OTC]** *see* Salicylic Acid *on page 1002*
♦ **Palmitate-A® [OTC]** *see* Vitamin A *on page 1151*
♦ **2-PAM** *see* Pralidoxime *on page 922*
♦ **Pamelor®** *see* Nortriptyline *on page 822*

Pamidronate (pa mi DROE nate)

U.S. Brand Names Aredia®
Synonyms Aminohydroxypropylidene Diphosphonate; APD
(Continued)

Pamidronate *(Continued)*

Therapeutic Category Antidote, Hypercalcemia; Bisphosphonate Derivative

Generic Available Yes

Use Symptomatic treatment of moderate to severe Paget's disease; hypercalcemia associated with malignancy; treatment of osteolytic bone lesions associated with multiple myeloma or metastatic breast cancer

Investigation use: Inhibit bone resorption in severe osteogenesis imperfecta

Pregnancy Risk Factor D

Contraindications Hypersensitivity to pamidronate or any component; pregnancy; severe renal impairment

Warnings Leukopenia has been observed with oral pamidronate; monitoring of white blood cell counts is suggested; vein irritation and thrombophlebitis may occur with I.V. infusions; due to increased potential for renal toxicity, single doses should not exceed 90 mg; monitor serum creatinine prior to each dose; avoid use in patients with severe renal impairment; in patients receiving pamidronate for bone metastases who experience deterioration in renal function, hold treatment until renal function returns to baseline

Precautions Use with caution in patients with renal impairment; maintain adequate hydration and urinary output during treatment; use with caution with other potentially nephrotoxic drugs

Adverse Reactions

Cardiovascular: Tachycardia, hypertension, syncope

Central nervous system: Malaise, fever, fatigue, somnolence, insomnia, seizures

Dermatologic: Rash

Endocrine & metabolic: Hypocalcemia, hypophosphatemia, hypothyroidism, hypokalemia, hypomagnesemia, fluid overload

Gastrointestinal: Nausea, anorexia, constipation, GI hemorrhage, abdominal pain, occult blood in stools, abnormal taste

Hematologic: Leukopenia, anemia

Local: Vein irritation, thrombophlebitis

Neuromuscular & skeletal: Bone pain, myalgia

Ocular: Scleritis, uveitis, conjunctivitis

Renal: Uremia

Respiratory: Rales, rhinitis

Miscellaneous: Moniliasis (associated with 90 mg dosage)

Stability Reconstituted solution stable for 24 hours at room temperature or refrigerated; incompatible with calcium-containing I.V. fluids (ie, Ringer's solution)

Mechanism of Action Pamidronate, a biphosphonate, lowers serum calcium concentrations by binding to bone and inhibiting osteoclast-mediated calcium resorption; this agent does not appear to produce any significant effect on renal tubular calcium handling

Pharmacodynamics

Onset of hypocalcemic action: 24-48 hours

Maximum effect: 5-7 days

Pharmacokinetics

Absorption: Poorly from the GI tract; pharmacokinetic studies are lacking

Distribution half-life: 1.6 hours

Bone half-life: 300 days

Half-life, unmetabolized: 2.5 hours

Elimination: Biphasic; ~50% excreted unchanged in urine within 72 hours

Usual Dosage

Hypercalcemia: I.V.: **Note:** Due to increased risk of nephrotoxicity, doses should not exceed 90 mg

Children (limited experience): 0.5-1 mg/kg

Adults: Dosage based upon serum calcium measurement:

Serum calcium 12-13.5 mg/dL: 60-90 mg

Serum calcium >13.5 mg/dL: 90 mg

Consider retreatment if the serum calcium becomes elevated again; allow a minimum of 7 days between each treatment to allow for a full response to the initial treatment

Osteogenesis imperfecta:

Children (limited experience): 0.5-3 mg/kg/day for 3 days; may repeat in 4- to 6-month intervals; or as an alternative 10-30 mg/m^2 monthly

Osteopenia in nonambulatory children with cerebral palsy: Limited experience (Henderson, 2002); 1 mg/kg/day for 3 days; each dose not <15 mg/day or >30 mg/day; repeat at 3-month intervals

Osteolytic bone lesions of breast cancer or multiple myeloma: Adults: 90 mg/month

Paget's disease: Adults: 30 mg for 3 consecutive days

Administration Reconstitute each vial with 10 mL SWI; dilute further in 250-1000 mL D_5W, $\frac{1}{2}NS$, or NS; do not mix with calcium-containing solutions (eg, LR); infuse over 2-24 hours; longer infusions (>2 hours) may reduce the risk for renal toxicity, particularly in patients with pre-existing renal insufficiency

Monitoring Parameters Monitor serum creatinine prior to each dose; serum calcium, phosphate, potassium, magnesium, hemoglobin, hematocrit, CBC with differential; in addition (Paget's disease) serum alkaline phosphatase, urinary hydroxyproline excretion

Dosage Forms

Injection, powder for reconstitution, lyophilized, as disodium (Aredia®): 30 mg, 90 mg
Injection, solution: 3 mg/mL (10 mL); 6 mg/mL (10 mL); 9 mg/mL (10 mL)

References

Falk MJ, Heeger S, Lynch KA, et al, "Intravenous Bisphosphonate Therapy in Children With Osteogenesis Imperfecta," *Pediatrics*, 2003, 111(3):573-8.
Glorieux FH, Bishop NH, Plotkin H, et al, "Cyclic Administration of Pamidronate in Children With Severe Osteogenesis Imperfecta," *N Engl J Med*, 1998, 339(14):947-52.
Henderson RC, Lark RK, Kecskemethy HH, et al, "Bisphosphonates to Treat Osteopenia in Children With Quadriplegic Cerebral Palsy: A Randomized, Placebo-Controlled Clinical Trial," *J Pediatr*, 2002, 141(5):644-51.
Lteif AN and Zimmerman D, "Bisphosphonates for Treatment of Childhood Hypercalcemia," *Pediatrics*, 1998, 102(4 Pt 1):990-3.

♦ **Pan-2400**™ **[OTC]** *see* Pancreatin *on page 855*

♦ **Pancrease**® *see* Pancrelipase *on page 856*

♦ **Pancrease**® **MT** *see* Pancrelipase *on page 856*

Pancreatin (PAN kree a tin)

U.S. Brand Names Hi-Vegi-Lip® [OTC]; Kutrase®; Ku-Zyme®; Pan-2400™ [OTC]; Pancreatin 4X 600 mg [OTC]; Pancreatin 8X 900 mg [OTC]; Veg-Pancreatin 4X [OTC]

Therapeutic Category Enzyme, Pancreatic; Pancreatic Enzyme

Generic Available Yes

Use Replacement therapy in symptomatic treatment of malabsorption syndrome caused by pancreatic enzyme insufficiency

Pregnancy Risk Factor C

Contraindications Hypersensitivity to pancreatin, any component, or to bovine or pork protein; acute pancreatitis; acute exacerbations of chronic pancreatic diseases

Warnings Pancreatin is inactivated by acids; use microencapsulated products whenever possible, since these products permit better dissolution of enzymes in the duodenum and protect the enzyme preparations from acid degradation in the stomach; these products are not bioequivalent, do not substitute without consulting a physician or pharmacist; do not substitute generic pancreatic enzymes for brand name products

Colonic strictures have been reported in several pediatric patients. There is a possible association between the development of strictures and a high lipase intake (mean >16,000 units/kg/meal). Patients receiving doses >2500 lipase units/kg/meal or 4000 lipase units/g fat/day should be re-evaluated or titrated downward to lowest effective dose.

Precautions Do not spill powder on hands as is a skin irritant; inhalation of powder may produce an asthmatic attack

Adverse Reactions

Dermatologic: Rash
Endocrine & metabolic: Hyperuricemia
Gastrointestinal: Nausea, abdominal cramps, constipation, diarrhea, colonic strictures, mouth irritation, greasy stools, perianal irritation/inflammation, flatulence
Ocular: Lacrimation
Renal: Hyperuricosuria
Respiratory: Sneezing, bronchospasm
Miscellaneous: Hypersensitivity reactions

Drug Interactions Calcium carbonate, magnesium hydroxide may decrease effectiveness of enzymes; pancreatin may decrease the response to oral iron therapy; H_2 antagonists (eg, ranitidine, cimetidine) increase effectiveness of pancreatic enzymes

Food Interactions Avoid placing contents of opened capsules on alkaline foods (pH >5.5), such as dairy products (milk, custard, or ice cream); see Administration

Mechanism of Action Replaces endogenous pancreatic enzymes to assist in digestion of protein, starch and fats

Pharmacokinetics

Absorption: Not absorbed, acts locally in the GI tract
Elimination: In feces
(Continued)

Pancreatin *(Continued)*

Usual Dosage Oral: The following dosage recommendations are only an approximation for initial dosages. The actual dosage will depend on the digestive requirements of the individual patient. Adjust dose based upon body weight and stool fat content. Oral: Total daily dose in children and adults is divided into 3 meals/day plus 2-3 snacks/day with half the meal-time dose given with the snack:

Infants: 2000-4000 lipase units/120 mL (4 ounce) formula

Children ≤4 years: 1000 lipase units/kg/meal (maximum: 2500 lipase units/kg), with ½ dose with each snack

Children >4 years and Adults: 400-500 lipase units/kg/meal (maximum: 2500 lipase units/kg), with ½ dose with each snack

Administration Oral: Swallow capsules/tablets whole; retention in the mouth before swallowing may cause mucosal irritation and stomatitis; administer before or with meals; when administering to infants, may open capsule and spread over acidic foods (applesauce, mashed fruits, rice cereal) in a rubber-tipped teaspoon (use mixture immediately, do not make ahead of time). Place mixture onto the middle of the infant's tongue and then give bottle or breast. As an alternative, the parent may dip a clean finger into the food/enzyme mixture and then place finger into the infant's mouth and allow infant to suck on. Check infant's mouth after eating for lodged enzyme beads and remove.

Monitoring Parameters Stool fat content

Additional Information Concomitant administration of conventional pancreatin enzymes with an H_2-receptor antagonist has been used to decrease acid inactivation of enzyme activity.

Dosage Forms See table.

Pancreatin

Product	Dosage Form	Lipase USP Units	Amylase USP Units	Protease USP Units	Pancreatin mg
Hi-Vegi-Lip®	Tablet	4800	60,000	60,000	2400
Kutrase®	Capsule	2400	30,000	30,000	
Ku-Zyme®	Capsule	1200	15,000	15,000	
Pan-2400™	Capsule	9816	75,900	60,214	2400
Pancreatin 4X 600 mg; Veg-Pancreatin	Tablet	1200	60,000	60,000	2400
Pancreatin 8X 900 mg	Tablet	22,500	180,000	180,000	7200

References

Pettei MJ, Leonidas JC, Levinne JJ, et al, "Pancolonic Disease in Cystic Fibrosis and High-Dose Pancreatic Enzyme Therapy," *J Pediatr*, 1994, 125(4):587-9.

Taylor CJ, "Colonic Strictures in Cystic Fibrosis," *Lancet*, 1994, 343(8898):615-6.

♦ **Pancreatin 4X 600 mg [OTC]** *see* Pancreatin *on page 855*

♦ **Pancreatin 8X 900 mg [OTC]** *see* Pancreatin *on page 855*

♦ **Pancrecarb® MS** *see* Pancrelipase *on page 856*

Pancrelipase *(pan kre LI pase)*

Related Information

Pancreatin *on page 855*

U.S. Brand Names Cotazym® [DSC]; Cotazym-S® [DSC]; Creon®; Ku-Zyme® HP; Lipram™ 4500; Lipram™-CR; Lipram™-PN; Lipram™-UL; Pancrease®; Pancrease® MT; Pancrecarb® MS; Pangestyme™ CN; Pangestyme™ EC; Pangestyme™ MT; Pangestyme™ UL; Ultrase®; Ultrase® MT; Viokase®

Synonyms Lipancreatin

Therapeutic Category Enzyme, Pancreatic; Pancreatic Enzyme

Generic Available Yes

Use Replacement therapy in symptomatic treatment of malabsorption syndrome caused by pancreatic enzyme insufficiency; open occluded feeding tubes

Pregnancy Risk Factor C

Contraindications Hypersensitivity to pancrelipase, any component, or to pork protein; acute pancreatitis; acute exacerbations of chronic pancreatic diseases

Warnings Pancrelipase is inactivated by acids; use microencapsulated products whenever possible, since these products permit better dissolution of enzymes in the duodenum and protect the enzyme preparations from acid degradation in the stomach; products are not bioequivalent, do not substitute without consulting a physician or pharmacist; do not substitute generic enzymes for brand name products

Colonic strictures have been reported in several pediatric patients. There is a possible association between the development of strictures and a high lipase intake (mean >16,000 units/kg/meal). Patients receiving doses >2500 lipase units/kg/meal or 4000 lipase units/g fat/day should be re-evaluated or titrated downward to lowest effective dose.

Precautions Do not spill powder on hands as is skin irritant; inhalation of powder may produce an asthmatic attack

Adverse Reactions

Dermatologic: Rash

Endocrine & metabolic: Hyperuricemia

Gastrointestinal: Nausea, abdominal cramps, constipation, diarrhea, colonic strictures, mouth irritation, greasy stools, perianal irritation/inflammation, flatulence

Ocular: Lacrimation

Renal: Hyperuricosuria

Respiratory: Sneezing, bronchospasm

Miscellaneous: Hypersensitivity reactions

Pancrelipase

Product	Dosage Form	Lipase USP Units	Amylase USP Units	Protease USP Units
Cotazym® [DSC] Ku-Zyme® HP	Capsule	8000	30,000	30,000
Cotazym®-S [DSC]	Capsule, enteric coated spheres	5000	20,000	20,000
Creon® 5	Capsule, delayed release, enteric coated microspheres	5000	16,600	18,750
Creon® 10	Capsule, delayed release, enteric coated microspheres	10,000	33,200	37,500
Creon® 20	Capsule, delayed release, enteric coated microspheres	20,000	66,400	75,000
Lipram™ 4500	Capsule, delayed release, enteric coated microspheres	4500	20,000	25,000
Lipram™-PN 16	Capsule, delayed release, enteric coated microspheres	16,000	48,000	48,000
Lipram™-PN 10	Capsule, delayed release, enteric coated microspheres	10,000	30,000	30,000
Lipram™-CR 10	Capsule, delayed release, enteric coated microspheres	10,000	33,200	37,500
Lipram™-CR 20	Capsule, delayed release, enteric coated microspheres	20,000	66,400	75,000
Lipram™-UL 12	Capsule, delayed release, enteric coated microspheres	12,000	39,000	39,000
Lipram™-UL 18	Capsule, delayed release, enteric coated microspheres	18,000	58,500	58,500
Lipram™-UL 20	Capsule, delayed release, enteric coated microspheres	20,000	65,000	65,000
Pancrease®	Capsule, enteric coated microspheres	4500	20,000	25,000
Pancrease® MT 4	Capsule, enteric coated microtablets	4000	12,000	12,000
Pancrease® MT 10	Capsule, enteric coated microtablets	10,000	30,000	30,000
Pancrease® MT 16	Capsule, enteric coated microtablets	16,000	48,000	48,000

(Continued)

Pancrelipase *(Continued)*

Product	Dosage Form	Lipase USP Units	Amylase USP Units	Protease USP Units
Pancrease® MT 20	Capsule, enteric coated microtablets	20,000	56,000	44,000
Pancrecarb® MS-4	Buffered, enteric coated microspheres	4000	25,000	25,000
Pancrecarb® MS-8	Buffered, enteric-coated microspheres	8000	40,000	45,000
Pangestyme™ CN-10	Capsule, delayed release	10,000	33,200	37,500
Pangestyme™ CN-20	Capsule, delayed release	20,000	66,400	75,000
Pangestyme™ EC	Capsule, enteric coated microspheres	4500	20,000	25,000
Pangestyme™ MT 16	Capsule, enteric coated microtablets	16,000	48,000	48,000
Pangestyme™ UL 12	Capsule, enteric coated microtablets	12,000	39,000	39,000
Pangestyme™ UL 18	Capsule, enteric coated microtablets	18,000	58,500	58,500
Pangestyme™ UL 20	Capsule, enteric coated microtablets	20,000	65,000	65,000
Ultrase®	Capsule, enteric coated microspheres	4500	20,000	25,000
Ultrase® MT 12	Capsule, enteric coated minitablets	12,000	39,000	39,000
Ultrase® MT 18	Capsule, enteric coated minitablets	18,000	58,500	58,500
Ultrase® MT 20	Capsule, enteric coated minitablets	20,000	65,000	65,000
Viokase®	Powder	16,800 (per 0.7 g)	70,000 (per 0.7 g)	70,000 (per 0.7 g)
Viokase® 8	Tablet	8000	30,000	30,000
Viokase® 16	Tablet	16,000	60,000	60,000

Drug Interactions Calcium carbonate, magnesium hydroxide may decrease effectiveness of enzymes; may decrease the response to oral iron therapy; H_2 antagonists (eg, ranitidine, cimetidine) may increase effectiveness of pancreatic enzymes

Food Interactions Avoid placing contents of opened capsules on alkaline foods (pH >5.5), such as dairy products (milk, custard, or ice cream); see Administration

Mechanism of Action Replaces endogenous pancreatic enzymes to assist in digestion of protein, starch and fats

Pharmacokinetics
  Absorption: Not absorbed, acts locally in the GI tract
  Elimination: In feces

Usual Dosage The following dosage recommendations are only an approximation for initial dosages. The actual dosage will depend on the digestive requirements of the individual patient. Adjust dose based upon body weight and stool fat content. Oral: Total daily dose in children and adults is divided into 3 meals/day plus 2-3 snacks/day with half the meal-time dose given with the snack:
  Infants: 2000-4000 lipase units/120 mL (4 ounce) formula
  Children ≤4 years: 1000 lipase units/kg/meal (maximum: 2500 lipase units/kg), with ½ dose with each snack
  Children >4 years and Adults: 400-500 lipase units/kg/meal (maximum: 2500 lipase units/kg), with ½ dose with each snack
  Occluded feeding tubes: Children and Adults: One tablet of Viokase® crushed with one 325 mg tablet of sodium bicarbonate (to activate the Viokase®) in 5 mL of water can be instilled into the nasogastric tube and clamped for 5 minutes; then flushed with 50 mL of water

Administration Oral: Swallow tablets and capsules whole; do not chew the microspheres or microtablets; retention in the mouth before swallowing may cause mucosal irritation and stomatitis; administer before or with meals; when administering to infants, may open capsule and spread over acidic foods (applesauce, mashed fruits, rice cereal) in a rubber-tipped teaspoon (use mixture immediately, do not make ahead of time). Place mixture onto the middle of the infant's tongue and then give bottle or breast. As an alternative, the parent may dip a clean finger into the food/enzyme mixture and then place finger into the infant's mouth and allow infant to suck on. Check infant's mouth after eating for lodged enzyme beads and remove.

Monitoring Parameters Stool fat content

Additional Information Concomitant administration of conventional pancreatin enzymes with an H_2-receptor antagonist has been used to decrease acid inactivation of enzyme activity. Colonic strictures have been reported in several pediatric patients. There is a possible association between the development of strictures and a high lipase intake (mean >16,000 units/kg/meal). Patients receiving doses >2500 lipase units/kg/meal or 4000 lipase units/g fat/day should be re-evaluated or titrated downward to lowest effective dose

Dosage Forms See tables on pages 857 and 858.

References

Pettei MJ, Leonidas JC, Levinne JJ, et al, "Pancolonic Disease in Cystic Fibrosis and High-Dose Pancreatic Enzyme Therapy," *J Pediatr*, 1994, 125(4):587-9.

Taylor CG, "Colonic Strictures in Cystic Fibrosis," *Lancet*, 1994, 343(8898):615-6.

Pancuronium (pan kyoo ROE nee um)

Therapeutic Category Neuromuscular Blocker Agent, Nondepolarizing; Skeletal Muscle Relaxant, Paralytic

Generic Available Yes

Use Produces skeletal muscle relaxation during surgery after induction of general anesthesia, increases pulmonary compliance during assisted mechanical respiration, facilitates endotracheal intubation

Pregnancy Risk Factor C

Contraindications Hypersensitivity to pancuronium, bromide, or any component (see Warnings)

Warnings Ventilation must be supported during neuromuscular blockade; electrolyte imbalance alters blockade; contains benzyl alcohol which may cause allergic reactions in susceptible individuals; large amounts of benzyl alcohol (≥99 mg/kg/day) have been associated with a potentially fatal toxicity ("gasping syndrome") in neonates; the "gasping syndrome" consists of metabolic acidosis, respiratory distress, gasping respirations, CNS dysfunction (including convulsions, intracranial hemorrhage), hypotension and cardiovascular collapse; *in vitro* and animal studies have shown that benzoate, a metabolite of benzyl alcohol, displaces bilirubin from protein binding sites; avoid use of benzyl alcohol containing products in neonates

Precautions Use with caution and decrease dose in patients with decreased renal function; many clinical conditions may affect the response to neuromuscular blockade, see table.

Clinical Conditions Affecting Neuromuscular Blockade

Potentiation	Antagonism
Electrolyte abnormalities	Alkalosis
Severe hyponatremia	Hypercalcemia
Severe hypocalcemia	Demyelinating lesions
Severe hypokalemia	Peripheral neuropathies
Hypermagnesemia	Diabetes mellitus
Neuromuscular diseases	
Acidosis	
Acute intermittent porphyria	
Renal failure	
Hepatic failure	

Adverse Reactions Most frequent adverse reactions are related to prolongation of pharmacologic actions

Cardiovascular: Tachycardia, hypertension
Dermatologic: Rash, erythema
Gastrointestinal: Excessive salivation
Local: Burning sensation along the vein
Neuromuscular & skeletal: Muscle weakness
Respiratory: Wheezes, bronchospasm
Miscellaneous: Hypersensitivity reactions

Drug Interactions See table on next page.

Stability Refrigerate; however, stable for up to 6 months at room temperature; compatible with D_5W, NS, D_5NS, and LR injections

Mechanism of Action Nondepolarizing neuromuscular blocker which blocks acetylcholine from binding to receptors on motor endplate thus inhibiting depolarization

(Continued)

Pancuronium (Continued)

Potential Drug Interactions

Potentiation	Antagonism
Inhalation anesthetics	Calcium
Desflurane, sevoflurane, enflurane and	Carbamazepine
isoflurane > halothane > nitrous	Phenytoin
oxide	Steroids (chronic administration)
Antibiotics	Theophylline
Aminoglycosides, polymyxins,	Anticholinesterases*
clindamycin, vancomycin, tetracycline	Neostigmine, pyridostigmine,
Magnesium	edrophonium, echothiophate
Antiarrhythmics	ophthalmic solution
Quinidine, procainamide, bretylium, and	Caffeine
possibly lidocaine	Azathioprine
Diuretics	
Furosemide, mannitol, thiazides	
Amphotericin B (secondary to hypokalemia)	
Local anesthetics	
Dantrolene (directly depresses skeletal muscle)	
Beta blockers	
Calcium channel blockers	
Ketamine	
Lithium	
Succinylcholine (when administered prior to nondepolarizing neuromuscular-blocking agent)	
Cyclosporine	

*Can prolong the effects of acetylcholine

Pharmacodynamics
Maximum effect: I.V. injection: Within 2-3 minutes
Duration: 40-60 minutes (dose dependent)

Pharmacokinetics
Distribution: V_d: Adult: 0.23 L/kg
Protein binding: 87%
Metabolism: 30% to 40% metabolized in liver
Half-life: 110 minutes
Elimination: Primarily in urine (60%) as unchanged drug and bile (40%)
Clearance: Adult: 1.9 mL/kg/minute

Usual Dosage I.V.:
Neonates and Infants: 0.1 mg/kg every 30-60 minutes as needed or as continuous infusion of 0.02-0.04 mg/kg/hour or 0.4-0.6 mcg/kg/minute
Children: 0.15 mg/kg every 30-60 minutes as needed or as continuous infusion 0.03-0.1 mg/kg/hour or 0.5-1.7 mcg/kg/minute
Adolescents and Adults: 0.15 mg/kg every 30-60 minutes as needed or as a continuous infusion 0.02-0.04 mg/kg/hour or 0.4-0.6 mcg/kg/minute
Dosing adjustment in renal impairment:
Cl_{cr} 10-50 mL/minute: Administer 50% of normal dose
Cl_{cr} <10 mL/minute: Do not use

Administration Parenteral: May be administered undiluted by rapid I.V. injection; for continuous infusion, dilute to 0.01-0.8 mg/mL in D_5NS, D_5W, LR, or NS.

Monitoring Parameters Heart rate, blood pressure, assisted ventilation status, peripheral nerve stimulator measuring twitch response

Nursing Implications Does not alter the patient's state of consciousness; addition of sedation and analgesia are recommended

Additional Information Patients with hepatic and biliary disease have a larger V_d which may result in a higher total initial dose and possibly a slower onset of effect; the duration of neuromuscular blocking effects may be prolonged in patients with hepatic, biliary, or renal dysfunction

Dosage Forms Injection, solution, as bromide: 1 mg/mL (10 mL); 2 mg/mL (2 mL, 5 mL) [may contain benzyl alcohol]

References
Martin LD, Bratton SL, and O'Rourke PP, "Clinical Uses and Controversies of Neuromuscular Blocking Agents in Infants and Children," *Crit Care Med*, 1999, 27(7):1358-68.

♦ **Pandel**® see Hydrocortisone on page 573

- **Pangestyme™ CN** *see* Pancrelipase *on page 856*
- **Pangestyme™ EC** *see* Pancrelipase *on page 856*
- **Pangestyme™ MT** *see* Pancrelipase *on page 856*
- **Pangestyme™ UL** *see* Pancrelipase *on page 856*
- **Panglobulin®** *see* Immune Globulin (Intravenous) *on page 598*
- **PanOxyl®** *see* Benzoyl Peroxide *on page 165*
- **PanOxyl®-AQ** *see* Benzoyl Peroxide *on page 165*
- **PanOxyl® Aqua Gel** *see* Benzoyl Peroxide *on page 165*
- **PanOxyl® Bar [OTC]** *see* Benzoyl Peroxide *on page 165*
- **Panto™ IV (Can)** *see* Pantoprazole *on page 861*
- **Pantoloc™ (Can)** *see* Pantoprazole *on page 861*

Pantoprazole (pan TOE pra zole)

U.S. Brand Names Protonix®

Canadian Brand Names Panto™ IV; Pantoloc™

Therapeutic Category Gastric Acid Secretion Inhibitor; Gastrointestinal Agent, Gastric or Duodenal Ulcer Treatment; Proton Pump Inhibitor

Generic Available No

Use

Oral: Treatment and maintenance of healing of erosive esophagitis associated with gastroesophageal reflux disease (GERD); treatment of pathological hypersecretory conditions including Zollinger-Ellison syndrome; adjunctive therapy of duodenal ulcers associated with *Helicobacter pylori* (unlabeled use)

I.V.: Short-term treatment (7-10 days) of patients with GERD with a history of erosive esophagitis; an alternative to oral therapy in patients who are unable to continue taking oral pantoprazole

Pregnancy Risk Factor B

Contraindications Hypersensitivity to pantoprazole, esomeprazole, omeprazole, lansoprazole, or any component

Warnings In long-term (2-year) studies in rodents, pantoprazole was carcinogenic and caused rare types of gastrointestinal tumors. While available endoscopic evaluations and histologic examinations of biopsy specimens from human stomachs have not detected a risk from short-term exposure to pantoprazole, further human data on the effect of sustained hypochlorhydria and hypergastrinemia are needed to rule out the possibility of an increased risk for the development of tumors in humans receiving long-term therapy.

Adverse Reactions

Cardiovascular: Chest pain, tachycardia, angina, palpitations, hypertension, hypotension, syncope

Central nervous system: Headache, dizziness, vertigo, insomnia, anxiety, fever, nervousness, confusion, depression, emotional lability, hallucinations

Dermatologic: Urticaria, pruritus, acne, alopecia, dry skin, maculopapular rash

Endocrine & metabolic: Hyperglycemia, hyperlipemia, goiter, gout

Gastrointestinal: Diarrhea, nausea, abdominal pain, vomiting, constipation, flatulence, dyspepsia, eructation, xerostomia, anorexia, dysgeusia, duodenitis, dysphagia, glossitis, halitosis, abnormal stools, tongue discoloration, ulcerative colitis, taste perversion

Genitourinary: Urinary frequency, UTI

Hematologic: Thrombocytopenia, leukopenia, leukocytosis, anemia

Hepatic: Hepatitis, elevated liver function tests, cholestatic jaundice, biliary pain, hyperbilirubinemia

Local: I.V.: Thrombophlebitis, abscess

Neuromuscular & skeletal: Muscle cramps, myalgia, arthralgia, neck pain, hypertonia, back pain, paresthesias, decreased reflexes, leg cramps, bone pain, bursitis

Ocular: Amblyopia, diplopia, extraocular palsy, glaucoma

Otic: Ear pain, tinnitus

Renal: Hematuria, pyuria, proteinuria, glycosuria

Respiratory: Rhinitis, bronchitis, cough, dyspnea, pharyngitis, sinusitis, URI

Miscellaneous: Anaphylaxis (I.V. formulation), flu-like syndrome, infection

Drug Interactions Cytochrome P450 isoenzyme CYP1A2 and CYP3A4 inducer; isoenzyme CYP2C19, CYP3A4, CYP2D6, and CYP2C9 substrate

The full potential for drug interactions remains to be determined; due to profound and long-lasting inhibition of gastric acid secretion, pantoprazole may decrease the absorption of ketoconazole, itraconazole, iron salts, and ampicillin esters

Stability Protect from light; store tablets at room temperature; refrigerate powder for injection (36°F to 46°F). Reconstituted injection is stable at room temperature for 2 hours; do not freeze; after further dilution with I.V. fluid, the solution is stable at room temperature for 12 hours. Neither the reconstituted solution or diluted solution need

(Continued)

Pantoprazole *(Continued)*

be protected from light. Pantoprazole stability is a function of pH; it is rapidly degraded in acidic media, but has acceptable stability under alkaline conditions. Each tablet of pantoprazole is enteric coated to prevent degradation by gastric acidity.

Mechanism of Action Suppresses gastric acid secretion by inhibiting the parietal cell membrane enzyme (H+/K+)-ATPase or proton pump; demonstrates antimicrobial activity against *Helicobacter pylori*

Pharmacodynamics Acid secretion: Oral:

Onset of action: 2.5 hours

Duration: 7 days

Pharmacokinetics

Distribution: V_d: Adults: 11-23.6 L

Protein binding: 98%

Metabolism: Extensive liver metabolism; no evidence of active metabolites

Bioavailability: ~77%

Half-life: Adults: 1 hour; prolonged half-life (3.5-10 hours) in slow metabolizers

Time to peak serum concentration: Oral: 2.5 hours

Elimination: Renal: 71% (as metabolites); biliary/fecal: 18%

Clearance: Adults: 7.6-14 L/hour

Dialysis: Not appreciably removed by hemodialysis

Usual Dosage

Erosive esophagitis associated with GERD:

Children: Oral: Limited data; 20 mg once daily (0.5-1 mg/kg/day) was used in 15 children, 6-13 years of age (20-40 kg) for 28 days (Madrazo-De La Garza, 2003)

Adults: Treatment and maintenance:

Oral: 40 mg/day for up to 8 weeks; in mild GERD, 20 mg/day has been effective

I.V.: 40 mg/day for 7-10 days

Hypersecretory conditions (including Zollinger-Ellison syndrome): Adults:

Oral: Initial: 40 mg twice daily; adjust dose based on patient response; doses up to 240 mg/day have been used

I.V.: Initial: 80 mg twice daily; adjust dosage to maintain acid output below 10 mEq/hour; doses up to 80 mg every 8 hours have been used

Adjunctive therapy of duodenal ulcers associated with *Helicobacter pylori* (in combination with antibiotic therapy) (unlabeled use): Adults: Oral: 40 mg once or twice daily

Administration

I.V.: Reconstitute powder for injection with 10 mL NS; further dilute in NS, D_5W, or LR to a final concentration 0.4-0.8 mg/mL; infuse over 15 minutes at a rate not to exceed 6 mg/minute; must use in-line filter (manufacturer provides 1.2 micron filter; however, filters ranging in pore size from 0.22-5 microns have been used); not for I.M. or S.C. use

Oral: Administer without regard to food; tablet should be swallowed whole, do not chew or crush; may be administered with antacids

Patient Information May cause dry mouth; do not chew or crush tablets

Dosage Forms

Injection, powder for reconstitution: 40 mg

Tablet, enteric coated: 20 mg, 40 mg

Extemporaneous Preparations A 2 mg/mL oral liquid may be prepared by first removing the Protonix® imprint from twenty 40 mg tablets by gently rubbing the tablets on a paper towel dampened with alcohol; allow to air dry; (this eliminates dark flecks in final product). Crush the tablets; place coarse powder in 600 mL beaker and add 340 mL SWI. Place beaker on a magnetic stirrer. While stirring, add 16.8 g sodium bicarbonate powder and stir for about 20 minutes until the tablet remnants have disintegrated and the coating has dissolved. While continuing to stir, add another 16.8 g sodium bicarbonate powder and stir for an additional 5 minutes until the powder dissolves. Add enough SWI to bring the final volume to 400 mL. Mix well. Stable 62 days refrigerated and protected from light. Label "shake well."

Dentinger PJ, Swenson CF, and Anaizi NH, "Stability of Pantoprazole in an Extemporaneously Compounded Oral Liquid," *Am J Health Syst Pharm*, 2002, 59(10):953-6.

References

Madrazo-De La Garza A, Dibildox M, Vargas A, et al, "Efficacy and Safety of Oral Pantoprazole 20 mg Given Once Daily for Reflux Esophagitis in Children," *J Pediatr Gastroenterol Nutr*, 2003, 36(2):261-5.

Papaverine *(pa PAV er een)*

Therapeutic Category Antimigraine Agent; Vasodilator

Generic Available Yes

Use Relief of peripheral and cerebral ischemia associated with arterial spasm; investigationally for prophylaxis of migraine headache; intracavernosal injection for impotence

Pregnancy Risk Factor C

Contraindications Hypersensitivity to papaverine or any component; complete atrioventricular block; Parkinson's disease

Precautions Use with caution in patients with glaucoma; administer I.V. slowly and with caution since arrhythmias and apnea may occur with rapid I.V. use; should **not** be used in neonates due to the increased risk of drug-induced cerebral vasodilation and possibility of an intracranial bleed

Adverse Reactions

Cardiovascular: Flushing of the face, tachycardia, hypotension, arrhythmias with rapid I.V. use

Central nervous system: Depression, dizziness, vertigo, drowsiness, sedation, lethargy, headache

Dermatologic: Pruritus

Gastrointestinal: Xerostomia, nausea, constipation

Hepatic: Hepatic hypersensitivity

Local: Thrombosis at the I.V. administration site

Respiratory: Apnea with rapid I.V. use

Miscellaneous: Diaphoresis

Drug Interactions Cytochrome P450 isoenzyme CYP2D6 substrate

Additive effects with CNS depressants or morphine; papaverine decreases the effects of levodopa

Stability Protect from heat or freezing; do not refrigerate injection; solutions should be clear to pale yellow; precipitates with LR

Mechanism of Action Smooth muscle spasmolytic producing a generalized smooth muscle relaxation including vasodilatation, GI sphincter relaxation, bronchiolar muscle relaxation, and potentially a depressed myocardium

Pharmacodynamics Onset of action: Oral: Rapid

Pharmacokinetics

Protein binding: 90%

Metabolism: Rapid in the liver

Bioavailability: Oral: ~54%

Half-life: 30-120 minutes

Elimination: Primarily as metabolites in urine

Usual Dosage

Children: I.M., I.V.: 1.5 mg/kg 4 times/day

Migraine prophylaxis: 6-15 years: Oral: Initial: 5 mg/kg/day given once daily; range: 5-10 mg/kg/day divided into 2-3 doses/day

Adults:

Oral: 75-300 mg 3-5 times/day

Oral, sustained release: 150-300 mg every 12 hours

I.M., I.V.: 30-120 mg every 3 hours as needed

Administration

Oral: Administer after or with meals, milk or antacids to decrease nausea; swallow sustained release capsule whole, do not crush or chew

Parenteral: Rapid I.V. administration may result in arrhythmias and fatal apnea; administer slow I.V. over 1-2 minutes

Monitoring Parameters Liver enzymes; intraocular pressure in glaucoma patients

Patient Information May cause dizziness, flushing, headache; may cause drowsiness and impair ability to perform activities requiring mental alertness or physical coordination; may cause dry mouth

Additional Information Evidence of therapeutic value of systemic use for relief of peripheral and cerebral ischemia related to arterial spasm is lacking

Further studies are needed to determine the benefit of adding papaverine (60 mg/500 mL) to arterial catheter infusions containing NS or ½NS and heparin 1 unit/mL. One investigation showed a lower risk of arterial catheter failure and longer duration of arterial catheter function in patients 7 months to 5.5 years of age who received papaverine in their arterial catheter solutions; these results should be verified by additional studies before the addition of papaverine to arterial catheter solutions can be recommended.

Dosage Forms

Capsule, sustained release, as hydrochloride: 150 mg

Injection, solution, as hydrochloride: 30 mg/mL (2 mL, 10 mL)

References

Heulitt MJ, Farrington EA, O'Shea TM, et al, "Double-Blind, Randomized, Controlled Trial of Papaverine-Containing Infusions to Prevent Failure of Arterial Catheters in Pediatric Patients," *Crit Care Med*, 1993, 21(6):825-9.

(Continued)

Papaverine *(Continued)*

Sillanpää M and Koponen M, "Papaverine in the Prophylaxis of Migraine and Other Vascular Headache in Children," *Acta Paediatr Scand*, 1978, 67(2):209-12.

♦ **Paracetamol** *see Acetaminophen on page 36*

♦ **Parafon Forte® DSC** *see Chlorzoxazone on page 266*

♦ **Paraplatin®** *see Carboplatin on page 215*

Paregoric (par e GOR ik)

Related Information
Carbohydrate and Alcohol Content of Liquid Medications for Use in Patients Receiving Ketogenic Diets *on page 1431*
Overdose and Toxicology *on page 1388*

Synonyms Camphorated Tincture of Opium

Therapeutic Category Analgesic, Narcotic; Antidiarrheal

Generic Available Yes

Use Treatment of diarrhea or relief of pain; neonatal abstinence syndrome (neonatal opiate withdrawal)

Restrictions C-III

Pregnancy Risk Factor B (D when used for long-term or in high-doses)

Contraindications Hypersensitivity to opium or any component (see Warnings and Additional Information); diarrhea caused by poisoning until the toxic material has been removed

Warnings Abrupt discontinuation after prolonged use may result in symptoms of withdrawal; paregoric contains benzoic acid; benzoic acid (benzoate) is a metabolite of benzyl alcohol; large amounts of benzyl alcohol (≥99 mg/kg/day) have been associated with a potentially fatal toxicity ("gasping syndrome") in neonates; the "gasping syndrome" consists of metabolic acidosis, respiratory distress, gasping respirations, CNS dysfunction (including convulsions, intracranial hemorrhage), hypotension and cardiovascular collapse; use paregoric products containing benzoic acid with caution in neonates; *in vitro* and animal studies have shown that benzoate displaces bilirubin from protein binding sites

Precautions Use with caution in patients with respiratory, hepatic or renal dysfunction, severe prostatic hypertrophy, or history of narcotic abuse; opium shares the toxic potential of opiate agonists, usual precautions of opiate agonist therapy should be observed; infants <3 months of age are more susceptible to respiratory depression, use with caution and in reduced doses in this age group

Adverse Reactions
Cardiovascular: Hypotension, bradycardia, vasodilation
Central nervous system: CNS depression, elevated intracranial pressure, drowsiness, dizziness, sedation
Endocrine & metabolic: Antidiuretic hormone release
Gastrointestinal: Nausea, vomiting, constipation, biliary tract spasm
Genitourinary: Urinary tract spasm, urinary retention
Ocular: Miosis
Respiratory: Respiratory depression
Miscellaneous: Physical and psychological dependence, histamine release

Drug Interactions CNS depressants (eg, alcohol, narcotics, benzodiazepines, tricyclic antidepressants, MAO inhibitors, phenothiazines) may increase effects/toxicity

Stability Store in light-resistant, tightly closed container; protect from freezing

Mechanism of Action Increases smooth muscle tone in GI tract, decreases motility and peristalsis, diminishes digestive secretions

Pharmacokinetics
Metabolism: Opium is metabolized in the liver
Elimination: In urine, primarily as morphine glucuronide conjugates and as parent compound (morphine, codeine, papaverine, etc)

Usual Dosage Oral:
Neonates (full term): (See Additional Information): Neonatal abstinence syndrome (opiate withdrawal): Initial: 0.1 mL/kg or 2 drops/kg with feedings every 3-4 hours; increase dosage by 0.1 mL/kg or 2 drops/kg every 3-4 hours until withdrawal symptoms are controlled; it is rare to exceed 0.7 mL/dose. Stabilize withdrawal symptoms for 3-5 days, then gradually decrease the dosage (keeping the same dosing interval) over a 2- to 4-week period.
Children: 0.25-0.5 mL/kg 1-4 times/day
Adults: 5-10 mL 1-4 times/day

Administration Oral: May administer with food to decrease GI upset; shake well before use

Monitoring Parameters Respiratory rate, blood pressure, heart rate, level of sedation; neonatal abstinence syndrome (opiate withdrawal): Monitor for resolution of withdrawal symptoms (such as irritability, high-pitched cry, stuffy nose, rhinorrhea, vomiting, poor feeding, diarrhea, sneezing, yawning, etc) and signs of over treatment (such as bradycardia, lethargy, hypotonia, irregular respirations, respiratory depression, etc); an abstinence scoring system (eg, Finnegan abstinence scoring system) can be used to more objectively assess neonatal opiate withdrawal symptoms and the need for dosage adjustment

Patient Information Avoid alcohol; may cause drowsiness and impair ability to perform activities requiring mental alertness or physical coordination; may be habit-forming; avoid abrupt discontinuation after prolonged use

Additional Information Do **not** confuse this product with opium tincture which is 25 times **more** potent; each 5 mL of paregoric contains 2 mg morphine equivalent, 0.02 mL anise oil, 20 mg benzoic acid, 20 mg camphor, 0.2 mL glycerin and alcohol; final alcohol content 45%; paregoric also contains papaverine and noscapine; because all of these additives may be harmful to neonates, **a 25-fold dilution of opium tincture** is often preferred for treatment of neonatal abstinence syndrome (opiate withdrawal); see Opium Tincture *on page 836*

Dosage Forms Liquid: 2 mg morphine equivalent/5 mL (473 mL) [equivalent to 20 mg opium powder; contains 45% alcohol and benzoic acid; licorice flavor]

References

Kraus DM and Pham JT, "Neonatal Therapy," *Applied Therapeutics: The Clinical Use of Drugs*, 7th ed, Koda-Kimble MA, Young LY, eds, Baltimore, MD: Lippincott Williams & Wilkins, 2001.

Levy M and Spino M, "Neonatal Withdrawal Syndrome: Associated Drugs and Pharmacologic Management," *Pharmacotherapy*, 1993, 13(3):202-11.

"Neonatal Drug Withdrawal. American Academy of Pediatrics Committee on Drugs," *Pediatrics*, 1998, 101(6):1079-88.

♦ **Parenteral Nutrition (PN)** *see page 1262*

Paromomycin (par oh moe MYE sin)

U.S. Brand Names Humatin®

Therapeutic Category Amebicide

Generic Available Yes

Use Treatment of acute and chronic intestinal amebiasis due to susceptible *Entamoeba histolytica* (not effective in the treatment of extraintestinal amebiasis); tapeworm infestations; adjunctive management of hepatic coma; treatment of cryptosporidial diarrhea

Pregnancy Risk Factor C

Contraindications Hypersensitivity to paromomycin or any component; intestinal obstruction

Warnings May result in overgrowth of nonsusceptible organisms

Precautions Use with caution in patients with impaired GI motility or possible or proven ulcerative bowel lesions; use with caution in patients with impaired renal function

Adverse Reactions

Central nervous system: Headache, vertigo

Dermatologic: Exanthema, rash, pruritus

Endocrine & metabolic: Hypocholesterolemia

Gastrointestinal: Diarrhea, abdominal cramps, nausea, vomiting, anorexia, steatorrhea, secondary enterocolitis, pancreatitis

Hematologic: Eosinophilia

Otic: Ototoxicity

Renal: Hematuria

Drug Interactions May decrease digoxin level; increased effect of oral anticoagulants

Food Interactions Paromomycin may cause malabsorption of xylose, sucrose, and fats

Mechanism of Action Acts directly on ameba in the intestinal lumen; interferes with bacterial protein synthesis by binding to 30S ribosomal subunit of susceptible bacteria

Pharmacokinetics

Absorption: Poor from the GI tract

Elimination: Excreted unchanged in feces; portion of oral dose that may be absorbed is excreted in urine

Usual Dosage Oral:

Children:

Intestinal amebiasis (*Entamoeba histolytica*): 25-35 mg/kg/day divided every 8 hours for 7 days

Dientamoeba fragilis infection: 25-30 mg/kg/day divided every 8 hours for 7 days

Tapeworm:

T. saginata, T. solium, D. latum: 11 mg/kg/dose every 15 minutes for 4 doses

H. nana: 45 mg/kg/day once daily for 5-7 days

(Continued)

Paromomycin *(Continued)*

Adults:

Intestinal amebiasis (*Entamoeba histolytica*): 25-35 mg/kg/day divided every 8 hours for 7 days

Dientamoeba fragilis infection: 25-30 mg/kg/day divided every 8 hours for 7 days

Tapeworm:

T. saginata, T. solium, D. latum: 1 g every 15 minutes for 4 doses

H. nana: 45 mg/kg/day once daily for 5-7 days

Hepatic coma: 4 g/day in 2-4 divided doses for 5-6 days

Cryptosporidial diarrhea: 1.5-2 g/day in 3-4 divided doses for 10-14 days

Administration Oral: Administer with or after meals

Monitoring Parameters Periodic urinalysis and renal function tests; be alert to ototoxicity

Patient Information Notify physician if ringing in ears, hearing loss, or dizziness occurs

Additional Information With the treatment of cestodiasis caused by *T. solium*, paromomycin may cause disintegration of worm segments and release of viable eggs resulting in an increased risk for the development of cysticercosis

Dosage Forms Capsule, as sulfate: 250 mg

References

Danziger LH, Kanyok TP, and Novak RM, "Treatment of Cryptosporidial Diarrhea in an AIDS Patient With Paromomycin," *Ann Pharmacother*, 1993, 27(12):1460-2.

Liu LX and Weller PF, "Antiparasitic Drugs," *N Engl J Med*, 1996, 334(18):1178-84.

Paroxetine *(pa ROKS e teen)*

Related Information

Comparison of Adverse Effects of Antidepressants *on page 1210*

Comparison of Usual Adult Dosage and Mechanism of Action of Antidepressants *on page 1209*

Serotonin Syndrome *on page 1420*

U.S. Brand Names Paxil®; Paxil® CR™

Therapeutic Category Antidepressant, Selective Serotonin Reuptake Inhibitor (SSRI)

Generic Available No

Use Treatment of depression, obsessive compulsive disorder, panic disorder, social anxiety disorder, generalized anxiety disorder, and post-traumatic stress disorder

Paxil® CR™: Treatment of depression and panic disorder

Pregnancy Risk Factor C

Contraindications Hypersensitivity to paroxetine or any component; use of MAO inhibitors within 14 days (potentially fatal reactions may occur, see Drug Interactions); concurrent use of thioridazine

Warnings Avoid abrupt discontinuation; taper dosage gradually in patients receiving >20 mg/day as withdrawal symptoms (sweating, nausea, agitation, anxiety, dizziness, paresthesia, abnormal dreams, confusion, and tremor) have been reported following abrupt discontinuation

Precautions Use with caution in patients with a history of seizures, mania, renal disease, cardiac disease, or hepatic disease and in suicidal patients, children, or during breast-feeding in lactating women; modify dosage in patients with renal or hepatic impairment; may cause hyponatremia, use with caution in patients with volume depletion or diuretic use; may cause abnormal bleeding (eg, ecchymosis, purpura); use with caution in patients with impaired platelet aggregation; no clinical studies have assessed the combined use of paroxetine and electroconvulsive therapy

Adverse Reactions

Cardiovascular: Palpitations, tachycardia, vasodilation, postural hypotension, bradycardia, hypotension

Central nervous system: Headache, somnolence, dizziness, insomnia, nervousness, agitation, anxiety, migraine

Dermatologic: Alopecia, purpura, ecchymosis

Endocrine & metabolic: Hyponatremia (volume-depleted patients), SIADH, sexual dysfunction

Gastrointestinal: Nausea, xerostomia, constipation, vomiting, diarrhea, anorexia, flatulence, gastritis

Hematologic: Anemia, leukopenia

Neuromuscular & skeletal: Weakness, tremor, arthritis, paresthesia, asthenia

Ocular: Eye pain

Otic: Ear pain

Respiratory: Asthma

Miscellaneous: Diaphoresis, thirst, bruxism, akinesia

Drug Interactions Cytochrome P450 isoenzyme CYP2D6 substrate (minor); CYP2D6, CYP1A2 (high dose) (weak), and CYP3A3/4 (weak) isoenzyme inhibitor

Decreased effect with phenobarbital, phenytoin (may also decrease phenytoin levels)

Increased effect/toxicity with alcohol, cimetidine, ritonavir, MAO inhibitors (potential fatal serotonin syndrome: hypertension, hyperthermia, mental status change, myoclonus, hyperpyrexic crisis), dextromethorphan (serotonin syndrome); phenothiazines, type 1C antiarrhythmics; the herbal medicine St John's wort (*Hypericum perforatum*) may increase serious side effects, it use is **not** recommended

Increased effect/toxicity of tricyclic antidepressants, fluoxetine, sertraline, theophylline, warfarin, thioridazine (paroxetine may inhibit the metabolism of thioridazine and increase the risk of serious cardiac effects such as prolongation of the QT$_c$ interval, ventricular arrhythmias, torsade de pointes, and sudden death; concurrent use of thioridazine and paroxetine is contraindicated)

Cyproheptadine may decrease or antagonize effects of paroxetine; use with sumatriptan may cause weakness, incoordination, and hyper-reflexia; paroxetine may decrease the AUC of digoxin by 15%; tryptophan, which can be metabolized to serotonin, may increase serious serotonin side effects and its use is **not** recommended; the combination of paroxetine and pimozide resulted in an oculogyric crisis in a 9-year old boy (Horrigan, 1994); paroxetine may increase or worsen lysergic acid diethylamide (LSD) flashbacks

Food Interactions Tryptophan supplements may increase serious side effects

Immediate release: Food or milk does not significantly affect extent of absorption; food may slightly increase AUC (by 6%), increase peak concentration by 29%, and decrease time to peak from 6.4 hours to 4.9 hours postdose

Controlled release: Bioavailability is not affected by food

Stability

Oral suspension and controlled release tablet: Store ≤77°F (25°C)

Immediate release tablet: Store between 59°F to 86°F (15°C to 30°C)

Mechanism of Action Paroxetine is a selective serotonin reuptake inhibitor (SSRI), chemically unrelated to tricyclic, tetracyclic, or other antidepressants; the inhibition of serotonin reuptake from CNS neuronal synapses potentiates serotonin activity in the brain

Pharmacodynamics

Onset of action: Antidepressant effects: Within 1-4 weeks

Anti-obsessional and antipanic effects: Up to several weeks

Pharmacokinetics

Absorption: Oral: Well absorbed

Distribution: V_d (adults): Mean: 8.7 L/kg; range: 3-28 L/kg

Protein binding: 95%

Metabolism: Extensive by cytochrome P450 enzymes via oxidation and methylation followed by glucuronide and sulfate conjugation; nonlinear kinetics may be seen with higher doses and longer duration of therapy due to saturation of P450 2D6 (CYP2D6), an enzyme partially responsible for metabolism

Bioavailability: Immediate release tablet and oral suspension have equal bioavailability

Half-life: Adults: Mean: 21 hours; range: 3-65 hours

Time to peak serum concentration:

Immediate release tablet: Mean: 5.2 hours

Controlled release tablet: 6-10 hours

Elimination: Metabolites are excreted in urine and bile; 2% of drug excreted unchanged in urine

Usual Dosage Oral: **Note:** For maintenance therapy, use lowest effective dose and periodically reassess need for continued treatment

Children and Adolescents: Limited information is available

Depression: Paroxetine was shown to be effective and generally well tolerated in a recent randomized, double-blind, placebo-controlled parallel-design study; 275 adolescents (12-18 years of age) with major depression were randomized to receive paroxetine, imipramine, or placebo; 93 patients (mean age: 14.8 ± 1.6 years) received paroxetine at initial doses of 20 mg/day given in the morning; doses were increased if needed at week 5 to 30 mg/day (given in divided doses) and at weeks 6-8 to 40 mg/day (given in divided doses); 48% of patients remained at the initial starting dose of 20 mg/day; mean optimal daily dose: 28 ± 8.54 mg (Keller, 2001). Paroxetine was also shown to be effective and well tolerated in an open label clinical trial in 45 children <14 years of age (mean age: 10.7 ± 2 years) with major depression (Rey-Sanchoz, 1997); doses were initiated at 10 mg/day and adjusted upward on an individual basis with a mean dose of 16.2 mg/day used for an average of 8.4 months. Further studies are needed.

Self-injurious behavior: A 15-year old autistic male with self-injurious behavior was successfully treated with paroxetine 20 mg/day (Snead, 1994). Further studies are needed.

(Continued)

Paroxetine *(Continued)*

Social phobia: A small case series reported the effective use of paroxetine in 5 pediatric patients with social phobia [2 children (7 and 11 years of age) and 3 adolescents (16, 17, and 18 years of age)]; comorbid diagnoses (obsessive compulsive disorder and/or dysthymia) existed in 3 patients; doses were adjusted on an individual basis; the 7-year old was started on 2.5 mg/day and increased to 5 mg/day after 4 weeks; the 11-year old was started on 5 mg/day and the dose was titrated upwards by 5 mg/day increments every 3-4 weeks to 15 mg/day; adolescents were started on ≤20 mg/day (see Mancini, 1999); further studies are needed

Adults:

Depression: Initial: 20 mg/day given once daily preferably in the morning; increase if needed by 10 mg/day increments at intervals of at least 1 week; maximum dose: 50 mg/day

Paxil® CR™: Initial: 25 mg/day given once daily preferably in the morning; increase if needed by 12.5 mg/day increments at intervals of at least 1 week; maximum dose: 62.5 mg/day

Obsessive compulsive disorder: Initial: 20 mg/day given once daily preferably in the morning; increase by 10 mg/day increments at intervals of at least 1 week; recommended dose: 40 mg/day; range: 20-60 mg/day; maximum dose: 60 mg/day

Panic disorder: Initial: 10 mg/day given once daily preferably in the morning; increase by 10 mg/day increments at intervals of at least 1 week; recommended dose: 40 mg/day; range: 10-60 mg/day; maximum dose: 60 mg/day

Paxil® CR™: Initial: 12.5 mg/day given once daily preferably in the morning; increase if needed by 12.5 mg/day increments at intervals of at least 1 week; maximum dose: 75 mg/day

Social anxiety disorder: Initial: 20 mg/day given once daily preferably in the morning; recommended dose: 20 mg/day; range: 20-60 mg/day; doses >20 mg may not have additional benefit

Generalized anxiety disorder: Initial: 20 mg/day given once daily preferably in the morning; recommended dose: 20 mg/day; range: 20-50 mg/day; doses >20 mg may not have additional benefit

Post-traumatic stress disorder: Initial: 20 mg/day given once daily preferably in the morning; recommended dose: 20 mg/day; range: 20-50 mg/day; doses of 40 mg/day have not been shown to be of greater benefit than 20 mg/day; if indicated, increase dose by 10 mg/day increments at intervals of at least 1 week

Dosing adjustment in severe hepatic or renal impairment: Adults: Initial: 10 mg/day; increase if needed by 10 mg/day increments at intervals of at least 1 week; maximum dose: 40 mg/day

Paxil® CR™: Initial: 12.5 mg/day; increase if needed by 12.5 mg/day increments at intervals of at least 1 week; maximum dose: 50 mg/day

Administration May be administered without regard to meals; administration with food may decrease GI side effects; shake suspension well before use; do not chew or crush controlled release tablet, swallow whole

Monitoring Parameters Blood pressure, heart rate, liver and renal function

Patient Information Avoid alcohol, tryptophan supplements, and the herbal medicine St John's wort; may cause dizziness or drowsiness and impair ability to perform activities requiring mental alertness or physical coordination; may cause dry mouth; avoid abrupt discontinuation; inform physician if taking or planning to take other medications, supplements, or herbal products

Additional Information Paroxetine is more potent and more selective than other SSRIs (eg, fluoxetine, fluvoxamine, sertraline, and clomipramine) in the inhibition of serotonin reuptake; if used for an extended period of time, long-term usefulness of paroxetine should be periodically re-evaluated for an individual patient; Paxil® CR™ tablets contain a degradable polymeric matrix (that controls the dissolution rate over ~4-5 hours) and an entering coating (that delays drug release until tablets leave the stomach); a recent report describes 5 children (age: 8-15 years) who developed epistaxis (n=4) or bruising (n=1) while receiving SSRI therapy (sertraline) (Lake, 2000). Another recent report describes the SSRI discontinuation syndrome in 6 children; the syndrome was similar to that reported in adults (see Diler, 2002).

Dosage Forms Note: Available as paroxetine hydrochloride; mg strength refers to paroxetine

Suspension, oral (Paxil®): 10 mg/5 mL (250 mL) [orange flavor]

Tablet (Paxil®): 10 mg, 20 mg, 30 mg, 40 mg

Tablet, controlled release (Paxil® CR™): 12.5 mg, 25 mg, 37.5 mg

References

Diler RS and Avci A, "Selective Serotonin Reuptake Inhibitor Discontinuation Syndrome in Children: Six Case Reports," *Current Therapeutic Research*, 2002, 63(3):188-97.

Findling RL, Reed MD, and Blumer JL, "Pharmacological Treatment of Depression in Children and Adolescents," *Paediatr Drugs*, 1999, 1(3):161-82.

Horrigan JP and Barnhill LJ, "Paroxetine-Pimozide Drug Interactions," *J Am Acad Child Adolesc Psychiatry*, 1994, 33(7):1060-1.

Keller MB, Ryan ND, Strober M, et al, "Efficacy of Paroxetine in the Treatment of Adolescent Major Depression: A Randomized, Controlled Trial," *J Am Acad Child Adolesc Psychiatry*, 2001, 40(7):762-72.

Lake MB, Birmaher B, Wassick S, et al, "Bleeding and Selective Serotonin Reuptake Inhibitors in Childhood and Adolescence," *J Child Adolesc Psychopharmacol*, 2000, 10(1):35-8.

Mancini C, Van Ameringen M, Oakman JM, et al, "Serotonergic Agents in the Treatment of Social Phobia in Children and Adolescents: A Case Series," *Depress Anxiety*, 1999, 10(1):33-9.

Markel H, Lee A, Holmes RD, et al, "LSD Flashback Syndrome Exacerbated by Selective Serotonin Reuptake Inhibitor Antidepressants in Adolescents," *J Pediatr*, 1994, 125(5 Pt 1):817-9.

Rey-Sanchez F and Guitierrez-Cassares JR, "Paroxetine in Children With Major Depressive Disorder: An Open Trial," *J Am Acad Child Adolesc Psychiatry*, 1997, 36(10):1443-7.

Snead RW, Boon F, and Presberg J, "Paroxetine for Self-Injurious Behavior," *J Am Acad Child Adolesc Psychiatry*, 1994, 33(6):909-10.

- **Parvolex® (Can)** see Acetylcysteine on page 43
- **Pathocil® (Can)** see Dicloxacillin on page 376
- **Paxil®** see Paroxetine on page 866
- **Paxil® CR™** see Paroxetine on page 866
- **PCA** see Procainamide on page 934
- **PCE®** see Erythromycin on page 448
- **Pectin and Kaolin** see Kaolin and Pectin on page 637
- **PediaCare® Decongestant, Infants [OTC]** see Pseudoephedrine on page 958
- **Pediaflor®** see Fluoride on page 500
- **Pediamist® [OTC]** see Sodium Chloride on page 1027
- **Pediapred®** see PrednisoLONE on page 925
- **Pediatric ALS Algorithm, Bradycardia** see page 1179
- **Pediatric ALS Algorithm, Pulseless Arrest** see page 1180
- **Pediatric ALS Algorithm, Tachycardia - Rapid Rhythm and Adequate Perfusion** see page 1181
- **Pediatric ALS Algorithm, Tachycardia - Rapid Rhythm and Evidence of Poor Perfusion** see page 1182
- **Pediatric HIV** see page 1323
- **Pediatrix (Can)** see Acetaminophen on page 36
- **Pediazole®** see Erythromycin and Sulfisoxazole on page 451
- **Pedi-Boro® [OTC]** see Aluminum Acetate on page 73
- **Pedi-Dri®** see Nystatin on page 827
- **Pediotic®** see Neomycin, (Bacitracin) Polymyxin B, and Hydrocortisone on page 802
- **Pedisilk® [OTC]** see Salicylic Acid on page 1002
- **Pedtrace-4®** see Trace Metals on page 1106

Pegaspargase (peg AS par jase)

Related Information
Emetogenic Potential of Single Chemotherapeutic Agents on page 1286

U.S. Brand Names Oncaspar®

Synonyms PEG-L-Asparaginase

Therapeutic Category Antineoplastic Agent, Miscellaneous

Generic Available No

Use
Induction treatment of acute lymphoblastic leukemia in combination with other chemotherapeutic agents in patients who have developed hypersensitivity to native forms of L-asparaginase derived from *E. coli* and/or *Erwinia chrysanthemia*; treatment of lymphoma

Pregnancy Risk Factor C

Contraindications
Pancreatitis; patients who have had significant hemorrhagic events associated with prior L-asparaginase therapy; patients who have had previous serious allergic reactions to pegaspargase

Warnings
The FDA currently recommends that procedures for proper handling and disposal of antineoplastic agents be considered; inhalation of vapors and contact with skin, eyes, or mucous membranes must be avoided; be prepared to treat anaphylaxis at each administration

Precautions
Use with caution in patients receiving anticoagulation therapy, aspirin, or NSAIDs; use with caution in patients with hepatic dysfunction or in patients receiving hepatotoxic agents

Adverse Reactions
Cardiovascular: Hypotension, chest pain, tachycardia

Central nervous system: Somnolence, confusion, seizures, fever, chills, headache, dizziness, malaise, coma, mental status changes

(Continued)

Pegaspargase *(Continued)*

Dermatologic: Rash, pruritus, urticaria

Endocrine & metabolic: Hyperglycemia, transient diabetes mellitus, hyperammonemia, hyperuricemia

Gastrointestinal: Protracted nausea and vomiting, abdominal pain, diarrhea, anorexia, pancreatitis

Genitourinary: Hemorrhagic cystitis

Hematologic: Leukopenia; prolonged prothrombin, thrombin and partial thromboplastin times; decreased fibrinogen; thrombosis; hemorrhage

Hepatic: Hepatotoxicity

Neuromuscular & skeletal: Paresthesia, weakness

Renal: Elevated BUN, elevated serum creatinine, renal failure

Respiratory: Cough, bronchospasm, epistaxis

Miscellaneous: Anaphylaxis

Drug Interactions Methotrexate (decreases antineoplastic effect if given immediately prior to MTX); vincristine (increases toxicity if given concomitantly); prednisone (increases hyperglycemic effect); may increase toxicity of highly protein bound drugs; may increase bleeding in patients receiving warfarin, heparin, aspirin, NSAID, or dipyridamole

Stability Store vials in refrigerator; do not freeze; do not administer if there is any indication that the drug has been frozen; avoid excessive agitation, do not shake; do not use if cloudy or if precipitate is present; use of a 0.2 micron filter may result in some loss of potency

Mechanism of Action Hydrolyzes asparagine to aspartic acid and ammonia depleting the exogenous asparagine supply needed by leukemic cells for protein synthesis

Pharmacokinetics

Absorption: Not absorbed from the GI tract; therefore, requires parenteral administration

Distribution: Apparent V_d: Plasma volume

Half-life: 5.73 days; patients who have had a hypersensitivity reaction to asparaginase have a decreased half-life

Elimination: Clearance is unaffected by age, renal function, or hepatic function; not detected in urine

Usual Dosage Refer to individual protocols; Children and Adults:

I.M., I.V.: 2500 units/m²/dose every 14 days; for children with BSA <0.6 m²: 82.5 units/kg every 14 days

Administration

I.M.: Preferred route of administration due to the lower incidence of hepatotoxicity, coagulopathy, and GI and renal disorders compared to the I.V. route; for I.M. administration, limit the volume at a single injection site to 2 mL; if the volume to be administered is >2 mL, use multiple injection sites

I.V.: Infusion in 100 mL of D_5W or NS over a period of 1-2 hours

Monitoring Parameters Vital signs during administration, CBC, urinalysis, serum amylase, liver enzymes, bilirubin, prothrombin time, renal function tests, urine glucose, blood glucose

Patient Information Notify physician if fever, sore throat, painful/burning urination, bruising, bleeding, or shortness of breath occurs

Nursing Implications Patients should be observed for 1 hour following injection; appropriate agents for maintenance of an adequate airway and treatment of a hypersensitivity reaction (antihistamine, epinephrine, oxygen, I.V. corticosteroids) should be readily available

Dosage Forms Injection, solution [preservative free]: 750 units/mL (5 mL)

References

Asselin BL, Whitin JC, Cappola DJ, et al, "Comparative Pharmacokinetic Studies of Three Asparaginase Preparations," *J Clin Oncol*, 1993, 11(9):1780-6.

Capizzi RL, "Asparaginase Revisited," *Leuk Lymphoma*, 1993, 10(Suppl):147-50.

♦ **PEG-L-Asparaginase** *see* Pegaspargase *on page 869*

♦ **Peglyte™ (Can)** *see* Polyethylene Glycol-Electrolyte Solution *on page 914*

♦ **PemADD™** *see* Pemoline *on page 870*

♦ **PemADD™ CT** *see* Pemoline *on page 870*

Pemoline *(PEM oh leen)*

Related Information

Carbohydrate and Alcohol Content of Liquid Medications for Use in Patients Receiving Ketogenic Diets *on page 1431*

U.S. Brand Names Cylert®; PemADD™; PemADD™ CT

Synonyms Phenylisohydantoin

Therapeutic Category Central Nervous System Stimulant, Nonamphetamine

Generic Available Yes

Use Attention-deficit/hyperactivity disorder (ADHD) (not first-line therapy, see Warnings); narcolepsy

Restrictions C-IV

Pregnancy Risk Factor B

Contraindications Hypersensitivity to pemoline or any component; liver disease; children <6 years of age; Tourette's syndrome

Warnings Life-threatening acute hepatic failure may occur; 15 cases of acute hepatic failure were reported to the FDA since 1975; this is 4 to 17 times the expected rate; 12 of the 15 cases resulted in death or liver transplantation; therefore, pemoline is not considered as first-line drug therapy for ADHD. Initiate pemoline only in patients without liver dysfunction/disease and only with normal baseline liver function tests; monitor serum ALT (SGPT) at baseline and every 2 weeks; discontinue drug if serum ALT increases ≥2 times the upper limit of normal, or to a clinically significant level, or if patient develops signs and symptoms of liver failure. Written informed consent (consent form provided by manufacturer; 847-937-7302) should be obtained prior to starting therapy; therapy should be withdrawn if no significant clinical benefit is seen within 3 weeks after completion of dose titration. Abrupt discontinuation may result in withdrawal symptoms or seizures.

Precautions Use with caution in patients with renal dysfunction, hypertension, or history of drug abuse; may cause growth suppression in children (monitor carefully); may decrease seizure threshold; may exacerbate thought disorder and behavior disturbance in psychotic children

Adverse Reactions
Central nervous system: Insomnia, seizures, precipitation of Tourette's syndrome, dizziness, hallucinations, headache
Dermatologic: Skin rashes
Endocrine & metabolic: Suppression of linear growth
Gastrointestinal: Stomach ache, nausea, diarrhea, anorexia, weight loss
Hematologic: Aplastic anemia (rare)
Hepatic: Elevated liver enzymes (usually reversible upon discontinuation), jaundice, fatal hepatic failure
Neuromuscular & skeletal: Movement disorders
Miscellaneous: Physical and psychological dependence

Drug Interactions CNS stimulants, CNS depressants, sympathomimetics; may alter insulin requirements in diabetics

Mechanism of Action Blocks the reuptake mechanism of dopaminergic neurons, appears to act at the cerebral cortex and subcortical structures; CNS and respiratory stimulant with weak sympathomimetic effects

Pharmacodynamics
Maximum effect: 4 hours; significant benefit on hyperactivity may not be evident until 3rd or 4th week of administration
Duration: 8 hours

Pharmacokinetics
Protein binding: 50%
Metabolism: In the liver
Half-life:
Children: 7-8.6 hours
Adults: 12 hours
Elimination: 43% to 50% excreted unchanged in the urine

Usual Dosage Children ≥6 years: Oral: Initial: 37.5 mg given once daily in the morning, increase by 18.75 mg/day at weekly intervals; effective dose range: 56.25-75 mg/day; maximum dose: 112.5 mg/day; dosage range: 0.5-3 mg/kg/24 hours

Administration Oral: Administer medication in the morning

Monitoring Parameters Liver enzymes (see Warnings); for ADHD: Height, weight

Patient Information Avoid alcohol; avoid caffeine; chewable tablet should be chewed; may cause dizziness and impair ability to perform activities requiring mental alertness or physical coordination; may be habit-forming; avoid abrupt discontinuation after prolonged use; drug may cause liver failure; inform physician immediately of any signs of liver dysfunction such as dark urine, yellow skin, lack of appetite, GI complaints, general feeling of weakness; comply with blood testing of liver function

Additional Information Treatment of ADHD should include "Drug Holidays" or periodic discontinuation of stimulant medication in order to assess the patient's requirements, to decrease tolerance, and limit suppression of linear growth and weight

Dosage Forms
Tablet (Cylert®, PemADD™): 18.75 mg, 37.5 mg, 75 mg
Tablet, chewable (Cylert®, PemADD™ CT): 37.5 mg
(Continued)

Pemoline *(Continued)*

References

Adcock KG, MacElroy DE, Wolford ET, et al, "Pemoline Therapy Resulting in Liver Transplantation," *Ann Pharmacother*, 1998, 32(4):422-5.

Greenhill LL, Pliszka S, Dulcan MK, et al, "Practice Parameter for the Use of Stimulant Medications in the Treatment of Children, Adolescents, and Adults," *J Am Acad Child Adolesc Psychiatry*, 2002, 41(2 Suppl):26S-49S.

Marotta PJ and Roberts EA, "Pemoline Hepatotoxicity in Children," *J Pediatr*, 1998, 132(5):894-7.

Rosh JR, Dellert SF, Narkewicz M, et al, "Four Cases of Severe Hepatotoxicity Associated With Pemoline: Possible Autoimmune Pathogenesis," *Pediatrics*, 1998, 101(5):921-3.

◆ **Pen G** *see* Penicillin G (Parenteral/Aqueous) *on page 875*

Penicillamine *(pen i SIL a meen)*

Related Information

Overdose and Toxicology *on page 1388*

U.S. Brand Names Cuprimine®; Depen®

Synonyms D-3-Mercaptovaline; β,β-Dimethylcysteine; D-Penicillamine

Therapeutic Category Antidote, Copper Toxicity; Antidote, Lead Toxicity; Chelating Agent, Oral

Generic Available No

Use Treatment of Wilson's disease, cystinuria, adjunct in the treatment of severe rheumatoid arthritis; lead poisoning, primary biliary cirrhosis (as adjunctive therapy following initial treatment with calcium EDTA or BAL)

Pregnancy Risk Factor D

Contraindications Hypersensitivity to penicillamine, any component, and possibly penicillin; patients with renal insufficiency; patients with previous penicillamine-related aplastic anemia or agranulocytosis; concomitant administration with other hematopoietic-depressant drugs (eg, gold, immunosuppressants, antimalarials, phenylbutazone), pregnancy, breast-feeding

Warnings Penicillamine has been associated with fatalities due to agranulocytosis, aplastic anemia, thrombocytopenia, Goodpasture's syndrome, and myasthenia gravis; patients should be warned to promptly report any symptoms suggesting toxicity; interruption of continuous therapy for Wilson's disease or cystinuria even for a few days has been associated with sensitivity reactions upon reinstitution of therapy; approximately 33% of patients will experience an allergic reaction

Precautions Patients on penicillamine for Wilson's disease or cystinuria should receive pyridoxine supplementation 25-50 mg/day; when treating rheumatoid arthritis, daily pyridoxine supplementation is also recommended

Adverse Reactions

Cardiovascular: Edema of the face, feet, or lower legs

Central nervous system: Fever, chills, myasthenic syndrome, fatigue

Dermatologic: Rash, pruritus, pemphigus, increased friability of the skin, exfoliative dermatitis, alopecia, angioedema

Endocrine & metabolic: Iron deficiency, hypoglycemia, thyroiditis

Gastrointestinal: Oral lesions, nausea, vomiting (in children with doses >60 mg/kg/day), epigastric pain, colitis, dysgeusia, ageusia, pancreatitis, sore throat, weight gain

Genitourinary: Urinary incontinence, bloody or cloudy urine

Hematologic: Leukopenia, thrombocytopenia, eosinophilia, aplastic anemia, agranulocytosis, hemolytic anemia

Hepatic: Hepatic dysfunction

Neuromuscular & skeletal: Arthralgia, dermatomyositis, polymyositis, peripheral neuropathy

Ocular: Optic neuritis

Otic: Tinnitus

Renal: Nephrotic syndrome, renal vasculitis, Goodpasture's syndrome, proteinuria, hematuria

Respiratory: Obliterative bronchiolitis, pulmonary fibrosis, interstitial pneumonitis, coughing, wheezing

Miscellaneous: Lymphadenopathy, allergic reactions, SLE-like syndrome, white spots on lips or mouth

Drug Interactions Gold, antimalarials, immunosuppressants, phenylbutazone are associated with similar serious hematologic reactions; iron salts, zinc salts, and antacids decrease penicillamine absorption; decreases serum digoxin levels

Food Interactions Do not administer with milk or food; iron and zinc may decrease drug action; increase dietary intake of pyridoxine; for Wilson's disease, decrease copper in diet and omit chocolate, nuts, shellfish, mushrooms, liver, raisins, broccoli, and molasses; for lead poisoning, decrease calcium in diet

Mechanism of Action Chelates with lead, copper, mercury, iron, and other heavy metals to form stable, soluble complexes that are excreted in the urine; depresses circulating IgM rheumatoid factor levels and *in vitro*, depresses T-cell but not B-cell activity; combines with cystine to form a more soluble compound which prevents the formation of cystine calculi

Pharmacokinetics

Absorption: 40% to 70%

Protein binding: 80% bound to albumin

Metabolism: In the liver

Half-life: 1.7-3.2 hours

Time to peak serum concentration: Within 1-2 hours

Elimination: Primarily (30% to 60%) in urine as unchanged drug

Usual Dosage Oral:

Rheumatoid arthritis:

Children: Initial: 3 mg/kg/day (≤250 mg/day) for 3 months, then 6 mg/kg/day (≤500 mg/day) in 2 divided doses for 3 months to a maximum of 10 mg/kg/day (≤1-1.5 g/day) in 3-4 divided doses

Adults: 125-250 mg/day, may increase dose at 1- to 3-month intervals up to 1-1.5 g/day; doses >500 mg/day should be given in divided doses

Wilson's disease (doses titrated to maintain urinary copper excretion >1 mg/day):

Infants and Children: 20 mg/kg/day in 2-4 doses; maximum dose: 1 g/day

Adults: 1 g/day in 4 divided doses; maximum dose: 2 g/day

Cystinuria (doses titrated to maintain urinary cystine excretion at <100-200 mg/day):

Children: 30 mg/kg/day in 4 divided doses; maximum dose: 4 g/day

Adults: Initial: 2 g/day divided every 6 hours (range: 1-4 g/day)

Lead poisoning (continue until blood lead level is <15 µg/dL; treatment duration varies from 4-12 weeks):

Children: 20-30 mg/kg/day in 3-4 divided doses; initiating treatment at 25% of this dose and gradually increasing to the full dose over 2-3 weeks may minimize adverse reactions; maximum dose: 1.5 g/day; a reduced dosage of 15 mg/kg/day in 2 divided doses has been shown to be effective in the treatment of mild to moderate lead poisoning (blood lead concentration 20-40 mcg/dL) with a reduction in adverse effects (Shannon, 2000)

Adults: 1-1.5 g/day in 3-4 divided doses; initiating treatment at 25% of this dose and gradually increasing to the full dose over 2-3 weeks may minimize adverse reactions

Primary biliary cirrhosis: Adults: 250 mg/day to start, increase by 250 mg every 2 weeks up to a maintenance dose of 1 g/day, as 250 mg 4 times/day

Arsenic poisoning: Children: 100 mg/kg/day divided every 6 hours for 5 days; not to exceed 1 g/day

Dosing adjustment in renal impairment: Cl_cr <50 mL/minute: Avoid use

Administration Oral: Administer on an empty stomach 1 hour before or 2 hours after meals; patients unable to swallow capsules may mix contents of capsule with fruit juice or chilled pureed fruit; patients with cystinuria should drink copious amounts of water

Monitoring Parameters Urinalysis, CBC with differential, hemoglobin, platelet count, liver function tests; weekly measurements of urinary and blood concentrations of the intoxicating metal is indicated (3 months has been tolerated); annual x-ray for renal stones; Wilson's disease: 24-hour urinary copper excretion; quantitative 24-hour urine protein at 1- to 2-week intervals initially (first 2-3 months); urinalysis

Patient Information Possible severe allergic reaction if patient allergic to penicillin; notify physician if unusual bleeding or bruising, or persistent fever, sore throat, or fatigue occur. Report any unexplained cough, shortness of breath, or rash; loss of taste may occur; do not skip or miss doses or discontinue without notifying physician.

Dosage Forms

Capsule (Cuprimine®): 125 mg, 250 mg

Tablet (Depen®): 250 mg

Extemporaneous Preparations A 50 mg/mL suspension may be made by mixing sixty 250 mg capsules with 3 g carboxymethylcellulose, 150 g sucrose, 300 mg citric acid, parabens (methylparaben 120 mg, propylparaben 12 mg, propylene glycol qsad to 100 mL), and purified water to a total volume of 300 mL; cherry flavor may be added. Stability is 30 days refrigerated.

DeCastro FJ, Jaeger RQ, and Rolfe UT, "An Extemporaneously Prepared Penicillamine Suspension Used to Treat Lead Intoxication," *Hosp Pharm*, 1977, 2:446-8.

References

Shannon MW and Townsend MK, "Adverse Effects of Reduced-Dose d-Penicillamine in Children With Mild-to-Moderate Lead Poisoning," *Ann Pharmacother*, 2000, 34(1):15-8.

Penicillin G Benzathine (pen i SIL in jee BENZ a theen)

U.S. Brand Names Bicillin® L-A; Permapen® Isoject®

Synonyms Benzathine Benzylpenicillin; Benzathine Penicillin G; Benzylpenicillin Benzathine

Therapeutic Category Antibiotic, Penicillin

Generic Available No

Use Active against most gram-positive organisms and some spirochetes; used only for the treatment of mild to moderately severe infections (ie, *Streptococcus* pharyngitis) caused by organisms susceptible to low concentrations of penicillin G, or for prophylaxis of infections caused by these organisms such as rheumatic fever prophylaxis

Pregnancy Risk Factor B

Contraindications Hypersensitivity to penicillin or any component

Precautions Use with caution in patients with impaired renal function, impaired cardiac function, pre-existing seizure disorder, or hypersensitivity to cephalosporins

Adverse Reactions

Central nervous system: Convulsions, confusion, lethargy, fever, dizziness

Dermatologic: Rash

Hematologic: Hemolytic anemia

Local: Pain at injection site

Neuromuscular & skeletal: Myoclonus

Renal: Interstitial nephritis

Miscellaneous: Jarisch-Herxheimer reaction, hypersensitivity reactions, anaphylaxis

Drug Interactions Probenecid increases serum concentration of penicillin; antibacterial activity with aminoglycosides is synergistic; tetracyclines, chloramphenicol, and erythromycin may antagonize the activity of penicillin

Stability Store in the refrigerator; avoid freezing

Mechanism of Action Inhibits bacterial cell wall synthesis by binding to one or more of the penicillin-binding proteins; inhibits the final transpeptidation step of peptidoglycan synthesis in bacterial cell wall

Pharmacokinetics

Absorption: I.M.: Slow

Distribution: Minimal concentrations attained in CSF with inflamed or uninflamed meninges

Time to peak serum concentration: Within 12-24 hours; serum levels are usually detectable for 1-4 weeks depending on the dose; larger doses result in more sustained levels rather than higher levels

Elimination: Penicillin G is detected in urine for up to 12 weeks after a single I.M. injection; renal clearance is delayed in neonates, young infants, and patients with impaired renal function

Usual Dosage I.M. (dosage frequency depends on infection being treated):

Neonates >1200 g: Asymptomatic congenital syphilis: 50,000 units/kg for 1 dose

Infants and Children:

Group A streptococcal upper respiratory infection: 25,000-50,000 units/kg as a single dose; maximum dose: 1.2 million units/dose **or**

Children <27 kg: 300,000-600,000 units as a single dose

Children ≥27 kg: 900,000 units as a single dose

Prophylaxis of recurrent rheumatic fever: 25,000-50,000 units/kg every 3-4 weeks; maximum dose: 1.2 million units/dose

Congenital syphilis: 50,000 units/kg every week for 3 weeks; maximum dose: 2.4 million units/dose

Syphilis of more than 1-year duration: 50,000 units/kg every week for 3 successive weeks; maximum dose: 2.4 million units/dose

Adults:

Group A streptococcal upper respiratory infection: 1.2 million units as a single dose

Prophylaxis of recurrent rheumatic fever: 1.2 million units every 3-4 weeks or 600,000 units twice monthly

Early syphilis: 2.4 million units as a single dose in 2 injection sites

Syphilis of more than 1-year duration: 2.4 million units (in 2 injection sites) once weekly for 3 doses

Administration Parenteral: I.M.: Give undiluted injection; administer by deep I.M. injection in the upper outer quadrant of the buttock (adolescents and adults) or into the midlateral muscle of the thigh (infants and children); do **not** give I.V., intra-arterially or S.C.; inadvertent I.V. administration has resulted in thrombosis, severe neurovascular damage, cardiac arrest, and death

Monitoring Parameters CBC, urinalysis, renal function tests

Test Interactions Positive Coombs' [direct], false-positive urinary and/or serum proteins

Nursing Implications S.C. administration may cause pain and induration; avoid repeated I.M. injections into the anterolateral thigh in neonates and infants since quadriceps femoris fibrosis and atrophy may occur

Additional Information Use a penicillin G benzathine/penicillin G procaine combination (ie, Bicillin® C-R) to achieve early peak levels in acute infections

Dosage Forms

Injection, suspension [prefilled syringe]:
Bicillin® L-A: 600,000 units/mL (1 mL, 2 mL, 4 mL) [contains povidone]
Permapen® Isoject®: 600,000 units/mL (2 mL) [contains povidone]

References

Kaplan EL, Berrios X, Speth J, et al, "Pharmacokinetics of Benzathine Penicillin G: Serum Levels During the 28 Days After Intramuscular Injection of 1,200,000 Units," *J Pediatr*, 1989, 115(1):146-50.

Paryani SG, Vaughn AJ, Crosby M, et al, "Treatment of Asymptomatic Congenital Syphilis: Benzathine Versus Procaine Penicillin G Therapy," *J Pediatr*, 1994, 125(3):471-5.

WHO Study Group, "Rheumatic Fever and Rheumatic Heart Disease," *World Health Organ Tech Rep Ser*, 1988, 764:1-58.

Penicillin G (Parenteral/Aqueous)

(pen i SIL in jee, pa REN ter al, AYE kwee us)

U.S. Brand Names Pfizerpen®

Synonyms Crystalline Penicillin; Pen G

Therapeutic Category Antibiotic, Penicillin

Generic Available Yes

Use Treatment of sepsis, meningitis, pericarditis, endocarditis, pneumonia, and other infections due to susceptible gram-positive organisms (except *Staphylococcus aureus*), some gram-negative organisms such as *Neisseria gonorrhoeae*, or *N. meningitidis* and some anaerobes and spirochetes

Pregnancy Risk Factor B

Contraindications Hypersensitivity to penicillin or any component

Precautions Use with caution in patients with renal impairment, hypersensitivity to cephalosporins, or pre-existing seizure disorder; dosage modification required in patients with renal impairment; further dosage reduction recommended in patients with impaired hepatic and renal function

Adverse Reactions

Central nervous system: Convulsions, confusion, lethargy, fever, dizziness
Dermatologic: Rash, urticaria
Endocrine & metabolic: Electrolyte imbalance
Gastrointestinal: Diarrhea
Hematologic: Hemolytic anemia, neutropenia
Local: Thrombophlebitis
Neuromuscular & skeletal: Myoclonus
Renal: Acute interstitial nephritis
Miscellaneous: Jarisch-Herxheimer reaction, hypersensitivity reactions, anaphylaxis

Drug Interactions Probenecid increases serum concentration of penicillin; antibacterial activity with aminoglycosides is synergistic; tetracyclines, chloramphenicol, and erythromycin may antagonize the activity of penicillin

Food Interactions Food or milk decreases absorption

Stability Reconstituted parenteral solution is stable for 7 days when refrigerated; incompatible with aminoglycosides; inactivated in acidic or alkaline solutions

Mechanism of Action Inhibits bacterial cell wall synthesis by binding to one or more of the penicillin-binding proteins; inhibits the final transpeptidation step of peptidoglycan synthesis in bacterial cell wall

Pharmacokinetics

Absorption: Oral: <30%
Distribution: Penetration across the blood-brain barrier is poor with uninflamed meninges; crosses the placenta; appears in breast milk
Protein binding: 65%
Metabolism: In the liver (10% to 30%) to penicilloic acid
Half-life:
Neonates:
<6 days: 3.2-3.4 hours
7-13 days: 1.2-2.2 hours
>14 days: 0.9-1.9 hours
Infants and Children: 0.5-1.2 hours
Adults: 0.5-0.75 hours with normal renal function
Time to peak serum concentration:
Oral: Within 30-60 minutes
I.M.: Within 30 minutes
Elimination: Penicillin G and its metabolites are excreted in urine mainly by tubular secretion
(Continued)

Penicillin G (Parenteral/Aqueous) *(Continued)*

Dialysis: Moderately dialyzable (20% to 50%)

Usual Dosage

Neonates: I.M., I.V.:

Postnatal age ≤7 days:

≤2000 g: 50,000 units/kg/day in divided doses every 12 hours

Meningitis: 100,000 units/kg/day in divided doses every 12 hours

>2000 g: 75,000 units/kg/day in divided doses every 8 hours

Meningitis: 150,000 units/kg/day in divided doses every 8 hours

Congenital syphilis: 100,000 units/kg/day in divided doses every 12 hours

Group B streptococcal meningitis: 250,000-450,000 units/kg/day in divided doses every 8 hours

Postnatal age >7 days:

<1200 g: 50,000 units/kg/day in divided doses every 12 hours

Meningitis: 100,000 units/kg/day in divided doses every 12 hours

1200-2000 g: 75,000 units/kg/day in divided doses every 8 hours

Meningitis: 150,000 units/kg/day in divided doses every 8 hours

>2000 g: 100,000 units/kg/day in divided doses every 6 hours

Meningitis: 200,000 units/kg/day in divided doses every 6 hours

Congenital syphilis: 150,000 units/kg/day in divided doses every 8 hours

Group B streptococcal meningitis: I.V.: 450,000 units/kg/day in divided doses every 6 hours

Infants and Children:

I.M., I.V.: 100,000 to 250,000 units/kg/day in divided doses every 4-6 hours

Severe infections: 250,000-400,000 units/kg/day in divided doses every 4-6 hours; maximum dose: 24 million units/day

Adults: I.M., I.V.: 2-24 million units/day in divided doses every 4-6 hours

Dosing interval in renal impairment:

Cl_{cr} 10-30 mL/minute: Administer normal dose every 8-12 hours

Cl_{cr} <10 mL/minute: Administer normal dose every 12-18 hours

Administration Parenteral: Administer by I.V. intermittent infusion over 15-60 minutes at a final concentration for administration of 100,000-500,000 units/mL. A final concentration of 50,000 units/mL infused over 15-30 minutes is recommended for neonates and infants. The potassium or sodium content of the dose should be considered when determining the infusion rate.

Monitoring Parameters Periodic serum electrolytes, renal and hematologic function tests

Test Interactions False-positive or negative urinary glucose determination using Clinitest®; positive Coombs' [direct]; false-positive urinary and/or serum proteins

Additional Information

Penicillin G potassium: 1.7 mEq of potassium and 0.3 mEq of sodium per 1 million units of penicillin G

Penicillin G sodium: 2 mEq of sodium per 1 million units of penicillin G

Dosage Forms

Infusion, as **potassium** [premixed iso-osmotic dextrose solution, frozen]: 1 million units (50 mL), 2 million units (50 mL), 3 million units (50 mL)

Injection, powder for reconstitution, as **potassium** (Pfizerpen®): 5 million units, 20 million units

Injection, powder for reconstitution, as **sodium**: 5 million units

References

American Academy of Pediatrics Committee on Infectious Diseases, "Treatment of Bacterial Meningitis," *Pediatrics*, 1988, 81(6):904-7.

Prober CG, Stevenson DK, and Benitz WE, "The Use of Antibiotics in Neonates Weighing Less Than 1200 Grams," *Pediatr Infect Dis J*, 1990, 9(2):111-21.

Penicillin G Procaine (pen i SIL in jee PROE kane)

U.S. Brand Names Wycillin®

Canadian Brand Names Pfizerpen-AS®

Synonyms APPG; Aqueous Procaine Penicillin G; Procaine Benzylpenicillin; Procaine Penicillin G

Therapeutic Category Antibiotic, Penicillin

Generic Available No

Use Moderately severe infections due to *Treponema pallidum* and other penicillin G-sensitive microorganisms that are susceptible to low but prolonged serum penicillin concentrations

Pregnancy Risk Factor B

Contraindications Hypersensitivity to penicillin, procaine, or any component (see Warnings)

Warnings Some formulations contain sulfites which may cause allergic reactions in susceptible individuals

Precautions Use with caution in patients with renal impairment, hypersensitivity to cephalosporins, or history of seizures; modify dosage in patients with severe renal impairment

Adverse Reactions

Cardiovascular: Myocardial depression, vasodilation, conduction disturbances

Central nervous system: Seizures, confusion, lethargy, dizziness, disorientation, agitation, hallucinations

Hematologic: Hemolytic anemia

Local: Sterile abscess and pain at injection site

Neuromuscular & skeletal: Myoclonus

Renal: Interstitial nephritis

Miscellaneous: Pseudoanaphylactic reactions, Jarisch-Herxheimer reaction, hypersensitivity reactions

Drug Interactions Probenecid increases serum concentration of penicillin; antibacterial activity with aminoglycosides is synergistic; tetracyclines, chloramphenicol, and erythromycin may antagonize the activity of penicillin

Stability Store in refrigerator

Mechanism of Action Inhibits bacterial cell wall synthesis by binding to one or more of the penicillin-binding proteins; inhibits the final transpeptidation step of peptidoglycan synthesis in bacterial cell wall

Pharmacokinetics

Absorption: I.M.: Slow

Distribution: Penetration across the blood-brain barrier is poor, despite inflamed meninges; appears in breast milk

Time to peak serum concentration: Within 1-4 hours and can persist within the therapeutic range for 15-24 hours

Elimination: Renal clearance is delayed in neonates, young infants, and patients with impaired renal function

Dialysis: Moderately dialyzable (20% to 50%)

Usual Dosage I.M.:

Neonates ≥1200 g: Avoid using in this age group since sterile abscesses and procaine toxicity occur more frequently with neonates than older patients

Congenital syphilis: 50,000 units/kg/day once daily for 10 days; if more than 1 day of therapy is missed, the entire course should be restarted

Infants and Children: 25,000-50,000 units/kg/day in divided doses every 12-24 hours; not to exceed 4.8 million units/24 hours

Congenital syphilis: 50,000 units/kg/day once daily for 10 days; if more than 1 day of therapy is missed, the entire course should be restarted

Adults: 0.6-4.8 million units/day in divided doses every 12-24 hours

When used in conjunction with an aminoglycoside for the treatment of endocarditis caused by susceptible S. viridans: 1.2 million units every 6 hours for 2-4 weeks

Neurosyphilis: 2.4 million units once daily for 10 days with probenecid 500 mg every 6 hours

Administration Parenteral: **Do not give I.V., intra-arterially, or S.C.;** procaine suspension for deep I.M. injection only; inadvertent I.V. administration has resulted in neurovascular damage; in infants and children it is preferable to administer I.M. into the midlateral muscles of the thigh; in adults, administer into the gluteus maximus or into the midlateral muscles of the thigh

Monitoring Parameters Periodic renal and hematologic function tests with prolonged therapy

Test Interactions Positive Coombs' [direct], false-positive urinary and/or serum proteins

Nursing Implications Avoid repeated I.M. injections into the anterolateral thigh in neonates and infants since quadriceps femoris fibrosis and atrophy may occur

Dosage Forms Injection, suspension: 600,000 units/mL (1 mL, 2 mL)

References

Paryani SG, Vaughn AJ, Crosby M, et al, "Treatment of Asymptomatic Congenital Syphilis: Benzathine Versus Procaine Penicillin G Therapy," J Pediatr, 1994, 125(3):471-5.

Penicillin V Potassium (pen i SIL in vee poe TASS ee um)

Related Information

Carbohydrate and Alcohol Content of Liquid Medications for Use in Patients Receiving Ketogenic Diets on page 1431

U.S. Brand Names Veetids®

Canadian Brand Names Apo®-Pen VK; Nadopen-V®; Novo-Pen-VK®; Nu-Pen-VK®; PVF® K

Synonyms Phenoxymethyl Penicillin

(Continued)

Penicillin V Potassium *(Continued)*

Therapeutic Category Antibiotic, Penicillin

Generic Available Yes

Use Treatment of mild to moderately severe susceptible bacterial infections involving the upper respiratory tract, skin, and urinary tract; prophylaxis of pneumococcal infections and rheumatic fever

Pregnancy Risk Factor B

Contraindications Hypersensitivity to penicillin or any component

Warnings Oral solution contains sodium benzoate; benzoic acid (benzoate) is a metabolite of benzyl alcohol; large amounts of benzyl alcohol (≥99 mg/kg/day) have been associated with a potentially fatal toxicity ("gasping syndrome") in neonates; the "gasping syndrome" consists of metabolic acidosis, respiratory distress, gasping respirations, CNS dysfunction (including convulsions, intracranial hemorrhage), hypotension and cardiovascular collapse; use oral solution containing sodium benzoate with caution in neonates; *in vitro* and animal studies have shown that benzoate displaces bilirubin from protein binding sites

Precautions Use with caution in patients with renal impairment, hypersensitivity to cephalosporins, or history of seizures; dosage adjustment may be necessary in patients with renal impairment; oral solution may contain aspartame which is metabolized to phenylalanine and must be avoided (or used with caution) in patients with phenylketonuria

Adverse Reactions

Central nervous system: Convulsions, fever

Dermatologic: Rash

Gastrointestinal: Nausea, diarrhea, vomiting, black hairy tongue, pseudomembranous colitis

Hematologic: Hemolytic anemia

Renal: Acute interstitial nephritis

Miscellaneous: Hypersensitivity reactions, anaphylaxis

Drug Interactions Probenecid (higher, prolonged penicillin serum concentration)

Food Interactions Food or milk may decrease absorption

Stability Refrigerate suspension after reconstitution; discard after 14 days

Mechanism of Action Interferes with bacterial cell wall synthesis during active multiplication by binding to one or more of the penicillin-binding proteins; inhibits the final transpeptidation step of peptidoglycan synthesis causing cell wall death and resultant bactericidal activity against susceptible bacteria

Pharmacokinetics

Absorption: Oral: 60% to 73% from the GI tract

Distribution: Widely distributed to kidneys, liver, skin, tonsils, and into synovial, pleural, and pericardial fluids; appears in breast milk

Protein binding: 80%

Metabolism: 10% to 30%

Half-life: 30 minutes and is prolonged in patients with renal impairment

Time to peak serum concentration: Within 30-60 minutes

Elimination: Penicillin V and its metabolites are excreted in urine mainly by tubular secretion

Usual Dosage Oral:

Systemic infections:

Children <12 years: 25-50 mg/kg/day in divided doses every 6-8 hours; maximum dose: 3 g/day

Children ≥12 years and Adults: 125-500 mg every 6-8 hours

Primary prevention of rheumatic fever (treatment of streptococcal tonsillopharyngitis):

Children: 250 mg 2-3 times/day for 10 days

Adolescents and Adults: 500 mg 2-3 times/day for 10 days

Prophylaxis of pneumococcal infections in children with sickle cell disease and functional or anatomic asplenia: Children:

<2 months to 3 years: 125 mg twice daily

>3-5 years: 250 mg twice daily; may discontinue penicillin prophylaxis after 5 years of age in children who have not experienced invasive pneumococcal infection and have received recommended pneumococcal immunizations

Recurrent rheumatic fever, prophylaxis: Children and Adults: 250 mg twice daily

Administration Oral: Administer with water on an empty stomach 1 hour before or 2 hours after meals; may be administered with food to decrease GI upset

Monitoring Parameters Periodic renal and hematologic function tests during prolonged therapy

Test Interactions False-positive or negative urinary glucose determination using Clinitest®; positive Coombs' [direct]; false-positive urinary and/or serum proteins

Additional Information 0.7 mEq of potassium/250 mg penicillin V; 250 mg = 400,000 units of penicillin

Dosage Forms

Powder for oral solution: 125 mg/5 mL (100 mL, 200 mL); 250 mg/5 mL (100 mL, 200 mL) [may contain phenylalanine (as aspartame) and/or sodium benzoate]

Tablet: 250 mg, 500 mg

Tablet, film coated: 250 mg, 500 mg

References

"American Academy of Pediatrics. Committee on Infectious Diseases. Policy Statement: Recommendations for the Prevention of Pneumococcal Infections, Including the Use of Pneumococcal Conjugate Vaccine (Prevnar™), Pneumococcal Polysaccharide Vaccine, and Antibiotic Prophylaxis," *Pediatrics*, 2000, 106(2 Pt 1):362-6.

Dajani A, Taubert K, Ferrieri P, et al, "Treatment of Acute Streptococcal Pharyngitis and Prevention of Rheumatic Fever: A Statement for Health Professionals. Committee on Rheumatic Fever, Endocarditis, and Kawasaki Disease of the Council on Cardiovascular Disease in the Young, the American Heart Association," *Pediatrics*, 1995, 96(4 Pt 1):758-64.

◆ **Penicilloyl-polylysine** *see* Benzylpenicilloyl-polylysine *on page 167*

◆ **Pentam-300®** *see* Pentamidine *on page 879*

Pentamidine (pen TAM i deen)

U.S. Brand Names NebuPent®; Pentam-300®

Therapeutic Category Antibiotic, Miscellaneous; Antiprotozoal

Generic Available Yes (injection)

Use Treatment and prevention of pneumonia caused by *Pneumocystis carinii* in patients who cannot tolerate or who fail to respond to sulfamethoxazole and trimethoprim; treatment of African trypanosomiasis; treatment of visceral leishmaniasis caused by *L. donovani*

Pregnancy Risk Factor C

Contraindications Hypersensitivity to pentamidine isethionate or any component (inhalation and injection); do not use concomitantly with didanosine since both drugs can cause pancreatitis

Warnings Healthcare personnel who administer aerosolized pentamidine inhalation therapy, a cough-producing procedure, should be aware of the possibility of secondary exposure to tuberculosis or other infections from patients with undiagnosed pulmonary disease

Precautions Use with caution in patients with diabetes mellitus, renal or hepatic dysfunction, hypertension or hypotension; adjust dose in renal impairment

Adverse Reactions

Cardiovascular: Hypotension, tachycardia, cardiac arrhythmias

Central nervous system: Dizziness, fever, fatigue, delirium

Dermatologic: Rash, itching

Endocrine & metabolic: Hypoglycemia, hyperglycemia, hypocalcemia, hyperkalemia

Gastrointestinal: Nausea, vomiting, metallic taste, pancreatitis

Hematologic: Megaloblastic anemia, neutropenia, leukopenia, thrombocytopenia

Hepatic: Mild hepatic injury

Local: Pain at injection site, thrombophlebitis, sterile abscess, erythema

Renal: Nephrotoxicity, elevated BUN, elevated serum creatinine

With aerosolized pentamidine: Irritation of the airway, cough, transient arterial desaturation, bronchospasm, fatigue, conjunctivitis

Miscellaneous: Jarisch-Herxheimer-like reaction

Drug Interactions Cytochrome P450 isoenzyme CYP2C19 substrate

Aminoglycosides, amphotericin B, cisplatin and vancomycin (additive nephrotoxicity); didanosine (additive toxicity)

Stability Reconstituted solution is stable for 48 hours at room temperature when protected from light; do not refrigerate due to the possibility of crystallization

Mechanism of Action Interferes with RNA/DNA, phospholipids and protein synthesis through inhibition of oxidative phosphorylation and/or interference with incorporation of nucleotides and nucleic acids into RNA and DNA, in protozoa

Pharmacokinetics

Absorption: I.M.: Well absorbed; limited systemic absorption following pentamidine inhalation therapy

Distribution: Binds to tissues and plasma protein; high concentrations are found in the liver, kidney, adrenals, spleen, lungs and pancreas; poor penetration into CNS; following oral inhalation, high concentrations are found in bronchoalveolar fluid

Half-life, terminal: 6.4-9.4 hours; half-life may be prolonged in patients with severe renal impairment

Elimination: 33% to 66% in urine as unchanged drug

Dialysis: Not appreciably removed by hemodialysis or peritoneal dialysis

(Continued)

Pentamidine (Continued)

Usual Dosage

Children:

Treatment of *Pneumocystis carinii* pneumonia: I.M., I.V. (I.V. preferred): 4 mg/kg/day once daily for 14-21 days

Prophylaxis for *Pneumocystis carinii* pneumonia (See **Note** in Additional Information):

I.M., I.V.: 4 mg/kg/dose every 2-4 weeks **or**

Inhalation: Every month via Respirgard® II nebulizer

Infants <1 year: Aerosolized pentamidine is administered at doses adjusted for minute ventilation and weight

Infant dose = 2.27 mg/kg x nebulizer output (L/minute) x wt (kg) divided by alveolar ventilation (L/minute)

Children <5 years: Some institutions have used a dose of 8 mg/kg

Children ≥5 years: 300 mg/dose

Treatment of trypanosomiasis: I.M.: 4 mg/kg/day once daily for 10 days

Treatment of visceral leishmaniasis: I.M.: 2-4 mg/kg/day once daily or every 2 days for up to 15 doses

Adults:

Treatment: I.M., I.V. (I.V. preferred): 4 mg/kg/day once daily for 14 days

Prevention: Inhalation: 300 mg every 4 weeks via Respirgard® II nebulizer

Dosing adjustment in renal impairment:

Cl_{cr} 10-30 mL/min: Administer normal dose once every 36 hours

Cl_{cr} <10 mL/min: Administer normal dose once every 48 hours

Administration

Oral inhalation: Safe and effective administration via nebulization in children is dependent on patients wearing an appropriately sized pediatric face mask

Parenteral: May administer deep I.M. or by slow I.V. infusion; rapid I.V. administration can cause severe hypotension; infuse I.V. slowly over a period of at least 60 minutes at a final concentration for administration not to exceed 6 mg/mL

Monitoring Parameters Liver function tests, renal function tests, blood glucose, serum potassium and calcium, CBC with differential and platelet count, EKG, blood pressure

Patient Information Maintain adequate fluid intake; notify physician if fever, cough, or shortness of breath occurs; avoid alcohol

Nursing Implications Patients should receive parenteral pentamidine while lying down and blood pressure should be monitored closely during administration and after completion of the infusion until blood pressure is stabilized; if hypotension occurs due to rapid I.V. administration, slow infusion rate to administer dose over 1-2 hours

Additional Information

Note: Guidelines for prophylaxis of *Pneumocystis carinii* pneumonia: Initiate PCP prophylaxis for the following patients: All HIV-exposed children at 4-6 weeks of age and continue through the first year of life or until HIV infection has been reasonably excluded; children 1-5 years of age with CD4+ count <500 or CD4+ percentage <15%; children 6-12 years of age with CD4+ count <200 or CD4+ percentage <15%; for children who had a CD4+ count <750 or a CD4+ percentage <15% in the first year of life, prophylaxis should be continued until 2 years of age

1 mg pentamidine: 1.74 mg pentamidine isethionate

Dosage Forms

Injection, powder for reconstitution, lyophilized, as isethionate (Pentam-300®): 300 mg

Powder for nebulization, lyophilized, as isethionate (NebuPent®): 300 mg

References

Hand IL, Wiznia AA, Porricolo M, et al, "Aerosolized Pentamidine for Prophylaxis of *Pneumocystis carinii* Pneumonia in Infants With Human Immunodeficiency Virus Infection," *Pediatr Infect Dis J*, 1994, 13(2):100-4.

Hughes WT, "*Pneumocystis carinii* Pneumonia: New Approaches to Diagnosis, Treatment, and Prevention," *Pediatr Infect Dis J*, 1991, 10(5):391-9.

"1999 USPHS/IDSA Guidelines for the Prevention of Opportunistic Infections in Persons Infected With Human Immunodeficiency Virus," *MMWR Morb Mortal Wkly Rep*, 1999, 48(RR-10):1-66.

♦ **Pentamycetin® (Can)** see Chloramphenicol on page 255

♦ **Pentasa®** see Mesalamine on page 723

Pentazocine (pen TAZ oh seen)

Related Information

Compatibility of Medications Mixed in a Syringe on page 1412

Narcotic Analgesics Comparison on page 1223

U.S. Brand Names Talwin®; Talwin® NX

Synonyms Pentazocine and Naloxone

Therapeutic Category Analgesic, Narcotic; Opiate Partial Agonist; Sedative

Generic Available Yes (tablet)

Use Relief of moderate to severe pain; a sedative prior to surgery; supplement to surgical anesthesia

Restrictions C-IV

Pregnancy Risk Factor B (D if used for prolonged periods or in high doses at term)

Contraindications Hypersensitivity to pentazocine or any component (see Warnings)

Warnings Pentazocine may precipitate opiate withdrawal symptoms in patients who have been receiving opiates regularly; injection may contain sodium bisulfite which may cause allergic reactions in susceptible individuals

Precautions Use with caution in seizure-prone patients, acute MI, patients undergoing biliary tract surgery, patients with renal and hepatic dysfunction, and patients with a history of prior opioid dependence or abuse; decrease dosage in patients with decreased hepatic or renal function

Adverse Reactions

Cardiovascular: Palpitations, hypotension, tachycardia, peripheral vasodilation

Central nervous system: CNS depression, drowsiness, sedation, dizziness, euphoria, lightheadedness (more frequently than morphine), hallucinations, confusion, disorientation, elevated intracranial pressure; seizures may occur in seizure-prone patients especially with large I.V. doses

Dermatologic: Pruritus, rash

Endocrine & metabolic: Antidiuretic hormone release

Gastrointestinal: Nausea (more frequently than morphine), vomiting, constipation, biliary tract spasm

Genitourinary: Urinary tract spasm

Local: Tissue damage and irritation with I.M./S.C. use

Ocular: Miosis

Respiratory: Respiratory depression, laryngospasm

Miscellaneous: Physical and psychological dependence, histamine release

Drug Interactions Cytochrome P450 isoenzyme CYP2D6 substrate

May potentiate or reduce analgesic effect of opiate agonist (ie, morphine), depending on patient's tolerance to opiates; additive effects seen with other CNS depressants; tripelennamine potentiates pentazocine effects and lethality and the two have been abused in combination (Ts and blues) I.V. to provide effects similar to heroin

Stability Store injection at room temperature; do not mix injection with barbiturates, precipitation will occur

Mechanism of Action Binds to opiate receptors in the CNS, causing inhibition of ascending pain pathways, altering the perception of and response to pain; produces generalized CNS depression

Pharmacodynamics

Onset of action:

Oral, I.M., S.C.: Within 15-30 minutes

I.V.: Within 2-3 minutes

Duration:

Oral: 4-5 hours

Parenteral: 2-3 hours

Pharmacokinetics

Protein binding: 60%

Metabolism: In the liver via oxidative and glucuronide conjugation pathways

Bioavailability: Oral: ~20% due to large first-pass effect; increased oral bioavailability to 60% to 70% in patients with cirrhosis

Half-life: Increased half-life with decreased hepatic function

Children 4-8 years (mean ± SD): 3 ± 1.5 hours

Adults: 2-3 hours

Elimination: Small amounts excreted unchanged in urine

Usual Dosage

Children <14 years: Limited information available:

I.M. doses of 15 mg for children 5-8 years of age and 30 mg for children 9-14 years of age to treat postoperative pain have been used (n=30) (Waterworth, 1974)

In 300 children (1-14 years) I.M. doses ranging from approximately 0.45-1.5 mg/kg in children <27 kg to 0.65-1.9 mg/kg in children >27 kg were used preoperatively (Rita, 1970)

I.V.: Intraoperative: Titrating doses of 0.5 mg/kg every 30-45 minutes as needed for analgesia have been given in 50 children 5-9 years of age; total dose required: 1-1.5 mg/kg (Ray, 1993)

Children >14 years and Adults: Oral: 50 mg every 3-4 hours; may increase to 100 mg/dose if needed; maximum dose: 600 mg/day

Adults:

I.M., S.C.: 30-60 mg every 3-4 hours; maximum: 360 mg/day

(Continued)

Pentazocine *(Continued)*

I.V.: 30 mg every 3-4 hours; maximum: 360 mg/day

Dosing adjustment in renal impairment: Children and Adults:

Cl_{cr} 10-50 mL/minute: Administer 75% of normal dose

Cl_{cr} <10 mL/minute: Administer 50% of normal dose

Administration

Oral: May be administered with food or milk to decrease GI upset

Parenteral: S.C. route not advised due to tissue damage; rotate injection site for I.M., S.C. use; avoid intra-arterial injection

Monitoring Parameters Respiratory and cardiovascular status; level of pain relief and sedation; blood pressure

Patient Information Avoid alcohol; may cause drowsiness and impair ability to perform activities requiring mental alertness or physical coordination; may be habit-forming; avoid abrupt discontinuation after prolonged use; will cause narcotic withdrawal symptoms in patients currently dependent on narcotics

Additional Information Use only in patients who are not tolerant to or physically dependent upon narcotics

Talwin® NX tablet (pentazocine hydrochloride with naloxone) was formulated to decrease abuse potential of dissolving tablets in water and using as injection

Dosage Forms

Injection, solution, as lactate (Talwin®): 30 mg/mL (1 mL, 2 mL, 10 mL) [multidose vial and prefilled syringe contain sodium bisulfite]

Tablet, scored (Talwin® NX): Pentazocine hydrochloride 50 mg and naloxone hydrochloride 0.5 mg

References

Hanunen K, Olkkola KT, Seppala T, et al, "Pharmacokinetics and Pharmacodynamics of Pentazocine in Children," *Pharmacol Toxicol*, 1993, 73(2):120-3.

Ray AD and Gupta M, "Clinical Trial of Pentazocine as Analgesic in Pediatric Cases," *J Indian Med Assoc*, 1994, 92(3):77-9.

Rita L, Seleny FL, and Levin RM, "A Comparison of Pentazocine and Morphine for Pediatric Premedication," *Anesth Analg*, 1970, 49(3):377-82.

Waterworth TA, "Pentazocine (Fortal) as Postoperative Analgesic in Children," *Arch Dis Child*, 1974, 49(6):488-90.

♦ Pentazocine and Naloxone *see* Pentazocine *on page 880*

Pentobarbital *(pen toe BAR bi tal)*

Related Information

Compatibility of Medications Mixed in a Syringe *on page 1412*

Laboratory Detection of Drugs in Urine *on page 1400*

Overdose and Toxicology *on page 1388*

Preprocedure Sedatives in Children *on page 1367*

U.S. Brand Names Nembutal®

Therapeutic Category Anticonvulsant, Barbiturate; Barbiturate; General Anesthetic; Hypnotic; Sedative

Generic Available No

Use Preoperative sedation; high-dose barbiturate coma for treatment of increased intracranial pressure or status epilepticus unresponsive to other therapy

Restrictions C-II

Pregnancy Risk Factor D

Contraindications Hypersensitivity to barbiturates or any component; marked liver function impairment or latent porphyria; chronic or acute pain

Warnings Abrupt discontinuation after prolonged use may result in withdrawal symptoms or seizures; commercially available injection contains 40% propylene glycol

Precautions Use with caution in patients with hypovolemic shock, CHF, or hepatic impairment

Adverse Reactions

Cardiovascular: Arrhythmias, bradycardia, hypotension

Central nervous system: Drowsiness, lethargy, CNS excitation or depression, impaired judgment, hypothermia

Dermatologic: Rash

Gastrointestinal: Nausea, vomiting

Local: Arterial spasm, gangrene with inadvertent intra-arterial injection, thrombophlebitis

Renal: Oliguria

Respiratory: Laryngospasm, respiratory depression, apnea (especially with rapid I.V. use)

Miscellaneous: Physical and psychological dependency with chronic use

Drug Interactions Barbiturates are enzyme inducers (monitor patient closely for decreased effect of concomitantly administered medications or increased effect when barbiturates are discontinued); carbamazepine, chloramphenicol, cimetidine, cortico-steroids, CNS depressants, alcohol, doxycycline, warfarin, valproic acid

Food Interactions High doses of pyridoxine may decrease drug effect; barbiturates may increase the metabolism of vitamins D and K; dietary requirements of vitamins D, K, C, B$_{12}$, folate, and calcium may be increased with long-term use

Stability Protect from light; aqueous solutions are not stable; low pH may cause precipitate; use only clear solution

Mechanism of Action Short-acting barbiturate with sedative, hypnotic, and anticon-vulsant properties; depresses CNS activity by binding to barbiturate site at GABA-receptor complex enhancing GABA activity; depresses reticular activating system; higher doses may be gabamimetic

Pharmacodynamics
Onset of action:
I.M.: Within 10-15 minutes
I.V.: Within 1 minute
Duration: I.V.: 15 minutes

Pharmacokinetics
Distribution: V$_d$:
Children: 0.8 L/kg
Adults: 1 L/kg
Protein binding: 35% to 55%
Metabolism: Extensive in the liver via hydroxylation and oxidation pathways
Half-life, terminal:
Children: 25 hours
Normal adults: 22 hours; range: 35-50 hours
Elimination: <1% excreted unchanged renally

Usual Dosage
Infants ≥6 months and Children: (**Note:** Limited information is available for infants <6 months of age):
Preoperative/preprocedure sedation:
I.M.: 2-6 mg/kg; maximum dose: 100 mg/dose
I.V.: 1-3 mg/kg to a maximum of 100 mg until asleep
Children:
Hypnotic: I.M.: 2-6 mg/kg; maximum dose: 100 mg/dose
Conscious sedation prior to a procedure: Children >18 months: I.V.: Initial: 2 mg/kg, additional doses of 1-2 mg/kg may be given every 5-10 minutes until adequate sedation is achieved; maximum total dose: 6 mg/kg or 150-200 mg; mean total dose required (for CT scan sedation): 3.3-4.5 mg/kg
Adolescents: Conscious sedation: I.V.: 100 mg prior to a procedure
Children and Adults: Pentobarbital coma: I.V. (see Additional Information):
Loading dose: 10-15 mg/kg given slowly over 1-2 hours; monitor blood pressure and respiratory rate
Maintenance infusion: Initial: 1 mg/kg/hour; may increase to 2-3 mg/kg/hour; main-tain burst suppression on EEG
Adults:
Hypnotic:
I.M.: 150-200 mg
I.V.: Initial: 100 mg, may repeat every 1-3 minutes up to 200-500 mg total
Preoperative sedation: I.M.: 150-200 mg

Administration
Parenteral: I.V.: Do not inject >50 mg/minute; rapid I.V. injection may cause respira-tory depression, apnea, laryngospasm, bronchospasm, and hypotension; admin-ister over 10-30 minutes; maximum concentration: 50 mg/mL for slow I.V. push; may dilute in D$_5$W, D$_{10}$W, NS, 1/2NS, LR, Ringer's injection, D$_5$LR, and dextrose/saline combinations for continuous infusion

Monitoring Parameters Vital signs, respiratory status (includes pulse oximetry for conscious sedation), cardiovascular status, CNS status; monitor ICP and cerebral perfusion pressure (CPP) (CPP = MAP - ICP) when using pentobarbital coma to reduce ICP

Reference Range Therapeutic:
Sedation: 1-5 µg/mL (SI: 4-22 µmol/L)
Sleep: 5-15 µg/mL (SI: 22-66 µmol/L)
Coma: 20-40 µg/mL (SI: 88-177 µmol/L)

Patient Information Avoid alcohol; limit caffeine; may be habit-forming; avoid abrupt discontinuation after prolonged use; may cause drowsiness and impair ability to perform activities requiring mental alertness or physical coordination

Nursing Implications Parenteral solutions are very alkaline; avoid extravasation; avoid intra-arterial injection
(Continued)

Pentobarbital *(Continued)*

Additional Information Tolerance to hypnotic effect can occur; taper dose to prevent withdrawal; **Note:** Loading doses of 15-35 mg/kg (given over 1-2 hours) have been utilized in pediatric patients for pentobarbital coma but these higher loading doses often cause hypotension requiring vasopressor therapy

I.V. continuous infusions of pentobarbital using initial bolus doses of 1-2 mg/kg followed by initial continuous infusions of 1-2 mg/kg/hour have been used for PICU sedation in six intubated, mechanically ventilated infants (age: 2-17 months) who "failed" sedation with fentanyl and midazolam infusions; doses were titrated to effect and supplemental boluses were administered as needed; further studies are needed (see Tobias, 1995)

Dosage Forms Injection, solution, as sodium: 50 mg/mL (20 mL, 50 mL) [contains 10% alcohol]

References

Fischer JH and Raineri DL, "Pentobarbital Anesthesia for Status Epilepticus," *Clin Pharm*, 1987, 6(8):601-2.

Hubbard AM, Markowitz RI, Kimmel B, et al, "Sedation for Pediatric Patients Undergoing CT and MRI," *J Comput Assist Tomogr*, 1992, 16(1):3-6.

Pereira JK, Burrows PE, Richards HM, et al, "Comparison of Sedation Regimens for Pediatric Outpatient CT," *Pediatr Radiol*, 1993, 23(5):341-4.

Schaible DH, Cupit GC, Swedlow DB, et al, "High-Dose Pentobarbital Pharmacokinetics in Hypothermic Brain-Injured Children," *J Pediatr*, 1982, 100(4):655-60.

Tobias JD, Deshpande JK, Pietsch JB, et al, "Pentobarbital Sedation for Patients in the Pediatric Intensive Care Unit," *South Med J*, 1995, 88(3):290-4.

♦ **Pentothal**® *see* Thiopental *on page 1084*

Pentoxifylline *(pen toks I fi leen)*

U.S. Brand Names Pentoxil®; Trental®

Canadian Brand Names Albert® Pentoxifylline; Apo®-Pentoxifylline SR; Nu-Pentoxifylline SR; ratio-Pentoxifylline

Synonyms Oxpentifylline

Therapeutic Category Blood Viscosity Reducer Agent

Generic Available Yes

Use Symptomatic management of peripheral vascular disease, mainly intermittent claudication

Investigational use: AIDS patients with increased tumor necrosis factor, cerebrovascular accidents, cerebrovascular diseases, new onset type I diabetes mellitus, diabetic atherosclerosis, diabetic neuropathy, gangrene, cutaneous polyarteritis nodosa, hemodialysis shunt thrombosis, cerebral malaria, septic shock, sepsis in premature neonates, sickle cell syndromes, vasculitis, Kawasaki disease, Raynaud's syndrome, cystic fibrosis, bone marrow transplant-related toxicities (ie, graft-versus-host disease, veno-occlusive disease, and interstitial pneumonitis), and persistent pulmonary hypertension of the newborn

Pregnancy Risk Factor C

Contraindications Hypersensitivity to pentoxifylline, any component, or other xanthine derivatives (eg, caffeine, theophylline, theobromine); recent cerebral or retinal hemorrhage

Warnings Use with caution in patients with renal or hepatic impairment, insulin-treated diabetics, chronic occlusive arterial disease of the limbs, recent surgery, or peptic ulcerations

Adverse Reactions

Cardiovascular: Mild hypotension, angina

Central nervous system: Headache, dizziness, agitation

Gastrointestinal: Dyspepsia, nausea, vomiting

Ocular: Blurred vision

Drug Interactions Cimetidine may increase plasma concentrations of pentoxifylline; pentoxifylline may increase the effect of antihypertensive agents, warfarin, heparin; pentoxifylline may increase serum theophylline levels and toxicity (monitor closely, dosage adjustment of theophylline may be needed)

Food Interactions Food may decrease rate but not extent of absorption

Mechanism of Action Mechanism of action remains unclear; is thought to reduce blood viscosity and improve blood flow by altering the rheology of red blood cells; inhibits production of tumor necrosis factor-alpha; inhibits neutrophil activation and adhesion; increases tissue oxygen levels in patients with peripheral arterial disease; inhibits platelet aggregation

Pharmacodynamics Onset of action: 2-4 weeks with multiple doses

Pharmacokinetics

Absorption: Oral: Well absorbed

Metabolism: Undergoes first-pass in the liver, dose-related (nonlinear) pharmacokinetics

Half-life, apparent:
Parent drug: 24-48 minutes
Metabolites: 60-96 minutes

Time to peak serum concentration: Within 2-4 hours

Elimination: Metabolites excreted in urine; 0% eliminated unchanged in the urine

Usual Dosage Oral:

Children: Minimal information available; one investigation (Furukawa, 1994) found a lower incidence of coronary artery lesions in 22 children (mean age 2 years) treated for acute Kawasaki disease with versus without pentoxifylline 20 mg/kg/day (given in 3 divided doses); all patients received aspirin and I.V. gamma globulin therapy; a lower dose (10 mg/kg/day) was not effective; higher doses have been used investigationally for the treatment of cystic fibrosis (Aronoff 1994)

Adults: 400 mg 3 times/day with meals; decrease to 400 mg twice daily if CNS or GI side effects occur

Administration Administer with food or antacids to decrease GI upset. Do not crush, break, or chew extended or controlled release tablet, swallow whole.

Test Interactions False positive theophylline level

Patient Information Limit caffeine; if GI or CNS side effects continue, contact physician; while beneficial effects may be seen in 2-4 weeks, continue treatment for at least 8 weeks

Dosage Forms

Tablet, controlled release (Trental®): 400 mg
Tablet, extended release (Pentoxil®): 400 mg

References

Aronoff SC, Quinn FJ, Carpenter LS, et al, "Effects of Pentoxifylline on Sputum Neutrophil Elastase and Pulmonary Function in Patients With Cystic Fibrosis: Preliminary Observations," *J Pediatr*, 1994, 125(6 Pt 1):992-7.

Berman W Jr, Berman N, Pathak D, et al, "Effects of Pentoxifylline (Trental®) on Blood Flow, Viscosity, and Oxygen Transport in Young Adults With Inoperable Cyanotic Congenital Heart Disease," *Pediatr Cardiol*, 1994, 15(2):66-70.

Furukawa S, Matsubara T, Umezawa Y, et al, "Pentoxifylline and Intravenous Gamma Globulin Combination Therapy for Acute Kawasaki Disease," *Eur J Pediatr*, 1994, 153(9):663-7.

Lauterbach R, "Pentoxifylline Treatment of Persistent Pulmonary Hypertension of Newborn," *Eur J Pediatr*, 1993, 152(5):460. (I.V. use)

Lauterbach R, Pawlik D, Tomaszczyk B, et al, "Pentoxifylline Treatment of Sepsis of Premature Infants; Preliminary Clinical Observations," *Eur J Pediatr*, 1994, 153(9):672-4. (I.V. use)

MacDonald MJ, Shahidi NT, Allen DB, et al, "Pentoxifylline in the Treatment of Children With New-Onset Type I Diabetes Mellitus," *JAMA*, 1994, 271(1):27-8.

Permethrin *(per METH rin)*

U.S. Brand Names A200® Lice [OTC]; Acticin®; Elimite®; Nix® [OTC]; Rid® Spray [OTC]

Canadian Brand Names Kwellada-P™

Therapeutic Category Antiparasitic Agent, Topical; Pediculocide; Scabicidal Agent
(Continued)

Permethrin *(Continued)*

Generic Available Yes (except spray)

Use Single application treatment of infestation with *Pediculus humanus capitis* (head louse) and its nits; treatment of *Sarcoptes scabiei* (scabies)

Pregnancy Risk Factor B

Contraindications Hypersensitivity to pyrethroid, pyrethrin, any component, or to chrysanthemums

Precautions For external use only; do not use near the eyes or on mucous membranes such as inside the nose, mouth, or vagina

Adverse Reactions
Dermatologic: Pruritus, erythema, rash of the scalp
Local: Burning, stinging, pain, edema, tingling, numbness, scalp discomfort

Mechanism of Action Inhibits sodium ion influx through nerve cell membrane channels in parasites resulting in delayed repolarization, paralysis, and death of organism

Pharmacokinetics
Absorption: Topical: Minimal (<2%)
Metabolism: By ester hydrolysis to inactive metabolites

Usual Dosage Topical: Children >2 months and Adults:
Head lice: After hair has been washed with shampoo, rinsed with water and towel dried, apply a sufficient volume of creme rinse to saturate the hair and scalp; also apply behind the ears and at the base of the neck; leave on hair for 10 minutes before rinsing off with water; remove remaining nits. May repeat in 1 week if lice or nits still present; in areas of head lice resistance to 1% permethrin, 5% permethrin has been applied to clean, dry hair and left on overnight (8-14 hours) under a shower cap.
Scabies: Apply cream from head to toe; leave on for 8-14 hours before washing off with water; for infants, also apply on the hairline, neck, scalp, temple, and forehead; may reapply in 1 week if live mites appear. Permethrin 5% cream was shown to be safe and effective when applied to an infant <1 month of age with neonatal scabies; time of application was limited to 6 hours before rinsing with soap and water.

Administration Topical: Avoid contact with eyes during application; shake creme rinse well before using

Patient Information Clothing and bedding should be washed in hot water or by dry cleaning to kill the scabies mite

Nursing Implications
To remove nits: Comb hair with a fine-toothed nit comb and apply a damp towel to the scalp for 30-60 minutes
For infestation of eyelashes: Apply petroleum ointment to eyelashes 3-4 times/day for 8-10 days; remove nits mechanically from the eyelashes
For scabies: Itching may continue for several weeks despite successful treatment; oral antihistamines and/or topical corticosteroids may be helpful in relieving symptoms

Additional Information Topical cream formulation contains formaldehyde which is a contact allergen

Dosage Forms
Cream topical (Acticin®, Elimite®): 5% (60 g) [contains formaldehyde]
Liquid, topical (Nix®): 1% (60 mL) [contains 20% isopropyl alcohol and propylene glycol; creme rinse formulation]
Lotion, topical: 1% (60 mL)
Shampoo (A200® Lice): 0.33% (60 mL, 120 mL) [contains benzyl alcohol]
Solution, spray [for bedding and furniture]:
A200® Lice: 0.5% (180 mL)
Nix®: 0.25% (148 mL)
Rid®: 0.5% (150 mL)

References
"Drugs for Head Lice," *Med Lett Drugs Ther*, 1997, 39(992):6-7.
Hogan DJ, Schachner L, Tanglertsampan C, "Diagnosis and Treatment of Childhood Scabies and Pediculosis," *Pediatr Clin North Am*, 1991, 38(4):941-57.
Krowchuk DP, Tunnessen WW Jr, and Hurwitz S, "Pediatric Dermatology Update," *Pediatrics*, 1992, 90(2 Pt 1):259-64.
Quarterman MJ and Lesher JL, "Neonatal Scabies Treated With Permethrin 5% Cream," *Pediatr Dermatol*, 1994, 11(3):264-6.

♦ **Pernox® Scrub Cleanser [OTC]** *see* Sulfur and Salicylic Acid *on page 1058*
♦ **Peroxide** *see* Hydrogen Peroxide *on page 577*
♦ **Peroxyl® [OTC]** *see* Hydrogen Peroxide *on page 577*
♦ **Persantine®** *see* Dipyridamole *on page 397*
♦ **Pertussin® DM [OTC]** *see* Dextromethorphan *on page 365*
♦ **Pethidine** *see* Meperidine *on page 717*

- **Pexicam® (Can)** see Piroxicam on page 910
- **PFA** see Foscarnet on page 520
- **Pfizerpen®** see Penicillin G (Parenteral/Aqueous) on page 875
- **Pfizerpen-AS® (Can)** see Penicillin G Procaine on page 876
- **PGE₁** see Alprostadil on page 66
- **Phanasin [OTC]** see Guaifenesin on page 550
- **Pharmaflur®** see Fluoride on page 500
- **Pharmaflur® 1.1** see Fluoride on page 500
- **Phazyme® Quick Dissolve [OTC]** see Simethicone on page 1020
- **Phazyme® Ultra Strength [OTC]** see Simethicone on page 1020
- **Phenaphen® With Codeine** see Acetaminophen and Codeine on page 39
- **Phenazo™ (Can)** see Phenazopyridine on page 887

Phenazopyridine (fen az oh PEER i deen)

U.S. Brand Names Azo-Gesic® [OTC]; Azo-Standard® [OTC]; Prodium® [OTC]; Pyridium®; ReAzo [OTC]; Uristat® [OTC]; UTI Relief® [OTC]

Canadian Brand Names Phenazo™

Synonyms Phenylazo Diamino Pyridine

Therapeutic Category Analgesic, Urinary; Local Anesthetic, Urinary

Generic Available Yes

Use Symptomatic relief of urinary burning, itching, frequency and urgency in association with urinary tract infection, or following urologic procedures

Pregnancy Risk Factor B

Contraindications Hypersensitivity to phenazopyridine or any component; liver or kidney disease (do not use in patients with Cl_{cr} <50 mL/minute)

Warnings Does not treat infection, acts only as an analgesic; drug should be discontinued if skin or sclera develop a yellow color. Pyridium® contains sodium benzoate; benzoic acid (benzoate) is a metabolite of benzyl alcohol; large amounts of benzyl alcohol (≥99 mg/kg/day) have been associated with a potentially fatal toxicity ("gasping syndrome") in neonates; in vitro and animal studies have shown that benzoate displaces bilirubin from protein binding sites; avoid use of Pyridium® in neonates

Precautions Use with caution in patients with renal impairment (Cl_{cr} 50-80 mL/minute)

Adverse Reactions
Central nervous system: Vertigo, headache
Dermatologic: Skin pigmentation, rash, pruritus
Gastrointestinal: Stomach cramps
Genitourinary: Discoloration of urine (orange or red)
Hematologic: Methemoglobinemia, hemolytic anemia
Hepatic: Hepatitis
Renal: Transient acute renal failure

Mechanism of Action Exerts local topical anesthetic or analgesic action on urinary tract mucosa through an unknown mechanism

Pharmacokinetics
Metabolism: In the liver and other tissues
Elimination: In urine (where it exerts its action); renal excretion (as unchanged drug) is rapid and accounts for 65% of the drug's elimination

Usual Dosage Oral:
Children: 12 mg/kg/day in 3 divided doses for 2 days if used concomitantly with an antibacterial agent for UTI
Adults: 100-200 mg 3-4 times/day for 2 days if used concomitantly with an antibacterial agent for UTI
Dosing interval in renal impairment:
Cl_{cr} 50-80 mL/minute: Administer every 8-16 hours
Cl_{cr} <50 mL/minute: Avoid use

Administration Oral: Administer with food to decrease GI distress

Test Interactions False-negative Clinistix®, Tes-Tape®, Ictotest®, Acetest®, Ketostix®, urinalysis based upon spectrometry or color reactions

Patient Information May discolor urine orange or red; may stain contact lenses and fabric; not an antibiotic and does not treat infection; contact physician for antibiotic therapy

Dosage Forms
Tablet, as hydrochloride: 100 mg, 200 mg
Azo-Gesic®, Azo-Standard®, Prodium®, Uristat®: 95 mg
Pyridium®: 100 mg, 200 mg [contains sodium benzoate]
ReAzo: 97 mg
UTI Relief®: 97.2 mg
(Continued)

Phenazopyridine *(Continued)*

Extemporaneous Preparations A 10 mg/mL suspension may be made by crushing three 200 mg tablets. Mix with a small amount of distilled water or glycerin. Add 20 mL Cologel® and levigate until a uniform mixture is obtained. Add sufficient 2:1 simple syrup/cherry syrup mixture to make a final volume of 60 mL. Store in an amber container. Label "shake well". Stability is 60 days refrigerated.

Handbook on Extemporaneous Formulations, Bethesda MD: American Society of Hospital Pharmacists, 1987.

◆ **Phenergan® (Can)** *see* Promethazine *on page 941*

◆ **Phenergan® With Codeine** *see* Promethazine and Codeine *on page 942*

Phenobarbital *(fee noe BAR bi tal)*

Related Information

Antiepileptic Drugs *on page 1374*

Blood Level Sampling Time Guidelines *on page 1386*

Carbohydrate and Alcohol Content of Liquid Medications for Use in Patients Receiving Ketogenic Diets *on page 1431*

Drugs and Breast-Feeding *on page 1404*

Laboratory Detection of Drugs in Urine *on page 1400*

Overdose and Toxicology *on page 1388*

U.S. Brand Names Luminal® Sodium

Synonyms Phenobarbitone; Phenylethylmalonylurea

Therapeutic Category Anticonvulsant, Barbiturate; Barbiturate; Hypnotic; Sedative

Generic Available Yes

Use Management of generalized tonic-clonic (grand mal) and partial seizures; neonatal seizures; febrile seizures in children; sedation; may also be used for prevention and treatment of neonatal hyperbilirubinemia and lowering of bilirubin in chronic cholestasis

Restrictions C-IV

Pregnancy Risk Factor D

Contraindications Hypersensitivity to phenobarbital or any component; pre-existing CNS depression, severe uncontrolled pain, porphyria, severe respiratory disease with dyspnea or obstruction

Warnings Abrupt withdrawal may precipitate status epilepticus

Precautions Use with caution in patients with renal or hepatic impairment

Adverse Reactions

Cardiovascular: Hypotension, circulatory collapse

Central nervous system: Drowsiness, paradoxical excitement, hyperkinetic activity, cognitive impairment, defects in general comprehension, short-term memory deficits, decreased attention span, ataxia

Dermatologic: Skin eruptions, skin rash, exfoliative dermatitis

Hematologic: Megaloblastic anemia

Hepatic: Hepatitis

Respiratory: Respiratory depression, apnea (especially with rapid I.V. use)

Miscellaneous: Psychological and physical dependence

Drug Interactions Cytochrome P450 isoenzyme CYP1A2, CYP2B6, CYP2C8, CYP2C9, CYP2C18, CYP2C19, CYP3A3/4, and CYP3A5-7 inducer

Phenobarbital may decrease the serum concentration or effect of lamotrigine, ritonavir, saquinavir, delavirdine, ethosuximide, warfarin, oral contraceptives, chloramphenicol, griseofulvin, doxycycline, beta-blockers, theophylline, corticosteroids, teniposide, etoposide, doxorubicin, vincristine, methotrexate, tricyclic antidepressants, cyclosporin, quinidine, haloperidol, and phenothiazines

Valproic acid, methylphenidate, chloramphenicol, felbamate, and propoxyphene may inhibit the metabolism of phenobarbital with resultant increase in phenobarbital serum concentration; ritonavir may affect the metabolism of phenobarbital; phenobarbital and benzodiazepines or other CNS depressants may increase CNS and respiratory depression (especially with I.V. loading doses of phenobarbital)

Food Interactions High doses of pyridoxine may decrease drug effect; barbiturates may increase the metabolism of vitamins D and K; dietary requirements of vitamins D, K, C, B$_{12}$, folate, and calcium may be increased with long-term use

Stability Protect elixir from light; not stable in aqueous solutions; use only clear solutions; do not add to acidic solutions, precipitation may occur

Mechanism of Action Depresses CNS activity by binding to barbiturate site at GABA-receptor complex enhancing GABA activity; depresses reticular activating system; higher doses may be gabamimetic

Pharmacodynamics Hypnosis:

Onset of action:

Oral: Within 20-60 minutes

I.V.: Within 5 minutes
Maximum effect: I.V.: Within 30 minutes
Duration:
Oral: 6-10 hours
I.V.: 4-10 hours

Pharmacokinetics
Absorption: Oral: 70% to 90%
Distribution: V_d:
Neonates: 0.8-1 L/kg
Infants: 0.7-0.8 L/kg
Children: 0.6-0.7 L/kg
Protein binding: 35% to 50%, decreased protein binding in neonates
Metabolism: In the liver via hydroxylation and glucuronide conjugation
Half-life:
Neonates: 45-200 hours
Infants: 20-133 hours
Children: 37-73 hours
Adults: 53-140 hours
Time to peak serum concentration: Oral: Within 1-6 hours
Elimination: 20% to 50% excreted unchanged in urine; clearance can be increased
with alkalinization of urine or with oral multiple-dose activated charcoal
Dialysis: Moderately dialyzable (20% to 50%)

Usual Dosage
Anticonvulsant: Status epilepticus: **Loading dose:** I.V.:
Neonates: 15-20 mg/kg in a single or divided dose
Infants, Children, and Adults: 15-18 mg/kg in a single or divided dose; usual
maximum loading dose: 20 mg/kg
Note: In select patients, may give additional 5 mg/kg/dose every 15-30 minutes
until seizure is controlled or a total dose of 30 mg/kg is reached; be prepared to
support respirations
Anticonvulsant **maintenance dose:** Oral, I.V. (**Note:** Maintenance dose usually starts
12 hours after loading dose):
Neonates: 3-4 mg/kg/day given once daily; assess serum concentrations; increase
to 5 mg/kg/day if needed (usually by second week of therapy)
Infants: 5-6 mg/kg/day in 1-2 divided doses
Children:
1-5 years: 6-8 mg/kg/day in 1-2 divided doses
5-12 years: 4-6 mg/kg/day in 1-2 divided doses
>12 years and adults: 1-3 mg/kg/day in 1-2 divided doses
Children:
Sedation: Oral: 2 mg/kg 3 times/day
Hypnotic: I.M., I.V., S.C.: 3-5 mg/kg at bedtime
Hyperbilirubinemia: <12 years: Oral: 3-8 mg/kg/day in 2-3 divided doses; doses up
to 12 mg/kg/day have been used
Preoperative sedation: Oral, I.M., I.V.: 1-3 mg/kg 1-1.5 hours before procedure
Adults:
Sedation: Oral, I.M.: 30-120 mg/day in 2-3 divided doses
Hypnotic: Oral, I.M., I.V., S.C.: 100-320 mg at bedtime
Hyperbilirubinemia: Oral: 90-180 mg/day in 2-3 divided doses
Preoperative sedation: I.M.: 100-200 mg 1-1.5 hours before procedure

Administration
Oral: Administer elixir with water, milk, or juice
Parenteral: Do not inject I.V. faster than 1 mg/kg/minute with a maximum of 30 mg/
minute for infants and children and 60 mg/minute for adults >60kg; do not administer intra-arterially; avoid extravasation; use only powder for injection for S.C. use,
not solutions for injection

Monitoring Parameters CNS status, seizure activity, liver enzymes, CBC with differential, renal function, serum concentrations; I.V. use: Respiratory rate, heart rate,
blood pressure; hyperbilirubinemia: bilirubin (total and direct)

Reference Range
Therapeutic: 15-40 µg/mL (SI: 65-172 µmol/L)
Potentially toxic: >40 µg/mL (SI: >172 µmol/L)
Coma: >50 µg/mL (SI: >215 µmol/L)
Potentially lethal: >80 µg/mL (SI: >344 µmol/L)

Patient Information Avoid alcohol; limit caffeine; may be habit-forming; avoid abrupt
discontinuation after prolonged use; may cause dizziness or drowsiness and impair
ability to perform activities requiring mental alertness or physical coordination

Nursing Implications Parenteral solutions are very alkaline

Additional Information Injectable solutions contain propylene glycol
(Continued)

Phenobarbital *(Continued)*

A recent study (Relling, 2000) demonstrated that enzyme-inducing antiepileptic drugs (AEDs) (carbamazepine, phenobarbital, and phenytoin) increased systemic clearance of antileukemic drugs (teniposide and methotrexate) and were associated with a worse event-free survival, CNS relapse, and hematologic relapse (ie, lower efficacy), in B-lineage ALL children receiving chemotherapy; the authors recommend using nonenzyme-inducing AEDs in patients receiving chemotherapy for ALL.

Dosage Forms

Elixir: 20 mg/5 mL (5 mL, 7.5 mL, 15 mL, 473 mL, 946 mL, 4000 mL) [contains alcohol]

Injection, solution, as sodium: 60 mg/mL (1 mL); 130 mg/mL (1 mL) [contains alcohol]

Luminal® Sodium: 60 mg/mL (1 mL); 130 mg/mL (1 mL) [contains 10% alcohol]

Tablet: 15 mg, 30 mg, 32 mg, 60 mg, 65 mg, 100 mg

References

Relling MV, Pui CH, Sandlund JT, et al, "Adverse Effect of Anticonvulsants on Efficacy of Chemotherapy for Acute Lymphoblastic Leukaemia," *Lancet*, 2000, 356(9226):285-90.

♦ **Phenobarbital, Hyoscyamine, Atropine, and Scopolamine** *see* Hyoscyamine, Atropine, Scopolamine, and Phenobarbital *on page 587*

♦ **Phenobarbitone** *see* Phenobarbital *on page 888*

♦ **Phenoptic®** *see* Phenylephrine *on page 892*

Phenoxybenzamine (fen oks ee BEN za meen)

Related Information

Overdose and Toxicology *on page 1388*

U.S. Brand Names Dibenzyline®

Therapeutic Category Alpha-Adrenergic Blocking Agent, Oral; Antihypertensive Agent; Vasodilator

Generic Available No

Use Symptomatic management of hypertension and sweating in patients with pheochromocytoma

Pregnancy Risk Factor C

Contraindications Hypersensitivity to phenoxybenzamine or any component (see Warnings); shock

Warnings Capsule contains benzyl alcohol which may cause allergic reactions in susceptible individuals; large amounts of benzyl alcohol (≥99 mg/kg/day) have been associated with a potentially fatal toxicity ("gasping syndrome") in neonates; avoid use of phenoxybenzamine products containing benzyl alcohol in neonates; *in vitro* and animal studies have shown that benzoate, a metabolite of benzyl alcohol, displaces bilirubin from protein binding sites

Precautions Use with caution in patients with renal dysfunction, cerebral or coronary arteriosclerosis

Adverse Reactions

Cardiovascular: Postural hypotension, tachycardia, syncope, shock

Central nervous system: Lethargy, headache, dizziness

Gastrointestinal: Vomiting, nausea, diarrhea

Neuromuscular & skeletal: Weakness

Ocular: Miosis

Respiratory: Nasal congestion

Drug Interactions Antagonizes effects of alpha-adrenergic stimulating sympathomimetic agents

Mechanism of Action Produces long-lasting noncompetitive alpha-adrenergic blockade of postganglionic synapses in exocrine glands and smooth muscle

Pharmacodynamics Oral:

Onset of action: Within 2 hours

Maximum effect: Within 4-6 hours

Duration: Effects can continue for up to 4 days

Pharmacokinetics

Absorption: Oral: ~20% to 30%

Distribution: Distributes to and may accumulate in adipose tissues

Half-life: Adults: 24 hours

Elimination: Primarily in urine and bile

Usual Dosage Oral:

Children: Initial: 0.2 mg/kg once daily; maximum dose: 10 mg/dose; increase every 4 days by 0.2 mg/kg/day increments; usual maintenance dose: 0.4-1.2 mg/kg/day every 6-8 hours; maximum doses of up to 2-4 mg/kg/day have been recommended

Adults: Initial: 10 mg twice daily; increase dose every other day to usual dose of 10-40 mg every 8-12 hours; higher doses may be needed

Administration Oral: May administer with milk to decrease GI upset

Monitoring Parameters Blood pressure, orthostasis, heart rate

Patient Information Avoid alcohol; may cause dizziness; avoid sudden changes in posture; may cause nasal congestion and constricted pupils; avoid cough, cold, or allergy medications containing sympathomimetics

Dosage Forms Capsule, as hydrochloride: 10 mg [contains benzyl alcohol]

Extemporaneous Preparations

A 2 mg/mL oral liquid preparation made from capsules and with 1% propylene glycol and 0.15% citric acid in distilled water was stable for 7 days when stored in amber glass prescription bottles under refrigeration (4°C). The vehicle is made by dissolving 150 mg of citric acid in a minimal amount of distilled water; then 1 mL of propylene glycol is added and the solution is mixed well; qsad to 100 mL with distilled water. Grind the contents of two 10 mg capsules in a mortar into a fine powder; add a small amount of the vehicle and mix well; transfer to a graduated cylinder and qsad with vehicle to 10 mL; transfer to an amber glass prescription bottle with tight-fitting cap; label "shake well" and "refrigerate" (Lim, 1997).

A stock solution of 10 mg/mL in propylene glycol was stable for 30 days when stored under refrigeration (4°C); when this stock solution was diluted 1:4 (v/v) with syrup (66.7% sucrose) to 2 mg/mL, the preparation was stable for 1 hour at 4°C (see Lim, 1997). **Note:** Although the stock solution is stable for 30 days, it **must be diluted** before administration to decrease the amount of propylene glycol delivered to the patient.

Lim LY, Tan LL, Chan EW, et al "Stability of Phenoxybenzamine Hydrochloride in Various Vehicles," *Am J Health Syst Pharm*, 1997, 54(18):2073-8.

♦ **Phenoxymethyl Penicillin** *see* Penicillin V Potassium *on page 877*

Phentolamine (fen TOLE a meen)

Related Information

Extravasation Treatment *on page 1240*
Overdose and Toxicology *on page 1388*

Canadian Brand Names Regitine®

Therapeutic Category Alpha-Adrenergic Blocking Agent, Parenteral; Antidote, Extravasation; Antihypertensive Agent; Diagnostic Agent, Pheochromocytoma; Vasodilator

Generic Available Yes

Use Diagnosis of pheochromocytoma; treatment of hypertension associated with pheochromocytoma or other causes of excess sympathomimetic amines; local treatment of dermal necrosis after extravasation of drugs with alpha-adrenergic effects (dobutamine, dopamine, epinephrine, metaraminol, norepinephrine, phenylephrine)

Pregnancy Risk Factor C

Contraindications Hypersensitivity to phentolamine or any component; renal impairment; coronary or cerebral arteriosclerosis; MI

Precautions Use with caution in patients with gastritis, peptic ulcer; history of cardiac arrhythmias; MI, cerebrovascular spasm, and cerebrovascular occlusion may occur

Adverse Reactions

Cardiovascular: Hypotension, tachycardia, angina, arrhythmias
Central nervous system: Dizziness, headache
Gastrointestinal: Nausea, vomiting, diarrhea, exacerbation of peptic ulcer
Neuromuscular & skeletal: Weakness
Respiratory: Nasal congestion

Stability Reconstituted solution is stable for 48 hours at room temperature and 1 week when refrigerated

Mechanism of Action Competitively blocks alpha-adrenergic receptors to produce brief antagonism of circulating epinephrine and norepinephrine; reduces hypertension caused by alpha effects of catecholamines; also has positive inotropic and chronotropic effects on the heart

Pharmacodynamics

Onset of action:
I.M.: Within 15-20 minutes
I.V.: Immediate
Maximum effect:
I.M.: Within 20 minutes
I.V.: Within 2 minutes
Duration:
I.M.: 30-45 minutes
I.V.: Within 15-30 minutes

Pharmacokinetics

Metabolism: In the liver
Half-life: Adults: 19 minutes
Elimination: 10% to 13% excreted in urine as unchanged drug

(Continued)

891

Phentolamine *(Continued)*

Usual Dosage
Treatment of alpha-adrenergic drug extravasation: S.C.:

Neonates: Infiltrate area with a small amount (eg, 1 mL) of solution (made by diluting 2.5-5 mg in 10 mL of preservative free NS) within 12 hours of extravasation; do not exceed 0.1 mg/kg or 2.5 mg total

Infants, Children, and Adults: Infiltrate area with a small amount (eg, 1 mL) of solution (made by diluting 5-10 mg in 10 mL of NS) within 12 hours of extravasation; do not exceed 0.1-0.2 mg/kg or 5 mg total

Diagnosis of pheochromocytoma: I.M., I.V.:

Children: 0.05-0.1 mg/kg/dose, maximum single dose: 5 mg

Adults: 5 mg

Hypertension (prior to surgery for pheochromocytoma): I.M., I.V.:

Children: 0.05-0.1 mg/kg/dose given 1-2 hours before pheochromocytomectomy; repeat as needed to control blood pressure; maximum single dose: 5 mg

Adults: 5 mg given 1-2 hours before pheochromocytomectomy; repeat as needed to control blood pressure

Hypertensive crisis due to MAO inhibitor/sympathomimetic amine interaction: I.M., I.V.: Adults: 5-20 mg

Administration
Parenteral: Treatment of extravasation: Infiltrate area of extravasation with multiple small injections of a diluted solution (see Usual Dosage); use 27- or 30-gauge needles and change needle between each skin entry; do not inject a volume such that swelling of the extremity or digit with resultant compartment syndrome occurs

Monitoring Parameters
Blood pressure, heart rate, orthostasis; treatment of extravasation: site of extravasation, skin color, local perfusion

Nursing Implications
When drugs with alpha-adrenergic effects extravasate, they cause local vasoconstriction which causes blanching of the skin and a pale, cold, hard appearance; S.C. phentolamine blocks the alpha-adrenergic receptors and reverses the vasoconstriction; the extravasation area should "pink up" and return to normal skin color; monitor the site of extravasation closely, as repeat doses of S.C. phentolamine may be needed

Additional Information
Injection contains mannitol 25 mg/vial

Dosage Forms
Injection, powder for reconstitution, lyophilized, as mesylate: 5 mg

♦ **Phenylalanine Mustard** *see Melphalan on page 716*

♦ **Phenylazo Diamino Pyridine** *see Phenazopyridine on page 887*

♦ **4-Phenylbutyric Acid Sodium** *see Sodium Phenylbutyrate on page 1028*

Phenylephrine *(fen il EF rin)*

Related Information
Extravasation Treatment *on page 1240*
OTC Cough & Cold Preparations, Pediatric *on page 1225*
Promethazine and Phenylephrine *on page 944*

U.S. Brand Names
AK-Dilate®; AK-Nefrin®; Formulation R™ [OTC]; Medicone® [OTC]; Mydfrin®; Neo-Synephrine® Extra Strength [OTC]; Neo-Synephrine® Mild [OTC]; Neo-Synephrine® Ophthalmic; Neo-Synephrine® Regular Strength [OTC]; Nostril® [OTC]; Phenoptic®; Prefrin™ [DSC]; Relief® [OTC]; Vicks® Sinex® Nasal Spray [OTC]; Vicks® Sinex® UltraFine Mist [OTC]

Canadian Brand Names
Dionephrine®

Therapeutic Category
Adrenergic Agonist Agent; Adrenergic Agonist Agent, Ophthalmic; Alpha-Adrenergic Agonist; Hemorrhoidal Treatment Agent; Nasal Agent, Vasoconstrictor; Ophthalmic Agent, Mydriatic; Sympathomimetic

Generic Available
Yes (except nasal spray and drops)

Use
Treatment of hypotension and vascular failure in shock; supraventricular tachycardia; as a vasoconstrictor in regional analgesia; symptomatic relief of nasal and nasopharyngeal mucosal congestion; as a mydriatic in ophthalmic procedures and treatment of wide-angle glaucoma; symptomatic relief of hemorrhoidal symptoms (rectal cream and ointment)

Pregnancy Risk Factor
C

Contraindications
Hypersensitivity to phenylephrine or any component (see Warnings); pheochromocytoma, severe hypertension, ventricular tachycardia; acute pancreatitis, hepatitis; peripheral or mesenteric vascular thrombosis, myocardial disease, severe coronary disease, narrow-angle glaucoma (ophthalmic preparation)

Warnings
Do not use if solution turns brown or contains a precipitate. Injection and ophthalmic agents may contain sulfites which may cause allergic reactions in susceptible individuals. Formulation R™ (rectal ointment) contains sodium benzoate; benzoic acid (benzoate) is a metabolite of benzyl alcohol; large amounts of benzyl alcohol (≥99 mg/kg/day) have been associated with a potentially fatal toxicity ("gasping

syndrome") in neonates; *in vitro* and animal studies have shown that benzoate displaces bilirubin from protein binding sites; avoid use of benzyl alcohol containing products in neonates

Precautions Use as pressor therapy for treatment of hypotension and vascular failure is **not** a substitute for replacement of blood, plasma, and body fluids; use with caution in patients with hyperthyroidism, bradycardia, partial heart block, myocardial disease, or severe arteriosclerosis; infuse into large veins to prevent extravasation which may cause severe necrosis

Adverse Reactions

Cardiovascular: Hypertension, angina, reflex severe bradycardia, arrhythmias, peripheral vasoconstriction

Central nervous system: Restlessness, excitability, headache, anxiety, nervousness, dizziness

Dermatologic: Pilomotor response, skin blanching

Local: Necrosis if extravasation occurs

Neuromuscular & skeletal: Tremor

Ocular: (Ophthalmic preparation): Transient stinging, browache, blurred vision, photophobia, lacrimation

Respiratory: Respiratory distress, rebound nasal congestion, sneezing, burning, stinging, dryness

Drug Interactions With alpha- and beta-adrenergic blocking agents, may see decreased actions; with oxytocic drugs, may see increased actions; with sympathomimetics and halogenated hydrocarbon anesthetics, tachycardia or arrhythmias may occur; with MAO inhibitors, guanethidine, and bretylium, actions may be potentiated

Stability Compatible when admixed with dextrose, dextrose-saline, Ringer's, LR, NS, and 1/6 M sodium lactate injection

Mechanism of Action Potent, direct-acting alpha-adrenergic stimulator with weak beta-adrenergic activity; causes vasoconstriction of the arterioles of the nasal mucosa and conjunctiva; activates the dilator muscle of the pupil to cause contraction; produces systemic arterial vasoconstriction

Pharmacodynamics

Onset of action:

I.M.: Within 10-15 minutes

I.V.: Following parenteral injection, effects occur immediately

S.C.: 10-15 minutes

Duration:

I.M.: 30 minutes to 2 hours

I.V.: 15-20 minutes

S.C.: 1 hour

Pharmacokinetics

Metabolism: In the liver and intestine by the enzyme monoamine oxidase

Half-life: 2.5 hours

Elimination: Metabolites, routes, and rates of excretion have not been identified

Usual Dosage

Ophthalmic procedures:

Infants <1 year: Instill 1 drop of 2.5% 15-30 minutes before procedures

Children and Adults: Instill 1 drop of 2.5% or 10% solution, may repeat in 10-60 minutes as needed

Nasal decongestant (therapy should not exceed 3-5 days): **Note:** 0.16% and 0.125% nasal solutions/sprays are no longer commercially available; may dilute 0.25% or 0.5% with NS to achieve desired concentration:

Infants >6 months: 1-2 drops of 0.16% every 3 hours

Children:

1-6 years: 2-3 drops every 4 hours of 0.125% solution as needed

6-12 years: 2-3 drops every 4 hours of 0.25% solution as needed

Children >12 years and Adults: 2-3 drops or 1-2 sprays every 4 hours of 0.25% to 0.5% solution as needed; 1% solution may be used in adults in cases of extreme nasal congestion

Hypotension/shock:

Children:

I.M., S.C.: 0.1 mg/kg/dose every 1-2 hours as needed (maximum dose: 5 mg)

I.V. bolus: 5-20 mcg/kg/dose every 10-15 minutes as needed

I.V. infusion: 0.1-0.5 mcg/kg/minute, titrate to desired effect

Adults:

I.M., S.C.: 2-5 mg/dose every 1-2 hours as needed (initial dose should not exceed 5 mg)

I.V. bolus: 0.1-0.5 mg/dose every 10-15 minutes as needed (initial dose should not exceed 0.5 mg)

I.V. infusion: 100-180 mcg/minute, titrate to desired effect; once stabilized, a maintenance rate of 40-60 mcg/minute is usually effective

(Continued)

Phenylephrine *(Continued)*

Paroxysmal supraventricular tachycardia: I.V.:
Children: 5-10 mcg/kg over 20-30 seconds
Adults: 0.25-0.5 mg over 20-30 seconds
Treatment of hemorrhoidal symptoms: Children ≥12 years and Adults: Apply to rectal area or by applicator into rectum up to 4 times/day

Administration

Intranasal: Spray or apply drops into each nostril while gently occluding the other

Ophthalmic: Instill drops into conjunctival sac of affected eye(s); avoid contact of bottle tip with skin or eye; finger pressure should be applied to the lacrimal sac during and for 1-2 minutes after instillation to decrease risk of absorption and systemic reactions

Parenteral: For direct I.V. administration, dilute to 1 mg/mL by adding 1 mL to 9 mL of SWI, then administer dose over 20-30 seconds; continuous infusion concentrations are usually 20-60 mcg/mL by adding 5 mg to 250 mL I.V. solution (20 mcg/mL) or 15 mg to 250 mL (60 mcg/mL); rate of infusion (mL/hour) = dose (mcg/kg/minute) x weight (kg) x 60 minutes/hour divided by concentration (mcg/mL); administer into a large vein to prevent the possibility of extravasation; use infusion device to control rate of flow; administration into an umbilical arterial catheter is **not** recommended

Rectal: Apply to clean and dry rectal area at night, in the morning, or after each bowel movement; when using applicator, remove protective cover from applicator and attach to tube. Lubricate applicator well, then gently insert into rectum. Thoroughly cleanse applicator after each use and replace protective cover.

Monitoring Parameters Heart rate, blood pressure, central venous pressure, arterial blood gases (hypotension/shock treatment)

Nursing Implications Extravasant; avoid I.V. infiltration; extravasation may be treated with local infiltration of phentolamine 5-10 mg diluted in 10-15 mL NS solution

Dosage Forms

Cream, rectal (Formulation R™): 0.25% (30 g, 60 g) [contains sodium benzoate]

Injection, solution, as hydrochloride: 1% [10 mg/mL] (1 mL) [may contain sodium metabisulfite]

Ointment, rectal (Formulation R™): 0.25% (30 g, 60 g) [contains benzoic acid]

Solution, intranasal **drops**, as hydrochloride:
Neo-Synephrine® Extra Strength: 1% (15 mL)
Neo-Synephrine® Regular Strength: 0.5% (15 mL)

Solution, intranasal spray, as hydrochloride:
Neo-Synephrine® Extra Strength: 1% (15 mL)
Neo-Synephrine® Mild: 0.25% (15 mL)
Neo-Synephrine® Regular Strength: 0.5% (15 mL)
Nostril®: 0.25% (15 mL); 0.5% (15 mL)
Vicks® Sinex®, Vicks® Sinex® UltraFine Mist: 0.5% (15 mL)

Solution, ophthalmic, as hydrochloride: 2.5% (2 mL, 3 mL, 5 mL, 15 mL) [may contain sodium bisulfite]
AK-Dilate®: 2.5% (2 mL, 15 mL); 10% (5 mL)
AK-Nefrin®: 0.12% (15 mL)
Mydfrin®: 2.5% (3 mL, 5 mL) [contains sodium bisulfite]
Neo-Synephrine®: 2.5% (15 mL); 10% (5 mL)
Neo-Synephrine® Viscous: 10% (5 mL)
Phenoptic®: 2.5% (15 mL)
Prefrin™ [DSC], Relief®: 0.12% (15 mL)

Suppository, rectal: 0.25% (12s)
Medicone®: 0.25% (18s, 24s)

♦ **Phenylephrine and Cyclopentolate** *see* Cyclopentolate and Phenylephrine *on page 320*

♦ **Phenylephrine and Promethazine** *see* Promethazine and Phenylephrine *on page 944*

♦ **Phenylephrine, Promethazine, and Codeine** *see* Promethazine, Phenylephrine, and Codeine *on page 945*

♦ **Phenylethylmalonylurea** *see* Phenobarbital *on page 888*

♦ **Phenylisohydantoin** *see* Pemoline *on page 870*

♦ **Phenytek™** *see* Phenytoin *on page 894*

Phenytoin *(FEN i toyn)*

Related Information

Adult ACLS Algorithm, Stable Ventricular Tachycardia *on page 1191*
Antiepileptic Drugs *on page 1374*
Blood Level Sampling Time Guidelines *on page 1386*

Carbohydrate and Alcohol Content of Liquid Medications for Use in Patients Receiving Ketogenic Diets *on page 1431*
Fosphenytoin *on page 522*
Overdose and Toxicology *on page 1388*

U.S. Brand Names Dilantin®; Phenytek™

Synonyms Diphenylhydantoin; DPH

Therapeutic Category Antiarrhythmic Agent, Class I-B; Anticonvulsant, Hydantoin

Generic Available Yes (except chewable tablet and extended capsule)

Use Management of generalized tonic-clonic (grand mal), simple partial and complex partial seizures; prevention of seizures following head trauma/neurosurgery; ventricular arrhythmias, including those associated with digitalis intoxication, prolonged QT interval and surgical repair of congenital heart diseases in children; epidermolysis bullosa

Pregnancy Risk Factor D

Contraindications Hypersensitivity to phenytoin or any component; heart block, sinus bradycardia

Warnings Dilantin® 30 mg capsule and oral suspension contain sodium benzoate; benzoic acid (benzoate) is a metabolite of benzyl alcohol; large amounts of benzyl alcohol (≥99 mg/kg/day) have been associated with a potentially fatal toxicity ("gasping syndrome") in neonates; the "gasping syndrome" consists of metabolic acidosis, respiratory distress, gasping respirations, CNS dysfunction (including convulsions, intracranial hemorrhage), hypotension and cardiovascular collapse; use phenytoin products containing sodium benzoate with caution in neonates; *in vitro* and animal studies have shown that benzoate displaces bilirubin from protein binding sites. Injection contains 40% propylene glycol and 10% alcohol.

Precautions Use with caution in patients with porphyria; discontinue if rash or lymphadenopathy occurs; modify dosage in patients with hepatic or renal dysfunction

Adverse Reactions
Dose-related:
Central nervous system: Slurred speech, dizziness, drowsiness, lethargy, coma, ataxia, dyskinesias
Ocular: Nystagmus, blurred vision, diplopia

Cardiovascular: I.V.: Hypotension, bradycardia, arrhythmias, cardiovascular collapse (especially with rapid I.V. use)
Central nervous system: Fever, mood changes
Dermatologic: Hirsutism, coarsening of facial features, Stevens-Johnson syndrome, rash, exfoliative dermatitis
Endocrine & metabolic: Folic acid depletion, hyperglycemia
Gastrointestinal: Nausea, vomiting, gingival hyperplasia, gum tenderness
Hematologic: Blood dyscrasias, pseudolymphoma, lymphoma
Hepatic: Hepatitis
Local: Venous irritation and pain, thrombophlebitis
Neuromuscular & skeletal: Peripheral neuropathy, osteomalacia
Miscellaneous: Lymphadenopathy, SLE-like syndrome

Drug Interactions Cytochrome P450 isoenzyme CYP2C9 and CYP2C19 substrate; CYP1A2, CYP2B6, CYP2C8, CYP2C9, CYP2C18, CYP2C19, CYP3A3/4, and CYP3A5-7 isoenzyme inducer
Phenytoin may decrease the serum concentration or effectiveness of lamotrigine, ritonavir, saquinavir, delavirdine, felbamate, valproic acid, ethosuximide, primidone, warfarin, oral contraceptives, corticosteroids, teniposide, etoposide, doxorubicin, vincristine, methotrexate, cyclosporine, theophylline, chloramphenicol, rifampin, doxycycline, quinidine, mexiletine, disopyramide, dopamine, or nondepolarizing skeletal muscle relaxants; protein binding of phenytoin can be affected by valproic acid or salicylates; serum phenytoin concentrations may be increased by cimetidine, chloramphenicol, felbamate, zidovudine, isoniazid, trimethoprim, or sulfonamides and decreased by rifampin, zidovudine, cisplatin, vinblastine, bleomycin, antacids (concurrent administration), folic acid, or continuous NG feeds; suspected interaction with nevirapine (monitor closely); ritonavir may affect the metabolism of phenytoin

Food Interactions Food may effect absorption of phenytoin, depending on product formulation; a high fat meal decreases the rate, but not the extent of absorption of 100 mg Dilantin® Kapseals (Cook, 2001); a high fat meal decreased the bioavailability of a generic extended phenytoin sodium capsule (Mylan) by 13% compared to Dilantin® Kapseals; when taken with a high fat meal, substituting the generic product for Dilantin® could result in a 37% decrease in serum phenytoin concentrations; substituting Dilantin® for the generic could result in a 102% increase in plasma phenytoin concentrations; thus, when taking phenytoin sodium with food, switching products may result in decreased efficacy or increased toxicity (see Wilder, 2001)
(Continued)

Phenytoin *(Continued)*

Tube feedings decrease phenytoin bioavailability; to avoid decreased serum levels with continuous NG feeds, hold feedings for 2 hours prior to and 2 hours after phenytoin administration, if possible; phenytoin may increase the metabolism of vitamins D and K; dietary requirements of vitamins D, K, B_{12}, folate, and calcium may be increased with long-term use; high doses of folate may decrease bioavailability of phenytoin; avoid giving calcium or magnesium supplements at the same time as phenytoin, space administration by ≥2 hours

Stability Parenteral solution may be used as long as there is no precipitate and it is not hazy; slightly yellowed solution may be used; refrigeration may cause precipitate, sometimes the precipitate is resolved by allowing the solution to reach room temperature again; drug may precipitate with pH ≤11.5; do not mix with other medications. I.V. intermittent infusion: No consensus exists in the literature regarding phenytoin stability in I.V. solutions; due to a low solubility, phenytoin may precipitate in aqueous solutions; some centers have successfully used dilutions of 1-10 mg/mL in NS or LR; infusions should begin as soon as possible after preparation (eg, within 1 hour); diluted solutions should **not** be refrigerated; inspect for particulate matter; discard 4 hours after preparation (see Gannaway, 1983).

Mechanism of Action Stabilizes neuronal membranes and decreases seizure activity by increasing efflux or decreasing influx of sodium ions across cell membranes in the motor cortex during generation of nerve impulses; prolongs effective refractory period and suppresses ventricular pacemaker automaticity, shortens action potential in the heart

Pharmacokinetics

Absorption: Oral: Slow, variable; dependent on product formulation (see Food Interactions); decreased in neonates

Distribution: V_d:

Neonates:

Premature: 1-1.2 L/kg

Full-term: 0.8-0.9 L/kg

Infants: 0.7-0.8 L/kg

Children: 0.7 L/kg

Adults: 0.6-0.7 L/kg

Protein binding: Adults: 90% to 95%; increased free fraction (decreased protein binding) in neonates (up to 20% free), infants (up to 15% free), and patients with hyperbilirubinemia, hypoalbuminemia, renal dysfunction, or uremia

Metabolism: Follows dose-dependent (Michaelis-Menten) pharmacokinetics; "apparent" or calculated half-life is dependent upon serum concentration, therefore, metabolism is best described in terms of K_m and V_{max}; V_{max} is increased in infants >6 months and children compared to adults; major metabolite (via oxidation) HPPA undergoes enterohepatic recycling and elimination in urine as glucuronides

Bioavailability: Formulation dependent

Time to peak serum concentration: Oral: Dependent upon formulation

Extended release capsule: Within 4-12 hours

Immediate release preparation: Within 2-3 hours

Elimination: <5% excreted unchanged in urine; increased clearance and decreased serum concentrations with febrile illness; highly variable clearance, dependent upon intrinsic hepatic function and dose administered

Usual Dosage

Status epilepticus: I.V.:

Loading dose:

Neonates: 15-20 mg/kg in a single or divided dose;

Infants, Children, and Adults: 15-18 mg/kg in a single or divided dose

Maintenance dose, anticonvulsant (**Note:** Maintenance dose usually starts 12 hours after the loading dose):

Neonates: Initial: 5 mg/kg/day in 2 divided doses; usual: 5-8 mg/kg/day in 2 divided doses; some patients may require dosing every 8 hours

Infants and Children: Initial: 5 mg/kg/day in 2-3 divided doses; usual doses:

0.5-3 years: 8-10 mg/kg/day

4-6 years: 7.5-9 mg/kg/day

7-9 years: 7-8 mg/kg/day

10-16 years: 6-7 mg/kg/day

Some patients require every 8 hours dosing due to fast apparent half-life

Adults: Usual: 300 mg/day or 4-6 mg/kg/day in 2-3 divided doses

Anticonvulsant: Infants, Children and Adults: Oral:

Loading dose: 15-20 mg/kg; based on phenytoin serum concentrations and recent dosing history; administer oral loading dose in 3 divided doses given every 2-4 hours to decrease GI adverse effects and to ensure complete oral absorption

Maintenance dose: Same as I.V. maintenance dose/day listed above. Divide daily dose into 3 doses/day when using suspension, chewable tablets or nonextended release preparations. Extended release preparations may be dosed in adults every 12 or 24 hours if patient is not receiving concomitant enzyme-inducing drugs and apparent half-life is sufficiently long.

Arrhythmias:

Children and Adults: Loading dose: I.V.: 1.25 mg/kg every 5 minutes, may repeat up to total loading dose: 15 mg/kg

Children: Maintenance dose: Oral, I.V.: 5-10 mg/kg/day in 2-3 divided doses

Adults: Loading dose: Oral: 250 mg 4 times/day for 1 day, 250 mg twice daily for 2 days, then maintenance at 300-400 mg/day in divided doses 1-4 times/day

Administration

Oral: To ensure consistent absorption, phenytoin should be administered at the same time with regards to meals; may administer with food or milk to decrease GI upset; 100 mg Dilantin® Kapseals may be administered without regard to meals; shake oral suspension well prior to each dose; separate administration of antacids or tube feedings and oral phenytoin by 2 hours

Parenteral: I.V.: Neonates: Do not exceed I.V. infusion rate of 0.5 mg/kg/minute; Infants, Children, Adults: Do not exceed I.V. infusion rate of 1-3 mg/kg/minute, maximum rate: 50 mg/minute; I.V. injections should be followed by NS flushes through the same needle or I.V. catheter to avoid local irritation of the vein; I.V. intermittent infusion: Dilute with NS to a concentration of 1-10 mg/mL (see Stability), use an in-line 0.22 micron filter; avoid extravasation; avoid I.M. use due to erratic absorption, pain on injection, and precipitation of drug at injection site

Monitoring Parameters Serum concentrations, CBC with differential, liver enzymes; blood pressure with I.V. use; free and total serum concentrations in patients with hyperbilirubinemia, hypoalbuminemia, renal dysfunction, or uremia

Reference Range

Neonates: Therapeutic: 8-15 µg/mL

Children and Adults:

Therapeutic: 10-20 µg/mL (SI: 40-79 µmol/L); toxicity is measured clinically, some patients require levels outside the suggested therapeutic range

Toxic: >20 µg/mL (SI: >79 µmol/L)

Lethal: >100 µg/mL (SI: >400 µmol/L)

Commonly accepted therapeutic free (unbound) concentration: 1-2 µg/mL

Patient Information Avoid alcohol; do not change brand or dosage without consulting physician; maintain good oral hygiene

Additional Information The 30 mg/5 mL oral suspension is no longer made; possible permanent cerebellum damage may occur with chronic toxic serum concentrations

A recent study (Relling, 2000) demonstrated that enzyme-inducing antiepileptic drugs (AEDs) (carbamazepine, phenobarbital, and phenytoin) increased systemic clearance of antileukemic drugs (teniposide and methotrexate) and were associated with a worse event-free survival, CNS relapse, and hematologic relapse, (ie, lower efficacy), in B-lineage ALL children receiving chemotherapy; the authors recommend using nonenzyme-inducing AEDs in patients receiving chemotherapy for ALL.

Dosage Forms

Capsule, extended, as sodium:

Dilantin®: 30 mg [contains sodium benzoate], 100 mg

Phenytek™: 200 mg, 300 mg

Capsule, prompt, as sodium: 100 mg

Injection, solution, as sodium: 50 mg/mL (2 mL, 5 mL) [contains alcohol]

Suspension, oral (Dilantin®): 125 mg/5 mL (240 mL) [contains ≤0.6% alcohol and sodium benzoate; orange-vanilla flavor]

Tablet, chewable (Dilantin®): 50 mg

References

Bauer LA and Blouin RA, "Phenytoin Michaelis-Menten Pharmacokinetics in Caucasian Pediatric Patients," *Clin Pharmacokinet*, 1983, 8(6):545-9.

Chiba K, Ishizaki T, Miura H, et al, "Michaelis-Menten Pharmacokinetics of Diphenylhydantoin and Application in the Pediatric Age Patient," *J Pediatr*, 1980, 96(3 Pt 1):479-84.

Cook J, Randinitis E, and Wilder BJ, "Effect of Food on the Bioavailability of 100-mg Dilantin® Kapseals," *Neurology*, 2001, 57(4):698-700.

Gannaway WL, Wilding DC, Siepler JK, et al, "Clinical Use of Intravenous Phenytoin Sodium Infusions," *Clin Pharm*, 1983, 2(2):135-8.

Relling MV, Pui CH, Sandlund JT, et al, "Adverse Effect of Anticonvulsants on Efficacy of Chemotherapy for Acute Lymphoblastic Leukaemia," *Lancet*, 2000, 356(9226):285-90.

Suzuki Y, Mimaki T, Cox S, et al, "Phenytoin Age-Dose-Concentration Relationship in Children," *Ther Drug Monit*, 1994, 16(2):145-50.

Wilder BJ, Leppik I, Hietpas TJ, et al, "Effect of Food on Absorption of Dilantin® Kapseals and Mylan Extended Phenytoin Sodium Capsules," *Neurology*, 2001, 57(4):582-9.

♦ **Phillips'® Milk of Magnesia [OTC]** *see* Magnesium Supplements *on page 701*

♦ **Phillips'® M-O [OTC]** *see* Magnesium Supplements *on page 701*

◆ **Phillips'®** **Stool Softener Laxative [OTC]** *see* Docusate *on page 402*

◆ **pHisoHex®** *see* Hexachlorophene *on page 562*

◆ **Phos-Flur®** *see* Fluoride *on page 500*

◆ **Phos-Flur® Rinse [OTC]** *see* Fluoride *on page 500*

◆ **PhosLo® Posture® [OTC]** *see* Calcium Supplements *on page 200*

Phosphate Supplements (FOS fate SUP la ments)

U.S. Brand Names Fleet® Enema [OTC]; Fleet® Phospho®-Soda [OTC]; K-Phos® M.F.; K-Phos® Neutral; K-Phos® No. 2; K-Phos® Original; Neutra-Phos® [OTC]; Neutra-Phos®-K [OTC]; Uro-KP-Neutral®

Available Salts Potassium Acid Phosphate; Potassium Phosphate; Potassium Phosphate and Sodium Phosphate; Sodium Phosphate

Therapeutic Category Electrolyte Supplement, Oral; Electrolyte Supplement, Parenteral; Laxative, Saline; Phosphate Salt; Potassium Salt; Sodium Salt; Urinary Acidifying Agent

Generic Available Yes (enema and injection)

Use Treatment and prevention of hypophosphatemia; short-term treatment of constipation (oral/rectal); evacuation of the colon for rectal and bowel exams; source of phosphate in large volume I.V. fluids; urinary acidifier (potassium acid phosphate) for reduction in formation of calcium stones

Pregnancy Risk Factor C

Contraindications Hypersensitivity to phosphate (salts) or any component; hyperphosphatemia, hyperkalemia (potassium salt form), hypocalcemia, hypomagnesemia, hypernatremia (sodium salt form), severe renal impairment, severe tissue trauma, heat cramps, CHF, abdominal pain (rectal forms), fecal impaction (rectal forms); patients with phosphate kidney stones

Warnings Parenteral **potassium** salt forms: should be administered only in patients with adequate urine flow; must be diluted before I.V. use and infused slowly (see Administration), and patients must be on a cardiac monitor during intermittent infusions. Use of >45 mL/day oral sodium phosphate solution as a bowel preparation in adults has been associated with significant electrolyte changes resulting in symptomatic dehydration, renal failure, metabolic acidosis, tetany and death; consider obtaining baseline and post-treatment electrolytes in patients receiving >45 mL/day of sodium phosphate solution

Precautions Use with caution in patients with renal impairment, patients receiving potassium-sparing drugs (potassium salt forms), patients with adrenal insufficiency, cirrhosis

Adverse Reactions

Cardiovascular: Hypotension, edema; **potassium salt form:** arrhythmias, heart block, cardiac arrest

Central nervous system: Tetany, mental confusion, seizures, dizziness, headache

Endocrine & metabolic: Hyperphosphatemia, hyperkalemia **(potassium salt form)**, hypocalcemia, hypernatremia **(sodium salt form)**

Gastrointestinal: Nausea, vomiting, diarrhea, flatulence (oral use)

Local: Phlebitis (parenteral forms)

Neuromuscular & skeletal: Paresthesia, bone and joint pain, arthralgia, weakness, muscle cramps

Renal: Acute renal failure

Drug Interactions Do not give orally at the same time as aluminum- and magnesium-containing antacids or sucralfate which can act as phosphate binders; use of potassium phosphate with potassium-sparing diuretics, ACE inhibitors, or salt substitutes may result in hyperkalemia

Food Interactions Avoid giving with oxalate (ie, berries, nuts, chocolate, beans, celery, tomatoes) or phytate-containing foods (ie, bran, whole wheat)

Stability Phosphate salts may precipitate when mixed with calcium salts; solubility is improved in amino acid parenteral nutrition solutions; check with a pharmacist to determine compatibility

Mechanism of Action Phosphorus participates in bone deposition, calcium metabolism, utilization of B complex vitamins, and as a buffer in acid-base equilibrium; as a laxative, exerts osmotic effect in the small intestine by drawing water into the lumen of the gut, producing distension, promoting peristalsis, and evacuation of the bowel

Pharmacodynamics Onset of action (catharsis):

Oral: 3-6 hours

Rectal: 2-5 minutes

Pharmacokinetics

Absorption: Oral: 1% to 20%

Elimination: Oral forms excreted in feces; I.V. forms are excreted in the urine with over 80% of dose reabsorbed by the kidney

Usual Dosage Note: Phosphate supplements are either sodium or potassium salt forms. Consider the contribution of these electrolytes also when determining appropriate phosphate replacement.

Phosphorus: Oral: See table.

Phosphorus - Recommended Daily Allowance (RDA) and Estimated Average Requirement (EAR)

Age	RDA (mmol/day)	EAR (mmol/day)
0-6 mo	–	3.2*
7-12 mo	–	8.9*
1-3 y	14.8	12.3
4-8 y	16.1	13.1
9-18 y	40.3	34
19-30 y	22.6	18.7

*Adequate intake (AI)

I.V. doses should be incorporated into the patient's maintenance I.V. fluids; intermittent I.V. infusion should be reserved for severe depletion situations; requires continuous cardiac monitoring (for potassium salts). **Note:** Doses listed as mmol of **phosphate**:

Hypophosphatemia: Intermittent I.V. infusion: Treatment: It is difficult to provide concrete guidelines for the treatment of severe hypophosphatemia because the extent of total body deficits and response to therapy are difficult to predict. Aggressive doses of phosphate may result in a transient serum elevation followed by redistribution into intracellular compartments or bone tissue. It is recommended that repletion of severe hypophosphatemia be done I.V. because large doses of oral phosphate may cause diarrhea and intestinal absorption may be unreliable
Children:
Low dose: 0.08 mmol/kg over 6 hours; use if losses are recent and uncomplicated
Intermediate dose: 0.16-0.24 mmol/kg over 4-6 hours; use if serum phosphorus level 0.5-1 mg/dL
High dose: 0.36 mmol/kg over 6 hours; use if serum phosphorus <0.5 mg/dL
Adults: Varying dosages: 0.15-0.3 mmol/kg/dose over 12 hours; may repeat as needed to achieve desired serum level **or**
15 mmol/dose over 2 hours; use if serum phosphorus <2 mg/dL **or**
Low dose: 0.16 mmol/kg over 4-6 hours; use if serum phosphorus level 2.3-3 mg/dL
Intermediate dose: 0.32 mmol/kg over 4-6 hours; use if serum phosphorus level 1.6-2.2 mg/dL
High dose: 0.64 mmol/kg over 8-12 hours; use if serum phosphorus <1.5 mg/dL
Maintenance:
Children:
I.V.: 0.5-1.5 mmol/kg/day
Oral: 2-3 mmol/kg/day in divided doses
Adults:
I.V.: 50-70 mmol/day
Oral: 50-150 mmol/day in divided doses
Laxative: Oral
Neutra-Phos®, Neutra-Phos®-K, or Uro-KP-Neutral®:
Children <4 years: 1 capsule or packet (250 mg phosphorus/8 mmol) 4 times/day; dilute as instructed
Children >4 years and Adults: 1-2 capsules or packets (250-500 mg phosphorus/8-16 mmol) 4 times/day; dilute as instructed
Fleet® Phospho®-Soda:® Oral:
Children 5-9 years: 5 mL as a single dose
Children 10-12 years: 10 mL as a single dose
Children ≥12 years and Adults: 20-30 mL as a single dose
Laxative: Rectal:
Fleet® Enema:
Children 2-11 years: Contents of one 2.25 oz pediatric enema as a single dose, may repeat
Children ≥12 years and Adults: Contents of one 4.5 oz enema as a single dose, may repeat
Urinary acidification: Adults: Oral (K-Phos® Original): 2 tablets 4 times/day
(Continued)

Phosphate Supplements *(Continued)*

Administration

Oral: Administer with food to reduce the risk of diarrhea; contents of 1 packet should be diluted in 75 mL water before administration; administer tablets with a full glass of water; maintain adequate fluid intake; dilute oral solution with an equal volume of cool water; K-Phos® Original tablets (urinary acidifier) should be dissolved in 6-8 ounces of water before administration

Parenteral: For intermittent I.V. infusion: Peripheral line: Dilute to a maximum concentration of 0.05 mmol/mL; Central line: Dilute to a maximum concentration of 0.12 mmol/mL (maximum concentrations were determined with consideration for maximum sodium or potassium concentrations); maximum rate of infusion: 0.06 mmol/kg/hour; do **not** infuse with calcium containing I.V. fluids

Monitoring Parameters Serum potassium (potassium salt forms), sodium (sodium salt forms), calcium, phosphorus, renal function, reflexes; cardiac monitor (when intermittent infusion or high-dose I.V. replacement of potassium salts needed), stool output (laxative use)

Reference Range Phosphorus:

Newborns: 4.2-9 mg/dL

6 weeks to 18 months: 3.8-6.7 mg/dL

18 months to 3 years: 2.9-5.9 mg/dL

3-15 years: 3.6-5.6 mg/dL

>15 years: 2.5-5 mg/dL

Dosage Forms

Enema: Monobasic sodium phosphate 19 g and dibasic sodium phosphate 7 g per 118 mL delivered dose (133 mL)

Fleet® Enema: Monobasic sodium phosphate 19 g and dibasic sodium phosphate 7 g per 118 mL delivered dose (133 mL)

Fleet® Enema for Children: Monobasic sodium phosphate 9.5 g and dibasic sodium phosphate 3.5 g per 59 mL delivered dose (66 mL)

Injection, solution, as **potassium phosphate**: Phosphate 3 mmol and potassium 4.4 mEq per mL (5 mL, 15 mL, 50 mL)

Injection, solution, as **sodium phosphate**: Phosphate 3 mmol and sodium 4 mEq per mL (5 mL, 15 mL, 50 mL)

Powder:

Neutra-Phos®: Phosphorus 250 mg [8 mmol], potassium 278 mg [7.125 mEq], and sodium 164 mg [7.125 mEq] per packet (100s)

Neutra-Phos®-K: Phosphorus 250 mg [8 mmol] and potassium 556 mg [14.25 mEq] per packet (100s) [sodium free]

Solution, oral (Fleet® Phospho®-Soda): Phosphate 4 mmol and sodium 4.82 mEq per mL (45 mL, 90 mL) [equivalent to monobasic sodium phosphate monohydrate 2.4 g and dibasic sodium phosphate heptahydrate 0.9 g per 5 mL; ginger-lemon or unflavored]

Tablet:

K-Phos® M.F.: Phosphorus 125.6 mg [4 mmol], potassium 44.5 mg [1.1 mEq], and sodium 67 mg [2.9 mEq]

K-Phos® Neutral: Phosphorus 250 mg [8 mmol], potassium 45 mg [1.1 mEq], and sodium 298 mg [13 mEq] per tablet

K-Phos® No. 2: Phosphorus 250 mg [8 mmol], potassium 88 mg [2.3 mEq], and sodium 134 mg [5.8 mEq]

K-Phos® Original: Phosphorus 114 mg [3.7 mmol] and potassium 144 mg [3.7 mEq] per tablet [sodium free]

Uro-KP-Neutral®: Phosphorus 258 mg [8 mmol], potassium 49.4 mg [1.27 mEq], and sodium 262.4 mg [10.9 mEq]

References

Clark CL, Sacks GS, Dickerson RN, et al, "Treatment of Hypophosphatemia in Patients Receiving Specialized Nutrition Support Using a Graduated Dosing Scheme: Results From a Prospective Clinical Trial," *Crit Care Med*, 1995, 23(9):1504-11.

"Dietary Reference Intakes for Calcium, Phosphorus, Magnesium, Vitamin D, and Fluoride. Standing Committee on the Scientific Evaluation of Dietary Reference Intakes, Food and Nutrition Board, Institute of Medicine," National Academy of Sciences, Washington, DC: National Academy Press, 1997.

Lentz RD, Brown BM, and Kjellstrand CM, "Treatment of Severe Hypophosphatemia," *Ann Intern Med*, 1978, 89(6):941-4.

Lloyd CW and Johnson CE, "Management of Hypophosphatemia," *Clin Pharm*, 1988, 7(2):123-8.

Rosen GH, Boullata JI, O'Rangers EA, et al, "Intravenous Phosphate Repletion Regimen for Critically Ill Patients With Moderate Hypophosphatemia," *Crit Care Med*, 1995, 23(7):1204-11.

♦ **Phosphonoformate** *see* Foscarnet *on page 520*

♦ **Phosphonoformic Acid** *see* Foscarnet *on page 520*

♦ **3-Phosphoryloxymethyl Phenytoin Disodium** *see* Fosphenytoin *on page 522*

♦ **Phoxal-timolol (Can)** *see* Timolol *on page 1095*

◆ *p*-Hydroxyampicillin *see* Amoxicillin *on page 94*
◆ Phylloquinone *see* Phytonadione *on page 902*

Physostigmine (fye zoe STIG meen)

Related Information
Overdose and Toxicology *on page 1388*
Canadian Brand Names Eserine®; Isopto® Eserine
Synonyms Eserine
Therapeutic Category Antidote, Anticholinergic Agent; Cholinergic Agent; Cholinergic Agent, Ophthalmic
Generic Available Yes
Use Reverse toxic CNS and cardiac effects caused by anticholinergics and tricyclic antidepressants
Pregnancy Risk Factor C
Contraindications Hypersensitivity to physostigmine or any component (see Warnings); GI or GU obstruction, asthma, diabetes mellitus, gangrene, severe cardiovascular disease; patients receiving depolarizing neuromuscular blockers (eg, succinylcholine)
Warnings Because physostigmine has the potential for producing severe adverse effects, (ie, seizures, bradycardia), routine use as an antidote is controversial; atropine should be readily available to treat severe adverse effects. Injection contains benzyl alcohol and bisulfite which may cause allergic reactions in susceptible individuals; large amounts of benzyl alcohol (≥99 mg/kg/day) have been associated with a potentially fatal toxicity ("gasping syndrome") in neonates; the "gasping syndrome" consists of metabolic acidosis, respiratory distress, gasping respirations, CNS dysfunction (including convulsions, intracranial hemorrhage), hypotension and cardiovascular collapse; *in vitro* and animal studies have shown that benzoate, a metabolite of benzyl alcohol, displaces bilirubin from protein-binding sites; use injection with caution in neonates.
Precautions Use with caution in patients with epilepsy, narrow-angle glaucoma, marked vagotonia, parkinsonism, bradycardia
Adverse Reactions
Cardiovascular: Palpitations, bradycardia
Central nervous system: Restlessness, hallucinations, seizures, nervousness
Dermatologic: Burning, redness
Gastrointestinal: Nausea, vomiting, epigastric pain, salivation, diarrhea
Neuromuscular & skeletal: Weakness, muscle twitching
Ocular: Miosis, lacrimation
Respiratory: Dyspnea, bronchospasm, respiratory paralysis, pulmonary edema
Miscellaneous: Diaphoresis
Drug Interactions Additive cholinergic activity with bethanechol and methacholine; succinylcholine
Mechanism of Action Inhibits destruction of acetylcholine by acetylcholinesterase which prolongs the central and peripheral effects of acetylcholine
Pharmacodynamics Parenteral:
Onset of action: Within 3-8 minutes
Duration: 30 minutes to 1 hour
Pharmacokinetics
Distribution: Widely distributed throughout the body; crosses into the CNS
Half-life: 1-2 hours
Elimination: Via hydrolysis by cholinesterases
Usual Dosage
Reversal of toxic anticholinergic effects:
Children: Reserve for life-threatening situations only: I.V.: 0.01-0.03 mg/kg/dose; may repeat after 15-20 minutes to a maximum total dose of 2 mg
Adults: I.M., I.V., S.C.: 0.5-2 mg initially, repeat every 20 minutes until response or adverse effect occurs; repeat 1-4 mg every 30-60 minutes as life-threatening signs (arrhythmias, seizures, deep come) recur
Preanesthetic reversal: Children and Adults:
I.M., I.V.: Give twice the dose, on a weight basis, of the anticholinergic drug (atropine, scopolamine)
Administration Parenteral: Infuse slowly I.V. without additional dilution at a maximum rate of 0.5 mg/minute in children or 1 mg/minute in adults
Monitoring Parameters Heart rate, respiratory rate
Dosage Forms Injection, solution, as salicylate: 1 mg/mL (2 mL) [contains benzyl alcohol and sodium metabisulfite]

◆ Phytomenadione *see* Phytonadione *on page 902*

Phytonadione (fye toe na DYE one)

U.S. Brand Names AquaMEPHYTON®; Mephyton®

Canadian Brand Names Konakion

Synonyms Methylphytyl Napthoquinone; Phylloquinone; Phytomenadione; Vitamin K₁

Therapeutic Category Nutritional Supplement; Vitamin, Fat Soluble

Generic Available Yes (injection)

Use Prevention and treatment of hypoprothrombinemia caused by vitamin K deficiency or anticoagulant-induced hypoprothrombinemia; hemorrhagic disease of the newborn

Pregnancy Risk Factor C

Contraindications Hypersensitivity to phytonadione or any component (see Warnings)

Warnings Ineffective in hereditary hypoprothrombinemia and hypoprothrombinemia caused by severe liver disease; severe hemolytic anemia and hyperbilirubinemia has been reported rarely in neonates following large doses (10-20 mg) of phytonadione. Injection contains 0.9% benzyl alcohol which may cause allergic reactions in susceptible individuals; large amounts of benzyl alcohol (≥99 mg/kg/day) have been associated with a potentially fatal toxicity ("gasping syndrome") in neonates; the "gasping syndrome" consists of metabolic acidosis, respiratory distress, gasping respirations, CNS dysfunction (including convulsions, intracranial hemorrhage), hypotension and cardiovascular collapse; *in vitro* and animal studies have shown that benzoate, a metabolite of benzyl alcohol, displaces bilirubin from protein-binding sites; injection is safe in neonates when used in appropriate doses.

Precautions Severe reactions resembling anaphylaxis or hypersensitivity have occurred rarely during or immediately after I.V. administration (even with proper dilution and rate of administration) and with I.M. administration; restrict I.V. and I.M. administration for situations where the subcutaneous route is not feasible

Adverse Reactions See Warnings and Precautions

Cardiovascular: Flushing, hypotension, cyanosis

Central nervous system: Dizziness

Gastrointestinal: GI upset, dysgeusia, hyperbilirubinemia (neonates)

Hematologic: Hemolysis

Local: Pain, edema, tenderness at injection site

Miscellaneous: Anaphylactoid reactions, diaphoresis

Respiratory: Dyspnea

Drug Interactions Antagonizes action of warfarin; mineral oil decreases phytonadione absorption

Mechanism of Action Cofactor in the liver synthesis of clotting factors (II, VII, IX, X)

Pharmacodynamics Onset of action: Blood coagulation factors increase within 6-12 hours after oral doses and within 1-2 hours following parenteral administration; after parenteral administration prothrombin time may become normal after 12-14 hours

Pharmacokinetics

Absorption: Oral: From the intestines in the presence of bile

Metabolism: Rapidly in the liver

Elimination: In bile and urine

Usual Dosage S.C. route is preferred; I.V. and I.M. routes should be restricted for situations when the S.C. route is not feasible

Hemorrhagic disease of the newborn: Neonates: S.C., I.M.:

Prophylaxis: 0.5-1 mg within 1 hour of birth; may repeat if necessary 6-8 hours later

Treatment: 1-2 mg/day

Oral anticoagulant overdose:

Infants and Children:

No bleeding, rapid reversal needed, patient will require further oral anticoagulant therapy: S.C., I.V.: 0.5-2 mg

No bleeding, rapid reversal needed, patient will **not** require further oral anticoagulant therapy: S.C., I.V.: 2-5 mg

Significant bleeding, not life-threatening: S.C., I.V.: 0.5-2 mg

Significant bleeding, life-threatening: I.V.: 5 mg

Adults: S.C., I.V.: 2.5-10 mg/dose (rarely up to 25-50 mg has been used); may repeat in 6-8 hours if given by S.C., I.V. route; may repeat 12-48 hours after oral route

Vitamin K deficiency due to drugs, malabsorption, or decreased synthesis of vitamin K:

Infants and Children:

Oral: 2.5-5 mg/24 hours

S.C., I.M., I.V.: 1-2 mg/dose as a single dose

Adults:

Oral: 2.5-25 mg/24 hours

S.C., I.M., I.V.: 10 mg

Minimum daily requirement: Oral: Not well established

Infants: 1-5 mcg/kg/day
Adults: 0.03 mcg/kg/day

Administration
Oral: May be administered with or without food
Parenteral: S.C. administration is the preferred method (see Precautions); for I.V. administration, dilute in 5-10 mL I.V. fluid (D$_5$W or NS) (maximum concentration: 10 mg/mL); infuse over 15-30 minutes; maximum rate of infusion: 1 mg/minute

Monitoring Parameters PT

Additional Information Phytonadione is more effective and is preferred to other vitamin K preparations in the presence of impending hemorrhage; oral absorption depends on the presence of bile salts

Dosage Forms
Injection, aqueous colloidal (AquaMEPHYTON®): 2 mg/mL (0.5 mL); 10 mg/mL (1 mL) [contains benzyl alcohol]
Tablet (Mephyton®): 5 mg

Extemporaneous Preparations A 1 mg/mL suspension may be made by crushing six 5 mg tablets, add 5 mL purified water and 5 mL 1% methylcellulose, mix well, add 70% sorbitol to a total volume of 30 mL; shake well, refrigerate, expected stability: 3 days.
Nahata MC and Hipple TF, *Pediatric Drug Formulations*, 4th ed, Cincinnati, OH: Harvey Whitney Books Co, 2000.

References
Michelson AD, Bovill E, Monagle P, et al, "Antithrombic Therapy in Children," *Chest*, 1998, 114(5 Suppl):748S-69S.

♦ **Pilocar**® *see Pilocarpine* *on page 903*

Pilocarpine (pye loe KAR peen)

U.S. Brand Names Isopto® Carpine; Ocusert Pilo-20® [DSC]; Ocusert Pilo-40® [DSC]; Pilocar®; Pilopine HS®; Piloptic®; Salagen®

Canadian Brand Names Diocarpine

Therapeutic Category Cholinergic Agent; Cholinergic Agent, Ophthalmic; Ophthalmic Agent, Miotic

Generic Available Yes (solution)

Use
Ophthalmic: Management of chronic simple glaucoma, chronic and acute angle-closure glaucoma; counter effects of cycloplegics
Oral: Symptomatic treatment of xerostomia caused by salivary gland hypofunction resulting from radiotherapy for cancer of the head and neck; and in Sjögren's syndrome

Pregnancy Risk Factor C

Contraindications Hypersensitivity to pilocarpine or any component; when cholinergic effects such as constriction are undesirable, eg, acute inflammatory disease of anterior chamber, acute iritis; severe hepatic impairment (oral use)

Warnings Reduce dosage in hepatic impairment

Precautions Use with caution in patients with pre-existing retinal disease, CHF, asthma, peptic ulcer, urinary tract obstruction, Parkinson's disease, corneal abrasion, or those predisposed to retinal tears; may occasionally precipitate angle closure by increased resistance to aqueous flow from the posterior to anterior eye chamber

Adverse Reactions
Cardiovascular: Rare hypertension, tachycardia, flushing
Central nervous system: Headache, chills, dizziness
Gastrointestinal (rare): Nausea, vomiting, diarrhea, salivation
Genitourinary: Polyuria
Local: Stinging, burning
Neuromuscular & skeletal: Weakness
Ocular: Ophthalmic formulation: Miosis, ciliary spasm, blurred vision, retinal detachment, photophobia, acute iritis, keratitis, corneal opacities, lacrimation, browache, conjunctival and ciliary congestion early in therapy
Otic: Tinnitus
Respiratory: Rhinitis
Miscellaneous: Hypersensitivity reactions, diaphoresis

Drug Interactions Topical NSAIDs may decrease pilocarpine effect; increased toxicities when combined with other parasympathomimetics; decreased effectiveness with anticholinergics; use with β-blockers may increase risk of conduction disturbances

Food Interactions High fat meals decrease the rate of oral absorption and maximum serum concentration; the time to reach maximum concentrations is also increased

Mechanism of Action Directly stimulates cholinergic receptors in the eye causing miosis (by contraction of the iris sphincter), loss of accommodation (by constriction of (Continued)

Pilocarpine (Continued)

ciliary muscle), and lowering of intraocular pressure (with decreased resistance to aqueous humor outflow)

Pharmacodynamics

Ophthalmic solution instillation: Miosis:
Onset of action: Within 10-30 minutes
Duration: 4-8 hours
Intraocular pressure reduction:
Onset of action: 1 hour
Duration: 4-12 hours
Oral: Increased salivary flow
Onset of action: 20 minutes
Maximum effect: 1 hour
Duration: 3-5 hours

Pharmacokinetics Adults:

Half-life, elimination: Oral: 0.76-1.35 hours
Mild to moderate hepatic impairment: 2.1 hours
Elimination: Urine

Usual Dosage

Ophthalmic: Children and Adults:
Gel: 0.5" (1.3 cm) ribbon applied to lower conjunctival sac once daily at bedtime; adjust dosage as required to control elevated intraocular pressure
Solution: Instill 1-2 drops up to 6 times/day; adjust the concentration and frequency as required to control elevated intraocular pressure
To counteract the mydriatic effects of sympathomimetic agents: Instill 1 drop of a 1% solution in the affected eye
Xerostomia: Adults: Oral:
Following head and neck cancer: 5 mg 3 times/day, titration up to 10 mg 3 times/day may be considered for patients who have not responded adequately; not to exceed 10 mg/dose
Sjögren's syndrome: 5 mg 4 times/day

Dosage adjustment in hepatic impairment: Adults: Oral: Patients with moderate impairment 5 mg 2 times/day regardless of indication; avoid use in severe hepatic impairment

Administration

Ophthalmic gel: Instill gel into affected eye(s); close the eye for 1-2 minutes and instruct patient to roll the eyeball in all directions; avoid contact of bottle tip with eye or skin
Ophthalmic solution: Shake well before use; instill into affected eye(s); apply finger pressure to lacrimal sac during and for 1-2 minutes after instillation to decrease drainage into the nose and throat and minimize possible systemic absorption
Oral: May be administered with or without food; avoid administration with high fat meal

Monitoring Parameters Intraocular pressure, funduscopic exam, visual field testing; salivation (xerostomia treatment)

Patient Information May sting on instillation; notify physician of sweating, urinary retention; usually causes difficulty in dark adaptation; use caution when driving at night or doing hazardous activities in poor light

Dosage Forms

Gel, ophthalmic, as hydrochloride (Pilopine HS®): 4% (3.5 g)
Ocular therapeutic system:
Ocusert® Pilo-20: Releases 20 mcg per hour for 1 week (8s) [DSC]
Ocusert® Pilo-40: Releases 40 mcg per hour for 1 week (8s) [DSC]
Solution, ophthalmic, as hydrochloride: 1% (15 mL); 2% (15 mL); 4% (15 mL); 6% (15 mL)
Isopto® Carpine: 1% (15 mL); 2% (15 mL, 30 mL); 4% (15 mL, 30 mL); 6% (15 mL); 8% (15 mL)
Pilocar®: 0.5% (15 mL); 1% (1 mL, 15 mL); 2% (1 mL, 15 mL); 3% (15 mL); 4% (1 mL, 15 mL); 6% (15 mL)
Piloptic®: 0.5% (15 mL); 1% (15 mL); 2% (15 mL); 3% (15 mL); 4% (15 mL); 6% (15 mL)
Tablet, as hydrochloride (Salagen®): 5 mg

♦ **Pilopine HS®** see Pilocarpine on page 903
♦ **Piloptic®** see Pilocarpine on page 903
♦ **Pima®** see Potassium Iodide on page 918

Pimecrolimus (pim e KROE li mus)

U.S. Brand Names Elidel®

Synonyms SDZ ASM 981

Therapeutic Category Immunomodulating Agent, Topical

Generic Available No

Use Mild to moderate atopic dermatitis in nonimmunocompromised patients

Pregnancy Risk Factor C

Contraindications Hypersensitivity to pimecrolimus or any component; Netherton's syndrome due to potential for increased systemic absorption; application to site with active cutaneous viral infection (treat and clear infection prior to the start of therapy)

Warnings Pimecrolimus therapy may be associated with an increased risk for eczema herpeticum, varicella zoster, or herpes simplex virus infection; consider discontinuing therapy in patients who develop lymphadenopathy or in patients who have skin papillomas which worsen. Cream contains benzyl alcohol which may cause allergic reactions in susceptible individuals; large amounts of benzyl alcohol (≥99 mg/kg/day) have been associated with a potentially fatal toxicity ("gasping syndrome") in neonates; the "gasping syndrome" consists of metabolic acidosis, respiratory distress, gasping respirations, CNS dysfunction (including convulsions, intracranial hemorrhage), hypotension and cardiovascular collapse.

Precautions Use with caution in immunocompromised patients and in patients who have experienced adverse effects to topical cyclosporine or tacrolimus.

Adverse Reactions

Central nervous system: Headache

Dermatologic: Pruritus, acne, infected hair follicles

Gastrointestinal: Nausea

Local: Burning sensation, stinging

Drug Interactions Cytochrome P450 isoenzyme CYP3A3/4 substrate

No drug interactions have been reported with topical pimecrolimus. However, patients with erythrodermic disease who may experience increased absorption of pimecrolimus should be monitored for evidence of pimecrolimus toxicity when coadministered with a CYP3A4 inhibitor such as erythromycin, itraconazole, keto-conazole, fluconazole, cimetidine, or calcium channel blockers.

Stability Store at room temperature; do not freeze

Mechanism of Action Binds with high affinity to macrophilin-12 (FKBP-12) inhibiting the calcium-dependent phosphatase activity of calcineurin. Inhibits T-cell activation by blocking the transcription and synthesis in human T-cells of early cytokines inter-leukin-2, interferon gamma (T_h1-type), interleukin-4, and interleukin-10 (T_h2-type). Prevents the release of inflammatory cytokines and mediators from mast cells after stimulation by antigen/IgE.

Pharmacodynamics Onset of action: Time to significant improvement: 8 days

Pharmacokinetics

Absorption: Topical: Low systemic absorption; blood concentration of pimecrolimus was routinely <2 ng/mL with treatment of atopic dermatitis in adult patients (13% to 62% BSA involvement); blood concentration of pimecrolimus was <3 ng/mL in 26 pediatric patients 2-14 years of age with atopic dermatitis (20% to 69% BSA involvement)

Protein binding: 74% to 87%

Metabolism: In the liver by the cytochrome P450 3A4 system

Half-life: Terminal: 30-40 hours

Time to peak serum concentration: Topical: 2-6 hours

Elimination: Primarily in the feces as metabolites

Usual Dosage Infants ≥3 months of age, Children and Adults: Topical: Apply twice daily; continue therapy for as long as symptoms persist; re-evaluate patient at 6 weeks

Administration Topical: Avoid contact with eyes, nose, mouth, and cut, scraped, or infected skin areas. Wash hands with soap and water prior to and after cream application. Apply thin layer of cream by gently rubbing it in over affected skin surfaces which may include head and neck areas. The use of occlusive dressings is not recommended.

Monitoring Parameters Check skin for signs of worsening condition (increase in pruritus, erythema, excoriation, and lichenification)

Patient Information Avoid exposure to sunlight and artificial light sources (sunlamps, tanning booth/bed); wear protective clothing, wide-brimmed hats, and lip sunscreen (SPF ≥15); use a sunscreen [broad-spectrum sunscreen or physical sunscreen (preferred) or sunblock with SPF ≥15]; contact physician if any signs of serious infection occurs

Dosage Forms Cream, topical: 1% (15 g, 30 g, 100 g) [contains benzyl alcohol and propylene glycol]

(Continued)

Pimecrolimus *(Continued)*

References

Eichenfield LF, Lucky AW, Boguniewicz M, et al, "Safety and Efficacy of Pimecrolimus (ASM 981) Cream 1% in the Treatment of Mild and Moderate Atopic Dermatitis in Children and Adolescents," *J Am Acad Dermatol*, 2002, 46(4):495-504.

Wahn U, Bos JD, Goodfield M, et al, "Efficacy and Safety of Pimecrolimus Cream in the Long-Term Management of Atopic Dermatitis in Children," *Pediatrics*, 2002, 110(1 Pt 1):e2.

Wellington K and Jarvis B, "Topical Pimecrolimus: A Review of Its Clinical Potential in the Management of Atopic Dermatitis," *Drugs*, 2002, 62(5):817-40.

♦ **Pin-X® [OTC]** *see* Pyrantel Pamoate *on page 960*

Piperacillin *(pi PER a sil in)*

U.S. Brand Names Pipracil®

Therapeutic Category Antibiotic, Penicillin (Antipseudomonal)

Generic Available No

Use Treatment of serious infections caused by susceptible strains of gram-positive, gram-negative, and anaerobic bacilli; where aerobic-anaerobic bacterial infections or empiric antibiotic therapy in granulocytopenic patients. Primary use is in the treatment of serious carbenicillin-resistant or ticarcillin-resistant *Pseudomonas aeruginosa* infections susceptible to piperacillin.

Pregnancy Risk Factor B

Contraindications Hypersensitivity to piperacillin, penicillins, or any component

Warnings Superinfection has been reported in up to 6% to 8% of patients receiving an extended spectrum penicillin; piperacillin therapy has been associated with an increased incidence of fever and rash in cystic fibrosis patients

Precautions Use with caution in patients with hypersensitivity to cephalosporins; dosage modification required in patients with impaired renal function

Adverse Reactions

Central nervous system: Seizures, fever, headache, dizziness, confusion, drowsiness

Dermatologic: Rash, exfoliative dermatitis

Endocrine & metabolic: Hypokalemia

Gastrointestinal: Diarrhea, vomiting

Hematologic: Hemolytic anemia, eosinophilia, neutropenia, prolonged bleeding time, thrombocytopenia

Hepatic: Elevated liver enzymes, cholestatic hepatitis

Local: Thrombophlebitis

Neuromuscular & skeletal: Myoclonus

Renal: Acute interstitial nephritis

Miscellaneous: Hypersensitivity reactions, anaphylaxis, serum sickness-like reaction

Drug Interactions Aminoglycosides (antibacterial activity is synergistic), probenecid (increases serum concentration of piperacillin), vecuronium (prolongs neuromuscular blockade)

Stability Reconstituted piperacillin solution is stable for 24 hours at room temperature and 7 days when refrigerated; incompatible with aminoglycosides

Mechanism of Action Inhibits bacterial cell wall synthesis by binding to one or more of the penicillin-binding proteins; inhibits the final transpeptidation step of peptidoglycan synthesis in bacterial cell walls

Pharmacokinetics

Absorption: I.M.: 70% to 80%

Distribution: Crosses the placenta; distributes into breast milk at low concentrations; penetration across the blood-brain barrier is poor when meninges are uninflamed; good biliary concentration (30-60 times higher than serum concentration)

Protein binding: 22%

Metabolism: 5% to 10%

Half-life: Prolonged with moderately severe renal or hepatic impairment

Neonates:

1-5 days: 3.6 hours

>6 days: 2.1-2.7 hours

Children:

1-6 months: 0.5-1 hours

6 months to 12 years: 0.39-0.5 hours

Adults: 36-80 minutes (dose-dependent)

Time to peak serum concentration: I.M.: Within 30-50 minutes

Elimination: Principally in urine and partially in feces (via bile)

Dialysis: Dialyzable (20% to 50%)

Usual Dosage Safety and efficacy in children <12 years of age has not been established

I.M., I.V.:

Neonates:

≤7 days: 150 mg/kg/day divided every 8 hours

>7 days: 200 mg/kg/day divided every 6 hours

Infants and Children: 200-300 mg/kg/day in divided doses every 4-6 hours; maximum dose: 24 g/day

Higher doses have been used in cystic fibrosis: 350-500 mg/kg/day in divided doses every 4 hours

Adults: 2-4 g/dose every 4-8 hours; maximum dose: 24 g/day

Dosing interval in renal impairment:

Cl_{cr} 20-40 mL/minute: Administer every 8 hours

Cl_{cr} <20 mL/minute: Administer every 12 hours

Administration Parenteral:

I.M.: Reconstitute each gram of piperacillin with at least 2 mL of SWI, NS, or 0.5% or 1% lidocaine hydrochloride (without epinephrine) to make a 400 mg/mL solution; administer by deep I.M. injection into the gluteus maximus

I.V. push: Administer over 3-5 minutes at a maximum concentration of 200 mg/mL

I.V. intermittent infusion: Administer over 30-60 minutes at a final concentration ≤20 mg/mL

Monitoring Parameters Serum electrolytes, bleeding time especially in patients with renal impairment; periodic tests of renal, hepatic and hematologic function

Test Interactions False-positive urinary and serum proteins, positive Coombs' [direct]

Nursing Implications If the patient is on concurrent aminoglycoside therapy, separate piperacillin administration from the aminoglycoside by at least 30-60 minutes

Additional Information Sodium content of 1 g: 1.85 mEq

Dosage Forms Injection, powder for reconstitution, as sodium: 2 g, 3 g, 4 g

References

Placzek M, Whitelaw A, Want S, et al, "Piperacillin in Early Neonatal Infection," *Arch Dis Child*, 1983, 58(12):1006-9.

Prince AS and Neu HC, "Use of Piperacillin, A Semisynthetic Penicillin, in the Therapy of Acute Exacerbations of Pulmonary Disease in Patients With Cystic Fibrosis," *J Pediatr*, 1980, 97(1):148-51.

Thirumoorthi MC, Asmar BI, Buckley JA, et al, "Pharmacokinetics of Intravenously Administered Piperacillin in Preadolescent Children," *J Pediatr*, 1983, 102(6):941-6.

Piperacillin and Tazobactam (pi PER a sil in & ta zoe BAK tam)

U.S. Brand Names Zosyn®

Canadian Brand Names Tacozin®

Synonyms Tazobactam and Piperacillin

Therapeutic Category Antibiotic, Beta-lactam and Beta-lactamase Combination; Antibiotic, Penicillin (Antipseudomonal)

Generic Available No

Use Treatment of sepsis, gynecologic, intra-abdominal infections, and infections involving skin and skin structures, the lower respiratory tract, and urinary tract caused by piperacillin-resistant, beta-lactamase producing strains that are piperacillin/tazobactam susceptible. Tazobactam expands activity of piperacillin to include beta-lactamase producing strains of *S. aureus*, *H. influenzae*, *B. fragilis*, *Klebsiella*, *E. coli*, and *Acinetobacter*.

Pregnancy Risk Factor B

Contraindications Hypersensitivity to piperacillin, tazobactam, penicillins, or any component

Warnings Prolonged use may result in superinfection; abnormal platelet aggregation and prolonged bleeding have been reported in patients with renal failure; piperacillin therapy has been associated with an increased incidence of fever and rash in cystic fibrosis patients

Precautions Use with caution in patients with hypersensitivity to cephalosporins or other beta-lactamase inhibitors; use with caution in patients with renal impairment or pre-existing seizure disorder; dosage modification required in patients with impaired renal function

Adverse Reactions

Cardiovascular: Hypertension, hypotension, edema

Central nervous system: Insomnia, headache, dizziness, agitation, confusion, fever, convulsions

Dermatologic: Rash, pruritus, erythema multiforme, Stevens-Johnson syndrome

Endocrine & metabolism: Hypokalemia

Gastrointestinal: Diarrhea, constipation, nausea, vomiting, dyspepsia, melena, pseudomembranous colitis

Hematologic: Leukopenia, thrombocytopenia, neutropenia, decrease in hemoglobin/hematocrit, eosinophilia, prolonged prothrombin time, hemolytic anemia

Hepatic: Elevated AST, ALT, bilirubin; hepatitis, cholestatic jaundice

Local: Phlebitis, pain

(Continued)

Piperacillin and Tazobactam *(Continued)*

Renal: Elevated BUN, elevated serum creatinine, interstitial nephritis

Miscellaneous: Hypersensitivity reactions, anaphylaxis

Drug Interactions Probenecid prolongs half-life of piperacillin/tazobactam; vecuronium (prolongs neuromuscular blockade); aminoglycosides (antibacterial activity is synergistic); may decrease renal clearance of methotrexate

Stability Reconstituted piperacillin/tazobactam solution is stable for 24 hours at room temperature and 2 days when refrigerated; incompatible with LR solution and aminoglycosides

Mechanism of Action Inhibits bacterial cell wall synthesis by binding to one or more of the penicillin-binding proteins; inhibits the final transpeptidation step of peptidoglycan synthesis in bacterial cell walls; tazobactam prevents degradation of piperacillin by binding to beta-lactamases

Pharmacokinetics Both AUC and peak concentrations are dose proportional

Distribution: Widely distributed into tissues and body fluids including lungs, intestinal mucosa, female reproductive tissues, interstitial fluid, gallbladder, and bile; penetration into CSF is poor when meninges are uninflamed; piperacillin is excreted into breast milk

Protein binding:

Piperacillin: ~26% to 33%

Tazobactam: 31% to 32%

Metabolism:

Piperacillin: 6% to 9%

Tazobactam: ~22%

Bioavailability: I.M.:

Piperacillin: 71%

Tazobactam: 84%

Half-life:

Piperacillin:

Infants 2-5 months: 1.4 hours

Children 6-23 months: 0.9 hour

Children 2-12 years: 0.7 hour

Adults: 0.7-1.2 hours

Metabolite: 1-1.5 hours

Tazobactam:

Infants 2-5 months: 1.6 hours

Children 6-23 months: 1 hour

Children 2-12 years: 0.8-0.9 hour

Adults: 0.7-0.9 hour

Elimination: Piperacillin and tazobactam are both eliminated by renal tubular secretion and glomerular filtration

Piperacillin: 50% to 70% eliminated unchanged in urine

Tazobactam: Found in urine at 24 hours, with 22% as the inactive metabolite

Dialysis: Hemodialysis removes 30% to 40% of a piperacillin/tazobactam dose; peritoneal dialysis removes 21% of tazobactam and 6% of piperacillin; hepatic impairment does not affect the kinetics of piperacillin or tazobactam significantly

Usual Dosage Safety and efficacy in children <12 years of age has not been established. Zosyn™ (piperacillin and tazobactam) is a combination product; each 3.375 g vial contains 3 g piperacillin sodium and 0.375 g tazobactam sodium in a 8:1 ratio. Dosage recommendations are based on the **piperacillin** component.

Infants <6 months of age: I.V.: 150-300 mg of piperacillin component/kg/day in divided doses every 6-8 hours

Infants and Children ≥6 months: I.V.: 240 mg of piperacillin component/kg/day in divided doses every 8 hours; higher doses have been used for serious pseudomonal infections: 300-400 mg of piperacillin component/kg/day in divided doses every 6 hours; maximum dose: 18 g of piperacillin component/day

Adults: I.V.: 3.375 g (3 g piperacillin/0.375 g tazobactam) every 6 hours; maximum dose: 18 g of piperacillin component/day

Dosing interval in renal impairment:

Cl_{cr} 20-40 mL/minute: Decrease dose by 30% and administer every 6 hours

Cl_{cr} <20 mL/minute: Decrease dose by 30% and administer every 8 hours

Hemodialysis: Adults: Administer 2.25 g every 8 hours with an additional dose of 0.75 g after each dialysis

Administration Parenteral: I.V. intermittent infusion: May administer over 30 minutes at a maximum concentration of 200 mg/mL (piperacillin component); however, concentrations ≤20 mg/mL are preferred. If the patient is on concurrent aminoglycoside therapy, separate piperacillin and tazobactam administration from the aminoglycoside by at least 30-60 minutes.

Monitoring Parameters Serum electrolytes, bleeding time especially in patients with renal impairment; periodic tests of renal, hepatic, and hematologic function

Test Interactions Positive Coombs' [direct], false-positive urinary and serum proteins; false-positive urine glucose using Clinitest®

Additional Information Sodium content of 1 g piperacillin component: 2.35 mEq

Dosage Forms Note: 8:1 ratio of piperacillin sodium to tazobactam sodium

    Infusion [premixed iso-osmotic solution in dextrose; frozen]:
        Piperacillin sodium 2 g and tazobactam sodium 0.25 g (50 mL)
        Piperacillin sodium 3 g and tazobactam sodium 0.375 g (50 mL)
        Piperacillin sodium 4 g and tazobactam sodium 0.5 g (50 mL)

    Injection, powder for reconstitution, as sodium salts:
        Piperacillin 2 g and tazobactam 0.25 g
        Piperacillin 3 g and tazobactam 0.375 g
        Piperacillin 4 g and tazobactam 0.5 g
        Piperacillin 36 g and tazobactam 4.5 g [bulk pharmacy vial]

References

Bryson HM and Brogden RN, "Piperacillin/Tazobactam. A Review of its Antibacterial Activity, Pharmacokinetic Properties, and Therapeutic Potential," *Drugs*, 1994, 47(3):506-35.

Reed MD, Goldfarb J, Yamashita T, et al, "Single-Dose Pharmacokinetics of Piperacillin and Tazobactam in Infants and Children," *Antimicrob Agents Chemother*, 1994, 38(12):2817-26.

Piperazine [DSC] (PI per a zeen)

U.S. Brand Names Vermizine® [DSC]

Canadian Brand Names Entacyl®

Therapeutic Category Anthelmintic

Use Treatment of pinworm (*Enterobius vermicularis*) and roundworm (*Ascaris lumbricoides*) infections; used as an alternative to first-line agents mebendazole or pyrantel pamoate for the treatment of these infections

Pregnancy Risk Factor B

Contraindications Hypersensitivity to piperazine or any component; seizure disorders, liver or kidney impairment

Precautions Use with caution in patients with anemia or malnutrition or patients receiving chlorpromazine; avoid prolonged or repeated piperazine use in children due to potential neurotoxicity

Adverse Reactions

    Central nervous system: Dizziness, vertigo, seizures, EEG changes, headache
    Gastrointestinal: Nausea, vomiting, diarrhea, abdominal cramps
    Hematologic: Hemolytic anemia
    Neuromuscular & skeletal: Tremor, weakness
    Ocular: Visual impairment, nystagmus
    Respiratory: Cough
    Miscellaneous: Hypersensitivity reactions (urticaria, erythema multiforme, photodermatitis, fever, arthralgia, bronchospasm)

Drug Interactions Pyrantel pamoate (antagonistic mode of action)

Mechanism of Action Causes muscle paralysis of the roundworm by blocking the effects of acetylcholine at the neuromuscular junction

Pharmacokinetics

    Absorption: Well absorbed from the GI tract
    Time to peak serum concentration: 1 hour
    Elimination: In urine as metabolites and unchanged drug

Usual Dosage Oral:

    Pinworms: Children and Adults: 65 mg/kg/day as a single daily dose for 7 days; in severe infections, repeat course after a 1-week interval; not to exceed 2.5 g/day
    Roundworms:
        Children: 75 mg/kg/day as a single daily dose for 2 days; maximum dose: 3.5 g/day; in severe infections, repeat course after a 1-week interval
        Adults: 3.5 g/day for 2 days (in severe infections, repeat course, after a 1-week interval)

Administration Oral: In the case of partial or complete intestinal obstruction due to a heavy roundworm load, administer dose as a solution through a GI tube

Monitoring Parameters Stool exam for worms and ova

Nursing Implications Cure rates may be decreased with massive infections or in patients with hypermotility of the GI tract

Dosage Forms

    Tablet, as citrate: 250 mg [DSC]

♦ **Pipracil®** *see* Piperacillin *on page 906*

Pirbuterol (peer BYOO ter ole)

U.S. Brand Names Maxair™; Maxair™ Autohaler™

Therapeutic Category Adrenergic Agonist Agent; Antiasthmatic; Beta₂-Adrenergic Agonist Agent; Bronchodilator; Sympathomimetic

Generic Available No

Use Prevention and treatment of bronchospasm in patients with reversible airway obstruction due to asthma or COPD

Pregnancy Risk Factor C

Contraindications Hypersensitivity to pirbuterol or or any component

Warnings Paradoxical bronchospasm may occur, especially with the first use of a new cannister

Precautions Use with caution in patients with hyperthyroidism, diabetes mellitus, cardiovascular disorders (including coronary insufficiency or hypertension); excessive or prolonged use can lead to tolerance

Adverse Reactions

Cardiovascular: Tachycardia, palpitations, hypertension, chest pain

Central nervous system: Nervousness, CNS stimulation, anxiety, syncope, hyperactivity, insomnia, dizziness, depression, lightheadedness, drowsiness, headache

Dermatologic: Rash, pruritus, alopecia

Endocrine & metabolic: Hypokalemia

Gastrointestinal: GI upset, xerostomia, glossitis, abdominal pain, vomiting, nausea, unusual taste, hoarseness

Neuromuscular & skeletal: Tremor, weakness, muscle cramping

Respiratory: Irritation of oropharynx, cough, paradoxical bronchospasm

Miscellaneous: Diaphoresis

Drug Interactions Action of pirbuterol is antagonized by beta-adrenergic blocking agents such as propranolol; cardiovascular effects are potentiated in patients also receiving MAO inhibitors or tricyclic antidepressants; concomitant administration of sympathomimetics may result in enhanced cardiovascular effects

Stability Store at room temperature

Mechanism of Action Relaxes bronchial smooth muscle by action on beta₂-adrenergic receptors with little effect on heart rate

Pharmacodynamics

Onset of action: 5 minutes

Maximum effect: 30-60 minutes

Duration: 5 hours

Pharmacokinetics

Metabolism: Liver (by sulfate conjugation)

Half-life: 2-3 hours

Elimination: 51% excreted in the urine as pirbuterol plus its sulfate conjugate

Usual Dosage Oral inhalation:

Children ≥12 years and Adults: 1-2 inhalations (0.2-0.4 mg) every 4-6 hours; do not exceed 12 inhalations/day

Administration Oral inhalation: Shake well before administration; use spacer for children <8 years of age (Maxair™ Inhaler only); Maxair™ Autohaler™ is breath activated; after sealing lips around mouthpiece, inhale deeply with steady, moderate force; inhalation triggers the release "puff" of medication; do not stop inhalation when puff occurs, but continue to take a deep, full breath; hold breath for 10 seconds, then exhale slowly

Monitoring Parameters Serum potassium, heart rate, pulmonary function tests, respiratory rate; arterial or capillary blood gases (if patient's condition warrants)

Patient Information Do not exceed recommended dosage; may cause dry mouth; rinse mouth with water following each inhalation to help with dry throat and mouth; if more than one inhalation is necessary, wait at least 1 full minute between inhalations; notify physician if palpitations, tachycardia, chest pain, muscle tremors, dizziness, headache, flushing occur, or if breathing difficulty persists

Dosage Forms

Aerosol for oral inhalation, as acetate:

Maxair™ Autohaler™: 0.2 mg/inhalation (2.8 g) [80 inhalations]; (14 g) [400 inhalations]

Maxair™ Inhaler: 0.2 mg/inhalation (25.6 g) [300 inhalations]

References

"National Asthma Education and Prevention Program. Expert Panel Report: Guidelines for the Diagnosis and Management of Asthma Update on Selected Topics--2002," *J Allergy Clin Immunol*, 2002, 110(5 Suppl):S141-219.

Piroxicam (peer OKS i kam)

Related Information

Overdose and Toxicology *on page 1388*

U.S. Brand Names Feldene®

Canadian Brand Names Apo®-Piroxicam; Gen-Piroxicam; Novo-Pirocam®; Nu-Pirox; Pexicam®

Therapeutic Category Analgesic, Non-narcotic; Anti-inflammatory Agent; Nonsteroidal Anti-inflammatory Drug (NSAID), Oral

Generic Available Yes

Use Management of inflammatory diseases and rheumatoid disorders; dysmenorrhea

Pregnancy Risk Factor B (D if used in 3rd trimester)

Contraindications Hypersensitivity to piroxicam, any component, aspirin, or other NSAIDs; active GI bleeding, ulcer disease; patients with the "aspirin triad" [asthma, rhinitis (with or without nasal polys), and aspirin intolerance] (fatal asthmatic and anaphylactoid reactions may occur in these patients)

Precautions Use with caution in patients with impaired cardiac function, hypertension, impaired renal function, GI disease and patients receiving anticoagulants

Adverse Reactions

Cardiovascular: Edema

Central nervous system: Dizziness, headache

Dermatologic: Rash, phototoxic skin eruptions, photosensitivity

Gastrointestinal: Nausea, epigastric distress, anorexia, abdominal discomfort, vomiting, GI bleeding, ulcers, perforation

Hematologic: Reduction in hemoglobin and hematocrit, inhibition of platelet aggregation

Hepatic: Hepatitis

Renal: Acute renal failure, elevated BUN, elevated serum creatinine

Drug Interactions Cytochrome P450 isoenzyme CYP2C9 and CYP2C18 substrate

May increase serum concentrations of lithium; aspirin may decrease piroxicam serum concentrations; GI irritants (eg, potassium supplements) may increase GI adverse effects; piroxicam may decrease antihypertensive effects of ACE inhibitors or angiotensin II antagonists; drug interactions similar to other NSAIDs may also occur; concurrent use of piroxicam with ritonavir is not recommended

Food Interactions Food may decrease the rate but not the extent of absorption

Mechanism of Action Inhibits prostaglandin synthesis by decreasing the activity of the enzyme, cyclooxygenase, which results in decreased formation of prostaglandin precursors

Pharmacodynamics Analgesia:

Onset of action: Oral: Within 1 hour

Maximum effect: 3-5 hours

Pharmacokinetics

Protein binding: 99%

Metabolism: In the liver

Half-life: 45-50 hours

Elimination: Excreted as metabolites and unchanged drug (~5% to 10%) in the urine; small amount excreted in feces

Usual Dosage Oral:

Children: 0.2-0.3 mg/kg/day once daily; maximum dose: 15 mg/day

Adults: 10-20 mg/day once daily; although associated with increase in GI adverse effects, doses >20 mg/day have been used (ie, 30-40 mg/day)

Administration Oral: May administer with food or milk to decrease GI upset

Monitoring Parameters CBC, BUN, serum creatinine, liver enzymes; periodic ophthalmologic exams with chronic use

Patient Information Avoid alcohol. May cause photosensitivity reactions (eg, exposure to sunlight may cause severe sunburn, skin rash, redness, or itching); avoid exposure to sunlight and artificial light sources (sunlamps, tanning booth/bed); wear protective clothing, wide-brimmed hats, sunglasses, and lip sunscreen (SPF ≥15); use a sunscreen [broad-spectrum sunscreen or physical sunscreen (preferred) or sunblock with SPF ≥15]; contact physician if reaction occurs.

Dosage Forms Capsule: 10 mg, 20 mg

- **PMPA** *see* Tenofovir *on page 1067*
- **PMS-Amantadine (Can)** *see* Amantadine *on page 73*
- **PMS-Amitriptyline (Can)** *see* Amitriptyline *on page 89*
- **PMS-Atenolol (Can)** *see* Atenolol *on page 137*
- **PMS-Baclofen (Can)** *see* Baclofen *on page 158*
- **PMS-Bethanechol (Can)** *see* Bethanechol *on page 171*
- **PMS-Buspirone (Can)** *see* BusPIRone *on page 191*
- **PMS-Captopril® (Can)** *see* Captopril *on page 207*
- **PMS-Carbamazepine (Can)** *see* Carbamazepine *on page 209*
- **PMS-Cefaclor (Can)** *see* Cefaclor *on page 223*
- **PMS-Chloral Hydrate (Can)** *see* Chloral Hydrate *on page 252*
- **PMS-Cholestyramine (Can)** *see* Cholestyramine Resin *on page 267*
- **PMS-Cimetidine (Can)** *see* Cimetidine *on page 272*
- **PMS-Clonazepam (Can)** *see* Clonazepam *on page 292*
- **PMS-Deferoxamine (Can)** *see* Deferoxamine *on page 346*
- **PMS-Desipramine (Can)** *see* Desipramine *on page 349*
- **PMS-Dexamethasone (Can)** *see* Dexamethasone *on page 354*
- **PMS-Diclofenac (Can)** *see* Diclofenac *on page 374*
- **PMS-Diclofenac SR (Can)** *see* Diclofenac *on page 374*
- **PMS-Diphenhydramine (Can)** *see* DiphenhydrAMINE *on page 393*
- **PMS-Dipivefrin (Can)** *see* Dipivefrin *on page 396*
- **PMS-Docusate Calcium (Can)** *see* Docusate *on page 402*
- **PMS-Docusate Sodium (Can)** *see* Docusate *on page 402*
- **PMS-Erythromycin (Can)** *see* Erythromycin *on page 448*
- **PMS-Fluorometholone (Can)** *see* Fluorometholone *on page 502*
- **PMS-Fluoxetine (Can)** *see* Fluoxetine *on page 505*
- **PMS-Gabapentin (Can)** *see* Gabapentin *on page 527*
- **PMS-Glyburide (Can)** *see* GlyBURIDE *on page 540*
- **PMS-Haloperidol LA (Can)** *see* Haloperidol *on page 554*
- **PMS-Hydromorphone (Can)** *see* Hydromorphone *on page 577*
- **PMS-Hydroxyzine (Can)** *see* HydrOXYzine *on page 584*
- **PMS-Ipratropium (Can)** *see* Ipratropium *on page 620*
- **PMS-Isoniazid (Can)** *see* Isoniazid *on page 629*
- **PMS-Lactulose (Can)** *see* Lactulose *on page 649*
- **PMS-Levobunolol (Can)** *see* Levobunolol *on page 665*
- **PMS-Lindane (Can)** *see* Lindane *on page 677*
- **PMS-Lithium Carbonate (Can)** *see* Lithium *on page 684*
- **PMS-Lithium Citrate (Can)** *see* Lithium *on page 684*
- **PMS-Loperamine (Can)** *see* Loperamide *on page 687*
- **PMS-Metformin (Can)** *see* Metformin *on page 729*
- **PMS-Methylphenidate (Can)** *see* Methylphenidate *on page 744*
- **PMS-Metoprolol (Can)** *see* Metoprolol *on page 752*
- **PMS-Nizatidine (Can)** *see* Nizatidine *on page 819*
- **PMS-Nortriptyline (Can)** *see* Nortriptyline *on page 822*
- **PMS-Nystatin (Can)** *see* Nystatin *on page 827*
- **PMS-Oxybutynin (Can)** *see* Oxybutynin *on page 843*
- **PMS-Pseudoephedrine (Can)** *see* Pseudoephedrine *on page 958*
- **PMS-Ranitidine (Can)** *see* Ranitidine *on page 972*
- **PMS-Salbutamol (Can)** *see* Albuterol *on page 54*
- **PMS-Sodium Polystyrene Sulfonate (Can)** *see* Sodium Polystyrene Sulfonate *on page 1029*
- **PMS-Sotalol (Can)** *see* Sotalol *on page 1032*
- **PMS-Sucralate (Can)** *see* Sucralfate *on page 1046*
- **PMS-Theophylline (Can)** *see* Theophylline *on page 1076*
- **PMS-Timolol (Can)** *see* Timolol *on page 1095*
- **PMS-Tobramycin (Can)** *see* Tobramycin *on page 1097*
- **PMS-Trazodone (Can)** *see* Trazodone *on page 1110*
- **PMS-Valproic Acid (Can)** *see* Valproic Acid and Derivatives *on page 1131*
- **PMS-Valproic Acid E.C. (Can)** *see* Valproic Acid and Derivatives *on page 1131*

Pneumococcal Polysaccharide Vaccine
(noo moe KOK al vak SEEN)

U.S. Brand Names Pneumovax® 23; Pnu-Imune® 23

Synonyms Pneumococcal Polysaccharide Vaccine, Polyvalent

Therapeutic Category Vaccine, Inactivated Bacteria

Generic Available No

Use Immunocompetent patients 2-64 years of age with a chronic illness (CHF, sickle cell disease, cardiomyopathy, COPD, diabetes mellitus, chronic liver disease, or CSF leak) or with functional or anatomic asplenia; immunocompromised patients ≥2 years of age with the following conditions: HIV, leukemia, lymphoma, Hodgkin's disease, generalized malignancy, chronic renal failure, nephrotic syndrome or conditions associated with immunosuppression (ie, organ transplantation or long-term corticosteroid therapy); adults ≥65 years of age

Contraindications Hypersensitivity to the vaccine or thimerosal; acute febrile illness; children <2 years of age (antibody response to the vaccine is poor in this age group); pregnancy

Warnings Epinephrine injection (1:1000) must be immediately available in case of anaphylaxis; may cause relapse in patients with stable idiopathic thrombocytopenia purpura

Adverse Reactions

Central nervous system: Low grade fever, Guillain-Barré syndrome

Dermatologic: Rash, urticaria

Neuromuscular & skeletal: Arthralgia

Local: Soreness at the injection site, erythema

Drug Interactions Decreased effect with immunosuppressive agents, live vaccines, immunoglobulin; initiate vaccine at least 2 weeks prior to immunosuppressive therapy and avoid during chemotherapy or radiation therapy

Stability Refrigerate

Usual Dosage I.M., S.C.: Children ≥2 years and Adults: 0.5 mL; if an elective splenectomy is planned, administer dose 2 weeks prior to surgery

Revaccination schedule:

Persons 2-64 years of age with functional or anatomic asplenia or immunocompromised persons:

Patients ≤10 years of age: Single revaccination 3-5 years after the previous dose

Patients >10 years of age: Single revaccination ≥5 years after the previous dose

Patients ≥65 years of age: Single revaccination if first dose was ≥5 years ago and patient was <65 years at the time

Administration Parenteral: I.M., S.C.: Do not inject I.V.; avoid intradermal administration; administer S.C. or I.M. into the deltoid muscle or lateral midthigh; pneumococcal vaccine may be given concurrently with other vaccines including MMR, DTP, poliovirus, H. influenzae type b, hepatitis B, or influenza vaccine

Patient Information Vaccination does not guarantee protection from fulminant pneumococcal disease in patient's with functional or anatomic asplenia

Nursing Implications Federal law requires that the date of administration, the vaccine manufacturer, lot number of the vaccine, and the administering person's name, title, and address be entered into the patient's permanent medical record

Dosage Forms

Injection, solution [prefilled syringe]:

Pneumovax® 23: 25 mcg of each type of capsular polysaccharide per 0.5 mL (0.5 mL)

Pnu-Imune® 23: 25 mcg of each type of capsular polysaccharide per 0.5 mL (0.5 mL) [contains thimerosol]

Injection, solution [vial]:

Pneumovax®: 25 mcg of each type of capsular polysaccharide/0.5 mL (0.5 mL, 2.5 mL)

Pnu-Imune®: 25 mcg of each type of capsular polysaccharide/0.5 mL (0.5 mL, 2.5 mL) [contains thimerosol]

References

Advisory Committee on Immunization Practices, "Prevention of Pneumococcal Disease," *MMWR Morb Mortal Wkly Rep*, 1997, 46(RR-8):1-31.

♦ **Pneumococcal Polysaccharide Vaccine, Polyvalent** *see* Pneumococcal Polysaccharide Vaccine *on page 913*

♦ **Pneumococcal Vaccine** *see page 1333*

♦ **Pneumovax® 23** *see* Pneumococcal Polysaccharide Vaccine *on page 913*

♦ **PNU-100766** *see* Linezolid *on page 678*

♦ **Pnu-Imune® 23** *see* Pneumococcal Polysaccharide Vaccine *on page 913*

♦ **Podocon-25®** *see* Podophyllum Resin *on page 914*

♦ **Podofilm® (Can)** *see* Podophyllum Resin *on page 914*

Podophyllum Resin (po DOF fil um REZ in)

U.S. Brand Names Podocon-25®

Canadian Brand Names Podofilm®

Therapeutic Category Keratolytic Agent

Generic Available No

Use Topical treatment of benign growths including external genital and perianal warts (condylomata acuminata), papillomas, fibroids

Pregnancy Risk Factor X

Contraindications Not to be used on birthmarks, moles, or warts with hair growth; cervical, urethral, oral warts; not to be used by diabetic patients or patients with poor circulation; pregnant women; do not apply to normal tissue

Warnings Avoid contact with the eyes as it can cause severe corneal damage; 25% solution should not be applied to or near mucous membranes; podophyllum resin has caused teratogenic effects (skin tags, polyneuritis, limb malformations, septal heart defects) and fetal death when used during pregnancy

Precautions Topical application to large areas or in excessive amounts for prolonged periods should be avoided

Adverse Reactions

Central nervous system: Confusion, lethargy, hallucinations, ataxia, apnea, agitation, seizures

Dermatologic: Pruritus, erythema, scarring

Gastrointestinal: Nausea, vomiting, abdominal pain, diarrhea

Hematologic: Leukopenia, thrombocytopenia

Hepatic: Hepatotoxicity

Local: Pain, local edema

Neuromuscular & skeletal: Peripheral neuropathy, weakness

Renal: Renal failure

Stability Protect from light; avoid exposure to excessive heat

Mechanism of Action Directly affects epithelial cell metabolism by arresting mitosis through binding to a protein subunit of spindle microtubules (tubulin)

Usual Dosage Children and Adults: Topical: 10% to 25% solution in compound benzoin tincture; use 1 drop at a time allowing drying between drops until area is covered; total volume should be limited to <0.5 mL to an area <10 cm^2 for genital or perianal warts or <2 cm^2 for vaginal warts per treatment session; therapy may be repeated once weekly for up to 4 applications for the treatment of genital or perianal warts; use 10% solution when applied to or near mucous membranes

Verrucae: 25% solution is applied directly to the wart; remove drug from area of application within 6 hours

Administration Topical: Shake well before using; use protective occlusive dressing around warts to prevent contact with unaffected skin; apply drug to dry surface of affected area

Patient Information Notify physician if undue skin irritation develops

Nursing Implications Solution should be washed off within 1-4 hours for genital and perianal warts and within 1-2 hours for accessible meatal warts

Dosage Forms Liquid, topical: 25% in compound benzoin tincture (15 mL)

References

Goldfarb MT, Gupta AK, Gupta MA, et al, "Office Therapy for Human Papillomavirus Infection in Nongenital Sites," *Dermatol Clin*, 1991, 9(2):287-96.

"1993 Sexually Transmitted Diseases Treatment Guidelines," *MMWR Morb Mortal Wkly Rep*, 1993, 42(RR-14):1-102.

- ♦ **Polaramine® [DSC]** see Chlorpheniramine on page 262
- ♦ **Poliovirus Vaccine, Live, Inactivated** see page 1333
- ♦ **Poliovirus Vaccine, Live, Trivalent, Oral** see page 1333
- ♦ **Polycidin® Ophthalmic Ointment (Can)** see Bacitracin and Polymyxin B on page 157
- ♦ **Polycitra®** see Citrate and Citric Acid on page 282
- ♦ **Polycitra K®** see Citrate and Citric Acid on page 282
- ♦ **Polycitra-LC®** see Citrate and Citric Acid on page 282

Polyethylene Glycol-Electrolyte Solution

(pol i ETH i leen GLY kol ee LEK troe lite soe LOO shun)

U.S. Brand Names CoLyte®; GoLYTELY®; MiraLax™; NuLYTELY®; OCL® [DSC]

Canadian Brand Names Klean-Prep®; Lyteprep™; Peglyte™

Synonyms Colonic Lavage Solution; Electrolyte Lavage Solution

Therapeutic Category Laxative, Bowel Evacuant; Laxative, Osmotic

Generic Available No

Use Bowel cleansing prior to GI examination (products containing electrolyte supplements only); treatment of occasional constipation (MiraLax™)

Pregnancy Risk Factor C

Contraindications Hypersensitivity to polyethylene glycol or any component; GI obstruction, gastric retention, bowel perforation, toxic colitis, megacolon

Warnings Do not add flavorings as additional ingredients before use

Precautions May interfere with barium coating of intestinal wall using the double contrast technique; use with caution in patients with ulcerative colitis; use with caution in patients with impaired gag reflex or those who are otherwise prone to regurgitation or aspiration during administration; treatment duration for occasional constipation should not exceed 2 weeks

Adverse Reactions

Dermatologic: Irritative perineal rashes

Endocrine & metabolic: Mild metabolic acidosis with prolonged irrigation periods, electrolyte disturbances

Gastrointestinal: Nausea, cramps, vomiting, abdominal distention, bloating

Drug Interactions Increased peristalsis may decrease absorption of oral medications given within 1 hour of beginning lavage solution

Mechanism of Action Induces catharsis by strong electrolyte and osmotic effects

Pharmacodynamics Onset of action: Bowel cleansing: Within 1-2 hours; constipation: 2-4 days

Usual Dosage

Bowel cleansing (to prevent excessive fluid and electrolyte changes, use only products containing supplemental electrolytes for bowel cleansing): Patient should fast at least 2 hours (preferably 3-4 hours) prior to ingestion:

Children: Oral, nasogastric: 25-40 mL/kg/hour until rectal effluent is clear (usually in 4-10 hours)

Adults:

Oral: Drink 240 mL (8 oz) every 10 minutes until 4 liters are consumed or the rectal effluent is clear

Nasogastric: 20-30 mL/minute (1.2-1.8 L/hour) until 4 liters are administered

Occasional constipation: MiraLax™: Adults: Oral: 17 g (~1 heaping tablespoon) daily

Administration Oral: Add tap water to "fill-line" for reconstitution of powder for solution; no solid foods for 2 hours prior to initiation of therapy; rapid drinking is preferred to drinking small amounts continuously; chilled solution often more palatable; do not add flavorings as additional ingredients before use; MiraLax™ 17 g (dose may be measured using bottle cap) added to 8 oz of water

Monitoring Parameters Electrolytes, BUN, serum glucose, urine osmolality

Patient Information Chilled solution is often more palatable

Nursing Implications First bowel movement should occur in 1 hour

Dosage Forms

Powder for oral solution:

CoLytely®: PEG 3350 227.1 g, sodium sulfate 21.5 g, sodium bicarbonate 6.36 g, sodium chloride 5.53 g and potassium chloride 2.82 g (18 oz) [regular and pineapple flavors]

CoLytely®-Flavored: PEG 3350 240 g, sodium sulfate 22.72 g, sodium bicarbonate 6.72 g, sodium chloride 5.84 g and potassium chloride 2.98 g (4000 mL) [available with cherry, citrus berry, lemon lime, and pineapple flavor packets]

GoLytely®: PEG 3350 227 g, sodium sulfate 21.5 g, sodium bicarbonate 6.36 g, sodium chloride 5.53 g and potassium chloride 2.82 g per packet (4000 mL)

GoLytely®: PEG 3350 236 g, sodium sulfate 22.74 g, sodium bicarbonate 6.74 g, sodium chloride 5.86 g and potassium chloride 2.97 g (4000 mL) [regular and pineapple flavors]

MiraLax™: PEG 3350 14 oz (255 g), 27 oz (527 g)

NuLYTELY®: PEG 3350 420 g, sodium bicarbonate 5.72 g, sodium chloride 11.2 g and potassium chloride 1.48 g (4000 mL) [also available in cherry, lemon-lime, or orange flavors]

Solution, oral (OCL®): PEG 3350 6 g, sodium sulfate decahydrate 1.29 g, sodium bicarbonate 168 mg, potassium chloride 75 mg, and polysorbate 80 30 mg per 100 mL (1500 mL) [DSC]

References

Sondheimer JM, Sokol RJ, Taylor SF, et al, "Safety, Efficacy and Tolerance of Intestinal Lavage in Pediatric Patients Undergoing Diagnostic Colonoscopy," *J Pediatr*, 1991, 119(1):148-52.

Tuggle DW, Hoelzer DJ, Tunell WP, et al, "The Safety and Cost-Effectiveness of Polyethylene Glycol Electrolyte Solution Bowel: Preparation in Infants and Children," *J Pediatr Surg*, 1987, 22(6):513-5.

♦ **Polygam® S/D** *see* Immune Globulin (Intravenous) *on page 598*

♦ **Poly-Iron 150 [OTC]** *see* Iron Supplements (Oral/Enteral) *on page 623*

Polymyxin B (pol i MIKS in bee)

U.S. Brand Names Poly-Rx

Therapeutic Category Antibiotic, Ophthalmic; Antibiotic, Urinary Irrigation; Antibiotic, Miscellaneous

Generic Available Yes

Use Topically for wound irrigation and bladder irrigation against *Pseudomonas aeruginosa*; used occasionally for gut decontamination. Parenteral use of polymyxin B has mainly been replaced by less toxic antibiotics. Reserved for life-threatening infections caused by organisms resistant to the preferred drugs; used as inhalation therapy for gram-negative respiratory infections resistant to preferred drugs; used intrathecally for meningeal infections due to susceptible organisms which are resistant to less toxic antibiotics

Pregnancy Risk Factor B

Contraindications Hypersensitivity to polymyxin or any component

Warnings Polymyxin B can cause serious nephrotoxicity and or neurotoxicity; neurotoxic reactions may be manifested by irritability, weakness, drowsiness, ataxia, perioral paresthesia, numbness of the extremities and blurring of vision. These reactions are usually associated with high serum levels found in patients with impaired renal function or nephrotoxicity. Avoid concurrent or sequential use of other nephrotoxic and neurotoxic drugs, particularly bacitracin, kanamycin, streptomycin, paromomycin, colistin, tobramycin, neomycin, gentamicin, and amikacin. The drug's neurotoxicity can result in respiratory paralysis from neuromuscular blockade, especially when the drug is given soon after anesthesia or muscle relaxants. Polymyxin B sulfate is toxic when given parenterally; **avoid parenteral use whenever possible**.

Precautions Use with caution in patients with myasthenia gravis, patients receiving neuromuscular blocking agents or anesthetics, and in patients with impaired renal function; modify dosage in patients with renal impairment; **I.M. use is not recommended in infants and children due to severe pain at injection site**

Adverse Reactions
Cardiovascular: Facial flushing
Central nervous system: Drowsiness, ataxia, fever, dizziness
Dermatologic: Rash, urticaria
Endocrine & metabolic: Hypocalcemia, hyponatremia, hypokalemia, hypochloremia
Local: Pain at injection site, thrombophlebitis
Neuromuscular & skeletal: Neuromuscular blockade, paresthesia
Ocular: Diplopia
Renal: Nephrotoxicity (hematuria, proteinuria, azotemia)
Respiratory: Respiratory arrest
Miscellaneous: Hypersensitivity reactions

Drug Interactions Neuromuscular blocking agents, anesthetics (increase skeletal muscle relaxation); aminoglycosides, colistin, sodium citrate, parenteral quinidine

Stability Protect from light; incompatible with calcium, magnesium, cephalothin, chloramphenicol, heparin, penicillins; inactivated by acidic or alkaline solutions

Mechanism of Action Binds to phospholipids, alters permeability and damages the bacterial cytoplasmic membrane permitting leakage of intracellular constituents

Pharmacokinetics
Absorption: Well absorbed from the peritoneum; minimal absorption (<10%) from the GI tract (except in neonates), from mucous membranes or intact skin
Distribution: Widely distributed to body tissues in the liver, kidneys, heart, muscle; does not penetrate into CSF or synovial fluid; does not cross the placenta
Half-life: 4.5-6 hours, increased with reduced renal function
Time to peak serum concentration: I.M.: Within 2 hours
Elimination: Primarily as unchanged drug (>60%) in urine via glomerular filtration
Dialysis: Not removed by hemodialysis

Usual Dosage Note: Avoid parenteral use when possible
Infants <2 years:
  I.M.: 25,000-40,000 units/kg/day divided every 6 hours
  I.V.: 15,000-45,000 units/kg/day by continuous I.V. infusion or divided every 12 hours
  Intrathecal: 20,000 units once daily for 3-4 days or 25,000 units once every other day; continue 25,000 units once every other day for at least 2 weeks after cultures of the CSF are negative
Children ≥2 years and Adults:
  I.M.: 25,000-30,000 units/kg/day divided every 6 hours
  I.V.: 15,000-25,000 units/kg/day divided every 12 hours or by continuous infusion; total daily dose should not exceed 2,000,000 units/day
  Bladder irrigation: Continuous irrigation of the urinary bladder for up to 10 days using 20 mg (equal to 200,000 units) added to 1 L of NS; usually no more than 1

L of irrigant is used per day unless urine flow rate is high; administration rate is adjusted to patient's urine output

Topical irrigation or topical solution: 0.1% to 0.3% solution used to irrigate infected wounds; should not exceed 2 million units/day in adults

Gut sterilization: Oral: 100,000-200,000 units/kg/day divided every 6-8 hours

Inhalation: 2-2.5 mg/kg/day divided every 6 hours; final concentration for administration should not exceed 10 mg/mL

Intrathecal: 50,000 units once daily for 3-4 days, then reduce to once every other day for at least 2 weeks after cultures of the CSF are negative

Dosing adjustment in renal impairment:

Cl_{cr} 5-20 mL/minute: Administer 50% of usual daily dose divided every 12 hours

Cl_{cr} <5 mL/minute: Administer 15% of the usual daily dose divided every 12 hours

Administration Parenteral (avoid parenteral use whenever possible):

I.M.: Not recommended for routine use in infants and children because of the severe pain which occurs with I.M. injection; administer I.M. injections deep into the upper outer quadrant of the gluteal muscles at a final concentration of 250,000 units/mL

I.V.: Infuse slowly over 60-90 minutes or by continuous infusion at a concentration of 1000-1667 units/mL in D_5W

Intrathecal: Reconstitute vial with 10 mL NS without preservatives to provide a final concentration of 50,000 units/mL

Monitoring Parameters WBC, serum electrolytes, renal function tests, serum drug concentration, urine output

Reference Range Serum concentration >5 µg/mL are toxic in adults

Additional Information 1 mg = 10,000 units; neuromuscular blockade may be reversed with calcium chloride

Dosage Forms

Injection, powder for reconstitution, lyophilized, as sulfate: 500,000 units

Powder [for prescription compounding] (Poly-Rx): 100 million units (13 g)

♦ **Polymyxin B and Bacitracin** see Bacitracin and Polymyxin B on page 157

♦ **Polymyxin B and Neomycin** see Neomycin and Polymyxin B on page 802

♦ **Polymyxin B, Neomycin, and Bacitracin** see Neomycin, Polymyxin B, and Bacitracin on page 804

♦ **Polymyxin B, Neomycin, and Prednisolone** see Neomycin, Polymyxin B, and Prednisolone on page 804

♦ **Polymyxin B, Neomycin, (Bacitracin), and Hydrocortisone** see Neomycin, (Bacitracin) Polymyxin B, and Hydrocortisone on page 802

♦ **Poly-Pred® Liquifilm®** see Neomycin, Polymyxin B, and Prednisolone on page 804

♦ **Poly-Rx** see Polymyxin B on page 916

♦ **Polysporin® Ophthalmic** see Bacitracin and Polymyxin B on page 157

♦ **Polysporin® Topical [OTC]** see Bacitracin and Polymyxin B on page 157

♦ **Polytar® [OTC]** see Coal Tar on page 299

♦ **Poly-Vi-Sol®** see page 1213

♦ **Pontocaine®** see Tetracaine on page 1073

Poractant Alfa (por AKT ant AL fa)

U.S. Brand Names Curosurf®

Synonyms Porcine Lung Surfactant

Therapeutic Category Lung Surfactant

Generic Available No

Use Treatment of respiratory distress syndrome (RDS) in premature infants

Warnings Rapidly affects oxygenation and lung compliance and should be restricted to a highly supervised use in a clinical setting with immediate availability of clinicians experienced with intubation and ventilatory management of premature infants; if transient episodes of bradycardia and decreased oxygen saturation occur, discontinue the dosing procedure and initiate measures to alleviate the condition; produces rapid improvements in lung oxygenation and compliance that may require immediate reductions in ventilator settings and FiO_2.

Precautions Correction of acidosis, hypotension, anemia, hypoglycemia, and hypothermia is recommended prior to administration

Adverse Reactions

Cardiovascular: Transient bradycardia, hypotension

Local: Endotracheal tube blockage

Respiratory: Oxygen desaturation

Stability Store in refrigerator; protect from light; prior to administration, allow to slowly warm to room temperature; artificial warming methods should **not** be used; unused, unopened vials warmed to room temperature may be returned to the refrigerator within 24 hours of warming only once

(Continued)

Poractant Alfa *(Continued)*

Mechanism of Action Poractant alfa, an extract of natural porcine lung surfactant, replaces deficient or ineffective endogenous lung surfactant in neonates with respiratory distress syndrome (RDS); surfactant prevents the alveoli from collapsing during expiration by lowering surface tension between air and alveolar surfaces

Usual Dosage Neonates: Intratracheal: Initial: 2.5 mL/kg/dose (200 mg/kg/dose); may repeat 1.25 mL/kg/dose (100 mg/kg/dose) at 12-hour intervals for up to 2 additional doses; maximum total dose: 5 mL/kg

Administration Intratracheal: For intratracheal administration only; suction infant prior to administration; inspect solution to verify complete mixing of the suspension; do not shake; gently turn vial upside-down to obtain uniform suspension; administer intratracheally by instillation through a 5-French end-hole catheter inserted into the infant's endotracheal tube; each dose should be administered as two aliquots, with each aliquot administered into one of the two main bronchi by positioning the infant with either the right or left side dependent; alternatively, it may be administered through a secondary lumen of a dual lumen endotracheal tube as a single dose administered over 1 minute without interrupting mechanical ventilation

Monitoring Parameters Continuous heart rate and transcutaneous O_2 saturation should be monitored during administration; frequent ABG sampling is necessary to prevent postdosing hyperoxia and hypocarbia

Dosage Forms Suspension for intratracheal instillation: 80 mg/mL (1.5 mL, 3 mL)

♦ **Porcine Lung Surfactant** *see* Poractant Alfa *on page 917*

♦ **Pork Regular Iletin® II** *see* Insulin Preparations *on page 609*

♦ **Post Peel Healing Balm [OTC]** *see* Hydrocortisone *on page 573*

♦ **Potassium Acetate** *see* Potassium Supplements *on page 919*

♦ **Potassium Acid Phosphate** *see* Phosphate Supplements *on page 898*

♦ **Potassium Bicarbonate** *see* Potassium Supplements *on page 919*

♦ **Potassium Chloride** *see* Potassium Supplements *on page 919*

♦ **Potassium Citrate** *see* Potassium Supplements *on page 919*

♦ **Potassium Gluconate** *see* Potassium Supplements *on page 919*

Potassium Iodide *(poe TASS ee um EYE oh dide)*

Related Information

Carbohydrate and Alcohol Content of Liquid Medications for Use in Patients Receiving Ketogenic Diets *on page 1431*

U.S. Brand Names Iostat™ [OTC]; Pima®; SSKI®

Synonyms KI; Lugol's Solution; Strong Iodine Solution

Therapeutic Category Antithyroid Agent; Expectorant

Generic Available Yes

Use Facilitate bronchial drainage and cough; reduce thyroid vascularity prior to thyroidectomy; manage thyrotoxic crisis; block thyroidal uptake of radioactive isotopes of iodine in a radiation emergency; treat cutaneous sporotrichosis

Pregnancy Risk Factor D

Contraindications Hypersensitivity to iodides or any component; hyperkalemia, tuberculosis, acute bronchitis, hypothyroidism, Addison's disease, acute dehydration, heat cramps

Warnings Prolonged use can lead to hypothyroidism

Precautions Use with caution in patients with cystic fibrosis (may have exaggerated susceptibility to goitrogenic effects); may cause flare-up of acne; use with caution in patients with a history of thyroid disease and in patients with cardiac disease or renal failure

Adverse Reactions

Cardiovascular: Arrhythmia

Central nervous system: Fever, headache, confusion

Dermatologic: Urticaria, acne, angioedema, cutaneous hemorrhage

Endocrine & metabolic: Goiter with hypothyroidism, thyroid adenoma, acute parotitis

Gastrointestinal: Metallic taste, GI upset, GI bleeding, soreness of teeth and gums, cutaneous and mucosal hemorrhage

Hematologic: Eosinophilia

Neuromuscular & skeletal: Arthralgia, numbness, paresthesia

Respiratory: Rhinitis

Miscellaneous: Lymph node enlargement

Drug Interactions Potassium-containing medications, ACE inhibitors, and potassium-sparing diuretics may increase serum potassium; lithium and antithyroid drugs may potentiate hypothyroid and goitrogenic effects

Stability Store at room temperature; cold temperatures result in crystallization; warming with shaking will redissolve crystals

Mechanism of Action Reduces viscosity of mucus by increasing respiratory tract secretions; inhibits the release and synthesis of thyroid hormone; blocks the thyroidal uptake of radioactive iodine species to provide effective protection against thyroid cancer

Pharmacodynamics Antithyroid effects:

Onset of action: 24-48 hours

Maximum effect: 10-15 days after continuous therapy

Duration: May persist up to 6 weeks

Usual Dosage Oral:

Expectorant:

Children: 60-250 mg 4 times/day; maximum single dose: 500 mg

Adults: 300-650 mg 3-4 times/day

Preoperative thyroidectomy: Children and Adults: Given 10-14 days before surgery: 50-250 mg (1-5 drops, 1 g/mL SSKI®) 3 times/day **or** 0.1-0.3 mL (3-5 drops) strong iodine (Lugol's solution) 3 times/day

Graves' disease in neonates: 1 drop strong iodine (Lugol's solution) 3 times/day

Thyrotoxic crisis:

Infants <1 year: 150-250 mg (3-5 drops, 1 g/mL SSKI®) 3 times/day

Children and Adults: 300-500 mg (6-10 drops 1 g/mL SSKI®) 3 times/day **or** 1 mL strong iodine (Lugol's solution) 3 times/day

Cutaneous Sporotrichosis: Oral:

Children: 250-500 mg (5-10 drops, 1 g/mL SSKI®) 3 times/day; increase gradually to a maximum of 1.25-2 g (25-40 drops SSKI®)

Adults: 250-500 mg (5-10 drops, 1 g/mL SSKI®) 3 times/day; increase gradually to a maximum of 2-2.5 g (40-50 drops SSKI®)

Note: Therapy is continued at the maximum tolerated dosage until the cutaneous lesions have resolved, usually 6-12 weeks

Prevention of thyroidal uptake of radioactive isotopes of iodine:

Infants <1 month: 16 mg once daily

Infants 1 month to Children 3 years: 32 mg once daily

Children 3-18 years (≤150 lbs): 65 mg once daily

>18 years (>150 lbs) to Adults (including pregnant and lactating women): 130 mg once daily

Note: Treatment should continue until the risk of exposure has passed and/or until other measures (evacuation, sheltering, control of the food and milk supply) have been successfully implemented.

Administration Oral: Administer after meals with food or milk or dilute with a large quantity of water, fruit juice, milk, or broth

Monitoring Parameters Thyroid function tests

Additional Information 10 drops SSKI® = potassium iodide 500 mg

Dosage Forms

Solution, oral:

SSKI®: 1 g/mL (30 mL, 240 mL)

Lugol's solution, strong iodine: Potassium iodide 100 mg and iodine 50 mg per mL (15 mL, 473 mL)

Syrup (Pima®): 325 mg/5 mL (473 mL) [black raspberry flavor]

Tablet: 65 mg [equivalent to 50 mg iodine]

Iostat™: 130 mg

♦ **Potassium Phosphate** *see* Phosphate Supplements *on page 898*

♦ **Potassium Phosphate and Sodium Phosphate** *see* Phosphate Supplements *on page 898*

Potassium Supplements (poe TASS ee um SUP la ments)

Related Information

Carbohydrate and Alcohol Content of Liquid Medications for Use in Patients Receiving Ketogenic Diets *on page 1431*

U.S. Brand Names Effer-K™; K+8; K+10; K-99™ [OTC]; Kaochlor®; Kaochlor® SF; Kaon®; Kaon-Cl®; Kay Ciel®; K+ Care; K+ Care ET; K-Dur®; K-Lor™; Klor-Con®; Klor-Con® 8; Klor-Con® 10; Klor-Con/25®; Klor-Con® EF; Klor-Con® M; Klotrix®; K-Lyte®; K-Lyte/Cl®; K-Lyte DS; K-Tab®; K-Vescent® Potassium Chloride; Micro-K®; Rum-K®; Slow-K® [DSC]; Tri-K®

Synonyms KCl (Potassium Chloride)

Available Salts Potassium Acetate; Potassium Bicarbonate; Potassium Chloride; Potassium Citrate; Potassium Gluconate

Therapeutic Category Electrolyte Supplement, Oral; Electrolyte Supplement, Parenteral; Potassium Salt

Generic Available Yes

Use Potassium deficiency; treatment or prevention of hypokalemia

Pregnancy Risk Factor C

(Continued)

Potassium Supplements *(Continued)*

Contraindications Hypersensitivity to any component of the potassium supplement (see Warnings); severe renal impairment, untreated Addison's disease, heat cramps, hyperkalemia, severe tissue trauma; solid oral dosage forms are contraindicated in patients in whom there is a structural, pathological, and/or pharmacologic cause for delay or arrest in passage through the GI tract; an oral liquid potassium preparation should be used in patients with esophageal compression or delayed gastric emptying time

Warnings Potassium injections should be administered only in patients with adequate urine flow; injection must be diluted before I.V. use and infused slowly (see Administration); some oral products contain tartrazine which may cause allergic reactions in susceptible individuals

Precautions Use with caution in patients with cardiac disease, patients receiving potassium-sparing drugs; patients should be on a cardiac monitor during intermittent infusions for doses >0.5 mEq/kg/hour

Adverse Reactions

Cardiovascular (with rapid I.V. administration): Arrhythmias and cardiac arrest, heart block, hypotension

Central nervous system: Mental confusion

Endocrine & metabolic: Hyperkalemia, metabolic alkalosis (acetate salt)

Gastrointestinal (with oral administration): Nausea, vomiting, diarrhea, abdominal pain, GI lesions, flatulence

Local: Pain at the site of injection, phlebitis

Neuromuscular & skeletal: Muscle weakness, paresthesia, flaccid paralysis

Drug Interactions Potassium-sparing diuretics, salt substitutes, and ACE inhibitors may result in increased serum potassium

Mechanism of Action Potassium is the major cation of intracellular fluid and is essential for the conduction of nerve impulses in heart, brain, and skeletal muscle; contraction of cardiac, skeletal, and smooth muscles; and maintenance of normal renal function, acid-base balance (acetate form), carbohydrate metabolism, and gastric secretion

Pharmacokinetics

Absorption: Well from upper GI tract; enters cells via active transport from extracellular fluid

Elimination: Largely by the kidneys

Usual Dosage I.V. doses should be incorporated into the patient's maintenance I.V. fluids; intermittent I.V. potassium administration should be reserved for severe depletion situations; continuous EKG monitoring should be used for intermittent doses >0.5 mEq/kg/hour. Doses listed as mEq of **potassium**. When using microencapsulated or wax matrix formulations, use no more than 20 mEq as a single dose.

Normal daily requirement: Oral, I.V.:

Neonates and Infants: 2-6 mEq/kg/day

Children: 2-3 mEq/kg/day

Adults: 40-80 mEq/day

Prevention of hypokalemia during diuretic therapy: Oral:

Neonates, Infants, and Children: 1-2 mEq/kg/day in 1-2 divided doses

Adults: 20-40 mEq/day in 1-2 divided doses

Treatment of hypokalemia: Oral, I.V.:

Neonates, Infants, and Children: 2-5 mEq/kg/day in divided doses

Adults: 40-100 mEq/day in divided doses

Treatment of hypokalemia: I.V. intermittent infusion (must be diluted prior to administration):

Neonates, Infants, and Children: 0.5-1 mEq/kg/dose (maximum dose: 30 mEq) to infuse at 0.3-0.5 mEq/kg/hour (maximum dose: 1 mEq/kg/hour)

Adults: 10-20 mEq/dose (maximum dose: 40 mEq/dose) to infuse over 2-3 hours (maximum dose: 40 mEq over 1 hour)

Administration

Oral: Sustained release and wax matrix tablets should be swallowed whole, do not crush or chew; effervescent tablets must be dissolved in water before use; administer with food; granules can be diluted or dissolved in water or juice; do not administer liquid full strength, must be diluted in 2-6 parts of water or juice

Parenteral: Potassium must be diluted prior to parenteral administration; maximum recommended concentration (peripheral line): 80 mEq/L; maximum recommended concentration (central line): 150 mEq/L or 15 mEq/100 mL; in severely fluid-restricted patients (with central lines): 200 mEq/L or 20 mEq/100 mL has been used; maximum rate of infusion, see Usual Dosage, I.V. intermittent infusion

Monitoring Parameters Serum potassium, glucose, chloride, pH, urine output (if indicated), cardiac monitor (if intermittent I.V. infusion or potassium I.V. infusion rates >0.5 mEq/kg/hour)

Dosage Forms

Potassium acetate:

Injection, solution: 2 mEq/mL (20 mL, 50 mL, 100 mL); 4 mEq/mL (50 mL)

Potassium chloride:

Capsule, controlled release:
  Micro-K®: 600 mg [8 mEq]
  Micro-K® 10: 750 mg [10 mEq]
Capsule, extended release: 750 mg [10 mEq]
Infusion, premixed:
  10 mEq in water for injection (50 mL, 100 mL)
  10 mEq in D_5W and 1/4 sodium chloride (500 mL, 1000 mL)
  10 mEq in D_5W and 1/2 sodium chloride (500 mL, 1000 mL)
  10 mEq in D_5W and 1/3 sodium chloride (500 mL)
  20 mEq in water for injection (50 mL, 100 mL)
  20 mEq in D_5W (1000 mL)
  20 mEq in D_5W and 1/4 sodium chloride (1000 mL)
  20 mEq in D_5W and 1/2 sodium chloride (1000 mL)
  20 mEq in D_5W and 1/3 sodium chloride (1000 mL)
  20 mEq in D_5W and NS (1000 mL)
  20 mEq in D_5W and LR (1000 mL)
  20 mEq in NS (1000 mL)
  30 mEq in water for injection (100 mL)
  30 mEq in D_5W (1000 mL)
  30 mEq in D_5W and 1/4 sodium chloride (1000 mL)
  30 mEq in D_5W and 1/2 sodium chloride (1000 mL)
  40 mEq in water for injection (100 mL)
  40 mEq in D_5W (1000 mL)
  40 mEq in D_5W and 1/4 sodium chloride (1000 mL)
  40 mEq in D_5W and 1/2 sodium chloride (1000 mL)
  40 mEq in D_5W and NS (1000 mL)
  40 mEq in D_5W and LR (1000 mL)
  40 mEq in NS (1000 mL)
Injection, solution, **concentrate**: 2 mEq/mL (5 mL, 10 mL, 15 mL, 20 mL, 30 mL, 250 mL)
Liquid:
  Kaochlor® 10%: 20 mEq/15 mL (480 mL) [contains 5% alcohol and tartrazine]
  Kaocholor® SF 10%: 20 mEq/15 mL (480 mL) [sugar free; contains 5% alcohol and benzoic acid; mixed fruit flavor]
  Kaon-Cl® 20%: 40 mEq/15 mL (480 mL) [contains 5% alcohol; cherry flavor]
Powder for oral solution: 20 mEq per packet (30s, 100s, 1000s)
  K+ Care: 20 mEq per packet (30s, 100s) [fruit and orange flavors]
  K-Lor™: 20 mEq per packet (30s, 100s)
  K-Vescent® Potassium Chloride: 20 mEq per packet (30s) [orange flavor]
  Kay Ciel®: 20 mEq per packet (30s, 100s) [sugar free]
  Klor-Con®: 20 mEq per packet (30s, 100s) [sugar free; fruit flavor]
  Klor-Con/25®: 25 mEq per packet (30s, 100s) [sugar free; fruit flavor]
Solution: 10%: 20 mEq/15 mL (500 mL, 3840 mL) [contains alcohol]; 20%: 40 mEq/ 15 mL (500 mL) [contains alcohol]
  Kay Ciel®: 10 mEq/15 mL (120 mL, 480 mL) [sugar free; contains 4% alcohol]
  Rum-K®: 30 mEq/15 mL (480 mL) [alcohol and sugar free; butter rum flavor]
Tablet, controlled release:
  Klotrix®: 750 mg [10 mEq]
Tablet, extended release: 750 mg [10 mEq]
  K+8, Klor-Con® 8, Micro-K®, Slow-K® [DSC]: 600 mg [8 mEq]
  K+10, Kaon-Cl®, K-Dur®, K-Tab®, Klor-Con® 10, Klor-Con® M 10, Micro-K® 10: 750 mg [10 mEq]
  K-Dur® 20, Klor-Con® M 20: 1500 mg [20 mEq]

Potassium gluconate:

Elixir (Kaon®): 20 mEq/15 mL (480 mL) [contains 5% alcohol; grape/lemon flavor]
Tablet: 500 mg
  K-99™: 595 mg

Potassium bicarbonate:

Tablet for oral solution (K+Care ET): 25 mEq [may contain tartrazine]

Potassium bicarbonate and potassium chloride:

Tablet for solution:
  K-Lyte/Cl®: 25 mEq potassium [citrus and fruit punch flavors]
  K-Lyte/Cl® 50: 50 mEq potassium [citrus and fruit punch flavors]

(Continued)

Potassium Supplements *(Continued)*

Potassium bicarbonate and potassium citrate:
Tablet for solution:
Effer-K™, K-Lyte®: 25 mEq potassium [effervescent tablets; orange and lime flavors]
Klor-Con® EF: 25 mEq [effervescent tablets; sugar free; orange flavor]
K-Lyte® DS: 50 mEq potassium [effervescent tablets; orange and lime flavors]

Potassium acetate, potassium bicarbonate, and potassium citrate:
Solution (Tri-K®): 15 mEq potassium/5 mL (480 mL)

References
Hamill RJ, Robinson LM, Wexler HR, et al, "Efficacy and Safety of Potassium Infusion Therapy in Hypokalemic Critically Ill Patients," *Crit Care Med*, 1991, 19(5):694-9.
Khilnani P, "Electrolyte Abnormalities in Critically Ill Children," *Crit Care Med*, 1992, 20(2):241-50.

♦ **PPL** *see Benzylpenicilloyl-polylysine on page 167*

Pralidoxime *(pra li DOKS eem)*

U.S. Brand Names Protopam®
Synonyms 2-PAM; 2-Pyridine Aldoxime Methochloride
Therapeutic Category Antidote, Anticholinesterase; Antidote, Organophosphate Poisoning
Generic Available No
Use Reverse muscle paralysis associated with toxic exposure to organophosphate anticholinesterase pesticides and chemicals; control of overdosage by anticholinesterase drugs used to treat myasthenia gravis (neostigmine, pyridostigmine)
Pregnancy Risk Factor C
Contraindications Hypersensitivity to pralidoxime or any component; poisonings due to phosphorus, inorganic phosphates, or organic phosphates without anticholinesterase activity
Warnings Not indicated as an antidote for carbamate classes of pesticides and may increase toxicity of carbaryl
Precautions Use with caution in patients with myasthenia gravis; dosage modification required in patients with impaired renal function; use with caution in patients receiving theophylline, succinylcholine, phenothiazines, respiratory depressants (eg, narcotic, barbiturates); rapid I.V. infusion has been associated with tachycardia, laryngospasm, and muscle rigidity
Adverse Reactions
Cardiovascular: Tachycardia (after rapid I.V. infusion), hypertension
Central nervous system: Dizziness, headache, drowsiness
Dermatologic: Rash
Gastrointestinal: Nausea
Local: Pain at injection site after I.M. use
Neuromuscular & skeletal: Muscular weakness, muscle rigidity (after rapid I.V. infusion), transient elevated CPK
Ocular: Blurred vision, diplopia
Respiratory: Hyperventilation, laryngospasm (after rapid I.V. administration)
Drug Interactions Barbiturates potentiated by anticholinesterases
Mechanism of Action Reactivates cholinesterase that had been inactivated by phosphorylation as a result of exposure to organophosphate pesticides; removes the phosphoryl group from the active site of the inactivated enzyme
Pharmacokinetics
Half-life: 74-77 minutes
Time to peak serum concentration: I.V.: Within 5-15 minutes
Elimination: 80% to 90% excreted unchanged in urine 12 hours after administration
Usual Dosage
Organophosphate poisoning:
Children: I.M., I.V. (use in conjunction with atropine): 20-50 mg/kg/dose; repeat in 1-2 hours if muscle weakness has not been relieved, then at 10- to 12-hour intervals if cholinergic signs recur
Adults: I.M., I.V. (use in conjunction with atropine): 1-2 g; repeat in 1-2 hours if muscle weakness has not been relieved, then at 10- to 12-hour intervals if cholinergic signs recur
Treatment of toxicity from medications used to treat myasthenia gravis: Adults: I.V.: 1-2 g followed by increments of 250 mg every 5 minutes
Administration Parenteral: Reconstitute with 20 mL SWI (preservative free) resulting in 50 mg/mL solution; dilute in NS to 20 mg/mL and infuse over 15-30 minutes; if a more rapid onset of effect is desired or in a fluid-restricted situation, the maximum concentration is 50 mg/mL; the maximum rate of infusion is over 5 minutes and not exceeding 200 mg/minute

Monitoring Parameters Heart rate, respiratory rate, blood pressure, continuous EKG, muscle strength

Dosage Forms Injection, powder for reconstitution, as chloride: 1 g

♦ **Prandase® (Can)** see Acarbose on page 35
♦ **Prax® [OTC]** see Hemorrhoidal Preparations on page 556

Praziquantel (pray zi KWON tel)

U.S. Brand Names Biltricide®

Therapeutic Category Anthelmintic

Generic Available No

Use Treatment of all stages of schistosomiasis caused by *Schistosoma* species pathogenic to humans; also active in the treatment of clonorchiasis, opisthorchiasis, cysticercosis, and many intestinal tapeworm and trematode infections

Pregnancy Risk Factor B

Contraindications Hypersensitivity to praziquantel or any component; ocular cysticercosis, spinal cysticercosis

Precautions Use with caution in patients with severe hepatic disease and in patients with a history of seizures

Adverse Reactions

Central nervous system: Dizziness, drowsiness, fever, headache, vertigo, malaise, CSF reaction syndrome in patients being treated for neurocysticercosis (syndrome includes headache, seizures, intracranial hypertension, elevated CSF protein concentrations, hyperthermia)

Dermatologic: Urticarial rash, itching

Gastrointestinal: Abdominal pain, nausea, vomiting, anorexia, diarrhea

Hematologic: Eosinophilia

Miscellaneous: Diaphoresis

Drug Interactions Alcohol may increase CNS depression; phenytoin and carbamazepine may induce metabolism of praziquantel and decrease its activity; cimetidine increases praziquantel serum concentrations

Mechanism of Action Increases the cell permeability to calcium in schistosomes; causes strong contractions and paralysis of worm musculature leading to detachment of suckers from the blood vessel walls and to dislodgment

Pharmacokinetics

Absorption: Oral: ~80%

Distribution: CSF concentration is 14% to 20% of plasma concentration; excreted in breast milk

Protein binding: ~80%

Metabolism: Extensive first-pass effect; metabolized by the liver to hydroxylated and conjugated metabolites

Half-life: 0.8-1.5 hours

Metabolites: 4.5 hours

Time to peak serum concentration: Within 1-3 hours

Elimination: Praziquantel and metabolites excreted mainly in urine (99% as metabolites)

Usual Dosage Children and Adults: Oral:

Schistosomiasis:

S. mansoni, S. haematobium: 20 mg/kg/dose twice daily for 1 day

S. japonicum, S. mekongi: 20 mg/kg/dose 3 times/day for 1 day at 4- to 6-hour intervals

Flukes:

Liver, intestine: 75 mg/kg/day divided every 8 hours for 1 day

Lung: 75 mg/kg/day divided every 8 hours for 2 days

Nanophyetus salmincola: 60 mg/kg/day divided every 8 hours for 1 day

Cysticercosis: 50 mg/kg/day divided every 8 hours for 15 days (adjunctive therapy with dexamethasone is recommended for patients with numerous cysts and for those in whom neurologic symptoms or intracranial hypertension develops); for neurocysticercosis, steroids should be administered **prior** to starting praziquantel

Tapeworms: 5-10 mg/kg as a single dose (25 mg/kg for *H. nana*)

Administration Oral: Administer with food; tablets can be halved or quartered; do not chew tablets due to bitter taste

Patient Information Avoid alcohol (increased CNS depression); may cause drowsiness and impair ability to perform activities requiring mental alertness or physical coordination

Dosage Forms Tablet, film coated, tri-scored: 600 mg

References

King CH and Mahmoud AA, "Drug Five Years Later: Praziquantel," *Ann Intern Med*, 1989, 110(4):290-6.
Liu LX and Weller PF, "Antiparasitic Drug," *N Engl J Med*, 1996, 334(18):1178-84.

Prazosin (PRA zoe sin)

Related Information
Overdose and Toxicology *on page 1388*

U.S. Brand Names Minipress®

Canadian Brand Names Apo®-Prazo; Novo-Prazin; Nu-Prazo

Synonyms Furazosin

Therapeutic Category Alpha-Adrenergic Blocking Agent, Oral; Antihypertensive Agent; Vasodilator

Generic Available Yes

Use Management of hypertension; severe CHF (in conjunction with diuretics and cardiac glycosides)

Pregnancy Risk Factor C

Contraindications Hypersensitivity to prazosin, quinazolines, or any component

Precautions Marked orthostatic hypotension, syncope, and loss of consciousness may occur with first dose ("first dose phenomenon"). This reaction is more likely to occur in patients receiving beta-blockers, diuretics, low sodium diets or larger first doses (ie, >1 mg/dose in adults); avoid rapid increase in dose; use with caution in patients with renal impairment.

Adverse Reactions
Cardiovascular: Orthostatic hypotension, syncope, palpitations, tachycardia, edema
Central nervous system: Dizziness, lightheadedness, nightmares, drowsiness, headache, hypothermia
Dermatologic: Rash
Endocrine & metabolic: Fluid retention, sexual dysfunction
Gastrointestinal: Nausea, xerostomia
Genitourinary: Urinary frequency
Neuromuscular & skeletal: Weakness
Respiratory: Nasal congestion

Drug Interactions Diuretics and antihypertensive medications (especially beta-blockers) may increase prazosin's hypotensive effect

Food Interactions Avoid natural licorice (causes sodium and water retention and increases potassium loss); food has variable effects on absorption

Mechanism of Action Competitively inhibits postsynaptic alpha-adrenergic receptors which results in vasodilation of veins and arterioles and a decrease in total peripheral resistance and blood pressure

Pharmacodynamics Hypotensive effect:
Onset of action: Within 2 hours
Maximum decrease: 2-4 hours
Duration: 10-24 hours

Pharmacokinetics
Distribution: V_d: 0.5 L/kg (hypertensive adults)
Protein-binding: 92% to 97%
Metabolism: Extensive in the liver, metabolites may be active
Bioavailability, oral: 43% to 82%
Half-life, adults: 2-4 hours, increased half-life with CHF
Elimination: 6% to 10% excreted renally as unchanged drug

Usual Dosage Oral:
Children: Initial: 5 mcg/kg/dose (to assess hypotensive effects); usual dosing interval every 6 hours; increase dosage gradually up to 25 mcg/kg/dose every 6 hours; maximum daily dose: 15 mg or 0.4 mg/kg/day (400 mcg/kg/day); may be divided in 2 or 3 doses/day for treatment of hypertension
Adults: Initial: 1 mg/dose 2-3 times/day; usual maintenance dose: 3-15 mg/day in divided doses 2-4 times/day; maximum daily dose: 20 mg

Administration Oral: Administer in a consistent manner with respect to meals

Monitoring Parameters Blood pressure (standing and sitting or supine)

Test Interactions False positive screening tests for pheochromocytoma (increases urinary VMA by 17%; increases norepinephrine metabolite by 42%)

Patient Information Avoid alcohol; rise slowly from sitting or lying position; may cause dizziness or drowsiness and impair ability to perform activities requiring mental alertness or physical coordination; may cause dry mouth

Nursing Implications Be aware of "first-dose phenomenon" (see Precautions); syncope may occur usually within 90 minutes of initial dose

Dosage Forms Capsule, as hydrochloride: 1 mg, 2 mg, 5 mg

References
Friedman WF and George BL, "New Concepts and Drugs in the Treatment of Congestive Heart Failure," *Pediatr Clin North Am*, 1984, 31(6):1197-227.
Sinaiko AR, "Pharmacologic Management of Childhood Hypertension," *Pediatr Clin North Am*, 1993, 40(1):195-212.

♦ **Precose®** *see Acarbose on page 35*
♦ **Pred Forte®** *see PrednisoLONE on page 925*
♦ **Pred-G®** *see Prednisolone and Gentamicin on page 927*
♦ **Pred Mild®** *see PrednisoLONE on page 925*

PrednisoLONE (pred NIS oh lone)

Related Information
Asthma Guidelines *on page 1376*
Carbohydrate and Alcohol Content of Liquid Medications for Use in Patients Receiving Ketogenic Diets *on page 1431*
Corticosteroids Comparison, Systemic *on page 1211*

U.S. Brand Names AK-Pred®; Econopred®; Econopred® Plus; Inflamase® Forte; Inflamase® Mild; Orapred®; Pediapred®; Pred Forte®; Pred Mild®; Prelone®

Canadian Brand Names Diopred®; Hydeltra T.B.A.®; Novo-Prednisolone®; Ophtho-Tate®

Synonyms Deltahydrocortisone; Metacortandralone

Therapeutic Category Adrenal Corticosteroid; Antiasthmatic; Anti-inflammatory Agent; Anti-inflammatory Agent, Ophthalmic; Corticosteroid, Ophthalmic; Corticosteroid, Systemic; Glucocorticoid

Generic Available Yes

Use Treatment of endocrine disorders, rheumatic disorders, collagen diseases, dermatologic diseases, allergic states, ophthalmic diseases, respiratory diseases, hematologic disorders, neoplastic diseases, edematous states, and GI diseases

Ophthalmic: Treatment of palpebral and bulbar conjunctivitis; corneal injury from chemical, radiation, thermal burns, or foreign body penetration

Pregnancy Risk Factor C

Contraindications Hypersensitivity to prednisolone or any component (see Warnings); acute superficial herpes simplex keratitis; systemic fungal infections; varicella

Warnings Hypothalamic pituitary adrenal (HPA) suppression may occur; acute adrenal insufficiency may occur with abrupt withdrawal after long term use or with stress; withdrawal or discontinuation of corticosteroids should be done carefully. Immunosuppression may occur. Corticosteroids may mask signs of infection.

Ophthalmic suspension may contain sodium bisulfite which may cause allergic reactions in susceptible individuals; tablets and Orapred® oral solution contain sodium benzoate and Prelone® syrup contains benzoic acid; benzoic acid (benzoate) is a metabolite of benzyl alcohol; large amounts of benzyl alcohol (≥99 mg/kg/day) have been associated with a potentially fatal toxicity ("gasping syndrome") in neonates; the "gasping syndrome" consists of metabolic acidosis, respiratory distress, gasping respirations, CNS dysfunction (including convulsions, intracranial hemorrhage), hypotension and cardiovascular collapse; use prednisolone products containing sodium benzoate or benzoic acid with caution in neonates; *in vitro* and animal studies have shown that benzoate displaces bilirubin from protein binding sites

Precautions Avoid using higher than recommended doses; suppression of HPA axis, suppression of linear growth, or hypercorticism (Cushing's syndrome) may occur; use with caution in patients with hypothyroidism, cirrhosis, ocular herpes simplex, peptic ulcer disease, osteoporosis, myasthenia gravis, hypertension, CHF, nonspecific ulcerative colitis, thromboembolic disorders, and renal dysfunction

Adverse Reactions
Cardiovascular: Edema, hypertension, CHF
Central nervous system: Vertigo, seizures, psychoses, pseudotumor cerebri, headache
Dermatologic: Acne, skin atrophy, impaired wound healing, petechiae, bruising
Endocrine & metabolic: Cushing's syndrome, pituitary-adrenal axis suppression, growth suppression, glucose intolerance, hypokalemia, alkalosis, sodium and water retention
Gastrointestinal: Peptic ulcer, nausea, vomiting
Genitourinary: Menstrual irregularities
Neuromuscular & skeletal: Muscle weakness, osteoporosis, fractures
Ocular: Cataracts, elevated IOP, glaucoma

Drug Interactions Cytochrome P450 isoenzyme CYP3A3/4 substrate and inducer
Barbiturates, phenytoin, rifampin, salicylates, toxoids, NSAIDs, diuretics (potassium depleting); caffeine and alcohol may increase risk for GI ulcer; live virus vaccines (increase risk of viral infection); vaccines may have decreased effects

Food Interactions Systemic use of corticosteroids may require a diet with increased potassium, vitamins A, B_6, C, D, folate, calcium, zinc, and phosphorus and decreased sodium
(Continued)

PrednisoLONE *(Continued)*

Stability Dispense oral liquid formulations in tight, light-resistant containers. Storage: Prelone® syrup: Store at room temperature, do not refrigerate; Pediapred® oral solution: Store at 4°C to 24°C (39°F to 77°F), may be refrigerated; Orapred® oral solution: Store in refrigerator [2°C to 8°C (36°F to 46°F)]

Mechanism of Action Decreases inflammation by suppression of migration of polymorphonuclear leukocytes and reversal of increased capillary permeability; suppresses the immune system by reducing activity and volume of the lymphatic system

Pharmacokinetics

Absorption: Oral: Well absorbed

Protein binding: 70% to 90% (concentration dependent)

Metabolism: Primarily in the liver, but also metabolized in most tissues, to inactive compounds

Half-life: Adults (serum): 2-4 hours

Elimination: In urine, principally as glucuronide and sulfate-conjugated metabolites

Usual Dosage Dose depends upon condition being treated and response of patient; dosage for infants and children should be based on disease severity and patient response rather than by rigid adherence to dosage guidelines by age, weight, or body surface area. Consider alternate day therapy for long-term therapy. Discontinuation of long-term therapy requires gradual withdrawal by tapering the dose.

NIH Asthma Guidelines (NAEPP, 2002): Oral:

Children ≤12 years:

Asthma exacerbations (emergency care or hospital doses): 1 mg/kg every 6 hours for 48 hours; then 1-2 mg/kg/day (maximum: 60 mg/day) in divided doses given twice daily until peak expiratory flow is 70% of predicted or personal best

Short-course "burst" (acute asthma): 1-2 mg/kg/day in divided doses 1-2 times/day for 3-10 days; longer treatment may be required; usually given for 5 days; maximum dose: 60 mg/day

Long-term treatment: 0.25-2 mg/kg/day given as a single dose in the morning or every other day as needed for asthma control; maximum dose: 60 mg/day

Children >12 years and Adults:

Asthma exacerbations (emergency care or hospital doses): 120-180 mg/day in divided doses 3-4 times/day for 48 hours; then 60-80 mg in divided doses given twice daily until peak expiratory flow is 70% of predicted or personal best

Short-course "burst" (acute asthma): 40-60 mg/day in divided doses 1-2 times/day for 3-10 days; longer treatment may be required; usually given for 5 days

Long-term treatment: 7.5-60 mg daily given as a single dose in the morning or every other day as needed for asthma control

Children: Oral:

Anti-inflammatory or immunosuppressive dose: 0.1-2 mg/kg/day in divided doses 1-4 times/day

Nephrotic syndrome:

Pediatric Nephrology Panel recommendations (Hogg, 2000):

Initial: 2 mg/kg/day or 60 mg/m²/day given every day in 1-3 divided doses (maximum dose: 80 mg/day) until urine is protein free for 4-6 weeks; followed by maintenance dose: 2 mg/kg/dose or 40 mg/m²/dose given every other day in the morning; gradually taper and discontinue after 4-6 weeks; **Note:** 6-week daily therapy followed by 6-week alternate day therapy may induce a higher rate of long remission compared to the standard of 4 weeks of daily therapy followed by 4 weeks of alternate day therapy; however, a higher incidence of adverse effects may be seen with the longer regimen and the clinical benefit may be variable

Relapse: Use high-dose daily steroid regimen (listed above) until urine is protein free for 3 days; follow with maintenance-tapering course of alternative therapy (maintenance dose listed above) for 4-6 weeks; subsequent therapy is determined by individual's response and number of relapses (see Hogg, 2000)

British Pediatric Nephrology Consensus Statement (Report of a Workshop by the British Association for Paediatric Nephrology and Research Unit, 1994):

First 3 episodes: Initial: 2 mg/kg/day or 60 mg/m²/day given every day (maximum dose: 80 mg/day) until urine is protein free for 3 consecutive days (maximum dose: 28 days); followed by 1-1.5 mg/kg/dose or 40 mg/m²/dose (maximum: 60 mg/dose) given every other day for 4 weeks

Frequent relapses (long-term maintenance dose): 0.5-1 mg/kg/dose given every other day for 3-6 months

Adults: Oral: 5-60 mg/day

926

Children and Adults: Ophthalmic suspension: Instill 1-2 drops into conjunctival sac every hour during day, every 2 hours at night until favorable response is obtained, then use 1 drop every 4 hours

Administration

Oral: Administer after meals or with food or milk to decrease GI upset

Ophthalmic: Shake suspension well before use; instill drops into affected eye(s); avoid contact of container tip with skin or eye; apply finger pressure to lacrimal sac during and for 1-2 minutes after instillation to decrease risk of absorption and systemic effects

Monitoring Parameters Blood pressure, weight, electrolytes, serum glucose; children's height and growth

Test Interactions Skin tests

Patient Information Avoid alcohol; limit caffeine; do not decrease dose or discontinue without physician's approval; avoid exposure to chicken pox or measles, if exposed, seek medical advice without delay

Additional Information Prelone® syrup also contains propylene glycol

Dosage Forms

Solution, ophthalmic, as **sodium phosphate**: 1% (5 mL, 10 mL, 15 mL)
AK-Pred®: 1% (5 mL, 15 mL)
Inflamase® Forte: 1% (5 mL, 10 mL, 15 mL)
Inflamase® Mild: 0.125% (5 mL, 10 mL)

Solution, oral, as **sodium phosphate**: 5 mg prednisolone base/5 mL (120 mL)
Orapred®: 20 mg/5 mL (240 mL) **[equivalent to 15 mg/5 mL prednisolone base**; dye free; contains 2% alcohol and sodium benzoate); grape flavor]
Pediapred®: 6.7 mg/5 mL (120 mL) **[equivalent to 5 mg/5 mL prednisolone base**; dye free; raspberry flavor]

Suspension, ophthalmic, as **acetate**: 1% (5 mL, 10 mL, 15 mL)
Econopred®: 0.125% (5 mL, 10 mL)
Econopred® Plus: 1% (5 mL, 10 mL)
Pred Forte®: 1% (1 mL, 5 mL, 10 mL, 15 mL) [contains sodium bisulfite]
Pred Mild®: 0.12% (5 mL, 10 mL) [contains sodium bisulfite]

Syrup, as **base**: 5 mg/5 mL (120 mL); 15 mg/5 mL (240 mL, 480 mL)
Prelone®: 5 mg/5 mL (120 mL) [dye and sugar free; contains ≤0.4% alcohol and 0.1% benzoic acid; wild cherry flavor]; 15 mg/5 mL (240 mL, 480 mL) [contains 5% alcohol and 0.1% benzoic acid; wild cherry flavor]

Tablet, as **base**: 5 mg [contains sodium benzoate]

References

Hogg RJ, Portman RJ, Milliner D, et al, "Evaluation and Management of Proteinuria and Nephrotic Syndrome in Children: Recommendations From a Pediatric Nephrology Panel Established at the National Kidney Foundation Conference on Proteinuria, Albuminuria, Risk, Assessment, Detection, and Elimination (PARADE)," *Pediatrics*, 2000, 105(6):1242-9.

"National Asthma Education and Prevention Program. Expert Panel Report: Guidelines for the Diagnosis and Management of Asthma Update on Selected Topics--2002," *J Allergy Clin Immunol*, 2002, 110(5 Suppl):S141-219.

Report of a Workshop by the British Association for Paediatric Nephrology and Research Unit, Royal College of Physicians, "Consensus Statement on Management and Audit Potential for Steroid Responsive Nephrotic Syndrome," *Arch Dis Child*, 1994, 70(2):151-7.

Prednisolone and Gentamicin (pred NIS oh lone & jen ta MYE sin)

U.S. Brand Names Pred-G®

Synonyms Gentamicin and Prednisolone

Therapeutic Category Antibiotic, Ophthalmic; Corticosteroid, Ophthalmic

Generic Available No

Use Treatment of steroid responsive inflammatory conditions and superficial ocular infections due to strains of microorganisms susceptible to gentamicin such as *Staphylococcus*, *E. coli*, *H. influenzae*, *Klebsiella*, *Neisseria*, *Pseudomonas*, *Proteus*, and *Serratia* species

Pregnancy Risk Factor C

Contraindications Hypersensitivity to prednisolone, gentamicin, or any component; dendritic keratitis, fungal diseases, vaccinia, varicella, most other viral infections, and mycobacterial infection of the eye. Contraindicated after uncomplicated removal of a corneal foreign body.

Warnings Prolonged use may result in glaucoma, damage to the optic nerve, defects in visual acuity, posterior subcapsular cataract formation, and secondary ocular infections

Adverse Reactions

Local: Burning, stinging, redness

Ocular: Elevation of intraocular pressure, glaucoma, infrequent optic nerve damage, posterior subcapsular cataract formation, superficial punctate keratitis, increased lacrimation

(Continued)

Prednisolone and Gentamicin *(Continued)*

Miscellaneous: Development of secondary infection, allergic sensitization, delayed wound healing

Mechanism of Action See individual monographs for Prednisolone *on page 925* and Gentamicin *on page 533*

Usual Dosage Children and Adults: Ophthalmic: Instill 1 drop 2-4 times/day; during the initial 24-48 hours, the dosing frequency may be increased if necessary, up to 1 drop every hour; or small amount ($1/_2$" ribbon) of ointment can be applied into the conjunctival sac 1-3 times/day

Administration Suspension: Shake well before using; instill drop into affected eye; avoid contacting bottle tip with skin or eye; apply finger pressure to lacrimal sac during and for 1-2 minutes after instillation to decrease risk of absorption and systemic effects

Monitoring Parameters With use >10 days, monitor intraocular pressure

Dosage Forms

Ointment, ophthalmic: Prednisolone acetate 0.6% and gentamicin sulfate 0.3% (3.5 g)

Suspension, ophthalmic: Prednisolone acetate 1% and gentamicin sulfate 0.3% (2 mL, 5 mL, 10 mL)

♦ **Prednisolone, Neomycin, and Polymyxin B** *see* Neomycin, Polymyxin B, and Prednisolone *on page 804*

PredniSONE *(PRED ni sone)*

Related Information

Antiepileptic Drugs *on page 1374*

Asthma Guidelines *on page 1376*

Carbohydrate and Alcohol Content of Liquid Medications for Use in Patients Receiving Ketogenic Diets *on page 1431*

Corticosteroids Comparison, Systemic *on page 1211*

U.S. Brand Names Deltasone®; Prednisone Intensol™; Sterapred®; Sterapred® DS

Canadian Brand Names Apo®-Prednisone; Winpred™

Synonyms Deltacortisone; Deltadehydrocortisone

Therapeutic Category Adrenal Corticosteroid; Antiasthmatic; Anti-inflammatory Agent; Corticosteroid, Systemic; Glucocorticoid

Generic Available Yes

Use Management of adrenocortical insufficiency; used for its anti-inflammatory or immunosuppressant effects

Pregnancy Risk Factor C

Contraindications Hypersensitivity to prednisone or any component; serious infections, except septic shock or tuberculous meningitis; systemic fungal infections; varicella

Warnings Hypothalamic pituitary adrenal (HPA) suppression may occur; acute adrenal insufficiency may occur with abrupt withdrawal after long term use or with stress; withdrawal or discontinuation of corticosteroids should be done carefully. Immunosuppression may occur. Corticosteroids may mask signs of infection.

Oral solution contains sodium benzoate; benzoic acid (benzoate) is a metabolite of benzyl alcohol; large amounts of benzyl alcohol (≥99 mg/kg/day) have been associated with a potentially fatal toxicity ("gasping syndrome") in neonates; the "gasping syndrome" consists of metabolic acidosis, respiratory distress, gasping respirations, CNS dysfunction (including convulsions, intracranial hemorrhage), hypotension and cardiovascular collapse; use prednisone products containing sodium benzoate with caution in neonates; *in vitro* and animal studies have shown that benzoate displaces bilirubin from protein binding sites

Precautions Avoid using higher than recommended doses; suppression of HPA axis, suppression of linear growth, or hypercorticism (Cushing's syndrome) may occur; use with caution in patients with hypothyroidism, cirrhosis, ocular herpes simplex, peptic ulcer disease, osteoporosis, myasthenia gravis, hypertension, CHF, nonspecific ulcerative colitis, thromboembolic disorders, and renal dysfunction

Adverse Reactions

Cardiovascular: Edema, hypertension, CHF

Central nervous system: Vertigo, seizures, psychoses, pseudotumor cerebri, headache

Dermatologic: Acne, skin atrophy, impaired wound healing, petechiae, bruising

Endocrine & metabolic: Cushing's syndrome, pituitary-adrenal axis suppression, growth suppression, glucose intolerance, hypokalemia, alkalosis, sodium and water retention

Gastrointestinal: Peptic ulcer, nausea, vomiting

Genitourinary: Menstrual irregularities

Neuromuscular & skeletal: Muscle weakness, osteoporosis, fractures

Ocular: Cataracts, elevated IOP, glaucoma

Drug Interactions Cytochrome P450 isoenzyme CYP3A3/4 substrate and inducer
Barbiturates, phenytoin, rifampin, salicylates, toxoids, NSAIDs, diuretics (potassium depleting); caffeine and alcohol may increase risk for GI ulcer; live virus vaccines (increase risk of viral infection); vaccines may have decreased effects

Food Interactions Systemic use of corticosteroids may require a diet with increased potassium, vitamins A, B$_6$, C, D, folate, calcium, zinc, and phosphorus and decreased sodium

Mechanism of Action Decreases inflammation by suppression of migration of polymorphonuclear leukocytes and reversal of increased capillary permeability; suppresses the immune system by reducing activity and volume of the lymphatic system

Pharmacokinetics Converted rapidly in the liver to prednisolone (active)

Usual Dosage Dose depends upon condition being treated and response of patient; dosage for infants and children should be based on disease severity and patient response rather than by rigid adherence to dosage guidelines by age, weight, or body surface area. Consider alternate day therapy for long-term therapy. Discontinuation of long-term therapy requires gradual withdrawal by tapering the dose. Oral:

NIH Asthma Guidelines (NAEPP, 2002):

Children ≤12 years:

Asthma exacerbations (emergency care or hospital doses): 1 mg/kg every 6 hours for 48 hours; then 1-2 mg/kg/day (maximum: 60 mg/day) in divided doses given twice daily until peak expiratory flow is 70% of predicted or personal best

Short-course "burst" (acute asthma): 1-2 mg/kg/day in divided doses 1-2 times/day for 3-10 days; longer treatment may be required; usually given for 5 days; maximum dose: 60 mg/day

Long-term treatment: 0.25-2 mg/kg/day given as a single dose in the morning or every other day as needed for asthma control; maximum dose: 60 mg/day

Children >12 years and Adults:

Asthma exacerbations (emergency care or hospital doses): 120-180 mg/day in divided doses 3-4 times/day for 48 hours; then 60-80 mg in divided doses given twice daily until peak expiratory flow is 70% of predicted or personal best

Short-course "burst" (acute asthma): 40-60 mg/day in divided doses 1-2 times/day for 3-10 days; longer treatment may be required; usually given for 5 days

Long-term treatment: 7.5-60 mg daily given as a single dose in the morning or every other day as needed for asthma control

Children:

Alternative asthma dosing by age:

Short-course "burst" (acute asthma):

<1 year: 10 mg every 12 hours

1-4 years: 20 mg every 12 hours

5-13 years: 30 mg every 12 hours

>13 years: 40 mg every 12 hours

Long-term treatment:

<1 year: 10 mg every other day

1-4 years: 20 mg every other day

5-13 years: 30 mg every other day

>13 years: 40 mg every other day

Anti-inflammatory or immunosuppressive: 0.05-2 mg/kg/day divided 1-4 times/day

Nephrotic syndrome:

Pediatric Nephrology Panel recommendations (Hogg, 2000):

Initial: 2 mg/kg/day or 60 mg/m^2/day given every day in 1-3 divided doses (maximum dose: 80 mg/day) until urine is protein free for 4-6 weeks; followed by maintenance dose: 2 mg/kg/dose or 40 mg/m^2/dose given every other day in the morning; gradually taper and discontinue after 4-6 weeks; **Note:** 6-week daily therapy followed by 6-week alternative day therapy may induce a higher rate of long remission compared to the standard of 4 weeks of daily therapy followed by 4 weeks of alternative day therapy; however, a higher incidence of adverse effects may be seen with the longer regimen and the clinical benefit may be variable

Relapse: Use high-dose daily steroid regimen (listed above) until urine is protein free for 3 days; follow with maintenance-tapering course of alternative therapy (maintenance dose listed above) for 4-6 weeks; subsequent therapy is determined by individual's response and number of relapses (see Hogg, 2000)

(Continued)

PredniSONE *(Continued)*

British Pediatric Nephrology Consensus Statement (Report of a Workshop by the British Association for Paediatric Nephrology and Research Unit, 1994):

First 3 episodes: Initial: 2 mg/kg/day or 60 mg/m²/day given every day (maximum dose: 80 mg/day) until urine is protein free for 3 consecutive days (maximum dose: 28 days); followed by 1-1.5 mg/kg/dose or 40 mg/m²/dose (maximum: 60 mg/dose) given every other day for 4 weeks

Frequent relapses (long-term maintenance dose): 0.5-1 mg/kg/dose given every other day for 3-6 months

Children and Adults: Physiologic replacement: 4-5 mg/m²/day

Adults: 5-60 mg/day in divided doses 1-4 times/day

Administration Oral: Administer after meals or with food or milk to decrease GI upset

Monitoring Parameters Blood pressure, weight, serum electrolytes, glucose; children's height and growth

Test Interactions Skin tests

Patient Information Avoid alcohol; limit caffeine; do not decrease dose or discontinue without physician's approval

Additional Information Oral solution also contains polysorbate 80 and propylene glycol; Prednisone Intensol™ also contains propylene glycol

Dosage Forms

Solution, oral: 5 mg/5 mL (5 mL, 120 mL, 500 mL) [contains 5% alcohol and sodium benzoate; vanilla flavor]

Solution, oral **concentrate** (Prednisone Intensol™): 5 mg/mL (30 mL) [contains 30% alcohol]

Tablet: 1 mg, 2.5 mg, 5 mg, 10 mg, 20 mg, 50 mg

Deltasone®: 2.5 mg, 5 mg, 10 mg, 20 mg, 50 mg

Sterapred®: 5 mg [supplied as 21 tablet 6-day unit dose package or 48 tablet 12-day unit dose package]

Sterapred® DS: 10 mg [supplied as 21 tablet 6-day unit dose package or 48 tablet 12-day unit dose package]

References

Hogg RJ, Portman RJ, Milliner D, et al, "Evaluation and Management of Proteinuria and Nephrotic Syndrome in Children: Recommendations From a Pediatric Nephrology Panel Established at the National Kidney Foundation Conference on Proteinuria, Albuminuria, Risk, Assessment, Detection, and Elimination (PARADE)," *Pediatrics*, 2000, 105(6):1242-9.

Murphy CM, Coonce SL, and Simon PA, "Treatment of Asthma in Children," *Clin Pharm*, 1991, 10(9):685-703.

"National Asthma Education and Prevention Program. Expert Panel Report: Guidelines for the Diagnosis and Management of Asthma Update on Selected Topics--2002," *J Allergy Clin Immunol*, 2002, 110(5 Suppl):S141-219.

Report of a Workshop by the British Association for Paediatric Nephrology and Research Unit, Royal College of Physicians, "Consensus Statement on Management and Audit Potential for Steroid Responsive Nephrotic Syndrome," *Arch Dis Child*, 1994, 70(2):151-7.

Primaquine (PRIM a kween)
Therapeutic Category Antimalarial Agent
Generic Available Yes
Use In conjunction with a blood schizonticidal agent to provide radical cure of *P. vivax* or *P. ovale* malaria after a clinical attack has been confirmed by blood smear or serologic titer; prevention of relapse of *P. ovale* or *P. vivax* malaria; malaria postexposure prophylaxis
Pregnancy Risk Factor C
Contraindications Acutely ill patients who have a tendency to develop granulocytopenia (rheumatoid arthritis, SLE); patients receiving other drugs capable of depressing the bone marrow; patients receiving quinacrine
Precautions Use with caution in patients with G-6-PD deficiency or NADH methemoglobin reductase deficiency
Adverse Reactions
Cardiovascular: Arrhythmias, hypertension
Central nervous system: Headache
Dermatologic: Pruritus
Gastrointestinal: Nausea, vomiting, abdominal cramps
Hematologic: Hemolytic anemia, methemoglobinemia, leukocytosis, leukopenia, agranulocytosis
Ocular: Interference with visual accommodation
Drug Interactions Quinacrine (increased toxicity of primaquine)
Stability Protect from light
Mechanism of Action Eliminates the primary tissue exoerythrocytic forms of *P. falciparum, P. malariae, P. ovale,* and *P. vivax*; interferes with plasmodial DNA
Pharmacokinetics
Absorption: Oral: Well absorbed
Metabolism: Liver metabolism to carboxyprimaquine, an active metabolite
Half-life: 3.7-9.6 hours
Time to peak serum concentration: Within 6 hours
Elimination: Small amount of unchanged drug excreted in urine
Usual Dosage Oral:
Children: 0.3 mg base/kg/day once daily for 14 days not to exceed 15 mg base/day, or 0.9 mg base/kg once weekly for 8 weeks not to exceed 45 mg base/week
Adults: 15 mg/day (base) once daily for 14 days or 45 mg base once weekly for 8 weeks
Administration Oral: Administer with meals to decrease adverse GI effects; drug has a bitter taste
Monitoring Parameters Periodic CBC, visual color check of urine, hemoglobin
Patient Information Notify physician if a darkening of the urine occurs
Dosage Forms Tablet, as phosphate: 26.3 mg [15 mg base]
References
Lynk A and Gold R, "Review of 40 Children With Imported Malaria," *Pediatr Infect Dis J*, 1989, 8(11):745-50.
Wyler DJ, "Malaria Chemoprophylaxis for the Traveler," *N Engl J Med*, 1993, 329(1):31-7.

♦ **Primatene® Mist [OTC]** *see* Epinephrine *on page 439*
♦ **Primaxin®** *see* Imipenem and Cilastatin *on page 595*

Primidone (PRI mi done)
Related Information
Antiepileptic Drugs *on page 1374*
Carbohydrate and Alcohol Content of Liquid Medications for Use in Patients Receiving Ketogenic Diets *on page 1431*
Drugs and Breast-Feeding *on page 1404*
U.S. Brand Names Mysoline®
Canadian Brand Names Apo®-Primidone
Therapeutic Category Anticonvulsant, Barbiturate; Barbiturate
Generic Available Yes
Use Management of generalized tonic-clonic (grand mal), complex partial and simple partial (focal) seizures
Pregnancy Risk Factor D
Contraindications Hypersensitivity to primidone or any component; porphyria
Warnings Generic tablet may contain sodium benzoate; benzoic acid (benzoate) is a metabolite of benzyl alcohol; large amounts of benzyl alcohol (≥99 mg/kg/day) have been associated with a potentially fatal toxicity ("gasping syndrome") in neonates; the "gasping syndrome" consists of metabolic acidosis, respiratory distress, gasping respirations, CNS dysfunction (including convulsions, intracranial hemorrhage), hypotension and cardiovascular collapse; avoid use of primidone products containing
(Continued)

Primidone *(Continued)*

sodium benzoate in neonates; *in vitro* and animal studies have shown that benzoate displaces bilirubin from protein binding sites

Precautions Use with caution in patients with renal or hepatic impairment; abrupt discontinuation may precipitate status epilepticus

Adverse Reactions

Central nervous system: Drowsiness, vertigo, lethargy, behavior change, ataxia

Dermatologic: Rash

Gastrointestinal: Nausea, vomiting

Hematologic: Leukopenia, malignant lymphoma-like syndrome, megaloblastic anemia

Ocular: Diplopia, nystagmus

Miscellaneous: Systemic lupus-like syndrome

Drug Interactions Cytochrome P450 isoenzyme CYP1A2, CYP2B6, CYP2C, CYP2C8, CYP3A3/4, and CYP3A5-7 inducer

Primidone may decrease serum concentrations of ethosuximide, valproic acid, griseofulvin; methylphenidate may increase primidone serum concentrations; phenytoin may decrease primidone serum concentrations; valproic acid may increase phenobarbital concentrations derived from primidone

Food Interactions May increase the metabolism of vitamins D and K; dietary requirements of vitamins D, K, B_{12}, folate, and calcium may be increased with long-term use

Mechanism of Action Decreases neuron excitability, raises seizure threshold similar to phenobarbital

Pharmacokinetics

Distribution: V_d: Adults: 2-3 L/kg

Protein-binding: 99%

Metabolism: In the liver to phenobarbital (active) and phenylethylmalonamide (PEMA)

Bioavailability: 60% to 80%

Half-life:

Primidone: 10-12 hours

PEMA: 16 hours

Phenobarbital: 52-118 hours (age-dependent)

Time to peak serum concentration: Oral: Within 4 hours

Elimination: Urinary excretion of both active metabolites and unchanged primidone (15% to 25%)

Usual Dosage Oral:

Neonates: 12-20 mg/kg/day in divided doses 2-4 times/day; start with lower dosage and titrate upward

Children <8 years: Initial: 50-125 mg/day given at bedtime; increase by 50-125 mg/day increments every 3-7 days; usual dose: 10-25 mg/kg/day in divided doses 3-4 times/day

Children ≥8 years and Adults: Initial: 125-250 mg/day at bedtime; increase by 125-250 mg/day every 3-7 days; usual dose: 750-1500 mg/day in divided doses 3-4 times/day with maximum dosage of 2 g/day

Administration Oral: Administer with food to decrease GI upset

Monitoring Parameters Serum primidone and phenobarbital concentrations; CBC with differential; neurological status, seizure frequency, duration, severity

Reference Range Monitor both primidone and phenobarbital concentrations (see Phenobarbital *on page 888*); Primidone:

Therapeutic: 5-12 µg/mL (SI: 23-55 µmol/L)

Toxic effects rarely present with levels <10 µg/mL (SI: 46 µmol/L) if phenobarbital concentrations are low

Toxic: >15 µg/mL (SI: >69 µmol/L)

Patient Information Avoid alcohol; limit caffeine; may cause drowsiness and impair ability to perform activities requiring mental alertness or physical coordination; do not abruptly discontinue or change dose without physician approval

Additional Information Mysoline® suspension was discontinued in February 2001

Dosage Forms Tablet: 50 mg, 250 mg [generic tablet may contain sodium benzoate]

Probenecid (proe BEN e sid)

Canadian Brand Names Benuryl™

Therapeutic Category Adjuvant Therapy, Penicillin Level Prolongation; Antigout Agent; Uric Acid Lowering Agent; Uricosuric Agent

Generic Available Yes

Use Prevention of gouty arthritis; hyperuricemia; prolong serum levels of penicillin/ cephalosporin

Pregnancy Risk Factor B

Contraindications Hypersensitivity to probenecid or any component; high dose aspirin therapy; moderate to severe renal impairment (Cl$_{cr}$ <10 mL/minute); children <2 years of age, blood dyscrasias, uric acid kidney stones

Precautions Use with caution in patients with peptic ulcer; hematuria, renal colic; formation of uric acid stones associated with the use of probenecid may be prevented by liberal fluid intake and alkalinization of urine; may not be effective when Cl$_{cr}$ 10-30 mL/minute

Adverse Reactions

Cardiovascular: Flushing

Central nervous system: Dizziness, headache

Dermatologic: Rash

Gastrointestinal: Anorexia, nausea, vomiting, sore gums

Genitourinary: Urinary frequency

Hematologic: Anemia, leukopenia, aplastic anemia, hemolytic anemia (possibly related to G-6-PD deficiency)

Hepatic: Hepatic necrosis

Renal: Nephrotic syndrome, renal colic, uric acid stones

Miscellaneous: Hypersensitivity reactions

Drug Interactions Salicylates and probenecid inhibit the uricosuric actions of each other; probenecid may increase the plasma levels of acyclovir, penicillins, ciprofloxacin, ganciclovir, cephalosporins, methotrexate, dapsone, NSAIDs, and zidovudine; benzodiazepines and thiopental may have prolonged effects; sulfonylureas may have an increase in half-life; clofibrate may have an increased accumulation of its active metabolite; avoid concomitant use with ketorolac since its half-life is increased twofold and levels and toxicity are significantly increased; niacin may inhibit uricosuric effects of probenecid

Mechanism of Action Competitively inhibits the reabsorption of uric acid at the proximal convoluted tubule, thereby promoting its excretion and reducing serum uric acid levels; increases plasma levels of weak organic acids (penicillins, cephalosporins, or other beta-lactam antibiotics) by competitively inhibiting their renal tubular secretion

Pharmacodynamics Exerts maximal effects on penicillin levels after 2 hours; produces maximal renal clearance of uric acid in 30 minutes

Pharmacokinetics

Absorption: Rapid and complete from GI tract

Protein binding: 85% to 95%

Metabolism: In the liver

Half-life: 4-17 hours

Time to peak serum concentration: Within 2-4 hours

Usual Dosage Oral:

Prolongation of penicillin serum levels:

Children 2-14 years: Initial: 25 mg/kg/dose or 0.7 g/m^2/dose as a single dose; maintenance: 40 mg/kg/day or 1.2 g/m^2/day in 4 divided doses (maximum single dose: 500 mg)

Adults: 500 mg 4 times/day

Hyperuricemia: Adults: Initial: 250 mg twice daily for 1 week; increase to 500 mg twice daily; may increase in 500 mg increments every 4 weeks if needed to a maximum of 2-3 g/day; begin therapy 2-3 weeks after an acute gouty attack

Gonorrhea: Adults: 1 g 30 minutes before penicillin, ampicillin, or amoxicillin

Dosing adjustment in renal impairment: Cl$_{cr}$ <50 mL/minute: Avoid use

Administration Oral: Administer with food or antacids to minimize GI effects

Monitoring Parameters Uric acid, renal function, CBC

Test Interactions False-positive glucosuria with Clinitest®; falsely elevated serum theophylline level (Schack & Waxler technique); inhibits renal excretion of phenosulfonphthalein (PSP), 17-ketosteroids, and sulfobromophthalein (BSP)

Patient Information Drink plenty of fluids to reduce the risk of uric acid stones; the frequency of acute gouty attacks may increase during the first 6-12 months of therapy; avoid taking large doses of aspirin or other salicylates; avoid alcohol

Dosage Forms Tablet: 500 mg

Procainamide (proe kane A mide)

Related Information

Adult ACLS Algorithm, Narrow-Complex Supraventricular Tachycardia *on page 1190*

Adult ACLS Algorithm, Stable Ventricular Tachycardia *on page 1191*

Adult ACLS Algorithm, V. Fib and Pulseless VT *on page 1185*

CPR Pediatric Drug Dosages *on page 1175*

Pediatric ALS Algorithm, Tachycardia - Rapid Rhythm and Adequate Perfusion *on page 1181*

Pediatric ALS Algorithm, Tachycardia - Rapid Rhythm and Evidence of Poor Perfusion *on page 1182*

U.S. Brand Names Procanbid®; Pronestyl®; Pronestyl-SR®

Canadian Brand Names Apo®-Procainamide; Procan® SR

Synonyms PCA; Procaine Amide

Therapeutic Category Antiarrhythmic Agent, Class I-A

Generic Available Yes (except tablet)

Use Treatment of ventricular tachycardia, premature ventricular contractions, paroxysmal atrial tachycardia, and atrial fibrillation; to prevent recurrence of ventricular tachycardia, paroxysmal supraventricular tachycardia, atrial fibrillation or flutter; **Note:** Due to proarrhythmic effects, use should be reserved for life-threatening arrhythmias

Pregnancy Risk Factor C

Contraindications Hypersensitivity to procainamide, procaine, related drugs, or any component (see Warnings); complete heart block; second or third degree heart block without pacemaker; "torsade de pointes" (twisting of the points), an unusual ventricular tachycardia; pre-existing QT prolongation; myasthenia gravis; SLE

Warnings Serious blood dyscrasias may occur (see Adverse Reactions); long-term administration leads to the development of a positive antinuclear antibody (ANA) test in 50% of patients which may lead to a lupus erythematosus-like syndrome (in 20% to 30% of patients); assess relative benefits and risks if ANA titer becomes positive and consider alternative agent; discontinue procainamide if SLE symptoms develop and change to alternative agent; do not use sustained release preparation for initial therapy; some tablets contain tartrazine and injection contains sulfites both of which may cause allergic reactions in susceptible individuals

The 100 mg/mL injection may contain benzyl alcohol which may cause allergic reactions in susceptible individuals; large amounts of benzyl alcohol (≥99 mg/kg/day) have been associated with a potentially fatal toxicity ("gasping syndrome") in neonates; the "gasping syndrome" consists of metabolic acidosis, respiratory distress, gasping respirations, CNS dysfunction (including convulsions, intracranial hemorrhage), hypotension and cardiovascular collapse; use procainamide products containing benzyl alcohol with caution in neonates; *in vitro* and animal studies have shown that benzoate, a metabolite of benzyl alcohol, displaces bilirubin from protein binding sites

Precautions Use with caution in patients with marked A-V conduction disturbances, bundle-branch block or severe cardiac glycoside intoxication, ventricular arrhythmias in patients with organic heart disease or coronary occlusion, CHF, supraventricular tachyarrhythmias unless digitalis glycoside levels are adequate to prevent marked increases in ventricular rates; drug may accumulate in patients with renal or hepatic dysfunction, dosage adjustment required

Adverse Reactions

Cardiovascular: Hypotension, tachycardia, arrhythmias, A-V block, QT prolongation, widening QRS complex

Central nervous system: Confusion, disorientation, drug fever

Gastrointestinal: Nausea, vomiting, GI complaints

Hematologic: Agranulocytosis, neutropenia, thrombocytopenia, hypoplastic anemia

Hepatic: Hepatomegaly, elevated liver enzymes

Miscellaneous: Lupus-like syndrome (arthralgia, positive Coombs' test, thrombocytopenia, rash, myalgia, fever, pericarditis, pleural effusion)

Drug Interactions Cimetidine, ranitidine, amiodarone, beta-blocking agents, trimethoprim may increase plasma procainamide and NAPA concentrations, procainamide dosage adjustment may be required; procainamide may potentiate skeletal muscle relaxants; anticholinergic drugs may have enhanced effects

Food Interactions Procanbid® extended release tablets: A high fat meal may increase extent of absorption by ~20%

Stability Use only clear or slightly yellow solutions; stability of parenteral admixture with D$_5$W at room temperature (25°C) is 24 hours but 7 days at refrigerated temperature (2°C to 8°C)

Mechanism of Action Class IA antiarrhythmic with anticholinergic and local anesthetic effects; decreases myocardial excitability and conduction velocity and depresses myocardial contractility, by increasing the electrical stimulation threshold of ventricle, His-Purkinje system and through direct cardiac effects

Pharmacodynamics Onset of action: I.M. 10-30 minutes

Pharmacokinetics

Absorption: Oral: Well absorbed; ProcanBid®: Absorption is sustained over 12 hours

Distribution: V_d (decreased with CHF or shock):

Children: 2.2 L/kg

Adults: 2 L/kg

Protein binding: 15% to 20%

Metabolism: By acetylation in the liver to produce N-acetyl procainamide (NAPA) (active metabolite)

Bioavailability, oral: 75% to 95%

Half-life:

Procainamide (dependent upon hepatic acetylator phenotype, cardiac function, and renal function):

Children: 1.7 hours

Adults with normal renal function: 2.5-4.7 hours

NAPA (dependent upon renal function):

Children: 6 hours

Adults with normal renal function: 6-8 hours

Time to peak serum concentration:

Oral (capsule): Within 45 minutes to 2.5 hours

I.M.: 15-60 minutes

Elimination: Urinary excretion (25% as NAPA)

Dialysis: Moderately dialyzable by hemodialysis (20% to 50%), but not dialyzable by peritoneal dialysis

Usual Dosage Must be titrated to patient's response

Children:

Oral: 15-50 mg/kg/day divided every 3-6 hours; maximum 4 g/day

I.M.: 20-30 mg/kg/day divided every 4-6 hours; maximum 4 g/day

I.V.:

Loading dose: 3-6 mg/kg/dose over 5 minutes, not to exceed 100 mg/dose; may repeat every 5-10 minutes to maximum total loading dose of 15 mg/kg; do not exceed 500 mg in 30 minutes

Maintenance: Continuous I.V. infusion: 20-80 mcg/kg/minute; maximum dose: 2 g/day

PALS Guidelines 2000 (for perfusing tachycardias): **Note:** Do not routinely administer together with amiodarone:

I.V., I.O.: Loading dose: 15 mg/kg infused over 30-60 minutes; monitor EKG continuously and blood pressure frequently; stop the infusion if hypotension occurs or QRS complex widens by >50% of baseline

Adults:

Oral: Immediate release products: 250-500 mg/dose every 3-6 hours; sustained release: 500 mg to 1 g every 6 hours; extended release (Procanbid®): 1-2 g every 12 hours; usual dose: 50 mg/kg/day or 2-4 g/day

I.V.:

Loading dose: 50-100 mg/dose, repeated every 5-10 minutes until patient controlled; or load with 15-18 mg/kg; maximum loading dose: 1-1.5 g

Maintenance: Continuous I.V. infusion: 3-4 mg/minute; range: 1-6 mg/minute; monitor levels and do not exceed 3 mg/minute for >24 hours in patients with renal failure

Refractory ventricular fibrillation:

Loading dose: 30 mg/minute up to a total of 17 mg/kg

I.V. maintenance infusion: 1-4 mg/minute; monitor levels and do not exceed 3 mg/minute for >24 hours in adults with renal failure

ACLS guidelines 2000:

I.V.: Loading dose: Infuse 20 mg/minute until arrhythmia is controlled, hypotension occurs, QRS complex widens by 50% of its original width, or total of 17 mg/kg is given

I.V. maintenance infusion: 1-4 mg/minute

Dosing interval in renal dysfunction:

Cl_{cr} 10-50 mL/minute: Administer normal dose every 6-12 hours

Cl_{cr} <10 mL/minute: Administer normal dose every 8-24 hours

Administration

Oral: Administer with water on an empty stomach; if GI distress occurs may administer with food or milk to decrease GI upset; swallow extended and sustained release tablets whole, do not chew, break, or crush

Parenteral: I.V.: Do not administer faster than 20-30 mg/minute; severe hypotension can occur with rapid I.V. administration; administer I.V. push over at least 5 minutes; administer I.V. loading doses and intermittent infusions over 25-30

(Continued)

Procainamide *(Continued)*

minutes; use concentration of 20-30 mg/mL for loading dose and 2-4 mg/mL for maintenance infusions; rate of infusion (mL/hour) = dose (mcg/kg/minute) x weight (kg) x 60 minutes/hour divided by the concentration

Monitoring Parameters EKG, blood pressure, CBC with differential, platelet count, antinuclear antibody test (ANA); serum drug concentrations, procainamide and NAPA, especially in patients with renal failure or those receiving higher maintenance doses (eg, adults: >3 mg/minute) for >24 hours

Reference Range

Therapeutic:

Procainamide: 4-10 µg/mL (SI: 15-37 µmol/L)

Sum of procainamide and N-acetyl procainamide: 10-30 µg/mL (SI: <110 µmol/L)

Optimal ranges must be ascertained for individual patients, with EKG monitoring

Toxic (procainamide): >10-12 µg/mL (SI: >37-44 µmol/L)

Patient Information Limit alcohol; some sustained release tablets have a wax core that slowly releases the drug, this wax core is not absorbed and will be eliminated in the stool; inform physician if symptoms such as fever, sore throat, chills, bruising, or bleeding occur

Dosage Forms

Capsule, as hydrochloride: 250 mg, 500 mg

Pronestyl®: 250 mg

Injection, solution, as hydrochloride: 100 mg/mL (10 mL); 500 mg/mL (2 mL) [contains sodium metabisulfite]

Pronestyl®: 100 mg/mL (10 mL) [contains benzyl alcohol and sodium bisulfite]

Tablet, as hydrochloride (Pronestyl®): 250 mg, 375 mg, 500 mg [contains tartrazine]

Tablet, extended release, as hydrochloride: 750 mg, 1000 mg

Procanbid®: 500 mg, 1000 mg

Pronestyl-SR®: 500 mg

Extemporaneous Preparations Note: Several formulations have been described, some being more complex; for all formulations, the pH must be 4-6 to prevent degradation; some preparations require adjustment of pH; **label all preparations "shake well before use"**

A 50 mg/mL oral liquid preparation made from the contents of capsules and 3 different vehicles (cherry syrup, a 1:1 mixture of Ora-Sweet® and Ora-Plus®, or a 1:1 mixture of Ora-Sweet® SF and Ora-Plus®) was stable for 60 days when stored in amber plastic prescription bottles in the dark at room temperature (25°C) or under refrigeration (5°C); empty the contents of twenty-four 250 mg capsules into a mortar; break up the powder and pulverize it; add 20 mL of the vehicle and mix well to form a uniform paste; mix while adding the vehicle in geometric proportions to **almost** 120 mL; transfer to a calibrated bottle and qsad with vehicle to 120 mL; label "protect from light" (Allen, 1996)

A suspension of 50 mg/mL can be made with the capsules, distilled water, and a 2:1 simple syrup/cherry syrup mixture; stability 2 weeks under refrigeration (ASHP, 1987)

Concentrations of 5, 50, and 100 mg/mL oral liquid preparations, (made with the capsules, sterile water for irrigation and cherry syrup) stored at 4°C to 6°C (pH 6) were stable for at least 6 months (Metras, 1992)

A sucrose-based syrup (procainamide 50 mg/mL) made with capsules, distilled water, simple syrup, parabens, and cherry flavoring had a calculated stability of 456 days at 25°C and measured stability of 42 days at 40°C (pH ~5) while a maltitol-based syrup (procainamide 50 mg/mL) made with capsules, distilled water, Lycasin® (a syrup vehicle with 75% w/w maltitol), parabens, sodium bisulfate, saccharin, sodium acetate, pineapple and apricot flavoring, FD & C yellow number 6, (pH adjusted to 5 with glacial acetic acid) had a calculated stability of 97 days at 25°C and a measured stability of 94 days at 40°C. The maltitol-based syrup was more stable than the sucrose-based syrup when temperature was >37°C, but the sucrose-based syrup was more stable at temperatures <37°C (Alexander, 1993)

Alexander KS, Pudipeddi M, and Parker GA, "Stability of Procainamide Hydrochloride Syrups Compounded From Capsules," *Am J Hosp Pharm*, 1993, 50(4):693-8.

Allen LV and Erickson MA, "Stability of Ketoconazole, Metolazone, Metronidazole, Procainamide Hydrochloride, and Spironolactone in Extemporaneously Compounded Oral Liquids," *Am J Health Syst Pharm*, 1996, 53(17):2073-8.

Handbook in Extemporaneous Formulations, Bethesda, MD: American Society of Hospital Pharmacists, 1987.

Metras JI, Swenson CF, and MacDermott MP, "Stability of Procainamide Hydrochloride in an Extemporaneously Compounded Oral Liquid," *Am J Hosp Pharm*, 1992, 49(7):1720-4.

Swenson CF, "Importance of Following Instructions When Compounding," *Am J Hosp Pharm*, 1993, 50(2):261.

References

"Guidelines 2000 for Cardiopulmonary Resuscitation and Emergency Cardiovascular Care, Part 6: Advanced Cardiovascular Life Support, The American Heart Association in Collaboration With the International Liaison Committee on Resuscitation," *Circulation*, 2000, 102(8 Suppl):I86-171.

"Guidelines 2000 for Cardiopulmonary Resuscitation and Emergency Cardiovascular Care, Part 10: Pediatric Advanced Life Support, The American Heart Association in Collaboration With the International Liason Committee on Resuscitation," *Circulation*, 2000, 102(8 Suppl): I291-342.

Singh S, Gelband H, Mehta AV, et al, "Procainamide Elimination Kinetics in Pediatric Patients," *Clin Pharmacol Ther*, 1982, 32(5):607-11.

♦ **Procaine Amide** *see* Procainamide *on page 934*

♦ **Procaine Benzylpenicillin** *see* Penicillin G Procaine *on page 876*

♦ **Procaine Penicillin G** *see* Penicillin G Procaine *on page 876*

♦ **Procanbid®** *see* Procainamide *on page 934*

♦ **Procan® SR (Can)** *see* Procainamide *on page 934*

Procarbazine (proe KAR ba zeen)

Related Information
  Emetogenic Potential of Single Chemotherapeutic Agents *on page 1286*

U.S. Brand Names Matulane®

Canadian Brand Names Natulan®

Synonyms Ibenzmethyzin

Therapeutic Category Antineoplastic Agent, Miscellaneous

Generic Available No

Use Treatment of Hodgkin's disease, non-Hodgkin's lymphoma, brain tumor, bronchogenic carcinoma

Pregnancy Risk Factor D

Contraindications Hypersensitivity to procarbazine or any component; pre-existing bone marrow aplasia

Warnings The FDA currently recommends that procedures for proper handling and disposal of antineoplastic agents be considered; procarbazine is a carcinogen which may cause a secondary acute nonlymphocytic leukemia; procarbazine may cause infertility and is potentially teratogenic

Precautions May potentiate CNS depression when used with phenothiazine derivatives, barbiturates, narcotics, alcohol, tricyclic antidepressants, methyldopa; use with caution in patients with pre-existing renal or hepatic impairment; reduce dosage in patients with marrow disorders, renal impairment (serum creatinine >2 mg/dL and/or a blood urea nitrogen >40 mg/dL), or decreased hepatic function (total bilirubin >3 mg/dL)

Adverse Reactions
  Central nervous system: CNS depression, somnolence, confusion, nervousness, irritability, cerebellar ataxia, hallucinations, seizures, nightmares, headache, chills, fever, dizziness
  Dermatologic: Dermatitis, alopecia, hypersensitivity rash, pruritus
  Endocrine & metabolic: Disulfiram-like reaction, amenorrhea
  Gastrointestinal: Nausea, vomiting, diarrhea, stomatitis, anorexia
  Genitourinary: Azoospermia, ovarian failure
  Hematologic: Myelosuppression, thrombocytopenia, pancytopenia, hemolysis
  Neuromuscular & skeletal: Arthralgia, myalgia, tremor, neuropathy, weakness
  Ocular: Nystagmus, diplopia, photophobia
  Miscellaneous: Flu-like syndrome

Drug Interactions Alcohol (disulfiram-like reaction with nausea, vomiting, headache, sedation, and visual disturbances); MAO inhibitors, tricyclic antidepressants, ephedrine, epinephrine, isoproterenol (hypertensive crisis, tremor, excitation, cardiac palpitations, angina); narcotics, phenothiazines, barbiturates, methyldopa (additive CNS depression); phenytoin, phenobarbital (increases cytotoxic activity of procarbazine)

Food Interactions Avoid food with high tyramine content (cheese, tea, dark beer, coffee, cola drinks, wine, bananas) as hypertensive crisis, tremor, excitation, cardiac palpitations, and angina may occur

Stability Unstable in water or aqueous solution; avoid contact of the drug with moisture

Mechanism of Action Inhibits DNA, RNA, and protein synthesis; may damage DNA directly via free-radical formation and suppress mitosis

Pharmacokinetics
  Absorption: Oral: Well absorbed
  Distribution: Crosses the blood-brain barrier and distributes into CSF, liver, kidney, intestine, and skin
  Metabolism: In the liver; first-pass conversion to cytotoxic metabolites
  Half-life: 10 minutes
  (Continued)

Procarbazine *(Continued)*

Time to peak serum concentration: Within 1 hour

Elimination: In urine (<5% as unchanged drug) and 70% as metabolites

Usual Dosage Oral (refer to individual protocols; base dosage on ideal body weight):

Children:

Hodgkin's disease: 50-100 mg/m^2/day once daily for 10-14 days of a 28-day cycle

BMT aplastic anemia conditioning regimen: 12.5 mg/kg/dose every other day for 4 doses

Brain tumor: 75 mg/m^2 at hour 1 on day 1; repeat cycle every 2-4 weeks if tolerated; or 100 mg/m^2 on days 1-14 of a treatment course

Neuroblastoma and medulloblastoma: Doses as high as 100-200 mg/m^2/day once daily have been used

Adults: Initial: 2-4 mg/kg/day in single or divided doses for 7 days then increase dose to 4-6 mg/kg/day until response is obtained or leukocyte count decreases to <4000/mm^3 or the platelet count decreases to <100,000/mm^3; maintenance: 1-2 mg/kg/day

Administration Oral: Administer with food or after meals; total daily dose may be administered at a single time or in divided doses throughout the day to minimize GI toxicity

Monitoring Parameters CBC with differential, platelet count, and reticulocyte count; urinalysis, liver function test, renal function test

Patient Information Notify physician of fever, sore throat, bleeding, or bruising; avoid alcohol (disulfiram-like reaction with nausea, vomiting, headache, sedation, and visual disturbances)

Additional Information Myelosuppressive effects:

WBC: Moderate

Platelets: Moderate

Onset (days): 14

Nadir (days): 21

Recovery (days): 28

Dosage Forms Capsule, as hydrochloride: 50 mg

References

Longo DL, Young RC, Wesley M, et al, "Twenty Years of MOPP Therapy for Hodgkin's Disease," *J Clin Oncol*, 1986, 4(9):1295-306.

Rodriguez LA, Prados M, Silver P, et al, "Re-evaluation of Procarbazine for the Treatment of Recurrent Malignant Central Nervous System Tumors," *Cancer*, 1989, 64(12):2420-3.

♦ **Procardia**® *see NIFEdipine on page 811*

♦ **Procardia XL**® *see NIFEdipine on page 811*

Prochlorperazine *(proe klor PER a zeen)*

Related Information

Carbohydrate and Alcohol Content of Liquid Medications for Use in Patients Receiving Ketogenic Diets *on page 1431*

Compatibility of Medications Mixed in a Syringe *on page 1412*

Overdose and Toxicology *on page 1388*

U.S. Brand Names Compazine®; Compro™

Canadian Brand Names Apo®-Prochlorperazine; Nu-Prochlor; Stemetil®

Therapeutic Category Antiemetic; Antipsychotic Agent; Phenothiazine Derivative

Generic Available Yes (injection, suppository, and tablet)

Use Management of nausea and vomiting; acute and chronic psychosis; treatment of intractable migraine headaches

Pregnancy Risk Factor C

Contraindications Hypersensitivity to prochlorperazine or any component (see Warnings); cross-sensitivity with other phenothiazines may exist; avoid use in patients with narrow-angle glaucoma; bone marrow suppression; severe liver or cardiac disease, severe toxic CNS depression or coma

Warnings High incidence of extrapyramidal reactions especially in children, reserve use in children <5 years of age to those who are unresponsive to other antiemetics; incidence of extrapyramidal reactions is increased with acute illnesses such as chicken pox, measles, CNS infections, gastroenteritis, and dehydration; injection contains sulfites which may cause allergic reactions in susceptible individuals; injection contains benzyl alcohol which may cause allergic reactions in susceptible individuals; large amounts of benzyl alcohol (≥99 mg/kg/day) have been associated with a potentially fatal toxicity ("gasping syndrome") in neonates; the "gasping syndrome" consists of metabolic acidosis, respiratory distress, gasping respirations, CNS dysfunction (including convulsions, intracranial hemorrhage), hypotension and cardiovascular collapse; avoid use of injection in neonates; syrup contains sodium benzoate; *in vitro* and animal studies have shown that benzoate, a metabolite of benzyl alcohol, displaces bilirubin from protein binding sites; avoid use of syrup in neonates; lowers seizure threshold, use cautiously in patients with seizure history; some products contain tartrazine which may cause allergic reactions in susceptible individuals; discontinue use at least 48 hours before myelography and do not resume until 24 hours post myelography

Precautions Safety and efficacy have not been established in children <9 kg or <2 years of age

Adverse Reactions Incidence of extrapyramidal reactions are higher with prochlorperazine than chlorpromazine

Cardiovascular: Hypotension (especially with I.V. use); orthostatic hypotension; tachycardia, arrhythmias, sudden death

Central nervous system: Sedation, drowsiness, restlessness, anxiety; extrapyramidal reactions which include dystonic reactions such as spasm of neck muscles, torticollis, extensor rigidity of back muscles, opisthotonos, trismus, and mandibular tics; pseudoparkinsonian signs and symptoms, tardive dyskinesia, neuroleptic malignant syndrome, seizures, altered central temperature regulation

Dermatologic: Hyperpigmentation, pruritus, rash, photosensitivity

Endocrine & metabolic: Amenorrhea, galactorrhea, gynecomastia, abnormal glucose tolerance

Gastrointestinal: GI upset, xerostomia, constipation, weight gain

Genitourinary: Impotence, urinary retention

Hematologic: Agranulocytosis, leukopenia (usually in patients with large doses for prolonged periods), thrombocytopenia, hemolytic anemia, eosinophilia

Hepatic: Cholestatic jaundice

Ocular: Retinal pigmentation, blurred vision

Miscellaneous: Anaphylactoid reactions

Drug Interactions Phenothiazines inhibit the ability of bromocriptine to lower serum prolactin concentrations; benztropine (and other anticholinergics) may inhibit the therapeutic response to prochlorperazine; sulfadoxine-pyrimethamine, propranolol, and chloroquine may increase prochlorperazine concentrations; cigarette smoking may enhance the hepatic metabolism of prochlorperazine; concurrent use of prochlorperazine and antihypertensives may produce additive hypotensive effects; antihypertensive effects of guanethidine and guanadrel may be inhibited by prochlorperazine; concurrent use with TCAs may produce increased toxicity or altered therapeutic response; prochlorperazine may inhibit the antiparkinsonian effect of levodopa; prochlorperazine plus lithium may rarely produce neurotoxicity; barbiturates may reduce prochlorperazine concentrations; prochlorperazine and CNS depressants (ethanol, narcotics) may produce additive CNS depressant effects; prochlorperazine and trazodone may produce additive hypotensive effects; use with cisapride may increase the risk of malignant arrhythmias

Food Interactions Increase dietary intake of riboflavin

Stability Protect from light; clear or slightly yellow solutions may be used; incompatible with aminophylline, amphotericin B, ampicillin, calcium salts, cephalothin, foscarnet (Y-site), furosemide, hydrocortisone, hydromorphone, methohexital, midazolam, penicillin G, pentobarbital, phenobarbital, thiopental

Mechanism of Action Blocks postsynaptic mesolimbic dopaminergic receptors in the brain, including the medullary chemoreceptor trigger zone; exhibits a strong alpha-adrenergic blocking effect and depresses the release of hypothalamic and hypophyseal hormones

Pharmacodynamics

Onset of action:
Oral: 30-40 minutes
I.M.: Within 10-20 minutes
Rectal: Within 60 minutes

Duration:
I.M., oral extended release: 12 hours
Rectal, oral immediate release: 3-4 hours

Usual Dosage

Antiemetic:

Children >10 kg:
Oral, rectal: 0.4 mg/kg/day in 3-4 divided doses; **or** as an alternative:
10-14 kg: 2.5 mg every 12-24 hours as needed; maximum dose: 7.5 mg/day
15-18 kg: 2.5 mg every 8-12 hours as needed; maximum dose: 10 mg/day
19-39 kg: 2.5 mg every 8 hours or 5 mg every 12 hours as needed; maximum dose: 15 mg/day

I.M.: 0.1-0.15 mg/kg/dose; usual: 0.13 mg/kg/dose; change to oral as soon as possible

I.V.: Not recommended

Adults:
Oral: 5-10 mg 3-4 times/day; usual maximum dose: 40 mg/day

(Continued)

Prochlorperazine *(Continued)*

Oral, extended release: 10 mg twice daily or 15 mg once daily

I.M.: 5-10 mg every 3-4 hours; usual maximum dose: 40 mg/day

I.V.: 2.5-10 mg; maximum 10 mg/dose or 40 mg/day; may repeat dose every 3-4 hours as needed

Rectal: 25 mg twice daily

Treatment of intractable migraine headaches (limited information available): I.V.: Children: 0.15 mg/kg as a single dose in 20 children between the ages of 8-17 years combined with I.V. hydration has been used (Kabbouche, 2001)

Treatment of psychoses:

Children 2-12 years:

Oral, rectal: 2.5 mg 2-3 times/day, increase dosage as needed to a maximum daily dose of 20 mg for 2-5 years and 25 mg for 6-12 years

I.M.: 0.13 mg/kg/dose, change to oral as soon as possible

Adults:

Oral: 5-10 mg 3-4 times/day, increase as needed to a daily maximum dose of 150 mg

I.M.: 10-20 mg every 4 hours as needed, change to oral as soon as possible

Administration

Oral: Administer with food or water

Parenteral: I.M. is preferred; avoid I.V. administration; if necessary, may be administered by direct I.V. injection at a maximum rate of 5 mg/minute; do not administer by S.C. route (tissue damage may occur)

Monitoring Parameters CBC with differential and periodic ophthalmic exams (if chronically used)

Test Interactions False-positives for phenylketonuria, urinary amylase, uroporphyrins, urobilinogen

Patient Information Limit caffeine; may cause drowsiness and impair ability to perform activities requiring mental alertness or physical coordination; may cause dry mouth. May cause photosensitivity reactions (eg, exposure to sunlight may cause severe sunburn, skin rash, redness, or itching); avoid exposure to sunlight and artificial light sources (sunlamps, tanning booth/bed); wear protective clothing, wide-brimmed hats, sunglasses, and lip sunscreen (SPF ≥15); use a sunscreen [broad-spectrum sunscreen or physical sunscreen (preferred) or sunblock with SPF ≥15]; contact physician if reaction occurs.

Nursing Implications Avoid skin contact with oral solution or injection, contact dermatitis has occurred

Additional Information Use lowest possible dose in pediatric patients to try to decrease incidence of extrapyramidal reactions

Dosage Forms

Capsule, sustained release, as **maleate** (Compazine®): 10 mg, 15 mg

Injection, solution, as **edisylate**: 5 mg/mL (2 mL)

Compazine®: 5 mg/mL (2 mL, 10 mL) [contains benzyl alcohol]

Suppository, rectal: 2.5 mg (12s), 5 mg (12s), 25 mg (12s)

Compazine®: 2.5 mg (12s), 5 mg (12s), 25 mg (12s)

Compro™: 25 mg (12s)

Syrup, as **edisylate** (Compazine®): 5 mg/5 mL (120 mL) [contains sodium benzoate; fruit flavor]

Tablet, as **maleate** (Compazine®): 5 mg, 10 mg

References

Kabbouche MA, Vockell AL, LeCates SL, et al, "Tolerability and Effectiveness of Prochlorperazine for Intractable Migraine in Children," *Pediatrics*, 2001, 107(4):E62, www.pediatrics.org/cgi/content/full/107/4/e62.

Promethazine (proe METH a zeen)

Related Information
Compatibility of Medications Mixed in a Syringe *on page 1412*
Overdose and Toxicology *on page 1388*
Promethazine and Phenylephrine *on page 944*
Canadian Brand Names Phenergan®
Therapeutic Category Antiemetic; Phenothiazine Derivative; Sedative
Generic Available Yes
Use Symptomatic treatment of various allergic conditions and motion sickness; sedative; antiemetic
Pregnancy Risk Factor C
Contraindications Hypersensitivity to promethazine or any component (cross reactivity with other phenothiazines may occur); severe toxic CNS depression or coma
Warnings Do not give S.C. or intra-arterially, necrotic lesions may occur; rapid I.V. administration may produce a transient fall in blood pressure; slow I.V. administration may produce a slightly elevated blood pressure. Neuroleptic malignant syndrome (NMS) has been reported with promethazine when used alone or in combination with antipsychotic drugs. Children with dehydration are at increased risk for development of dystonic reactions; not for S.C. administration due to severe local reactions including necrosis
Precautions Use with caution in patients with cardiovascular disease, narrow-angle glaucoma, prostatic hypertrophy, GI or GU obstruction, bone marrow depression, impaired liver function, asthma, peptic ulcer, sleep apnea, and hypertensive crisis; avoid in patients with suspected Reye's syndrome; promethazine may lower the seizure threshold; use with caution in patients with seizure disorders or receiving other medications which may also lower the seizure threshold

Adverse Reactions
Cardiovascular: Tachycardia, bradycardia, hypotension (rapid I.V. administration), hypertension (slow I.V. administration), palpitations
Central nervous system: Sedation (pronounced), drowsiness, confusion, fatigue, excitation, extrapyramidal reactions, dystonia, tardive dyskinesia, NMS, hallucinations
Dermatologic: Photosensitivity, rash, angioedema
Gastrointestinal: Xerostomia, GI upset, increased appetite, weight gain, abdominal pain, diarrhea, nausea
Genitourinary: Urinary retention
Hematologic: Thrombocytopenia, leukopenia, agranulocytosis (rare)
Hepatic: Cholestatic jaundice, hepatitis
Ocular: Blurred vision
Neuromuscular & skeletal: Arthralgia, tremor, paresthesia, myalgia
Respiratory: Thickening of bronchial secretions, pharyngitis, respiratory depression
Miscellaneous: Allergic reactions

Drug Interactions Cytochrome P450 isoenzyme CYP2D6 enzyme substrate
Phenothiazines inhibit the ability of bromocriptine to lower serum prolactin concentrations; benztropine (and other anticholinergics) may inhibit the therapeutic response to promethazine; sulfadoxine-pyrimethamine, propranolol, and chloroquine may increase promethazine concentrations; cigarette smoking may enhance the hepatic metabolism of promethazine; concurrent use of promethazine with an antihypertensive may produce additive hypotensive effects; antihypertensive effects of guanethidine and guanadrel may be inhibited by promethazine; concurrent use with TCA may produce increased toxicity or altered therapeutic response; promethazine may inhibit the antiparkinsonian effect of levodopa; promethazine plus lithium may rarely produce neurotoxicity; barbiturates may reduce promethazine concentrations; promethazine may reverse the pressor effects of epinephrine; promethazine and CNS depressants (ethanol, narcotics) may produce additive CNS depressant effects; promethazine and trazodone may produce additive hypotensive effects; use with cisapride may increase the risk of malignant arrhythmias; additive effects when used with anticholinergic medications; increased extrapyramidal effects when used with MAO inhibitors
Food Interactions Increase dietary intake of riboflavin
Stability Protect from light; store at controlled room temperature; **compatible** (when comixed in the same syringe) with atropine, chlorpromazine, diphenhydramine, droperidol, fentanyl, glycopyrrolate, hydromorphone, hydroxyzine hydrochloride, meperidine, midazolam, nalbuphine, pentazocine, prochlorperazine, scopolamine; **incompatible** when mixed with aminophylline, cefoperazone (Y-site), chloramphenicol, dimenhydrinate (same syringe), foscarnet (Y-site), furosemide, heparin, hydrocortisone, methohexital, penicillin G, pentobarbital, phenobarbital, thiopental
Mechanism of Action Blocks postsynaptic mesolimbic dopaminergic receptors in the brain; exhibits a strong alpha-adrenergic blocking effect and depresses the release of
(Continued)

Promethazine *(Continued)*

hypothalamic and hypophyseal hormones; competes with histamine for the H_1-receptor

Pharmacodynamics

Onset of action:
Oral, I.M.: Within 20 minutes
I.V.: 3-5 minutes
Duration: Oral: 4-6 hours

Pharmacokinetics

Absorption: 88%
Bioavailability: 25% (due to first pass metabolism)
Half-life: 16-19 hours
Metabolism: In the liver
Elimination: Principally as inactive metabolites in the urine and in the feces

Usual Dosage

Children:
Antihistamine: Oral: 0.1 mg/kg/dose (not to exceed 12.5 mg) every 6 hours during the day and 0.5 mg/kg/dose (not to exceed 25 mg) at bedtime as needed
Antiemetic: Oral, I.M., I.V., rectal: 0.25-1 mg/kg (not to exceed 25 mg) 4-6 times/day as needed
Motion sickness: Oral, rectal: 0.5 mg/kg (not to exceed 25 mg) 30 minutes to 1 hour before departure, then every 12 hours as needed
Sedation: Oral, I.M., I.V., rectal: 0.5-1 mg/kg/dose (not to exceed 50 mg) every 6 hours as needed

Adults:
Antihistamine:
Oral, rectal: 6.25-12.5 mg 3 times/day and 25 mg at bedtime
I.M., I.V.: 25 mg, may repeat in 2 hours when necessary; switch to oral route as soon as feasible
Antiemetic: Oral, I.M., I.V., rectal: 12.5-25 mg every 4 hours as needed
Motion sickness: Oral: 25 mg twice daily with the first dose 30 minutes to 1 hour before departure, then repeat 8-12 hours later as needed
Sedation: Oral, I.M., I.V., rectal: 25-50 mg/dose; repeat every 4-6 hours if needed

Administration

Oral: Administer with food, water, or milk to decrease GI distress
Parenteral: I.M. administration is preferred; avoid I.V. use (see Warnings); in selected patients, promethazine has been administered I.V. diluted to a maximum concentration of 25 mg/mL and infused at a maximum rate of 25 mg/minute; not for S.C. administration, promethazine is a chemical irritant which may produce necrosis

Test Interactions Alters the flare response in intradermal allergen tests; false negative and positive reactions with pregnancy tests relying on immunological reactions between hCG and anti-hCG

Patient Information May cause drowsiness and impair ability to perform activities requiring mental alertness or physical coordination; notify physician of involuntary movements or feelings of restlessness; may cause dry mouth. May cause photosensitivity reactions (eg, exposure to sunlight may cause severe sunburn, skin rash, redness, or itching); avoid exposure to sunlight and artificial light sources (sunlamps, tanning booth/bed); wear protective clothing, wide-brimmed hats, sunglasses, and lip sunscreen (SPF ≥15); use a sunscreen [broad-spectrum sunscreen or physical sunscreen (preferred) or sunblock with SPF ≥15]; contact physician if reaction occurs.

Additional Information Although promethazine has been used in combination with meperidine and chlorpromazine as a premedication (lytic cocktail), this combination may have a higher rate of adverse effects compared to alternative sedative/analgesics

Dosage Forms

Injection, solution, as hydrochloride: 25 mg/mL (1 mL); 50 mg/mL (1 mL)
Suppository, rectal, as hydrochloride: 25 mg, 50 mg
Syrup, as hydrochloride: 6.25 mg/5 mL (120 mL, 480 mL) [contains alcohol]
Tablet, as hydrochloride: 25 mg, 50 mg

References

Strenkoski-Nix LC, Ermer J, DeCleene S, et al, "Pharmacokinetics of Promethazine Hydrochloride After Administration of Rectal Suppositories and Oral Syrup to Healthy Subjects," *Am J Health Syst Pharm*, 2000, 57(16):1499-505.

Promethazine and Codeine *(proe METH a zeen & KOE deen)*

U.S. Brand Names Phenergan® With Codeine
Synonyms Codeine and Promethazine
Therapeutic Category Antitussive; Cough Preparation; Phenothiazine Derivative
Generic Available Yes

Use Temporary relief of coughs and upper respiratory symptoms associated with allergy or the common cold

Restrictions C-V

Pregnancy Risk Factor C

Contraindications Hypersensitivity to promethazine, codeine, or any component; cross reactivity with other phenothiazines may occur; lower respiratory tract symptoms, including asthma; concurrent use of MAO inhibitors

Warnings Phenergan® With Codeine contains sodium benzoate; benzoic acid (benzoate) is a metabolite of benzyl alcohol; large amounts of benzyl alcohol (≥99 mg/kg/day) have been associated with a potentially fatal toxicity ("gasping syndrome") in neonates; *in vitro* and animal studies have shown that benzoate displaces bilirubin from protein binding sites; avoid its use in neonates. Neuroleptic malignant syndrome (NMS) has been reported with promethazine when used alone or in combination with antipsychotic drugs. Children with dehydration are at increased risk for development of dystonic reactions.

Precautions Use with caution in patients with cardiovascular disease, narrow-angle glaucoma, prostatic hypertrophy, GI or GU obstruction, bone marrow depression, impaired liver function, asthma, peptic ulcer, sleep apnea, and hypertensive crisis; avoid in patients with suspected Reye's syndrome; promethazine may lower the seizure threshold; use with caution in patients with seizure disorders or receiving other medications which may also lower the seizure threshold; use with caution in patients with hypersensitivity reactions to morphine, hydrocodone, hydromorphone, levorphanol, oxycodone, oxymorphone

Adverse Reactions

Promethazine:

Cardiovascular: Tachycardia, bradycardia, palpitations

Central nervous system: Sedation (pronounced), confusion, drowsiness, restlessness, anxiety, extrapyramidal reactions, tardive dyskinesia, seizures, hallucinations, NMS

Dermatologic: Rash, photosensitivity

Endocrine & metabolic: Antidiuretic hormone release

Gastrointestinal: GI upset, xerostomia, constipation

Genitourinary: Urinary retention

Hematologic: Agranulocytosis, leukopenia (rare), thrombocytopenia

Hepatic: Cholestatic jaundice, hepatitis

Neuromuscular & skeletal: Arthralgia, tremor, paresthesia, myalgia

Ocular: Blurred vision

Respiratory: Thickening of bronchial secretions, pharyngitis

Miscellaneous: Allergic reactions

Codeine:

Cardiovascular: Palpitations, orthostatic hypotension, tachycardia or bradycardia, peripheral vasodilation

Central nervous system: CNS depression, dizziness, sedation, euphoria, hallucination, seizures

Dermatologic: Pruritus

Gastrointestinal: Nausea, vomiting, constipation, biliary tract spasm

Genitourinary: Urinary tract spasm

Ocular: Miosis

Respiratory: Respiratory depression

Miscellaneous: Physical and psychological dependence, histamine release, allergic reactions

Drug Interactions See Promethazine *on page 941* and Codeine *on page 301*

Food Interactions Increase fluids, fiber intake, and riboflavin in diet

Mechanism of Action See individual monographs for Codeine *on page 301* and Promethazine *on page 941*

Usual Dosage Oral (**in terms of codeine**):

Children: 1-1.5 mg/kg/day divided every 4 hours as needed; maximum dose: 30 mg/day **or**

2-6 years: 1.25-2.5 mL every 4-6 hours as needed or 2.5-5 mg/dose every 4-6 hours as needed; maximum dose: 30 mg codeine/day

6-12 years: 2.5-5 mL every 4-6 hours as needed or 5-10 mg/dose every 4-6 hours as needed; maximum dose: 60 mg codeine/day

Adults: 10-20 mg/dose every 4-6 hours as needed; maximum dose: 120 mg codeine/day; or 5-10 mL every 4-6 hours as needed

Administration Oral: Administer with food or water to decrease GI upset

Test Interactions Alters the flare response in intradermal allergen tests; false negative and positive reactions with pregnancy tests relying on immunological reactions between hCG and anti-hCG

(Continued)

Promethazine and Codeine *(Continued)*

Patient Information May cause drowsiness and impair ability to perform activities requiring mental alertness or physical coordination; may cause dry mouth; may be habit-forming; do not discontinue abruptly. May cause photosensitivity reactions (eg, exposure to sunlight may cause severe sunburn, skin rash, redness, or itching); avoid exposure to sunlight and artificial light sources (sunlamps, tanning booth/bed); wear protective clothing, wide-brimmed hats, sunglasses, and lip sunscreen (SPF ≥15); use a sunscreen [broad-spectrum sunscreen or physical sunscreen (preferred) or sunblock with SPF ≥15]; contact physician if reaction occurs.

Dosage Forms

Syrup: Promethazine hydrochloride 6.25 mg and codeine phosphate 10 mg per 5 mL (120 mL, 473 mL, 3840 mL) [contains alcohol]

Phenergan® With Codeine: Promethazine hydrochloride 6.25 mg and codeine phosphate 10 mg per 5 mL (120 mL) [contains 7% alcohol and sodium benzoate]

Promethazine and Phenylephrine (proe METH a zeen & fen il EF rin)

Synonyms Phenylephrine and Promethazine

Therapeutic Category Antihistamine/Decongestant Combination

Generic Available Yes

Use Temporary relief of upper respiratory symptoms associated with allergy or the common cold

Pregnancy Risk Factor C

Contraindications Hypersensitivity to promethazine, phenylephrine, or any component; cross reactivity with other phenothiazines may occur; asthma, peripheral vascular disease, severe hypertension, cardiovascular disease, liver disease, patients receiving MAO inhibitors

Warnings Neuroleptic malignant syndrome (NMS) has been reported with promethazine when used alone or in combination with antipsychotic drugs. Children with dehydration are at increased risk for development of dystonic reactions.

Precautions Use with caution in patients with cardiovascular disease, narrow-angle glaucoma, prostatic hypertrophy, GI or GU obstruction, bone marrow depression, impaired liver function, asthma, peptic ulcer, sleep apnea, and hypertensive crisis; avoid in patients with suspected Reye's syndrome; promethazine may lower the seizure threshold; use with caution in patients with seizure disorders or receiving other medications which may also lower the seizure threshold

Adverse Reactions

Promethazine:

Cardiovascular: Hypertension, hypotension, tachycardia

Central nervous system: Sedation (pronounced), drowsiness, confusion, fatigue, excitation, extrapyramidal reactions, dystonia, tardive dyskinesia, hallucinations, NMS

Dermatologic: Photosensitivity, rash, angioedema

Gastrointestinal: Xerostomia, GI upset, increased appetite, weight gain, abdominal pain, diarrhea, nausea

Genitourinary: Urinary retention

Hematologic: Thrombocytopenia, leukopenia, agranulocytosis (rare)

Hepatic: Cholestatic jaundice, hepatitis

Ocular: Blurred vision

Neuromuscular & skeletal: Arthralgia, tremor, paresthesia, myalgia

Respiratory: Thickening of bronchial secretions, pharyngitis

Miscellaneous: Allergic reactions

Phenylephrine:

Cardiovascular: Hypertension, angina, reflex severe bradycardia, arrhythmias, peripheral vasoconstriction

Central nervous system: Restlessness, excitability, headache, anxiety, nervousness, dizziness

Dermatologic: Pilomotor response, skin blanching

Neuromuscular & skeletal: Tremor

Respiratory: Respiratory distress, rebound nasal congestion, sneezing, burning, stinging, dryness

Drug Interactions See Promethazine *on page 941* and Phenylephrine *on page 892*

Food Interactions Increase dietary intake of riboflavin

Usual Dosage Oral:

Children:

2-6 years: 1.25 mL every 4-6 hours, not to exceed 7.5 mL in 24 hours

6-12 years: 2.5 mL every 4-6 hours, not to exceed 15 mL in 24 hours

Children >12 years and Adults: 5 mL every 4-6 hours, not to exceed 30 mL in 24 hours

Administration Oral: Administer with food, water, or milk to decrease GI distress

Test Interactions Alters the flare response in intradermal allergen tests; false negative and positive reactions with pregnancy tests relying on immunological reactions between hCG and anti-hCG

Patient Information May cause drowsiness and impair ability to perform activities requiring mental alertness or physical coordination; may cause dry mouth. May cause photosensitivity reactions (eg, exposure to sunlight may cause severe sunburn, skin rash, redness, or itching); avoid exposure to sunlight and artificial light sources (sunlamps, tanning booth/bed); wear protective clothing, wide-brimmed hats, sunglasses, and lip sunscreen (SPF ≥15); use a sunscreen [broad-spectrum sunscreen or physical sunscreen (preferred) or sunblock with SPF ≥15]; contact physician if reaction occurs.

Dosage Forms Syrup: Promethazine hydrochloride 6.25 mg and phenylephrine hydrochloride 5 mg per 5 mL (120 mL, 480 mL, 4000 mL) [contains alcohol]

Promethazine, Phenylephrine, and Codeine
(proe METH a zeen, fen il EF rin, & KOE deen)

Synonyms Codeine, Promethazine, and Phenylephrine; Phenylephrine, Promethazine, and Codeine

Therapeutic Category Antihistamine/Decongestant Combination; Antitussive; Cough Preparation

Generic Available Yes

Use Temporary relief of coughs and upper respiratory symptoms including nasal congestion

Restrictions C-V

Pregnancy Risk Factor C

Contraindications Hypersensitivity to promethazine, codeine, phenylephrine, or any component; cross reactivity with other phenothiazines may occur; asthma, peripheral vascular disease; patients receiving MAO inhibitors

Warnings See individual monographs for Promethazine *on page 941*, Phenylephrine *on page 892*, and Codeine *on page 301*

Precautions See individual monographs for Promethazine *on page 941*, Phenylephrine *on page 892*, and Codeine *on page 301*

Adverse Reactions See individual monographs for Promethazine *on page 941*, Phenylephrine *on page 892*, and Codeine *on page 301*

Drug Interactions See individual monographs for Promethazine *on page 941*, Phenylephrine *on page 892*, and Codeine *on page 301*

Food Interactions Increase fluids, fiber intake, and riboflavin in diet

Usual Dosage Oral: Not recommended for children <2 years of age

Children (**dose expressed in terms of codeine**): 1-1.5 mg/kg/day divided every 4-6 hours, maximum dose: 30 mg/day **or**

<6 years:

Weight 25 lb: 1.25-2.5 mL every 4-6 hours, not to exceed 6 mL/24 hours
Weight 30 lb: 1.25-2.5 mL every 4-6 hours, not to exceed 7 mL/24 hours
Weight 35 lb: 1.25-2.5 mL every 4-6 hours, not to exceed 8 mL/24 hours
Weight 40 lb: 1.25-2.5 mL every 4-6 hours, not to exceed 9 mL/24 hours
6-11 years: 2.5-5 mL every 4-6 hours, not to exceed 15 mL/24 hours

Children ≥12 years and Adults: 5 mL every 4-6 hours, not to exceed 30 mL/24 hours

Administration Oral: Administer with food or water to decrease GI upset

Patient Information May cause dry mouth. May cause photosensitivity reactions (eg, exposure to sunlight may cause severe sunburn, skin rash, redness, or itching); avoid exposure to sunlight and artificial light sources (sunlamps, tanning booth/bed); wear protective clothing, wide-brimmed hats, sunglasses, and lip sunscreen (SPF ≥15); use a sunscreen [broad-spectrum sunscreen or physical sunscreen (preferred) or sunblock with SPF ≥15]; contact physician if reaction occurs.

Dosage Forms Syrup: Promethazine hydrochloride 6.25 mg, phenylephrine hydrochloride 5 mg, and codeine phosphate 10 mg per 5 mL (120 mL, 480 mL) [contains 7% alcohol]

♦ **Pronestyl®** *see Procainamide on page 934*
♦ **Pronestyl-SR®** *see Procainamide on page 934*
♦ **Propaderm® (Can)** *see Beclomethasone on page 160*
♦ **Propanthel™ (Can)** *see Propantheline on page 945*

Propantheline (proe PAN the leen)
Canadian Brand Names Propanthel™

Therapeutic Category Anticholinergic Agent; Antispasmodic Agent, Gastrointestinal; Antispasmodic Agent, Urinary

Generic Available Yes

(Continued)

Propantheline *(Continued)*

Use Adjunctive treatment of peptic ulcer, irritable bowel syndrome, pancreatitis, ureteral and urinary bladder spasm; to reduce duodenal motility during diagnostic radiologic procedures

Pregnancy Risk Factor C

Contraindications Hypersensitivity to propantheline or any component; narrow-angle glaucoma; ulcerative colitis; toxic megacolon; obstructive disease of the GI or urinary tract

Warnings Infants, patients with Down's syndrome, and children with spastic paralysis or brain damage may be hypersensitive to antimuscarinic effects

Precautions Use with caution in febrile patients, patients with hyperthyroidism, hepatic, cardiac, or renal disease, hypertension, GI infections, diarrhea, reflux esophagitis

Adverse Reactions
Cardiovascular: Tachycardia, palpitations, flushing
Central nervous system: Insomnia, drowsiness, dizziness, nervousness, headache
Dermatologic: Rash, dry skin
Endocrine & metabolic: Suppression of lactation
Gastrointestinal: Xerostomia, nausea, vomiting, constipation, dry throat, dysphagia
Genitourinary: Impotence, urinary retention
Ocular: Mydriasis, blurred vision
Neuromuscular & skeletal: Weakness
Respiratory: Dry nose
Miscellaneous: Allergic reactions, diaphoresis (decreased)

Drug Interactions May increase potential of potassium chloride wax-matrix preparations to cause intestinal lesions due to decreased peristalsis; increased effect/toxicity with anticholinergics, disopyramide, narcotic analgesics, bretylium, type I antiarrhythmics, antihistamines, phenothiazines, tricyclic antidepressants, corticosteroids (increased IOP), CNS depressants (sedation), adenosine, amiodarone, beta-blockers, amoxapine

Mechanism of Action Competitively blocks the action of acetylcholine at postganglionic parasympathetic receptor sites

Pharmacodynamics
Onset of action: Within 30-45 minutes
Duration: 4-6 hours

Pharmacokinetics
Metabolism: In the liver and GI tract
Elimination: In urine, bile, and other body fluids

Usual Dosage Oral:
Antisecretory:
Children: 1-2 mg/kg/day in 3-4 divided doses
Adults: 15 mg 3 times/day before meals or food and 30 mg at bedtime; for mild manifestations: 7.5 mg 3 times/day
Antispasmodic:
Children: 2-3 mg/kg/day in divided doses every 4-6 hours and at bedtime
Adults: 15 mg 3 times/day before meals or food and 30 mg at bedtime

Administration Oral: Administer 30 minutes before meals and at bedtime

Patient Information May cause drowsiness and impair ability to perform activities requiring mental alertness or physical coordination; notify physician if skin rash, flushing, or eye pain occurs; or if difficulty in urinating, constipation, or sensitivity to light becomes severe or persists; may cause dry mouth; maintain good oral hygiene habits, because lack of saliva may increase chance of cavities

Dosage Forms Tablet, as bromide: 15 mg

♦ **Propa pH [OTC]** *see Salicylic Acid on page 1002*

Proparacaine *(proe PAR a kane)*

U.S. Brand Names Alcaine®; Ophthetic®

Synonyms Proxymetacaine

Therapeutic Category Local Anesthetic, Ophthalmic

Generic Available Yes

Use Local anesthesia for tonometry, gonioscopy; suture removal from cornea; removal of corneal foreign body; cataract extraction, glaucoma surgery; short operative procedure involving the cornea and conjunctiva

Pregnancy Risk Factor C

Contraindications Hypersensitivity to proparacaine or any component

Precautions Use with caution in patients with cardiac disease, hyperthyroidism

Adverse Reactions
Dermatologic: Allergic contact dermatitis

Local: Irritation, stinging, sensitization

Ocular: Keratitis, iritis, erosion of the corneal epithelium, conjunctival congestion and hemorrhage, corneal opacification

Stability Refrigerate and protect from light

Mechanism of Action Local anesthetic; prevents initiation and transmission of impulse at the nerve cell membrane by decreasing ion permeability

Pharmacodynamics
Onset of action: Within 20 seconds of instillation

Duration: 15-20 minutes

Usual Dosage Children and Adults:

Ophthalmic surgery: Instill 1 drop of 0.5% solution in eye every 5-10 minutes for 5-7 doses

Tonometry, gonioscopy, suture removal: Instill 1-2 drops of 0.5% solution in eye just prior to procedure

Administration Ophthalmic: Instill drops into affected eye(s); avoid contact of bottle tip with skin or eye

Patient Information Do not rub eye until anesthesia has worn off

Dosage Forms Solution, ophthalmic, as hydrochloride: 0.5% (15 mL)

♦ **Propine**® *see* Dipivefrin *on page 396*

♦ **Proplex**® **T** *see* Factor IX Complex (Human) *on page 471*

Propofol (PROE po fole)
U.S. Brand Names Diprivan®

Therapeutic Category General Anesthetic

Generic Available Yes

Use Induction of anesthesia in children ≥3 years and adults; maintenance of anesthesia in children ≥2 months and adults; initiation and maintenance of monitored anesthesia care sedation in adults; continuous sedation of adult intensive care unit patients

Pregnancy Risk Factor B

Contraindications Hypersensitivity to propofol or any component (see Warnings); patients who are not intubated or mechanically ventilated; other contraindications to general anesthesia or sedation apply

Warnings Diprivan® contains disodium edetate and egg lecithin, the generic product contains sodium metabisulfite and egg yolk phospholipid, and both products contain soybean oil, any of which may cause allergic reactions in susceptible individuals.

Not recommended for induction of anesthesia in children <3 years or for maintenance of anesthesia in infants <2 months of age; not recommended for monitored anesthesia care sedation in children; **not recommended for sedation of PICU patients. Note: The FDA is very concerned about the safety of propofol in PICU patients.** The results of a manufacturer's randomized controlled clinical trial (n=327) revealed an increase in the number of deaths in PICU patients treated with Diprivan® versus other standard sedative agents. Diprivan® was administered at initial infusion rates of 5.5 mg/kg/hour and titrated to maintain a standardized level of sedation. Twenty-one of the 25 deaths occurred in patients who received propofol. The FDA's review of the data did not find a correlation of the deaths with an underlying disease state, nor did the review identify a definite pattern to the causes of death. A new clinical trial will be conducted to address this issue (see http://www.FDA.gov/medwatch/safety/2001/dipvivan_deardoc.pdf). The use of propofol in PICU patients, especially at high doses for prolonged periods of time may be associated with certain toxicities; metabolic acidosis with fatal cardiac failure has occurred in several children (4 weeks to 11 years of age) who received propofol infusions at average rates of infusion of 4.5-10 mg/kg/hour for 66-115 hours (maximum rates of infusion 6.2-11.5 mg/kg/hour); see Parke, 1992; Strickland, 1995; and Bray, 1995.

Patients require continuous monitoring and airway management; cardiovascular and respiratory resuscitation equipment should be available; decrease the dose in ASA III or IV, elderly, debilitated, or hypovolemic patients; not recommended for use in obstetrics, cesarean deliveries, lactating women, patients with increased ICP or impaired cerebral circulation. Abrupt discontinuation may result in rapid awakening, anxiety, agitation, and resistance to mechanical ventilation. Although products contain preservatives, rapid growth of micro-organisms can occur; failure to use aseptic technique can result in microbial contamination and fever, sepsis, infection, life-threatening illnesses, or death; discard I.V. tubing and unused portions after 12 hours; **do not use if microbial contamination is suspected.**
(Continued)

Propofol *(Continued)*

Propofol should be administered by qualified healthcare professionals trained in advanced cardiac life support and anesthetic drug use (when used for general anesthesia and monitored anesthesia care sedation) or management of critically ill patients (when used for sedation in intensive care patient).

Precautions Use with caution in patients with seizures or history of epilepsy, or severe cardiac or respiratory disease; I.V. injection may produce transient local pain; perioperative myoclonia may occur; decrease dose and rate of infusion for elderly, debilitated, or ASA III/IV patients. Abrupt discontinuation in pediatric patients may cause agitation, hyperirritability, tremulousness, and flushing of hands and feet. Increased frequency of bradycardia, jitteriness, and agitation have also been observed.

Diprivan® contains disodium edetate which can chelate trace metals, including zinc; as much as 10 mg of elemented zinc may be lost per day when calcium disodium edetate is used in gram doses to treat heavy metal poisonings; no reports of zinc deficiency or low zinc levels have been reported with Diprivan®, however, the manufacturer recommends that Diprivan® not be infused for >5 days without giving a "drug holiday"; during this time off of Diprivan®, replacement of estimated or measured urine zinc losses is recommended.

Adverse Reactions
Cardiovascular: Hypotension (dose related), bradycardia, myocardial depression, flushing
Central nervous system: Fever, headache, dizziness
Dermatologic: Rash, pruritus
Endocrine & metabolic: Hyperlipidemia; fatal metabolic acidosis has been reported
Gastrointestinal: Nausea, vomiting, abdominal cramping
Genitourinary: Discoloration of urine (green)
Local: Pain at injection site (especially when administered via small vein); **Note:** Dilution with D_5W or administration of lidocaine pretreatment may decrease local pain
Neuromuscular & skeletal: Myalgia, twitching, clonic/myoclonic movement
Respiratory: Respiratory acidosis, respiratory depression, apnea
Miscellaneous: Anaphylaxis, anaphylactoid reactions

Drug Interactions Theophylline may antagonize the CNS effects of propofol; propofol may increase serum concentrations of alfentanil; increased toxicity may occur with acetazolamide (cardiorespiratory instability), CNS depressants, atracurium (anaphylaxis), phenothiazines, fentanyl (increased concentration of propofol), guanabenz, MAO inhibitors, narcotic analgesics, vecuronium (increased neuromuscular blockade); in pediatric patients, concurrent use of propofol with fentanyl may cause serious bradycardia

Stability Does not require refrigeration; protect from light; do not use if there is evidence of separation of phases of emulsion, particulate matter, or discoloration; discard unused portions at end of surgical procedure; ICU use: Discard tubing and unused portions after 12 hours; dilute with D_5W only; do not dilute to <2 mg/mL; diluted emulsion is more stable in glass; stability in plastic: 95% potency after 2 hours; may administer with D_5W, LR, D_5LR, $D_5/^1/_2NS$, $D_5/^1/_4NS$; do not administer with blood or blood products through the same I.V. catheter; do not mix with other drugs

Mechanism of Action Propofol is a hindered phenolic compound with intravenous general anesthetic properties. The drug is unrelated to any of the currently used barbiturate, opioid, benzodiazepine, arylcyclohexylamine, or imidazole intravenous anesthetic agents.

Pharmacodynamics
Onset of anesthesia: Within 30 seconds after bolus infusion
Duration: ~3-10 minutes depending on the dose, rate and duration of administration; with prolonged use (eg, 10 days ICU sedation), propofol accumulates in tissues and redistributes into plasma when the drug is discontinued, so that the time to awakening (duration of action) is increased; however, if dose is titrated on a daily basis, so that the minimum effective dose is utilized, time to awakening may be within 10-15 minutes even after prolonged use

Pharmacokinetics
Distribution: Large volume of distribution; highly lipophilic
V_d (apparent): Children 4-12 years: 5-10 L/kg
V_{dss}:
Adults: 170-350 L
Adults (10-day infusion): 60 L/kg
Protein binding: 97% to 99%
Metabolism: In the liver via glucuronide and sulfate conjugation
Half-life (three-compartment model):
Alpha: 2-8 minutes
Beta (second distribution): ~40 minutes

Terminal: ~200 minutes; range: 300-700 minutes
Terminal (after 10-day infusion): 1-3 days
Elimination: ~90% excreted in urine as metabolites and <1% as unchanged drug

Usual Dosage Dosage must be individualized based on total body weight and titrated to the desired clinical effect; wait at least 3-5 minutes between dosage adjustments to clinically assess drug effects; smaller doses are required when used with narcotics; the following are general dosing guidelines:

General anesthesia:

I.V. induction: (See "Symbols and Abbreviations Used in This Handbook" in front section of this book for explanation of ASA classes):

Children ≥3 years, ASA I or II: 2.5-3.5 mg/kg; use a lower dose for children ASA III or IV

Adults, ASA I or II, <55 years: 2-2.5 mg/kg (~40 mg every 10 seconds until onset of induction)

Elderly, debilitated, hypovolemic, or ASA III or IV: 1-1.5 mg/kg (~20 mg every 10 seconds until onset of induction)

Cardiac anesthesia: 0.5-1.5 mg/kg (~20 mg every 10 seconds until onset of induction)

Neurosurgical patients: 1-2 mg/kg (~20 mg every 10 seconds until onset of induction)

Maintenance: I.V. infusion:

Infants ≥2 months to Children 16 years, ASA I or II: Initial: 200-300 mcg/kg/minute; decrease dose after 30 minutes if clinical signs of light anesthesia are absent; usual infusion rate: 125-150 mcg/kg/minute; younger pediatric patients may require larger infusion rates compared to older children

Adults, ASA I or II, <55 years: Initial: 150-200 mcg/kg/minute for 10-15 minutes; decrease by 30% to 50% during first 30 minutes of maintenance; usual infusion rate: 100-200 mcg/kg/minute

Elderly, debilitated, hypovolemic, ASA III or IV: 50-100 mcg/kg/minute

Cardiac anesthesia:

Low dose propofol with primary opioid: 50-100 mcg/kg/minute (see manufacturer's labeling)

Primary propofol with secondary opioid: 100-150 mcg/kg/minute

Neurosurgical patients: 100-200 mcg/kg/minute

Maintenance: I.V. intermittent bolus: Adults, ASA I or II, <55 years: 20-50 mg increments as needed

Monitored Anesthesia Care sedation:

Initiation:

Adults, ASA I or II, <55 years: Slow I.V. infusion: 100-150 mcg/kg/minute for 3-5 minutes; slow injection: 0.5 mg/kg over 3-5 minutes

Elderly, debilitated, neurosurgical, or ASA III or IV patients: Use similar doses to healthy adults; avoid rapid I.V. boluses

Maintenance:

Adults, ASA I or II, <55 years: I.V. infusion using variable rates (preferred over intermittent boluses): 25-75 mcg/kg/minute; incremental bolus doses: 10 mg or 20 mg

Elderly, debilitated, neurosurgical, or ASA III or IV patients: Use 80% of healthy adult dose; **do not** use rapid bolus doses (single or repeated)

ICU sedation in intubated mechanically ventilated patients: Avoid rapid bolus injection; individualize dose and titrate to response

Adults: Continuous infusion: Initial: 0.3 mg/kg/hour; increase by 0.3-0.6 mg/kg/hour every 5-10 minutes until desired sedation level is achieved; usual maintenance: 0.3-3 mg/kg/hour or higher; reduce dose by 80% in elderly, debilitated, and ASA III or IV patients; reduce dose after adequate sedation established and adjust to response (ie, evaluate frequently to use minimum dose for sedation)

Administration Parenteral: I.V.: Shake injection well before use; administer pediatric induction doses over 20-30 seconds; do not administer via filter with <5-micron pore size

Monitoring Parameters Respiratory rate, blood pressure, heart rate, oxygen saturation, ABGs, depth of sedation; serum lipids or triglycerides with use >24 hours

Nursing Implications May change urine color to green

Additional Information Due to poor water solubility, the I.V. formulation is an isotonic oil-in-water emulsion and contains soybean oil, glycerol, egg lecithin, and sodium hydroxide (for pH adjustment); the brand name and generic product differ in the preservative used; Diprivan® contains 0.005% disodium edetate, while the generic product contains sodium metabisulfite (0.25 mg/mL); propofol injection contains ~0.1 g of fat/mL (1.1 kcal/mL)

(Continued)

Propofol *(Continued)*

Dosage Forms

Injection, emulsion: 10 mg/mL (20 mL, 50 mL, 100 mL) [contains EDTA, egg yolk phospholipid, sodium metabisulfite, and soybean oil]

Diprivan®: 10 mg/mL (20 mL, 50 mL, 100 mL) [contains EDTA, egg lecithin, and soybean oil]

References

Bray RJ, "Fatal Myocardial Failure Associated With a Propofol Infusion in a Child," *Anaesthesia*, 1995, 50(1):94.

Parke TJ, Stevens JE, Rice ASC, et al, "Metabolic Acidosis and Fatal Myocardial Failure After Propofol Infusion in Children: Five Case Reports," *BMJ*, 1992, 305(6854):613-6.

Strickland RA and Murray MJ, "Fatal Metabolic Acidosis in a Pediatric Patient Receiving an Infusion of Propofol in the Intensive Care Unit: Is There a Relationship?" *Crit Care Med*, 1995, 23(2):405-9.

Propoxyphene *(proe POKS i feen)*

Related Information

Overdose and Toxicology *on page 1388*

U.S. Brand Names Darvon®; Darvon-N®

Canadian Brand Names 642® Tablet

Synonyms Dextropropoxyphene

Therapeutic Category Analgesic, Narcotic

Generic Available Yes (capsule)

Use Management of mild to moderate pain

Restrictions C-IV

Pregnancy Risk Factor C (D if used for prolonged periods)

Contraindications Hypersensitivity to propoxyphene or any component

Warnings Do not exceed recommended dosage; abrupt discontinuation after prolonged use may result in withdrawal symptoms

Precautions Use with caution in patients with renal or hepatic dysfunction, or when substituting propoxyphene for opiates in narcotic dependent patients; reduce dose in patients with hepatic dysfunction; avoid use in patients with Cl_{cr} <10 mL/minute

Adverse Reactions

Central nervous system: Dizziness, lightheadedness, sedation, paradoxical excitement and insomnia, headache

Dermatologic: Rashes

Gastrointestinal: GI upset, nausea, vomiting, constipation

Hepatic: Elevated liver enzymes

Neuromuscular & skeletal: Weakness

Miscellaneous: Psychologic and physical dependence

Drug Interactions Cytochrome P450 isoenzyme CYP2C9, CYP2D6, CYP3A3/4, and CYP3A5-7 inhibitor

CNS depressants, alcohol, MAO inhibitors, may potentiate adverse effects; propoxyphene may inhibit the metabolism and increase the serum concentrations of carbamazepine, phenobarbital, tricyclic antidepressants, and warfarin; concurrent use of propoxyphene with ritonavir is not recommended

Food Interactions Food may decrease rate of absorption, but may slightly increase bioavailability

Mechanism of Action Binds to opiate receptors in the CNS, causing inhibition of ascending pain pathways, altering the perception of and response to pain; produces generalized CNS depression

Pharmacodynamics

Onset of action: Oral: Within 30-60 minutes

Duration: 4-6 hours

Pharmacokinetics

Metabolism: In the liver to an active metabolite (norpropoxyphene) and inactive metabolites

Bioavailability: Oral: 30% to 70% due to first-pass effect

Half-life, adults: 8-24 hours (mean: ~15 hours)

Norpropoxyphene, adults: 34 hours

Dialysis: Not dialyzable (0% to 5%)

Usual Dosage Oral:

Children: Dose not well established; doses of propoxyphene hydrochloride of 2-3 mg/kg/day divided every 6 hours have been used

Adults:

Hydrochloride: 65 mg every 3-4 hours as needed for pain; maximum dose: 390 mg/day

Napsylate: 100 mg every 4 hours as needed for pain; maximum dose: 600 mg/day

Dosing adjustment in renal impairment: Cl_{cr} <10 mL/minute: Avoid use

Dosing adjustment in hepatic impairment: Reduced doses should be used

Administration Oral: May administer with food to decrease GI upset

Monitoring Parameters Pain relief, respiratory rate, blood pressure, mental status; liver enzymes with long-term use

Test Interactions False-positive methadone test

Patient Information Avoid alcohol; may be habit-forming; avoid abrupt discontinuation after prolonged use; may cause dizziness or drowsiness and impair ability to perform activities requiring mental alertness or physical coordination

Additional Information Propoxyphene does not possess any anti-inflammatory or antipyretic actions; it possesses little, if any, antitussive effects; propoxyphene napsylate 100 mg is equivalent to 65 mg of propoxyphene hydrochloride; several cases utilizing propoxyphene in children for opioid detoxification have been reported (see References)

Dosage Forms

Capsule, as **hydrochloride** (Darvon®): 65 mg

Tablet, as **napsylate** (Darvon-N®): 100 mg

References

Hasday JD and Weintraub M, "Propoxyphene in Children With Iatrogenic Morphine Dependence," *Am J Dis Child,* 1983, 137(8):745-8.

Propoxyphene and Acetaminophen

(proe POKS i feen & a seet a MIN oh fen)

Related Information

Narcotic Analgesics Comparison *on page 1223*

Overdose and Toxicology *on page 1388*

U.S. Brand Names Darvocet-N® 50; Darvocet-N® 100

Synonyms Acetaminophen and Propoxyphene

Therapeutic Category Analgesic, Narcotic

Generic Available Yes

Use Management of mild to moderate pain

Restrictions C-IV

Pregnancy Risk Factor C

Contraindications Hypersensitivity to propoxyphene, acetaminophen, or any component

Warnings Do not exceed recommended dosage; abrupt discontinuation after prolonged use may result in withdrawal symptoms

Precautions Use with caution in patients with renal or hepatic dysfunction or when substituting propoxyphene for opiates in narcotic dependent patients

Adverse Reactions

Propoxyphene:

Central nervous system: Dizziness, lightheadedness, sedation, paradoxical excitement, insomnia, headache

Dermatologic: Rashes

Gastrointestinal: GI upset, nausea, vomiting, constipation

Hepatic: Elevated liver enzymes

Neuromuscular & skeletal: Weakness

Miscellaneous: Psychologic and physical dependence

Acetaminophen:

Dermatologic: Rash

Hematologic: Blood dyscrasias (neutropenia, pancytopenia, leukopenia)

Hepatic: Hepatic necrosis with overdose

Renal: Renal injury with chronic use

Miscellaneous: Hypersensitivity reactions (rare)

Drug Interactions See Propoxyphene *on page 950* and Acetaminophen *on page 36*

Food Interactions Food may decrease rate of absorption of propoxyphene, but may slightly increase bioavailability; the rate of absorption of acetaminophen may be decreased when given with food high in carbohydrates

Pharmacodynamics See individual monographs for Propoxyphene *on page 950* and Acetaminophen *on page 36*

Pharmacokinetics See individual monographs for Propoxyphene *on page 950* and Acetaminophen *on page 36*

Usual Dosage Adults: Oral:

Darvocet-N® 50: 1-2 tablets every 4 hours as needed; maximum: 600 mg propoxyphene napsylate/day

Darvocet-N® 100: 1 tablet every 4 hours as needed; maximum: 600 mg propoxyphene napsylate/day

Administration Oral: Administer with water on an empty stomach; may administer with food to decrease GI upset

(Continued)

Propoxyphene and Acetaminophen *(Continued)*

Monitoring Parameters Pain relief, respiratory rate, blood pressure, mental status; liver enzymes with long-term use

Test Interactions False-positive methadone test

Patient Information Avoid alcohol; may be habit-forming; avoid abrupt discontinuation after prolonged use; may cause dizziness or drowsiness and impair ability to perform activities requiring mental alertness or physical coordination

Additional Information Propoxyphene napsylate 100 mg is equivalent to 65 mg of propoxyphene hydrochloride; Wygesic® tablets were discontinued in May 2001

Dosage Forms
  Tablet: Propoxyphene **hydrochloride** 65 mg and acetaminophen 650 mg; propoxyphene **napsylate** 100 mg and acetaminophen 650 mg
  Darvocet-N® 50: Propoxyphene **napsylate** 50 mg and acetaminophen 325 mg
  Darvocet-N® 100: Propoxyphene **napsylate** 100 mg and acetaminophen 650 mg

Propranolol *(proe PRAN oh lole)*

Related Information
  Carbohydrate and Alcohol Content of Liquid Medications for Use in Patients Receiving Ketogenic Diets *on page 1431*
  Overdose and Toxicology *on page 1388*

U.S. Brand Names Inderal®; Inderal® LA; Propranolol Intensol™

Canadian Brand Names Apo®-Propranolol; Nu-Propranolol

Therapeutic Category Antianginal Agent; Antiarrhythmic Agent, Class II; Antihypertensive Agent; Antimigraine Agent; Beta-Adrenergic Blocker

Generic Available Yes (except capsule)

Use Management of hypertension, angina pectoris, pheochromocytoma, essential tremor, tetralogy of Fallot cyanotic spells, and arrhythmias (such as atrial fibrillation and flutter, A-V nodal re-entrant tachycardias, and catecholamine-induced arrhythmias); prevention of MI, migraine headache; symptomatic treatment of hypertrophic subaortic stenosis; short-term adjunctive therapy of thyrotoxicosis

Pregnancy Risk Factor C

Contraindications Hypersensitivity to propranolol or any component; uncompensated CHF, cardiogenic shock, bradycardia or heart block, asthma, hyperactive airway disease, chronic obstructive lung disease, Raynaud's syndrome

Warnings In patients with angina pectoris, exacerbation of angina and, in some cases, MI occurred following abrupt discontinuance of therapy; hypoglycemia may occur, particularly in infants and children (whether the patient has diabetes mellitus or not), especially during fasting before surgery; hypoglycemia may also occur after prolonged physical exertion and in patients with renal dysfunction

Precautions Propranolol may block hypoglycemia-induced tachycardia and blood pressure changes, use with caution in patients with diabetes mellitus; acute elevations in blood pressure have been reported after insulin-induced hypoglycemia in patients receiving propranolol; use with caution in patients with renal or hepatic dysfunction; avoid I.V. use in patients receiving calcium channel blockers (eg, verapamil) (effects may be potentiated); patients receiving beta blockers who have a history of anaphylactic reactions, may be more reactive to a repeated allergen challenge and may not be responsive to the usual epinephrine doses used to treat an allergic reaction

Adverse Reactions
  Cardiovascular: Hypotension, impaired myocardial contractility, CHF, bradycardia, worsening of A-V conduction disturbances
  Central nervous system: Lightheadedness, insomnia, vivid dreams, lethargy, depression
  Endocrine & metabolic: Hypoglycemia [also blunts warning signs of hypoglycemia (eg, tachycardia)], hyperglycemia
  Gastrointestinal: Nausea, vomiting, diarrhea, GI distress
  Hematologic: Agranulocytosis
  Neuromuscular & skeletal: Weakness
  Respiratory: Bronchospasm
  Miscellaneous: Cold extremities

Drug Interactions Cytochrome P450 isoenzyme CYP1A2, CYP2C18, CYP2C19, and CYP2D6 substrate
  Phenobarbital, rifampin may increase propranolol clearance and may decrease its activity; cimetidine may reduce propranolol clearance and may increase its effects; aluminum-containing antacid may reduce GI absorption of propranolol; flecainide, hydralazine, quinidine, verapamil may increase cardiovascular adverse effects; abrupt withdrawal of clonidine while receiving beta-blockers may result in an exaggerated hypertensive crisis

Food Interactions Avoid natural licorice (causes sodium and water retention and increases potassium loss); protein-rich foods may increase bioavailability; a change in diet from high carbohydrate/low protein to low carbohydrate/high protein may result in increased oral clearance

Stability Injection is compatible in D_5W, NS, D_5/NS, $D_5/^1/_2NS$, $^1/_2NS$, LR; incompatible with bicarbonate; protect injection from light

Mechanism of Action Nonselective beta-adrenergic blocker (class II antiarrhythmic); competitively blocks response to beta$_1$ and beta$_2$-adrenergic stimulation which results in decrease in heart rate, myocardial contractility, blood pressure, and myocardial oxygen demand

Pharmacodynamics Beta blockade: Oral:
  Onset of action: Within 1-2 hours
  Duration: ~6 hours

Pharmacokinetics
  Distribution: V_d: Adults: 3.9 L/kg; crosses the placenta; small amounts appear in breast milk
  Protein-binding (Alpha$_1$-acid glycoprotein and albumin):
    Newborns: 60% to 68%
    Adults: 93%
  Metabolism: Extensive first-pass effect, metabolized in the liver to active and inactive compounds
  Bioavailability: 30% to 40%; oral bioavailability may be increased in Down syndrome children
  Half-life (prolonged with hepatic dysfunction):
    Neonates and Infants: Possible increased half-life
    Children: 3.9-6.4 hours
    Adults: 4-6 hours
  Elimination: Metabolites are excreted primarily in urine (96% to 99%); <1% excreted in urine as unchanged drug
  Dialysis: Not dialyzable: (0% to 5%)

Usual Dosage
  Neonates:
    Oral: Initial: 0.25 mg/kg/dose every 6-8 hours; increase slowly as needed to maximum of 5 mg/kg/day
    I.V.: Initial: 0.01 mg/kg slow I.V. push over 10 minutes; may repeat every 6-8 hours as needed; increase slowly to maximum of 0.15 mg/kg/dose every 6-8 hours
  Arrhythmias:
    Oral:
      Children: Initial: 0.5-1 mg/kg/day in divided doses every 6-8 hours; titrate dosage upward every 3-5 days; usual dose: 2-4 mg/kg/day; higher doses may be needed; do not exceed 16 mg/kg/day or 60 mg/day
      Adults: Initial: 10-20 mg/dose every 6-8 hours, increase gradually; usual range: 40-320 mg/day
    I.V.:
      Children: 0.01-0.1 mg/kg slow I.V. over 10 minutes; maximum dose: 1 mg (infants); 3 mg (children)
      Adults: 1 mg/dose slow I.V.; repeat every 5 minutes up to a total of 5 mg
  Hypertension: Oral:
      Children: Initial: 0.5-1 mg/kg/day in divided doses every 6-12 hours; increase gradually every 3-5 days; usual dose: 1-5 mg/kg/day; maximum dose: 8 mg/kg/day
      Adults: Initial: 40 mg twice daily or 60-80 mg once daily as sustained release capsules; increase dosage every 3-5 days; usual dose: ≤320 mg divided in 2-3 doses/day or once daily as sustained release; maximum daily dose: 640 mg
  Migraine headache prophylaxis: Oral:
      Children: 0.6-1.5 mg/kg/day divided every 8 hours; maximum dose: 4 mg/kg/day **or**
        ≤35 kg: 10-20 mg 3 times/day
        >35 kg: 20-40 mg 3 times/day
      Adults: Initial: 80 mg divided every 6-8 hours (or once daily as sustained release capsule); increase by 20-40 mg/dose every 3-4 weeks to a maximum of 160-240 mg/day given in divided doses every 6-8 hours (or once daily as sustained release capsules)
  Tetralogy spells: Infants and Children:
      Oral: Usual: 1-2 mg/kg/dose every 6 hours, may initiate at $^1/_2$ the usual dose; may increase by 1 mg/kg/day every 24 hours to maximum of 5 mg/kg/day; if refractory may increase slowly to a maximum of 10-15 mg/kg/day but must carefully monitor heart rate, heart size, and cardiac contractility (Garson, 1981).
      I.V.: 0.15-0.25 mg/kg/dose slow I.V.; may repeat in 15 minutes
(Continued)

Propranolol *(Continued)*

Thyrotoxicosis:

Neonates: Oral: 2 mg/kg/day in divided doses every 6-12 hours; occasionally higher doses may be required

Adolescents and Adults: Oral: 10-40 mg/dose every 6 hours

Adults: I.V.: 1-3 mg/dose slow I.V. as a single dose

Administration

Oral: Administer with food; do not chew or crush sustained release capsules, swallow whole; mix concentrated oral solution with water, fruit juice, liquid, or semisolid food before administration

Parenteral: I.V. administration should not exceed 1 mg/minute; administer slow I.V. over 10 minutes in children; maximum concentration for injection: 1 mg/mL

Monitoring Parameters EKG, blood pressure

Reference Range Therapeutic: 50-100 ng/mL (SI: 190-390 nmol/L) at end of dosing interval

Patient Information Avoid alcohol; do not discontinue abruptly; may mask fast heart rate of hypoglycemia, but sweating will still occur

Nursing Implications The I.V. dose is much smaller than oral dose

Additional Information Not indicated for hypertensive emergencies; do not abruptly discontinue therapy, taper dosage gradually over 2 weeks

Dosage Forms

Capsule, sustained release, as hydrochloride (Inderal® LA): 60 mg, 80 mg, 120 mg, 160 mg

Injection, solution, as hydrochloride (Inderal®): 1 mg/mL (1 mL)

Solution, oral, as hydrochloride: 4 mg/mL (5 mL, 500 mL); 8 mg/mL (500 mL) [alcohol free; strawberry-mint flavor]

Solution, oral **concentrate**, as hydrochloride (Propranolol Intensol™): 80 mg/mL (30 mL)

Tablet, as hydrochloride (Inderal®): 10 mg, 20 mg, 40 mg, 60 mg, 80 mg

References

Garson A Jr, Gillette PC, and McNamara DG, "Propranolol: The Preferred Palliation for Tetralogy of Fallot," *Am J Cardiol*, 1981, 47(5):1098-104.

Lai CW, Ziegler DK, Lansky LL, et al, "Hemiplegic Migraine in Childhood: Diagnostic and Therapeutic Aspects," *J Pediatr*, 1982, 101(5):696-9.

Pickoff AS, Zies L, Ferrer PL, et al, "High-Dose Propranolol Therapy in the Management of Supraventricular Tachycardia," *J Pediatr*, 1979, 94(1):144-6.

Rasoulpour M and Marinelli KA, "Systemic Hypertension," *Clin Perinatol*, 1992, 19(1):121-37.

Sinaiko AR, "Pharmacologic Management of Childhood Hypertension," *Pediatr Clin North Am*, 1993, 40(1):195-212.

♦ **Propranolol Intensol™** *see* Propranolol *on page 952*

♦ **Propulsid®** *see* Cisapride *U.S. - Available Via Limited-Access Protocol Only on page 277*

♦ **2-Propylpentanoic Acid** *see* Valproic Acid and Derivatives *on page 1131*

Propylthiouracil *(proe pil thye oh YOOR a sil)*

Canadian Brand Names Propyl-Thyracil®

Synonyms PTU

Therapeutic Category Antithyroid Agent

Generic Available Yes

Use Palliative treatment of hyperthyroidism; adjunct to ameliorate hyperthyroidism in preparation for surgical treatment or radioactive iodine therapy; management of thyrotoxic crisis

Pregnancy Risk Factor D

Contraindications Hypersensitivity to propylthiouracil or any component

Warnings May cause agranulocytosis, thyroid hyperplasia, thyroid carcinoma (usage >1 year); discontinue in the presence of agranulocytosis, aplastic anemia, ANCA-positive vasculitis, hepatitis, unexplained fever, or exfoliative dermatitis

Precautions Use with caution in patients receiving other drugs known to cause agranulocytosis

Adverse Reactions

Cardiovascular: Edema, cutaneous vasculitis

Central nervous system: Drowsiness, vertigo, dizziness, headache, drug fever

Dermatologic: Rash, urticaria, pruritus, exfoliative dermatitis, alopecia, skin pigmentation

Gastrointestinal: Nausea, vomiting, ageusia, sialadenopathy, constipation

Hematologic: Agranulocytosis, leukopenia, thrombocytopenia, bleeding, hypoprothrombinemia

Hepatic: Jaundice, hepatitis

Neuromuscular & skeletal: Arthralgia, paresthesia, neuritis

Renal: Nephritis
Respiratory: Interstitial pneumonitis
Miscellaneous: Lymphadenopathy

Drug Interactions Anticoagulants (enhanced anticoagulant activity); correction of hyperthyroidism may alter the disposition of beta-blockers, digoxin, and theophylline, necessitating a dose reduction in these agents

Mechanism of Action Inhibits the synthesis of thyroid hormones by blocking the oxidation of iodine in the thyroid gland; blocks synthesis of thyroxine and triiodothyronine

Pharmacodynamics For significant therapeutic effects 24-36 hours are required; remission of hyperthyroidism usually does not occur before 4 months of continued therapy

Pharmacokinetics
Distribution: Breast milk to plasma ratio: 0.1
Protein binding: 75% to 80%
Metabolism: Hepatic
Bioavailability: 80% to 95%
Half-life: 1.5-5 hours
End-stage renal disease: 8.5 hours
Time to peak serum concentration: Oral: Within 1 hour; persists for 2-3 hours
Elimination: 35% excreted in urine

Usual Dosage Oral:
Neonates: 5-10 mg/kg/day in divided doses every 8 hours
Children: 5-7 mg/kg/day in divided doses every 8 hours **or**
6-10 years: 50-150 mg/day divided every 8 hours
≥10 years: 150-300 mg/day divided every 8 hours
Maintenance: $1/3$-$2/3$ of the initial dose in divided doses every 8-12 hours; this begins usually after 2 months on an effective initial dosage
Adults: Initial: 300-450 mg/day in divided doses every 8 hours (doses of 600-1200 mg/day are sometimes needed); maintenance: 100-150 mg/day in divided doses every 8-12 hours

Dosing adjustment in renal impairment: Adjustment is not necessary

Administration Oral: Administer with food

Monitoring Parameters CBC with differential, liver function tests, platelets, thyroid function tests (TSH, T_3, T_4), prothrombin time

Reference Range See normal values for thyroid function in Normal Laboratory Values for Children on page 1353

Patient Information Do not exceed prescribed dosage; take at regular intervals around-the-clock; notify physician or pharmacist if fever, sore throat, unusual bleeding or bruising, headache, or general malaise occurs

Dosage Forms Tablet: 50 mg

Extemporaneous Preparations A 5 mg/mL oral suspension may be made by crushing twenty 50 mg propylthiouracil tablets; add by geometric proportions 1:1 mixture of Ora-Plus® and Ora-Sweet® to a final volume of 200 mL; stable 91 days at 4°C and 70 days at 25°C

Nahata MC, Morosco RS, and Trowbridge JM, "Stability of Propylthiouracil in Extemporaneously Prepared Oral Suspensions at 4 and 25 Degrees C," *Am J Health Syst Pharm*, 2000, 57(12):1141-3.

References
Raby C, Lagorce JF, Jambut-Absil AC, et al, "The Mechanism of Action of Synthetic Antithyroid Drugs: Iodine Complexation During Oxidation of Iodide," *Endocrinology*, 1990, 126(3):1683-91.

♦ **Propyl-Thyracil® (Can)** see Propylthiouracil on page 954
♦ **2-Propylvaleric Acid** see Valproic Acid and Derivatives on page 1131
♦ **Prostaglandin E₁** see Alprostadil on page 66
♦ **Prostigmin®** see Neostigmine on page 805
♦ **Prostin VR Pediatric®** see Alprostadil on page 66

Protamine (PROE ta meen)

Therapeutic Category Antidote, Heparin

Generic Available Yes

Use Treatment of heparin overdosage; neutralize heparin during surgery or dialysis procedures

Pregnancy Risk Factor C

Contraindications Hypersensitivity to protamine or any component

Warnings Heparin rebound associated with anticoagulation and bleeding has been reported to occur occasionally; symptoms typically occur 8-9 hours after protamine administration, but may occur as long as 18 hours later
(Continued)

Protamine *(Continued)*

Precautions Use with caution in patients allergic to fish, with prior history of vasectomy, patients receiving protamine-containing insulin or previous protamine therapy

Adverse Reactions

Cardiovascular: Hypotension, bradycardia, flushing, pulmonary hypertension

Central nervous system: Lassitude

Gastrointestinal: Nausea, vomiting

Neuromuscular & skeletal: Back pain

Respiratory: Dyspnea

Miscellaneous: Hypersensitivity reactions

Stability Refrigerate; stable for at least 2 weeks at room temperature

Mechanism of Action Combines with strongly acidic heparin to form a stable complex (salt) neutralizing the anticoagulant activity of both drugs

Pharmacodynamics Onset of action: Heparin neutralization occurs within 5 minutes following I.V. injection

Pharmacokinetics Elimination: Unknown

Usual Dosage I.V.: Protamine dosage is determined by the most recent dosage of heparin or low molecular weight heparin (LMWH); 1 mg of protamine neutralizes 90 USP units of heparin (lung), 115 USP units of heparin (intestinal), and 1 mg (100 units) LMWH; maximum dose: 50 mg

Heparin overdosage: Since blood heparin concentrations decrease rapidly **after** heparin administration, adjust the protamine dosage depending upon the duration of time since heparin administration as follows (see table):

Time Since Last Heparin Dose (min)	Dose of Protamine (mg) to Neutralize 100 units of Heparin
<30	1
30-60	0.5-0.75
60-120	0.375-0.5
>120	0.25-0.375

If heparin is administered by deep S.C. injection, use 1-1.5 mg protamine per 100 units heparin; this may be done by administering a portion of the dose (eg, 25-50 mg) slowly I.V. followed by the remaining portion as a continuous infusion over 8-16 hours (the expected absorption time of the S.C. heparin dose)

LMWH overdosage: If most recent LMWH dose has been administered within the last 4 hours, use 1 mg protamine per 1 mg (100 units) LMWH; a second dose of 0.5 mg protamine per 1 mg (100 units) LMWH may be given if APTT remains prolonged 2-4 hours after the first dose

Administration Parenteral: Reconstitute vial with 5 mL SWI; if using protamine in neonates, reconstitute with preservative free SWI; resulting solution equals 10 mg/mL; inject without further dilution over 10 minutes not to exceed 5 mg/minute; maximum of 50 mg in any 10-minute period

Monitoring Parameters Coagulation tests, APTT or ACT, cardiac monitor, and blood pressure monitor required during administration

Dosage Forms Injection, solution, as sulfate [preservative free]: 10 mg/mL (5 mL, 25 mL)

References

Monagle P, Michelson AD, Bovill E, et al, "Antithrombic Therapy in Children," *Chest*, 2001, 119:344S-70S.

♦ **Protein C (Activated), Human Recombinant** *see* Drotrecogin Alfa (Activated) *on page 420*

Protirelin *(proe TYE re lin)*

U.S. Brand Names Thyrel® TRH

Canadian Brand Names Relefact® TRH

Synonyms Lopremone

Therapeutic Category Diagnostic Agent, Thyroid Function

Generic Available No

Use Adjunct in the diagnostic assessment of thyroid function, and an adjunct to other diagnostic procedures in assessment of patients with pituitary or hypothalamic dysfunction; also causes release of prolactin from the pituitary and is used to detect defective control of prolactin secretion.

Pregnancy Risk Factor C

Contraindications Hypersensitivity to protirelin or any component

Warnings Due to transient changes in blood pressure (both increases and decreases), monitor blood pressure frequently during and at frequent intervals during first 15

minutes after administration; patient should be supine before, during, and immediately after administration; do not administer to patients in whom marked changes in blood pressure may cause serious risk

Precautions Thyroid hormones reduce TSH response to protirelin; when using diagnostically, discontinue thyroid hormones (liothyronine 7 days prior to testing and levothyroxine 14 days prior to testing); do not discontinue thyroid hormones when using protirelin to evaluate the effectiveness of thyroid suppression by thyroid hormone in patients with nodular or diffuse goiter or for an adjustment of thyroid hormone dosage in primary hypothyroidism

Adverse Reactions

Cardiovascular: Marked changes in blood pressure (hypotension or hypertension), flushing, chest tightness

Central nervous system: Lightheadedness, anxiety, seizures (rare), drowsiness, headache

Endocrine & metabolic: Breast enlargement

Gastrointestinal: Nausea, dysgeusia, abdominal discomfort, xerostomia

Genitourinary: Urinary frequency

Miscellaneous: Diaphoresis

Drug Interactions Aspirin in therapeutic doses, pharmacologic doses of steroids, levodopa, and thyroid hormones reduce TSH response to protirelin

Mechanism of Action Increases release of thyroid stimulating hormone (TSH) and prolactin from the anterior pituitary

Pharmacodynamics Maximum TSH levels occur in 20-30 minutes; TSH returns to baseline after about 3 hours

Pharmacokinetics Mean plasma half-life: 5 minutes

Usual Dosage I.V.:

Infants and Children: 7 mcg/kg to a maximum dose of 500 mcg

Adults: 500 mcg (range 200-500 mcg)

Administration Parenteral: Administer undiluted direct I.V. over 15-30 seconds with the patient remaining supine for an additional 15 minutes (see Warnings)

Monitoring Parameters Blood pressure, prolactin, TSH (drawn immediately prior to injection and 30 minutes after), T_4, and T_3

Reference Range

Characterization Based on Serum TSH Levels at Baseline and 30 Minutes After Protirelin

	Baseline Serum TSH (μU/mL)	Change of Serum TSH (μU/mL) at 30 minutes
Euthyroidism (normal thyroid function)	≤10 (usually ≤6); 20% have <1.5 μU/mL)	≥2 (usually 6-30)
Hyperthyroidism	≤10 (usually ≤4)	<2
Primary Hypothyroidism (Thyroidal)	>10 (usually 15-100)	≥2 (usually ≥20)
Secondary Hypothyroidism (Pituitary)	≤10 (usually ≤6)	<2 (59%) 2-50 (41%)
Tertiary Hypothyroidism (Hypoalamic)	≤10 (often <2)	≥2

Patient Information May cause dry mouth; fast or eat low fat meal before test

Nursing Implications Keep patient supine during drug administration; have patient urinate prior to administration

Additional Information TSH response is reduced by repetitive protirelin administration; do not repeat test for at least 7 days

Dosage Forms Injection, solution: 500 mcg/mL (1 mL)

♦ **Prozac® Weekly™** *see* Fluoxetine *on page 505*
♦ **Prudoxin™** *see* Doxepin *on page 411*

Pseudoephedrine (soo doe e FED rin)

Related Information
　OTC Cough & Cold Preparations, Pediatric *on page 1225*
U.S. Brand Names Biofed [OTC]; Decofed® [OTC]; Dimetapp® 12-Hour Non-Drowsy Extentabs® [OTC]; Dimetapp® Decongestant [OTC]; Dimetapp® Decongestant Infant Drops; Genaphed® [OTC]; Kidkare Decongestant [OTC]; Kodet SE [OTC]; Oranyl [OTC]; PediaCare® Decongestant, Infants [OTC]; Silfedrine®, Children's [OTC]; Sudafed® [OTC]; Sudafed® 12 Hour [OTC]; Sudafed® 24 Hour [OTC]; Sudafed®, Children's [OTC]; Sudodrin [OTC]; Triaminic® Allergy Congestion [OTC]
Canadian Brand Names Balminil® Decongestant; Contac® Cold 12 Hour Relief Non Drowsy; Drixoral® ND; Eltor®; PMS-Pseudoephedrine; Pseudofrin; Robidrine®
Synonyms *d*-Isoephedrine
Therapeutic Category Adrenergic Agonist Agent; Decongestant; Sympathomimetic
Generic Available Yes (syrup and tablet)
Use Temporary symptomatic relief of nasal congestion due to common cold, upper respiratory allergies, and sinusitis; also promotes nasal or sinus drainage
Pregnancy Risk Factor C
Contraindications Hypersensitivity to pseudoephedrine or any component; MAO inhibitor therapy, severe hypertension, severe coronary artery disease
Warnings Some products contain sodium benzoate; benzoic acid (benzoate) is a metabolite of benzyl alcohol; large amounts of benzyl alcohol (≥99 mg/kg/day) have been associated with a potentially fatal toxicity ("gasping syndrome") in neonates; *in vitro* and animal studies have shown that benzoate displaces bilirubin from protein binding sites; avoid use of sodium benzoate containing products in neonates
Precautions Use with caution in patients with hyperthyroidism, diabetes mellitus, prostatic hypertrophy, mild-moderate hypertension, arrhythmias. Chewable tablets contain phenylalanine; avoid or use with caution in patients with phenylketonuria.
Adverse Reactions
　Cardiovascular: Tachycardia, palpitations, arrhythmias
　Central nervous system: Nervousness, excitability, dizziness, insomnia, drowsiness, headache, seizures, hallucinations
　Gastrointestinal: Nausea, vomiting
　Neuromuscular & skeletal: Tremor, weakness
　Miscellaneous: Diaphoresis
Drug Interactions Additive effects with other sympathomimetics; hypertensive crisis with MAO inhibitors; phenothiazines and tricyclic antidepressants potentiate pressor effects; propranolol (beta-blockers)
Mechanism of Action Directly stimulates alpha-adrenergic receptors of respiratory mucosa causing vasoconstriction; directly stimulates beta-adrenergic receptors causing bronchial relaxation, increased heart rate and contractility
Pharmacodynamics
　Onset of action: Oral: Decongestant effects occur within 15-30 minutes
　Duration: 4-6 hours (up to 12 hours with extended release formulation administration)
Pharmacokinetics
　Distribution: Children: V_d: 2.4-2.6 L/kg; breast milk to plasma ratio: 2.6-3.3
　Metabolism: Incomplete in the liver to inactive metabolite
　Half-life:
　　Children 3.1 hours
　　Adults: 9-16 hours
　Elimination: 55% to 75% of dose excreted unchanged in urine
　　Clearance:
　　　Children: 9.2-10.3 mL/minute/kg
　　　Adults: 7.3-7.6 mL/minute/kg
Usual Dosage Oral:
　Children:
　　<2 years: 4 mg/kg/day in divided doses every 6 hours
　　2-5 years: 15 mg every 6 hours; maximum dose: 60 mg/24 hours
　　6-12 years: 30 mg every 6 hours; maximum dose: 120 mg/24 hours
　Children >12 years and Adults: 60 mg every 6 hours; maximum dose: 240 mg/day; using extended release products: 120 mg every 12 hours or 240 mg once daily
Administration Oral: Administer with water or milk to decrease GI distress; swallow timed release tablets or capsules whole, do not chew or crush
Test Interactions False-positive test for amphetamines by EMIT assay
Dosage Forms
　Gelcap (Dimetapp® Decongestant): 30 mg

Liquid, as hydrochloride:
Children's Silfedrine®: 15 mg/5 mL (120 mL, 480 mL) [alcohol and sugar free; grape flavor]
Children's Sudafed®: 15 mg/5 mL (120 mL) [alcohol and sugar free; contains sodium benzoate; grape flavor]
Triaminic® Allergy Congestion: 15 mg/5 mL (120 mL) [contains benzoic acid]
Solution, oral **drops**, as hydrochloride:
Dimetapp® Decongestant Infant Drops: 7.5 mg/0.8 mL (15 mL) [alcohol free]
Kidkare Decongestant: 7.5 mg/0.8 mL (30 mL)
Infants PediaCare® Decongestant: 7.5 mg/0.8 mL (15 mL) [contains benzoic acid and sodium benzoate; fruit flavor]
Syrup, as hydrochloride: 30 mg/5 mL (120 mL, 480 mL)
Biofed: 30 mg/5 mL (120 mL, 240 mL, 480 mL, 3840 mL) [alcohol free; contains sodium benzoate]
Decofed®: 30 mg/5 mL (120 mL, 480 mL) [raspberry flavor]
Tablet, as hydrochloride: 30 mg, 60 mg
Genaphed®, Kodet SE, Oranyl, Sudafed®, Sudodrin: 30 mg
Tablet, chewable, as hydrochloride:
Children's Sudafed®: 15 mg [sugar free; contains 0.78 mg phenylalanine (as aspartame)/tablet; orange flavor]
Triaminic® Allergy Congestion: 15 mg [contains 17.6 mg phenylalanine (as aspartame)/tablet]
Tablet, extended release, as hydrochloride:
Dimetapp® 12-Hour Non-Drowsy Extentabs®: 120 mg
Sudafed® 12 Hour: 120 mg
Sudafed® 24 Hour: 240 mg

References
Simons FE, Gu X, Watson WT, et al, "Pharmacokinetics of the Orally Administered Decongestants Pseudoephedrine and Phenylpropanolamine in Children," *J Pediatr*, 1996, 129(5):729-34.

♦ **Pseudoephedrine and Brompheniramine** *see* Brompheniramine and Pseudoephedrine *on page 182*

♦ **Pseudoephedrine and Carbinoxamine** *see* Carbinoxamine and Pseudoephedrine *on page 214*

♦ **Pseudoephedrine and Triprolidine** *see* Triprolidine and Pseudoephedrine *on page 1122*

♦ **Pseudofrin (Can)** *see* Pseudoephedrine *on page 958*

♦ **Pseudomonic Acid A** *see* Mupirocin *on page 783*

♦ **Psorigel® [OTC]** *see* Coal Tar *on page 299*

Psyllium (SIL i yum)

U.S. Brand Names Fiberall®; Genfiber® [OTC]; Hydrocil® [OTC]; Konsyl® [OTC]; Konsyl-D® [OTC]; Konsyl® Easy Mix [OTC]; Konsyl® Orange [OTC]; Metamucil® [OTC]; Metamucil® Smooth Texture [OTC]; Modane® Bulk [OTC]; Perdium Fiber® Therapy [OTC]; Reguloid® [OTC]; Serutan® [OTC]
Canadian Brand Names Novo-Mucilax
Synonyms Plantago Seed; Plantain Seed; Psyllium Hydrophilic Mucilloid
Therapeutic Category Laxative, Bulk-Producing
Generic Available Yes (powder)
Use Treatment of chronic atonic or spastic constipation and in constipation associated with rectal disorders; management of irritable bowel syndrome; adjunctive treatment with low cholesterol and saturated fat diet to reduce risk of coronary artery disease
Pregnancy Risk Factor B
Contraindications Hypersensitivity to psyllium or any component; fecal impaction, GI obstruction
Warnings Inhalation of psyllium powder may produce allergic reactions in susceptible individuals
Precautions Use with caution in patients with esophageal strictures, ulcers, stenosis, or intestinal adhesions. Products may contain aspartame which is metabolized to phenylalanine and must be avoided (or used with caution) in patients with phenylketonuria.
Adverse Reactions
Gastrointestinal: Esophageal or bowel obstruction, diarrhea, constipation, abdominal cramps
Respiratory: Bronchospasm
Miscellaneous: Rhinoconjunctivitis, anaphylaxis upon inhalation in susceptible individuals
Drug Interactions Decreased effect of warfarin, digitalis, potassium-sparing diuretics, salicylates, tetracyclines, nitrofurantoin
(Continued)

Psyllium *(Continued)*

Mechanism of Action Adsorbs water in the intestine to form a viscous liquid which promotes peristalsis and reduces transit time

Pharmacodynamics
Onset of action: 12-24 hours
Maximum effect: May take 2-3 days

Pharmacokinetics Absorption: Oral: Generally not absorbed; small amounts of grain extract present in the preparation have been reportedly absorbed following colonic hydrolysis

Usual Dosage Oral (3.4 g psyllium hydrophilic mucilloid/7 g powder is equivalent to a rounded teaspoonful or 1 packet or 1 wafer):
Constipation:
Children 6-11 years: $1/2$-1 rounded teaspoonful in 4 oz glass of liquid 1-3 times/day
Adults: 1-2 rounded teaspoonfuls or 1-2 packets or 1-2 wafers 1-4 times/day; 5 capsules up to 3 times/day
Fiber supplementation: Children ≥12 years and Adults: 2-6 capsules up to 3 times/day

Administration Oral: Granules and powder must be mixed in an 8 ounce glass of water or juice; drink a 8 ounce glass of liquid with each dose of wafers or capsules

Monitoring Parameters Stool output and frequency

Patient Information Each dose must be taken with an 8 ounce glass of water; inadequate fluid intake may result in throat swelling and choking

Nursing Implications Inhalation of psyllium dust may cause sensitivity to psyllium (runny nose, watery eyes, wheezing)

Dosage Forms
Capsules (Metamucil®): 0.52 g [provides 3 g dietary fiber per 6 capsules]
Granules:
Perdiem Fiber® Therapy: 4 g/5 mL (250 g)
Serutan®: 2.5 g/5 mL (510 g) [contains sodium benzoate]
Powder: 3.4 g/dose (unit dose packets, 397 g)
Fiberall®: 3.54 g/dose (454 g) [sugar free; contains phenylalanine; orange flavor]
Genfiber®: 3.4 g/dose (397 g, 595 g) [regular and orange flavors]
Hydrocil® Instant: 3.5 g/dose (300 g)
Konsyl®: 6 g/dose (6 g unit dose packets, 300 g, 450 g) [sodium and sugar free; regular and orange flavors]
Konsyl-D®: 3.4 g/dose (6.5 unit dose packets, 325 g, 500 g)
Konsyl® Easy Mix: 6 g/dose (6 g unit dose packets, 250 g) [sodium and sugar free]
Konsyl® Orange: 3.4 g/dose (12 g unit dose packets, 425 g, 538 g) [contains sucrose]
Metamucil®: 3.4 g/dose (390 g, 570 g, 870 g, 1254 g) [regular or orange flavor]
Metamucil® Smooth Texture: 3.4 g/dose (unit dose packets, 609 g, 912 g, 1368 g) [orange flavor]
Metamucil® Smooth Texture: 3.4 g/dose (unit dose packets, 300 g, 450 g, 660 g, 699 g) [sugar free; contains 25 mg phenylalanine (as aspartame)/5 mL; regular or orange flavor]
Modane® Bulk: 3.4 g/dose (390 g)
Reguloid®: 3.4 g/dose (300 g, 390 g, 450 g, 570 g) [regular and orange flavor; also available sugar free]
Wafers (Metamucil®): 3.4 g/dose (24s) [apple crisp and cinnamon spice flavors]

♦ **Psyllium Hydrophilic Mucilloid** *see* Psyllium *on page 959*
♦ **P.T.E.-4®** *see* Trace Metals *on page 1106*
♦ **P.T.E.-5®** *see* Trace Metals *on page 1106*
♦ **Pteroylglutamic Acid** *see* Folic Acid *on page 516*
♦ **PTU** *see* Propylthiouracil *on page 954*
♦ **Pulmicort® Respules®** *see* Budesonide *on page 183*
♦ **Pulmicort® Turbuhaler®** *see* Budesonide *on page 183*
♦ **Pulmophylline (Can)** *see* Theophylline *on page 1076*
♦ **Pulmozyme®** *see* Dornase Alfa *on page 406*
♦ **Puralube® [OTC]** *see* Ocular Lubricant *on page 831*
♦ **Purge® [OTC]** *see* Castor Oil *on page 222*
♦ **Purinethol®** *see* Mercaptopurine *on page 720*
♦ **PVF® K (Can)** *see* Penicillin V Potassium *on page 877*

Pyrantel Pamoate *(pi RAN tel PAM oh ate)*

U.S. Brand Names Pin-X® [OTC]; Reese's® Pinworm Medicine [OTC]
Canadian Brand Names Combantrin™
Therapeutic Category Anthelmintic
Generic Available No

Use Roundworm (*Ascaris lumbricoides*), pinworm (*Enterobius vermicularis*), and hookworm (*Ancylostoma duodenale* and *Necator americanus*) infestations, and trichostrongyliasis

Pregnancy Risk Factor C

Contraindications Hypersensitivity to pyrantel pamoate or any component

Warnings Pin-X® contains sodium benzoate; benzoic acid (benzoate) is a metabolite of benzyl alcohol; large amounts of benzyl alcohol (≥99 mg/kg/day) have been associated with a potentially fatal toxicity ("gasping syndrome") in neonates; the "gasping syndrome" consists of metabolic acidosis, respiratory distress, gasping respirations, CNS dysfunction (including convulsions, intracranial hemorrhage), hypotension and cardiovascular collapse; avoid use of pyrantel pamoate products containing sodium benzoate in neonates; *in vitro* and animal studies have shown that benzoate displaces bilirubin from protein binding sites

Precautions Use with caution in patients with liver impairment, anemia, malnutrition

Adverse Reactions
Central nervous system: Dizziness, drowsiness, insomnia, headache, fever
Dermatologic: Rash
Gastrointestinal: Nausea, vomiting, anorexia, diarrhea, abdominal cramps, tenesmus
Hepatic: Elevated liver enzymes
Neuromuscular & skeletal: Weakness

Drug Interactions Piperazine (antagonist)

Stability Protect from light

Mechanism of Action Promotes release of acetylcholine and inhibits cholinesterase causing neuromuscular paralysis of susceptible helminths

Pharmacokinetics
Absorption: Oral: Poor
Metabolism: Undergoes partial hepatic metabolism
Time to peak serum concentration: Within 1-3 hours
Elimination: In feces (50% as unchanged drug) and urine (7% as unchanged drug)

Usual Dosage Children and Adults: Oral:
Roundworm, pinworm, or trichostrongyliasis: 11 mg/kg administered as a single dose; maximum dose: 1 g; dosage should be repeated after 2 weeks for pinworm infection
Hookworm: 11 mg/kg/day once daily for 3 days
Maximum daily dose: 1 g

Administration Oral: May mix drug with milk or fruit juice; may administer with or without food; shake suspension well before use

Monitoring Parameters Stool for presence of eggs, worms, and occult blood; serum AST and ALT

Patient Information Hygienic precaution is essential to prevent reinfection

Nursing Implications Fasting or purgation is not required prior to administration

Dosage Forms
Suspension, oral, as pamoate:
Pin-X®: 50 mg/mL (as pyrantel) (30 mL, 60 mL) [contains sodium benzoate; caramel flavor]
Reese's® Pinworm Medicine: 50 mg/mL (as pyrantel) (30 mL)
Tablet, as pamoate (Reese's® Pinworm Medicine): 62.5 mg (as pyrantel)

Pyrazinamide (peer a ZIN a mide)

Canadian Brand Names Tebrazid™

Synonyms Pyrazinoic Acid Amide

Therapeutic Category Antitubercular Agent

Generic Available Yes

Use In combination with other antituberculosis agents in the treatment of *Mycobacterium* tuberculosis infection (especially useful in disseminated and meningeal tuberculosis); CDC currently recommends a 3 or 4 multidrug regimen which includes pyrazinamide, rifampin, INH, and at times ethambutol or streptomycin for the treatment of tuberculosis

Pregnancy Risk Factor C

Contraindications Hypersensitivity to pyrazinamide or any component; severe hepatic damage

Warnings Two-month rifampin-pyrazinamide regimen for the treatment of latent tuberculosis infection has been associated with severe and fatal liver injuries. Pyrazinamide maximum dose is 20 mg/kg/day not to exceed 2 g/day in patients receiving the rifampin-pyrazinamide 2-month treatment regimen.

Precautions Use with caution in patients with renal failure, gout, diabetes mellitus, patients receiving concurrent medications associated with liver injury (particularly with rifampin), or in patients with a history of alcoholism
(Continued)

Pyrazinamide *(Continued)*

Adverse Reactions

Central nervous system: Malaise, fever

Dermatologic: Urticaria, rash, photosensitivity

Endocrine & metabolic: Gout, hyperuricemia

Gastrointestinal: Nausea, vomiting, anorexia, abdominal pain

Hepatic: Hepatotoxicity (increased incidence with doses >30 mg/kg/day), jaundice

Neuromuscular & skeletal: Arthralgia

Drug Interactions Isoniazid (decreased INH serum levels); combination therapy with rifampin has been associated with severe and fatal hepatotoxic reactions

Mechanism of Action Converted to pyrazinoic acid in susceptible strains of *Mycobacterium* which lowers the pH of the environment

Pharmacokinetics

Absorption: Oral: Well absorbed

Distribution: Widely distributed into body tissues and fluids including the liver, lung, and CSF

Protein binding: 50%

Metabolism: In the liver

Half-life: 9-10 hours, prolonged with reduced renal or hepatic function

Time to peak serum concentration: Within 2 hours

Elimination: In urine (4% as unchanged drug)

Usual Dosage Oral:

Infants, Children, and Adolescents: 20-40 mg/kg/day in divided doses every 12-24 hours for the first 2 months of active treatment; daily dose not to exceed 2 g; **or** daily pyrazinamide for 2 weeks followed by directly observed therapy of 50 mg/kg/ dose twice weekly to a maximum of 2 g/dose for 6 weeks

Adults: 15-30 mg/kg/day in 1-4 divided doses for the first 2 months of active treatment; maximum daily dose: 3 g/day; or daily pyrazinamide for 2 weeks followed by directly observed therapy of 50-70 mg/kg/dose twice weekly to a maximum of 4 g/ dose for 6 weeks

Monitoring Parameters Periodic liver function tests, serum uric acid

Patient Information Notify physician if fatigue, weakness, nausea, abdominal pain, jaundice, vomiting, or joint pain and swelling occur. May cause photosensitivity reactions (eg, exposure to sunlight may cause severe sunburn, skin rash, redness, or itching); avoid exposure to sunlight and artificial light sources (sunlamps, tanning booth/bed); wear protective clothing, wide-brimmed hats, sunglasses, and lip sunscreen (SPF ≥15); use a sunscreen [broad-spectrum sunscreen or physical sunscreen (preferred) or sunblock with SPF ≥15]; contact physician if reaction occurs.

Dosage Forms Tablet, scored: 500 mg

Extemporaneous Preparations

Pyrazinamide suspension can be compounded with simple syrup or 0.5% methylcellulose with simple syrup at a concentration of 100 mg/mL; the suspension is stable for 2 months at 4°C or 25°C when stored in glass or plastic bottles

To prepare pyrazinamide suspension in 0.5% methylcellulose with simple syrup: Crush 200 pyrazinamide 500 mg tablets and mix with a suspension containing 500 mL of 1% methylcellulose and 500 mL simple syrup. Add to this a suspension containing 140 crushed pyrazinamide tablets in 350 mL of 1% methylcellulose and 350 mL of simple syrup to make 1.7 L of suspension containing pyrazinamide 100 mg/mL in 0.5% methylcellulose with simple syrup.

Nahata MC, Morosco RS, and Peritre SP, "Stability of Pyrazinamide in Two Suspensions," *Am J Health-Syst Pharm*, 1995, 52:1558-60.

References

Ad Hoc Committee of the Scientific Assembly on Microbiology, Tuberculosis and Pulmonary Infections, "Treatment of Tuberculosis and Tuberculosis Infection in Adults and Children," *Clin Infect Dis*, 1995, 21:9-27.

American Academy of Pediatrics, Committee on Infectious Diseases, "Chemotherapy for Tuberculosis in Infants and Children," *Pediatrics*, 1992, 89(1):161-5.

"Update: Fatal and Severe Liver Injuries Associated With Rifampin and Pyrazinamide for Latent Tuberculosis Infection, and Revisions in American Thoracic Society/CDC Recommendations - United States, 2001," *MMWR Morb Mortal Wkly Rep*, 2001, 50(34):733-5.

Starke JR, "Multidrug Therapy for Tuberculosis in Children," *Pediatr Infect Dis J*, 1990, 9(11):785-93.

Starke JR and Correa AG, "Management of Mycobacterial Infection and Disease in Children," *Pediatr Infect Dis J*, 1995, 14(6):455-70.

♦ **Pyrazinoic Acid Amide** *see* Pyrazinamide *on page 961*

♦ **2-Pyridine Aldoxime Methochloride** *see* Pralidoxime *on page 922*

♦ **Pyridium®** *see* Phenazopyridine *on page 887*

Pyridostigmine *(peer id oh STIG meen)*

Related Information

Overdose and Toxicology *on page 1388*

U.S. Brand Names Mestinon®; Mestinon® Timespan®; Regonol® [DSC]

Canadian Brand Names Mestinon®-SR

Therapeutic Category Antidote, Neuromuscular Blocking Agent; Cholinergic Agent

Generic Available Yes (tablet)

Use Symptomatic treatment of myasthenia gravis by improving muscle strength; reversal of effects of nondepolarizing neuromuscular blocking agents; pretreatment for Soman nerve gas exposure (military use only)

Pregnancy Risk Factor B

Contraindications Hypersensitivity to pyridostigmine, bromides, or any component (see Warnings); GI or GU obstruction

Warnings Overdosage may result in cholinergic crisis, this must be distinguished from myasthenic crisis; adequate facilities should be available for cardiopulmonary resuscitation when testing and adjusting dose for myasthenia gravis; have atropine and epinephrine ready to treat hypersensitivity reactions; neonates of myasthenic mothers may have transient difficulties in swallowing, sucking, and breathing; use of pyridostigmine may be of benefit; use edrophonium test to assess neonate with these symptoms

Injection (Regonol®) contains benzyl alcohol which may cause allergic reactions in susceptible individuals; large amounts of benzyl alcohol (≥99 mg/kg/day) have been associated with a potentially fatal toxicity ("gasping syndrome") in neonates; the "gasping syndrome" consists of metabolic acidosis, respiratory distress, gasping respirations, CNS dysfunction (including convulsions, intracranial hemorrhage), hypotension and cardiovascular collapse; avoid use of this injection in neonates; the syrup contains sodium benzoate; *in vitro* and animal studies have shown that benzoate, a metabolite of benzyl alcohol, displaces bilirubin from protein-binding sites; avoid use of the syrup in neonates

Pretreatment with pyridostigmine alone will not protect against exposure to Soman nerve gas; its efficacy is dependent upon the rapid use of atropine and pralidoxime after exposure. Discontinue use of pyridostigmine after exposure.

Precautions Use with caution in patients with epilepsy, asthma, bradycardia, hyperthyroidism, arrhythmias, recent coronary occlusion, vagotonia, or peptic ulcer; use with caution and modify dosage in patients with renal disease

Adverse Reactions

Cardiovascular: Bradycardia, hypotension, arrhythmias, A-V block, syncope

Central nervous system: Headache, convulsions, drowsiness, dizziness

Dermatologic: Rash, dry skin

Gastrointestinal: Nausea, vomiting, diarrhea, increased peristalsis, abdominal cramps, dysphagia, salivation

Genitourinary: Urinary frequency, dysmenorrhea

Local: Thrombophlebitis (after I.V. administration)

Neuromuscular & skeletal: Muscle cramps, weakness, myalgia

Ocular: Miosis, lacrimation, diplopia, conjunctival hyperemia

Respiratory: Increased bronchial secretions, bronchospasm, laryngospasm, dyspnea, epistaxis

Miscellaneous: Diaphoresis

Drug Interactions Corticosteroids and magnesium may decrease effect of pyridostigmine; increases effects of depolarizing neuromuscular blocking agents (eg, succinylcholine); decreases the effects of nondepolarizing neuromuscular blocking agents (eg, pancuronium); may prolong neuromuscular blockade associated with aminoglycoside antibiotics; additive effects with beta-blockers; atropine is direct antagonist; additive effects with anticholinesterase drugs

Stability Protect from light; tablets are extremely moisture sensitive; do not remove desiccant and keep bottle closed tightly. Store 30 mg tablets in refrigerator; stable at room temperature for 3 months

Mechanism of Action Competitively inhibits destruction of acetylcholine by acetylcholinesterase which facilitates transmission of impulses across myoneural junction producing generalized cholinergic responses such as miosis, increased tonus of skeletal and intestinal musculature, bronchial and ureteral constriction, bradycardia, and increased salivary and sweat gland production

Pharmacodynamics

Onset of action:

Oral: 30-45 minutes

I.M.: <15 minutes

I.V.: Within 2-5 minutes

Duration:

Oral: 3-6 hours

I.M., I.V.: 2-3 hours

(Continued)

Pyridostigmine (Continued)

Pharmacokinetics
Absorption: Oral: Very poor (10% to 20%) from the GI tract
Distribution: Adults: V_d: 19 ± 12 L
Metabolism: In the liver and at tissue site by cholinesterases
Bioavailability: 10% to 20%
Half-life: Adults: 3 hours
Elimination: Clearance: Adults: 830 mL/minute

Usual Dosage
Myasthenia gravis (dosage should be adjusted so patient takes larger doses prior to time of greatest fatigue)

Oral:
Neonates: 5 mg every 4-6 hours
Children: 7 mg/kg/day in 5-6 divided doses
Adults: Initial: 60 mg 3 times/day with maintenance dose ranging from 60 mg to 1.5 g/day (incremental increases every 48 hours or more if needed) or as sustained release tablet (Mestinon® Timespan®) 180-540 mg (1-3 tablets) once or twice daily (the interval between doses should be at least 6 hours)

I.M., I.V.:
Neonates and Children: 0.05-0.15 mg/kg/dose (maximum single dose: 10 mg)
Adults: 2 mg every 2-3 hours (or 1/30th of oral dose)

Reversal of nondepolarizing neuromuscular blocker: I.V.:
Children: 0.1-0.25 mg/kg/dose preceded by atropine or glycopyrrolate
Adults: 10-20 mg preceded by atropine or glycopyrrolate

Pretreatment for Soman nerve gas exposure: Oral: Adults: 30 mg every 8 hours beginning several hours before exposure; discontinue after exposure to nerve gas (treatment with atropine and pralidoxime are indicated after exposure)

Administration
Parenteral: Administer direct I.V. slowly over 2-4 minutes; patients receiving large parenteral doses should be pretreated with atropine
Oral: Swallow sustained release tablets whole, do not chew or crush

Monitoring Parameters
Muscle strength, heart rate, vital capacity

Dosage Forms
Injection, solution, as bromide:
Mestinon®: 5 mg/mL (2 mL)
Regonol®: 5 mg/mL (2 mL, 5 mL) [contains 1% benzyl alcohol] [DSC]
Syrup, as bromide (Mestinon®): 60 mg/5 mL (480 mL) [contains 5% alcohol and sodium benzoate; raspberry flavor]
Tablet, as bromide: 30 mg [blister pack of 21], 60 mg
Mestinon®: 60 mg
Tablet, sustained release, as bromide (Mestinon® Timespan®): 180 mg

Pyridoxine (peer i DOKS een)

Related Information
Antiepileptic Drugs on page 1374

U.S. Brand Names
Aminoxin® [OTC]

Synonyms
Vitamin B_6

Therapeutic Category
Antidote, Cycloserine Toxicity; Antidote, Hydrazine Toxicity; Antidote, Mushroom Toxicity; Drug-induced Neuritis, Treatment Agent; Nutritional Supplement; Vitamin, Water Soluble

Generic Available
Yes

Use
Prevention and treatment of vitamin B_6 deficiency, pyridoxine-dependent seizures in infants; treatment of drug-induced deficiency (eg, isoniazid or hydralazine); treatment of acute intoxication of isoniazid, cycloserine, hydrazine, mushroom (genus Gyromitra)

Pregnancy Risk Factor
A (C if dose exceeds RDA recommendation)

Contraindications
Hypersensitivity to pyridoxine or any component

Adverse Reactions
Central nervous system: Sensory neuropathy (after chronic administration of large doses), seizures (following I.V. administration of very large doses), headache
Gastrointestinal: Nausea
Hematologic: Decreased serum folic acid concentration
Hepatic: Elevated AST
Local: Burning or stinging at injection site
Neuromuscular & skeletal: Paresthesia
Respiratory: Respiratory distress
Miscellaneous: Allergic reactions have been reported

Drug Interactions
Decreases levodopa effectiveness when used without carbidopa; decreases serum levels of phenobarbital and phenytoin

Mechanism of Action Precursor to pyridoxal and pyridoxamine which function as cofactors in the metabolism of proteins, carbohydrates, and fats; also aids in the release of liver and muscle stored glycogen and in the synthesis of GABA (within the CNS) and heme

Pharmacokinetics
Absorption: Readily from the GI tract; primarily in jejunum
Metabolism: Converted to pyridoxal (active form in liver)
Half-life, biologic: 15-20 days
Elimination: By liver metabolism

Usual Dosage
Adequate intake: Oral: Infants:
<6 months: 0.1 mg (0.01 mg/kg)
6-12 months: 0.3 mg (0.03 mg/kg)
Recommended daily allowance: Oral:
1-3 years: 0.5 mg
4-8 years: 0.6 mg
9-13 years: 1 mg
14-19 years:
Male: 1.3 mg
Female: 1.2 mg
20-50 years: 1.3 mg
>50 years:
Male: 1.7 mg
Female: 1.5 mg
Pyridoxine-dependent seizures: Oral, I.M., I.V.:
Neonates and Infants: Initial: 10-100 mg; maintenance: Oral: 50-100 mg/day
Dietary deficiency: Oral:
Children: 5-25 mg/day for 3 weeks, then 1.5-2.5 mg/day in multivitamin product
Adults: 2.5-10 mg/day until clinical signs are corrected, then 2-5 mg/day (dosage found in multivitamin products)
Drug-induced neuritis (eg, isoniazid, hydralazine, penicillamine, cycloserine): Oral:
Children:
Treatment: 10-50 mg/day
Prophylaxis: 1-2 mg/kg/day
Adults:
Cycloserine: Treatment 100-300 mg/day in divided doses
Isoniazid or penicillamine: Treatment: 100-200 mg/day for 3 weeks; prophylaxis: 25-100 mg/day
Acute intoxication: Children and Adults:
Hydrazine: 25 mg/kg: $\frac{1}{3}$ dose I.M. and $\frac{2}{3}$ dose I.V. infusion over 3 hours
Isoniazid: Dose equal to isoniazid ingested given as a first dose of 1-4 g I.V., followed by 1 g I.M. every 30 minutes until total dosage completed
Mushroom ingestion (genus *Gyromitra*): I.V.: 25 mg/kg; repeat as necessary to a maximum total dose of 15-20 g

Administration
Parenteral: Administer slow I.V.
Oral: Administer without regard to meals

Monitoring Parameters When administering large I.V. doses, monitor respiratory rate, heart rate, and blood pressure

Reference Range 30-80 ng/mL

Test Interactions False positive urobilinogen spot test using Ehrlich's reagent

Dosage Forms
Capsule, as hydrochloride: 250 mg
Injection, solution, as hydrochloride: 100 mg/mL (1 mL)
Tablet, as hydrochloride: 25 mg, 50 mg, 100 mg, 250 mg, 500 mg
Tablet, enteric coated, as hydrochloride (Aminoxin®): 20 mg

Extemporaneous Preparations A 1 mg/mL oral solution has an expected stability of 30 days when refrigerated when compounded as follows: Withdraw 100 mg (1 mL of a 100 mg/mL injection) from a vial with a needle and syringe, add to 99 mL of simple syrup in an amber bottle; keep in refrigerator
Nahata MC and Hipple TF, *Pediatric Drug Formulations*, 4th ed, Cincinnati, OH: Harvey Whitney Books Co, 2000.

Pyrimethamine (peer i METH a meen)

U.S. Brand Names Daraprim®
Therapeutic Category Antimalarial Agent
Generic Available No
Use Used in combination with sulfadiazine for treatment of toxoplasmosis; used in combination with dapsone as primary or secondary prophylaxis for *Pneumocystis*
(Continued)

Pyrimethamine *(Continued)*

carinii in HIV-infected patients; pyrimethamine has been used for chemoprophylaxis of malaria, however, due to severe adverse reactions and reports of resistance to pyrimethamine, other antimalarial agents are now generally preferred

Pregnancy Risk Factor C

Contraindications Hypersensitivity to pyrimethamine, chloroguanide, or any component; megaloblastic anemia; resistant malaria and patients with seizure disorders

Precautions Use with caution in patients with impaired renal or hepatic function and in patients with possible folate deficiency

Adverse Reactions

Cardiovascular: Shock

Central nervous system: Seizures, fever, fatigue, ataxia, headache

Dermatologic: Rash, photosensitivity

Endocrine & metabolic: Folic acid deficiency

Gastrointestinal: Anorexia, abdominal cramps, vomiting, atrophic glossitis, diarrhea

Hematologic: Megaloblastic anemia, leukopenia, thrombocytopenia, agranulocytosis, pancytopenia, pulmonary eosinophilia

Neuromuscular & skeletal: Tremor

Renal: Hematuria

Respiratory: Respiratory failure

Drug Interactions Para-aminobenzoic acid, sulfonamides

Mechanism of Action Inhibits parasitic dihydrofolate reductase resulting in inhibition of tetrahydrofolic acid synthesis

Pharmacokinetics

Absorption: Oral: Well absorbed

Distribution: V_d: Adults: 2.9 L/kg; appears in breast milk; distributed to the kidneys, lung, liver, and spleen

Protein binding: 80% to 87%

Half-life: 111 hours (range: 54-148 hours)

Time to peak serum concentration: Within 2-6 hours

Elimination: Pyrimethamine and metabolites are excreted in urine

Usual Dosage Oral:

Toxoplasmosis (with sulfadiazine):

Newborns and Infants: Initial: 2 mg/kg/day divided every 12 hours for 2 days, then 1 mg/kg/day once daily given with sulfadiazine for the first 6 months; next 6 months: 1 mg/kg/day 3 times/week with sulfadiazine; oral folinic acid 5-10 mg 3 times/week should be administered to prevent hematologic toxicity

Children: 2 mg/kg/day divided every 12 hours for 3 days followed by 1 mg/kg/day (maximum: 25 mg/day) once daily or divided twice daily for 4 weeks given with sulfadiazine; oral folinic acid 5-10 mg 3 times/week should be administered to prevent hematologic toxicity

Adults: 50-75 mg/day together with 1-4 g of a sulfonamide plus oral folinic acid 5-10 mg 3 times/week for 1-3 weeks depending on patient's tolerance and response, then reduce dose by 50% and continue for 4-5 weeks **or** 25-50 mg/day for 3-4 weeks

Prophylaxis for first episode of *Toxoplasma gondii*:

Children ≥1 month of age: 1 mg/kg/day once daily with dapsone plus oral folinic acid 5 mg every 3 days

Adolescents and Adults: 50 mg once weekly with dapsone plus oral folinic acid 25 mg once weekly

Prophylaxis for recurrence of *Toxoplasma gondii*:

Children ≥1 month of age: 1 mg/kg/day once daily given with sulfadiazine or clindamycin, plus oral folinic acid 5 mg every 3 days

Adolescents and Adults: 25-75 mg once daily in combination with sulfadiazine or clindamycin, plus oral folinic acid 10-25 mg daily

Prophylaxis for first episode or recurrence of *Pneumocystis carinii*:

Adolescents and Adults: 50-75 mg once weekly in combination with dapsone plus oral folinic acid 25 mg once weekly

Administration Oral: Administer with meals to minimize vomiting

Monitoring Parameters CBC including platelet counts

Patient Information Notify physician if rash, sore throat, pallor, or glossitis occurs. May cause photosensitivity reactions (eg, exposure to sunlight may cause severe sunburn, skin rash, redness, or itching); avoid exposure to sunlight and artificial light sources (sunlamps, tanning booth/bed); wear protective clothing, wide-brimmed hats, sunglasses, and lip sunscreen (SPF ≥15); use a sunscreen [broad-spectrum sunscreen or physical sunscreen (preferred) or sunblock with SPF ≥15]; contact physician if reaction occurs.

Additional Information Folinic acid may be given in a dosage of 3-9 mg/day for 3 days, or 5 mg every 3 days, or as required to reverse symptoms or to prevent hematologic problems due to pyrimethamine-induced folic acid deficiency

Dosage Forms Tablet, scored: 25 mg

Extemporaneous Preparations Pyrimethamine tablets may be crushed to prepare oral suspensions of the drug in a 1:1 mixture of simple syrup and 1% methylcellulose to yield a suspension with a pyrimethamine concentration of 2 mg/mL; stable for at least 91 days when stored in plastic or glass prescription bottles at 4°C or 25°C

Nahata MC, Morosco RS, and Hipple TF, "Stability of Pyrimethamine in a Liquid Dosage Formulation Stored for Three Months," *Am J Health-Syst Pharm*, 1997, 54:2714-6.

References
"1997 USPHS/IDSA Guidelines for the Prevention of Opportunistic Infections in Persons Infected With Human Immunodeficiency Virus," *MMWR Morb Mortal Wkly Rep*, 1997, 46(RR-12):1-46.

Van Voorhis WC, "Therapy and Prophylaxis of Systemic Protozoan Infections," *Drugs*, 1990, 40(2):176-202.

♦ **Pyrimethamine and Sulfadoxine** *see* Sulfadoxine and Pyrimethamine *on page 1051*

♦ **Quelicin®** *see* Succinylcholine *on page 1044*

♦ **Questran®** *see* Cholestyramine Resin *on page 267*

♦ **Questran® Light** *see* Cholestyramine Resin *on page 267*

♦ **Quibron®-T** *see* Theophylline *on page 1076*

♦ **Quibron®-T/SR** *see* Theophylline *on page 1076*

♦ **Quinaglute® Dura-Tabs®** *see* Quinidine *on page 967*

♦ **Quinalbarbitone** *see* Secobarbital *on page 1011*

♦ **Quinate® (Can)** *see* Quinidine *on page 967*

♦ **Quinidex® Extentabs®** *see* Quinidine *on page 967*

Quinidine (KWIN i deen)

U.S. Brand Names Quinaglute® Dura-Tabs®; Quinidex® Extentabs®

Canadian Brand Names Apo®-Quin-G; Apo®-Quinidine; BioQuin® Durules™; Novo-Quinidin; Quinate®

Therapeutic Category Antiarrhythmic Agent, Class I-A

Generic Available Yes

Use Prophylaxis after cardioversion of atrial fibrillation and/or flutter to maintain normal sinus rhythm; also used to prevent reoccurrence of paroxysmal supraventricular tachycardia, paroxysmal A-V junctional rhythm, paroxysmal ventricular tachycardia, paroxysmal atrial fibrillation, and atrial or ventricular premature contractions; also has activity against *Plasmodium falciparum* malaria

Pregnancy Risk Factor C

Contraindications Hypersensitivity to quinidine, any component, or cinchona derivatives; patients with complete A-V block with an A-V junctional or idioventricular pacemaker; patients with intraventricular conduction defects (marked widening of QRS complex); patients with cardiac glycoside-induced A-V conduction disorders

Warnings May cause syncope, most likely due to ventricular tachycardia or fibrillation; syncope may subside spontaneously, but occasionally may be fatal; discontinue quinidine if syncope occurs

Precautions Use with caution in patients with myocardial depression, sick sinus syndrome, incomplete A-V block, cardiac glycoside intoxication, hepatic and/or renal insufficiency, myasthenia gravis; hemolysis may occur in patients with G-6-PD deficiency; quinidine-induced hepatotoxicity, including granulomatous hepatitis, increased serum AST and alkaline phosphatase concentrations, and jaundice may occur; use with caution in nursing women; adjust dose with severe renal impairment

Adverse Reactions

Cardiovascular: Syncope, hypotension, tachycardia, heart block, ventricular fibrillation, vascular collapse, severe hypotension with rapid I.V. administration

Central nervous system: Fever, headache

Dermatologic: Angioedema, rash; photosensitivity (rare)

Gastrointestinal: GI disturbances, nausea, vomiting, cramps

Hematologic: Blood dyscrasias, thrombotic thrombocytopenic purpura

Hepatic: Elevated AST; elevated alkaline phosphatase, jaundice, granulomatous hepatitis

Respiratory: Respiratory depression

Miscellaneous: Cinchonism (nausea, tinnitus, headache, impaired hearing or vision, vomiting, abdominal pain, vertigo, confusion, delirium, syncope)

Drug Interactions Cytochrome P450 isoenzyme CYP3A3/4 substrate; CYP2D6 (potent) and CYP3A3/4 (weak) isoenzyme inhibitor

(Continued)

Quinidine *(Continued)*

Quinidine potentiates nondepolarizing and depolarizing muscle relaxants; diltiazem, verapamil, delavirdine, saquinavir, amiodarone, alkalinizing agents, and cimetidine may increase quinidine serum concentrations; phenobarbital, phenytoin, and rifampin may decrease quinidine serum concentrations. Quinidine may increase plasma concentration of digoxin; closely monitor digoxin concentrations; digoxin dosage may need to be reduced (by one-half) when quinidine is initiated; new steady-state digoxin plasma concentrations occur in 5-7 days. Beta-blockers plus quinidine may increase bradycardia; quinidine may enhance coumarin anticoagulants; potential interaction with ritonavir, concurrent use is not recommended

Food Interactions Excessive intake of fruit juices or vitamin C may decrease urine pH and result in increased clearance of quinidine with decreased serum concentration; alkaline foods may result in increased quinidine serum concentrations; food has a variable effect on absorption of extended release formulation. Grapefruit juice delays absorption of quinidine, decreases quinidine clearance, inhibits cytochrome P450 CYP3A4 mediated metabolism of quinidine to 3-hydroxyquinidine (major metabolite of quinidine), and significantly decreases the AUC of 3-hydroxyquinidine (although the clinical significance of the quinidine-grapefruit juice interaction is unknown, grapefruit juice should be avoided). A decrease in dietary salt intake may increase serum quinidine concentrations.

Stability Do not use discolored parenteral solution

Mechanism of Action Class IA antiarrhythmic with anticholinergic, local anesthetic, and mild negative inotropic effects; depresses phase 0 of the action potential; decreases myocardial excitability, conduction velocity, and myocardial contractility by decreasing sodium influx during depolarization and potassium efflux in repolarization; also reduces calcium transport across cell membrane

Pharmacokinetics

Distribution: V_d: Adults: 2-3.5 L/kg, decreased V_d with CHF, malaria; increased V_d with cirrhosis; crosses the placenta; appears in breast milk

Protein-binding:

Newborns: 60% to 70%

Adults: 80% to 90%

Decreased protein binding with cyanotic congenital heart disease, cirrhosis, or acute MI

Metabolism: Extensive in the liver (50% to 90%) to inactive compounds

Bioavailability:

Gluconate: 70%

Sulfate: 80%

Half-life, plasma (increased half-life with cirrhosis and CHF):

Children: 2.5-6.7 hours

Adults: 6-8 hours

Elimination: In urine (15% to 25% as unchanged drug)

Dialysis: Slightly dialyzable (5% to 20%) by hemodialysis; not removed by peritoneal dialysis

Usual Dosage Note: Dose expressed in terms of the salt: 267 mg of quinidine gluconate = 200 mg of quinidine sulfate

Children: Test dose (for idiosyncratic reaction, intolerance, syncope, thrombocytopenia) (**sulfate**, oral or **gluconate**, I.M.): 2 mg/kg or 60 mg/m²

Oral (**quinidine sulfate**): Usual: 30 mg/kg/day or 900 mg/m²/day given in 5 daily doses or 6 mg/kg every 4-6 hours; range: 15-60 mg/kg/day in 4-5 divided doses

I.V. (**quinidine gluconate**): 2-10 mg/kg/dose every 3-6 hours as needed (I.V. route **not** recommended)

Adults: Test dose (for idiosyncratic reaction, intolerance, syncope, thrombocytopenia): 200 mg administered several hours before full dosage

Oral (**sulfate**): 100-600 mg/dose every 4-6 hours; begin at 200 mg/dose and titrate to desired effect

Oral (**gluconate**): 324-972 mg every 8-12 hours

I.M.: 400 mg/dose every 4-6 hours

I.V.: 200-400 mg/dose diluted and given at a rate ≤10 mg/minute

Dosing adjustment in renal impairment: Children and Adults: Cl_{cr} <10 mL/minute: Administer 75% of normal dose

Administration

Oral: Administer with water on an empty stomach, but may administer with food or milk to decrease GI upset; best to administer in a consistent manner with regards to meals; avoid administration with grapefruit juice; swallow extended release tablets whole, do not chew or crush

Parenteral: I.V.: Maximum rate of infusion: 10 mg/minute; maximum concentration: 16 mg/mL; I.V. tubing length should be minimized (quinidine may be significantly adsorbed to polyvinyl chloride tubing)

Monitoring Parameters CBC with differential, platelet count, liver and renal function tests, and serum concentrations should be routinely performed during long-term administration

Reference Range Optimal therapeutic level is method dependent
Therapeutic: 2-7 µg/mL (SI: 6.2-15.4 µmol/L)
Toxic: >8 µg/mL (SI: >18 µmol/L)

Patient Information Notify physician if fever, rash, unusual bruising or bleeding, visual disturbances, or ringing in the ears occurs; avoid grapefruit juice; avoid excessive intake of fruit juices or vitamin C. May rarely cause photosensitivity reactions; avoid exposure to sunlight and artificial light sources (sunlamps, tanning booth/bed); use a sunscreen; contact physician if reaction occurs.

Additional Information Use of extended release products is not recommended in children. Formation of a concretion of tablets or bezoar in the stomach has been reported following tablet ingestion by a 16-month old infant; diagnostic or therapeutic endoscopy may be required in patients with massive overdose and prolonged elevated serum quinidine concentrations

Dosage Forms
Injection, solution, as **gluconate**: 80 mg/mL (10 mL) [equivalent to 50 mg quinidine base]
Tablet, as **sulfate**: 200 mg, 300 mg
Tablet, extended release, as **gluconate** (Quinaglute® Dura-Tabs®): 324 mg [equivalent to 202 mg quinidine base]
Tablet, extended release, as **sulfate** (Quinidex® Extentabs®): 300 mg [equivalent to 249 mg quinidine base]

Extemporaneous Preparations
A 10 mg/mL quinidine sulfate oral liquid preparation made from tablets and 3 different vehicles (cherry syrup, a 1:1 mixture of Ora-Sweet® and Ora-Plus®, or a 1:1 mixture of Ora-Sweet® SF and Ora-Plus®) was stable for 60 days when stored in amber plastic prescription bottles in the dark at room temperature (25°C) or under refrigeration (5°C); Grind six 200 mg tablets in a mortar into a fine powder; add 15 mL of the vehicle and mix well to form a uniform paste; mix while adding the vehicle in geometric proportions to **almost** 120 mL; transfer to a calibrated bottle and qsad to 120 mL; label "shake well" and "protect from light" (Allen 1998).

Allen LV and Erickson MA, "Stability of Bethanechol Chloride, Pyrazinamide, Quinidine Sulfate, Rifampin, and Tetracycline in Extemporaneously Compounded Oral Liquids," *Am J Health Syst Pharm*, 1998, 55(17):1804-9.

References
Pickoff AS, Singh S, and Gelband H, *The Medical Management of Cardiac Arrhythmias in Cardiac Arrhythmias in the Neonate, Infant and Child*, Roberts NK and Gelband H, ed, Norwalk, CT: Appleton-Century-Crofts, 1983.
Szefler SJ, Pieroni DR, Gingell RL, et al, "Rapid Elimination of Quinidine in Pediatric Patients," *Pediatrics*, 1982, 70(3):370-5.

Quinine (KWYE nine)

Canadian Brand Names Quinine-Odan™

Therapeutic Category Antimalarial Agent; Skeletal Muscle Relaxant, Miscellaneous

Generic Available Yes

Use Suppression or treatment of chloroquine-resistant *P. falciparum* malaria (inactive against sporozoites, pre-erythrocytic or exoerythrocytic forms of plasmodia); treatment of *Babesia microti* infection; prevention and treatment of nocturnal recumbency leg muscle cramps

Pregnancy Risk Factor D

Contraindications Hypersensitivity to quinine or any component; tinnitus, optic neuritis, G-6-PD deficiency; history of black water fever; pregnancy

Precautions Use with caution in patients with cardiac arrhythmias (quinine has quinidine-like activity), in patients with myasthenia gravis, and in patients with impaired liver function

Adverse Reactions
Cardiovascular: Flushing of the skin, anginal symptoms, conduction disturbances, ventricular tachycardia
Central nervous system: Fever, headache, confusion
Dermatologic: Rash, pruritus
Endocrine & metabolic: Hypoglycemia
Gastrointestinal: Nausea, vomiting, epigastric pain
Hematologic: Hemolysis, thrombocytopenia
Hepatic: Hepatitis
Ocular: Visual disturbances
Otic: Tinnitus, impaired hearing
(Continued)

Quinine *(Continued)*

Miscellaneous: Hypersensitivity reactions, cinchonism (nausea, tinnitus, headache, impaired hearing or vision, vomiting, abdominal pain, vertigo, confusion, delirium, syncope)

Drug Interactions Cytochrome P450 isoenzyme CYP3A3/4 substrate and inhibitor

Quinine may decrease the clearance of digoxin or digitoxin leading to increased plasma concentrations of these cardiac glycosides; cimetidine (prolongs half-life of quinine), aluminum-containing antacids (decreases quinine absorption); quinine may potentiate the effects of neuromuscular blocking agents; oral anticoagulants, urinary alkalinizers (may increase quinine toxicity); mefloquine (additive cardiotoxicity); ritonavir, verapamil, and amiodarone may increase serum quinine concentrations

Stability Protect from light

Mechanism of Action Depresses oxygen uptake and carbohydrate metabolism; intercalates into DNA, disrupting the parasite's replication and transcription; affects calcium distribution within muscle fibers and decreases the excitability of the motor end-plate region

Pharmacokinetics

Absorption: Oral: Readily absorbed, mainly from the upper small intestine

Distribution: Widely distributed to body tissues and fluids including small amounts into bile and CSF; crosses the placenta; excreted into breast milk

V_d (children): 0.8 L/kg

V_d (adults): 1.9 L/kg

Protein binding: 70% to 90%

Metabolism: Primarily in the liver via hydroxylation pathways

Half-life:

Children: 6-12 hours

Adults: 8-14 hours

Time to peak serum concentration: Within 1-3 hours

Elimination: In bile and saliva with <5% excreted unchanged in urine

Dialysis: Not effectively removed by peritoneal dialysis, removed by hemodialysis

Usual Dosage Oral:

Children:

Treatment of chloroquine-resistant malaria: 30 mg/kg/day in divided doses every 8 hours for 3-7 days in conjunction with another agent; maximum dose: 2 g/day

Babesiosis: 25 mg/kg/day, divided every 8 hours for 7 days; maximum dose: 650 mg/dose

Adults:

Treatment of chloroquine-resistant malaria: 650 mg every 8 hours for 3-7 days in conjunction with another agent

Suppression of malaria: 325 mg twice daily and continued for 6 weeks after exposure

Babesiosis: 650 mg every 6-8 hours for 7 days

Leg cramps: 200-300 mg at bedtime

Administration Oral: Do not crush tablets or capsule to avoid bitter taste

Monitoring Parameters CBC with platelet count, liver function tests, blood glucose, ophthalmologic examination

Patient Information Report to physician if tinnitus, hearing loss, rash, or visual disturbances occur during therapy

Additional Information Parenteral form of quinine (dihydrochloride) is no longer available from the CDC; quinidine gluconate should be used instead; the FDA has banned over-the-counter (OTC) drug products containing quinine sold for treatment and/or prevention of malaria, as well as, products labeled for treatment or prevention of nocturnal leg cramps

Dosage Forms

Capsule, as sulfate: 200 mg, 260 mg, 325 mg

Tablet, as sulfate: 260 mg

References

Schulbe DE, "Quinine Ban Signals Change for Pharmacists, APhA," *Pharmacy Today*, 1995, 1(12):6.

♦ **Quinine-Odan™ (Can)** *see* Quinine *on page 969*

♦ **Quintasa® (Can)** *see* Mesalamine *on page 723*

Quinupristin/Dalfopristin (kwi NYOO pris tin/dal FOE pris tin)

U.S. Brand Names Synercid®

Synonyms Pristinamycin; RP59500

Therapeutic Category Antibiotic, Streptogramin

Generic Available No

Use Treatment of serious or life-threatening infections caused by vancomycin-resistant *Enterococcus faecium*; treatment of complicated skin and skin structure infections caused by *Staphylococcus aureus* (methicillin-susceptible and methicillin-resistant strains) or *Streptococcus pyogenes*

Pregnancy Risk Factor B

Contraindications Hypersensitivity to quinupristin, dalfopristin, other streptogramins (pristinamycin or virginiamycin), or to any component

Warnings Quinupristin/dalfopristin inhibit cytochrome P450 3A4 metabolism of cyclosporine, midazolam, nifedipine, and terfenadine. There was a 77% increase in cyclosporine's half-life with a 63% increase in the AUC. Cyclosporine levels should be closely monitored in patients who are receiving quinupristin/dalfopristin therapy concomitantly. Coadministration of quinupristin/dalfopristin with cytochrome P450 3A4 substrates with narrow therapeutic ranges require serum concentration monitoring of these drugs. Concurrent use with astemizole, terfenadine, and cisapride is not recommended. Superinfections and pseudomembranous colitis have been reported with the use of quinupristin/dalfopristin. Resistance to quinupristin/dalfopristin has been reported in a few cases of *Enterococcus faecium* infections.

Precautions Use with caution in patients with hepatic or renal dysfunction; dosage reduction may be necessary in patients with hepatic cirrhosis; may cause pain and phlebitis when infused through a peripheral line; episodes of severe arthralgia and myalgia have been reported which improve with a dose frequency reduction to "q12h" or discontinuation of quinupristin/dalfopristin

Adverse Reactions

Central nervous system: Headache

Dermatologic: Rash, pruritus, urticaria

Hepatic: Elevated AST, ALT, bilirubin

Local: Pain, edema, inflammation at infusion site; thrombophlebitis

Neuromuscular & skeletal: Arthralgia, myalgia

Miscellaneous: Superinfection

Drug Interactions Cytochrome P450 isoenzyme CYP3A4 inhibitor

Quinupristin/dalfopristin may increase plasma concentration of cyclosporine, tacrolimus, astemizole, terfenadine, delavirdine, nevirapine, indinavir, ritonavir, vinca alkaloids, docetaxel, paclitaxel, midazolam, diazepam, dihydropyridines, verapamil, diltiazem, HMG-CoA reductase inhibitors, cisapride, methylprednisolone, carbamazepine, quinidine, lidocaine, disopyramide (see Warnings)

Stability Unopened vials should be stored in a refrigerator at 2°C to 8°C; reconstituted drug is stable for 1 hour at room temperature; infusion bag is stable for 5 hours at room temperature and for 54 hours if refrigerated at 2°C to 8°C; incompatible with NS and heparin; compatible with aztreonam, ciprofloxacin, fluconazole, haloperidol, metoclopramide, morphine, and potassium chloride during Y-site administration

Mechanism of Action Inhibits bacterial protein synthesis by binding to the 50S bacterial ribosomal subunit resulting in peptide chain elongation inhibition and peptidyl transferase inhibition

Pharmacokinetics

Distribution:

V_d: Quinupristin: 0.45 L/kg

V_d: Dalfopristin: 0.24 L/kg

Protein binding:

Quinupristin: 23% to 32%

Dalfopristin: 50% to 56%

Metabolism: Quinupristin is conjugated with glutathione and cysteine to active metabolites; dalfopristin is hydrolyzed to an active metabolite

Half-life:

Quinupristin: 0.85 hour

Dalfopristin: 0.7 hour

Elimination: 75% to 77% excreted in the bile and feces

Usual Dosage Dosage is expressed in terms of combined "mg" of quinupristin plus dalfopristin: I.V.:

Children: Limited information is available; quinupristin/dalfopristin has been used in a limited number of pediatric patients under a compassionate use protocol

Treatment of vancomycin-resistant *Enterococcus faecium* infection: 7.5 mg/kg/dose every 8 hours

Treatment of vancomycin-resistant *Enterococcus faecium* CNS shunt infection: 7.5 mg/kg/dose every 8 hours (plus 1 mg intrathecal dose daily at the time of shunt tap was used in an 8-month old infant for 28 days in one case report; 1 or 2 mg doses every day for 5-33 days have been administered intrathecally in 6 patients)

Treatment of complicated skin and skin structure infection: 7.5 mg/kg/dose every 12 hours for at least 7 days

(Continued)

Quinupristin/Dalfopristin *(Continued)*

Adolescents ≥16 years and Adults:

Treatment of vancomycin-resistant *Enterococcus faecium* infection: 7.5 mg/kg/dose every 8 hours

Treatment of complicated skin and skin structure infection: 7.5 mg/kg/dose every 12 hours

Dosage adjustment in hepatic impairment: Dosage adjustment may be necessary, but exact recommendations cannot be made at this time

Administration Parenteral: Reconstitute vial by slowly adding 5 mL D_5W or SWI to make a 100 mg/mL solution; gently swirl the vial contents without shaking to minimize foam formation; further dilute the reconstituted solution with D_5W to a final maximum concentration for administration via peripheral line of 2 mg/mL; maximum concentration for administration via a central line is 5 mg/mL; if an injection site reaction occurs, the dose can be further diluted to a final concentration of <1 mg/mL; administer infusion over 60 minutes; following infusion of quinupristin/dalfopristin, the infusion line should be flushed with D_5W to minimize venous irritation; **DO NOT FLUSH** with saline or heparin solutions due to incompatibility

Monitoring Parameters CBC, liver function test; monitor infusion site closely

Nursing Implications If moderate to severe venous irritation occurs following peripheral quinupristin/dalfopristin administration, consider increasing the infusion volume, changing infusion sites, or establishing central venous access; administration of hydrocortisone or diphenhydramine did not decrease infusion site reactions

Dosage Forms Injection, powder for reconstitution, lyophilized: 500 mg vial (150 mg quinupristin and 350 mg dalfopristin)

References

Gransden WR, King A, Marossy D, et al, "Quinupristin/Dalfopristin in Neonatal *Enterococcus faecium* Meningitis," *Arch Dis Child Fetal Neonatal Ed*, 1998, 78(3):F235-6.

Gray JW, Darbyshire PJ, Beath SV, et al, "Experience With Quinupristin/Dalfopristin in Treating Infections With Vancomycin-Resistant *Enterococcus faecium* in Children," *Pediatr Infect Dis J*, 2000, 19(3):234-8.

Nachman SA, Verma R, and Egnor M, "Vancomycin-Resistant *Enterococcus faecium* Shunt Infection in an Infant: An Antibiotic Cure," *Microb Drug Resist*, 1995, 1(1):95-6

♦ **Quixin™** *see* Levofloxacin *on page 667*

♦ **QVAR® 40 mcg** *see* Beclomethasone *on page 160*

♦ **QVAR® 80 mcg** *see* Beclomethasone *on page 160*

♦ **Rabies Immune Globulin, Human** *see page 1333*

♦ **Rabies Virus Vaccine, Human Diploid** *see page 1333*

♦ **Racemic Epinephrine** *see* Epinephrine *on page 439*

♦ **rAHF** *see* Antihemophilic Factor (Recombinant) *on page 119*

♦ **R-albuterol** *see* Levalbuterol *on page 663*

Ranitidine *(ra NI ti deen)*

Related Information

Carbohydrate and Alcohol Content of Liquid Medications for Use in Patients Receiving Ketogenic Diets *on page 1431*

U.S. Brand Names Zantac®; Zantac® 75 [OTC]; Zantac® EFFERdose®

Canadian Brand Names Alti-Ranitidine; Apo®-Ranitidine; Gen-Ranidine; Novo-Ranitidine; Nu-Ranit; PMS-Ranitidine; Rhoxal-ranitidine

Therapeutic Category Gastrointestinal Agent, Gastric or Duodenal Ulcer Treatment; Histamine H_2 Antagonist

Generic Available Yes (except injection and effervescent granules and tablets)

Use Short-term treatment of active duodenal ulcers and benign gastric ulcers; long-term prophylaxis of duodenal ulcer and gastric hypersecretory states; gastroesophageal reflux disease (GERD); recurrent postoperative ulcer; treatment and prophylaxis of erosive esophagitis; upper GI bleeding, prevention of acid-aspiration pneumonitis during surgery, and prevention of stress-induced ulcers; over-the-counter (OTC) formulation for use in the relief of heartburn, acid indigestion, and sour stomach

Pregnancy Risk Factor B

Contraindications Hypersensitivity to ranitidine or any component or other H_2 antagonists; patients with history of acute porphyria (may precipitate an acute attack)

Warnings Zantac® EFFERdose® tablets and granules contain sodium benzoate; benzoic acid (benzoate) is a metabolite of benzyl alcohol; large amounts of benzyl alcohol (≥99 mg/kg/day) have been associated with a potentially fatal toxicity ("gasping syndrome") in neonates; *in vitro* and animal studies have shown that benzoate displaces bilirubin from protein binding sites; avoid use in neonates

Precautions Use with caution in patients with liver and renal impairment; dosage modification required in patients with renal impairment. Zantac® 150 EFFERdose® tablets and Zantac® 150 EFFERdose® granules contain phenylalanine; use with caution in patients with phenylketonuria.

Adverse Reactions
Cardiovascular: Bradycardia, tachycardia, vasculitis (rare)

Central nervous system: Dizziness, sedation, malaise, mental confusion, headache, hallucinations, anxiety

Dermatologic: Rash, alopecia (rare), erythema multiforme (rare)

Endocrine & metabolic: Gynecomastia

Gastrointestinal: Constipation, nausea, vomiting, abdominal discomfort, pancreatitis (rare)

Hematologic: Thrombocytopenia, aplastic anemia (rare), granulocytopenia, leukopenia

Hepatic: Hepatitis

Local: Transient pain at injection site

Neuromuscular & skeletal: Arthralgias

Renal: Elevated serum creatinine

Drug Interactions
Cytochrome P450 isoenzyme CYP2D6 and 3A3/4 inhibitor

Variable effects on warfarin; antacids may decrease absorption of ranitidine; ranitidine decreases the absorption of ketoconazole and itraconazole

Stability
Protect injection from light; stable for 48 hours at room temperature or 30 days when frozen in D_5W or NS; stable for 24 hours in TPN solutions; stable for 24 hours in 3-in-1 total nutrient admixture

Mechanism of Action
Competitive inhibition of histamine at H_2-receptors of the gastric parietal cells, which inhibits gastric acid secretion

Pharmacokinetics
Distribution: Minimally penetrates the blood-brain barrier; breast milk to plasma ratio: 1.9-6.7

V_d:
Children: 1-1.3 L/kg
Adults: 1.4 L/kg

Protein binding: 15%

Metabolism: In the liver

Bioavailability: Oral: ~50%

Half-life:
Neonates (receiving ECMO): 6.6 hours
Infants: 3.5 hours
Children 3.5-16 years: 1.8-2 hours
Adults:
Normal renal and hepatic function: 2-2.5 hours
Decreased renal function (Cl_{cr} 25-35 mL/minute): 4.8 hours

Time to peak serum concentration:
Oral: 1-3 hours
I.M.: 15 minutes

Elimination: 30% (oral) or 70% (I.V.) eliminated as unchanged drug in the urine and in feces

Dialysis: Hemodialysis: Slightly dialyzable (5% to 20%)

Usual Dosage
Premature and Term Infants <2 weeks:
Oral: 2 mg/kg/day divided every 12 hours
I.V.: 1.5 mg/kg/dose as loading dose, then 12 hours later maintenance dose of 1.5-2 mg/kg/day divided every 12 hours
Continuous infusion: 1.5 mg/kg/dose as loading dose followed by 0.04-0.08 mg/kg/hour infusion (or 1-2 mg/kg/day)

Children ≥1 month to 16 years:
Gastric/duodenal ulcer:
Oral:
Treatment: 2-4 mg/kg/day divided twice daily; maximum: 300 mg/day
Maintenance: 2-4 mg/kg/day divided twice daily; maximum: 150 mg/day
I.V.: 2-4 mg/kg/day divided every 6-8 hours; maximum: 200 mg/day
GERD and erosive esophagitis:
Oral: 4-10 mg/kg/day divided twice daily; maximum: GERD: 300 mg/day; erosive esophagitis: 600 mg/day
I.V.: 2-4 mg/kg/day divided every 6-8 hours; maximum: 200 mg/day **or as an alternative**
Continuous infusion: Initial: 1 mg/kg/dose for one dose followed by infusion of 0.08-0.17 mg/kg/hour or 2-4 mg/kg/day

Children ≥16 years and Adults:
Treatment of duodenal or gastric ulcers, GERD, maintenance of erosive esophagitis: Oral: 150 mg/dose twice daily or 300 mg at bedtime
Prophylaxis of recurrent duodenal ulcer: Oral: 150 mg at bedtime
Gastric hypersecretory conditions:
Oral: 150 mg twice daily; maximum: 600 mg/day

(Continued)

Ranitidine *(Continued)*

I.M., I.V.: 50 mg/dose every 6-8 hours (dose not to exceed 400 mg/day)

Continuous I.V. infusion: Initial 50 mg I.V. followed by 6.25 mg/hour titrated to gastric pH >4.0 for prophylaxis or >7.0 for treatment; **continuous I.V. infusion is preferred in patients with active bleeding**

Erosive esophagitis: Oral: 150 mg 4 times/day

Pathologic hypersecretory conditions (eg, Zollinger-Ellison syndrome):

Continuous I.V. infusion: Initial 50 mg I.V. followed by 1 mg/kg/hour infusion; titrate dosage in 0.5 mg/kg/hour increments to maintain gastric acid output at <10 mEq/hour; doses up to 2.5 mg/kg/hour (220 mg/hour) have been used

Oral: 150 mg twice daily; more frequent administration may be indicated depending upon response; doses up to 6.3 g/day have been used in severe cases

Relief of heartburn, acid indigestion, sour stomach (OTC use): Oral: 75 mg 30-60 minutes before eating; no more than 2 tablets/day

Dosing adjustment in renal impairment:

Children and Adults (Aronoff, 1999):

Cl_{cr} 10-50 mL/minute: Reduce dose to 50% of dose recommended for indication

Cl_{cr} <10 mL/minute: Reduce dose to 25% of dose recommended for indication

or as an alternative per manufacturer's recommendations:

Adults: Cl_{cr} <50 mL/minute:

Oral: 150 mg every 24 hours; adjust dose cautiously if needed

I.V.: 50 mg every 18-24 hours; adjust dose cautiously if needed

Hemodialysis: Adjust dose schedule to administer dose at the end of dialysis

Administration

Oral: Administer with meals and at bedtime; EFFERdose® tablets and granules must be dissolved in 6-8 ounces of water before use

Parenteral: Intermittent I.V. infusion preferred over direct injection to decrease risk of bradycardia; for intermittent infusion, infuse over 15-30 minutes, at a usual concentration of 0.5 mg/mL; for direct I.V. injection, administer over a period of at least 5 minutes, not to exceed 10 mg/minute (4 mL/minute) at a final concentration not to exceed 2.5 mg/mL; For I.M., administer undiluted (25 mg/mL)

Monitoring Parameters AST, ALT, serum creatinine; when used to prevent stress-related GI bleeding, measure the intragastric pH and try to maintain pH >4; gastric acid secretion (<10 mEq/hour)

Reference Range Serum level necessary to inhibit basal acid secretion:

Children: 90% suppression: 40-60 ng/mL

Adults: 50% suppression: 36-94 ng/mL

Test Interactions False-positive urine protein using Multistix®; gastric acid secretion test, skin test allergen extracts

Patient Information Avoid excessive amounts of coffee and aspirin; when self-medicating, if symptoms of heartburn, acid indigestion, or sour stomach persist after 2 weeks of continuous use of the drug, consult a clinician.

Additional Information Causes fewer CNS adverse reactions and drug interactions compared to cimetidine; safety and efficacy of full-dose therapy extending beyond 8 weeks have not been determined; Zantac® EFFERdose® 150 mg tablets and granules contain 7.55 mEq sodium

Dosage Forms

Capsule, as hydrochloride: 150 mg, 300 mg

Granules, effervescent, as hydrochloride (Zantac® EFFERdose®): 150 mg (60s) [contains 16.84 mg phenylalanine (as aspartame)/tablet, 7.55 mEq sodium/tablet, and sodium benzoate] [DSC]

Infusion, as hydrochloride [preservative free; premixed in NaCl 0.45%] (Zantac®): 50 mg (50 mL)

Injection, solution, as hydrochloride (Zantac®): 25 mg/mL (2 mL, 6 mL, 40 mL)

Syrup, as hydrochloride: 15 mg/mL (10 mL) [contains 7.5% alcohol; peppermint flavor]

Zantac®: 15 mg/mL (473 mL) [contains 7.5% alcohol; peppermint flavor]

Tablet, as hydrochloride: 75 mg [OTC], 150 mg, 300 mg

Zantac®: 150 mg, 300 mg

Zantac® 75: 75 mg

Tablet, effervescent, as hydrochloride (Zantac® EFFERdose®): 150 mg [contains 16.84 mg phenylalanine (as aspartame)/tablet, 7.55 mEq sodium/tablet, and sodium benzoate]

References

Blumer JL, Rothstein FC, Kaplan BS, et al, "Pharmacokinetic Determination of Ranitidine Pharmacodynamics in Pediatric Ulcer Disease," *J Pediatr,* 1985, 107(2):301-6.

Drug Prescribing in Renal Failure: Dosing Guidelines for Adults, 4th ed, Aronoff GR, et al, eds, Philadelphia, PA: American College of Physicians, 1999, 71.

Eddleston JM, Booker PD, and Green JR, "Use of Ranitidine in Children Undergoing Cardiopulmonary Bypass," *Crit Care Med,* 1989, 17(1):26-9.

Fontana M, Massironi E, Rossi A, et al, "Ranitidine Pharmacokinetics in Newborn Infants," *Arch Dis Child*, 1993, 68(5 Spec No):602-3.

Lopez-Herce J, Albajara L, Codoceo R, et al, "Ranitidine Prophylaxis in Acute Gastric Mucosal Damage in Critically Ill Pediatric Patients," *Crit Care Med*, 1988, 16(6):591-93.

Morris DL, Markham SJ, Beechey A, et al, "Ranitidine-Bolus or Infusion Prophylaxis for Stress Ulcer," *Crit Care Med*, 1988, 16(3):229-32.

Roberts CJ, "Clinical Pharmacokinetics of Ranitidine," *Clin Pharmacokinet*, 1984, 9(3):211-21.

Rasburicase (ras BYOOR i kayse)

U.S. Brand Names Elitek™

Synonyms Urate oxidase

Therapeutic Category Uric Acid Lowering Agent

Generic Available No

Use Initial management of plasma uric acid levels in pediatric patients with leukemia, lymphoma, and solid tumor malignancies who are receiving anti-cancer therapy expected to result in tumor lysis and subsequent elevation of plasma uric acid

Pregnancy Risk Factor C

Contraindications Hypersensitivity to rasburicase (see Warnings) or any component; patients with G-6-PD deficiency

Warnings Rasburicase may cause severe allergic reactions, including anaphylaxis; **discontinue immediately and permanently** in any patient exhibiting signs and symptoms of severe allergy, including chest pain, dyspnea, hypotension, and/or urticaria; rasburicase is immunogenic and can elicit antibodies that inhibit its activity (time to detection of antibodies after exposure to rasburicase varied from 1-6 weeks in normal, healthy volunteers); due to the potential for developing hypersensitivity reactions, rasburicase is indicated only for a single course of treatment.

Because hydrogen peroxide is one of the major byproducts of the conversion of uric acid to allantoin, rasburicase may cause severe hemolytic reactions in patients with G-6-PD deficiency; patients at high risk for G-6-PD deficiency should be screened prior to treatment with rasburicase; **discontinue treatment immediately and permanently** in any patient developing hemolysis; rasburicase has been associated with methemoglobinemia; **discontinue treatment immediately** in any patient developing methemoglobinemia

Precautions Rasburicase may interfere with uric acid measurements (see Test Interactions); patients receiving rasburicase should receive I.V. hydration as appropriate for the management of tumor lysis syndrome

Adverse Reactions

Cardiovascular: Arrhythmias, CHF, cardiac arrest, chest pain, cyanosis, flushing, MI, thrombosis, cerebrovascular disorder

Central nervous system: Fever, seizures, headache

Dermatologic: Rash, cellulitis

Gastrointestinal: Mucositis, diarrhea, ileus, intestinal obstruction, nausea, abdominal pain, constipation, vomiting

Hematologic: Hemolysis (see Warnings), neutropenia, pancytopenia, methemoglobinemia (see Warnings)

Neuromuscular & skeletal: Paresthesia

Ophthalmic: Retinal hemorrhages

Renal: Acute renal failure

Respiratory: Respiratory distress, bronchospasm, pulmonary edema, pulmonary hypertension

Miscellaneous: Severe hypersensitivity reactions, including anaphylaxis (see Warnings), sepsis

Drug Interactions None have as yet been identified

Stability Store rasburicase and diluent in the refrigerator; protect from light and do not freeze; reconstituted solution and final dilution (see Administration) are stable refrigerated, but must be used within 24 hours due to the lack of a preservative

Mechanism of Action Rasburicase is a recombinant urate-oxidase enzyme that catalyzes the enzymatic oxidation of uric acid into an inactive and soluble metabolite, allantoin; it does not inhibit the formation of uric acid

Pharmacokinetics

Distribution: V_d: Children: 110-127 mL/kg

Half-life: Children: 18 hours

Usual Dosage I.V.: Children: 0.15-0.2 mg/kg/dose once daily for up to 5 days

Administration I.V.: Dilute each vial with 1 mL of provided diluent; gently swirl, do not shake; further dilute desired dose in NS to a final volume of 50 mL; infuse over 30 minutes, do not bolus; do not filter or mix with other medications; chemotherapy may be initiated 4-24 hours after the first dose of rasburicase

Monitoring Parameters Uric acid (See Test Interactions); BUN, serum creatinine, phosphorus, urine output, CBC with differential

(Continued)

Rasburicase *(Continued)*

Test Interactions Rasburicase will cause enzymatic degradation of the uric acid within blood samples when left at room temperature, resulting in spuriously low uric acid levels; to avoid this interaction, blood must be collected into prechilled tubes containing heparin anticoagulant and immediately immersed and maintained in an ice water bath; plasma samples should be assayed within 4 hours of collection

Dosage Forms Injection, powder for reconstitution, lyophilized: 1.5 mg [packaged with three 1 mL ampules of diluent]

References

Goldman SC, Holcenberg JS, Finklestein JZ, et al, "A Randomized Comparison Between Rasburicase and Allopurinol in Children With Lymphoma or Leukemia at High Risk for Tumor Lysis," *Blood*, 2001, 97(10):2998-3003.

Pui CH, Mahmoud HH, Wiley JM, et al, "Recombinant Urate Oxidase for the Prophylaxis or Treatment of Hyperuricemia in Patients With Leukemia or Lymphoma," *J Clin Oncol*, 2001, 19(3):697-704.

◆ **ratio-Acyclovir (Can)** *see* Acyclovir *on page 45*
◆ **ratio-AmoxiClav (Can)** *see* Amoxicillin and Clavulanic Acid *on page 96*
◆ **ratio-Colchicine (Can)** *see* Colchicine *on page 303*
◆ **ratio-Diltiazem CD (Can)** *see* Diltiazem *on page 388*
◆ **ratio-Famotidine (Can)** *see* Famotidine *on page 473*
◆ **ratio-Glyburide (Can)** *see* GlyBURIDE *on page 540*
◆ **ratio-Inspra-Sal (Can)** *see* Albuterol *on page 54*
◆ **ratio-Lovastatin (Can)** *see* Lovastatin *on page 697*
◆ **ratio-Methotrexate (Can)** *see* Methotrexate *on page 737*
◆ **ratio-Morphine SR (Can)** *see* Morphine Sulfate *on page 778*
◆ **ratio-Pentoxifylline (Can)** *see* Pentoxifylline *on page 884*
◆ **ratio-Salbutamol (Can)** *see* Albuterol *on page 54*
◆ **ratio-Sertraline (Can)** *see* Sertraline *on page 1016*
◆ **ratio-Theo-Bronc (Can)** *see* Theophylline *on page 1076*
◆ **Reactine™ (Can)** *see* Cetirizine *on page 249*
◆ **ReAzo [OTC]** *see* Phenazopyridine *on page 887*
◆ **Rebetol®** *see* Ribavirin *on page 981*
◆ **Recombinant Human Activated Protein C** *see* Drotrecogin Alfa (Activated) *on page 420*
◆ **Recombinant Human α-L-Iduronidase** *see* Laronidase *on page 658*
◆ **Recombinant Human Deoxyribonuclease** *see* Dornase Alfa *on page 406*
◆ **Recombinate™** *see* Antihemophilic Factor (Recombinant) *on page 119*
◆ **Redutemp® [OTC]** *see* Acetaminophen *on page 36*
◆ **Reese's® Pinworm Medicine [OTC]** *see* Pyrantel Pamoate *on page 960*
◆ **ReFacto®** *see* Antihemophilic Factor (Recombinant) *on page 119*
◆ **Refresh PM® [OTC]** *see* Ocular Lubricant *on page 831*
◆ **Regitine® (Can)** *see* Phentolamine *on page 891*
◆ **Reglan®** *see* Metoclopramide *on page 749*
◆ **Regonol® [DSC]** *see* Pyridostigmine *on page 962*
◆ **Regulex® (Can)** *see* Docusate *on page 402*
◆ **Reguloid® [OTC]** *see* Psyllium *on page 959*
◆ **Rejuva-A® (Can)** *see* Tretinoin *on page 1111*
◆ **Relefact® TRH (Can)** *see* Protirelin *on page 956*
◆ **Relief® [OTC]** *see* Phenylephrine *on page 892*
◆ **Remicade®** *see* Infliximab *on page 608*
◆ **Remular® S** *see* Chlorzoxazone *on page 266*
◆ **Renova®** *see* Tretinoin *on page 1111*
◆ **Resectisol®** *see* Mannitol *on page 706*
◆ **Respa-DM®** *see* Guaifenesin and Dextromethorphan *on page 553*
◆ **Respa-GF** *see* Guaifenesin *on page 550*
◆ **RespiGam®** *see* Respiratory Syncytial Virus Immune Globulin (Intravenous) *on page 976*

Respiratory Syncytial Virus Immune Globulin (Intravenous)

(RES peer rah tor ee sin SISH al VYE rus i MYUN GLOB yoo lin in tra VEE nus)

U.S. Brand Names RespiGam®

Synonyms RSV-IGIV; RSV-IVIG

Therapeutic Category Immune Globulin

Generic Available No

Use Prevention of serious lower respiratory tract infection caused by RSV in children <24 months of age with BPD who are receiving supplemental oxygen; history of prematurity (≤32 weeks gestation); prophylaxis of infants with severe immune deficiency exposed to RSV; prophylaxis of infants and children with severe immunosuppression (eg, BMT patient exposed to RSV)

Pregnancy Risk Factor C

Contraindications Hypersensitivity to any component; history of a severe reaction associated with the administration of RSV-IGIV or other human immunoglobulin preparations; patients with IgA deficiency

Warnings Renal dysfunction and/or acute renal failure has been reported with the administration of IVIG; 88% of the cases were associated with the administration of sucrose-containing IVIG products. Since RespiGam® contains sucrose, ensure that patients are not volume depleted prior to the initiation of an infusion to decrease risk of renal dysfunction or failure. Adverse reactions may be related to the rate of administration; loop diuretics should be available for the management of patients who are at risk for fluid overload; epinephrine and diphenhydramine should be available for treatment of acute hypersensitivity reactions. Aseptic meningitis syndrome (onset of several hours to 2 days following RSV-IGIV administration: Symptoms of severe headache, drowsiness, fever, photophobia, painful eye movements, muscle rigidity, nausea and vomiting with pleocytosis and elevated protein levels in CSF have occurred in 3 patients in the PREVENT trial); (see Additional Information)

Precautions Use with caution in patients with underlying pulmonary disease since these patients are sensitive to extra fluid volume; use with caution in patients at increased risk for developing acute renal failure (patients with pre-existing renal insufficiency, diabetes mellitus, volume depletion, sepsis, paraproteinemia, and concomitant nephrotoxic drugs); immunization with MMR and varicella vaccines should be deferred for 9 months after the last RSV-IGIV dose

Adverse Reactions

Cardiovascular: Tachycardia, hypertension, edema, hypotension, heart murmur, cyanosis

Central nervous system: Fever/pyrexia (6%), dizziness, anxiety, aseptic meningitis syndrome

Dermatologic: Rash, eczema, pruritus

Gastrointestinal: Vomiting (6%), diarrhea, gastroenteritis

Local: Injection site inflammation

Respiratory: Respiratory distress, wheezing, rales, hypoxia, tachypnea, cyanosis, cough, rhinorrhea, dyspnea

Drug Interactions Live virus vaccine (ie, MMR, measles, varicella) when given during or within 10 months after RSV-IGIV administration; antibody response to DPT, DTaP, OPV, and *H. influenzae* b vaccine may be lower

Stability Refrigerate; do not freeze; do not shake vials; compatible with dextrose 5% through dextrose 20% with or without sodium chloride

Pharmacokinetics Half-life: 22-28 days

Usual Dosage I.V. infusion: Infants and Young Children: 750 mg/kg once monthly during RSV season (starting November with the last infusion in April).

Administration Infusion should start within 6 hours and be completed by 12 hours after vial entry; an in-line filter is not necessary, but if one is used, the pore size should be larger than 15 µM; if dilution is needed, a dilution of no greater than 1:2 should be used.

The infusion schedule is as follows:

Initial infusion rate for the first 15 minutes: 1.5 mL/kg/hour

15 minutes to end of infusion: 3.6 mL/kg/hour

Maximum infusion rate: 3.6 mL/kg/hour

Monitoring Parameters Heart rate, blood pressure, temperature, respiratory rate; observe for retractions and rales

Additional Information PREVENT (Prophylaxis of RSV in elevated-risk neonates trial) was a multicenter, randomized, double-blind, placebo-controlled trial (n=250 RSV-IGIV, n=260 placebo) among infants ≤24 months, born prematurely (≤35 weeks gestation), or children with BPD and a requirement for supplemental oxygen within the past 6 months. Each patient received a monthly infusion from November through April. The trial showed that children treated with RSV-IGIV had less RSV hospitalizations (20 days vs. 35 days, p=0.047); fewer RSV hospital days per 100 days (60 days vs. 129 days, p=0.045); fewer RSV hospital days with supplemental oxygen (34 days vs. 85 days, p=0.007). There was no difference between the two groups for ICU admissions, RSV ICU days per 100 children, RSV mechanical ventilation or days of ventilation per 100 children. (Groothius, 1993)

RSV-IGIV is a sterile liquid without preservatives purified using Cohn-Oncley cold ethanol fractionation and further treatment with a solvent-detergent partitioning (Continued)

Respiratory Syncytial Virus Immune Globulin (Intravenous) *(Continued)*

method; contains trace amounts of IgA and IgM, sucrose and albumin; sodium content: 20-30 mEq/L

Dosage Forms Injection, solution [preservative free]: 50 mg/mL (50 mL)

References

American Academy of Pediatrics Committee on Infectious Diseases, Committee on Fetus and Newborn, "Respiratory Syncytial Virus Immune Globulin Intravenous: Indications for Use," *Pediatrics*, 1997, 99(4):645-50.

Ellenberg SS, Epstein JS, Fratantoni JC, et al, "A Trial of RSV Immune Globulin in Infants and Young Children: The FDA's View," *N Engl J Med*, 1994, 331(3):203-5.

Groothuis JR, Simoes EA, Levin MJ, et al, "Prophylactic Administration of Respiratory Syncytial Virus Immune Globulin to High-Risk Infants and Young Children. The Respiratory Syncytial Virus Immune Globulin Study Group," *N Engl J Med*, 1993, 329(21):1524-30.

- ◆ **Restasis™** *see* CycloSPORINE *on page 324*
- ◆ **Retin-A®** *see* Tretinoin *on page 1111*
- ◆ **Retin-A® Micro** *see* Tretinoin *on page 1111*
- ◆ **Retinoic Acid** *see* Tretinoin *on page 1111*
- ◆ **Retinova® (Can)** *see* Tretinoin *on page 1111*
- ◆ **Retrovir®** *see* Zidovudine *on page 1163*
- ◆ **Reversol®** *see* Edrophonium *on page 426*
- ◆ **Revitalose C-1000® (Can)** *see* Ascorbic Acid *on page 131*
- ◆ **R-Gene®** *see* Arginine *on page 130*
- ◆ **rGM-CSF** *see* Sargramostim *on page 1007*
- ◆ **Rheumatrex®** *see* Methotrexate *on page 737*
- ◆ **RhIG** *see* Rhₒ(D) Immune Globulin *on page 978*
- ◆ **Rhinalar® (Can)** *see* Flunisolide *on page 497*
- ◆ **Rhinocort® [DSC]** *see* Budesonide *on page 183*
- ◆ **Rhinocort® Aqua™** *see* Budesonide *on page 183*
- ◆ **Rho-Clonazepam (Can)** *see* Clonazepam *on page 292*
- ◆ **Rhodacine® (Can)** *see* Indomethacin *on page 606*

Rhₒ(D) Immune Globulin *(ar aych oh (dee) i MYUN GLOB yoo lin)*

U.S. Brand Names BayRho-D® Full-Dose; BayRho-D® Mini-Dose; MICRhoGAM®; RhoGAM®; WinRho SDF®

Synonyms RhIG; Rhₒ(D) Immune Globulin (Human); RhₒIGIV; RhₒIVIM

Therapeutic Category Immune Globulin

Generic Available No

Use

Suppression of Rh isoimmunization: Use in the following situations when an Rhₒ(D)-negative individual is exposed to Rhₒ(D)-positive blood: During delivery of an Rhₒ(D)-positive infant; abortion; amniocentesis; chorionic villus sampling; ruptured tubal pregnancy; abdominal trauma; transplacental hemorrhage. Used when the mother is Rhₒ(D) negative, the father of the child is either Rhₒ(D) positive or Rhₒ(D) unknown, the baby is either either Rhₒ(D) positive or Rhₒ(D) unknown.

Transfusion: Suppression of Rh isoimmunization in Rhₒ(D)-negative female children and female adults in their childbearing years transfused with Rhₒ(D) antigen-positive RBCs or blood components containing Rhₒ(D) antigen-positive RBCs

Treatment of idiopathic thrombocytopenic purpura (ITP): **I.V. formulation only:** Used in the following nonsplenectomized Rhₒ(D) positive individuals: Children with acute or chronic ITP, adults with chronic ITP, children and adults with ITP secondary to HIV infection

Pregnancy Risk Factor C

Contraindications Hypersensitivity to immune globulin, thimerosal (RhoGAM® formulation) or any component; IgA deficiency; Rhₒ(D)-positive mother or pregnant woman; transfusion of Rhₒ(D)-positive blood in previous 3 months; prior sensitization to Rhₒ(D); mothers whose Rh group or immune status is uncertain

Warnings Use only the I.V. formulation when treating ITP; when using the I.V. formulation (WinRho SDF®) to treat ITP, a decrease in hemoglobin concentration as a result of destruction of Rhₒ(D)-positive red blood cells can be expected; reduce WinRho SDF® dosage in ITP patients with Hgb <10 g/dL (see Usual Dosage) to minimize the risk of increasing the severity of anemia. These patients should be monitored for signs and/or symptoms of intravascular hemolysis, clinically compromising anemia, and renal insufficiency

When used to suppress Rh isoimmunization, the drug is administered to the mother **not** the infant; anaphylactic hypersensitivity reactions can occur; studies indicate that there is no discernible risk of transmitting HIV or hepatitis B; not intended for use as immunoglobulin replacement therapy for immune deficiency syndromes

Precautions Use with caution in patients with thrombocytopenia or bleeding disorders or in patients with hemoglobin concentrations <8 g/dL

Adverse Reactions

Cardiovascular: Hypotension, pallor, vasodilation (I.V. formulation)

Central nervous system: Fever, headache, chills, dizziness, somnolence, lethargy

Dermatologic: Rash, pruritus

Gastrointestinal: Abdominal pain, diarrhea, splenomegaly

Genitourinary: Hemoglobinuria

Hematologic: Hemolysis (hemoglobin decrease >2 g/dL in 5% to 10% of ITP patients)

Hepatic: Elevated bilirubin

Local: Discomfort and swelling at injection site

Neuromuscular & skeletal: Back pain, myalgia, hyperkinesia, arthralgia, weakness, hyperkinesia

Miscellaneous: Hypersensitivity reactions, diaphoresis

Drug Interactions May interfere with the immune response to live virus vaccines (allow 3 months after administration of vaccine)

Stability Refrigerate, do not freeze; reconstituted powder (WinRho SDF®) is stable 12 hours at room temperature; solution (RhoGAM®, BayRho-D®) may be stable for up to 30 days at room temperature

Mechanism of Action The Rh$_o$(D) antigen is responsible for most cases of Rh sensitization, which occurs when Rh-positive fetal RBCs enter the maternal circulation of an Rh-negative woman. Injection of anti-D globulin results in opsonization of the fetal RBCs, which are then phagocytized in the spleen, preventing immunization of the mother. Injection of anti-D into an Rh-positive patient with ITP coats the patient's own D-positive RBCs with antibody and, as they are cleared by the spleen, they saturate the capacity of the spleen to clear antibody-coated cells, sparing antibody-coated platelets. Other proposed mechanisms involve the generation of cytokines following the interaction between antibody-coated RBCs and macrophages.

Pharmacodynamics

Onset of action:

Rh isoimmunization: I.V.: 8 hours

ITP: I.V.: 1-2 days

Maximum effect: ITP: 7-14 days

Duration:

ITP (single dose): I.V.: 30 days

Passive anti-Rh$_o$(D) antibodies (after 120 mcg dose): I.V.: 6 weeks

Pharmacokinetics

Distribution: Appears in breast milk, however, not absorbed by the nursing infant

Half-life, elimination:

I.M.: 30 days

I.V.: 24 days

Time to peak serum concentration:

I.M.: 5-10 days

I.V.: 2 hours

Usual Dosage

ITP: Children and Adults: **I.V. only:**

Initial:

Hemoglobin ≥10 g/dL: 50 mcg/kg (250 international units/kg) as single dose or divided into 2 doses given on separate days

Hemoglobin <10 g/dL: 25-40 mcg/kg (125-200 international units/kg) as single dose or divided into 2 doses given on separate days

Hemoglobin <8 g/dL: Use with caution (see Warnings and Precautions)

Maintenance (usage dependent upon clinical response, platelet count, hemoglobin, red blood cell counts, and reticulocyte levels)

Response to initial dose: 25-60 mcg/kg (125-300 international units/kg) as single dose

Nonresponse to initial therapy:

Hemoglobin >10 g/dL: 50-60 mcg/kg (250-300 international units/kg) as single dose

Hemoglobin 8-10 g/dL: 25-40 mcg/kg (125-200 international units/kg) as single dose

Hemoglobin <8 g/dL: Use with caution (see Warnings and Precautions)

Suppression of RH isoimmunization: **Adult female:** I.V., I.M.: See table on next page.

Note: One "full dose" (300 mcg) provides enough antibody to prevent Rh sensitization if the volume of fetal RBCs entering the maternal circulation is ≤15 mL. When >15 mL is suspected, a fetal red cell count should be performed to determine the appropriate dose.

(Continued)

Rh₀(D) Immune Globulin *(Continued)*

Rh₀D Immune Globulin Dosage in Pregnancy and Obstetrical Conditions

Condition	WinRho SDF® Dosage I.V. or I.M.	BayRho-D® or RhoGAM® Dosage I.M.
Pregnancy	300 mcg (1500 international units) at 28 weeks gestation; repeat every 12 weeks throughout pregnancy	300 mcg at 28 weeks and following delivery, preferably within 72 hours of delivery
Postpartum (if newborn Rh-positive)	120 mcg (600 international units) as soon as possible, preferably <72 hours, after delivery; if baby's Rh status is not known by 72 hours administer as soon as possible up to 28 days after delivery	300 mcg as soon as possible, preferably within 72 hours of delivery
Threatened abortion at any time	300 mcg (1500 international units) as soon as possible within 72 hours	300 mcg as soon as possible
Amniocentesis and chronic villus sampling	Before 34 weeks gestation: 300 mcg (1500 international units) administered immediately; repeat every 12 weeks throughout pregnancy After 34 weeks gestation: 120 mcg (600 international units) administered immediately or within 72 hours	At 15-18 weeks gestation or during the 3rd trimester: 300 mcg; if given between 13-18 weeks, repeat at 26-28 weeks and within 72 hours of delivery
Abortion, miscarriage, termination of ectopic pregnancy	After 34 weeks gestation: 120 mcg (600 international units) administered immediately or within 72 hours	<13 weeks gestation: 50 mcg ≥13 weeks gestation: 300 mcg administered immediately or within 72 hours
Abdominal trauma, manipulation	After 34 weeks gestation: 120 mcg (600 international units) administered immediately or within 72 hours	During the 2nd or 3rd trimester: 300 mcg; if given between 13-18 weeks, repeat at 26-28 weeks and within 72 hours of delivery

Treatment of exposure to incompatible blood transfusion or massive fetal hemorrhage, within 72 hours of event:

WinRho SDF®: Children and Adults:

Exposed to Rh₀(D) positive whole blood:

I.M.: 12 mcg (60 international units)/mL blood; administer in 1200 mcg (6000 international units) aliquots every 12 hours until the total calculated dose is administered

I.V.: 9 mcg (45 international units)/mL blood; administer in 600 mcg (3000 international units) aliquots every 8 hours until the total calculated dose is administered

Exposed to Rh₀(D) positive red blood cells:

I.M.: 24 mcg (120 international units)/mL cells administer in 1200 mcg (6000 international units) aliquots every 12 hours until the total calculated dose is administered

I.V.: 18 mcg (90 international units)/mL cells; administer in 600 mcg (3000 international units) aliquots every 8 hours until the total calculated dose is administered

BayRho-D®, RhoGAM®: Adults: I.M.: Multiply the volume of Rh-positive whole blood administered by the hematocrit of the donor unit to equal the volume of RBCs transfused. The volume of RBCs is then divided by 15 mL, resulting in the number of 300 mcg doses to administer. If the dose calculated results in a fraction, round up to the next higher whole 300 mcg dose.

Administration Parenteral: WinRho SDF® is the only immune globulin product available that can be administered both I.M. and I.V.; however, **for the treatment of ITP, it must be administered I.V.**

I.M.: Administer into the deltoid muscle of upper arm or the anterolateral aspect of the upper thigh; the gluteal region is not recommended for routine administration due to the potential risk of sciatic nerve injury; if gluteal area is used, administer only in the upper, outer quadrant. The total volume can be given in divided doses at different sites at one time or may be divided and given at intervals provided the total dosage is given within 72 hours of the fetomaternal hemorrhage or transfusion

WinRho SDF®: Reconstitute 120 mcg and 300 mcg vials with 1.25 mL NS and the 100 mcg vial with 8.5 mL NS; gently swirl vial; do not shake

I.V.: WinRho SDF®: Reconstitute 120 mcg and 300 mcg vials with 2.5 mL NS and 8.5 mL NS for the 1000 mcg vial; gently swirl vial; do not shake; infuse over 3-5 minutes

Monitoring Parameters ITP: Signs and symptoms of intravascular hemolysis, CBC, reticulocytes, UA, renal function, platelets

Additional Information WinRho SDF® 1 mcg = 5 international units

Treatment of ITP in Rh-positive patients with an intact spleen appears to be about as effective as IVIG.

Dosage Forms

Injection, powder for reconstitution [preservative free] (WinRho SDF®): 120 mcg [600 international units], 300 mcg [1500 international units], 1000 mcg [5000 international units] [for I.M. or I.V. use]

Injection, solution [preservative free]:
BayRho-D® Full-Dose, RhoGAM®: 300 mcg [for I.M. use only]
BayRho-D® Mini-Dose, MICRhoGAM®: 50 mcg [for I.M. use only]

References

Gaines AR, "Acute Onset Hemoglobinemia and/or Hemoglobinuria and Sequelae Following Rh(o)(D) Immune Globulin Intravenous Administration in Immune Thrombocytopenic Purpura Patients," *Blood*, 2000, 95(8):2523-9.

Ribavirin (rye ba VYE rin)

U.S. Brand Names Copegus™; Rebetol®; Virazole®

Synonyms ICN-1299; RTCA; Tribavirin

Therapeutic Category Antiviral Agent, Inhalation Therapy

Generic Available No

Use Treatment of patients with RSV infections; specially indicated for treatment of severe lower respiratory tract RSV infections in patients with an underlying compromising condition (prematurity, BPD and other chronic lung conditions, congenital heart disease, immunodeficiency, immunosuppression), and recent transplant recipients; may also be used in other viral infections including influenza A and B and adenovirus

Pregnancy Risk Factor X

Contraindications Females of childbearing age

Warnings Ribavirin is potentially mutagenic, tumor-promoting, and gonadotoxic; there is evidence that ribavirin is teratogenic in small animals

Precautions Use with caution in patients requiring assisted ventilation because precipitation of the drug in the respiratory equipment may interfere with safe and effective patient ventilation; carefully monitor patients with COPD and asthma for deterioration of respiratory function

Adverse Reactions
Cardiovascular: Hypotension, cardiac arrest
Central nervous system: Headache
Dermatologic: Rash, skin irritation
Hematologic: Anemia
Ocular: Conjunctivitis
Respiratory: Mild bronchospasm, worsening of respiratory function, nasal and throat irritation

Drug Interactions Ribavirin antagonizes the antiviral activity of zidovudine and zalcitabine against HIV

Stability Reconstituted solution is stable for 24 hours at room temperature
(Continued)

Ribavirin *(Continued)*

Mechanism of Action Inhibits replication of RNA and DNA viruses; inhibits influenza virus RNA polymerase activity and interferes with the expression of messenger RNA resulting in inhibition of viral protein synthesis

Pharmacokinetics

Absorption: Systemically absorbed from the respiratory tract following nasal and oral inhalation; absorption is dependent upon respiratory factors and method of drug delivery; maximal absorption occurs with the use of the aerosol generator via an endotracheal tube

Distribution: Highest concentrations are found in the respiratory tract and erythrocytes

Metabolism: Occurs intracellularly and may be necessary for drug action; metabolized by the liver to deribosylated ribavirin (active metabolite)

Half-life:

Respiratory tract secretions: ~2 hours

Plasma:

Children: 6.5-11 hours

Adults: 24 hours; half-life is much longer in the erythrocyte (16-40 days), which can be used as a marker for intracellular metabolism

Time to peak serum concentration: Aerosol inhalation: At the end of the inhalation period

Elimination: Hepatic metabolism is the major route of elimination with 40% of the drug cleared renally as unchanged drug and metabolites

Usual Dosage Infants, Children, and Adults: Aerosol inhalation:

Use with Viratek® small particle aerosol generator (SPAG-2) at a concentration of 20 mg/mL (6 g reconstituted with 300 mL of sterile water without preservatives); 6 g ribavirin vial has also been diluted with 300 mL of sterile NS solution rather than sterile water to achieve a near isotonic solution.

Note: Dose actually delivered to the patient will depend on patient's minute ventilation

Continuous aerosolization: 12-18 hours/day for 3 days, or up to 7 days in length

Intermittent aerosolization (high-dose, short-duration aerosol): 2 g over 2 hours 3 times/day at a concentration of 60 mg/mL (6 g reconstituted with 100 mL of sterile water without preservatives) in **non-mechanically ventilated** patients for 3-7 days has been used to permit easier accessibility for patient care and limit environmental exposure of healthcare worker. Due to apparent increased potential for crystallization of the high-dose 60 mg/mL solution around areas of turbulent flow such as bends in tubing or connector pieces, use of high-dose therapy in individuals with an endotracheal tube in place is **not** recommended.

Administration Ribavirin should be administered in well-ventilated rooms (at least 6 air changes/hour)

Mechanically ventilated patients: Ribavirin can potentially be deposited in the ventilator delivery system depending on temperature, humidity, and electrostatic forces; this deposition can lead to malfunction or obstruction of the expiratory valve, resulting in inadvertently high positive end-expiratory pressures. The use of one-way valves in the inspiratory lines, a breathing circuit filter in the expiratory line, and frequent monitoring and filter replacement have been effective in preventing these problems.

Monitoring Parameters Respiratory function, hemoglobin, reticulocyte count, CBC, I & O

Nursing Implications Healthcare workers who are pregnant or who may become pregnant should be advised of the potential risks of exposure and counseled about risk reduction strategies including alternate job responsibilities; limit contact by visitors with patients receiving ribavirin; ribavirin may adsorb to contact lenses

Additional Information RSV season is usually December to April; viral shedding period for RSV is usually 3-8 days

Dosage Forms

Capsule (Rebetol®): 200 mg

Powder for aerosol, lyophilized (Virazole®): 6 g

Tablet (Copegus™): 200 mg

References

American Academy of Pediatrics Committee on Infectious Diseases, "Reassessment of the Indications for Ribavirin Therapy in Respiratory Syncytial Virus Infections," *Pediatrics*, 1996, 97(1):137-40.

Englund JA, Piedra PA, Ahn Y-M, et al, "High-Dose, Short-Duration Ribavirin Aerosol Therapy Compared With Standard Ribavirin Therapy in Children With Suspected Respiratory Syncytial Virus Infection," *J Pediatr*, 1994, 125:635-41.

Janai HK, Marks MI, Zaleska M, et al, "Ribavirin: Adverse Drug Reactions 1986 to 1988," *Pediatr Infect Dis J*, 1990, 9(3):209-11.

Meert KL, Sarnaik AP, Gelmini MJ, et al, "Aerosolized Ribavirin in Mechanically Ventilated Children With Respiratory Syncytial Virus Lower Respiratory Tract Disease: A Prospective, Double-Blind, Randomized Trial," *Crit Care Med*, 1994, 22(4):566-72.

Smith DW, Frankel LR, Mathers LH, et al, "A Controlled Trial of Aerosolized Ribavirin in Infants Receiving Mechanical Ventilation for Severe Respiratory Syncytial Virus Infection," *N Engl J Med*, 1991, 325(1):24-9.

Riboflavin (RYE boe flay vin)

Synonyms Lactoflavin; Vitamin B_2; Vitamin G

Therapeutic Category Nutritional Supplement; Vitamin, Water Soluble

Generic Available Yes

Use Prevention of riboflavin deficiency and treatment of ariboflavinosis; microcytic anemia associated with glutathione reductase deficiency

Pregnancy Risk Factor A (C if dose exceeds RDA recommendation)

Contraindications Hypersensitivity to riboflavin or any component

Adverse Reactions Genitourinary: Discoloration of urine (bright yellow) with large doses

Drug Interactions Probenecid

Food Interactions Food increases the extent of GI absorption

Stability Protect from light

Mechanism of Action Converted to coenzymes which act as hydrogen-carrier molecules, which are necessary for normal tissue respiration; also needed for activation of pyridoxine and conversion of tryptophan to niacin

Pharmacokinetics

Absorption: Readily via GI tract; GI absorption is decreased in patients with hepatitis, cirrhosis, or biliary obstruction

Metabolism: Metabolic fate unknown

Half-life, biologic: 66-84 minutes

Elimination: 9% eliminated unchanged in urine

Usual Dosage Oral:

Riboflavin deficiency:

Children: 3-10 mg/day in divided doses

Adults: 5-30 mg/day in divided doses

Adequate intake: Infants:

<6 months: 0.3 mg (0.04 mg/kg)

6-12 months: 0.4 mg (0.04 mg/kg)

Recommended daily allowance (RDA):

Children:

1-3 years: 0.5 mg

4-8 years: 0.6 mg

9-13 years: 0.9 mg

14-18 years:

Male: 1.3 mg

Female: 1 mg

19-70 years:

Male: 1.3 mg

Female: 1.1 mg

Microcytic anemia associated with glutathione reductase deficiency: Adults: 10 mg daily for 10 days

Administration Oral: Administer with food

Monitoring Parameters CBC and reticulocyte counts (if anemic when treating deficiency)

Test Interactions Large doses may interfere with urinalysis based on spectrometry; may cause false elevations in fluorometric determinations of catecholamines and urobilinogen

Patient Information Large doses may cause bright yellow urine

Dosage Forms

Capsule: 100 mg

Tablet: 25 mg, 50 mg, 100 mg

♦ **Rid-a-Pain-HP® [OTC]** *see* Capsaicin *on page 206*

♦ **Ridaura®** *see* Auranofin *on page 147*

♦ **Rid® Spray [OTC]** *see* Permethrin *on page 885*

Rifabutin (rif a BYOO tin)

U.S. Brand Names Mycobutin®

Synonyms Ansamycin

Therapeutic Category Antibiotic, Miscellaneous; Antitubercular Agent

Generic Available No

Use Prevention of disseminated *Mycobacterium avium* complex (MAC) in patients with advanced HIV infection; utilized in multiple drug regimens for treatment of MAC

Pregnancy Risk Factor B

Contraindications Hypersensitivity to rifabutin, any component, or other rifamycin; rifabutin is contraindicated in patients with a WBC <1000/mm³ or a platelet count
(Continued)

Rifabutin *(Continued)*

<50,000 mm^3; coadministration of rifabutin with delavirdine or ritonavir (see Drug Interactions)

Warnings Rifabutin as a single agent must not be administered to patients with active tuberculosis since its use may lead to the development of tuberculosis that is resistant to both rifabutin and rifampin; rifabutin should be discontinued in patients with AST >500 international units/L or if total bilirubin is >3 mg/dL. Tiny, asymptomatic peripheral and central corneal deposits have been observed during routine ophthalmologic exams in HIV-positive patients receiving rifabutin.

Precautions Use with caution in patients with liver or renal impairment; modify dose in patients with Cl$_{cr}$ <30 mL/minute. Rifabutin is a CYP3A3/4 isoenzyme inducer which may reduce the plasma concentrations of itraconazole, clarithromycin, and saquinavir. CYP3A3/4 isoenzyme inhibitors such as fluconazole and clarithromycin may elevate levels of rifabutin increasing the risk of adverse reactions. Monitor patients, and in some cases, reduce the rifabutin dose when coadministered with fluconazole or clarithromycin (see Drug Interactions).

Adverse Reactions
Central nervous system: Fever, headache, seizures, confusion, insomnia
Dermatologic: Rash, staining of skin (brown-orange)
Gastrointestinal: Abdominal pain, diarrhea, dyspepsia, nausea, anorexia, vomiting, dysgeusia, flatulence
Genitourinary: Discoloration of urine (brown-orange)
Hematologic: Thrombocytopenia, anemia, leukopenia, neutropenia
Hepatic: Elevated liver enzymes
Neuromuscular & skeletal: Arthralgia, myositis
Ocular: Uveitis, corneal deposits
Miscellaneous: Discoloration of body fluids (brown-orange)

Drug Interactions Cytochrome P450 isoenzyme CYP3A3/4 inducer
May decrease the serum concentration or effect of dapsone, verapamil, methadone, ketoconazole, digoxin, theophylline, barbiturates, itraconazole, clarithromycin, protease inhibitors, non-nucleoside reverse transcriptase inhibitors, anticoagulants, corticosteroids, zidovudine, cyclosporine, quinidine, and oral contraceptives (alternative form of contraception should be considered); indinavir and ritonavir increase rifabutin concentrations (decrease daily rifabutin dose by 50% if given with indinavir or nelfinavir; decrease rifabutin adult dose to 150 mg 2-3 times per week if given with ritonavir); protease inhibitors, erythromycin, clarithromycin, delavirdine, ketoconazole, fluconazole, and itraconazole may increase serum concentration of rifabutin

Food Interactions High-fat meal may decrease the rate but not the extent of absorption

Mechanism of Action Inhibits DNA-dependent RNA polymerase at the beta subunit which prevents chain initiation

Pharmacokinetics
Absorption: Oral: Readily absorbed
Distribution: To body tissues including the lungs, liver, spleen, eyes, and kidneys
V$_d$: Adults: 9.3 ± 1.5 L/kg
Protein binding: 85%
Metabolism: To active and inactive metabolites
Bioavailability: Adults: 20% in HIV patients
Half-life, terminal: Adults: 45 hours (range: 16-69 hours)
Time to peak serum concentration: 2-4 hours
Elimination: Renal and biliary clearance of unchanged drug is 10%; 30% excreted in feces

Usual Dosage Oral:
Children: Efficacy and safety of rifabutin have not been established in children; a limited number of HIV-positive children with MAC (n=22) have been given rifabutin for MAC prophylaxis; dosages of up to 75 mg/day have been given to children <4 years of age (~5-6 mg/kg/day)
Infants and Children: Prophylaxis for first episode of MAC in HIV-infected patients:
Children <6 years: 5 mg/kg once daily
Children ≥6 years: 300 mg once daily
Infants and Children: Prophylaxis for recurrence of MAC in HIV-infected patients: 5 mg/kg (maximum dose: 300 mg) once daily in combination with clarithromycin
Adolescents and Adults:
Prophylaxis for first episode of MAC in HIV-infected patient: 300 mg once daily; for patients who experience GI upset, rifabutin can be administered 150 mg twice daily with food
Prophylaxis for recurrence of MAC in HIV-infected patient: 300 mg once daily as a component of a multiple drug regimen

Dosage adjustment in renal impairment: Cl_{cr} <30 mL/minute: Reduce dose by 50%

Administration Oral: May administer with or without food or mix with applesauce; administer with food to decrease GI upset

Monitoring Parameters Periodic liver function tests, CBC with differential, platelet count, hemoglobin, hematocrit, ophthalmologic exam

Patient Information May discolor skin, urine, tears, perspiration, or other body fluids to a brown-orange color; soft contact lenses may be permanently stained. Notify physician of any severe flu-like symptoms, nausea, vomiting, dark urine, unusual bleeding or bruising, or any eye problems

Dosage Forms Capsule: 150 mg

Extemporaneous Preparations A 20 mg/mL rifabutin suspension is made by placing the powder from eight 150 mg rifabutin capsules into a glass mortar, levigating with 20 mL of a 1:1 vehicle of Ora-Sweet® and Ora-Plus® and triturating the mixture to make a paste. Additional vehicle is added in geometric proportion levigating until a uniform mixture is obtained; qsad to 60 mL with vehicle. Stable for 12 weeks at 4°C, 25°C, 30°C, and 40°C. Label "shake well before using."

Haslam JL, Egodage KL, Chen Y, et al, "Stability of Rifabutin in Two Extemporaneously Compounded Oral Liquids," *Am J Health Syst Pharm*, 1999, 56(4):333-6.

References
Kaplan JE, Masur H, and Holmes KK, "Guidelines for Preventing Opportunistic Infections Among HIV-Infected Persons - 2002 Recommendations of the USPHS and IDSA," *MMWR*, 2002, 51(RR-8):1-46.

Krause PJ, Hight DW, Schwartz AN, et al, "Successful Management of *Mycobacterium intracellulare* Pneumonia in a Child," *Pediatr Infect Dis*, 1986, 5(2):269-71.

Levin RH and Bolinger AM, "Treatment of Nontuberculous Mycobacterial Infections in Pediatric Patients," *Clin Pharm*, 1988, 7(7):545-51.

Starke JR and Correa AG, "Management of Mycobacterial Infection and Disease in Children," *Pediatr Infect Dis J*, 1995, 14(6):455-70.

♦ **Rifadin®** *see* Rifampin *on page 985*

♦ **Rifampicin** *see* Rifampin *on page 985*

Rifampin (RIF am pin)

U.S. Brand Names Rifadin®; Rimactane®
Canadian Brand Names Rofact™
Synonyms Rifampicin
Therapeutic Category Antibiotic, Miscellaneous; Antitubercular Agent
Generic Available Yes

Use Used in combination with other antitubercular drugs for the treatment of active tuberculosis; elimination of meningococci from asymptomatic carriers; prophylaxis in contacts of patients with *Haemophilus influenzae* type B infection; used in combination with other anti-infectives in the treatment of staphylococcal infections

Pregnancy Risk Factor C

Contraindications Hypersensitivity to rifampin, rifamycins, or any component; concurrent use with amprenavir

Warnings Two month rifampin-pyrazinamide regimen for the treatment of latent tuberculosis infection has been associated with severe and fatal liver injuries.

Precautions Use with caution in patients with liver impairment, patients receiving concurrent medications associated with liver injury (particularly with pyrazinamide), or in patients with a history of alcoholism; modification of dosage should be considered in patients with severe liver impairment

Adverse Reactions

Central nervous system: Drowsiness, fatigue, confusion, ataxia, fever, headache, dizziness

Dermatologic: Rash, pruritus, urticaria

Gastrointestinal: Nausea, vomiting, diarrhea, stomatitis, anorexia

Hematologic: Eosinophilia, blood dyscrasias (leukopenia, thrombocytopenia), hemolytic anemia

Hepatic: Hepatitis, cholestatic jaundice, elevated liver enzymes

Local: Irritation at the I.V. site

Neuromuscular & skeletal: Myalgias, arthralgia, weakness

Renal: Renal failure, interstitial nephritis

Miscellaneous: Flu-like syndrome; discoloration of body fluids (red-orange)

Drug Interactions Cytochrome P450 isoenzyme CYP3A4 substrate; isoenzyme CYP1A2, CYP2C9, CYP2C18, CYP2C19, CYP3A3/4, and CYP3A5-7 inducer

Rifampin induces liver enzymes which may decrease the plasma concentration of the following drugs: verapamil, diltiazem, nifedipine, methadone, digoxin, cyclosporine, tacrolimus, benzodiazepines, corticosteroids, oral anticoagulants, theophylline, barbiturates, chloramphenicol, ketoconazole, oral contraceptives (alternate form of contraception should be considered), protease inhibitors, non-nucleoside reverse transcriptase inhibitors, and quinidine; halothane, pyrazinamide, or isoniazid (additive hepatotoxic effects)

(Continued)

Rifampin *(Continued)*

Food Interactions Food may delay and reduce the amount of rifampin absorbed

Stability Reconstituted I.V. solution is stable for 24 hours at room temperature; once the reconstituted rifampin I.V. solution is further diluted, it is stable for 4 hours in D_5W and up to 24 hours in NS. However, 11% to 13% rifampin decomposition has been reported to occur in 24 hours for solutions diluted in NS. Administer rifampin I.V. solution within 4 hours after preparation to avoid potential for precipitation and decomposition beyond this period.

Mechanism of Action Inhibits bacterial RNA synthesis by binding to the beta subunit of DNA-dependent RNA polymerase, blocking RNA transcription

Pharmacokinetics

Absorption: Oral: Well absorbed

Distribution: Highly lipophilic; crosses the blood-brain barrier and is widely distributed into body tissues and fluids such as the liver, lungs, gallbladder, bile, tears, and breast milk; distributes into CSF when meninges are inflamed

Protein binding: 80%

Metabolism: Undergoes enterohepatic recycling; metabolized in the liver to a deacetylated metabolite (active)

Half-life: 3-4 hours, prolonged with hepatic impairment

Time to peak serum concentration: Oral: Within 2-4 hours

Elimination: Principally in feces (60% to 65%) and urine (~30%)

Dialysis: Plasma rifampin concentrations are not significantly affected by hemodialysis or peritoneal dialysis

Usual Dosage Oral (I.V. infusion dose is the same as for the oral route):

Tuberculosis:

Infants and Children: 10-20 mg/kg/day in divided doses every 12-24 hours

Adults: 10 mg/kg/day administered once daily; maximum dose: 600 mg/day

American Thoracic Society and CDC currently recommend twice weekly therapy as part of a short-course regimen which follows 1-2 months of daily treatment of uncomplicated pulmonary tuberculosis in the compliant patient

Children: 10-20 mg/kg/dose (up to 600 mg) twice weekly under supervision to ensure compliance

Adults: 10 mg/kg (up to 600 mg) twice weekly

H. influenzae prophylaxis:

Neonates <1 month: 10 mg/kg/day every 24 hours for 4 days

Infants and Children: 20 mg/kg/day every 24 hours for 4 days, not to exceed 600 mg/dose

Adults: 600 mg every 24 hours for 4 days

Meningococcal prophylaxis:

<1 month: 10 mg/kg/day in divided doses every 12 hours for 2 days

Infants and Children: 20 mg/kg/day in divided doses every 12 hours for 2 days, not to exceed 600 mg/dose

Adults: 600 mg every 12 hours for 2 days

Nasal carriers of *Staphylococcus aureus*:

Children: 15 mg/kg/day divided every 12 hours for 5-10 days in combination with other antibiotics

Adults: 600 mg once daily for 5-10 days in combination with other antibiotics

Synergy for *Staphylococcus aureus* infections:

Neonates: 5-20 mg/kg/day in divided doses every 12 hours with other antibiotics

Adults: 300-600 mg twice daily with other antibiotics

Administration

Oral: Administer 1 hour before or 2 hours after a meal on an empty stomach; may administer with food to decrease GI distress; may mix contents of capsule with applesauce or jelly

Parenteral: Do not administer I.M. or S.C.; administer I.V. preparation once daily by slow I.V. infusion over 30 minutes to 3 hours at a final concentration not to exceed 6 mg/mL

Monitoring Parameters Periodic monitoring of liver function (AST, ALT); bilirubin, CBC, platelet count

Test Interactions Positive Coombs' reaction [direct], rifampin inhibits standard assay's ability to measure serum folate and vitamin B_{12}

Patient Information May discolor urine, tears, sweat, or other body fluids to a red-orange color; soft contact lenses may be permanently stained. Notify physician of any severe or persistent flu-like symptoms, nausea, vomiting, dark urine, or unusual bleeding or bruising

Nursing Implications The compounded oral suspension must be shaken well before using. Extravasation may cause local irritation and inflammation.

Dosage Forms

Capsule: 150 mg, 300 mg

Rifadin®: 150 mg, 300 mg
Rimactane®: 300 mg
Injection, powder for reconstitution (Rifadin®): 600 mg

Extemporaneous Preparations Rifampin oral suspension can be compounded with simple syrup or wild cherry syrup at a concentration of 10 mg/mL; the suspension is stable for 4 weeks at room temperature or in a refrigerator when stored in a glass amber prescription bottle. However, there are some experts who do not recommend using rifampin syrup formulated from capsules due to conflicting reports indicating that the product is unstable (14.5% to 68% of labeled potency after preparation). It may be preferable to perform trituration, rather than simple mixing in syrup when preparing rifampin oral suspension.

Nahata MC, Morosco RS, and Hipple TF, "Effect of Preparation Method and Storage on Rifampin Concentration in Suspensions," *Ann Pharmacother*, 1994, 28(2):182-5.

References
American Academy of Pediatrics Committee on Infectious Diseases, "Chemotherapy for Tuberculosis in Infants and Children," *Pediatrics*, 1992, 89(1):161-5.
Starke JR, "Modern Approach to the Diagnosis and Treatment of Tuberculosis in Children," *Pediatr Clin North Am*, 1988, 35(3):441-64.
Starke JR, "Multidrug Therapy for Tuberculosis in Children," *Pediatr Infect Dis J*, 1990, 9(11):785-93.
Tan TQ, Mason EO Jr, Ou CN, et al, "Use of Intravenous Rifampin in Neonates With Persistent Staphylococcal Bacteremia," *Antimicrob Agents Chemother*, 1993, 37(11):2401-6.

♦ **rIFN-α** see Interferon Alfa-2a *on page 614*

♦ **rIFN-α2** see Interferon Alfa-2b *on page 616*

♦ **Rimactane®** see Rifampin *on page 985*

Rimantadine (ri MAN ta deen)

U.S. Brand Names Flumadine®
Therapeutic Category Antiviral Agent, Oral
Generic Available Yes (tablet)
Use Prophylaxis (adults and children) and treatment (adults) of influenza A viral infection
Pregnancy Risk Factor C
Contraindications Hypersensitivity to rimantadine, amantadine, or any component
Precautions Use with caution in patients with liver disease, epilepsy, history of recurrent eczematoid dermatitis, uncontrolled psychosis, severe psychoneurosis, and in patients receiving CNS stimulant drugs; modify dosage in patients with renal impairment, severe hepatic dysfunction, or active seizure disorder

Adverse Reactions
Cardiovascular: Orthostatic hypotension, edema
Central nervous system: Dizziness, confusion, headache, insomnia, difficulty in concentrating, anxiety, restlessness, irritability, hallucinations; CNS adverse effects are less than with amantadine
Gastrointestinal: Nausea, vomiting, xerostomia
Genitourinary: Urinary retention

Drug Interactions Anticholinergic agents, CNS stimulants may possibly increase adverse effects
Food Interactions Food does not affect rate or extent of absorption
Mechanism of Action Blocks the uncoating of influenza A viral RNA and prevents penetration of the virus into host cell; inhibits M_2 protein in the assembly of progeny virions

Pharmacokinetics
Absorption: Oral: Well absorbed
Distribution: Adults: 17-25 L/kg
Protein binding: ~40%
Metabolism: Extensively in the liver via hydroxylation and glucuronidation
Half-life:
Children 4-8 years: 13-38 hours
Adults: 24-36 hours
Elimination: <25% excreted unchanged in the urine
Dialysis: Hemodialysis: Negligible effect

Usual Dosage Oral: (See Additional Information for duration of therapy)
Prophylaxis:
Children <10 years: 5 mg/kg once daily; maximum dose: 150 mg/day
Children >10 years and Adults: 100 mg twice daily (see Note)
Treatment: Adults: 100 mg twice daily (see Note)
Note: Patients with severe hepatic or renal dysfunction or elderly nursing home patients: 100 mg/day
Administration Oral: May administer with food
(Continued)

Rimantadine *(Continued)*

Patient Information May cause dizziness or confusion and impair ability to perform activities requiring mental alertness or physical coordination; may cause dry mouth

Additional Information Not active against influenza B; treatment or prophylaxis in immunosuppressed patients has not been fully evaluated

Duration of treatment: 5-7 days; optimal duration not established

Duration of prophylactic therapy: For at least 10 days after known exposure; usually for 6-8 weeks during influenza A season or local outbreak (or until vaccine produces sufficient antibody titers)

Duration of fever and other symptoms can be reduced if rimantadine therapy is started within the first 48 hours of influenza A illness

During an outbreak of influenza, administer rimantadine prophylaxis for 2-3 weeks after influenza vaccination until vaccine antibody titers are sufficient to provide protection

Dosage Forms

Syrup, as hydrochloride: 50 mg/5 mL (240 mL) [raspberry flavor]

Tablet, as hydrochloride: 100 mg

♦ **Riopan® Plus [OTC]** *see Antacid Preparations on page 112*
♦ **Riphenidate (Can)** *see Methylphenidate on page 744*
♦ **Risperdal®** *see Risperidone on page 988*

Risperidone *(ris PER i done)*

U.S. Brand Names Risperdal®

Therapeutic Category Antipsychotic Agent, Atypical; Antipsychotic Agent, Benzisoxazole

Generic Available No

Use Management of schizophrenia; has also been used to treat Tourette's syndrome, bipolar disorder, pervasive developmental disorders, autism, and aggressive behavior in patients with various psychiatric diagnoses

Pregnancy Risk Factor C

Contraindications Hypersensitivity to risperidone or any component (see Warnings)

Warnings May cause neuroleptic malignant syndrome (symptoms include hyperpyrexia, altered mental status, muscle rigidity, autonomic instability, acute renal failure, rhabdomyolysis, and elevated CPK). May cause extrapyramidal reactions, including pseudoparkinsonism, acute dystonic reactions, akathisia, and tardive dyskinesia (risk of these reactions is low relative to other neuroleptics, and is dose-dependent; to decrease risk of tardive dyskinesia: use smallest dose and shortest duration possible; evaluate continued need periodically). May lengthen the QT interval; other medications that prolong the QT interval may result in torsade de pointes (a life-threatening arrhythmia); risk factors for torsade de pointes include: Presence of congenital prolongation of QT, concurrent use with other drugs that prolong the QT interval, electrolyte imbalance, and bradycardia

Oral solution contains benzoic acid; benzoic acid (benzoate) is a metabolite of benzyl alcohol; large amounts of benzyl alcohol (≥99 mg/kg/day) have been associated with a potentially fatal toxicity ("gasping syndrome") in neonates; avoid use of risperidone products containing benzoic acid in neonates; *in vitro* and animal studies have shown that benzoate displaces bilirubin from protein binding sites

Precautions Use with caution and decrease the dose in patients with renal or hepatic impairment. Use with caution in patients with seizure disorders (seizures have been rarely reported), concomitant illnesses that may effect hepatic metabolism or hemodynamic responses (eg, unstable cardiac disease, recent MI), breast cancer or other prolactin-dependent tumors (risperidone elevates prolactin levels), in suicidal patients and in those at risk of aspiration pneumonia (esophageal dysmotility and aspiration have been associated with antipsychotic agents)

May cause orthostatic hypotension with resultant dizziness, tachycardia, or syncope (especially during initial dose titration); use with caution in patients with cardiovascular disease (conduction abnormalities, heart failure, past MI, or myocardia ischemia), cerebrovascular disease, dehydration, hypovolemia, or other conditions which may predispose patients to hypotension; may cause hypotension when used with antihypertensive agents. May cause somnolence (dose-related), priapism (rarely), alteration of temperature regulation (use with caution in patients exposed to temperature extremes); may mask diseases or toxicity of other drugs due to antiemetic effects; may rarely cause hyperglycemia (use with caution in patients with diabetes or other disorders of glucose regulation)

Adverse Reactions

Cardiovascular: Hypotension (especially orthostatic), tachycardia, syncope (0.2%); prolongation of QT interval

Central nervous system: Insomnia, agitation, anxiety, headache, dizziness, somnolence, restlessness, extrapyramidal reactions (dose dependent), dystonic reactions, pseudoparkinsonism, tardive dyskinesia, neuroleptic malignant syndrome, fever, altered central temperature regulation, seizures (0.3 %)

Dermatologic: Rash, dry skin

Endocrine & metabolic: Weight gain, elevated serum prolactin, amenorrhea, galactorrhea, gynecomastia, sexual dysfunction, hyperglycemia (rare)

Gastrointestinal: Constipation, nausea, xerostomia, dyspepsia, vomiting, abdominal pain, anorexia

Genitourinary: Polyuria, nocturnal enuresis, priapism (rare)

Hepatic: Hepatotoxicity (rare) (see Kumra, 1997 and McDougle, 2000)

Neuromuscular & skeletal: Arthralgia

Ocular: Abnormal vision

Respiratory: Rhinitis, coughing, pharyngitis, sinusitis, dyspnea

Drug Interactions Cytochrome P450 isoenzyme CYP2D6 and CYP3A4 substrate; isoenzyme CYP2D6 inhibitor (weak)

Risperidone may enhance the hypotensive effects of antihypertensive agents; may antagonize the effects of levodopa and dopamine agonists; use with valproic acid may result in generalized edema (case report); CNS depressants, alcohol may potentiate the adverse effects of risperidone; the herbal medicine St John's wort (*Hypericum perforatum*), may increase serious side effects (its use is **not** recommended)

Carbamazepine and other enzyme inducers may increase the clearance of risperidone, reducing its effectiveness; drugs that inhibit cytochrome P450 CYP2D6 may inhibit the metabolism of risperidone (monitor for increased effect or toxicity); clozapine may decrease the clearance of risperidone; fluoxetine may increase the serum concentration of risperidone; venlafaxine may increase serum concentrations of risperidone, but does not significantly alter the disposition of the total active moiety [risperidone plus 9-hydroxyrisperidone (active metabolite)]

Food Interactions Food does not affect rate or extent of absorption; oral solution is not compatible with cola or tea

Stability Store at controlled room temperature 15°C to 25°C (59°F to 77°F); protect from light; protect tablets from moisture; protect oral solution from freezing

Mechanism of Action Atypical antipsychotic (benzisoxazole derivative); highly potent serotonin and dopamine receptor antagonist; binds to 5-HT$_2$-receptors in the CNS and in the periphery with a very high affinity; binds to dopamine-D$_2$ receptors, but with less affinity (~20 times lower). The addition of serotonin antagonism to dopamine antagonism (classic neuroleptic mechanism) is thought to improve negative symptoms of psychoses and reduce the incidence of extrapyramidal side effects. Alpha$_1$, alpha$_2$ adrenergic, and histaminergic receptors are also antagonized with high affinity. Risperidone has low to moderate affinity for 5-HT$_{1c}$, 5-HT$_{1D}$, and 5-HT$_{1A}$ receptors, weak affinity for D$_1$ and no affinity for cholinergic muscarinic or beta$_1$ and beta$_2$ receptors

Pharmacokinetics

Absorption: Well absorbed

Distribution: Distributes into breast milk; breast milk to plasma ratio (n=1): Risperidone: 0.42; 9-hydroxyrisperidone: 0.24 (Hill, 2000)

Protein binding: Risperidone: ~90%, plasma protein binding increases with increasing concentrations of alpha$_1$-acid glycoprotein; 9-hydroxyresperidone: 77%; **Note:** Risperidone free fraction may be increased by ~35% in patients with hepatic impairment due to decreased concentrations of albumin and alpha$_1$-acid glycoprotein

Metabolism: Extensive in the liver via cytochrome P450 CYP2D6 to 9-hydroxyrisperidone (major active metabolite); also undergoes N-dealkylation (minor pathway); **Note:** 9-hydroxyrisperidone is the predominant circulating form and is approximately equal to risperidone in receptor binding activity; clinical effects are from combined concentrations of risperidone and 9-hydroxyrisperidone; clinically important differences between CYP2D6 poor and extensive metabolizers are not expected (pharmacokinetics of the sum of risperidone and 9-hydroxyrisperidone were similar in poor and extensive metabolizers)

Bioavailability: Oral: 70%; tablet (relative to solution): 94%

Half-life (apparent): Adults:

Risperidone: Extensive metabolizers: 3 hours; poor metabolizers: 20 hours

9-hydroxyrisperidone: Extensive metabolizers: 21 hours; poor metabolizers: 30 hours

Sum of risperidone and 9-hydroxyrisperidone: Overall mean: 20 hours

Time to peak serum concentration:

Risperidone: 1 hour

9-hydroxyrisperidone: Extensive metabolizers: 3 hours; poor metabolizers: 17 hours

(Continued)

Risperidone *(Continued)*

Elimination:

Clearance: Moderate to severe renal impairment (sum of risperidone and 9-hydroxyrisperidone): Decreased by 60%

Usual Dosage Oral:

Children and Adolescents:

Aggressive behavior in patients with various psychiatric diagnoses: Limited information is available. In a randomized, double-blind, placebo-controlled study, 10 children and adolescents 6-14 years of age (mean: 9.2 ± 2.9 years) with conduct disorder and prominent aggressive behavior received risperidone in the following doses: Patients <50 kg: Initial: 0.25 mg once daily; doses were increased as needed by 0.25 mg/day increments each week to a maximum of 1.5 mg/day; patients $\geq$50 kg: Initial: 0.5 mg once daily; doses were increased as needed by 0.5 mg/day increments each week to a maximum of 3 mg/day; doses were given once daily in the morning in all but one patient (who received twice daily dosing); 6 of 10 patients completed the 10-week study; final dose: 0.75-1.5 mg/day; mean: 0.028 ± 0.004 mg/kg/day; risperidone was more effective than placebo in decreasing aggressive behavior (Findling, 2000). In another randomized, double-blind, placebo-controlled study, 19 adolescents (mean age: 14 ± 1.5 years; 7 with borderline IQ and 6 with mild mental retardation) who were hospitalized for treatment of psychiatric disorders associated with aggressive behavior, received initial risperidone doses of 0.5 mg twice daily; doses were increased as needed by 1 mg/day increments up to a planned maximum of 5 mg twice daily; final doses: Range: 1.5-4 mg/day (0.019-0.08 mg/kg/day); mean: 2.9 mg/day (0.044 mg/kg/day); risperidone was more effective than placebo in decreasing aggressive behavior; although the initial dose was well tolerated by all patients, the authors recommend the following initial doses for clinical practice: Patients <25 kg: 0.25 mg/day; patients $\geq$25 kg: 0.5 mg/day (Buitelaar, 2001).

In an open trial, 26 children and adolescents 10-18 years of age (mean: 15 ± 1.9 years) with a borderline IQ (n=19) or mild mental retardation (n=5), who were hospitalized for treatment of psychiatric disorders associated with aggressive behavior, received initial risperidone doses of 0.5 mg/day; doses were increased by 0.5-1 mg/day increments every 3 days up to a planned maximum of 6 mg/day and given in twice daily doses; final dose: 0.5-4 mg/day; mean: 2.1 ± 1 mg/day; a marked reduction in aggressive behavior was observed in 14 of 26 patients (54%); **Note:** Four subjects who discontinued therapy after 8 weeks had received higher doses (mean: 3.3 ± 1 mg/day) than those who continued on medication (mean: 1.9 ± 0.9 mg/day) (Buitelaar, 2000). Eleven children and adolescents 5.5-16 years of age (mean: 9.8 years) with mood disorders and aggressive behavior received risperidone in titrated doses in an open trial; final dose: 0.75-2.5 mg/day given in 2-3 divided doses; a decrease in aggressive behavior was observed in 8 of 11 patients (Schreier, 1998).

Autism and pervasive developmental disorders (PDDs): A recent multi-center double-blind, placebo-controlled trial of risperidone in children and adolescents 5-17 years of age (mean: 8.8 ± 2.7 years) with autism and serious behavioral problems demonstrated the short-term efficacy of risperidone for the treatment of aggression, tantrums, or self-injurious behavior. The following doses were used: Children 15-20 kg: Initial: 0.25 mg/day. Children 20-45 kg: Initial: 0.5 mg at bedtime on days 1-3 and 0.5 mg twice daily on day 4; dose was gradually increased in 0.5 mg increments to a maximum dose of 2.5 mg/day (given as 1 mg in the morning and 1.5 mg at bedtime) by day 29. Children >45 kg: A "slightly accelerated dose schedule" was used; maximum dose: 3.5 mg/day (given as 1.5 mg in the morning and 2 mg at bedtime). Doses were titrated to effect; mean effective dose: 1.8 ± 0.7 mg/day (range: 0.5-3.5 mg/day). **Note:** This study did **not** identify the minimal effective dose (McCraken, 2002).

In an open-labeled prospective study, 10 boys 4.5-10.8 years of age (mean: 7.2 ± 2.2 years) with autistic disorder were started on risperidone 0.5 mg/day; doses were titrated as needed by increments of $\leq$0.5 mg/day at intervals of $\geq$7 days; final dose (at 12 weeks): Range: 1-2.5 mg/day (0.03-0.08 mg/kg/day); mean: 1.3 $\pm$ 0.5 mg/day (0.05 ± 0.2 mg/kg/day); 8 of 10 children responded (Nicolson, 1998). In an open clinical trial, 6 children 5-9 years of age (mean: 7.33 years) with autistic disorder were started on risperidone monotherapy 0.25 mg at bedtime; doses were titrated as needed by 0.25 mg increments at intervals of $\geq$7 days and dosed twice daily; final doses (at week 8): Range: 0.75-1.5 mg/day (0.03-0.06 mg/kg/day); mean: 1.1 mg (0.04 mg/kg/day); improvement was noted in all 6 patients (Findling, 1997).

In a prospective open-labeled study, 18 children and adolescents 5-18 years of age (mean 10.2 ± 3.7 years) were treated for PDDs (11 with autistic disorder) with initial doses of 0.5 mg at night; doses were increased as needed by 0.5 mg/day increments every week and dosed twice daily; optimal dose: 1-4 mg/day (mean: 1.8 ± 1 mg/day); 12 of 18 patients responded (McDougle, 1997). Fourteen children and adolescents 9-17 years of age (mean: 12.7 ± 4 years) were treated in an open case series, for PDDs (4 with autistic disorder) with initial doses of 0.25 mg twice daily; doses were increased as needed by 0.25 mg/day increments every 5-7 days; optimal dose: 0.75-1.5 mg/day given in divided doses; 13 of 14 patients showed a beneficial response (Fisman, 1996). In an open trial, 6 children and adolescents 7-14 years of age (mean: 10.7 ± 3.3 years) were treated for PDDs (5 with autistic disorder; all 6 with severe behavioral problems) with initial doses of 0.5 mg once or twice daily; doses were increased as needed by 0.5 mg/day increments every few days; optimal dose: 1-6 mg/day (mean 2.7 ± 2.2 mg/day); significant benefit was seen in 5 of the 6 patients (Perry, 1997). Twenty children and adolescents (age: 8-17 years) with developmental disorders refractory to previous psychotropic agents were treated in an open clinical trial with risperidone; doses were increased as needed slowly over several weeks; final doses (n=20): 1.5-10 mg/day; responders (n=13): 1-4 mg/day; nonresponders: 4.5-10 mg/day (Hardan, 1996). Further studies are needed.

Bipolar disorder: Very limited information is available. In a retrospective chart review, 28 children and adolescents 4-17 years of age (mean: 10.4 ± 3.8 years) were treated for bipolar disorder; risperidone doses were titrated as needed; optimal mean dose: 1.7 ± 1.3 mg/day; 82% of patients showed improvement in their manic and aggressive symptoms (Frazier 1999). Further studies are needed.

Schizophrenia: Limited information is available. In a prospective, open-labeled pilot study, 10 children and adolescents 11-18 years of age (mean: 15.1 years) were treated for schizophrenia with initial doses of 1 mg twice daily; doses were increased as needed by 1 mg/day increments every 2 days up to a maximum of 10 mg/day and given twice daily; final dose: Range: 4-10 mg/day (0.05-0.17 mg/kg/day); mean: 6.6 mg/day (0.095 mg/kg/day) (Armenteros, 1997). In a retrospective study, 16 children and adolescents 9-20 years of age (mean 14.9 ± 2.73 years) were treated for psychotic disorders (13 with schizophrenia) with initial doses of 1 mg twice daily; doses were increased as needed by 1 mg increments every 3-4 days; optimal dose: 2-10 mg/day (mean 5.9 ± 2.8 mg/day) divided and given in 2-3 doses/day; 15 of 16 patients responded (Grcevich, 1996). Further studies are needed.

Tourette's syndrome: Limited information is available. In a multi-center, double-blind, parallel-group comparative study, 50 patients 11-50 years of age were treated for Tourette's syndrome with risperidone (n=26; median age: 20 years; 10 patients <18 years of age) versus pimozide (n=24); a fixed-dose titration of risperidone from 0.5 mg/day to 2 mg/day was used for the first week of therapy; this was followed by a flexible dosing period of 7 weeks; doses were increased by ≤1 mg/week up to a maximum of 6 mg/day and were given once daily; final dose: 0.5-6 mg/day (mean: 3.8 mg/day); both drugs significantly improved tics; although there was no difference in efficacy between drugs, risperidone was better tolerated; the authors suggest that the average dose in this study is high compared to their clinical experience and that the fixed-dose titration during the first week may have been too rapid; a slower dosing schedule and lower long-term doses (eg, 1-2 mg/day) may be needed (Bruggeman, 2001).

Seven children and adolescents 11-16 years of age (mean: 12.9 ± 1.9 years) were treated in a prospective open-labeled trial for chronic tic disorders (5 with Tourette's syndrome) with initial doses of 0.5 mg at bedtime; doses were increased in 5 of the 7 patients by 0.5 mg/day increments every 5 days as tolerated to a maximum of 2.5 mg/day and given in twice daily doses (doses were increased more rapidly in 2 patients); final dose: 1-2.5 mg/day; a decrease in tic severity was seen in all patients; the authors recommend initial doses of 0.5 mg/day and increases of 0.5 mg/day every 5-7 days (Lombroso, 1995). In a retrospective review, 28 children and adolescents 5-18 years of age (mean 11.1 ± 3.6 years) with Tourette's syndrome and aggressive behavior were treated with risperidone; final dose: 0.5-9 mg/day (mean: 2 mg/day); a decrease in aggression scores occurred in 22 of 28 patients (78.5%); frequency and severity of tics were decreased in 17 patients (61.7%) (Sandor, 2000). Further studies are needed.

Adults: **Schizophrenia: Note:** May be administered once or twice daily. Patients who may be predisposed to hypotension or in whom hypotension would be a risk, and debilitated or elderly patients should use the dose listed below for renal or hepatic (Continued)

Risperidone *(Continued)*

impairment; monitor carefully; debilitated or elderly patients should receive twice daily dosing for 2-3 days at the target dose before switching to once daily dosing.

Earlier short-term studies used the following: Initial: 1 mg twice daily; increase (as tolerated) in increments of 1 mg twice daily on day 2 and 3, to a target dose of 3 mg twice daily by day 3; slower titration may be required in some patients; doses up to 8 mg once daily have also been shown to be safe and effective; if needed, further changes may be made at intervals of ≥7 days, in small increments or decrements of 1-2 mg; maximal effect: 4-8 mg/day; for twice daily dosing, doses >6 mg/day did not appear to be more effective than lower doses and were associated with more adverse effects (eg, extrapyramidal symptoms); doses >3 mg twice daily are generally not recommended; safety of doses >16 mg/day has not been assessed. Use lowest effective dose; reassess periodically for continued need.

Maintenance therapy: A long-term controlled trial in patients who were clinically stable for at least 4 weeks on antipsychotic medication used initial risperidone doses of 1 mg once daily; doses were increased to 2 mg once daily on day 2, and to a target dose of 4 mg once daily on day 3; maximum dose: 8 mg/day; patients were observed for relapse for 1-2 years; risperidone patients had a significantly longer time to relapse versus the comparator drug

Dosing adjustment in renal or hepatic impairment: Adults: Initial: 0.5 mg twice daily; increase (as tolerated) in increments of ≤0.5 mg twice daily; increases above 1.5 mg twice daily should be made at intervals of ≥7 days; slower titration may be required in some patients

Administration May be administered without regard to meals. May mix oral solution with water, coffee, orange juice, or low-fat milk; do not mix with cola or tea

Monitoring Parameters Orthostatic blood pressure and heart rate, especially during dosage titration; weight; liver enzymes in children (especially obese children or those who are rapidly gaining weight while receiving therapy); EKG

Patient Information May cause dizziness or drowsiness and impair ability to perform activities requiring mental alertness or physical coordination; may cause dry mouth; may cause postural hypotension, especially during initial dose titration (use caution when changing position from lying or sitting to standing); report the use of other medications, nonprescription medications and herbal or natural products to your physician and pharmacist; avoid alcohol and the herbal medicine, St John's wort; report persistent CNS effects (eg, trembling fingers, altered gait or balance, excessive sedation, seizures, unusual muscle or skeletal movements), rapid heartbeat, palpitations, severe dizziness, fainting, swelling or pain in breasts (male and female), altered menstrual pattern, changes in urinary patterns, vision changes, skin rash, difficulty breathing, or worsening of condition to your physician

Nursing Implications May need to assist patient in rising slowly from lying or sitting to standing position [orthostatic blood pressure changes, tachycardia and syncope (rare) may occur (see Warnings and Monitoring Parameters)]

Additional Information Long-term usefulness of risperidone should be periodically re-evaluated in patients receiving the drug for extended periods of time.

Dosage Forms

Solution, oral: 1 mg/mL (30 mL) [contains benzoic acid; calibrated pipette is marked in milligrams and milliliters from 0.25 to 3 mL]

Tablet: 0.25 mg, 0.5 mg, 1 mg, 2 mg, 3 mg, 4 mg

References

Armenteros JL, Whitaker AH, Welikson M, et al, "Risperidone in Adolescents With Schizophrenia: An Open Pilot Study," *J Am Acad Child Adolesc Psychiatry*, 1997, 36(5):694-700.

Bruggeman R, van der Linden C, Buitelaar JK, et al, "Risperidone Versus Pimozide in Tourette's Disorder: A Comparative Double-Blind Parallel-Group Study," *J Clin Psychiatry*, 2001, 62(1):50-6.

Buitelaar JK, "Open-Label Treatment With Risperidone of 26 Psychiatrically-Hospitalized Children and Adolescents With Mixed Diagnoses and Aggressive Behavior," *J Child Adolesc Psychopharmacol*, 2000, 10(1):19-26.

Buitelaar JK, van der Gaag RJ, Cohen-Kettenis P, et al, "A Randomized Controlled Trial of Risperidone in the Treatment of Aggression in Hospitalized Adolescents With Subaverage Cognitive Abilities," *J Clin Psychiatry*, 2001, 62(4):239-48.

Findling RL, Maxwell K, and Wiznitzer M, "An Open Clinical Trial of Risperidone Monotherapy in Young Children With Autistic Disorder," *Psychopharmacol Bull*, 1997, 33(1):155-9.

Findling RL, McNamara NK, Branicky LA, et al, "A Double-Blind Pilot Study of Risperidone in the Treatment of Conduct Disorder," *J Am Acad Child Adolesc Psychiatry*, 2000, 39(4):509-16.

Fisman S and Steele M, "Use of Risperidone in Pervasive Developmental Disorders: A Case Series," *J Child Adolesc Psychopharmacol*, 1996, 6(3):177-90.

Frazier JA, Meyer MC, Biederman J, et al, "Risperidone Treatment for Juvenile Bipolar Disorder: A Retrospective Chart Review," *J Am Acad Child Adolesc Psychiatry*, 1999, 38(8):960-5.

Grcevich SJ, Findling RL, Rowane WA, et al, "Risperidone in the Treatment of Children and Adolescents With Schizophrenia: A Retrospective Study," *J Child Adolesc Psychopharmacol*, 1996, 6(4):251-7.

Hardan A, Johnson K, Johnson C, et al, "Case Study: Risperidone Treatment of Children and Adolescents With Developmental Disorders," *J Am Acad Child Adolesc Psychiatry*, 1996, 35(11):1551-6.

Hill RC, McIvor RJ, Wojnar-Horton RE, et al, "Risperidone Distribution and Excretion Into Human Milk: Case Report and Estimated Infant Exposure During Breast-Feeding," *J Clin Psychopharmacol*, 2000, 20(2):285-6.

Kumra S, Herion D, Jacobsen LK, et al, "Case Study: Risperidone-Induced Hepatotoxicity in Pediatric Patients," *J Am Acad Child Adolesc Psychiatry*, 1997, 36(5):701-5.

Lombroso PJ, Scahill L, King RA, et al, "Risperidone Treatment of Children and Adolescents With Chronic Tic Disorders: A Preliminary Report," *J Am Acad Child Adolesc Psychiatry*, 1995, 34(9):1147-52.

McCracken JT, McGough J, Shah B, et al, "Risperidone in Children With Autism and Serious Behavioral Problems," *N Engl J Med*, 2002, 347(5):314-21.

McDougle CJ, Holmes JP, Bronson MR, et al, "Risperidone Treatment of Children and Adolescents With Pervasive Developmental Disorders: A Prospective Open-Label Study," *J Am Acad Child Adolesc Psychiatry*, 1997, 36(5):685-93.

McDougle CJ, Scahill L, McCracken JT, et al, "Research Units on Pediatric Psychopharmacology (RUPP) Autism Network. Background and Rationale for an Initial Controlled Study of Risperidone," *Child Adolesc Psychiatr Clin N Am*, 2000, 9(1):201-24.

Nicolson R, Awad G, and Sloman L, "An Open Trial of Risperidone in Young Autistic Children," *J Am Acad Child Adolesc Psychiatry*, 1998, 37(4):372-6.

Perry R, Pataki C, Munoz-Silva DM, et al, "Risperidone in Children and Adolescents With Pervasive Developmental Disorder: Pilot Trial and Follow-Up," *J Child Adolesc Psychopharmacol*, 1997, 7(3):167-79.

Sandor P and Stephens RJ, "Risperidone Treatment of Aggressive Behavior in Children With Tourette Syndrome," *J Clin Psychopharmacol*, 2000, 20(6):710-2.

Schreier HA, "Risperidone for Young Children With Mood Disorders and Aggressive Behavior," *J Child Adolesc Psychopharmacol*, 1998, 8(1):49-59.

♦ **Ritalin®** *see* Methylphenidate *on page 744*

♦ **Ritalin® LA** *see* Methylphenidate *on page 744*

♦ **Ritalin-SR®** *see* Methylphenidate *on page 744*

Ritonavir (rit ON uh veer)

Related Information

Adult and Adolescent HIV *on page 1327*
Pediatric HIV *on page 1323*

U.S. Brand Names Norvir®

Canadian Brand Names Norvir® SEC

Therapeutic Category Antiretroviral Agent; HIV Agents (Anti-HIV Agents); Protease Inhibitor

Generic Available No

Use Treatment of HIV infection in combination with other antiretroviral agents. (**Note:** HIV regimens consisting of **three** antiretroviral agents are strongly recommended)

Pregnancy Risk Factor B

Contraindications Hypersensitivity to ritonavir or any component; do not breast-feed while receiving ritonavir

Warnings Ritonavir is a potent CYP3A enzyme inhibitor which interacts with numerous drugs. Due to potential serious and/or life-threatening drug interactions, the following drugs should not be coadministered with ritonavir: amiodarone, astemizole, bepridil, bupropion, cisapride, clozapine, dihydroergotamine, ergotamine, ergonovine, methylergonovine, flecainide, encainide, meperidine, lovastatin, simvastatin, pimozide, piroxicam, propafenone, propoxyphene, quinidine, rifabutin, terfenadine, alprazolam, clorazepate, diazepam, estazolam, flurazepam, midazolam, triazolam, and zolpidem (see Drug Interactions); the herbal medicine St John's wort (*Hypericum perforatum*) may lead to loss of virologic response and/or resistance (avoid concurrent use). Spontaneous bleeding episodes have been reported in patients with hemophilia type A and B. New onset diabetes mellitus, exacerbation of diabetes, and hyperglycemia have been reported in HIV-infected patients receiving protease inhibitors.

Precautions Fat redistribution and accumulation [ie, central obesity, peripheral wasting, facial wasting, breast enlargement, dorsocervical fat enlargement (buffalo hump), and cushingoid appearance] have been observed in patients receiving antiretroviral agents (causal relationship not established). Use caution in patients with hepatic insufficiency; ritonavir oral solution contains 43% alcohol by volume; accidental ingestion could result in alcohol-related toxicity

Adverse Reactions

Central nervous system: Headache, confusion

Endocrine & metabolic: Elevated triglycerides and cholesterol, elevated creatine phosphokinase; rare: hyperglycemia, diabetes, ketoacidosis; redistribution of body fat to cause protease paunch, buffalo hump, facial atrophy, and breast enlargement

Gastrointestinal: Nausea, vomiting, diarrhea, taste perversion, abdominal pain, anorexia, pancreatitis

Hematologic: Rare: Spontaneous bleeding episodes in hemophiliacs

Hepatic: Elevated liver enzymes, hepatitis

Neuromuscular & skeletal: Circumoral and peripheral paresthesias, weakness

Miscellaneous: Allergic reaction (urticaria, rash, bronchospasm, angioedema)

(Continued)

Ritonavir *(Continued)*

Drug Interactions Cytochrome P450 isoenzyme CYP1A2, CYP2A6, CYP2C9, CYP2C19, CYP2E1, and CYP3A/4 substrate; isoenzyme CYP2D6 substrate (minor); isoenzyme CYP1A2 inducer; isoenzyme CYP2A6, CYP2C9, CYP1A2, CYP2C19, CYP2D6, CYP2E1, and CYP3A/4 inhibitor

Increases plasma concentration of amiodarone, astemizole, warfarin (monitor antico-agulant effect), bepridil, bupropion, cisapride, clozapine, dihydroergotamine, ergo-novine, methylergonovine, encainide, ergotamine, flecainide, meperidine, pimozide, piroxicam, propafenone, propoxyphene, quinidine, lovastatin, simva-statin, rifabutin, and terfenadine; inhibits metabolism of alprazolam, clorazepate, diazepam, estazolam, flurazepam, midazolam, triazolam, and zolpidem resulting in profound and prolonged sedation; 77% increase in clarithromycin AUC (decrease clarithromycin dose in patients with renal impairment); 145% increase in desipra-mine AUC (consider dosage reduction); 13% decrease in didanosine AUC (if patient is on concurrent ritonavir and didanosine therapy, doses should be spaced 2.5 hours apart); 40% decrease in ethinyl estradiol AUC (consider alternative contraceptive measures); 43% decrease in theophylline AUC (monitor theophylline levels); metronidazole (disulfiram-like reaction); inhibits indinavir and saquinavir metabolism; coadministration with nelfinavir increases concentration of nelfinavir; ritonavir decreases methadone serum concentrations; the herbal medicine St John's wort (*Hypericum perforatum*) may significantly decrease concentrations of ritonavir and is **not** recommended for concurrent use; rifampin decreases concen-trations of ritonavir; fluoxetine (serotonin syndrome)

Stability Refrigerate capsules; liquid formulation is stable for 30 days at room tempera-ture; liquid formulation should be stored in the original container; protect from light

Mechanism of Action A protease inhibitor which acts on an enzyme late in the HIV replication process after the virus has entered into the cell's nucleus preventing cleavage of protein precursors essential for HIV infection of new cells and viral replication. Saquinavir- and zidovudine-resistant HIV isolates are generally suscep-tible to ritonavir but strains resistant to ritonavir are usually cross-resistant to indinavir and saquinavir.

Pharmacokinetics

Absorption: Well absorbed

Distribution: High concentrations in serum and lymph nodes

Protein binding: 98% to 99%

Metabolism: In the liver by the cytochrome P450 enzyme 3A (CYP3A) to an active and inactive metabolite

Half-life:

Children: 2-4 hours

Adults: 3-5 hours

Time to peak serum concentration: 2-4 hours

Elimination: Renal clearance is negligible

Usual Dosage Oral:

Neonates: Under investigation in PACTG 354

Children ≤12 years: Initial: 250 mg/m^2/dose twice daily; titrate upward by 50 mg/m^2/dose twice daily increments over 5 days, up to 400 mg/m^2/dose twice daily; dosage range: 350-400 mg/m^2/dose twice daily (every 12 hours); maximum dose: 600 mg/dose twice daily

Adolescents and Adults: 600 mg twice daily; may use a dose titration schedule to reduce adverse events (nausea/vomiting) by initiating therapy at 300 mg twice daily; increase dose by 100 mg twice daily increments over 5 days up to a maximum dose of 600 mg twice daily

Administration Administer with food to increase absorption; consider reserving liquid formulation for use in patients receiving tube feeding due to its bad taste. May mix liquid formulation with milk, chocolate milk, vanilla or chocolate pudding or ice cream, or a liquid nutritional supplement. Other techniques used to increase tolerance in children include dulling the taste buds by chewing ice, giving popsicles or spoonfuls or partially frozen orange or grape juice concentrates before administration of ritonavir; coating the mouth with peanut butter to eat before the dose; administration of strong-tasting foods such as maple syrup, cheese, or strong-flavored chewing gum immediately after a dose.

Monitoring Parameters Liver function tests, blood glucose levels, CD4 cell count, plasma levels of HIV RNA

Patient Information Ritonavir is not a cure for HIV. Avoid the herbal medicine St John's wort; if dose is missed, take the next dose as soon as possible; however, if a dose is skipped, do not double the next dose. Notify physician if you have an increase in thirst and/or frequent urination, nausea, vomiting, or abdominal pain

HIV medications may cause changes in body fat, including an increase in fat in the upper back and neck, breasts, and trunk; a loss of fat from the face, arms, and legs may also occur.

Dosage Forms

Capsule, liquid-filled: 100 mg [contains alcohol and polyoxyl 35 castor oil]

Solution: 80 mg/mL (240 mL) [contains alcohol, polyoxyl 35 castor oil, and propylene glycol; peppermint and caramel flavors]

References

Danner SA, Carr A, Leonard JM, et al, "A Short-Term Study of the Safety, Pharmacokinetics, and Efficacy of Ritonavir, an Inhibitor of HIV-1 Protease. European-Australian Collaborative Ritonavir Study Group," *N Engl J Med*, 1995, 333(23):1528-33.

DeSilva KE, Le Flore DB, Marston BJ, et al, "Serotonin Syndrome in HIV-Infected Individuals Receiving Antiretroviral Therapy and Fluoxetine," *AIDS*, 2001, 15(10)1281-5.

Mueller BU, Nelson RP Jr, Sleasman J, et al, "A Phase I/II Study of the Protease Inhibitor Ritonavir in Children With Human Immunodeficiency Virus Infection," *Pediatrics*, 1998, 101(3 Pt 1):335-43.

Working Group on Antiretroviral Therapy and Medical Management of HIV-Infected Children, "Guidelines for the Use of Antiretroviral Agents in Pediatric HIV Infection," December 14, 2001, http://www.aidsinfo.nih.gov.

Rocuronium (roe kyoor OH nee um)

U.S. Brand Names Zemuron®

Therapeutic Category Neuromuscular Blocker Agent, Nondepolarizing; Skeletal Muscle Relaxant, Paralytic

Generic Available No

Clinical Conditions Affecting Neuromuscular Blockade

Potentiation	Antagonism
Electrolyte abnormalities	Alkalosis
Severe hyponatremia	Hypercalcemia
Severe hypocalcemia	Demyelinating lesions
Severe hypokalemia	Peripheral neuropathies
Hypermagnesemia	Diabetes mellitus
Neuromuscular diseases	
Acidosis	
Acute intermittent porphyria	
Renal failure	
Hepatic failure	

(Continued)

Rocuronium *(Continued)*

Use Produces skeletal muscle relaxation during surgery after induction of general anesthesia, increases pulmonary compliance during assisted mechanical respiration, facilitates endotracheal intubation

Pregnancy Risk Factor C

Contraindications Hypersensitivity to rocuronium or any component

Warnings Dosage adjustment needed in patients with severe hepatic disease; ventilation must be supported during neuromuscular blockade; rocuronium should only be used by individuals who are experienced in the maintenance of an adequate airway and respiratory support

Precautions Many clinical conditions may potentiate or antagonize neuromuscular blockade, see table on previous page.

Increased sensitivity in patients with myasthenia gravis, Eaton-Lambert syndrome; resistance to neuromuscular blockade in burn patients (>30% of body) for period of 5-70 days postinjury; resistance to neuromuscular blockade in patients with muscle trauma, denervation, immobilization, infection

Adverse Reactions Most frequent adverse reactions are associated with prolongation of its pharmacologic actions

Cardiovascular: Hypotension, hypertension, arrhythmias, tachycardia

Dermatologic: Rash, pruritus

Gastrointestinal: Vomiting

Local: Injection site edema

Neuromuscular & skeletal: Muscle weakness

Respiratory: Bronchospasm

Miscellaneous: Hiccups, hypersensitivity reactions

Drug Interactions See table.

Potential Drug Interactions

Potentiation	Antagonism
Inhalation anesthetics	Calcium
Desflurane, sevoflurane, enflurane and	Carbamazepine
isoflurane > halothane > nitrous	Phenytoin
oxide	Steroids (chronic administration)
Antibiotics	Theophylline
Aminoglycosides, polymyxins,	Anticholinesterases*
clindamycin, vancomycin, tetracycline	Neostigmine, pyridostigmine,
Magnesium	edrophonium, echothiophate
Antiarrhythmics	ophthalmic solution
Quinidine, procainamide, bretylium, and	Caffeine
possibly lidocaine	Azathioprine
Diuretics	
Furosemide, mannitol, thiazides	
Amphotericin B (secondary to hypokalemia)	
Local anesthetics	
Dantrolene (directly depresses skeletal muscle)	
Beta blockers	
Calcium channel blockers	
Ketamine	
Lithium	
Succinylcholine (when administered prior to nondepolarizing neuromuscular-blocking agent)	
Cyclosporine	

*Can prolong the effects of acetylcholine

Stability Refrigerate; unopened vials are stable 60 days at room temperature; open vials are stable for 30 days at room temperature; compatible with NS and D$_5$W; do not mix with alkaline solutions

Mechanism of Action Nondepolarizing neuromuscular blocking agent which blocks neural transmission at the myoneural junction by binding with cholinergic receptor sites

Pharmacodynamics

Maximum effect:

Children: 30 seconds to 1 minute

Adults: 1-3.7 minutes
Duration:
Children:
3-12 months: 40 minutes
1-12 years: 26-30 minutes
Adults: 20-94 minutes (dose-related) (most prolonged in elderly ≥65 years of age)

Pharmacokinetics
Distribution: V_d:
Children: 0.21-0.3 L/kg
Adults: 0.22-0.26 L/kg
Hepatic dysfunction: 0.53 L/kg
Renal dysfunction: 0.34 L/kg
Protein binding: ~30%
Half-life:
Alpha elimination: 1-2 minutes
Beta elimination:
Children:
3-12 months: 1.3 ± 0.5 hours
1 <3 years: 1.1 ± 0.7 hours
3 to <8 years: 0.8 ± 0.3 hours
Adults: 1.4-2.4 hours
Hepatic dysfunction: 4.3 hours
Renal dysfunction: 2.4 hours
Elimination: Primarily biliary excretion (70%); up to 30% of dose excreted unchanged in urine
Clearance: Children:
3 to <12 months: 0.35 L/kg/hour
1 to <3 years: 0.32 L/kg/hour
3 to <8 years: 0.44 L/kg/hour

Usual Dosage I.V. (dosage based upon actual body weight even if the patient is obese):
Infants: 0.5 mg/kg/dose repeat every 20-30 minutes as needed
Children: Initial: 0.6 mg/kg/dose with repeat doses of 0.075-0.125 mg/kg every 20-30 minutes as determined by clinical response
Adolescents and Adults:
Rapid sequence intubation: 0.6-1.2 mg/kg
Tracheal intubation: 0.6 mg/kg with repeated doses of 0.1-0.2 mg/kg every 20-30 minutes as determined by clinical response
Children and Adults: Continuous infusion: 10-12 mcg/kg/minute (effective range reported to be 4-16 mcg/kg/minute)
Note: While I.V. administration is preferred, I.M. administration in single doses of 1 mg/kg (infants) and 1.8 mg/kg (children) has been used successfully (Kaplan, 1999).

Administration Parenteral: May be administered undiluted by rapid I.V. injection; for continuous infusion, dilute with NS, D_5W, or LR to a concentration of 0.5-1 mg/mL

Monitoring Parameters Peripheral nerve stimulator measuring twitch response, heart rate, blood pressure, assisted ventilation status

Nursing Implications Does not alter the patient's state of consciousness; addition of sedation and analgesia are recommended

Dosage Forms Injection, solution, as bromide: 10 mg/mL (5 mL, 10 mL)

References
Kaplan RF, Uejima T, Lobel G, et al, "Intramuscular Rocuronium in Infants and Children: A Multicenter Study to Evaluate Tracheal Intubating Conditions, Onset, and Duration of Action," *Anesthesiology*, 1999, 91(3):633-8.
Martin LD, Bratton SL, and O'Rourke PP, "Clinical Uses and Controversies of Neuromuscular Blocking Agents in Infants and Children," *Crit Care Med*, 1999, 27(7):1358-68.
Reynolds LM, Lau M, Brown R, et al, "Bioavailability of Intramuscular Rocuronium in Infants and Children," *Anesthesiology*, 1997, 87(5):1096-105.
Willets LS, "Rocuronium for Tracheal Intubation," *Ped Pharmacotherapy*, 2000, 6(10):1-6.

♦ **Rofact™ (Can)** *see* Rifampin *on page 985*
♦ **Roferon-A®** *see* Interferon Alfa-2a *on page 614*
♦ **Rogaine® Extra Strength for Men [OTC]** *see* Minoxidil *on page 768*
♦ **Rogaine® for Men [OTC]** *see* Minoxidil *on page 768*
♦ **Rogaine® for Women [OTC]** *see* Minoxidil *on page 768*
♦ **Rolaids® [OTC]** *see* Calcium Supplements *on page 200*
♦ **Rolaids® Extra Strength [OTC]** *see* Calcium Supplements *on page 200*
♦ **Romazicon®** *see* Flumazenil *on page 495*
♦ **Romilar® AC** *see* Guaifenesin and Codeine *on page 551*
♦ **Rondec® Drops** *see* Carbinoxamine and Pseudoephedrine *on page 214*

+ **Rondec® Syrup** *see* Brompheniramine and Pseudoephedrine *on page 182*
+ **Rondec® Tablets** *see* Carbinoxamine and Pseudoephedrine *on page 214*
+ **Rondec-TR® Tablets** *see* Carbinoxamine and Pseudoephedrine *on page 214*

Ropivacaine (roe PIV a kane)

U.S. Brand Names Naropin™

Synonyms LEA-103

Therapeutic Category Local Anesthetic, Injectable

Generic Available No

Use Production of local or regional anesthesia for surgery, obstetrical procedures, and for acute pain management: peripheral nerve block, local infiltration, sympathetic block, caudal or epidural block

Pregnancy Risk Factor B

Contraindications Hypersensitivity to ropivacaine hydrochloride, any anesthetic of the amide type (eg, bupivacaine, lidocaine, mepivacaine), or any component; not recommended for I.V. regional anesthesia (Bier block)

Warnings Convulsions due to systemic toxicity leading to cardiac arrest have been reported, presumably following unintentional I.V. injection; should be administered in small incremental doses; not for use in emergency situations when rapid onset of surgical anesthesia is necessary; not for use for the production of obstetrical paracervical block anesthesia, retrobulbar block, or spinal anesthesia (subarachnoid block)

Precautions Use with caution in patients with liver disease, impaired cardiovascular function, particularly CHF, hypotension, and neurological or psychiatric disorders. For epidural use, it is recommended that a test dose of either a local anesthetic with rapid onset or ropivacaine in combination with epinephrine be administered prior to ropivacaine to detect unintentional intravascular or intrathecal injection which would result in systemic toxicity (CNS or cardiovascular)

Adverse Reactions

Cardiovascular: Cardiac arrest, hypotension, bradycardia, fetal bradycardia (during epidural anesthesia for cesarean section), arrhythmias, hypertension, tachycardia, chest pain

Central nervous system: Headache, restlessness, anxiety, agitation, lightheadedness, dizziness, tinnitus, seizures, fever

Dermatologic: Pruritus, rash

Endocrine & metabolic: Hypomagnesemia, hypokalemia

Gastrointestinal: Nausea, vomiting, fecal incontinence, tenesmus

Genitourinary: Urinary retention

Hepatic: Jaundice

Local: Pain at injection site

Neuromuscular & skeletal: Weakness, back pain, paresthesia

Ocular: Vision abnormalities

Otic: Tinnitus

Respiratory: Dyspnea, rhinitis

Miscellaneous: Shivering, chills, rigor, fetal disorders including tachycardia, fetal distress, tachypnea, fever, and vomiting

Drug Interactions Cytochrome P450 isoenzyme CYP1A2 and CYP3A4 substrate Fluvoxamine decreases ropivacaine clearance

Stability Store at controlled room temperature; preservative-free, discard promptly after use; do not mix with alkaline solutions as precipitation will occur

Mechanism of Action Blocks both the initiation and conduction of nerve impulses by decreasing the neuronal membrane's permeability to sodium ions, which results in inhibition of depolarization with resultant blockade of conduction

Pharmacodynamics

Onset of anesthetic action (dependent on dose and route of administration):

Epidural block (100-200 mg): T10 sensory block: 10 minutes (range: 5-13 minutes)

Epidural block, Cesarean section (up to 150 mg): T6 sensory block: 11-26 minutes

Duration (dependent upon dose and route of administration):

Epidural block (100-200 mg): 4 hours (range: 3-5 hours)

Epidural block, Cesarean section (up to 150 mg):

Sensory block: 1.7-3.2 hours

Motor block: 1.4-2.9 hours

Pharmacokinetics

Absorption: Well absorbed systemically following epidural administration; addition of epinephrine has no affect on the absorption of ropivacaine

Distribution: Distributes into breast milk

V_d:

Children: 2.1-4.2 L/kg

Adults: 36-60 L

Protein binding: 94%

Metabolism: In the liver via cytochrome P450 isoenzyme, predominantly CYP1A2 and CYP3A4 (10 metabolites with 2 active)

Bioavailability: 87% to 98% (epidural)

Half-life: Epidural:
Children: 4.9 hours (range: 3-6.7 hours)
Adults: 3.6-6 hours

Time to peak serum concentration (dose and route dependent):
Caudal (children): 0.33-2.05 hours
Cesarian section: 14-65 minutes
Epidural (adults): 17-97 minutes

Elimination: 1% to 2% excreted unchanged in urine

Usual Dosage Dose varies with procedure, depth of anesthesia, vascularity of tissues, duration of anesthesia,and condition of patient
Caudal block: Children (limited data): 2 mg/kg
Epidural block (other than caudal block): Children: 1.7 mg/kg
Lumbar epidural surgery: Adults: 75-150 mg (maximum: 200 mg)
Lumbar epidural Cesarean section: Adults: 100-150 mg
Epidural continuous infusion:
Children 4 months to 7 years (limited data) (Hansen, 2000): 1 mg/kg loading dose followed by 0.4 mg/kg/hour continuous **epidural** infusion
Adults: 10-14 mg loading dose (5-7 mL 0.2%) followed by 12-28 mg/hour (6-14 mL/ hour 0.2%) continuous **epidural** infusion
Major nerve block (eg, brachial plexus block): Adults: 75-300 mg
Minor nerve block and infiltration: Adults: 5-200 mg

Administration Parenteral: Administer in small incremental doses with frequent aspirations before and during the injection to avoid intravascular injection

Monitoring Parameters After epidural or subarachnoid administration: Blood pressure, heart rate, respiration, signs of CNS toxicity (lightheadedness, dizziness, tinnitus, restlessness, drowsiness, circumoral paresthesia)

Patient Information Temporary loss of sensation and motor activity in the anesthetized part of the body may occur following proper administration of lumbar epidural anesthesia.

Dosage Forms Injection, as hydrochloride [preservative free]: 0.2% [2 mg/mL] (10 mL, 20 mL); 0.5% [5 mg/mL] (10 mL, 20 mL, 30 mL); 0.75% [7.5 mg/mL] (10 mL, 20 mL); 1% [10 mg/mL] (10 mL, 20 mL)

References

Hansen TG, Ilett KF, Lim SI, et al, "Pharmacokinetics and Clinical Efficacy of Long-Term Epidural Ropivacaine Infusion in Children," *Br J Anaesth*, 2000, 85(3):347-53.

Hansen TG, Ilett KF, Reid C, et al, "Caudal Ropivacaine in Infants: Population Pharmacokinetics and Plasma Concentrations," *Anesthesiology*, 2001, 94(4):579-84.

Lonnqvist PA, Westrin P, Larsson BA, et al, "Ropivacaine Pharmacokinetics After Caudal Block in 1-8 Year Old Children," *Br J Anaesth*, 2000, 85(4):506-11.

Wulf H, Peters C, and Behnke H, "The Pharmacokinetics of Caudal Ropivacaine 0.2% in Children. A Study of Infants Aged Less Than 1 Year and Toddlers Aged 1-5 Years Undergoing Inguinal Hernia Repair," *Anaesthesia*, 2000, 55(8):757-60.

Rosiglitazone (ROSE i gli ta zone)

U.S. Brand Names Avandia®

Therapeutic Category Antidiabetic Agent, Oral; Antidiabetic Agent, Thiazolidinedione

Generic Available No

Use Type 2 diabetes mellitus (noninsulin-dependent, NIDDM) when diet and exercise alone do not result in adequate glycemic control; may be used in combination with metformin, sulfonylurea, or insulin

Pregnancy Risk Factor C

Contraindications Hypersensitivity to rosiglitazone or any component; moderate to severe liver disease (transaminases >2.5 times the upper limit of normal at baseline); patients who experienced jaundice during troglitazone therapy; type 1 diabetes mellitus; diabetic ketoacidosis

Warnings Used alone or in combination with insulin, rosiglitazone can cause fluid retention which can exacerbate or lead to CHF; patients should be closely monitored for signs and symptoms of CHF; discontinue use if any deterioration of cardiac function occurs; avoid use in patients with NYHA class 3 or 4 heart failure

A dose-related weight gain has been reported with rosiglitazone which may be due to a combination of fluid retention and fat accumulation over time; a more rapid onset of weight gain may be suggestive of excessive edema and heart failure; idiosyncratic hepatotoxicity has been reported with another thiazolidinedione agent (troglitazone); two cases of hepatocellular injury (Forman, et al and Al-Salman, 2000) have been reported occurring within 2-3 weeks after initiation of rosiglitazone therapy; LFTs in these patients revealed severe hepatocellular injury which responded with rapid
(Continued)

Rosiglitazone *(Continued)*

improvement of liver function and resolution of symptoms upon discontinuation of rosiglitazone; monitoring should include periodic determinations of liver function

Precautions Use with extreme caution in patients with heart failure or edema (see Warnings); use with caution in patients with elevated transaminases (AST or ALT) and in patients with anemia or depressed leukocyte counts (may reduce hemoglobin, hematocrit, and/or WBC)

Adverse Reactions

Cardiovascular: Edema, CHF

Central nervous system: Headache, fatigue

Endocrine & metabolic: Weight gain, elevated total LDL and HDL cholesterol, hyperglycemia, hypoglycemia

Gastrointestinal: Diarrhea

Hematologic: Anemia

Hepatic: Elevated transaminases, elevated bilirubin

Neuromuscular & skeletal: Back pain

Respiratory: Upper respiratory tract infection, sinusitis

Miscellaneous: Injury

Drug Interactions Cytochrome P450 isoenzyme CYP2C8 substrate; isoenzyme CYP2C9 (minor)

Food Interactions Peak concentrations are lower by 28% and delayed when administered with food; these effects are not believed to be clinically significant

Mechanism of Action Thiazolidinedione antidiabetic agent that lowers blood glucose by improving target cell response to insulin, without increasing pancreatic insulin secretion; this mechanism of action is dependent on the presence of insulin for activity

Pharmacodynamics Maximum effect: Up to 12 weeks

Pharmacokinetics

Distribution: V_{dss} (apparent): 17.6 L

Protein binding: 99%

Metabolism: Hepatic (99%), metabolism by cytochrome P450 isoenzyme CYP2C8, minor metabolism via CYP2C9

Bioavailability: 99%

Half-life: 3-4 hours

Time to peak serum concentration: 1 hour

Elimination: As metabolites, in urine (64%) and feces (23%)

Usual Dosage Adults: Oral: Initial: 4 mg in single or divided doses twice daily; after 8-12 weeks of treatment the dosage may be increased to 8 mg daily in single or divided doses twice daily. **Note:** When changing patients from troglitazone to rosiglitazone, a 1-week washout is recommended before initiating therapy with rosiglitazone

Dosage adjustment in renal impairment: No dosage adjustment is required

Dosage comment in hepatic impairment: Clearance is significantly lower in hepatic impairment. Therapy should not be initiated if the patient exhibits active liver disease with increased transaminases (>2.5 times the upper limit of normal) at baseline (see Contraindications and Warnings)

Administration Oral: May be taken without regard to meals

Monitoring Parameters Signs and symptoms of hypoglycemia and heart failure, fasting blood glucose, hemoglobin A_{1c}; liver enzymes: baseline, every 2 months for the first 12 months of therapy, and periodically thereafter; patients with an elevation in ALT >3 times the upper limit of normal should be rechecked as soon as possible; if the ALT levels remain >3 times the upper limit of normal, therapy with rosiglitazone should be discontinued

Reference Range Target range:

Blood glucose: Fasting and preprandial: 80-120 mg/dL; bedtime: 100-140 mg/dL

Glycosylated hemoglobin (hemoglobin A_{1c}): <7%

Patient Information Follow directions of prescriber; if dose is missed at the usual meal, take it with next meal; do not double dose if daily dose is missed completely; more frequent monitoring is required during periods of stress, trauma, surgery, pregnancy, increased activity, or exercise; avoid alcohol; report an unusually rapid increase in weight, edema, or shortness of breath immediately to your physician; also report chest pain, rapid heartbeat or palpitations, abdominal pain, fever, rash, hypoglycemic reactions, yellowing of skin or eyes, dark urine or light stool, or unusual fatigue or nausea/vomiting.

Dosage Forms Tablet: 2 mg, 4 mg, 8 mg

References

Al-Salman J, Arjomand H, Kemp DG, et al, "Hepatocellular Injury in a Patient Receiving Rosiglitazone. A Case Report," *Ann Intern Med*, 2000, 132(2):121-4.

DeFronzo RA, "Pharmacologic Therapy for Type 2 Diabetes Mellitus," *Ann Intern Med*, 1999, 131(4):281-303.

Forman LM, Simmons DA, and Diamond RH, "Hepatic Failure in a Patient Taking Rosiglitazone," *Ann Intern Med*, 2000, 132(2):118-21.

- **Rowasa®** *see* Mesalamine *on page 723*
- **Roxanol™** *see* Morphine Sulfate *on page 778*
- **Roxanol™ 100** *see* Morphine Sulfate *on page 778*
- **Roxanol™ T** *see* Morphine Sulfate *on page 778*
- **Roxicet®** *see* Oxycodone and Acetaminophen *on page 847*
- **Roxicet® 5/500** *see* Oxycodone and Acetaminophen *on page 847*
- **Roxicodone™** *see* Oxycodone *on page 845*
- **Roxicodone™ Intensol™** *see* Oxycodone *on page 845*
- **RP59500** *see* Quinupristin/Dalfopristin *on page 970*
- **RS61443** *see* Mycophenolate *on page 785*
- **R-salbutamol** *see* Levalbuterol *on page 663*
- **RSV-IGIV** *see* Respiratory Syncytial Virus Immune Globulin (Intravenous) *on page 976*
- **RSV-IVIG** *see* Respiratory Syncytial Virus Immune Globulin (Intravenous) *on page 976*
- **RTCA** *see* Ribavirin *on page 981*
- **Rubella Virus Vaccine, Live** *see page 1333*
- **Rubex®** *see* DOXOrubicin *on page 413*
- **Rubidomycin** *see* DAUNOrubicin *on page 344*
- **Rum-K®** *see* Potassium Supplements *on page 919*
- **Rythmodan® (Can)** *see* Disopyramide *on page 399*
- **Rythmodan®-LA (Can)** *see* Disopyramide *on page 399*
- **S₂® [OTC]** *see* Epinephrine *on page 439*
- **SAB-Gentamicin (Can)** *see* Gentamicin *on page 533*

Sacrosidase (sak RO se dase)

U.S. Brand Names Sucraid®

Therapeutic Category Sucrase Deficiency, Treatment Agent

Generic Available No

Use Oral replacement therapy in congenital sucrase-isomaltase deficiency (CSID)

Pregnancy Risk Factor C

Contraindications Hypersensitivity to sacrosidase or any component, yeast and yeast products and glycerol

Warnings Hypersensitivity reactions to sacrosidase, including bronchospasm, have been reported; administer initial doses in a setting where acute hypersensitivity reactions may be treated within a few minutes; skin testing may be performed prior to administration to potentially identify patients at risk for hypersensitivity reactions.

Precautions Use with caution in CSID patients with diabetes mellitus, as Sucraid® will improve absorption of the products of sucrose hydrolysis (glucose and fructose); diet and/or insulin dosage may need to be adjusted

Adverse Reactions
  Central nervous system: Insomnia, headache, nervousness
  Endocrine & metabolic: Dehydration
  Gastrointestinal: Abdominal pain, vomiting, nausea, diarrhea, constipation
  Respiratory: Bronchospasm
  Miscellaneous: Hypersensitivity reactions (see Warnings)

Drug Interactions None as yet have been identified

Food Interactions May be inactivated or denatured if administered with fruit juice, warm or hot food or liquids; since isomaltase deficiency is not affected by sacrosidase, adherence to a low-starch diet may be required to decrease symptomatology

Stability Refrigerate at 4°C to 8°C (36°F to 46°F); protect from light; discard 4 weeks after opening

Mechanism of Action Sacrosidase is a naturally occurring GI enzyme which breaks down the disaccharide sucrose into its monosaccharide components; this hydrolysis is necessary to allow absorption of these nutrients

Pharmacokinetics Metabolism: Sacrosidase is metabolized in the GI tract to individual amino acids which are systemically absorbed

Usual Dosage Oral:
  Infants and Children ≤15 kg: 8500 international units (1 mL) per meal or snack
  Children >15 kg and Adults: 17,000 international units (2 mL) per meal or snack

Administration Oral: Dilute in 2-4 ounces of water, milk, or formula; approximately ½ of the dose may be taken before, and the remainder of the dose at the completion of, (Continued)

Sacrosidase *(Continued)*

each meal or snack; do not administer with fruit juices, warm or hot food or liquids (see Food Interactions)

Monitoring Parameters Breath hydrogen test, oral sucrose tolerance test, urinary disaccharides, intestinal disaccharidases (measured from small bowel biopsy)
CSID symptomatology: Diarrhea, abdominal pain, gas and bloating

Additional Information 1 mL = 22 drops from sacrosidase container tip

Dosage Forms Solution, oral: 8500 international units/mL (118 mL)

References

Treem WR, McAdams L, Stanford L, et al, "Sacrosidase Therapy for Congenital Sucrose-Isomaltase Deficiency," *J Pediatr Gastroenterol Nutr*, 1999, 28(2):137-42.

- ♦ **Safe Tussin® 30 [OTC]** *see* Guaifenesin and Dextromethorphan *on page 553*
- ♦ **Saizen®** *see* Human Growth Hormone *on page 564*
- ♦ **SalAc® [OTC]** *see* Salicylic Acid *on page 1002*
- ♦ **Sal-Acid®** *see* Salicylic Acid *on page 1002*
- ♦ **Salactic® [OTC]** *see* Salicylic Acid *on page 1002*
- ♦ **Salagen®** *see* Pilocarpine *on page 903*
- ♦ **Salazopyrin® (Can)** *see* Sulfasalazine *on page 1055*
- ♦ **Salazopyrin En-Tabs® (Can)** *see* Sulfasalazine *on page 1055*
- ♦ **Salbu-2 (Can)** *see* Albuterol *on page 54*
- ♦ **Salbu-4 (Can)** *see* Albuterol *on page 54*
- ♦ **Salbutamol** *see* Albuterol *on page 54*
- ♦ **Salicylazosulfapyridine** *see* Sulfasalazine *on page 1055*

Salicylic Acid *(sal i SIL ik AS id)*

U.S. Brand Names Compound W® [OTC]; Compound W® One Step Wart Remover [OTC]; DHS™ Sal [OTC]; Dr. Scholl's® Callus Remover [OTC]; Dr. Scholl's® Clear Away [OTC]; Duofilm® [OTC]; Duoplant® [OTC] [DSC]; Freezone® [OTC]; Fung-O® [OTC]; Gordofilm® [OTC]; Hydrisalic™ [OTC]; Ionil® [OTC]; Ionil® Plus [OTC]; Keralyt® [OTC]; Lupicare™ Dandruff [OTC]; Lupicare™ II Psoriasis [OTC]; Lupicare™ Psoriasis [OTC]; Mediplast® [OTC]; MG 217 Sal-Acid® [OTC]; Mosco® Corn and Callus Remover [OTC]; NeoCeuticals™ Acne Spot Treatment [OTC]; Neutrogena® Acne Wash [OTC]; Neutrogena® Body Clear™ [OTC]; Neutrogena® Clear Pore [OTC]; Neutrogena® Clear Pore Shine Control [OTC]; Neutrogena® Healthy Scalp [OTC]; Neutrogena® Maximum Strength T/Sal® [OTC]; Neutrogena® On The Spot® Acne Patch [OTC]; Occlusal®-HP [OTC]; Oxy Balance® [OTC]; Oxy Balance® Deep Pore [OTC]; Palmer's® Skin Success Acne Cleanser [OTC]; Pedisilk® [OTC]; Propa pH [OTC]; SalAc® [OTC]; Sal-Acid®; Salactic® [OTC]; Sal-Plant® [OTC]; Stridex® [OTC]; Stridex® Body Focus [OTC]; Stridex® Facewipes To Go™ [OTC]; Stridex® Maximum Strength [OTC]; Tinamed® [OTC]; Tiseb® [OTC]; Trans-Ver-Sal® [OTC]; Wart-Off® Maximum Strength [OTC]; Zapzyt® Acne Wash [OTC]; Zapzyt® Pore Treatment [OTC]

Canadian Brand Names Duoforte® 27; Occlusal™; Sebcur®; Soluver®; Soluver® Plus; Trans-Plantar®

Therapeutic Category Keratolytic Agent

Generic Available Yes (gel and soap)

Use Topically for its keratolytic effect in controlling seborrheic dermatitis or psoriasis of body and scalp, dandruff, and other scaling dermatoses; to remove warts, corns, calluses; also used in the treatment of acne

Pregnancy Risk Factor C

Contraindications Hypersensitivity to salicylic acid or any component (see Warnings); children <2 years of age

Warnings Should not be used systemically due to severe irritating effect on GI mucosa; prolonged use over large areas, especially in children, may result in salicylate toxicity; do not apply on irritated, reddened, or infected skin; do not use on moles, birthmarks, warts with hair growing from them, or genital warts; topical liquid may contain tartrazine which may cause allergic reactions in susceptible individuals

Precautions For external use only; avoid contact with eyes, face, and other mucous membranes

Adverse Reactions

Dermatologic: Facial scarring, erythema, scaling

Local: Irritation, burning

Mechanism of Action Produces desquamation of hyperkeratotic epithelium; increases hydration of the stratum corneum causing the skin to swell, soften, and desquamate

Pharmacokinetics

Absorption: Topical: Readily absorbed

Time to peak serum concentration: Within 5 hours when applied with an occlusive dressing

Elimination: Salicyluric acid (52%), salicylate glucuronides (42%), and salicylic acid (6%) are the major metabolites identified in urine after percutaneous absorption

Usual Dosage Children ≥2 years and Adults: Topical:

Lotion, cream, gel: Apply a thin layer to the affected area once or twice daily

Plaster: Cut to size that covers the corn or callus, apply and leave in place for 48 hours; do not exceed 5 applications over a 14-day period

Shampoo: Initial: Use daily or every other day; apply to wet hair and massage vigorously into the scalp; rinse hair thoroughly after shampooing; 1-2 treatments/week will usually maintain control

Solution: Apply a thin layer directly to wart using brush applicator once daily as directed for 1 week or until the wart is removed

Administration Topical: For external use only; when applying in concentrations >10%, protect surrounding normal tissue with petrolatum

Monitoring Parameters Signs and symptoms of salicylate toxicity: Nausea, vomiting, dizziness, tinnitus, loss of hearing, lethargy, diarrhea, psychic disturbances

Nursing Implications For warts: Before applying product, soak area in warm water for 5 minutes; dry area thoroughly, then apply medication

Dosage Forms

Cream:

Lupicare® Dandruff, Lupicare® Psoriasis: 2.5% (120 g, 240 g) [contains alcohol]

Lupicare® II Psoriasis: 2.5% (60 g, 240 g) [contains alcohol]

Neutrogena® Acne Wash: 2% (200 mL) [contains alcohol]

Cloths (Neutrogena® Acne Wash): 2% (30s) [disposable cloths]

Foam:

Neutrogena® Acne Wash: 2% (150 mL) [foaming cleanser]

SalAc®: 2% (100 g)

Gel: 17% (15 g)

Compound W®: 17% (7 g) [contains alcohol]

DuoPlant®: 17% (15 g) [DSC]

Hydrisalic™: 6% (28 g) [contains alcohol]

Keralyt®: 6% (30 g) [contains alcohol]

NeoCeuticals™ Acne Spot Treatment: 2% (15 g) [contains alcohol]

Neutrogena® Clear Pore: 2% (60 g) [contains alcohol]

Neutrogena® Clear Pore Shine Control: 0.5% (10 g)

Oxy Balance®: 2% (240 mL) [shower gel]

Sal-Plant®: 17% (14 g) [contains alcohol]

Stridex® Body Focus™: 2% (300 mL)

Zapzyt® Acne Wash: 2% (190 g) [alcohol free]

Zapzyt® Pore Treatment: 2% (23 g) [alcohol free]

Liquid, topical:

Compound W®: 17% (9 mL) [contains alcohol]

DuoFilm®: 17% (15 mL) [contains alcohol]

Freezone®: 17.6% (9.3 mL) [contains alcohol]

Fung-O®: 17% (15 mL)

Gordofilm®: 16.7% (15 mL)

Mosco® Corn and Callus Remover: 17.6% (10 mL)

NeoCeuticals™ Acne Spot Treatment: 2% (60 mL) [contains alcohol]

Neutrogena® Acne Wash: 2% (180 mL) [contains tartrazine]

Neutrogena® Body Clear™: 2% (250 mL) [body scrub with microbeads; contains tartrazine]

Neutrogena® Body Clear™: 2% (250 mL) [body wash; contains tartrazine]

Occlusal®-HP: 17% (10 mL)

Palmer's Skin Success Acne Cleanser: 0.5% (240 mL)

Pedisilk®: 17% (15 mL)

Propa pH: 2% (80 mL) [alcohol free]

SalAc®: 2% (180 mL)

Salactic®: 17% (15 mL) [contains alcohol]

Tinamed®: 17% (15 mL)

Wart-Off® Maximum Strength: 17% (13 mL) [contains alcohol]

Ointment (MG217 Sal-Acid®): 3% (56 g) [contains vitamin E]

Pads:

Oxy Balance®, Oxy Balance® Deep Pore: 0.5% (55s, 90s) [contains alcohol]

Stridex®: 0.5% (55s)

Stridex® Facewipes To Go™: 0.5% (32s) [contains alcohol]

Stridex® Maximum Strength: 2% (32s, 55s, 90s)

Patch, transdermal:

Compound W® One Step Wart Remover: 40% (12s, 14s)

Dr. Scholl's® Callus Remover: 40% (4s)

(Continued)

Salicylic Acid (Continued)

    Dr. Scholl's® Clear Away: 40% (14s, 16s, 18s, 24s)
    DuoFilm®: 40% (18s)
    Neutrogena® On The Spot® Acne Patch: 2% (27s)
    Trans-Ver-Sal®: 15% [6 mm PediaPatch, 12 mm AdultPatch, 20 mm PlantarPatch]
      (10s, 12s, 15s, 25s, 40s)
  Plaster:
    Mediplast®: 40% (25s)
    Sal-Acid®: 40% (14s)
    Tinamed®: 40% (24s)
  Shampoo:
    DHS™ Sal: 3% (120 mL)
    Ionil®: 2% (240 mL, 480 mL, 960 mL)
    Ionil® Plus: 2% (240 mL) [conditioning shampoo]
    Lupicare® Dandruff, Lupicare® Psoriasis: 2% (120 mL, 240 mL)
    Neutrogena® Healthy Scalp: 1.8% (90 mL, 180 mL)
    Neutrogena® Maximum Strength T/Sal®: 3% (135 mL)
    Tiseb®: 2% (240 mL)
  Soap: 2% (114 g)

♦ **Salicylic Acid and Sulfur** *see* Sulfur and Salicylic Acid *on page 1058*
♦ **SalineX® [OTC]** *see* Sodium Chloride *on page 1027*

Salmeterol (sal ME te role)

Related Information
  Asthma Guidelines *on page 1376*
U.S. Brand Names Serevent®; Serevent® Diskus®
Therapeutic Category Adrenergic Agonist Agent; Antiasthmatic; Beta$_2$-Adrenergic Agonist Agent; Bronchodilator
Generic Available No
Use Maintenance treatment of asthma; prevention of bronchospasm in patients with reversible obstructive airway disease; prevention of exercise-induced bronchospasm
Pregnancy Risk Factor C
Contraindications Hypersensitivity to salmeterol, adrenergic amines, or any component
Warnings Cardiovascular effects are not common with salmeterol when used in recommended doses. Salmeterol is not meant to relieve acute asthmatic symptoms. Acute episodes should be treated with short-acting beta$_2$ agonist. Do not increase the frequency of salmeterol use. Paroxysmal bronchospasm (which can be fatal) has been reported with this and other inhaled agents. If this occurs, discontinue treatment; most commonly occurs with first use of a new canister or vial

GlaxoSmithKline (GSK), in association with the Food and Drug Administration (FDA), has issued a letter to healthcare professionals concerning the recently suspended Salmeterol Multi-center Asthma Research Trial (SMART) study. The objective of this study was to compare salmeterol to placebo and evaluate the incidence of respiratory-related deaths and life-threatening experiences. The eligible study population included children >12 years. An interim analysis was conducted when enrollment reached half of the anticipated total (25,858 patients were included). Due to a low incidence of primary events, the findings of the interim analysis were not conclusive.

Although statistically significant differences for the primary endpoints were not established, a higher number of asthma-related, life-threatening experiences (including death) were reported in the treatment group. Specific subpopulations were also evaluated. It was noted that African-American patients receiving salmeterol experienced a higher number of primary events and asthma-related events (including death) as compared to patients receiving placebo. Of note, these events occurred in <1% of all African-Americans enrolled. In contrast to the overall results, the difference observed in the African-American population was statistically significant. However, it has been noted that characteristics of this subpopulation [including a greater severity of asthma at baseline and a lower rate (38% vs 50% in Caucasians) of inhaled corticosteroid use], may have contributed to the observed differences. Of note, the low inhaled corticosteroid use across the study population at baseline (47%) was considered to be inconsistent with current NAEPP asthma management guidelines. The study was not designed to provide robust results within or between subpopulations. The SMART study was terminated after the review concluded it was not likely to answer the questions which were raised by the interim analysis.

Precautions Use with caution in patients with cardiovascular disorders, convulsive disorders, thyrotoxicosis, or others who are sensitive to the effects of sympathomimetic amines

Adverse Reactions

Cardiovascular: Prolonged QT_c interval (large doses), tachycardia, palpitations, arrhythmias

Central nervous system: Dizziness, headache, nervousness, hyperactivity, insomnia, malaise

Dermatologic: Rash, pruritus

Endocrine & metabolic: Hypokalemia

Gastrointestinal: GI upset, diarrhea, nausea, oropharyngeal irritation

Neuromuscular & skeletal: Joint and back pain, tremors, muscle cramps

Respiratory: Respiratory arrest, cough, pharyngitis, paradoxical bronchospasm (see Warnings)

Miscellaneous: Hypersensitivity reactions, tachyphylaxis

Drug Interactions Cytochrome P450 isoenzyme CYP3A3/4 substrate

Additive effects with beta-adrenergic agents; MAO inhibitors and tricyclic antidepressants potentiate cardiovascular effects; beta-blocking agents antagonize effects; increased potassium losses with diuretics

Stability The therapeutic effect may decrease when the cannister is cold, therefore, the canister should remain at room temperature. Do not store at temperatures >120°F. Serevent® Diskus® is stable for 6 weeks after protective foil is removed.

Mechanism of Action Relaxes bronchial smooth muscle by selective action on beta$_2$-receptors with little effect on heart rate

Pharmacodynamics

Onset of action: 10-20 minutes

Maximum effect: 3 hours

Duration: Up to 12 hours

Pharmacokinetics

Protein binding: 94% to 95%

Metabolism: Extensive via hydroxylation

Half-life: 3-4 hours

Usual Dosage Children >4 years and Adults:

Maintenance and prevention of asthma, COPD

Inhalation, oral:

Serevent®: 42 mcg (2 actuations/puffs) twice daily, 12 hours apart

Serevent® Diskus®: 50 mcg (1 actuation/puff) twice daily, 12 hours apart

Prevention of exercise-induced asthma: Inhalation: Serevent®42 mcg (2 actuations/puffs) 30-60 minutes prior to exercise; additional doses should not be used for 12 hours; patients who are using salmeterol twice daily should **not** use an additional salmeterol dose prior to exercise; if twice daily use is not effective during exercise, consider other appropriate therapy

Administration Inhalation:

Serevent®: Shake well before use; before using inhaler for first time or if unused for more than 4 weeks, "test spray" 4 times into the air; use Serevent® with spacer device in children <8 years of age

Serevent® Diskus®: May not be used with a spacer

Monitoring Parameters Pulmonary function tests

Patient Information Do not use to treat acute symptoms; do not exceed the prescribed dose of salmeterol; do not stop using inhaled or oral corticosteroids without medical advice even if feeling better; avoid spraying in eyes; remove the cannister and rinse the plastic case and cap under warm water and dry daily. Store cannister with nozzle end down.

Additional Information When salmeterol is initiated in patients previously receiving a short-acting beta agonist, instruct the patient to discontinue the regular use of the short-acting beta agonist and to utilize the shorter-acting agent for symptomatic or acute episodes only. Although each puff delivers 25 mcg the amount delivered through the mouthpiece is actually 21 mcg per puff.

Dosage Forms

Aerosol for oral inhalation, as xinafoate (Serevent®): 25 mcg/actuation (6.5 g) [delivers 21 mcg/inhalation; 60 inhalations], (13 g) [delivers 21 mcg/inhalation; 120 inhalations]

Powder for oral inhalation, as xinafoate (Serevent® Diskus®): 50 mcg (28s, 60s) [delivers 46 mcg/inhalation]

References

Meyer JM, Wenzel CL, and Kradjan WA, "Salmeterol: A Novel, Long-Acting Beta$_2$-Agonist," *Ann Pharmacother*, 1993, 27(12):1478-87.

"National Asthma Education and Prevention Program. Expert Panel Report: Guidelines for the Diagnosis and Management of Asthma Update on Selected Topics--2002," *J Allergy Clin Immunol*, 2002, 110(5 Suppl):S141-219.

♦ **Salofalk® (Can)** *see* Mesalamine *on page 723*

♦ **Sal-Plant® [OTC]** *see* Salicylic Acid *on page 1002*

♦ **Salt Poor Albumin**   *see Albumin on page 52*

♦ **Sal-Tropine**™   *see Atropine on page 144*

♦ **Sandimmune**®   *see CycloSPORINE on page 324*

♦ **Sandostatin**®   *see Octreotide Acetate on page 828*

♦ **Sandostatin LAR**®   *see Octreotide Acetate on page 828*

♦ **Sani-Supp**® **[OTC]**   *see Glycerin on page 543*

Saquinavir (sa KWIN a veer)

Related Information
Adult and Adolescent HIV *on page 1327*

U.S. Brand Names Fortovase®; Invirase®

Therapeutic Category Antiretroviral Agent;   HIV Agents (Anti-HIV Agents); Protease Inhibitor

Generic Available No

Use Treatment of HIV infection in combination with other antiretroviral agents; **(Note:** HIV regimens consisting of **three** antiretroviral agents are strongly recommended); in a randomized, double-blind study of 297 patients, a triple drug combination of saquinavir, zalcitabine, and zidovudine reduced HIV-1 replication, increased CD4+ cell counts, and decreased levels of activation markers in serum more than did treatment with zidovudine and either saquinavir or zalcitabine; postexposure chemoprophylaxis following occupational exposure to HIV

Pregnancy Risk Factor B

Contraindications Hypersensitivity to saquinavir or any component; concurrent therapy with astemizole, terfenadine, cisapride, midazolam, triazolam, ergot derivatives, simvastatin, or lovastatin

Warnings Spontaneous bleeding episodes have been reported in patients with hemophilia receiving an HIV protease inhibitor; new onset diabetes mellitus, exacerbation of diabetes and hyperglycemia have been reported in HIV-infected patients receiving protease inhibitors. Redistribution or accumulation of body fat has been reported in patients taking protease inhibitors. Due to potential serious and/or life-threatening drug interactions, certain drugs are contraindicated (see Contraindications and Drug Interactions).

Precautions Fat redistribution and accumulation [ie, central obesity, peripheral wasting, facial wasting, breast enlargement, dorsocervical fat enlargement (buffalo hump), and cushingoid appearance] have been observed in patients receiving antiretroviral agents (causal relationship not established). Use with caution in patients with diabetes mellitus, hepatic impairment or in patients receiving drugs which induce or are substrates of cytochrome P450 3A

Adverse Reactions
Cardiovascular: Cyanosis, heart murmur, hypotension, hypertension, syncope

Central nervous system: Confusion, ataxia, headache, dizziness, seizures, fever, hallucinations, asthenia, agitation, fatigue

Dermatologic: Rash, photosensitivity, acne

Endocrine & metabolic: Hypoglycemia, elevated creatine phosphokinase; rare: hyperglycemia, diabetes, ketoacidosis; central redistribution of body fat: Central obesity, buffalo hump, facial atrophy, and breast enlargement

Gastrointestinal: Diarrhea, abdominal discomfort, nausea, vomiting, stomatitis

Hematologic: Hemolytic anemia, pancytopenia, thrombocytopenia, microhemorrhages; rare: spontaneous bleeding episodes in hemophiliacs

Hepatic: Elevated ALT, AST, bilirubin, and amylase

Neuromuscular & skeletal: Parethesias, peripheral neuropathy, tremor, arthralgia

Respiratory: Cough

Drug Interactions Cytochrome P450 isoenzyme CYP3A3/4 substrate and inhibitor

Rifampin decreases saquinavir concentrations by 80%; rifabutin, nevirapine, phenobarbital, phenytoin, dexamethasone, carbamazepine may decrease saquinavir concentrations; saquinavir may increase concentrations of calcium channel blockers, clindamycin, sildenafil, dapsone, quinidine, astemizole, terfenadine, cisapride, ergot alkaloid derivatives, midazolam, triazolam, lovastatin, simvastatin, cerivastatin, and atorvastatin; ketoconazole, delavirdine, clarithromycin, indinavir, nelfinavir, ritonavir may increase saquinavir levels; saquinavir decreases delavirdine levels; the herbal medicine St John's wort (*Hypericum perforatum*) decreases AUC and plasma concentration of saquinavir

Food Interactions Presence of a high fat meal maximizes bioavailability of saquinavir; grapefruit juice may increase saquinavir levels

Stability
Fortovase®: Store capsules in refrigerator; stable for 3 months if stored at room temperature

Invirase®: Store at room temperature in tightly closed bottles

Mechanism of Action Saquinavir is an HIV protease inhibitor which acts late in the life cycle of the virus inside the cell by blocking the cleavage of a polyprotein precursor into structural proteins required for the assembly of infectious virions in lymphocytes and monocytes

Pharmacokinetics

Distribution: CSF concentration is negligible when compared to concentrations from matched plasma samples; partitions into tissues

Protein binding: 98%

Metabolism: Extensive first-pass effect; hepatic metabolism by cytochrome P450 3A system to inactive metabolites

Bioavailability:

Invirase®: 4% (increased in the presence of food)

Fortovase®: Relative to Invirase® is ~331%

Half-life: Adults: 13 hours

Elimination: 88% of dose eliminated in feces; 1% excreted in urine

Usual Dosage Oral:

Children: Safety and efficacy in children and adolescents <16 years of age have not been established; Fortovase®: 50 mg/kg/dose 3 times/day is under study in Pediatric AIDS Clinical Trials Group protocol 397

Adults:

Invirase®: 600 mg 3 times/day; lower doses (<1800 mg/day) have not shown effective antiviral activity

Fortovase®: 1200 mg 3 times/day

Note: Invirase® and Fortovase® capsules are not bioequivalent and cannot be used interchangeably. Fortovase® is the recommended formulation to be used for the initiation of saquinavir therapy since it provides greater bioavailability than Invirase®. In rare circumstances, Invirase® may be considered if it is to be used with antiretrovirals that significantly inhibit its metabolism.

Administration Oral: Administer within 2 hours after a full meal to increase absorption; avoid taking saquinavir with grapefruit juice

Monitoring Parameters Liver function tests, triglyceride levels, blood glucose levels, CD4 cell count, plasma levels of HIV RNA

Patient Information Saquinavir is not a cure for HIV infection; if a dose is missed, take the next dose as soon as possible; however, if a dose is skipped, do not double the next dose; notify physician if numbness, tingling, persistent severe abdominal pain, nausea, or vomiting occurs. Report the use of other medications, nonprescription medications, and herbal or natural products to your physician and pharmacist; avoid the herbal medicine St John's wort. May cause photosensitivity reactions (eg, exposure to sunlight may cause severe sunburn, skin rash, redness, or itching); avoid exposure to sunlight and artificial light sources (sunlamps, tanning booth/bed); wear protective clothing, wide-brimmed hats, sunglasses, and lip sunscreen (SPF ≥15); use a sunscreen [broad-spectrum sunscreen or physical sunscreen (preferred) or sunblock with SPF ≥15]; contact physician if reaction occurs. Do not breast-feed while receiving antiretroviral medications.

HIV medications may cause changes in body fat, including an increase in fat in the upper back and neck, breasts, and trunk; a loss of fat from the face, arms, and legs may also occur.

Dosage Forms

Capsule, as **mesylate** (Invirase®): 200 mg

Capsule, soft gelatin, liquid filled, as **base** (Fortovase®): 200 mg

References

Collier AC, Coombs RW, Schoenfeld DA, et al, "Treatment of Human Immunodeficiency Virus Infection With Saquinavir, Zidovudine, and Zalcitabine," *N Engl J Med*, 1996, 334(16):1011-7.

Mueller BU, "Antiviral Chemotherapy," *Curr Opin Pediatr*, 1997, 9(2):178-83.

Working Group on Antiretroviral Therapy and Medical Management of HIV-Infected Children, "Guidelines for the Use of Antiretroviral Agents in Pediatric HIV Infection," January 7, 2000, http://www.aidsinfo.nih.gov.

♦ **Sarafem**™ *see* Fluoxetine *on page 505*

Sargramostim (sar GRAM oh stim)

U.S. Brand Names Leukine®

Synonyms GM-CSF; Granulocyte Macrophage Colony Stimulating Factor; rGM-CSF

Therapeutic Category Colony-Stimulating Factor

Generic Available No

Use Accelerates myeloid recovery in patients undergoing autologous or allogeneic BMT; mobilize hematopoietic progenitor cells into peripheral blood for collection by leukapheresis; accelerate myeloid engraftment following autologous peripheral blood progenitor cell transplantation; increase neutrophil counts in patients with malignancies receiving myelosuppressive chemotherapy; increase leukocyte counts in patients with severe aplastic anemia; neonatal neutropenia

(Continued)

Sargramostim *(Continued)*

Pregnancy Risk Factor C

Contraindications Hypersensitivity to GM-CSF, yeast-derived products, or any component (see Warnings); excessive leukemic myeloid blasts in bone marrow or peripheral blood ≥10%; history of idiopathic thrombocytopenic purpura

Warnings Injection solution contains benzyl alcohol which may cause allergic reactions in susceptible individuals; large amounts of benzyl alcohol (≥99 mg/kg/day) have been associated with a potentially fatal toxicity ("gasping syndrome") in neonates; the "gasping syndrome" consists of metabolic acidosis, respiratory distress, gasping respirations, CNS dysfunction (including convulsions, intracranial hemorrhage), hypotension and cardiovascular collapse; use sargramostim injection products containing benzyl alcohol with caution in neonates; *in vitro* and animal studies have shown that benzoate, a metabolite of benzyl alcohol, displaces bilirubin from protein binding sites

Precautions Use with caution in patients with autoimmune or chronic inflammatory disease, hypertension, cardiovascular disease, pulmonary disease, or renal or hepatic impairment

Rapid increase in peripheral blood counts: If ANC is >20,000/mm^3 or platelets >500,000/mm^3, decrease dose by 50% or discontinue drug (counts will fall to normal within 3-7 days after discontinuing drug)

Growth factor potential: Caution with myeloid malignancies; do **not** administer within 24 hours prior to or after chemotherapy or 12 hours prior to or after radiation therapy

Adverse Reactions

Cardiovascular: Hypotension, tachycardia, flushing, pericardial effusion, fluid retention, venous thrombosis

Central nervous system: Malaise, fever, headache, chills

Dermatologic: Rash

Endocrine & metabolic: Polydipsia

Gastrointestinal: Nausea, vomiting, diarrhea, stomatitis, GI hemorrhage

Hepatic: Elevated liver function tests

Neuromuscular & skeletal: Bone pain, myalgia, rigors, weakness

Respiratory: Dyspnea

Miscellaneous: "First dose" reaction (fever, hypotension, tachycardia, rigors, flushing, nausea, vomiting, dyspnea)

Drug Interactions Lithium and corticosteroids may potentiate myeloproliferative effects of sargramostim

Stability Store vial in the refrigerator; stable after reconstitution for 6 hours at room temperature; use only NS to prepare I.V. infusion solution; GM-CSF at a concentration ≥10 mcg/mL is compatible with TPN during Y-site administration

Mechanism of Action Stimulates proliferation, differentiation and functional activity of neutrophils, eosinophils, monocytes and macrophages

Pharmacodynamics

Onset of action: Increase in WBC in 7-14 days

Duration: WBC will return to baseline within 1 week after discontinuing drug

Pharmacokinetics

Half-life: 2 hours

Time to peak serum concentration: S.C.: Within 3 hours

Usual Dosage I.V., S.C.:

Neonates: 10 mcg/kg/day once daily for 5 days has been administered to preterm neonates at high risk of both neutropenia and sepsis

Children (no dosing for children has been FDA approved): 250 mcg/m^2/day once daily for 21 days to begin 2-4 hours after the marrow infusion on day 0 of BMT or not less than 24 hours after chemotherapy. If significant adverse effects or "first dose" reaction is seen at this dose, discontinue the drug until toxicity resolves, then restart at a reduced dose of 125 mcg/m^2/day

Aplastic anemia: 8-32 mcg/kg/day once daily

Cancer chemotherapy recovery: 3-15 mcg/kg/day once daily for 14-21 days; maximum dose: 30 mcg/kg/day or 1500 mcg/m^2/day

Adults: 250 mcg/m^2/day once daily for 21 days to begin 2-4 hours after BMT, or not less than 24 hours after chemotherapy (to minimize first dose reaction, start with low doses and increase gradually)

Aplastic anemia: 15-480 mcg/m^2 once daily

Cancer chemotherapy recovery: 3-15 mcg/kg/day once daily for 10 days

Administration Parenteral:

I.V.: Administer as a 30-minute, 2-hour, or 6-hour I.V. infusion or by continuous I.V. infusion. Do not shake solution to avoid foaming. Dilute in NS; if the final concentration of GM-CSF in NS is <10 mcg/mL, then add 1 mg albumin per mL of I.V. fluid.

Albumin acts as a carrier molecule to prevent drug adsorption to the I.V. tubing. Albumin should be added to NS prior to addition of GM-CSF.

S.C.: Reconstituted 250 mcg/mL or 500 mcg/mL solution may be administered without further dilution; rotate injection sites

Monitoring Parameters CBC with differential, platelets; renal/liver function tests, especially with previous dysfunction; vital signs, weight; pulmonary function

Reference Range Excessive leukocytosis (WBC >50,000 cells/mm^3, ANC >20,000 cells/mm^3)

Patient Information Possible bone pain may occur

Nursing Implications Can premedicate with analgesics and antipyretics; control bone pain with non-narcotic analgesics

Additional Information Produced by recombinant DNA technology using a yeast-derived expression system

Dosage Forms

Injection, powder for reconstitution: 250 mcg

Injection, solution: 500 mcg/mL (1 mL) [contains benzyl alcohol]

References

Carr R, Modi N, Dore CJ, et al, "A Randomized, Controlled Trial of Prophylactic Granulocyte-Macrophage Colony-Stimulating Factor in Human Newborns Less Than 32 Weeks Gestation," *Pediatrics*, 1999, 103(4 Pt 1):796-802.

Lieschke GJ and Burgess AW, "Granulocyte Colony-Stimulating Factor and Granulocyte-Macrophage Colony-Stimulating Factor," (1) *N Engl J Med*, 1992, 327(1):28-35.

Lieschke GJ and Burgess AW, "Granulocyte Colony-Stimulating Factor and Granulocyte-Macrophage Colony-Stimulating Factor," (2) *N Engl J Med*, 1992, 327(2):99-106.

Stute N, Furman WL, Schell M, et al, "Pharmacokinetics of Recombinant Human Granulocyte - Macrophage Colony - Stimulating Factor in Children After Intravenous and Subcutaneous Administration," *J Pharm Sci*, 1995, 84(7):824-8.

Trissel LA, Bready BB, Kwan JW, et al, "Visual Compatibility of Sargramostim With Selected Antineoplastic Agents, Anti-infectives, or Other Drugs During Simulated Y-Site Injection," *Am J Hosp Pharm*, 1992, 49(2):402-6.

♦ **Sarna® HC (Can)** *see* Hydrocortisone *on page 573*

♦ **Sarnol®-HC [OTC]** *see* Hydrocortisone *on page 573*

♦ **SCH 52365** *see* Temozolomide *on page 1065*

♦ **Scheinpharm B12 (Can)** *see* Cyanocobalamin *on page 316*

♦ **Scopace™** *see* Scopolamine *on page 1009*

Scopolamine (skoe POL a meen)

Related Information

Overdose and Toxicology *on page 1388*

U.S. Brand Names Isopto® Hyoscine; Scopace™; Transderm Scop®

Canadian Brand Names Transderm-V®

Synonyms Hyoscine

Therapeutic Category Anticholinergic Agent; Anticholinergic Agent, Ophthalmic; Anticholinergic Agent, Transdermal; Ophthalmic Agent, Mydriatic

Generic Available Yes

Use Preoperative medication to produce amnesia and decrease salivary and respiratory secretions; to produce cycloplegia and mydriasis (ophthalmic formulation); treatment of iridocyclitis (ophthalmic formulation); prevention of motion sickness (oral and transdermal formulations) and prevention of postoperative nausea and vomiting (transdermal formulation)

Pregnancy Risk Factor C

Contraindications Hypersensitivity to scopolamine or any component; patients hypersensitive to belladonna or barbiturates may be hypersensitive to scopolamine; narrow-angle glaucoma, GI or GU obstruction, thyrotoxicosis, tachycardia secondary to cardiac insufficiency, paralytic ileus, myasthenia gravis

Warnings Drug withdrawal symptoms such as nausea, vomiting, headache, dizziness, and equilibrium disturbance have been reported following removal of transdermal system, primarily in patients using the system for more than 3 days

Precautions Use with caution with hepatic or renal dysfunction since adverse CNS effects occur more often in these patients; use with caution in infants and children since they may be more susceptible to adverse effects of scopolamine; use with caution in patients with cardiac disease, seizures, or psychoses

Adverse Reactions

Cardiovascular: Tachycardia, palpitations

Central nervous system: Disorientation, drowsiness, hallucinations, confusion, psychosis, delirium, excitement, restlessness, dizziness

Gastrointestinal: Xerostomia, constipation, nausea, vomiting, dysphagia, dysgeusia

Genitourinary: Urinary retention

Ocular: Blurred vision, cycloplegia, mydriasis, photophobia, elevated intraocular pressure

(Continued)

Scopolamine *(Continued)*

Miscellaneous: Anaphylaxis, allergic reactions

Note: Systemic adverse effects have been reported with both the topical and ophthalmic preparations

Drug Interactions Additive adverse effects with other anticholinergic agents and amantadine; GI absorption of the following drugs may be affected: acetaminophen, levodopa, ketoconazole, digoxin (tablets only), riboflavin, KCl wax-matrix preparations; additive CNS effects with other CNS depressants, alcohol

Stability Physically compatible when mixed in the same syringe with atropine, butorphanol, chlorpromazine, dimenhydrinate, diphenhydramine, droperidol, fentanyl, glycopyrrolate, hydromorphone, hydroxyzine, meperidine, metoclopramide, morphine, pentazocine, pentobarbital, perphenazine, prochlorperazine, promazine, promethazine, or thiopental

Mechanism of Action Blocks the action of acetylcholine at parasympathetic sites in smooth muscle, secretory glands and the CNS, resulting in anticholinergic activity (inhibition of secretion of saliva and sweat, decreased GI motility and secretions, dilated pupils, increased heart rate, drowsiness, depressed motor function); antagonizes histamine and serotonin

Pharmacodynamics

Onset of action:

Oral, I.M.: 30 minutes to 1 hour

I.V.: 10 minutes

Transdermal: 4 hours

Duration:

Oral, I.M.: 4-6 hours

I.V.: 2 hours

Transdermal: 72 hours

Pharmacokinetics

Absorption: Well absorbed by all routes of administration

Metabolism: In the liver

Half-life: 9.5 hours

Excretion: <5% excreted unchanged in the urine

Usual Dosage

Preoperatively and antiemetic:

I.M., I.V., S.C.:

Children: 6 mcg/kg/dose (maximum dose: 0.3 mg/dose); may be repeated every 6-8 hours

Adults: 0.3-0.65 mg; may be repeated 3-4 times/day

Transdermal: Adults: Apply 1 disc behind the ear the evening before surgery; if prior to cesarean section, apply 1 hour prior to minimize exposure to infant

Motion sickness:

Oral: Children >12 years and Adults: 1-2 tablets 1 hour prior to exposure; may repeat after 8 hours of continued exposure

Transdermal: Children >12 years and Adults: Apply 1 disc behind the ear at least 4 hours prior to exposure every 3 days as needed

Ophthalmic:

Refraction:

Children: Instill 1 drop of 0.25% to eye(s) twice daily for 2 days before procedure

Adults: Instill 1-2 drops of 0.25% to eye(s) 1 hour before procedure

Iridocyclitis:

Children: Instill 1 drop of 0.25% to eye(s) up to 3 times/day

Adults: Instill 1-2 drops of 0.25% to eye(s) up to 3 times/day

Administration

Oral: May be administered without regard to food

Parenteral: I.V.: Dilute with an equal volume of SWI and administer by direct I.V. injection over 2-3 minutes

Transdermal: Apply patch to hairless area behind one ear; wash hands before and after application; if becomes dislodged, replace with fresh patch; if usage >72 hours, replace with new patch (see Usual Dosage for time of administration)

Ophthalmic: Instill drops to conjunctival sac of affected eye(s); avoid contact of bottle tip with skin or eye; finger pressure should be applied to lacrimal sac during and for 1-2 minutes after instillation to decrease risk of absorption and systemic reactions

Patient Information May cause drowsiness and impair ability to perform activities requiring mental alertness or physical coordination; may cause dry mouth; avoid alcohol; wash hands thoroughly with soap and water after handling the patch as dilation of pupils and blurred vision may occur if contact with eye; dispose of patches properly to avoid contact with children or pets; remove patch immediately if experiencing difficulty urinating or pain and reddening of eyes accompanied by dilated pupils

Additional Information Transdermal disc is programmed to deliver *in vivo* 0.5 mg over 3 days

Dosage Forms
Injection, solution, as hydrobromide: 0.4 mg/mL (1 mL)
Solution, ophthalmic, as hydrobromide (Isopto® Hyoscine): 0.25% (5 mL, 15 mL)
Tablet, soluble, as hydrobromide (Scopace™): 0.4 mg
Transdermal system (Transderm Scop®): 1.5 mg (4s) [releases ~1 mg over 72 hours]

◆ **Scopolamine, Hyoscyamine, Atropine, and Phenobarbital** *see* Hyoscyamine, Atropine, Scopolamine, and Phenobarbital *on page 587*

◆ **Scot-Tussin® Allergy Relief [OTC]** *see* DiphenhydrAMINE *on page 393*

◆ **Scot-Tussin DM® Cough Chasers [OTC]** *see* Dextromethorphan *on page 365*

◆ **Scot-Tussin® Sugar Free Expectorant [OTC]** *see* Guaifenesin *on page 550*

◆ **SDZ ASM 981** *see* Pimecrolimus *on page 905*

◆ **SeaMist® [OTC]** *see* Sodium Chloride *on page 1027*

◆ **Seba-Gel™** *see* Benzoyl Peroxide *on page 165*

◆ **Sebcur® (Can)** *see* Salicylic Acid *on page 1002*

◆ **Sebex® [OTC]** *see* Sulfur and Salicylic Acid *on page 1058*

◆ **Sebulex® [OTC]** *see* Sulfur and Salicylic Acid *on page 1058*

Secobarbital (see koe BAR bi tal)

Related Information
Laboratory Detection of Drugs in Urine *on page 1400*

U.S. Brand Names Seconal®

Synonyms Quinalbarbitone

Therapeutic Category Barbiturate; Hypnotic; Sedative

Generic Available No

Use Short-term treatment of insomnia; preanesthetic agent

Restrictions C-II

Pregnancy Risk Factor D

Contraindications Hypersensitivity to secobarbital or any component; pre-existing CNS depression, severe uncontrolled pain, porphyria, severe respiratory disease with dyspnea or obstruction

Precautions Use with caution in patients with hypovolemic shock, CHF, hepatic impairment, respiratory dysfunction or depression, previous addiction to the sedative/hypnotic group, chronic or acute pain, renal dysfunction; tolerance or psychological and physical dependence may occur with prolonged use; abrupt discontinuation after prolonged use may result in withdrawal symptoms

Adverse Reactions
Cardiovascular: Hypotension, cardiac arrhythmias, bradycardia
Central nervous system: Dizziness, lightheadedness, drowsiness, "hangover" effect, lethargy, impaired judgment, CNS depression or paradoxical excitation, hypothermia, nightmares, hallucinations
Dermatologic: Rash, exfoliative dermatitis, Stevens-Johnson syndrome
Gastrointestinal: Nausea, vomiting, constipation
Hematologic: Megaloblastic anemia, thrombocytopenia, agranulocytosis
Respiratory: Respiratory depression, apnea
Miscellaneous: Psychological and physical dependence with prolonged use

Drug Interactions Cytochrome P450 isoenzyme CYP2A6, CYP2C9, and CYP3A3/4 inducer
Barbiturates are enzyme inducers (monitor patients closely for decreased effect of concomitantly administered medications or increased effect when barbiturates are discontinued)
Secobarbital may decrease the serum concentration or effect of ethosuximide, warfarin, oral contraceptives, chloramphenicol, griseofulvin, doxycycline, beta-blockers, cyclophosphamide, theophylline, corticosteroids, tricyclic antidepressants, quinidine, haloperidol, and phenothiazines. Secobarbital given with other CNS depressants may increase CNS and respiratory depression. Chloramphenicol, valproic acid, and chlorpropamide may inhibit the metabolism of secobarbital with a resultant increase in secobarbital serum concentration.

Food Interactions High doses of pyridoxine may decrease drug effect; barbiturates may increase the metabolism of vitamins D and K

Mechanism of Action Depresses CNS activity by binding to barbiturate site at GABA-receptor complex enhancing GABA activity; depresses reticular activating system; higher doses may be gabamimetic

Pharmacodynamics
Onset of action: Hypnosis: Oral: 15-30 minutes
Duration: Hypnosis: Oral: 3-4 hours with 100 mg dose
(Continued)

Secobarbital *(Continued)*

Pharmacokinetics
Absorption: Oral: Well absorbed (90%)
Distribution: V_d: Adult: 1.5 L/kg; crosses the placenta; appears in breast milk
Protein binding: 45% to 60%
Metabolism: In the liver by the microsomal enzyme system
Half-life:
Children: 2-13 years: 2.7-13.5 hours
Adults: 15-40 hours; mean 28 hours
Time to peak serum concentration: Oral: Within 2-4 hours
Elimination: Renally as inactive metabolites and small amounts as unchanged drug
Dialysis: Hemodialysis: Slightly dialyzable (5% to 20%)

Usual Dosage Oral:
Children:
Preoperative sedation: 2-6 mg/kg (maximum dose: 100 mg/dose) 1-2 hours before procedure
Sedation: 6 mg/kg/day divided every 8 hours
Adults:
Hypnotic: Usual: 100 mg/dose at bedtime; range 100-200 mg/dose
Preoperative sedation: 100-300 mg 1-2 hours before procedure

Monitoring Parameters Blood pressure, heart rate, respiratory rate, pulse oximetry, CNS status

Patient Information Avoid alcohol and other CNS depressants; may be habit-forming; avoid abrupt discontinuation after prolonged use; may cause dizziness or drowsiness and impair ability to perform activities requiring mental alertness or physical coordination

Additional Information Effectiveness for insomnia decreases greatly after 2 weeks of use; alkalinization of urine does not significantly increase excretion; withdraw slowly over 5-6 days after prolonged use to avoid sleep disturbances and rapid eye movement (REM) rebound

Dosage Forms Capsule, as sodium: 100 mg

References
Levine HL, Cohen ME, Duffner PK, et al, "Rectal Absorption and Disposition of Secobarbital in Epileptic Children," *Pediatr Pharmacol (New York)*, 1982, 2(1):33-8.
Nahata MC, Starling S, and Edwards RC, "Prolonged Sedation Associated With Secobarbital in Newborn Infants Receiving Ventilatory Support," *Am J Perinatol*, 1991, 8(1):35-6.
Wolfert RR and Cox RM, "Room Temperature Stability of Drug Products Labeled for Refrigerated Storage," *Am J Hosp Pharm*, 1975, 32(6):585-7.

♦ **Seconal**® *see* Secobarbital *on page 1011*

♦ **SecreFlo**™ *see* Secretin *on page 1012*

Secretin *(SEE kre tin)*

U.S. Brand Names SecreFlo™

Therapeutic Category Diagnostic Agent, Pancreatic Exocrine Insufficiency; Diagnostic Agent, Gastrinoma (Zollinger-Ellison Syndrome)

Generic Available No

Use Diagnosis of gastrinoma (Zollinger-Ellison syndrome) and diagnosis of pancreatic exocrine dysfunction (chronic pancreatitis); facilitation of endoscopic retrograde cholangiopancreatography (ERCP) visualization

Pregnancy Risk Factor C

Contraindications Hypersensitivity to secretin or any component; do not give to patients with acute pancreatitis until attack has subsided

Precautions Patients with a history of hypersensitivity, allergy or asthma should receive an I.V. test dose of 0.2 mcg; use with caution in patients who are highly nervous or have an excessive gag reflex; patients receiving anticholinergics, patients who have had a vagotomy, or patients with inflammatory bowel disease may have a reduced response to secretin; patients with alcoholic or other liver diseases may have an increased response to secretin

Adverse Reactions
Cardiovascular: Hypotension, bradycardia (mild)
Central nervous system: Headache, fever
Gastrointestinal: Abdominal discomfort and cramps, vomiting, diarrhea, nausea
Respiratory: Transient decrease in oxygen saturation, respiratory distress
Miscellaneous: Hypersensitivity reactions, diaphoresis

Drug Interactions Anticholinergics may reduce response to secretin

Stability Store in freezer (-20°C); should be used immediately after reconstitution

Mechanism of Action Secretin is a naturally-occurring hormone secreted by cells in the duodenal and upper jejunal mucosa which increases the volume and bicarbonate content of pancreatic juice; when used as a diagnostic agent, synthetic porcine secretin stimulates an increase in gastrin release in patients with Zollinger-Ellison syndrome when compared with normal patients; gastrin bicarbonate concentration is reduced in patients with chronic pancreatitis when compared with a normal patient's response to secretin

Pharmacodynamics
Maximum output of pancreatic secretions: Within 30 minutes
Duration: At least 2 hours

Pharmacokinetics
Distribution: V_d: 2 L (approximately)
Protein binding: 40%
Inactivated by proteolytic enzymes if administered orally
Metabolism: Metabolic fate is thought to be hydrolysis to smaller peptides
Half-life: 27 minutes
Elimination: Clearance: 487 ± 136 mL/minute

Usual Dosage Children and Adults: I.V.:
Diagnostic agent for pancreatic function: 0.2 mcg/kg as single dose
Diagnostic agent for gastrinoma (Zollinger-Ellison): 0.4 mcg/kg as single dose
Facilitation of ERCP visualization: 0.2 mcg/kg as a single dose

Administration Parenteral: Reconstitute with 8 mL of NS resulting in a 2 mcg/mL solution; shake vigorously to ensure dissolution; use immediately by direct I.V. injection slowly over 1 minute

Monitoring Parameters Peak bicarbonate concentration of duodenal fluid aspirate (chronic pancreatitis); serum gastrin (gastrinoma)

Reference Range
Peak gastric bicarbonate concentration:
Normal: 94-134 mEq/L
Chronic pancreatitis: <80 mEq/L
Severe pancreatitis: <50 mEq/L
Serum gastrin:
Normal: ≤110 pg/mL
Gastrinoma: >110 pg/mL

Nursing Implications Patients should fast at least 12 hours before testing for Zollinger-Ellison syndrome

Additional Information Available currently as an orphan drug by contacting the manufacturer Repligen; a double-blind crossover study of secretin 0.2 cU/kg versus placebo in 56 autistic children revealed no significant differences between the 2 groups (Owley, 2001)

Dosage Forms Injection, powder for reconstitution: 16 mcg

References
Owley T, McMahon W, Cook EH, et al, "Multisite, Double-Blind, Placebo-Controlled Trial of Porcine Secretin in Autism," *J Am Acad Child Adolesc Psychiatry*, 2001, 40(11):1293-9.

♦ **Selax® (Can)** *see Docusate on page 402*
♦ **Selenium** *see Trace Metals on page 1106*

Selenium Sulfide (se LEE nee um SUL fide)

U.S. Brand Names Exsel® [DSC]; Head & Shoulders® Intensive Treatment [OTC]; Selsun®; Selsun Blue® 2-in-1 Treatment [OTC]; Selsun Blue® Balanced Treatment [OTC]; Selsun Blue® Medicated Treatment [OTC]; Selsun Blue® Moisturizing Treatment [OTC]

Canadian Brand Names Versel®

Therapeutic Category Antiseborrheic Agent, Topical; Shampoos

Generic Available Yes

Use To treat itching and flaking of the scalp associated with dandruff; to control scalp seborrheic dermatitis; treatment of tinea versicolor

Pregnancy Risk Factor C

Contraindications Hypersensitivity to selenium or any component

Warnings Safety in infants has not been established; avoid use in children <2 years of age

Precautions Do not use on damaged skin to avoid any systemic toxicity

Adverse Reactions
Central nervous system: Lethargy
Dermatologic: Alopecia, discoloration of hair
Gastrointestinal: Vomiting following long-term use on damaged skin, abdominal pain, garlic breath
Local: Local irritation
Neuromuscular & skeletal: Tremor
Miscellaneous: Perspiration

Mechanism of Action May block the enzymes involved in growth of epithelial tissue
(Continued)

Selenium Sulfide *(Continued)*

Pharmacokinetics Absorption: Not absorbed topically through intact skin, but can be absorbed topically through damaged skin

Usual Dosage Children ≥ 2 years and Adults: Topical:

Dandruff, seborrhea: Massage 5-10 mL into wet scalp, leave on scalp 2-3 minutes, rinse thoroughly and repeat application; alternatively, 5-10 mL of shampoo is applied and allowed to remain on scalp for 5-10 minutes before being rinsed off thoroughly without a repeat application; shampoo twice weekly for 2 weeks initially, then use once every 1-4 weeks as indicated depending upon control

Tinea versicolor: Apply the 2.5% lotion in a thin layer covering the body surface from the face to the knees; leave on skin for 30 minutes, then rinse thoroughly; apply every day for 7 days; then follow with monthly applications for 3 months to prevent recurrences

Administration Topical: For external use only; avoid contact with eyes or acutely inflamed skin

Patient Information Remove all jewelry before using the lotion; wash hands thoroughly following application of the lotion; may discolor hair

Dosage Forms

Lotion, topical, as sulfide: 2.5% (120 mL)
Selsun®: 2.5% (120 mL)
Shampoo, topical, as sulfide: 1% (210 mL)
Head & Shoulders® Intensive Treatment: 1% (400 mL)
Selsun®: 2.5% (120 mL)
Selsun Blue® Balanced Treatment, Selsun Blue® Medicated Treatment, Selsun Blue® Moisturizing Treatment, Selsun Blue® 2-in-1 Treatment: 1% (120 mL, 210 mL, 330 mL)

References

Lester RS, "Topical Formulary for the Pediatrician," *Pediatr Clin North Am*, 1983, 30(4):749-65.

- ◆ **Selepen®** *see* Trace Metals *on page 1106*
- ◆ **Selsun®** *see* Selenium Sulfide *on page 1013*
- ◆ **Selsun Blue® 2-in-1 Treatment [OTC]** *see* Selenium Sulfide *on page 1013*
- ◆ **Selsun Blue® Balanced Treatment [OTC]** *see* Selenium Sulfide *on page 1013*
- ◆ **Selsun Blue® Medicated Treatment [OTC]** *see* Selenium Sulfide *on page 1013*
- ◆ **Selsun Blue® Moisturizing Treatment [OTC]** *see* Selenium Sulfide *on page 1013*
- ◆ **Senexon® [OTC]** *see* Senna *on page 1014*

Senna *(SEN na)*

Related Information

Carbohydrate and Alcohol Content of Liquid Medications for Use in Patients Receiving Ketogenic Diets *on page 1431*

U.S. Brand Names Agoral® Maximum Strength Laxative [OTC]; Evac-u-gen [OTC]; ex-lax® [OTC]; ex-lax® Maximum Strength [OTC]; Fletcher's® Castoria® [OTC]; Senexon® [OTC]; Senna-Gen® [OTC]; Sennatural™ [OTC]; Senokot® [OTC]; Senokot®, Children's [OTC]; SenokotXTRA® [OTC]; X-Prep® [OTC]

Therapeutic Category Laxative, Stimulant

Generic Available Yes (tablet)

Use Short-term treatment of constipation; evacuate the colon for bowel or rectal examinations

Pregnancy Risk Factor C

Contraindications Hypersensitivity to senna or any component; nausea and vomiting; undiagnosed abdominal pain, appendicitis, intestinal obstruction or perforation

Warnings Concentrated liquid contains sodium benzoate which may cause allergic reactions in susceptible individuals; use products containing sodium benzoate with caution in neonates; *in vitro* and animal studies have shown that benzoate displaces bilirubin from protein binding sites

Precautions Avoid prolonged use (>1 week); chronic use may lead to dependency, fluid and electrolyte imbalance, vitamin and mineral deficiencies

Adverse Reactions

Endocrine & metabolic: Electrolyte and fluid imbalance
Gastrointestinal: Nausea, vomiting, diarrhea, abdominal cramps, perianal irritation, discoloration of feces
Genitourinary: Discoloration of urine

Drug Interactions Docusate may enhance the absorption of senna

Mechanism of Action Active metabolite (aglycone) acts as a local irritant on the colon, stimulates Auerbach's plexus to produce peristalsis

Pharmacodynamics Onset of action:
Oral: Within 6-24 hours
Rectal: Evacuation occurs in 30 minutes to 2 hours

Pharmacokinetics
Metabolism: In the liver
Elimination: In the feces (via bile) and in urine

Usual Dosage Oral:
Constipation:
Infants 1 month to 2 years: Syrup: 1.25-2.5 mL (2.2-4.4 mg sennosides) at bedtime, not to exceed 5 mL (8.8 mg sennosides)/day
Children:
Granules:
2 to <6 years: ¼ teaspoonful (3.75 mg sennosides) at bedtime, not to exceed ½ teaspoonful (7.5 mg sennosides) twice daily
6-12 years: ½ teaspoonful (7.5 mg sennosides) at bedtime, not to exceed 1 teaspoonful (15 mg sennosides) twice daily
Syrup:
2 to <6 years: 2.5-3.75 mL (4.4-6.6 mg sennosides) at bedtime, not to exceed 3.75 mL (6.6 mg sennosides) twice daily
6-12 years: 5-7.5 mL (8.8-13.2 mg sennosides) at bedtime, not to exceed 7.5 mL (13.2 mg sennosides) twice daily
Tablet:
2 to <6 years: ½ tablet (4.3 mg sennosides) at bedtime, not to exceed 1 tablet (8.6 mg sennosides) twice daily
6-12 years: 1 tablet (8.6 mg sennosides) at bedtime, not to exceed 2 tablets (17.2 mg sennosides) twice daily
Children ≥12 years and Adults:
Granules: 1 teaspoonful (15 mg sennosides) at bedtime, not to exceed 2 teaspoonfuls (30 mg sennosides) twice daily
Syrup: 10-15 mL (17.6-26.4 mg sennosides) at bedtime, not to exceed 15 mL (26.4 mg sennosides) twice daily
Tablet: 2 tablets (17.2 mg sennosides) at bedtime, not to exceed 4 tablets (34.4 mg sennosides) twice daily
Bowel evacuation: Children ≥12 years and Adults: 130 mg sennosides (X-Prep® 75 mL) between 2:00 PM to 4:00 PM on the day prior to procedure

Administration Oral: Administer with water; syrup can be taken with juice or milk or mixed with ice cream to mask taste. Granules may be sprinkled onto food, eaten plain, or mixed into food or drinks.

Monitoring Parameters I & O, frequency of bowel movements, serum electrolytes if severe diarrhea occurs

Patient Information May discolor urine or feces; drink plenty of fluids

Dosage Forms
Granules (Senokot®): 15 mg sennosides/teaspoon (60 g, 180 g, 360 g) [cocoa flavor]
Liquid:
Agoral® Maximum Strength Laxative: 25 mg sennosides/15 mL (480 mL) [contains 19.6 mg sodium/15 mL; marshmallow and raspberry flavors]
X-Prep®: 8.8 mg sennosides/5 mL (75 mL) [alcohol free; available alone or in a kit; contains 50 g sugar/75 mL]
Liquid, **concentrate** (Fletcher's® Castoria®): 3 mg sennosides/mL (75 mL) [alcohol free; contains sodium benzoate; root beer flavor]
Syrup:
Senokot®: 8.8 mg sennosides/5 mL (240 mL) [alcohol free; cocoa flavor]
Children's Senokot®: 8.8 mg sennosides/5 mL (74 mL) [alcohol free; chocolate flavor]
Tablet: 8.6 mg sennosides
ex-lax®: 15 mg sennosides USP [contains sodium benzoate]
ex-lax® Maximum Strength: 25 mg sennosides USP [contains sodium benzoate]
Sennatural™, Senokot®, Senexon®, Senna-Gen®: 8.6 mg sennosides
SenokotXTRA®: 17 mg sennosides
Tablet, chewable:
ex-lax®: 15 mg sennosides USP [chocolate flavor]
Evac-u-gen: 10 mg sennosides

References
Perkin JM, "Constipation in Childhood: A Controlled Comparison Between Lactulose and Standardized Senna," *Curr Med Res Opin*, 1977, 4(8):540-3.

♦ **Senna-Gen® [OTC]** *see* Senna *on page 1014*
♦ **Sennatural™ [OTC]** *see* Senna *on page 1014*
♦ **Senokot® [OTC]** *see* Senna *on page 1014*
♦ **Senokot®, Children's [OTC]** *see* Senna *on page 1014*

- **SenokotXTRA® [OTC]** *see* Senna *on page 1014*
- **Sensorcaine®** *see* Bupivacaine *on page 189*
- **Sensorcaine-MPF®** *see* Bupivacaine *on page 189*
- **Septra®** *see* Sulfamethoxazole and Trimethoprim *on page 1052*
- **Septra® DS** *see* Sulfamethoxazole and Trimethoprim *on page 1052*
- **Septra® Injection (Can)** *see* Sulfamethoxazole and Trimethoprim *on page 1052*
- **Serevent®** *see* Salmeterol *on page 1004*
- **Serevent® Diskus®** *see* Salmeterol *on page 1004*
- **Seromycin® Pulvules®** *see* CycloSERINE *on page 323*
- **Serostim®** *see* Human Growth Hormone *on page 564*
- **Serotonin Syndrome** *see page 1420*

Sertraline (SER tra leen)

U.S. Brand Names Zoloft®

Canadian Brand Names Apo®-Sertraline; Gen-Sertraline; Novo-Sertraline; ratio-Sertraline; Rhoxal-sertraline

Therapeutic Category Antidepressant, Selective Serotonin Reuptake Inhibitor (SSRI)

Generic Available No

Use Treatment of major depression, obsessive-compulsive disorder, panic disorder (with or without agoraphobia), post-traumatic stress disorder, premenstrual dysphoric disorder, social anxiety disorder

Pregnancy Risk Factor C

Contraindications Hypersensitivity to sertraline or any component; use of MAO inhibitors within 14 days (potentially fatal reactions may occur, see Drug Interactions); concurrent use of pimozide; oral concentrate is contraindicated in patients receiving disulfiram (contains 12% alcohol)

Precautions Use with caution in patients with seizure disorders, concomitant illnesses that may effect hepatic metabolism or hemodynamic responses (eg, unstable cardiac disease, recent MI), and in suicidal patients; use with caution and decrease dose in patients with hepatic dysfunction; may result in hyponatremia, SIADH, significant weight loss, decrease in serum uric acid (mild uricosuric effect, use with caution in patient at risk of uric acid nephropathy), activation of mania/hypomania, or abnormal platelet function; dropper for oral concentrate contains dry natural rubber, use with caution in patients with latex allergy

Adverse Reactions

Central nervous system: Agitation, dizziness, headache, insomnia, nervousness, fatigue, somnolence, fever, impaired concentration, activation of mania or hypomania, emotional lability, abnormal thinking, seizures

Dermatologic: Rash

Endocrine & metabolic: Weight loss; SIADH, hyponatremia (volume-depleted patients); decreased serum uric acid, sexual dysfunction, decreased libido; weight gain has also been reported

Gastrointestinal: Nausea, vomiting, diarrhea, loose stools, xerostomia, constipation, anorexia, dyspepsia

Hematologic: Altered platelet function, purpura

Neuromuscular & skeletal: Tremor, paresthesia, hyperkinesia, twitching, malaise

Ocular: Abnormal vision

Respiratory: Epistaxis

Miscellaneous: Diaphoresis

Drug Interactions Cytochrome P450 isoenzyme CYP3A3/4 and CYP2D6 (minor) substrate; isoenzyme CYP2C9, CYP2C19, and CYP3A3/4 inhibitor; weak inhibitor of CYP1A2 and CYP2D6

Use within 2 weeks of MAO inhibitors may result in fever, tremors, rigidity, myoclonus, autonomic instability, rapid fluctuations in vital signs, irritability, confusion, extreme agitation, delirium, and coma (use of sertraline within 14 days of MAO inhibitors is contraindicated); sertraline may increase serum concentrations of pimozide by ~40% and potentially cause serious adverse effects (concurrent use of pimozide and sertraline is contraindicated); sertraline may displace highly protein bound drugs and cause adverse effects; may increase prothrombin time in patients receiving warfarin; use with sumatriptan may cause weakness, incoordination, and hyper-reflexia; although lithium levels were not significantly affected in one study, monitoring of lithium levels and appropriate dosage adjustments is recommended in patients initiating sertraline therapy. Tryptophan (which can be metabolized to serotonin) and the herbal medicine St John's wort (*Hypericum perforatum*) may increase serious side effects; use of these agents is **not recommended.**

Sertraline may decrease the metabolism of tricyclic antidepressants, tolbutamide, diazepam, flecainide, propafenone, and other drugs metabolized by CYP enzymes (monitoring of serum drug concentrations and dosage reduction of these agents may be required); cimetidine may increase sertraline concentrations; the following drugs may increase the risk of serotonin syndrome if given with selective serotonin reuptake inhibitors: Amitriptyline, amphetamines, buspirone, dihydroergotamine, erythromycin, fentanyl, meperidine, nefazodone, ritonavir, sumatriptan, sympathomimetics, tramadol

Food Interactions Tryptophan supplements may increase serious side effects; grapefruit juice may significantly increase sertraline serum concentrations

Tablets: Food may slightly increase AUC, increase peak concentrations by 25% and shorten the time to peak plasma concentrations

Oral concentrate: Food may prolong the rate, but does not effect the extent of absorption

Stability Store at room temperature

Mechanism of Action Selective inhibitor of CNS neuronal serotonin uptake; minimal effects on reuptake of norepinephrine or dopamine; does not significantly bind to alpha-adrenergic, benzodiazepine, cholinergic, dopamine, GABA, histamine, or serotonin receptors; may therefore be useful in patients at risk from sedation, hypotension and anticholinergic effects of tricyclic antidepressants; does not inhibit monoamine oxidase

Pharmacodynamics Maximum effect may take several weeks

Pharmacokinetics

Protein binding: 98%

Metabolism: Significant first pass effect; undergoes N-demethylation to N-desmethyl-sertraline (significantly less active than sertraline); both parent and metabolite undergo oxidative deamination, followed by reduction, hydroxylation and conjugation with glucuronide (**Note:** Children 6-17 years may metabolize sertraline slightly better than adults, as pediatric AUCs and peak concentrations were 22% lower than adults when adjusted for weight; however, lower doses are recommended for younger pediatric patients to avoid excessive drug levels)

Bioavailability: Tablets approximately equal to oral solution

Half-life: Parent: Mean: 26 hours; metabolite (N-desmethylsertraline): 62-104 hours

Children: 6-12 years: Mean: 26.2 hours

Children: 13-17 years: Mean: 27.8 hours

Adults: 18-45 years: Mean: 27.2 hours

Elimination: 40% to 45% of dose eliminated in urine (none as unchanged drug); 40% to 45% eliminated in feces (12% to 14% as unchanged drug)

Clearance: May be decreased in patients with hepatic impairment

Dialysis: Not likely to remove significant amount of drug due to large V_d

Usual Dosage Oral: (**Note:** See Additional Information)

Children 6-12 years:

Depression: Initial: 25 mg once daily; titrate dose upwards if clinically needed; may increase by 25-50 mg/day increments at intervals of at least 1 week; mean final dose in 21 children (8-18 years of age) was 100 ± 53 mg or 1.6 mg/kg/day (n=11); range: 25-200 mg/day; maximum dose: 200 mg/day (see Tierney, 1995); avoid excessive dosing

Obsessive-compulsive disorder: Initial: 25 mg once daily; titrate dose upwards if clinically needed; increase by 25-50 mg/day increments at intervals of at least 1 week; range: 25-200 mg/day; maximum dose: 200 mg/day; avoid excessive dosing

Adolescents 13-17 years:

Depression: Initial 50 mg once daily; titrate dose upwards if clinically needed; may increase by 50 mg/day increments at intervals of at least 1 week; mean final dose in 13 adolescents was 110 ± 50 mg or about 2 mg/kg/day (see McConville, 1996); in another study using a slower titration, the mean dose at week 6 was 93 mg (n=41) and at week 10 was 127 mg (n=34) (see Ambrosini, 1999)

Obsessive-compulsive disorder: Initial: 50 mg once daily; titrate dose upwards if clinically needed; increase by 50 mg/day increments at intervals of at least 1 week; range: 25-200 mg/day; maximum dose: 200 mg/day

Adults:

Depression and obsessive-compulsive disorder: Initial: 50 mg once daily; titrate dose upwards if clinically needed; increase by 50 mg/day increments at intervals of at least 1 week; range: 50-200 mg/day; maximum dose: 200 mg/day

Panic disorder, post-traumatic stress disorder, and social anxiety disorder: Initial: 25 mg once daily; increase dose after 1 week to 50 mg once daily; titrate dose further if clinically needed; increase by 50 mg/day increments at intervals of at least 1 week; range: 50-200 mg/day; maximum dose: 200 mg/day

Premenstrual dysphoric disorder: Initial: 50 mg/day given daily throughout the menstrual cycle **or** only during the luteal phase of the menstrual cycle (depending

(Continued)

Sertraline *(Continued)*

on assessment of physician); may increase if needed by 50 mg increments per menstrual cycle; maximum dose when using daily dosing throughout the menstrual cycle: 150 mg/day; maximum dose when dosing only during the luteal phase of the menstrual cycle: 100 mg/day. **Note:** If using a 100 mg/day dose with luteal phase dosing, use a 50 mg/day titration step for 3 days at the beginning of each luteal phase dosing period.

Dosing adjustment in renal impairment: None needed

Dosing adjustment in hepatic impairment: Use with caution and in reduced doses

Administration Oral: May be administered without regard to food; avoid administration with grapefruit juice; administer once daily dosage in morning or evening. Must dilute oral concentrate before use; measure dose with dropper provided and mix with 4 ounces of water, orange juice, lemonade, ginger ale, or lemon/lime soda; do not mix with other liquids; take dose immediately after mixing, do not mix ahead of time; sometimes a slight haze may be seen after mixing (this is normal)

Monitoring Parameters Weight and growth in children if long-term therapy; uric acid, CBC, liver function, serum sodium, urine output

Patient Information May cause dizziness or drowsiness and impair ability to perform activities requiring mental alertness or physical coordination; may cause dry mouth; report the use of other medications, nonprescription medications, and herbal or natural products to your physician and pharmacist; avoid alcohol, grapefruit juice, tryptophan supplements, and the herbal medicine St John's wort

Nursing Implications If patient experiences somnolence, administer dose at bedtime; if patient experiences insomnia, administer dose in morning

Additional Information Two larger studies of children and adolescents with depression and obsessive-compulsive disorder utilized a forced upward dosage titration of sertraline to 200 mg/day; these studies conclude that the adult dosage titration regimen can be used in children ≥6 years and adolescents (see Alderman, 1998 and March, 1998); however, other studies in adults (see Fabre, 1995) demonstrate that lower sertraline doses (50 mg/day) are as effective as higher doses with fewer adverse effects and discontinuations of therapy. Further studies are needed in pediatric patients to identify optimal doses; clinically, doses should be individually titrated based on patient response and adverse effects.

A recent report (Lake, 2000) describes 5 children (age 8-15 years) who developed epistaxis (n=4) or bruising (n=1) while receiving sertraline therapy. Another recent report describes the SSRI discontinuation syndrome in 6 children; the syndrome was similar to that reported in adults (see Diler, 2002). Due to limited long-term studies, the clinical usefulness of sertraline should be periodically re-evaluated in patients receiving the drug for extended intervals; effects of long term use of sertraline on pediatric growth, development, and maturation have not been directly assessed.

Dosage Forms Note: Available as sertraline hydrochloride; mg strength refers to sertraline

Solution, oral **concentrate:** 20 mg/mL (60 mL) [contains 12% alcohol]

Tablet: 25 mg, 50 mg, 100 mg

References

Alderman J, Wolkow R, Chung M, et al, "Sertraline Treatment of Children and Adolescents With Obsessive-Compulsive Disorder or Depression: Pharmacokinetics, Tolerability, and Efficacy," *J Am Acad Child Adolesc Psychiatry*, 1998, 37(4):386-94.

Ambrosini PJ, Wagner KD, Biederman J, et al, "Multicenter Open-Label Sertraline Study in Adolescent Outpatients With Major Depression," *J Am Acad Child Adolesc Psychiatry*, 1999, 38(5):566-72.

Diler R and Avci A, "Selective Serotonin Reuptake Inhibitor Discontinuation Syndrome in Children: Six Case Reports," *Current Therapeutic Research*, 2002, 63(3):188-97.

Fabre LF, Abuzzahab FS, Amin M, et al, "Sertraline Safety and Efficacy in Major Depression: A Double-Blind Fixed-Dose Comparison With Placebo," *Biol Psychiatry*, 1995, 38(9):592-602.

Findling RL, Reed MD, and Blumer JL, "Pharmacological Treatment of Depression in Children and Adolescents," *Paediatr Drugs*, 1999, 1(3):161-82.

Lake MB, Birmaher B, Wassick S, et al, "Bleeding and Selective Serotonin Reuptake Inhibitors in Childhood and Adolescence," *J Child Adolesc Psychopharmacol*, 2000, 10(1):35-8.

March JS, Biederman J, Wolkow R, et al, "Sertraline in Children and Adolescents With Obsessive-Compulsive Disorder: A Multicenter Randomized Controlled Trial," *JAMA*, 1998, 280(20):1752-6.

McConville BJ, Minnery KL, Sorter MT, et al, "An Open Study of the Effects of Sertraline on Adolescent Major Depression," *J Child Adolesc Psychopharmacol*, 1996, 6(1):41-51.

Thomsen PH, "Obsessive-Compulsive Disorder: Pharmacological Treatment," *Eur Child Adolesc Psychiatry*, 2000, 9 Suppl 1:I76-84.

Tierney E, Joshi PT, Llinas JF, et al, "Sertraline for Major Depression in Children and Adolescents: Preliminary Clinical Experience," *J Child Adolesc Psychopharmacol*, 1995; 5(1):13-27.

♦ **Silapap®, Infant's [OTC]** *see* Acetaminophen *on page 36*
♦ **Silexin® [OTC]** *see* Guaifenesin and Dextromethorphan *on page 553*
♦ **Silfedrine®, Children's [OTC]** *see* Pseudoephedrine *on page 958*
♦ **Silphen DM® [OTC]** *see* Dextromethorphan *on page 365*
♦ **Silvadene®** *see* Silver Sulfadiazine *on page 1019*

Silver Nitrate (SIL ver NYE trate)

Therapeutic Category Ophthalmic Agent, Miscellaneous; Topical Skin Product
Generic Available Yes
Use Cauterization of wounds and sluggish ulcers, removal of granulation tissue and warts
Pregnancy Risk Factor C
Contraindications Hypersensitivity to silver nitrate or any component; not for use on broken skin or cuts
Warnings Do not use applicator sticks on the eyes
Adverse Reactions
    Dermatologic: Staining of the skin
    Hematologic: Methemoglobinemia
    Local: Burning and skin irritation
    Ocular: Cauterization of the cornea, blindness, chemical conjunctivitis
Stability Store applicator sticks in a dry place since moisture causes the oxidized film to dissolve; protect from light
Mechanism of Action Free silver ions precipitate bacterial proteins by combining with chloride in tissue forming silver chloride; coagulates cellular protein to form an eschar
Pharmacokinetics Absorption: Not readily absorbed from mucous membranes
Usual Dosage Children and Adults:
    Sticks: Apply to mucous membranes and other moist surfaces only on area to be treated 2-3 times/week for 2-3 weeks
    Topical solution: Apply a cotton applicator dipped in solution on the affected area 2-3 times/week for 2-3 weeks
Monitoring Parameters With prolonged use, monitor methemoglobin levels
Patient Information Discontinue topical preparation if redness or irritation develop; silver nitrate solution may stain skin
Nursing Implications Silver nitrate solutions stain skin and utensils
Dosage Forms
    Applicator sticks, topical: Silver nitrate 75% and potassium nitrate 25% (6", 12", 18")
    Ointment, topical: 10% (30 g)
    Solution, topical: 10% (30 mL); 25% (30 mL); 50% (30 mL)
References
    Cushing AH and Smith S, "Methemoglobinemia With Silver Nitrate Therapy of a Burn: Report of a Case," *J Pediatr*, 1969, 74(4):613-5.

Silver Sulfadiazine (SIL ver sul fa DYE a zeen)

U.S. Brand Names Silvadene®; SSD®; SSD® AF; Thermazene®
Canadian Brand Names Dermazin™; Flamazine®
Therapeutic Category Antibiotic, Topical
Generic Available Yes
Use Adjunct in the prevention and treatment of infection in second and third degree burns
Pregnancy Risk Factor C
Contraindications Hypersensitivity to silver sulfadiazine or any component; premature infants or neonates <2 months of age since sulfas may displace bilirubin from protein binding sites and cause kernicterus
Precautions Use with caution in patients with G-6-PD deficiency and renal impairment; sulfadiazine may accumulate in patients with impaired hepatic or renal function
Adverse Reactions
    Dermatologic: Itching, rash, erythema multiforme, discoloration of skin
    Hematologic: Hemolytic anemia, leukopenia, agranulocytosis, aplastic anemia, thrombocytopenia
    Hepatic: Hepatitis
    Local: Pain, burning
    Renal: Interstitial nephritis
    Miscellaneous: Serum hyperosmolality (due to propylene glycol component in the cream), hypersensitivity reactions to sulfas
Drug Interactions Topical proteolytic enzymes (silver may inactivate enzymes)
Stability Discard if cream is darkened (reacts with heavy metals resulting in release of silver)
    (Continued)

Silver Sulfadiazine *(Continued)*

Mechanism of Action Acts upon the bacterial cell wall and cell membrane

Pharmacokinetics

Absorption: Significant percutaneous absorption of sulfadiazine can occur especially when applied to extensive burns

Half-life: 10 hours and is prolonged in patients with renal insufficiency

Time to peak serum concentration: Within 3-11 days of continuous topical therapy

Elimination: ~50% excreted unchanged in urine

Usual Dosage Children and Adults: Topical: Apply once or twice daily with a sterile gloved hand; apply to a thickness of $^1/_{16}$"; burned area should be covered with cream at all times

Administration Topical: Apply to cleansed, debrided burned areas

Monitoring Parameters Serum electrolytes, UA, renal function test, CBC in patients with extensive burns on long-term treatment

Patient Information For external use only; may discolor skin

Additional Information Contains methylparaben and propylene glycol

Dosage Forms

Cream, topical: 1% [10 mg/g] (25 g, 85 g, 400 g) [contains propylene glycol]

Silvadene®, Thermazene®: 1% (20 g, 50 g, 85 g, 400 g, 1000 g)

SSD®: 1% (25 g, 50 g, 85 g, 400 g)

SSD® AF: 1% (50 g, 400 g)

References

Kulick MI, Wong R, Okarma TB, et al, "Prospective Study of Side Effects Associated With the Use of Silver Sulfadiazine in Severely Burned Patients," *Ann Plast Surg*, 1985, 14(5):407-18.

Lockhart SP, Rushworth A, Azmy AA, et al, "Topical Silver Sulfadiazine: Side Effects and Urinary Excretion," *Burns Incl Therm Inj*, 1983, 10(1):9-12.

Simethicone *(sye METH i kone)*

Related Information

Carbohydrate and Alcohol Content of Liquid Medications for Use in Patients Receiving Ketogenic Diets *on page 1431*

U.S. Brand Names Alka-Seltzer® Gas Relief [OTC]; Baby Gasz [OTC]; Flatulex® [OTC]; Gas-X® [OTC]; Gas-X® Extra Strength [OTC]; Genasyme® [OTC]; Mylanta Gas® [OTC]; Mylanta Gas® Maximum Strength [OTC]; Mylicon®, Infants [OTC]; Phazyme® Quick Dissolve [OTC]; Phazyme® Ultra Strength [OTC]

Canadian Brand Names Ovol®

Synonyms Activated Dimethicone; Activated Methylpolysiloxane

Therapeutic Category Antiflatulent

Generic Available Yes (suspension and tablet)

Use Relieve flatulence, functional gastric bloating, and postoperative gas pains

Pregnancy Risk Factor C

Contraindications Hypersensitivity to simethicone or any component

Warnings Mylicon® Infant drops contain sodium benzoate; benzoic acid (benzoate) is a metabolite of benzyl alcohol; large amounts of benzyl alcohol (≥99 mg/kg/day) have been associated with a potentially fatal toxicity ("gasping syndrome") in neonates; *in vitro* and animal studies have shown that benzoate displaces bilirubin from protein binding sites; avoid use of Mylicon® Infant drops in neonates.

Precautions Phazyme® Quick Dissolve contains phenylalanine; avoid use or use with caution in phenylketonurics

Food Interactions Avoid gas-forming foods

Mechanism of Action Spreads on surface of aqueous liquids forming a film of low surface tension which collapses foam bubbles; allows mucous-surrounded gas bubbles to coalesce and be expelled

Pharmacokinetics Elimination: In feces

Usual Dosage Oral:

Infants and Children <2 years: 20 mg 4 times/day

Children 2-12 years: 40 mg 4 times/day

Children >12 years and Adults: 40-250 mg after meals and at bedtime as needed, not to exceed 500 mg/day

Administration Oral: Administer after meals or at bedtime; chew tablets thoroughly before swallowing; mix with water, infant formula or other liquids

Patient Information Avoid carbonated beverages

Dosage Forms

Softgels:

Alka-Seltzer® Gas Relief, Gas-X® Extra Strength, Mylanta Gas® Maximum Strength: 125 mg

Phazyme® Ultra Strength: 180 mg

Suspension, oral **drops**: 40 mg/0.6 mL (30 mL)

Baby Gasz, Genasym®: 40 mg/0.6 mL (30 mL)

Flatulex®: 40 mg/0.6 mL (30 mL) [fruit flavor]

Infants Mylicon®: 40 mg/0.6 mL (30 mL) [alcohol free; contains sodium benzoate; available in nonstaining formula]

Tablet, chewable: 80 mg, 125 mg

Gas-X®: 80 mg [peppermint creme and sodium free cherry creme flavors]

Gas-X® Extra Strength: 125 mg [cherry creme and peppermint creme flavors]

Genasym®: 80 mg

Mylanta® Gas: 80 mg [mint flavor]

Mylanta® Gas Maximum Strength: 125 mg [cherry and mint flavors]

Phazyme® Quick Dissolve: 125 mg [contains 0.4 mg phenylalanine (as aspartame)/ tablet; mint flavor]

♦ **Simply Allergy®** [OTC] *see* DiphenhydrAMINE *on page 393*

♦ **Simply Cough™** [OTC] *see* Dextromethorphan *on page 365*

♦ **Simply Saline™** [OTC] *see* Sodium Chloride *on page 1027*

♦ **Simply Sleep®** [OTC] *see* DiphenhydrAMINE *on page 393*

Simvastatin (SIM va stat in)

U.S. Brand Names Zocor®

Therapeutic Category Antilipemic Agent; HMG-CoA Reductase Inhibitor

Generic Available No

Use Hyperlipidemia: Adjunct to dietary therapy to decrease elevated serum total and low density lipoprotein cholesterol (LDL-C), apolipoprotein B (apo-B), and triglyceride levels, and to increase high density lipoprotein cholesterol (HDL-C) in patients with primary hypercholesterolemia (heterozygous, familial and nonfamilial) and mixed dyslipidemia (Fredrickson types IIa and IIb); treatment of homozygous familial hypercholesterolemia; treatment of isolated hypertriglyceridemia (Fredrickson type IV) and type III hyperlipoproteinemia

"Secondary prevention" in patients with coronary heart disease and hypercholesterolemia to reduce the risk of total mortality by reducing coronary death; reduce the risk of nonfatal MI; reduce the risk of undergoing myocardial revascularization procedures; and reduce the risk of stroke or TIA

Pregnancy Risk Factor X

Contraindications Hypersensitivity to simvastatin or any component; active liver disease; unexplained persistent elevations of serum transaminases; pregnancy

Warnings Rhabdomyolysis with or without acute renal failure secondary to myoglobinuria has occurred rarely. Risk is increased with increasing doses (0.02% at 20 mg, 0.07% at 40 mg, and 0.3% at 80 mg) and with concurrent use of amiodarone, clarithromycin, danazol, diltiazem, fluvoxamine, indinavir, nefazodone, nelfinavir, ritonavir, verapamil, troleandomycin, cyclosporine, fibric acid derivatives, erythromycin, niacin, or azole antifungals. Assess the risk versus benefit before combining any of these medications with simvastatin. A lowered dosage of simvastatin is recommended when used with these medications (see Usual Dosage). Temporarily discontinue simvastatin in any patient experiencing an acute or serious condition predisposing to renal failure secondary to rhabdomyolysis.

Precautions Persistent increases in serum transaminases have occurred; liver function must be monitored by laboratory assessment at the initiation of therapy and periodically thereafter for the first year of treatment or until one year after the last elevation in dose. Patients titrated to the 80 mg dose should receive an additional test at 3 months of therapy. Use with caution in patients with diabetes mellitus and renal impairment (may be at increased risk for developing rhabdomyolysis)

Adverse Reactions

Cardiovascular: Angina, transient symptomatic hypotension, sinus tachycardia

Central nervous system: Dizziness, headache, vertigo, fatigue, insomnia, depression, tremor, memory loss, psychic disturbances, anxiety

Dermatologic: Eczema, pruritus, rash, lichen planus, photosensitivity, alopecia, Stevens-Johnson syndrome, skin discoloration, dry skin

Endocrine & metabolic: Gynecomastia, thyroid function abnormalities

Gastrointestinal: Constipation, dyspepsia, flatulence, abdominal pain, diarrhea, nausea, pancreatitis

Hematologic: Thrombocytopenia

Hepatic: Elevated serum transaminases, hepatitis (including chronic active hepatitis), cholestatic jaundice

Neuromuscular & skeletal: Elevated CPK, myalgia, muscle cramps, myopathy, peripheral neuropathy, paresthesias, rhabdomyolysis, arthralgias, dysfunction of certain cranial nerves (including alteration of taste, impairment of extraocular movement, and facial paresis)

Ocular: Cataracts, ophthalmoplegia, diplopia

Renal: Acute renal failure

(Continued)

Simvastatin *(Continued)*

Respiratory: Upper respiratory infections

Miscellaneous: Hypersensitivity syndrome (including one or more of the following features: Anaphylaxis, angioedema, lupus erythematous-like syndrome, polymyalgia rheumatica, dermatomyositis, vasculitis, purpura, leukopenia, hemolytic anemia, erythema multiforme, toxic epidermal necrolysis)

Drug Interactions Cytochrome P450 isoenzyme CYP3A3/4 enzyme substrate

Plasma concentrations may be decreased when given with magnesium-aluminum hydroxide containing antacids; cholestyramine reduces absorption; clofibrate, fenofibrate, gemfibrozil, niacin (≥1 g/day), amiodarone, and cyclosporine may increase the risk of myopathy and rhabdomyolysis (see Warnings); CYP3A3/4 inhibitors (clarithromycin, cyclosporine, danazol, diltiazem, fluconazole, fluvoxamine, erythromycin, indinavir, itraconazole, ketoconazole, miconazole, nefazodone, nelfinavir, ritonavir, saquinavir, indinavir, amprenavir, troleandomycin, and verapamil) increase simvastatin blood levels and may increase the risk of simvastatin-induced myopathy and rhabdomyolysis (see Warnings); simvastatin increases the hypoprothrombinemic response to warfarin; may increase digoxin serum level

Food Interactions Simvastatin serum concentration may be increased when taken with large quantities (>1 quart/day) of grapefruit juice; avoid concurrent use

Stability Tablets should be stored in well closed containers at temperatures between 5°C to 30°C (41°F to 86°F)

Mechanism of Action Simvastatin is a methylated derivative of lovastatin that acts by competitively inhibiting 3-hydroxy-3-methylglutaryl-coenzyme A (HMG-CoA) reductase, the enzyme that catalyzes the rate-limiting step in cholesterol biosynthesis

Pharmacodynamics

Onset of action: >3 days

Maximum effect: After 2 weeks

Average LDL-C reduction: 18% to 55%

Average HDL-C increase: 5% to 15%

Average triglyceride reduction: 7% to 30%

Pharmacokinetics

Absorption: Oral: Although 85% is absorbed following administration, <5% reaches the general circulation due to an extensive first-pass effect

Time to peak serum concentration: 1.3-2.4 hours

Protein binding: ~95%

Elimination: 13% excreted in urine and 60% in feces

Usual Dosage Oral:

Hyperlipidemia: Limited data in 32 children (<17 years of age) enrolled in compassionate use study (Ducobu, 1992):

Children <10 years: 5 mg once daily in the evening increasing to 10 mg once daily after 4 weeks and to 20 mg once daily after 8 weeks as tolerated

Children ≥10 years: 10 mg once daily in the evening increasing to 20 mg once daily after 6 weeks and to 40 mg once daily after 12 weeks as tolerated

Adults:

Initial: 20 mg once daily in the evening; patients who require only a moderate reduction of LDL-C may be started at 10 mg once daily; patients who require a reduction of >45% in LDL-C may be started at 40 mg once daily

Maintenance: Recommended dosage range: 5-80 mg/day as a single dose in the evening; doses should be adjusted at intervals of at least 4 weeks

Heterozygous familial hypercholesterolemia: Adolescents 10-17 years: 10 mg once daily in the evening; increase in intervals of 4 weeks or more to a maximum of 40 mg/day

Homozygous familial hypercholesterolemia: Adults: 40 mg in the evening or 80 mg/day in 3 divided doses of 20 mg, 20 mg, and an evening dose of 40 mg.

Dosage adjustment in patients who are concomitantly receiving cyclosporine: Adults: Initial: 5 mg, not to exceed 10 mg/day

Dosage adjustment in patients receiving concomitant fibrates or niacin: Adults: Dose should not exceed 10 mg/day

Dosage adjustment in patients receiving concomitant amiodarone or verapamil: Adults: Dose should not exceed 20 mg/day

Dosing adjustment in renal impairment: Adults: Because simvastatin does not undergo significant renal excretion, modification of dose should only be necessary in patients with severe renal impairment: Cl$_{cr}$ <10 mL/minute: Initial: 5 mg/day

Administration Oral: May be taken without regard to meals. Administration with the evening meal or at bedtime has been associated with somewhat greater LDL-C reduction

Monitoring Parameters Serum cholesterol (total and fractionated), CPK; liver function tests (see Precautions)

Reference Range Hypercholesterolemia: See table below; Desired: HDL-C <40 mg/dL

Classification of Blood Cholesterol, LDL-C, and Triglyceride Concentrations*

Classification	Cholesterol (mg/dL)		LDL-C (mg/dL)		Triglycerides (mg/dL)
	Children	Adults	Children	Adults	Adults
Acceptable/optimal	<170	<200	<110	<100	<150
Above optimal	†	†	†	100-129	†
Borderline high	170-199	200-239	110-129	130-159	150-199
High	≥200	≥240	≥130	160-189	200-499
Very high	†	†	†	≥190	≥500

*Adapted from American Academy of Pediatrics Committee on Nutrition, "Cholesterol in Childhood," *Pediatrics*, 1998, 101(1 Pt 1):141-7 and "Third Report of the National Cholesterol Education Program Expert Panel on Detection, Evaluation, and Treatment of High Blood Cholesterol in Adults (Adult Treatment Panel III)," May 2001, www.nhlbi.gov/guidelines/cholesterol.

†Lack of specific type of classification in either pediatric or adult recommendations.

Patient Information May rarely cause photosensitivity reactions (eg, exposure to sunlight may cause severe sunburn, skin rash, redness, or itching); avoid direct exposure to sunlight. Report severe and unresolved gastric upset, any vision changes, muscle pain and weakness, changes in color of urine or stool, yellowing of skin or eyes, and any unusual bruising. Female patients of childbearing age must be counseled to use 2 effective forms of contraception simultaneously, unless absolute abstinence is the chosen method; this drug may cause severe fetal defects.

Additional Information The current recommendation for treatment of hypercholesterolemia in children is limited to children ≥10 years of age who, after a 6-month to 1-year trial of diet therapy, continue to have LDL-C concentrations ≥190 mg/dL alone, or LDL-C concentrations ≥160 mg/dL and a family history of premature coronary artery disease or two or more other coronary artery disease risk factors (AAP Committee on Nutrition, 1998). For more specific risk assessment and treatment recommendations for adults, see the NIH Guidelines, 2001.

Dosage Forms Tablet: 5 mg, 10 mg, 20 mg, 40 mg, 80 mg

References

American Academy of Pediatrics Committee on Nutrition, "Cholesterol in Childhood," *Pediatrics*, 1998, 101(1 Pt 1):141-7.

American Academy of Pediatrics, "National Cholesterol Education Program: Report of the Expert Panel on Blood Cholesterol Levels in Children and Adolescents," *Pediatrics*, 1992, 89(3 Pt 2):525-84.

DeJongh S, et al, "Efficacy, Safety, and Tolerability of Simvastatin in Children With Familial Hypercholesterolemia," *Clin Drug Invest*, 2002, 22(8): 533-40.

Ducobu J, Brasseur D, Chaudron JM, et al, "Simvastatin Use in Children," *Lancet*, 1992, 339(8807):1488.

Duplaga BA, "Treatment of Childhood Hypercholesterolemia With HMG-CoA Reductase Inhibitors," *Ann Pharmacother*, 1999, 33(11):1224-7.

"Third Report of the National Cholesterol Education Program Expert Panel on Detection, Evaluation, and Treatment of High Blood Cholesterol in Adults (Adult Treatment Panel III)," May 2001, www.nhlbi.nih.gov/guidelines/cholesterol.

♦ **Sinequan**® *see* Doxepin *on page 411*

♦ **Singulair**® *see* Montelukast *on page 777*

♦ **Sleepinal**® **[OTC]** *see* DiphenhydrAMINE *on page 393*

♦ **Slo-Niacin**® **[OTC]** *see* Niacin *on page 809*

♦ **Slow FE**® **[OTC]** *see* Iron Supplements (Oral/Enteral) *on page 623*

♦ **Slow-K**® **[DSC]** *see* Potassium Supplements *on page 919*

♦ **Slow-Mag**® **[OTC]** *see* Magnesium Supplements *on page 701*

♦ **SM-7338** *see* Meropenem *on page 722*

♦ **SMX-TMP** *see* Sulfamethoxazole and Trimethoprim *on page 1052*

♦ **Snake (Pit Vipers) Antivenin** *see* Crotalidae Polyvalent Antivenin (Equine) *on page 313*

♦ **Sodium 2-Mercaptoethane Sulfonate** *see* Mesna *on page 725*

♦ **Sodium 4-Phenylbutyrate** *see* Sodium Phenylbutyrate *on page 1028*

Sodium Acetate (SOW dee um AS e tate)

Therapeutic Category Alkalinizing Agent, Parenteral; Electrolyte Supplement, Parenteral; Sodium Salt

Generic Available Yes

Use Sodium salt replacement; correction of acidosis through conversion of acetate to bicarbonate

Pregnancy Risk Factor C

Contraindications Hypersensitivity to sodium acetate or any component; alkalosis, hypocalcemia, edema, cirrhosis, excessive chloride losses, hypernatremia

(Continued)

Sodium Acetate *(Continued)*

Warnings Avoid extravasation

Precautions Use with caution in patients with hepatic failure, CHF or other sodium-retaining conditions

Adverse Reactions

Cardiovascular: Thrombosis, hypervolemia, edema, cerebral hemorrhage

Endocrine & metabolic: Hypernatremia, hypokalemic metabolic alkalosis, hypocalcemia

Local: Extravasant, local cellulitis

Respiratory: Pulmonary edema

Stability Protect from light, heat, and from freezing; **incompatible** with acids, acidic salts, catecholamines, atropine

Mechanism of Action Sodium is the principal extracellular cation; functions in fluid and electrolyte balance, osmotic pressure control, and water distribution; acetate is metabolized to bicarbonate which neutralizes hydrogen ion concentration and raises blood and urinary pH

Usual Dosage Sodium acetate is metabolized to bicarbonate on an equimolar basis outside the liver; administer in large volume I.V. fluids as a sodium source. Dosage is dependent upon the clinical condition, fluid, electrolytes and acid-base balance of the patient.

Maintenance sodium requirements: I.V.:

Neonates, Infants, and Children: 3-4 mEq/kg/day; maximum dose: 100-150 mEq/day

Adults: 154 mEq/day

Metabolic acidosis: If sodium acetate is desired over sodium bicarbonate, the amount of acetate may be dosed utilizing the equation found in the sodium bicarbonate monograph as each mEq acetate is converted to a mEq of HCO_3; see Sodium Bicarbonate *on page 1025*

Administration Parenteral: Must be diluted prior to I.V. administration; infuse hypertonic solutions (>154 mEq/L) via a central line; maximum rate of administration: 1 mEq/kg/hour

Monitoring Parameters Serum electrolytes including calcium, arterial blood gases (if indicated)

Additional Information Sodium and acetate content of 1 g: 7.3 mEq

Dosage Forms Injection, solution: 2 mEq/mL (20 mL, 50 mL, 100 mL, 250 mL); 4 mEq/mL (50 mL, 100 mL)

♦ **Sodium Acid Carbonate** *see Sodium Bicarbonate on page 1025*

Sodium Benzoate *(SOW dee um BENZ oh ate)*

Therapeutic Category Ammonium Detoxicant; Hyperammonemia Agent; Urea Cycle Disorder (UCD) Treatment Agent

Generic Available Yes

Use Adjunctive therapy for the prevention and treatment of hyperammonemia due to suspected or proven urea cycle disorders

Precautions Use with caution in patients with Reye's syndrome, propionic or methylmalonic acidemia. *In vitro* and animal studies have shown that benzoate, a metabolite of benzyl alcohol, displaces bilirubin from protein binding sites; use cautiously in neonates, particularly those with hyperbilirubinemia.

Adverse Reactions

Endocrine & metabolic: Metabolic acidosis

Gastrointestinal: Nausea, vomiting

Mechanism of Action Assists in lowering serum ammonia levels by activation of a nonurea cycle pathway (the benzoate-hippurate pathway); ammonia in the presence of benzoate will conjugate with glycine to form hippurate which is excreted by the kidney

Pharmacokinetics

Half-life: 0.75-7.4 hours

Elimination: Clearance is largely attributable to metabolism with urinary excretion of hippurate, the major metabolite

Usual Dosage Investigational use (not FDA approved): Oral, I.V.:

Infants and Children: 0.25 g/kg bolus followed by 0.25 g/kg/day as continuous infusion or divided every 6-8 hours

Adolescents and Adults: Initial 5.5 g/m^2 bolus followed by 5.5 g/m^2/day as continuous I.V. infusion or divided every 6-8 hours

Administration Not available commercially

Oral: Must be compounded using chemical powder

I.V.: I.V. solutions must also be compounded and tested for sterility and pyrogenicity prior to use; infuse bolus (with sodium phenylacetate) over 90 minutes in 25-35 mL/kg $D_{10}W$

Monitoring Parameters Plasma ammonia and amino acids

Additional Information Used to treat urea cycle enzyme deficiency in combination with arginine; a maximum of 1 mole nitrogen is removed for every 1 mole of benzoate administered

Dosage Forms Powder: 500 g

References

Batshaw ML, "Hyperammonemia," *Curr Probl Pediatr*, 1984, 14(11):1-69.

Batshaw ML and Brusilow SW, "Treatment of Hyperammonemic Coma Caused by Inborn Errors of Urea Synthesis," *J Pediatr*, 1980, 97(6):893-900.

Batshaw ML, MacArthur RB, and Tuchman M, "Alternative Pathway Therapy for Urea Cycle Disorders: Twenty Years Later," *J Pediatr*, 2001, 138(1 Suppl):S46-54.

Green TP, Marchessault RP, and Freese DK, "Disposition of Sodium Benzoate in Newborn Infants With Hyperammonemia," *J Pediatr*, 1983, 102(5):785-90.

Maestri NE, Hauser ER, Bartholomew D, et al, "Prospective Treatment of Urea Cycle Disorders," *J Pediatr*, 1991, 119(6):923-8.

Summar M, "Current Strategies for the Management of Neonatal Urea Cycle Disorders," *J Pediatr*, 2001, 138(1 Suppl):S30-9.

Sodium Bicarbonate (SOW dee um bye KAR bun ate)

Related Information

Adult ACLS Algorithm, Asystole *on page 1187*
Adult ACLS Algorithm, Pulseless Electrical Activity *on page 1186*
Antacid Preparations *on page 112*
CPR Pediatric Drug Dosages *on page 1175*

U.S. Brand Names Brioschi® [OTC]; Neut®

Synonyms Baking Soda; $NaHCO_3$; Sodium Acid Carbonate; Sodium Hydrogen Carbonate

Therapeutic Category Alkalinizing Agent, Oral; Alkalinizing Agent, Parenteral; Antacid; Electrolyte Supplement, Oral; Electrolyte Supplement, Parenteral; Sodium Salt

Generic Available Yes

Use Management of metabolic acidosis; antacid; alkalinization of urine; stabilization of acid base status in cardiac arrest (see Warnings) and treatment of life-threatening hyperkalemia

Pregnancy Risk Factor C

Contraindications Hypersensitivity to sodium bicarbonate or any component; alkalosis, hypocalcemia, hypernatremia; unknown abdominal pain, inadequate ventilation during cardiopulmonary resuscitation; excessive chloride losses

Warnings Avoid extravasation, tissue necrosis can occur due to the hypertonicity of $NaHCO_3$; use of I.V. $NaHCO_3$ should be reserved for documented metabolic acidosis and for life-threatening hyperkalemia; routine use in cardiac arrest is not recommended; patient should be adequately ventilated before administering in cardiac arrest; administration of excessive amounts of sodium bicarbonate may result in metabolic alkalosis which decreases the delivery of oxygen to tissues; monitor use closely

Precautions Use with caution in patients with CHF or other sodium-retaining conditions, renal insufficiency

Adverse Reactions

Cardiovascular: Edema, cerebral hemorrhage (especially with rapid injection of the hyperosmotic $NaHCO_3$ solution in infants)

Central nervous system: Tetany, intracranial acidosis

Endocrine & metabolic: Metabolic alkalosis, hypernatremia, hypokalemia, hypocalcemia, hyperosmolality

Gastrointestinal: Gastric distention, flatulence may occur with oral administration

Local: Tissue necrosis, ulceration after I.V. extravasation

Respiratory: Pulmonary edema

Drug Interactions Chlorpropamide, lithium, methotrexate, salicylates, and tetracycline have increased renal clearance with alkaline urine; anorexiants, flecainide, mecamylamine, quinidine, and sympathomimetics have decreased renal clearance with alkaline urine; concurrent doses with iron may decrease iron absorption

Stability Do not mix $NaHCO_3$ with calcium salts, catecholamines, atropine

Mechanism of Action Dissociates to provide bicarbonate ion which neutralizes hydrogen ion concentration and raises blood and urinary pH

Pharmacodynamics

Onset of action:

Oral, as antacid: 15 minutes

I.V.: Rapid

(Continued)

Sodium Bicarbonate *(Continued)*

Duration:
Oral: 1-3 hours
I.V.: 8-10 minutes

Pharmacokinetics

Absorption: Oral: Well absorbed
Elimination: Reabsorbed by kidney and <1% is excreted in urine

Usual Dosage

Cardiac arrest: See Warnings; patient should be adequately ventilated before administering $NaHCO_3$

Infants: 1 mEq/kg slow IVP initially; may repeat with 0.5 mEq/kg in 10 minutes one time, or as indicated by the patient's acid-base status

Children and Adults: 1 mEq/kg IVP initially; may repeat with 0.5 mEq/kg in 10 minutes one time, or as indicated by the patient's acid-base status

Metabolic acidosis: Dosage should be based on the following formula if blood gases and pH measurements are available:

Neonates, Infants and Children: $HCO_3^-(mEq) = 0.3$ x weight (kg) x base deficit (mEq/L) **or** $HCO_3^-(mEq) = 0.5$ x weight (kg) x [24 - serum $HCO_3^-(mEq/L)$]

Adults: $HCO_3^-(mEq) = 0.2$ x weight (kg) x base deficit (mEq/L) **or** $HCO_3^-(mEq) = 0.5$ x weight (kg) x [24 - serum $HCO_3^-(mEq/L)$]

If acid-base status is not available: Dose for older Children and Adults: 2-5 mEq/kg I.V. infusion over 4-8 hours; subsequent doses should be based on patient's acid-base status

Prevention of hyperuricemia secondary to tumor lysis syndrome (urinary alkalinization) (refer to individual protocols):

Infants and Children:

I.V.: 120-200 $mEq/m^2/day$ diluted in maintenance I.V. fluids of 3000 $mL/m^2/day$; titrate to maintain urine pH between 6-7

Oral: 12 $g/m^2/day$ divided into 4 doses; titrate to maintain urine pH between 6-7

Chronic renal failure: Oral: Initiate when plasma HCO_3^- <15 mEq/L:

Children: 1-3 mEq/kg/day in divided doses

Adults: 20-36 mEq/day in divided doses

Renal tubular acidosis: Oral:

Distal:

Children: 2-3 mEq/kg/day in divided doses

Adults: 0.5-2 mEq/kg/day given in 4-5 divided doses

Proximal: Children and Adults: Initial: 5-10 mEq/kg/day in divided doses; maintenance: Increase as required to maintain serum bicarbonate in the normal range

Urine alkalinization: Oral:

Children: 1-10 mEq (84-840 mg)/kg/day in divided doses; dose should be titrated to desired urinary pH

Adults: 48 mEq (4 g) initially, then 12-24 mEq (1-2 g) every 4 hours; dose should be titrated to desired urinary pH; doses up to 16 g/day have been used

Antacid: Oral: Adults: 325 mg to 2 grams 1-4 times/day

Administration

Oral: Administer 1-3 hours after meals

Parenteral: For direct I.V. administration: in neonates and infants, use the 0.5 mEq/mL solution or dilute the 1 mEq/mL solution 1:1 with **SWI**; in children and adults, the 1 mEq/mL solution may be used; administer slowly (maximum rate in neonates and infants: 10 mEq/minute); for infusion, dilute to a maximum concentration of 0.5 mEq/mL in dextrose solution and infuse over 2 hours (maximum rate of administration: 1 mEq/kg/hour)

Monitoring Parameters Serum electrolytes including calcium, urinary pH, arterial blood gases (if indicated)

Additional Information 1 mEq $NaHCO_3$ is equivalent to 84 mg; each g of $NaHCO_3$ provides 12 mEq each of sodium and bicarbonate ions; the osmolarity of 0.5 mEq/mL is 1000 mOsm/L and 1 mEq/mL is 2000 mOsm/L

Dosage Forms

Granules, effervescent (Brioschi®): 6 g, 120 g, 240 g [lemon flavor]

Injection, solution: 4.2% [42 mg/mL = 5 mEq/10 mL] (10 mL); 5% (500 mL); 7.5% [75 mg/mL = 8.92 mEq/10 mL] (50 mL); 8.4% [84 mg/mL = 10 mEq/10 mL] (10 mL, 50 mL)

Neut®: 4% [40 mg/mL = 2.4 mEq/5 mL] (5 mL)

Infusion [premixed in sterile water]: 5% (500 mL)

Powder: 120 g, 480 g

Tablet: 325 mg [3.8 mEq]; 650 mg [7.6 mEq]

Sodium Chloride (SOW dee um KLOR ide)

U.S. Brand Names Altamist [OTC]; Ayr® Baby Saline [OTC]; Ayr® Saline [OTC]; Ayr® Saline Mist [OTC]; Breathe Right® Saline [OTC]; Broncho® Saline [OTC]; Entsol® [OTC]; HuMIST® [OTC]; Muro 128® [OTC]; NaSal™ [OTC]; Nasal Moist® [OTC]; Na-Zone® [OTC]; Ocean [OTC]; Pediamist® [OTC]; Pretz® Irrigation [OTC]; SalineX® [OTC]; SeaMist® [OTC]; Simply Saline™ [OTC]; Wound Wash Saline™ [OTC]

Synonyms NaCl; Normal Saline; NS; ½NS

Therapeutic Category Electrolyte Supplement, Oral; Electrolyte Supplement, Parenteral; Lubricant, Ocular; Sodium Salt

Generic Available Yes

Use Prevention of muscle cramps and heat prostration; restoration of sodium ion in hyponatremia; restores moisture to nasal membranes; reduction of corneal edema; source of electrolytes and water for expansion of the extracellular fluid compartment

Pregnancy Risk Factor C

Contraindications Hypersensitivity to sodium chloride or any component; hypertonic uterus, hypernatremia, fluid retention

Warnings Sodium toxicity is almost exclusively related to how fast a sodium deficit is corrected; both rate and magnitude of correction are extremely important

Precautions Use with caution in patients with CHF, renal insufficiency, cirrhosis, hypertension

Adverse Reactions
Cardiovascular: Edema, thrombosis, hypervolemia
Endocrine & metabolic: Hypernatremia, dilution of serum electrolytes, overhydration
Gastrointestinal: Nausea, vomiting (oral use)
Local: Phlebitis (with concentrations >0.9%)
Respiratory: Pulmonary edema

Mechanism of Action Principal extracellular cation; functions in fluid and electrolyte balance, osmotic pressure control and water distribution

Pharmacokinetics
Absorption: Oral, I.V.: Rapid
Distribution: Widely distributed
Elimination: Mainly in urine but also in sweat, tears, and saliva

Usual Dosage Dosage depends upon clinical condition, fluid, electrolyte and acid-base balance of patient; hypertonic solutions (>0.9%) should only be used for the initial treatment of acute serious symptomatic hyponatremia; see Fluid and Electrolyte Requirements in Children *on page 1258*

Maintenance sodium requirements: Oral, I.V.:
Premature neonates: 2-8 mEq/kg/day
Term neonates: 1-4 mEq/kg/day
Infants and Children: 3-4 mEq/kg/day; maximum dose: 100-150 mEq/day
Adults: 154 mEq/day
Nasal: Children and Adults: Use as often as needed
Heat cramps: Adults: Oral: 0.5-1 g, up to 5-10 times/day (5 g/day maximum)
Ophthalmic, ointment: Children and Adults: Apply once daily or more often as needed
To correct acute, serious hyponatremia: mEq sodium = [desired sodium (mEq/L) - actual sodium (mEq/L)] x 0.6 x wt (kg); for acute correction use 125 mEq/L as the desired serum sodium; acutely correct serum sodium in 5 mEq/L/dose increments; more gradual correction in increments of 10 mEq/L/day is indicated in the asymptomatic patient

Administration
Nasal: Spray into 1 nostril while gently occluding other
Ophthalmic: Apply to affected eye(s); avoid contact of bottle tip with eye or skin
Oral: Administer with full glass of water
Parenteral: Infuse hypertonic solutions (>0.9% saline) via central line only; maximum rate of administration: 1 mEq/kg/hour

Monitoring Parameters Serum sodium, chloride, I & O, weight

Reference Range Serum/plasma sodium levels:
Premature neonates: 132-140 mEq/L
Full-term neonates: 133-142 mEq/L
Infants ≥2 months to Adults: 135-145 mEq/L

Nursing Implications Bacteriostatic NS should not be used for diluting or reconstituting drugs for administration in neonates

Additional Information Normal saline (0.9%) = 154 mEq/L; 3% NaCl = 513 mEq/L; 5% NaCl = 855 mEq/L

Dosage Forms
Gel, nasal (Nasal Moist®): 0.65% (30 g)
Injection, solution: 0.45% (25 mL, 50 mL, 100 mL, 250 mL, 500 mL, 1000 mL, 1500 mL, 2000 mL); 0.9% (1 mL, 2 mL, 3 mL, 5 mL, 10 mL, 20 mL, 25 mL, 30 mL, 50 mL, (Continued)

Sodium Chloride *(Continued)*

100 mL, 150 mL, 250 mL, 500 mL, 1000 mL); 2.5% (250 mL); 3% (500 mL); 5% (500 mL)

Injection, solution, bacteriostatic: 0.9% (10 mL, 20 mL, 30 mL)

Injection, solution, **concentrate**: 14.6% (2.5 mEq/mL) (20 mL, 40 mL, 250 mL); 23.4% (4 mEq/mL) (30 mL, 50 mL, 100 mL, 200 mL, 250 mL)

Ointment, ophthalmic (Muro 128®): 5% (3.5 g)

Powder for nasal solution (Entsol®): 3% (10.5 g)

Solution for inhalation: 0.45% (3 mL, 5 mL); 0.9% (3 mL, 5 mL, 15 mL); 3% (15 mL); 10% (15 mL)

Broncho® Saline: 0.9% (90 mL, 240 mL)

Solution for irrigation: 0.45% (2000 mL); 0.9% (250 mL, 500 mL, 1000 mL, 1500 mL, 2000 mL, 3000 mL, 4000 mL, 5000 mL)

Wound Wash Saline™: 0.9% (90 mL, 210 mL)

Solution, intranasal: 0.65% (45 mL)

Altamist: 0.65% (60 mL) [spray]

Ayr® Saline: 0.65% (50 mL) [drops]

Ayr® Saline Mist: 0.65% (50 mL) [spray]

Ayr® Baby Saline: 0.65% (30 mL) [spray/drops]

Breathe Right® Saline: 0.65% (44 mL) [spray]

Entsol®: 3% (100 mL) [preservative free spray]

Entsol® Mist: 3% (30 mL) [spray]

Entsol® Single Use: 3% (240 mL) [preservative free nasal wash]

HuMIST®: 0.65% (45 mL) [spray]

Na-Zone®: 0.75% (60 mL) [spray]

NaSal™: 0.65% (15 mL) [drops], (30 mL) [spray]

Nasal Moist®: 0.65% (15 mL, 45 mL) [spray]

Ocean®: 0.65% (45 mL) [spray/drops]

Pediamist®: 0.5% (15 mL) [spray]

Pretz® Irrigation: 0.75% (240 mL)

Salinex®: 0.4% (15 mL) [drops]; (50 mL) [spray]

Sea Mist®: 0.65% (15 mL) [spray]

Simply Saline™: 0.9% (44 mL) [mist]

Solution, ophthalmic: 5% (15 mL)

Muro-128®: 2% (15 mL); 5% (15 mL, 30 mL)

Tablet: 1 g (17 mEq)

♦ **Sodium Edetate** *see* Edetate Disodium *on page 425*

♦ **Sodium Etidronate** *see* Etidronate Disodium *on page 467*

♦ **Sodium Ferric Gluconate** *see* Iron Supplements (Parenteral) *on page 626*

♦ **Sodium Hydrogen Carbonate** *see* Sodium Bicarbonate *on page 1025*

♦ **Sodium Hyposulfate** *see* Sodium Thiosulfate *on page 1030*

Sodium Phenylbutyrate (SOW dee um fen il BYOO ti rate)

U.S. Brand Names Buphenyl®

Synonyms Ammonapse; 4-Phenylbutyric Acid Sodium; Sodium 4-Phenylbutyrate

Therapeutic Category Ammonium Detoxicant; Hyperammonemia Agent; Urea Cycle Disorder (UCD) Treatment Agent

Use Adjunctive therapy in the chronic management of patients with urea cycle disorder involving deficiencies of carbamoylphosphate synthetase, ornithine transcarbamylase, or argininosuccinic acid synthetase; provides an alternative pathway for waste nitrogen excretion

Pregnancy Risk Factor C

Contraindications Hypersensitivity to phenylbutyrate, or any component; patients with severe hypertension, heart failure or renal dysfunction; **phenylbutyrate is not indicated in the treatment of acute hyperammonemia**

Precautions Use cautiously in patients with renal or hepatic dysfunction and in patients who must maintain a low sodium diet as each gram of drug contains 125 mg sodium

Adverse Reactions

Cardiovascular: Edema, arrhythmias, syncope

Central nervous system: Headache, depression

Dermatologic: Rash

Endocrine & metabolic: Amenorrhea, menstrual dysfunction, acidosis, alkalosis, hyperchloremia, hyperuricemia, hypokalemia, hypernatremia, hyperphosphatemia

Gastrointestinal: Anorexia, abnormal taste, abdominal pain, nausea, vomiting, weight gain, gastritis; rare: peptic ulcer, rectal bleeding, pancreatitis

Hematologic: Anemia, leukopenia, leukocytosis, thrombocytopenia, aplastic anemia

Hepatic: Hypoalbuminemia, elevated liver enzymes, elevated bilirubin

Renal: Renal tubular acidosis

Miscellaneous: Offensive body odor

Drug Interactions Haloperidol, valproic acid and corticosteroids increase ammonia concentrations and may decrease effectiveness of sodium phenylbutyrate; probenecid may decrease urinary excretion

Food Interactions Avoid mixing with acidic-type beverages (eg, colas, lemonade, grape juice) since drug may precipitate

Stability Store at room temperature (59°F to 86°F); after opening, containers should be kept tightly closed

Mechanism of Action Sodium phenylbutyrate is a prodrug that, when given orally, is rapidly converted to phenylacetate. Phenylacetate is conjugated with glutamine to form the active compound phenylacetylglutamine. Phenylacetylglutamine serves as a substitute for urea and is excreted in the urine carrying with it 2 moles nitrogen (equivalent to urea) per mole of phenylacetylglutamine thus assisting in the clearance of nitrogenous waste in patients with urea cycle disorders.

Pharmacokinetics

Distribution: V_d: 0.2 L/kg

Metabolism: conjugation to phenylacetylglutamine (active form); undergoes nonlinear Michaelis-Menten elimination kinetics

Half-life: 0.8 hours (parent compound); 1.2 hours (phenylacetate)

Time to peak serum concentration:

Powder: 1 hour

Tablet: 1.35 hours

Elimination: 80% of metabolite excreted in urine in 24 hours

Usual Dosage Oral:

Neonates, Infants, and Children <20 kg: 450-600 mg/kg/day divided four to six times daily; maximum daily dose 20 g/day

Children >20 kg and Adults: 9.9-13 g/m²/day, divided four to six times daily; maximum daily dose 20 g/day

Administration Oral: Administer with meals or feedings; mix powder with food or drink; avoid mixing with acidic beverages (eg, most fruit juices or colas)

Monitoring Parameters Plasma ammonia and glutamine concentrations, serum electrolytes, proteins, hepatic and renal function tests, physical signs/symptoms of hyperammonemia (ie, lethargy, ataxia, confusion, vomiting, seizures, and memory impairment)

Patient Information It is important to follow the dietary restrictions required when treating this disorder, the medication must be taken in strict accordance with the prescribed regimen; avoid altering the dosage without the prescriber's knowledge; the powder formulation has a very salty taste

Additional Information Teaspoon and tablespoon measuring devices are provided with the powder; each 1 g powder contains 0.94 g sodium phenylbutyrate = 125 mg sodium; each tablet contains 0.5 g sodium phenylbutyrate = 62 mg sodium

Dosage Forms

Powder: 3.2 g [sodium phenylbutyrate 3 g] per **teaspoon or** 9.1 g [sodium phenylbutyrate 8.6 g] per **tablespoon**

Tablet: 500 mg

References

Batshaw ML, MacArthur RB, and Tuchman M, "Alternative Pathway Therapy for Urea Cycle Disorders: Twenty Years Later," *J Pediatr*, 2001, 138(1 Suppl):S46-S55.

Berry GT and Steiner RD, "Long-Term Management of Patients With Urea Cycle Disorders," *J Pediatr*, 2001, 138(1 Suppl):S56-60.

Brusilow SW, "Phenylacetylglutamine May Replace Urea as a Vehicle for Waste Nitrogen Excretion," *Pediatr Res*, 1991, 29(2):147-50.

Maestri NE, Brusilow SW, Clissold DB, et al, "Long-Term Treatment of Girls With Ornithine Trans-carbamylase Deficiency," *N Engl J Med*, 1996, 335(12):855-9.

♦ **Sodium Phosphate** *see* Phosphate Supplements *on page 898*

Sodium Polystyrene Sulfonate

(SOW dee um pol ee STYE reen SUL fon ate)

Related Information

Carbohydrate and Alcohol Content of Liquid Medications for Use in Patients Receiving Ketogenic Diets *on page 1431*

U.S. Brand Names Kayexalate®; Kionex™; SPS®

Canadian Brand Names PMS-Sodium Polystyrene Sulfonate

Therapeutic Category Antidote, Hyperkalemia

Generic Available Yes

Use Treatment of hyperkalemia

Pregnancy Risk Factor C

Contraindications Hypersensitivity to sodium polystyrene sulfonate or any component; hypernatremia; intestinal obstruction or perforation (oral use)

(Continued)

Sodium Polystyrene Sulfonate *(Continued)*

Warnings Treatment with this drug alone may be insufficient to rapidly correct severe hyperkalemia; other more rapidly effective appropriate measures should be used; enema will reduce the serum potassium faster than oral administration, but the oral route will result in a greater reduction over several hours.

Precautions Use with caution in patients with severe CHF, hypertension, or edema; small amounts of magnesium and calcium may also be lost in binding

Adverse Reactions

Endocrine & metabolic: Hypokalemia, hypocalcemia, hypomagnesemia, hypernatremia

Gastrointestinal: Anorexia, nausea, vomiting, constipation, intestinal necrosis

Drug Interactions Cation-donating antacids (such as magnesium hydroxide or calcium carbonate)

Food Interactions Never mix in orange juice

Mechanism of Action Removes potassium by exchanging sodium ions for potassium ions in the intestine before the resin is passed from the body

Pharmacodynamics Onset of action: Within 2-24 hours

Pharmacokinetics Elimination: Remains in the GI tract to be completely excreted in the feces (primarily as potassium polystyrene sulfonate)

Usual Dosage

Children:

Oral: 1 g/kg/dose every 6 hours

Rectal: 1 g/kg/dose every 2-6 hours

Adults:

Oral: 15 g 1-4 times/day

Rectal: 30-50 g every 6 hours

Administration

Oral or NG: Shake commercially available suspension well before use; when using powder, dilute in 3-4 mL fluid per g of resin; 10% sorbitol, water, or syrup may be used as diluent

Enema: Shake commercially available suspension well before use; when using powder, dilute in water or 25% sorbitol at a concentration of 0.3-0.5 g/mL; retain enema in colon for at least 30-60 minutes or several hours, if possible

Monitoring Parameters Serum sodium, potassium, calcium, magnesium, EKG (if applicable)

Additional Information 1 g of resin binds ~1 mEq of potassium; 4.1 mEq sodium per g of powder; 1 level teaspoon contains 3.5 g polystyrene sulfonate

Dosage Forms Oral or rectal:

Powder for suspension:

Kionex™: 454 g

Kayexalate®: 480 g

Suspension (SPS®): 15 g/60 mL [with sorbitol and alcohol] (60 mL, 120 mL, 200 mL, 500 mL)

♦ **Sodium Sulamyd® (Can)** *see* Sulfacetamide *on page 1048*

Sodium Thiosulfate *(SOW dee um thye oh SUL fate)*

U.S. Brand Names Versiclear™

Synonyms Disodium Thiosulfate Pentahydrate; Sodium Hyposulfate; Thiosulfuric Acid

Therapeutic Category Antidote, Cisplatin; Antidote, Cyanide; Antidote, Extravasation; Antifungal Agent, Topical

Generic Available Yes (injection)

Use

Parenteral: Used alone or with sodium nitrite or amyl nitrite in cyanide poisoning or arsenic poisoning; reduce the risk of nephrotoxicity associated with cisplatin therapy; local infiltration (in diluted form) of selected chemotherapy extravasation

Topical: Treatment of tinea versicolor, acne

Pregnancy Risk Factor C

Contraindications Hypersensitivity to sodium thiosulfate or any component

Precautions Discontinue if irritation or sensitivity occurs; rapid I.V. infusion has caused transient hypotension and EKG changes in dogs

Adverse Reactions

Cardiovascular: Hypotension

Central nervous system: Coma, CNS depression secondary to thiocyanate intoxication, psychosis, confusion

Dermatologic: Contact dermatitis

Local: Local irritation

Neuromuscular & skeletal: Weakness

Otic: Tinnitus

Stability Stable diluted in NS or D₅W at concentrations of 1.5% and 9.76% sodium thiosulfate for 24 hours

Mechanism of Action

Prevention of cyanide toxicity: By providing an extra sulfur group to the enzyme rhodanase, it increases the rate of detoxification of cyanide

Prevention of cisplatin nephrotoxicity: Complexes with cisplatin to form a compound that is nontoxic to either normal or cancerous cells

Pharmacokinetics

Half-life, elimination: 0.65 hours

Elimination: 28.5% excreted unchanged in the urine

Usual Dosage

Cyanide and nitroprusside antidote: I.V.: See Usual Dosage in Cyanide Antidote Kit on page 109

Prevention of cisplatin nephrotoxicity: Adults: I.V.: 12 g over 6 hours in association with cisplatin **or** 9 g/m² I.V. bolus then 1.2 g/m²/hour for 6 hours; should be administered before or during cisplatin administration

Chemotherapy infiltration: Children and Adults: Dilute 10% sodium thiosulfate 4-8 mL with 6 mL SWI to make ⅛ to ⅓ molar solution; as local infiltration for the following chemotherapy agents:

Mechlorethamine: Use 2 mL for each mg infiltrated

Cis-platinum: 2 mL for each 100 mg infiltrated; use only for large infiltrates (>20 mL) and concentrations >0.5 mg/mL of cis-platinum

Topical use (antifungal, acne): Children and Adults: 25% solution: Apply thin film twice daily to affected areas for several weeks to months

Administration

Parenteral: I.V.: Inject slowly, over at least 10 minutes; rapid administration may cause hypotension

Topical: Do not apply topically to or near eyes; thoroughly cleanse and dry affects areas prior to application

Dosage Forms

Injection, solution [preservative free]: 100 mg/mL (10 mL); 250 mg/mL (50 mL)

Lotion (Versiclear™): Sodium thiosulfate 25% and salicylic acid 1% (120 mL) [contains 10% isopropyl alcohol]

References

Hall AH and Rumack BH, "Hydroxocobalamin/Sodium Thiosulfate as a Cyanide Antidote," *J Emerg Med*, 1987, 5(2):115-21.

Naughton M, "Acute Cyanide Poisoning," *Anaesth Intensive Care*, 1974, 2(4):351-6.

- **Soflax**™ **(Can)** *see* Docusate *on page 402*
- **Solaraze**™   *see* Diclofenac *on page 374*
- **Solarcaine**® **[OTC]** *see* Benzocaine *on page 163*
- **Solarcaine**® **Aloe Extra Burn Relief [OTC]** *see* Lidocaine *on page 671*
- **Solganal**® *see* Aurothioglucose *on page 148*
- **Solu-Cortef**® *see* Hydrocortisone *on page 573*
- **Solugel**® **(Can)** *see* Benzoyl Peroxide *on page 165*
- **Solu-Medrol**® *see* MethylPREDNISolone *on page 747*
- **Solurex**® *see* Dexamethasone *on page 354*
- **Solurex L.A.**® *see* Dexamethasone *on page 354*
- **Soluver**® **(Can)** *see* Salicylic Acid *on page 1002*
- **Soluver**® **Plus (Can)** *see* Salicylic Acid *on page 1002*
- **Somatrem** *see* Human Growth Hormone *on page 564*
- **Somatropin** *see* Human Growth Hormone *on page 564*
- **Sominex**® **[OTC]** *see* DiphenhydrAMINE *on page 393*
- **Sominex**® **Maximum Strength [OTC]** *see* DiphenhydrAMINE *on page 393*
- **Somnote**™ *see* Chloral Hydrate *on page 252*

Sorbitol (SOR bi tole)

Therapeutic Category Laxative, Hyperosmolar; Laxative, Osmotic

Generic Available Yes

Use Humectant; sweetening agent; hyperosmotic laxative; facilitates the passage of sodium polystyrene sulfonate or a charcoal-toxin complex through the intestinal tract

Contraindications Anuria

Adverse Reactions

Endocrine & metabolic: Fluid and electrolyte losses, lactic acidosis

Gastrointestinal: Diarrhea, abdominal distress, nausea, vomiting

Mechanism of Action A polyalcoholic sugar with osmotic cathartic actions

(Continued)

Sorbitol *(Continued)*

Pharmacodynamics

Onset of action: Oral: Mean time to first stool in patients receiving a charcoal-sorbitol slurry:

Children (ingestions):

6.4 hours (dose: 1.5 g/kg in 4 patients)

8.48 hours (dose: 2 g/kg in 33 patients)

Adults:

Nonpoisoned volunteers: 1.6 hours (dose: 2 g/kg)

Ingestion: 7.2 hours (14 adults; dose not specified)

Pharmacokinetics

Absorption: Oral, rectal: Poor

Metabolism: Mainly in the liver to fructose

Usual Dosage Hyperosmotic laxative (as single dose, at infrequent intervals):

Children 2-11 years:

Oral: 2 mL/kg (as 70% solution)

Rectal enema: 30-60 mL as 25% to 30% solution

Children ≥12 years and Adults:

Oral: 30-150 mL (as 70% solution)

Rectal enema: 120 mL as 25% to 30% solution

Adjunct to sodium polystyrene sulfonate: 15 mL as 70% solution orally until diarrhea occurs (10-20 mL/2 hours) or 20-100 mL as an oral vehicle for the sodium polystyrene sulfonate resin

When administered with charcoal: Oral:

Children: 4.3 mL/kg of 35% sorbitol with 1 g/kg of activated charcoal or maximum dose: 2 g/kg sorbitol with activated charcoal

Adults: 4.3 mL/kg of 70% sorbitol with 1 g/kg of activated charcoal

Monitoring Parameters Serum electrolytes, I & O

Dosage Forms

Solution, irrigation: 3% (3000 mL, 5000 mL); 3.3% (2000 mL, 4000 mL)

Solution, oral: 70% (480 mL, 3840 mL)

References

Charney EB and Bodurtha JN, "Intractable Diarrhea Associated With the Use of Sorbitol," *J Pediatr*, 1981, 98:157-8.

James LP, Nichols MH, and King WD, "A Comparison of Cathartics in Pediatric Ingestions," *Pediatrics*, 1995, 96(2 Pt 1):235-8.

Kumar A, Weatherly MR, and Beaman DC, "Sweeteners, Flavorings, and Dyes in Antibiotic Preparations," *Pediatrics*, 1991, 87(3):352-60.

♦ **Sorine™** *see Sotalol on page 1032*

♦ **Sotacor® (Can)** *see Sotalol on page 1032*

Sotalol *(SOE ta lol)*

U.S. Brand Names Betapace®; Betapace AF™; Sorine™

Canadian Brand Names Alti-Sotalol; Apo®-Sotalol; Gen-Sotalol; Lin-Sotalol; Novo-Sotalol; Nu-Sotalol; PMS-Sotalol; Rho®-Sotalol; Sotacor®

Therapeutic Category Antiarrhythmic Agent, Class II; Antiarrhythmic Agent, Class III; Beta-Adrenergic Blocker

Generic Available Yes (for Betapace® and Sorine™)

Use

Betapace®, Sorine™, generic: Treatment of life-threatening ventricular arrhythmias (eg, sustained ventricular tachycardia)

Betapace AF™: Maintenance of normal sinus rhythm in patients who have highly symptomatic atrial fibrillation and atrial flutter, but who are currently in normal sinus rhythm [not usually for use in patients with paroxysmal atrial fibrillation/flutter that is easily reversed (eg, by Valsalva maneuver)]

Note: Do not substitute Betapace AF™ for other products (and vice versa); significant differences in FDA approved labeling exist [eg, dosage and administration, safety information and patient package insert (Betapace AF™ labeling contains a patient package insert specific for atrial fibrillation/flutter)]

Pregnancy Risk Factor B

Contraindications Hypersensitivity to sotalol or any component; sinus bradycardia; heart block greater than first degree (except in patients with a functioning artificial pacemaker); congenital or acquired long QT syndromes; uncontrolled CHF; cardiogenic shock; asthma. Betapace AF™ is also contraindicated in patients with sick sinus syndrome (except in patients with a functioning artificial pacemaker), a baseline QT interval >450 msec, hypokalemia (serum potassium <4 mEq/L), or significantly reduced renal function (Cl$_{cr}$ <40 mL/minute).

Warnings Initiation, reinitiation, and dosage increases of sotalol must occur in a hospital facility that can provide continuous EKG monitoring, recognition and treatment of life-threatening arrhythmias, and CPR. Patients must be monitored with continuous EKG for a minimum of 3 days (on their maintenance dose). Use with caution and adjust the dose in patients with renal impairment; creatinine clearance must be calculated prior to dosing.

May cause serious and life-threatening proarrhythmias [may cause or worsen ventricular arrhythmias (eg, sustained ventricular tachycardia, torsade de pointes, ventricular fibrillation)]; risk factors for torsade de pointes include: Higher sotalol doses, presence of sustained VT, female gender, excessive prolongation of the QT_c interval, history of CHF or cardiomegaly, decreased renal function, hypokalemia, hypomagnesemia, and bradycardia; monitor EKG for proarrhythmic effects; adjust dose to prevent QT_c prolongation; correct electrolyte imbalances (especially hypokalemia and hypomagnesemia) before initiating sotalol

Bradycardia and heart block may occur; consider pre-existing conditions such as sick sinus syndrome before initiating; may cause or worsen CHF (use with caution in patients with compensated CHF); use with caution and titrate dose carefully within the first 2 weeks post-MI (experience is limited); use with caution in patients with peripheral vascular disease (may aggravate arterial insufficiency); concomitant use with other drugs that prolong the QT interval or prolong refractoriness is not recommended (see Drug Interactions)

Exacerbation of angina, arrhythmias, and in some cases MI may occur following abrupt discontinuation of beta-blockers; avoid abrupt discontinuation, wean slowly, monitor for signs and symptoms of ischemia. Beta-blockers should generally be avoided in patients with bronchospastic disease; if administered, use the lowest possible dose and monitor patients carefully. Patients receiving beta-blockers, who have a history of anaphylactic reactions, may be more reactive to a repeated allergen challenge and may not be responsive to the usual epinephrine doses used to treat an allergic reaction. Beta-blockers may block hypoglycemia-induced tachycardia and blood pressure changes; use with caution in patients with diabetes mellitus. May mask signs of thyrotoxicosis. Use caution with anesthetic agents that decrease myocardial function.

Precautions Use with caution in patients receiving calcium channel blockers (see Drug Interactions)

Adverse Reactions

Cardiovascular: Bradycardia, chest pain, palpitations, CHF, peripheral vascular disorders, edema, abnormal EKG, proarrhythmias, QT interval prolongation, torsade de pointes, heart block, hypotension, syncope, sinus pauses

Central nervous system: Fatigue, dizziness, lightheadedness, confusion, anxiety, headache, insomnia, depression, mood change

Dermatologic: Rash

Endocrine & metabolic: Weight change, sexual dysfunction; hyperglycemia in diabetic patients

Gastrointestinal: Diarrhea, nausea, vomiting, dyspepsia, abdominal pain, abdominal distention, flatulence, appetite disorder

Hematologic: Bleeding

Neuromuscular & skeletal: Weakness, paresthesia, extremity pain, back pain

Ocular: Vision problems

Respiratory: Dyspnea, upper respiratory tract problems, cough, asthma

Miscellaneous: Sweating

Drug Interactions Drugs that prolong the QT interval (eg, class I and class III antiarrhythmics, phenothiazines, TCAs, astemizole, bepridil, and certain quinolone and oral macrolide antibiotics) may increase adverse cardiac effects (concomitant use of these drugs is not recommended); class I or III antiarrhythmics should be withheld for ≥3 half-lives prior to starting sotalol; in clinical studies, sotalol was not given to patients who were treated with oral amiodarone for >1 month in the previous 3 months; do not initiate sotalol after discontinuation of amiodarone until the QT interval is normalized; concomitant use with drugs that prolong refractoriness [class Ia (eg, disopyramide, quinidine, procainamide) and other class III (eg, amiodarone) antiarrhythmics] is not recommended; use with other beta-blockers may potentiate cardiovascular effects; calcium channel blockers may have additive effects on AV conduction, ventricular function, or blood pressure (use with caution)

Catecholamine-depleting drugs, such as reserpine, may have additive effects (hypotension, bradycardia); abrupt withdrawal of clonidine while receiving beta-blockers may result in an exaggerated hypertensive crisis; myocardial depressant general anesthetics may have additive effects with beta-blockers. Concomitant administration of magnesium- and aluminum-containing antacids will significantly decrease the oral absorption of sotalol (administer antacids 2 hours after sotalol); bronchodilation (Continued)

Sotalol (Continued)

effects of beta$_2$-adrenergic agonists may be antagonized by sotalol (increased doses of beta$_2$ agonists may be needed)

Food Interactions Food decreases oral absorption by ~20% compared to fasting

Stability Store at controlled room temperature 25°C (77°F); dispense in tight, light-resistant container

Mechanism of Action Beta-blocker with both class II antiarrhythmic (beta-adrenergic blockade) and class III antiarrhythmic (prolongation of the cardiac action potential duration) properties; does not possess partial agonist or membrane stabilizing activity. Class II effects: Nonselective beta-blockade; competitively blocks response to beta$_1$- and beta$_2$-adrenergic stimulation; decreases heart rate and AV nodal conduction; increases AV nodal refractoriness. Class III effects: Prolongs atrial and ventricular monophasic action potentials; prolongs the effective refractory period of atrial muscle, ventricular muscle, and AV accessory pathways (if present) in both antegrade and retrograde directions. Significant beta-blocking effects may be seen at lower doses (children: ≥90 mg/m^2/day; adults: 25 mg); class III electrophysiologic effects are seen at higher doses (children: 210 mg/m^2/day; adults: ≥160 mg/day). Sotalol is available as a racemic mixture; both isomers (d- and l-sotalol) have similar class III antiarrhythmic effects; the l-isomer is responsible for almost all of the beta-adrenergic blocking activity

Pharmacokinetics

Distribution: Poor penetration across blood-brain barrier; distributes into breast milk; breast milk to plasma ratio: 2.2-8.8 (mean: 5.4) (O'Hare, 1980)

Protein binding: Sotalol is not protein bound

Metabolism: Sotalol is not metabolized

Bioavailability: Oral: 90% to 100%

Half-life (mean):

Neonates ≤1 month: 8.4 hours

Infants and children >1 month to 24 months: 7.4 hours

Children >2 years to <7 years: 9.1 hours

Children 7-12 years: 9.2 hours

Adults: 12 hours

Adults with renal failure (anuric): Up to 69 hours

Time to peak serum concentration:

Children 4 days to 12 years: Mean: 2-3 hours

Adults: 2.5-4 hours

Elimination: Primarily as unchanged drug via the kidney

Clearance (apparent):

Neonates ≤1 month: 11 mL/minute

Infants and children >1 month to 24 months: 32 mL/minute

Children >2 years to <7 years: 63 mL/minute

Children 7-12 years: 95 mL/minute

Dialysis: Partially removed by hemodialysis; partial rebound in serum concentrations may occur following dialysis

Usual Dosage Oral: **Note:** Dosage must be adjusted to individual response and tolerance; doses should be initiated or increased in a hospital facility that can provide continuous EKG monitoring, recognition and treatment of life-threatening arrhythmias, and CPR (see Warnings):

Neonates, Infants, and Children: **Note:** Safety and efficacy in pediatric patients have not been established; manufacturer's dosing recommendations are based on doses per m^2 (that are equivalent to the doses recommended in adults) and on pediatric pharmacokinetic and pharmacodynamic studies (see Saul, 2001 and Saul, 2001a). BSA, rather than body weight, better predicted apparent clearance of sotalol; however, for a given dose per m^2, a larger drug exposure (larger AUC) and greater pharmacologic effects were observed in smaller subjects (ie, those with BSA <0.33 m^2 versus those with BSA ≥0.33 m^2). For infants and children ≤2 years of age, the manufacturer recommends a dosage reduction based on an age factor determined from a graph (see next page).

Manufacturer's recommendations: **Note:** Use with extreme caution if QT$_c$ is >500 msec while receiving sotalol; reduce the dose or discontinue drug if QT$_c$ >550 msec

Neonates, infants, and children ≤2 years: The pediatric dosage listed below must be reduced by an age-related factor that is obtained from the graph (see graph). First, obtain the patient's age in months; use the graph to determine where the patient's age (on the logarithmic scale) intersects the age factor curve; read the age factor from the Y-axis ; then multiply the age factor by the pediatric dose listed below (ie, the dose for children >2 years); this will result in the proper reduction in dose for age. For example, the age factor for an infant 1 month of age is 0.68, so the initial dosage would be (0.68 x 30 mg/m²/dose) = 20 mg/m²/dose given 3 times daily. Similar calculations should be made for dosage titrations; increase dosage gradually, if needed; allow adequate time between dosage increments to achieve new steady-state and to monitor clinical response, heart rate and QT_c intervals; half-life is prolonged with decreasing age (<2 years), so time to reach new steady-state will increase; for example, the time to reach steady-state in a neonate may be ≥1 week

Sotalol Age Factor Nomogram for Patients ≤2 Years of Age

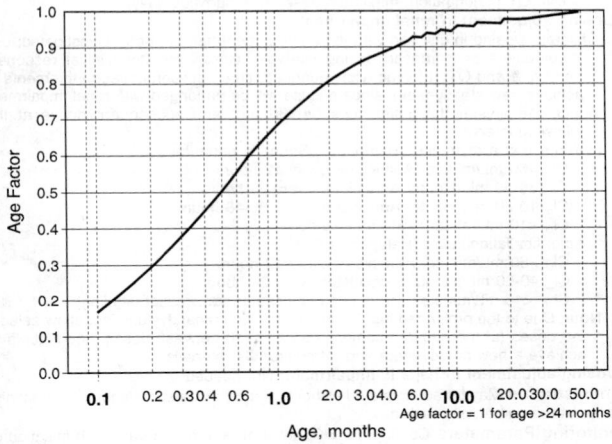

Adapted from U.S. Food and Drug Administration.
http://www.fda.gov/cder/foi/label/2001/2115s3lbl.PDF

Children >2 years: Initial: 30 mg/m²/dose given 3 times daily; increase dosage gradually if needed; allow at least 36 hours between dosage increments to achieve new steady-state and to monitor clinical response, heart rate, and QT_c intervals; may increase gradually to a maximum of 60 mg/m²/dose given 3 times daily

Alternative pediatric dosing: Initial: 2 mg/kg/day divided in 2-3 doses/day; if needed, increase dosage gradually by 1-2 mg/kg/day increments, allow 3 days between dosage increments to achieve new steady-state and to monitor clinical response, heart rate and QT_c intervals; maximum: 8 mg/kg/day (Pfammatter, 1997); do not exceed adult doses; **Note:** Although clinical studies have not assessed the relationship between mg/kg/day doses and age, it appears that the mean effective mg/kg/day dose for infants is less than in older children (see Tipple, 1991; Maragnes, 1992; Colloridi, 1992; Pfammatter, 1995; Beaufort-Krol, 1997).

Adults:

Ventricular arrhythmias (Betapace®, Sorine™, generic) (**Note:** Use with extreme caution if QT_c is >500 msec while receiving sotalol; reduce the dose or discontinue drug if QT_c >550 msec):

Initial: 80 mg twice daily; increase dosage gradually if needed; allow 3 days between dosage increments to achieve new steady-state and to determine maximum effects on QT interval; may increase gradually to 240-320 mg/day in 2 divided doses; usual effective dose: 160-320 mg/day given in 2-3 divided doses; **Note:** Doses as high as 480-640 mg/day may be required in some patients with life-threatening refractory ventricular arrhythmias; however, potential benefit must outweigh increased risk of adverse effects (eg, proarrhythmias).

Atrial fibrillation or atrial flutter (Betapace AF™): [**Note:** If baseline QT interval is >450 msec, do not initiate therapy (see Contraindications). During initiation and dose titration, if the QT interval is ≥500 msec, reduce the dose or discontinue the

(Continued)

1035

Sotalol *(Continued)*

drug. During maintenance therapy, monitor the QT interval regularly; if the QT interval is ≥520 msec, reduce the dose or discontinue the drug]:

Initial: 80 mg twice daily; increase dosage gradually after 3 days, if needed [ie, if frequency of relapses of atrial fibrillation/flutter is not reduced and the dose is tolerated without excessive QT prolongation (ie, if QT interval is <520 msec)]; allow 3 days between dosage increments to achieve new steady-state and to determine maximum effects on QT interval; reduce the dose or discontinue the drug if the QT interval is ≥500 msec; dose may be increased to 120 mg twice daily (usual effective dose); the dosage may be further increased to 160 mg twice daily if response is inadequate and the dose is tolerated without excessive QT prolongation; maximum dose: 160 mg twice daily.

Dosing adjustment in renal impairment:

Children: Dosing in children with renal impairment has not been investigated; use lower doses or increased dosing intervals; closely monitor clinical response, heart rate and QT$_c$ interval; allow adequate time between dosage increments to achieve new steady-state, since half-life will be prolonged with renal impairment

Adults: Administer the initial dose (ie, 80 mg) and subsequent doses at the following intervals:

Ventricular arrhythmias (Betapace®, Sorine™, generic):

Cl$_{cr}$ >60 mL/minute: Administer every 12 hours

Cl$_{cr}$ 30-59 mL/minute: Administer every 24 hours

Cl$_{cr}$ 10-29 mL/minute: Administer every 36-48 hours

Cl$_{cr}$ <10 mL/minute: Individualize dose

Atrial fibrillation/flutter (Betapace AF™):

Cl$_{cr}$ >60 mL/minute: Administer every 12 hours

Cl$_{cr}$ 40-60 mL/minute: Administer every 24 hours

Cl$_{cr}$ <40 mL/minute: Use is contraindicated (per product labeling)

Note: Due to the prolonged half-life in patients with renal dysfunction, allow at least 5-6 doses (at the above recommended interval) between dosage increments to achieve a new steady-state and to monitor QT intervals

Dosing adjustment in hepatic impairment: Not needed

Administration May be administered without regard to meals, but should be administered at the same time each day

Monitoring Parameters Continuous EKG for a minimum of 3 days with initiation of therapy or dosage increase, QT interval, heart rate, renal function, serum potassium and magnesium

Betapace AF™: In addition, during initiation and dosage titration, monitor the QT interval 2-4 hours after each dose

Test Interactions May falsely elevate urinary metanephrine values when fluorimetric or photometric methods are used; does not interact with HPLC assay with solid phase extraction for determination of urinary catecholamines

Patient Information Take sotalol every day as prescribed; do not change dose or discontinue without physician's advice; if a dose is missed, do not double the next dose, take the next dose at the usual time. Avoid abrupt discontinuation; if sotalol is to be discontinued, physician will advise how to slowly taper the dose over 1-2 weeks. May cause drowsiness and impair ability to perform activities requiring mental alertness or physical coordination. Regular cardiac checkups, EKGs, and blood tests will be needed while taking this medication. Report the use of other medications, nonprescription medications, and herbal or natural products to your physician and pharmacist; do not start new medications without checking with your physician and pharmacist; tell your dentist and physician that you are taking sotalol before you have dental surgery or an operation (sotalol may interact with certain anesthetic agents). Report fast heartbeats, dizziness, or fainting immediately to your physician or go to an emergency room (these may be signs of an abnormal heartbeat); report severe diarrhea, unusual sweating, vomiting, increased thirst, or decreased appetite immediately to your physician (these may be things that make an abnormal heartbeat more likely to occur); report chest pain, fast heartbeat, swelling of ankles or legs, difficulty breathing or unusual cough to your physician (these may be serious side effects of the medication).

Nursing Implications Be prepared to recognize and treat cardiac arrhythmias; lidocaine and other resuscitative measures should be available (see Warnings)

Additional Information Betapace AF™: Do not discharge patients from the hospital within 12 hours of electrical or pharmacological conversion from atrial fibrillation/flutter to normal sinus rhythm.

Dosage Forms

Tablet, as hydrochloride: 80 mg, 120 mg, 160 mg, 240 mg

Betapace®, Sorine™: 80 mg, 120 mg, 160 mg, 240 mg

Betapace AF™: 80 mg, 120 mg, 160 mg

Extemporaneous Preparations A 5 mg/mL syrup of sotalol hydrochloride made from Betapace® or Betapace AF™ tablets and Simple Syrup containing 0.1% sodium benzoate (Syrup, NF) is stable for 3 months when stored at controlled room temperature (15°C to 30°C; 59°F to 86°F) and ambient humidity; place 120 mL of Syrup, NF into a 6 ounce amber plastic (polyethylene terephthalate) prescription bottle; add five Betapace® or Betapace AF™ 120 mg tablets; shake the bottle to wet the tablets; allow tablets to hydrate for at least 2 hours; then shake intermittently over ≥2 hours until the tablets are completely disintegrated; a dispersion of fine particles (water-insoluble inactive ingredients) in syrup should be obtained (**Note:** To simplify the disintegration process, tablets can hydrate overnight; tablets may also be crushed, carefully transferred into the bottle and shaken well until a dispersion of fine particles in syrup is obtained); label "shake well" [Betapace® and Betapace AF™ tablets (package inserts), 2001].

A 5 mg/mL liquid formulation of sotalol hydrochloride made from 160 mg tablets [Sotocor® (from Canada)] and a suspending vehicle (300 mL of Simple Syrup and 700 mL of a methylcellulose 1% gel containing sodium benzoate) was stable and had no evidence of microbial growth for 8 weeks when stored in amber glass bottles under refrigeration (4°C); **Note:** Microbial growth was observed in samples stored at room temperature; to prepare the methylcellulose 1% gel and the suspending vehicle, see reference; label "shake well" and "refrigerate" (Dupuis, 1988).

Betapace® and Betapace AF™ (package inserts), Wayne, NJ: Berlex Laboratories; 2001

Dupuis LL, James G, and Bacola G, "Stability of Sotalol Hydrochloride Oral Liquid Formulation," *Canadian Journal of Hospital Pharmacy*, 1988, 41(3):121-3.

References

Beaufort-Krol GC and Bink-Boelkens MT, "Effectiveness of Sotalol for Atrial Flutter in Children After Surgery for Congenital Heart Disease," *Am J Cardiol*, 1997, 79(1):92-4.

Colloridi V, Perri C, Ventriglia F, et al, "Oral Sotalol in Pediatric Atrial Ectopic Tachycardia," *Am Heart J*, 1992, 123(1):254-6.

Maragnes P, Tipple M, and Fournier A, "Effectiveness of Oral Sotalol for Treatment of Pediatric Arrhythmias," *Am J Cardiol*, 1992, 69(8):751-4.

O'Hare MF, Murnaghan GA, Russell CJ, et al, "Sotalol as a Hypotensive Agent in Pregnancy," *Br J Obstet Gynaecol*, 1980, 87(9):814-20.

Pfammatter JP and Paul T, "New Antiarrhythmic Drug in Pediatric Use: Sotalol," *Pediatr Cardiol*, 1997, 18(1):28-34.

Pfammatter JP, Paul T, Lehmann C, et al, "Efficacy and Proarrhythmia of Oral Sotalol in Pediatric Patients," *J Am Coll Cardiol*, 1995, 26(4):1002-7.

Saul JP, Ross B, Schaffer MS, et al, "Pharmacokinetics and Pharmacodynamics of Sotalol in a Pediatric Population With Supraventricular and Ventricular Tachyarrhythmia," *Clin Pharmacol Ther*, 2001, 69(3):145-57.

Saul JP, Schaffer MS, Karpawich PP, et al, "Single-Dose Pharmacokinetics of Sotalol in a Pediatric Population With Supraventricular and/or Ventricular Tachyarrhythmia," *J Clin Pharmacol*, 2001a, 41(1):35-43.

Tanel RE, Walsh EP, Lulu JA, et al, "Sotalol for Refractory Arrhythmias in Pediatric and Young Adult Patients: Initial Efficacy and Long-Term Outcome," *Am Heart J*, 1995, 130(4):791-7.

Tipple M and Sandor G, "Efficacy and Safety of Oral Sotalol in Early Infancy," *Pacing Clin Electrophysiol*, 1991, 14(11 Pt 2):2062-5.

- ◆ **Spacol** *see Hyoscyamine on page 585*
- ◆ **Spacol T/S** *see Hyoscyamine on page 585*
- ◆ **Spectazole®** *see Econazole on page 423*
- ◆ **SpectroGram 2™ (Can)** *see Chlorhexidine Gluconate on page 257*
- ◆ **SpectroTar Skin Wash™ (Can)** *see Coal Tar on page 299*

Spironolactone (speer on oh LAK tone)

U.S. Brand Names Aldactone®

Canadian Brand Names Novo-Spiroton

Therapeutic Category Antihypertensive Agent; Diuretic, Potassium Sparing

Generic Available Yes

Use Management of edema associated with CHF, cirrhosis of the liver accompanied by edema or ascites, and nephrotic syndrome; treatment of essential hypertension, primary hyperaldosteronism, hypokalemia, and hirsutism

Pregnancy Risk Factor C

Contraindications Hypersensitivity to spironolactone or any component; renal failure, anuria, hyperkalemia

Warnings Spironolactone has been shown to be tumorigenic in toxicity studies using 25-250 times the usual human dose in rats; use in combination with ACE inhibitors, potassium, and NSAIDs may result in severe hyperkalemia; monitor potassium levels closely

Precautions Use with caution in patients with dehydration, hyponatremia, impaired renal clearance (Cl_{cr} <50 mL/minute) or hepatic dysfunction; patients receiving other potassium-sparing diuretics or potassium supplements

(Continued)

Spironolactone *(Continued)*

Adverse Reactions

Cardiovascular: Arrhythmia

Central nervous system: Lethargy, headache, mental confusion, fever, ataxia

Dermatologic: Rash, urticaria

Endocrine & metabolic: Hyperkalemia, dehydration, hyponatremia, hyperchloremic metabolic acidosis, postmenopausal bleeding, amenorrhea, gynecomastia (in males); breast tenderness, deepening of voice, and increased hair growth (in females)

Gastrointestinal: Anorexia, nausea, vomiting, diarrhea, gastritis, cramping, gastric bleeding

Genitourinary: Dysuria

Hematologic: Agranulocytosis

Neuromuscular & skeletal: Weakness, numbness or paresthesia in hands, feet or lips, lower back or side pain

Renal: Decreased renal function (including renal failure)

Respiratory: Cough, shortness of breath, dyspnea, hoarseness

Drug Interactions Potassium, other potassium-sparing diuretics, NSAIDs, and ACE inhibitors (eg, captopril) may additively increase the serum potassium; may decrease digoxin clearance and attenuate its inotropic effect; decreased hypoprothrombinemic effect of oral anticoagulants; decreases vascular response to norepinephrine; salicylates may interfere with natriuretic action of spironolactone

Food Interactions Avoid natural licorice (causes sodium and water retention and increases potassium loss) and salt substitutes; avoid diets high in potassium

Mechanism of Action Competes with aldosterone for receptor sites in the distal renal tubules, increasing sodium chloride and water excretion while conserving potassium and hydrogen ions; may block the effect of aldosterone on arteriolar smooth muscle as well

Pharmacokinetics

Distribution: V_d: Breast milk to plasma ratio: 0.51-0.72

Protein binding: 91% to 98%

Metabolism: In the liver to multiple metabolites, including canrenone (active)

Half-life:

Spironolactone: 78-84 minutes

Canrenone: 13-24 hours

Time to peak serum concentration: Within 1-3 hours (primarily as the active metabolite)

Elimination: Urinary and biliary

Usual Dosage Oral:

Neonates: Diuretic: 1-3 mg/kg/day every 12-24 hours

Children:

Diuretic, hypertension: 1.5-3.3 mg/kg/day or 60 mg/m²/day in divided doses every 6-24 hours

Diagnosis of primary aldosteronism: 100-400 mg/m²/day in 1-2 divided doses

Adults:

Edema, hypertension, hypokalemia: 25-200 mg/day in 1-2 divided doses

Diagnosis of primary aldosteronism: 400 mg/day; if a positive diagnosis is established, continue treatment; 100-400 mg/day in 1-2 divided doses

Hirsutism in women: 50-200 mg/day in 1-2 divided doses

CHF: Patients with severe heart failure already using an ACE inhibitor and a loop diuretic ± digoxin: 25 mg/day, increase or reduce depending on individual response and evidence of hyperkalemia

Dosing interval in renal impairment:

Cl_{cr} 10-50 mL/minute: Administer every 12-24 hours

Cl_{cr} <10 mL/minute: Avoid use

Administration Oral: Administer with food

Monitoring Parameters Serum potassium, sodium, and renal function

Test Interactions May cause false elevation in serum digoxin concentrations measured by RIA

Patient Information May cause drowsiness and impair ability to perform activities requiring mental alertness or physical coordination

Dosage Forms Tablet: 25 mg, 50 mg, 100 mg

Extemporaneous Preparations

A 1 mg/mL suspension may be compounded by crushing ten 25 mg tablets, add a small amount of water and soak for 5 minutes; add 50 mL 1.5% carboxymethylcellulose, 100 mL syrup NF, and mix; use a sufficient quantity of purified water to a total volume of 250 mL; stable at room temperature or refrigerated for 3 months (Nahata, 1993)

A 2.5 mg/mL suspension may be made by crushing twelve 25 mg tablets, levigating with a small amount of distilled water or glycerin; dilute with cherry syrup to make a final volume of 120 mL; stable 28 days when refrigerated (Mathur, 1989)

A 5 mg/mL suspension may be made by crushing twenty-four 25 mg tablets, levigating with a small amount of distilled water or glycerin; dilute with cherry syrup to a total volume of 120 mL; stable 28 days refrigerated (Mathur, 1989)

A 25 mg/mL suspension may be made by crushing one-hundred twenty-five 25 mg tablets, add in geometric proportions a 1:1 mixture of Ora-Sweet® and Ora-Plus® or Ora-Sweet® SF and Ora-Plus® to a total volume of 120 mL; stable 60 days refrigerated stored in amber bottles; shake well (Allen, 1996)

Allen LV and Erickson MA, "Stability of Labetalol Hydrochloride, Metoprolol Tartrate, Verapamil Hydrochloride, and Spironolactone With Hydrochlorothiazide in Extemporaneously Compounded Oral Liquids," *Am J Health Syst Pharm*, 1996, 53(19):2304-9.

Mathur LK and Wickman A, "Stability of Extemporaneously Compounded Spironolactone Suspensions," *Am J Hosp Pharm*, 1989, 46(10):2040-2.

Nahata MC, Morosco RS, and Hipple TF, "Stability of Spironolactone in an Extemporaneously Prepared Suspension at Two Temperatures," *Ann Pharmacother*, 1993, 27:1198-9.

♦ **Spironolactone and Hydrochlorothiazide** *see* Hydrochlorothiazide and Spironolactone *on page 570*

♦ **Sporanox®** *see* Itraconazole *on page 634*

♦ **SPS®** *see* Sodium Polystyrene Sulfonate *on page 1029*

♦ **SSD®** *see* Silver Sulfadiazine *on page 1019*

♦ **SSD® AF** *see* Silver Sulfadiazine *on page 1019*

♦ **SSKI®** *see* Potassium Iodide *on page 918*

♦ **Stagesic®** *see* Hydrocodone and Acetaminophen *on page 571*

♦ **Stan-gard®** *see* Fluoride *on page 500*

♦ **Statex® (Can)** *see* Morphine Sulfate *on page 778*

♦ **Staticin®** *see* Erythromycin *on page 448*

♦ **Stat Touch 2® [OTC] [DSC]** *see* Chlorhexidine Gluconate *on page 257*

Stavudine (STAV yoo deen)

Related Information
Adult and Adolescent HIV *on page 1327*
Pediatric HIV *on page 1323*

U.S. Brand Names Zerit®

Synonyms d4T; 2',3'-didehydro-3'-deoxythymidine

Therapeutic Category Antiretroviral Agent; HIV Agents (Anti-HIV Agents); Nucleoside Reverse Transcriptase Inhibitor (NRTI)

Generic Available No

Use Treatment of HIV infection in combination with other antiretroviral agents. (**Note:** HIV regimens consisting of **three** antiretroviral agents are strongly recommended)

Pregnancy Risk Factor C

Contraindications Hypersensitivity to stavudine or any component

Warnings The major clinical toxicity of stavudine is peripheral neuropathy which has occurred in 15% to 21% of patients in controlled trials; lactic acidosis and severe hepatomegaly with steatosis is a rare but potentially life-threatening toxicity associated with the use of NRTIs. Risk may be increased in obesity, prolonged nucleoside exposure, or in female patients. Severe motor weakness (resembling Guillain-Barré syndrome) has been reported, usually in association with lactic acidosis; manufacturer recommends prompt suspension of all antiretroviral therapy in suspected cases of lactic acidosis with or without neuromuscular weakness. Fatal and nonfatal pancreatitis has occurred during combination therapy which included didanosine with or without hydroxyurea.

Precautions Fat redistribution and accumulation [ie, central obesity, peripheral wasting, facial wasting, breast enlargement, dorsocervical fat enlargement (buffalo hump), and cushingoid appearance] have been observed in patients receiving antiretroviral agents (causal relationship not established). Use with caution in patients with a history of peripheral neuropathy, or hepatic or renal impairment; dosage adjustment required in patients with impaired renal function

Adverse Reactions
Central nervous system: Headache, fever, insomnia, malaise, dizziness, nervousness, increased energy, mania

Dermatologic: Rash, pruritus

Endocrine & metabolic: Lactic acidosis; redistribution of body fat to cause buffalo hump, facial atrophy, and breast enlargement

(Continued)

Stavudine *(Continued)*

Gastrointestinal: Abdominal pain, diarrhea, nausea, vomiting, anorexia, pancreatitis

Hematologic: Anemia, leukopenia, thrombocytopenia

Hepatic: Elevated AST and ALT, hepatic steatosis, hepatitis, elevated bilirubin

Neuromuscular & skeletal: Peripheral neuropathy (tingling, burning, pain, numbness of hands or feet), weakness, myalgia

Otic: Ear pain

Respiratory: Rhinitis, cough

Drug Interactions Drugs associated with peripheral neuropathy (chloramphenicol, cisplatin, dapsone, ethionamide, gold, hydralazine, iodoquinol, isoniazid, lithium, metronidazole, nitrofurantoin, pentamidine, phenytoin, ribavirin, vincristine) may increase risk for stavudine peripheral neuropathy; drugs that decrease renal function could decrease clearance of stavudine; stavudine should not be administered in combination with zidovudine (poor antiretroviral effect); concurrent use with didanosine and hydroxyurea may increase risk of pancreatitis, lactic acidosis, and severe hepatomegaly; methadone may decrease stavudine levels by 27% (no dosage adjustment needed)

Stability

Capsules: Store in tightly closed containers at room temperature

Oral solution: Reconstitute powder for oral solution according to manufacturer's instructions; keep refrigerated; solution is stable for 30 days

Mechanism of Action Antiviral activity is dependent on intracellular conversion of stavudine to the active metabolite d4-triphosphate; Inhibits replication of retroviruses by competing with thymidine triphosphate for viral RNA-directed DNA polymerase and incorporation into DNA

Pharmacokinetics

Distribution: Penetrates into the CSF achieving 16% to 97% of concomitant plasma concentrations; distributes into extravascular spaces

V_d: Children: 18.5 ± 9.2 L/m^2

Metabolism: Converted intracellularly to active triphosphate form

Bioavailability: Children: 61% to 78%; adults: 80%

Half-life, elimination: Children: 1.1 hours; adults: 1.2-1.45 hours

Time to peak serum concentration: 0.5-0.75 hours

Elimination: 24% to 57% is excreted unchanged in the urine

Usual Dosage Oral:

Neonates: Under investigation in PACTG 332

Children <30 kg: 1 mg/kg/dose every 12 hours; do not exceed adult doses

Adolescent and Adults:

30-59 kg: 30 mg every 12 hours

≥60 kg: 40 mg every 12 hours

Dosing adjustment in renal impairment:

Cl_{cr} 26-50 mL/minute: Decrease dose by 50% (eg, ≥60 kg: administer 20 mg every 12 hours)

Cl_{cr} <10-25 mL/minute: Decrease dose by 75% (eg, ≥60 kg: administer 20 mg every 24 hours)

Dosing adjustment in hepatic impairment: no data

Administration Oral: Administer with or without food; shake solution well before using

Monitoring Parameters Periodic CBC with differential, hemoglobin, renal function, liver enzymes, serum amylase, CD4 cell count, HIV RNA plasma levels, signs/symptoms of peripheral neuropathy

Patient Information Stavudine is not a cure for HIV. Avoid alcohol. Notify physician if tingling, burning, pain, numbness of hands or feet, abdominal discomfort, nausea, vomiting, fatigue, dyspnea, or motor weakness occurs

HIV medications may cause changes in body fat, including an increase in fat in the upper back and neck, breasts, and trunk; a loss of fat from the face, arms, and legs may also occur.

Dosage Forms

Capsule: 15 mg, 20 mg, 30 mg, 40 mg

Powder for oral solution: 1 mg/mL (200 mL) [dye free; fruit flavor]

References

Kline MW, Dunkle LM, Church JA, et al, "A Phase I/II Evaluation of Stavudine (d4T) in Children With Human Immunodeficiency Virus Infection," *Pediatrics*, 1995, 96(2 Pt 1):247-52.

Working Group on Antiretroviral Therapy and Medical Management of HIV-Infected Children, "Guidelines for the Use of Antiretroviral Agents in Pediatric HIV Infection," December 14, 2001, http://www.aidsinfo.nih.gov.

◆ **Stemetil®** *(Can)* *see* Prochlorperazine *on page 938*
◆ **Sterapred®** *see* PredniSONE *on page 928*
◆ **Sterapred® DS** *see* PredniSONE *on page 928*

- **Stimate®** *see Desmopressin on page 352*
- **St. Joseph Pain Reliever [OTC]** *see Aspirin on page 134*
- **Stop®** *see Fluoride on page 500*
- **Strattera™** *see Atomoxetine on page 138*
- **Streptase®** *see Streptokinase on page 1041*

Streptokinase (strep toe KYE nase)

Related Information
Antithrombotic Therapy in Children *on page 1316*

U.S. Brand Names Streptase®

Therapeutic Category Thrombolytic Agent; Thrombotic Occlusion (Central Venous Catheter), Treatment Agent

Generic Available No

Use Thrombolytic agent used in treatment of recent severe or massive deep vein thrombosis, pulmonary emboli, MI, arterial thrombosis or embolism, and occluded arteriovenous cannulas

Pregnancy Risk Factor C

Contraindications Hypersensitivity to streptokinase or any component; recent streptococcal infection; any internal bleeding; CVA or intracranial or intraspinal surgery (within 2 months); severe uncontrolled hypertension; brain carcinoma

Warnings Bleeding may occur; avoid I.M. injections

Precautions Relative contraindications: major surgery within the last 10 days, GI bleeding, recent trauma, severe hypertension

Adverse Reactions
Cardiovascular: Hypotension, arrhythmias, flushing
Central nervous system: Fever
Dermatologic: Itching, urticaria, angioneurotic edema
Hematologic: Surface bleeding, internal bleeding, cerebral hemorrhage
Neuromuscular & skeletal: Musculoskeletal pain
Respiratory: Bronchospasm

Drug Interactions Anticoagulants, antiplatelet agents, antifibrinolytic agents

Stability Store unopened vials at room temperature; store reconstituted solutions in refrigerator and use within 24 hours

Mechanism of Action Promotes thrombolysis; activates the conversion of plasminogen to plasmin by forming a complex, exposing plasminogen-activating site, and cleaving a peptide bond that converts plasminogen to plasmin; plasmin degrades fibrin, fibrinogen and other procoagulant proteins into soluble fragments; effective both outside and within the formed thrombus/embolus

Pharmacodynamics
Onset of action: Activation of plasminogen: Almost immediate
Duration:
Fibrinolytic effects: Only a few hours
Anticoagulant effects: 12-24 hours

Pharmacokinetics
Half-life, biologic: 83 minutes
Elimination: By circulating antibodies and via the reticuloendothelial system

Usual Dosage
Children: Safety and efficacy not established
Thromboses: I.V.: *Chest*, 2001 recommendations: Initial (loading dose): 2000 units/kg followed by 2000 units/kg/hour for 6-12 hours; some patients may require longer or shorter courses of treatment; dose should be individualized based on response
Clotted catheter: **Note: Not recommended** due to possibility of allergic reactions with repeated doses: 10,000-25,000 units diluted in NS to a final volume equivalent to catheter volume; instill into catheter and leave in place for 1 hour, then aspirate contents out of catheter and flush catheter with NS
Adults:
Thromboses: I.V.: 250,000 units to start, then 100,000 units/hour for 24-72 hours depending on location
Cannula occlusion: **Note:** Not recommended due to possibility of allergic reactions with repeated doses: 250,000 units into cannula, clamp for 2 hours, then aspirate contents out of catheter and flush with NS; **Note:** Serious adverse effects (hypersensitivity reactions, hypotension, apnea, and bleeding), some of which were life-threatening, have been reported with this use and dose; lower doses of 3000 units/hour for 12-24 hours infused into each lumen have been successfully used (see Phelps, 2001)

Administration Parenteral: I.V.: Dilute in NS (preferred) or D_5W; maximum concentration: 1.5 million units/50 mL
(Continued)

Streptokinase *(Continued)*

Monitoring Parameters For systemic therapy: Blood pressure, thrombin clotting time, PTT, APTT, fibrinogen level, fibrin/fibrinogen degradation products, D-dimers, platelet count, hemoglobin, hematocrit, signs of bleeding

Nursing Implications For intravenous or intracoronary use only; avoid I.M. injections

Additional Information Best results are realized if used within 5-6 hours of MI; antibodies to streptokinase remain for 3-6 months after initial dose, use another thrombolytic enzyme (ie, urokinase) if repeat thrombolytic therapy is indicated

Failure of thrombolytic agents in newborns/neonates may occur due to the low plasminogen concentrations (~50% to 70% of adult levels); streptokinase- induced clot lysis may be more impaired than urokinase or TPA in these patients; supplementing plasminogen (via administration of fresh frozen plasma) may possibly help

Dosage Forms Injection, powder for reconstitution, lyophilized: 250,000 units; 750,000 units; 1,500,000 units

References

Andrew M, Brooker L, Leaker M, et al,"Fibrin Clot Lysis by Thrombolytic Agents Is Impaired in Newborns Due to a Low Plasminogen Concentration," *Thromb Haemost*, 1992, 68(3):325-30.

Kothari SS, Varma S, and Wasir HS, "Thrombolytic Therapy in Infants and Children," *Am Heart J*, 1994, 127(3):651-7.

Monagle P, Michelson AD, Bovill E, et al, "Antithrombotic Therapy in Children," *Chest*, 2001, 119:344S-70S.

Nowak-Göttl U, Auberger K, Halimeh S, et al, "Thrombolysis in Newborns and Infants," *Thromb Haemost*, 1999, 82(Suppl 1):112-6.

Phelps KC and Verazino KC, "Alternatives to Urokinase for the Management of Central Venous Catheter Occlusion," *Hospital Pharmacy*, 2001, 36(3): 265-74.

Streptomycin *(strep toe MYE sin)*

Related Information

Overdose and Toxicology *on page 1388*

Therapeutic Category Antibiotic, Aminoglycoside; Antitubercular Agent

Generic Available Yes

Use Combination therapy of active tuberculosis; used in combination with other agents for treatment of streptococcal or enterococcal endocarditis, mycobacterial infections, plague, tularemia, and brucellosis

Pregnancy Risk Factor D

Contraindications Hypersensitivity to streptomycin or any component

Warnings Aminoglycosides are associated with significant nephrotoxicity or ototoxicity; the ototoxicity is directly proportional to the amount of drug given and the duration of treatment; tinnitus or vertigo are indications of vestibular injury and impending bilateral irreversible deafness; renal damage is usually reversible

Precautions Use with caution in patients with pre-existing vertigo, tinnitus, hearing loss, neuromuscular disorders, or renal impairment; modify dosage in patients with renal impairment

Adverse Reactions

Cardiovascular: Myocarditis, cardiovascular collapse

Central nervous system: Dizziness, vertigo, headache, ataxia

Dermatologic: Toxic epidermal necrolysis

Gastrointestinal: Vomiting

Hematologic: Bone marrow suppression

Neuromuscular & skeletal: Neuromuscular blockade

Otic: Ototoxicity, hearing loss

Renal: Nephrotoxicity

Miscellaneous: Hypersensitivity reactions, serum sickness

Drug Interactions Additive nephrotoxicity with acyclovir, amphotericin B, cisplatin, vancomycin; additive ototoxicity with ethacrynic acid, furosemide, urea, mannitol; potentiates neuromuscular blocking action of succinylcholine, tubocurarine

Stability Streptomycin injection should be stored in the refrigerator

Mechanism of Action Inhibits bacterial protein synthesis by binding directly to the 30S ribosomal subunits causing faulty peptide sequence to form in the protein chain

Pharmacokinetics

Distribution: Distributes into most body tissues and fluids except the brain; small amounts enter the CSF only with inflamed meninges; crosses the placenta; small amounts appear in breast milk

Protein binding: 34%

Half-life (prolonged with renal impairment):

Newborns: 4-10 hours

Adults: 2-4.7 hours

Time to peak serum concentration: I.M.: Within 1-2 hours

Elimination: 30% to 90% of dose excreted as unchanged drug in urine, with small amount (1%) excreted in bile, saliva, sweat, and tears

Usual Dosage I.M. (I.V. in patients who cannot tolerate I.M. injections):
Newborns: 10-20 mg/kg/day once daily
Infants: 20-30 mg/kg/day in divided doses every 12 hours
Children:
Tuberculosis: 20-40 mg/kg/day once daily, not to exceed 1 g/day; **or** 20-40 mg/kg/dose twice weekly under direct observation, not to exceed 1.5 g/dose; usually discontinued after 2-3 months of therapy or as soon as isoniazid and rifampin susceptibility is established
Other infections: 20-40 mg/kg/day in combination with other antibiotics divided every 6-12 hours
Plague: 30 mg/kg/day divided every 8-12 hours
Adults:
Tuberculosis: 15 mg/kg/day once daily, not to exceed 1 g/day; **or** 25-30 mg/kg/dose twice weekly under direct observation, not to exceed 1.5 g/dose
Enterococcal endocarditis: 1 g every 12 hours for 2 weeks, then 500 mg every 12 hours for 4 weeks in combination with penicillin
Streptococcal endocarditis: 1 g every 12 hours for 1 week, then 500 mg every 12 hours for 1 week
Tularemia: 1-2 g/day in divided doses for 7-10 days or until patient is afebrile for 5-7 days
Plague: 2 g/day in divided doses until the patient is afebrile for at least 3 days
Dosing adjustment in renal impairment:
Cl_{cr} 50-80 mL/minute: Administer 7.5 mg/kg/dose every 24 hours
Cl_{cr} 10-50 mL/minute: Administer 7.5 mg/kg/dose every 24-72 hours
Cl_{cr} <10 mL/minute: Administer 7.5 mg/kg/dose every 72-96 hours
Administration Parenteral:
I.M.: Inject deep I.M. into a large muscle mass; administer at a concentration not to exceed 500 mg/mL; rotate injection sites
I.V.: I.V. infusion through a peripheral or central line; 12-15 mg/kg/dose is diluted in 100 mL of NS; infuse over 30-60 minutes
Monitoring Parameters Hearing (audiogram), BUN, creatinine; serum concentration of the drug should be monitored in patients with renal impairment; eighth cranial nerve damage is usually preceded by high-pitched tinnitus, roaring noises, sense of fullness in ears, or impaired hearing and may persist for weeks after drug is discontinued
Reference Range Therapeutic serum concentrations: Peak: 15-40 µg/mL; trough: <5 µg/mL
Test Interactions False-positive urine glucose with Benedict's solution
Additional Information For use by patients with active tuberculosis that is resistant to isoniazid and rifampin or patients with active tuberculosis in areas where resistance is common and whose drug susceptibility is not yet known. Pfizer will distribute streptomycin directly to physicians and health clinics at no charge. Call Pfizer at 1-800-254-4445.
Dosage Forms
Injection, powder for reconstitution, as sulfate: 1 g
References
Ad Hoc Committee of the Scientific Assembly on Microbiology, Tuberculosis, and Pulmonary Infections, "Treatment of Tuberculosis and Tuberculosis Infection in Adults and Children," *Clin Infect Dis*, 1995, 21:9-27.
American Academy of Pediatrics Committee on Infectious Diseases, "Chemotherapy for Tuberculosis in Infants and Children," *Pediatrics* 1992, 89(1):161-5.
Arguedas AG and Wehrle PP, "New Concepts for Antimicrobial Use in Central Nervous System Infections," *Semin Pediatr Infect Dis*, 1991, 2(1):36-42.
Lorin MI, Hsu KH, and Jacob SC, "Treatment of Tuberculosis in Children," *Pediatr Clin North Am*, 1983, 30(2):333-48.

♦ **Stridex® [OTC]** see Salicylic Acid on page 1002
♦ **Stridex® Body Focus [OTC]** see Salicylic Acid on page 1002
♦ **Stridex® Facewipes To Go™ [OTC]** see Salicylic Acid on page 1002
♦ **Stridex® Maximum Strength [OTC]** see Salicylic Acid on page 1002
♦ **Strifon Forte® (Can)** see Chlorzoxazone on page 266
♦ **Strong Iodine Solution** see Potassium Iodide on page 918
♦ **Sublimaze®** see Fentanyl on page 479

Succimer (SUKS i mer)
U.S. Brand Names Chemet®
Synonyms DMSA
Therapeutic Category Antidote, Lead Toxicity; Chelating Agent, Oral
Generic Available No
Use Treatment of lead poisoning in children with blood levels >45 mcg/dL; not indicated for prophylaxis of lead poisoning in a lead-containing environment
(Continued)

Succimer *(Continued)*

Pregnancy Risk Factor C

Contraindications Hypersensitivity to succimer or any component

Warnings Elevated blood lead levels and associated symptoms may return rapidly after discontinuation due to redistribution of lead from bone stores to soft tissues and blood; monitor blood lead levels for "rebound" after therapy; mild to moderate neutropenia has been reported; monitor CBC with differential prior to and during therapy; discontinue treatment if ANC <1200/µL

Precautions Use with caution in patients with renal or hepatic impairment; adequate hydration should be maintained during therapy

Adverse Reactions The most common events attributable to succimer have been observed in about 10% of patients treated

Central nervous system: Headache, fatigue, dizziness

Dermatologic: Rash, pruritus

Gastrointestinal: Nausea, vomiting, diarrhea, appetite loss, metallic taste, hemorrhoidal symptoms, sulfurous odor to breath, sore throat

Hematologic: Thrombocytosis, eosinophilia, reversible neutropenia

Hepatic: Transiently elevated AST, ALT, alkaline phosphatase, and serum cholesterol

Neuromuscular & skeletal: Paresthesia, sensorimotor neuropathy, back, rib, kneecap, and leg pains

Ocular: Watery eyes, cloudy film in eye

Renal: Sulfurous odor to urine, decreased urination, proteinuria

Respiratory: Rhinorrhea, nasal congestion

Miscellaneous: Flu-like symptoms, mucocutaneous hypersensitivity reactions (with repeat administration)

Drug Interactions Not recommended to be used concomitantly with edetate calcium disodium or penicillamine

Mechanism of Action Forms stable water-soluble complexes with lead resulting in increased urinary excretion; also chelates other toxic heavy metals such as arsenic and mercury

Pharmacokinetics

Absorption: Oral: Rapid, variable

Metabolism: Extensive to mixed succimer-cysteine disulfides

Half-life, elimination: 2 days

Time to peak serum concentration: ~1-2 hours

Elimination: ~25% in urine with peak urinary excretion occurring between 2-4 hours after dosing; of the total amount of succimer eliminated in urine, 90% is eliminated as mixed succimer-cysteine disulfide conjugates; 10% is excreted unchanged; fecal excretion of succimer probably represents unabsorbed drug

Dialysis: Succimer is dialyzable but lead chelates are not

Usual Dosage Children and Adults: Oral: 10 mg/kg/dose (or 350 mg/m²/dose) every 8 hours for 5 days followed by 10 mg/kg/dose (or 350 mg/m²/dose) every 12 hours for 14 days

Note: Concomitant iron therapy has been reported in a small number of children without the formation of a toxic complex with iron (as seen with dimercaprol); courses of therapy may be repeated if indicated by weekly monitoring of blood lead levels; lead levels should be stabilized to <15 mcg/dL; 2 weeks between courses is recommended unless more timely treatment is indicated by lead levels; patients who have received calcium disodium EDTA with or without BAL may be treated with succimer after at least 4 weeks have passed since treatment

Dosing adjustment in renal/hepatic impairment: Administer with caution and monitor closely

Administration Oral: Ensure adequate patient hydration; for patients who cannot swallow the capsule, sprinkle the medicated beads on a small amount of soft food or administer with a fruit juice to mask the odor

Monitoring Parameters Blood lead levels; liver enzymes and CBC with differential (prior to therapy and weekly during therapy)

Test Interactions Falsely decreased CPK; false-positive urine ketones with Ketostix®, falsely decreased uric acid measurements

Dosage Forms Capsule: 100 mg

References

Mann KV and Travers JD, "Succimer, An Oral Lead Chelator," *Clin Pharm*, 1991, 10(12):914-22.

Succinylcholine *(suks in il KOE leen)*

U.S. Brand Names Anectine® [DSC]; Quelicin®

Synonyms Suxamethonium

Therapeutic Category Neuromuscular Blocker Agent, Depolarizing; Skeletal Muscle Relaxant, Paralytic

Generic Available Yes

Use Used to produce skeletal muscle relaxation in procedures of short duration such as endotracheal intubation or endoscopic exams

Pregnancy Risk Factor C

Contraindications Hypersensitivity to succinylcholine chloride or any component; history of decreased concentration and/or decreased activity of plasma pseudocholinesterase; malignant hyperthermia; myopathies associated with elevated serum creatinine values; narrow-angle glaucoma; penetrating eye injuries

Warnings Malignant hyperthermia may be triggered by succinylcholine use; monitor closely for signs/symptoms; avoid use in patients with serum potassium >5.5 mEq/L; if sudden cardiac arrest occurs immediately after administration of succinylcholine, consider hyperkalemia as potential etiology and manage accordingly

Precautions As rare reports of acute rhabdomyolysis with hyperkalemia followed by ventricular dysrhythmias, cardiac arrest, and death have been reported in children with undiagnosed skeletal muscle myopathy, use with caution in patients recovering from severe trauma; use with caution in patients with pre-existing hyperkalemia, paraplegia, extensive or severe burns, extensive denervation of skeletal muscle because of disease or injury to the CNS or with degenerative or dystrophic neuromuscular disease

Adverse Reactions

Cardiovascular: Bradycardia, hypotension, cardiac arrhythmias, flushing, cardiac arrest, hypertension, tachycardia

Central nervous system: Malignant hyperthermia

Dermatologic: Rash

Endocrine & metabolic: Hyperkalemia, myoglobinemia

Gastrointestinal: Elevated intragastric pressure, salivation

Neuromuscular & skeletal: Myalgia due to muscle fasciculations, muscle weakness

Ocular: Elevated intraocular pressure

Renal: Myoglobinuria

Respiratory: Apnea, bronchospasm, respiratory depression

Drug Interactions Decreased neuromuscular blockade with diazepam; increased neuromuscular blockade with promazine, cyclophosphamide, oral contraceptives, glucocorticoids, MAO inhibitors, oxytocin, phenothiazines, quinidine, beta-blocking agents, procainamide, lidocaine, lithium, trimethaphan, furosemide, magnesium, chloroquine, acetylcholine, anticholinesterases, amphotericin B, and thiazide diuretics (due to electrolyte imbalances); cyclophosphamide, aminoglycosides, clindamycin may increase bradycardia; narcotic analgesics and inhalation anesthetics may increase the risk of sinus arrest; increased arrhythmias with digoxin (due to potassium changes)

Stability Injection is incompatible with alkaline solutions; store in refrigerator; stability at room temperature is product specific; check with each manufacturer

Mechanism of Action Acts similarly to acetylcholine, produces depolarization of the motor endplate at the myoneural junction which causes sustained flaccid skeletal muscle paralysis

Pharmacodynamics

I.M.:

Onset of action: 2-3 minutes

Duration: 10-30 minutes

I.V.:

Onset of action: Within 30-60 seconds

Duration: ~4-6 minutes

Pharmacokinetics

Metabolism: Succinylcholine is rapidly hydrolyzed by plasma pseudocholinesterase

Elimination: 10% excreted unchanged in urine

Usual Dosage

Children:

I.M.: 2.5-4 mg/kg (maximum dose: 150 mg)

I.V.: Initial: 1-2 mg/kg (maximum dose: 150 mg); maintenance: 0.3-0.6 mg/kg every 5-10 minutes as needed; because of the risk of malignant hyperthermia, use of continuous infusions is **not** recommended in infants and children

Adults: I.M., I.V.: 0.6 mg/kg (range: 0.3-1.1 mg/kg), up to 150 mg total dose; maintenance: 0.04-0.07 mg/kg every 5-10 minutes as needed

Continuous infusion: 2.5 mg/minute (range: 0.5-10 mg/minute)

Note: Pretreatment with atropine may reduce occurrence of bradycardia

Dosing adjustment in hepatic impairment: Dose should be decreased in patients with severe liver disease

Administration Parenteral: I.V.: May be administered by rapid I.V. injection without further dilution; continuous infusion: Dilute 1-2 mg/mL in NS or D_5W; I.M.: Injection should be made deeply

(Continued)

Succinylcholine *(Continued)*

Monitoring Parameters Heart rate, serum potassium, assisted ventilator status, peripheral nerve stimulator measuring twitch response

Dosage Forms

Injection, solution, as chloride: 20 mg/mL (10 mL)

Anectine®: 20 mg/mL (10 mL) [DSC]

Quelicin®: 20 mg/mL (5 mL, 10 mL); 50 mg/mL (10 mL); 100 mg/mL (10 mL)

♦ **Sucraid**® *see* Sacrosidase *on page 1001*

Sucralfate *(soo KRAL fate)*

Related Information

Carbohydrate and Alcohol Content of Liquid Medications for Use in Patients Receiving Ketogenic Diets *on page 1431*

U.S. Brand Names Carafate®

Canadian Brand Names Apo®-Sucralate; Novo-Sucralate; Nu-Sucralate; PMS-Sucralate

Synonyms Aluminum Sucrose Sulfate, Basic

Therapeutic Category Gastrointestinal Agent, Gastric or Duodenal Ulcer Treatment

Generic Available Yes

Use Short-term management of duodenal ulcers

Unlabeled use: Gastric ulcers; suspension may be used topically for treatment of stomatitis due to cancer chemotherapy or other causes of esophageal, gastric, and rectal erosions; treatment of NSAID mucosal damage; prevention of stress ulcers

Pregnancy Risk Factor B

Contraindications Hypersensitivity to sucralfate or any component

Warnings Because of the potential for sucralfate to alter the absorption of some drugs, separate administration times (administer other medications 2 hours before or after sucralfate) should be considered when alterations in bioavailability are believed to be critical

Precautions Use with caution in renal failure due to accumulation of aluminum

Adverse Reactions

Cardiovascular: Facial edema

Central nervous system: Dizziness, sleepiness, vertigo, headache

Dermatologic: Rash, pruritus, angioedema

Gastrointestinal: Constipation, diarrhea, nausea, gastric discomfort, indigestion, xerostomia, flatulence

Neuromuscular & skeletal: Back pain

Respiratory: Laryngospasm, rhinitis, respiratory difficulty

Drug Interactions Absorption of cimetidine colistin, digoxin, gentamicin, ketoconazole, L-thyroxine, phenytoin, quinidine, quinolones, ranitidine, sodium and potassium phosphate salts, tetracycline, and sustained release theophylline may be decreased (separate administration by 2 hours); aluminum-containing antacids may increase total body burden of aluminum; antacids, cimetidine, and ranitidine when administered concomitantly may decrease sucralfate's activity (gastric acidity is required for sucralfate to form its protective barrier)

Food Interactions Interferes with absorption of vitamin A, vitamin D, vitamin E, and vitamin K

Mechanism of Action Aluminum salt of sulfated sucrose which in the presence of acid pH (gastric acid) forms a complex, paste-like substance that adheres to the damaged mucosal area. This selectively forms a protective coating that protects the lining against peptic acid, pepsin, and bile salts.

Pharmacodynamics GI protection effect:

Acid neutralizing capacity: 14-17 mEq/1 g dose of sucralfate

Onset of action: 1-2 hours

Duration: Up to 6 hours

Pharmacokinetics

Absorption: Oral: <5%

Metabolism: Not metabolized

Elimination: 90% excreted in stool; small amounts that are absorbed are excreted in the urine as unchanged compounds

Usual Dosage Oral:

Children: Dose not established; doses of 40-80 mg/kg/day divided every 6 hours have been used

Stomatitis: 5-10 mL (1 g/10 mL); swish and spit or swish and swallow 4 times/day

Adults:

Stress ulcer prophylaxis: 1 g 4 times/day

Stress ulcer treatment: 1 g every 4 hours

Duodenal ulcer:
    Treatment: 1 g 4 times/day for 4-8 weeks, or alternatively 2 g twice daily; treatment is recommended for 4-8 weeks in adults
    Maintenance: Prophylaxis: 1 g twice daily
Stomatitis: 1 g/10 mL suspension, swish and spit or swish and swallow 4 times/day
Proctitis: Rectal enema: 2 g/20 mL once or twice daily
Dosage comment in renal impairment: Aluminum salt is minimally absorbed (<5%), however, may accumulate in renal failure

Administration

Oral: Administer on an empty stomach 1 hour before meals and at bedtime (see Warnings); tablet may be broken or dissolved in water before ingestion; do not administer antacids within 30 minutes of administration; shake suspension well before use

Rectal: May administer oral suspension as rectal enema; shake suspension well before use

Patient Information May cause dry mouth; separate times of administration with other medications (see Drug Interactions) by at least 2 hours

Additional Information There is approximately 14-16 mEq acid neutralizing capacity per 1g sucralfate

Dosage Forms

Suspension, oral: 1 g/10 mL (10 mL)
    Carafate®: 1 g/10 mL (420 mL)
Tablet (Carafate®): 1 g

References

Melko GP, Turco TF, Phelan TF, et al, "Treatment of Radiation-Induced Proctitis With Sucralfate Enemas," *Ann Pharmacother*, 1999, 33(12):1274-6.

♦ **Sucrets® [OTC]** *see* Dyclonine *on page 422*
♦ **Sudafed® [OTC]** *see* Pseudoephedrine *on page 958*
♦ **Sudafed® 12 Hour [OTC]** *see* Pseudoephedrine *on page 958*
♦ **Sudafed® 24 Hour [OTC]** *see* Pseudoephedrine *on page 958*
♦ **Sudafed®, Children's [OTC]** *see* Pseudoephedrine *on page 958*
♦ **Sudodrin [OTC]** *see* Pseudoephedrine *on page 958*
♦ **Sufenta®** *see* Sufentanil *on page 1047*

Sufentanil (soo FEN ta nil)

Related Information

Overdose and Toxicology *on page 1388*

U.S. Brand Names Sufenta®

Therapeutic Category Analgesic, Narcotic; General Anesthetic

Generic Available Yes

Use Analgesia; analgesia adjunct; anesthetic agent

Restrictions C-II

Pregnancy Risk Factor C

Contraindications Hypersensitivity to sufentanil or any component; increased intracranial pressure; severe respiratory depression

Warnings May cause severe respiratory depression; rapid I.V. infusion may result in skeletal muscle and chest wall rigidity, impaired ventilation, respiratory distress, apnea, bronchoconstriction, laryngospasm, arrest; inject slowly over 3-5 minutes; nondepolarizing skeletal muscle relaxant may be required; abrupt discontinuation after prolonged use may result in withdrawal symptoms

Precautions Use with caution in patients with head injuries, hepatic impairment, pulmonary disease, or with use of MAO inhibitors within past 14 days; sufentanil shares the toxic potential of opiate agonists, precautions of opiate agonist therapy should be observed

Adverse Reactions

Cardiovascular: Bradycardia, hypotension, peripheral vasodilation
Central nervous system: CNS depression, drowsiness, dizziness, sedation
Dermatologic: Erythema, pruritus, rash
Endocrine & metabolic: ADH release
Gastrointestinal: Nausea, vomiting, constipation, biliary tract spasm
Genitourinary: Urinary tract spasm
Neuromuscular & skeletal: Skeletal and thoracic muscle rigidity, especially after rapid I.V. administration
Ocular: Miosis, blurred vision
Respiratory: Respiratory depression, apnea
Miscellaneous: Physical and psychological dependence with prolonged use

Drug Interactions Cytochrome P450 isoenzyme CYP3A3/4 substrate
(Continued)

Sufentanil *(Continued)*

CNS depressants, phenothiazines, MAO inhibitors, tricyclic antidepressants may potentiate adverse effects of opiates; beta-blocker therapy may potentiate sufentanil bradycardia

Mechanism of Action Binds with stereospecific receptors at many sites within the CNS, increases pain threshold, alters pain reception, inhibits ascending pain pathways; ultra short-acting narcotic

Pharmacodynamics

Onset of action: 1-3 minutes

Duration: Dose dependent; anesthesia adjunct doses: 5 minutes

Pharmacokinetics

Distribution: V_{dss}:

Children 2-8 years: 2.9 ± 0.6 L/kg

Adults: 1.7 ± 0.2 L/kg

Protein binding (alpha$_1$-acid glycoprotein):

Neonates: 79%

Adults:

Male: 93%

Postpartum women: 91%

Metabolism: Primarily by the liver via demethylation and dealkylation

Half-life, elimination:

Neonates: 382-1162 minutes

Children 2-8 years: 97 ± 42 minutes

Adolescents 10-15 years: 76 ± 33 minutes

Adults: 164 ± 22 minutes

Elimination: ~2% excreted unchanged in the urine; 80% of dose excreted in urine (mostly as metabolites) within 24 hours

Clearance:

Children 2-8 years: 30.5 ± 8.8 mL/minute/kg

Adolescents: 12.8 ± 12 mL/minute/kg

Adults: 12.7 ± 0.8 mL/minute/kg

Usual Dosage Doses should be titrated to appropriate effects; wide range of doses, dependent upon desired degree of analgesia or anesthesia; use lean body weight to dose patients who are >20% above ideal body weight

Children <12 years: Anesthesia: I.V.: Initial: 10-25 mcg/kg; maintenance: Up to 25-50 mcg as needed

Adults: I.V.:

Adjunct to general anesthesia:

Low dose: Initial: 0.5-1 mcg/kg; maintenance: 10-25 mcg as needed

Moderate dose: Initial: 2-8 mcg/kg; maintenance: 10-50 mcg as needed

Anesthesia: Initial: 8-30 mcg/kg; maintenance: 10-50 mcg as needed

Administration Parenteral: I.V.: Slow I.V. injection or by infusion

Monitoring Parameters Respiratory rate, blood pressure, heart rate, oxygen saturation, neurological status (for degree of analgesia/anesthesia)

Patient Information May be habit-forming; avoid abrupt discontinuation after prolonged use

Nursing Implications Patient may develop rebound respiratory depression postoperatively

Dosage Forms Injection, solution, as citrate [preservative free]: 50 mcg/mL (1 mL, 2 mL, 5 mL)

References

Guay J, Gaudreault P, Tang A, et al, "Pharmacokinetics of Sufentanil in Normal Children," *Can J Anaesth*, 1992, 39(1):14-20.

Seguin JH, Erenberg A, and Leff RD, "Safety and Efficacy of Sufentanil Therapy in the Ventilated Infant," *Neonatal Netw*, 1994, 13(4):37-40.

♦ **Sulbactam and Ampicillin** *see* Ampicillin and Sulbactam *on page 105*

♦ **Sulf-10**® *see* Sulfacetamide *on page 1048*

Sulfacetamide *(sul fa SEE ta mide)*

U.S. Brand Names AK-Sulf®; Bleph®-10; Carmol® Scalp; Klaron®; Ocusulf-10; Ovace™; Sulf-10®

Canadian Brand Names Cetamide™; Diosulf™; Sodium Sulamyd®

Therapeutic Category Antibiotic, Ophthalmic; Antibiotic, Sulfonamide Derivative

Generic Available Yes (ointment and solution)

Use

Ophthalmic: Treatment and prophylaxis of conjunctivitis, corneal ulcers, and other superficial ocular infections due to susceptible organisms; adjunctive treatment with systemic sulfonamides for therapy of trachoma

Topical: Treatment of acne vulgaris, seborrheic dermatitis, seborrhea sicca, and secondary bacterial infections of the skin due to susceptible organisms

Pregnancy Risk Factor C

Contraindications Hypersensitivity to sulfacetamide, any component (see Warnings), or sulfonamides; infants <2 months of age; epithelial herpes simplex keratitis, vaccinia, varicella, and other viral diseases of the cornea and conjunctiva; fungal diseases of the ocular structures

Warnings Antibacterial activity may be decreased in the presence of purulent exudates containing para-aminobenzoic acid (PABA); nonsusceptible organisms such as fungi may proliferate with prolonged or repeated use of sulfonamide preparations; hemolysis may occur in patients with G-6-PD deficiency. Hypersensitivity reactions may occur when a sulfonamide is readministered, irrespective of the route of administration. Stevens-Johnson syndrome has been reported following the use of sulfacetamide topically. At the first sign of hypersensitivity, skin rash, or other reactions, inform physician and discontinue use. Some products contain sulfites which may cause allergic reactions in susceptible individuals

Precautions Use with caution in patients with severe dry eye or G-6-PD deficiency

Adverse Reactions
Central nervous system: Headache, fever
Dermatologic: Stevens-Johnson syndrome, exfoliative dermatitis, toxic epidermal necrolysis, rash, photosensitivity, erythema, pruritus, scaling of the skin
Hematologic: Bone marrow suppression
Local: Irritation, stinging and burning (especially with 30% solution), itching
Ocular: Blurred vision, transient epithelial keratitis, reactive hyperemia, conjunctival edema
Miscellaneous: Hypersensitivity reactions, syndrome resembling systemic lupus erythematosus

Drug Interactions Silver, gentamicin (antagonism)

Stability Protect from light; discolored or cloudy solutions should not be used; incompatible with silver and zinc sulfate; sulfacetamide is inactivated by blood or purulent exudates

Mechanism of Action Interferes with bacterial growth by inhibiting bacterial folic acid synthesis through competitive antagonism of PABA

Pharmacodynamics Onset of action: Improvement of conjunctivitis is usually seen within 3-6 days

Pharmacokinetics
Distribution: Excreted in breast milk
Half-life: 7-13 hours
Elimination: When absorbed, excreted primarily in urine as unchanged drug

Usual Dosage Children >2 months and Adults:
Ophthalmic:
Ointment: Apply to lower conjunctival sac 1-4 times/day and at bedtime or apply ½" to 1" into the conjunctival sac at night in conjunction with the use of drops during the day
Solution: Instill 1-2 drops into the lower conjunctival sac every 1-3 hours according to severity of infection during the waking hours and less frequently at night; **Note:** 30% solution is used for more severe infections
Trachoma (30% solution): 2 drops every 2 hours (concomitant use of systemic sulfonamide therapy is recommended)
Topical: Children and Adults:
Lotion: Apply to affected areas twice daily
Scalp lotion: Apply at bedtime. For severe cases with crusting, heavy scaling and inflammation, apply twice daily. Once eruption subsides, apply once or twice weekly or every other week to prevent reoccurrence.
Wash: Wash affected areas twice daily. If skin dryness occurs, use less frequently.

Administration
Ophthalmic: Avoid contact of tube or bottle tip with skin or eye; solution: Apply finger pressure to lacrimal sac during and for 1-2 minutes after instillation to decrease risk of absorption and systemic effects
Topical: For external use only
Lotion: Shake lotion well before using; apply a thin film to affected area.
Scalp lotion: Wash hair and scalp prior to application. Part hair a section at a time and apply a small quantity of lotion. Completely moisten scalp and gently rub in lotion with the fingertips. Then brush hair thoroughly for 2-3 minutes.
Wash: Wet skin and apply wash liberally to areas to be cleansed. Massage gently into skin working into a lather; rinse thoroughly and pat dry.

Monitoring Parameters Response to therapy

Patient Information Eye drops may burn and sting when first instilled; may cause sensitivity to bright light.
(Continued)

Sulfacetamide *(Continued)*

Dosage Forms

Lotion, as sodium:
Carmol® Scalp: 10% (85 g)
Klaron®: 10% (120 mL) [contains sodium metabisulfite]
Ovace™: 10% (180 mL, 360 mL)
Ointment, ophthalmic, as sodium (AK-Sulf®, Bleph®-10): 10% (3.5 g)
Solution, ophthalmic, as sodium: 10% (15 mL)
Bleph®-10: 10% (2.5 mL, 5 mL, 15 mL)
Ocusulf-10: 10% (15 mL)
Sulf-10®: 10% (1 mL) [contains thimerosal]

References

Lohr JA, Austin RD, Grossman M, et al, "Comparison of Three Topical Antimicrobials for Acute Bacterial Conjunctivitis," *Pediatr Infect Dis J,* 1988, 7(9):626-9.

SulfaDIAZINE *(sul fa DYE a zeen)*

Therapeutic Category Antibiotic, Sulfonamide Derivative

Generic Available Yes

Use Adjunctive treatment in toxoplasmosis; treatment of urinary tract infections and nocardiosis; rheumatic fever prophylaxis in penicillin-allergic patient; uncomplicated attack of malaria

Pregnancy Risk Factor B (D at term)

Contraindications Hypersensitivity to any sulfa drug or any component; porphyria; infants <2 months of age due to competition with bilirubin for protein-binding sites (unless indicated for the treatment of congenital toxoplasmosis); pregnant women during third trimester

Precautions Use with caution in patients with impaired hepatic function or impaired renal function, urinary obstruction, blood dyscrasia, G-6-PD deficiency; dosage modification required in patients with renal impairment

Adverse Reactions

Cardiovascular: Vasculitis
Central nervous system: Dizziness, fever, headache
Dermatologic: Rash, exfoliative dermatitis, Stevens-Johnson syndrome, photosensitivity, urticaria
Gastrointestinal: Nausea, vomiting, abdominal pain
Genitourinary: Crystalluria
Hematologic: Granulocytopenia, leukopenia, thrombocytopenia, aplastic anemia, hemolytic anemia
Hepatic: Jaundice, hepatitis
Renal: Acute nephropathy, hematuria
Miscellaneous: Serum sickness-like reactions

Drug Interactions PABA, procaine; tetracaine antagonizes antibacterial action of sulfonamides; paraldehyde increases potential for crystalluria; displaces agents from protein binding sites: coumarin anticoagulants increase bleeding, MTX increases toxicity, sulfonylurea antidiabetic agents (hypoglycemia)

Food Interactions Supplemental folinic acid should be administered to reverse symptoms or prevent problems due to folic acid deficiency; avoid large quantities of vitamin C or acidifying agents (cranberry juice) to prevent crystalluria

Stability Protect from light

Mechanism of Action Interferes with bacterial growth by inhibiting bacterial folic acid synthesis through competitive antagonism of PABA

Pharmacokinetics

Absorption: Oral: Well absorbed
Distribution: Excreted in breast milk; diffuses into CSF with higher concentrations reached when meninges are inflamed; distributed into most body tissues
Protein binding: 32% to 56%
Metabolism: Metabolized by N-acetylation
Half-life: 10 hours
Time to peak serum concentration: Within 4 hours
Elimination: In urine as metabolites (15% to 40%) and as unchanged drug (43% to 60%)

Usual Dosage Oral:

Congenital toxoplasmosis: Newborns: 100 mg/kg/day divided every 12 hours for 12 months in conjunction with pyrimethamine 1 mg/kg/day once daily and supplemental folinic acid 5 mg every 3 days for first 6 months, then pyrimethamine 1 mg/kg/day 3 times/week and folinic acid 10 mg 3 times/week for the next 6 months
Toxoplasmosis:
Children: 120-200 mg/kg/day divided every 6 hours in conjunction with pyrimethamine 2 mg/kg/day divided every 12 hours for 3 days followed by 1 mg/kg/day

once daily (maximum dose: 25 mg/day) with supplemental folinic acid 5-10 mg every 3 days

Adults: 2-8 g/day divided every 6 hours in conjunction with pyrimethamine 25 mg/day and with supplemental folinic acid 5-10 mg every 3 days

Prophylaxis of recurrent rheumatic fever:

≤30 kg: 500 mg once daily

>30 kg: 1 g once daily

Administration Oral: Administer with water on an empty stomach

Monitoring Parameters CBC, renal function tests, urinalysis

Patient Information Drink plenty of fluids; limit alcohol; notify physician if rash, sore throat, fever, arthralgia, shortness of breath, or jaundice occurs. May cause photosensitivity reactions (eg, exposure to sunlight may cause severe sunburn, skin rash, redness, or itching); avoid exposure to sunlight and artificial light sources (sunlamps, tanning booth/bed); wear protective clothing, wide-brimmed hats, sunglasses, and lip sunscreen (SPF ≥15); use a sunscreen [broad-spectrum sunscreen or physical sunscreen (preferred) or sunblock with SPF ≥15]; contact physician if reaction occurs.

Dosage Forms Tablet: 500 mg

Extemporaneous Preparations Tablets may be crushed to prepare oral suspension of the drug in water or with a sucrose-containing solution; aqueous suspension with concentrations of 100 mg/mL should be stored in the refrigerator and used within 7 days

References

Frenkel JK, "Toxoplasmosis," *Pediatr Clin North Am*, 1985, 32(4):917-32.

Sulfadoxine and Pyrimethamine

(sul fa DOKS een & peer i METH a meen)

U.S. Brand Names Fansidar®

Synonyms Pyrimethamine and Sulfadoxine

Therapeutic Category Antimalarial Agent

Generic Available No

Use Treatment of *Plasmodium falciparum* malaria in patients in whom chloroquine resistance is suspected; malaria prophylaxis for travelers to areas where chloroquine-resistant malaria is endemic

Pregnancy Risk Factor C

Contraindications Hypersensitivity to any sulfa drug, pyrimethamine, or any component; porphyria, megaloblastic anemia, severe renal insufficiency; children <2 months of age due to competition with bilirubin for protein binding sites; pregnant women at term; do not use for treatment of malaria acquired in Southeast Asia or the Amazon Basin since resistance to sulfadoxine and pyrimethamine has been reported

Warnings Fatalities associated with sulfonamides, although rare, have occurred due to severe reactions including Stevens-Johnson syndrome, toxic epidermal necrolysis, hepatic necrosis, agranulocytosis, aplastic anemia and other blood dyscrasias; discontinue use at first sign of rash or any sign of adverse reaction; hemolysis may occur in patients with G-6-PD deficiency

Precautions Use with caution in patients with renal or hepatic impairment, patients with possible folate deficiency, patients with bronchial asthma, and patients with seizure disorders

Adverse Reactions

Cardiovascular: Vasculitis

Central nervous system: Seizures, headache, insomnia, ataxia, fatigue, hyperesthesia

Dermatologic: Erythema multiforme, Stevens-Johnson syndrome, toxic epidermal necrolysis, rash, photosensitivity, urticaria, pruritus

Endocrine & metabolic: Folic acid deficiency

Gastrointestinal: Anorexia, vomiting, gastritis, glossitis, diarrhea, abdominal cramps

Hematologic: Megaloblastic anemia, leukopenia, thrombocytopenia, pancytopenia, agranulocytosis, pulmonary eosinophilia

Hepatic: Hepatic necrosis; jaundice; elevated ALT, AST

Neuromuscular & skeletal: Tremor

Respiratory: Respiratory failure

Drug Interactions Para-aminobenzoic acid, folic acid

Stability Protect from light

Mechanism of Action Sulfadoxine interferes with bacterial folic acid synthesis and growth via competitive inhibition of para-aminiobenzoic acid; pyrimethamine inhibits microbial dihydrofolate reductase, resulting in inhibition of tetrahydrofolic acid synthesis

Pharmacokinetics

Absorption: Oral: Well absorbed

(Continued)

Sulfadoxine and Pyrimethamine *(Continued)*

Distribution: Excreted in breast milk; pyrimethamine is distributed to kidneys, lungs, liver, and spleen; sulfadoxine is widely distributed in the body

Protein binding:
Pyrimethamine: 80% to 87%
Sulfadoxine: 90% to 95%

Half-life:
Pyrimethamine: 111 hours
Sulfadoxine: 169 hours

Time to peak serum concentration: Within 2-8 hours

Elimination: In urine as parent compounds and several unidentified metabolites

Usual Dosage Children ≥ 2 months and Adults: Oral:

Treatment of acute attack of malaria: A single dose of the following number of Fansidar® tablets is used in sequence with quinine on last day of quinine therapy:
2-11 months: 1/4 tablet
1-3 years: 1/2 tablet
4-8 years: 1 tablet
9-14 years: 2 tablets
>14 years: 3 tablets
Adults: 3 tablets on last day of quinine therapy

Malaria prophylaxis (for areas where chloroquine-resistant *P. falciparum* exists):
Short-term travel (≤3 weeks): Travelers should carry pyrimethamine-sulfadoxine for use as presumptive self-treatment if a febrile illness develops while taking chloroquine for prophylaxis. Take single dose in the event of febrile illness when medical attention is not immediately available:
2-11 months: 1/4 tablet
1-3 years: 1/2 tablet
4-8 years: 1 tablet
9-14 years: 2 tablets
>14 years and Adults: 3 tablets

Administration Oral: Administer with meals

Monitoring Parameters Liver function tests, CBC including platelet counts, renal function tests and urinalysis should be performed periodically

Patient Information Drink plenty of fluids; notify physician if rash, sore throat, pallor, glossitis, fever, arthralgia, cough, shortness of breath, or jaundice occurs; limit alcohol. May cause photosensitivity reactions (eg, exposure to sunlight may cause severe sunburn, skin rash, redness, or itching); avoid exposure to sunlight and artificial light sources (sunlamps, tanning booth/bed); wear protective clothing, wide-brimmed hats, sunglasses, and lip sunscreen (SPF ≥15); use a sunscreen [broad-spectrum sunscreen or physical sunscreen (preferred) or sunblock with SPF ≥15]; contact physician if reaction occurs.

Additional Information Leucovorin should be administered to reverse signs and symptoms of folic acid deficiency

Dosage Forms Tablet, scored: Sulfadoxine 500 mg and pyrimethamine 25 mg

References
Lynk A and Gold R, "Review of 40 Children With Imported Malaria," *Pediatr Infect Dis J*, 1989, 8(11):745-50.
Randall JS and Seidel JS, "Malaria," *Pediatr Clin North Am*, 1985, 32(4):893-916.

♦ **Sulfalax®** [OTC] *see* Docusate *on page 402*

Sulfamethoxazole and Trimethoprim

(sul fa meth OKS a zole & trye METH oh prim)

Related Information
Carbohydrate and Alcohol Content of Liquid Medications for Use in Patients Receiving Ketogenic Diets *on page 1431*

U.S. Brand Names Bactrim™; Bactrim™ DS; Septra®; Septra® DS; Sulfatrim® Pediatric

Canadian Brand Names Apo®-Sulfatrim; Novo-Trimel; Novo-Trimel D.S.; Nu-Cotrimox®; Septra® Injection

Synonyms Co-Trimoxazole; SMX-TMP; TMP-SMX; Trimethoprim and Sulfamethoxazole

Therapeutic Category Antibiotic, Sulfonamide Derivative

Generic Available Yes

Use Treatment of urinary tract infections caused by susceptible *E. coli*, *Klebsiella*, *Enterobacter*, *Proteus mirabilis*, *Proteus* (indole positive); acute otitis media due to amoxicillin-resistant *H. influenzae*, *S. pneumoniae*, and *M. catarrhalis*; acute exacerbations of chronic bronchitis; prophylaxis and treatment of *Pneumocystis carinii* pneumonitis (PCP); treatment of susceptible shigellosis, typhoid fever, *Nocardia asteroides* infection, and *Xanthomonas maltophilia* infection; the I.V. preparation is used for treatment of *Pneumocystis carinii* pneumonitis, *Shigella*, and severe urinary tract infections

Pregnancy Risk Factor C

Contraindications Hypersensitivity to any sulfa drug, trimethoprim, or any component (see Warnings); porphyria; megaloblastic anemia due to folate deficiency; infants <2 months of age (for exception, see Additional Information)

Warnings Fatalities associated with sulfonamides, although rare, have occurred due to severe reactions including Stevens-Johnson syndrome, toxic epidermal necrolysis, hepatic necrosis, agranulocytosis, aplastic anemia, and other blood dyscrasias; discontinue use at first sign of rash or any sign of adverse reaction

Oral suspension may contain sodium benzoate and injection contains propylene glycol, benzyl alcohol, and sodium metabisulfites; propylene glycol may be toxic to newborns in high doses; sodium benzoate, benzyl alcohol and sodium metabisulfites may cause allergic reactions in susceptible individuals; large amounts of benzyl alcohol (≥99 mg/kg/day) have been associated with a potentially fatal toxicity ("gasping syndrome") in neonates; the "gasping syndrome" consists of metabolic acidosis, respiratory distress, gasping respirations, CNS dysfunction (including convulsions, intracranial hemorrhage), hypotension and cardiovascular collapse; use products containing benzyl alcohol with caution in neonates; *in vitro* and animal studies have shown that benzoate, a metabolite of benzyl alcohol, displaces bilirubin from protein binding sites

Precautions Use with caution in patients with G-6-PD deficiency, impaired renal or hepatic function; adjust dosage in patients with renal impairment

Adverse Reactions

Cardiovascular: Allergic myocarditis, hypotension

Central nervous system: Confusion, depression, hallucinations, seizures, fever, ataxia, kernicterus in neonates, aseptic meningitis, headache, insomnia

Dermatologic: Rash (more common in patients taking large dosages or in patients with AIDS), erythema multiforme, epidermal necrolysis, Stevens-Johnson syndrome, pruritus, urticaria

Endocrine & metabolic: Hyperkalemia

Gastrointestinal: Nausea, vomiting, glossitis, stomatitis, diarrhea, pseudomembranous colitis, pancreatitis, splenomegaly, anorexia

Hematologic: Thrombocytopenia, megaloblastic anemia, granulocytopenia, aplastic anemia, hemolysis (with G-6-PD deficiency)

Hepatic: Hepatitis, cholestatic jaundice

Local: Local irritation, pain, phlebitis

Neuromuscular & skeletal: Arthralgia, myalgia, rhabdomyolysis

Renal: Interstitial nephritis, renal tubular acidosis

Respiratory: Shortness of breath, cough, pulmonary infiltrates

Miscellaneous: Serum sickness, angioedema

Drug Interactions Cytochrome P450 isoenzyme CYP2C9 inhibitor

Sulfamethoxazole and trimethoprim decreases the clearance of warfarin; methotrexate (displaced from protein binding sites); increases the effect of sulfonylureas, phenytoin, digoxin, and thiopental; decreases serum cyclosporine concentrations

Stability Do not refrigerate concentrate for injection; for I.V. administration, a 1:25 dilution is stable for 48 hours in D_5W or NS; 1:20 dilution is stable for 24 hours in D_5W or 14 hours in NS; 1:15 dilution is stable for 4 hours in D_5W or 2 hours in NS; 1:10 dilution is stable for 1 hour in D_5W or NS; do not mix with other drugs or solutions

Mechanism of Action Sulfamethoxazole interferes with bacterial folic acid synthesis and growth via inhibition of dihydrofolic acid formation from para-aminobenzoic acid; trimethoprim inhibits dihydrofolic acid reduction to tetrahydrofolate resulting in sequential inhibition of enzymes of the folic acid pathway

Pharmacokinetics

Absorption: Oral: Almost completely (90% to 100%)

Distribution: Crosses the placenta; distributes into breast milk, joint fluid, sputum, middle ear fluid, bile, and CSF

Protein binding:
TMP: 45%
SMX: 68%

Metabolism:
TMP: Metabolized to oxide and hydroxylated metabolites
SMX: N-acetylated and glucuronidated

Half-life:
TMP: 6-11 hours, prolonged in renal failure
SMX: 9-12 hours, prolonged in renal failure

Time to peak serum concentration: Oral: Within 1-4 hours

Elimination: Both excreted in urine as metabolites and unchanged drug

(Continued)

Sulfamethoxazole and Trimethoprim *(Continued)*

Usual Dosage Oral, I.V. **(dosage recommendations are based on the trimethoprim (TMP) component):**

Children >2 months and Adults:

Mild-moderate infections: 6-12 mg TMP/kg/day in divided doses every 12 hours

Serious infection/*Pneumocystis*: 15-20 mg TMP/kg/day in divided doses every 6-8 hours

Prophylaxis of *Pneumocystis* (see **Note** in Additional Information): 150 mg TMP/m^2/day in divided doses every 12 hours 3 days/week on consecutive days; acceptable alternative dosage schedules include 150 mg TMP/m^2/day as a single daily dose 3 times/week on consecutive days or 150 mg TMP/m^2/day in divided doses every 12 hours administered 7 days/week, or 150 mg TMP/m^2/day in divided doses every 12 hours administered 3 times/week on alternate days; dose should not exceed 320 mg trimethoprim and 1600 mg sulfamethoxazole/day

Urinary tract infection prophylaxis: 2 mg TMP/kg/dose daily or 5 mg TMP/kg/dose twice weekly

Adults:

Urinary tract infection/chronic bronchitis: 1 double strength tablet every 12 hours for 10-14 days

Prophylaxis of *Pneumocystis*: One double-strength tablet daily or an acceptable alternative is 1 single-strength tablet daily

Dosing adjustment in renal impairment (frequency may need to be adjusted):

Cl_{cr} 15-30 mL/minute: Reduce dose by 50%

Cl_{cr} <15 mL/minute: Not recommended

Administration

Oral: May administer with water on an empty stomach; shake suspension well before use

Parenteral: Infuse I.V. sulfamethoxazole and trimethoprim over 60-90 minutes; must be further diluted 1:25 (5 mL drug to 125 mL diluent, ie, D_5W); in patients who require fluid restriction, a 1:15 dilution (5 mL drug to 75 mL diluent, ie, D_5W) or a 1:10 dilution (5 mL drug to 50 mL diluent, ie, D_5W) may be administered; see Stability

Monitoring Parameters CBC, renal function test, liver function test, urinalysis; observe for change in bowel frequency

Patient Information Maintain adequate fluid intake

Additional Information Note: Guidelines for prophylaxis of *Pneumocystis carinii* pneumonia: Initiate PCP prophylaxis in the following patients: Children born to HIV-infected mothers should be given prophylaxis with TMP/SMZ beginning at 4-6 weeks of age and continue through the first year of life or until HIV infection has been reasonably excluded; children 1-5 years of age with CD4+ count <500 or CD4+ percentage <15%; children 6-12 years of age with CD4+ count <200 or CD4+ percentage <15%; adolescents and adults with CD4+ count <200 or oropharyngeal candidiasis. Folinic acid should be given if bone marrow suppression occurs.

Dosage Forms The 5:1 ratio (SMX to TMP) remains constant in all dosage forms:

Injection, solution: Sulfamethoxazole 80 mg and trimethoprim 16 mg per mL (5 mL, 10 mL, 30 mL)

Septra®: Sulfamethoxazole 80 mg and trimethoprim 16 mg per mL (10 mL, 20 mL) [contains 10% alcohol, 1% benzyl alcohol, 40% propylene glycol, and sodium metabisulfite]

Suspension, oral: Sulfamethoxazole 200 mg and trimethoprim 40 mg per 5 mL (20 mL, 100 mL, 150 mL, 200 mL, 480 mL)

Septra®: Sulfamethoxazole 200 mg and trimethoprim 40 mg per 5 mL (100 mL, 480 mL) [contains 0.26% alcohol and 0.1% sodium benzoate; cherry and grape flavors]

Sulfatrim® Pediatric: Sulfamethoxazole 200 mg and trimethoprim 40 mg per 5 mL (20 mL, 100 mL, 480 mL) [contains 0.5% alcohol; cherry and fruit-licorice flavors]

Tablet (Bactrim™, Septra®): Sulfamethoxazole 400 mg and trimethoprim 80 mg

Tablet, double strength (Bactrim™ DS, Septra® DS): Sulfamethoxazole 800 mg and trimethoprim 160 mg

References

Jarosinki PF, Kennedy PE, and Gallelli JF, "Stability of Concentrated Trimethoprim-Sulfamethoxazole Admixtures," *AJHP*, 1989, 46(4):732-7.

Hughes WT, "*Pneumocystis carinii* Pneumonia: New Approaches to Diagnosis, Treatment, and Prevention," *Pediatr Infect Dis J*, 1991, 10(5):391-9.

"1999 USPHS/IDSA Guidelines for the Prevention of Opportunistic Infections in Persons Infected With Human Immunodeficiency Virus. USPHS/IDSA Prevention of Opportunistic Infections Working Group," *MMWR Morb Mortal Wkly Rep*, 1999, 48(RR-10):1-66.

♦ **Sulfamylon®** *see* Mafenide *on page 700*

Sulfasalazine (sul fa SAL a zeen)

Related Information
Drugs and Breast-Feeding *on page 1404*

U.S. Brand Names Azulfidine®; Azulfidine® EN-tabs®

Canadian Brand Names Alti-Sulfasalazine; Salazopyrin®; Salazopyrin En-Tabs®

Synonyms Salicylazosulfapyridine

Therapeutic Category 5-Aminosalicylic Acid Derivative; Anti-inflammatory Agent

Generic Available Yes (tablet)

Use Management of ulcerative colitis; treatment of active Crohn's disease and juvenile rheumatoid arthritis

Pregnancy Risk Factor B (D at term)

Contraindications Hypersensitivity to sulfasalazine, sulfa drugs, or any component; porphyria, GI or GU obstruction; hypersensitivity to salicylates; children <2 years of age

Precautions Use with caution in patients with renal impairment, G-6-PD deficiency, blood dyscrasias, or bronchial asthma

Adverse Reactions Incidence of adverse effects increase with dosage >4 g/day and in slow acetylators of sulfapyridine

Cardiovascular: Vasculitis

Central nervous system: Headache, fever, convulsions, vertigo, malaise, mood changes

Dermatologic: Rash, toxic epidermal necrolysis, urticaria, Stevens-Johnson syndrome, photosensitivity, staining of skin (orange-yellow)

Gastrointestinal: Nausea, vomiting, diarrhea, pancreatitis, anorexia

Genitourinary: Crystalluria, infertility (oligospermia), discoloration of urine (orange-yellow)

Hematologic: Hemolytic anemia, agranulocytosis, neutropenia, leukopenia

Hepatic: Elevated liver enzymes, jaundice, cholestatic jaundice, cirrhosis, liver necrosis/failure

Otic: Tinnitus

Renal: Nephrotoxicity

Respiratory: Fibrosing alveolitis, pulmonary eosinophilia

Miscellaneous: Serum sickness-like reaction

Drug Interactions
Decreased effect of iron, digoxin, folic acid, and PABA or PABA metabolites of drugs (ie, procaine, proparacaine, tetracaine)

Increased effect of oral anticoagulants, methotrexate, and oral hypoglycemic agents (as with other sulfa drugs)

Food Interactions Need to increase dietary intake of iron; since sulfasalazine impairs folate absorption, consider providing 1 mg/day folate supplement

Mechanism of Action Acts locally in the colon to decrease the inflammatory response and interfere with secretion by inhibiting prostaglandin synthesis; therapeutic effect may result from antibacterial action with change in intestinal flora

Pharmacodynamics Onset of action:

JRA: Minimum trial of 3 months is necessary

Ulcerative colitis: >3-4 weeks

Pharmacokinetics
Absorption: Oral: 10% to 15% as unchanged drug from the small intestine; upon administration, the drug is split into sulfapyridine and 5-aminosalicylic acid (5-ASA) in the colon

Distribution: Breast milk to plasma ratio: 0.09-0.17

Metabolism: Both components are metabolized in the liver; slow acetylators have higher plasma sulfapyridine concentrations

Half-life:

Sulfasalazine:

Single dose: 5.7 hours

Multiple doses: 7.6 hours

Sulfapyridine:

Single dose: 8.4 hours

Multiple doses: 10.4 hours

Time to peak serum concentration:

Serum sulfasalazine: Within 1.5-6 hours

Serum sulfapyridine (active metabolite): Within 6-24 hours

Elimination: Primarily in urine (as unchanged drug, components, and acetylated metabolites); small amounts appear in feces

Usual Dosage Oral:

Children ≥2 years:

Ulcerative colitis:

Mild exacerbation: 40-50 mg/kg/day divided every 6 hours

(Continued)

Sulfasalazine *(Continued)*

Moderate-severe exacerbation: 50-75 mg/kg/day divided every 4-6 hours, not to exceed 6 g/day

Maintenance dose: 30-50 mg/kg/day divided every 4-8 hours; not to exceed 2 g/day

Juvenile rheumatoid arthritis (JRA): Initial: 10 mg/kg/day; increase weekly by 10 mg/kg/day; usual dose: 30-50 mg/kg/day in 2 divided doses; maximum dose: 2 g/day

Adults: 1 g 3-4 times/day divided every 4-6 hours, not to exceed 6 g/day; maintenance: 2 g/day divided every 6-12 hours

Administration Oral: Administer after meals or with food; do not administer with antacids

Monitoring Parameters Stool frequency, hematocrit, reticulocyte count, CBC, urinalysis, renal function tests, liver function tests

Patient Information Maintain adequate fluid intake; may cause orange-yellow discoloration of urine and skin; may stain soft contact lenses yellow. May cause photosensitivity reactions (eg, exposure to sunlight may cause severe sunburn, skin rash, redness, or itching); avoid exposure to sunlight and artificial light sources (sunlamps, tanning booth/bed); wear protective clothing, wide-brimmed hats, sunglasses, and lip sunscreen (SPF ≥15); use a sunscreen [broad-spectrum sunscreen or physical sunscreen (preferred) or sunblock with SPF ≥15]; contact physician if reaction occurs.

Additional Information Good response to sulfasalazine for JRA is most likely to occur in HLA B27-positive boys who are older than 9 years of age at onset of arthritis

Dosage Forms

Tablet (Azulfidine®): 500 mg

Tablet, delayed release, enteric coated (Azulfidine® EN-tabs®): 500 mg

References

American College of Rheumatology Ad Hoc Committee on Clinical Guidelines, "Guidelines for the Management of Rheumatoid Arthritis," *Arthritis Rheum*, 1996, 39(5):713-22.

Giannini EH and Cawkwell GD, "Drug Treatment in Children With Juvenile Rheumatoid Arthritis," *Pediatr Clin North Am*, 1995, 42(5):1099-125.

Kirschner BS, "Inflammatory Bowel Disease in Children," *Pediatr Clin North Am*, 1988, 35(1):189-208.

♦ **Sulfatrim® Pediatric** *see* Sulfamethoxazole and Trimethoprim *on page 1052*

SulfiSOXAZOLE *(sul fi SOKS a zole)*

Related Information

Carbohydrate and Alcohol Content of Liquid Medications for Use in Patients Receiving Ketogenic Diets *on page 1431*

U.S. Brand Names Gantrisin®

Canadian Brand Names Novo-Soxazole®; Sulfizole®

Synonyms Sulphafurazole

Therapeutic Category Antibiotic, Sulfonamide Derivative

Generic Available Yes (tablet)

Use Treatment of uncomplicated urinary tract infections, otitis media, *Chlamydia*; nocardiosis; treatment of acute pelvic inflammatory disease in prepubertal children

Pregnancy Risk Factor B (D at term)

Contraindications Hypersensitivity to any sulfa drug or any component; porphyria; infants <2 months of age (sulfas compete with bilirubin for protein binding sites which may result in kernicterus in newborns); patients with urinary obstruction; pregnant women during third trimester; nursing mothers

Precautions Use with caution in patients with G-6-PD deficiency (hemolysis may occur), hepatic or renal impairment; dosage modification required in patients with renal impairment; risk of crystalluria should be considered in patients with impaired renal function

Adverse Reactions

Cardiovascular: Vasculitis

Central nervous system: Dizziness, headache, fever, vertigo, disorientation

Dermatologic: Rash, Stevens-Johnson syndrome, photosensitivity, exfoliative dermatitis

Gastrointestinal: Nausea, vomiting, anorexia, stomatitis, pseudomembranous colitis

Genitourinary: Crystalluria (rare)

Hematologic: Thrombocytopenia, leukopenia, agranulocytosis, aplastic anemia, hemolytic anemia, neutropenia

Hepatic: Jaundice, hepatitis

Renal: Nephrotoxicity

Miscellaneous: Hypersensitivity reactions

Drug Interactions Methotrexate, tolbutamide, chlorpropamide, oral anticoagulants (displaced from protein binding sites); PABA (antagonizes the antibacterial activity of sulfas); thiopental (competes for plasma protein binding)

Food Interactions Interferes with folate absorption

Stability Protect from light

Mechanism of Action Interferes with bacterial growth by inhibiting bacterial folic acid synthesis through competitive antagonism of PABA

Pharmacokinetics

Absorption: Sulfisoxazole acetyl is hydrolyzed in the GI tract to sulfisoxazole which is readily absorbed

Distribution: Crosses the placenta; excreted into breast milk; distributes into extracellular space; CSF concentration ranges from 8% to 57% of blood concentration in patients with normal meninges

Protein binding: 85% to 88%

Metabolism: In the liver by acetylation and glucuronide conjugation to inactive compounds

Half-life: 4-8 hours, prolonged with renal impairment

Time to peak serum concentration: Within 2-4 hours

Elimination: Primarily in urine (95% within 24 hours), 40% to 60% as unchanged drug

Dialysis: >50% removed by hemodialysis

Usual Dosage

Infants ≥2 months and Children: Oral: Initial: 75 mg/kg for 1 dose, followed by 120-150 mg/kg/day in divided doses every 4-6 hours; not to exceed 6 g/day

Pelvic inflammatory disease: 100 mg/kg/day in divided doses every 6 hours; used in combination with ceftriaxone

Chlamydia trachomatis: 100 mg/kg/day divided every 6 hours; maximum dose: 2 g/day

Prophylaxis of UTI: 10-20 mg/kg/day divided every 12 hours

Prophylaxis of recurrent acute otitis media: 35-75 mg/kg/day once daily at bedtime

Adults: Oral: 2-4 g stat, followed by 4-8 g/day in divided doses every 4-6 hours

Children and Adults: Ophthalmic: Solution: Instill 1-2 drops to conjunctiva of affected eye every 2-3 hours

Dosing interval in renal impairment:

Cl_{cr} 10-50 mL/minutes: Administer every 8-12 hours

Cl_{cr} <10 mL/minute: Administer every 12-24 hours

Administration

Ophthalmic: Avoid contact of bottle tip with skin or eye; apply finger pressure to lacrimal sac during and for 1-2 minutes after instillation of drops to decrease risk of absorption and systemic effects

Oral: Administer with a glass of water on an empty stomach; shake suspension well before use

Monitoring Parameters CBC, urinalysis, renal function tests

Test Interactions False-positive protein in urine; false-positive urine glucose with Clinitest®

Patient Information Report to physician any sore throat, mouth sores, rash, unusual bleeding, or fever; limit alcohol. May cause photosensitivity reactions (eg, exposure to sunlight may cause severe sunburn, skin rash, redness, or itching); avoid exposure to sunlight and artificial light sources (sunlamps, tanning booth/bed); wear protective clothing, wide-brimmed hats, sunglasses, and lip sunscreen (SPF ≥15); use a sunscreen [broad-spectrum sunscreen or physical sunscreen (preferred) or sunblock with SPF ≥15]; contact physician if reaction occurs.

Nursing Implications Maintain adequate patient fluid intake

Dosage Forms

Suspension, oral, pediatric, as acetyl (Gantrisin®): 500 mg/5 mL (480 mL) [contains 0.3% alcohol; raspberry flavor]

Tablet: 500 mg

References

Erramouspe J and Heyneman CA, "Treatment and Prevention of Otitis Media," *Ann Pharmacother*, 2000, 34(12):1452-68.

Klein JO, "Protecting the Therapeutic Advantage of Antimicrobial Agents Used for Otitis Media," *Pediatr Infect Dis J*, 1998, 17(6):571-5.

"Practice Parameter: The Diagnosis, Treatment, and Evaluation of the Initial Urinary Tract Infection in Febrile Infants and Young Children. American Academy of Pediatrics. Committee on Quality Improvement. Subcommittee on Urinary Tract Infection," *Pediatrics*, 1999, 103(4 Pt 1):843-52.

Thoene DE and Johnson CE, "Pharmacotherapy of Otitis Media," *Pharmacotherapy*, 1991, 11(3):212-21.

♦ **Sulfisoxazole and Erythromycin** *see* Erythromycin and Sulfisoxazole *on page 451*

♦ **Sulfizole® (Can)** *see* SulfiSOXAZOLE *on page 1056*

Sulfur and Salicylic Acid (SUL fur & sal i SIL ik AS id)

U.S. Brand Names Meted® [OTC]; MG 217 Medicated Tar-Free [OTC]; Pernox® Scrub Cleanser [OTC]; Sebex® [OTC]; Sebulex® [OTC]

Synonyms Salicylic Acid and Sulfur

Therapeutic Category Antiseborrheic Agent, Topical

Generic Available Yes (soap)

Use Therapeutic shampoo for dandruff and seborrheal dermatitis; acne skin cleanser

Contraindications Hypersensitivity to sulfur, salicylic acid, or any component

Warnings For external use only; avoid contact with eyes; discontinue use if skin irritation develops

Precautions Infants are more sensitive to sulfur than adults; do not use in children <2 years of age

Adverse Reactions Topical preparations containing 2% to 5% sulfur generally are well tolerated; concentration >15% is very irritating to the skin; higher concentrations (eg, 10% or higher) may cause systemic toxicity

Cardiovascular: Collapse (with sulfur concentration >10%)

Central nervous system: Dizziness, headache

Gastrointestinal: Vomiting

Local: Irritation

Neuromuscular & skeletal: Muscle cramps

Stability Preparations containing sulfur may react with metals including silver and copper, resulting in discoloration of the metal

Mechanism of Action Salicylic acid works synergistically with sulfur in its keratolytic action to break down keratin and promote skin peeling

Pharmacokinetics Absorption: 1% of topically applied sulfur is absorbed; sulfur is reduced to hydrogen sulfide

Usual Dosage Children ≥2 years and Adults: Topical:

Shampoo: Initial: Massage onto wet scalp; leave lather on scalp for 5 minutes, rinse, repeat application, then rinse thoroughly; use daily or every other day; 1-2 treatments/week will usually maintain control

Soap: Use daily or every other day

Administration Topical: Avoid contact with the eyes; for external use only

Patient Information Contact physician if condition worsens or rash or irritation develops

Dosage Forms

Cleanser, topical (Pernox® Scrub Cleanser): Sulfur 2% and salicylic acid 1.5% (60 mL, 120 mL)

Shampoo, topical:

Meted®, Sebex®: Sulfur 5% and salicylic acid 3% (120 mL)

MG217 Medicated Tar-Free: Colloidal sulfur 5% and salicylic acid 3% (120 mL, 240 mL)

Sebulex®: Sulfur 2% and salicylic acid 2% (120 mL, 240 mL)

Soap, topical: Precipitated sulfur 5% and salicylic acid 3% (116 g)

Sulindac (sul IN dak)

Related Information

Overdose and Toxicology *on page 1388*

U.S. Brand Names Clinoril®

Canadian Brand Names Apo®-Sulin; Novo-Sundac; Nu-Sundac

Therapeutic Category Analgesic, Non-narcotic; Anti-inflammatory Agent; Nonsteroidal Anti-inflammatory Drug (NSAID), Oral

Generic Available Yes

Use Management of inflammatory disease, rheumatoid disorders; acute gouty arthritis

Pregnancy Risk Factor B (D in 3rd trimester or near delivery)

Contraindications Hypersensitivity to sulindac, any component, aspirin, or other NSAIDs; active GI bleeding, ulcer disease; patients who have acute asthmatic attacks, urticaria, or rhinitis that are precipitated by aspirin or other NSAIDs; patients with the "aspirin triad" [asthma, rhinitis (with or without nasal polyps), and aspirin intolerance] (fatal asthmatic and anaphylactoid reactions may occur in these patients)

Precautions Use with caution in patients with peptic ulcer disease, GI bleeding, bleeding abnormalities, impaired renal or hepatic function, CHF, hypertension, and patients receiving anticoagulants

Adverse Reactions

Cardiovascular: Edema

Central nervous system: Dizziness, nervousness, headache

Dermatologic: Rash, pruritus

Gastrointestinal: Abdominal pain; GI bleeding, ulcer, perforation; nausea; vomiting; diarrhea; constipation

Hematologic: Thrombocytopenia, agranulocytosis, inhibition of platelet aggregation, bone marrow suppression

Hepatic: Hepatitis

Otic: Tinnitus

Renal: Renal impairment

Respiratory: Bronchospasm

Drug Interactions Cytochrome P450 isoenzyme CYP2C9 inhibitor

Sulindac may potentiate effects of warfarin; probenecid may increase serum concentration of sulindac; dimethyl sulfoxide or ASA may decrease sulindac serum concentration; sulindac may increase methotrexate serum concentrations and may increase cyclosporin nephrotoxicity; potassium supplements and other GI irritants may increase GI adverse effects; effects of antihypertensive agents, furosemide, thiazides may be decreased; drug interactions similar to other NSAIDs may also occur

Food Interactions Food may decrease rate and extent of absorption

Mechanism of Action Inhibits prostaglandin synthesis by decreasing the activity of the enzyme, cyclooxygenase, which results in decreased formation of prostaglandin precursors

Usual Dosage Oral:

Children: Limited information exists; some centers use the following: 2-4 mg/kg/day in 2 divided doses; maximum: 6 mg/kg/day; do not exceed 400 mg/day (Skeith, 1991; Giannini, 1995)

Adults: 150-200 mg twice daily; not to exceed 400 mg/day

Administration Oral: Administer with food or milk to decrease GI upset

Monitoring Parameters Liver enzymes, BUN, serum creatinine, CBC with differential, platelet count; periodic ophthalmologic exams with chronic use

Patient Information Avoid alcohol; may cause dizziness; do not take with aspirin

Dosage Forms Tablet: 150 mg, 200 mg

References

Giannini EH and Cawkwell GD, "Drug Treatment in Children With Juvenile Rheumatoid Arthritis. Past, Present, and Future," *Pediatr Clin North Am*, 1995, 42(5):1099-125.

Skeith KJ and Jamali F, "Clinical Pharmacokinetics of Drugs Used in Juvenile Arthritis," *Clin Pharmacokinet*, 1991, 21(2):129-49.

♦ **Sulphafurazole** *see* SulfiSOXAZOLE *on page 1056*

Sumatriptan (SOO ma trip tan)

Related Information

Serotonin Syndrome *on page 1420*

U.S. Brand Names Imitrex®

Therapeutic Category Antimigraine Agent

Generic Available No

Use

Injection, intranasal, and tablets: Acute treatment of migraine with or without aura

Injection: Acute treatment of cluster headaches

Pregnancy Risk Factor C

Contraindications Hypersensitivity to sumatriptan or any component; I.V. administration (coronary vasospasm may occur); ischemic heart disease, Prinzmetal angina, cerebrovascular or peripheral vascular syndromes (eg, stroke, TIA, ischemic bowel disease), severe hepatic impairment, patients with signs or symptoms of ischemic heart disease, MI, silent MI, uncontrolled hypertension; concomitant use of ergotamine derivatives (within last 24 hours), vasoconstrictive drugs, methysergide, or MAO inhibitors; use of MAO inhibitors within past 2 weeks; management of hemiplegic or basilar migraine

Warnings Life-threatening or fatal hypersensitivity reactions may occur; rarely, serious coronary events including acute MI, life-threatening arrhythmias, and death, may occur; avoid use in patients with risk factors for coronary artery disease, unless cardiovascular disease can be ruled out; consider administering first dose under close supervision to patients at high risk for coronary disease; EKG should be performed if angina-like symptoms occur; periodically evaluate cardiovascular system in patients with risk factors for coronary artery disease

Precautions Temporary increases in peripheral vascular resistance and blood pressure may occur; use with caution in patients with impaired hepatic or renal function, epilepsy; cross-hypersensitivity to sulfonamides is possible; other potentially serious neurological conditions should be ruled out prior to acute migraine therapy; sumatriptan (given at five times the maximum oral single dose) has caused corneal opacities in dogs; other animal studies suggest it may bind to the melanin of the eye; human studies are not available

(Continued)

Sumatriptan *(Continued)*

Adverse Reactions

Cardiovascular: Hypertension; flushing; chest tightness, pressure, pain; coronary artery vasospasm; vascular ischemia; colonic ischemia; rarely: acute MI, life-threatening arrhythmias

Central nervous system: Dizziness, drowsiness, headache

Gastrointestinal: Nausea, vomiting, abdominal discomfort; bad or unusual taste (with intranasal use)

Local: Injection site reaction (59%), pain, redness at injection site

Neuromuscular & skeletal: Weakness, myalgia, neck pain with stiffness

Miscellaneous: Atypical sensations of tingling, heat, flushing, burning, heaviness, pressure, tightness, numbness; jaw, mouth, tongue discomfort; diaphoresis; rarely: hypersensitivity reactions (potentially fatal anaphylaxis or anaphylactoid reactions)

Drug Interactions Use with ergot-containing drugs may result in prolonged vasospasm reactions; vasoconstrictive drugs; methysergide; MAO inhibitors (MAO inhibitors may significantly increase sumatriptan serum concentrations; use of MAO inhibitors is contraindicated); selective serotonin reuptake inhibitors (may cause weakness, incoordination, hyper-reflexia; monitor patients carefully)

Food Interactions Food slightly delays the rate but not the extent of oral absorption

Stability Store at 2°C to 20°C (36°F to 86°F); protect from light

Mechanism of Action Selective agonist for serotonin ($5\text{-}HT_1$) receptor in cranial arteries; causes vasoconstriction and reduces sterile inflammation associated with antidromic neuronal transmission correlating with relief of migraine

Pharmacodynamics Migraine pain relief:

Onset of action:

Oral: 1-1.5 hours

S.C.: 10 minutes to 2 hours

Maximum effect: Oral: 2-4 hours

Pharmacokinetics

Distribution: Adults:

V_d (central): 50 L;

V_d (apparent): 2.4 L/kg

Protein binding: 14% to 21%

Metabolism: In the liver to an indole acetic acid metabolite (inactive) which then undergoes ester glucuronide conjugation; may be metabolized by monoamine oxidase (MAO)

Bioavailability:

Oral: ~15%; may be significantly increased with liver disease

Intranasal: 17% (compared to S.C.)

S.C.: 97%

Half-life:

Distribution: 15 minutes

Terminal: 2 hours; range: 1-4 hours

Time to peak serum concentration:

Oral: Healthy adults: 2 hours; during migraine attacks: 2.5 hours

S.C.: Range: 5-20 minutes; mean: 12 minutes

Elimination: 60% of an oral dose is renally excreted (primarily as metabolites), 40% is eliminated via the feces, and only 3% as unchanged drug; 42% of an intranasal dose is excreted as the indole acetic acid metabolite with 3% excreted in the urine unchanged; 22% of a S.C. dose is excreted in urine unchanged and 38% as the indole acetic acid metabolite

Usual Dosage

Children and Adolescents <18 years: Use not recommended:

Intranasal: A randomized, double-blind, placebo-controlled, single-attack study in adolescent migraine patients (12-17 years of age) used sumatriptan nasal spray in doses of 5 mg (n=128), 10 mg (n=133), and 20 mg (n=118). Compared to placebo, the percent of patients with headache relief (reduction in headache pain) at 1 hour postdose was significantly greater for the 10 mg and 20 mg group and at 2 hours postdose was significantly greater for the 5 mg group. The percent of patients with **complete** headache relief at 2 hours was significantly greater for the 20 mg group. Younger patients (12-14 years of age) had higher efficacy rates at lower doses, but patients 15-17 years of age had the highest efficacy with the 20 mg doses (Winner, 2000); a small retrospective review of 10 younger children, 5-12 years of age (mean: 9.9 years) used intranasal doses of 5 mg (n=2) or 20 mg (n=8) to treat 57 headaches; 82.5% of headaches responded to sumatriptan (Hershey, 2001); additional studies are needed

Oral: Efficacy of oral sumatriptan was **not** established in placebo-controlled trials in patients 12-17 years of age (n=701) with doses of 25-100 mg; adverse events were similar to adults; frequency of adverse events was dose- and age-dependent (increased frequency of adverse events in younger patients); postmarketing reports include the occurrence of MI in a 14-year-old male after oral sumatriptan with symptoms occurring within 1 day of drug use

S.C.: An open-labeled prospective trial in 17 children 6-16 years of age with juvenile migraine used S.C. doses of 6 mg in 15 children 30-70 kg, and 3 mg/ dose in two children who weighed 22 kg and 30 kg (MacDonald, 1994); additional studies are needed

Adults:

Intranasal: Initial single dose: 5 mg, 10 mg, or 20 mg administered in one nostril, given as soon as possible after the onset of migraine; 10 mg dose may be administered as 5 mg in each nostril; may repeat after 2 hours; maximum: 40 mg/ day

Oral: Initial single dose: 25 mg given as soon as possible after the onset of a migraine; range: 25-100 mg/dose; maximum single dose: 100 mg; may repeat after 2 hours; maximum: 200 mg/day

S.C.: 6 mg given as soon as possible after the onset of a migraine; a second injection (≤6 mg) may be administered at least 1 hour after the initial dose; maximum dose: 12 mg/24 hours

Dosing adjustment in hepatic dysfunction: Adults: Oral: Maximum single dose: 50 mg

Administration

Intranasal: Each nasal spray unit is preloaded with 1 dose; **do not** test the spray unit before use; remove unit from plastic pack when ready to use; while sitting down, gently blow nose to clear nasal passages; keep head upright and close one nostril gently with index finger; hold container with other hand, with thumb supporting bottom and index and middle fingers on either side of nozzle; insert nozzle into nostril about $1/2$ inch; close mouth; take a breath through nose while releasing spray into nostril by pressing firmly on blue plunger; remove nozzle from nostril; keep head level for 10-20 seconds and gently breathe in through nose and out through mouth; **do not breathe deeply**

Oral: Administer with fluids

Parenteral: S.C. use only; do **not** administer I.M.; do **not** administer I.V. (may cause coronary vasospasm)

Patient Information If pain or tightness in chest or throat occurs, notify physician; females should avoid pregnancy; pain at injection site lasts <1 hour

Additional Information Safety of treating >4 headaches per month is not established; sumatriptan is **not** indicated for migraine prophylaxis

Dosage Forms Note: Injection and tablets are available as succinate; mg strength for all products refers to sumatriptan

Injection, solution, as succinate: 12 mg/mL (0.5 mL)

Solution, nasal spray: 5 mg (100 µL unit dose spray device); 20 mg (100 µL unit dose spray device)

Tablet, as succinate: 25 mg, 50 mg, 100 mg

Extemporaneous Preparations A 5 mg/mL oral liquid preparation made from tablets and 3 different vehicles (Ora-Sweet®, Ora-Sweet® SF, or Syrpalta® syrups) was stable for 21 days when stored in amber glass bottles in the dark under refrigeration (4°C); **Note:** Preparations with Ora-Sweet® and Ora-Sweet® SF used Ora-Plus® as a suspending vehicle; grind nine 100 mg tablets in a mortar into a fine powder; add 40 mL of Ora-Plus® Suspending Vehicle, 5 mL at a time, and mix thoroughly between each addition; **Note:** The suspending vehicle helps to facilitate dispersion of the tablets and is used only if Ora-Sweet® or Ora-Sweet® SF is the vehicle to be used (ie, suspending vehicle is not used if preparation uses Syrpalta® syrup as the vehicle); transfer to a calibrated amber glass bottle; rinse mortar and pestle 5 times with 10 mL of Ora-Plus® suspension vehicle pouring into bottle each time; qsad with appropriate syrup (Ora-Sweet® or Ora-Sweet® SF) to 180 mL; label "shake well," "refrigerate," and "protect from light"; (**Note:** This study also tested microbial growth on days 0 and 28; no growth of bacteria or fungus occurred) (Fish, 1997)

Fish DN, Beall HD, Goodwin SD, et al, "Stability of Sumatriptan Succinate in Extemporaneously Prepared Oral Liquids," *Am J Health Syst Pharm*, 1997, 54(14):1619-22.

References

Hershey AD, Powers SW, LeCates S, et al, "Effectiveness of Nasal Sumatriptan in 5- to 12-Year-Old Children," *Headache*, 2001, 41(7):693-7.

MacDonald JT, "Treatment of Juvenile Migraine With Subcutaneous Sumatriptan," *Headache*, 1994, 34(10):581-2.

Scott AK, "Sumatriptan Clinical Pharmacokinetics," *Clin Pharmacokinet*, 1994, 27(5):337-44.

Winner P, Rothner AD, Saper J, et al, "A Randomized, Double-Blind, Placebo-Controlled Study of Sumatriptan Nasal Spray in the Treatment of Acute Migraine in Adolescents," *Pediatrics*, 2000, 106(5):989-97.

♦ **Summer's Eve® SpecialCare™ Medicated Anti-Itch Cream [OTC]** *see* Hydrocortisone *on page 573*

- **Sumycin®** *see* Tetracycline *on page 1074*
- **Superdophilus® [OTC]** *see* Lactobacillus acidophilus and Lactobacillus bulgaricus *on page 648*
- **Supeudol® (Can)** *see* Oxycodone *on page 845*
- **Suprax® [DSC]** *see* Cefixime [DSC] *on page 229*
- **Surfak® [OTC]** *see* Docusate *on page 402*
- **Survanta®** *see* Beractant *on page 168*
- **Sustiva®** *see* Efavirenz *on page 428*
- **Suxamethonium** *see* Succinylcholine *on page 1044*
- **Symax SL** *see* Hyoscyamine *on page 585*
- **Symax SR** *see* Hyoscyamine *on page 585*
- **Symmetrel®** *see* Amantadine *on page 73*
- **Synacthen** *see* Cosyntropin *on page 310*
- **Synagis®** *see* Palivizumab *on page 852*
- **Synalar®** *see* Fluocinolone *on page 498*
- **Syn-Diltiazem® (Can)** *see* Diltiazem *on page 388*
- **Synercid®** *see* Quinupristin/Dalfopristin *on page 970*
- **Synthetic Lung Surfactant** *see* Colfosceril [DSC] *on page 304*
- **Synthroid®** *see* Levothyroxine *on page 669*
- **T₃** *see* Liothyronine *on page 680*
- **T₄ Thyroxine** *see* Levothyroxine *on page 669*
- **642® Tablet (Can)** *see* Propoxyphene *on page 950*
- **Tac™-3 [DSC]** *see* Triamcinolone *on page 1112*
- **Tacozin® (Can)** *see* Piperacillin and Tazobactam *on page 907*

Tacrolimus (ta KROE li mus)

U.S. Brand Names Prograf®; Protopic®
Synonyms FK506
Therapeutic Category Immunosuppressant Agent
Generic Available No
Use
> Oral/injection: Immunosuppressant used with corticosteroids to prevent graft versus host disease in patients who have received organ transplants and are not responding to cyclosporine
> Topical: Moderate to severe atopic dermatitis in patients not responsive to conventional therapy or when conventional therapy is not appropriate

Pregnancy Risk Factor C
Contraindications Hypersensitivity to tacrolimus, polyoxyl 60 hydrogenated castor oil, or any component
Warnings Avoid use with other immunosuppressants; immunosuppression with tacrolimus may result in increased susceptibility to infection and the possible development of lymphoma; insulin-dependent post-transplant diabetes mellitus was reported in 11% to 20% of transplant patients; risk increases in African-American and Hispanic kidney transplant patients. Neurotoxicity and nephrotoxicity have been reported especially when used in high doses. To avoid excess nephrotoxicity, do not administer simultaneously with cyclosporine. Adequate airway, supportive measures, and agents for treating anaphylaxis should be available when tacrolimus is administered I.V.
Precautions Use with caution and modify dosage in patients with hepatic or renal impairment
Adverse Reactions
> Cardiovascular: Hypertension, hypotension, peripheral edema, chest pain, myocardial hypertrophy, angina pectoris, palpitations, CHF, arrhythmias, hypertrophic obstructive cardiomyopathy, thrombosis
> Central nervous system: Encephalopathy, headache, hallucinations, agitation, pain, fever, seizures, altered mental status, insomnia, dizziness, depression
> Dermatologic: Pruritus, rash, Stevens-Johnson syndrome, photosensitivity
> Endocrine & metabolic: Hyperkalemia, hyperglycemia, hypomagnesemia, hypophosphatemia, hypercalcemia, hypercholesterolemia, Cushing's syndrome
> Gastrointestinal: Diarrhea, nausea, vomiting, constipation, dyspepsia, pancreatitis, GI hemorrhage
> Genitourinary: Dysuria, hematuria, albuminuria, nocturia, cystitis, oliguria
> Hematologic: Anemia, thrombocytopenia, leukocytosis, eosinophilia
> Hepatic: Hepatotoxicity; elevated AST, ALT, and LDH
> Neuromuscular & skeletal: Tremor, paresthesia, back pain, arthralgia, myalgia
> Ocular: Abnormal vision
> Otic: Tinnitus, deafness

Renal: Nephrotoxicity, elevated BUN and serum creatinine, oliguria
Respiratory: Pleural effusion, respiratory distress, cough
Miscellaneous: Increased susceptibility to infections, lymphoproliferative disorders, anaphylaxis (may be due to polyoxyl 60 hydrogenated castor oil injectable vehicle), hemolytic-uremic syndrome

Topical:
Cardiovascular: Peripheral edema
Central nervous system: Headache, fever, hyperesthesia, pain
Dermatologic: Skin burning, pruritus, erythema, acne, urticaria, rash
Endocrine & metabolic: Dysmenorrhea
Gastrointestinal: Diarrhea, abdominal pain, nausea
Respiratory: Cough, rhinitis

Drug Interactions Cytochrome P450 isoenzyme CYP3A3/4 substrate

Diltiazem, verapamil, nifedipine, fluconazole, itraconazole, ketoconazole, cimetidine, clarithromycin, erythromycin, methylprednisolone, omeprazole, nefazodone, cisapride, protease inhibitors, metoclopramide, cyclosporine, and oral clotrimazole increase tacrolimus serum concentrations; antacids, cholestyramine, sodium polystyrene sulfonate, carbamazepine, phenobarbital, primidone, phenytoin, rifabutin, rifampin, and St John's wort decrease tacrolimus serum concentrations; additive nephrotoxicity when used with NSAIDs, cisplatin, nephrotoxic antibiotics, amphotericin B, or cyclosporine

Food Interactions Food reduces the rate and extent of absorption by ~27%; grapefruit juice may increase tacrolimus blood concentration

Stability Reconstitution: Stable for 24 hours when mixed in D_5W or NS in glass or polyolefin containers; 24-hour stability in plastic syringes stored at 24°C; no need to protect from light; do not store in polyvinyl chloride containers since the polyoxyl 60 hydrogenated castor oil injectable vehicle may leach phthalates from polyvinyl chloride containers; polyvinyl-containing administration sets adsorb drug and may lead to a lower dose being delivered to the patient; tacrolimus is unstable in alkaline media; do not mix with acyclovir or ganciclovir

Mechanism of Action Binds to an intracellular protein forming a complex which inhibits phosphatase activity of calcineurin resulting in the inhibition of T-cell activation

Pharmacokinetics
Absorption: Erratic and incomplete oral absorption (5% to 67%)
Distribution: Distributes to erythrocytes, breast milk, lung, kidneys, pancreas, liver, placenta, heart, and spleen; V_d: 5-65 L/kg (V_d is increased in pediatric patients versus adults)
Protein binding: 99% to alpha-acid glycoprotein (some binding to albumin)
Metabolism: Hepatic metabolism through the cytochrome P450 system (CYP3A) to eight possible metabolites (major metabolite: 31-demethyl tacrolimus has same activity as tacrolimus in vitro)
Bioavailability:
Oral:
Children: 10% to 52%
Adults: 7% to 28%
Topical: <0.5%
Half-life, elimination: 3.5-40.5 hours (mean: 8.7 hours)
Time to peak serum concentration: Oral: 1-4 hours
Elimination: Primarily in bile; <1% excreted unchanged in urine
Clearance: 7-103 mL/minute/kg (average: 30 mL/minute/kg); clearance may be higher in children

Usual Dosage
Children:
Oral: 0.15-0.4 mg/kg/day divided every 12 hours; children generally require higher maintenance dosages on a mg/kg basis than adults
Liver transplant: Initial: 0.15-0.2 mg/kg/day divided every 12 hours
I.V. continuous infusion: 0.03-0.15 mg/kg/day
Children ≥2 years: Topical: Moderate to severe atopic dermatitis: Apply 0.03% ointment to affected area twice daily; continue applications for 1 week after symptoms have cleared
Adults:
Oral: 0.15-0.3 mg/kg/day divided every 12 hours
Liver transplant: Initial: 0.1-0.15 mg/kg/day divided every 12 hours
Kidney transplant: Initial: 0.2 mg/kg/day divided every 12 hours
I.V. continuous infusion: 0.03-0.1 mg/kg/day
Dosing adjustment in renal or hepatic impairment: Patients with renal or hepatic impairment should receive the lowest dose in the recommended dosage range; further reductions in dose below these ranges may be required
(Continued)

Tacrolimus *(Continued)*

Hemodialysis: Not removed by hemodialysis

Administration

Oral: Administer on an empty stomach; use oral syringe or glass container (not plastic or foam cup) when administering this medication; do not administer with grapefruit juice; do not administer within 2 hours before or after antacids

Parenteral: May administer by I.V. continuous infusion; I.V. concentrate for injection must be diluted to 0.004-0.02 mg/mL in NS or D_5W prior to administration; PVC-free administration tubing should be used to minimize the potential for significant drug absorption onto the tubing; begin no sooner than 6-hours post-transplant; continue only until oral medication can be tolerated

Topical: For external use only; do not cover with occlusive dressings; rub ointment in gently and completely onto clean, dry skin

Monitoring Parameters Liver enzymes, BUN, serum creatinine, glucose, potassium, magnesium, phosphorus, blood tacrolimus concentrations, CBC with differential; blood pressure, neurologic status, EKG

Reference Range Limited data correlating serum level to therapeutic efficacy/toxicity:
Trough (whole blood ELISA): 5-20 ng/mL
Trough (HPLC): 0.5-1.5 ng/mL

Patient Information Administer dose at the same time each day; you will be susceptible to infection (avoid crowds and people with infections); notify physician if you develop increased urination, thirst, chest pain, acute headache or dizziness, symptoms of respiratory infection, rash, unusual bruising or bleeding. May cause photosensitivity reactions (eg, exposure to sunlight may cause severe sunburn, skin rash, redness, or itching); avoid exposure to sunlight and artificial light sources (sunlamps, tanning booth/bed); wear protective clothing, wide-brimmed hats, sunglasses, and lip sunscreen (SPF ≥15); use a sunscreen [broad-spectrum sunscreen or physical sunscreen (preferred) or sunblock with SPF ≥15]; contact physician if reaction occurs.

Nursing Implications Patients receiving I.V. tacrolimus should be under continuous observation for at least the first 30 minutes following dosage initiation; adequate airway, supportive measures, and agents for treating anaphylaxis should be available when tacrolimus is administered I.V.

Additional Information Tacrolimus should be initiated no sooner than 6 hours after transplant; convert I.V. tacrolimus to oral form as soon as possible or within 2-3 days (the oral formulation should be started 8-12 hours after stopping the I.V. infusion); when switching a patient from cyclosporine to tacrolimus, allow at least 24 hours after discontinuing cyclosporine before initiating tacrolimus therapy to minimize the risk of nephrotoxicity

Additional dosing considerations:

Switch from I.V. to oral therapy: Approximately three-fold increase in dose compared to I.V.

Pediatric patients: Approximately two times higher dose compared to adults

Dosage Forms

Capsule (Prograf®): 0.5 mg, 1 mg, 5 mg

Injection, solution (Prograf®): 5 mg/mL (1 mL) [contains 80% dehydrated alcohol and polyoxyl 60 hydrogenated castor oil]

Ointment, topical (Protopic®): 0.03% (30 g, 60g); 0.1% (30 g, 60 g)

Extemporaneous Preparations A 0.5 mg/mL suspension has been prepared by mixing the contents of six 5 mg tacrolimus capsules with equal amounts of Ora-Plus® and Simple Syrup, NF to make a final volume of 60 mL. When compounding tacrolimus oral suspension, protect hands with latex gloves. The suspension is stable for 56 days when stored at room temperature in either glass or plastic amber prescription bottles. Label "shake well before using."

Jacobson PA, Johnson CE, West NJ, et al, "Stability of Tacrolimus in an Extemporaneously Compounded Oral Liquid," *Am J Health Sys Pharm* , 1997, 54(2):178-80.

References

Asante-Korang A, Boyle GJ, Webber SA, et al, "Experience of FK506 Immune Suppression in Pediatric Heart Transplantation: A Study of Long-Term Adverse Effects," *J Heart Lung Transplant*, 1996, 15(4):415-22.

McDiarmid SV, Colonna JO, Shaked A, et al, "Differences in Oral FK506 Dose Requirements Between Adults and Pediatric Liver Transplant Patients," *Transplantation*, 1993, 55(6):1328-32.

Menegaux F, Keeffe EB, Andrews BT, et al, "Neurological Complications of Liver Transplantation in Adult Versus Pediatric Patients," *Transplantation*, 1994, 58(4):447-50.

♦ **Tagamet®** *see* Cimetidine *on page 272*

♦ **Tagamet®-HB [OTC]** *see* Cimetidine *on page 272*

♦ **Tagamet®-HB 200 [OTC]** *see* Cimetidine *on page 272*

♦ **Talwin®** *see* Pentazocine *on page 880*

♦ **Talwin® NX** *see* Pentazocine *on page 880*

+ **Tambocor**™ *see* Flecainide *on page 486*
+ **Tamiflu**® *see* Oseltamivir *on page 838*
+ **TAO**® *see* Troleandomycin *on page 1123*
+ **Tapazole**® *see* Methimazole *on page 734*
+ **Targel**® **(Can)** *see* Coal Tar *on page 299*
+ **Tarka**® **(Can)** *see* Verapamil *on page 1144*
+ **Taro-Carbamazepine Chewable (Can)** *see* Carbamazepine *on page 209*
+ **Taro-Sone**® **(Can)** *see* Betamethasone *on page 169*
+ **Taro-Warfarin (Can)** *see* Warfarin *on page 1156*
+ **Tavist**® **Allergy [OTC]** *see* Clemastine *on page 287*
+ **Taxol**® *see* Paclitaxel *on page 851*
+ **Tazicef**® *see* Ceftazidime *on page 238*
+ **Tazidime**® *see* Ceftazidime *on page 238*
+ **Tazobactam and Piperacillin** *see* Piperacillin and Tazobactam *on page 907*
+ **3TC** *see* Lamivudine *on page 650*
+ **3TC, Abacavir, and AZT** *see* Abacavir, Lamivudine, and Zidovudine *on page 32*
+ **3TC, Abacavir, and ZDV** *see* Abacavir, Lamivudine, and Zidovudine *on page 32*
+ **3TC, Abacavir, and Zidovudine** *see* Abacavir, Lamivudine, and Zidovudine *on page 32*
+ **3TC, ABC, and AZT** *see* Abacavir, Lamivudine, and Zidovudine *on page 32*
+ **3TC, ABC, and ZDV** *see* Abacavir, Lamivudine, and Zidovudine *on page 32*
+ **3TC and AZT** *see* Lamivudine and Zidovudine *on page 652*
+ **3TC and ZDV** *see* Lamivudine and Zidovudine *on page 652*
+ **T-Cell Growth Factor** *see* Aldesleukin *on page 56*
+ **TCGF** *see* Aldesleukin *on page 56*
+ **TCN** *see* Tetracycline *on page 1074*
+ **Tears Naturale**® **PM [OTC]** *see* Ocular Lubricant *on page 831*
+ **Tears Renewed**® **[OTC]** *see* Ocular Lubricant *on page 831*
+ **Tebrazid**™ **(Can)** *see* Pyrazinamide *on page 961*
+ **Tegopen**® *see* Cloxacillin *on page 298*
+ **Tegretol**® *see* Carbamazepine *on page 209*
+ **Tegretol**®**-XR** *see* Carbamazepine *on page 209*
+ **Tegrin**® **[OTC]** *see* Coal Tar *on page 299*
+ **Temodal**™ **(Can)** *see* Temozolomide *on page 1065*
+ **Temodar**® *see* Temozolomide *on page 1065*

Temozolomide (te mo ZOLE oh mide)

U.S. Brand Names Temodar®
Canadian Brand Names Temodal™
Synonyms SCH 52365
Therapeutic Category Antineoplastic Agent, Alkylating Agent
Generic Available No
Use Treatment of refractory anaplastic astrocytoma with relapse after initial therapy with a nitrosourea and procarbazine; active against primary and recurrent grade 3 and 4 gliomas and metastatic melanoma
Pregnancy Risk Factor D
Contraindications Hypersensitivity to temozolomide, dacarbazine, or any component; pregnancy
Warnings The FDA currently recommends that procedures for proper handling and disposal of antineoplastic agents be considered. Thrombocytopenia and neutropenia are dose-limiting toxicities which occur late in the treatment cycle and usually resolve within 14 days; prior to therapy initiation patients must have an absolute neutrophil count (ANC) ≥1.5 x 10^9 and a platelet count ≥100 x 10^9/L; obtain a CBC on day 22 and weekly until the ANC >1.5 x 10^9 and platelet count >100 x 10^9; may cause fetal harm so pregnancy should be avoided during therapy
Precautions Use with caution in patients with severe renal or hepatic impairment; since it is unknown whether temozolomide is excreted in breast milk, patients receiving temozolomide should discontinue nursing
Adverse Reactions
  Cardiovascular: Peripheral edema, thromboembolism
  Central nervous system: Headache, dizziness, fatigue, anxiety, confusion, depression, amnesia, insomnia, convulsions, hemiparesis, lethargy, fever
  Dermatologic: Rash, pruritus, alopecia
  Gastrointestinal: Nausea, vomiting, anorexia, diarrhea, abdominal pain, constipation, mucositis, dysphagia
  (Continued)

Temozolomide *(Continued)*

Genitourinary: Urinary tract infection, urinary frequency

Hematologic: Thrombocytopenia, leukopenia, anemia, lymphopenia

Hepatic: Hepatotoxicity, elevated liver enzymes

Neuromuscular & skeletal: Myalgia, ataxia

Ocular: Diplopia, visual changes

Miscellaneous: Secondary tumors or malignancy, anaphylaxis (rare)

Drug Interactions Valproic acid may decrease temozolomide clearance by 5%

Food Interactions Food reduces the rate and extent of absorption

Stability Store capsules at room temperature.

Mechanism of Action Prodrug which is hydrolyzed to MTIC and exerts its effect by site-specific DNA cross-linking resulting from the methylation of the O^6 and N^7 positions of guanine.

Pharmacokinetics

Absorption: Oral: Rapidly and completely absorbed

Distribution: Penetrates CNS at ~30% of plasma levels

V_d: Adults: 17-28 L/m^2

Protein binding: 14%

Bioavailability: 100%

Metabolism: At a neutral or alkaline pH, hydrolyzes to MTIC (3-methyl-(triazen-1-yl) imidazole-4-carboxamide) and temozolomide acid metabolite; MTIC is further metabolized to 5-amino-imidazole-4-carboxamide (AIC) and methylhydrazine (active alkylating agent)

Half-life:

Children: 1.7 hours

Adults: 1.6-1.8 hours

Time to peak serum concentration: Oral: 1 hour

Elimination: <1% excreted in feces; 5% to 7% of unchanged temozolomide excreted renally

Clearance: 5.5 L/hour/m^2

Usual Dosage Oral (refer to individual protocols):

Children: In a Phase I study to determine the maximum tolerated dose of temozolomide in pediatric solid tumor patients with prior craniospinal irradiation (CSI) therapy and those without prior CSI (n=53; age range: 1-19 years), 100-240 mg/m^2/day was administered; the maximum tolerated dose was 215 mg/m^2/day for 5 days in patients without prior CSI and 180 mg/m^2/day for 5 days in patients with prior CSI with subsequent courses to begin on day 28 (Nicholson, 1998)

Adults: Initial: 150 mg/m^2/day for 5 consecutive days of a 28-day cycle; subsequent doses are adjusted based on nadir platelet count and ANC during the previous cycle (day 22) and ANC and platelet count on day 29; treatment cycle should be held until ANC >1500/µL and platelet count >100,000/µL

Minimum dose: 100 mg/m^2/day once daily for 5 days every 4 weeks; maintenance dose: 200 mg/m^2/day once daily for 5 days every 4 weeks; treatment can be continued until there is disease progression, but optimum duration of therapy is unknown

Dose modification:

If ANC <1000/µL or the platelet count is <50,000/µL, postpone therapy until ANC >1500/µL and platelet count >100,000/µL; reduce dose by 50 mg/m^2 for subsequent cycle.

If ANC 1000-1500/µL or platelets 50,000-100,000/µL, postpone therapy until ANC >1500/µL and platelet count >100,000/µL; maintain initial dose.

If ANC >1500/µL and platelet count >100,000/µL, increase dose to, or maintain dose at 200 mg/m^2/day for 5 days for subsequent cycle.

Administration Oral: Swallow capsule intact with a glass of water; do not chew; if patient is unable to swallow capsule, open capsule and dissolve in apple juice or applesauce taking precautions to avoid exposure to the cytotoxic agent; administer on an empty stomach to reduce the incidence of nausea and vomiting; may administer with food as long as food intake and administration time are performed in a consistent manner to ensure consistent bioavailability; bedtime administration may be preferred

Monitoring Parameters CBC with ANC (absolute neutrophil count) and platelet count

Patient Information Instruct patient to take all the capsules in a single dose package for that day of the cycle (each day's dose is packaged separately); advise women and men to avoid pregnancy

Nursing Implications Avoid opening capsules; if capsules are accidentally opened, avoid inhalation or contact with skin or mucous membranes

Additional Information To minimize the risk of a wrong dose error, each day's dose should be packaged separately and labeled as day 1, day 2, day 3, day 4, and day 5.

Dosage Forms Capsule: 5 mg, 20 mg, 100 mg, 250 mg

References

Friedman HS, Kerby T, and Calvert H, "Temozolomide and Treatment of Malignant Glioma," *Clin Cancer Res*, 2000, 6(7):2585-97.

Middleton MR, Grob JJ, Aaronson N, et al, "Randomized Phase III Study of Temozolomide Versus Dacarbazine in the Treatment of Patients With Advanced Metastatic Malignant Melanoma," *J Clin Oncol*, 2000, 18(1):158-66.

Nicholson HS, Krailo M, Ames MM, et al, "Phase I Study of Temozolomide in Children and Adolescents With Recurrent Solid Tumors: A Report From the Children's Cancer Group," *J Clin Oncol*, 1998, 16(9):3037-43.

♦ **Tempra® (Can)** *see* Acetaminophen *on page 36*

Tenofovir (te NOE fo veer)

U.S. Brand Names Viread™

Synonyms PMPA

Therapeutic Category Antiretroviral Agent; HIV Agents (Anti-HIV Agents); Nucleotide Reverse Transcriptase Inhibitor (NRTI)

Generic Available No

Use Treatment of HIV-1 infection in combination with other antiretroviral agents. **(Note:** HIV regimens consisting of **three** antiretroviral agents are strongly recommended)

Pregnancy Risk Factor B

Contraindications Hypersensitivity to tenofovir or any component

Warnings Cases of lactic acidosis, severe hepatomegaly with steatosis and death have been reported in patients receiving nucleoside analogues; most of these cases have been in women; prolonged nucleoside use, obesity, and prior liver disease may be risk factors; use with extreme caution in patients with other risk factors for liver disease; discontinue therapy in patients who develop laboratory or clinical evidence of lactic acidosis or pronounced hepatotoxicity. Avoid use in patients with renal impairment (Cl_{cr} <60 mL/minute); tenofovir is renally eliminated and pharmacokinetic data in patients with renal impairment is not available; renal dysfunction, including hypophosphatemia may occur (especially in patients with renal disease, underlying systemic disease, or those taking nephrotoxic medications); avoid tenofovir in patients with concomitant or recent use of nephrotoxic agents

Precautions Use with caution in patients with hepatic impairment (tenofovir pharmacokinetics may be altered); fat redistribution and accumulation [ie, central obesity, peripheral wasting, facial wasting, breast enlargement, dorsocervical fat enlargement (buffalo hump), and cushingoid appearance] have been observed in patients receiving antiretroviral agents (causal relationship not established). Bone toxicity (osteomalacia and reduced bone mineral density) and renal toxicity (increased S_{cr}, BUN, calciuria, phosphaturia, glucosuria, proteinuria, and hypophosphatemia) have been observed in animal studies; long term effects in humans is not known; monitor for potential bone and renal toxicities during therapy.

Adverse Reactions

Central nervous system: Headache, dizziness

Dermatologic: Rash

Endocrine & metabolic: Hypophosphatemia, lactic acidosis

Gastrointestinal: Nausea, diarrhea, vomiting, flatulence, anorexia, pancreatitis

Hepatic: Elevated liver enzymes

Neuromuscular & skeletal: Asthenia

Renal: Renal impairment, elevated serum creatinine, kidney failure, Fanconi syndrome

Respiratory: Dyspnea

Drug Interactions Cytochrome P450 isoenzyme CYP1A2 inhibitor (minor)

Tenofovir significantly increases didanosine peak concentrations and AUC, potentially increasing didanosine-related adverse effects, such as pancreatitis and neuropathy; use didanosine with great caution in patients receiving tenofovir; monitor patients closely; discontinue didanosine if adverse effects/toxicity develop; **Note:** Some centers make an emperic reduction in the didanosine dosage when used with tenofovir (further studies are needed). Tenofovir may decrease peak serum concentrations of lamivudine by 24% and indinavir by 11%; tenofovir may decrease peak concentrations and AUC of lopinavir and ritonavir. Indinavir may increase tenofovir peak concentrations by 14%; lopinavir/ritonavir may increase serum concentrations and AUC of tenofovir. Drugs that are excreted by active tubular secretion (eg, acyclovir, cidofovir, ganciclovir, valacyclovir, valganciclovir) may compete with tenofovir for elimination and may result in an increase in serum concentrations of tenofovir or these coadministered drugs (monitor for dose-related toxicities); drugs that impair renal function may decrease the renal elimination of tenofovir and result in increased tenofovir serum concentrations

(Continued)

Tenofovir *(Continued)*

Food Interactions A high-fat meal increases oral bioavailability (AUC) by 40% and increases peak serum concentrations by 14%; food delays the time to peak concentrations by 1 hour

Mechanism of Action Tenofovir disoproxil fumarate (TDF) is a prodrug of tenofovir; *in vivo*, TDF undergoes diester hydrolysis to tenofovir; tenofovir is an acyclic nucleoside phosphate (nucleotide) analog of adenosine 5'-monophosphate; tenofovir undergoes phosphorylation by cellular enzymes to the active tenofovir diphosphate, which serves as an alternative substrate to deoxyadenosine 5'-triphosphate, a natural substrate for cellular DNA polymerase and reverse transcriptase; tenofovir diphosphate inhibits HIV viral reverse transcriptase by competing with natural deoxyadenosine 5'-triphosphate and by becoming incorporated into viral DNA causing chain termination. **Note:** Tenofovir also has activity against the hepatitis B virus (studies are ongoing).

Pharmacokinetics

Distribution: Mean V_d: Adults: 1.2-1.3 L/kg

Protein binding: Minimal (7.2% to serum proteins)

Metabolism: Not metabolized by CYP isoenzymes; tenofovir disoproxil fumarate (a prodrug) undergoes diester hydrolysis to tenofovir; tenofovir undergoes phosphorylation to the active tenofovir diphosphate

Bioavailability: 25% (fasting); high-fat meals will increase AUC by 40%

Half-life: Adults: Serum: 17 hours; intracellular: 10-50 hours

Time to peak serum concentration: Fasting: 1 hour

Elimination: Excreted via glomerular filtration and active tubular secretion; after I.V. administration: 70% to 80% is excreted in the urine as unchanged drug within 72 hours; after multiple oral doses (administered with food): 32% ± 10% is excreted in the urine within 24 hours

Dialysis: Effects of hemodialysis and peritoneal dialysis are not known

Usual Dosage Oral:

Note: Clinical trials previously excluded patients <18 years of age; a phase I open-label, dose escalation study in children (4 to <18 years of age) is currently enrolling patients; call 301-496-7308 for patient enrollment eligibility

Adolescents ≥18 years and Adults: 300 mg once daily with a meal

Dosing adjustment in renal impairment: Cl_{cr} <60 mL/minute: Not recommended; avoid use, no dosage guidelines are available.

Administration Administer with meals to increase absorption

Monitoring Parameters CBC with differential, hemoglobin, MCV, reticulocyte count, liver enzymes, bilirubin, CD4 cell count, HIV RNA plasma levels, renal and hepatic function tests. Monitor for potential bone and renal abnormalities; consider monitoring for alterations in S_{cr} and serum phosphorus in patients at risk or with a history of renal dysfunction.

Patient Information Tenofovir is not a cure for HIV; take tenofovir every day as prescribed, with a meal (this will help increase the amount of tenofovir in the blood); do not change dose or discontinue without physician's advice; if a dose is missed, take it as soon as possible, then return to normal dosing schedule; if a dose is skipped, do **not** double the next dose; report the use of other medications, nonprescription medications and herbal or natural products to your physician and pharmacist; long-term effects are not known; notify physician if persistent severe abdominal pain, nausea, or vomiting occurs

HIV medications may cause changes in body fat, including an increase in fat in the upper back and neck, breasts, and trunk; a loss of fat from the face, arms, and legs may also occur.

Additional Information Clinical trials involved the addition of tenofovir (versus placebo) to stable antiretroviral regimens in treatment-experienced adults who had evidence of HIV replication despite therapy; the risk:benefit ratio in treatment-naive patients has not been determined. Patients who received tenofovir showed significant reductions in viral load; long term studies demonstrating a decrease of clinical progression of HIV are needed.

Consider tenofovir in patients with HIV strains that would be susceptible as assessed by treatment history or laboratory tests. Mutation of reverse transcriptase at the 65 codon (K65R mutation) confers *in vitro* resistance to tenofovir; the K65R mutation is selected in some patients after treatment with didanosine, zalcitabine, or abacavir; thus, cross-resistance may occur. Multiple nucleoside mutations with a T69S double insertion showed decreased *in vitro* susceptibility to tenofovir; patients with HIV strains that had ≥3 zidovudine-associated mutations that included M41L or L210W showed decreased responses to tenofovir (but these responses were still better than placebo); patients with mutations at K65R, or L74V without zidovudine-associated mutations seemed to have a decreased response to tenofovir

Dosage Forms Tablet, as disoproxil fumarate: 300 mg [equivalent to 245 mg tenofovir disoproxil]

References

Center for Disease Control and Prevention, "Guidelines for Using Antiretroviral Agents Among HIV-Infected Adults and Adolescents. Recommendations of the Panel on Clinical Practices for Treatment of HIV," *MMWR*, 2002, 51(RR-7):1-55.

Deeks SG, Barditch-Crovo P, Lietman PS, et al, "Safety, Pharmacokinetics, and Antiretroviral Activity of Intravenous 9-[2-(R)-(Phosphonomethoxy)propyl]adenine, a Novel Anti-human Immunodeficiency Virus (HIV) Therapy, in HIV-Infected Adults," *Antimicrob Agents Chemother*, 1998, 42(9):2380-4.

Panel on Clinical Practices for Treatment of HIV Infection. "Guidelines for the Use of Antiretroviral Agents in HIV-Infected Adults and Adolescents," February 4, 2002, http://www.aidsinfo.nih.gov.

Robbins BL, Srinivas RV, Kim C, et al, "Anti-human Immunodeficiency Virus Activity and Cellular Metabolism of a Potential Prodrug of the Acyclic Nucleoside Phosphonate 9-R-(2-phosphonomethoxypropyl)adenine (PMPA), Bis(Isopropyloxymethyl-carbonyl)PMPA," *Antimicrob Agents Chemother*, 1998, 42(3):612-7.

Srinivas RV and Fridland A, "Antiviral Activities of 9-R-2-Phosphonomethoxypropyl adenine (PMPA) and Bis(Isopropyloxymethylcarbonyl)PMPA Against Various Drug-Resistant Human Immunodeficiency Virus Strains," *Antimicrob Agents Chemother*, 1998, 42(6):1484-7.

♦ **Tenolin (Can)** *see* Atenolol *on page 137*

♦ **Tenormin**® *see* Atenolol *on page 137*

Terbutaline (ter BYOO ta leen)

Related Information

Asthma Guidelines *on page 1376*

U.S. Brand Names Brethine®

Canadian Brand Names Bricanyl® [DSC]

Therapeutic Category Adrenergic Agonist Agent; Antiasthmatic; Beta$_2$-Adrenergic Agonist Agent; Bronchodilator; Sympathomimetic; Tocolytic Agent

Generic Available Yes (tablet)

Use Bronchodilator for relief of reversible bronchospasm in patients with asthma, bronchitis, and emphysema

Pregnancy Risk Factor B

Contraindications Hypersensitivity to terbutaline, other sympathomimetic amines, or any component

Warnings Paradoxical bronchoconstriction may occur with excessive use; if it occurs, discontinue terbutaline immediately

Precautions Use with caution in patients with diabetes mellitus, hypertension, hyperthyroidism, history of seizures, or cardiac disease; excessive or prolonged use may lead to tolerance

Adverse Reactions

Cardiovascular: Tachycardia, hypertension, arrhythmias, flushing, prolonged QT$_c$ interval, elevated CPK isoenzyme

Central nervous system: Drowsiness, headache, nervousness, seizures, dizziness

Endocrine & metabolic: Hyperglycemia, hypokalemia

Gastrointestinal: Nausea, vomiting, dysgeusia

Neuromuscular & skeletal: Tremor

Otic: Tinnitus

Respiratory: Dyspnea, bronchospasm (with excessive use), pharyngitis, dry throat, chest tightness

Miscellaneous: Diaphoresis

Drug Interactions Additive effects with other sympathomimetics; increased pressor response with methyldopa, MAO inhibitors, oxytocic drugs, and tricyclic antidepressants

Mechanism of Action Relaxes bronchial smooth muscle and muscles of peripheral vasculature by action on beta$_2$-receptors with less effect on heart rate

Pharmacodynamics

Onset of action:

Oral: 30 minutes

Oral inhalation: 5-30 minutes

S.C.: 6-15 minutes

Duration:

Oral: 4-8 hours

Oral inhalation: 3-6 hours

S.C.: 1.5-4 hours

Pharmacokinetics

Absorption: 33% to 50%

Distribution: Breast milk to plasma ratio: <2.9

Metabolism: Possible first-pass metabolism after oral use

Half-life: 5.7 hours (range: 2.9-14 hours)

Time to peak serum concentration: S.C.: 0.5 hours

Elimination: Primarily (60%) unchanged in urine after parenteral use

(Continued)

Terbutaline *(Continued)*

Usual Dosage

Children <12 years:

Oral: Initial: 0.05 mg/kg/dose every 8 hours, increase gradually, up to 0.15 mg/kg/dose; maximum daily dose: 5 mg

S.C.: 0.005-0.01 mg/kg/dose to a maximum of 0.4 mg/dose every 15-20 minutes for 3 doses; may repeat every 2-6 hours as needed

Note: Continuous I.V. infusion has been used successfully in children with asthma; a 2-10 mcg/kg loading dose followed by an 0.08-0.4 mcg/kg/minute continuous infusion; depending upon the clinical response, the dosage may require titration in increments of 0.1-0.2 mcg/kg/minute every 30 minutes; doses as high as 10 mcg/kg/minute have been used.

Children ≥12 years and Adults:

Oral: 2.5-5 mg/dose every 6-8 hours; maximum daily dose:

12-15 years: 7.5 mg

>15 years: 15 mg

S.C.: 0.25 mg/dose repeated in 20 minutes for 3 doses; a total dose of 0.75 mg should not be exceeded

Nebulization: Children and Adults: 0.01-0.03 mL/kg (1 mg = 1 mL using injection); minimum dose: 0.1 mL; maximum dose: 2.5 mL every 4-6 hours

Administration

Oral: May administer without regard to food

Parenteral: May administer undiluted, direct I.V. over 5-10 minutes; for continuous infusion, dilute to a maximum concentration of 1 mg/mL in D_5W or NS

Inhalation: Nebulization: Dilute dose with 1-2 mL NS

Monitoring Parameters Heart rate, blood pressure, respiratory rate, serum potassium, arterial or capillary blood gases (if applicable)

Dosage Forms

Injection, solution, as sulfate: 1 mg/mL (1 mL)

Tablet, as sulfate: 2.5 mg, 5 mg

Extemporaneous Preparations A 1 mg/mL suspension made from terbutaline tablets in simple syrup NF is stable 30 days when refrigerated

Horner RK and Johnson CE, "Stability of An Extemporaneously Compounded Terbutaline Sulfate Oral Liquid," *Am J Hosp Pharm*, 1991, 48(2):293-5.

References

Bohn D, Kalloghlian A, Jenkins J, et al, "Intravenous Salbutamol in the Treatment of Status Asthmaticus in Children," *Crit Care Med*, 1984, 12(10):892-6.

Canny GJ and Levison H, "Aerosols - Therapeutic Use and Delivery in Childhood Asthma," *Ann Allergy*, 1988, 60(1):11-9.

Fuglsang G, Pedersen S, and Borgstrom L, "Dose-Response Relationships of I.V. Administered Terbutaline in Children With Asthma," *J Pediatr*, 1989, 114(2):315-20.

Goldenhersh N and Rachelefsky GS, "Childhood Asthma: Management," *Pediatr Rev*, 1989, 10(9):259-67.

Expert Panel Report 2, "Guidelines for the Diagnosis and Management of Asthma," *Clinical Practice Guidelines*, National Institutes of Health, National Heart, Lung, and Blood Institute, NIH Publication No. 94-4051, April, 1997.

"National Asthma Education and Prevention Program. Expert Panel Report: Guidelines for the Diagnosis and Management of Asthma Update on Selected Topics--2002," *J Allergy Clin Immunol*, 2002, 110(5 Suppl):S141-219.

Rachelefsky GS and Siegel SC, "Asthma in Infants and Children - Treatment of Childhood Asthma: Part II," *J Allergy Clin Immunol*, 1985, 76(3):409-25.

Tipton WR and Nelson HS, "Frequent Parenteral Terbutaline in the Treatment of Status Asthmaticus in Children," *Ann Allergy*, 1987, 58(4):252-6.

♦ **TESPA** *see* Thiotepa *on page 1087*

♦ **Testim™** *see* Testosterone *on page 1070*

♦ **Testoderm®** *see* Testosterone *on page 1070*

♦ **Testoderm® TTS [DSC]** *see* Testosterone *on page 1070*

♦ **Testoderm® With Adhesive** *see* Testosterone *on page 1070*

♦ **Testopel®** *see* Testosterone *on page 1070*

Testosterone *(tes TOS ter one)*

U.S. Brand Names Androderm®; AndroGel®; Delatestryl®; Depo®-Testosterone; Testim™; Testoderm®; Testoderm® TTS [DSC]; Testoderm® With Adhesive; Testopel®

Canadian Brand Names Andriol®; Andropository; Depotest® 100; Everone® 200; Virilon® IM

Synonyms Aqueous Testosterone

Therapeutic Category Androgen

Generic Available No

Use Testosterone replacement therapy in males for conditions associated with a deficiency or absence of endogenous testosterone; primary hypogonadism (congenital or acquired) and hypogonadotropic hypogonadism (congenital or acquired)

Restrictions C-III

Pregnancy Risk Factor X

Contraindications Hypersensitivity to testosterone or any component including testosterone USP that is chemically synthesized from soy (see Warnings); severe renal, hepatic, or cardiac disease; male patients with prostatic or breast cancer, hypercalcemia, pregnancy; use in women

Warnings May accelerate bone maturation without producing compensating gain in linear growth; perform radiographic examination of the hand and wrist every 6 months to determine the rate of bone maturation (when using in prepubertal children). Depo®-Testosterone contains benzyl alcohol which may cause allergic reactions in susceptible individuals; large amounts of benzyl alcohol ($\geq$99 mg/kg/day) have been associated with a potentially fatal toxicity ("gasping syndrome") in neonates; the "gasping syndrome" consists of metabolic acidosis, respiratory distress, gasping respirations, CNS dysfunction (including convulsions, intracranial hemorrhage), hypotension and cardiovascular collapse; *in vitro* and animal studies have shown that benzoate, a metabolite of benzyl alcohol, displaces bilirubin from protein binding sites; avoid use of Depo®-Testosterone in neonates. In the event that unwashed or unclothed skin of a pregnant woman comes in direct contact with testosterone gel, wash with soap and water. Long-term therapy has been associated with serious hepatic adverse effects (hepatitis, hepatic neoplasms, cholestatic hepatitis, jaundice).

Precautions Use with caution in patients with hepatic, cardiac, or renal dysfunction; virilization of female sexual partners has been reported with male use of topical testosterone; may decrease blood glucose and insulin requirements in diabetics; may cause fluid retention; use with caution in patients with mild to moderate cardiovascular disease or other edematous conditions

Adverse Reactions

Cardiovascular: Flushing, edema, hypertension, tachycardia

Central nervous system: Excitation, aggressive behavior, sleeplessness, anxiety, mental depression, headache, nervousness

Dermatologic: Acne, hirsutism, urticaria

Endocrine & metabolic: Gynecomastia, hypercalcemia, hypoglycemia, elevated serum cholesterol, hyperlipemia, hyponatremia, increased or decreased libido

Gastrointestinal: Nausea, abdominal pain, diarrhea

Genitourinary: Epididymitis, priapism, bladder irritability

Hematologic: Leukopenia, suppression of clotting factors, polycythemia

Hepatic: Cholestatic hepatitis, peliosis hepatitis, hepatocellular carcinoma (high doses), elevated liver function tests

Local: Inflammation and itching at injection site

Neuromuscular & skeletal: Myalgia

Respiratory: Sleep apnea

Drug Interactions Cytochrome P450 isoenzyme CYP3A3/4 and CYP3A5-7 substrate Potentiates effects of oral anticoagulants; increases propranolol clearance

Stability Store at room temperature; protect from light; drug reservoirs for transdermals may burst due to excessive pressure or heat

Mechanism of Action Principal endogenous androgen responsible for promoting the growth and development of the male sex organs and maintaining secondary sex characteristics in androgen-deficient males

Pharmacodynamics Duration: Based upon the route of administration and the specific testosterone ester used; the cypionate and enanthate esters have the longest duration, up to 2-4 weeks after I.M. administration; pellets 3-4 months

Pharmacokinetics

Absorption: Transdermal gel: 10%

Protein binding: 98%

Metabolism: Inactivation in liver

Half-life: Cypionate: I.M.: 8 days

Elimination: 90% excreted in urine as metabolites

Usual Dosage

Children: I.M.:

Male hypogonadism: Testosterone cypionate or enanthate:

Initiation of pubertal growth: 40-50 mg/m^2/dose monthly until the growth rate falls to prepubertal levels

Terminal growth phase: 100 mg/m^2/dose monthly until growth ceases

Maintenance virilizing dose: 100 mg/m^2/dose twice monthly

Delayed puberty: 40-50 mg/m^2/dose monthly for 6 months

Adults: Hypogonadism:

Testosterone cypionate or enanthate: I.M.: 50-400 mg every 2-4 weeks

(Continued)

Testosterone *(Continued)*

Transdermal: 5-6 mg/day initially (use 4 mg/day if scrotal area cannot accommodate 6 mg/day system); adjust dosage in 3-4 weeks depending upon testosterone level

Testosterone pellets: S.C.: Dosage depends on the minimum daily requirements of testosterone propionate [each 25 mg testosterone propionate weekly equals 150 mg (2 pellets)]; usual dose (testosterone pellets): 150-450 mg (2-6 pellets) every 3 months

AndroGel®: Transdermal gel: Males >18 years: Initial: 5 g applied once daily (preferably in the morning); may increase as needed to a maximum of 10 g once daily

Adults: Postpubertal cryptorchism: Testosterone or testosterone propionate: I.M.: 10-25 mg 2-3 times/week

Administration

Parenteral: Administer deep I.M.; not for I.V. administration; pellets only are for S.C. administration

Topical:

Androderm® or Testoderm® TTS: The adhesive side of system should be applied to clean, dry area of the skin on the back, abdomen, upper arms or thighs; avoid application over boney prominences or on a part of the body that may be subject to prolonged pressure; **do not apply to the scrotum**; rotate sites every 7 days

AndroGel®: Apply AndroGel® to clean, dry, intact skin of the shoulder and upper arms and/or abdomen. Upon opening the packet(s), the entire contents should be squeezed into the palm of the hand and immediately applied to the application site(s). Application sites should be allowed to dry for a few minutes prior to dressing. Hands should be washed with soap and water after application. Wait at least 1 hour, preferably 5-6 hours, after application before showering or swimming. **Do not apply AndroGel® to the genitals**

Testoderm®: Apply Testoderm® or Testoderm® with Adhesive transdermal system to scrotum; skin should be clean and dry, scrotal hair should be dry-shaved; do not use chemical depilatories; apply transdermal system firmly for 10 seconds. If system should fall off <12 hours from initial application, it may be reapplied; if >12 hours, apply new system at the next scheduled time.

Monitoring Parameters Periodic liver function tests, radiologic examination of wrist and hand every 6 months (when using in prepubertal children); hemoglobin, hematocrit, testosterone level, serum electrolytes, HDL cholesterol, prostate-specific antigen (PSA)

Reference Range Testosterone, Urine:

Male: 100-1500 ng/24 hours

Female: 100-500 ng/24 hours

Patient Information See Administration. Notify physician if penile erections are too frequent or prolonged; notify physician if nausea, vomiting, yellow skin (jaundice), ankle swelling, or breathing problems develop and in particular if sleeping or difficulty with urination occurs.

Nursing Implications 0.1% triamcinolone cream may be applied to skin under Androderm® to decrease irritation; do not use ointment formulations for pretreatment; they may significantly reduce testosterone absorption

Additional Information Testosterone 5% cream, not available commercially (must be compounded), has been effective in the treatment of microphallus when applied topically for 21 days

Dosage Forms

Gel, topical:

AndroGel®: 2.5 g [25 mg] (30s); 5 g [50 mg] (30s)

Testim™: 5 g [50 mg] (30s)

Injection, in oil, as **cypionate** (Depo® Testosterone): 100 mg/mL (10 mL); 200 mg/mL (1 mL, 10 mL) [contains benzyl alcohol and benzyl benzoate]

Injection, in oil, as **enanthate** (Delatestryl®): 200 mg/mL (1 mL [prefilled syringe], (5 mL) [multidose vial])

Pellet, for subcutaneous implantation (Testopel®): 75 mg (1 pellet/vial)

Transdermal system:

Androderm®: 2.5 mg/day (60s); 5 mg/day (30s)

Testoderm®: 4 mg/day (30s); 6 mg/day (30s)

Testoderm® TTS [DSC]: 5 mg/day (30s) [contains alcohol]

Testoderm® with Adhesive: 6 mg/day (30s)

♦ **Tetanus Immune Globulin, Human** *see page 1333*

♦ **Tetanus Toxoid, Adsorbed** *see page 1333*

♦ **Tetanus Toxoid, Fluid** *see page 1333*

Tetracaine (TET ra kane)

U.S. Brand Names AK-T-Caine™; Cepacol Viractin® [OTC]; Opticaine®; Pontocaine®

Canadian Brand Names Ametop™

Synonyms Amethocaine

Therapeutic Category Analgesic, Topical; Local Anesthetic, Injectable; Local Anesthetic, Ophthalmic; Local Anesthetic, Oral; Local Anesthetic, Topical

Generic Available Yes (ophthalmic solution)

Use Local anesthesia in the eye for various diagnostic and examination purposes; spinal anesthesia; local anesthesia for mucous membranes

Pregnancy Risk Factor C

Contraindications Hypersensitivity to tetracaine or any component (see Warnings); patients with liver disease; CNS disease, meningitis (if used for epidural or spinal anesthesia); myasthenia gravis, impaired cardiac conduction; eye infection (ophthalmic) formulation

Warnings Parenteral form may contain sulfites which may cause allergic reactions in susceptible individuals

Precautions Use with caution in patients with cardiac disease and hyperthyroidism

Adverse Reactions

Cardiovascular: Cardiac arrest, bradycardia, myocardial depression, cardiac arrhythmias, hypotension

Central nervous system: Anxiety, apprehension, nervousness, disorientation, seizures, drowsiness, unconsciousness

Dermatologic: Urticaria

Gastrointestinal: Nausea, vomiting

Local: Stinging, burning at injection site

Ocular: Lacrimation, photophobia, corneal epithelial erosion, keratitis, corneal opacification, miosis

Otic: Tinnitus

Respiratory: Respiratory arrest

Drug Interactions Inhibits sulfonamide activity; enhances CNS depression of other CNS depressants

Mechanism of Action Blocks both the generation and conduction of sensory, motor, and autonomic nerve fibers by decreasing the neuronal membrane's permeability to sodium ions, which results in decreasing the rate of depolarization of the nerve membrane

Pharmacodynamics

Onset of action:

Ophthalmic instillation: Anesthetic effects occur within 60 seconds

Topical: Within 3 minutes when applied to mucous membranes

Duration: 1.5-3 hours

Pharmacokinetics

Metabolism: By the liver

Elimination: Metabolites are renally excreted

Usual Dosage

Children: Safety and efficacy have not been established

Adults:

Cream: Apply to affected area as needed

Injection: Dosage varies with the anesthetic procedure, the degree of anesthesia required, and the individual patient response; it is administered by subarachnoid injection for spinal anesthesia. High, medium, low, or saddle blocks use 0.2% or 0.3% solution. Prolonged effect (2-3 hours): Use 1% solution (a 1% solution should be diluted with an equal volume of CSF before administration)

Perineal anesthesia: 5 mg

Perineal and lower extremities: 10 mg

Anesthesia extending up to the costal margin: 15-20 mg

Low spinal anesthesia (saddle block): 2-5 mg

Ophthalmic: Solution: Instill 1-2 drops

Topical solution (mucous membranes): Apply 2% solution as needed; do not exceed 20 mg (1 mL) per application

Administration

Ophthalmic: Apply drops to conjunctiva of affected eye(s); avoid contact of bottle tip with skin or eye; finger pressure should be applied to lacrimal sac during and for 1-2 minutes after instillation to decrease risk of absorption and systemic reactions

Parenteral: Subarachnoid administration by experienced individuals only

Patient Information Do not touch or rub eye until anesthesia (if ophthalmic) has worn off

Nursing Implications Not for prolonged use topically

(Continued)

Tetracaine *(Continued)*

Dosage Forms

Gel, as hydrochloride (Cepacol Viractin®): 2% (7.1 g)

Injection, solution, as hydrochloride (Pontocaine®): 1% [10 mg/mL] (2 mL) [contains sodium bisulfite]

Injection, solution, as hydrochloride [premixed in 6% dextrose] (Pontocaine®): 0.3% [3 mg/mL] (5 mL)

Injection, powder for reconstitution, as hydrochloride (Pontocaine®): 20 mg

Solution, ophthalmic, as hydrochloride: 0.5% [5 mg/mL] (15 mL)

AK-T-Caine™, Opticaine®: 0.5% (15 mL)

Pontocaine®: 0.5% (15 mL, 59 mL)

Solution, topical, as hydrochloride (Pontocaine®): 2% [20 mg/mL] (30 mL, 118 mL)

♦ **Tetracosactide** *see* Cosyntropin *on page 310*

Tetracycline *(tet ra SYE kleen)*

Related Information

Carbohydrate and Alcohol Content of Liquid Medications for Use in Patients Receiving Ketogenic Diets *on page 1431*

U.S. Brand Names Sumycin®

Canadian Brand Names Apo®-Tetra; Novo-Tetra; Nu-Tetra

Synonyms TCN

Therapeutic Category Acne Products; Antibiotic, Ophthalmic; Antibiotic, Tetracycline Derivative; Antibiotic, Topical

Generic Available Yes (capsule)

Use

Children, Adolescents and Adults: Treatment of Rocky Mountain spotted fever caused by susceptible *Rickettsia* or brucellosis

Adolescents and Adults: Presumptive treatment of chlamydial infection in patients with gonorrhea

Children >8 years, Adolescents and Adults: Treatment of moderate to severe inflammatory acne vulgaris, Lyme disease, mycoplasmal disease or *Legionella*

Pregnancy Risk Factor D; B (topical)

Contraindications Hypersensitivity to tetracycline or any component; pregnancy; children ≤8 years; use of tetracyclines during tooth development may cause permanent discoloration of the teeth, enamel hypoplasia and retardation of skeletal development and bone growth with risk being greatest for children <4 years and in those receiving high doses

Warnings Photosensitivity reaction may occur with this drug; avoid prolonged exposure to sunlight or tanning equipment; prolonged use may result in superinfection

Precautions Use with caution in patients with renal and liver impairment; dosage modification required in patients with renal impairment

Adverse Reactions

Central nervous system: Pseudotumor cerebri, fever

Dermatologic: Rash, exfoliative dermatitis, photosensitivity, angioedema, discoloration of nails

Gastrointestinal: Nausea, vomiting, diarrhea, stomatitis, glossitis, antibiotic-associated pseudomembranous colitis, esophagitis, oral candidiasis

Hematologic: Hemolytic anemia

Hepatic: Hepatotoxicity

Neuromuscular & skeletal: Injury to growing bones and teeth

Renal: Renal damage, Fanconi-like syndrome

Respiratory: Pulmonary infiltrates with eosinophilia

Miscellaneous: Hypersensitivity reactions, candidal superinfection

Drug Interactions Calcium-, magnesium- or aluminum-containing antacids; iron, zinc; kaolin-, pectin-, or bismuth-containing antidiarrheals decrease tetracycline absorption. Tetracycline enhances the hypoprothrombinemic effect of warfarin; methoxyflurane increases chance of nephrotoxicity; concomitant use with isotretinoin has been associated with cases of pseudotumor cerebri

Food Interactions Tetracyclines decrease absorption of magnesium, zinc, calcium, dairy products, iron, and amino acids; calcium, dairy products, iron supplements decrease tetracycline absorption

Stability Protect from light; outdated tetracyclines have caused a Fanconi-like syndrome

Mechanism of Action Inhibits bacterial protein synthesis by binding to the 30S and possibly the 50S ribosomal subunit(s) of susceptible bacteria preventing additions of amino acids to the growing peptide chain; may also cause alterations in the cytoplasmic membrane

Pharmacokinetics

Distribution: Widely distributed to most body fluids and tissues including ascitic, synovial and pleural fluids; bronchial secretions; appears in breast milk; poor penetration into CSF

Absorption:
Oral: 75%
I.M.: Poor, with less than 60% of dose absorbed

Protein binding: 30% to 60%

Half-life: 6-12 hours with normal renal function and is prolonged with renal impairment

Time to peak serum concentration: Within 2-4 hours

Elimination: Primary route is the kidney, with 60% of a dose excreted as unchanged drug in urine, small amounts appear in bile

Dialysis: Slightly dialyzable (5% to 20%)

Usual Dosage

Children >8 years:
Oral: 25-50 mg/kg/day in divided doses every 6 hours; not to exceed 3 g/day
Ophthalmic:
Ointment: Apply every 2-12 hours
Suspension: Instill 1-2 drops 2-4 times/day

Adolescents and Adults:
Oral: 250-500 mg/dose every 6-12 hours
Ophthalmic:
Ointment: Apply every 2-12 hours
Suspension: Instill 1-2 drops 2-4 times/day
Topical:
Ointment: Apply small amount of ointment to cleansed area 2-3 times daily
Solution: Acne: Apply each morning and evening

Dosing adjustment in renal impairment:
Cl_{cr} 50-80 mL/minute: Administer every 8-12 hours
Cl_{cr} 10-50 mL/minute: Administer every 12-24 hours
Cl_{cr} <10 mL/minute: Administer every 24 hours

Administration

Oral: Administer 1 hour before or 2 hours after meals with adequate amounts of fluid; avoid taking antacids, calcium, iron, dairy products, or milk formulas within 3 hours of tetracyclines; shake suspension well before use

Ophthalmic: Avoid contact of tube or bottle tip with skin or eye; instill ointment or drops in the lower conjunctival sac; apply finger pressure to lacrimal sac during and for 1-2 minutes after instillation of drops to decrease risk of absorption and systemic effects; shake suspension well before use

Topical: Acne: Topical solution should be applied to cleansed affected area; reconstitute topical solution by inserting the plastic applicator unit containing the powder into the bottle containing the diluent; apply solution by tilting the bottle and rubbing applicator tip over the skin while gently applying pressure

Monitoring Parameters Renal, hepatic, and hematologic function tests

Test Interactions False-negative urine glucose with Clinistix®

Patient Information May discolor nails. May cause photosensitivity reactions (eg, exposure to sunlight may cause severe sunburn, skin rash, redness, or itching); avoid exposure to sunlight and artificial light sources (sunlamps, tanning booth/bed); wear protective clothing, wide-brimmed hats, sunglasses, and lip sunscreen (SPF ≥15); use a sunscreen [broad-spectrum sunscreen or physical sunscreen (preferred) or sunblock with SPF ≥15]; contact physician if reaction occurs.

Dosage Forms

Capsule, as hydrochloride: 250 mg, 500 mg

Suspension, oral, as hydrochloride (Sumycin®): 125 mg/5 mL (480 mL) [contains sodium benzoate and sodium metabisulfite; fruit flavor]

Tablet, film coated, as hydrochloride (Sumycin®): 250 mg, 500 mg

References

American Academy of Pediatrics. Committee on Drugs. "Requiem for Tetracyclines," *Pediatrics*, 1975, 55(1):142-3.

♦ **Theo-Dur®** **(Can)** see Theophylline on page 1076
♦ **Theolair™** see Theophylline on page 1076
♦ **Theolair-SR® [DSC]** see Theophylline on page 1076

Theophylline (thee OF i lin)

Related Information

Asthma Guidelines on page 1376
Blood Level Sampling Time Guidelines on page 1386
Carbohydrate and Alcohol Content of Liquid Medications for Use in Patients Receiving Ketogenic Diets on page 1431
Overdose and Toxicology on page 1388

U.S. Brand Names Elixophyllin®; Quibron®-T; Quibron®-T/SR; Theo-24®; Theochron®; Theolair™; Theolair-SR® [DSC]; T-Phyl®; Uniphyl®

Canadian Brand Names Apo®-Theo LA; Novo-Theophyl SR; PMS-Theophylline; Pulmophylline; ratio-Theo-Bronc; Theochron® SR; Theo-Dur®; Uniphyl® SRT

Therapeutic Category Antiasthmatic; Bronchodilator; Respiratory Stimulant; Theophylline Derivative

Generic Available Yes (elixir, extended release tablet, infusion, and solution)

Use Treatment of symptoms and reversible airway obstruction due to chronic asthma, chronic bronchitis, or COPD; treatment of idiopathic apnea of prematurity in neonates

Pregnancy Risk Factor C

Contraindications Hypersensitivity to theophylline or any component

Warnings If a patient develops signs and symptoms of theophylline toxicity (eg, persistent, repetitive vomiting), a serum theophylline level should be measured and subsequent doses held; due to potential saturation of theophylline clearance at serum levels within or (in some patients) less than the therapeutic range, dosage adjustments should be made in small increments (maximum dosage adjustment: 25%); due to wide interpatient variability, theophylline serum level measurements must be used to optimize therapy and prevent serious toxicity

Precautions Use with caution in patients with peptic ulcer, hyperthyroidism, seizure disorders, hypertension, and patients with cardiac arrhythmias (excluding bradyarrhythmias)

Adverse Reactions See table.

Theophylline Serum Levels (μg/mL)*	Adverse Reactions
15-25	GI upset, GE reflux, diarrhea, nausea, vomiting, abdominal pain, nervousness, headache, insomnia, agitation, dizziness, muscle cramp, tremor
25-35	Tachycardia, occasional PVC
>35	Ventricular tachycardia, frequent PVC, seizure

*Adverse effects do not necessarily occur according to serum levels. Arrhythmia and seizure can occur without seeing the other adverse effects.

Drug Interactions Cytochrome P450 isoenzyme CYP1A2, CYP2E1, and CYP3A3/4 substrate

Decreases adenosine, esmolol, benzodiazepine, and pancuronium effects; increases lithium clearance; increases CNS side effects with ephedrine; increases risk of cardiac arrhythmias with halothane; decreases zafirlukast serum levels; for medications which alter theophylline clearance, see tables on next page.

Food Interactions Food does not appreciably affect the absorption of liquid, fast-release products and most sustained release products; however, food may induce a sudden release (dose-dumping) of once-daily sustained release products resulting in an increase in serum drug levels and potential toxicity; avoid excessive amounts of caffeine; avoid extremes of dietary protein and carbohydrate intake; limit charcoal-broiled foods and caffeinated beverages

Mechanism of Action Competitively inhibits two isoenzymes of the enzyme phosphodiesterase resulting in increased levels of cyclic adenine monophosphate (cAMP) which may be responsible for most of theophylline's effects; effects on the myocardium and neuromuscular transmission may be due to the intracellular translocation of ionized calcium; overall, theophylline produces the following effects: relaxation of the smooth muscle of the respiratory tract, suppression of the response of airways to stimuli, increases the force of contraction of diaphragmatic muscles; pulmonary, coronary, and renal artery dilation; CNS stimulation, diuresis, stimulation of catecholamine release, gastric acid secretion, and relaxation of biliary and GI smooth muscle

Clinical Factors Reported to Affect Theophylline Clearance

Decreased Theophylline Level	Increased Theophylline Level
Smoking (cigarettes, marijuana)	Acute pulmonary edema
High protein/low carbohydrate diet	Cessation of smoking (after chronic use)
Charcoal broiled beef	Cor pulmonale
	Congestive heart failure
	Hypothyroidism
	Fever (≥102° for 24 hours or more, or lesser temperature elevations for longer periods)
	Hepatic cirrhosis/acute hepatitis
	Renal failure in infants <3 mo of age
	Sepsis with multisystem organ failure
	Shock
	Viral illness

Medications Affecting Theophylline Clearance Resulting in Either Increased or Decreased Serum Levels

Decreased Theophylline Level	Increased Theophylline Level
Aminoglutethimide	Alcohol
Carbamazepine	Allopurinol (>600 mg/day)
Isoproterenol (I.V.)	Beta-blockers
Isoniazid*	Calcium channel blockers
Ketoconazole	Cimetidine
Loop diuretics*	Ciprofloxacin
Nevirapine	Clarithromycin
Phenobarbital	Corticosteroids
Phenytoin	Disulfiram
Rifampin	Ephedrine
Ritonavir	Erythromycin
Sulfinpyrazone	Esmolol
Sympathomimetics	Influenza virus vaccine
	Interferon, human recombinant alpha 2-a and 2-b
	Isoniazid*
	Loop diuretics*
	Methotrexate
	Mexiletine
	Oral contraceptives
	Propafenone
	Propranolol
	Tacrine
	Thiabendazole
	Thyroid hormones
	Troleandomycin (TAO®)
	Verapamil
	Zileuton

*Both increased and decreased theophylline levels have been reported.

Pharmacokinetics

Absorption: Oral: Rapid and complete with up to 100% absorption depending upon the formulation used

Distribution: V_d: 0.45 L/kg; distributes into breast milk; breast milk to plasma ratio: 0.67; crosses the placenta and into the CSF

Protein binding: 40%; decreased protein binding in neonates (due to a greater percentage of fetal albumin), hepatic cirrhosis, uncorrected acidemia, women in third trimester of pregnancy, and geriatric patients

Metabolism: In the liver by demethylation and oxidation; theophylline is metabolized to caffeine (active); in neonates this theophylline-derived caffeine accumulates (due to decreased hepatic metabolism) and significant concentrations of caffeine may occur; a substantial decrease in serum caffeine concentrations occurs after 40 weeks postconceptional age

Half-life: See table on next page.

Elimination: In urine; children >3 months and adults excrete 10% in urine as unchanged drug; neonates excrete approximately 50% of the dose unchanged in urine

(Continued)

1077

Theophylline *(Continued)*

Theophylline Clearance and Half-Life With Respect to Age and Altered Physiological States*

Patient Group	Mean Clearance (mL/kg/min)	Mean Half-life (h)
Premature infants		
postnatal age 3-15 d	0.29	30
postnatal age 25-57 d	0.64	20
Term infants		
postnatal age 1-2 d	Not reported†	25
postnatal age 3-30 wk‡	Not reported†	11
Children		
1-4 y	1.7	3.4
4-12 y	1.6	Not reported†
13-15 y	0.9	Not reported†
16-17 y	1.4	3.7 (range: 1.5-5.9)
Adults		
16-60 (nonsmoking)	0.65	8.2
>60 y (nonsmoking, healthy)	0.41	9.8
Acute pulmonary edema	0.33	19
Cystic fibrosis (14-28 y)	1.25	6
Liver disease		
acute hepatitis	0.35	19.2
cholestasis	0.65	14.4
cirrhosis	0.31	32
Sepsis with multiorgan failure	0.46	18.8
Hypothyroid	0.38	11.6
Hyperthyroid	0.8	4.5
COPD >60 y, nonsmoking >1 y	0.54	11

*From Hendeles L, 1995

†Either not reported or not reported in a comparable format

‡Maturation of clearance in premature infants and term infants is most closely related to postconceptional age (PCA); adult clearance values are reached at approximately 55 weeks PCA and higher pediatric values at approximately 60 weeks PCA (Kraus, 1993).

Maintenance Dose for Acute Symptoms

Population Group	Oral Theophylline (mg/kg/day)
Premature infant or newborn to 6 wk (for apnea/bradycardia)	4*
6 wk to 6 mo	10*
Infants 6 mo to 1 y	12-18*
Children 1-9 y	20-24
Children 9-12 y, adolescent daily smokers of cigarettes or marijuana, and otherwise healthy adult smokers <50 y	16
Adolescents 12-16 y (nonsmokers)	13
Otherwise healthy nonsmoking adults (including elderly patients)	10 (not to exceed 900 mg/day)
Cardiac decompensation, cor pulmonale, and/or liver dysfunction	5 (not to exceed 400 mg/day)
*Alternative dosing regimen for full-term infants <1 year of age:	

*Alternative dosing regimen for full-term infants <1 year of age:

Total daily dose (mg) = [(0.2 x age in weeks) + 5] x weight (kg)

Postnatal Age <26 weeks: Total daily dose divided every 8 hours

Postnatal Age >26 weeks: Total daily dose divided every 6 hours

Usual Dosage Oral (see Aminophylline *on page 81* for I.V. doses):

Loading dose:

Neonates: Apnea of prematurity: 4 mg/kg/dose

Infants and Children: Treatment of acute bronchospasm: (to achieve a serum level of about 10 mcg/mL; loading doses should be given using a rapidly absorbed oral product **not** a sustained release product):

If no theophylline has been administered in the previous 24 hours: 5 mg/kg theophylline

If theophylline has been administered in the previous 24 hours: 2.5 mg/kg theophylline may be given in emergencies when serum levels are not available

A modified loading dose (mg/kg) may be calculated (when the serum level is known) by: [Blood level desired - blood level measured] divided by 2 (for every 1 mg/kg theophylline given, the blood level will rise by approximately 2 mcg/mL)

Maintenance dose: See table on previous page.

These recommendations, based on mean clearance rates for age or risk factors, were calculated to achieve a serum level of 10 mcg/mL (5 mcg/mL for newborns with apnea/bradycardia). In newborns and infants, a fast-release oral product can be used. The total daily dose can be divided every 12 hours in newborns and every 6-8 hours in infants. In children and healthy adults, a slow-release product can be used. The total daily dose can be divided every 8-12 hours.

Use ideal body weight for obese patients

Dose should be further adjusted based on serum levels. Guidelines for drawing theophylline serum levels are shown in the table.

Guidelines for Drawing Theophylline Serum Levels

Dosage Form	Time to Draw Level*
I.V. bolus	30 min after end of 30-min infusion
I.V. continuous infusion	12-24 h after initiation of infusion
P.O. liquid, fast-release formulation	Peak: 1 h postdose after at least 1 day of therapy Trough: Just before a dose after at least 1 day of therapy

*The time to achieve steady-state serum levels is prolonged in patients with longer half-lives (eg, premature neonates, infants, and adults with cardiac or liver failure (see theophylline half-life table). In these patients, serum theophylline levels should be drawn after 48-72 hours of therapy; serum levels may need to be done prior to steady-state to assess the patient's current progress or evaluate potential toxicity.

Administration

Oral: Sustained release preparations should be administered with a full glass of water, whole or cut by half only; do not crush; sustained release capsule forms may be opened and sprinkled on soft foods; do not chew or crush beads

Parenteral: Premade I.V. infusion bags for continuous infusion usage; rate of infusion dependent upon dosage; loading doses using I.V. infusion should be administered over 20-30 minutes

Monitoring Parameters Respiratory rate, heart rate, serum theophylline level, arterial or capillary blood gases (if applicable); number and severity of apnea spells (apnea of prematurity)

Reference Range

Therapeutic levels:

Asthma: 10-15 µg/mL (peak level)

Apnea of prematurity: 6-14 µg/mL

Toxic concentration: >20 µg/mL

Test Interactions May elevate uric acid levels

Patient Information Contact physician whenever nausea, vomiting, persistent headache, or irregular heartbeats occur; notify physician if a new illness develops (especially if high fevers); do not alter time, dose, or frequency of administration without physician knowledge; avoid drinking or eating of large quantities of caffeine-containing beverages or food

Additional Information Due to improved theophylline clearance during the first year of life, serum concentration determinations and dosage adjustments may be needed to optimize therapy

Dosage Forms

Capsule, extended release (Theo-24®): 100 mg, 200 mg, 300 mg, 400 mg **[24 hours]**

Elixir (Elixophyllin®): 80 mg/15 mL (480 mL) [contains 20% alcohol; fruit flavor]

Infusion [premixed in D_5W]: 0.8 mg/mL (500 mL, 1000 mL); 1.6 mg/mL (250 mL, 500 mL); 2 mg/mL (100 mL); 3.2 mg/mL (250 mL); 4 mg/mL (50 mL, 100 mL)

Solution, oral: 80 mg/15 mL (15 mL, 18.75 mL, 500 mL) [dye and sugar free; contains 0.4% alcohol and benzoic acid; orange flavor]

(Continued)

Theophylline *(Continued)*

Tablet, immediate release:
Quibron®-T: 300 mg
Theolair™: 125 mg, 250 mg
Tablet, controlled release:
T-Phyl®: 200 mg **[12 hours**; contains cetostearyl alcohol]
Uniphyl®: 400 mg, 600 mg **[24 hours**; contains cetostearyl alcohol]
Tablet, extended release: 100 mg, 200 mg, 300 mg, 450 mg
Theochron®: 100 mg, 200 mg, 300 mg **[12-24 hours]**
Tablet, sustained release (Quibron®-T/SR): 300 mg **[8-12 hours]**
Tablet, timed release (Theolair-SR®): 300 mg, 500 mg **[8-24 hours]** [DSC]

References

Bhatt-Mehta V and Schumacher RE, "Treatment of Apnea of Prematurity," *Paediatr Drugs*, 2003, 5(3):195-210.

Hendeles L, Jenkins J, and Temple R, "Revised FDA Labeling Guideline for Theophylline Oral Dosage Forms," *Pharmacotherapy*, 1995, 15(4):409-427.

Kearney TE, Manoguerra AS, Curtis GP, et al, "Theophylline Toxicity and the Beta-Adrenergic System," *Ann Intern Med*, 1985, 102(6):766-9.

Kraus DM, Fischer JH, Reitz SJ, et al, "Alterations in Theophylline Metabolism During the First Year of Life," *Clin Pharmacol Ther*, 1993, 54(4):351-9.

"National Asthma Education and Prevention Program. Expert Panel Report: Guidelines for the Diagnosis and Management of Asthma Update on Selected Topics--2002," *J Allergy Clin Immunol*, 2002, 110(5 Suppl):S141-219.

Upton RA, "Pharmacokinetic Interactions Between Theophylline and Other Medication (Part I)," *Clin Pharmacokinet*, 1991, 20(1):66-80.

♦ **Theophylline Ethylenediamine** *see* Aminophylline *on page 81*

♦ **Theracort® [OTC]** *see* Hydrocortisone *on page 573*

♦ **Thera-Flur-N®** *see* Fluoride *on page 500*

♦ **Theramycin™ Z** *see* Erythromycin *on page 448*

♦ **TheraPatch® Warm [OTC]** *see* Capsaicin *on page 206*

♦ **Thermazene®** *see* Silver Sulfadiazine *on page 1019*

Thiabendazole *(thye a BEN da zole)*

U.S. Brand Names Mintezol®

Synonyms Tiabendazole

Therapeutic Category Anthelmintic

Generic Available No

Use Treatment of strongyloidiasis, cutaneous larva migrans, visceral larva migrans, dracunculosis, trichinosis, and mixed helminthic infections

Pregnancy Risk Factor C

Contraindications Hypersensitivity to thiabendazole or any component; pregnancy. Contraindicated as prophylactic treatment for pinworm infestation.

Warnings Abnormal sensation in eyes, blurred vision, xanthopsia, drying of mucous membranes, and Sicca syndrome have been reported in patients receiving thiabendazole; ocular adverse effect may persist beyond one year in some cases

Precautions Use with caution in patients with renal or hepatic impairment, malnutrition, anemia, or dehydration

Adverse Reactions

Cardiovascular: Flushing, hypotension, bradycardia
Central nervous system: Dizziness, drowsiness, vertigo, seizures, fever, malaise, headache, chills, hallucinations
Dermatologic: Rash, Stevens-Johnson syndrome, erythema multiforme, pruritus
Endocrine & metabolic: Hyperglycemia
Gastrointestinal: Nausea, vomiting, diarrhea, anorexia, abdominal pain
Genitourinary: Malodor of the urine
Hematologic: Leukopenia
Hepatic: Hepatotoxicity, jaundice, cholestasis
Neuromuscular & skeletal: Paresthesia, numbness
Ocular: Blurred vision, Sicca syndrome
Otic: Tinnitus
Renal: Nephrotoxicity, hematuria
Miscellaneous: Hypersensitivity reactions, lymphadenopathy

Drug Interactions Increases serum theophylline concentrations (monitor serum theophylline level in patients receiving both drugs concomitantly)

Mechanism of Action Inhibits helminth-specific mitochondrial fumarate reductase

Pharmacokinetics

Absorption: From the GI tract and through the skin
Metabolism: Extensive in the liver via hydroxylation and conjugation with sulfuric and/or glucuronic acid
Time to peak serum concentration: Within 1-2 hours

Elimination: In feces (5%) and urine (87%), primarily as conjugated metabolites

Usual Dosage

Oral:

Children and Adults: 50 mg/kg/day divided every 12 hours (maximum dose: 3 g/day)

Strongyloidiasis: For 2 consecutive days (5 days or longer for disseminated disease)

Cutaneous larva migrans: For 2-5 consecutive days

Visceral larva migrans: For 5-7 consecutive days

Trichinosis: For 2-4 consecutive days

Angiostrongylosis: 50-75 mg/kg/day divided every 8-12 hours for 3 days

Dracunculosis: 50-75 mg/kg/day divided every 12 hours for 3 days

Topical: Cutaneous larva migrans: Instead of oral therapy, thiabendazole 10% to 15% suspension or a 10% ointment in white petrolatum has been applied topically to lesions 4-6 times/day

Administration Oral: Administer after meals; chew tablet well before swallowing; shake suspension well before use

Monitoring Parameters Periodic renal and hepatic function tests, serum glucose

Patient Information May cause drowsiness and impair ability to perform activities requiring mental alertness or physical coordination

Nursing Implications Purgation is not required prior to use

Dosage Forms

Suspension, oral: 500 mg/5 mL (120 mL)

Tablet, chewable, scored: 500 mg [orange flavor]

References

Walden J, "Parasitic Diseases. Other Roundworms. *Trichuris*, Hookworm, and *Strongyloides*," *Prim Care*, 1991, 18(1):53-74.

Zygmunt DJ, "*Strongyloides stearcoralis*," *Infect Control Hosp Epidemiol*, 1990, 11(9):495-7.

♦ **Thiamazole** *see* Methimazole *on page 734*

♦ **Thiamilate® [OTC]** *see* Thiamine *on page 1081*

Thiamine (THYE a min)

U.S. Brand Names Thiamilate® [OTC]

Canadian Brand Names Betaxin®

Synonyms Aneurine; Thiaminium; Vitamin B₁

Therapeutic Category Nutritional Supplement; Vitamin, Water Soluble

Generic Available Yes

Use Treatment of thiamine deficiency including beriberi, Wernicke's encephalopathy syndrome, and peripheral neuritis associated with pellagra; alcoholic patients with altered sensorium; various genetic metabolic disorders

Pregnancy Risk Factor A (C if dose exceeds RDA recommendation)

Contraindications Hypersensitivity to thiamine or any component

Warnings Large doses should be given in divided doses for better oral absorption

Precautions Use parenteral route cautiously, see Adverse Reactions

Adverse Reactions

Cardiovascular: Cardiovascular collapse and death (primarily following repeated I.V. administration), warmth

Dermatologic: Rash, angioedema

Genitourinary: Discoloration of urine (bright yellow) with large doses

Neuromuscular & skeletal: Paresthesia

Drug Interactions I.V. dextrose solutions increase thiamine requirement; thiamine may enhance the effects of neuromuscular blocking agents

Food Interactions High carbohydrate diets may increase thiamine requirement

Stability Unstable with alkaline or neutral solutions

Mechanism of Action An essential coenzyme in carbohydrate metabolism; combines with adenosine triphosphate to form thiamine pyrophosphate

Pharmacokinetics

Absorption:

Oral: Poor

I.M.: Rapid and complete

Metabolism: In the liver

Elimination: Renally as unchanged drug only after body storage sites become saturated

Usual Dosage

Adequate intake: Oral: Infants:

<6 months: 0.2 mg (0.03 mg/kg)

6-12 months: 0.3 mg (0.03 mg/kg)

(Continued)

Thiamine *(Continued)*

Recommended daily allowance (RDA): Oral:
  1-3 years: 0.5 mg
  4-8 years: 0.6 mg
  9-13 years: 0.9 mg
  14-18 years:
    Male: 1.2 mg
    Female: 1 mg
  ≥19 years:
    Male: 1.2 mg
    Female: 1.1 mg
Dietary supplement (depends on caloric or carbohydrate content of the diet)
  Oral:
    Infants: 0.3-0.5 mg/day
    Children: 0.5-1 mg/day
    Adults: 1-2 mg/day
Note: The above doses can be found in multivitamin preparations
Thiamine deficiency (beriberi):
  Children: 10-25 mg/dose I.M. or I.V. daily (if critically ill), or 10-50 mg/dose orally every day for 2 weeks, then 5-10 mg/dose orally daily for 1 month
  Adults: 5-30 mg/dose I.M. or I.V. 3 times/day (if critically ill); then orally 5-30 mg/day in single or divided doses 3 times/day for 1 month
  Wernicke's encephalopathy: Adults: Initial: 100 mg I.V., then 50-100 mg/day I.M. or I.V. until consuming a regular, balanced diet
  Metabolic disorders: Oral: Adults: 10-20 mg/day (dosages up to 4 g/day in divided doses have been used)

Administration
Oral: May administer with or without food
Parenteral: Administer by slow I.V. injection or I.M.

Reference Range Normal values: 1.6-4 mg/dL

Test Interactions False-positive for uric acid using the phosphotungstate method and for urobilinogen using the Ehrlich's reagent; large doses may interfere with the spectrophotometric determination of serum theophylline concentration

Patient Information May color urine bright yellow

Additional Information Dietary sources include legumes, pork, beef, whole grains, yeast, fresh vegetables; a deficiency state can occur in as little as 3 weeks following total dietary absence

Dosage Forms
Injection, solution, as hydrochloride: 100 mg/mL (2 mL)
Tablet, as hydrochloride: 50 mg, 100 mg, 250 mg, 500 mg
Tablet, enteric coated, as hydrochloride (Thiamilate®): 20 mg

♦ **Thiaminium** *see* Thiamine *on page 1081*

Thiethylperazine *(thye eth il PER a zeen)*

Related Information
Overdose and Toxicology *on page 1388*

U.S. Brand Names Torecan®

Therapeutic Category Antiemetic; Phenothiazine Derivative

Generic Available No

Use Relief of nausea and vomiting

Pregnancy Risk Factor X

Contraindications Hypersensitivity to thiethylperazine or any component (see Warnings); pregnancy; severe CNS depression, comatose states

Warnings Safety and efficacy in children <12 years of age have not been established; postural hypotension may occur after I.M. injection; the injectable form contains sulfite and tablets contain tartrazine both of which may cause allergic reactions in susceptible individuals; avoid use in children and adolescents whose signs and symptoms are suggestive of Reye's syndrome

Adverse Reactions
Cardiovascular: Hypotension, peripheral edema
Central nervous system: Drowsiness, extrapyramidal effects, seizures, fever, headache, neuroleptic malignant syndrome
Dermatologic: Photosensitivity
Gastrointestinal: Xerostomia
Hepatic: Cholestatic jaundice (occasional)
Neuromuscular & skeletal: Trigeminal neuralgia
Ocular: Blurred vision
Respiratory: Dryness of mucous membranes

Drug Interactions Additive effects with anticholinergic agents and other phenothiazines; additive CNS depression with sedatives and antihistamines

Mechanism of Action Blocks postsynaptic mesolimbic dopaminergic receptors in the
brain including the medullary chemoreceptor trigger zone; exhibits a strong alpha-
adrenergic blocking effect and depresses the release of hypothalamic and hypophyseal hormones

Pharmacodynamics
Onset of action: Oral, I.M.: Antiemetic effects occur within 30 minutes
Duration: ~4 hours

Usual Dosage Children >12 years and Adults: Oral, I.M.: 10 mg 1-3 times/day as
needed

Administration Parenteral: Inject I.M. deeply into large muscle mass, patient should
be lying down and remain so for at least 1 hour; I.V. and S.C. routes of administration
are not recommended

Patient Information May cause drowsiness and impair ability to perform activities
requiring mental alertness or physical coordination; may cause dry mouth. May rarely
cause photosensitivity reactions (eg, exposure to sunlight may cause severe
sunburn, skin rash, redness, or itching); avoid direct exposure to sunlight.

Dosage Forms
Injection, solution, as maleate [DSC]: 5 mg/mL (2 mL) [contains sodium metabisulfite]
Tablet, as maleate: 10 mg [contains sodium benzoate and tartrazine]

Thioguanine (thye oh GWAH neen)

Related Information
Emetogenic Potential of Single Chemotherapeutic Agents *on page 1286*

Synonyms 2-Amino-6-mercaptopurine; TG; 6-TG; 6-Thioguanine; Tioguanine

Therapeutic Category Antineoplastic Agent, Antimetabolite

Generic Available Yes

Use Remission induction in acute myelogenous (nonlymphocytic) leukemia; treatment
of chronic myelogenous leukemia and acute lymphocytic leukemia

Pregnancy Risk Factor D

Contraindications Hypersensitivity to thioguanine or any component; history of
previous therapy resistance with thioguanine and in patients resistant to mercaptopurine

Warnings The FDA currently recommends that procedures for proper handling and
disposal of antineoplastic agents be considered; thioguanine is potentially carcinogenic and teratogenic

Precautions Use with caution and reduce dose of thioguanine in patients with renal or
hepatic impairment

Adverse Reactions
Central nervous system: Neurotoxicity
Dermatologic: Skin rash, photosensitivity, staining of skin or eyes (yellow)
Endocrine & metabolic: Hyperuricemia
Gastrointestinal: Mild nausea or vomiting, anorexia, stomatitis, diarrhea
Hematologic: Myelosuppression (leukopenia, thrombocytopenia, anemia)
Hepatic: Hepatitis, jaundice, veno-occlusive hepatic disease
Neuromuscular & skeletal: Unsteady gait

Drug Interactions Busulfan (increases busulfan toxicity)

Food Interactions Enhanced absorption if administered between meals

Mechanism of Action Purine analog that is incorporated into DNA and RNA resulting
in the inhibition of synthesis and utilization of purine nucleotides

Pharmacokinetics
Absorption: Oral: 30% (variable and incomplete)
Distribution: Crosses the placenta; does not appear to cross into CSF
Metabolism: Rapid and extensive hepatic metabolism by methylation of thioguanine
to 2-amino-6-methylthioguanine (active) and inactive compounds
Half-life, terminal: 11 hours
Time to peak serum concentration: Within 8-12 hours
Elimination: Metabolites excreted in urine

Usual Dosage Oral (refer to individual protocols):
Infants <3 years: Combination drug therapy for ANLL: 3.3 mg/kg/day in divided doses
twice daily for 4 days
Children and Adults:
Single agent chemotherapy for ANLL: 2-3 mg/kg/day once daily calculated to
nearest 20 mg
Induction of remission in patients with acute leukemia (combination therapy): 75-
200 mg/m²/day in 1-2 divided doses for 5-7 days or until remission is attained

Administration Oral: Administer between meals on an empty stomach
(Continued)

Thioguanine *(Continued)*

Monitoring Parameters CBC with (differential, platelet count), liver function tests, hemoglobin, hematocrit, serum uric acid

Patient Information Notify physician if fever, sore throat, bleeding, bruising, yellow discoloration of skin or eyes, or leg swelling occurs. May cause photosensitivity reactions (eg, exposure to sunlight may cause severe sunburn, skin rash, redness, or itching); avoid exposure to sunlight and artificial light sources (sunlamps, tanning booth/bed); wear protective clothing, wide-brimmed hats, sunglasses, and lip sunscreen (SPF ≥15); use a sunscreen [broad-spectrum sunscreen or physical sunscreen (preferred) or sunblock with SPF ≥15]; contact physician if reaction occurs.

Nursing Implications Ensure adequate patient hydration, alkalinization of the urine, and/or administration of allopurinol to prevent hyperuricemia

Additional Information Myelosuppressive effects:
WBC: Moderate
Platelets: Moderate
Onset (days): 7-10
Nadir (days): 14
Recovery (days): 21

Dosage Forms Tablet, scored: 40 mg

References
Culbert SJ, Shuster JJ, Land VJ, et al, "Remission Induction and Continuation Therapy in Children With Their First Relapse of Acute Lymphoid Leukemia: A Pediatric Oncology Group Study," *Cancer,* 1991, 67(1):37-42.
Steuber CP, Civin C, Krischer J, et al, "A Comparison of Induction and Maintenance Therapy for Acute Nonlymphocytic Leukemia in Childhood: Results of a Pediatric Oncology Group Study," *J Clin Oncol,* 1991, 9(2):247-58.

♦ **6-Thioguanine** *see* Thioguanine *on page 1083*

Thiopental *(thye oh PEN tal)*

Related Information
Preprocedure Sedatives in Children *on page 1367*

U.S. Brand Names Pentothal®

Therapeutic Category Anticonvulsant, Barbiturate; Barbiturate; General Anesthetic; Hypnotic; Sedative

Generic Available Yes

Use Induction of anesthesia; adjunct for intubation in head injury patients; control of convulsive states; treatment of elevated intracranial pressure

Restrictions C-III

Pregnancy Risk Factor C

Contraindications Hypersensitivity to thiopental, pentobarbital, any component, or other barbiturates; porphyria (variegate or acute intermittent)

Precautions Use with caution in patients with asthma or pharyngeal infections because cough, laryngospasm, or bronchospasms may occur; use with caution in patients with hypotension, severe cardiovascular disease, hepatic or renal dysfunction; avoid extravasation or intra-arterial injection which may cause necrosis due to pH of 10.6; ensure patient has intravenous access

Adverse Reactions
Cardiovascular: Decreased cardiac output, hypotension
Local: Necrosis with I.V. extravasation
Renal: Decreased urine output
Respiratory: Cough, laryngospasm, bronchospasm, respiratory depression, apnea
Miscellaneous: Anaphylaxis

Drug Interactions Barbiturates are enzyme inducers (monitor patients closely for decreased effect of concomitantly administered medications or increased effect when barbiturates are discontinued); CNS depressants

Stability Solutions are alkaline and incompatible with drugs with acidic pH, such as succinylcholine, atropine sulfate

Mechanism of Action Ultra-short-acting barbiturate; depresses CNS activity by binding to barbiturate site at GABA-receptor complex enhancing GABA activity; depresses reticular activating system; higher doses may be gabamimetic

Pharmacodynamics Anesthesia effects:
Onset of action: I.V.: 30-60 seconds
Duration: 5-30 minutes

Pharmacokinetics
Distribution: V_d: Adults: 1.4 L/kg
Protein binding: 72% to 86%
Metabolism: In the liver primarily to inactive metabolites but pentobarbital is also formed
Half-life, adults: 3-11.5 hours (shorter half-life in children)

Usual Dosage
Induction anesthesia: I.V.:
  Neonates: 3-4 mg/kg
  Infants: 5-8 mg/kg
  Children 1-12 years: 5-6 mg/kg
  Children >12 years and Adults: 3-5 mg/kg
Maintenance anesthesia: I.V.:
  Children: 1 mg/kg as needed
  Adults: 25-100 mg as needed
Increased intracranial pressure: Children: I.V.: 1.5-5 mg/kg/dose; repeat as needed to control intracranial pressure; larger doses (30 mg/kg) to induce coma after hypoxic-ischemic injury do not appear to improve neurologic outcome
Seizures: I.V.:
  Children: 2-3 mg/kg/dose, repeat as needed
  Adults: 75-250 mg/dose, repeat as needed
Sedation: Rectal:
  Children: 5-10 mg/kg/dose
  Adults: 3-4 g/dose

Administration Parenteral: Avoid rapid I.V. injection (may cause hypotension or decreased cardiac output); may administer by intermittent infusion over 10-60 minutes at a maximum concentration of 50 mg/mL

Monitoring Parameters Respiratory rate, heart rate, blood pressure

Reference Range
Therapeutic:
  Hypnotic: 1-5 μg/mL (SI: 4.1-20.7 μmol/L)
  Coma: 30-100 μg/mL (SI: 124-413 μmol/L)
  Anesthesia: 7-130 μg/mL (SI: 29-536 μmol/L)

Nursing Implications Avoid extravasation, necrosis may occur

Additional Information Accumulation may occur with chronic dosing due to lipid solubility; prolonged recovery occurs due to redistribution of thiopental from fat stores; therefore, thiopental is usually not used for procedures lasting >15-20 minutes; sodium content, injection: 4.9 mEq/g

Dosage Forms
Injection, powder for reconstitution, as sodium: 500 mg, 2.5 g, 5 g
Pentothal®: 250 mg, 400 mg, 500 mg, 1g, 2.5 g, 5 g

♦ **Thioplex®** see Thiotepa on page 1087

Thioridazine (thye oh RID a zeen)

Related Information
Overdose and Toxicology on page 1388

U.S. Brand Names Mellaril® [DSC]; Thioridazine Intensol™

Canadian Brand Names Apo®-Thioridazine

Therapeutic Category Antipsychotic Agent; Phenothiazine Derivative

Generic Available Yes

Use Due to prolongation of the QT_c interval (see Warnings), thioridazine is currently indicated only for the treatment of refractory schizophrenic patients; in the past, the drug had been used for management of psychotic disorders; depressive neurosis; dementia in elderly; severe behavioral problems in children

Pregnancy Risk Factor C

Contraindications Hypersensitivity to thioridazine or any component; cross-sensitivity to other phenothiazines may exist; concurrent therapy with propranolol, pindolol, fluvoxamine, fluoxetine, paroxetine, drugs that inhibit cytochrome P450 isoenzyme CYP2D6, drugs that prolong the QT_c interval, and patients with reduced levels of CYP2D6, a history of cardiac arrhythmias, congenital long QT syndrome, or a QT_c interval >450 msec (adults); severe CNS depression; avoid use in patients with narrow-angle glaucoma, blood dyscrasias, severe liver or cardiac disease

Warnings Prolongation of the QT_c interval may occur and may be associated with torsade de pointes arrhythmias and sudden death; tablets may contain sodium benzoate; benzoic acid (benzoate) is a metabolite of benzyl alcohol; large amounts of benzyl alcohol (≥99 mg/kg/day) have been associated with a potentially fatal toxicity ("gasping syndrome") in neonates; avoid use of thioridazine products containing sodium benzoate in neonates; in vitro and animal studies have shown that benzoate displaces bilirubin from protein binding sites

Precautions Use with caution in patients with severe cardiovascular disorder or seizures

Adverse Reactions Sedation and anticholinergic effects are more pronounced than extrapyramidal effects; EKG changes and retinal pigmentation are more common than with chlorpromazine
Cardiovascular: Hypotension, orthostatic hypotension, tachycardia, arrhythmias
(Continued)

Thioridazine *(Continued)*

Central nervous system: Sedation, drowsiness, restlessness, anxiety, extrapyramidal reactions, pseudoparkinsonian signs and symptoms, tardive dyskinesia, neuroleptic malignant syndrome, seizures, altered central temperature regulation

Dermatologic: Hyperpigmentation, pruritus, rash, contact dermatitis, photosensitivity (rare)

Endocrine & metabolic: Amenorrhea, galactorrhea, gynecomastia

Gastrointestinal: GI upset, xerostomia, constipation, weight gain

Genitourinary: Urinary retention

Hematologic: Agranulocytosis, leukopenia (usually in patients with large doses for prolonged periods)

Hepatic: Cholestatic jaundice

Ocular: Retinal pigmentation (usually in patients receiving larger than recommended doses), blurred vision, brownish coloring of vision, decreased night vision, decreased visual acuity (may be irreversible)

Miscellaneous: Anaphylactoid reactions

Drug Interactions Cytochrome P450 isoenzyme CYP1A2 and CYP2D6 substrate; CYP2D6 isoenzyme inhibitor

Additive effects with alcohol and other CNS depressants; concurrent use with lithium has caused acute encephalopathy-like syndrome (rare); increased cardiac arrhythmias with tricyclic antidepressants; epinephrine may cause hypotension; drugs that inhibit the metabolism of thioridazine (eg, fluoxetine, fluvoxamine, paroxetine) or drugs that prolong the QT_c interval may increase the risk of serious adverse effects, such as QT_c prolongation, serious ventricular arrhythmias (eg, torsade de pointes) and sudden death (such drugs are contraindicated; see Contraindications); mixing liquid thioridazine with carbamazepine suspension will result in precipitation of an orange rubbery mass (see also Contraindications)

Food Interactions May increase dietary requirements for riboflavin; liquid thioridazine formulations may precipitate with enteral formulas

Mechanism of Action Blocks postsynaptic mesolimbic dopaminergic receptors in the brain; exhibits a strong alpha-adrenergic blocking effect and depresses the release of hypothalamic and hypophyseal hormones

Pharmacokinetics

Protein binding: 99%

Metabolism: In the liver to active and inactive metabolites

Bioavailability: 25% to 33%

Half-life: Adults: 9-30 hours

Dialysis: Not dialyzable: (0% to 5%)

Usual Dosage Oral:

Children >2 years: Initial: 0.5 mg/kg/day in 2-3 divided doses; range: 0.5-3 mg/kg/day; usual: 1 mg/kg/day in 2-3 divided doses; maximum dose: 3 mg/kg/day

Behavior problems: Initial: 10 mg 2-3 times/day, increase gradually

Severe psychoses: Initial: 25 mg 2-3 times/day, increase gradually

Children >12 years and Adults:

Schizophrenia/psychoses: Initial: 25-100 mg 3 times/day with gradual increments as needed and tolerated; maximum daily dose: 800 mg/day in 2-4 divided doses; maintenance: 10-200 mg/dose 2-4 times/day

Depressive disorders, dementia: Initial: 25 mg 3 times/day; maintenance dose: 20-200 mg/day

Administration Oral: Administer with water, food, or milk to decrease GI upset; dilute the oral concentrate with water or juice before administration; do not administer liquid thioridazine simultaneously with carbamazepine suspension (see Drug Interactions); do not mix liquid thioridazine with enteric formulas (see Food Interactions)

Monitoring Parameters Baseline and periodic EKG and serum potassium; periodic eye exam, CBC with differential, blood pressure, liver enzyme tests

Test Interactions False-positives for phenylketonuria, urinary amylase, uroporphyrins, urobilinogen

Patient Information Avoid alcohol; may cause drowsiness and impair ability to perform activities requiring mental alertness or physical coordination; may cause dry mouth; avoid skin contact with oral liquid preparations, may cause contact dermatitis; do not discontinue or alter dose without physician approval. May rarely cause photosensitivity reactions; avoid exposure to sunlight and artificial light sources (sunlamps, tanning booth/bed); use a sunscreen; contact physician if reaction occurs

Additional Information In cases of overdoses, cardiovascular monitoring and continuous EKG monitoring should be performed; avoid drugs (such as quinidine, disopyramide, and procainamide) that may further prolong the QT interval

Note: All Mellaril® (brand name) products have been discontinued; Mellaril® suspension was discontinued October, 2000; oral concentrate 100 mg/mL was discontinued

March 2001; tablets and 30 mg/mL oral concentrate were discontinued in January 2002.

Dosage Forms

Solution, oral **concentrate**, as hydrochloride (Thioridazine Intensol™): 30 mg/mL (120 mL); 100 mg/mL (120 mL) [contains <0.5% alcohol; fruit-mint flavor]

Mellaril®: 30 mg/mL (120 mL) [contains 3% alcohol; fruit-mint flavor]; 100 mg/mL (120 mL) [contains 4.2% alcohol; fruit-mint flavor] [DSC]

Tablet, as hydrochloride: 10 mg, 15 mg, 25 mg, 50 mg, 100 mg, 150 mg, 200 mg

Mellaril®: 10 mg, 15 mg, 25 mg, 50 mg, 100 mg, 150 mg, 200 mg [all tablets contain sodium benzoate except 15 mg] [DSC]

References

Aman MG, Marks RE, Turbott SH, et al, "Clinical Effects of Methylphenidate and Thioridazine in Intellectually Subaverage Children," *J Am Acad Child Adolesc Psychiatry*, 1991, 30(2):246-56.

♦ **Thioridazine Intensol™** *see* Thioridazine *on page 1085*

♦ **Thiosulfuric Acid** *see* Sodium Thiosulfate *on page 1030*

Thiotepa (thye oh TEP a)

Related Information

Emetogenic Potential of Single Chemotherapeutic Agents *on page 1286*

U.S. Brand Names Thioplex®

Synonyms TESPA; Triethylenethiophosphoramide; TSPA

Therapeutic Category Antineoplastic Agent, Alkylating Agent

Generic Available Yes

Use Treatment of superficial tumors of the bladder; palliative treatment of adenocarcinoma of breast or ovary; lymphomas and sarcomas; meningeal neoplasms; control of pleural, pericardial or peritoneal effusions caused by metastatic tumors; high-dose regimens with autologous bone marrow transplantation

Pregnancy Risk Factor D

Contraindications Hypersensitivity to thiotepa or any component; severe myelosuppression with leukocyte count <3000/mm³ or platelet count <150,000 mm³; pregnancy

Warnings The FDA currently recommends that procedures for proper handling and disposal of antineoplastic agents be considered. The drug is potentially mutagenic, carcinogenic, teratogenic, and may cause fertility impairment.

Precautions Reduce dosage in patients with hepatic, renal, or bone marrow dysfunction

Adverse Reactions

Central nervous system: Dizziness, fever, headache, confusion, somnolence

Dermatologic: Alopecia, rash, pruritus, hyperpigmentation of skin with high-dose therapy

Endocrine & metabolic: Amenorrhea, hyperuricemia, azoospermia

Gastrointestinal: Nausea, vomiting, stomatitis, esophagitis, anorexia, mucositis

Genitourinary: Rarely hemorrhagic cystitis

Hematologic: Leukopenia (nadir: 7-10 days), anemia, thrombocytopenia (nadir: 3 weeks), granulocytopenia

Hepatic: Elevated liver transaminase and bilirubin (high-dose therapy)

Local: Pain at injection site

Renal: Hematuria

Miscellaneous: Anaphylaxis

Drug Interactions Succinylcholine (thiotepa inhibits pseudocholinesterase activity; prolongs muscular paralysis); other alkylating agents (intensifies toxicity)

Stability Refrigerate, protect from light; the reconstituted 10 mg/mL solution is chemically stable for 5 days when stored in the refrigerator; since it contains no preservatives use within 8 hours; unstable in acid medium. Thiotepa is stable for 24 hours at a concentration of 1-5 mg/mL in NS when stored at room temperature; at 0.5 mg/mL, thiotepa is stable for 8 hours at room temperature; stability decreases significantly at concentrations <0.5 mg/mL (1 hour).

Mechanism of Action Polyfunctional alkylating agent that reacts with DNA phosphate groups to produce cross-linking of DNA strands leading to inhibition of DNA, RNA, and protein synthesis

Pharmacokinetics

Absorption: Variable absorption through serous membranes and from I.M. injection sites; bladder mucosa: 10% to 100% and is increased with mucosal inflammation or tumor infiltration

Distribution: V_{dss}: 0.7-1.6 L/kg; distributes into CSF

Protein binding: 8% to 13%

Metabolism: In the liver via oxidative desulfuration (cytochrome P450 microsomal enzyme system) primarily to TEPA (active metabolite)

Half-life, terminal:

Thiotepa: 109 minutes (51.6-212 minutes) with dose-dependent clearance

(Continued)

Thiotepa *(Continued)*

TEPA: 10-21 hours

Elimination: Very little thiotepa or active metabolite are excreted unchanged in urine (1.5% of thiotepa dose)

Usual Dosage Refer to individual protocols

Children: I.V.: Sarcomas: 25-65 mg/m^2 as a single dose every 3-4 weeks

High-dose thiotepa with ABMT: One regimen uses 300 mg/m^2/dose over 3 hours; repeat every 24 hours for a total of 3 doses; maximum tolerated dose over 3 days: 900-1125 mg/m^2

Adults:

I.V.: 0.3-0.4 mg/kg at 1- to 4-week intervals or 0.2 mg/kg (6 mg/m^2)/day for 4-5 days, repeat at 2- to 4-week intervals; continuous infusion: 15-35 mg/m^2 over 48 hours

Intracavitary: 0.6-0.8 mg/kg; dose should not be repeated more frequently than at a 1 week interval

Administration

Bladder instillation: Prepare with 30-60 mg diluted in 30-60 mL sterile water and instill by catheter and retain for 2 hours

Intrapleural or pericardial: Dose is further diluted to a volume of 10-20 mL in NS or D$_5$W;

Intraperitoneal: Administration requires dilution in larger volumes (up to 2 L)

I.V.: Filter through a 0.22 micron filter (Millex-GS) prior to administration; administer direct I.V. over 5 minutes at a final concentration of 10 mg/mL; administer I.V. intermittent or continuous infusion at a final concentration for administration of 1 mg/mL (thiotepa may be further diluted in D$_5$W, NS, or LR)

Monitoring Parameters CBC with differential and platelet count, uric acid, urinalysis

Patient Information Notify physician if fever, sore throat, bleeding, or bruising occurs

Nursing Implications If thiotepa solution comes in contact with skin or mucosa, the affected area should be washed with soap and water immediately or affected mucosa should be rinsed thoroughly with water.

Additional Information Myelosuppressive effects:

WBC: Moderate

Platelets: Severe

Onset (days): 7-10

Nadir (days): 14-20

Recovery (days): 28

Dosage Forms Injection, powder for reconstitution: 15 mg

References

Grovas AC, Boyett JM, Lindsley K, et al, "Regimen-Related Toxicity of Myeloablative Chemotherapy With BCNU, Thiotepa, and Etoposide Followed by Autologous Stem Cell Rescue for Children With Newly Diagnosed Glioblastoma Multiforme: Report From the Children's Cancer Group," *Med Pediatr Oncol*, 1999, 33(2):83-7.

Heideman R, Cole D, Balis F, et al, "Phase I and Pharmacokinetic Evaluation of Thiotepa in the Cerebrospinal Fluid and Plasma of Pediatric Patients: Evidence for Dose-Dependent Plasma Clearance of Thiotepa," *Cancer Res*, 1989, 49(3):736-41.

Herzig GP, "Phase I-II Studies of High-Dose Thiotepa and Autologous BMT in Patients With Refractory Malignancies," *Adv Cancer Chemotherapy*, 1987, 17-29 (proceedings of a symposium, Oct 1986)

Saarinen UM, Hovi L, and Makipern CA, "High Dose Thiotepa With Autologous Bone Marrow Rescue in Pediatric Solid Tumors," *Proc Am Soc Clin Oncol*, 1989, 8:303.

Thiothixene *(thye oh THIKS een)*

Related Information

Overdose and Toxicology *on page 1388*

U.S. Brand Names Navane®

Therapeutic Category Antipsychotic Agent; Phenothiazine Derivative

Generic Available Yes

Use Management of schizophrenia; also used for management of psychotic disorders

Pregnancy Risk Factor C

Contraindications Hypersensitivity to thiothixene or any component; cross-sensitivity with other phenothiazines may exist; patients with CNS depression, comatose states, circulatory collapse, or blood dyscrasias; avoid use in patients with narrow-angle glaucoma, bone marrow suppression, severe liver or cardiac disease

Warnings Tardive dyskinesias and neuroleptic malignant syndrome may occur

Precautions Use with caution in patients with cardiovascular disease or seizures

Adverse Reactions Sedation and extrapyramidal effects occur more often

Cardiovascular: Hypotension (especially with parenteral use), orthostatic hypotension, tachycardia, arrhythmias

Central nervous system: Sedation, drowsiness, restlessness, anxiety, insomnia, extrapyramidal reactions, tardive dyskinesia, neuroleptic malignant syndrome, seizures, altered central temperature regulation

Dermatologic: Rash, photosensitivity
Endocrine & metabolic: Amenorrhea, galactorrhea, gynecomastia
Gastrointestinal: GI upset, xerostomia, constipation, weight gain
Genitourinary: Urinary retention
Hematologic: Agranulocytosis, leukopenia
Ocular: Retinal pigmentation, blurred vision

Drug Interactions Cytochrome P450 isoenzyme CYP1A2 substrate
Alcohol and other CNS depressants, anticholinergics, or hypotensive agents may increase adverse effects

Food Interactions May cause increase in dietary riboflavin requirements

Mechanism of Action Elicits antipsychotic activity by postsynaptic blockade of CNS dopamine receptors resulting in inhibition of dopamine-mediated effects; also has alpha-adrenergic blocking activity

Usual Dosage Oral:
Children ≤12 years: Dose not well established (use not recommended); 0.25 mg/kg/day in divided doses
Children >12 years and Adults: Initial: 2 mg 3 times/day, up to 20-30 mg/day; maximum dose: 60 mg/day

Administration Oral: Administer with food or water

Monitoring Parameters Periodic eye exam, CBC with differential, blood pressure, liver enzyme tests

Patient Information Avoid alcohol; limit caffeine; may cause drowsiness and impair ability to perform activities requiring mental alertness or physical coordination; may cause dry mouth. May cause photosensitivity reactions (eg, exposure to sunlight may cause severe sunburn, skin rash, redness, or itching); avoid exposure to sunlight and artificial light sources (sunlamps, tanning booth/bed); wear protective clothing, wide-brimmed hats, sunglasses, and lip sunscreen (SPF ≥15); use a sunscreen [broad-spectrum sunscreen or physical sunscreen (preferred) or sunblock with SPF ≥15]; contact physician if reaction occurs.

Dosage Forms
Capsule: 1 mg, 2 mg, 5 mg, 10 mg
Navane®: 1 mg, 2 mg, 5 mg, 10 mg, 20 mg
Solution, oral **concentrate**, as hydrochloride: 5 mg/mL (120 mL) [fruit flavor]

References
Wiener JM, "Psychopharmacology in Childhood Disorders," *Psychiatr Clin North Am*, 1984, 7(4):831-43.

♦ **Thorazine**® *see* ChlorproMAZINE *on page 263*
♦ **Thrombin-JMI**® *see* Thrombin (Topical) *on page 1089*

Thrombin (Topical) (THROM bin, TOP i kal)

U.S. Brand Names Thrombin-JMI®; Thrombogen®
Canadian Brand Names Thrombostat™
Therapeutic Category Hemostatic Agent
Generic Available No
Use Hemostasis whenever minor bleeding from capillaries and small venules is accessible

Pregnancy Risk Factor C
Contraindications Hypersensitivity to thrombin, any component, or material of bovine origin

Warnings For topical use only - do not inject; injection may result in extensive intravascular clotting and death. Use of topical thrombin has been associated with abnormalities in hemostasis ranging from asymptomatic alterations in PT and PTT to severe bleeding or thrombosis which have rarely been fatal. These hemostatic effects may be related to formation of antibodies against bovine thrombin and/or factor V which in some cases may cross react with human factor V resulting in factor V deficiency; patients with antibodies to bovine thrombin should not receive topical thrombin again

Adverse Reactions
Central nervous system: Fever
Miscellaneous: Allergic reactions

Stability Following reconstitution, use immediately; stable 3 hours refrigerated; stable frozen (reconstituted) for 48 hours

Mechanism of Action Catalyzes the conversion of fibrinogen to fibrin

Usual Dosage Topical: Apply powder directly to the site of bleeding or on oozing surfaces or use 1000-2000 units/mL of solution where bleeding is profuse; use 100 units/mL for bleeding from skin or mucosal surfaces

Administration Not for injection
Topical: May be applied directly as a powder or as reconstituted solution; the most effective hemostasis results when the thrombin mixes freely with blood as it
(Continued)

Thrombin (Topical) *(Continued)*

appears; use sterile water or NS to reconstitute powder to 1000-2000 units/mL concentration; for profuse bleeding, 1000 units/mL may be required; for use in dental extractions, plastic surgery, or skin grafting 100 units/mL is frequently used. The recipient surface should be sponged (not wiped) free of blood before application; do not sponge **treated** surfaces to assure that clot remains securely in place

Additional Information One unit is amount required to clot 1 mL of standardized fibrinogen solution in 15 seconds

Dosage Forms

Powder for reconstitution, topical:

Thrombin-JMI®: 1000 units, 5000 units, 10,000 units, 20,000 units, 50,000 units

Thrombin-JMI® Spray Kit: 5000 unit, 10,000 units, 20,000 units

Thrombin-JMI® Syringe Spray Kit: 10,000 units, 20,000 units

Thrombogen®: 5000 units, 20,000 units

Thrombogen® Spray Kit: 10,000 units, 20,000 units

♦ **Thrombogen®** *see* Thrombin (Topical) *on page 1089*

♦ **Thrombostat™ (Can)** *see* Thrombin (Topical) *on page 1089*

♦ **Thymocyte Stimulating Factor** *see* Aldesleukin *on page 56*

♦ **Thyrel® TRH** *see* Protirelin *on page 956*

♦ **Tiabendazole** *see* Thiabendazole *on page 1080*

Tiagabine *(tye AG a bene)*

U.S. Brand Names Gabitril®

Therapeutic Category Anticonvulsant, Miscellaneous

Generic Available No

Use Adjunctive therapy of partial epilepsy

Pregnancy Risk Factor C

Contraindications Hypersensitivity to tiagabine or any component

Warnings Do not abruptly discontinue therapy, withdraw gradually to lessen chance for increased seizure frequency (unless a more rapid withdrawal is required due to safety concerns); exacerbation of EEG abnormalities associated with CNS adverse events (cognitive and neuropsychiatric) may occur in patients with an EEG history of spike and wave discharges and may require dosage adjustment; nonconvulsant status epilepticus has also been reported and may respond to dosage reduction or discontinuation

Precautions Use with caution in patients with hepatic impairment; possible long-term ophthalmologic effects exist (more studies are needed); use with caution with alcohol or other CNS depressants

Adverse Reactions

Central nervous system: Impaired concentration, speech/language problems, confusion, somnolence, fatigue, dizziness, nervousness, depression, ataxia, insomnia, emotional lability, headache

Gastrointestinal: Nausea, abdominal pain, diarrhea

Neuromuscular & skeletal: Asthenia, tremor

Drug Interactions Cytochrome P450 isoenzyme CYP3A substrate, may also be metabolized by CYP1A2, 2D6, or 2C19

Tiagabine may decrease valproic acid concentrations by ~10%; carbamazepine, phenytoin, primidone, and phenobarbital may increase tiagabine clearance by 60%; naproxen, salicylates, and valproic acid may decrease tiagabine protein binding and increase the free concentration

Food Interactions Food may decrease the rate but not the extent of absorption

Stability Protect from moisture and light; store at room temperature

Mechanism of Action Exact mechanism unknown; thought to potentiate the action of GABA (an inhibitory neurotransmitter) by selectively binding to the GABA uptake carrier and blocking GABA uptake into presynaptic neurons. This allows more GABA to be available at its site of action to bind to postsynaptic neuronal receptors.

Pharmacokinetics

Absorption: Rapid and nearly complete (>95%)

Distribution: Mean V_d:

Children 3-10 years: 2.4 L/kg

Adults: 1.3-1.6 L/kg

Note: V_d values are more similar between children and adults when expressed as L/m^2 (see Gustavson, 1997)

Protein binding: 96%, mainly to albumin and alpha$_1$-acid glycoprotein

Metabolism: Extensive in the liver via oxidation and glucuronidation; undergoes enterohepatic recirculation

Bioavailability: 90%

Diurnal effect: Trough concentrations and AUC are lower in the evening versus morning

Half-life:
  Children 3-10 years: Mean: 5.7 hours (range: 2-10 hours)
  Children 3-10 years receiving enzyme-inducing AEDs: Mean: 3.2 hours (range: 2-7.8 hours)
  Adults (normal volunteers): 7-9 hours
  Adults receiving enzyme-inducing AEDs: 4-7 hours

Time to peak serum concentration: Fasting state: ~45 minutes

Elimination: ~2% excreted unchanged in urine; 25% excreted in urine and 63% excreted in feces as metabolites

Clearance:
  Children 3-10 years: 4.2 ± 1.6 mL/minute/kg
  Children 3-10 years receiving enzyme-inducing AEDs: 8.6 ± 3.3 mL/minute/kg
  Adults (normal volunteers): 109 mL/minute
  Adult patients: 1.9 ± 0.5 mL/minute/kg
  Adults receiving enzyme-inducing AEDs: 6.3 ± 3.5 mL/minute/kg
  Note: Clearance values are more similar between children and adults when expressed as mL/minute/m^2 (see Gustavson, 1997)
    Hepatic impairment: Clearance of unbound drug is decreased by 60%

Usual Dosage Oral: **Note:** Doses were determined in patients receiving enzyme-inducing AEDs; lower doses or slower titration may be required in patients not receiving enzyme-inducing agents

Children <12 years: Only limited preliminary information is available; dosing guidelines are not established (see Adkins, 1998 and Pellock, 1999)

Children 12-18 years: Initial: 4 mg once daily for 1 week, then 8 mg/day given in 2 divided doses for 1 week, then increase weekly by 4-8 mg/day; administer in 2-4 divided doses per day; titrate dose to response; maximum dose: 32 mg/day (doses >32 mg/day have been used in select adolescent patients for short periods of time)

Adults: Initial: 4 mg once daily for 1 week, then increase weekly by 4-8 mg/day; administer in 2-4 divided doses per day; titrate dose to response; maximum dose: 56 mg/day. **Note:** Twice daily dosing may not be well tolerated and dosing 3 times/day is the currently favored dosing frequency (see Kalviainen, 1998).

Dosing adjustment in renal impairment: None needed

Dosing adjustment in hepatic impairment: Reduced doses and longer dosing intervals may be required

Administration Oral: Administer with food (to avoid rapid increase in plasma concentrations and adverse CNS effects)

Monitoring Parameters Seizure frequency, duration, and severity

Reference Range Not established

Patient Information May cause dizziness or drowsiness and impair ability to perform activities requiring mental alertness or physical coordination

Additional Information Population pharmacokinetic analysis suggests that tiagabine may be administered at similar doses without adjustment for age, gender, or body weight in epilepsy patients ≥11 years of age (see Samara, 1998)

Note: On August 24, 2001, the new manufacturer of Gabitril® (Cephalon, Inc.) announced changes in the product labeling and appearance of Gabitril® tablets. The word "Filmtab" has been removed from the Gabitril® product name and from all product labeling and prescribing information. In addition, the Abbott logo on the tablets has been replaced with the Cephalon logo. Healthcare providers should be aware of these changes, since patients may become concerned by the change in appearance of the tablets. A letter detailing this announcement can be found at http://www.fda.gov/medwatch/safety/2001/safety01.htm#gabitr.

Dosage Forms Tablet, as hydrochloride: 2 mg, 4 mg, 12 mg, 16 mg

References

Adkins JC and Noble S, "Tiagabine. A Review of Its Pharmacodynamic and Pharmacokinetic Properties and Therapeutic Potential in the Management of Epilepsy," *Drugs*, 1998, 55(3):437-60.

Gustavson LE, Boellner SW, Granneman GR, et al, "A Single-Dose Study to Define Tiagabine Pharmacokinetics in Pediatric Patients With Complex Partial Seizures," *Neurology*, 1997, 48(4):1032-7.

Kalviainen R, Brodie MJ, Duncan J, et al, "A Double-Blind, Placebo-Controlled Trial of Tiagabine Given Three-Times Daily as Add-On Therapy for Refractory Partial Seizures. Northern European Tiagabine Study Group," *Epilepsy Res*, 1998, 30(1):31-40.

Leach JP and Brodie MJ, "Tiagabine," *Lancet*, 1998, 351(9097):203-7.

Pellock JM, "Managing Pediatric Epilepsy Syndromes With New Antiepileptic Drugs," *Pediatrics*, 1999, 104(5 Pt 1):1106-16.

Samara EE, Gustavson LE, El-Shourbagy T, et al, "Population Analysis of the Pharmacokinetics of Tiagabine in Patients With Epilepsy," *Epilepsy*, 1998, 39(8):868-73.

◆ **Tiamol® (Can)** see Fluocinonide on page 499
◆ **Tiazac®** see Diltiazem on page 388
◆ **Ticar®** see Ticarcillin on page 1092

Ticarcillin (tye kar SIL in)

U.S. Brand Names Ticar®

Therapeutic Category Antibiotic, Penicillin (Antipseudomonal)

Generic Available No

Use Treatment of infections such as septicemia, acute and chronic respiratory tract infections, skin and soft tissue infections, and urinary tract infections due to susceptible strains of *Pseudomonas*, *Proteus*, *Escherichia coli*, and *Enterobacter*

Pregnancy Risk Factor B

Contraindications Hypersensitivity to ticarcillin, any component, or penicillins

Warnings Prolonged use may result in superinfection

Precautions Use with caution in patients with CHF due to ticarcillin's high sodium content; dosage modification required in patients with impaired renal and/or hepatic function

Adverse Reactions

Central nervous system: Seizures, headache, fever

Dermatologic: Rash

Endocrine & metabolic: Hypernatremia, hypokalemia, metabolic alkalosis

Gastrointestinal: Diarrhea, pseudomembranous colitis, stomatitis, nausea

Genitourinary: Cystitis, hematuria

Hematologic: Inhibition of platelet aggregation, leukopenia, neutropenia, eosinophilia, prolonged prothrombin time, bleeding diathesis, hemolytic anemia, decreased hemoglobin and hematocrit

Hepatic: Elevated AST and ALT, hepatitis

Local: Phlebitis

Renal: Elevated BUN, elevated serum creatinine

Miscellaneous: Hypersensitivity reactions including anaphylaxis; superinfection

Drug Interactions Aminoglycosides (antibacterial activity is synergistic), probenecid (increases serum concentration of ticarcillin); may alter renal elimination of lithium

Stability Reconstituted ticarcillin solution 200-300 mg/mL is stable for 24 hours at room temperature or 72 hours when refrigerated; incompatible with aminoglycosides

Mechanism of Action Inhibits bacterial cell wall synthesis by binding to one or more of the penicillin-binding proteins; inhibits the final transpeptidation step of peptidoglycan synthesis in bacterial cell walls

Pharmacokinetics

Absorption: I.M.: 86%

Distribution: V_d: Neonates: 0.42-0.76 L/kg; distributed into breast milk at low concentrations; attains high concentrations in bile; minimal concentrations attained in CSF with uninflamed meninges

Protein binding: 45% to 65%

Metabolism: 10%

Half-life, adults: 1-1.3 hours, prolonged with renal impairment and/or hepatic impairment

Neonates:

<1 week: 3.5-5.6 hours

1-8 weeks: 1.3-2.2 hours

Children 5-13 years: 0.9 hours

Time to peak serum concentration: I.M.: Within 30-75 minutes

Elimination: Almost entirely in urine as unchanged drug and its metabolites with small amounts excreted in feces (3.5%)

Dialysis: Moderately dialyzable (20% to 50%)

Usual Dosage Ticarcillin is generally only given I.M. for the treatment of uncomplicated urinary tract infections

Neonates: I.V.:

Postnatal age ≤7 days:

≤2000 g: 150 mg/kg/day in divided doses every 12 hours

>2000 g: 225 mg/kg/day in divided doses every 8 hours

Postnatal age >7 days:

<1200 g: 150 mg/kg/day in divided doses every 12 hours

1200-2000 g: 225 mg/kg/day in divided doses every 8 hours

>2000 g: 300 mg/kg/day in divided doses every 6-8 hours

Infants and Children:

I.M.: 50-100 mg/kg/day in divided doses every 6-8 hours

I.V.: 200-300 mg/kg/day in divided doses every 4-6 hours; doses as high as 400 mg/kg/day divided every 4-6 hours have been used in acute pulmonary exacerbations of cystic fibrosis

Maximum dose: 24 g/day

Adults:

I.M.: 1 g every 6 hours

I.V.: 1-4 g every 4-6 hours; maximum dose: 24 g/day

Dosing interval in renal impairment:
Cl_{cr} 10-30 mL/minute: Administer every 8 hours

Cl_{cr} 10-30 mL/minute: Administer every 8 hours

Cl_{cr} <10 mL/minute: Administer every 12 hours

Administration Parenteral:

I.M.: Reconstitute each gram of ticarcillin with 2 mL SWI or 1% lidocaine hydrochloride injection (without epinephrine) to make a 385 mg/mL solution; administer by deep I.M. injection into a large muscle mass

I.V.: Ticarcillin may be administered I.V. push over 10-20 minutes or by I.V. intermittent infusion over 30-120 minutes at a final concentration not to exceed 100 mg/mL; concentrations ≤50 mg/mL are preferred for peripheral intermittent infusions to avoid vein irritation; if the patient is on concurrent aminoglycoside therapy, separate ticarcillin administration from the aminoglycoside by at least 30-60 minutes

Monitoring Parameters Serum electrolytes, bleeding time, and periodic tests of renal, hepatic, and hematologic function

Test Interactions False-positive urinary or serum protein, positive Coombs' [direct]

Additional Information Sodium content of 1 g: 5.2-6.5 mEq

Dosage Forms Injection, powder for reconstitution, as disodium: 3 g, 20 g

References

Brogden RN, Heel RC, Speight TM, et al, "Ticarcillin: A Review of Its Pharmacological Properties and Therapeutic Efficacy," *Drugs*, 1980, 20(5):325-52.

Nelson JD, Kusmiesz H, Shelton S, et al, "Clinical Pharmacology and Efficacy of Ticarcillin in Infants and Children," *Pediatrics*, 1978, 61(6):858-63.

Ticarcillin and Clavulanate Potassium

(tye kar SIL in & klav yoo LAN ate poe TASS ee um)

U.S. Brand Names Timentin®

Synonyms Clavulanate Potassium and Ticarcillin

Therapeutic Category Antibiotic, Beta-lactam and Beta-lactamase Combination; Antibiotic, Penicillin (Antipseudomonal)

Generic Available No

Use Treatment of infections caused by susceptible organisms involving the lower respiratory tract, urinary tract, skin and skin structures, bone and joint, and septicemia. Clavulanate expands activity of ticarcillin to include beta-lactamase producing strains of *S. aureus, H. influenzae, Moraxella catarrhalis, B. fragilis, Klebsiella,* and *Proteus* species

Pregnancy Risk Factor B

Contraindications Hypersensitivity to ticarcillin, clavulanate, or penicillin

Warnings Abnormal platelet aggregation and prolonged bleeding have been reported in patients with renal impairment receiving high doses; prolonged use may result in superinfection

Precautions Use with caution and modify dosage in patients with renal impairment; use with caution in patients with CHF due to high sodium content of the formulation

Adverse Reactions

Central nervous system: Seizures, headache, fever

Dermatologic: Rash, erythema multiforme, toxic epidermal necrolysis, Stevens-Johnson syndrome

Endocrine & metabolic: Hypernatremia, hypokalemia, metabolic alkalosis

Gastrointestinal: Diarrhea, stomatitis, nausea, pseudomembranous colitis

Genitourinary: Cystitis, hematuria

Hematologic: Eosinophilia, leukopenia, decreased hemoglobin and hematocrit, inhibition of platelet aggregation, prolongation of bleeding time, neutropenia, hemolytic anemia

Hepatic: Elevated ALT and AST, hepatitis

Local: Thrombophlebitis

Renal: Elevated BUN, elevated serum creatinine

Miscellaneous: Hypersensitivity reactions including anaphylaxis; superinfection

Drug Interactions Aminoglycosides (antibacterial activity is synergistic), probenecid (increases serum concentration of ticarcillin)

Stability Reconstituted 200 mg/mL solution is stable for 6 hours at room temperature and 72 hours when refrigerated; darkening of drug indicates loss of potency of clavulanate potassium; incompatible with sodium bicarbonate and aminoglycosides

Mechanism of Action Ticarcillin inhibits bacterial cell wall synthesis by binding to one or more of the penicillin-binding proteins; inhibits the final transpeptidation step of peptidoglycan synthesis in bacterial cell walls; clavulanic acid inhibits degradation of ticarcillin by binding to beta-lactamases

(Continued)

Ticarcillin and Clavulanate Potassium *(Continued)*

Pharmacokinetics

Distribution: Ticarcillin is distributed into tissue, interstitial fluid, pleural fluid, bile, and breast milk; low concentrations of ticarcillin distribute into the CSF but increase when meninges are inflamed

V_{dss} ticarcillin: 0.22 L/kg

V_{dss} clavulanic acid: 0.4 L/kg

Protein binding:

Ticarcillin: 45% to 65%

Clavulanic acid: 9% to 30%

Metabolism: Clavulanic acid is metabolized in the liver

Half-life: In patients with normal renal function

Neonates:

Clavulanic acid: 1.9 hours

Ticarcillin: 4.4 hours

Children (1 month to 9.3 years):

Clavulanic acid: 54 minutes

Ticarcillin: 66 minutes

Adults:

Clavulanic acid: 66-90 minutes

Ticarcillin: 66-72 minutes

Clavulanic acid does not affect the clearance of ticarcillin

Elimination:

Children: 71% of the ticarcillin and 50% of the clavulanic acid dose are excreted unchanged in the urine over 4 hours

Adults: 45% of clavulanate is excreted unchanged in urine, whereas 60% to 90% of ticarcillin is excreted unchanged in urine

Dialysis: Removed by hemodialysis

Usual Dosage I.V.: (**Note:** Timentin® (ticarcillin/clavulanate) is a combination product; each 3.1 g vial contains 3 g ticarcillin disodium and 0.1 g clavulanic acid. Dosage recommendations are based on **ticarcillin** component):

Term neonates and Infants <3 months: 200-300 mg ticarcillin component/kg/day divided every 6-8 hours

Infants ≥3 months and Children:

Mild to moderate infection: 200 mg ticarcillin component/kg/day divided every 6 hours

Severe infections that occur outside the CNS: 300 mg ticarcillin component/kg/day in divided doses every 4-6 hours; maximum dose: 400 mg/kg/day not to exceed 18-24 g/day

Adults: 3 g ticarcillin component every 4-6 hours; maximum dose: 18-24 g/day

Urinary tract infections: 3 g ticarcillin component every 6-8 hours

Dosing interval in renal impairment:

Cl_{cr} 10-30 mL/minute: Administer every 8 hours

Cl_{cr} <10 mL/minute: Administer every 12 hours

Dosing interval in hepatic impairment and a Cl_{cr} <10 mL/minute: Administer every 24 hours

Administration Parenteral: Administer by I.V. intermittent infusion over 30 minutes; final concentration for administration should not exceed 100 mg/mL of ticarcillin; however, concentrations ≤50 mg/mL are preferred; if the patient is on concurrent aminoglycoside therapy, separate ticarcillin and clavulanate potassium administration from the aminoglycoside by at least 30-60 minutes

Monitoring Parameters Serum electrolytes, periodic renal, hepatic and hematologic function tests

Test Interactions Positive Coombs' [direct], false-positive urinary and serum proteins

Additional Information

Sodium content of 1 g: 4.75 mEq

Potassium content of 1 g: 0.15 mEq

Dosage Forms

Infusion [premixed, frozen]: Ticarcillin disodium 3 g and clavulanic acid 0.1 g (100 mL)

Injection, powder for reconstitution: Ticarcillin disodium 3 g and clavulanic acid 0.1 g (3.1 g, 31 g)

References

Begue P, Quiniou F, Quinet B, "Efficacy and Pharmacokinetics of Timentin® in Paediatric Infections," *J Antimicrob Chemother*, 1986, 17(Suppl C):81-91.

Reed MD, Yamashita TS, and Blumer JL, "Pharmacokinetic-Based Ticarcillin/Clavulanic Acid Dose Recommendations for Infants and Children," *J Clin Pharmacol*, 1995, 35(7):658-65.

Stutman HR and Marks MI, "Review of Pediatric Antimicrobial Therapies," *Semin Pediatr Infect Dis*, 1991, 2:3-17.

♦ **Tigan**® *see* Trimethobenzamide *on page 1119*

- **Tilade®** *see Nedocromil on page 798*
- **Tim-AK (Can)** *see Timolol on page 1095*
- **Timentin®** *see Ticarcillin and Clavulanate Potassium on page 1093*

Timolol (TYE moe lole)

Related Information
Overdose and Toxicology *on page 1388*

U.S. Brand Names Betimol®; Blocadren®; Timoptic®; Timoptic® OcuDose®; Timoptic-XE®

Canadian Brand Names Alti-Timolol; Apo®-Timol; Apo®-Timop; Gen-Timolol; Nu-Timolol; Phoxal-timolol; PMS-Timolol; Tim-AK

Therapeutic Category Antihypertensive Agent; Antimigraine Agent; Beta-Adrenergic Blocker; Beta-Adrenergic Blocker, Ophthalmic

Generic Available Yes (except hemihydrate and preservative free maleate ophthalmic solutions)

Use
Ophthalmic: Treatment of elevated intraocular pressure such as glaucoma or ocular hypertension
Oral: Treatment of hypertension and angina; prevention of MI and migraine headaches

Pregnancy Risk Factor C

Contraindications Hypersensitivity to timolol or any component; uncompensated CHF, cardiogenic shock, bradycardia or heart block, bronchial asthma, severe chronic obstructive pulmonary disease or history of asthma, CHF or bradycardia

Warnings Severe CNS, cardiovascular and respiratory adverse effects have been seen following ophthalmic use

Precautions Similar to other beta-blockers; use with caution in patients with decreased renal or hepatic function (dosage adjustment required); use with a miotic in angle-closure or narrow-angle glaucoma; use with caution in patients with diabetes mellitus, may block hypoglycemia-induced tachycardia and blood pressure changes

Adverse Reactions
Cardiovascular: Bradycardia, arrhythmia, hypotension, syncope
Central nervous system: Dizziness, headache
Dermatologic: Rash
Gastrointestinal: Diarrhea, nausea
Local (ocular): Irritation, conjunctivitis, keratitis, visual disturbances; transient (30 seconds to 5 minutes) blurred vision after instillation of ophthalmic gel
Respiratory: Bronchospasm
Miscellaneous: Hypersensitivity reactions, anaphylaxis

Drug Interactions Cytochrome P450 isoenzyme CYP2D6 substrate
Verapamil, nifedipine, diltiazem, digitalis, quinidine may increase adverse cardiac effects; NSAIDs may decrease antihypertensive effects of timolol; patients receiving beta blockers, who have a history of anaphylactic reactions, may be more reactive to a repeated allergen challenge and may not be responsive to the usual epinephrine doses used to treat an allergic reaction; abrupt withdrawal of clonidine while receiving beta-blockers may result in an exaggerated hypertensive crisis; drug interactions similar to other beta-blockers may occur

Stability Ophthalmic: Store at room temperature; do not freeze; protect from light

Mechanism of Action Blocks both beta$_1$- and beta$_2$-adrenergic receptors; reduces intraocular pressure by reducing aqueous humor production or possibly outflow; reduces blood pressure by blocking adrenergic receptors and decreasing sympathetic outflow; produces negative chronotropic and negative inotropic activity

Pharmacodynamics Hypotensive effects:
Onset of action: Oral: Within 15-45 minutes
Maximum effect: 30-150 minutes
Duration:
Oral: 4 hours
Ophthalmic (intraocular effects): 24 hours

Pharmacokinetics
Protein binding: <10%
Metabolism: Extensively in the liver, extensive first-pass effect
Bioavailability: Oral: ~60%
Half-life: Adults: 2-4 hours; prolonged with reduced renal function
Elimination: Urinary excretion (15% to 20% as unchanged drug)
Dialysis: Not readily dialyzable

Usual Dosage
Ophthalmic:
Gel (Timoptic-XE®): Adults: 0.25% or 0.5% gel, instill 1 drop once daily; do not exceed 1 drop once daily of 0.5% gel
(Continued)

Timolol *(Continued)*

Solution (Timoptic®): Children and Adults: Initial: 0.25% solution, instill 1 drop twice daily; increase to 0.5% solution if response not adequate; decrease to 1 drop/day if controlled; do not exceed 1 drop twice daily of 0.5% solution (see Additional Information)

Oral:

Children: No information regarding pediatric dose is currently available in literature

Adults:

Hypertension: Initial: 10 mg twice daily, increase gradually every 7 days, usual dosage: 20-40 mg/day in 2 divided doses; maximum dose: 60 mg/day

Prevention of MI: 10 mg twice daily initiated within 1-4 weeks after infarction

Migraine headache: Initial: 10 mg twice daily, increase to maximum of 30 mg/day

Administration

Ophthalmic: Apply gentle pressure to lacrimal sac during and immediately following instillation (1 minute) or instruct patient to gently close eyelid after administration, to decrease systemic absorption of ophthalmic drops; avoid contact of bottle tip with skin or eye. Remove contact lenses prior to administration (ophthalmic solution contains benzalkonium chloride which may adsorb to soft contact lenses); lenses may be inserted 15 minutes after administration. Gel: Invert container, shake once before use; administer other topical ophthalmic medications at least 10 minutes before Timoptic-XE®

Oral: May be administered without regard to food

Monitoring Parameters

Heart rate, blood pressure; liver enzymes, BUN, serum creatinine with long-term oral use; monitor IOP with ophthalmic use; monitor respiratory rate, CNS status, and cardiovascular status with ophthalmic use in patients at risk for adverse effects (eg, asthmatics, CHF patients, etc)

Patient Information

Potential visual disturbances from ophthalmic use may impair ability to perform hazardous duties such as driving or operating machinery

Nursing Implications

Discontinue medication if breathing difficulty occurs

Additional Information

Ophthalmic: Use lowest effective dose in pediatric patients. Children had higher plasma concentrations vs adults following ophthalmic use; some achieved therapeutic levels; this may result in increased adverse systemic effects. The concurrent use of 2 ophthalmic beta blockers is not recommended.

Dosage Forms

Gel forming solution, ophthalmic, as **maleate** (Timoptic-XE®): 0.25% (2.5 mL, 5 mL); 0.5% (2.5 mL, 5 mL)

Solution, ophthalmic, as **hemihydrate** (Betimol®): 0.25% (5 mL, 10 mL, 15 mL); 0.5% (5 mL, 10 mL, 15 mL)

Solution, ophthalmic, as **maleate**: 0.25% (5 mL, 10 mL, 15 mL); 0.5% (5 mL, 10 mL, 15 mL)

Timoptic®: 0.25% (5 mL, 10 mL); 0.5% (5 mL, 10 mL)

Solution, ophthalmic, as **maleate** [preservative free] (Timoptic® OcuDose®): 0.25% (0.2 mL); 0.5% (0.2 mL) [single use]

Tablet, as **maleate** (Blocadren®): 5 mg, 10 mg, 20 mg

References

Hoskins HD, Hetherington J Jr, Magee SD, et al, "Clinical Experience With Timolol in Childhood Glaucoma," *Arch Ophthalmol*, 1985, 103(8):1163-5.

Passo MS, Palmer EA, and Van Buskirk EM, "Plasma Timolol in Glaucoma Patients," *Ophthalmology*, 1984, 91(11):1361-3.

Tobramycin (toe bra MYE sin)

Related Information
Blood Level Sampling Time Guidelines *on page 1386*
Overdose and Toxicology *on page 1388*

U.S. Brand Names AKTob®; Nebcin®; TOBI®; Tobrex®; Tomycine™ [DSC]

Canadian Brand Names PMS-Tobramycin

Therapeutic Category Antibiotic, Aminoglycoside; Antibiotic, Ophthalmic

Generic Available Yes (ophthalmic solution and solution for injection)

Use Treatment of documented or suspected infections caused by susceptible gram-negative bacilli including *Pseudomonas aeruginosa*; nonpseudomonal enteric bacillus infection which is more sensitive to tobramycin than gentamicin based on susceptibility tests; susceptible organisms in lower respiratory tract infections, septicemia; intra-abdominal, skin, bone, and urinary tract infections; empiric therapy in cystic fibrosis and immunocompromised patients; used topically to treat superficial ophthalmic infections caused by susceptible bacteria; inhalation therapy management of cystic fibrosis patients with *P. aeruginosa*

Pregnancy Risk Factor D

Contraindications Hypersensitivity to tobramycin, any component (see Warnings), or aminoglycosides

Warnings I.M., I.V.: Aminoglycosides are associated with significant nephrotoxicity or ototoxicity; the ototoxicity is directly proportional to the amount of drug given and the duration of treatment; tinnitus, vertigo, ataxia, or dizziness are indications of vestibular injury and impending irreversible bilateral deafness; renal damage is usually reversible. Some formulations contain sulfites which may cause allergic reactions in susceptible individuals; transient tinnitus and hearing loss have been reported in tobramycin inhalation-treated patients; bronchospasm can occur with inhalation of tobramycin. Aminoglycosides can cause fetal harm when administered to a pregnant woman; aminoglycosides have been associated with several reports of total, irreversible, bilateral congenital deafness in pediatric patients exposed *in utero*

Precautions Use with caution in patients with renal impairment, pre-existing auditory or vestibular impairment, patients receiving anesthetics or neuromuscular blocking agents, and in patients with neuromuscular disorders; dosage modification required in patients with impaired renal function

Adverse Reactions

Central nervous system: Vertigo, gait instability, fever, ataxia, dizziness, headache

Dermatologic: Allergic contact dermatitis, rash

Endocrine & metabolic: Hypomagnesemia

Gastrointestinal: Nausea, vomiting

Hematologic: Granulocytopenia, thrombocytopenia, eosinophilia

Hepatic: Elevated AST and ALT

Local: Thrombophlebitis

Neuromuscular & skeletal: Neuromuscular blockade, paresthesia, tremor, weakness

Ocular: Ophthalmic use: Lacrimation, itching, edema of the eyelid, keratitis

Otic: Ototoxicity (may be associated with high serum aminoglycoside concentrations persisting for prolonged periods or with high peak serum concentrations following rapid I.V. bolus administration) with tinnitus, hearing loss; early toxicity usually affects high-pitched sound

Renal: Nephrotoxicity (high trough levels) with proteinuria, reduction in glomerular filtration rate, elevated serum creatinine, decrease in urine specific gravity, casts in urine and possible electrolyte wasting

Respiratory: With inhalation therapy: Voice alteration, bronchospasm, dyspnea, increased cough, pharyngitis, hoarseness

Drug Interactions Increased toxicity: Concurrent use of amphotericin B, cephalosporins, penicillins, loop diuretics, urea, mannitol, vancomycin, cisplatin, indomethacin; potentiates effect of neuromuscular blocking agents and botulinum toxin

Stability Incompatible with penicillins, cephalosporins, heparin

Inhalation solution: Store in refrigerator; upon removal from the refrigerator, the solution may be stored at room temperature for up to 28 days; do not use solution if it is cloudy or contains particles; a darkened yellow solution does not indicate loss of potency; protect from intense light; incompatible with dornase alfa (may precipitate)

Mechanism of Action Inhibits cellular initiation of bacterial protein synthesis by binding to 30S and 50S ribosomal subunits resulting in a defective bacterial cell membrane

Pharmacokinetics

Absorption:

Oral: Poor

I.M.: Rapid and complete

(Continued)

Tobramycin *(Continued)*

Inhalation: Low systemic bioavailability although peak tobramycin serum concentration 1 hour after inhalation ranges between 0.95-1.05 mg/mL

Distribution: Crosses the placenta; distributes primarily in the extracellular fluid volume; poor penetration into the CSF and into bronchial secretions; drug accumulates in the renal cortex; small amounts distribute into bile, sputum, saliva, tears, and breast milk

V_d: Increased by fever, edema, ascites, fluid overload, and in neonates; V_d is decreased in patients with dehydration

Neonates: 0.45 ± 0.1 L/kg

Infants: 0.4 ± 0.1 L/kg

Children: 0.35 ± 0.15 L/kg

Adolescents: 0.3 ± 0.1 L/kg

Adults: 0.2-0.3 L/kg

Protein binding: <30%

Half-life:

Neonates:

≤1200 g: 11 hours

>1200 g: 2-9 hours

Infants: 4 ± 1 hour

Children: 2 ± 1 hour

Adolescents: 1.5 ± 1 hour

Adults with normal renal function: 2-3 hours, directly dependent upon glomerular filtration rate; impaired renal function: 5-70 hours

Time to peak serum concentration:

I.M.: Within 30-60 minutes

I.V.: 30 minutes after a 30-minute infusion

Elimination: With normal renal function, ~90% to 95% of dose excreted in urine within 24 hours

Dialysis: Dialyzable (50% to 100%)

Usual Dosage Dosage should be based on an estimate of ideal body weight except in neonates (neonatal dosage should be based on actual weight unless the patient has hydrocephalus or hydrops fetalis)

Neonates: I.M., I.V.:

Preterm neonates <1000 g: 3.5 mg/kg/dose every 24 hours

0-4 weeks, <1200 g: 2.5 mg/kg/dose every 18 hours

Postnatal age ≤7 days:

1200-2000 g: 2.5 mg/kg/dose every 12 hours

>2000 g: 2.5 mg/kg/dose every 12 hours

Postnatal age >7 days:

1200-2000 g: 2.5 mg/kg/dose every 8-12 hours

>2000 g: 2.5 mg/kg/dose every 8 hours

Infants and Children <5 years: I.M., I.V.: 2.5 mg/kg/dose every 8 hours*

Pulmonary infection in cystic fibrosis: 2.5-3.3 mg/kg/dose every 6-8 hours

Patients on hemodialysis: 1.25-1.75 mg/kg/dose postdialysis

Children ≥5 years: I.M., I.V.: 2-2.5 mg/kg/dose every 8 hours*

Pulmonary infection in cystic fibrosis: 2.5-3.3 mg/kg/dose every 6-8 hours

Patients on hemodialysis: 1.25-1.75 mg/kg/dose postdialysis

*Note: Some patients may require larger or more frequent doses if serum levels document the need (ie, cystic fibrosis, patients undergoing continuous hemofiltration, patients with major burns, or febrile granulocytopenic patients); modify dose based on individual patient requirements as determined by renal function, serum drug concentrations, and patient-specific clinical parameters.

Children and Adults: Ophthalmic:

Ointment: Apply 0.5" ribbon into the affected eye 2-3 times/day; for severe infections, apply ointment every 3-4 hours

Solution:

Mild to moderate infections: Instill 1-2 drops every 4 hours

Severe infections: instill 2 drops every 30-60 minutes initially, then reduce to less frequent intervals

Inhalation:

Standard aerosolized tobramycin:

Children: 40-80 mg 2-3 times/day

Adults: 60-80 mg 3 times/day

High dose regimen: Children ≥6 years and Adults: 300 mg every 12 hours (do not administer doses less than 6 hours apart); administer in repeated cycles of 28 days on drug followed by 28 days off drug

Adults: I.M., I.V.: 3-6 mg/kg/day in 3 divided doses; studies of once daily dosing have used I.V. doses of 4-6.6 mg/kg once daily

Patients on hemodialysis: 0.5-0.7 mg/kg/dose postdialysis
Dosing in Renal Impairment:
Children and Adults: 2.5 mg/kg (2-3 serum level measurements should be obtained after the initial dose to measure the half-life in order to determine the frequency of subsequent doses)

Administration
Inhalation (high-dose regimen): Use a PARI LC Plus™ reusable nebulizer and a DeVilbiss Pulmo-Aide® air compressor for administration of tobramycin by inhalation; patient should be sitting or standing upright and breathing normally through the mouthpiece of the nebulizer

Ophthalmic: Avoid contact of tube or bottle tip with skin or eye; apply finger pressure to lacrimal sac during and for 1-2 minutes after instillation of drops to decrease risk of absorption and systemic effects

Parenteral: Administer by I.M., I.V. slow intermittent infusion over 30-60 minutes or by direct injection over 15 minutes; final I.V. concentration for administration should not exceed 10 mg/mL; administer other antibiotics such as penicillins and cephalosporins at least 1 hour before or after tobramycin

Monitoring Parameters Urinalysis, urine output, BUN, serum creatinine, peak and trough serum tobramycin levels; be alert to ototoxicity, audiograms

Not all pediatric patients who receive aminoglycosides require monitoring of serum aminoglycoside concentrations. Indications for use of aminoglycoside serum concentration monitoring include:
Treatment course >5 days
Patients with decreased or changing renal function
Patients with a poor therapeutic response
Infants <3 months of age
Atypical body constituency (obesity, expanded extracellular fluid volume)
Clinical need for higher doses or shorter intervals (cystic fibrosis, burns, endocarditis, meningitis, relatively resistant organism)
Patients on hemodialysis or chronic ambulatory peritoneal dialysis
Signs of nephrotoxicity or ototoxicity
Concomitant use of other nephrotoxic agents
Patients on high-dose aerosolized tobramycin: Peak tobramycin level obtained 1 hour following inhalation to identify patients who are significant absorbers

Reference Range
Peak: 4-12 µg/mL; peak values are 2-3 times greater with once daily dosing regimens
Trough: 0.5-2 µg/mL

Test Interactions Aminoglycoside serum levels measured in blood taken from Silastic® central line catheters can sometimes give falsely high readings

Patient Information Report any dizziness or sensation of ringing or fullness in ears to the physician

Nursing Implications Obtain serum concentration after the third dose except in neonates or patients with rapidly changing renal function in whom levels need to be measured sooner; peak tobramycin serum concentrations are drawn 30 minutes after the end of a 30-minute infusion, immediately on completion of a 1-hour I.V. infusion or 1 hour after an intramuscular injection; the trough is drawn just before the next dose; provide optimal patient hydration and perfusion

Dosage Forms
Injection, powder for reconstitution, as sulfate (Nebcin®): 1.2 g
Injection, solution, as sulfate: 10 mg/mL (2 mL, 6 mL, 8 mL); 40 mg/mL (2 mL, 30 mL, 50 mL) [may contain sodium metabisulfite]
Nebcin®: 40 mg/mL (2 mL, 3 mL) [contains sodium bisulfite]
Nebcin® Pediatric: 10 mg/mL (2 mL) [contains sodium bisulfite]
Ointment, ophthalmic (Tobrex®): 0.3% (3 mg/g) (3.5 g)
Solution for nebulization [preservative free] (TOBI®): 60 mg/mL (5 mL)
Solution, ophthalmic (AKTob®, Tobrex®, Tomycine™ [DSC]): 0.3% [3 mg/mL] (5 mL)

References
Gilbert DN, "Once-Daily Aminoglycoside Therapy," *Antimicrob Agents Chemother*, 1991, 35(3):399-405.
Green TP, Mirkin BL, Peterson PK, et al, "Tobramycin Serum Level Monitoring in Young Patients With Normal Renal Function," *Clin Pharmacokinet*, 1984, 9(5):457-68.
Nahata MC, Powell DA, Durrell DE, et al, "Effect of Gestational Age and Birth Weight on Tobramycin Kinetics in Newborn Infants," *J Antimicrob Chemother*, 1984, 14(1):59-65.
Ramsey BW, Burns J, Smith A, et al, "Safety and Efficacy of Tobramycin for Inhalation in Patients With Cystic Fibrosis: The Results of Two Phase III Placebo Controlled Clinical Trials," *Pediatr Pulmonol*, 1997, (Suppl 14):137-8, S10.3.
Ramsey BW, Dorkin HL, Eisenberg JD, et al, "Efficacy of Aerosolized Tobramycin in Patients With Cystic Fibrosis," *N Engl J Med*, 1993, 328(24):1740-6.
Shaw PK, Braun TL, Liebergen A, et al, "Aerosolized Tobramycin Pharmacokinetics in Cystic Fibrosis Patients," *J Pediatr Pharm Pract*, 1997, 2(1):23-6.

♦ **Tobrex®** *see* Tobramycin *on page 1097*
♦ **Tofranil®** *see* Imipramine *on page 597*

♦ **Tofranil-PM®** *see* Imipramine *on page 597*

Tolazoline [DSC] (tole AZ oh leen)

Related Information
  Overdose and Toxicology *on page 1388*

U.S. Brand Names Priscoline® [DSC]

Synonyms Benzazoline

Therapeutic Category Alpha-Adrenergic Blocking Agent, Parenteral; Antihypertensive Agent; Vasodilator

Generic Available No

Use Persistent pulmonary hypertension of the newborn (PPHN), also known as persistent fetal circulation (PFC); peripheral vasospastic disorders

Pregnancy Risk Factor C

Contraindications Hypersensitivity to tolazoline or any component; known or suspected coronary artery disease

Warnings May activate stress ulcers via stimulation of gastric secretions

Precautions Use with caution in patients with mitral stenosis, gastritis, peptic ulcers; use with caution and decrease dose in patients with renal dysfunction

Adverse Reactions
  Cardiovascular: Hypotension, flushing, tachycardia, arrhythmias
  Endocrine & metabolic: Hypochloremic alkalosis
  Gastrointestinal: Increased secretions, nausea, vomiting, diarrhea, epigastric discomfort, GI bleeding
  Hematology: Agranulocytosis, thrombocytopenia, pancytopenia
  Ocular: Mydriasis
  Renal: Oliguria
  Respiratory: Pulmonary hemorrhage
  Miscellaneous: Increased pilomotor activity

Drug Interactions A paradoxical decrease in blood pressure followed by a significant rebound increase in blood pressure can be seen when epinephrine or norepinephrine is administered with tolazoline; a disulfiram reaction may possibly be seen with concomitant ethanol use

Stability Compatible in D_5W, $D_{10}W$ and saline solutions; do not mix with other drugs

Mechanism of Action Competitively blocks alpha-adrenergic receptors to produce brief antagonism of circulating epinephrine and norepinephrine; reduces hypertension caused by catecholamines and causes vascular smooth muscle relaxation (direct action); results in peripheral vasodilation and decreased peripheral resistance; GI adverse effects and peripheral vasodilation mediated via histamine-like action

Pharmacodynamics Maximum effect: Within 30 minutes

Pharmacokinetics
  Distribution: V_d: Neonates: 1.6 L/kg
  Half-life, neonates: 3-10 hours; increased half-life with decreased renal function, oliguria
  Elimination: Rapid in urine primarily as unchanged drug

Usual Dosage
  Neonates: I.V.:
    Initial: 1-2 mg/kg over 10-15 minutes via scalp vein or upper extremity
    Maintenance: I.V. continuous infusion: 1-2 mg/kg/hour; **Note:** Some neonatal centers use lower maintenance doses (eg, 0.15-0.3 mg/kg/hour or 0.5-1 mg/kg/hour)
    Acute vasospasm "cath toes": 0.25 mg/kg/hour (no load)
  Adults: Peripheral vasospastic disorder: I.M., I.V., S.C.: 10-50 mg 4 times/day
  Dosing adjustment in renal dysfunction: Neonates: Urine output <0.9 mL/kg/hour: Decrease dose by 50%

Administration Parenteral: I.V.: Usual maximum concentration: 0.1 mg/mL

Monitoring Parameters Heart rate, blood pressure, respiratory rate, blood gases, serum chloride and bicarbonate

Additional Information Little experience with infusions >48 hours; acidosis may decrease tolazoline's effects

Dosage Forms Injection, solution, as hydrochloride: 25 mg/mL (4 mL) [DSC]

References
Ward RM, Daniel CH, Kendig JW, et al, "Oliguria and Tolazoline Pharmacokinetics in the Newborn," *Pediatrics*, 1986, 77(3):307-15.

♦ **Tolectin®** *see* Tolmetin *on page 1101*
♦ **Tolectin® DS** *see* Tolmetin *on page 1101*

Tolmetin (TOLE met in)

Related Information
Overdose and Toxicology *on page 1388*

U.S. Brand Names Tolectin®; Tolectin® DS

Therapeutic Category Analgesic, Non-narcotic; Nonsteroidal Anti-inflammatory Drug (NSAID), Oral

Generic Available Yes

Use Treatment of inflammatory and rheumatoid disorders, including juvenile rheumatoid arthritis

Pregnancy Risk Factor C (D in 3rd trimester or near delivery)

Contraindications Hypersensitivity to tolmetin, any component, aspirin, or other NSAIDs; active GI bleeding, ulcer disease; patients with the "aspirin triad" [asthma, rhinitis (with or without nasal polyps), and aspirin intolerance] (fatal asthmatic and anaphylactoid reactions may occur in these patients)

Precautions Use with caution in patients with upper GI disease, impaired renal function, CHF, hypertension, and patients receiving anticoagulants; although rare, anaphylactoid reactions occur more commonly with tolmetin than other NSAIDs

Adverse Reactions
Cardiovascular: Edema
Central nervous system: Dizziness, nervousness, drowsiness, headache
Dermatologic: Rash, urticaria
Gastrointestinal: Nausea, abdominal pain, dyspepsia, diarrhea, constipation; GI bleeding, ulcer, perforation
Hematologic: Anemia, leukopenia, prolongation of bleeding time
Hepatic: Hepatitis
Otic: Tinnitus
Renal: Acute renal failure, renal dysfunction

Drug Interactions Tolmetin may potentiate the effects of warfarin and may increase prothrombin time and bleeding; aspirin may decrease tolmetin serum concentration; tolmetin may increase serum concentrations of methotrexate; tolmetin may decrease antihypertensive effects of ACE inhibitors or angiotensin II antagonists; drug interactions similar to other NSAIDs may also occur

Food Interactions Food or milk may decrease the extent of oral absorption

Mechanism of Action Inhibits prostaglandin synthesis by decreasing the activity of the enzyme, cyclooxygenase, which results in decreased formation of prostaglandin precursors

Pharmacokinetics
Absorption: Oral: Well absorbed
Protein binding: 99%
Metabolism: In the liver via oxidation and conjugation
Half-life, elimination: 5 hours
Time to peak serum concentration: Within 30-60 minutes
Elimination: Excreted in the urine as metabolites or conjugates

Usual Dosage Oral:
Children ≥2 years:
Anti-inflammatory: Initial: 20 mg/kg/day in 3-4 divided doses, then 15-30 mg/kg/day in 3-4 divided doses; maximum dose: 30 mg/kg/day in 4 divided doses; do not exceed 1800 mg/day
Analgesic: 5-7 mg/kg/dose every 6-8 hours
Adults: 400 mg 3 times/day; usual dose: 600 mg to 1.8 g/day; maximum dose: 2 g/day

Administration Oral: May administer with food, milk, or antacids to decrease GI adverse effects

Monitoring Parameters CBC with differential, liver enzymes, occult blood loss, BUN, serum creatinine; periodic ophthalmologic exams

Patient Information Avoid alcohol; may cause dizziness or drowsiness and impair ability to perform activities requiring mental alertness or physical coordination

Dosage Forms
Capsule, as sodium (Tolectin® DS): 400 mg
Tablet, as sodium (Tolectin®): 600 mg

References
Berde C, Ablin A, Glazer J, et al, "American Academy of Pediatrics Report of the Subcommittee on Disease-Related Pain in Childhood Cancer," *Pediatrics*, 1990, 86(5 Pt 2):818-25.
Giannini EH and Cawkwell GD, "Drug Treatment in Children With Juvenile Rheumatoid Arthritis. Past, Present, and Future," *Pediatr Clin North Am*, 1995, 42(5):1099-125.
Hollingworth P, "The Use of Non-Steroidal Anti-inflammatory Drugs in Paediatric Rheumatic Diseases," *Br J Rheumatol*, 1993, 32(1):73-7.
Rose CD and Doughty RA, "Pharmacological Management of Juvenile Rheumatoid Arthritis," *Drugs*, 1992, 43(6):849-63.

Tolnaftate (tole NAF tate)

U.S. Brand Names Absorbine Jr.® Antifungal [OTC]; Aftate® Antifungal [OTC]; Fungi-Guard® [OTC]; Tinactin® Antifungal [OTC]; Tinactin® Jock Itch [OTC]; Tinaderm [OTC]; Ting® [OTC]

Canadian Brand Names Pitrex

Therapeutic Category Antifungal Agent, Topical

Generic Available Yes (cream, powder, and solution)

Use Treatment of tinea pedis, tinea cruris, tinea corporis, tinea manuum caused by *Trichophyton rubrum*, *T. mentagrophytes*, *T. tonsurans*, *M. canis*, *M. audouinii*, and *E. floccosum*; also effective in the treatment of tinea versicolor infections due to *Malassezia furfur*

Pregnancy Risk Factor C

Contraindications Hypersensitivity to tolnaftate or any component; nail and scalp infections

Adverse Reactions
Dermatologic: Pruritus, contact dermatitis
Local: Irritation, stinging
Miscellaneous: Hypersensitivity reaction, sensitization to butylated hydroxytoluene component of cream, solution, and aerosol powder

Mechanism of Action Distorts the hyphae and stunts mycelial growth in susceptible fungi

Pharmacodynamics Onset of action: Response may be seen 24-72 hours after initiation of therapy

Usual Dosage Children and Adults: Topical: Apply 1-3 drops of solution or a small amount of cream or powder and rub into the affected areas 2-3 times/day for 2-4 weeks

Administration Topical: Wash and dry affected area before drug application; avoid contact with eyes

Monitoring Parameters Resolution of skin infection

Patient Information Avoid contact with the eyes; apply to clean dry area; consult the physician if a skin irritation develops or if the skin infection worsens or does not improve after 10 days of therapy

Additional Information Usually not effective alone for the treatment of infections involving hair follicles or nails

Dosage Forms
Aerosol, liquid, topical:
Aftate®: 1% (120 mL) [contains alcohol]
Tinactin® Antifungal: 1% (120 mL) [contains alcohol]
Ting®: 1% (90 mL)
Aerosol, powder, topical:
Aftate®: 1% (105 g) [contains alcohol]
Tinactin® Antifungal: 1% (45 g, 90 g, 100 g, 150 g) [contains alcohol]
Tinactin® Antifungal Jock Itch: 1% (100 g) [contains alcohol]
Ting®: 1% (90 g)
Cream, topical: 1% (15 g, 30 g)
Fungi-Guard®: 1% (15 g)
Tinactin® Antifungal: 1% (15 g, 30 g) [contains propylene glycol]
Tinactin® Antifungal Jock Itch: 1% (15 g) [contains propylene glycol]
Gel, topical (Absorbine Jr.® Antifungal): 1% (21 g)
Powder, topical: 1% (45 g)
Solution, topical: 1% (10 mL)
Absorbine Jr.® Antifungal: 1% (60 mL)
Tinaderm: 1% (10 mL)

♦ **Tolu-Sed® DM [OTC]** *see* Guaifenesin and Dextromethorphan *on page 553*

♦ **Tomoxetine** *see* Atomoxetine *on page 138*

♦ **Tomycine™ [DSC]** *see* Tobramycin *on page 1097*

♦ **Topamax®** *see* Topiramate *on page 1102*

♦ **Topicaine® [OTC]** *see* Lidocaine *on page 671*

♦ **Topilene® (Can)** *see* Betamethasone *on page 169*

Topiramate (toe PYE ra mate)

U.S. Brand Names Topamax®

Therapeutic Category Anticonvulsant, Miscellaneous

Generic Available No

Use Adjunctive treatment of primary generalized tonic-clonic seizures or partial onset seizures in children 2-16 years of age and adults; treatment of seizures associated with Lennox-Gastaut syndrome in patients ≥2 years of age; may potentially be useful in infantile spasms

Pregnancy Risk Factor C

Contraindications Hypersensitivity to topiramate or any component

Warnings An ocular syndrome (characterized by secondary acute angle closure glaucoma and acute myopia) has been reported in adult and pediatric patients. Symptoms generally occur within 1 month of treatment initiation and include an acute decrease in visual acuity and/or ocular pain. Ophthalmologic findings may include increased IOP, anterior chamber shallowing, ocular hyperemia, mydriasis, and supracilliary effusion with anterior displacement of lens and iris. Patients experiencing blurred vision and/or eye pain should contact their physician immediately. Primary treatment of this syndrome is discontinuation of topiramate as soon as possible, based on physician judgment. If left untreated, this syndrome may cause serious damage to the eye, including permanent vision loss.

Do not abruptly discontinue therapy, withdraw gradually to lessen chance for increased seizure frequency; CNS adverse effects are common (see Adverse Reactions); avoid use with alcohol, CNS depressants, or carbonic anhydrase inhibitors (see Drug Interactions)

Precautions Use with caution and decrease the dose in patients with renal dysfunction; use with caution in patients allergic to sulfa drugs and in patients with hepatic impairment

Adverse Reactions
Central nervous system: Ataxia, difficulty in concentrating, dizziness, memory difficulties, fatigue, nervousness, somnolence, psychomotor slowing, speech/language problems, confusion, depression, anxiety, cognitive problems; irritability and sleep disturbances (reported in children); Note: Somnolence and fatigue are the most common CNS adverse effects in children
Gastrointestinal: Weight loss, anorexia, nausea
Hematologic: Purpura
Neuromuscular & skeletal: Paresthesia, tremor
Ocular: Nystagmus, diplopia, abnormal vision, ocular syndrome (see Warnings)
Renal: Nephrolithiasis
Respiratory: Epistaxis

Drug Interactions Cytochrome P450 isoenzyme CYP2C19 substrate and inhibitor
Phenytoin and carbamazepine may significantly decrease topiramate serum concentrations (topiramate dosage increase may be needed); valproic acid may decrease topiramate concentrations; topiramate may decrease serum concentrations of valproic acid, digoxin, and ethinyl estradiol (may decrease the efficacy of oral contraceptives); alcohol or other CNS depressants may increase adverse CNS effects; carbonic anhydrase inhibitors may increase the risk of nephrolithiasis or paresthesia; topiramate may increase phenytoin serum concentrations by 25% in some patients

Food Interactions Food may decrease the rate but not the extent of absorption

Stability Protect from moisture; store at room temperature

Mechanism of Action Exact mechanism unknown; thought to decrease the spread of seizure activity by blockade of sodium channels, potentiation of GABA (an inhibitory neurotransmitter) and antagonism of kainate activation of glutamate (an excitatory amino acid) subtype receptors; also inhibits carbonic anhydrase (minor effect)

Pharmacokinetics Note: Sprinkle capsule is bioequivalent to tablet
Absorption: Rapid
Distribution: V_d: Adults: 0.6-0.8 L/kg
Protein binding: 13% to 17%
Metabolism: Minor amounts metabolized in liver via hydroxylation, hydrolysis, and glucuronidation; percentage of dose metabolized in liver and clearance are increased in patients receiving enzyme inducers
Bioavailability: Tablet: 80% (relative to a prepared solution)
Half-life:
Adults: 19-23 hours (mean 21 hours)
Adults with renal impairment: 59 ± 11 hours (n=7)
Time to peak serum concentration: 2 hours; range: 1.4-4.3 hours
Elimination: 70% of dose excreted unchanged in urine; may undergo renal tubular reabsorption
Clearance:
Children 4-17 years: ~50% higher than adults (per kg)
Adults: 20-30 mL/minute
Renal impairment: Reduced
Hepatic impairment: May be reduced
(Continued)

Topiramate *(Continued)*

Dialysis: Significantly hemodialyzed; dialysis clearance: 120 mL/minute (4-6 times higher than in adults with normal renal function); supplemental doses may be required

Usual Dosage Oral:

Children 2-16 years:

Partial onset seizures or Lennox-Gastaut syndrome: Initial: 1-3 mg/kg/day (maximum: 25 mg) given nightly for 1 week; increase at 1- to 2-week intervals by 1-3 mg/kg/day given in 2 divided doses; titrate dose to response; usual maintenance: 5-9 mg/kg/day given in 2 divided doses

Primary generalized tonic-clonic seizures: Use initial dose as listed above, but use slower initial titration rate; titrate to 6 mg/kg/day by the end of 8 weeks

Adolescents ≥17 years and Adults:

Partial onset seizures: Initial: 25-50 mg/day given daily for 1 week; increase at weekly intervals by 25-50 mg/day; titrate dose to response; usual maintenance: 200 mg twice daily; maximum dose: 1600 mg/day

Primary generalized tonic-clonic seizures: Use initial dose as listed above, but use slower initial titration rate; titrate upwards to recommended dose by the end of 8 weeks

Dosing adjustment in renal impairment: Cl_{cr} <70 mL/minute/1.73 m^2: Administer 50% of the usual dose; titrate more slowly due to prolonged half-life

Dosing adjustment in hepatic impairment: Carefully adjust dose as plasma concentrations may be increased if normal dosing is used

Administration May be administered without regard to food; broken tablets have a bitter taste; tablets may be crushed, mixed with water, and administered immediately. Swallow sprinkle capsules whole or open and sprinkle contents on small amount of soft food (eg, 1 teaspoonful of applesauce); swallow sprinkle/food mixture immediately; do not chew; do not store for later use; drink fluids after dose to make sure mixture is completely swallowed

Monitoring Parameters Seizure frequency, duration, and severity; renal function

Reference Range Not applicable; plasma topiramate concentrations have not been shown to correlate with clinical efficacy

Patient Information Contact physician immediately if blurred vision or eye pain occur; ensure adequate fluid intake to avoid kidney stone formation; may cause dizziness or drowsiness and impair ability to perform activities requiring mental alertness or physical coordination; avoid alcohol

Dosage Forms

Capsule, sprinkle: 15 mg, 25 mg

Tablet: 25 mg, 100 mg, 200 mg

References

Doose DR, Walker SA, Gisclon LG, et al, "Single-Dose Pharmacokinetics and Effect of Food on the Bioavailability of Topiramate, a Novel Antiepileptic Drug," *J Clin Pharmacol*, 1996, 36(10):884-91.

Glauser TA, "Preliminary Observations on Topiramate in Pediatric Epilepsies," *Epilepsia*, 1997, 38(Suppl 1):S37-41.

Glauser TA, "Topiramate Use in Pediatric Patients," *Can J Neurol Sci*, 1998, 25(3):S8-12.

Glauser TA, Clark PO, and Strawsburg R, "A Pilot Study of Topiramate in the Treatment of Infantile Spasms," *Epilepsia*, 1998, 39(12):1324-8.

Pellock JM, "Managing Pediatric Epilepsy Syndromes With New Antiepileptic Drugs," *Pediatrics*, 1999, 104(5 Pt 1):1106-16.

Sachdeo RC, "Topiramate. Clinical Profile in Epilepsy," *Clin Pharmacokinet*, 1998, 34(5):335-46.

♦ **Topisone® (Can)** *see* Betamethasone *on page 169*

♦ **Toposar®** *see* Etoposide *on page 469*

♦ **Toprol XL®** *see* Metoprolol *on page 752*

♦ **Topsyn® (Can)** *see* Fluocinonide *on page 499*

♦ **Toradol®** *see* Ketorolac *on page 641*

♦ **Torecan®** *see* Thiethylperazine *on page 1082*

♦ **Tornalate® [DSC]** *see* Bitolterol *on page 176*

Torsemide *(TOR se mide)*

U.S. Brand Names Demadex®

Therapeutic Category Antihypertensive Agent; Diuretic, Loop

Generic Available No

Use Management of edema associated with CHF and hepatic or renal disease; used alone or in combination with antihypertensives in treatment of hypertension

Pregnancy Risk Factor B

Contraindications Hypersensitivity to torsemide, any component, or other sulfonylureas; anuria

Warnings Loop diuretics are potent diuretics, excess amounts can lead to profound diuresis with fluid and electrolyte loss; close medical supervision and dose evaluation is required

Adverse Reactions
Cardiovascular: Orthostatic hypotension, EKG abnormality, chest pain, atrial fibrillation, ventricular tachycardia, syncope

Central nervous system: Headache, dizziness, insomnia, nervousness

Dermatologic: Rash, photosensitivity

Endocrine & metabolic: Hyponatremia, hypokalemia, hypochloremia, alkalosis, hypocalcemia, dehydration, hyperuricemia, gout

Gastrointestinal: Diarrhea, nausea, constipation, dyspepsia, GI hemorrhage, stomach cramps, pancreatitis

Genitourinary: Excessive urination

Hematologic: Agranulocytosis, anemia

Neuromuscular & skeletal: Myalgia, arthralgia, weakness

Otic: Ototoxicity

Renal: Prerenal azotemia, interstitial nephritis, nephrocalcinosis

Drug Interactions Cytochrome P450 isoenzyme CYP2C9 substrate
Increased risk of ototoxicity with aminoglycosides and cis-platinum; increased anticoagulant effects of warfarin; increased risk of digoxin toxicity when used alone or combined with other medications which cause increased potassium losses (eg, corticosteroids, amphotericin B); decreased glucose tolerance which may result in increased requirements of sulfonylureas and other antidiabetic agents; decreased diuretic effects of torsemide when combined with NSAIDs; increased lithium serum levels; increased salicylate levels with potential toxicity (with high dose salicylates)

Stability Stable for 24 hours at room temperature when mixed with D_5W or NS

Mechanism of Action Inhibits reabsorption of sodium and chloride in the ascending loop of Henle and distal renal tubule, interfering with the chloride-binding cotransport system, thus causing increased excretion of water, sodium, chloride, magnesium, and calcium

Pharmacodynamics
Onset of action:
Oral: 60 minutes
I.V.: 10 minutes
Maximum effect:
Oral: 60-120 minutes
I.V.: Within 60 minutes
Duration: Oral, I.V.: 6-8 hours

Pharmacokinetics
Absorption: Oral: Rapid
Distribution: V_d: 12-15 L (adults)
Protein binding: Plasma: ~97% to 99%
Metabolism: Hepatic by cytochrome P450, 80%
Bioavailability: 80% to 90%
Half-life: 3.5 hours (range 2-4 hours); 7-8 hours in cirrhosis (dose modification appears unnecessary)
Time to peak serum concentration: Oral: 1 hour
Elimination: 20% eliminated unchanged in urine

Usual Dosage Adults: Oral, I.V.:
Edema: 10-20 mg once daily; titrate upward as needed (maximum dose: 200 mg/day)
Hepatic cirrhosis: 5-10 mg once daily
Hypertension: Initial: 5 mg once daily; increase to 10 mg if ineffective after 4-6 weeks of therapy

Administration
Oral: May be administered with food or milk
Parenteral: May be administered undiluted direct I.V. over 3-5 minutes

Monitoring Parameters Renal function, serum electrolytes, and fluid intake and output, blood pressure

Patient Information Rise slowly from a lying or sitting position to minimize dizziness, lightheadedness or fainting; also use extra care when exercising, standing for long periods of time. Take last dose of day early in the evening to prevent nocturia. May cause photosensitivity reactions (eg, exposure to sunlight may cause severe sunburn, skin rash, redness, or itching); avoid exposure to sunlight and artificial light sources (sunlamps, tanning booth/bed); wear protective clothing, wide-brimmed hats, sunglasses, and lip sunscreen (SPF ≥15); use a sunscreen [broad-spectrum sunscreen or physical sunscreen (preferred) or sunblock with SPF ≥15]; contact physician if reaction occurs.

Additional Information 10-20 mg torsemide is approximately equivalent to:
Furosemide 40 mg
(Continued)

Torsemide *(Continued)*

Bumetanide 1 mg

Dosage Forms

Injection, solution: 10 mg/mL (2 mL, 5 mL)

Tablet: 5 mg, 10 mg, 20 mg, 100 mg

♦ **Total Blood Volume** *see page 1319*

♦ **Touro® DM** *see Guaifenesin and Dextromethorphan on page 553*

♦ **Touro Ex®** *see Guaifenesin on page 550*

♦ **t-PA** *see Alteplase on page 67*

♦ **T-Phyl®** *see Theophylline on page 1076*

♦ **Trace Elements** *see Trace Metals on page 1106*

Trace Metals *(trase MET als)*

Related Information

Parenteral Nutrition (PN) *on page 1262*

U.S. Brand Names Iodopen®; Molypen®; M.T.E.-4®; M.T.E.-5®; M.T.E.-6®; M.T.E.-7®; Multitrace™-4; Multitrace™-4 Neonatal; Multitrace™-4 Pediatric; Multitrace™-5; Neotrace-4®; Pedtrace-4®; P.T.E.-4®; P.T.E.-5®; Selepen®

Synonyms Multiple Trace Metals; Neonatal Trace Metals; Selenium; Trace Elements

Available Salts Ammonium Molybdate; Chromium Chloride; Copper Sulfate; Cupric Chloride; Iodine Sodium; Manganese Chloride; Manganese Sulfate; Zinc Chloride; Zinc Sulfate

Therapeutic Category Mineral, Parenteral; Trace Element, Parenteral; Trace Element, Multiple, Neonatal

Generic Available Yes

Use Prevent and correct trace metal deficiencies

Pregnancy Risk Factor C

Contraindications Hypersensitivity to a specific trace metal or component of the trace metal solution (see Warnings); do not give by direct injection because of potential for phlebitis, tissue irritation, and potential to increase renal loss of minerals from a bolus injection

Warnings Metals may accumulate in conditions of renal failure or biliary obstruction; consider reduction in dosage or deletion of copper and manganese in patients with biliary obstruction; avoid copper use in patients with Wilson's disease; administration of copper in the absence of zinc or zinc in the absence of copper may cause decreases in their respective plasma levels; molybdenum promotes the utilization of copper and increases its excretion; excessive amounts of molybdenum may produce copper deficiency; multiple trace metal solutions present a risk of overdosage when the need for one trace element is appreciably higher than for others in the formulation; utilization of individual trace metal solutions may be needed. Consider reduction in dosage or deletion of selenium and chromium in patients with renal dysfunction.

Some products contain benzyl alcohol which may cause allergic reactions in susceptible individuals; large amounts of benzyl alcohol (≥99 mg/kg/day) have been associated with a potentially fatal toxicity ("gasping syndrome") in neonates; the "gasping syndrome" consists of metabolic acidosis, respiratory distress, gasping respirations, CNS dysfunction (including convulsions, intracranial hemorrhage), hypotension and cardiovascular collapse; *in vitro* and animal studies have shown that benzoate, a metabolite of benzyl alcohol, displaces bilirubin from protein-binding sites; use benzyl alcohol-containing products with caution in neonates.

Precautions Chromic chloride contains aluminum which may accumulate with prolonged use, particularly in patients with decreased renal function; use cautiously in neonates and other patients with decreased renal function

Adverse Reactions The following describe the symptomatology associated with excess trace metals:

Chromium: Nausea, vomiting, GI ulcers, renal and hepatic dysfunction, convulsions, coma

Copper: Prostration, behavioral changes, diarrhea, progressive marasmus, hypotonia, photophobia, hepatic dysfunction, peripheral edema

Manganese: Irritability, speech disturbances, abnormal gait, headache, anorexia, apathy, impotence, cholestatic jaundice, movement disorders

Molybdenum: Gout-like syndrome with elevated blood levels of uric acid and xanthine oxidase

Selenium: Alopecia, weak nails, dermatitis, dental defects, GI disorders, nervousness, mental depression, metallic taste, garlic odor of breath and sweat

Zinc: Profuse diaphoresis, decreased consciousness, blurred vision, tachycardia, hypothermia

Mechanism of Action

Chromium: Part of glucose tolerance factor, an essential activator of insulin-mediated reactions; helps maintain normal glucose metabolism and peripheral nerve function

Copper: Cofactor for serum ceruloplasmin, helps maintain normal rates of red and white cell formation

Manganese: Activator for several enzymes including manganese-dependent super-oxide dismutase and pyruvate carboxylase; activates glycosyl transferases involved in mucopolysaccharide synthesis

Molybdenum: Constituent of the enzymes xanthine oxidase, sulfite oxidase, and aldehyde oxidase

Selenium: Part of glutathione peroxidase which protects cell components from oxidative damage due to peroxides produced in cellular metabolism

Zinc: A cofactor for >70 different enzymes; facilitates wound healing, helps maintain normal growth rates, normal skin hydration, and the senses of taste and smell

Pharmacokinetics

Chromium: 10% to 20% oral absorption; excretion primarily via kidneys and bile

Copper: 30% oral absorption; 80% elimination via bile; intestinal wall 16% and urine 4%

Manganese: 10% oral absorption; excretion primarily via bile; ancillary routes via pancreatic secretions or reabsorption into the intestinal lumen occur during periods of biliary obstruction

Molybdenum: 30% to 70% oral absorption; primarily renal excretion; some biliary excretion associated with an enterohepatic cycle

Selenium: Very poor oral absorption; 75% excretion via kidneys, remainder via feces, lung, and skin

Zinc: 20% to 30% oral absorption; 90% excretion in stools, remainder via urine and perspiration

Usual Dosage See table.

Trace Mineral Daily Requirements*

	Infants	Children (≥3 mo to ≤5 y)	Older Children, Adolescents, and Adults
Chromium†	0.2 mcg/kg	0.14-0.2 mcg/kg (max: 5 mcg)	10-15 mcg
Copper‡	20 mcg/kg	20 mcg/kg (max: 300 mcg)	0.3-0.5 mg
Iodide§	1 mcg/kg	1 mcg/kg	1 mcg/kg
Manganese‡	1 mcg/kg	2-10 mcg/kg (max: 50 mcg)	60-150 mcg
Selenium†¶	2-3 mcg/kg	2-3 mcg/kg (max: 30 mcg)	20-60 mcg
Zinc	400 mcg/kg (preterm) 300 mcg/kg (term <3 mo)	100 mcg/kg (max: 5 mg)	2.5-5 mg

*Recommended intakes of trace elements cannot be achieved through the use of a commercially available combination trace element product. Only through the use of individualized trace element products can recommended intakes be achieved.

†Omit in patients with renal dysfunction.

‡Omit in patients with impaired biliary excretion or cholestatic liver disease.

§Percutaneous absorption from protein-bound iodine may be adequate.

¶Indicated for use in long-term parenteral nutrition patients.

Administration Parenteral: Must be diluted prior to use and infused as component of parenteral nutrition or parenteral solutions

Reference Range

Chromium: 0.18-0.47 ng/mL (SI: 35-90 nmol/L); some laboratories report much higher

*Copper: ~0.7-1.5 µg/mL (SI: 11-24 µmol/L); levels are higher in pregnant women and children

Manganese: 18-30 µg/dL (SI: 2.3-3.8 µmol/L)

Selenium: 95-165 ng/mL (SI: 120-209 nmol/L)

Zinc: 70-120 µg/dL (SI: 10-18.4 µmol/L)

*May not be a meaningful measurement of body stores

Additional Information Persistent diarrhea or excessive GI fluid losses from ostomy sites may grossly increase zinc losses

Dosage Forms See table on next page.

(Continued)

Trace Metals *(Continued)*

Multiple Trace Metal Parenteral Solutions

	Content per mL					
	Chromium (mcg)	Copper (mg)	Iodide (mcg)	Manganese (mg)	Selenium (mcg)	Zinc (mg)
Pedtrace-4® (3 mL, 10 mL) [preservative free]	0.85	0.1	—	0.025	—	0.5
Neotrace-4® (2 mL) [preservative free]	0.85	0.1	—	0.025	—	1.5
P.T.E.-4® (3 mL) [preservative free]	1	0.1	—	0.025	—	1
M.T.E.-4® (3 mL, 10 mL, 30 mL) [30 mL contains benzyl alcohol]	4	0.4	—	0.1	—	1
M.T.E.-4® concentrate (1 mL, 10 mL) [10 mL contains benzyl alcohol]	10	1	—	0.5	—	5
PTE-5® (3 mL) [preservative free]	1	0.1	—	0.025	15	1
M.T.E.-5® (10 mL) [preservative free]	4	0.4	—	0.1	20	1
M.T.E.-5® concentrate (1 mL, 10 mL) [10 mL contains benzyl alcohol]	10	1	—	0.5	60	5
M.T.E.-6® (10 mL) [preservative free]	4	0.4	25	0.1	20	1
M.T.E.-7®* (10 mL) [preservative free]	4	0.4	25	0.1	20	1
M.T.E.-6® concentrate (10 mL) [contains benzyl alcohol]	10	1	75	0.5	60	5
Multitrace™-4 (10 mL) [contains benzyl alcohol]	4	0.4		0.1		1
Multitrace™-4 Neonatal (2 mL)	0.85	0.1		0.025		1.5
Multitrace™-4 Pediatric (3 mL)	1	0.1		0.025		1
Multitrace™-4 Concentrate (1 mL, 10 mL) [10 mL contains benzyl alcohol]	10	1		0.5		5
Multitrace™-5 (10 mL) [contains benzyl alcohol]	4	0.4		0.1	20	1
Multitrace™-5 Concentrate (1 mL, 10 mL) [10 mL contains benzyl alcohol]	10	1		0.5	60	5
Trace elements pediatric (10 mL) [contains benzyl alcohol]	1	0.1		0.03		0.5

*With 25 mcg molybdenum.

Injection, solution [elemental equivalence]:

Chromium, as chromic chloride (hexahydrate): 0.0205 mg/mL [0.004 mg/mL] (10 mL) [preservative free]

Copper, as cupric chloride: 1.07 mg/mL [0.4 mg/mL] (10 mL)

Iodine, as iodine sodium (Iodopen®): 0.118 mg/mL [0.1 mg/mL] (10 mL)

Manganese:
As chloride: 0.36 mg/mL [0.1 mg/mL] (10 mL)
As sulfate: 0.31 mg/mL [0.1 mg/mL] (10 mL) [preservative free]

Molybdenum, as ammonium molybdate (tetrahydrate) (Molypen®): 46 mcg/mL [25 mcg/mL] (10 mL)

Selenium, as selenious acid: 0.0654 mg/mL [0.04 mg/mL] (10 mL)
Selepen®: 0.0654 mg/mL [0.04 mg/mL] (10 mL, 30 mL) [30 mL contains benzyl alcohol]

Zinc:
As chloride: 2.09 mg/mL [1 mg/mL] (10 mL, 50 mL)
As sulfate, anhydrous: 2.46 mg/mL [1 mg/mL] (10 mL) [preservative free]
As sulfate, anhydrous, **concentrate**: 12.32 mg/mL [5 mg/mL] (5 mL) [preservative free]

References

Dahlstrom KA, Ament ME, Medhin MG, et al, "Serum Trace Elements in Children Receiving Long-Term Parenteral Nutrition," *J Pediatr*, 1986, 109(4):625-30.

Fell JM, Reynolds AP, Meadows N, et al, "Manganese Toxicity in Children Receiving Long-Term Parenteral Nutrition," *Lancet*, 1996, 347(9010):1218-21.

Greene HL, Hambridge KM, Schanler R, et al, "Guidelines for the Use of Vitamins, Trace Elements, Calcium, Magnesium and Phosphorus in Infants and Children Receiving Total Parenteral Nutrition: Report of the Subcommittee on Pediatric Nutrient Requirements From the Committee on Clinical Practice Issues of The American Society for Clinical Nutrition," *Am J Clin Nutr*, 1988, 48(5):1324-42.

"Guidelines for the Use of Parenteral and Enteral Nutrition in Adult and Pediatric Patients. ASPEN Board of Directors and The Clinical Guidelines Task Force," *JPEN J Parenter Enteral Nutr*, 2002, 26(1 Suppl):1-138SA.

Litov RE, and Combs GF Jr, "Selenium in Pediatric Nutrition," *Pediatrics*, 1991, 87(3):339-51.

♦ **Tracrium**® *see* Atracurium *on page 142*
♦ **Trandate**® *see* Labetalol *on page 645*

Tranexamic Acid (tran eks AM ik AS id)

U.S. Brand Names Cyklokapron®

Synonyms AMCA; CL-65336; transAMCA

Therapeutic Category Antihemophilic Agent

Generic Available No

Use Prevention of excessive bleeding after tonsillectomy; short-term use (2-8 days) in hemophilia patients during and following tooth extraction; primary menorrhagia; prevention of GI hemorrhage and hemorrhage following ocular trauma; recurrent epistaxis; hereditary angioneurotic edema

Pregnancy Risk Factor B

Contraindications Hypersensitivity to tranexamic acid or any component; subarachnoid hemorrhage; acquired defective color vision, active intravascular clotting process

Warnings Patients receiving therapy for a long duration should have baseline and frequent ophthalmologic exams; do not administer concomitantly with factor IX complex concentrates or anti-inhibitor coagulant concentrates due to increased risk of thrombosis

Precautions Dosage modification required in patients with renal impairment; use with caution in patients with cardiovascular, renal, cerebrovascular disease, or transurethral prostatectomy

Adverse Reactions

Cardiovascular: Hypotension (with rapid I.V. administration), thromboembolic events (eg, deep vein thrombosis, pulmonary embolism, acute cortical necrosis)

Central nervous system: Cerebral ischemia and infarction (when used in the treatment of subarachnoid hemorrhage), headache, hydrocephalus, giddiness

Gastrointestinal: Nausea, diarrhea, vomiting

Hematologic: Thrombocytopenia, coagulation defects, abnormal bleeding times

Ocular: Visual abnormalities (focal areas of retinal degeneration have been seen in animals), central venous stasis retinopathy

Drug Interactions Chlorpromazine

Stability Incompatible with solutions containing penicillin; compatible with dextrose, saline, and electrolyte solutions

Mechanism of Action Forms a reversible complex that displaces plasminogen from fibrin resulting in inhibition of fibrinolysis; it also inhibits the proteolytic activity of plasmin

Pharmacokinetics

Distribution: Breast milk levels are 1% of serum; CSF levels are 10% of plasma
  V_d: Adults: 9-12 L

Protein binding: 3%

Bioavailability:
  Oral: 33% to 35%
  I.M.: 100%

Half-life: 2 hours

Time to peak serum concentration:
  Oral: 3 hours
  I.M.: 1 hour
  I.V.: 5 minutes

Elimination: Elimination characteristics differ by route of administration: after I.V. administration 95% excreted as unchanged drug in urine vs 39% after oral administration

Usual Dosage Dental extraction in hemophiliacs: Children and Adults: 10 mg/kg I.V. immediately before surgery, then 25 mg/kg/dose orally 3-4 times/day for 2-8 days

Alternatives:
  I.V.: 10 mg/kg/dose 3-4 times/day (if unable to take orally)
  Oral: 25 mg/kg/dose 3-4 times/day beginning 1 day prior to surgery

Menorrhagia: Oral: Adolescents and Adults: 1-1.5 g (12-25 mg/kg/dose) 3-4 times daily for 3-4 days

(Continued)

Tranexamic Acid *(Continued)*

Adults: Oral:
Epistaxis: 1.5 g 3 times/day
Ocular trauma: 1 g 3 times/day
Dosing adjustment in renal impairment: Adults: See table.

Tranxemic Acid Dosage Adjustments in Renal Impairment (Adult Data)

Serum Creatinine (mg/dL)	I.V. dose	Oral dose
1.36-2.83	10 mg/kg twice daily	15 mg/kg twice daily
>2.83-5.66	10 mg/kg once daily	15 mg/kg once daily
>5.66	10 mg/kg every 48 h or 5 mg/kg every 24 h	15 mg/kg every 48 h or 7.5 mg/kg every 24 h

Administration
Parenteral: May be administered by direct I.V. injection at a maximum rate of 100 mg/minute (1 mL/minute)
Oral: May be administered with food
Monitoring Parameters Ophthalmologic exams (baseline and at regular intervals) of chronic therapy
Reference Range 5-10 µg/mL is required to decrease fibrinolysis
Additional Information Tablets available in U.S. only for individual patients by contacting manufacturer (Pharmacia) directly.
Dosage Forms
Injection, solution: 100 mg/mL (10 mL)
Tablet: 500 mg

♦ **transAMCA** *see* Tranexamic Acid *on page 1109*
♦ **Transderm-Nitro® (Can)** *see* Nitroglycerin *on page 815*
♦ **Transderm Scop®** *see* Scopolamine *on page 1009*
♦ **Transderm-V® (Can)** *see* Scopolamine *on page 1009*
♦ **Trans-Plantar® (Can)** *see* Salicylic Acid *on page 1002*
♦ *trans*-**Retinoic Acid** *see* Tretinoin *on page 1111*
♦ **Trans-Ver-Sal® [OTC]** *see* Salicylic Acid *on page 1002*
♦ **Tranxene® SD™** *see* Clorazepate *on page 296*
♦ **Tranxene® SD™-Half Strength** *see* Clorazepate *on page 296*
♦ **Tranxene® T-Tab®** *see* Clorazepate *on page 296*
♦ **Trasylol®** *see* Aprotinin *on page 128*

Trazodone *(TRAZ oh done)*

Related Information
Comparison of Adverse Effects of Antidepressants *on page 1210*
Comparison of Usual Adult Dosage and Mechanism of Action of Antidepressants *on page 1209*
Drugs and Breast-Feeding *on page 1404*
Serotonin Syndrome *on page 1420*
U.S. Brand Names Desyrel®
Canadian Brand Names Alti-Trazodone; Apo®-Trazodone; Apo®-Trazodone D; Gen-Trazodone; Novo-Trazodone; Nu-Trazodone; PMS-Trazodone
Therapeutic Category Antidepressant
Generic Available Yes
Use Treatment of depression
Pregnancy Risk Factor C
Contraindications Hypersensitivity to trazodone or any component
Warnings Monitor closely and use with extreme caution in patients with cardiac disease or arrhythmias
Adverse Reactions Possesses fewer anticholinergic and cardiac adverse effects than tricyclic antidepressants
Cardiovascular: Postural hypotension (5%), arrhythmias
Central nervous system: Drowsiness (20% to 50%), sedation, dizziness, insomnia, confusion, agitation, seizures, extrapyramidal reactions, headache
Gastrointestinal: Xerostomia, constipation, nausea, vomiting
Genitourinary: Prolonged priapism (1:6000), urinary retention (rare)

Hepatic: Hepatitis
Neuromuscular & skeletal: Weakness
Ocular: Blurred vision (15% to 30%)

Drug Interactions Cytochrome P450 isoenzyme CYP2D6 and CYP3A3/4 substrate
May antagonize the antihypertensive effects of clonidine and methyldopa; may increase the serum concentrations of phenytoin or digoxin; effects may be additive with other CNS depressants, alcohol; fluoxetine may increase trazodone serum concentration

Food Interactions Food may decrease the rate but not the extent of absorption

Mechanism of Action Inhibits reuptake of serotonin; minimal or no effect on reuptake of norepinephrine or dopamine; possesses little if any anticholinergic effects; alpha-adrenergic blockade thought to be responsible for orthostatic hypotension and dry mouth

Pharmacodynamics Maximum antidepressant effect: ~2-6 weeks

Pharmacokinetics
Protein binding: 85% to 95%
Metabolism: In the liver via hydroxylation and oxidation
Half-life, elimination: 5-9 hours, prolonged in obese patients
Elimination: Primarily in urine (74%) with ~21% excreted in feces

Usual Dosage Oral:
Children 6-18 years: Initial: 1.5-2 mg/kg/day in divided doses; increase gradually every 3-4 days as needed; maximum dose: 6 mg/kg/day in 3 divided doses
Adolescents: Initial: 25-50 mg/day; increase to 100-150 mg/day in divided doses
Adults: Initial: 150 mg/day in 3 divided doses (may increase by 50 mg/day every 3-7 days); maximum dose: 600 mg/day

Administration Oral: Administer after meals or a snack to decrease lightheadedness, sedation, and postural hypotension

Monitoring Parameters Blood pressure, mental status, liver enzymes

Reference Range
Therapeutic: 0.5-2.5 µg/mL (SI: 1-6 µmol/L)
Potentially toxic: >2.5 µg/mL (SI: >6 µmol/L)
Toxic: >4 µg/mL (SI: >10 µmol/L)

Patient Information Avoid alcohol; may cause drowsiness and impair ability to perform activities requiring mental alertness or physical coordination; may cause dry mouth

Additional Information Mean doses of ~5 mg/kg/day were used in 22 children 5-12 years of age to treat severe behavioral disorders (Zubieta, 1992). Doses of 1 mg/kg/ day given in 3 divided doses were used for migraine prophylaxis in 40 patients 7-18 years of age (Battistella, 1993). Further studies are needed before trazodone can be recommended in children for these indications.

Dosage Forms Tablet, as hydrochloride: 50 mg, 100 mg, 150 mg, 300 mg

References
Battistella PA, Ruffilli R, Cernetti R, et al, "A Placebo-Controlled Crossover Trial Using Trazodone in Pediatric Migraine," *Headache*, 1993, 33(1):36-9.
Zubieta JK and Alessi NE, "Acute and Chronic Administration of Trazodone in the Treatment of Disruptive Behavior Disorders in Children," *J Clin Psychopharmacol*, 1992, 12(5):346-51.

♦ **Trecator®-SC** *see* Ethionamide *on page 463*
♦ **Trental®** *see* Pentoxifylline *on page 884*

Tretinoin (TRET i noyn)

U.S. Brand Names Altinac™; Avita®; Renova®; Retin-A®; Retin-A® Micro
Canadian Brand Names Rejuva-A®; Retinova®
Synonyms Retinoic Acid; *trans*-Retinoic Acid; Vitamin A Acid
Therapeutic Category Acne Products; Retinoic Acid Derivative; Vitamin, Topical
Generic Available Yes (cream and gel)
Use Treatment of acne vulgaris, photodamaged skin, and some skin cancers
Pregnancy Risk Factor C
Contraindications Hypersensitivity to tretinoin or any component; sunburn
Warnings Avoid contact with abraded skin, mucous membranes, eyes, mouth, angles of the nose; avoid excessive exposure to sunlight or sunlamps
Precautions Use with caution in patients with eczema
Adverse Reactions
Cardiovascular: Edema
Dermatologic: Excessive dryness, erythema, scaling of the skin, hyperpigmentation or hypopigmentation, photosensitivity, initial acne flare-up
Local: Stinging, blistering
Drug Interactions Sulfur, benzoyl peroxide, salicylic acid, and resorcinol potentiate adverse reactions seen with tretinoin
(Continued)

Tretinoin *(Continued)*

Food Interactions Avoid excessive intake of vitamin A

Mechanism of Action Keratinocytes in the sebaceous follicle become less adherent which allows for easy removal; inhibits microcomedone formation and eliminates lesions already present

Pharmacodynamics
Onset of action: 2-3 weeks
Maximum effect: May require 6 weeks or longer

Pharmacokinetics
Absorption: Topical: Minimum absorption
Metabolism: In the liver
Elimination: In bile and urine

Usual Dosage Children >12 years and Adults: Topical: Begin therapy with a weaker formulation of tretinoin (0.025% cream or 0.01% gel) and increase the concentration as tolerated; apply once daily before retiring or on alternate days; if stinging or irritation develop, decrease frequency of application

Administration Topical: Apply to dry skin (wait at least 15-30 minutes to apply after cleansing); avoid contact with eyes, mucous membranes, mouth, or open wounds

Patient Information May cause photosensitivity reactions (eg, exposure to sunlight may cause severe sunburn, skin rash, redness, or itching); avoid exposure to sunlight and artificial light sources (sunlamps, tanning booth/bed); wear protective clothing, wide-brimmed hats, sunglasses, and lip sunscreen (SPF ≥15); use a sunscreen [broad-spectrum sunscreen or physical sunscreen (preferred) or sunblock with SPF ≥15]; contact physician if reaction occurs. Avoid washing face more frequently than 2-3 times/day; avoid using topical preparations with high alcoholic content during treatment period.

Additional Information Liquid preparation generally is more irritating

Dosage Forms
Cream, topical: 0.025% (20 g, 45 g); 0.05% (20 g, 45 g); 0.1% (20 g, 45 g)
Altinac™: 0.025% (20 g, 45 g); 0.05% (20 g, 45 g); 0.1% (20 g, 45 g)
Avita®: 0.025% (20 g, 45 g)
Renova®: 0.02% (40 g); 0.05% (40 g, 60 g)
Retin-A®: 0.025% (20 g, 45 g); 0.05% (20 g, 45 g); 0.1% (20 g, 45 g)
Gel, topical: 0.025% (15 g, 45 g)
Avita®: 0.025% (15 g, 45 g)
Retin-A®: 0.01% (15 g, 45 g); 0.025% (15 g, 45 g) [contains denatured alcohol]
Retin-A® Micro: 0.04% (20 g, 45 g); 0.1% (20 g, 45 g) [contains benzyl alcohol and propylene glycol]
Liquid, topical (Retin-A®): 0.05% (28 mL) [contains denatured alcohol and polyethylene glycol]

References
Winston MH, Shalita AR, "Acne Vulgaris, Pathogenesis and Treatment," *Pediatr Clin North Am*, 1991, 38(4):889-903.

♦ **Trexall**™ *see* Methotrexate *on page 737*

♦ **Triacetyloleandomycin** *see* Troleandomycin *on page 1123*

Triamcinolone *(trye am SIN oh lone)*

Related Information
Asthma Guidelines *on page 1376*
Corticosteroids Comparison, Topical *on page 1212*
Estimated Comparative Daily Dosages for Inhaled Corticosteroids *on page 1382*

U.S. Brand Names Aristocort®; Aristocort® A; Aristocort® Forte; Aristospan®; Azmacort®; Kenalog®; Kenalog-10®; Kenalog-40®; Kenalog® in Orabase®; Nasacort®; Nasacort® AQ; Tac™-3 [DSC]; Triderm®; Tri-Nasal®

Canadian Brand Names Oracort

Therapeutic Category Adrenal Corticosteroid; Antiasthmatic; Anti-inflammatory Agent; Corticosteroid, Inhalant (Oral); Corticosteroid, Intranasal; Corticosteroid, Systemic; Corticosteroid, Topical; Glucocorticoid

Generic Available Yes (cream, lotion, and ointment)

Use
Oral inhalation: Long-term (chronic) control of persistent bronchial asthma; **NOT** indicated for the relief of acute bronchospasm. Also used to help reduce or discontinue oral corticosteroid therapy for asthma.
Intranasal: Management of seasonal and perennial allergic rhinitis
Systemic: Immunosuppression; relief of severe inflammation
Topical: Relief of inflammation and pruritus associated with corticosteroid-responsive dermatoses

Topical (dental paste): Adjunctive treatment and temporary relief of symptoms related to oral inflammatory lesions and ulcerative lesions due to trauma

Pregnancy Risk Factor C

Contraindications Hypersensitivity to triamcinolone or any component (see Warnings); primary treatment of status asthmaticus; systemic fungal infections; serious infections, except septic shock or tuberculous meningitis; topical: Local fungal, viral, or bacterial infections

Warnings Fatalities have occurred due to adrenal insufficiency in asthmatic patients during and after switching from systemic corticosteroids to aerosol steroids; several months may be required for full recovery of the adrenal glands; patients receiving higher doses of systemic corticosteroids (eg, adults receiving ≥20 mg of prednisone per day) may be at greater risk; during this period of adrenal suppression, aerosol steroids do **not** provide the systemic corticosteroid needed to treat patients requiring stress doses (ie, patients with major stress such as trauma, surgery, or infections); when used at high doses hypothalamic - pituitary - adrenal (HPA) suppression may occur; use with inhaled or systemic corticosteroids (even alternate-day dosing) may increase risk of HPA suppression; withdrawal and discontinuation of corticosteroids should be done carefully. Immunosuppression may occur.

Injection contains and cream may contain benzyl alcohol which may cause allergic reactions in susceptible individuals; tablet contains sodium benzoate; benzoic acid (benzoate) is a metabolite of benzyl alcohol; large amounts of benzyl alcohol (≥99 mg/kg/day) have been associated with a potentially fatal toxicity ("gasping syndrome") in neonates; the "gasping syndrome" consists of metabolic acidosis, respiratory distress, gasping respirations, CNS dysfunction (including convulsions, intracranial hemorrhage), hypotension and cardiovascular collapse; avoid use of triamcinolone products containing benzyl alcohol or sodium benzoate in neonates; *in vitro* and animal studies have shown that benzoate displaces bilirubin from protein binding sites

Precautions Avoid using higher than recommended doses; suppression of HPA function, suppression of linear growth, or hypercorticism (Cushing's syndrome) may occur; use with extreme caution in patients with respiratory tuberculosis, untreated systemic infections, or ocular herpes simplex

Adverse Reactions

Cardiovascular: Facial edema, hypertension

Central nervous system: Fatigue

Dermatologic: Itching, hypertrichosis, skin atrophy, hyperpigmentation, hypopigmentation, acne

Endocrine & metabolic: Cushingoid state, sodium retention, pituitary-adrenal axis suppression, potential growth suppression, glucose intolerance, hypokalemia

Gastrointestinal: Oral candidiasis, dry throat, xerostomia, peptic ulcer

Local: Burning, sterile abscesses

Neuromuscular & skeletal: Osteoporosis

Ocular: Cataracts

Respiratory: Hoarseness, wheezing, cough

Drug Interactions Cytochrome P450 isoenzyme CYP3A3/4 inducer

Barbiturates, phenytoin, rifampin increase the metabolism of triamcinolone; salicylates; NSAIDs, caffeine and alcohol may increase risk of GI ulcer; live virus vaccines (increase risk of viral infection); vaccines may have decreased effects

Food Interactions Systemic use of corticosteroids may require a diet with increased potassium, vitamins A, B_6, C, D, folate, calcium, zinc, and phosphorus and decreased sodium

Mechanism of Action Controls the rate of protein synthesis, depresses the migration of polymorphonuclear leukocytes and fibroblasts, reverses capillary permeability, and stabilizes lysosomal membranes at the cellular level to prevent or control inflammation

Pharmacokinetics

Half-life: 88 minutes

Time to peak serum concentration: I.M.: Within 8-10 hours

Usual Dosage

I.M. (as acetonide or hexacetonide): Children: 6-12 years: 0.03-0.2 mg/kg at 1- to 7-day intervals

Intra-articular (as hexacetonide): Children >12 years and Adults: 2-20 mg every 3-4 weeks

Intra-articular, intrabursal, or tendon-sheath injection: Children: 6-12 years: 2.5-15 mg, repeat as needed

Intra-articular, intrasynovial, intralesional (as diacetate or acetonide): Children >12 years and Adults: 2.5-40 mg, repeat as needed when signs and symptoms recur

(Continued)

Triamcinolone *(Continued)*

Intralesional, sublesional (as diacetate or acetonide): Children >12 years and Adults: Up to 1 mg per injection site and may be repeated 1 or more times weekly; multiple sites may be injected if they are 1 cm or more apart, not to exceed 30 mg

Intranasal:

Nasacort®:

Children 6-11 years: Initial: 2 sprays in each nostril once daily; titrate to lowest effective dose once symptoms are controlled

Children >12 years and Adults: Initial: 2 sprays in each nostril once daily; may increase after 4-7 days up to 4 sprays in each nostril once daily, 2 sprays in each nostril twice daily, or 1 spray in each nostril 4 times/day

Nasacort AQ®: Children >12 years and Adults: Initial: 2 sprays in each nostril once daily; titrate to lowest effective dose once symptoms are controlled; usual maintenance dose: 1 spray in each nostril once daily

Tri-Nasal®: Children >12 years and Adults: Initial: 2 sprays in each nostril once daily; may increase to maximum dose of 4 sprays in each nostril once daily or 2 sprays in each nostril twice daily; may initiate at maximum doses if faster relief of symptoms is required; titrate to lowest effective dose once symptoms are controlled

Oral: Children >12 years and Adults: 4-100 mg/day in 1-4 divided doses

Oral inhalation: Doses should be titrated to the lowest effective dose once asthma is controlled; maintenance doses may be given twice daily. Manufacturer recommendation:

Children: 6-12 years: 1-2 puffs given 3-4 times/day; maximum dose: 12 puffs/day

Children >12 years and Adults: 2 puffs given 3-4 times/day; for severe asthma: 12-16 puffs/day divided into 3-4 doses/day; maximum dose: 16 puffs/day

NIH Asthma Guidelines (NAEPP, 2002; NIH, 1997) [give in divided doses 3-4 times/day]:

Children ≤12 years:

"Low" dose: 400-800 mcg/day (4-8 puffs/day)

"Medium" dose: 800-1200 mcg/day (8-12 puffs/day)

"High" dose: >1200 mcg/day (>12 puffs/day)

Children >12 years and Adults:

"Low" dose: 400-1000 mcg/day (4-10 puffs/day)

"Medium" dose: 1000-2000 mcg/day (10-20 puffs/day)

"High" dose: >2000 mcg/day (>20 puffs/day)

Topical: Children and Adults: Apply a thin film 2-3 times/day

Topical (dental): Adults: Press a small amount (~1/4 inch) to the lesion until a thin film develops; some lesions may require a larger quantity; apply once daily at bedtime; more severe lesions may require application 2-3 times/day (preferably after meals)

Administration

Oral: May administer with meals to decrease GI upset

Oral inhalant: Shake canister well before use; use a spacer device for children <8 years of age; do not spray in eyes

Intranasal: Shake container well before use; clear nasal passages by blowing nose prior to use; do not spray in eyes

Parenteral: Avoid S.C. use; **do not inject I.V.**; acetonide or hexacetonide may be administered I.M.; see Usual Dosage for other parenteral routes of administration

Topical: Apply sparingly to affected area, gently rub in until disappears; avoid application on face; do not occlude area unless directed; do not use on open skin; avoid contact with eyes

Topical (dental): Apply sparingly; do not rub in; spreading the paste may result in a granular, gritty sensation and crumbling; apply at bedtime to allow contact of the medication with the lesion overnight.

Monitoring Parameters Oral inhalation: Check mucus membranes for signs of fungal infection; monitor growth in pediatric patients

Patient Information Notify physician if condition being treated persists or worsens; do not decrease dose or discontinue without physician approval; avoid exposure to chicken pox or measles, if exposed seek medical advice without delay; may cause dry mouth; avoid alcohol

Oral inhalant: Rinse mouth with water without swallowing to decrease chance of oral candidiasis; report sore mouth or mouth lesions to physician

Nursing Implications Once daily oral doses should be given in the morning

Additional Information Oral inhalation: If bronchospasm with wheezing occurs after use, a fast-acting bronchodilator may be used

Dosage Forms

Aerosol for nasal inhalation, as **acetonide** (Nasacort®): 55 mcg/inhalation (10 g) [100 doses]

Aerosol, nasal spray, as **acetonide**:
Nasacort® AQ: 55 mcg/inhalation (16.5 g) [120 doses]
Tri-Nasal®: 50 mcg/inhalation (15 mL) [120 doses]
Aerosol for oral inhalation, as **acetonide** (Azmacort®): 100 mcg per actuation (20 g) [240 actuations]
Aerosol, topical, as **acetonide** (Kenalog®): 0.2 mg/2-second spray (63 g)
Cream, as **acetonide**: 0.025% (15 g, 80 g); 0.1% (15 g, 30 g, 80 g, 454 g, 2270 g); 0.5% (15 g)
Aristocort® A: 0.025% (15 g, 60 g); 0.1% (15 g, 60 g); 0.5% (15 g) [contains benzyl alcohol]
Kenalog®: 0.1% (15 g, 60 g, 80 g); 0.5% (20 g)
Triderm®: 0.1% (30 g, 85 g)
Injection, suspension, as **acetonide**:
Kenalog-10®: 10 mg/mL (5 mL) [contains benzyl alcohol]
Kenalog-40®: 40 mg/mL (1 mL, 5 mL, 10 mL) [contains benzyl alcohol]
Tac™-3: 3 mg/mL (5 mL) [DSC]
Injection, suspension, as **diacetate**:
Aristocort®: 25 mg/mL (5 mL) [contains benzyl alcohol]
Aristocort® Forte: 40 mg/mL (1 mL, 5 mL) [contains benzyl alcohol]
Injection, suspension, as **hexacetonide** (Aristospan®): 5 mg/mL (5 mL); 20 mg/mL (1 mL, 5 mL) [contains benzyl alcohol]
Lotion, as **acetonide**: 0.025% (60 mL); 0.1% (60 mL)
Ointment, topical, as **acetonide**: 0.025% (80 g); 0.1% (15 g, 80 g)
Aristocort® A, Kenalog®: 0.1% (15 g, 60 g)
Paste, oral, topical, as **acetonide** (Kenalog® in Orabase®): 0.1% (5 g)
Tablet (Aristocort®): 4 mg [contains sodium benzoate]

References

Expert Panel Report 2, "Guidelines for the Diagnosis and Management of Asthma," *Clinical Practice Guidelines*, National Institutes of Health, National Heart, Lung, and Blood Institute, NIH Publication No. 94-4051, April, 1997.

"National Asthma Education and Prevention Program. Expert Panel Report: Guidelines for the Diagnosis and Management of Asthma Update on Selected Topics--2002," *J Allergy Clin Immunol*, 2002, 110(5 Suppl):S141-219.

♦ **Triaminic® Allergy Congestion [OTC]** *see* Pseudoephedrine *on page 958*

Triamterene (trye AM ter een)

U.S. Brand Names Dyrenium®
Therapeutic Category Antihypertensive Agent; Diuretic, Potassium Sparing
Generic Available No
Use Used alone or in combination with other diuretics to treat edema and hypertension; decreases potassium excretion caused by kaliuretic diuretics
Pregnancy Risk Factor B
Contraindications Hypersensitivity to triamterene or any component; severe renal or hepatic impairment, hyperkalemia
Precautions Use with caution in patients with impaired hepatic or renal function, history of renal calculi, diabetes mellitus; patients receiving other potassium-sparing diuretics or potassium supplements
Adverse Reactions
Cardiovascular: Hypotension
Central nervous system: Dizziness, headache
Endocrine & metabolic: Hyperkalemia, hyponatremia, hypomagnesemia, hyperchloremia, hyperuricemia, metabolic acidosis
Dermatologic: Photosensitivity
Gastrointestinal: Nausea, vomiting, diarrhea, xerostomia
Genitourinary: Slight alkalinization of urine
Hematologic: Blood dyscrasias, thrombocytopenia, megaloblastic anemia
Hepatic: Abnormal liver function
Neuromuscular & skeletal: Muscle cramps, weakness
Renal: Prerenal azotemia, nephrolithiasis (rare), reversible acute renal failure
Miscellaneous: Allergic reactions have been reported
Drug Interactions Increased risk of hyperkalemia if given together with other potassium-sparing diuretics (ie, spironolactone); may increase risk of hyperkalemia with ACE inhibitors, (ie, captopril, enalapril); concomitant administration of triamterene and indomethacin may increase nephrotoxicity; increased risk of hyperkalemia with potassium-containing preparations; may increase lithium toxicity by decreasing lithium clearance; may increase amantadine toxicity possibly by decreasing its renal excretion
Food Interactions Avoid salt substitutes and diets with increased potassium

(Continued)

Triamterene *(Continued)*

Mechanism of Action Interferes with potassium/sodium exchange (active transport) in the distal tubule, cortical collecting tubule and collecting duct by inhibiting sodium, potassium-ATPase; decreases calcium excretion; increases magnesium loss

Pharmacodynamics
Onset of action: Diuresis occurs within 2-4 hours
Duration: 7-9 hours
Note: Maximum therapeutic effect may not occur until after several days of therapy

Pharmacokinetics
Absorption: Oral: Unreliably absorbed
Metabolism: Hepatic conjugation
Half-life: 100-150 minutes
Elimination: 21% excreted unchanged in urine

Usual Dosage Oral:
Children: 2-4 mg/kg/day in 1-2 divided doses; maximum dose: 6 mg/kg/day and not to exceed 300 mg/day
Adults: 25-100 mg/day in 1-2 divided doses; maximum dose: 300 mg/day

Administration Oral: Administer with food to avoid GI upset

Monitoring Parameters Electrolytes (sodium, potassium, magnesium, HCO_3, chloride), CBC, BUN, creatinine, platelets

Test Interactions Interferes with fluorometric assay of quinidine

Patient Information May cause dry mouth. May cause photosensitivity reactions (eg, exposure to sunlight may cause severe sunburn, skin rash, redness, or itching); avoid exposure to sunlight and artificial light sources (sunlamps, tanning booth/bed); wear protective clothing, wide-brimmed hats, sunglasses, and lip sunscreen (SPF ≥15); use a sunscreen [broad-spectrum sunscreen or physical sunscreen (preferred) or sunblock with SPF ≥15]; contact physician if reaction occurs.

Additional Information Abrupt discontinuation of therapy may result in rebound kaliuresis; taper off gradually

Dosage Forms Capsule: 50 mg, 100 mg [contains benzyl alcohol]

- ◆ **Triatec-8 (Can)** *see* Acetaminophen and Codeine *on page 39*
- ◆ **Triatec-8 Strong (Can)** *see* Acetaminophen and Codeine *on page 39*
- ◆ **Triatec-30 (Can)** *see* Acetaminophen and Codeine *on page 39*
- ◆ **Triaz®** *see* Benzoyl Peroxide *on page 165*
- ◆ **Triaz® Cleanser** *see* Benzoyl Peroxide *on page 165*

Triazolam *(trye AY zoe lam)*

Related Information
Overdose and Toxicology *on page 1388*

U.S. Brand Names Halcion®

Canadian Brand Names Apo®-Triazo; Gen-Triazolam

Therapeutic Category Benzodiazepine; Hypnotic; Sedative

Generic Available Yes

Use Short-term treatment of insomnia

Restrictions C-IV

Pregnancy Risk Factor X

Contraindications Hypersensitivity to triazolam or any component; cross-sensitivity with other benzodiazepines may occur; severe uncontrolled pain; pre-existing CNS depression; narrow-angle glaucoma; not to be used in pregnancy or lactation

Warnings Abrupt discontinuation after prolonged use may result in withdrawal symptoms or rebound insomnia; tablet contains sodium benzoate; benzoic acid (benzoate) is a metabolite of benzyl alcohol; large amounts of benzyl alcohol (≥99 mg/kg/day) have been associated with a potentially fatal toxicity ("gasping syndrome") in neonates; avoid use of triazolam products containing sodium benzoate in neonates; *in vitro* and animal studies have shown that benzoate displaces bilirubin from protein binding sites

Adverse Reactions
Central nervous system: Drowsiness, anterograde amnesia, confusion, bizarre behavior, agitation, dizziness, hallucinations, nightmares, headache, ataxia
Gastrointestinal: Xerostomia, nausea, vomiting
Hepatic: Cholestatic jaundice
Miscellaneous: Physical and psychological dependence

Drug Interactions Cytochrome P450 isoenzyme CYP3A3/4 and CYP3A5-7 substrate CNS depressants, alcohol may increase CNS adverse effects; cimetidine, erythromycin may decrease and enzyme inducers may increase the metabolism of triazolam; protease inhibitors (indinavir, nelfinavir, lopinavir, ritonavir, saquinavir) and delavirdine may potentially decrease triazolam's metabolism and increase triazolam serum concentrations; concurrent use of triazolam with protease inhibitors or delavirdine is not recommended; ketoconazole, itraconazole may increase intensity and duration of triazolam effects

Food Interactions Food may decrease the rate, but not the extent of absorption; grapefruit juice significantly increases the bioavailability of oral triazolam

Mechanism of Action Depresses all levels of the CNS, including the limbic and reticular formation, by binding to the benzodiazepine site on the gamma-aminobutyric acid (GABA) receptor complex and modulating GABA, which is a major inhibitory neurotransmitter in the brain

Pharmacodynamics Hypnotic effects:
Onset of action: Within 15-30 minutes
Duration: 6-7 hours

Pharmacokinetics
Distribution: V_d: 0.8-1.8 L/kg
Protein binding: 89%
Metabolism: Extensive in the liver
Half-life: 1.7-5 hours
Elimination: In urine as unchanged drug and metabolites

Usual Dosage Oral:
Children <18 years: Dosage not established; investigational doses of 0.02 mg/kg given as an elixir have been used in children (n=20) for sedation prior to dental procedures; further studies are needed before this dose can be recommended
Adults: 0.125-0.25 mg at bedtime

Administration Oral: Administer dose in bed, since onset of hypnotic effect is rapid; do not administer with grapefruit juice

Monitoring Parameters Liver enzymes with prolonged use

Patient Information Avoid alcohol and grapefruit juice; may be habit-forming; avoid abrupt discontinuation with prolonged use; may cause drowsiness and impair ability to perform activities requiring mental alertness or physical coordination; take dose in bed at bedtime; may also cause daytime drowsiness; may cause dry mouth

Additional Information Onset of action is rapid, patient should be in bed when taking medication

Dosage Forms Tablet: 0.125 mg, 0.25 mg [contains sodium benzoate]

References
Meyer ML, Mourino AP, and Farrington FH, "Comparison of Triazolam to a Chloral Hydrate/Hydroxyzine Combination in the Sedation of Pediatric Dental Patients," *Pediatr Dent*, 1990, 12(5):283-7.

♦ **Tribavirin** *see* Ribavirin *on page 981*

♦ **Trichloroacetaldehyde Monohydrate** *see* Chloral Hydrate *on page 252*

♦ **Tricosal®** *see* Choline Magnesium Trisalicylate *on page 268*

♦ **Triderm®** *see* Triamcinolone *on page 1112*

Triethanolamine Polypeptide Oleate-Condensate
(trye eth a NOLE a meen pol i PEP tide OH lee ate-KON den sate)

U.S. Brand Names Cerumenex®

Therapeutic Category Otic Agent, Cerumenolytic

Generic Available No

Use Removal of ear wax (cerumen)

Pregnancy Risk Factor C

Contraindications Hypersensitivity to triethanolamine polypeptide oleate-condensate or any component; perforated tympanic membrane or otitis media

Warnings Discontinue if sensitization or irritation occurs

Precautions Avoid undue exposure to skin during administration and the flushing out of ear canal; exposure of ear canal to otic solution should be limited to 15-30 minutes

Adverse Reactions Local: Localized dermatitis, mild erythema and pruritus, severe eczematoid reactions involving the external ear and periauricular tissue

Mechanism of Action Emulsifies and disperses accumulated cerumen for easier removal

Pharmacodynamics Onset of action: Produces slight disintegration of very hard ear wax by 24 hours

Usual Dosage Children and Adults: Otic: Fill ear canal, insert cotton plug; allow to remain 15-30 minutes; flush ear with lukewarm water as a single treatment; if a second application is needed for unusually hard impactions, repeat the procedure

Monitoring Parameters Evaluate hearing before and after instillation of medication

Patient Information For external use in the ear only; warm to body temperature before using to improve effect

Nursing Implications Avoid undue exposure of the drug to the periaural skin

Dosage Forms Solution, otic: 10% (6 mL, 12 mL) [contains propylene glycol]
(Continued)

Triethanolamine Polypeptide Oleate-Condensate
(Continued)

References
Mehta AK, "An *In Vitro* Comparison of the Disintegration of Human Ear Wax by Five Cerumenolytics Commonly Used in General Practice," *Br J Clin Pract*, 1985, 39(5):200-3.

◆ **Triethylenethiophosphoramide** *see* Thiotepa *on page 1087*

◆ **Trifluorothymidine** *see* Trifluridine *on page 1118*

Trifluridine (trye FLURE i deen)
U.S. Brand Names Viroptic®

Synonyms F_3T; Trifluorothymidine

Therapeutic Category Antiviral Agent, Ophthalmic

Generic Available Yes

Use Treatment of primary keratoconjunctivitis and recurrent epithelial keratitis caused by herpes simplex virus types I and II

Pregnancy Risk Factor C

Contraindications Hypersensitivity to trifluridine or any component

Adverse Reactions
Cardiovascular: Hyperemia
Local: Burning, stinging
Ocular: Palpebral edema, epithelial keratopathy, keratitis, stromal edema, elevated intraocular pressure
Miscellaneous: Hypersensitivity reactions

Stability Store in refrigerator; storage at room temperature may result in a solution with altered pH which could result in ocular discomfort upon administration and/or decreased potency

Mechanism of Action Interferes with viral replication by incorporating into viral DNA in place of thymidine, inhibiting thymidylate synthetase resulting in the formation of defective proteins

Pharmacodynamics Onset of action: Response to treatment occurs within 2-7 days; epithelial healing is complete in 1-2 weeks

Pharmacokinetics Absorption: Ophthalmic: Systemic absorption is negligible, while corneal penetration is adequate

Usual Dosage Children and Adults: Ophthalmic: Instill 1 drop into affected eye every 2 hours while awake, to a maximum of 9 drops/day, until re-epithelialization of corneal ulcer occurs; then use 1 drop every 4 hours for another 7 days; do **not** exceed 21 days of treatment

Administration Ophthalmic: Avoid contact of bottle tip with skin or eye; instill drops onto the cornea of the affected eye(s); apply finger pressure to lacrimal sac during and for 1-2 minutes after instillation to decrease risk of absorption and systemic effects

Monitoring Parameters Ophthalmologic exam (test for corneal staining with fluorescein or rose Bengal)

Additional Information Found to be effective in 138 of 150 patients unresponsive or intolerant to idoxuridine or vidarabine

Dosage Forms
Solution, ophthalmic: 1% (7.5 mL)
Viroptic®: 1% (7.5 mL) [contains thimerosal]

◆ **Triglycerides, Medium Chain** *see* Medium Chain Triglycerides *on page 711*

Trihexyphenidyl (trye heks ee FEN i dil)
Related Information
Overdose and Toxicology *on page 1388*

Canadian Brand Names Apo®-Trihex

Synonyms Benzhexol

Therapeutic Category Anticholinergic Agent; Antidote, Drug-induced Dystonic Reactions; Anti-Parkinson's Agent

Generic Available Yes

Use Adjunctive treatment of Parkinson's disease; also used in treatment of drug-induced extrapyramidal effects and acute dystonic reactions

Pregnancy Risk Factor C

Contraindications Hypersensitivity to trihexyphenidyl or any component; children younger than 3 years of age; patients with narrow-angle glaucoma, GI or GU obstruction; myasthenia gravis, achalasia

Precautions Use with caution in patients with hyperthyroidism, renal or hepatic dysfunction, hypertension, hiatal hernia, tachycardia, cardiac arrhythmias, peptic ulcer, esophageal reflux; use with caution in hot weather or during exercise

Adverse Reactions

Cardiovascular: Tachycardia

Central nervous system: Dizziness, nervousness, drowsiness, agitation, delirium, headache

Dermatologic: Rash

Gastrointestinal: Xerostomia, nausea, constipation

Genitourinary: Urinary hesitancy or retention

Neuromuscular & skeletal: Weakness

Ocular: Blurred vision, mydriasis, elevated intraocular tension

Drug Interactions May increase gastric degradation of levodopa and decrease the amount of levodopa absorbed by delaying gastric emptying; antagonizes the therapeutic effects of cholinergic agents (tacrine, donepezil) and neuroleptics; increases central and/or peripheral anticholinergic effects when administered with amantadine, rimantadine, narcotic analgesics, phenothiazines and other antipsychotics (especially with high anticholinergic activity), tricyclic antidepressants, quinidine and some other antiarrhythmics, and antihistamines

Mechanism of Action Presumed to act by blocking excess acetylcholine at cerebral synapses; many of its effects are due to its pharmacologic similarities with atropine

Pharmacodynamics

Onset of action: 1 hour

Maximum effect: 2-3 hours

Duration: 6-12 hours

Pharmacokinetics

Metabolism: Metabolic fate undetermined

Bioavailability: 100%

Half-life: 5.6-10.2 hours

Elimination: Some urinary excretion

Usual Dosage Adults: Oral:

Extrapyramidal: 5-15 mg/day in 3-4 divided doses

Parkinsonism: 1 mg daily; increase by 2 mg increments every 3-5 days to 6-10 mg/day (maximum daily dosage: 12-15 mg); doses >10 mg/day should be divided into 3-4 doses

Administration Oral: Administer with food or water to decrease GI irritation

Monitoring Parameters Intraocular pressure monitoring (baseline and at regular intervals)

Patient Information May cause drowsiness and impair ability to perform activities requiring mental alertness or physical coordination; may cause dry mouth

Dosage Forms

Elixir, as hydrochloride: 2 mg/5 mL (480 mL)

Tablet, as hydrochloride: 2 mg, 5 mg

◆ **Tri-K®** *see* Potassium Supplements *on page 919*

◆ **Trileptal®** *see* Oxcarbazepine *on page 841*

◆ **Trilisate®** *see* Choline Magnesium Trisalicylate *on page 268*

Trimethobenzamide (trye meth oh BEN za mide)

Related Information

Compatibility of Medications Mixed in a Syringe *on page 1412*

U.S. Brand Names Tigan®

Therapeutic Category Antiemetic

Generic Available Yes (capsule and injection)

Use Control of postoperative nausea and vomiting and nausea associated with gastroenteritis

Pregnancy Risk Factor C

Contraindications Hypersensitivity to trimethobenzamide, any component, or benzocaine (contained in suppository); suppositories are contraindicated in premature infants and neonates; injection is contraindicated in children

Precautions Use cautiously in infants and children; may mask emesis due to Reye's syndrome or mimic CNS effects of Reye's syndrome in patients with emesis of other etiologies

Adverse Reactions

Cardiovascular: Hypotension (especially after I.M. use)

Central nervous system: Drowsiness, sedation, extrapyramidal symptoms, dizziness, seizures, coma, depression, opisthotonos

Dermatologic: Hypersensitivity skin reactions

Gastrointestinal: Diarrhea

Hematologic: Blood dyscrasias

Hepatic: Jaundice

Local: Pain, stinging, burning at I.M. injection site

(Continued)

Trimethobenzamide *(Continued)*

Ocular: Blurred vision

Mechanism of Action Acts centrally to inhibit stimulation of the medullary chemoreceptor trigger zone

Pharmacodynamics

Onset of action:
Oral: 10-40 minutes
I.M.: 15-35 minutes
Duration:
Oral: 3-4 hours
I.M.: 2-3 hours

Pharmacokinetics

Metabolism: Not well determined
Bioavailability: Oral dose is ~60% of I.M. dose
Half-life: Adults: 7-9 hours
Elimination: 20% excreted unchanged in urine in 24 hours

Usual Dosage Do not use rectally in neonates and infants

Children:
Oral, rectal: 15-20 mg/kg/day (400-500 mg/m^2/day) divided into 3-4 doses; **or as an alternative**
<13.6 kg (30 lbs): 100 mg 3-4 times/day
13.6-41 kg (30-90 lbs): 100-200 mg 3-4 times/day
I.M.: Not recommended
Adults:
Oral: 250-300 mg 3-4 times/day
I.M., rectal: 200 mg 3-4 times/day

Administration

Oral: May administer without regard to food
Parenteral: I.M. use only by deep injection into upper outer quadrant of gluteal region; **not** for I.V. use

Patient Information May cause drowsiness and impair ability to perform activities requiring mental alertness or physical coordination

Additional Information Note: Less effective than phenothiazines but may be associated with fewer side effects

Dosage Forms

Capsule, as hydrochloride: 250 mg
Tigan®: 300 mg
Injection, solution, as hydrochloride: 100 mg/mL (2 mL)
Tigan®: 100 mg/mL (2 mL, 20 mL)
Suppository, rectal, as hydrochloride (Tigan®): 100 mg, 200 mg [contains benzocaine]

Trimethoprim *(trye METH oh prim)*

Related Information

Blood Level Sampling Time Guidelines *on page 1386*

U.S. Brand Names Primsol®; Proloprim®

Canadian Brand Names Apo®-Trimethoprim

Synonyms TMP

Therapeutic Category Antibiotic, Miscellaneous

Generic Available Yes (tablet)

Use Treatment of urinary tract infections caused by susceptible *Escherichia coli*, *Proteus mirabilis*, *Klebsiella pneumoniae*, *Enterobacter* species, and coagulase-negative *Staphylococcus* (including *S. saprophyticus*); prophylaxis of urinary tract infections; in combination with other agents for treatment of *Pneumocystis carinii* pneumonia; treatment of otitis media caused by susceptible *Streptococcus pneumoniae* and *Haemophilus influenzae* (not indicated for *Moraxella catarrhalis* due to consistent resistance); not indicated for prolonged administration or prophylaxis of otitis media

Pregnancy Risk Factor C

Contraindications Hypersensitivity to trimethoprim or any component; megaloblastic anemia due to folate deficiency

Warnings May cause folate deficiencies with subsequent bone marrow suppression and blood dyscrasias; monitor patients for fever, sore throat, purpura, or pallor; discontinue trimethoprim if bone marrow depression occurs; leucovorin (folinic acid) may be needed to restore normal hematopoiesis

Oral solution contains propylene glycol and sodium benzoate; benzoic acid (benzoate) is a metabolite of benzyl alcohol; large amounts of benzyl alcohol (≥99 mg/kg/day) have been associated with a potentially fatal toxicity ("gasping syndrome") in neonates; the "gasping syndrome" consists of metabolic acidosis, respiratory distress, gasping respirations, CNS dysfunction (including convulsions, intracranial hemorrhage), hypotension and cardiovascular collapse; avoid use of trimethoprim products containing sodium benzoate in neonates; *in vitro* and animal studies have shown that benzoate displaces bilirubin from protein binding sites

Precautions Use with caution in patients with impaired renal or hepatic function or with possible folate deficiency; decrease dose in patients with renal dysfunction; safety is not established in infants <2 months of age; effectiveness for treatment of acute otitis media is not established in infants <6 months of age

Adverse Reactions

Central nervous system: Fever, headache, aseptic meningitis (rare)

Dermatologic: Rash, pruritus, phototoxic skin eruptions, exfoliative dermatitis (rare), erythema multiforme (rare), Stevens-Johnson syndrome (rare), toxic epidermal necrolysis (rare)

Endocrine & metabolic: Hyperkalemia, hyponatremia

Hematologic: Megaloblastic anemia, neutropenia, leukopenia, thrombocytopenia, methemoglobinemia

Hepatic: Elevated liver enzymes, cholestatic jaundice

Gastrointestinal: Nausea, vomiting, epigastric distress, glossitis

Renal: Elevated BUN and serum creatinine

Miscellaneous: Anaphylaxis, hypersensitivity reactions

Drug Interactions Cytochrome P450 isoenzyme CYP2C8 and CYP2C9 inhibitor

Use with other folate antagonists (methotrexate, pyrimethamine) may increase risk of megaloblastic anemia; trimethoprim may decrease the metabolism of phenytoin resulting in increased phenytoin serum concentrations; cyclosporine, dapsone, procainamide, rifampin, warfarin

Food Interactions May cause folic acid deficiency, supplements may be needed

Stability Store tablets and solution at 15°C to 25°C (59°F to 77°F); protect from light

Mechanism of Action Binds to the enzyme dihydrofolate reductase in bacteria and inhibits conversion of dihydrofolic acid to tetrahydrofolate (functional form of folic acid). This results in depletion of folic acid, interference with bacterial biosynthesis of nucleic acids and protein production, and inhibition of microbial growth.

Pharmacokinetics

Absorption: Oral: Readily and extensively absorbed (90% to 100%)

Distribution: Penetrates into middle ear fluid with a mean peak middle ear fluid concentration in children 1-12 years of 2 mcg/mL after a single 4 mg/kg dose; crosses the placenta; excreted in breast milk

V_d:

Newborns: ~2.7 L/kg

Infants: 1.5 L/kg

Children 1-10 years: ~1 L/kg

Adults: 1.3-1.8 L/kg

Protein binding: 42% to 46%

Metabolism: Partially (10% to 20%) metabolized in the liver via demethylation, oxidation, and hydroxylation

Bioavailability: Similar for tablets and solution

Half-life (prolonged in renal dysfunction):

Newborns: ~19 hours

Infants 2 months to 1 year: 3-6 hours; mean: 4.6 hours

Children 1-10 years: 3-5.5 hours

Adults, normal renal function: 8-11 hours

Adults, anuric: 20-50 hours

Time to peak serum concentration: Within 1-4 hours

Elimination: Significantly excreted in urine (60% to 80%) as unchanged drug via glomerular filtration and tubular secretion; increased renal excretion with acidic urine

Dialysis: Moderately dialyzable (20% to 50%)

Usual Dosage Oral:

Infants ≥6 months and Children: Acute otitis media: 10 mg/kg/day in divided doses every 12 hours for 10 days

Infants and Children <12 years: Urinary tract infection: Treatment: 4-6 mg/kg/day in divided doses every 12 hours for 10 days

Children ≥12 years and Adults:

Urinary tract infection: Treatment: 100 mg every 12 hours or 200 mg every 24 hours for 10 days

Prophylaxis: 100 mg once daily

Pneumocystis carinii pneumonia treatment (given with dapsone): 15-20 mg/kg/day in 4 divided doses for 21 days

Dosing adjustment in renal impairment:

Cl$_{cr}$ 15-30 mL/minute: Administer 50% of normal dose

Cl$_{cr}$ <15 mL/minute: Avoid use

(Continued)

Trimethoprim *(Continued)*

Administration Oral: Administer on an empty stomach; may administer with milk or food if GI upset occurs

Monitoring Parameters CBC with differential, platelet count, liver enzyme tests, bilirubin, serum creatinine and BUN

Reference Range Therapeutic:
Peak: 5-15 mg/L
Trough: 2-8 mg/L

Test Interactions May falsely increase creatinine determination measured by the Jaffé alkaline picrate assay; may interfere with determination of serum methotrexate when measured by methods that use a bacterial dihydrofolate reductase as the binding protein (eg, the competitive binding protein technique); does **not** interfere with RIA for methotrexate

Patient Information Report any skin rash, persistent or severe fatigue, fever, sore throat, or unusual bleeding or bruising; complete full course of therapy

Additional Information Not effective versus *Pseudomonas* or *B. fragilis*; discontinue if bone marrow suppression occurs

Dosage Forms
Solution, oral, as hydrochloride (Primsol®): 50 mg base/5 mL (473 mL) [alcohol and dye free; contains propylene glycol and sodium benzoate; bubblegum flavor]
Tablet: 100 mg
Proloprim®: 100 mg, 200 mg

References
Hoppu K, "Age Differences in Trimethoprim Pharmacokinetics: Need for Revised Dosing in Children?" *Clin Pharmacol Ther*, 1987, 41(3):336-43.
Hoppu K, Koskimies O, and Vilska J, "Trimethoprim in the Treatment of Acute Urinary Tract Infections in Children," *Int J Clin Pharmacol Ther Toxicol*, 1988, 26(2):65-8.
Leff RD, Cho CT, and Reed MD, "Safety and Efficacy of Trimethoprim Hydrochloride Solution for the Treatment of Children With Otitis Media," *Journal of Pediatric Pharmacy Practice*, 1998, 3(1): 33-9.

♦ **Trimethoprim and Sulfamethoxazole** *see* Sulfamethoxazole and Trimethoprim *on page 1052*

♦ **Trimox®** *see* Amoxicillin *on page 94*

♦ **Tri-Nasal®** *see* Triamcinolone *on page 1112*

♦ **Triostat®** *see* Liothyronine *on page 680*

♦ **Triple Antibiotic®** *see* Neomycin, Polymyxin B, and Bacitracin *on page 804*

♦ **Triple Care® Antifungal [OTC]** *see* Miconazole *on page 759*

Triprolidine and Pseudoephedrine

(trye PROE li deen & soo doe e FED rin)

Related Information
OTC Cough & Cold Preparations, Pediatric *on page 1225*
Overdose and Toxicology *on page 1388*

U.S. Brand Names Actifed® Cold and Allergy [OTC]; Allerfrim® [OTC]; Allerphed® [OTC]; Aphedrid™ [OTC]; Aprodine® [OTC]; Genac® [OTC]; Silafed® [OTC]; Tri-Sudo® [OTC]; Uni-Fed® [OTC]

Synonyms Pseudoephedrine and Triprolidine

Therapeutic Category Antihistamine/Decongestant Combination; Sympathomimetic

Generic Available Yes

Use Temporary relief of nasal congestion, running nose, sneezing, itching of nose or throat and itchy, watery eyes due to common cold, hay fever or other upper respiratory allergies

Pregnancy Risk Factor C

Contraindications Hypersensitivity to triprolidine, pseudoephedrine, or any component; severe hypertension or coronary artery disease; MAO inhibitor therapy, GI or GU obstruction, narrow-angle glaucoma

Warnings Not recommended for use in children <4 months of age

Precautions Use with caution in patients with mild to moderate high blood pressure, heart disease, diabetes mellitus, asthma, thyroid disease, or prostatic hypertrophy

Adverse Reactions
Cardiovascular: Hypertension, tachycardia
Central nervous system: Sedation, CNS stimulation, headache
Gastrointestinal: Nausea, vomiting, xerostomia, anorexia

Drug Interactions MAO inhibitors, beta-blocking agents, other sympathomimetics, methyldopa, reserpine, alpha-blocking agents, CNS depressants

Usual Dosage Oral:
Children: May dose according to **pseudoephedrine** component: 4 mg/kg/day in divided doses 3-4 times/day **or**

4 months to 2 years: 1.25 mL 3-4 times/day
2-4 years: 2.5 mL 3-4 times/day
4-6 years: 3.75 mL 3-4 times/day
6-12 years: 5 mL or ½ tablet 3-4 times/day
Children >12 years and Adults: 10 mL or 1 tablet 3-4 times/day

Administration Oral: Administer with food or milk to decrease GI irritation

Patient Information May cause drowsiness and impair ability to perform activities requiring mental alertness or physical coordination; may cause dry mouth

Dosage Forms

Syrup: Triprolidine hydrochloride 1.25 mg and pseudoephedrine hydrochloride 30 mg per 5 mL (120 mL)

Allerfrim®: Triprolidine hydrochloride 1.25 mg and pseudoephedrine hydrochloride 30 mg per 5 mL (120 mL, 480 mL)

Allerphed®, Aprodine®: Triprolidine hydrochloride 1.25 mg and pseudoephedrine hydrochloride 30 mg per 5 mL (120 mL)

Silafed®: Triprolidine hydrochloride 1.25 mg and pseudoephedrine hydrochloride 30 mg per 5 mL (120 mL, 240 mL)

Tablet (Actifed® Cold and Allergy, Allerfrim®, Aphedrid™, Aprodine®, Genac®, Tri-Sudo®, Uni-Fed®): Triprolidine hydrochloride 2.5 mg and pseudoephedrine hydrochloride 60 mg

- **Tris Buffer** *see* Tromethamine *on page 1124*
- **Tris(hydroxymethyl)aminomethane** *see* Tromethamine *on page 1124*
- **Tri-Sudo® [OTC]** *see* Triprolidine and Pseudoephedrine *on page 1122*
- **Trivagizole-3® (Can)** *see* Clotrimazole *on page 297*
- **Tri-Vi-Flor®** *see page 1213*
- **Tri-Vi-Sol®** *see page 1213*
- **Tri-Vit** *see page 1213*
- **Tri-Vit With Fluoride** *see page 1213*
- **Trizivir®** *see* Abacavir, Lamivudine, and Zidovudine *on page 32*
- **Trocaine® [OTC]** *see* Benzocaine *on page 163*

Troleandomycin (troe lee an doe MYE sin)

U.S. Brand Names TAO®

Synonyms Triacetyloleandomycin

Therapeutic Category Antibiotic, Macrolide

Generic Available No

Use Adjunct in the treatment of severe corticosteroid-dependent asthma due to its steroid-sparing properties; obsolete antibiotic with spectrum of activity similar to erythromycin

Pregnancy Risk Factor C

Contraindications Hypersensitivity to troleandomycin or any component; concomitant administration of terfenadine, astemizole, pimozide, or cisapride with troleandomycin may result in QT interval prolongation, ventricular tachycardia, and torsade de pointes

Warnings Cholestatic hepatitis has been reported in patients who have received troleandomycin for 2 weeks or longer and in cases where repeated courses were administered

Precautions Use with caution in patients with impaired hepatic function

Adverse Reactions

Central nervous system: Fever

Dermatologic: Urticaria, rash

Gastrointestinal: Abdominal cramping, nausea, vomiting, diarrhea, rectal burning, esophagitis

Hepatic: Cholestatic hepatitis, jaundice

Drug Interactions Cytochrome P450 isoenzyme CYP3A3/4 substrate; isoenzyme CYP3A3/4 and CYP3A5-7 inhibitor

Troleandomycin inhibits the cytochrome P450 microsomal enzyme system decreasing clearance of theophylline (see Additional Information), cisapride, triazolam, pimozide, astemizole, and terfenadine; interferes with metabolism of ergotamine and carbamazepine potentiating their action; decreases methylprednisolone clearance from a linear first order decline to a nonlinear decline in plasma concentration

Food Interactions Food delays the rate, but not the extent of absorption

Mechanism of Action Troleandomycin has an undefined action independent of its effects on steroid elimination

Pharmacokinetics

Time to peak serum concentration: Oral: Within 2 hours

(Continued)

Troleandomycin (Continued)

Elimination: 10% to 25% excreted in urine as active drug; excreted in feces via bile

Usual Dosage Oral:

Children: 25-40 mg/kg/day divided every 6 hours

Adjunct in corticosteroid-dependent asthma: 14 mg/kg/day in divided doses every 6-12 hours not to exceed 250 mg every 6 hours; dose is tapered to once daily then alternate day dosing

Adults: 250-500 mg 4 times/day

Monitoring Parameters Hepatic function tests

Patient Information Report any prodromal symptoms of hepatitis (fatigue, weakness, nausea, vomiting, dark urine, or yellowing of eyes)

Additional Information For patients on both troleandomycin and theophylline: Troleandomycin can significantly reduce theophylline clearance resulting in higher serum theophylline concentrations; empiric reduction in theophylline dosage appears to be indicated with the initiation of troleandomycin

Dosage Forms Capsule: 250 mg

References

Brenner AM and Szefler SJ, "Troleandomycin in the Treatment of Severe Asthma," *Immunol Allergy Clin North Am*, 1991, 11(1):91-102.

Kamada AK, Hill MR, Brenner AM, et al, "Effect of Low-Dose Troleandomycin on Theophylline Clearance: Implications for Therapeutic Drug Monitoring," *Pharmacotherapy*, 1992, 12(2):98-102.

Spector SL, Katz FH, and Farr RS, "Troleandomycin: Effectiveness in Steroid-Dependent Asthma and Bronchitis," *J Allergy Clin Immunol*, 1974, 54(6):367-79.

Tromethamine (troe METH a meen)

U.S. Brand Names THAM®

Synonyms Tris Buffer; Tris(hydroxymethyl)aminomethane

Therapeutic Category Alkalinizing Agent, Parenteral

Generic Available No

Use Correction of metabolic acidosis associated with cardiac bypass surgery or cardiac arrest; to correct excess acidity of stored blood that is preserved with acid citrate dextrose (ACD); to prime the pump-oxygenator during cardiac bypass surgery; indicated in severe metabolic acidosis in patients in whom sodium or carbon dioxide elimination is restricted [eg, infants needing alkalinization after receiving maximum sodium bicarbonate (8-10 mEq/kg/24 hours)]

Pregnancy Risk Factor C

Contraindications Hypersensitivity to tromethamine or any component; uremia or anuria; chronic respiratory acidosis; salicylate intoxication

Warnings Avoid infusion via low-lying umbilical venous catheters due to associated risk of hepatocellular necrosis; due to osmotic effects, use of sodium bicarbonate for the treatment of acidotic neonates and infants with RDS may be preferred; rapid I.V. infusion may cause prolonged hypoglycemia

Precautions Reduce dose and monitor pH carefully in renal impairment

Adverse Reactions

Cardiovascular: Venospasm

Endocrine & metabolic: Hyperosmolality of serum, hyperkalemia, hypoglycemia (rapid administration)

Hepatic: Liver cell destruction from direct contact with tromethamine, hemorrhagic hepatic necrosis (when administered through umbilical vein at concentrations ≥1.2 M)

Local: Tissue irritation, necrosis with extravasation

Respiratory: Respiratory depression, apnea

Mechanism of Action Proton acceptor, which combines with hydrogen ions to form bicarbonate and buffer

Pharmacokinetics 30% of dose is not ionized; rapidly eliminated by kidneys

Usual Dosage I.V.: Dose depends on severity and progression of acidosis:

Neonates: Manufacturer's recommendation: 1 mL/kg for each pH unit below 7.4

Infants, Children, and Adults:

Empiric dosage based upon base deficit: Tromethamine mL of 0.3 M solution = body weight (kg) x base deficit (mEq/L); maximum: 500 mg/kg/dose = 13.9 mL/kg/dose using 0.3 M solution

Metabolic acidosis with cardiac arrest: Tromethamine mL of 0.3 M solution: 3.5-6 mL/kg/dose (126-216 mg/kg/dose); maximum: 500 mg/kg/dose = 13.9 mL/kg/dose using 0.3 M solution

Excess acidity of acid citrate dextrose priming blood: Tromethamine mL of 0.3 M solution: 14-70 mL added added to each 500 mL of blood

Acidosis during cardiac bypass surgery: Tromethamine mL of 0.3 M solution: 9 mL/kg (324 mg/kg/dose); maximum dose: 1000 mL (36 g) as single dose

Administration Parenteral: Maximum concentration: 0.3 molar; infuse slowly over at least 1 hour or 3-16 mL/kg/hour up to 33-40 mL/kg/day; administer into a central venous line

Monitoring Parameters Serum electrolytes, arterial blood gases, serum pH, blood sugar, EKG monitoring, renal function tests

Additional Information 1 mM = 120 mg = 3.3 mL = 1 mEq of THAM®

Dosage Forms Injection, solution (THAM®): 18 g [0.3 molar] (500 mL)

♦ Tronolane® [OTC] *see* Hemorrhoidal Preparations *on page 556*

♦ Tropicacyl® *see* Tropicamide *on page 1125*

Tropicamide (troe PIK a mide)

U.S. Brand Names Mydriacyl®; Opticyl®; Tropicacyl®

Canadian Brand Names Diotrope®

Synonyms Bistropamide

Therapeutic Category Ophthalmic Agent, Mydriatic

Generic Available Yes

Use Short-acting mydriatic used in diagnostic procedures; as well as preoperatively and postoperatively; treatment of some cases of acute iritis, iridocyclitis, and keratitis

Pregnancy Risk Factor C

Contraindications Hypersensitivity to tropicamide or any component; glaucoma, adhesions between the iris and the lens

Warnings Tropicamide may cause an increase in intraocular pressure

Precautions Use with caution in infants and children since tropicamide may cause potentially dangerous CNS disturbances and psychotic reactions

Adverse Reactions

Cardiovascular: Tachycardia, flushing

Central nervous system: Parasympathetic stimulation, drowsiness, headache, behavioral disturbances, psychotic reactions

Gastrointestinal: Xerostomia

Local: Transient stinging

Ocular: Blurred vision, photophobia, elevated intraocular pressure, follicular conjunctivitis

Miscellaneous: Allergic reactions

Stability Store at room temperature; do not refrigerate

Mechanism of Action Prevents the sphincter muscle of the iris and the muscle of the ciliary body from responding to cholinergic stimulation producing pupillary dilation and paralysis of accommodation

Pharmacodynamics

Maximum mydriatic effect: ~20-40 minutes

Duration: ~6-7 hours

Maximum cycloplegic effect:

Peak: 20-35 minutes

Duration: <6 hours

Usual Dosage Children and Adults: Ophthalmic:

Cycloplegia: Instill 1-2 drops (1%); may repeat in 5 minutes. The exam must be performed within 30 minutes after the repeat dose; if the patient is not examined within 20-30 minutes, instill an additional drop. Concentrations <1% are inadequate for producing satisfactory cycloplegia.

Mydriasis: Instill 1-2 drops (0.5%) 15-20 minutes before exam; may repeat every 30 minutes as needed

Administration Ophthalmic: To minimize systemic absorption, apply finger pressure on the lacrimal sac for 1-2 minutes following instillation of the ophthalmic solution; avoid contact of bottle tip with skin or eye

Patient Information May cause blurred vision; do not drive or engage in hazardous activities while the pupils are dilated; may cause sensitivity to light; may cause dry mouth

Dosage Forms

Solution, ophthalmic: 0.5% (15 mL); 1% (2 mL, 3 mL, 15 mL)

Mydriacyl®: 0.5% (15 mL); 1% (3 mL, 15 mL)

Opticyl®, Tropicacyl®: 0.5% (15 mL); 1% (15 mL)

References

Caputo AR and Schnitzer RE, "Systemic Response to Mydriatic Eyedrops in Neonates: Mydriatics in Neonates," *J Pediatr Ophthalmol Strabismus*, 1978, 15(2):109-22.

♦ Trusopt® *see* Dorzolamide *on page 407*

♦ TSPA *see* Thiotepa *on page 1087*

♦ T-Stat® *see* Erythromycin *on page 448*

♦ Tucks® [OTC] *see* Hemorrhoidal Preparations *on page 556*

- ◆ **Tumor Lysis Syndrome, Management** *see page 1315*
- ◆ **Tums®** [OTC] *see Antacid Preparations on page 112*
- ◆ **Tums®** [OTC] *see Calcium Supplements on page 200*
- ◆ **Tums® 500** [OTC] *see Calcium Supplements on page 200*
- ◆ **Tums® E-X** [OTC] *see Calcium Supplements on page 200*
- ◆ **Tums® Ultra®** [OTC] *see Calcium Supplements on page 200*
- ◆ **Tussi-Organidin® DM NR** *see Guaifenesin and Dextromethorphan on page 553*
- ◆ **Tussi-Organidin® NR** *see Guaifenesin and Codeine on page 551*
- ◆ **Tussi-Organidin® S-NR** *see Guaifenesin and Codeine on page 551*
- ◆ **Tusstat®** *see DiphenhydrAMINE on page 393*
- ◆ **Twice-A-Day®** [OTC] *see Oxymetazoline on page 849*
- ◆ **Tylenol®** [OTC] *see Acetaminophen on page 36*
- ◆ **Tylenol® Arthritis Pain** [OTC] *see Acetaminophen on page 36*
- ◆ **Tylenol®, Children's** [OTC] *see Acetaminophen on page 36*
- ◆ **Tylenol® Extra Strength** [OTC] *see Acetaminophen on page 36*
- ◆ **Tylenol®, Infants** [OTC] *see Acetaminophen on page 36*
- ◆ **Tylenol®, Junior Strength** [OTC] *see Acetaminophen on page 36*
- ◆ **Tylenol® Sore Throat** [OTC] *see Acetaminophen on page 36*
- ◆ **Tylenol® With Codeine** *see Acetaminophen and Codeine on page 39*
- ◆ **Tylox®** *see Oxycodone and Acetaminophen on page 847*
- ◆ **UCB-P071** *see Cetirizine on page 249*
- ◆ **UDCA** *see Ursodiol on page 1129*
- ◆ **UK109496** *see Voriconazole on page 1154*
- ◆ **Ultrase®** *see Pancrelipase on page 856*
- ◆ **Ultrase® MT** *see Pancrelipase on page 856*
- ◆ **Unasyn®** *see Ampicillin and Sulbactam on page 105*

Undecylenic Acid and Derivatives
(un de sil EN ik AS id & dah RIV ah tivs)
U.S. Brand Names Fungi-Nail® [OTC]; Undelenic®
Synonyms Zincundecate
Therapeutic Category Antifungal Agent, Topical
Generic Available No

Use Treatment of athlete's foot (tinea pedis), ringworm (except nails and scalp), prickly heat, jock itch (tinea cruris), diaper rash, and other minor skin irritations due to superficial dermatophytes

Contraindications Hypersensitivity to undecylenic acid and derivatives or any component; fungal infections of the scalp or nails

Warnings Do not apply to blistered, raw, or oozing areas of skin or over deep wounds or puncture wounds

Adverse Reactions
Dermatologic: Rash
Local: Skin irritation, stinging, sensitization

Mechanism of Action Undecylenic acid is a fatty acid with fungistatic activity that retards proliferation of the fungus by altering the conditions of growth; zinc undecylenate provides an astringent action that aids in the reduction of inflammation and irritation

Pharmacodynamics Onset of action: Improvement in erythema and pruritus may be seen within 1 week after initiation of therapy

Usual Dosage Children and Adults: Topical: Apply as needed twice daily for 2-4 weeks

Administration Topical: Clean and dry the affected area before topical application; if the solution is sprayed or applied onto the affected area, allow area to air dry; ointment or cream should be applied at night, the powder may be applied during the day or used alone when a drying effect is needed

Monitoring Parameters Resolution of skin infection

Patient Information For external use only; avoid contact with the eye; do not inhale the powder

Dosage Forms
Ointment, topical (Undelenic®): Undecylenic acid 10% and Chloroxylenol 0.5% (60 g, 454 g)
Solution, topical (Fungi-Nail®): Undecylenic acid 25% (29.57 mL)
Tincture (Undelenic®): Undecylenic acid 0.5% and zinc undecylenate 20% [total undecylenate 25%] (30 mL, 480 mL) [contains isopropyl alcohol and propylene glycol]

+ **Undelenic®** *see* Undecylenic Acid and Derivatives *on page 1126*
+ **Uni-Fed® [OTC]** *see* Triprolidine and Pseudoephedrine *on page 1122*
+ **Unipen® (Can)** *see* Nafcillin *on page 789*
+ **Uniphyl®** *see* Theophylline *on page 1076*
+ **Uniphyl® SRT (Can)** *see* Theophylline *on page 1076*
+ **Unisom® Maximum Strength SleepGels® [OTC]** *see* DiphenhydrAMINE *on page 393*
+ **Unithroid®** *see* Levothyroxine *on page 669*
+ **Urasal® (Can)** *see* Methenamine *on page 733*
+ **Urate oxidase** *see* Rasburicase *on page 975*
+ **Urea Peroxide** *see* Carbamide Peroxide *on page 212*
+ **Urecholine®** *see* Bethanechol *on page 171*
+ **Urex®** *see* Methenamine *on page 733*
+ **Uristat® [OTC]** *see* Phenazopyridine *on page 887*
+ **Urocit®-K** *see* Citrate and Citric Acid *on page 282*

Urokinase (yoor oh KIN ase)

Related Information
Antithrombotic Therapy in Children *on page 1316*

U.S. Brand Names Abbokinase®

Therapeutic Category Thrombolytic Agent; Thrombotic Occlusion (Central Venous Catheter), Treatment Agent

Generic Available No

Use Thrombolytic agent used in the treatment (lysis) of acute massive pulmonary emboli and pulmonary emboli with unstable hemodynamics (current labeled indications); also used in the treatment of recent severe or massive deep vein or arterial thrombosis, and occluded arteriovenous cannulas; **Note:** Urokinase was discontinued in 1999 due to problems in the manufacturing process; it was reintroduced into the market in October 2002, but its labeled indication was narrowed to only include pulmonary embolism (to speed the approval process); currently the product is labeled for I.V. infusion only

Pregnancy Risk Factor B

Contraindications Hypersensitivity to urokinase or any component; active internal bleeding; CVA or intracranial or intraspinal surgery within 2 months; recent trauma (including CPR); intracranial aneurysm, AV malformation, or intracranial neoplasm; known bleeding diatheses; severe uncontrolled arterial hypertension

Warnings Serious bleeding, including fatalities from intracranial and retroperitoneal bleeding, may occur; concurrent use with anticoagulants, other thrombolytic agents or drugs that inhibit platelet function may increase risk of serious bleed. Carefully monitor all potential bleeding sites (eg, catheter insertion sites, cutdown sites, arterial and venous puncture sites, other needle puncture sites); avoid nonessential handling of patient and I.M. injections; perform venipunctures carefully and only when necessary; if arterial puncture is necessary, use an upper extremity vessel that can be manually compressed. Discontinue urokinase if serious bleeding occurs.

Risk of bleeding may be increased for the following conditions (carefully weigh risks versus benefits before starting therapy): Recent (within 10 days) serious GI bleed, major surgery, organ biopsy, obstetrical delivery, previous puncture of noncompressible vessels; high likelihood of left heart thrombus (eg, mitral valve stenosis with atrial fibrillation); subacute bacterial endocarditis; hemostatic defects (eg, due to severe renal or hepatic disease); pregnancy; cerebrovascular disease; diabetic hemorrhagic retinopathy; other conditions where bleeding may constitute a significant hazard or be difficult to manage because of its location.

Hypersensitivity reactions, including anaphylaxis (and rarely death) have been reported. Rare cases of cholesterol embolization may occur. Urokinase is made from kidney cells that come from human neonates (postmortum harvesting) and is formulated in human albumin; products made from human sources carry a small risk of transmitting infectious agents (such as viruses), even when the proper manufacturing processes are followed.

Precautions Systemic use: Use with caution in patients with severe hypertension, recent lumbar puncture, patient receiving I.M. administration of medications. If indicated, febrile patients should receive antibiotics for at least 24 hours prior to urokinase therapy; obtain an echocardiogram in febrile patients prior to therapy to rule out intracardiac vegetations; pretreatment lab studies should include platelet count, PT/PTT, fibrinogen, fibrin degradation products, plasminogen, antithrombin III, protein S, protein C.
(Continued)

Urokinase *(Continued)*

Urokinase should only be used in hospital settings where appropriate diagnostic and monitoring techniques are available; patients must be monitored closely (see Monitoring Parameters); do not take blood pressure in lower extremities to avoid dislodgment of possible DVTs.

Adverse Reactions

Central nervous system: Fever, chills, rigor

Dermatologic: Rash

Hematologic: Hemorrhage (potentially fatal)

Local: Bleeding, hematoma at I.M. or L.P. sites

Respiratory: Bronchospasm, hypoxia, cyanosis, dyspnea

Miscellaneous: Allergic reactions, anaphylaxis, infusion reactions, cholesterol embolization (rare)

Drug Interactions Anticoagulants, thrombolytic agents, and drugs that inhibit platelet function (eg, aspirin, NSAIDs, dipyridamole) may potentiate the risk of serious bleeding (use with caution and closely monitor patients)

Stability Store unreconstituted vials in refrigerator at 2°C to 8°C (36°F to 46°F); avoid freezing. Reconstitute vials with **preservative free** SWI; do not use bacteriostatic water for injection; gently roll and tilt vial to reconstitute; **do not shake**; shaking may increase formation of filaments; thin translucent filaments may sometimes occur, but do **not** indicate a decrease in potency; after reconstitution, visually inspect for particulate matter or discoloration; reconstituted solution should be pale and straw-colored; do **not** use highly colored solutions. Does not contain preservative; vial should be reconstituted just prior to use; discard unused portion; reconstituted vial is stable for 24 hours under refrigeration

Mechanism of Action Promotes thrombolysis by directly activating plasminogen to plasmin, which degrades fibrin, fibrinogen, and other procoagulant plasma proteins

Pharmacodynamics

Onset of action: I.V.: Fibrinolysis occurs rapidly

Duration: 4 or more hours

Pharmacokinetics

Half-life: 10-20 minutes

Elimination: Cleared by the liver with a small amount excreted in the urine and the bile

Usual Dosage

Infants, Children, and Adults:

Arterial or venous thrombosis or pulmonary emboli: I.V.: Loading dose: 4400 units/kg over 10 minutes, followed by 4400 units/kg/hour for 6-12 hours; some patients may require longer (12-72 hours) or shorter courses of treatment; dose should be individualized based on response; continuous infusion doses of 4000-10,000 units/kg/hour have been used; reassess clot size every 12-24 hours

Occluded I.V. catheters:

5000 units/mL concentration; the volume to instill into the catheter is equal to the internal volume of the catheter; administer in each lumen over 1-2 minutes, leave in lumen for 1-4 hours, then **aspirate out of catheter**, flush catheter with NS; may repeat with 10,000 units in each lumen if 5000 units fails to clear the catheter; **do not infuse into the patient**

Continuous I.V. infusion: 150-200 units/kg/hour in each lumen for 8-48 hours; infuse at a rate of at least 20 mL/hour in children and adults

Dialysis patients: 5000 units is administered in each lumen over 1-2 minutes; leave urokinase in lumen for 1-2 days, then aspirate out of lumen

Adults: MI: Intracoronary: 6000 units/minute up to 2 hours

Administration Parenteral: I.V. infusion: Dilute reconstituted solution with NS or D_5W; usual final concentration: 1250-1500 units/mL; maximum concentration not yet defined. For adults, the manufacturer recommends administering the total dose (loading dose plus 12-hour infusion dose) in a final volume of 195 mL; this results in a range of final concentrations of 11,538 units/mL for adults weighing 37 kg to 32,051 units/mL for adults weighing ~114 kg.

Monitoring Parameters Vital signs and clinical response; CBC, reticulocyte, platelet count; fibrinogen level, plasminogen, fibrin/fibrinogen degradation products, D-dimer, PT, APTT, thrombin clotting time, ATIII, protein C, ACT, urinalysis

Reference Range Systemic thrombolysis: Usual desired pediatric lower limit for fibrinogen level is 100 mg/dL

Nursing Implications Use 0.22 or 0.45 micron filter during I.V. systemic therapy. Infusion reactions usually occur within 1 hour of starting infusion. Do not take blood pressure in lower extremities to avoid dislodgment of possible DVTs.

Additional Information Failure of thrombolytic agents in newborns/neonates may occur due to the low plasminogen concentrations (~50% to 70% of adult levels); higher doses of urokinase may be needed, supplementing plasminogen (via administration of fresh frozen plasma) may possibly help

After the use of I.V. urokinase, the aPTT should be less than twice the normal control value before (re)starting anticoagulants; if heparin is used, do **not** give a heparin loading dose; treatment of PE should be followed by oral anticoagulant. **Note:** Coagulation tests and measures of fibrinolytic activity do not reliably predict efficacy or risk of bleeding for patients receiving urokinase.

Two forms of urokinase exist; the forms differ in molecular weight, but have similar clinical effects; Abbokinase® contains the low molecular weight form; it consists of an A chain of 2000 daltons linked by a sulfhydryl bond to a B chain of 30,400 daltons.

Dosage Forms Injection, powder for reconstitution [preservative free]: 250,000 units [contains 250 mg human albumin, 25 mg mannitol, and 50 mg sodium chloride]

References
Andrew M, Brooker L, Leaker M, et al, "Fibrin Clot Lysis by Thrombolytic Agents Is Impaired in Newborns Due to a Low Plasminogen Concentration," *Thromb Haemost*, 1992, 68(3):325-30.

Bagnall HA, Gomperts E, and Atkinson JB, "Continuous Infusion of Low-Dose Urokinase in the Treatment of Central Venous Catheter Thrombosis in Infants and Children," *Pediatrics*, 1989, 83(6):963-6.

Kothari SS, Varma S, and Wasir HS, "Thrombolytic Therapy in Infants and Children," *Am Heart J*, 1994, 127(3):651-7.

Manco-Johnson MJ, Nuss R, Hays T, et al, "Combined Thrombolytic and Anticoagulant Therapy for Venous Thrombosis in Children," *J Pediatr*, 2000, 136(4):446-53.

Monagle P, Michelson AD, Bovill E, et al, "Antithrombotic Therapy in Children," *Chest*, 2001, 119:334S-70S.

Nowak-Gottl U, Auberger K, Halimeh S, et al, "Thrombolysis in Newborns and Infants," *Thromb Haemost*, 1999, 82 (Suppl 1):112-6.

Phelps KC and Verazino KC, "Alternatives to Urokinase for the Management of Central Venous Catheter Occlusion," *Hospital Pharmacy*, 2001, 36(3): 265-74.

Ursodiol (ER soe dye ole)

U.S. Brand Names Actigall™; Urso®
Synonyms UDCA; Ursacol; Ursodeoxycholic Acid
Therapeutic Category Gallstone Dissolution Agent
Generic Available Yes (capsule)
Use Gallbladder stone dissolution; prevention of gallstone formation (obese patients experiencing rapid weight loss); primary biliary cirrhosis (Urso®)
Unlabeled use: facilitate bile excretion in infants with biliary atresia; treatment of cholestasis secondary to PN; improve the hepatic metabolism of essential fatty acids in patients with cystic fibrosis
Pregnancy Risk Factor B
Contraindications Hypersensitivity to ursodiol, bile acids, or any component; not to be used with calcified cholesterol stones, radiopaque stones, bile pigment stones, or stones larger than 20 mm in diameter; patients with compelling reasons for cholecystectomy (eg, unremitting acute cholecystitis, cholangitis, biliary obstruction)
Warnings Gallbladder stone dissolution may take several months of therapy; complete dissolution may not occur and recurrence of stones within 5 years has been observed in 50% of patients
Precautions Use with caution in patients with a nonvisualizing gallbladder and those with chronic liver disease
Adverse Reactions
Central nervous system: Headache, fatigue, anxiety, depression, sleep disorder
Dermatologic: Rash, pruritus, hair thinning
Gastrointestinal: Diarrhea, biliary pain, constipation, stomatitis, flatulence, nausea, vomiting, abdominal pain
Hepatic: Elevated liver enzymes
Neuromuscular & skeletal: Arthralgias, myalgia, back pain
Respiratory: Cough, rhinitis
Drug Interactions Decreased effect with aluminum-containing antacids, cholestyramine, colestipol, clofibrate, oral contraceptives (estrogens), activated charcoal
Stability Store at room temperature
Mechanism of Action Decreases the cholesterol content of bile and bile stones by reducing the secretion of cholesterol from the liver and the fractional reabsorption of cholesterol by the intestines; mechanism of action in primary biliary cirrhosis is not clearly defined
Pharmacokinetics
Absorption: 90%
(Continued)

Ursodiol (Continued)

Protein binding: 70%

Metabolism: Undergoes extensive enterohepatic recycling; following hepatic conjugation and biliary secretion, the drug is hydrolyzed to active ursodiol, where it is recycled or transformed to lithocholic acid by colonic microbial flora; during chronic administration, ursodiol becomes a major biliary and plasma bile acid constituting 30% to 50% of biliary and plasma bile acids

Half-life: 100 hours

Elimination: In feces via bile

Usual Dosage Oral:

Biliary atresia: Infants: 10-15 mg/kg/day once daily

Improvement in the hepatic metabolism of essential fatty acids in cystic fibrosis: Children: 30 mg/kg/day in 2 divided doses

TPN-induced cholestasis: Infants and Children: 30 mg/kg/day in 3 divided doses

Gallstone dissolution: Adults: 8-10 mg/kg/day in 2-3 divided doses; maintenance therapy: 250 mg/day at bedtime for 6 months to 1 year; use beyond 24 months is not established

Gallstone prevention: Adults: 300 mg twice daily

Primary biliary cirrhosis: Adults: 13-15 mg/kg/day in 4 divided doses

Administration Oral: Administer with food or, if a single dosage, at bedtime

Monitoring Parameters ALT, AST, sonogram, oral cholecystogram before therapy and every 6 months during therapy; obtain ultrasound images of gallbladder at 6-month intervals for the first year of therapy

Patient Information Frequent blood work necessary to follow drug effects; report any persistent nausea, vomiting, abdominal pain

Additional Information 30% to 50% of patients have stone recurrence after dissolution

Dosage Forms

Capsule (Actigall™): 300 mg

Tablet, film-coated (Urso®): 250 mg

Extemporaneous Preparations

A 20 mg/mL ursodiol suspension may be made by opening seventeen 300 mg capsules; add in geometric proportions a 1:1 mixture of Ora-Sweet®:Ora-Plus® or 1% methylcellulose:syrup NF to a total volume of 255 mL; stable 91 days refrigerated. (Nahata, 1999)

A 25 mg/mL ursodiol suspension may be made by opening ten 300 mg capsules; mix with 10 mL Glycerin, USP until smooth mixture is obtained. Add 60 mL Ora-Plus® and continue to levigate until a smooth mixture is achieved. Transfer mixture to a light-resistent bottle; add a small amount of Orange Syrup, NF to wash remaining drug from the mortar to bottle. Add additional syrup to make final volume of 120 mL. Label "shake well"; stable 60 days at room temperature or refrigerated. (Mallett MS)

A 50 mg/mL ursodiol suspension may be made by crushing twelve 250 mg tablets, add 30 mL Ora-Plus® and 30 mL either strawberry syrup or Ora-Sweet® SF; final volume 60 mL. Stable 90 days refrigerated. (Johnson, 2002)

A 60 mg/mL ursodiol suspension may be made in a similar method by opening twelve 300 mg capsules and wetting with sufficient glycerin and triturating to make a fine paste; gradually add simple syrup to make a final volume of 60 mL. Label "shake well"; stable 35 days in refrigerator. (Johnson, 1995)

Johnson CE and Nesbitt J, "Stability of Ursodiol in an Extemporaneously Compounded Oral Liquid," *Am J Health Syst Pharm*, 1995, 52(16):1798-800.

Johnson CE and Streetman DD, "Stability of Oral Suspension of Ursodiol Made From Tablets," *Am J Health Syst Pharm*, 2002, 59(4):361-3.

Mallett MS, Hagan RL, and Peters DA, "Stability of Ursodiol 25 mg/mL in an Extemporaneously Prepared Oral Liquid," *Am J Health-Syst Pharm*, 1997, 54(12):1401-4.

Nahata MC, Morosco RS, and Hipple TF, "Stability of Ursodiol in Two Extemporaneously Prepared Oral Suspensions," *J Appl Ther Res*, 1999, 3:221-4.

References

Colombo C, Setchell KD, Podda M, et al, "Effect of Ursodeoxycholic Acid Therapy for Liver Disease Associated With Cystic Fibrosis," *J Pediatr*, 1990, 117(3):482-9.

Lepage G, Paradis K, Lacaille F, et al, "Ursodeoxycholic Acid Improves the Hepatic Metabolism of Essential Fatty Acids and Retinol in Children With Cystic Fibrosis," *J Pediatr*, 1997, 130(1)52-8.

Spagnuolo MI, Iorio R, Vegnente A, et al, "Ursodeoxycholic Acid for Treatment of Cholestasis in Children on Long-Term Total Parenteral Nutrition - A Pilot Study," *Gastroenterology*, 1996, 111(3):716-9.

Ullrich D, Rating D, Schroter W, et al, "Treatment With Ursodeoxycholic Acid Renders Children With Biliary Atresia Suitable for Liver Transplantation," *Lancet*, 1987, 2(8571):1324.

♦ **UTI Relief®** **[OTC]** *see* Phenazopyridine *on page 887*

♦ **Vagifem®** *see* Estradiol *on page 456*

♦ **Valisone® Scalp Lotion (Can)** *see* Betamethasone *on page 169*

♦ **Valium®** *see Diazepam on page 369*

♦ **Valorin [OTC]** *see Acetaminophen on page 36*

♦ **Valorin Extra [OTC]** *see Acetaminophen on page 36*

Valproic Acid and Derivatives (val PROE ik AS id & dah RIV ah tivs)

Related Information

Antiepileptic Drugs *on page 1374*

Blood Level Sampling Time Guidelines *on page 1386*

Carbohydrate and Alcohol Content of Liquid Medications for Use in Patients Receiving Ketogenic Diets *on page 1431*

Serotonin Syndrome *on page 1420*

U.S. Brand Names Depacon®; Depakene®; Depakote®; Depakote®-ER; Depakote® Sprinkle®

Canadian Brand Names Alti-Divalproex; Apo®-Divalproex; Epival® ER; Epival® I.V.; Gen-Divalproex; Novo-Divalproex; Nu-Divalproex; PMS-Valproic Acid; PMS-Valproic Acid E.C.; Rhoxal-valproic

Synonyms Dipropylacetic Acid; DPA; 2-Propylpentanoic Acid; 2-Propylvaleric Acid; VPA

Therapeutic Category Anticonvulsant, Miscellaneous; Infantile Spasms, Treatment

Generic Available Yes (capsule, as valproic acid)

Use Management of simple and complex partial seizures, simple and complex absence seizures, mixed seizure types, myoclonic and generalized tonic-clonic (grand mal) seizures; may be effective in infantile spasms; divalproex sodium delayed-release tablets (Depakote®) are also indicated for the treatment of manic episodes of bipolar disorders (manic-depressive illness) in adults; divalproex sodium delayed-release tablet (Depakote®) and extended-release tablet (Depakote®-ER) are also both indicated for the prevention of migraine headaches in adults; I.V. formulation is indicated for patients in whom oral administration of valproate is temporarily not feasible (eg, NPO for an operative procedure) or in patients with absence status epilepticus

Pregnancy Risk Factor D

Contraindications Hypersensitivity to valproic acid or derivatives or any component; hepatic disease or significant hepatic dysfunction; urea cycle disorders

Warnings Hepatic failure resulting in death may occur; children <2 years of age (especially those on polytherapy, with congenital metabolic disorders, with seizure disorders and mental retardation, or with organic brain disease) are at considerable risk; monitor patients closely for appearance of malaise, loss of seizure control, weakness, facial edema, anorexia, jaundice and vomiting; hepatotoxicity has been reported after 3 days to 6 months of therapy; discontinue valproate if hepatotoxicity occurs. Pancreatitis resulting in death may occur; pancreatitis may be hemorrhagic and rapidly progress to death; onset has occurred shortly after starting therapy and after several years of treatment; monitor patients closely for nausea, vomiting, anorexia, and abdominal pain and evaluate promptly; discontinue valproate if pancreatitis occurs. Dose-related thrombocytopenia may occur. I.V. valproate is not recommended for the prophylaxis of post-traumatic seizures in patients with acute head trauma

Hyperammonemic encephalopathy, which was sometimes fatal, has been reported following initiation of valproate therapy in patients with known or suspected urea cycle disorders (UCD) (particularly ornithine transcarbamylase deficiency). Before valproate therapy is started, evaluation for UCD should be considered in patients with 1) a history of unexplained coma or encephalopathy, encephalopathy associated with a protein load, unexplained mental retardation, pregnancy-related encephalopathy, postpartum encephalopathy, or history of increased plasma ammonia or glutamine; 2) cyclical vomiting and lethargy, episodic extreme irritability, ataxia, low BUN, or protein avoidance; 3) family history of UCD or family history of unexplained infant deaths (especially males); 4) other signs and symptoms of UCD. Patients who develop symptoms of hyperammonemic encephalopathy during therapy with valproate should receive prompt treatment; valproate therapy should be discontinued, and patients should be evaluated for UCD.

Precautions Hyperammonemia may occur, even in the absence of liver enzyme abnormalities; asymptomatic elevations of ammonia require continued monitoring; discontinuation of valproate should be considered if elevations persist. Hyperammonemic encephalopathy should be considered in patients with unexplained lethargy, vomiting, or changes in mental status and serum ammonia should be measured; valproate should be discontinued in symptomatic patients with elevated serum ammonia; hyperammonemia should be treated and patients should be evaluated for UCD. Valproate may stimulate the replication of HIV and CMV *in vitro*; clinical effects are unknown

(Continued)

Valproic Acid and Derivatives *(Continued)*

Adverse Reactions

Central nervous system: Drowsiness, irritability, confusion, restlessness, hyperactivity, malaise, headache, ataxia, dizziness, asthenia; hyperammonemic encephalopathy (in patients with UCD)

Dermatologic: Alopecia, erythema multiforme

Endocrine & metabolic: Hyperammonemia, impaired fatty-acid oxidation, carnitine deficiency

Gastrointestinal: Nausea, vomiting, diarrhea, dyspepsia, constipation, pancreatitis (potentially fatal), weight gain, taste perversion (I.V.)

Hematologic: Thrombocytopenia [risk increases significantly with serum levels ≥110 mcg/mL (females) or ≥135 mcg/mL (males)], prolongation of bleeding time

Hepatic: Transiently elevated liver enzymes, liver failure (can be fatal)

Local: I.V.: Pain and local reaction at injection site

Neuromuscular & skeletal: Tremor

Ocular: Diplopia, blurred vision

Drug Interactions
Cytochrome P450 isoenzyme CYP2C19 substrate; CYP2C9 and CYP2D6 isoenzyme inhibitor, CYP3A3/4 isoenzyme inhibitor (weak)

Valproic acid may displace phenytoin and diazepam from protein binding sites. Aspirin may displace valproic acid from protein binding sites which may result in toxicity. Valproic acid may significantly increase phenobarbital serum concentrations in patients receiving phenobarbital or primidone. Valproic acid may increase zidovudine, amitriptyline, or nortriptyline concentrations; valproic acid may inhibit the metabolism of lamotrigine and phenytoin. Phenobarbital, primidone, phenytoin, carbamazepine, and meropenem may decrease serum levels of valproic acid; felbamate may increase plasma concentrations of valproic acid; antacids may increase the oral absorption of valproic acid. Use with risperidone may result in generalized edema (case report).

Food Interactions
Dietary carnitine requirements may be increased; food may decrease the rate but not the extent of absorption

Stability
Injection: Stable for 24 hours at room temperature when diluted in D_5W, NS, or LR; discard unused portion of vial (does not contain preservative)

Mechanism of Action
Causes increased availability of gamma-aminobutyric acid (GABA), an inhibitory neurotransmitter, to brain neurons or may enhance the action of GABA or mimic its action at postsynaptic receptor sites

Pharmacokinetics

Protein binding: 80% to 90% (dose dependent); decreased protein binding in neonates and patients with renal impairment or chronic hepatic disease

Distribution: Distributes into CSF at concentrations similar to unbound concentration in plasma (ie, ~10% of total plasma concentration)

Metabolism: Extensive in liver via glucuronide conjugation and oxidation

Bioavailability: Oral (all products except Depakote®-ER): Equivalent to I.V.; **Depakote®-ER tablets are not bioequivalent to Depakote® delayed release tablets;** mean bioavailability of Depakote®-ER tablets is 81% to 89%, relative to Depakote® delayed release tablets; recent studies in adults show that when Depakote®-ER is administered in doses 8% to 20% higher than the total daily dose of Depakote®, then the 2 products are bioequivalent

Half-life: Increased with liver disease

Newborns (exposed to VPA *in utero*): 30-60 hours

Newborns 1st week of life: 40-45 hours

Newborns <10 days: 10-67 hours

Children >2 months: 7-13 hours

Children 2-14 years: Mean: 9 hours; range: 3.5-20 hours

Adults: 8-17 hours

Time to peak serum concentration:

Oral: 1-4 hours; divalproex (enteric coated): 3-5 hours

I.V.: At the end of the infusion

Elimination: 2% to 3% excreted unchanged in urine; faster clearance in children who receive other antiepileptic drugs and those who are younger; age and polytherapy explain 80% of interpatient variability in total clearance; children >10 years of age have pharmacokinetic parameters similar to adults

Usual Dosage
Note: Use of Depakote®-ER in pediatric patients is not recommended; do not confuse Depakote®-ER with Depakote®. **Erroneous substitution of Depakote® (delayed release tablets) for Depakote®-ER has resulted in toxicities; only Depakote®-ER is intended for once daily administration.**

Seizures: Children and Adults:

Oral: Initial: 10-15 mg/kg/day in 1-3 divided doses; increase by 5-10 mg/kg/day at weekly intervals until therapeutic levels are achieved; maintenance: 30-60 mg/kg/day in 2-3 divided doses; Depakote® and Depakote® Sprinkle® can be given twice daily

Note: Children receiving more than 1 anticonvulsant (ie, polytherapy) may require doses up to 100 mg/kg/day in 3-4 divided doses. Due to differences in bioavailability, adult epilepsy patients receiving Depakote® may be switched to Depakote®-ER by using a once-daily Depakote®-ER dose that is 8% to 20% higher than the total daily dose of Depakote® (see Depakote®-ER package insert for details)

I.V.: Total daily I.V. dose is equivalent to the total daily oral dose, however, I.V. dose should be divided with a frequency of every 6 hours; if I.V. form is administered 2-3 times/day, close monitoring of trough levels is recommended; switch patients to oral product as soon as clinically possible (I.V. use has not been studied for >14 days)

Rectal: Dilute syrup 1:1 with water for use as a retention enema; loading dose: 17-20 mg/kg one time; maintenance: 10-15 mg/kg/dose every 8 hours

Prophylaxis of migraine headaches: Adults: Oral:

Depakote®: Initial: 250 mg twice daily; increase dose based on patient response; maximum dose: 1000 mg/day

Depakote®-ER: Initial: 500 mg once daily for 7 days; may increase if needed to 1000 mg once daily; range: 500-1000 mg/day; dose should be individualized; if smaller dosage adjustments are needed, use Depakote® delayed release tablets; may initiate treatment with lower dose of Depakote® delayed release tablet in patients who have GI upset

Mania: Adults: Oral: Depakote®: Initial: 750 mg/day in divided doses; adjust dose as rapidly as possible to desired clinical effect or plasma concentration; maximum recommended dose: 60 mg/kg/day

Dosing adjustment in renal impairment: Cl_{cr} <10 mL/minute: No dosage adjustment is needed for patients on hemodialysis (unbound clearance of valproate is reduced (27%) in these patients, but hemodialysis reduces valproate concentrations by ~20%)

Administration

Oral: May administer with food to decrease adverse GI effects; do not administer with carbonated drinks; do not administer tablet with milk; may mix contents of Depakote® Sprinkle® capsule with semisolid food (eg, applesauce, pudding, mashed potatoes) and swallow immediately, but do not crush or chew sprinkle beads; swallow delayed release and extended release tablets whole, do not crush, break, or chew

I.V.: Dilute dose with at least 50 mL of D_5W, NS, or LR; infuse over 60 minutes; maximum infusion rate: 20 mg/minute; **Note:** Rapid infusions may be associated with an increase in adverse effects; a limited number of patients have received infusions of ≤15 mg/kg administered over 5-10 minutes (1.5-3 mg/kg/minute); patients generally tolerated these faster infusion rates, but the study was not designed to directly compare adverse effects with the recommended 1 hour infusion rate, or to assess efficacy.

Monitoring Parameters Liver enzymes, bilirubin, serum ammonia, CBC with platelets, serum concentrations

Reference Range

Therapeutic: 50-100 µg/mL (SI: 350-690 µmol/L)

Toxic: >100-150 µg/mL (SI: >690-1040 µmol/L)

Seizure control may improve at levels >100 µg/mL (SI: >690 µmol/L), but toxicity may occur

Test Interactions False-positive result for urine ketones; altered thyroid function tests

Patient Information Avoid alcohol; may cause drowsiness and impair ability to perform activities requiring mental alertness and physical coordination; notify physician if nausea, vomiting, unexplained lethargy, change in mental status, general feeling of weakness, loss of appetite, abdominal pain, yellow skin, bleeding, or easy bruising occur

Nursing Implications Instruct patients/parents to report signs or symptoms of hepatotoxicity, pancreatitis, and hyperammonemic encephalopathy (see Warnings); GI side effects of divalproex may be less than valproic acid

Additional Information A valproic acid associated Reye's-like syndrome has been reported (see Hilmas, 2000). Acute intoxications: Naloxone may reverse the CNS depressant effects but may also block the action of other anticonvulsants; carnitine may reduce the ammonia level; multiple dosing of activated charcoal can enhance elimination.

Routine prophylactic use of carnitine in children receiving valproic acid to avoid carnitine deficiency and hepatotoxicity is probably not indicated (Freeman, 1994); a case of fatal hepatotoxic reaction has been reported in a child receiving valproic acid despite carnitine supplementation (Murphy, 1993)

(Continued)

Valproic Acid and Derivatives *(Continued)*

Sodium content of valproate sodium syrup: 5 mL = 23 mg (1 mEq of sodium); safety of I.V. form has not been well studied in children <2 years of age

Dosage Forms

Capsule, as **valproic acid** (Depakene®): 250 mg

Capsule, sprinkles, as **divalproex sodium** (Depakote® Sprinkle®): 125 mg

Injection, solution, as **sodium valproate** (Depacon®): 100 mg/mL (5 mL)

Syrup, as **sodium valproate**: 250 mg/5 mL (5 mL, 480 mL)

Depakene®: 250 mg/mL (480 mL)

Tablet, delayed release, as **divalproex sodium** (Depakote®): 125 mg, 250 mg, 500 mg

Tablet, extended release, as **divalproex sodium** (Depakote®-ER): 500 mg

References

Cloyd JC, Fischer JH, Kriel RL, et al, "Valproic Acid Pharmacokinetics in Children. IV. Effects of Age and Antiepileptic Drugs on Protein Binding and Intrinsic Clearance," *Clin Pharmacol Ther*, 1993, 53(1):22-9.

Cloyd JC, Kriel RL, Fischer JH, et al, "Pharmacokinetics of Valproic Acid in Children: I. Multiple Antiepileptic Drug Therapy," *Neurology*, 1983, 33(2):185-91.

Dreifuss FE, Santilli N, Langer DH, et al, "Valproic Acid Hepatic Fatalities: A Retrospective Review," *Neurology*, 1987, 37(3):379-85.

Freeman JM, Vining EP, Cost S, et al, "Does Carnitine Administration Improve the Symptoms Attributed to Anticonvulsant Medications?: A Double-Blinded, Crossover Study," *Pediatrics*, 1994, 93(6 Pt 1):893-5.

Hilmas E and Lee CK, "Valproic Acid-Related Reye's-Like Syndrome," *The Journal of Pediatric Pharmacy Practice*, 2000, 5(3):149-55.

Murphy JV, Groover RV and Hodge C, "Hepatotoxic Effects in a Child Receiving Valproate and Carnitine," *J Pediatr*, 1993, 123(2):318-20.

♦ **Vancenase® AQ 84 mcg [DSC]** *see* Beclomethasone *on page 160*

♦ **Vancenase® Pockethaler® [DSC]** *see* Beclomethasone *on page 160*

♦ **Vanceril® [DSC]** *see* Beclomethasone *on page 160*

♦ **Vancocin®** *see* Vancomycin *on page 1134*

Vancomycin *(van koe MYE sin)*

Related Information

Blood Level Sampling Time Guidelines *on page 1386*

Carbohydrate and Alcohol Content of Liquid Medications for Use in Patients Receiving Ketogenic Diets *on page 1431*

Endocarditis Prophylaxis *on page 1321*

U.S. Brand Names Vancocin®

Therapeutic Category Antibiotic, Miscellaneous

Generic Available Yes (injection)

Use

Parenteral: Treatment of patients with the following infections or conditions: Infections due to documented or suspected methicillin-resistant *S. aureus* or beta-lactam resistant coagulase negative *Staphylococcus*; serious or life-threatening infections (ie, endocarditis, meningitis, osteomyelitis) due to documented or suspected staphylococcal or streptococcal infections in patients who are allergic to penicillins and/or cephalosporins; empiric therapy of infections associated with central lines, VP shunts, hemodialysis shunts, vascular grafts, prosthetic heart valves

Oral: Treatment of staphylococcal enterocolitis or for antibiotic-associated pseudomembranous colitis produced by *C. difficile*

Pregnancy Risk Factor C

Contraindications Hypersensitivity to vancomycin or any component; avoid in patients with previous hearing loss

Warnings Use may result in superinfection

Precautions Use with caution in patients with renal impairment or those receiving other nephrotoxic or ototoxic drugs; dosage modification required in patients with impaired renal function

Adverse Reactions Rapid infusion associated with red neck or red man syndrome: Erythema multiforme-like reaction with intense pruritus, tachycardia, hypotension, rash involving face, neck, upper trunk, back and upper arms; red man or red neck syndrome usually develops during a rapid infusion of vancomycin or with doses ≥15-20 mg/kg/hour; reaction usually dissipates in 30-60 minutes

Cardiovascular: Cardiac arrest

Central nervous system: Fever, chills

Dermatologic: Red neck or red man syndrome, urticaria, macular skin rash

Gastrointestinal: Nausea

Hematologic: Neutropenia, eosinophilia

Local: Phlebitis

Neuromuscular & skeletal: Lower back pain

Otic: Ototoxicity associated with prolonged serum concentration >40 µg/mL

Renal: Nephrotoxicity (higher incidence with trough concentrations >10 µg/mL)

Miscellaneous: Hypersensitivity reactions

Drug Interactions Anesthetic agents (erythema, hypotension, hypothermia, and facial flushing); concurrent ototoxic or nephrotoxic drugs including loop diuretics, cisplatin, and aminoglycosides

Stability After the oral or parenteral solution is reconstituted, refrigerate and use within 2 weeks; incompatible with heparin, phenobarbital, and ceftazidime

Mechanism of Action Inhibits bacterial cell wall synthesis; alters bacterial-cell-membrane permeability; blocks glycopeptide polymerization of the phosphodisaccha-ride-pentapeptide complex in the second stage of cell wall synthesis by binding tightly to D-alanyl-D-alanine portion of cell wall precursor

Pharmacokinetics

Absorption:

Oral: Poor

I.M.: Erratic

Intraperitoneal administration can result in 38% systemic absorption

Distribution: Widely distributed in body tissues and fluids including pericardial, pleural, ascites, and synovial fluids; low concentration in CSF if meninges are inflamed

Protein binding: 55%

Metabolism: <3%

Half-life, biphasic: Prolonged significantly with reduced renal function

Terminal:

Newborns: 6-10 hours

3 months to 4 years: 4 hours

>3 years: 2.2-3 hours

Adults: 5-8 hours

Elimination: Primarily via glomerular filtration; excreted as unchanged drug in the urine (80% to 90%); oral doses are excreted primarily in the feces; presence of malignancy in children is associated with an increase in vancomycin clearance

Dialysis: Not dialyzable (0% to 5%)

Usual Dosage Initial dosage recommendation:

Neonates: I.V.:

Postnatal age ≤7 days:

<1200 g: 15 mg/kg/day given every 24 hours

1200-2000 g: 10-15 mg/kg/dose given every 12-18 hours

>2000 g: 10-15 mg/kg/dose given every 8-12 hours

Postnatal age >7 days:

<1200 g: 15 mg/kg/day given every 24 hours

1200-2000 g: 10-15 mg/kg/dose given every 8-12 hours

>2000 g: 15-20 mg/kg/dose given every 8 hours

Infants >1 month and Children: I.V.: 40 mg/kg/day in divided doses every 6-8 hours

Nonobese pediatric cancer patients with normal renal function (n=28, age range: 9 months to 13 years): initial dosage regimen of 60 mg/kg/day divided every 6 hours has been recommended

Staphylococcal CNS infection: I.V.: 60 mg/kg/day in divided doses every 6 hours; maximum dose: 1 g/dose

Adults (with normal renal function): I.V.: 0.5 g every 6 hours or 1 g every 12 hours; maximum dose: 4 g/day

Dosing interval in renal impairment:

Cl$_{cr}$ >90 mL/minute: Administer normal dose every 6 hours

Cl$_{cr}$ 70-89 mL/minute: Administer normal dose every 8 hours

Cl$_{cr}$ 46-69 mL/minute: Administer normal dose every 12 hours

Cl$_{cr}$ 30-45 mL/minute: Administer normal dose every 18 hours

Cl$_{cr}$ 15-29 mL/minute: Administer normal dose every 24 hours

Renal dysfunction, end stage renal disease, or on dialysis: 10-20 mg/kg; subsequent dosages and frequency of administration are best determined by measurement of serum levels and assessment of renal insufficiency

Intrathecal/intraventricular:

Neonates: 5-10 mg/day

Children: 5-20 mg/day

Adults: 20 mg/day

Oral (antibiotic-associated pseudomembraneous colitis: Metronidazole is the drug of initial choice per 2000 Red Book recommendations):

Children: 40 mg/kg/day in divided doses every 6 hours for 7-10 days; not to exceed 2 g/day

Adults: 0.5-2 g/day in divided doses every 6-8 hours

(Continued)

Vancomycin *(Continued)*

Prophylaxis of endocarditis in penicillin allergic patients: I.V.:
  GI or genitourinary procedures:
    Children: 20 mg/kg 1 hour prior to the procedure **plus** gentamicin 1.5 mg/kg 30 minutes prior to the procedure
    Adults: 1 g 1 hour prior to the procedure **plus** gentamicin 1.5 mg/kg (maximum dose: 120 mg) 30 minutes prior to the procedure

Administration

Oral: May further dilute the appropriate oral solution dose in water or with a flavoring syrup to improve the taste

Parenteral: Administer vancomycin by I.V. intermittent infusion over 60 minutes at a final concentration not to exceed 5 mg/mL; if a maculopapular rash appears on face, neck, trunk, and upper extremities, slow the infusion rate to administer dose over 1½ to 2 hours and increase the dilution volume; the reaction usually dissipates in 30-60 minutes; administration of antihistamines just before the infusion may also prevent or minimize this reaction

Intrathecal/Intraventricular: Dilute in NS without preservatives to a final concentration between 2-5 mg/mL

Monitoring Parameters Periodic renal function tests, urinalysis, serum vancomycin concentrations, WBC; audiogram (in patients who concurrently receive ototoxic chemotherapy)

Reference Range

Peak: 25-40 µg/mL
Trough: 5-10 µg/mL

Patient Information Report pain at infusion site; dizziness, fullness or ringing in ears with I.V. use

Nursing Implications Do not administer I.M.; peak levels are drawn 30 minutes to 1 hour after the completion of a 1-hour infusion; troughs are obtained just before the next dose

Dosage Forms

Capsule, as hydrochloride (Vancocin®): 125 mg, 250 mg

Infusion, as hydrochloride [premixed in iso-osmotic dextrose]: 500 mg (100 mL), 1 g (200 mL)

Injection, powder for reconstitution, lyophilized, as hydrochloride: 500 mg, 1 g, 5 g, 10 g
Vancocin®: 500 mg, 1 g, 10 g [all sizes DSC]

Powder for oral solution, as hydrochloride (Vancocin®): 1 g [provides 250 mg/5 mL when mixed]; 10 g [provides 500 mg/6 mL when mixed; contains alcohol]

References

American Academy of Pediatrics Committee on Infectious Diseases, "Treatment of Bacterial Meningitis," *Pediatrics*, 1998, 81(6):904-7.

Chang D, "Influence of Malignancy on the Pharmacokinetics of Vancomycin in Infants and Children," *Pediatr Infect Dis J*, 1995, 14(8):667-73.

Chang D, Liem L, and Malogolowkin M, "A Prospective Study of Vancomycin Pharmacokinetics and Dosage Requirements in Pediatric Cancer Patients," *Pediatr Infect Dis J*, 1994, 13(11):969-74.

Leonard MB, Koren G, Stevenson DK, et al, "Vancomycin Pharmacokinetics in Very Low Birth Weight Neonates," *Pediatr Infect Dis J*, 1989, 8(5):282-6.

Matzke GR, Zhanel GG, and Guay DRP, "Clinical Pharmacokinetics of Vancomycin," *Clin Pharmacokinet*, 1986, 11(4):257-82.

Rodvold KA, Everett JA, Pryka RD, and Kraus DM, "Pharmacokinetics and Administration Regimens of Vancomycin in Neonates, Infants and Children," *Clin Pharmacokinet*, 1997, 33(1):32-51.

Rybak MJ, Albrecht LM, Boike SC, et al, "Nephrotoxicity of Vancomycin, Alone and With an Aminoglycoside," *J Antimicrob Chemother*, 1990, 25(4):679-87.

♦ **Vantin®** *see* Cefpodoxime *on page 235*

♦ **Vaponefrin® (Can)** *see* Epinephrine *on page 439*

♦ **Varicella-Zoster Immune Globulin (Human)** *see page 1333*

♦ **VasoClear® [OTC]** *see* Naphazoline *on page 795*

♦ **Vasocon® (Can)** *see* Naphazoline *on page 795*

Vasopressin *(vay soe PRES in)*

Related Information

Adult ACLS Algorithm, Cardiac Arrest *on page 1183*
Adult ACLS Algorithm, Comprehensive ECC *on page 1184*
Adult ACLS Algorithm, V. Fib and Pulseless VT *on page 1185*

U.S. Brand Names Pitressin®

Canadian Brand Names Pressyn®

Synonyms ADH; Antidiuretic Hormone; 8-Arginine Vasopressin

Therapeutic Category Antidiuretic Hormone Analog; Hormone, Posterior Pituitary

Generic Available No

Use Treatment of diabetes insipidus; prevention and treatment of postoperative abdominal distention; differential diagnosis of diabetes insipidus; adjunct in the treatment of acute massive hemorrhage of GI tract or esophageal varices; treatment of ventricular fibrillation or tachycardia refractory to initial defibrillation (see Adult ACLS Algorithms *on page 1183*); treatment of vasodilatory shock with hypotension unresponsive to fluid resuscitation or exogenous catecholamines

Pregnancy Risk Factor B

Contraindications Hypersensitivity to vasopressin or any component

Warnings I.V. infiltration may lead to severe vasoconstriction and localized tissue necrosis

Precautions Use with caution in patients with seizure disorders, migraine, asthma, vascular disease, renal disease, cardiac disease, goiter with cardiac complications, arteriosclerosis, chronic nephritis with nitrogen retention; an increased risk of cardiac arrest has been reported in adults receiving I.V. infusions at rates >0.05 units/minute

Adverse Reactions
Cardiovascular: Circumoral pallor; with high doses: hypertension, bradycardia, arrhythmias, venous thrombosis, vasoconstriction, angina, heart block, cardiac arrest, distal limb ischemia (I.V. infusion rates >10 units/hour)
Central nervous system: Vertigo, fever, headache
Dermatologic: Urticaria
Endocrine & metabolic: Water intoxication, hyponatremia
Gastrointestinal: Abdominal cramps, nausea, vomiting, flatus, diarrhea
Local: Skin necrosis (after extravasation of I.V. infiltration)
Neuromuscular & skeletal: Tremor
Respiratory: Wheezing, bronchoconstriction
Miscellaneous: Diaphoresis

Drug Interactions
Decreased antidiuretic activity: Lithium, demeclocycline, large doses of epinephrine, heparin (therapeutic doses), alcohol
Increased antidiuretic activity: Chlorpropamide, carbamazepine, phenformin, tricyclic antidepressants, clofibrate, fludrocortisone

Mechanism of Action Increases cyclic adenosine monophosphate (cAMP) which increases water permeability at the distal convoluted tubule and collecting duct resulting in decreased urine volume and increased urine osmolality; causes peristalsis by directly stimulating the smooth muscle in the GI tract (in doses greater than those required for its antidiuretic action); causes vasoconstriction (primarily of capillaries and small arterioles); directly stimulates receptors in pituitary gland resulting in increased ACTH production

Pharmacodynamics I.M., S.C.:
Onset of action: 1 hour
Duration: 2-8 hours

Pharmacokinetics Destroyed by trypsin in GI tract, must be administered parenterally
Metabolism: Most of dose is rapidly metabolized in liver and kidney
Half-life: 10-35 minutes

Usual Dosage
Diabetes insipidus:
I.M., S.C.: (Highly variable dosage; titrate dosage based upon serum and urine sodium and osmolality in addition to fluid balance and urine output)
Children: 2.5-10 units 2-4 times/day
Adults: 5-10 units 2-4 times/day as needed (range: 5-60 units/day)
Continuous infusion: Children and Adults: Initial: 0.5 milliunit/kg/hour (0.0005 unit/kg/hour); double dosage as needed every 30 minutes to a maximum of 10 milliunit/kg/hour (0.01 units/kg/hour)
Abdominal distention: Adults: I.M.: 5 units initially, then repeated every 3-4 hours; dosage may be increased to 10 units if necessary
Ventricular fibrillation or tachycardia unresponsive to initial defibrillation: Adults: I.V.: 40 units as a single dose only (see Adult ACLS Algorithms *on page 1183*)
GI hemorrhage: I.V. continuous infusion (may also be infused directly into the superior mesenteric artery):
Children: Initial: 0.002-0.005 units/kg/minute; titrate dose as needed; maximum dose: 0.01 units/kg/minute;
or as an alternative: Initial: 0.1 units/minute; increase by 0.05 units/minute to a maximum of:
<5 years: 0.2 units/minute
5-12 years: 0.3 units/minute
>12 years: 0.4 units/minute
If bleeding stops for 12 hours, then taper off over 24-48 hours
(Continued)

Vasopressin *(Continued)*

Adults: Initial: I.V.: 0.2-0.4 unit/minute, then titrate dose as needed (maximum dose: 0.9 units/minute); if bleeding stops, continue at same dose for 12 hours, taper off over 24-48 hours

Vasodilatory shock with hypotension unresponsive to fluid resuscitation and exogenous catecholamines: **Note:** Optimal dosage has not been clearly established in any patient population: I.V.:

Infants and Children: Limited study in 11 infants and children treated for profound hypotension following cardiac surgery: Initial: 0.0003-0.002 units/kg/minute; titrate to effect (Rosenzweig, 1999)

Adults: Initial: 0.04-0.1 units/minute; titrate to effect (doses >0.05 units/minute have been associated with increased risk of cardiac arrest in some patients)

Note: Abrupt discontinuation of infusion may result in hypotension; to discontinue gradually taper infusion

Dosing adjustment in hepatic impairment: Some patients with cirrhosis respond to much lower doses

Administration Parenteral:

I.V.: Continuous infusion: Dilute in NS or D_5W to a final concentration of 0.1-1 unit/mL; see Usual Dosage for rate of infusion

I.M.: Administer without further dilution

Monitoring Parameters Fluid intake and output, urine specific gravity, urine and serum osmolality, serum and urine sodium; hemoglobin and hematocrit (GI bleeding)

Reference Range Vasopressin levels:

Basal: <4 pg/mL

Water deprivation: 10 pg/mL

Shock: 100-1000 pg/mL (biphasic response)

Patient Information Avoid alcohol

Dosage Forms

Injection, solution, aqueous: 20 pressor units/mL (0.5 mL, 1 mL, 10 mL)

Pitressin®: 20 pressor units/mL (1 mL)

References

Hodges BM and Fraser G, "Vasopressin for Vasodilatory Shock," *Hosp Pharm*, 2002, 37(11):1149-57.

Rosenzweig EB, Starc TJ, Chen JM, et al, "Intravenous Arginine-Vasopressin in Children With Vasodilatory Shock After Cardiac Surgery," *Circulation*, 1999, 100(19 Suppl):II182-6.

Tuggle DW, Bennett KG, Scott J, et al, "Intravenous Vasopressin and Gastrointestinal Hemorrhage in Children," *J Pediatr Surg*, 1988, 23(7):627-9.

◆ **Vasotec®** *see* Enalapril/Enalaprilat *on page 431*

◆ **Vasotec® I.V.** *see* Enalapril/Enalaprilat *on page 431*

◆ **VCR** *see* VinCRIStine *on page 1149*

Vecuronium (ve KYOO roe nee um)

U.S. Brand Names Norcuron®

Synonyms ORG NC 45

Therapeutic Category Neuromuscular Blocker Agent, Nondepolarizing; Skeletal Muscle Relaxant, Paralytic

Generic Available Yes

Use Adjunct to anesthesia, to facilitate endotracheal intubation, and provide skeletal muscle relaxation during surgery or mechanical ventilation

Pregnancy Risk Factor C

Contraindications Hypersensitivity to vecuronium or any component (see Warnings)

Clinical Conditions Affecting Neuromuscular Blockade

Potentiation	Antagonism
Electrolyte abnormalities	Alkalosis
Severe hyponatremia	Hypercalcemia
Severe hypocalcemia	Demyelinating lesions
Severe hypokalemia	Peripheral neuropathies
Hypermagnesemia	Diabetes mellitus
Neuromuscular diseases	
Acidosis	
Acute intermittent porphyria	
Renal failure	
Hepatic failure	

Warnings Ventilation must be supported during neuromuscular blockade; use only by individuals who are experienced in the maintenance of an adequate airway and respiratory support. Commercially supplied diluent contains benzyl alcohol which may cause allergic reactions in susceptible individuals; large amounts of benzyl alcohol (≥99 mg/kg/day) have been associated with a potentially fatal toxicity ("gasping syndrome") in neonates; the "gasping syndrome" consists of metabolic acidosis, respiratory distress, gasping respirations, CNS dysfunction (including convulsions, intracranial hemorrhage), hypotension and cardiovascular collapse; *in vitro* and animal studies have shown that benzoate, a metabolite of benzyl alcohol, displaces bilirubin from protein binding sites; avoid use of benzyl alcohol containing diluent in neonates; SWI may be used for reconstitution in neonates

Precautions Use with caution in patients with hepatic impairment, neuromuscular disease, myasthenia gravis; many clinical conditions may potentiate or antagonize neuromuscular blockade, see table on previous page.

Adverse Reactions Most frequent reactions are associated with prolongation of its pharmacologic effect

Cardiovascular: Arrhythmias, tachycardia, hypotension, hypertension

Dermatologic: Urticaria, rash

Neuromuscular & skeletal: Muscle weakness

Respiratory: Respiratory insufficiency, bronchospasm, apnea

Drug Interactions See table.

Potential Drug Interactions

Potentiation	Antagonism
Inhalation anesthetics	Calcium
Desflurane, sevoflurane, enflurane and	Carbamazepine
isoflurane > halothane > nitrous	Phenytoin
oxide	Steroids (chronic administration)
Antibiotics	Theophylline
Aminoglycosides, polymyxins,	Anticholinesterases*
clindamycin, vancomycin, tetracycline	Neostigmine, pyridostigmine,
Magnesium	edrophonium, echothiophate
Antiarrhythmics	ophthalmic solution
Quinidine, procainamide, bretylium, and	Caffeine
possibly lidocaine	Azathioprine
Diuretics	
Furosemide, mannitol, thiazides	
Amphotericin B (secondary to hypokalemia)	
Local anesthetics	
Dantrolene (directly depresses skeletal muscle)	
Beta blockers	
Calcium channel blockers	
Ketamine	
Lithium	
Succinylcholine (when administered prior to nondepolarizing neuromuscular-blocking agent)	
Cyclosporine	

*Can prolong the effects of acetylcholine

Stability Stable for 5 days at room temperature when reconstituted with bacteriostatic water; stable for 24 hours at room temperature when reconstituted with preservative free SWI or other compatible I.V. fluid (dextrose, NS, or LR) (avoid preservatives in neonates); do not mix with alkaline drugs

Mechanism of Action Nondepolarizing neuromuscular blocker which blocks acetylcholine from binding to receptors on motor endplate thus inhibiting depolarization

Pharmacodynamics

Onset of action: Within 1-3 minutes

Duration (dose dependent): 30-40 minutes

Pharmacokinetics

Distribution: V_d:

Infants: 0.36 L/kg

Children: 0.2 L/kg

Adults: 0.27 L/kg

Protein binding: 60% to 80%

Half-life, distribution: Adults: 4 minutes

(Continued)

Vecuronium *(Continued)*

Half-life, elimination:
Infants: 65 minutes
Children: 41 minutes
Adults: 65-75 minutes
Elimination: Vecuronium bromide and its metabolite(s) appear to be excreted principally in feces via biliary elimination (50%); the drug and its metabolite(s) are also excreted in urine (25%); the rate of elimination is appreciably reduced with hepatic dysfunction but not with renal dysfunction

Usual Dosage I.V.:
Neonates: 0.1 mg/kg/dose; maintenance: 0.03-0.15 mg/kg/dose every 1-2 hours as needed
Infants >7 weeks to 1 year: 0.1 mg/kg/dose; repeat every hour as needed; may be administered as a continuous infusion at 1-1.5 mcg/kg/minute (0.06-0.09 mg/kg/hour)
Children >1 year: 0.1 mg/kg/dose; repeat every hour as needed; may be administered as a continuous infusion at 1.5-2.5 mcg/kg/minute (0.09-0.15 mg/kg/hour)
Adults: 0.1 mg/kg/dose; repeat every hour as needed; may be administered as a continuous infusion at 1.5-2 mcg/kg/minute (0.09-0.12 mg/kg/hour)
Dosing adjustment in hepatic impairment: Dose reductions are necessary in patients with cirrhosis or cholestasis
Administration Parenteral: I.V.: Dilute vial to a maximum concentration of 2 mg/mL and administer by rapid direct injection; for continuous infusion, dilute to a maximum concentration of 1 mg/mL in D_5W, NS, or LR; use SWI instead of provided diluent (contains benzyl alcohol) in neonates (see Warnings)
Monitoring Parameters Assisted ventilation status, heart rate, blood pressure, peripheral nerve stimulator measuring twitch response
Nursing Implications Does not alter the patient's state of consciousness; addition of sedation and analgesia is recommended
Additional Information Produces minimal, if any, histamine release
Dosage Forms Injection, powder for reconstitution, lyophilized, as bromide: 10 mg, 20 mg [may be supplied with diluent containing benzyl alcohol]
References
Martin LD, Bratton SL, and O'Rourke PP, "Clinical Uses and Controversies of Neuromuscular Blocking Agents in Infants and Children," *Crit Care Med*, 1999, 27(7):1358-68.

♦ **Veetids®** *see* Penicillin V Potassium *on page 877*

♦ **Veg-Pancreatin 4X [OTC]** *see* Pancreatin *on page 855*

♦ **Velban® [DSC]** *see* VinBLAStine *on page 1148*

♦ **Velosef®** *see* Cephradine *on page 247*

♦ **Velosulin® BR Human (Buffered)** *see* Insulin Preparations *on page 609*

Venlafaxine *(VEN la faks een)*

U.S. Brand Names Effexor®; Effexor® XR
Therapeutic Category Antidepressant, Serotonin/Norepinephrine Reuptake Inhibitor
Generic Available No
Use Treatment of depression, generalized anxiety disorder, social anxiety disorder; prevention of recurrences/relapses of depression; has also been used to treat ADHD and autism in children and obsessive-compulsive disorder and chronic fatigue syndrome in adults
Pregnancy Risk Factor C
Contraindications Hypersensitivity to venlafaxine or any component; use of MAO inhibitors within 14 days (potentially fatal reactions may occur, see Drug Interactions); do not initiate MAO inhibitor within 7 days of discontinuing venlafaxine
Warnings May cause sustained increase in blood pressure (dose dependent; monitor blood pressure; dose reduction or discontinuation may be needed)
Precautions Use with caution and decrease the dose in patients with renal or hepatic impairment. Use with caution in patients with seizure disorders (seizures have been reported; discontinue if seizures occur), concomitant illnesses that may affect hepatic metabolism or hemodynamic responses (eg, unstable cardiac disease, recent MI), history of mania (may activate mania or hypomania), and in suicidal patients. Use with caution in patients receiving diuretics, those who are volume-depleted or elderly (may cause hyponatremia or SIADH); may cause mydriasis (use with caution and closely monitor patients with increased IOP or those at risk of acute narrow-angle glaucoma). May cause anxiety, nervousness, and insomnia; may cause anorexia and significant weight loss (use with caution in patients where weight loss is undesirable); may cause abnormal bleeding (eg, ecchymosis; use with caution in patients with abnormal platelet function); may cause tachycardia [use with caution in patients with underlying medical conditions (eg, recent MI, heart failure, hyperthyroidism) that may

worsen with tachycardia, especially at doses >200 mg/day in adults]. In adult studies of depression, Effexor® XR was associated with an increase in QT_c interval of 4.7 msec from baseline (versus a 1.9 msec decrease for placebo); clinical significance of this effect is not known.

Discontinuation symptoms (including agitation, dysphoria, anxiety, confusion, dizziness, hypomania, nightmares, and other symptoms) may occur if therapy is abruptly discontinued or dose reduced; risk of discontinuation symptoms may be increased at higher doses and with longer duration of therapy; to discontinue therapy in patients receiving venlafaxine for >1 week, taper the dose to minimize risks of discontinuation symptoms; to discontinue therapy in patients receiving venlafaxine for ≥6 weeks, taper the dose gradually over at least 2 weeks. **Note:** Clinical trials of Effexor® XR tapered the daily dose slowly at 1 week intervals by increments of 75 mg

Adverse Reactions

Cardiovascular system: Vasodilation, hypertension (dose-related), tachycardia, chest pain, postural hypotension

Central nervous system: Headache, somnolence, dizziness, insomnia, nervousness, anxiety, abnormal dreams, yawning, agitation, confusion, abnormal thinking, depersonalization, depression, manic reaction (0.5%), seizures (0.3%); **Note:** Increased hyperactivity (behavioral activation) was observed in several children treated for ADHD (see Olvera, 1996)

Dermatologic: Rash, pruritus

Endocrine & metabolic: Anorexia, weight loss (dose-related), hyponatremia, SIADH, hypercholesterolemia

Gastrointestinal: Nausea, xerostomia, constipation, diarrhea, vomiting, dyspepsia, flatulence, altered taste, abdominal pain

Genitourinary: Sexual dysfunction, urinary frequency, impaired urination, urinary retention; priapism (case report in an adolescent patient; see Samuel, 2000)

Hematologic: Abnormal bleeding, ecchymosis

Neuromuscular & skeletal: Asthenia, tremor, hypertonia, twitching, paresthesia

Ocular: Blurred vision, mydriasis

Otic: Tinnitus

Miscellaneous: Diaphoresis, chills

Drug Interactions Cytochrome P450 isoenzyme CYP2D6 (O-desmethylation), CYP2E1, and CYP3A3/4 (N-demethylation) enzyme substrate; CYP2D6 enzyme inhibitor (weak)

Use within 2 weeks of MAO inhibitors or use of MAO inhibitors within 7 days of discontinuing venlafaxine may result in hyperthermia (with features similar to neuroleptic malignant syndrome), tremors, myoclonus, nausea, vomiting, diaphoresis, flushing, dizziness, seizures, and death (see Contraindications). Concurrent use with buspirone, meperidine, TCAs, selective serotonin reuptake inhibitors (SSRIs) or serotonin agonists (eg, sumatriptan) may result in serotonin syndrome (concurrent use is best avoided). Tryptophan (which can be metabolized to serotonin) and the herbal medicine St John's wort (*Hypericum perforatum*), may increase serious side effects; use of these agents is **not** recommended.

Venlafaxine significantly increases haloperidol serum concentrations (increases AUC by 70%); may increase clozapine concentrations and result in adverse effects (eg, seizures); may increase PT, PTT, or INR in patients receiving warfarin. Concurrent use with imipramine may increase serum concentrations of desipramine and 2-OH-desipramine (metabolites of imipramine). Venlafaxine may increase serum concentrations of risperidone, but does not significantly alter the disposition of the total active moiety [risperidone plus 9-hydroxyrisperidone (active metabolite)]. **Note:** Interactions of venlafaxine with other CNS agents have not been evaluated (use such drugs with caution). Venlafaxine may decrease indinavir AUC by 28% and peak serum concentrations by 36%.

Drugs that inhibit cytochrome P450 CYP2D6, CYP2E1, or CYP3A4 may inhibit the metabolism of venlafaxine (monitor for increased effect or toxicity). Cimetidine increased venlafaxine serum concentrations, but did not affect ODV (active metabolite) concentrations; no dosage adjustment is needed for most patients; however, this interaction may be more pronounced in patients with hepatic dysfunction, hypertension, or in the elderly (use with caution and monitor in these patients). Enzyme inducers may increase the metabolism of venlafaxine, reducing its effectiveness.

Food Interactions Food does not affect bioavailability of venlafaxine or ODV (active metabolite); tryptophan supplements may increase serious side effects

Stability Tablets and capsules: Store at controlled room temperature, 20°C to 25°C (68°F to 77°F); Effexor® tablets: Store in a dry place, dispense in a tight container; Effexor® XR 37.5 mg capsules: Protect from light and dispense in light resistant container

(Continued)

Venlafaxine *(Continued)*

Mechanism of Action Venlafaxine and o-desmethylvenlafaxine (ODV) are potent inhibitors of CNS neuronal serotonin and norepinephrine reuptake and weak inhibitors of dopamine reuptake; venlafaxine and ODV do not significantly bind to alpha-adrenergic, histamine, or muscarinic cholinergic receptors (may therefore be useful in patients at risk from sedation, hypotension and anticholinergic effects of tricyclic antidepressants); venlafaxine and ODV do not inhibit monoamine oxidase

Pharmacokinetics

Absorption: Oral: ≥92%

Distribution: Distributes into breast milk; breast milk to plasma ratio: Venlafaxine: 2.8-4.8 (mean 4.1); ODV: 2.8-3.8 (mean 3.1) (Ilett, 1998)

Mean V_d (apparent): Adults:
  Venlafaxine: 7.5 ± 3.7 L/kg
  ODV: 5.7 ± 1.8 L/kg

Protein binding: Venlafaxine: 27%; ODV: 30%

Metabolism: Extensive in the liver, primarily via cytochrome P450 CYP2D6 to o-desmethylvenlafaxine (ODV; active metabolite); also metabolized to N-desmethylvenlafaxine, N,O-desmethylvenlafaxine, and other minor metabolites. **Note:** Clinically important differences between CYP2D6 poor and extensive metabolizers is not expected (sum of venlafaxine and ODV serum concentrations is similar in poor and extensive metabolizers; ODV is approximately equal in activity and potency to venlafaxine)

Bioavailability: Oral: 45%

Half-life:
  Adults: Venlafaxine: 5 ± 2 hours; ODV: 11 ± 2 hours
  Adults with cirrhosis: Venlafaxine: Half-life prolonged by ~30%; ODV: Half-life prolonged by ~60%
  Adults with renal impairment (GFR: 10-70 mL/minute): Venlafaxine: Half-life prolonged by ~50%; ODV: Half-life prolonged by ~40%
  Adults on dialysis: Venlafaxine: Half-life prolonged by ~180%; ODV: Half-life prolonged by 142%

Time to peak serum concentration:
  Immediate release: Venlafaxine: 2 hours; ODV: 3 hours
  Extended release: Venlafaxine: 5.5 hours; ODV: 9 hours

Elimination: ~87% of dose is excreted in urine within 48 hours; 5% as unchanged drug, 29% as unconjugated ODV, 26% as conjugated ODV, and 27% as other minor metabolites

Clearance:
  Adults with cirrhosis: Venlafaxine: Clearance is decreased by ~50%; ODV: Clearance is decreased by ~30%
  Adults with more severe cirrhosis: Venlafaxine: Clearance is decreased by ~90%
  Adults with renal impairment (GFR: 10-70 mL/minute): Venlafaxine: Clearance is decreased by ~24%; ODV: Clearance unchanged versus normal subjects
  Adults on dialysis: Venlafaxine: Clearance decreased by ~57%; ODV: Clearance decreased by ~56%

Dialysis: Not likely to significantly remove drug due to large volume of distribution

Usual Dosage Oral:

Children and Adolescents: Limited information is available:

ADHD: One open-label clinical trial and one case report are available; 16 children and adolescents (8-16 years of age; mean: 11.6 ± 2.3 years) were enrolled in a 5-week open trial of venlafaxine; doses were initiated at 12.5 mg/day for the first week; for children <40 kg, the daily dose was increased (if tolerated) by 12.5 mg each week to a maximum of 50 mg/day divided in 2 doses; for patients ≥40 kg, the daily dose was increased (if tolerated) by 25 mg each week to a maximum of 75 mg/day divided in 3 doses; mean dose: 60 mg/day (1.4 mg/kg/day) in 2-3 divided doses; 10 patients completed the study [2 were lost to follow-up; 5 discontinued therapy due to adverse effects (4 had an increase in hyperactivity; 1 had severe nausea)]; venlafaxine decreased behavioral symptoms (but not cognitive symptoms) in 7 of 16 subjects (44%) (Olvera, 1996). An initial dose of 37.5 mg given 3 times/day was used in an 11-year-old female with ADHD; the dose was slowly titrated to 100 mg given 3 times/day; after 6 weeks the patient showed moderate to marked improvement in symptoms, but developed hypertension; the dose was then decreased to 75 mg given 3 times/day with normalization of blood pressure (Pleak, 1995). Further studies are needed.

Autism: One retrospective report is available; 10 patients (3-21 years of age; mean 10.5 ± 5.6 years) with autism spectrum disorders (autism, Asperger's syndrome, and pervasive developmental disorders not otherwise specified) received initial doses of 12.5 mg/day administered once daily at breakfast; doses were gradually titrated based on clinical response and side effects; mean final dose: 24.4 mg/day range: 6.25-50 mg/day; 6 of the 10 patients were sustained-treatment responders (Hollander, 2000). Further studies are needed.

Depression: One double-blind, placebo-controlled, 6-week study is available; 33 children and adolescents (8-17 years of age) with major depression completed the trial (16 received venlafaxine; **Note:** One patient who did not complete the study, discontinued venlafaxine due to development of a manic episode requiring hospitalization and lithium therapy); for children 8-12 years, doses were initiated at 12.5 mg once daily for 3 days, then increased to 12.5 mg twice daily for 3 days, then increased to 12.5 mg given 3 times/day for the rest of the study; for adolescents 13-17 years, doses were initiated at 25 mg once daily for 3 days, then increased to 25 mg twice daily for 3 days, then increased to 25 mg given 3 times/day for the rest of the study; both venlafaxine and placebo patients improved over time; however, no significant difference in symptoms was noted between groups (ie, venlafaxine did not have a significant effect on symptoms or specific behaviors); the authors suggest this lack of efficacy may be due to the low doses used and short duration of treatment (Mandoki, 1997).

A large multicenter double-blind, placebo-controlled study of venlafaxine-ER in children and adolescents 7-17 years of age with major depression is ongoing; this study is using higher doses; initial: 37.5 mg/day for 1 week; with increases to 75 mg/day for weeks 2-8; results are not yet available (see Weller, 2000). One report of two 16-year-old patients used higher doses of venlafaxine (final doses: 112.5 mg/day and 150 mg/day) in combination with lithium to successfully treat major depression (see Walter, 1998). Further studies are needed.

Adults:

Immediate release: Depression: Initial: 75 mg/day in 2-3 divided doses; dose may be increased (if needed) by increments of up to 75 mg/day at intervals of ≥4 days as tolerated, up to 225 mg/day. **Note:** Doses >225 mg/day for outpatients (moderately depressed patients) were not more effective; more severely depressed patients may require 350 mg/day; maximum: 375 mg/day in 3 divided doses

Extended release:

Depression: Initial: Usual: 75 mg/day; may start with 37.5 mg/day for 4-7 days to allow patient to adjust to medication, then increase to 75 mg/day; dose may be increased (if needed) by increments of up to 75 mg/day at intervals of ≥4 days as tolerated, up to a maximum of 225 mg/day. **Note:** Although higher doses of the immediate release tablets have been used in more severely depressed inpatients (see above), experience with extended release capsule in doses >225 mg/day is very limited

Generalized anxiety disorder and social anxiety disorder: 75 mg/day; may start with 37.5 mg/day for 4-7 days to allow patient to adjust to medication, then increase to 75 mg/day. **Note:** Although a dose-response relationship has not been clearly established, certain patients may benefit from doses >75 mg/day; dose may be increased (if needed) by increments of up to 75 mg/day at intervals of ≥4 days as tolerated, up to a maximum of 225 mg/day

Dosing adjustment in renal impairment: Adults: GFR 10-70 mL/minute: Decrease total daily dose by 25% to 50%

Dosing adjustment in patients on dialysis: Decrease total daily dose by 50%; withhold dose until completion of dialysis treatment; further individualization of dose may be needed

Dosing adjustment in hepatic impairment: Moderate hepatic impairment: Decrease total daily dose dose by 50%; further individualization of dose may be needed

Administration

Immediate release tablet: Administer with food

Extended release capsule: Administer with food once daily at about the same time each day; swallow whole with fluid; do not crush, chew, divide, or place in water; capsule may be opened and entire contents sprinkled on spoonful of applesauce; swallow drug/food mixture immediately. Do not store for future use; do not chew contents (ie, pellets) of capsule; follow drug/food mixture with water to ensure complete swallowing of pellets.

Monitoring Parameters Monitor blood pressure regularly, especially in patients with high baseline blood pressure; monitor renal and hepatic function (for possible dose reductions), heart rate, weight, serum cholesterol and sodium

Patient Information May cause dizziness or drowsiness and impair ability to perform activities requiring mental alertness or physical coordination; may cause dry mouth; avoid abrupt discontinuation; report the use of other medications, nonprescription medications, and herbal or natural products to your physician and pharmacist; avoid alcohol, tryptophan supplements, and the herbal medicine, St John's wort; report skin rashes, hives, or allergic reactions to your physician

(Continued)

Venlafaxine (Continued)

Nursing Implications Mean increases in heart rate of 4 beats/minute and 8.5 beats/minute have been reported; when discontinuing therapy, dose must be tapered to minimize risk of discontinuation symptoms (see Precautions)

Additional Information Drug release from extended release capsules is not pH dependent (it is controlled by diffusion through the coating membrane on the spheroids); patients with depression who are receiving Effexor® may be switched to Effexor® XR using the nearest mg/day equivalent dose (dosing may need further individualization)

Long-term usefulness of venlafaxine should be periodically re-evaluated in patients receiving the drug for extended periods of time

Dosage Forms Available as venlafaxine hydrochloride; mg strength refers to venlafaxine

Capsule, extended release: 37.5 mg, 75 mg, 150 mg

Tablet: 25 mg, 37.5 mg, 50 mg, 75 mg, 100 mg

References

Hollander E, Kaplan A, Cartwright C, et al, "Venlafaxine in Children, Adolescents, and Young Adults With Autism Spectrum Disorders: An Open Retrospective Clinical Report," *J Child Neurol*, 2000, 15(2):132-5.

Ilett KF, Hackett LP, Dusci LJ, et al, "Distribution and Excretion of Venlafaxine and O-Desmethylvenlafaxine in Human Milk," *Br J Clin Pharmacol*, 1998, 45(5):459-62.

Mandoki MW, Tapia MR, Tapia MA, et al, "Venlafaxine in the Treatment of Children and Adolescents With Major Depression," *Psychopharmacol Bull*, 1997, 33(1):149-54.

Olvera RL, Pliszka SR, Luh J, et al, "An Open Trial of Venlafaxine in the Treatment of Attention-Deficit/Hyperactivity Disorder in Children and Adolescents," *J Child Adolesc Psychopharmacol*, 1996, 6(4):241-50.

Pleak RR and Gormly LJ, "Effects of Venlafaxine Treatment for ADHD in a Child," *Am J Psychiatry*, 1995, 152(7):1099.

Samuel RZ, "Priapism Associated With Venlafaxine Use," *J Am Acad Child Adolesc Psychiatry*, 2000, 39(1):16-7.

Walter G, Lyndon B, and Kubb R, "Lithium Augmentation of Venlafaxine in Adolescent Major Depression," *Aust N Z J Psychiatry* 1998, 32(3):457-9.

Weller EB, Weller RA, and Davis GP, "Use of Venlafaxine in Children and Adolescents: A Review of Current Literature," *Depress Anxiety*, 2000, 12(Suppl 1):85-9.

- ◆ **Venofer®** see Iron Supplements (Parenteral) on page 626
- ◆ **Venoglobulin®-S** see Immune Globulin (Intravenous) on page 598
- ◆ **Ventolin®** see Albuterol on page 54
- ◆ **Ventolin® Diskus (Can)** see Albuterol on page 54
- ◆ **Ventolin® HFA** see Albuterol on page 54
- ◆ **Ventrodisk (Can)** see Albuterol on page 54
- ◆ **VePesid®** see Etoposide on page 469

Verapamil (ver AP a mil)

U.S. Brand Names Calan®; Calan® SR; Covera-HS®; Isoptin® SR; Verelan®; Verelan® PM

Canadian Brand Names Alti-Verapamil; Apo®-Verap; Chronovera®; Covera®; Gen-Verapamil; Gen-Verapamil SR; Isoptin®; Isoptin® I.V.; Novo-Veramil; Novo-Veramil SR; Nu-Verap; Tarka®

Synonyms Iproveratril

Therapeutic Category Antianginal Agent; Antiarrhythmic Agent, Class IV; Antihypertensive Agent; Calcium Channel Blocker

Generic Available Yes

Use Orally for the treatment of angina and hypertension; I.V. for supraventricular tachyarrhythmias (PSVT, atrial fibrillation, atrial flutter)

Pregnancy Risk Factor C

Contraindications Hypersensitivity to verapamil or any component; sinus bradycardia; advanced heart block; ventricular tachycardia; cardiogenic shock; atrial fibrillation or flutter associated with accessory conduction pathways

Warnings Avoid I.V. use in neonates and young infants due to severe apnea, bradycardia, hypotensive reactions, and cardiac arrest; I.V. use is discouraged in children due to hypotension and myocardial depression; monitor EKG and blood pressure closely in patients receiving I.V. therapy; have I.V. calcium chloride 10 mg/kg available at bedside to treat hypotension. I.V. administration, hypertrophic cardiomyopathy, sick sinus syndrome, moderate to severe CHF, concomitant therapy with beta-blockers or digoxin can all increase the incidence of adverse effects.

Precautions Use with caution in patients with sick sinus syndrome, severe left ventricular dysfunction, hepatic or renal impairment, hypertrophic cardiomyopathy (especially obstructive), concomitant therapy with beta-blockers or digoxin; reduce dose in patients with severe renal dysfunction; verapamil may decrease neuromuscular transmission in patients with Duchenne's muscular dystrophy and may worsen myasthenia gravis

Adverse Reactions

Cardiovascular: Hypotension, bradycardia; first, second, or third degree A-V block, worsening heart failure

Central nervous system: Dizziness, fatigue, seizures (occasionally with I.V. use), headache

Gastrointestinal: Constipation, nausea, abdominal discomfort

Hepatic: Elevated hepatic enzymes

Otic: Tinnitus

Respiratory: May precipitate insufficiency of respiratory muscle function in Duchenne muscular dystrophy

Drug Interactions Cytochrome P450 isoenzyme CYP1A2, CYP2C8 (minor), CYP2C9 (minor), CYP2C18 (minor), and CYP3A3/4 substrate; CYP3A3/4 isoenzyme inhibitor

Increased cardiovascular adverse effects with beta-adrenergic blocking agents, digoxin, quinidine, and disopyramide. Verapamil may increase serum concentrations of caffeine, ethanol, digoxin, quinidine, carbamazepine, and cyclosporine necessitating a decrease in dosage. Combined use of verapamil with lovastatin or simvastatin may result in an increased risk of myopathy or rhabdomyolysis (dosage reduction of lovastatin and simvastatin is recommended); phenobarbital and rifampin may decrease verapamil serum concentrations by increasing hepatic metabolism. Enzyme inhibitors (eg, erythromycin, ritonavir) may increase verapamil serum concentration. Use with aspirin may increase bleeding time. Verapamil may prolong recovery from vecuronium. Avoid combination with disopyramide, discontinue disopyramide 48 hours before starting therapy, do not restart until 24 hours after verapamil has been discontinued. Verapamil may increase, decrease, or have no effect on lithium serum concentrations (monitor patients carefully).

Food Interactions Grapefruit juice may increase verapamil serum concentrations

Calan® SR and Isoptin® SR: Food may decrease bioavailability, but produces a narrow peak to trough ratio

Covera-HS®: A high fat meal does not affect absorption

Verelan®: Food does not affect rate or extent of absorption

Verelan® PM: A high fat meal slightly affects the rate, but not the extent of absorption

Stability Store injection at room temperature; protect from heat and from freezing; use only clear solutions; compatible in solutions of pH of 3-6, but may precipitate in solutions having a pH ≥6

Mechanism of Action Inhibits calcium ions from entering the "slow channels" or select voltage-sensitive areas of vascular smooth muscle and myocardium during depolarization; produces a relaxation of coronary vascular smooth muscle and coronary vasodilation; increases myocardial oxygen delivery in patients with vasospastic angina

Pharmacodynamics

Maximum effect:

Oral (nonsustained tablets): 2 hours

I.V.: 1-5 minutes

Duration:

Oral: 6-8 hours

I.V.: 10-20 minutes

Pharmacokinetics

Protein binding:

Neonates: ~60%

Adults: 90%

Metabolism: Extensive first-pass effect, metabolized in the liver to several inactive dealkylated metabolites; major metabolite is norverapamil which possesses weak hemodynamic effects

Bioavailability: Oral: 20% to 30%

Half-life:

Infants: 4.4-6.9 hours

Adults (single dose): 2-8 hours, increased up to 12 hours with multiple dosing

Increased half-life with hepatic cirrhosis

Elimination: 70% of dose excreted in urine (3% to 4% as unchanged drug), and 16% in feces

Usual Dosage

Infants <1 year: I.V.: **Not recommended** (see Warnings); administer with continuous EKG monitoring, have I.V. calcium available at bedside: 0.1-0.2 mg/kg (usual: 0.75-2 mg/dose) may repeat dose in 30 minutes if adequate response not achieved

Children 1-16 years: I.V.: 0.1-0.3 mg/kg/dose (**Note:** PALS 2000 guidelines recommend 0.1 mg/kg); maximum dose: 5 mg/dose; may repeat dose in 30 minutes if adequate response not achieved; maximum for second dose: 10 mg/dose

(Continued)

Verapamil *(Continued)*

Children: Oral (dose not well established):

4-8 mg/kg/day in 3 divided doses

or

1-5 years: 40-80 mg every 8 hours

>5 years: 80 mg every 6-8 hours

Note: A mean daily dose of ~5 mg/kg/day (range: 2.3-8.1 mg/kg/day) was used in 22 children 15 days to 17 years of age receiving chronic oral therapy for SVT (n=20) or hypertrophic cardiomyopathy (n=2) (Piovan)

Adults:

Oral: 240-480 mg/24 hours divided 3-4 times/day or divided 1-2 times/day for sustained release products or given once daily for extended release product (see Administration)

I.V. (ACLS 2000 guidelines): PSVT (narrow complex, unresponsive to vagal maneuvers and adenosine, in patients with preserved cardiac function): Initial: 2.5-5 mg; if no response in 15-30 minutes and no adverse effects seen, give 5-10 mg every 15-30 minutes to a maximum total dose of 20 mg

I.V.: 5-10 mg (0.075-0.15 mg/kg); may repeat 10 mg (0.15 mg/kg) 15-30 minutes after the initial dose if needed and if patient tolerated initial dose

I.V. continuous infusion: Loading dose: 5-10 mg; may repeat in 30 minutes if adequate response is not achieved; follow with continuous infusion: 5 mg/hour; titrate dose to ventricular rate; usual: 5-10 mg/hour; range: 4-24 mg/hour. **Note**: Previously recommended doses of 0.005 mg/kg/minute (5 mcg/kg/minute) will result in doses of ~20 mg/hour and may produce adverse effects such as hypotension; lower infusion rates (5-10 mg/hour) are effective in most adult patients.

Dosing adjustment in renal impairment: Children and Adults: Cl_{cr} <10 mL/minute: Administer 50% to 75% of normal dose

Administration

Oral: Do not administer with grapefruit juice; nonsustained-release tablets can be administered with or without food; swallow extended and sustained released preparations whole, do not chew or crush; administer Calan® SR and Isoptin® SR with food on a once daily or twice daily schedule; administer Covera-HS® and Verelan® PM once daily at bedtime. Administer Verelan® (sustained release capsules) once daily in the morning; capsule may be opened and contents sprinkled on a spoonful of applesauce; swallow immediately, do not chew; do not store for future use; follow with water to ensure complete swallowing of capsule pellets; do not divide capsule

Parenteral:

I.V.: Infuse I.V. dose over 2-3 minutes; infuse I.V. over 3-4 minutes if blood pressure is in the lower range of normal: Maximum concentration: 2.5 mg/mL

I.V. continuous infusion: Final concentration for administration: 0.5-2.5 mg/mL

Monitoring Parameters EKG, blood pressure, heart rate; hepatic enzymes with long-term use

Patient Information Avoid alcohol and grapefruit juice; limit caffeine

Dosage Forms

Caplet, sustained release (Calan® SR): 120 mg, 180 mg, 240 mg

Capsule, extended release, as hydrochloride: 120 mg, 180 mg, 240 mg

Verelan® PM: 100 mg, 200 mg, 300 mg

Capsule, sustained release, as hydrochloride: 120 mg, 180 mg, 240 mg

Verelan®: 120 mg, 180 mg, 240 mg, 360 mg

Injection, solution, as hydrochloride: 2.5 mg/mL (2 mL, 4 mL)

Tablet, as hydrochloride (Calan®): 40 mg, 80 mg, 120 mg

Tablet, extended release: 120 mg, 180 mg, 240 mg

Covera HS®: 180 mg, 240 mg

Tablet, sustained release, as hydrochloride (Isoptin® SR): 120 mg, 180 mg, 240 mg

Extemporaneous Preparations

A 50 mg/mL oral suspension may be made using twenty 80 mg verapamil tablets (regular, not sustained release), 3 mL of purified water USP, 8 mL of methylcellulose 1% and simple syrup qs ad to 32 mL; stability is 91 days under refrigeration; shake well before use (Nahata, 2000)

A 50 mg/mL oral liquid preparation made from tablets (regular, not sustained release) and 3 different vehicles (cherry syrup, a 1:1 mixture of Ora-Sweet® and Ora-Plus®, or a 1:1 mixture of Ora-Sweet® SF and Ora-Plus®) was stable for 60 days when stored in amber plastic prescription bottles in the dark at room temperature (25°C) or under refrigeration (5°C); grind seventy-five 80 mg tablets in a mortar into a fine powder; add 40 mL of the vehicle and mix well to form a uniform paste; mix while adding the vehicle in geometric proportions to **almost** 120 mL; transfer to a calibrated bottle and qsad with vehicle to make 120 mL; label "shake well" and "protect from light" (Allen, 1996).

Allen LV and Erickson MA, "Stability of Labetalol Hydrochloride, Metoprolol Tartrate, Verapamil Hydrochloride, and Spironolactone With Hydrochlorothiazide in Extemporaneously Compounded Oral Liquids," *Am J Health Syst Pharm*, 1996, 53(19):2304-9.

Nahata MC and Hipple TF, *Pediatric Drug Formulations*, 4th ed, Cincinnati, OH: Harvey Whitney Books Co, 2000.

References

Barbarash RA, Bauman JL, Lukazewski AA, et al, "Verapamil Infusions in the Treatment of Atrial Tachyarrhythmias," *Crit Care Med*, 1986, 14(10):886-8.

"Guidelines 2000 for Cardiopulmonary Resuscitation and Emergency Cardiovascular Care, Part 6: Advanced Cardiovascular Life Support, The American Heart Association in Collaboration With the International Liaison Committee on Resuscitation," *Circulation*, 2000, 102(8 Suppl):I86-171.

"Guidelines 2000 for Cardiopulmonary Resuscitation and Emergency Cardiovascular Care, Part 10: Pediatric Advanced Life Support, The American Heart Association in Collaboration With the International Liaison Committee on Resuscitation," *Circulation*, 2000, 102(8 Suppl): I291-342.

Piovan D, Padrini R, Svalato Moreolo G, et al, "Verapamil and Norverapamil Plasma Levels in Infants and Children During Chronic Oral Treatment," *Ther Drug Monit*, 1995, 17(1):60-7.

Sapire DW, O'Riordan AC, and Black IF, "Safety and Efficacy of Short- and Long-Term Verapamil Therapy in Children With Tachycardia," *Am J Cardiol*, 1981, 48(6):1091-7.

Shakibi JG, "Arrhythmias in Infants and Children," *Pediatrician*, 1981, 10(1-3):117-22.

- ◆ **Verelan®** *see* Verapamil *on page 1144*
- ◆ **Verelan® PM** *see* Verapamil *on page 1144*
- ◆ **Vermizine® [DSC]** *see* Piperazine [DSC] *on page 909*
- ◆ **Vermox®** *see* Mebendazole *on page 708*
- ◆ **Versed®** *see* Midazolam *on page 761*
- ◆ **Versel® (Can)** *see* Selenium Sulfide *on page 1013*
- ◆ **Versiclear™** *see* Sodium Thiosulfate *on page 1030*
- ◆ **VFEND®** *see* Voriconazole *on page 1154*
- ◆ **Viadur®** *see* Leuprolide *on page 662*
- ◆ **Vibramycin®** *see* Doxycycline *on page 415*
- ◆ **Vibra-Tabs®** *see* Doxycycline *on page 415*
- ◆ **Vicks® 44 Cough Relief [OTC]** *see* Dextromethorphan *on page 365*
- ◆ **Vicks® 44E [OTC]** *see* Guaifenesin and Dextromethorphan *on page 553*
- ◆ **Vicks® Pediatric Formula 44E [OTC]** *see* Guaifenesin and Dextromethorphan *on page 553*
- ◆ **Vicks® Sinex® 12 Hour Ultrafine Mist [OTC]** *see* Oxymetazoline *on page 849*
- ◆ **Vicks® Sinex® Nasal Spray [OTC]** *see* Phenylephrine *on page 892*
- ◆ **Vicks® Sinex® UltraFine Mist [OTC]** *see* Phenylephrine *on page 892*
- ◆ **Vicodin®** *see* Hydrocodone and Acetaminophen *on page 571*
- ◆ **Vicodin® ES** *see* Hydrocodone and Acetaminophen *on page 571*
- ◆ **Vicodin® HP** *see* Hydrocodone and Acetaminophen *on page 571*

Vidarabine (vye DARE a been)

U.S. Brand Names Vira-A® [DSC]

Synonyms Adenine Arabinoside; Ara-A; Arabinofuranosyladenine

Therapeutic Category Antiviral Agent, Ophthalmic

Generic Available No

Use Treatment of acute keratoconjunctivitis and epithelial keratitis due to herpes simplex virus

Pregnancy Risk Factor C

Contraindications Hypersensitivity to vidarabine or any component; concurrent application of a corticosteroid in the treatment of herpes simplex keratitis

Warnings Vidarabine is potentially mutagenic, teratogenic, and oncogenic

Adverse Reactions Ocular: Keratitis, photophobia, lacrimation, foreign body sensation, uveitis, stromal edema, blurred vision, burning

Stability Store at room temperature; avoid freezing

Mechanism of Action Inhibits viral DNA synthesis by blocking DNA polymerase or virus-induced ribonucleotide reductase

Pharmacokinetics

Absorption: Systemic absorption is not expected to occur following ophthalmic use

Distribution: Trace amounts detected in the aqueous humor if there is an epithelial defect in the cornea

Protein binding:

Vidarabine: 20% to 30%

Ara-hypoxanthine: 0% to 3%

Elimination: Following administration, rapidly deaminated by red cell adenosine deaminase to ara-hypoxanthine (active); excreted in urine as vidarabine (1% to 3%) and the active metabolite (40% to 53%)

(Continued)

Vidarabine *(Continued)*

Usual Dosage Children and Adults: Ophthalmic: Keratoconjunctivitis: Apply ½" of ointment in lower conjunctival sac 5 times/day every 3 hours while awake until complete re-epithelialization has occurred, then twice daily for an additional 7 days

Administration Ophthalmic: Instill 1 cm of ointment in lower conjunctival sac of the affected eye; avoid contact of tube tip with skin or eye

Patient Information Ophthalmic ointment may cause sensitivity to bright light; minimize light sensitivity by wearing sunglasses

Dosage Forms Ointment, ophthalmic, as monohydrate: 3% [30 mg/mL = 28 mg/mL base] (3.5 g) [DSC]

♦ **Videx®** *see* Didanosine *on page 377*
♦ **Videx® EC** *see* Didanosine *on page 377*

VinBLAStine *(vin BLAS teen)*

Related Information
Emetogenic Potential of Single Chemotherapeutic Agents *on page 1286*
Extravasation Treatment *on page 1240*

U.S. Brand Names Velban® [DSC]

Synonyms Vincaleukoblastine; VLB

Therapeutic Category Antineoplastic Agent, Mitotic Inhibitor

Generic Available Yes

Use Palliative treatment of Hodgkin's disease; advanced testicular germinal-cell cancers; non-Hodgkin's lymphoma, histiocytosis, and choriocarcinoma

Pregnancy Risk Factor D

Contraindications Hypersensitivity to vinblastine or any component (see Warnings); severe leukopenia

Warnings The FDA currently recommends that procedures for proper handling and disposal of antineoplastic agents be considered; vinblastine may cause fetal toxicity when administered to pregnant women; for I.V. use only; **intrathecal administration may result in death**

Injection (solution) contains benzyl alcohol which may cause allergic reactions in susceptible individuals; large amounts of benzyl alcohol ($\geq$99 mg/kg/day) have been associated with a potentially fatal toxicity ("gasping syndrome") in neonates; the "gasping syndrome" consists of metabolic acidosis, respiratory distress, gasping respirations, CNS dysfunction (including convulsions, intracranial hemorrhage), hypotension and cardiovascular collapse; avoid use of vinblastine products containing benzyl alcohol in neonates; *in vitro* and animal studies have shown that benzoate, a metabolite of benzyl alcohol, displaces bilirubin from protein binding sites

Precautions Avoid extravasation; dosage modification required in patients with impaired liver function or neurotoxicity; dosage should be reduced in patients with recent exposure to radiation therapy or chemotherapy

Adverse Reactions
Cardiovascular: Tachycardia, orthostatic hypotension
Central nervous system: Depression, malaise, seizures, headache
Dermatologic: Rashes, mild alopecia, photosensitivity
Endocrine & metabolic: Hyperuricemia
Gastrointestinal: Nausea, hemorrhagic enterocolitis, vomiting, constipation, abdominal pain, paralytic ileus, stomatitis
Genitourinary: Urinary retention
Hematologic: Myelosuppression: Leukopenia (nadir: 4-10 days), thrombocytopenia
Local: Severe tissue burn if infiltrated
Neuromuscular & skeletal: Jaw pain, myalgia, peripheral neuropathy, paresthesia

Drug Interactions Cytochrome P450 isoenzyme CYP3A3/4 and CYP3A5-7 substrate; isoenzyme CYP2D6 inhibitor
Concomitant administration with mitomycin has resulted in severe bronchospasm and shortness of breath; may decrease serum phenytoin concentrations

Stability Store in refrigerator; 1 mg/mL solutions prepared with preserved NS injection is stable for 30 days when refrigerated and protected from light. **Note:** Vinblastine must be dispensed in overwrap which bears the statement "Do not remove covering until the moment of injection. Fatal if given intrathecally. For I.V. use only."

Mechanism of Action Binds to microtubular protein of the mitotic spindle causing metaphase arrest

Pharmacokinetics
Distribution: Poor penetration into CSF; rapidly distributed into body tissues; V_{dss}: 27.3 L/kg
Protein binding: 75%
Metabolism: Extensive in the liver to a more active metabolite

Half-life, terminal: 24 hours
Elimination: Biliary excretion (95%)

Usual Dosage Vinblastine may be administered at intervals of every 7 days or greater and only after leukocyte count has returned to at least 4000/mm³; maintenance therapy should be titrated according to leukocyte count

I.V. (refer to individual protocols):
Children:
Hodgkin's disease: 2.5-6 mg/m²/day once every 1-2 weeks for 3-6 weeks; maximum weekly dose: 12.5 mg/m²
Histiocytosis: 0.4 mg/kg once ever 7-10 days
Germ cell tumor: 0.2 mg/kg on days 1 and 2 of cycle every 3 weeks times 4 cycles
Adults: 3.7-18.5 mg/m²/day every 7-10 days or 0.1-0.5 mg/kg/day once weekly or 1.4-1.8 mg/m²/day for 5 days given as an I.V. continuous infusion

Dosing adjustment in hepatic impairment: Children and Adults: Direct serum bilirubin concentration >3 mg/dL: Reduce dose 50%

Administration Parenteral: **Do not administer intrathecally, death may occur**; do not administer I.M. or S.C. since the drug is very irritating; may be administered IVP directly into the vein or through a Y-site of a freely running I.V. over a 1-minute period at a concentration for administration of 1 mg/mL; I.V. continuous infusion: Each day's dose may be diluted in 1000 mL of D₅W or NS; administer over 24 hours

Monitoring Parameters CBC with differential and platelet count, serum uric acid, hepatic function tests

Patient Information Report to physician any fever, sore throat, bleeding, or bruising; avoid contact with the eyes since the drug is very irritating and corneal ulceration may result. May cause photosensitivity reactions (eg, exposure to sunlight may cause severe sunburn, skin rash, redness, or itching); avoid exposure to sunlight and artificial light sources (sunlamps, tanning booth/bed); wear protective clothing, wide-brimmed hats, sunglasses, and lip sunscreen (SPF ≥15); use a sunscreen [broad-spectrum sunscreen or physical sunscreen (preferred) or sunblock with SPF ≥15]; contact physician if reaction occurs.

Nursing Implications Maintain adequate hydration. Allopurinol may be given to prevent uric acid nephropathy; stool softeners may be helpful in preventing constipation; vinblastine is a tissue irritant and can cause sloughing upon extravasation; check vein patency before drug administration; care should be taken to avoid extravasation. If extravasation occurs, local injection of hyaluronidase into the leading edge of the extravasation site and a warm compress can be used for treatment; apply warm pack immediately for 30-60 minutes, then alternate off/on every 15 minutes for 1 day. Refer to Extravasation Treatment *on page 1240*.

Additional Information Myelosuppressive effects:
Nadir (days): 4-10
Recovery (days): 7-14

Dosage Forms
Injection, solution, as sulfate: 1 mg/mL (10 mL) [contains benzyl alcohol]
Injection, powder for reconstitution, lyophilized, as sulfate: 10 mg

References

Balis FM, Holcenberg JS and Bleyer WA, "Clinical Pharmacokinetics of Commonly Used Anticancer Drugs," *Clin Pharmacokinet*, 1983, 8(3):202-32.

Crom WR, Glynn-Barnhart AM, Rodman JH, et al, "Pharmacokinetics of Anticancer Drugs in Children," *Clin Pharmacokinet*, 1987, 12(3):168-213.

Tannock I, Ehrlichman C, Perrault D, et al, "Failure of 5-Day Vinblastine Infusion in the Treatment of Patients With Advanced Refractory Breast Cancer," *Cancer Treat Rep*, 1982, 66(9):1783-4.

Yap HY, Blumenschein GR, Keating MJ, et al, "Vinblastine Given as a Continuous 5-Day Infusion in the Treatment of Refractory Breast Cancer," *Cancer Treat Rep*, 1980, 64(2-3):279-83.

♦ **Vincaleukoblastine** *see* VinBLAStine *on page 1148*

♦ **Vincasar PFS®** *see* VinCRIStine *on page 1149*

VinCRIStine (vin KRIS teen)

Related Information
Emetogenic Potential of Single Chemotherapeutic Agents *on page 1286*
Extravasation Treatment *on page 1240*

U.S. Brand Names Oncovin® [DSC]; Vincasar PFS®

Synonyms LCR; Leurocristine; VCR

Therapeutic Category Antineoplastic Agent, Mitotic Inhibitor

Generic Available Yes

Use Treatment of leukemias, Hodgkin's disease, neuroblastoma, malignant lymphomas, Wilms' tumor, and rhabdomyosarcoma

Pregnancy Risk Factor D

(Continued)

VinCRIStine *(Continued)*

Contraindications Hypersensitivity to vincristine or any component; patients with demyelinating form of Charcot-Marie-Tooth syndrome

Warnings The FDA currently recommends that procedures for proper handling and disposal of antineoplastic agents be considered; vincristine may cause fetal toxicity when administered to pregnant women; for I.V. use only; **intrathecal administration may result in death**.

Precautions Dosage modification required in patients with impaired hepatic function, patients receiving other neurotoxic drugs, or patients with pre-existing neuromuscular disease; avoid extravasation

Adverse Reactions

Cardiovascular: Orthostatic hypotension

Central nervous system: Neurotoxicity, seizures, CNS depression, cranial nerve paralysis

Dermatologic: Alopecia, rash

Endocrine & metabolic: Hyperuricemia, SIADH

Gastrointestinal: Constipation, paralytic ileus, nausea, vomiting, diarrhea, stomatitis

Local: Pain, cellulitis and tissue necrosis if infiltrated, phlebitis

Neuromuscular & skeletal: Jaw pain, leg pain, myalgia, numbness, motor difficulties, cramping, weakness

Ocular: Extraocular muscle paresis, photophobia

Respiratory: Dyspnea

Drug Interactions Cytochrome P450 isoenzyme CYP3A3/4 and CYP3A5-7 substrate; isoenzyme CYP2D6 inhibitor

Asparaginase may decrease vincristine clearance; acute pulmonary reactions may occur with concomitant use of mitomycin C; concurrent administration with itraconazole may result in an increased severity of neuromuscular side effects

Stability Store in refrigerator; injectable solution is stable for 1 month at room temperature. **Note:** Vincristine must be dispensed in overwrap which bears the statement "Do not remove covering until the moment of injection. Fatal if given intrathecally. For I.V. use only."

Mechanism of Action Binds to microtubular protein of the mitotic spindle causing metaphase arrest

Pharmacokinetics

Distribution: Poor penetration into the CSF; V_{dss}: 120 L/m^2

Protein binding: 75%

Metabolism: Extensive in the liver

Half-life, terminal: 24 hours

Elimination: Primarily in bile (~80%)

Clearance:

Infants: Vincristine clearance is more closely related to body weight than to body surface area

Children 2-18 years: 482 mL/minute/m^2 (faster clearance in children <10 years of age than in adolescents)

Usual Dosage I.V. (refer to individual protocols):

Children ≤10 kg or BSA <1 m^2: Initial therapy: 0.05 mg/kg once weekly then titrate dose; maximum single dose: 2 mg

Children >10 kg or BSA ≥1 m^2: 1-2 mg/m^2, may repeat once weekly for 3-6 weeks; maximum single dose: 2 mg

Neuroblastoma: I.V. continuous infusion with doxorubicin: 1 mg/m^2/day for 72 hours

Adults: 0.4-1.4 mg/m^2 up to 2 mg; may repeat every week

Dosing adjustment in hepatic impairment: Children and Adults: Direct serum bilirubin concentration >3 mg/dL: Dosage reduction of 50% is recommended

Administration Parenteral: **Do not administer intrathecally, death may occur**; do not administer I.M. or S.C. since the drug is very irritating; I.V.: Vincristine is administered IVP or through a Y-site of a freely running I.V. over a period of 1 minute at a concentration for administration of 1 mg/mL; may administer as a dilute I.V. infusion

Monitoring Parameters Serum electrolytes (sodium), hepatic function tests, neurologic examination, CBC, hemoglobin, serum uric acid

Patient Information Stool softener should be used for constipation prophylaxis; report to physician any fever, sore throat, bleeding, bruising, or shortness of breath

Nursing Implications Maintain adequate hydration. Allopurinol may be given to prevent uric acid nephropathy; vincristine is a tissue irritant; care should be taken to avoid extravasation. If extravasation occurs, local injection of hyaluronidase into the leading edge of the extravasation site and a warm compress can be used for treatment; apply warm pack immediately for 30-60 minutes, then alternate off/on every 15 minutes for 1 day; refer to Extravasation Treatment *on page 1240*. Avoid contact with the eye since vincristine is very irritating.

Dosage Forms Injection, solution, as sulfate: 1 mg/mL (1 mL, 2 mL)

References
Crom WR, deGraaf SS, Synold T, et al, "Pharmacokinetics of Vincristine in Children and Adolescents With Acute Lymphocytic Leukemia," *J Pediatr*, 1994, 125(4):642-9.
Woods WG, O'Leary M, and Nesbit ME, "Life-Threatening Neuropathy and Hepatotoxicity in Infants During Induction Therapy for Acute Lymphoblastic Leukemia," *J Pediatr*, 1981, 98(4):642-5.

Vitamin A (VYE ta min aye)

Related Information
Carbohydrate and Alcohol Content of Liquid Medications for Use in Patients Receiving Ketogenic Diets *on page 1431*

U.S. Brand Names Aquasol A®; Palmitate-A® [OTC]

Synonyms Oleovitamin A

Therapeutic Category Nutritional Supplement; Vitamin, Fat Soluble

Generic Available Yes (capsule)

Use Treatment and prevention of vitamin A deficiency; supplementation in children 6 months to 2 years with measles

Pregnancy Risk Factor A (X if dose exceeds RDA recommendation)

Contraindications Hypersensitivity to vitamin A or any component; hypervitaminosis A; pregnancy (dose exceeding RDA)

Warnings Patients receiving >25,000 units/day should be closely monitored for toxicity; polysorbates contained in parenteral vitamin A have been associated with thrombocytopenia, renal dysfunction, hepatomegaly, cholestasis, ascites, hypotension, and metabolic acidosis when administered to neonates (E-Ferol syndrome); avoid use in neonates

Adverse Reactions Seen only with doses exceeding physiologic replacement
Central nervous system: Irritability, drowsiness, vertigo, delirium, headache, coma, elevated intracranial pressure
Dermatologic: Erythema, peeling skin
Gastrointestinal: Vomiting, diarrhea
Ocular: Visual disturbances, papilledema

Drug Interactions Cholestyramine decreases absorption of vitamin A; neomycin and mineral oil may also interfere with vitamin A absorption; retinoids may have additive adverse effects; enhances hypoprothrombinemic effects of warfarin

Stability Protect injectable preparation from light

Mechanism of Action Needed for bone development, growth, visual adaptation to darkness, testicular and ovarian function, and as a cofactor in many biochemical processes

Pharmacokinetics
Absorption: Vitamin A in dosages **not** exceeding physiologic replacement is well absorbed after oral administration; water miscible preparations are absorbed more rapidly than oil preparations; large oral doses, conditions of fat malabsorption, low protein intake, or hepatic or pancreatic disease reduce oral absorption
Metabolism: Conjugated with glucuronide, undergoes enterohepatic circulation
Elimination: In feces via biliary elimination

Usual Dosage
Recommended daily allowance (RDA): Oral:
<1 year: 375 mcg* (1250 units)
1-3 years: 400 mcg* (1330 units)
4-6 years: 500 mcg* (1670 units)
7-10 years: 700 mcg* (2330 units)
>10 years: Female: 800 mcg* (2670 units); Male: 1000 mcg* (3330 units)
*mcg retinol equivalent (0.3 mcg retinol = 1 unit vitamin A)
Daily dietary supplement: Oral:
Infants up to 6 months: 1500 units
(Continued)

Vitamin A (Continued)

Children:
- 6 months to 3 years: 1500-2000 units
- 4-6 years: 2500 units
- 7-10 years: 3300-3500 units
- Children >10 years and Adults: 4000-5000 units

Vitamin A supplementation in measles (recommendation of the World Health Organization): Children: Oral: Give as a single dose; repeat the next day and at 4 weeks for children with ophthalmologic evidence of vitamin A deficiency:
- 6 months to 1 year: 100,000 units
- >1 year: 200,000 units

Note: Use of vitamin A in measles is recommended only for patients 6 months to 2 years of age hospitalized with measles and its complications **or** patients >6 months of age who have any of the following risk factors and who are not already receiving vitamin A: immunodeficiency, ophthalmologic evidence of vitamin A deficiency including night blindness, Bitot's spots or evidence of xerophthalmia, impaired intestinal absorption, moderate to severe malnutrition including that associated with eating disorders, or recent immigration from areas where high mortality rates from measles have been observed

Note: Monitor patients closely; dosages >25,000 units/kg have been associated with toxicity

Vitamin A deficiency (varying recommendations available):
Severe deficiency with xerophthalmia:
- Infants: I.M.: 7500-15,000 units/day followed by oral 5000-10,000 units/day for 10 days
- Children 1-8 years: Oral: 5000 units/kg/day for 5 days then 5000-10,000 units/day for 2 months; I.M.: 17,500-35,000 units/day for 10 days
- Children >8 years and Adults: Oral: 500,000 units/day for 3 days, then 50,000 units/day for 14 days; then 10,000-20,000 units/day for 2 months; I.M.: 100,000 units/day for 3 days; then 50,000 units/day for 14 days

Prophylactic therapy for children at risk for developing deficiency: Oral: Given every 4-6 months:
- Infants ≤1 year: 100,000 units
- Children >1 year: 200,000 units

Malabsorption syndrome (prophylaxis): Children >8 years and Adults: Oral: 10,000-50,000 units/day of water miscible product

Administration
Oral: Administer with food or milk
Parenteral: I.M. only

Additional Information 1 USP vitamin A unit = 0.3 mcg of all-*trans* isomer of retinol; 1 RE (retinol equivalent) = 1 mcg of all-*trans*-retinol

Dosage Forms
Capsule: 10,000 units, 25,000 units [softgel]
Injection, solution (Aquasol-A®): 50,000 units/mL (2 mL)
Tablet (Palmitate-A®): 5000 units, 15,000 units

References
Committee on Infectious Diseases, "Vitamin A in the Treatment of Measles," *Pediatrics*, 1993, 91(5):1014-5.

DeMaeyer EM, "The WHO Programme of Prevention and Control of Vitamin A Deficiency, Xerophthalmia, and Nutritional Blindness," *Nutr Health*, 1986, 4(2):105-12.

Hussey GD and Klein M, "A Randomized, Controlled Trial of Vitamin A in Children With Severe Measles," *N Engl J Med*, 1990, 323(3):160-4.

- ◆ **Vitamin A Acid** *see* Tretinoin *on page 1111*
- ◆ **Vitamin B₁** *see* Thiamine *on page 1081*
- ◆ **Vitamin B₂** *see* Riboflavin *on page 983*
- ◆ **Vitamin B₃** *see* Niacin *on page 809*
- ◆ **Vitamin B₆** *see* Pyridoxine *on page 964*
- ◆ **Vitamin B₁₂** *see* Cyanocobalamin *on page 316*
- ◆ **Vitamin B₁₂** *see* Hydroxocobalamin *on page 579*
- ◆ **Vitamin C** *see* Ascorbic Acid *on page 131*
- ◆ **Vitamin D₂** *see* Ergocalciferol *on page 445*

Vitamin E (VYE ta min ee)

Related Information
Carbohydrate and Alcohol Content of Liquid Medications for Use in Patients Receiving Ketogenic Diets *on page 1431*

U.S. Brand Names Aqua Gem E® [OTC]; Aquasol E® [OTC]; E-Gems® [OTC]; Key-E® [OTC]; Key-E® Kaps [OTC]

Synonyms d-Alpha Tocopherol; dl-Alpha Tocopherol

Therapeutic Category Nutritional Supplement; Vitamin, Fat Soluble; Vitamin, Topical

Generic Available Yes

Use Prevention and treatment of vitamin E deficiency

Pregnancy Risk Factor A (C if dose exceeds RDA recommendation)

Contraindications Hypersensitivity to vitamin E or any component

Warnings Necrotizing enterocolitis has been associated with oral administration of large dosages (eg, >200 units/day) of a hyperosmolar vitamin E preparation in low birth weight infants

Adverse Reactions

Central nervous system: Headache

Dermatologic: Rash

Endocrine & metabolic: Gonadal dysfunction; decreased serum thyroxine and triiodo-thyronine; elevated cholesterol and triglycerides

Gastrointestinal: Nausea, diarrhea, intestinal cramps, necrotizing enterocolitis (see Warnings)

Neuromuscular & skeletal: Weakness

Ocular: Blurred vision

Renal: Creatinuria and elevated serum creatinine kinase; elevated urinary estrogens and androgens

Drug Interactions Iron, mineral oil, warfarin

Mechanism of Action Antioxidant which prevents oxidation of vitamin A and C; protects polyunsaturated fatty acids in membranes from attack by free radicals and protects red blood cells against hemolysis by oxidizing agents

Pharmacokinetics

Absorption: Oral: Depends upon the presence of bile; absorption is reduced in conditions of malabsorption, in low birth weight premature infants, and as dosage increases; water miscible preparations are better absorbed than oil preparations

Metabolism: In the liver to glucuronides

Elimination: Primarily in bile

Usual Dosage 1 unit vitamin E = 1 mg *dl*-alpha-tocopherol acetate. Oral:

Vitamin E - Recommended Daily Allowance (RDA) and Estimated Average Requirement (EAR)

Age	RDA (mg/day)	EAR (mg/day)
0-6 mo	–	4 (6 units)
7-12 mo	–	6 (9 units)
1-3 y	6 (9 units)	5 (7.5 units)
4-8 y	7 (10.5 units)	6 (9 units)
9-13 y	11 (16.5 units)	9 (13.5 units)
≥14 y	15 (22.5 units)	12 (18 units)

Vitamin E deficiency:

Neonates, premature, low birth weight: 25-50 units/day results in normal levels within 1 week

Children (with malabsorption syndrome): 1 unit/kg/day of water miscible vitamin E (to raise plasma tocopherol concentrations to the normal range within 2 months and to maintain normal plasma concentrations)

Adults: 60-75 units/day

Prevention of vitamin E deficiency:

Neonates:

Low birth weight: 5 units/day

Full-term: 5 units/L of formula ingested

Adults: 30 units/day

Prevention of retinopathy of prematurity or BPD secondary to O_2 therapy: Neonates and Infants: (American Academy of Pediatrics considers this use investigational and routine use is not recommended): 15-30 units/kg/day to maintain plasma levels between 1.5-2 mcg/mL (may need as high as 100 units/kg/day)

Cystic fibrosis, beta-thalassemia, sickle cell anemia may require higher daily maintenance doses: Infants, Children, and Adolescents:

Cystic fibrosis: 100-400 units/day

Beta-thalassemia: 750 units/day

Sickle cell: 450 units/day

Topical: Apply a thin layer over affected area

Administration Oral: May administer with or without food

Monitoring Parameters Plasma tocopherol concentrations

(Continued)

1153

Vitamin E *(Continued)*

Reference Range Plasma tocopherol: 6-14 µg/mL
Dosage Forms
　Capsule: 100 units, 200 units, 400 units, 600 units, 1000 units
　　Aqua Gem E®: 200 units, 400 units
　　E-Gems®: 30 units, 100 units, 600 units, 800 units, 1000 units, 1200 units
　　Key-E® Kaps: 200 units, 400 units
　Cream: 100 units/g (60 g)
　　Key-E®: 30 units/g (60 g, 120 g, 480 g)
　Oil: 100 units/0.25 mL (60 mL); 1150 units/0.25 mL (30 mL, 60 mL, 120 mL)
　　E-Gem®: 100 units/10 drops (15 mL, 60 mL)
　Ointment (Key-E®): 30 units/g (60 g, 120 g, 480 g)
　Powder (Key-E®): 700 units/dose (15 g, 75 g, 1000 g)
　Solution, oral **drops** (Aquasol E®): 15 units/0.3 mL (12 mL, 30 mL)
　Spray (Key-E®): 30 units/3 seconds (105 g)
　Tablet: 100 units, 200 units, 400 units, 500 units, 800 units
　　Key-E®: 100 units, 200 units, 400 units
References
American Academy of Pediatrics Committee on Fetus and Newborn, "Vitamin E and the Prevention of Retinopathy of Prematurity," *Pediatrics,* 1985, 76(2):315-6.

- **Vitamin G** *see* Riboflavin *on page 983*
- **Vitamin K₁** *see* Phytonadione *on page 902*
- **Vitamins, Multiple** *see page 1213*
- **Vitrasert®** *see* Ganciclovir *on page 530*
- **Vivelle®** *see* Estradiol *on page 456*
- **Vivelle Dot®** *see* Estradiol *on page 456*
- **VLB** *see* VinBLAStine *on page 1148*
- **Volmax®** *see* Albuterol *on page 54*
- **Voltaren®** *see* Diclofenac *on page 374*
- **Voltaren Ophthalmic®** *see* Diclofenac *on page 374*
- **Voltaren Rapide® (Can)** *see* Diclofenac *on page 374*
- **Voltaren®-XR** *see* Diclofenac *on page 374*

Voriconazole *(vor i KOE na zole)*

U.S. Brand Names VFEND®
Synonyms UK109496
Therapeutic Category Antifungal Agent, Systemic; Antifungal Agent, Triazole
Generic Available No
Use Treatment of invasive aspergillosis, especially in immunocompromised patients; treatment of serious fungal infections caused by *Scedosporium apiospermum* or *Fusarium* spp (including *Fusarium solanae*) in patients intolerant of, or refractory to, conventional antifungal therapy
Pregnancy Risk Factor D
Contraindications Hypersensitivity to voriconazole or any component; concurrent therapy with rifampin, carbamazepine, phenobarbital, mephobarbital, sirolimus, terfenadine, astemizole, cisapride, pimozide, quinidine, ergot alkaloids, or rifabutin (see Drug Interactions).
Warnings Serious hepatic reactions including hepatitis, cholestasis, fulminant hepatic failure, and death have been reported. Liver function test abnormalities may be associated with higher plasma drug concentrations and/or doses; dosage adjustment or discontinuation of therapy may be required. Visual changes such as blurred vision, photophobia, changes in visual acuity and color have been reported in 30% of patients in clinical trials. Patients should be warned to avoid tasks which depend on vision, including operating machinery or driving; the effect on vision with long-term administration (beyond 28 days) is unknown and should be monitored. If used during pregnancy, the patient should be informed that voriconazole may cause fetal harm. Voriconazole tablets contain lactose; avoid use in patients with rare hereditary problems of galactose intolerance, Lapp lactase deficiency, or glucose-galactose malabsorption.

Voriconazole is metabolized by cytochrome P450 enzymes resulting in interactions with other drugs. Due to potential serious and/or life-threatening drug interactions, some drugs are contraindicated (see Contraindications and Drug Interactions).
Precautions Use with caution in patients with severe renal or hepatic impairment; avoid administration of voriconazole injection in patients with Cl$_{cr}$ <50 mL/minute
Adverse Reactions
　Cardiovascular: Arrhythmias, peripheral edema, tachycardia, hypertension, hypotension, vasodilation

Central nervous system: Headache, dizziness, fatigue, anxiety, confusion, depression, amnesia, insomnia, convulsions, hemiparesis, lethargy, fever, chills, hallucinations

Dermatologic: Rash, pruritus, alopecia; photosensitivity (occurs more frequently with long-term treatment)

Endocrine & metabolic: Hypokalemia, hypomagnesemia

Gastrointestinal: Nausea, vomiting, anorexia, diarrhea, abdominal pain, constipation, mucositis, dysphagia, xerostomia

Genitourinary: Urinary tract infection, urinary retention, hemorrhagic cystitis

Hematologic: Thrombocytopenia, leukopenia, anemia, lymphopenia

Hepatic: Elevated ALT, AST, alkaline phosphatase, and bilirubin; cholestatic jaundice, hepatitis, fulminant hepatic failure

Neuromuscular & skeletal: Myalgia, ataxia

Ocular: Photophobia, visual changes, color vision change, blurred vision (visual disturbance is reversible; incidence is dose-related; onset after 1st-2nd dose)

Renal: Elevated creatinine, acute renal failure

Respiratory: Cough, dyspnea

Miscellaneous: Anaphylaxis, anaphylactoid-type reaction (flushing, fever, sweating, tachycardia, chest tightness, dyspnea, faintness, nausea, pruritus and rash) may appear immediately after initiating the I.V. infusion

Drug Interactions Cytochrome P450 isoenzyme CYP2C9, CYP2C19, and CYP3A4 (minor) substrate; isoenzyme CYP2C9, CYP2C19, and CYP3A3/4 (minor) inhibitor.

May increase plasma levels of lovastatin, midazolam, triazolam, alprazolam, phenytoin, calcium channel blockers, sulfonylureas, saquinavir, amprenavir, nelfinavir, omeprazole, and vinca alkaloids; ritonavir, saquinavir, amprenavir, delavirdine, and efavirenz may inhibit voriconazole metabolism; rifabutin may decrease voriconazole serum concentrations and voriconazole may increase rifabutin serum levels (coadministration of rifabutin with voriconazole is contraindicated; see Warnings); increases plasma concentration of sirolimus, terfenadine, astemizole, cisapride, pimozide, ergot alkaloids, and quinidine (coadministration with voriconazole is contraindicated; see Warnings); increases prothrombin time with warfarin (monitor anticoagulation tests); increases plasma cyclosporine and tacrolimus levels (adjust dose and monitor blood levels); phenytoin decreases voriconazole plasma levels (adjust voriconazole dose and monitor phenytoin levels); synergistic with caspofungin; rifampin, carbamazepine, phenobarbital, and mephobarbital reduce plasma voriconazole concentrations (coadministration with voriconazole is contraindicated; see Warnings)

Food Interactions High fat meals reduce the extent of absorption by 24%.

Stability Store tablets and unreconstituted vials at room temperature; protect from light. Reconstituted 10 mg/mL I.V. solution should be used immediately after preparation since it contains no preservative. If not used immediately, the solution is stable for 24 hours at 2°C to 8°C. The reconstituted I.V. solution can be further diluted with NS, D_5W, LR, D_5LR, D_5W with 20 mEq KCl/liter, $D_5\frac{1}{2}NS$, D_5NS, or $\frac{1}{2}NS$; voriconazole is incompatible with TPN, blood products, sodium bicarbonate, and electrolyte supplement infusions.

Mechanism of Action Inhibits fungal cytochrome P450-dependent 14a-sterol demethylase, an essential enzyme in ergosterol biosynthesis resulting in the inhibition of fungal cell membrane formation

Pharmacokinetics

Absorption: Oral: Rapid and complete

Distribution: Extensive tissue distribution

V_d: Adults: 4.6 L/kg

Protein binding: 58%

Metabolism: Metabolized by cytochrome P450 enzymes to voriconazole N-oxide (minimal antifungal activity); CYP2C19 is significantly involved in metabolism of voriconazole; CYP2C19 exhibits genetic polymorphism (15% to 20% Asians may be poor metabolizers of voriconazole; 3% to 5% Caucasians and African Americans may be poor metabolizers)

Bioavailability: 96%

Half-life: Terminal (dose-dependent): Variable

Time to peak serum concentration: Oral: 1-2 hours

Elimination: <2% excreted unchanged in urine

Usual Dosage Children and Adults:

I.V.: Loading dose: 6 mg/kg/dose every 12 hours for 2 doses on day 1; maintenance dose: 4 mg/kg/dose every 12 hours

If patient is unable to tolerate I.V. therapy, reduce the dose to 3 mg/kg/dose every 12 hours.

(Continued)

Voriconazole *(Continued)*

Oral:
Patients <40 kg: Loading dose: 200 mg every 12 hours for 2 doses on day 1; maintenance dose: 100 mg every 12 hours

If patient response is inadequate, increase dose to 150 mg every 12 hours

If patient is unable to tolerate oral dose, decrease dose by 50 mg decrement to a minimum of 100 mg every 12 hours

Note: Limited information is currently available in the literature regarding oral voriconazole use in pediatric patients; some centers have used initial maintenance doses of 3-5 mg/kg/dose every 12 hours in patients <25 kg

Patients ≥40 kg: Loading dose: 400 mg every 12 hours for 2 doses on day 1; maintenance dose: 200 mg every 12 hours

If patient response is inadequate, increase dose to 300 mg every 12 hours

If patient is unable to tolerate oral dose, decrease dose by 50 mg decrement to a minimum of 200 mg every 12 hours

Dosing adjustment in renal impairment:

Oral: No adjustment is necessary

I.V.: Cl_{cr} <50 mL/minute: Switch patient to oral voriconazole (parenteral formulation contains the excipient sulfobutyl ether beta-cyclodextrin sodium which accumulates in patients with renal impairment)

Dialysis: No dosage adjustment needed after 4-hour hemodialysis session

Dosing adjustment in hepatic impairment:

Child-Pugh Class A and B: Use standard loading dose regimen; decrease maintenance dose by 50%

Child-Pugh Class C: Not recommended for use unless benefit outweighs the risk

Administration

Oral: Administer at least one hour before or one hour after a meal

Parenteral: I.V.: **Do not administer I.V. push;** voriconazole must be administered by I.V. infusion over 1-2 hours at a rate not to exceed 3 mg/kg/hour; final concentration for administration should be 5-5 mg/mL

Monitoring Parameters Periodic renal function (particularly serum creatinine), hepatic function tests, and bilirubin; monitor visual activity, visual field, and color perception

Patient Information Avoid driving at night or performing hazardous tasks while taking voriconazole; it may cause blurred vision and/or photophobia. May cause photosensitivity reactions (eg, exposure to sunlight may cause severe sunburn, skin rash, redness, or itching); avoid exposure to sunlight and artificial light sources (sunlamps, tanning booth/bed); wear protective clothing, wide-brimmed hats, sunglasses, and lip sunscreen (SPF ≥15); use a sunscreen [broad-spectrum sunscreen or physical sunscreen (preferred) or sunblock with SPF ≥15]; contact physician if reaction occurs.

Nursing Implications Stop voriconazole infusion if anaphylactoid-type reaction occurs

Dosage Forms

Injection, powder for reconstitution: 200 mg [contains sulfobutyl ether betacyclodextrin (SBECD)]

Tablet, film coated: 50 mg, 200 mg [contains povidone]

References

Romero AJ, Pogamp PL, Nilsson LG, et al, "Effect of Voriconazole on the Pharmacokinetics of Cyclosporine in Renal Transplant Patients," *Clin Pharmacol Ther*, 2002, 71(4):226-34.

Walsh TJ, Lutsar I, Driscoll T, et al, "Voriconazole in the Treatment of Aspergillosis, Scedosporiosis and Other Invasive Fungal Infections in Children," *Pediatr Infect Dis J*, 2002, 21(3):240-8.

Walsh TJ, Pappas P, Winston DJ, et al, "Voriconazole Compared With Liposomal Amphotericin B for Empirical Antifungal Therapy in Patients With Neutropenia and Persistent Fever," *N Engl J Med*, 2002, 346(4):225-34.

♦ VoSpire ER™ *see* Albuterol *on page 54*

♦ VP-16 *see* Etoposide *on page 469*

♦ VP-16-213 *see* Etoposide *on page 469*

♦ VPA *see* Valproic Acid and Derivatives *on page 1131*

Warfarin *(WAR far in)*

Related Information

Antithrombotic Therapy in Children *on page 1316*

Overdose and Toxicology *on page 1388*

U.S. Brand Names Coumadin®

Canadian Brand Names Apo®-Warfarin; Gen-Warfarin; Taro-Warfarin

Therapeutic Category Anticoagulant

Generic Available Yes (tablet)

Use Prophylaxis and treatment of venous thromboembolic disorder and pulmonary embolism; prevention and treatment of arterial thromboembolism in patients with prosthetic heart valves or atrial fibrillation; prevention of death, recurrent MI, and thromboembolic events such as systemic embolization or stroke after MI

Pregnancy Risk Factor X

Contraindications Hypersensitivity to warfarin or any component; severe liver or kidney disease; hemorrhagic tendencies or blood dyscrasias; recent or contemplated surgery of the CNS, eye, or traumatic surgery with large open wounds; active ulceration or overt bleeding of GI, GU, or respiratory tracts, cerebrovascular hemorrhage, cerebral aneurysms, dissecting aortic aneurysms, pericarditis and pericardial effusions, bacterial endocarditis; uncontrolled bleeding; spinal puncture; major regional or lumbar block anesthesia; neurosurgical procedures; malignant hypertension; pregnancy, threatened abortion, eclampsia, pre-eclampsia; inadequate laboratory facilities; unsupervised patients with senility, alcoholism, or psychoses or other lack of patient cooperation

Warnings Serious and potentially fatal hemorrhage or necrosis and/or gangrene of the skin and other tissues may occur. Dosage must be individualized for each patient. Systemic cholesterol microemboli (eg, "purple toes syndrome") and atheroemboli may occur. Concomitant use with vitamin K may decrease anticoagulant effect; monitor carefully; concomitant use with ethacrynic acid, indomethacin, NSAIDs, phenylbutazone, or aspirin increases warfarin's anticoagulant effect and may cause severe GI irritation; oral anticoagulant therapy is usually avoided in neonates due to a greater potential risk of bleeding (see Monagle, 2001)

Precautions Do not switch brands once desired therapeutic response has been achieved; use with caution in patients with active tuberculosis, diabetes mellitus, or heparin-induced thrombocytopenia with deep vein thrombosis; use with caution in patients with or at risk for hemorrhage, necrosis, or gangrene

Periodic monitoring of INR (preferred) or prothrombin time is essential. A large number of factors (alone or in combination), including travel, changes in diet, environment, physical state, medications, and herbal remedies, may influence the patient's response to warfarin; monitor patients more closely when these factors change.

Adverse Reactions

Central nervous system: Fever

Dermatologic: Skin lesions, skin necrosis; gangrene of skin; hair loss (rare in children)

Gastrointestinal: Anorexia, nausea, vomiting, diarrhea

Hematologic: Hemorrhage

Respiratory: Hemoptysis; tracheal calcification (rare in children)

Miscellaneous: Systemic cholesterol microembolization ("purple toes syndrome")

Drug Interactions Cytochrome P450 isoenzyme CYP1A2 substrate (minor), CYP2C8, CYP2C9, CYP2C18, CYP2C19, and CYP3A3/4 isoenzyme substrate; CYP2C9 and CYP2C19 isoenzyme inhibitor

Alcohol, alteplase, amiodarone, anabolic steroids, aspirin, amoxicillin, barbiturates, carbamazepine, cefaclor, chloral hydrate, chloramphenicol, chlordiazepoxide, cholestyramine, cimetidine, clofibrate, cloxacillin, disulfiram, erythromycin, fluconazole, griseofulvin, isoniazid, ketoconazole, metronidazole, miconazole (systemic or intravaginal use), nafcillin, omeprazole, phenylbutazone, phenytoin, phenobarbital, piroxicam, prednisone, propranolol, ranitidine, rifampin, salicylates, streptokinase, sucralfate, sulfamethoxazole and trimethoprim, sulfonamides, urokinase, vitamin K, zafirlukast, zileuton; ritonavir and delavirdine may decrease warfarin metabolism; concurrent use of delavirdine and warfarin is not recommended; suspected drug interaction with nevirapine (monitor closely)

Herbal remedies such as bromelains, danshen, dong quai, garlic, ginkgo biloba, and ginseng may increase the effects of warfarin; coenzyme Q$_{10}$ (ubidecarenone) and St John's wort (*Hypericum perforatum*) may decrease the effects of Coumadin®.

Food Interactions Vitamin K can reverse the anticoagulation effects of warfarin; large amounts of food high in vitamin K (such as green leafy vegetables) may reverse warfarin, decrease prothrombin time, and lead to therapeutic failure; a balanced diet with a consistent intake of vitamin K is essential; avoid large amounts of alfalfa, asparagus, broccoli, brussel sprouts, cabbage, cauliflower, green teas, kale, lettuce, spinach, turnip greens, watercress; avoid enteral feeds high in vitamin K. **Note:** Breast-fed infants may be more sensitive to warfarin due to low amounts of vitamin K in breast milk.

High doses of vitamin A, E, or C may alter PT; use caution with fish oils or omega 3 fatty acids; avoid fried or boiled onions as they may increase drug effect by increasing fibrinolytic activity; avoid herbal teas and remedies such as tonka beans, melilot, and woodruff as they contain natural coumarins and will increase effect of warfarin; avoid large amounts of liver, avocado, soy protein, soybean oil, papain.

Stability

Tablets and injection: Protect from light

(Continued)

Warfarin (Continued)

Injection: Use within 4 hours after reconstitution, do not refrigerate, discard unused portion (does not contain preservative)

Mechanism of Action Interferes with hepatic synthesis of vitamin K-dependent coagulation factors (II, VII, IX, X)

Pharmacodynamics Anticoagulation effects:
Onset of action: Within 36-72 hours
Maximum effect: Within 5-7 days

Pharmacokinetics
Absorption: Oral: Rapid
Metabolism: In the liver
Half-life: 42 hours, highly variable among individuals

Usual Dosage Oral:
Infants and Children: **To maintain an International Normalized Ratio (INR) between 2-3:**
Initial loading dose on day 1 (if baseline INR is 1-1.3): 0.2 mg/kg (maximum dose: 10 mg); use initial loading dose of 0.1 mg/kg if patient has liver dysfunction

Loading dose for days 2-4: doses are dependent upon patient's INR
if INR is 1.1-1.3, repeat the initial loading dose
if INR is 1.4-1.9, give 50% of the initial loading dose
if INR is 2-3, give 50% of the initial loading dose
if INR is 3.1-3.5, give 25% of the initial loading dose
if INR is >3.5, hold the drug until INR <3.5, then restart at 50% less than the previous dose

Maintenance dose guidelines for day 5 of therapy and beyond: doses are dependent upon patient's INR
if INR is 1.1-1.4, increase dose by 20% of previous dose
if INR is 1.5-1.9, increase dose by 10% of previous dose
if INR is 2-3, do not change the dose
if INR is 3.1-3.5, decrease dose by 10% of previous dose
if INR is >3.5, hold the drug and check INR daily until INR <3.5, then restart at 20% less than the previous dose

Usual maintenance dose: ~0.1 mg/kg/day; range: 0.05-0.34 mg/kg/day; the dose in mg/kg/day is inversely related to age; in one study (Andrew, 1994), to attain an INR of 2-3, children <12 months of age required a mean dose of 0.32 mg/kg/day, but children 11-18 years required a mean dose of 0.09 mg/kg/day; to attain an INR of 1.3-1.8, children <12 months (n=2) required 0.24 and 0.27 mg/kg/day, but children >1 year required a mean of 0.08 mg/kg/day (range: 0.03-0.17 mg/kg/day); consistent anticoagulation may be difficult to maintain in children <5 years of age

Adults: 5-15 mg/day for 2-5 days, then adjust dose according to results of INR or PT; usual maintenance dose ranges from 2-10 mg/day

I.V.: (For patients who cannot take oral form): I.V. dose is equal to oral dose

Administration
Oral: May administer on an empty or full stomach
Parenteral: I.V. use only; do not administer I.M.; reconstitute 5 mg vial with 2.7 mL SWI to produce 2 mg/mL solution; administer by slow I.V. injection over 1-2 minutes into peripheral vein

Monitoring Parameters INR (preferred) or prothrombin time; hemoglobin, hematocrit, signs and symptoms of bleeding

Reference Range The INR is now the standard test used to monitor warfarin anticoagulation; the desired INR is based upon indication; due to the lack of pediatric clinical trials assessing optimal INR ranges and clinical outcomes, the desired INR ranges for children are extrapolated from adult studies; the optimal therapeutic INR ranges may possibly be lower in children versus adults. Further pediatric studies are needed (see Monagle, 2001)

For pediatric patients, a target INR of 2.5 (range: 2-3) is recommended for the treatment of venous thromboembolisms. A target INR of 3.0 (range: 2.5-3.5) is recommended for children with mechanical prosthetic heart valves. Low-dose warfarin (INR target range: 1.4-1.9) is recommended for the following situations: Children with substantial risks for bleeding or when monitoring is not possible; initial treatment of children with an old thrombus or those who are at a significant risk for thromboembolism; following 3 months of therapeutic doses of warfarin in children with a new thrombus and a long-term predisposing cause for recurrent thromboembolism (see Monagle, 2001) (see Additional Information).

For Adults, an INR of 2-3 is recommended for most venous thrombotic diseases including prevention and treatment of DVT, treatment of PE, prevention of systemic embolism (due to atrial fibrillation, valvulvar heart disease, acute MI, and cardiac valve replacement with tissue valves). An INR of 2.5-3.5 is recommended for cardiac valve replacement with mechanical prosthetic valves (high risk), but for a bileaflet mechanical valve in the aortic position an INR of 2-3 is recommended. An INR of 2.5-3.5 is recommended in adults to prevent recurrent MI (Hirsh, 2001).

Note: If INR is not available, prothrombin time should be $1^1/_2$ to 2 times the control.

Patient Information Avoid alcohol; limit caffeine; report any signs of bleeding to physician at once (eg, gums bleeding, dark brown urine, black tar-like stools); avoid hazardous activities; use soft toothbrush; carry Medi-Alert® ID identifying drug use; be aware of other drugs, foods, and herbal remedies to avoid; report the use of other medications, nonprescription medications, and herbal or natural products to your physician and pharmacist

Nursing Implications Be aware of drug interactions, interactions with herbal remedies, and foods that contain vitamin K which can alter anticoagulant effects; avoid I.M. injections of drugs

Additional Information Usual duration of therapy: **First venous thrombotic event:** Treat for at least 3 months; after 3 months, low-dose warfarin (INR 1.5-1.8) or LMWH is recommended as an option in children with first time central venous line-related DVT until the central venous line is removed. **Recurrent central venous line related thromboembolic events:** After initial 3 months of warfarin therapy, low-dose warfarin (INR 1.5-1.8) or LMWH is recommended until removal of the central venous line; if thromboembolism recurs during low-dose therapy, increase to a therapeutic dose and continue until central venous line is removed or for at least 3 months. **Idiopathic thrombotic event:** Treat for at least 6 months. **Recurrent noncentral venous line related thrombotic event:** After initial 3 months of warfarin therapy (recommendation: 1-3 months), treat with therapeutic or low-dose warfarin (or LMWH) indefinitely. **Mechanical prosthetic heart valves:** Treat for life (see Monagle, 2001).

Overdoses of warfarin may be treated with vitamin K, to reverse warfarin's anticoagulation effect

Dosage Forms
Injection, powder for reconstitution, lyophilized, as sodium: 5 mg
Tablet, as sodium: 1 mg, 2 mg, 2.5 mg, 3 mg, 4 mg, 5 mg, 6 mg, 7.5 mg, 10 mg

References
Andrew M, Marzinotto V, Brooker LA, et al, "Oral Anticoagulation Therapy in Pediatric Patients: A Prospective Study," *Thromb Haemost*, 1994, 71(3):265-9.

David M and Andrew M, "Venous Thromboembolic Complications in Children," *J Pediatr*, 1993, 123(3):337-46.

Fihn SD "Aiming for Safe Anticoagulation," *N Engl J Med*, 1995, 333(1):54-5.

Hirsh J, Dalen JE, Anderson DR, et al, "Oral Anticoagulants. Mechanism of Action, Clinical Effectiveness, and Optimal Therapeutic Range," *Chest*, 2001, 119:8S-21S.

Monagle P, Michelson AD, Bovill E, et al, "Antithrombotic Therapy in Children," *Chest*, 2001, 119:344S-70S.

Wells PS, Holbrook AM, Crowther NR, et al, "Interactions of Warfarin With Drugs and Food," *Ann Intern Med*, 1994, 121(9):676-83.

Zafirlukast (za FIR loo kast)

Related Information
Asthma Guidelines *on page 1376*

U.S. Brand Names Accolate®

Therapeutic Category Antiasthmatic; Leukotriene Receptor Antagonist

Generic Available No

Use Prophylaxis and chronic treatment of asthma

Pregnancy Risk Factor B

Contraindications Hypersensitivity to zafirlukast or any component

Warnings Zafirlukast is not indicated for use in the reversal of bronchospasm in acute asthma attacks, including status asthmaticus. Therapy with zafirlukast can be continued during acute exacerbations of asthma. An increased proportion of zafirlukast patients (>55 years of age) reported infections as compared to placebo-treated patients; these infections were mostly mild or moderate in intensity, predominantly affected the respiratory tract, were dose-proportional to the total milligrams of zafirlukast exposure, and associated with coadministration of inhaled corticosteroids.

Precautions Use with caution in patients receiving warfarin (see Drug Interactions) and patients with liver disease; dosage reduction in patients with hepatic impairment may be needed; discontinue therapy if liver dysfunction occurs; where no other attributable cause of liver dysfunction is identified, do not resume zafirlukast therapy

Adverse Reactions
Central nervous system: Headache, dizziness, pain, fever, asthenia

Gastrointestinal: Nausea, diarrhea, abdominal pain, vomiting, dyspepsia, xerostomia

Hepatic: Elevated liver enzymes, hepatitis, hyperbilirubinemia

Neuromuscular & skeletal: Myalgia, weakness, arthralgia

Respiratory: Rhinitis, pharyngitis

Miscellaneous: Infections (primarily respiratory), hypersensitivity reactions

Drug Interactions Cytochrome P450 isoenzyme CYP2C9 substrate; CYP2C9 and CYP3A3/4 isoenzyme inhibitor

Erythromycin, terfenadine, and theophylline decrease zafirlukast serum levels; aspirin increases plasma levels of zafirlukast; coadministration of zafirlukast with warfarin results in a clinically significant increase in prothrombin time (PT)

Food Interactions Food decreases zafirlukast absorption by 40%

Stability Store tablets at controlled room temperature; protect from light and moisture; dispense in original airtight container

Mechanism of Action Zafirlukast is a selective and competitive leukotriene-receptor antagonist (LTRA) of cysteinyl leukotrienes C_4 (LTC_4), D_4 (LTD_4), and E_4 (LTE_4). This activity produces inhibition of the effects of these leukotrienes on bronchial smooth muscle resulting in the attenuation of bronchoconstriction and decreased vascular permeability, mucosal edema, and mucus production.

Pharmacodynamics Asthma symptom improvement:
Maximum effect: 2-6 weeks
Duration: 12 hours

Pharmacokinetics
Absorption: Rapid

Distribution: Extensively excreted into breast milk; breast milk to plasma ratio: 0.15

Protein binding: 99%, predominantly albumin

Metabolism: Extensively metabolized by liver via cytochrome P450 isoenzyme CYP2C9 pathway

Half-life, elimination: 10 hours

Time to peak serum concentration: 2-4 hours

Elimination: Fecal (90%) and urine (10%)

Usual Dosage Oral:
Children 7-11 years: 10 mg twice daily
Children ≥12 years and Adults: 20 mg twice daily

Dosing adjustment in hepatic impairment: In patients with hepatic impairment (ie, biopsy-proven cirrhosis), there is a 50% to 60% greater C_{max} and AUC compared to normal subjects; these patients should be monitored closely for adverse effects and dosage reductions made if indicated (see Precautions)

Administration Oral: Administer at least 1 hour before or 2 hours after a meal

Monitoring Parameters Pulmonary function tests (FEV-1, PEF), improvement in asthma symptoms, liver function tests

Reference Range Plasma levels not clinically indicated; plasma zafirlukast serum concentrations exceeding 5 ng/mL at 12-14 hours following oral doses have correlated with activity; mean trough serum levels at doses of 20 mg twice daily were 20 ng/mL

Patient Information Take regularly as prescribed, even during symptom-free periods. Do not use to treat acute episodes of asthma. Do not decrease the dose or stop taking any other asthma medications unless instructed by a physician. May cause dry mouth. Nursing women should not take zafirlukast.

Dosage Forms Tablet: 10 mg, 20 mg

References
"National Asthma Education and Prevention Program. Expert Panel Report: Guidelines for the Diagnosis and Management of Asthma Update on Selected Topics--2002," *J Allergy Clin Immunol*, 2002, 110(5 Suppl):S141-219.

Zalcitabine (zal SITE a been)

Related Information
Adult and Adolescent HIV *on page 1327*
Pediatric HIV *on page 1323*

U.S. Brand Names Hivid®

Synonyms ddC; Dideoxycytidine

Therapeutic Category Antiretroviral Agent; HIV Agents (Anti-HIV Agents); Nucleoside Reverse Transcriptase Inhibitor (NRTI)

Generic Available No

Use Treatment of HIV infection in combination with other antiretroviral agents. (**Note:** HIV regimens consisting of **three** antiretroviral agents are strongly recommended)

Pregnancy Risk Factor C

Contraindications Hypersensitivity to zalcitabine or any component

Warnings An accumulative dose-related, clinically disabling peripheral neuropathy (treatment-limiting), or fatal pancreatitis may occur; discontinue therapy in patients with symptoms of pancreatitis until pancreatitis can be ruled out; cases of fatal lactic acidosis and severe hepatomegaly with steatosis may occur; hepatic failure and death (which may be related to underlying hepatitis B) have been reported (rare); discontinue therapy in patients with clinical or laboratory signs suggestive of lactic acidosis or hepatotoxicity (eg, steatosis and hepatomegaly even without marked elevations of liver enzymes) or if liver function tests increase to >5 times the upper limit of normal

Precautions Use with extreme caution in patients with pre-existing peripheral neuropathy; avoid use in patients with moderate or severe peripheral neuropathy; use with caution in patients at risk for developing peripheral neuropathy [patients with low CD4 count (<50 cells/mm^2), diabetes mellitus, weight loss, concurrent therapy with other drugs that cause peripheral neuropathy]; zalcitabine may exacerbate existing liver dysfunction in patients with a previous history of liver disease or alcohol abuse; increased liver function tests were observed in patients on zalcitabine therapy; use with caution in patients with hepatic impairment; obtain CBC and clinical chemistry tests prior to and during therapy; obtain serum amylase and triglyceride levels and use with caution in patients with history of pancreatitis, increased amylase, ethanol abuse or patients receiving hyperalimentation; use with caution and adjust dose in patients with renal dysfunction; multiple potentially serious drug interactions exist (see Drug Interactions); fat redistribution and accumulation [ie, central obesity, peripheral wasting, facial wasting, breast enlargement, dorsocervical fat enlargement (buffalo hump), and cushingoid appearance] have been observed in patients receiving antiretroviral agents (causal relationship not established).

Adverse Reactions
Cardiovascular: Chest pain, edema, hypertension, palpitations, syncope, atrial fibrillation, tachycardia, CHF, heart racing
Central nervous system: Headache, dizziness, fever, malaise, fatigue, chest pain
Dermatologic: Pruritus, rash (may be erythematous, maculopapular, follicular or other)
Endocrine & metabolic: Lactic acidosis (rare, but potentially fatal), hyperglycemia, hypocalcemia, fat redistribution and accumulation (see Precautions)
Gastrointestinal: Oral ulcers, nausea, esophageal ulcers, dysphagia, anorexia, abdominal pain, vomiting, diarrhea, constipation, pancreatitis (1.1%; can be fatal), weight loss
Hematologic: Leukopenia, absolute neutrophil count alteration, anemia, granulocytosis, neutrophilia, thrombocytopenia
Hepatic: Jaundice, hepatitis; severe hepatomegaly with steatosis (can be fatal)
Neuromuscular & skeletal: Peripheral neuropathy (22% to 35%), myalgia, arthralgia, weakness, foot pain, myositis
Respiratory: Pharyngitis, epistaxis
Miscellaneous: Anaphylactoid reactions, hypersensitivity reactions, night sweats

Drug Interactions Magnesium- and aluminum-containing antacids and metoclopramide may decrease the bioavailability of zalcitabine; amphotericin, foscarnet, probenecid, cimetidine, and aminoglycosides may interfere with the renal elimination of zalcitabine and potentiate the risk of peripheral neuropathy or other zalcitabine toxicities; drugs associated with peripheral neuropathy (chloramphenicol, cisplatin, (Continued)

Zalcitabine *(Continued)*

dapsone, disulfiram, ethionamide, glutethimide, gold, hydralazine, iodoquinol, isoniazid, lithium, metronidazole, nitrofurantoin, pentamidine, phenytoin, ribavirin, and vincristine) may increase the risk for zalcitabine peripheral neuropathy; concomitant use of zalcitabine with didanosine is **not** recommended (increased risk of peripheral neuropathy); lamivudine and zalcitabine may inhibit the intracellular phosphorylation of each other (concurrent use of lamivudine and zalcitabine is **not** recommended); one case of fulminant pancreatitis associated with concomitant zalcitabine and pentamidine use has been reported; if I.V. pentamidine is required to treat *Pneumocystis carinii* pneumonia, treatment with zalcitabine should be interrupted; doxorubicin may decrease zalcitabine phosphorylation to the active metabolite (*in vitro* study; clinical relevance unknown)

Food Interactions Food decreases the rate and extent of absorption (AUC decreased by 14%)

Stability Tablets should be stored in tightly closed bottles at 59°F to 86°F

Mechanism of Action A nucleoside (pyrimidine) analogue that is converted within cells to the active metabolite dideoxycytidine triphosphate (ddCTP) which serves as an alternative substrate to deoxycytidine triphosphate (dCTP), a natural substrate for cellular DNA polymerase and reverse transcriptase; inhibits HIV viral enzyme reverse transcriptase and DNA synthesis causing chain termination

Pharmacokinetics

Distribution: V_{dss}:
Children: 9.3 L/m^2
Adults: 0.53 L/kg
CSF levels are 9% to 37% of serum levels (mean 20%)

Protein binding: Minimal, <4%

Metabolism: Converted intracellularly to active triphosphate form; minimal hepatic metabolism; primary identified metabolite is dideoxyuridine

Bioavailability:
Children: 29% to 100% (mean: 54%)
Adults: >80%

Half-life:
Children: Mean: 1.4 hours
Adults: 1-3 hours (mean: 2 hours)
Adults with Cl_{cr} <55 mL/minute: up to 8.5 hours

Elimination: Primarily renal with 60% of dose excreted unchanged in urine within 24 hours; elimination is prolonged in patients with renal dysfunction

Dialysis: Hemodialysis reduces plasma levels by 50%

Usual Dosage Oral: (Use in combination with other antiretroviral agents)

Neonates: Dose unknown

Infants and Children <13 years: Usual dose: 0.01 mg/kg every 8 hours; range: 0.005-0.01 mg/kg every 8 hours

Adolescents and Adults: 0.75 mg 3 times/day

Dosing adjustment in severe renal impairment: Adults:
Cl_{cr} 10-40 mL/minute: 0.75 mg every 12 hours
Cl_{cr} <10 mL/minute: 0.75 mg every 24 hours

Administration Oral: Administer on an empty stomach 1 hour before or 2 hours after a meal; do not administer concurrently with antacids

Monitoring Parameters Renal function, CD4 counts, viral load, CBC with differential, liver enzymes, serum chemistries, serum amylase, triglyceride, signs/symptoms of peripheral neuropathy

Patient Information Avoid alcohol; zalcitabine is not a cure; notify physician if numbness, tingling, persistent severe abdominal pain, nausea, or vomiting occurs; take zalcitabine every day as prescribed; do not change dose or discontinue without physician's advice; if a dose is missed, take it as soon as possible, then return to normal dosing schedule; if a dose is skipped, do **not** double the next dose

HIV medications may cause changes in body fat, including an increase in fat in the upper back and neck, breasts, and trunk; a loss of fat from the face, arms, and legs may also occur.

Additional Information Adverse events may be increased in patients with decreased CD4 cell counts; an oral 0.1 mg/mL zalcitabine raspberry syrup formulation is available on an investigational basis from Roche Pharmaceuticals as part of a U.S. pediatric compassionate use study (NV14610)

Dosage Forms Tablet: 0.375 mg, 0.75 mg

References

Adkins JC, Peters DH, and Faulds D, "Zalcitabine. An Update of Its Pharmacodynamic and Pharmacokinetic Properties and Clinical Efficacy in the Management of HIV Infection," *Drugs*, 1997, 53(6):1054-80.
Bakshi SS, Britto P, Capparelli E, et al, "Evaluation of Pharmacokinetics, Safety, Tolerance, and Activity of Combination of Zalcitabine and Zidovudine in Stable, Zidovudine-Treated Pediatric Patients With

Human Immunodeficiency Virus Infection. AIDS Clinical Trials Group Protocol 190 Team," *J Infect Dis*, 1997, 175(5):1039-50.

Center for Disease Control and Prevention, "Guidelines for Using Antiretroviral Agents Among HIV-Infected Adults and Adolescents. Recommendations of the Panel on Clinical Practices for Treatment of HIV," *MMWR*, 2002, 51(RR-7):1-55.

Chadwick EG, Nazareno LA, Nieuwenhuis TJ, et al, "Phase I Evaluation of Zalcitabine Administered to Human Immunodeficiency Virus-Infected Children," *J Infect Dis*, 1995, 172(6):1475-9.

Pizzo PA, Butler K, Balis F, et al, "Dideoxycytidine Alone and in an Alternating Schedule With Zidovudine in Children With Symptomatic Human Immunodeficiency Virus Infection," *J Pediatr*, 1990, 117(5):799-808.

Spector SA, "HIV Therapy Advances. Pediatric Antiretroviral Choices," *AIDS*, 1994, 8(Suppl 3):S15-8.

Spector SA, Blanchard S, Wara DW, et al, "Comparative Trial of Two Dosages of Zalcitabine in Zidovudine-Experienced Children With Advanced Human Immunodeficiency Virus Disease. Pediatric AIDS Clinical Trials Group," *Pediatr Infect Dis J*, 1997, 16(6):623-6.

Working Group on Antiretroviral Therapy and Medical Management of HIV-Infected Children, "Guidelines for the Use of Antiretroviral Agents in Pediatric HIV Infection," December 14, 2001, http://www.aidsinfo.nih.gov.

Working Group on Antiretroviral Therapy and Medical Management of HIV-Infected Children, "Guidelines for the Use of Antiretroviral Agents in Pediatric HIV Infection. Hyperlink Supplement I: Pediatric Antiretroviral Drug Information," December 14, 2001, http://www.aidsinfo.nih.gov.

- **Zantac®** *see* Ranitidine *on page 972*
- **Zantac® 75 [OTC]** *see* Ranitidine *on page 972*
- **Zantac® EFFERdose®** *see* Ranitidine *on page 972*
- **Zapzyt® [OTC]** *see* Benzoyl Peroxide *on page 165*
- **Zapzyt® Acne Wash [OTC]** *see* Salicylic Acid *on page 1002*
- **Zapzyt® Pore Treatment [OTC]** *see* Salicylic Acid *on page 1002*
- **Zarontin®** *see* Ethosuximide *on page 464*
- **Zaroxolyn®** *see* Metolazone *on page 750*
- **ZDV** *see* Zidovudine *on page 1163*
- **ZDV, Abacavir, and 3TC** *see* Abacavir, Lamivudine, and Zidovudine *on page 32*
- **ZDV, Abacavir, and Lamivudine** *see* Abacavir, Lamivudine, and Zidovudine *on page 32*
- **ZDV, ABC, and 3TC** *see* Abacavir, Lamivudine, and Zidovudine *on page 32*
- **Zeasorb®-AF [OTC]** *see* Miconazole *on page 759*
- **Zemuron®** *see* Rocuronium *on page 995*
- **Zenapax®** *see* Daclizumab *on page 334*
- **Zerit®** *see* Stavudine *on page 1039*
- **Zestril®** *see* Lisinopril *on page 682*
- **Zetar® [OTC]** *see* Coal Tar *on page 299*
- **Ziagen®** *see* Abacavir *on page 30*

Zidovudine (zye DOE vyoo deen)

Related Information
Adult and Adolescent HIV *on page 1327*
Carbohydrate and Alcohol Content of Liquid Medications for Use in Patients Receiving Ketogenic Diets *on page 1431*
Pediatric HIV *on page 1323*

U.S. Brand Names Retrovir®
Canadian Brand Names Apo®-Zidovudine; AZT™; Novo-AZT
Synonyms Azidothymidine; AZT; Compound S; ZDV
Therapeutic Category Antiretroviral Agent; HIV Agents (Anti-HIV Agents); Nucleoside Reverse Transcriptase Inhibitor (NRTI)
Generic Available No
Use Treatment of HIV infection in combination with other antiretroviral agents; (**Note:** HIV regimens consisting of **three** antiretroviral agents are strongly recommended); chemoprophylaxis after occupational exposure to HIV; chemoprophylaxis to reduce perinatal HIV transmission
Pregnancy Risk Factor C
Contraindications Life-threatening hypersensitivity to zidovudine or any component
Warnings Associated with hematologic toxicity including granulocytopenia and severe anemia requiring transfusions; zidovudine treatment should be stopped in children with an absolute neutrophil count <500 cells/mm^3 until marrow recovery is observed; use of erythropoietin, filgrastim, or reduced zidovudine dosage may be necessary in some patients; use has been associated with potentially fatal lactic acidosis and severe hepatomegaly with steatosis; zidovudine has been shown to be carcinogenic in rats and mice

Syrup contains sodium benzoate; benzoic acid (benzoate) is a metabolite of benzyl alcohol; large amounts of benzyl alcohol (≥99 mg/kg/day) have been associated with a potentially fatal toxicity ("gasping syndrome") in neonates; the "gasping syndrome" consists of metabolic acidosis, respiratory distress, gasping respirations, CNS (Continued)

Zidovudine *(Continued)*

dysfunction (including convulsions, intracranial hemorrhage), hypotension and cardiovascular collapse; use syrup containing sodium benzoate with caution in neonates; *in vitro* and animal studies have shown that benzoate displaces bilirubin from protein binding sites

Precautions Fat redistribution and accumulation [ie, central obesity, peripheral wasting, facial wasting, breast enlargement, dorsocervical fat enlargement (buffalo hump), and cushingoid appearance] have been observed in patients receiving antiretroviral agents (causal relationship not established). Use with caution in patients with bone marrow compromise or in patients with impaired renal or hepatic function; reduce dosage or interrupt therapy in patients with anemia and/or granulocytopenia, myopathy, renal or hepatic impairment

Adverse Reactions

Central nervous system: Malaise, dizziness, manic syndrome, seizures, confusion, fever, severe headache, insomnia, asthenia

Dermatologic: Rash, pigmentation of nails (blue)

Endocrine & metabolic: Lactic acidosis; central redistribution of body fat: Central obesity, buffalo hump, facial atrophy, and breast enlargement

Gastrointestinal: Nausea, diarrhea, vomiting, anorexia

Hematologic: Granulocytopenia, thrombocytopenia, leukopenia, anemia

Hepatic: Cholestatic hepatitis, hepatomegaly; elevated serum AST, LDH, and alkaline phosphatase

Neuromuscular & skeletal: Myalgia, tremor, weakness; unusual: myopathy, myositis

Drug Interactions Acyclovir; coadministration with drugs that increase zidovudine concentration (acetaminophen, atovaquone, methadone, valproic acid, cimetidine, indomethacin, lorazepam, fluconazole, probenecid, aspirin) may increase toxicity of zidovudine; flucytosine, pentamidine, and sulfamethoxazole and trimethoprim may increase hematologic side effects; didanosine, foscarnet, ganciclovir, zalcitabine (synergistic antiretroviral activity); ribavirin (antagonistic); coadministration with rifampin or rifabutin may increase metabolism of zidovudine; clarithromycin decreases zidovudine concentration by interfering with its absorption (administer doses 4 hours apart); do not administer in combination with stavudine (poor antiretroviral effect)

Food Interactions Folate or vitamin B_{12} deficiency increases zidovudine-associated myelosuppression

Stability Diluted I.V. zidovudine solution is stable for 24 hours when refrigerated

Mechanism of Action Zidovudine is a thymidine analog that enters the cell and is phosphorylated by cellular kinases to the active metabolite zidovudine triphosphate which serves as an alternative substrate to deoxythymidine triphosphate for incorporation by reverse transcriptase; inhibits HIV viral polymerases and DNA synthesis

Pharmacokinetics

Absorption: Oral: Well absorbed (66% to 70%)

Distribution: Significant penetration into the CSF; crosses the placenta

Protein binding: 25% to 38%

Metabolism: Extensive first-pass effect; metabolized in the liver via glucuronidation to inactive metabolites

Bioavailability:

Neonates <14 days: 89%

Infants: 60%

Half-life, terminal: 60 minutes

Premature neonate: 6.3 hours

Full-term neonates: 3.1 hours

Older infants: 1.9 hours

Time to peak serum concentration: Within 30-90 minutes

Elimination: Urinary excretion (63% to 95%)

Oral: 72% to 74% of drug excreted in urine as metabolites and 14% to 18% as unchanged drug

I.V.: 45% to 60% excreted in urine as metabolites and 18% to 29% as unchanged drug

Usual Dosage

Premature Infants: (Standard neonatal dose may be excessive in premature infants)
Under investigation in PACTG 331: Oral: 1.5 mg/kg/dose every 12 hours from birth to 2 weeks of age; then increase to 2 mg/kg/dose every 8 hours after 2 weeks of age

Neonates:

Oral: 2 mg/kg/dose every 6 hours

I.V.: 1.5 mg/kg/dose every 6 hours

Children:

Oral: 160 mg/m^2/dose every 8 hours; dosage range: 90 mg/m^2/dose to 180 mg/m^2/dose every 6-8 hours; some Working Group members use a dose of 180 mg/m^2 every 12 hours when using in drug combinations with other antiretroviral compounds, but data on this dosing in children is limited

I.V. continuous infusion: 20 mg/m^2/hour

I.V. intermittent infusion: 120 mg/m^2/dose every 6 hours

Dosing adjustment in children with zidovudine toxicity:

Hemoglobin <8 g/dL: Reduce zidovudine dose by 30%

Children >12 years and Adults:

Oral: 200 mg 3 times/day or 300 mg twice daily

HIV postexposure prophylaxis: 600 mg/day in divided doses (eg, 300 mg twice daily, 200 mg 3 times/day or 100 mg every 4 hours) in combination with lamivudine 150 mg twice daily and indinavir 800 mg 3 times/day are first-line agents for HIV postexposure prophylaxis

I.V.: 1-2 mg/kg/dose every 4 hours

Administration

Oral: May administer with food (although the manufacturer recommends administration 30 minutes before or 1 hour after a meal with a glass of water); the patient should be in an upright position while taking zidovudine capsules to minimize the risk of esophageal ulceration

Parenteral: Do not administer I.M.; do not administer I.V. push or by rapid infusion; infuse I.V. zidovudine over 1 hour at a final concentration not to exceed 4 mg/mL in D$_5$W

Monitoring Parameters CBC with differential, hemoglobin, MCV, reticulocyte count, serum creatine kinase, CD4 cell count, HIV RNA plasma levels, renal and hepatic function tests

Patient Information Zidovudine is not a cure for HIV. Take zidovudine as directed. Notify physician if muscle weakness, shortness of breath, headache, insomnia, signs of infection, unusual bleeding, or rash occur.

HIV medications may cause changes in body fat, including an increase in fat in the upper back and neck, breasts, and trunk; a loss of fat from the face, arms, and legs may also occur.

Additional Information Conversion from oral to I.V. dose: I.V. dose = ^{2}/$_3$ of the oral dose

Dosage Forms

Capsule: 100 mg

Injection, solution: 10 mg/mL (20 mL)

Syrup: 50 mg/5 mL (240 mL) [contains sodium benzoate; strawberry flavor]

Tablet, film coated: 300 mg

References

Carpenter CC, Fischel MA, Hammer SM, et al, "Antiretroviral Therapy for HIV Infection in 1997. Updated Recommendations of the International AIDS Society - USA Panel," *JAMA*, 1997, 277(24):1962-9.

CDC and the National Foundation for Infectious Disease, "Public Health Service Guidelines for the Management of Health-Care Worker Exposures to HIV and Recommendations for Postexposure Prophylaxis," *MMWR Morb Mortal Wkly Rep*, May 15, 1998/47 (RR-7):29-30.

Mueller BU, Jacobsen F, Butler KM, et al, "Combination Treatment With Azidothymidine and Granulocyte Colony-Stimulating Factor in Children With Human Immunodeficiency Virus Infection," *J Pediatr*, 1992, 121(5 Pt 1):797-802.

Volberding PA, Lagakos SW, Koch MA, et al, "Zidovudine in Asymptomatic Human Immunodeficiency Virus Infection. A Controlled Trial in Persons With Fewer Than 500 CD4-Positive Cells Per Cubic Millimeter. The AIDS Clinical Trials Group of the National Institute of Allergy and Infectious Diseases," *N Engl J Med*, 1990, 322(14):941-9.

Working Group on Antiretroviral Therapy and Medical Management of HIV-Infected Children, "Guidelines for the Use of Antiretroviral Agents in Pediatric HIV Infection," April 15, 1999, http://www.aidsinfo.nih.gov.

♦ **Zidovudine, Abacavir, and Lamivudine** *see* Abacavir, Lamivudine, and Zidovudine *on page 32*

♦ **Zidovudine and Lamivudine** *see* Lamivudine and Zidovudine *on page 652*

♦ **Zilactin®-B [OTC]** *see* Benzocaine *on page 163*

♦ **Zilactin® Baby [OTC]** *see* Benzocaine *on page 163*

♦ **Zilactin®-L [OTC]** *see* Lidocaine *on page 671*

Zileuton (zye LOO ton)

Related Information

Asthma Guidelines *on page 1376*

U.S. Brand Names Zyflo™

Therapeutic Category Antiasthmatic; Leukotriene Receptor Antagonist

Generic Available No

Use Prophylaxis and chronic treatment of asthma

Pregnancy Risk Factor C

(Continued)

Zileuton *(Continued)*

Contraindications Hypersensitivity to zileuton or any component; active liver disease or transaminase elevations greater than or equal to three times the upper limit of normal

Warnings Coadministration of zileuton with theophylline, propranolol, astemizole, and terfenadine is associated with significant increases in serum levels of these agents which may require reductions in dosage; elevated terfenadine and astemizole levels have been associated with severe cardiovascular effects including QT interval prolongation, ventricular tachycardia, ventricular fibrillation, death, cardiac arrest, hypotension, and palpitations; elevations of one or more liver function tests may occur during therapy; these laboratory abnormalities may progress, remain unchanged, or resolve with continued therapy; zileuton is **not** indicated for use in the reversal of bronchospasm in acute asthma attacks, including status asthmaticus; zileuton can be continued during acute exacerbations of asthma.

Precautions Use with caution in patients who consume substantial quantities of alcohol or have a past history of liver disease

Adverse Reactions

Cardiovascular: Chest pain

Central nervous system: Headache, pain, dizziness, fever, insomnia, fatigue, nervousness, somnolence

Gastrointestinal: Dyspepsia, nausea, abdominal pain, constipation, flatulence

Hematologic: Low white blood cell count

Hepatic: Elevated liver enzymes

Neuromuscular & skeletal: Myalgia, arthralgia, weakness, paresthesias, asthenia

Ocular: Conjunctivitis

Drug Interactions Cytochrome P450 isoenzyme CYP1A2, CYP2C9, and CYP3A3/4 substrate; CYP1A2 and CYP3A3/4 isoenzyme inhibitor

Increased toxicity: Coadministration of zileuton with propranolol or theophylline results in an approximate doubling of serum concentrations (propranolol or theophylline); coadministration of zileuton with warfarin results in a clinically significant increase in prothrombin time (PT); coadministration of zileuton with terfenadine or astemizole results in a decrease in clearance leading to an increase in terfenadine or astemizole serum levels (elevated serum levels have been associated with severe cardiovascular effects, see Warnings)

Mechanism of Action Specific inhibitor of 5-lipoxygenase and thus inhibits leukotriene (LTB1, LTC1, LTD1, and LTE1) formation. Leukotrienes are substances that induce numerous biological effects including augmentation of neutrophil and eosinophil migration, neutrophil and monocyte aggregation, leukocyte adhesion, increased capillary permeability and smooth muscle contraction.

Pharmacodynamics After discontinuation of zileuton therapy, 5-lipoxygenase activity (eg, return of leukotriene B4 levels to baseline) occurred in approximately 7 days. See table.

Zileuton Pharmacodynamic Parameters

Parameter	Inhibition of Leukotriene B4 Production	Increased FEV-1
Onset of effect	0.5-1 h	30 min
Peak effect	2-4 h	1 h
Maximal effect	5-8 h	4 wk

Pharmacokinetics

Absorption: Rapidly absorbed

Distribution: V_d: 1.2 L/kg

Protein binding: 93%

Metabolism: Several metabolites in plasma and urine; metabolized by the cytochrome P450 isoenzymes CYP1A2, CYP2C9, and CYP3A4

Half-life: 2.1-2.5 hours

Time to peak serum concentration: 1-3 hours

Elimination: Predominantly via metabolism; <0.5% excreted unchanged in urine

Clearance: 7 mL/minute/kg

Usual Dosage Oral: Children ≥12 years and Adults: 600 mg 4 times daily with meals and at bedtime

Dosing adjustment in hepatic impairment: Contraindicated in patients with active liver disease

Administration May administer without regard to meals

Monitoring Parameters Monitor serum ALT before treatment begins, once monthly for the first 3 months, every 2-3 months for the remainder of the first year and periodically thereafter for patients receiving long-term zileuton therapy; complete blood count periodically when on long-term therapy; pulmonary function tests, improvement in asthma symptoms

Patient Information Inform patients that zileuton is indicated for the chronic treatment of asthma and to take regularly as prescribed even during symptom-free periods. Zileuton is not a bronchodilator; do not use to treat acute episodes of asthma. When taking zileuton, do not decrease the dose or stop taking any other asthma medications unless instructed by a physician.

If experiencing signs or symptoms of liver dysfunction (right upper quadrant pain, nausea, fatigue, lethargy, pruritus, jaundice, or "flu-like" symptoms), contact a physician immediately.

Zileuton can interact with other drugs. While taking zileuton, consult a physician or pharmacist before starting or stopping any prescription or nonprescription medicines.

Dosage Forms Tablet: 600 mg

- ◆ **Zinacef®** *see* Cefuroxime *on page 242*
- ◆ **Zinc Acetate** *see* Zinc Supplements *on page 1167*
- ◆ **Zincate®** *see* Zinc Supplements *on page 1167*
- ◆ **Zinc Carbonate** *see* Zinc Supplements *on page 1167*
- ◆ **Zinc Chloride** *see* Trace Metals *on page 1106*
- ◆ **Zinc Chloride** *see* Zinc Supplements *on page 1167*
- ◆ **Zinc Gluconate** *see* Zinc Supplements *on page 1167*
- ◆ **Zincofax® (Can)** *see* Zinc Oxide *on page 1167*

Zinc Oxide (zingk OKS ide)

U.S. Brand Names Ammens® Medicated Deodorant [OTC]; Balmex® [OTC]; Boudreaux's® Butt Paste [OTC]; Critic-Aid Skin Care® [OTC]; Desitin® [OTC]; Desitin® Creamy [OTC]

Canadian Brand Names Zincofax®

Synonyms Lassar's Zinc Paste

Therapeutic Category Topical Skin Product

Generic Available Yes (ointment)

Use Protective coating for mild skin irritations and abrasions; soothing and protective ointment to promote healing of chapped skin, diaper rash

Contraindications Hypersensitivity to zinc oxide or any component

Stability Avoid prolonged storage at temperatures >30°C

Mechanism of Action Mild astringent, protective and weak antiseptic action

Usual Dosage Infants, Children, and Adults: Topical: Apply several times daily to affected area

Administration Topical: For external use only; do not use in the eyes

Patient Information Paste is easily removed with mineral oil

Dosage Forms
Ointment, topical: 20% (30 g, 60 g, 480 g)
  Balmex®: 11.3% (60 g, 120 g, 480 g)
  Desitin®: 40% (30 g, 60 g, 90 g, 120 g, 270 g, 480 g)
  Desitin® Creamy: 10% (60 g, 120 g)
Paste, topical:
  Boudreaux's® Butt Paste: 16% (30 g, 60 g, 120 g, 480 g) [contains castor oil, boric acid, mineral oil, and Peruvian balsam]
  Critic-Aid Skin Care®: 20% (71 g, 170 g)
Powder, topical (Ammens® Medicated Deodorant): 9.1% (187.5 g, 330 g) [original and shower fresh scent]

- ◆ **Zinc Sulfate** *see* Trace Metals *on page 1106*
- ◆ **Zinc Sulfate** *see* Zinc Supplements *on page 1167*

Zinc Supplements (zink SUP la ments)

U.S. Brand Names Cold-Eeze® [OTC]; Galzin™; Orazinc® [OTC]; Zincate®

Available Salts Zinc Acetate; Zinc Carbonate; Zinc Chloride; Zinc Gluconate; Zinc Sulfate

Therapeutic Category Antidote, Copper Toxicity; Mineral, Oral; Mineral, Parenteral

Generic Available Yes

Use Treatment and prevention of zinc deficiency states; may improve wound healing in those who are zinc deficient; maintenance treatment of Wilson's disease (zinc acetate)

Pregnancy Risk Factor C (A for zinc acetate)

(Continued)

Zinc Supplements *(Continued)*

Contraindications Hypersensitivity to zinc salts or any component

Warnings Do not administer undiluted by direct injection into a peripheral vein due to potential for phlebitis, tissue irritation, and potential increased renal loss of minerals from a bolus injection; administration of zinc in absence of copper may decrease plasma copper levels; excessive intake in healthy persons may be deleterious as decreases in HDL (high-density lipoproteins) and impairment of immune system function have been reported

Adverse Reactions

Cardiovascular: Hypotension, tachycardia (excessive doses)

Central nervous system: Hypothermia (excessive doses)

Gastrointestinal: Indigestion, nausea, vomiting

Hematologic: Neutropenia, leukopenia

Hepatic: Jaundice (excessive doses)

Ocular: Blurred vision (excessive doses)

Respiratory: Pulmonary edema (excessive doses)

Miscellaneous: Profuse diaphoresis

Drug Interactions Zinc may decrease penicillamine, tetracycline, and quinolone absorption; iron decreases zinc absorption; agents which increase gastric pH, such as H_2-blockers, may decrease zinc absorption

Food Interactions Coffee, foods high in phytate (eg, whole grain cereals & legumes), bran, and dairy products reduce zinc absorption; avoid foods high in calcium or phosphorus

Mechanism of Action A cofactor for more than 70 enzymes which are important to carbohydrate and protein metabolism, zinc helps to maintain normal growth and tissue repair, normal skin hydration, and senses of taste and smell; in Wilson's disease, zinc cation inhibits the absorption of dietary copper by inducing the synthesis of metallothionein, a metal-binding protein present in the intestinal mucosa. This protein binds metals, including copper, forming a nontoxic complex that is not absorbed systematically but excreted in the stool.

Pharmacokinetics

Absorption: pH dependent; poor from GI tract (20% to 30%); solubilized by conversion to zinc chloride in the presence of gastric acid

Distribution: Storage sites are liver and skeletal muscle; serum levels do not adequately reflect whole-body zinc status

Protein binding: 55% bound to albumin; 40% bound to alpha 1-macroglobulin

Elimination: 90% in feces with only traces appearing in urine and perspiration

Usual Dosage Clinical response may not occur for up to 6-8 weeks

RDA: Oral:

Neonates and Infants <12 months: 5 mg **elemental** zinc/day

Children 1-10 years: 10 mg **elemental** zinc/day

Children ≥11 years and Adults: Male: 15 mg **elemental** zinc/day; Female: 12 mg **elemental** zinc/day

Zinc deficiency: Oral:

Infants and Children: 0.5-1 mg **elemental** zinc/kg/day divided 1-3 times/day; larger doses may be needed if impaired intestinal absorption or an excessive loss of zinc (eg, excessive, prolonged diarrhea)

Adults: 25-50 mg **elemental** zinc/dose (110-220 mg zinc sulfate) 3 times/day

Supplement to parenteral nutrition solutions (clinical response may not occur for up to 6-8 weeks): (See Trace Metals): I.V. (all doses are mcg of **elemental** zinc):

Premature Infants: 400 mcg/kg/day

Term Infants <3 months: 300 mcg/kg/day

Infants ≥3 months and Children ≤5 years: 100 mcg/kg/day (maximum: 5 mg/day)

Children >5 years and Adolescents: 2.5-5 mg/day

Adults:

Stable metabolically: 2.5-4 mg **elemental** zinc/day; catabolic state: Increase by an additional 2 mg/day (eg, 4.5-6 mg **elemental** zinc/day)

Stable with fluid loss from small bowel: Additional 12.2 mg **elemental** zinc/L parenteral nutrition or 17.1 mg **elemental** zinc/kg of stool or ileostomy output

Wound healing: Oral: Adults: 50 mg **elemental** zinc (220 mg zinc sulfate) 3 times daily in patients with low serum zinc levels (<110 mcg/dL)

Maintenance treatment of Wilson's disease: **Zinc acetate:** Dose is in mg elemental zinc:

Children ≥10 years and Pregnant Women: 25 mg 3 times/day

Adults (nonpregnant): 50 mg 3 times/day

Note: Not indicated for initial treatment of Wilson's disease but for maintenance after initial therapy with a chelating agent (approximately 4-6 months)

Administration

Oral: Administer oral formulation with food if GI upset occurs; in patients with Wilson's disease, administer zinc acetate 1 hour before or after meals or beverage (except water); zinc acetate capsules should be swallowed whole; do not open or chew

Parenteral: Dilute as component of daily parenteral nutrition or maintenance fluids; do not give undiluted by direct injection into a peripheral vein due to potential for phlebitis and tissue irritation, and potential to increase renal losses of minerals from a bolus injection

Monitoring Parameters Patients on parenteral nutrition or chronic therapy should have periodic serum copper and serum zinc levels; alkaline phosphatase, taste acuity, mental depression, wound healing (if indicated), growth (if indicated), skin integrity; Wilson's disease: 24-hour urinary copper excretion, neuropsychiatric evaluations, LFTs

Reference Range

Serum: 70-130 µg/dL

Urinary copper (Wilson's disease patient **not** on chelation therapy): <125 g/24 hours (patients on chelation therapy will have increased urinary copper due to chelated copper)

Patient Information Do not exceed recommended dose

Dosage Forms

Zinc acetate:

Capsule (Galzin™): 25 mg elemental zinc, 50 mg elemental zinc

Zinc chloride:

Injection, solution: 1 mg elemental zinc/mL (10 mL, 50 mL)

Zinc, elemental:

Lozenges: 10 mg, 23 mg

Cold-Eeze®: 13.3 mg [bubblegum, citrus, cherry, menthol, and tropical fruit flavors]

Tablet: 30 mg, 60 mg

Zinc gluconate (14.3% zinc):

Tablet: 50 mg [elemental zinc 7 mg]; 100 mg [elemental zinc 14 mg]

Zinc sulfate (23% zinc):

Capsule (Orazinc®, Zincate®): 220 mg [elemental zinc 50 mg]

Injection, solution [preservative free]: 1 mg elemental zinc/mL (10 mL); 5 mg elemental zinc/mL (5 mL)

Tablet (Orazinc®): 110 mg [elemental zinc 25 mg]

References

Anderson LA, Hakojarvi SL, and Boudreaux SK, "Zinc Acetate Treatment in Wilson's Disease," *Ann Pharmacother*, 1998, 32:78-87.

Zonisamide (zoe NIS a mide)

U.S. Brand Names Zonegran®

Therapeutic Category Anticonvulsant, Miscellaneous

Generic Available No

Use Adjunctive treatment of partial seizures in adolescents >16 years of age and adults with epilepsy; has been used investigationally for the treatment of generalized epilepsies including, generalized tonic-clonic seizures, absence seizures, infantile spasms, myoclonic epilepsies, and Lennox-Gastaut syndrome (see Leppik, 1999 and Oommen, 1999)

Pregnancy Risk Factor C

Contraindications Hypersensitivity to zonisamide, sulfonamides, or any component

Warnings Zonisamide is a sulfonamide; although rare, severe, and life-threatening sulfonamide reactions may occur (eg, Stevens-Johnson syndrome, toxic epidermal necrolysis, aplastic anemia, agranulocytosis, other blood dyscrasias, and fulminant hepatic necrosis); discontinue zonisamide in patients with signs of hypersensitivity reaction or other serious reactions; consider discontinuation of zonisamide in any
(Continued)

Zonisamide *(Continued)*

patient who develops a rash or monitor very closely; deaths due to serious rashes have been reported; rashes usually appear within 2-16 weeks of starting therapy.

Oligohydrosis (decreased sweating) and hyperthermia have been reported in 40 pediatric patients; many cases occurred after exposure to elevated environmental temperatures; some cases resulted in heat stroke requiring hospitalization; pediatric patients may be at an increased risk; monitor patients, especially pediatric patients, for decreased sweating and hyperthermia, especially in warm or hot weather; use zonisamide with caution in patients receiving drugs that predispose to heat-related disorders (eg, anticholinergic agents, carbonic anhydrase inhibitors); safety and efficacy in pediatric patients <16 years of age has not been established.

Do not abruptly discontinue therapy; abrupt withdrawal may precipitate seizures; withdraw gradually to lessen chance for increased seizure frequency (unless a more rapid withdrawal is required due to safety concerns). CNS adverse effects may occur including fatigue or somnolence, psychiatric symptoms (eg, depression, psychosis), and cognitive symptoms [difficulty concentrating, speech or language problems (especially word-finding difficulties), and psychomotor slowing]; fatigue and somnolence usually occur within the first month of starting therapy, most commonly at higher doses (eg, in adults at doses of 300-500 mg/day).

Precautions Use with caution in patients with renal or hepatic dysfunction; do not use in patients with Cl_{cr} <50 mL/minute; zonisamide may cause kidney stones (ensure patients have adequate fluid intake); zonisamide may decrease GFR and increase serum creatinine and BUN; discontinue therapy in patients who develop acute renal failure or a persistent significant increase in serum creatinine or BUN

Adverse Reactions

Central nervous system: Somnolence, fatigue, dizziness, headache, agitation, irritability, tiredness, ataxia, confusion, memory impairment, depression, psychosis, difficulty concentrating, speech or language problems (especially word-finding difficulties), psychomotor slowing, insomnia, mental slowing, anxiety, nervousness, tremor, convulsion, hyperesthesia, incoordination; behavior disorders in children have been reported (Kimura, 1994)

Dermatologic: Rash, bruising, pruritus, Stevens-Johnson syndrome (rare), toxic epidermal necrolysis (rare)

Gastrointestinal: Anorexia, nausea, diarrhea, abdominal pain, dyspepsia, weight loss, constipation, dry mouth, taste perversion, vomiting

Hematologic: Aplastic anemia (rare), agranulocytosis (rare), other blood dyscrasias (rare)

Hepatic: Elevated alkaline phosphatase; elevated LDH and transaminases (rare)

Neuromuscular & skeletal: Paresthesia, abnormal gait

Ocular: Diplopia, nystagmus, amblyopia

Otic: Tinnitus

Renal: Elevated BUN and serum creatinine

Respiratory: Rhinitis, pharyngitis, increased cough

Miscellaneous: Flu-like syndrome; oligohydrosis and hyperthermia [pediatric patients may be at increased risk (see Warnings)]

Drug Interactions Cytochrome P450 isoenzyme CYP3A4 substrate

Enzyme inducers (eg, carbamazepine, phenobarbital, phenytoin) may increase the metabolism of zonisamide and decrease zonisamide serum concentrations; valproate may decrease the half-life of zonisamide. Lamotrigine may inhibit the clearance of zonisamide and increase zonisamide serum concentrations; enzyme inhibitors may increase zonisamide serum concentrations (monitor for increased effect/toxicity)

Zonisamide does **not** affect serum concentrations of carbamazepine, phenytoin, or valproate. Zonisamide may decrease serum concentrations of the carbamazepine epoxide metabolite in patients receiving carbamazepine. CNS depressants, including alcohol, may increase sedative effects (monitor for increased effect/toxicity).

Food Interactions Food decreases the rate, but not the extent of absorption.

Stability Store at controlled room temperature 25°C (77°C). Protect from moisture and light.

Mechanism of Action Exact mechanism of action is not known; may stabilize neuronal membranes and suppress neuronal hypersynchronization by blocking sodium channels and T-type calcium currents; does not affect GABA activity; possesses weak carbonic anhydrase inhibiting activity, but this in not thought to be a very significant component of its antiepileptic action

Pharmacokinetics

Absorption: Oral: Rapid and complete

Distribution: V_d (apparent): Adults: 1.45 L/kg; highly concentrated in erythrocytes; distributes into breast milk at a transfer rate of 41% to 57% (see Kawada, 2002)

Protein binding: 40%

Metabolism: Hepatic; undergoes acetylation to form N-acetyl zonisamide, and reduction via cytochrome P450 isoenzyme CYP3A4 to 2-sulfamoylacetylphenol (SMAP); SMAP then undergoes conjugation with glucuronide

Half-life: Adults: 63 hours (range: 50-68 hours)

Time to peak serum concentration: 2-6 hours

Elimination: Urine: 62% (35% as unchanged drug, 15% as N-acetyl zonisamide, 50% as SMAP glucuronide); feces (3%); **Note:** Of the dose recovered in Japanese patients, 28% is as unchanged drug, 52% is as N-acetyl zonisamide, and 19% is as SMAP glucuronide (Glauser, 2002)

Usual Dosage Oral:

Infants and Children: In a review article of 20 Japanese pediatric studies, the following doses were recommended (see Glauser, 2002): Initial: 1-2 mg/kg/day given in two divided doses/day; increase dose in increments of 0.5-1 mg/kg/day every 2 weeks; usual dose: 5-8 mg/kg/day.

Higher initial and maximum doses have been recommended by others (see Leppik, 1999 and Oommen, 1999): Initial: 2-4 mg/kg/day given in two divided doses/day; titrate dose upwards if needed every 2 weeks; usual dose: 4-8 mg/kg/day; maximum dose: 12 mg/kg/day

Infantile spasms: Several studies used a faster titration of zonisamide to control infantile spasms. Suzuki treated 11 newly diagnosed infants (mean age: ~6 months) with zonisamide monotherapy starting at doses of 3-5 mg/kg/day given in 2 divided doses/day; doses were increased every 4th day until seizures were controlled or a maximum dose of 10 mg/kg/day was attained; 4 of 11 patients responded at doses of 4-5 mg/kg/day (see Suzuki, 1997). Yanai treated 27 newly diagnosed infantile spasm patients with zonisamide add-on or monotherapy starting at doses of 2-4 mg/kg/day given in 2 divided doses/day; doses were increased by 2-5 mg/kg every 2-4 days until seizures were controlled or a maximum of 10-20 mg/kg/day was attained; 9 of 27 patients responded at a mean effective dose of 7.8 mg/kg/day (range: 5-12.5 mg/kg/day); non-responders received doses of 8-20 mg/kg/day (mean: 10.8 mg/kg/day) (see Yania, 1999). Suzuki treated 54 newly diagnosed infants (11 of which were previously reported) with zonisamide monotherapy starting at doses of 3-4 mg/kg/day given in 2 divided doses; doses were increased every 4th day until seizures were controlled or a maximum dose of 10-13 mg/kg/day was attained; 11 of 54 infants responded at a mean effective dose of 7.2 mg/kg/day (range: 4-12 mg/kg/day); the majority of infants who responded did so at a dose of 4-8 mg/kg/day and within 1-2 weeks of starting therapy (see Suzuki, 2001). Further studies are needed.

Adolescents >16 years and Adults: Initial: 100 mg once daily; dose may be increased to 200 mg/day after 2 weeks; further increases in dose should be made in increments of 100 mg/day and only after a minimum of 2 weeks between adjustments; usual effective dose: 100-600 mg/day. **Note:** There is no evidence of increased benefit with doses >400 mg/day. Steady-state serum concentrations fluctuate 27% with once daily dosing, and 14% with twice daily dosing; patients may benefit from divided doses given twice daily (Leppik, 1999)

Dosage adjustment in renal/hepatic impairment: Slower dosage titration and more frequent monitoring are recommended in patients with renal or hepatic disease. Do not use if Cl_{cr} <50 mL/minute.

Administration May be administered without regard to meals; swallow capsule whole; do not crush, chew, or break capsule

Monitoring Parameters Seizure frequency, duration, and severity; symptoms of CNS adverse effects; skin rash; BUN and serum creatinine; monitor patients, especially pediatric patients, for decreased sweating and hyperthermia, especially in warm or hot weather

Reference Range Monitoring of plasma concentrations may be useful; proposed therapeutic range: 10-20 mcg/mL; patients may benefit from higher concentrations (ie, up to 30 mcg/mL), but concentrations >30 mcg/mL have been associated with adverse effects (see Oommen, 1999 and Leppik, 1999)

Patient Information Inform prescriber if allergic to sulfa drugs (eg, Bactrim®, Septra®); do not abruptly discontinue therapy, an increase in seizure activity may result; may cause drowsiness and impair ability to perform activities that require mental alertness or physical coordination; report excessive drowsiness, unusual thoughts, depression, problems with concentrating or speaking, worsening of seizures, or any skin rashes to physician immediately; avoid alcohol; notify physician immediately if a child taking zonisamide is not sweating as usual or has elevated temperature; drink adequate amount of fluids and report any symptoms of kidney stones (eg, back pain, stomach pain, pain on urination, bloody urine); report any unusual symptoms, such as a bruises, sore throat, fever, or mouth ulcers to physician (Continued)

Zonisamide *(Continued)*

Dosage Forms Capsule: 100 mg

References

Glauser TA and Pellock JM, "Zonisamide in Pediatric Epilepsy: Review of the Japanese Experience," *J Child Neurol*, 2002, 17(2):87-96.

Kawada K, Itoh S, Kusaka T, et al, "Pharmacokinetics of Zonisamide in Perinatal Period," *Brain Dev*, 2002, 24(2):95-7.

Kimura S, "Zonisamide-Induced Behavior Disorder in Two Children," *Epilepsia*, 1994, 35(2):403-5.

Leppik IE, "Zonisamide," *Epilepsia*, 1999, 40(Suppl 5):S23-9.

Oommen KJ and Mathews S, "Zonisamide: A New Antiepileptic Drug," *Clin Neuropharmacol*, 1999, 22(4):192-200.

Suzuki Y, Nagai T, Ono J, et al, "Zonisamide Monotherapy in Newly Diagnosed Infantile Spasms," *Epilepsia*, 1997, 38(9):1035-8.

Suzuki Y, "Zonisamide in West Syndrome," *Brain Dev*, 2001, 23(7):658-61.

Yanai S, Hanai T, and Narazaki O, "Treatment of Infantile Spasms With Zonisamide," *Brain Dev*, 1999, 21(3):157-61.

- **ZORprin®** *see* Aspirin *on page 134*
- **Zostrix® [OTC]** *see* Capsaicin *on page 206*
- **Zostrix®-HP [OTC]** *see* Capsaicin *on page 206*
- **Zostrix® Sports [OTC]** *see* Capsaicin *on page 206*
- **Zosyn®** *see* Piperacillin and Tazobactam *on page 907*
- **Zovirax®** *see* Acyclovir *on page 45*
- **ZVD and 3TC** *see* Lamivudine and Zidovudine *on page 652*
- **Zydone®** *see* Hydrocodone and Acetaminophen *on page 571*
- **Zyflo™** *see* Zileuton *on page 1165*
- **Zyloprim®** *see* Allopurinol *on page 62*
- **Zyrtec®** *see* Cetirizine *on page 249*
- **Zyvox™** *see* Linezolid *on page 678*

APPENDIX TABLE OF CONTENTS

CPR PEDIATRIC DRUG DOSAGES

(PALS Medications for Cardiac Arrest and Symptomatic Arrhythmias)

Drug	Dose	Remarks
Adenosine	0.1 mg/kg Repeat dose: 0.2 mg/kg Maximum single dose: 12 mg	Rapid I.V., I.O. bolus Rapid flush to central circulation Monitor ECG during dose
Amiodarone for pulseless VF/VT	I.V., I.O.: 5 mg/kg	Rapid I.V. bolus
Amiodarone for perfusing tachycardias	Loading dose: I.V., I.O.: 5 mg/kg Maximum dose: 15 mg/kg/day	I.V. over 20-60 minutes Routine use in combination with drugs prolonging QT interval is **not** recommended; hypotension is most frequent side effect
Atropine sulfate*	I.V.: 0.02 mg/kg (minimum dose = 0.1 mg) Maximum single dose (may repeat once): Children: 0.5 mg Adolescents: 1 mg	May give I.V., I.O., or E.T. Tachycardia and pupil dilation may occur but **not** fixed dilated pupils
Calcium chloride 10% = 100 mg/mL (=27.2 mg/mL elemental Ca)	I.V., I.O.: 20 mg/kg (0.2 mL/kg)	Give slow I.V. push for hypocalcemia, hypermagnesemia, calcium channel blocker toxicity, preferably via central vein; monitor heart rate - bradycardia may occur
Calcium gluconate 10% = 100 mg/mL (=9 mg/mL elemental Ca)	I.V., I.O.: 60-100 mg/kg (0.6-1 mL/kg)	Give slow I.V. push for hypocalcemia, hypermagnesemia, calcium channel blocker toxicity, preferably via central vein
Epinephrine for symptomatic bradycardia*	I.V., I.O.: 0.01 mg/kg (1:10,000; 0.1 mL/kg) E.T.: 0.1 mg/kg (1:1000; 0.1 mL/kg)	Tachyarrhythmias, hypertension may occur

Epinephrine for pulseless arrest*	First dose:
	I.V., I.O.: 0.01 mg/kg (1:10,000; 0.1 mL/kg)
	E.T.: 0.1 mg/kg (1:1000; 0.1 mL/kg)
	
	Subsequent doses: Repeat initial dose or may increase up to 10 times (0.1 mg/kg, 1:1000, 0.1 mL/kg)
	
	    Administer epinephrine every 3-5 minutes
	
	    I.V., I.O., E.T. doses as high as 0.2 mg/kg of 1:1000 may be effective	

Epinephrine for **neonatal** resuscitation	I.V., E.T.: 0.01-0.03 mg/kg (1:10,000; 0.1-0.3 mL/kg) Repeat every 3-5 minutes as indicated	Data in neonates is not sufficient to recommend higher doses for E.T. route; I.O. route not commonly used in the newly born (umbilical vein is more accessible, smaller bones are fragile, I.O. space is small in premature infants), but may be used in neonate and older infant.
Glucose (10%, 25%, or 50%)	I.V., I.O.: 0.5-1 g/kg • 1-2 mL/kg 50% • 2-4 mL/kg 25% • 5-10 mL/kg 10%	For suspected hypoglycemia; avoid hyperglycemia
Lidocaine* Lidocaine infusion	I.V., I.O., E.T.: 1 mg/kg I.V., I.O. (start after a bolus): 20-50 mcg/kg/min	Rapid bolus 1-2.5 mL/kg/hour of 120 mg/100 mL solution or use "Rule of 6"

CPR PEDIATRIC DRUG DOSAGES *(Continued)*

Drug	Dose	Remarks
Magnesium sulfate (500 mg/mL)	I.V., I.O.: 25-50 mg/kg Maximum dose: 2 g/dose	Rapid I.V. infusion for torsades or suspected hypomagnesemia; 10- to 20-minute infusion for asthma that responds poorly to beta-adrenergic agonists
Naloxone*	≤5 years or ≤20 kg: 0.1 mg/kg >5 years or >20 kg: 2 mg	For total reversal of narcotic effect. Use small repeated doses (0.01-0.03 mg/kg) titrated to desired effect
Procainamide for perfusing tachycardias (100 mg/mL and 500 mg/mL)	Loading dose: I.V., I.O.: 15 mg/kg	Infusion over 30-60 minutes; routine use in combination with drugs prolonging QT interval is **not** recommended
Sodium bicarbonate (1 mEq/mL and 0.5 mEq/mL)	I.V., I.O.: 1 mEq/kg/dose	Infuse slowly and only if ventilation is adequate

I.V. = intravenous; I.O. = intraosseous; E.T. = endotracheal

*For endotracheal administration, use higher doses (2-10 times the I.V. dose); dilute medication with NS to a volume of 3-5 mL and follow with several positive-pressure ventilations.

Adapted with permission of Lippincott Williams & Wilkins, "Guidelines 2000 for Cardiopulmonary Resuscitation and Emergency Cardiovascular Care. Part 10: Pediatric Advanced Life Support. The American Heart Association in Collaboration With the International Liaison Committee on Resuscitation," *Circulation*, 2000, 102(8 Suppl):I308.

EMERGENCY PEDIATRIC DRIP CALCULATIONS

Drips

Drug	Dose	Calculation*	Rate & Dose
Dobutamine	5-20 mcg/kg/min	6 x body wt (kg) is the mg added to make 100 mL	1 mL/h = 1 mcg/kg/min
Dopamine	2-20 mcg/kg/min	6 x body wt (kg) is the mg added to make 100 mL	1 mL/h = 1 mcg/kg/min
Epinephrine	0.1-1 mcg/kg/min	0.6 x body wt (kg) is the mg added to make 100 mL	1 mL/h = 0.1 mcg/kg/min
Isoproterenol	0.1-1 mcg/kg/min	0.6 x body wt (kg) is the mg added to make 100 mL	1 mL/h = 0.1 mcg/kg/min
Lidocaine	20-50 mcg/kg/min	120 mg in 100 mL of D_5W	1 mL/kg/h = 20 mcg/kg/min

*Note: Patients ≥40 kg and those requiring fluid restriction may need more concentrated solutions in order to deliver less fluid per hour. In those cases, or as an alternative to the listed calculations above, use the following equation:

$$\text{Rate (mL/h)} = \frac{\text{dose (mcg/kg/min) x weight (kg) x 60 min/h}}{\text{concentration (mcg/mL)}}$$

NEONATAL RESUSCITATION ALGORITHM

Algorithm for Resuscitation of the Newly Born Infant

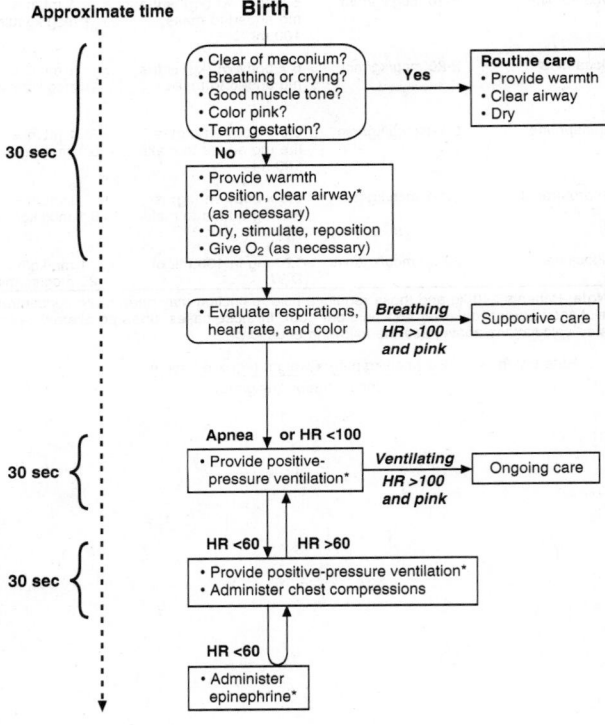

*Endotracheal intubation may be considered at several steps.

Epinephrine dose for neonatal resuscitation: I.V., E.T.: 0.01-0.03 mg/kg (1:10,000; 0.1-0.3 mL/kg). Repeat every 3-5 minutes as indicated. Data in neonates is not sufficient to recommend higher doses for E.T. route; I.O. route not commonly used in the newly born (umbilical vein is more accessible, smaller bones are fragile, I.O. space is small in premature infants), but may be used in neonate and older infant.

Adapted with permission of Lippincott Williams & Wilkins, "Guidelines 2000 for Cardiopulmonary Resuscitation and Emergency Cardiovascular Care, Part 11: Neonatal Resuscitation, the American Heart Association in Collaboration With the International Liaison Comittee in Resuscitation," *Circulation*, 2000, 102(8 Suppl):I349.

PEDIATRIC ALS ALGORITHMS

PALS Bradycardia Algorithm

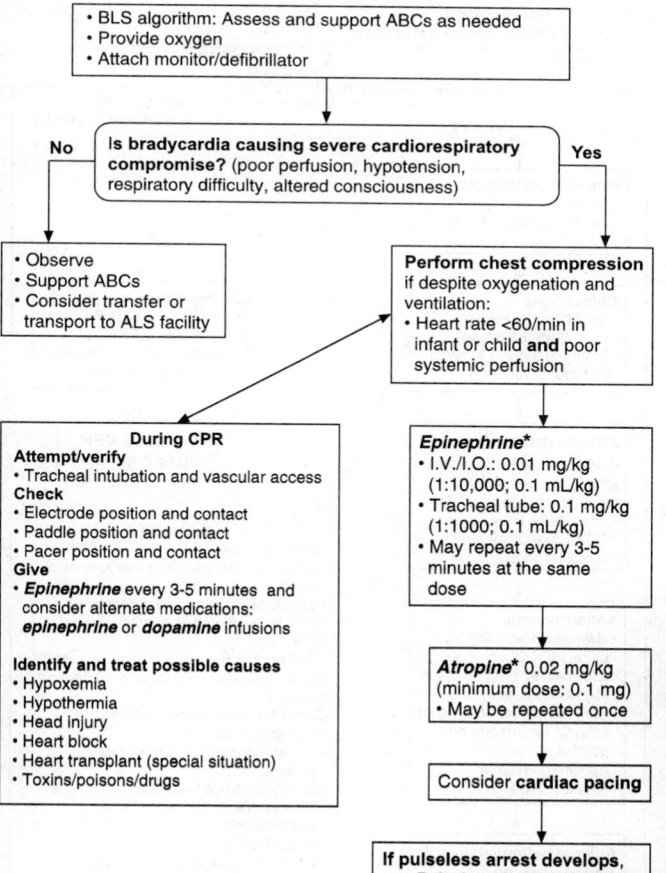

- BLS algorithm: Assess and support ABCs as needed
- Provide oxygen
- Attach monitor/defibrillator

Is bradycardia causing severe cardiorespiratory compromise? (poor perfusion, hypotension, respiratory difficulty, altered consciousness)

No

- Observe
- Support ABCs
- Consider transfer or transport to ALS facility

Yes

Perform chest compression if despite oxygenation and ventilation:
- Heart rate <60/min in infant or child **and** poor systemic perfusion

During CPR
Attempt/verify
- Tracheal intubation and vascular access
Check
- Electrode position and contact
- Paddle position and contact
- Pacer position and contact
Give
- *Epinephrine* every 3-5 minutes and consider alternate medications: *epinephrine* or *dopamine* infusions

Identify and treat possible causes
- Hypoxemia
- Hypothermia
- Head injury
- Heart block
- Heart transplant (special situation)
- Toxins/poisons/drugs

Epinephrine*
- I.V./I.O.: 0.01 mg/kg (1:10,000; 0.1 mL/kg)
- Tracheal tube: 0.1 mg/kg (1:1000; 0.1 mL/kg)
- May repeat every 3-5 minutes at the same dose

Atropine* 0.02 mg/kg (minimum dose: 0.1 mg)
- May be repeated once

Consider **cardiac pacing**

If pulseless arrest develops, *see* Pulseless Arrest Algorithm

*Give atropine first for bradycardia due to suspected increased vagal tone or primary AV block.

Adapted with permission of Lippincott Williams & Wilkins, "Guidelines 2000 for Cardio-pulmonary Resuscitation and Emergency Cardiovascular Care, Part 10: Pediatric Advanced Life Support, The American Heart Association in Collaboration With the International Liaison Committee on Resuscitation," *Circulation*, 2000, 102(8 Suppl):I313.

PEDIATRIC ALS ALGORITHMS *(Continued)*

PALS Pulseless Arrest Algorithm

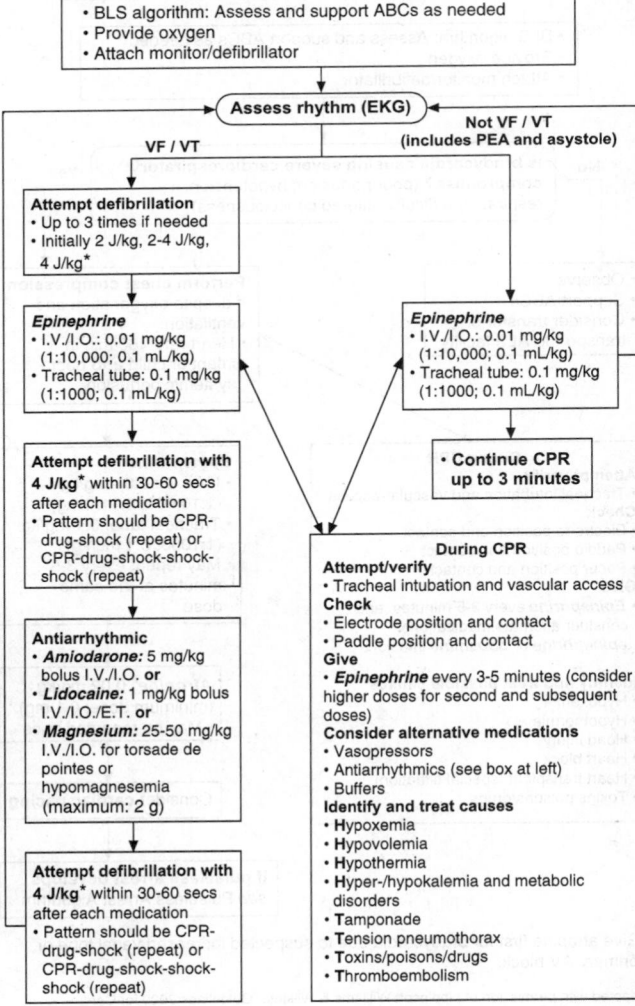

*Alternative waveforms and higher doses are Class Indeterminate for children.

Adapted with permission of Lippincott Williams & Wilkins, "Guidelines 2000 for Cardiopulmonary Resuscitation and Emergency Cardiovascular Care, Part 10: Pediatric Advanced Life Support, The American Heart Association in Collaboration With the International Liaison Committee on Resuscitation," *Circulation*, 2000, 102(8 Suppl):I311.

PALS Tachycardia Algorithm
for Infants and Children With Rapid Rhythm and Adequate Perfusion

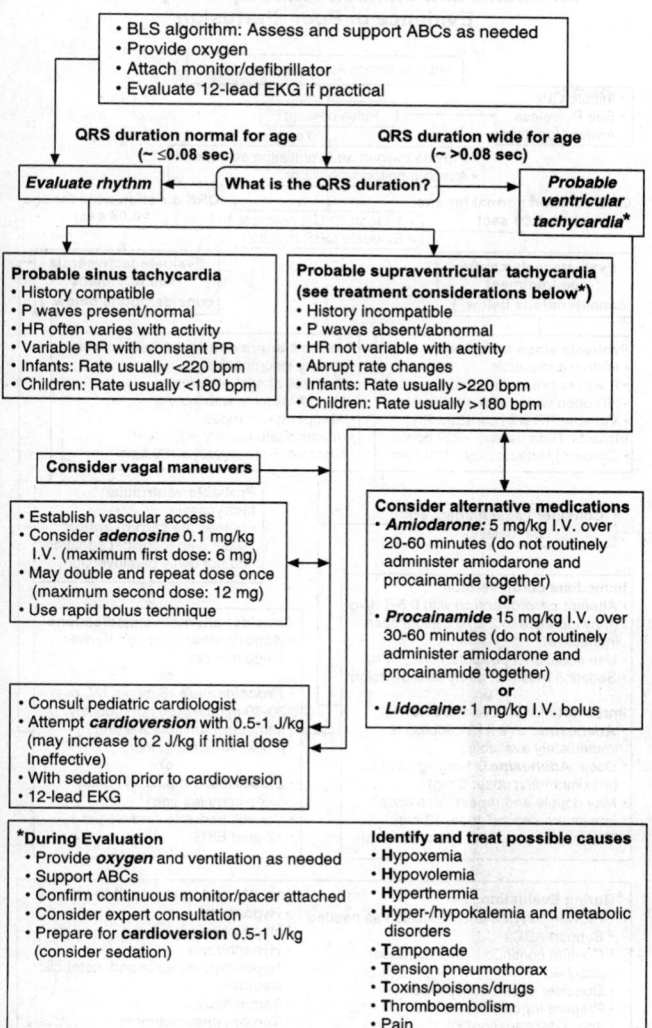

- BLS algorithm: Assess and support ABCs as needed
- Provide oxygen
- Attach monitor/defibrillator
- Evaluate 12-lead EKG if practical

QRS duration normal for age (~ ≤0.08 sec)

QRS duration wide for age (~ >0.08 sec)

Evaluate rhythm ← **What is the QRS duration?** → *Probable ventricular tachycardia**

Probable sinus tachycardia
- History compatible
- P waves present/normal
- HR often varies with activity
- Variable RR with constant PR
- Infants: Rate usually <220 bpm
- Children: Rate usually <180 bpm

Probable supraventricular tachycardia (see treatment considerations below*)
- History incompatible
- P waves absent/abnormal
- HR not variable with activity
- Abrupt rate changes
- Infants: Rate usually >220 bpm
- Children: Rate usually >180 bpm

Consider vagal maneuvers

- Establish vascular access
- Consider *adenosine* 0.1 mg/kg I.V. (maximum first dose: 6 mg)
- May double and repeat dose once (maximum second dose: 12 mg)
- Use rapid bolus technique

Consider alternative medications
- *Amiodarone:* 5 mg/kg I.V. over 20-60 minutes (do not routinely administer amiodarone and procainamide together)
  or
- *Procainamide* 15 mg/kg I.V. over 30-60 minutes (do not routinely administer amiodarone and procainamide together)
  or
- *Lidocaine:* 1 mg/kg I.V. bolus

- Consult pediatric cardiologist
- Attempt *cardioversion* with 0.5-1 J/kg (may increase to 2 J/kg if initial dose ineffective)
- With sedation prior to cardioversion
- 12-lead EKG

*During Evaluation
- Provide *oxygen* and ventilation as needed
- Support ABCs
- Confirm continuous monitor/pacer attached
- Consider expert consultation
- Prepare for **cardioversion** 0.5-1 J/kg (consider sedation)

Identify and treat possible causes
- Hypoxemia
- Hypovolemia
- Hyperthermia
- Hyper-/hypokalemia and metabolic disorders
- Tamponade
- Tension pneumothorax
- Toxins/poisons/drugs
- Thromboembolism
- Pain

Adapted with permission of Lippincott Williams & Wilkins, "Guidelines 2000 for Cardiopulmonary Resuscitation and Emergency Cardiovascular Care, Part 10: Pediatric Advanced Life Support, The American Heart Association in Collaboration With the International Liaison Committee on Resuscitation," Circulation, 2000, 102(8 Suppl):I315.

PEDIATRIC ALS ALGORITHMS (Continued)

PALS Tachycardia Algorithm for Infants and Children With Rapid Rhythm and Evidence of Poor Perfusion

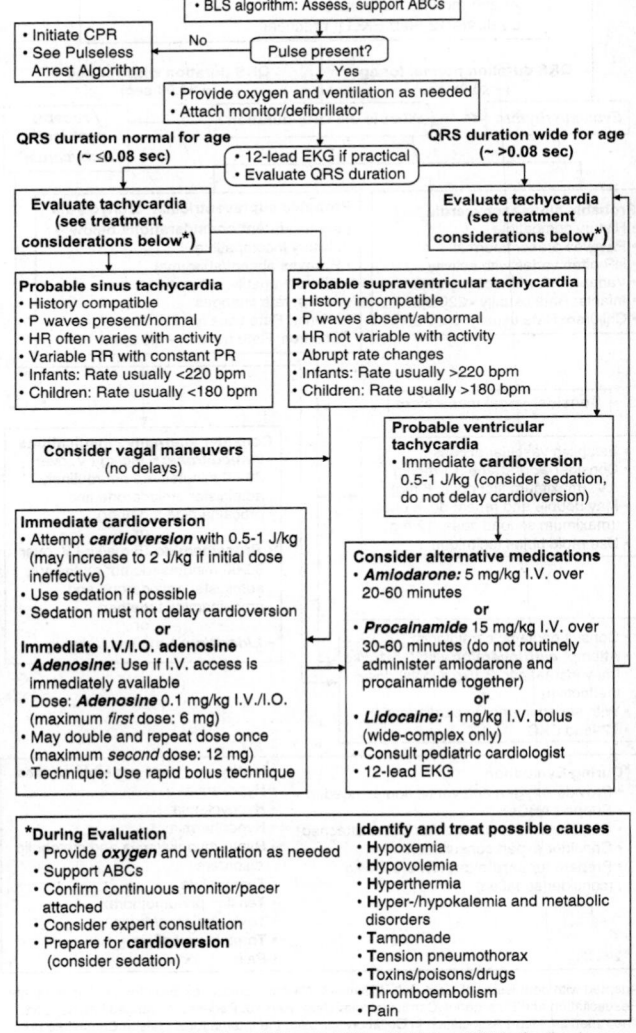

• BLS algorithm: Assess, support ABCs

Pulse present?

No → • Initiate CPR
• See Pulseless Arrest Algorithm

Yes ↓

• Provide oxygen and ventilation as needed
• Attach monitor/defibrillator

QRS duration normal for age (~ ≤0.08 sec)

QRS duration wide for age (~ >0.08 sec)

• 12-lead EKG if practical
• Evaluate QRS duration

Evaluate tachycardia (see treatment considerations below*)

Evaluate tachycardia (see treatment considerations below*)

Probable sinus tachycardia
• History compatible
• P waves present/normal
• HR often varies with activity
• Variable RR with constant PR
• Infants: Rate usually <220 bpm
• Children: Rate usually <180 bpm

Probable supraventricular tachycardia
• History incompatible
• P waves absent/abnormal
• HR not variable with activity
• Abrupt rate changes
• Infants: Rate usually >220 bpm
• Children: Rate usually >180 bpm

Probable ventricular tachycardia
• Immediate **cardioversion** 0.5-1 J/kg (consider sedation, do not delay cardioversion)

Consider vagal maneuvers (no delays)

Immediate cardioversion
• Attempt **cardioversion** with 0.5-1 J/kg (may increase to 2 J/kg if initial dose ineffective)
• Use sedation if possible
• Sedation must not delay cardioversion
or
Immediate I.V./I.O. adenosine
• **Adenosine**: Use if I.V. access is immediately available
• Dose: **Adenosine** 0.1 mg/kg I.V./I.O. (maximum *first* dose: 6 mg)
• May double and repeat dose once (maximum *second* dose: 12 mg)
• Technique: Use rapid bolus technique

Consider alternative medications
• **Amiodarone**: 5 mg/kg I.V. over 20-60 minutes
or
• **Procainamide** 15 mg/kg I.V. over 30-60 minutes (do not routinely administer amiodarone and procainamide together)
or
• **Lidocaine**: 1 mg/kg I.V. bolus (wide-complex only)
• Consult pediatric cardiologist
• 12-lead EKG

*During Evaluation
• Provide **oxygen** and ventilation as needed
• Support ABCs
• Confirm continuous monitor/pacer attached
• Consider expert consultation
• Prepare for **cardioversion** (consider sedation)

Identify and treat possible causes
• Hypoxemia
• Hypovolemia
• Hyperthermia
• Hyper-/hypokalemia and metabolic disorders
• Tamponade
• Tension pneumothorax
• Toxins/poisons/drugs
• Thromboembolism
• Pain

Adapted with permission of Lippincott Williams & Wilkins, "Guidelines 2000 for Cardiopulmonary Resuscitation and Emergency Cardiovascular Care, Part 10: Pediatric Advanced Life Support, The American Heart Association in Collaboration With the International Liaison Committee on Resuscitation," *Circulation*, 2000, 102(8 Suppl):I316.

ADULT ACLS ALGORITHMS

ILCOR Universal / International ACLS Algorithm

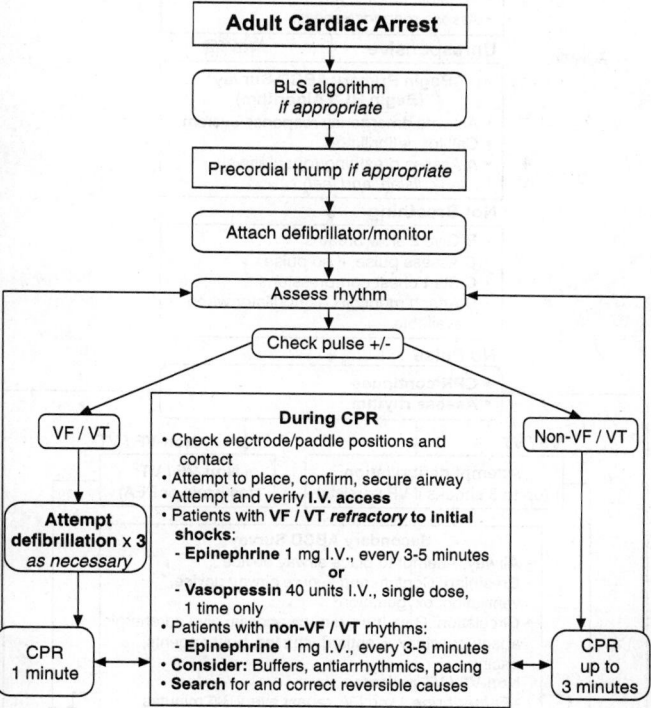

Consider causes that are potentially reversible

- Hypovolemia
- Hypoxia
- Hydrogen ion - acidosis
- Hyper-/hypokalemia, other metabolic
- Hypothermia

- "Tablets" (drug OD, accidents)
- Tamponade, cardiac (pericardiocentesis)
- Tension pneumothorax (decompress)
- Thrombosis, coronary (ACS); (fibrinolytics)
- Thrombosis, pulmonary (embolism, fibrinolytics, surgical evacuation)

Adapted with permission of Lippincott Williams & Wilkins, "Guidelines 2000 for Cardiopulmonary Resuscitation and Emergency Cardiovascular Care, Part 6: Advanced Cardiovascular Life Support, The American Heart Association in Collaboration With the International Liaison Committee on Resuscitation," *Circulation*, 2000, 102(8 Suppl):I143.

ADULT ACLS ALGORITHMS *(Continued)*

Comprehensive ECC Algorithm

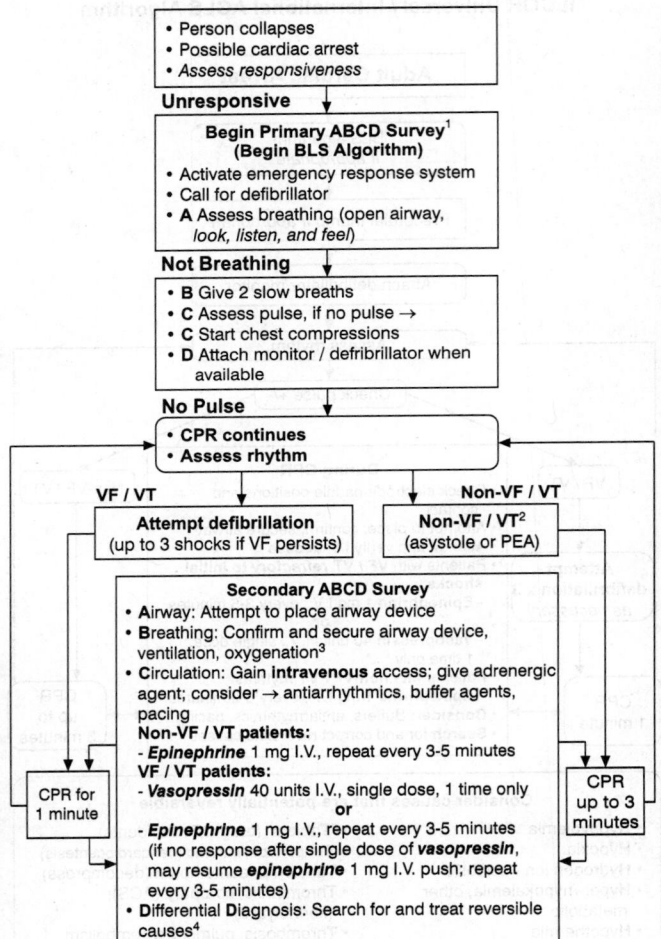

- Person collapses
- Possible cardiac arrest
- *Assess responsiveness*

Unresponsive

Begin Primary ABCD Survey[1]
(Begin BLS Algorithm)
- Activate emergency response system
- Call for defibrillator
- **A** Assess breathing (open airway,
  look, listen, and feel)

Not Breathing

- **B** Give 2 slow breaths
- **C** Assess pulse, if no pulse →
- **C** Start chest compressions
- **D** Attach monitor / defibrillator when
  available

No Pulse

- **CPR continues**
- **Assess rhythm**

VF / VT

Attempt defibrillation
(up to 3 shocks if VF persists)

Non-VF / VT

Non-VF / VT[2]
(asystole or PEA)

Secondary ABCD Survey
- **Airway:** Attempt to place airway device
- **Breathing:** Confirm and secure airway device,
  ventilation, oxygenation[3]
- **Circulation:** Gain **intravenous** access; give adrenergic
  agent; consider → antiarrhythmics, buffer agents,
  pacing
  Non-VF / VT patients:
  - *Epinephrine* 1 mg I.V., repeat every 3-5 minutes
  VF / VT patients:
  - *Vasopressin* 40 units I.V., single dose, 1 time only
  or
  - *Epinephrine* 1 mg I.V., repeat every 3-5 minutes
    (if no response after single dose of *vasopressin*,
    may resume *epinephrine* 1 mg I.V. push; repeat
    every 3-5 minutes)
- **Differential Diagnosis:** Search for and treat reversible
  causes[4]

CPR for 1 minute

CPR up to 3 minutes

[1]Do not attempt resuscitation if any objective indicators of DNAR status or clinical
indicators that resuscitation attempts are not indicated (eg, signs of death).
[2]Recommendation is to consider non-VF / VT rhythms as one rthythm when the patient
is in cardiac arrest.
[3]Use 2 methods to confirm tube placement: Primary physical examination criteria plus a
secondary device (qualitative and quantitative measures of end-tidal CO$_2$).
[4]Reversible causes: See ILCOR Universal / International ACLS Algorithm.

Adapted with permission of Lippincott Williams & Wilkins, "Guidelines 2000 for Cardiopulmonary
Resuscitation and Emergency Cardiovascular Care, Part 6: Advanced Cardiovascular Life
Support, The American Heart Association in Collaboration With the International Liaison
Committee on Resuscitation," *Circulation*, 2000, 102(8 Suppl):I144.

Ventricular Fibrillation / Pulseless VT Algorithm

Primary ABCD Survey[1]
Focus: Basic CPR and defibrillation

- **Check** responsiveness
- **Activate** emergency response system
- **Call** for defibrillator

A Airway: Open the airway
B Breathing: Provide positive-pressure ventilations
C Circulation: Give chest compressions
D Defibrillation: Assess for and shock VF / pulseless VT, up to 3 times
(200 J, 200-300 J, 360 J, or equivalent *biphasic*) if necessary

---

Rhythm after first 3 shocks?

Persistent or recurrent VF / VT

Secondary ABCD Survey
Focus: More advanced assessments and treatments

A Airway: Place airway device as soon as possible
B Breathing: Confirm airway device placement by exam plus confirmation device[2]
B Breathing: Secure airway device; purpose-made tube holders preferred[3]
B Breathing: Confirm effective oxygenation and ventilation[4]
C Circulation: Establish I.V. access
C Circulation: Identify rhythm → monitor
C Circulation: Administer drugs appropriate for rhythm and condition
D Differential Diagnosis: Search for and treat identified reversible causes

---

- *Epinephrine* 1 mg I.V. push, repeat every 3-5 minutes[5]
  or
- *Vasopressin* 40 units I.V., **single dose**, 1 time only[6]

Resume attempts to defibrillate
1 x 360 J (or equivalent *biphasic*) within 30-60 seconds

Consider antiarrhythmics:[7]

Amiodarone (IIb): 300 mg I.V. push. If VF/pulseless VT recurs, consider a second dose of 150 mg (maximum cumulative dose: 2.2 g over 24 hours)
Lidocaine (indeterminate): 1-1.5 mg/kg I.V. push. Consider repeat in 3-5 minutes to maximum cumulative dose of 3 mg/kg
Magnesium sulfate (IIb if hypomagnesemic state): 1-2 g I.V. in polymorphic VT (torsade de pointes) and suspected hypomagnesemic state
Procainamide (IIb for intermittent/recurrent VF / VT): 30 mg/min in refractory VF (maximum total dose: 17 mg/kg) - acceptable but not recommended due to prolonged administration time
Consider buffers

Resume attempts to defibrillate

---

[1]Do not attempt resuscitation if any objective indicators of DNAR status or clinical indicators that resuscitation attempts are not indicated (eg, signs of death).
[2]Consider continuous qualitative end-tidal CO_2 monitor (Class IIa - acceptable, probably effective).
[3]Commercial purpose-made tracheal tube holders recommended (Class IIb - acceptable, possibly effective).
[4]End-tidal CO_2 monitor and oxygen saturation monitor.
[5]If this fails, higher doses of epinephrine (up to 0.2 mg/kg) are acceptable (growing evidence of potential harm).
[6]No evidence about value of repeat vasopressin doses.
[7]Numbers in parentheses represent strength of recommendation (Class IIb - acceptable, possibly effective).

Adapted with permission of Lippincott Williams & Wilkins, "Guidelines 2000 for Cardiopulmonary Resuscitation and Emergency Cardiovascular Care, Part 6: Advanced Cardiovascular Life Support, The American Heart Association in Collaboration With the International Liaison Committee on Resuscitation," *Circulation*, 2000, 102(8 Suppl):I147.

ADULT ACLS ALGORITHMS *(Continued)*

Pulseless Electrical Activity Algorithm

(PEA = rhythm on monitor, without detectable pulse)

Primary ABCD Survey[1]
Focus: Basic CPR and defibrillation

- **Check** responsiveness
- **Activate** emergency response system
- **Call** for defibrillator

A Airway: Open the airway
B Breathing: Provide positive-pressure ventilations
C Circulation: Give chest compressions
D Defibrillation: Assess for and shock VF / pulseless VT

Secondary ABCD Survey
Focus: More advanced assessments and treatments

A Airway: Place airway device as soon as possible
B Breathing: Confirm airway device placement by exam plus confirmation device[2]
B Breathing: Secure airway device; purpose-made tube holders preferred[3]
B Breathing: Confirm effective oxygenation and ventilation[4]
C Circulation: Establish I.V. access
C Circulation: Identify rhythm → monitor
C Circulation: Administer drugs appropriate for rhythm and condition
C Circulation: Assess for occult blood flow ("pseudo-EMT")
D Differential Diagnosis: Search for and treat identified reversible causes

---

Review for most frequent causes[5]

- Hypovolemia
- Hypoxia
- Hydrogen ion - acidosis
- Hyper-/hypokalemia
- Hypothermia

- "Tablets" (drug OD, accidents)
- Tamponade, cardiac
- Tension pneumothorax
- Thrombosis, coronary (ACS)
- Thrombosis, pulmonary (embolism)

- ***Epinephrine*** 1 mg I.V. push, repeat every 3-5 minutes[6]

- ***Atropine*** 1 mg I.V. (if PEA rate is **slow**), repeat every 3-5 minutes as needed, to a total dose of 0.04 mg/kg

---

[1]Do not attempt resuscitation if any objective indicators of DNAR status or clinical indicators that resuscitation attempts are not indicated (eg, signs of death).
[2]Consider continuous qualitative end-tidal CO_2 monitor (Class IIa - acceptable, probably effective).
[3]Commercial purpose-made tracheal tube holders recommended (Class IIb - acceptable, possibly effective).
[4]End-tidal CO_2 monitor and oxygen saturation monitor.
[5]Sodium bicarbonate 1 mEq/kg recommended in the following:
Class I: If patient has known, preexisting hyperkalemia
Class IIa: Known, preexisting bicarbonate-responsive acidosis, in tricyclic antidepressant overdose, or to alkalinize the urine in aspirin or other drug overdoses
Class IIb: In intubated and ventilated patients with long arrest interval, or on return of circulation after a long arrest interval
Note: Ineffective or harmful in hypercarbic acidosis (Class III)
[6]If this fails, higher doses of epinephrine (up to 0.2 mg/kg) are acceptable (growing evidence of potential harm).

Adapted with permission of Lippincott Williams & Wilkins, "Guidelines 2000 for Cardiopulmonary Resuscitation and Emergency Cardiovascular Care, Part 6: Advanced Cardiovascular Life Support, The American Heart Association in Collaboration With the International Liaison Committee on Resuscitation," *Circulation*, 2000, 102(8 Suppl):I151.

Asystole: The Silent Heart Algorithm

Primary ABCD Survey[1]
Focus: Basic CPR and defibrillation

- **Check** responsiveness
- **Activate** emergency response system
- **Call** for defibrillator

A Airway: Open the airway
B Breathing: Provide positive-pressure ventilations
C Circulation: Give chest compressions
C Confirm true asystole
D Defibrillation: Assess for VF / pulseless VT; shock if indicated

Rapid scene survey: Any evidence personnel should **not** attempt resuscitation?

↓

Secondary ABCD Survey[2,3]
Focus: More advanced assessments and treatments

A Airway: Place airway device as soon as possible
B Breathing: Confirm airway device placement by exam plus confirmation device
B Breathing: Secure airway device; purpose-made tube holders preferred[4]
B Breathing: Confirm effective oxygenation and ventilation[5]
C Circulation: Confirm true asystole
C Circulation: Establish I.V. access
C Circulation: Identify rhythm → monitor
C Circulation: Administer drugs appropriate for rhythm and condition
C Circulation: Give medications appropriate for rhythm and condition
D Differential Diagnosis: Search for and treat identified reversible causes

↓

Transcutaneous pacing
If considered, perform immediately

↓

- ***Epinephrine*** 1 mg I.V. push, repeat every 3-5 minutes[6]

↓

- ***Atropine*** 1 mg I.V., repeat every 3-5 minutes up to a total of 0.04 mg/kg

↓

Asystole persists
Withhold or cease resuscitation efforts?
- Consider quality of resuscitation?
- Atypical clinical features present?
- Support for cease-efforts protocols in place?

[1] Do not attempt resuscitation if any objective indicators of DNAR status or clinical indicators that resuscitation attempts are not indicated (eg, signs of death).
[2] Confirm true asystole.
[3] Sodium bicarbonate 1 mEq/kg indicated for patients with tracheal intubation plus long arrest intervals, on return of spontaneous circulation if long arrest interval, tricyclic antidepressant overdose, to alkalinize urine (eg, ASA overdose). **Note:** Ineffective or harmful in hypercarbic acidosis.
[4] Commercial purpose-made tracheal tube holders recommended (Class IIb - acceptable, possibly effective).
[5] End-tidal CO_2 monitor and oxygen saturation monitor
[6] If this fails, higher doses of epinephrine (up to 0.2 mg/kg) are acceptable (growing evidence of potential harm).

Adapted with permission of Lippincott Williams & Wilkins, "Guidelines 2000 for Cardiopulmonary Resuscitation and Emergency Cardiovascular Care, Part 6: Advanced Cardiovascular Life Support, The American Heart Association in Collaboration With the International Liaison Committee on Resuscitation," *Circulation*, 2000, 102(8 Suppl):153.

ADULT ACLS ALGORITHMS *(Continued)*

Bradycardia Algorithm

Bradycardia
- **Slow** (absolute bradycardia = rate <60 bpm)

or

- **Relatively slow** (rate less than expected relative to underlying condition or cause)

Primary ABCD Survey
- Assess ABCs
- Secure airway noninvasively
- Ensure monitor / defibrillator is available

Secondary ABCD Survey
- Assess secondary ABCs (invasive airway management needed?)
- Oxygen - I.V. access - monitor - fluids
- Vital signs, pulse oximeter, monitor BP
- Obtain and review 12-lead EKG
- Obtain and review portable chest x-ray
- Problem-focused history
- Problem-focused physical examination
- Consider causes (differential diagnoses)

Serious signs or symptoms?[1]
Due to the bradycardia?

No / Yes

Type II second-degree AV block[2]
or
Third-degree AV block?

No / Yes

Observe

- Prepare for transvenous pacer[5]
- If symptoms develop, use transcutaneous pacemaker until transvenous pacer placed

Intervention sequence[3]
- *Atropine* 0.5-1 mg[4]
- *Transcutaneous pacing* if available
- *Dopamine* 5-20 mcg/kg/min
- *Epinephrine* 2-10 mcg/min

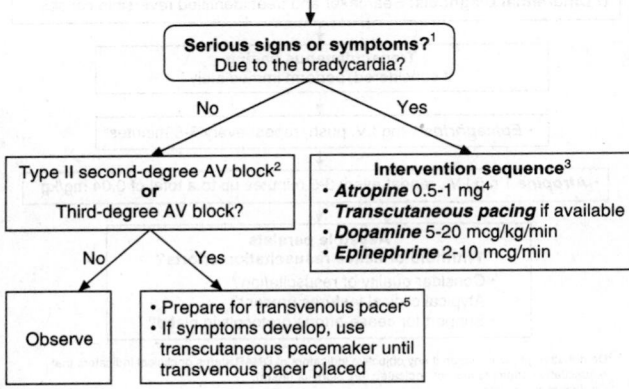

[1]Signs/symptoms must be attributable to slow rate. Manifestations include chest pain, shortness of breath, decreased LOC, hypotension, shock, CHF, pulmonary congestion.
[2]Never treat combination of third-degree heart block and ventricular escape beats with lidocaine (or any agent which suppresses ventricular escape rhythms).
[3]Do not delay transcutaneous pacing in symptomatic patients while waiting for I.V. access or for atropine to take effect; denervated transplanted hearts will not respond to atropine - go directly to catecholamine infusion or pacing.
[4]Atropine should be repeated every 3-5 minutes up to 0.03-0.04 mg/kg total dose; use every 3 minutes in severe clinical conditions.
[5]Verify patient tolerance and mechanical capture. Use analgesia and sedation as needed.
Adapted with permission of Lippincott Williams & Wilkins, "Guidelines 2000 for Cardiopulmonary Resuscitation and Emergency Cardiovascular Care, Part 6: Advanced Cardiovascular Life Support, The American Heart Association in Collaboration With the International Liaison Committee on Resuscitation," *Circulation*, 2000, 102(8 Suppl):I156.

Tachycardia Overview Algorithm

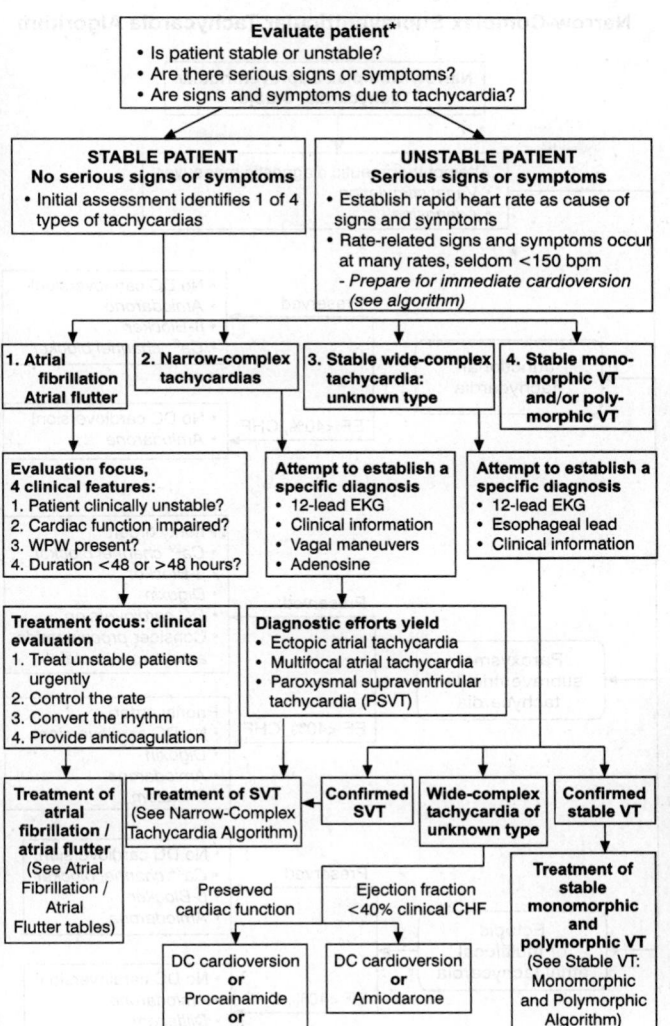

Evaluate patient*
- Is patient stable or unstable?
- Are there serious signs or symptoms?
- Are signs and symptoms due to tachycardia?

STABLE PATIENT
No serious signs or symptoms
- Initial assessment identifies 1 of 4 types of tachycardias

UNSTABLE PATIENT
Serious signs or symptoms
- Establish rapid heart rate as cause of signs and symptoms
- Rate-related signs and symptoms occur at many rates, seldom <150 bpm
  - *Prepare for immediate cardioversion (see algorithm)*

1. Atrial fibrillation Atrial flutter

2. Narrow-complex tachycardias

3. Stable wide-complex tachycardia: unknown type

4. Stable mono-morphic VT and/or poly-morphic VT

Evaluation focus, 4 clinical features:
1. Patient clinically unstable?
2. Cardiac function impaired?
3. WPW present?
4. Duration <48 or >48 hours?

Attempt to establish a specific diagnosis
- 12-lead EKG
- Clinical information
- Vagal maneuvers
- Adenosine

Attempt to establish a specific diagnosis
- 12-lead EKG
- Esophageal lead
- Clinical information

Treatment focus: clinical evaluation
1. Treat unstable patients urgently
2. Control the rate
3. Convert the rhythm
4. Provide anticoagulation

Diagnostic efforts yield
- Ectopic atrial tachycardia
- Multifocal atrial tachycardia
- Paroxysmal supraventricular tachycardia (PSVT)

Treatment of atrial fibrillation / atrial flutter
(See Atrial Fibrillation / Atrial Flutter tables)

Treatment of SVT
(See Narrow-Complex Tachycardia Algorithm)

Confirmed SVT

Wide-complex tachycardia of unknown type

Confirmed stable VT

Treatment of stable monomorphic and polymorphic VT
(See Stable VT: Monomorphic and Polymorphic Algorithm)

Preserved cardiac function

Ejection fraction <40% clinical CHF

DC cardioversion or Procainamide or Amiodarone

DC cardioversion or Amiodarone

*Unstable condition must be related to the tachycardia. Signs and symptoms may include chest pain, shortness of breath, decreased LOC, hypotension, shock, pulmonary congestion, CHF, and AMI.

Adapted with permission of Lippincott Williams & Wilkins, "Guidelines 2000 for Cardiopulmonary Resuscitation and Emergency Cardiovascular Care, Part 6: Advanced Cardiovascular Life Support, The American Heart Association in Collaboration With the International Liaison Committee on Resuscitation," *Circulation*, 2000, 102(8 Suppl):I159.

ADULT ACLS ALGORITHMS *(Continued)*

Narrow-Complex Supraventricular Tachycardia Algorithm

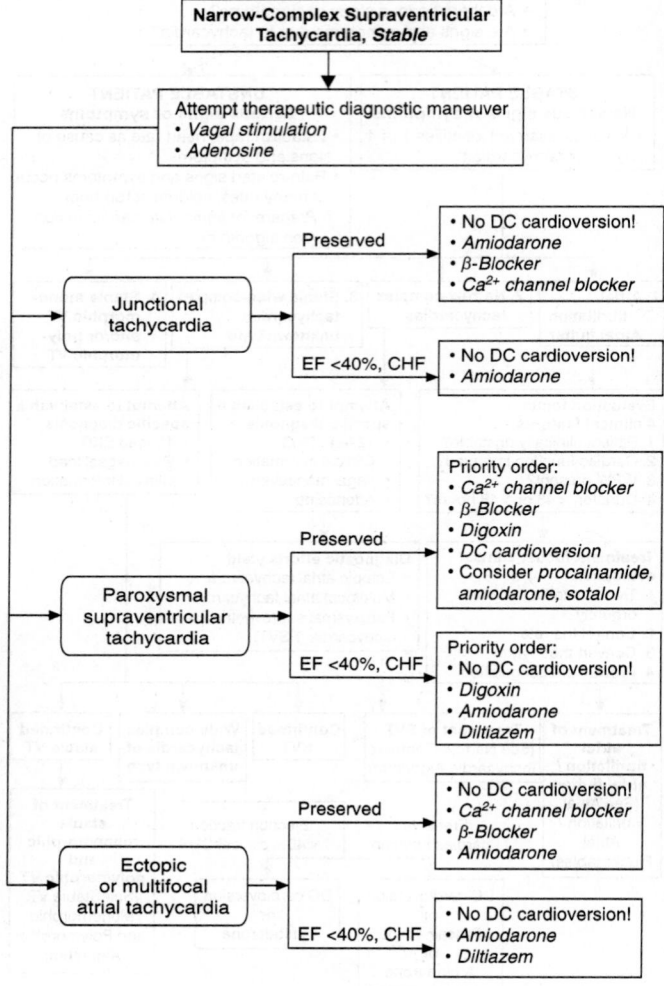

Adapted with permission of Lippincott Williams & Wilkins, "Guidelines 2000 for Cardiopulmonary Resuscitation and Emergency Cardiovascular Care, Part 6: Advanced Cardiovascular Life Support, The American Heart Association in Collaboration With the International Liaison Committee on Resuscitation," *Circulation*, 2000, 102(8 Suppl):I162.

Stable Ventricular Tachycardia
(Monomorphic or Polymorphic) Algorithm

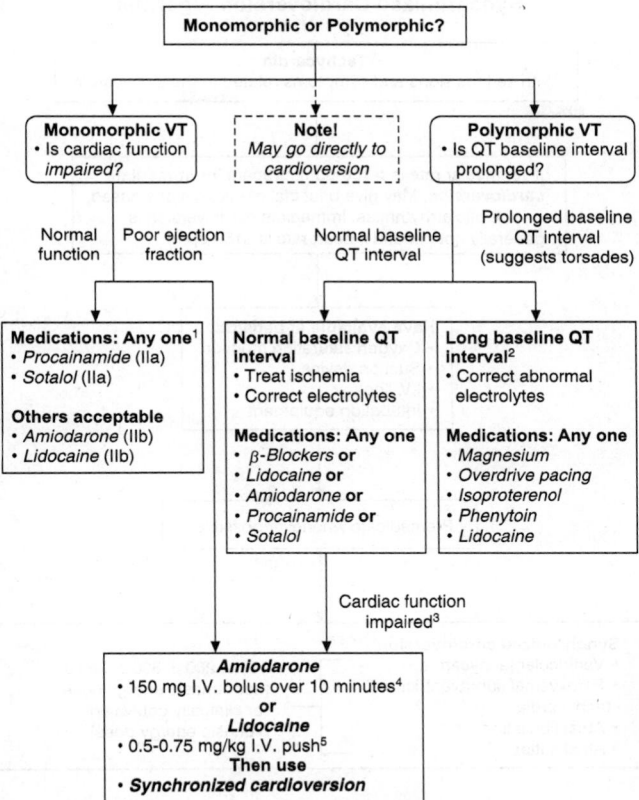

¹Use just one agent at a time. **Note:** Numbers in parentheses represent strength of recommendation, not antiarrhythmic classification.
²Stop/avoid treatments which prolong QT. Identify and treat any electrolyte abnormalities.
³Clinical signs suggestive of impaired LV function (EF <40% or CHF).
⁴Repeat 150 mg I.V. over 10 minutes every 10-15 minutes as needed. Alternative infusion: 360 mg over 6 hours, then 540 mg over the remaining 18 hours. Maximum total dose: 2.2 g in 24 hours.
⁵Repeat every 5-10 minutes, then infuse 1-4 mg/min. Maximum total dose: 3 mg/kg (or 300 mg) over 1 hour.
Note: Class IIa recommendation: Acceptable, probably effective;
Class IIb: Acceptable, possibly effective.

Adapted with permission of Lippincott Williams & Wilkins, "Guidelines 2000 for Cardiopulmonary Resuscitation and Emergency Cardiovascular Care, Part 6: Advanced Cardiovascular Life Support, The American Heart Association in Collaboration With the International Liaison Committee on Resuscitation," *Circulation*, 2000, 102(8 Suppl):I163.

ADULT ACLS ALGORITHMS *(Continued)*

Synchronized Cardioversion Algorithm

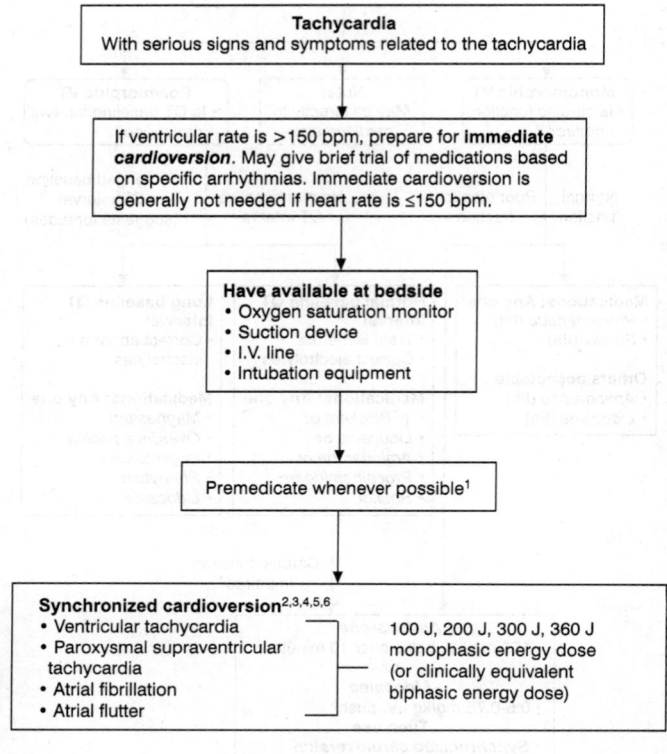

Tachycardia
With serious signs and symptoms related to the tachycardia

If ventricular rate is >150 bpm, prepare for **immediate cardioversion**. May give brief trial of medications based on specific arrhythmias. Immediate cardioversion is generally not needed if heart rate is ≤150 bpm.

Have available at bedside
- Oxygen saturation monitor
- Suction device
- I.V. line
- Intubation equipment

Premedicate whenever possible[1]

Synchronized cardioversion[2,3,4,5,6]
- Ventricular tachycardia
- Paroxysmal supraventricular tachycardia
- Atrial fibrillation
- Atrial flutter

100 J, 200 J, 300 J, 360 J monophasic energy dose (or clinically equivalent biphasic energy dose)

[1]Effective regimens have included a sedative (eg, *diazepam*, *midazolam*, *barbiturates*, *etomidate*, *ketamine*, *methohexital*) with or without an analgesic agent (eg, *fentanyl*, *morphine*, *meperidine*). Many experts recommend anesthesia if service is readily available.

[2]Both monophasic and biphasic waveforms are acceptable if documented as clinically equivalent to reports of monophasic shock success.

[3]Note possible need to resynchronize after each cardioversion.

[4]If delays in synchronization occur and clinical condition is critical, go immediately to unsynchronized shocks.

[5]Treat polymorphic ventricular tachycardia (irregular form and rate) like ventricular fibrillation: see ventricular fibrillation/pulseless ventricular tachycardia algorithm.

[6]Paroxysmal supraventricular tachycardia and atrial flutter often respond to lower energy levels (start with 50 J).

Adapted with permission of Lippincott Williams & Wilkins, "Guidelines 2000 for Cardiopulmonary Resuscitation and Emergency Cardiovascular Care, Part 6: Advanced Cardiovascular Life Support, The American Heart Association in Collaboration With the International Liaison Committee on Resuscitation," *Circulation*, 2000, 102(8 Suppl):I164.

ATRIAL FIBRILLATION / ATRIAL FLUTTER

Atrial Fibrillation / Atrial Flutter in
Normal Cardiac Function — Control of Rate and Rhythm

Control Rate		Convert Rhythm	
Heart Function Preserved	Impaired Heart Function EF <40% or CHF	Duration <48 Hours	Duration >48 Hours or Unknown
Note: AF >48-hours duration: Use agents to convert rhythm with extreme caution in patient not receiving adequate anticoagulation because of possible embolic complications Use only one of the following agents*: • Calcium channel blocker (Class I) • Beta blocker (Class I) • Other drugs (class IIb recommendations) eg, digoxin, amiodarone	Not applicable	**Consider:** • DC cardioversion Use only one of the following agents*: • Amiodarone (Class IIa) • Ibutilide (Class IIa) • Flecainide (Class IIa) • Propafenone (Class IIa) • Procainamide (Class IIa) • Other drugs (class IIb recommendations) eg, sotalol, disopyramide	**NO DC CARDIOVERSION!** **Note:** Conversion of AF to NSR with drugs or shock may cause embolization of atrial thrombi unless patient has adequate anticoagulation. Use antiarrhythmic agents with extreme caution (see Note above) if AF is >48-hours duration **OR** **Delayed cardioversion** Anticoagulation for 3 weeks at proper levels • Cardioversion, **then** • Anticoagulation for 4 more weeks **OR** **Early cardioversion** • Begin I.V. heparin at once • TEE to exclude atrial clot, **then** • Cardioversion within 24 hours, **then** • Anticoagulation for 4 more weeks

Legend: AF: Atrial fibrillation; Class I: Acceptable, definitely effective; Class IIa: Acceptable, probably effective; Class IIb: Acceptable, possibly effective; Class III: Not indicated, may be harmful; EF: Ejection fraction; NSR: Normal sinus rhythm; TEE: Transesophageal echocardiogram

*Occasionally, two of the named antiarrhythmic agents may be used, but use of these agents in combination may have proarrhythmic potential; classes listed represent the *Class of Recommendation* rather than the Vaughn-Williams classification of antiarrhythmics.

Adapted with permission from Lippincott Williams & Wilkins, "Guidelines 2000 for Cardiopulmonary Resuscitation and Emergency Cardiovascular Care. Part 6: Advanced Cardiovascular Life Support. The American Heart Association in Collaboration With the International Liaison Committee on Resuscitation", *Circulation*, 2000, 102(8 Suppl), I160-1.

ATRIAL FIBRILLATION / ATRIAL FLUTTER *(Continued)*

Atrial Fibrillation / Atrial Flutter in Impaired Heart Function (EF <40% or CHF) — Control of Rate and Rhythm

Heart Function Preserved	Control Rate — Impaired Heart Function EF <40% or CHF	Convert Rhythm — Duration <48 Hours	Convert Rhythm — Duration >48 Hours or Unknown
Not applicable	**Note:** AF >48-hours duration: Use agents to convert rhythm with extreme caution in patient not receiving adequate anticoagulation because of possible embolic complications. Use only one of the following agents*: • Digoxin (Class IIb) • Diltiazem (Class IIb) • Amiodarone (Class IIb)	**Consider:** • DC cardioversion OR • Amiodarone (Class IIb)	• **Anticoagulation** (as described in "Control of Rate and Rhythm - Normal Cardiac Function"), followed by • **DC Cardioversion**

Legend: AF: Atrial fibrillation; Class I: Acceptable, definitely effective; Class IIa: Acceptable, probably effective; Class IIb: Acceptable, possibly effective; Class III: Not indicated, may be harmful; EF: Ejection fraction; NSR: Normal sinus rhythm; TEE: Transesophageal echocardiogram

*Occasionally, two of the named antiarrhythmic agents may be used, but use of these agents in combination may have proarrhythmic potential; classes listed represent the *Class of Recommendation* rather than the Vaughn-Williams classification of antiarrhythmics.

Adapted with permission from Lippincott Williams & Wilkins, "Guidelines 2000 for Cardiopulmonary Resuscitation and Emergency Cardiovascular Care. Part 6: Advanced Cardiovascular Life Support. The American Heart Association in Collaboration With International Liaison Committee on Resuscitation," *Circulation*, 2000, 102(8 Suppl), I160-1.

Atrial Fibrillation / Atrial Flutter in
Wolff-Parkinson-White Syndrome — Control of Rate and Rhythm

Control Rate		Convert Rhythm	
Heart Function Preserved	Impaired Heart Function EF <40% or CHF	Duration <48 Hours	Duration >48 Hours or Unknown
Note: AF >48-hours duration: Use agents to convert rhythm with extreme caution in patient not receiving adequate anticoagulation because of possible embolic complications • DC Cardioversion **OR** • **Primary antiarrhythmic agents** Use only one of the following agents*: • Amiodarone (Class IIb) • Flecainide (Class IIb) • Procainamide (Class IIb) • Propafenone (Class IIb) • Sotalol (Class IIb) • **Class III** **(can be harmful)** • Adenosine • Beta-blockers • Calcium channel blockers • Digoxin	**Note:** AF >48-hours duration: Use agents to convert rhythm with extreme caution in patient not receiving adequate anticoagulation because of possible embolic complications • DC Cardioversion **OR** • Amiodarone (Class IIb)	• DC Cardioversion **OR** • **Primary antiarrhythmic agents** Use only one of the following agents*: • Amiodarone (Class IIb) • Flecainide (Class IIb) • Procainamide (Class IIb) • Propafenone (Class IIb) • Sotalol (Class IIb) • **Class III** **(can be harmful)** • Adenosine • Beta-blockers • Calcium channel blockers • Digoxin	• **Anticoagulation** (as described in "Control of Rate and Rhythm - Normal Cardiac Function"), followed by • **DC Cardioversion**

Legend: AF: Atrial fibrillation; Class I: Acceptable, definitely effective; Class IIa: Acceptable, probably effective; Class IIb: Acceptable, possibly effective; Class III: Not indicated, may be harmful; EF: Ejection fraction; NSR: Normal sinus rhythm; TEE: Transesophageal echocardiogram

*Occasionally, two of the named antiarrhythmic agents may be used, but use of these agents in combination may have proarrhythmic potential; classes listed represent the *Class of Recommendation* rather than the Vaughn-Williams classification of antiarrhythmics.

Adapted with permission from Lippincott Williams & Wilkins, "Guidelines 2000 for Cardiopulmonary Resuscitation and Emergency Cardiovascular Care. Part 6: Advanced Cardiovascular Life Support. The American Heart Association in Collaboration With the International Liaison Committee on Resuscitation," *Circulation*, 2000, 102(8 Suppl), I160-1.

NORMAL HEART RATES

Age	Mean Heart Rate (beats/minute)	Heart Rate Range (2nd – 98th percentile)
<1 d	123	93-154
1-2 d	123	91-159
3-6 d	129	91-166
1-3 wk	148	107-182
1-2 mo	149	121-179
3-5 mo	141	106-186
6-11 mo	134	109-169
1-2 y	119	89-151
3-4 y	108	73-137
5-7 y	100	65-133
8-11 y	91	62-130
12-15 y	85	60-119

Adapted from *The Harriet Lane Handbook*, 12th ed, Greene MG, ed, St Louis, MO: Mosby Yearbook, 1991.

Normal QRS Axes
(in degrees)

Age	Mean	Range
1 wk – 1 mo	+110	+30 to +180
1–3 mo	+70	+10 to +125
3 mo – 3 y	+60	+10 to +110
>3 y	+60	+20 to +120
Adults	+50	−30 to +105

INTERVALS AND SEGMENTS
OF AN EKG CYCLE

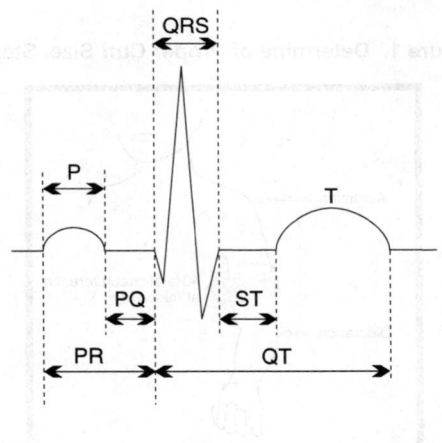

HEXAXIAL REFERENCE
SYSTEM

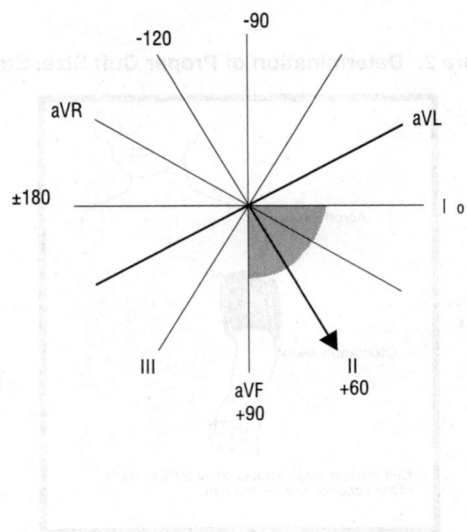

MEASURING PEDIATRIC BLOOD PRESSURE

Figure 1. Determine of Proper Cuff Size, Step 1

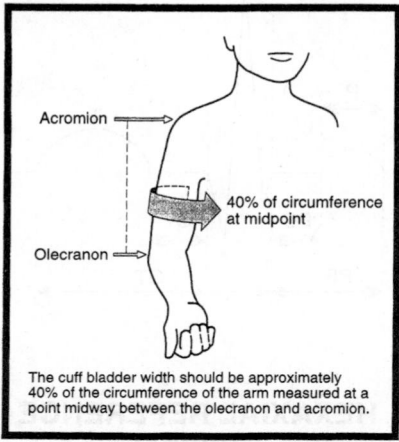

The cuff bladder width should be approximately 40% of the circumference of the arm measured at a point midway between the olecranon and acromion.

Figure 2. Determination of Proper Cuff Size, Step 2

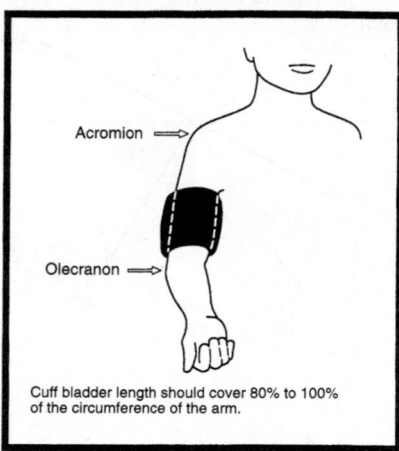

Cuff bladder length should cover 80% to 100% of the circumference of the arm.

Figure 3. Blood Pressure Measurement

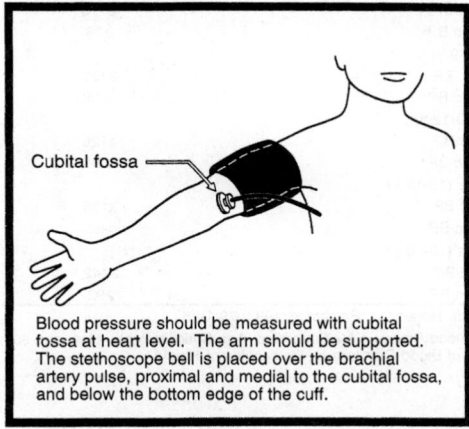

Cubital fossa

Blood pressure should be measured with cubital fossa at heart level. The arm should be supported. The stethoscope bell is placed over the brachial artery pulse, proximal and medial to the cubital fossa, and below the bottom edge of the cuff.

Used with permission: Perloff D, Grim C, Flack J, et al, "Human Blood Pressure Determination by Sphygmomanometry," *Circulation*, 1993, 88:2460-7.

HYPERTENSION, CLASSIFICATION BY AGE GROUP*

Age Group	Significant Hypertension (mm Hg)	Severe Hypertension (mm Hg)
Newborn (7 d)		
systolic BP	≥96	≥106
Newborn (8-30 d)		
systolic BP	≥104	≥110
Infant (<2 y)		
systolic BP	≥112	≥118
diastolic BP	≥74	≥82
Children (3-5 y)		
systolic BP	≥116	≥124
diastolic BP	≥76	≥84
Children (6-9 y)		
systolic BP	≥122	≥130
diastolic BP	≥78	≥86
Children (10-12 y)		
systolic BP	≥126	≥134
diastolic BP	≥82	≥90
Adolescents (13-15 y)		
systolic BP	≥136	≥144
diastolic BP	≥86	≥92
Adolescents (16-18 y)		
systolic BP	≥142	≥150
diastolic BP	≥92	≥98

Adapted from Horan MJ, *Pediatrics*, 1987, 79:1-25.

*See also Blood Pressure Measurement, Age Specific Percentiles, and 90th and 95th Percentiles of Blood Pressure by Percentiles of Height.

BLOOD PRESSURE IN PREMATURE INFANTS, NORMAL

(Birth weight 600-1750 g)*

Day	600-999 g		1000-1249 g	
	S (± 2SD)	D (± 2SD)	S (± 2SD)	D (± 2SD)
1	37.9 (17.4)	23.2 (10.3)	44 (22.8)	22.5 (13.5)
3	44.9 (15.7)	30.6 (12.3)	48 (15.4)	36.5 (9.6)
7	50 (14.8)	30.4 (12.4)	57 (14)	42.5 (16.5)
14	50.2 (14.8)	37.4 (12)	53 (30)	
28	61 (23.5)	45.8 (27.4)	57 (30)	

Day	1250-1499 g		1500-1750 g	
	S (± 2SD)	D (± 2SD)	S (± 2SD)	D (± 2SD)
1	48 (18)	27 (12.4)	47 (15.8)	26 (15.6)
3	59 (21.1)	40 (13.7)	51 (18.2)	35 (10)
7	68 (14.8)	40 (11.3)	66 (23)	41 (24)
14	64 (21.2)	36 (24.2)	76 (34.8)	42 (20.3)
28	69 (31.4)	44 (26.2)	73 (5.6)	50 (9.9)

*Blood pressure was obtained by the Dinamap method.

S = systolic; D = diastolic; SD = standard deviation.

Modified from Ingelfinger JR, Powers L, and Epstein MF, "Blood Pressure Norms in Low-Weight Infants: Birth Through Four Weeks", *Pediatr Res*, 1983, 17:319A.

BLOOD PRESSURE MEASUREMENTS, AGE-SPECIFIC PERCENTILES

Blood Pressure Measurements: Ages 0-12 Months, Boys

Korotkoff phase IV (K4) used for diastolic BP. Reproduced with permission from Horan MJ, *Pediatrics*, 1987, 79:11-25.

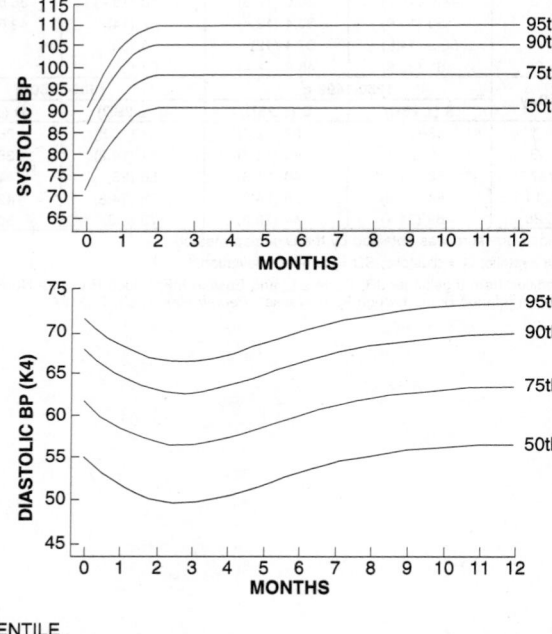

90th PERCENTILE													
SYSTOLIC BP	87	101	106	106	106	105	105	105	105	105	105	105	105
DIASTOLIC BP	68	65	63	63	63	65	66	67	68	68	69	69	69
HEIGHT CM	51	59	63	66	68	70	72	73	74	76	77	78	80
WEIGHT KG	4	4	5	5	6	7	8	9	9	10	10	11	11

Blood Pressure Measurements: Ages 0-12 Months, Girls

Korotkoff phase IV (K4) used for diastolic BP. Reproduced with permission from Horan MJ, *Pediatrics*, 1987, 79:11-25.

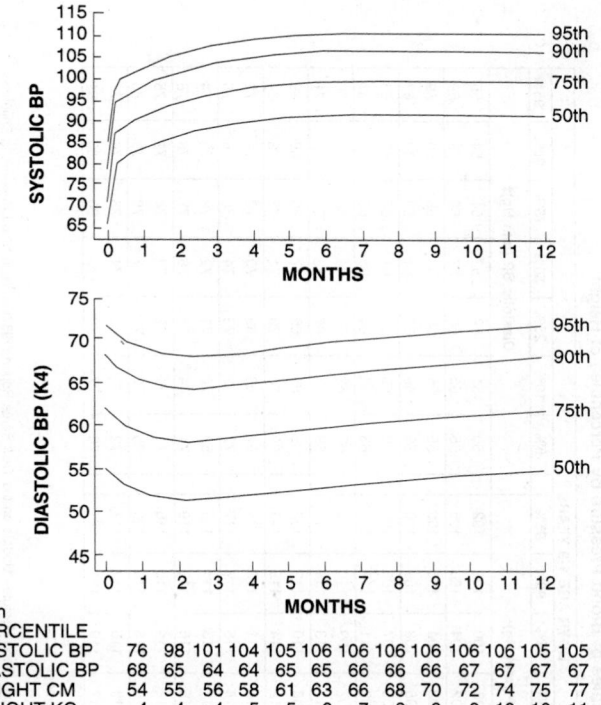

90th PERCENTILE												
SYSTOLIC BP	76	98	101	104	105	106	106	106	106	106	106	105	105
DIASTOLIC BP	68	65	64	64	65	65	66	66	66	67	67	67	67
HEIGHT CM	54	55	56	58	61	63	66	68	70	72	74	75	77
WEIGHT KG	4	4	4	5	5	6	7	8	9	9	10	10	11

BLOOD PRESSURE MEASUREMENTS, AGE-SPECIFIC PERCENTILES (Continued)

90th and 95th Percentiles of Blood Pressure by Percentiles of Height

BOYS AGE 1-9 YEARS

Height Percentiles* →	BP Percentiles† →	Systolic BP (mm Hg)							Diastolic BP (mm Hg)‡						
Age (y)	BP Percentiles†	5%	10%	25%	50%	75%	90%	95%	5%	10%	25%	50%	75%	90%	95%
1	90th	94	95	97	98	100	102	102	50	51	52	53	54	54	55
	95th	98	99	101	102	104	106	106	55	55	56	57	58	59	59
2	90th	98	99	100	102	104	105	106	55	55	56	57	58	59	59
	95th	101	102	104	106	108	109	110	59	59	60	61	62	63	63
3	90th	100	101	103	105	107	108	109	59	59	60	61	62	63	63
	95th	104	105	107	109	111	112	113	63	63	64	65	66	67	67
4	90th	102	103	105	107	109	110	111	62	62	63	64	65	66	66
	95th	106	107	109	111	113	114	115	66	67	67	68	69	70	71
5	90th	104	105	106	108	110	112	112	65	65	66	67	68	69	69
	95th	108	109	110	112	114	115	116	69	70	70	71	72	73	74
6	90th	105	106	108	110	111	113	114	67	68	69	70	70	71	72
	95th	109	110	112	114	115	117	117	72	72	73	74	75	76	76
7	90th	106	107	109	111	113	114	115	69	70	71	72	72	73	74
	95th	110	111	113	115	116	118	119	74	74	75	76	77	78	78
8	90th	107	108	110	112	114	115	116	71	71	72	73	74	75	75
	95th	111	112	114	116	118	119	120	75	76	76	77	78	79	80
9	90th	109	110	112	113	115	117	117	72	73	73	74	75	76	77
	95th	113	114	116	117	119	121	121	76	77	78	79	80	80	81

*Height percentile determined by standard growth curves.

† Blood pressure percentile determined by a single measurement

‡Korotkoff phase V (K5) used for diastolic BP

Source: National Institutes of Health, National Heart, Lung, and Blood Institute, "Update on the Task Force Report (1987) on High Blood Pressure in Children and Adolescents: A Working Group Report from the National High Blood Pressure Education Program," NIH No, 96-3790, 1996.

BOYS AGE 10-17 YEARS

Height Percentiles* →		5%	10%	25%	50%	75%	90%	95%	5%	10%	25%	50%	75%	90%	95%
Age (y)	BP Percentiles† →	Systolic BP (mm Hg)							Diastolic BP (mm Hg)‡						
10	90th	110	112	113	115	117	118	119	73	74	74	75	76	77	78
	95th	114	115	117	119	121	122	123	77	78	79	80	80	81	82
11	90th	112	113	115	117	119	120	121	74	74	75	76	77	78	78
	95th	116	117	119	121	123	124	125	78	79	79	80	81	82	83
12	90th	115	116	117	119	121	123	123	75	75	76	77	78	78	79
	95th	119	120	121	123	125	126	127	79	79	80	81	82	83	83
13	90th	117	118	120	122	124	125	126	75	76	76	77	78	79	80
	95th	121	122	124	126	128	129	130	79	80	81	82	83	83	84
14	90th	120	121	123	125	126	128	128	76	76	77	78	79	80	80
	95th	124	125	127	128	130	132	132	80	81	81	82	83	84	85
15	90th	123	124	125	127	129	131	131	77	77	78	79	80	81	81
	95th	127	128	129	131	133	134	135	81	82	83	83	84	85	86
16	90th	125	126	128	130	132	133	134	79	79	80	81	82	82	83
	95th	129	130	132	134	136	137	138	83	83	84	85	86	87	87
17	90th	128	129	131	133	134	136	136	81	81	82	83	84	85	85
	95th	132	133	135	136	138	140	140	85	85	86	87	88	89	89

*Height percentile determined by standard growth curves.

† Blood pressure percentile determined by a single measurement

‡Korotkoff phase V (K5) used for diastolic BP

Source: National Institutes of Health, National Heart, Lung, and Blood Institute. "Update on the Task Force Report (1987) on High Blood Pressure in Children and Adolescents: A Working Group Report from the National High Blood Pressure Education Program," NIH No, 96-3790, 1996.

BLOOD PRESSURE MEASUREMENTS, AGE-SPECIFIC PERCENTILES (Continued)

Height Percentiles* →		GIRLS AGE 1-9 YEARS															
Age (y)	BP Percentiles† ↓	Systolic BP (mm Hg)							Diastolic BP (mm Hg)‡							
		5%	10%	25%	50%	75%	90%	95%	5%	10%	25%	50%	75%	90%	95%
1	90th	97	98	99	100	102	103	104	53	53	53	54	55	56	56
	95th	101	102	103	104	105	107	107	57	57	57	58	59	60	60
2	90th	99	99	100	102	103	104	105	57	57	58	58	59	60	61
	95th	102	103	104	105	107	108	109	61	61	62	62	63	64	65
3	90th	100	100	102	103	104	105	106	61	61	61	62	63	63	64
	95th	104	104	105	107	108	109	110	65	65	65	66	67	67	68
4	90th	101	102	103	104	106	107	108	63	63	64	65	65	66	67
	95th	105	106	107	108	109	111	111	67	67	68	69	69	70	71
5	90th	103	103	104	106	107	108	109	65	66	66	67	68	68	69
	95th	107	107	108	110	111	112	113	69	70	70	71	72	72	73
6	90th	104	105	106	107	109	110	111	67	67	68	69	69	70	71
	95th	108	109	110	111	112	114	114	71	71	72	73	73	74	75
7	90th	106	107	108	109	110	112	112	69	69	69	70	71	72	72
	95th	110	110	112	113	114	115	116	73	73	73	74	75	76	76
8	90th	108	109	110	111	112	113	114	70	70	71	71	72	73	74
	95th	112	112	113	115	116	117	118	74	74	75	75	76	77	78
9	90th	110	110	112	113	114	115	116	71	72	72	73	74	74	75
	95th	114	114	115	117	118	119	120	75	76	76	77	78	78	79

*Height percentile determined by standard growth curves.

† Blood pressure percentile determined by a single measurement

‡Korotkoff phase V (K5) used for diastolic BP

Source: National Institutes of Health, National Heart, Lung, and Blood Institute, "Update on the Task Force Report (1987) on High Blood Pressure in Children and Adolescents: A Working Group Report from the National High Blood Pressure Education Program," NIH No, 96-3790, 1996.

GIRLS AGE 10-17 YEARS

Height Percentiles* →		Systolic BP (mm Hg)							Diastolic BP (mm Hg)						
Age (y)	BP Percentiles ↓	5%	10%	25%	50%	75%	90%	95%	5%	10%	25%	50%	75%	90%	95%
10	90th	112	112	114	115	116	117	118	73	73	73	74	75	76	76
	95th	116	116	117	119	120	121	122	77	77	77	78	79	80	80
11	90th	114	114	116	117	118	119	120	74	74	75	75	76	77	77
	95th	118	118	119	121	122	123	124	78	78	79	79	80	81	81
12	90th	116	116	118	119	120	121	122	75	75	76	76	77	78	78
	95th	120	120	121	123	124	125	126	79	79	80	80	81	82	82
13	90th	118	118	119	121	122	123	124	76	76	77	78	78	79	80
	95th	121	121	123	125	126	127	128	80	80	81	82	82	83	84
14	90th	119	120	121	122	124	125	126	77	77	78	79	79	80	81
	95th	123	124	125	126	128	129	130	81	81	82	83	83	84	85
15	90th	121	121	122	124	125	126	127	78	78	79	79	80	81	82
	95th	124	125	126	128	129	130	131	82	82	83	83	84	85	86
16	90th	122	122	123	125	126	127	128	79	79	79	80	81	82	82
	95th	125	126	127	128	130	131	132	83	83	83	84	85	86	86
17	90th	122	123	124	125	126	128	128	79	79	79	80	81	82	82
	95th	126	126	127	129	130	131	132	83	83	83	84	85	86	86

*Height percentile determined by standard growth curves.

† Blood pressure percentile determined by a single measurement

‡Korotkoff phase V (K5) used for diastolic BP

Source: National Institutes of Health, National Heart, Lung, and Blood Institute, "Update on the Task Force Report (1987) on High Blood Pressure in Children and Adolescents: A Working Group Report from the National High Blood Pressure Education Program," NIH No, 96-3790, 1996.

ANTIHYPERTENSIVE AGENTS BY CLASS

Alpha Adrenergic (Alpha 1 and Alpha 2) Antagonists
Phenoxybenzamine
Phentolamine
Tolazoline [DSC]

Alpha 1 Antagonists
Prazosin

Alpha 2 Agonists
Clonidine
Methyldopa

Beta Antagonists
Atenolol
Esmolol
Metoprolol
Nadolol
Propranolol
Timolol

Mixed Alpha / Beta Antagonists
Labetalol

Angiotensin Converting Enzyme Inhibitors
Captopril
Enalapril/Enalaprilat
Lisinopril

Calcium Channel Blockers
Amlodipine
Diltiazem
Nifedipine
Verapamil

Diuretics
Amiloride
Bumetanide
Chlorothiazide
Furosemide
Hydrochlorothiazide
Mannitol
Metolazone
Spironolactone
Torsemide
Triamterene

Ganglionic Blockers
Trimethaphan

Nitrates
Isosorbide dinitrate
Nitroglycerin

Vasodilators (Direct-acting)
Diazoxide
Hydralazine
Minoxidil
Nitroprusside

ANTIDEPRESSANT AGENTS

Comparison of Usual Adult Dosage and Mechanism of Action

Drug	Usual Adult Dosage (mg/d)	Reuptake Inhibition	
		Norepinephrine	Serotonin
First-Generation Antidepressants *Tricyclic Antidepressants*			
Amitriptyline (Elavil®, Endep®)	100-300	Moderate	High
Clomipramine† (Anafranil®)	100-250	Moderate	High
Desipramine (Norpramin®, Pertofrane®)	100-300	High	Low
Doxepin (Adapin®, Sinequan®)	100-300	Low	Moderate
Imipramine (Janimine®, Tofranil®)	100-300	Moderate	Moderate
Nortriptyline (Aventyl®, Pamelor®)	50-200	Moderate	Low
Protriptyline (Vivactil®)	15-60	Moderate	Low
Trimipramine (Surmontil®)	100-300	Low	Low
Monoamine Oxidase Inhibitors			
Phenelzine (Nardil®)	15-90	—	—
Tranylcypromine (Parnate®)	10-40	—	—
Second-Generation Antidepressants *Older Second-Generation Antidepressants*			
Amoxapine (Asendin®)	100-400	Moderate	Low
Maprotiline (Ludiomil®)	100-225	Moderate	Low
Trazodone (Desyrel®)	150-500	Very low	Moderate
Newer Second-Generation Antidepressants			
Bupropion (Wellbutrin®)	300-450‡	Very low§	Very low§
Third-Generation Antidepressants *Selective Serotonin Reuptake Inhibitors*			
Fluoxetine (Prozac®)	10-40	Very low	High
Fluvoxamine (Luvox®)	100-300	Very low	Very high
Paroxetine (Paxil®)	20-50	Very low	Very high
Sertraline (Zoloft®)	50-150	Very low	Very high
Serotonin/Norepinephrine Reuptake Inhibitors			
Venlafaxine (Effexor®)	75-375	Very high	Very high
Atypical Antidepressants with 5HT2 Receptor Antagonist Properties			
Mirtazapine (Remeron®)**	15-45	Very low	Very low
Nefazodone (Serzone®)**	300-600	Very low	High

†Not approved by FDA for depression.

‡Not to exceed 150 mg/dose to minimize seizure risk.

§Norepinephrine and serotonin reuptake inhibition is minimal, but inhibits dopamine reuptake.

**These agents work primarily through antagonizing the postsynaptic 5HT2 receptor.

ANTIDEPRESSANT AGENTS *(Continued)*

Comparison of Adverse Effects

Drug	ACH	Drowsiness	Orthostatic Hypotension	Cardiac Arrhythmias	GI Distress	Weight Gain
First-Generation Antidepressants *Tricyclic Antidepressants*						
Amitriptyline (Elavil®, Endep®)	4+	4+	4+	3+	0	4+
Clomipramine† (Anafranil®)	4+	4+	2+	3+	1+	4+
Desipramine (Norpramin®, Pertofrane®)	1+	2+	2+	2+	0	1+
Doxepin (Adapin®, Sinequan®)	3+	4+	2+	2+	0	4+
Imipramine (Janimine®, Tofranil®)	3+	3+	4+	3+	1+	4+
Nortriptyline (Aventyl®, Pamelor®)	2+	2+	1+	2+	0	1+
Protriptyline (Vivactil®)	2+	1+	2+	3+	0	0
Trimipramine (Surmontil®)	4+	4+	3+	3+	0	4+
Monoamine Oxidase Inhibitors						
Phenelzine (Nardil®)	2+	2+	2+	1+	1+	3+
Tranylcypromine (Parnate®)	2+	1+	2+	1+	1+	2+
Second-Generation Antidepressants *Older Second-Generation Antidepressants*						
Amoxapine (Asendin®)	2+	2+	2+	2+	0	2+
Maprotiline (Ludiomil®)	2+	3+	2+	2+	0	2+
Trazodone (Desyrel®)	0	4+	3+	1+	1+	2+
Newer Second-Generation Antidepressants						
Bupropion (Wellbutrin®)	0	0	0	1+	1+	0
Third-Generation Antidepressants *Selective Serotonin Reuptake Inhibitors*						
Fluoxetine (Prozac®)	0	0	0	0	3+¶	0
Fluvoxamine (Luvox®)	0	0	0	0	3+¶	0
Paroxetine (Paxil®)	1+	1+	0	0	3+¶	1+
Sertraline (Zoloft®)	0	0	0	0	3+¶	0
Serotonin/Norepinephrine Reuptake Inhibitors						
Venlafaxine# (Effexor®)	1+	1+	0	1+	3+¶	0
Atypical Antidepressants with 5HT2 Receptor Antagonist Properties						
Mirtazapine (Remeron®)	1+	2+	0	0	3+	0
Nefazodone (Serzone®)	1+	1+	0	0	1+	0

Key: ACH = anticholinergic effects (dry mouth, blurred vision, urinary retention, constipation); 0 - 4+ = absent or rare - relatively common.

†Not approved by FDA for depression.

¶Nausea is usually mild and transient.

#Comparative studies evaluating the adverse effects of venlafaxine in relation to other antidepressants have not been performed.

CORTICOSTEROIDS, SYSTEMIC

Relative Potencies and Equivalent Doses of Corticosteroids

(Glucocorticoid potency compared to hydrocortisone "mg" for "mg" basis)

Compound	Gluco-corticoid Potency	Mineralo-corticoid Potency	Equivalent Dose (mg)	Duration* of Action
Cortisone (Cortone®) Injection: 50 mg/mL suspension Tablet: 5 mg	0.8	++	25	S
Dexamethasone (Decadron®, Dexone®, Hexadrol®) Elixir: 0.5 mg/5 mL Injection: 4 mg/mL Intensol: 1 mg/mL Tablet: 0.25 mg, 0.5 mg, 0.75 mg, 1 mg, 1.5 mg, 2 mg, 4 mg	25-30	0	0.75	L
Fludrocortisone (Florinef®) Tablet: 0.1 mg	10	+++++		I
Hydrocortisone (Cortef®) Injection: 50 mg/mL Suspension: 10 mg/5 mL Tablet: 5 mg, 10 mg, 20 mg	1	++	20	S
Methylprednisolone (Medrol®, Solu-Medrol®, Depo-Medrol®) Injection: 40 mg, 125 mg, 500 mg, 1 g Injection, susp: 80 mg/mL Tablet: 2 mg, 4 mg, 16 mg, 24 mg	5	0	4	I
Prednisolone (Delta-Cortef®, Prelone® Syrup, Pediapred®) Liquid: 5 mg/5 mL Syrup: 15 mg/5 mL Tablet: 5 mg	4	+	5	I
Prednisone (Deltasone®, Liquid Pred®, Orasone®) Liquid: 5 mg/5 mL Tablet: 1 mg, 2.5 mg, 5 mg, 10 mg, 20 mg, 50 mg	4	+	5	I

*S = Short, 8-12 hours biologic activity.

I = Intermediate, 12-36 hours biologic activity.

L = Long, 36-54 hours biologic activity.

Reference

Knoben JE, and Anderson PO, *Handbook of Clinical Drug Data*, 6th ed, Drug Intelligence Pub, Inc, 1988.

CORTICOSTEROIDS, TOPICAL

The following topical corticosteroid preparations are grouped according to relative anti-inflammatory activity. Preparations in each group are approximately equivalent.

Drug	Dosage Form
Lowest Potency	
Hydrocortisone	0.5% cream, ointment
Hydrocortisone	1% cream, ointment
Hydrocortisone	2.5% cream, ointment
Hydrocortisone	1% solution
Hydrocortisone	1% lotion
Low Potency	
Alclometasone Dipropionate (Aclovate®)	0.05% cream, ointment
Desonide (Tridesilon®)	0.05% cream, ointment
Fluocinolone Acetonide (Synalar®)	0.01% cream
Low Intermediate Potency	
Flurandrenolide (Cordran®)*	0.025% cream, ointment
Hydrocortisone Valerate (Westcort®)	0.2% cream, ointment
Triamcinolone Acetonide (Kenalog®)	0.025% cream, ointment, lotion
High Intermediate Potency	
Betamethasone Valerate	0.1% cream, ointment, lotion
Desoximetasone (Topicort®)	0.05% gel
Fluocinolone Acetonide (Synalar®)*	0.025% cream, ointment
Flurandrenolide (Cordran®)*	0.05% cream, ointment, lotion
Halcinonide (Halog®)	0.025% cream
Triamcinolone Acetonide (Aristocort®, Kenalog®)	0.1% cream, ointment, lotion
High Potency	
Amcinonide (Cyclocort®)*	0.1% ointment
Betamethasone Dipropionate (Diprosone®)	0.05% cream, ointment, lotion
Desoximetasone (Topicort®)	0.25% cream, ointment
Diflorasone Diacetate	0.05% cream, ointment
Fluocinolone Acetonide (Synalar®-HP)	0.2% cream
Fluocinonide (Lidex®)	0.05% cream, ointment, solution
Halcinonide (Halog®)	0.1% cream, ointment, solution
Triamcinolone Acetonide (Aristocort®, Kenalog®)	0.5% cream, ointment

*Does not contain propylene glycol.

Reference
Modified from Cornell RC and Stoughton RB, "The Use of Topical Steroids in Psoriasis," *Dermatol Clin,* 1984, 2:397-407.

MULTIVITAMIN PRODUCTS

MULTIVITAMIN PRODUCTS (PARENTERAL)
Formulations for Neonates, Infants, and Children <11 Years of Age

Product	A (int. units)	B₁ (mg)	B₂ (mg)	B₆ (mg)	B₁₂ (mcg)	C (mg)	D (int. units)	E (int. units)	K (mcg)	Additional Information
Infuvite® Pediatric (per 5 mL)	2300	1.2	1.4	1	1	80	400	7	200	Supplied as one 4 mL vial and one 1 mL vial Biotin 20 mcg, folic acid 140 mcg, niacinamide 17 mg, dexpanthenol 5 mg
M.V.I.® Pediatric	2300	1.2	1.4	1	1	80	400	7	200	Biotin 20 mcg, folic acid 140 mcg, niacinamide 17 mg, dexpanthenol 5 mg

Legend: int. = international

MULTIVITAMIN PRODUCTS *(Continued)*

MULTIVITAMIN PRODUCTS (PARENTERAL)
Formulations for Children ≥11 Years to Adults

Product	A (int. units)	B₁ (mg)	B₂ (mg)	B₆ (mg)	B₁₂ (mcg)	C (mg)	D (int. units)	E (int. units)	K (mcg)	Additional Information
Infuvite® Adult (per 10 mL)	3300	6	3.6	6	5	200	200	10	150	Supplied as two 5 mL vials Biotin 60 mcg, folic acid 600 mcg, niacinamide 40 mg, dexpanthenol 15 mg
M.V.I.®-12 (per 10 mL)	3300	3	3.6	4	12.5	100	200	10	–	Supplied as two 5 mL vials or a single 2-chambered 10 mL vial Biotin 60 mcg, folic acid 400 mcg, niacinamide 40 mg, dexpanthenol 15 mg

Legend: int. = international

MULTIVITAMIN PRODUCTS (ORAL / ENTERAL)
Neonatal and Infant Formulations

Product	A (int. units)	B_1 (mg)	B_2 (mg)	B_6 (mg)	B_{12} (mcg)	C (mg)	D (int. units)	E (int. units)	Additional Information
					Drops				
ADEKs (per mL) [OTC]	1500	0.5	0.6	0.6	4	45	400	40	Beta carotene 1 mg, biotin 15 mcg, niacin 6 mg, vitamin K 0.1 mg, Zn 5 mg; alcohol free, dye free (60 mL)
Poly-Vi-Sol® (per mL) [OTC]	1500	0.5	0.6	0.4	2	35	400	5	Niacin 8 mg (50 mL)
Poly-Vi-Sol® With Iron (per mL) [OTC]	1500	0.5	0.6	0.4		35	400	5	Fe 10 mg, niacin 8 mg (50 mL)
Tri-Vi-Sol® (per mL) [OTC]	1500					35	400		Fruit flavor (50 mL)
Tri-Vi-Sol® With Iron (per mL) [OTC]	1500					35	400		Fe 10 mg; fruit flavor (50 mL)
Vi-Daylin® (per mL) [OTC]	1500	0.5	0.6	0.4	1.5	35	400	5	Niacin 8 mg; alcohol <0.5%, sugar free, fruit flavor (50 mL)
Vi-Daylin® + Iron (per mL) [OTC]	1500	0.5	0.6	0.4		35	400	5	Fe 10 mg, niacin 8 mg; alcohol <0.5%, sugar free, fruit flavor (50 mL)
Vi-Daylin® ADC (per mL) [OTC]	1500					35	400		Alcohol <0.5%, sugar free, fruit flavor (50 mL)
Vi-Daylin® ADC + Iron (per mL) [OTC]	1500					35	400		Fe 10 mg; benzoic acid, sugar free, fruit flavor (50 mL)

Legend: Ca = elemental calcium, Cr = chromium, Cu = copper, Fe = elemental iron, int. = international, Mg = magnesium, Mn = manganese, Mo = molybdenum, Zn = zinc.

MULTIVITAMIN PRODUCTS *(Continued)*

MULTIVITAMIN PRODUCTS (ORAL / ENTERAL)
Fluoride-Containing Neonatal and Infant Multivitamin Formulations

Product	A (int. units)	B₁ (mg)	B₂ (mg)	B₆ (mg)	B₁₂ (mcg)	C (mg)	D (int. units)	E (int. units)	Additional Information
					Drops				
Poly-Vi-Flor® 0.25 mg (per mL)	1500	0.5	0.6	0.4	2	35	400	5	**Fluoride 0.25 mg**, niacin 8 mg; fruit flavor (50 mL)
Poly-Vi-Flor® 0.5 mg (per mL)	1500	0.5	0.6	0.4	2	35	400	5	**Fluoride 0.5 mg**, niacin 8 mg; fruit flavor (50 mL)
Poly-Vi-Flor® With Iron 0.25 mg (per mL)	1500	0.5	0.6	0.4		35	400	5	**Fluoride 0.25 mg**, Fe 10 mg, niacin 8 mg; fruit flavor (50 mL)
Soluvite-F® (per 0.6 mL)	1500					35	400		**Fluoride 0.25 mg**; alcohol free, dye free, orange flavor (57 mL)
Tri-Vi-Flor® 0.25 mg (per mL)	1500					35	400		**Fluoride 0.25 mg**; fruit flavor (50 mL)
Tri-Vi-Flor® With Iron 0.25 mg (per mL)	1500					35	400		**Fluoride 0.25 mg**, Fe 10 mg; fruit flavor (50 mL)
Vi-Daylin®/F (per mL)	1500	0.5	0.6	0.4		35	400	5	**Fluoride 0.25 mg**, niacin 8 mg; alcohol <0.1%, benzoic acid, sugar free, fruit flavor (50 mL)
Vi-Daylin®/F + Iron (per mL)	1500	0.5	0.6	0.4		35	400	5	**Fluoride 0.25 mg**, Fe 10 mg, niacin 8 mg; alcohol <0.1%, benzoic acid, sugar free, fruit flavor (50 mL)
Vi-Daylin®/F ADC (per mL)	1500					35	400		**Fluoride 0.25 mg**; sugar free, fruit flavor (50 mL)
Vi-Daylin®/F ADC + Iron (per mL)	1500					35	400		**Fluoride 0.25 mg**, Fe 10 mg; sugar free, fruit flavor (50 mL)

Legend: Ca = elemental calcium, Cr = chromium, Cu = copper, elemental Fe = iron, int. = international, Mg = magnesium, Mn = manganese, Mo = molybdenum, Zn = zinc.

Pediatric Multivitamin Formulations

Product	A (int. units)	B₁ (mg)	B₂ (mg)	B₆ (mg)	B₁₂ (mcg)	C (mg)	D (int. units)	E (int. units)	Additional Information
Tablet, Chewable									
ADEKs® [OTC]	4000	1.2	1.3	1.5	12	60	400	150	Beta carotene 3 mg, biotin 50 mcg, folic acid 0.2 mg, niacin 10 mg, pantothenic acid 10 mg, vitamin K 150 mcg, Zn 7.5 mg; dye free
Centrum® Kids Rugrats™ Extra C [OTC]	5000	1.5	1.7	1	5	250	400	15	Ca 108 mg, Cu 0.5 mg, folic acid 0.3 mg, niacin 13.5 mg, phosphorus 50 mg, sodium 15 mg, Zn 4 mg; cherry, fruit punch, and orange flavors
Centrum® Kids Rugrats™ Extra Calcium [OTC]	5000	1.5	1.7	1	5	60	400	15	Ca 200 mg, Cu 0.5 mg, folic acid 0.3 mg, niacin 13.5 mg, phosphorus 50 mg, Zn 4 mg; cherry, fruit punch, and orange flavors
Centrum® Kids Rugrats™ Complete [OTC]	5000	1.5	1.7	2	6	60	400	30	Biotin 45 mcg, Ca 108 mg, Cr 20 mcg, Cu 2 mg, Fe 18 mg, folic acid 0.4 mg, iodine 150 mcg, Mg 40 mg, Mn 1 mg, Mo 20 mcg, niacin 20 mg, pantothenic acid 10 mg, phosphorus 50 mg, vitamin K 10 mg, Zn 15 mg; cherry, fruit punch, and orange flavors
Flintstones® Original [OTC]	2500	1.05	1.2	1.05	4.5	60	400	15	Folic acid 0.3 mg, niacin 13.5 mg
Flintstones® Complete [OTC]	5000	1.5	1.7	2	6	60	400	30	Biotin 40 mcg, Ca 100 mg, Cu 2 mg, Fe 18 mg, folic acid 0.4 mg, iodine 150 mcg, Mg 20 mg, niacin 20 mg, pantothenic acid 10 mg, phosphorus 100 mg, Zn 15 mg; **phenylalanine 4.56 mg**[*]; cherry, grape, and orange flavors
Flintstones® Plus Calcium [OTC]	2500	1.05	1.2	1.05	4.5	60	400	15	Ca 200 mg, folic acid 0.3 mg, niacin 13.5 mg; **phenylalanine <4 mg**[*]; cherry, grape, and orange flavors
Flintstones® Plus Extra C [OTC]	2500	1.05	1.2	1.05	4.5	250	400	15	Folic acid 0.3 mg, niacin 13.5 mg; grape, orange, peach-apricot, raspberry, and strawberry flavors
Flintstones® Plus Iron [OTC]	2500	1.05	1.2	1.05	4.5	60	400	15	Fe 15 mg, folic acid 0.3 mg, niacin 13.5 mg; grape, orange, peach-apricot, raspberry, and strawberry flavors

MULTIVITAMIN PRODUCTS (Continued)

Pediatric Multivitamin Formulations (continued)

Product	A (int. units)	B₁ (mg)	B₂ (mg)	B₆ (mg)	B₁₂ (mcg)	C (mg)	D (int. units)	E (int. units)	Additional Information
My First Flintstones® [OTC]	2500	1.05	1.2	1.05	4.5	60	400	15	Folic acid 0.3 mg, niacin 13.5 mg; cherry, grape, and orange flavors
One-A-Day® Kids Bugs Bunny and Friends Complete [OTC]	5000	1.5	1.7	2	6	60	400	30	Biotin 40 mcg, Ca 100 mg, Cu 2 mg, Fe 18 mg, folic acid 0.4 mg, iodine 150 mcg, Mg 20 mg, niacin 20 mg, pantothenic acid 10 mg, phosphorus 100 mg, Zn 15 mg; sugar free, fruity flavors
One-A-Day® Kids Bugs Bunny and Friends Plus Extra C [OTC]	2500	1.05	1.2	1.05	4.5	250	400	15	Folic acid 0.3 mg, niacin 13.5 mg, **phenylalanine***; sugar free, fruity flavors
One-A-Day® Kids Extreme Sports [OTC]	5000	1.5	1.2	2	6	60	400	30	Biotin 40 mcg, Ca 100 mg, Cu 2 mg, Fe 18 mg, folic acid 0.4 mg, iodine 150 mcg, Mg 20 mg, niacin 20 mg, pantothenic acid 10 mg, phosphorus 100 mg, Zn 15 mg
One-A-Day® Kids Scooby-Doo! Complete [OTC]	5000	1.5	1.7	2	6	60	400	30	Biotin 40 mcg, Ca 100 mg, Cu 2 mg, Fe 18 mg, folic acid 0.4 mg, iodine 150 mcg, Mg 20 mg, niacin 20 mg, pantothenic acid 10 mg, phosphorus 100 mg, Zn 15 mg; fruity flavors
One-A-Day® Kids Scooby-Doo! Plus Calcium [OTC]	2500	1.05	1.2	1.05	4.5	60	400	15	Ca 200 mg, folic acid 0.3 mg, niacin 13.5 mg; fruity flavors

Legend: Ca = elemental calcium, Cr = chromium, Cu = copper, Fe = elemental iron, int. = international, Mg = magnesium, Mn = manganese, Mo = molybdenum, Zn = zinc.
*Contains phenylalanine; use with caution in phenylketonurics

Adolescent and Adult Multivitamin Formulations

Product	A (int. units)	B_1 (mg)	B_2 (mg)	B_6 (mg)	B_{12} (mcg)	C (mg)	D (int. units)	E (int. units)	Additional Information
Liquid									
Centrum® (per 15 mL) [OTC]	2500	1.5	1.7	2	6	60	400	30	Biotin 300 mcg, Cr 25 mcg, Fe 9 mg, iodine 150 mcg, Mn 2 mg, Mo 25 mg, niacin 20 mg, pantothenic acid 10 mg, Zn 3 mg; alcohol 5.4%, sodium benzoate (240 mL)
Iberet® (per 5 mL) [OTC]		1.2	1.35	0.925	5.63	33.8			Fe 23.6 mg, niacin 6.8 mg, pantothenic acid 2.4 mg; alcohol (240 mL)
Iberet®-500 (per 5 mL) [OTC]		1.2	1.35	0.925	5.63	125			Fe 23.6 mg, niacin 6.8 mg, pantothenic acid 2.4 mg; alcohol (240 mL)
Vi-Daylin® (per 5 mL) [OTC]	2500	1.05	1.2	1.05	4.5	60	400	15	Niacin 13.5 mg; alcohol <0.5%, benzoic acid; lemon/orange flavor (240 mL, 480 mL)
Vi-Daylin® + Iron (per 5 mL) [OTC]	2500	1.05	1.2	1.05	4.5	60	400	15	Fe 10 mg, niacin 13.5 mg; alcohol <0.5%, benzoic acid; lemon/orange flavor (240 mL, 480 mL)
Caplet									
Theragran-M® Advanced Formula [OTC]	5000	3	3.4	6	12	90	400	60	Biotin 30 mcg, boron 150 mcg, Ca 40 mg, chloride 7.5 mg, Cr 50 mcg, Cu 2 mg, Fe 9 mg, folic acid 0.4 mg, iodine 150 mcg, Mg 100 mg, Mn 2 mg, Mo 75 mcg, niacin 20 mg, nickel 5 mcg, pantothenic acid 10 mg, phosphorus 31 mg, potassium 7.5 mg, Se 70 mcg, silicon 2 mg, tin 10 mcg, vanadium 10 mcg, vitamin K 28 mcg, Zn 15 mg
Capsule									
Vitacon Forte	8000	10	5	2	10	150		50	Folic acid 1 mg, Mg 70 mg, Mn 4 mg, niacinamide 25 mg, Zn 80 mg
Vicon Plus® [OTC]	3400	9.3	4.6	1.5		140		45	Mg 5 mg, Mn 1 mg, niacin 24 mg, pantothenic acid 11 mg, Zn 10 mg

MULTIVITAMIN PRODUCTS (Continued)

Adolescent and Adult Multivitamin Formulations (continued)

Product	A (int. units)	B₁ (mg)	B₂ (mg)	B₆ (mg)	B₁₂ (mcg)	C (mg)	D (int. units)	E (int. units)	Additional Information
					Tablet				
Centrum® [OTC]	5000	1.5	1.7	2	6	60	400	30	Biotin 30 mcg, boron 150 mcg, Ca 162 mg, chloride 72 mg, Cr 120 mcg, Cu 2 mg, Fe 18 mg, folic acid 0.4 mg, iodine 150 mcg, lutein 250 mcg, Mg 100 mg, Mn 2 mg, Mo 75 mcg, niacin 20 mg, nickel 5 mcg, pantothenic acid 10 mg, phosphorus 109 mg, potassium 80 mcg, Se 20 mcg, silicon 2 mg, tin 10 mcg, vanadium 10 mcg, vitamin K 25 mcg, Zn 15 mg
Centrum® Performance™ [OTC]	5000	4.5	5.1	6	18	120	400	60	Biotin 40 mcg, boron 60 mcg, chloride 72 mg, folic acid 0.4 mg, Ca 100 mg, Cr 120 mcg, Cu 2 mg, Fe 18 mg, iodine 150 mcg, Mg 40 mg, Mn 4 mg, Mo 75 mcg, niacin 40 mg, nickel 5 mcg, pantothenic acid 10 mg, phosphorus 48 mg, potassium 80 mg, Se 70 mcg, silicon 4 mg, tin 10 mcg, vanadium 10 mcg, vitamin K 25 mcg, Zn 15 mg
Iberet®-500 [OTC]		4.96	5.4	3.7	22.5	500			Fe 95 mg (controlled release), niacin 27.2 mg, pantothenic acid 8.28 mg, sodium 65 mg
Iberet-Folic-500® [OTC]		6	6	5	25	500			Fe 105 mg (controlled release), folic acid 0.8 mg, niacinamide 30 mg, pantothenic acid 10 mg
One-A-Day® Active Formula [OTC]	5000	4.5	5.1	6	18	120	400	60	American ginseng 55 mg, biotin 40 mcg, boron 150 mcg, Ca 110 mg, chloride 180 mg, Cr 100 mcg, Cu 2 mg, Fe 9 mg, folic acid 0.4 mg, iodine 150 mcg, Mg 40 mg, Mn 2 mg, Mo 25 mcg, niacin 40 mg, nickel 5 mcg, pantothenic acid 10 mg, phosphorus 48 mg, potassium 200 mg, Se 45 mcg, silicon 6 mg, tin 10 mcg, vanadium 10 mcg, vitamin K 25 mcg, Zn 15 mg
One-A-Day® Essential Formula [OTC]	5000	1.5	1.7	2	6	60	400	30	Folic acid 0.4 mg, niacin 20 mg, pantothenic acid 10 mg

Adolescent and Adult Multivitamin Formulations (continued)

Product	A (int. units)	B₁ (mg)	B₂ (mg)	B₆ (mg)	B₁₂ (mcg)	C (mg)	D (int. units)	E (int. units)	Additional Information
One-A-Day® Maximum Formula [OTC]	5000	1.5	1.7	2	6	60	400	30	Biotin 30 mcg, boron 150 mcg, Ca 162 mg, chloride 72 mg, Cr 65 mcg, Cu 2 mg, Fe 18 mg, folic acid 0.4 mg, iodine 150 mcg, Mg 100 mg, Mn 3.5 mg, Mo 160 mcg, niacin 20 mg, nickel 5 mcg, pantothenic acid 10 mg, phosphorus 109 mg, potassium 80 mg, Se 20 mcg, silicon 2 mg, tin 10 mcg, vanadium 10 mcg, vitamin K 25 mcg, Zn 15 mg
One-A-Day® Today [OTC]	3000	1.1	1.7	3	18	75	400	33	Biotin 30 mcg, Ca 240 mg, Cr 120 mcg, Cu 2 mg, folic acid 0.4 mg, Mg 120 mg, Mn 2 mg, niacin 14 mg, pantothenic acid 5 mg, potassium 100 mg, Se 70 mcg, soy extract 10 mg, vitamin K 20 mcg, Zn 15 mg
Tablet, Chewable									
Centrum® [OTC]	5000	1.5	1.7	2	6	60	400	30	Biotin 45 mcg, Ca 108 mg, Cr 20 mcg, Cu 2 mg, Fe 18 mg, folic acid 0.4 mg, iodine 150 mcg, Mg 40 mg, Mn 1 mg, Mo 20 mcg, niacin 20 mg, pantothenic acid 10 mg, Zn 15 mg

Legend: Ca = calcium, Cr = chromium, Cu = copper, Fe = iron, int. = international, Mg = magnesium, Mn = manganese, Mo = molybdenum, Se = selenium, Zn = zinc.

MULTIVITAMIN PRODUCTS *(Continued)*

Vitamin B Complex Formulations
Adolescent and Adult

Product	B₁ (mg)	B₂ (mg)	B₆ (mg)	B₁₂ (mcg)	C (mg)	E (int. units)	Additional Information
Caplet							
Allbee® with C [OTC]	15	10.2	5		300		Niacinamide 50 mg, pantothenic acid 10 mg
Allbee® C-800 [OTC]	15	17	25	12	800	45	Niacinamide 100 mg, pantothenic acid 25 mg
Allbee® C-800 + Iron [OTC]	15	17	25	12	800	45	Fe 27 mg, folic acid 0.4 mcg, niacinamide 100 mg, pantothenic acid 25 mg
Liquid							
Apatate® (per 5 mL) [OTC]	15		0.5	25			Cherry flavor (120 mL)
Gevrabon® (per 30 mL) [OTC]	5	2.5	1	1			Choline 10 mg, Fe 15 mg, iodine 100 mcg, Mg 2 mg, Mn 2 mg, niacinamide 60 mg, pantothenic acid 10 mg, Zn 2 mg; alcohol, benzoic acid; sherry wine flavor (480 mL)
Softgel							
Nephrocaps®	1.5	1.7	10	6	100		Biotin 150 mcg, folic acid 1 mcg, niacinamide 20 mg, pantothenic acid 5 mg
Tablet							
Nephro-Vite®	1.5	1.7	10	6	60		Biotin 300 mcg, folic acid 0.8 mcg, niacinamide 20 mg, pantothenic acid 10 mg
Nephro-Vite® Rx	1.5	1.7	10	6	60		Biotin 300 mcg, folic acid 1 mcg, niacinamide 20 mg, pantothenic acid 10 mg
Stresstabs® B-Complex [OTC]	10	10	5	12	500	30	Biotin 45 mcg, folic acid 0.4 mcg, niacinamide 100 mg, pantothenic acid 20 mg
Stresstabs® B-Complex + Iron [OTC]	10	10	5	12	500	30	Biotin 45 mcg, Fe 18 mg, folic acid 0.4 mcg, niacinamide 100 mg, pantothenic acid 20 mg
Stresstabs® B-Complex + Zinc [OTC]	10	10	5	12	500	30	Biotin 45 mcg, Cu 3 mg, folic acid 0.4 mcg, niacinamide 100 mg, pantothenic acid 20 mg, Zn 23.9 mg
Surbex-T® [OTC]	15	10	5	10	500		Ca 20 mg, niacinamide 100 mg
Z-Bec® [OTC]	15	10.2	10	6	600	45	Niacinamide 100 mg, pantothenic acid 25 mg, Zn 22.5 mg
Tablet, Chewable							
Apatate® [OTC]	15		0.5	25			Cherry flavor

Legend: Ca = calcium, Cu = copper, Fe = iron, int. = international, Mg = magnesium, Mn = manganese, Zn = zinc.

NARCOTIC ANALGESICS COMPARISON

Drug	Dosage Form	Onset (min)	Duration (h)	Equi-analgesic I.M. Dose (mg)	Equi-analgesic P.O. Dose (mg)	Parenteral Oral Ratio	Partial Antagonist
Alfentanil hydrochloride	Inj: 500 mcg/mL, 5 mL amp	Immediate (I.V.)	ND	ND	—	—	No
Codeine	Inj: 30 mg/mL as phosphate Tab: 15 mg, 30 mg as sulfate, 60 mg as phosphate	10-30 (I.M.)	4-6 (I.M.)	120	200	1/2-2/3	No
Fentanyl citrate (Sublimaze®)	Inj: 50 mcg/mL, 2 mL, 10 mL amp	7-8 (I.M.)	1-2 (I.M.); 0.5-1 (I.V.)	0.1-0.2	—	—	No
Hydrocodone and acetaminophen	Tab: 5 mg hydrocodone + 500 mg acetaminophen (Vicodin®)	ND	4-6 (P.O.)	—	ND	ND	No
Hydromorphone hydrochloride (Dilaudid®)	Inj: 2 mg/mL amp Tab: 2 mg	15-30 (I.M.)	4-5 (I.M.)	1.5	7.5	1/5	No
Meperidine hydrochloride (Demerol®)	Inj: 25 mg/0.5 mL, 50 mg/mL, 100 mg/mL amp Syrup: 10 mg/mL Tab: 50 mg	10-45 (I.M.)	2-4 (I.M.)	75-100	300	1/3-1/2	No
Methadone hydrochloride (Dolophine®)	Inj: 10 mg/mL amp Solution: 1 mg/mL Tab: 5 mg, 10 mg	30-60 (I.M.)	4-6 (I.M.); duration increases with repeated use due to cumulative effects	10	20	1/2	No

NARCOTIC ANALGESICS COMPARISON (Continued)

Drug	Dosage Form	Onset (min)	Duration (h)	Equi-analgesic I.M. Dose (mg)	Equi-analgesic P.O. Dose (mg)	Parenteral Oral Ratio	Partial Antagonist
Morphine sulfate	Inj: 10 mg/mL, 15 mg/mL amp, 2 mg/mL Carbuject®, 1 mg/mL 30 mL PCA syringe Inj, preservative free: 1 mg/mL, 10 mL vial, 5 mg/10 mL amp (Duramorph® PF) Solution: 10 mg/5 mL, 20 mg/5 mL Tab (soluble): 10 mg, 30 mg Tab (controlled release): 30 mg (MS Contin®)	15-60 (epidural or I.T.) 15-30 (S.C.)	4-5 (I.M.) (S.C.)	10	60	1/6; ratio decreases to 1/1.5-2.5 upon chronic dosing	No
Oxycodone hydrochloride and acetaminophen (P.O.) (Percodan®, Tylox®)	Cap: Oxycodone 5 mg + acetaminophen 500 mg Tab: Oxycodone (~5 mg) + acetaminophen 325 mg	15-30 (P.O.)	4-6 (P.O.)	—	30	—	No
Pentazocine (Talwin® NX)	Inj: 30 mg/mL as lactate, 1 mL, 1.5 mL, 2 mL uni-amp or Carbuject®, 10 mL vial Tab: 50 mg with 0.5 mg naloxone (Talwin® NX)	15-30 (I.M.) (P.O.)	2-3 (I.M) 4-5 (P.O.)	50	150	1/3	Yes
Propoxyphene and acetaminophen (P.O.) (Darvocet-N® 50, Darvocet-N® 100, Darvon®)	Cap: Propoxyphene HCl (Darvon®) 32 mg, 65 mg Tab: Propoxyphene napsylate 50 mg + acetaminophen 325 mg (Darvocet-N® 50); Propoxyphene napsylate 100 mg + acetaminophen 650 mg (Darvocet-N® 100)	30-60 (P.O.)	4-6 (P.O.)	—	HCl salt: 130 Napsylate salt: 200	—	No

ND = no data.

Note: These values are based on adult studies. Duration may be shorter in children due to faster elimination (in general) compared to adults.

OTC COUGH AND COLD PREPARATIONS, PEDIATRIC

Commonly Used Pediatric OTC Cough & Cold Preparations

Brand Name	Type of Preparation
Actifed® Cold & Allergy	Antihistamine/Decongestant
Actifed® Cold & Sinus	Antihistamine/Decongestant
Benadryl® Allergy, Children's	Antihistamine
Benadryl® Allergy & Sinus Children's Elixir	Antihistamine/Decongestant
Benadryl® Allergy & Cold Fastmelt	Antihistamine/Decongestant
Benylin® Pediatric	Antitussive
Benylin® Expectorant	Antitussive/Expectorant
Chlor-Trimeton®	Antihistamine
Dimetane® DX	Antihistamine/Decongestant/Expectorant
Dimetapp® Cold & Cough, Children's	Antihistamine/Antitussive/Decongestant
Dimetapp® Cold & Congestion	Antitussive/Decongestant/Expectorant
Dimetapp® Cold & Allergy	Antihistamine/Decongestant
Dimetapp® Elixir Cold & Allergy, Children's	Antihistamine/Decongestant
Dimetapp® Infant Drops	Decongestant
Dimetapp® Infant Drops Decongestant & Cough	Antitussive/Decongestant
Neo-Synephrine® 12-Hour Children's Nose Drops	Decongestant
Neo-Synephrine® Nose Drops/Nasal Spray	Decongestant
Organidin® NR	Expectorant
PediaCare® Cold & Allergy	Antihistamine/Decongestant
PediaCare® Decongestant Plus Cough Infant Drops	Antitussive/Decongestant
PediaCare® Infant Decongestant Drops	Decongestant
PediaCare® Multisymptom Cold	Antihistamine/Antitussive/Decongestant
PediaCare® "Night Rest" Cough & Cold	Antihistamine/Antitussive/Decongestant
Robitussin® Allergy & Cough	Antihistamine/Antitussive/Decongestant
Robitussin® Cold & Flu	Antitussive/Decongestant/Expectorant
Robitussin® Cough & Cold Infant Drops	Antitussive/Decongestant/Expectorant
Robitussin® DM	Antitussive/Expectorant
Robitussin® DM Drops	Antitussive/Expectorant
Robitussin® Flu	Antihistamine/Antitussive/Decongestant
Robitussin® Pediatric Cough Syrup	Antitussive
Robitussin® Pediatric Cough & Cold Syrup	Antitussive/Decongestant
Robitussin® Pediatric Night Relief	Antihistamine/Antitussive/Decongestant
Sudafed® Cold & Cough, Children's	Antitussive/Decongestant
Sudafed® Nasal Decongestant	Decongestant
Sudafed® Nasal Decongestant, Children's	Decongestant
Sudafed® Sinus & Allergy	Antihistamine/Decongestant
Simply Cough™	Antitussive
Simply Stuffy™	Decongestant
Triaminic® Cold & Cough	Antihistamine/Antitussive/Decongestant
Triaminic® Cold & Cough Soft Chews	Antihistamine/Antitussive/Decongestant
Triaminic Cold & Allergy Syrup® (orange)	Antihistamine/Decongestant
Triaminic® Cold, Cough, & Fever	Antihistamine/Antitussive/Decongestant
Triaminic® Cough & Sore Throat (dark red)	Antitussive/Decongestant
Tylenol® Cold, Children's	Antihistamine/Decongestant
Tylenol® Cold Concentrated Drops, Infants	Decongestant
Tylenol® Cold Plus Cough, Children's	Antihistamine/Antitussive/Decongestant
Tylenol® Cold Plus Cough Concentrated Drops, Infants	Antitussive/Decongestant
Tylenol® Flu, Children's	Antihistamine/Antitussive/Decongestant
Tylenol® Sinus, Children's	Decongestant
Vicks® Nyquil®, Children's	Antihistamine/Antitussive/Decongestant
Vicks® 44e® Cough & Chest Congestion Relief, Pediatric	Antitussive/Expectorant
Vicks® 44m® Cough & Cold Relief, Pediatric	Antihistamine/Antitussive/Decongestant

OTC COUGH AND COLD PREPARATIONS, PEDIATRIC
(Continued)

Content of Commonly Used Pediatric Cough & Cold Preparations

The following chart lists the contents of the more common OTC cough and cold preparations. Products are grouped by preparation type. For specific recommendations, see individual drug monographs.

Brand Name	Generic(s)	Strength	Other Information
Decongestants			
Dimetapp® Infant Drops	Pseudoephedrine	7.5 mg/0.8 mL	–
Neo-Synephrine® 12-Hour Children's Nose Drops	Oxymethazoline	0.05%	
Neo-Synephrine® Nose Drops/Nasal Spray	Phenylephrine	0.25% 0.25%-0.5%	≤6 y must be diluted prior to use (see Phenylephrine) >6 to 12 y use 0.25%
PediaCare® Decongestant Infant Drops	Pseudoephedrine	7.5 mg/0.8 mL	–
Simply Stuffy™	Pseudoephedrine	15 mg/5 mL	–
Sudafed® Nasal Decongestant	Pseudoephedrine	15 mg/5 mL 30 mg/5 mL 15 mg/tab 30 mg/tab 60 mg/tab 120 mg/tab or cap (timed release) 240 mg/tab (timed release)	–
Tylenol® Cold Concentrated Drops, Infants	Pseudoephedrine	15 mg/1.6 mL	Acetaminophen 160 mg/1.6 mL
Tylenol® Sinus, Children's	Pseudoephedrine	15 mg/5 mL 7.5 mg/tab	Acetaminophen 160 mg/5 mL 80 mg/tab
Antihistamines			
Benadryl® Allergy Children's	Diphenhydramine	12.5 mg/chew tab 12.5 mg/5 mL	Tablet contains aspartame
Chlor-Trimeton®	Chlorpheniramine	4 mg/tab 8 mg/tab 12 mg/tab	–
Expectorants			
Organidin® NR	Guaifenesin	100 mg/5 mL	–
Antitussives			
Benylin® Pediatric Syrup	Dextromethorphan	7.5 mg/5 mL	–
Robitussin® Pediatric Cough Syrup	Dextromethorphan HBr	7.5 mg/5 mL	–
Simply Cough™	Dextromethorphan	5 mg/5 mL	–
Antihistamine / Decongestants			
Actifed® Cold & Allergy	Triprolidine	1.25 mg/5 mL 2.5 mg/tab	–
	Pseudoephedrine	30 mg/5 mL 60 mg/tab	
Actifed® Cold & Sinus	Chlorpheniramine Pseudoephedrine	2 mg/tab 30 mg/tab	Acetaminophen 500 mg/tab
Benadryl® Allergy & Cold Fastmelt	Diphenhydramine citrate	19 mg/tab	Citrate salt equivalent to 12.5 mg diphenhydramine HCl
	Pseudoephedrine	30 mg/tab	Phenylalanine 4.6 mg/tab
Benadryl® Allergy & Sinus, Children's	Diphenhydramine Pseudoephedrine	12.5 mg/5 mL 30 mg/5 mL	–
Dimetapp® Cold & Allergy	Chlorpheniramine Phenylephrine	2 mg/tab 5 mg/tab	Acetaminophen 325 mg/tab
Dimetapp® Elixir Cold & Allergy, Children's	Brompheniramine Pseudoephedrine	1 mg/5 mL 15 mg/5 mL	–
PediaCare® Cold & Allergy	Brompheniramine Pseudoephedrine	1 mg/5 mL 15 mg/5 mL	–
Sudafed® Sinus & Allergy	Chlorpheniramine Pseudoephedrine	4 mg/tab 60 mg/tab	

Brand Name	Generic(s)	Strength	Other Information
Triaminic® Cold & Allergy (orange)	Chlorpheniramine Pseudoephedrine	1 mg/5 mL 15 mg/5 mL	–
Tylenol® Cold, Children's	Chlorpheniramine Pseudoephedrine	1 mg/5 mL 0.5 mg/tab 15 mg/5 mL 7.5 mg/tab	Acetaminophen 160 mg/5 mL 80 mg/tab
Antitussive / Decongestant			
Dimetapp® Infant Drops Decongestant & Cough	Dextromethorphan Pseudoephedrine	2.5 mg/0.8 mL 7.5 mg/0.8 mL	–
Dimetapp® Long-Acting Cough & Cold	Dextromethorphan Pseudoephedrine	7.5 mg/5 mL 15 mg/5 mL	–
PediaCare® Decongestant Plus Cough, Infant Drops	Dextromethorphan Pseudoephedrine	2.5 mg/0.8 mL 7.5 mg/0.8 mL	–
Robitussin® Pediatric Cough & Cold Syrup	Dextromethorphan Pseudoephedrine	7.5 mg/5 mL 15 mg/5 mL	–
Sudafed® Cold & Cough, Children's	Dextromethorphan Pseudoephedrine	5 mg/5 mL 15 mg/5 mL	–
Triaminic® Cough & Sore Throat	Dextromethorphan Pseudoephedrine	7.5 mg/5 mL 15 mg/5 mL	Acetaminophen 160 mg
Tylenol® Cold Plus Cough Concentrated Drops, Infants	Dextromethorphan Pseudoephedrine	5 mg/1.6 mL 15 mg/1.6 mL	Acetaminophen 160 mg/1.6 mL
Antitussive / Expectorant			
Benylin® Expectorant	Dextromethorphan Guaifenesin	5 mg/5 mL 100 mg/5 mL	–
Robitussin® DM	Dextromethorphan Guaifenesin	10 mg/5 mL 100 mg/5 mL	1.4% alcohol
Robitussin® DM Drops	Dextromethorphan Guaifenesin	5 mg/2.5 mL 100 mg/2.5 mL	–
Vicks® 44e® Cough & Chest Congestion Relief, Pediatric	Dextromethorphan Guaifenesin	3.3 mg/5 mL 33 mg/5 mL	–
Antihistamine / Antitussive / Decongestant			
Children's Dimetapp® DM Cold & Cough	Brompheniramine Dextromethorphan Pseudoephedrine	1 mg/5 mL 5 mg/5 mL 15 mg/5 mL	–
PediaCare® Multisymptom Cold	Chlorpheniramine Dextromethorphan Pseudoephedrine	1 mg/5 mL 5 mg/5 mL 15 mg/5 mL	–
PediaCare® "Night Rest" Cough & Cold	Chlorpheniramine Dextromethorphan Pseudoephedrine	1 mg/5 mL 7.5 mg/5 mL 15 mg/5 mL	–
Robitussin® Allergy & Cough	Brompheniramine Dextromethorphan Pseudoephedrine	2 mg/5 mL 10 mg/5 mL 30 mg/5 mL	–
Robitussin® Flu	Chlorpheniramine Dextromethorphan Pseudoephedrine	1 mg/5 mL 5 mg/5 mL 15 mg/5 mL	Acetaminophen 160 mg
Robitussin® Pediatric Night Relief	Chlorpheniramine Dextromethorphan Pseudoephedrine	1 mg/5 mL 7.5 mg/5 mL 15 mg/5 mL	–
Triaminic® Cold & Cough	Chlorpheniramine Dextromethorphan Pseudoephedrine	1 mg/5 mL 5 mg/5 mL 15 mg/5 mL	–
Triaminic® Cold & Cough Soft Chews	Chlorpheniramine Dextromethorphan Pseudoephedrine	1 mg/chew tab 5 mg/chew tab 15 mg/chew tab	–
Triaminic® Cold, Cough, & Fever	Chlorpheniramine Dextromethorphan Pseudoephedrine	1 mg/5 mL 7.5 mg/5 mL 15 mg/5 mL	Acetaminophen 160 mg
Tylenol® Cold Plus Cough, Children's	Chlorpheniramine Dextromethorphan Pseudoephedrine Chlorpheniramine Dextromethorphan Pseudoephedrine	1 mg/5 mL 5 mg/5 mL 15 mg/5 mL 0.5 mg/tab 2.5 mg/tab 7.5 mg/tab	Acetaminophen 160 mg/5 mL Acetaminophen 80 mg/tab
Tylenol® Flu, Children's	Chlorpheniramine Dextromethorphan Pseudoephedrine	1 mg/5 mL 7.5 mg/5 mL 15 mg/5 mL	Acetaminophen 160 mg
Vicks® Nyquil®, Children's	Chlorpheniramine Dextromethorphan Pseudoephedrine	0.67 mg/5 mL 5 mg/5 mL 10 mg/5 mL	–

OTC COUGH AND COLD PREPARATIONS, PEDIATRIC
(Continued)

Brand Name	Generic(s)	Strength	Other Information
Vicks® 44m® Cough & Cold Relief, Pediatric	Chlorpheniramine Dextromethorphan Pseudoephedrine	0.67 mg/5 mL 5 mg/5 mL 10 mg/5 mL	–
Antitussive / Decongestant / Expectorant			
Dimetane® DX	Brompheniramine Dextromethorphan Pseudoephedrine	2 mg/5 mL 10 mg/5 mL 30 mg/5 mL	0.95% alcohol
Dimetapp® Cold & Congestion	Dextromethorphan Pseudoephedrine Guaifenesin	10 mg/caplet 30 mg/caplet 200 mg/caplet	–
Robitussin® Cold & Cold Infant Drops	Dextromethorphan Pseudoephedrine Guaifenesin	5 mg/2.5 mL 15 mg/2.5 mL 100 mg/2.5 mL	–
Robitussin® Cold & Flu Caplets or Softgels	Dextromethorphan Pseudoephedrine Guaifenesin	10 mg/caplet/softgel 30 mg/caplet/softgel 200 mg/caplet/softgel	–

CONVERSIONS

Apothecary-Metric Exact Equivalents

1 gram (g)	=	15.43 grains	0.1 mg	=	1/600 gr
1 milliliter (mL)	=	16.23 minims	0.12 mg	=	1/500 gr
1 minim	=	0.06 mL	0.15 mg	=	1/400 gr
1 grain (gr)	=	64.8 milligrams	0.2 mg	=	1/300 gr
1 fluid ounce (fl. oz)	=	29.57 mL	0.3 mg	=	1/200 gr
1 pint (pt)	=	473.2 mL	0.4 mg	=	1/150 gr
1 ounce (oz)	=	28.35 grams	0.5 mg	=	1/120 gr
1 pound (lb)	=	453.6 grams	0.6 mg	=	1/100 gr
1 kilogram (kg)	=	2.2 pounds	0.8 mg	=	1/80 gr
1 quart (qt)	=	946.4 mL	1 mg	=	1/65 gr

Apothecary-Metric Approximate Equivalents*

Liquids			Solids		
1 teaspoonful	=	5 mL	1/4 grain	=	15 mg
1 tablespoonful	=	15 mL	1/2 grain	=	30 mg
			1 grain	=	60 mg
			1 1/2 grain	=	100 mg
			5 grains	=	300 mg
			10 grains	=	600 mg

*Use exact equivalents for compounding and calculations requiring a high degree of accuracy.

Pounds-Kilograms Conversion

1 pound = 0.45359 kilograms
1 kilogram = 2.2 pounds

Temperature Conversion

Celsius to Fahrenheit = (°C x 9/5) + 32 = °F
Fahrenheit to Celsius = (°F - 32) x 5/9 = °C

CYTOCHROME P450 ENZYMES AND DRUG METABOLISM

Background

The cytochrome P450 enzymes are a "superfamily" of enzymes that catalyze the biotransformation (metabolism) of endogenous and exogenous lipophilic substances. These enzymes are considered to be the most important of the phase I enzymes and account for the majority of drug metabolism in humans. Enzyme "families," known as isoenzymes, are located primarily in the liver. The nomenclature of this system has been standardized. Isoenzyme "families" are identified using a CYP prefix, followed by an Arabic number (eg, CYP1). Subfamilies are designated by a letter following the number (eg, CYP1A) and individual isoenzymes are numbered sequentially within the subfamily (eg, CYP1A2). Cytochrome P450 isoenzymes that are important in the metabolism of drugs in humans are primarily found in the CYP1, CYP2, and CYP3 families.

Enzymes may be inhibited (slowing metabolism through this pathway) or induced (increased in activity or number). Individual drugs metabolized by a specific enzyme are identified as substrates for the isoenzyme. Considerable effort has been expended in recent years to classify drugs metabolized by this system as either an inhibitor, inducer, or substrate of a specific isoenzyme. It should be noted that a drug may demonstrate complex activity within this scheme, acting as an inhibitor of one isoenzyme while serving as a substrate for another.

By recognizing that a substrate's metabolism may be dramatically altered by concurrent therapy with either an inducer or inhibitor, potential interactions may be identified and addressed. For example, a drug which inhibits CYP1A2 is likely to block metabolism of theophylline (a substrate for this isoenzyme). Because of this interaction, the dose of theophylline required to maintain a consistent level in the patient should be reduced when an inhibitor is added. Failure to make this adjustment may lead to supratherapeutic theophylline concentrations and potential toxicity.

This approach does have limitations. For example, the metabolism of specific drugs may have primary and secondary pathways. The contribution of secondary pathways to the overall metabolism may limit the impact of any given inhibitor. In addition, there may be up to a tenfold variation in the concentration of an isoenzyme across the broad population. In fact, a complete absence of an isoenzyme may occur in some genetic subgroups. Finally, the relative potency of inhibition, relative to the affinity of the enzyme for its substrate, demonstrates a high degree of variability. These issues make it difficult to anticipate whether a theoretical interaction will have a clinically relevant impact in a specific patient.

The details of this enzyme system continue to be investigated, and information is expanding daily. However, to be complete, it should be noted that other enzyme systems also influence a drug's pharmacokinetic profile. For example, a key enzyme system regulating the absorption of drugs is the p-glycoprotein system. Recent evidence suggests that some interactions originally attributed to the cytochrome system may, in fact, have been the result of inhibition of this enzyme.

The following tables represent an attempt to detail the available information with respect to isoenzyme activities. Within certain limits, they may be used to identify potential interactions. Of particular note, an effort has been made in each drug monograph to identify involvement of a particular isoenzyme in the drug's metabolism. These tables are intended to supplement the limited space available to list drug interactions in the monograph. Consequently, they may be used to define a greater range of both actual and potential drug interactions.

CYTOCHROME P450 ENZYMES AND RESPECTIVE METABOLIZED DRUGS

CYP1A2

Substrates

Acetaminophen
Acetanilid
Alosetron
Aminophylline
Amitriptyline (demethylation)
Antipyrine
Apomorphine
Betaxolol
Caffeine
Chlorpromazine
Clomipramine (demethylation)
Clozapine
Cyclobenzaprine (demethylation)
Desipramine (demethylation)
Estradiol
Estradiol and medroxyprogesterone
Fluvoxamine
Frovatriptan
Haloperidol (minor)
Imipramine (demethylation)
Levobupivacaine
Levomepromazine
Lidocaine
Maprotiline
Methadone

Metoclopramide
Mirtazapine (hydroxylation)
Nordiazepam
Nortriptyline
Olanzapine (demethylation, hydroxylation)
Ondansetron
Phenacetin
Phenothiazines
Pimozide (minor)
Propafenone
Propranolol
Riluzole
Ritonavir
Ropinirole
Ropivacaine
Tacrine
Theophylline
Thioridazine
Thiothixene
Trifluoperazine
Verapamil
Warfarin (R-warfarin, minor pathway)
Zileuton
Ziprasidone (minor)
Zopiclone

Inducers

Carbamazepine
Charbroiled foods
Cigarette smoke
Cruciferous vegetables (cabbage, brussels
  sprouts, broccoli, cauliflower)
Griseofulvin
Modafinil (weak)

Nicotine
Omeprazole
Phenobarbital
Phenytoin
Primidone
Rifampin
Ritonavir

Inhibitors

Albendazole (weak)
Anastrozole
Cimetidine
Ciprofloxacin
Citalopram (weak)
Clarithromycin
Diethyldithiocarbamate
Diltiazem
Enoxacin
Entacapone (high dose)
Erythromycin
Estradiol
Ethinyl estradiol
Fluoxetine (high dose)
Fluvoxamine
Grapefruit juice

Isoniazid
Ketoconazole
Lidocaine
Mexiletine
Mibefradil
Moricizine (possible)
Norfloxacin
Paroxetine (high dose)(weak)
Ritonavir
Sertraline (weak)
Tacrine
Tenofovir (minor)
Tertiary TCAs
Ticlopidine (possible)
Zileuton

CYTOCHROME P450 ENZYMES AND DRUG METABOLISM
(Continued)

CYP2A6

Substrates

Acetaminophen	Nicotine
Dexmedetomidine	Ritonavir
Letrozole	
Montelukast	Tolcapone

Inducers

Barbiturates

Inhibitors

Diethyldithiocarbamate	Methoxsalen
Entacapone (high dose)	Ritonavir
Letrozole	Tranylcypromine

CYP2B6

Substrates

Antipyrine	Erythromycin (minor)
Bupropion (hydroxylation)	Ifosfamide
Cyclophosphamide	Lidocaine
Diazepam	Nicotine
Efavirenz	Orphenadrine

Inducers

Modafinil (weak)	Phenytoin
Phenobarbital	Primidone

Inhibitors

Diethyldithiocarbamate   Orphenadrine

CYP2C
(Specific isozyme has not been identified)

Substrates

Antipyrine	Mephobarbital
Carvedilol	Mestranol
Clozapine (minor)	Ticrynafen

Inducers

Carbamazepine	Primidone
Phenobarbital	Rifampin
Phenytoin	Sulfinpyrazone

Inhibitors

Isoniazid	Ketoprofen
Ketoconazole	

CYP2C8

Substrates

Carbamazepine
Diazepam
Diclofenac
Ibuprofen
Mephobarbital
Naproxen (5-hydroxylation)
Omeprazole
Paclitaxel

Pioglitazone
Retinoic acid
Rifampin
Rosiglitazone
Tolbutamide
Verapamil (minor)
Warfarin (S-warfarin)

Inducers

Carbamazepine
Phenobarbital
Phenytoin

Primidone
Rifampin
Rifapentine

Inhibitors

Anastrozole
Nicardipine

Omeprazole
Trimethoprim

CYP2C9

Substrates

Acetaminophen
Alosetron
Amitriptyline (demethylation)
Amoxapine
Bosentan
Carvedilol
Celecoxib
Dapsone
Desogestrel
Diazepam
Diclofenac
Flurbiprofen
Fluvastatin
Glimepiride
Hexobarbital
Ibuprofen
Imipramine (demethylation)
Indomethacin
Irbesartan
Losartan
Mefenamic acid
Mestranol
Metronidazole

Mirtazapine
Montelukast
Naproxen (5-hydroxylation)
Nateglinide
Omeprazole
Phenytoin
Piroxicam
Quetiapine (minor pathway)
Repaglinide
Rifampin
Ritonavir
Rosiglitazone (minor)
Sildenafil citrate (minor pathway)
Tamoxifen
Tenoxicam
Tetrahydrocannabinol
Tolbutamide
Torsemide
Valdecoxib
Verapamil (minor)
Warfarin (S-warfarin)
Zafirlukast (hydroxylation)
Zileuton

Inducers

Bosentan
Carbamazepine
Fluconazole
Fluoxetine
Phenobarbital

Phenytoin
Rifampin
Rifapentine
Secobarbital

Inhibitors

Amiodarone
Anastrozole
Chloramphenicol
Cimetidine
Clopidogrel (high conc – in vitro)
Co-trimoxazole
Diclofenac
Disulfiram
Drospirenone
Efavirenz
Entacapone (high dose)
Fluconazole
Fluoxetine
Flurbiprofen
Fluvastatin
Fluvoxamine (potent)
Imatinib
Isoniazid
Ketoconazole (weak)
Ketoprofen
Leflunomide (in vitro only)

Metronidazole
Miconazole
Nateglinide
Nicardipine
Omeprazole
Phenylbutazone
Propoxyphene
Ritonavir
Sertraline
Sulfamethoxazole-trimethoprim
Sulfaphenazole
Sulfinpyrazone
Sulfonamides
Sulindac
Trimethoprim
Troglitazone
Valdecoxib (weak in vitro)
Valproic acid
Warfarin (R-warfarin)
Zafirlukast

CYTOCHROME P450 ENZYMES AND DRUG METABOLISM
(Continued)

CYP2C18

Substrates

Dronabinol	Propranolol
Naproxen	Retinoic acid
Omeprazole	Tolbutamide
Piroxicam	Warfarin
Proguanil	

Inducers

Carbamazepine	Phenytoin
Phenobarbital	Rifampin

Inhibitors

Cimetidine	Fluvastatin
Fluconazole	Isoniazid

CYP2C19

Substrates

Amitriptyline (demethylation)	Mephobarbital
Amoxapine	Moclobemide
Apomorphine	Olanzapine (minor)
Barbiturates	Omeprazole
Carisoprodol	Pantoprazole
Cilostazol (minor)	Pentamidine
Citalopram	Phenytoin
Clomipramine (demethylation)	Progesterone
Desmethyldiazepam	Proguanil
Desogestrel	Propranolol
Diazepam (N-demethylation, minor pathway)	Ritonavir
Divalproex sodium	Tolbutamide
Esomeprazole	Topiramate
Hexobarbital	Valproic acid
Imipramine (demethylation)	Verapamil (minor)
Lansoprazole	Warfarin (R-warfarin)
Mephenytoin	

Inducers

Carbamazepine	Phenytoin
Phenobarbital	Rifampin

Inhibitors

Cimetidine	Modafinil
Citalopram (weak)	Nicardipine
Diazepam	Omeprazole
Disulfiram	Oxcarbazepine
Drospirenone	Proguanil
Efavirenz	Ritonavir
Entacapone (high conc)	Sertraline
Ethinyl estradiol	Telmisartan
Felbamate	Teniposide
Fluconazole	Ticlopidine (potent)
Fluoxetine	Tolbutamide
Fluvastatin	Topiramate
Fluvoxamine	Tranylcypromine
Isoniazid	Troglitazone
Ketoconazole (weak)	Valdecoxib (moderate *in vitro*)
Letrozole	Warfarin (R-warfarin)

CYP2D6

Substrates

Acetaminophen
Almotriptan
Amitriptyline (hydroxylation)
Amoxapine
Amphetamine
Betaxolol
Bisoprolol
Brofaromine
Bufuronol
Captopril
Carvedilol
Cevimeline
Chlorpheniramine
Chlorpromazine
Cinnarizine
Clomipramine (hydroxylation)
Clozapine (minor pathway)
Codeine (hydroxylation, o-demethylation)
Cyclobenzaprine (hydroxylation)
Cyclophosphamide
Debrisoquin
Delavirdine
Desipramine
Dexfenfluramine
Dextromethorphan (o-demethylation)
Dihydrocodeine
Diphenhydramine
Dolasetron
Donepezil
Doxepin
Encainide
Ethylmorphine
Fenfluramine
Flecainide
Fluoxetine (minor pathway)
Fluphenazine
Galantamine
Halofantrine
Haloperidol (minor pathway)
Hydrocodone
Hydrocortisone
Hydroxyamphetamine
Imipramine (hydroxylation)
Labetalol
Lidocaine
Loratadine
Maprotiline

m-Chlorophenylpiperazine (m-CPP)
Meperidine
Methadone
Methamphetamine
Metoclopramide
Metoprolol
Mexiletine
Mianserin
Mirtazapine (hydroxylation)
Moclobemide
Molindone
Morphine
Nortriptyline (hydroxylation)
Olanzapine (minor, hydroxymethylation)
Ondansetron
Orphenadrine
Oxycodone
Papaverine
Paroxetine (minor pathway)
Penbutolol
Pentazocine
Perhexiline
Perphenazine
Phenformin
Pindolol
Promethazine
Propafenone
Propranolol
Quetiapine (minor pathway)
Remoxipride
Risperidone
Ritonavir (minor)
Ropivacaine
Selegiline
Sertindole
Sertraline (minor pathway)
Sparteine
Tamoxifen
Thioridazine[1]
Timolol
Tolterodine
Tramadol
Trazodone
Trimipramine
Tropisetron
Venlafaxine (o-desmethylation)
Yohimbine

Inducers

Rifampin

Inhibitors

Amiodarone
Celecoxib
Chloroquine
Chlorpromazine
Cimetidine
Citalopram
Clomipramine
Codeine
Delavirdine
Desipramine
Dextropropoxyphene
Diltiazem
Doxorubicin
Entacapone (high dose)
Fexofenadine (weak)
Fluoxetine
Fluphenazine
Fluvoxamine
Haloperidol
Imatinib
Labetalol
Lobeline
Lomustine
Methadone
Mibefradil

Moclobemide
Nicardipine
Norfluoxetine
Paroxetine
Perphenazine
Primaquine
Propafenone
Propoxyphene
Quinacrine
Quinidine (potent)
Ranitidine
Risperidone (weak)
Ritonavir
Sertindole
Sertraline (weak)
Thioridazine
Ticlopidine (weak)
Valdecoxib (weak at supratherapeutic doses)
Valproic acid
Venlafaxine (weak)
Vinblastine
Vincristine
Vinorelbine
Yohimbine

CYTOCHROME P450 ENZYMES AND DRUG METABOLISM
(Continued)

CYP2E1

Substrates

Acetaminophen
Acetone
Aniline
Benzene
Caffeine
Chloral hydrate
Chlorzoxazone
Clozapine
Dapsone
Dextromethorphan
Enflurane
Ethanol
Halothane

Isoflurane
Isoniazid
Methoxyflurane
Nitrosamine
Ondansetron
Phenol
Ritonavir
Sevoflurane
Styrene
Tamoxifen
Theophylline (minor pathway)
Venlafaxine

Inducers

Ethanol
Isoniazid

Mitoxantrone (weak)

Inhibitors

Diethyldithiocarbamate (disulfiram metabolite)
Dimethyl sulfoxide
Disulfiram

Entacapone (high dose)
Ritonavir

CYP3A3/4

Substrates

Acetaminophen
Alfentanil
Almotriptan
Alosetron
Alprazolam[1]
Amiodarone
Amitriptyline (minor)
Amlodipine
Amoxapine
Amprenavir
Anastrozole
Androsterone
Antipyrine
Apomorphine
Astemizole[1]
Atorvastatin
Benzphetamine
Bepridil
Bexarotene
Bosentan
Bromazepam
Bromocriptine
Budesonide
Buprenorphine HCl
Bupropion (minor)
Buspirone
Busulfan
Caffeine
Cannabinoids
Carbamazepine
Cevimeline
Chlordiazepoxide
Chlorpromazine
Cilostazol (major)
Cimetidine
Cisapride[1]
Citalopram
Clarithromycin
Clindamycin
Clofibrate

Clomipramine
Clonazepam
Clorazepate
Clozapine
Cocaine
Codeine (demethylation)
Cortisol
Cortisone
Cyclobenzaprine (demethylation)
Cyclophosphamide
Cyclosporine
Dapsone
Dehydroepiandrostendione
Delavirdine
Desmethyldiazepam
Dexamethasone
Dextromethorphan (minor, N-demethylation)
Diazepam (minor; hydroxylation,
    N-demethylation)
Digitoxin
Diltiazem
Disopyramide
Docetaxel
Dofetilide (minor)
Dolasetron
Domperidone
Donepezil
Doxorubicin
Doxycycline
Dronabinol
Drospirenone
Dutasteride
Efavirenz
Enalapril
Erythromycin
Esomeprazole
Estradiol
Estradiol and medroxyprogesterone
Ethinyl estradiol
Ethosuximide

Etonogestrel
Etoposide
Exemestane
Felodipine
Fentanyl
Fexofenadine
Finasteride
Fluoxetine
Flurazepam
Flutamide
Fluticasone
Galantamine
Gemfibrozil
Glyburide
Granisetron
Halofantrine
Haloperidol
Hydrocortisone
Hydroxyarginine
Ifosfamide
Imatinib
Imipramine
Indinavir
Isradipine
Itraconazole
Ketamine
Ketoconazole
Lansoprazole (minor)
Letrozole
Levobupivacaine
Levomethadyl acetate hydrochloride
Levonorgestrel
Lidocaine
Lopinavir
Loratadine
Losartan
Lovastatin
Methadone
Mibefradil
Miconazole
Midazolam
Mifepristone
Mirtazapine (N-demethylation)
Modafinil
Montelukast
Nateglinide
Navelbine
Nefazodone
Nelfinavir[1]
Nevirapine
Nicardipine
Nifedipine
Niludipine
Nimodipine
Nisoldipine
Nitrendipine
Norgestrel
Omeprazole (sulfonation)
Ondansetron
Oral contraceptives
Orphenadrine
Paclitaxel

Pantoprazole
Pimecrolimus (only if significantly absorbed)
Pimozide[1]
Pioglitazone
Pravastatin (minor)
Prednisolone
Prednisone
Progesterone
Proguanil
Propafenone
Quercetin
Quetiapine
Quinidine
Quinine
Repaglinide
Retinoic acid
Rifampin (major)
Risperidone
Ritonavir[1]
Salmeterol
Saquinavir
Sertindole
Sertraline
Sibutramine[2]
Sildenafil citrate
Simvastatin
Sirolimus
Sufentanil
Tacrolimus
Tamoxifen
Temazepam
Teniposide
Terfenadine[1]
Testosterone
Tetrahydrocannabinol
Theophylline
Tiagabine
Ticlopidine
Tolcapone
Tolterodine
Toremifene
Tramadol
Trazodone
Tretinoin
Triazolam[1]
Troglitazone
Troleandomycin
Valdecoxib
Venlafaxine (N-demethylation)
Verapamil
Vinblastine
Vincristine
Warfarin (R-warfarin)
Yohimbine
Zaleplon (minor pathway)
Zatosetron
Zidovudine
Zileuton
Ziprasidone
Zolpidem[1]
Zonisamide

Inducers

Bosentan
Carbamazepine
Dexamethasone
Ethosuximide
Glucocorticoids
Nafcillin
Nelfinavir
Nevirapine
Oxcarbazepine
Phenobarbital
Phenylbutazone

Phenytoin
Primidone
Rifabutin
Rifampin
Rifapentine
Rofecoxib (mild)
St John's wort
Sulfadimidine
Sulfinpyrazone
Troglitazone

CYTOCHROME P450 ENZYMES AND DRUG METABOLISM
(Continued)

Inhibitors

Amiodarone
Amprenavir
Anastrozole (high conc)
Cannabinoids
Cimetidine
Clarithromycin[1]
Clotrimazole
Cyclosporine
Danazol
Delavirdine
Dexamethasone
Diazepam
Diethyldithiocarbamate
Diltiazem
Dirithromycin
Disulfiram (and metabolite
    diethyldithiocarbamate
Drospirenone (weak)
Efavirenz
Entacapone (high dose)
Erythromycin[1]
Ethinyl estradiol (weak)
Fluconazole (weak)
Fluoxetine
Fluvoxamine[1]
Gestodene
Grapefruit juice
Imatinib (potent)
Indinavir
Isoniazid
Itraconazole[1]
Ketoconazole[1]

Metronidazole
Mibefradil[1]
Miconazole (moderate)
Mifepristone
Modafinil (minor)
Nefazodone[1]
Nelfinavir
Nevirapine
Nicardipine
Norfloxacin
Norfluoxetine
Omeprazole (weak)
Oxiconazole
Paroxetine (weak)
Propoxyphene
Quinidine (weak)
Quinine[1]
Quinupristin and dalfopristin
Ranitidine
Ritonavir[1]
Saquinavir
Sertindole
Sertraline
Troglitazone
Troleandomycin
Valdecoxib (weak in vitro)
Valproic acid (weak)
Verapamil
Vinorelbine
Zafirlukast
Zileuton

CYP3A4/5

Substrate

Argatroban (minor)

Progesterone

Inducer

Oxcarbazepine

CYP3A5-7

Substrates

Cortisol
Diazepam
Estradiol and medroxyprogesterone
Ethinyl estradiol
Nifedipine

Terfenadine
Testosterone
Triazolam
Vinblastine
Vincristine

Inducers

Phenobarbital
Phenytoin

Primidone
Rifampin

Inhibitors

Clotrimazole
Ketoconazole
Metronidazole

Propoxyphene
Troleandomycin

[1]**Contraindications:**
Terfenadine, astemizole, cisapride, and triazolam contraindicated with nefazodone
Pimozide contraindicated with CYP3A3/4 inhibitors
Alprazolam and triazolam contraindicated with ketoconazole and itraconazole
Terfenadine, astemizole, and cisapride contraindicated with fluvoxamine
Terfenadine contraindicated with mibefradil, ketoconazole, erythromycin, clarithromycin, troleando-
    mycin
Thioridazine contraindicated with CYP2D6 inhibitors

Ritonavir contraindicated with triazolam, zolpidem, astemizole, rifabutin, quinine, clarithromycin, troleandomycin
Mibefradil contraindicated with astemizole
Nelfinavir contraindicated with rifabutin

[2]Do not use with SSRIs, sumatriptan, lithium, meperidine, fentanyl, dextromethorphan, or pentazocine within 2 weeks of an MAOI.

References

Baker GB, Urichuk CJ, and Coutts RT, "Drug Metabolism and Metabolic Drug-Drug Interactions in Psychiatry," *Child Adolescent Psychopharm News (Suppl).*

DeVane CL, "Pharmacogenetics and Drug Metabolism of Newer Antidepressant Agents," *J Clin Psychiatry*, 1994, 55(Suppl 12):38-45.

Drug Interactions Analysis and Management. Cytochrome (CYP) 450 Isozyme Drug Interactions, Vancouver, WA: Applied Therapeutics, Inc, 523-7.

Ereshefsky L, "Drug-Drug Interactions Involving Antidepressants: Focus on Venlafaxine," *J Clin Psychopharmacol*, 1996, 16(3 Suppl 2):375-535.

Ereshefsky L, *Psychiatr Annal*, 1996, 26:342-50.

Fleishaker JC and Hulst LK, "A Pharmacokinetic and Pharmacodynamic Evaluation of the Combined Administration of Alprazolam and Fluvoxamine," *Eur J Clin Pharmacol*, 1994, 46(1):35-9.

Flockhart DA, et al, *Clin Pharmacol Ther*, 1996, 59:189.

Ketter TA, Flockhart DA, Post RM, et al, "The Emerging Role of Cytochrome P450 3A in Psychopharmacology," *J Clin Psychopharmacol*, 1995, 15(6):387-98.

Michalets EL, "Update: Clinically Significant Cytochrome P450 Drug Interactions," *Pharmacotherapy*, 1998, 18(1):84-112.

Nemeroff CB, DeVane CL, and Pollock BG, "Newer Antidepressants and the Cytochrome P450 System," *Am J Psychiatry*, 1996, 153(3):311-20.

Pollock BG, "Recent Developments in Drug Metabolism of Relevance to Psychiatrists," *Harv Rev Psychiatry*, 1994, 2(4):204-13.

Richelson E, "Pharmacokinetic Drug Interactions of New Antidepressants: A Review of the Effects on the Metabolism of Other Drugs," *Mayo Clin Proc*, 1997, 72(9):835-47.

Riesenman C, "Antidepressant Drug Interactions and the Cytochrome P450 System: A Critical Appraisal," *Pharmacotherapy*, 1995, 15(6 Pt 2):84S-99S.

Schmider J, Greenblatt DJ, von Moltke LL, et al, "Relationship of *In Vitro* Data on Drug Metabolism to *In Vivo* Pharmacokinetics and Drug Interactions: Implications for Diazepam Disposition in Humans," *J Clin Psychopharmacol*, 1996, 16(4):267-72.

Slaughter RL, *Pharm Times*, 1996, 7:6-16.

Watkins PB, "Role of Cytochrome P450 in Drug Metabolism and Hepatotoxicity," *Semin Liver Dis*, 1990, 10(4):235-50.

EXTRAVASATION TREATMENT

Medication Extravasated	Cold/Warm Pack	Antidote
VESICANTS		

Direct Cellular Toxins – Chemotherapeutic Agents

DNA Intercalators		
Amsacrine Daunorubicin Doxorubicin Epirubicin Idarubicin	Cold	None
Vinca alkaloids		
Paclitaxel* Vinblastine Vincristine Vindesine Vinorelbine	Warm	Hyaluronidase (Wydase®) 1. Add 1 mL NS to 150 units vial to make 150 units/mL concentration 2. Administer 0.2 mL injection subcutaneously or intradermally into the extravasation site at the leading edge **Note:** Some institutions utilize a 1:10 dilution in infants and children; prepare by mixing 0.1 mL of 150 units/mL solution with 0.9 mL NS in 1 mL syringe to make final concentration = 15 units/mL
Alkylating agents		
Cisplatin Mechlorethamine (Nitrogen mustard)	Cold	Sodium thiosulfate 1/6 molar solution: mix 4 mL of 10% sodium thiosulfate with 6 mL of sterile water; inject 2 mL for each mg mechlorethamine or 100 mg cisplatinum (use only for large cisplatinum infiltrates >20 mL and when using cisplatinum concentrations >0.5 mg/mL; no data for use in cisplatinum infusions in children)
Other vesicant chemotherapeutic agents		
Dactinomycin Mitomycin C Mitoxantrone Plicamycin	Cold	None
Ischemic Inducers		
Dobutamine Dopamine Epinephrine Metaraminol Norepinephrine Phenylephrine Vasopressin	None	Phentolamine (Regitine®) Mix 5 mg with 9 mL of NS Inject a small amount of this dilution into extravasated area. Blanching should reverse immediately. Monitor site. If blanching should recur, additional injections of phentolamine may be needed.
Other Direct Cellular Toxins		
Aminophylline Calcium Chlordiazepoxide Diazepam Digoxin Ethanol Nafcillin Nitroglycerin Phenytoin Propylene glycol Sodium thiopental Tetracycline	Cold	Hyaluronidase (Wydase®) As described above

(continued)

Medication Extravasated	Cold/Warm Pack	Antidote
Hyperosmotic Agents (>280 mOsm/L)		
Calcium	Cold	Hyaluronidase as described above
Contrast media		
Crystalline amino acids (>4.25%)		
Dextrose (>10%)		
Mannitol (>5%)		
Potassium chloride/acetate (>2 mEq/mL)		
Sodium bicarbonate (8.4%)		
Sodium chloride (>1%)		
IRRITANTS		
Arsenic trioxide	Cold	
Carboplatin ≥10 mg/mL		
Carmustine		
Cyclophosphamide		
Dacarbazine		
Daunorubicin citrate (liposomal)		
Dexrazoxane		
Doxorubicin, liposomal		
Etoposide		
Fluorouracil		
Gemcitabine		
Gemtuzumab		
Ifosfamide		
Irinotecan		
Oxaliplatin		
Teniposide		
Topotecan		

Note:

Extravasation: The unintentional leakage of pharmacologic and physiologic solutions into the perivascular, subcutaneous, or interstitial space.

Vesicants: Agents that cause redness, pain, and blistering when infiltrated and can progress to ulceration and tissue necrosis.

Irritants: Agents that cause redness at the injection site or along the vein and often include a mild pruritic allergic reaction related to histamine release. These reaction "flares" usually do not require intervention and subside in 30 minutes.

*Some references consider agent as an irritant instead of vesicant.

References

Camp-Sorrell D, "Developing Extravasation Protocols and Monitoring Outcomes," *J Intraven Nurs*, 1998, 21(4):232-9.

Kassner E, "Evaluation and Treatment of Chemotherapy Extravasation Injuries," *J Pediatr Oncol Nurs*, 2000, 17(3):135-48.

NIH, Standards of Practice: Care of the Patient Receiving IV Cytoxic or Biologic Agents, 2001.

BURN MANAGEMENT

Modified Lund-Browder Burn Assessment Chart
Estimation of Total Body Surface Area of Burn Involvement*
(% by site and age)

The total body surface area of burn involvement is determined by the sum of the percentages of each site.

Site†	0-1 years	1-4 years	5-9 years	10-14 years	15 years	Adult
Head	9.5	8.5	6.5	5.5	4.5	3.5
Neck	0.5	0.5	0.5	0.5	0.5	0.5
Trunk	13	13	13	13	13	13
Upper arm	2	2	2	2	2	2
Forearm	1.5	1.5	1.5	1.5	1.5	1.5
Hand	1.5	1.5	1.5	1.5	1.5	1.5
Perineum	1	1	1	1	1	1
Buttock (each)	2.5	2.5	2.5	2.5	2.5	2.5
Thigh	2.75	3.25	4	4.25	4.5	4.75
Leg	2.5	2.5	2.75	3	3.25	3.5
Foot	1.75	1.75	1.75	1.75	1.75	1.75

*Applies only to second- and third-degree burns

†Percentage for each site is only for **a single extremity with** anterior **OR** posterior involvement. Percentage should be **doubled if both anterior and posterior** involvement of a single extremity.

Adapted from Coren CV, "Burn Injuries in Children," *Pediatric Annals*, 1987, 16(4):328-39.

Parkland Fluid Replacement Formula

A guideline for replacement of deficits and ongoing losses (**Note:** For infants, maintenance fluids may need to be added to this): Administer 4 mL/kg/% burn of Ringer's lactate (glucose may be added but beware of stress hyperglycemia) over the first 24 hours; half of this total is given over the first 8 hours **calculated from the time of injury**; the remaining half is given over the next 16 hours. The second 24-hour fluid requirements average 50% to 75% of first day's requirement. Concentrations and rates best determined by monitoring weight, serum electrolytes, urine output, NG losses, etc.

Colloid may be added after 18-24 hours (1 g/kg/day of albumin) to maintain serum albumin >2 g/100 mL.

Potassium is generally withheld for the first 48 hours due to the large amount of potassium that is released from damaged tissues. To manage serum electrolytes, monitor urine electrolytes twice weekly and replace calculated urine losses.

ORAL CONTRACEPTIVES

Brand Name	Type	Progestin	Estrogen	Availability
Brevicon® Genora®0.5/35 Modicon® Nelova®0.5/35E	Combo	Norethindrone 0.5 mg	Ethinyl estradiol 35 mcg	21, 28
Demulen®1/35	Combo	Ethynodiol diacetate 1 mg	Ethinyl estradiol 35 mcg	21, 28
Demulen®1/50	Combo	Ethynodiol diacetate 1 mg	Ethinyl estradiol 50 mcg	21, 28
Desogen®	Combo	Desogestrel 0.15 mg	Ethinyl estradiol 30 mcg	28
Jenest™-28	Biphasic			
	1-7 d	Norethindrone 0.5 mg	Ethinyl estradiol 35 mcg	28
	8-21 d	Norethindrone 1 mg	Ethinyl estradiol 35 mcg	
	22-28 d	Inert	—	
Lo/Ovral®	Combo	Norgestrel 0.3 mg	Ethinyl estradiol 30 mcg	21, 28
Loestrin 21®1.5/30	Combo	Norethindrone acetate 1.5 mg	Ethinyl estradiol 30 mcg	21
Loestrin Fe 1.5/30	Combo/Iron 21-28 d	Norethindrone acetate 1.5 mg	Ethinyl estradiol 30 mcg	28
Loestrin 21® 1/20	Combo	Norethindrone acetate 1 mg	Ethinyl estradiol 20 mcg	21
Loestrin® Fe 1/20	Combo/Iron 21-28 d	Norethindrone acetate 1 mg	Ethinyl estradiol 20 mcg	28
Genora® 1/35 N.E.E.® 1/35 Nelova®1/35 E Norinyl®1+35 Ortho-Novum® 1/35	Combo	Norethindrone 1 mg	Ethinyl estradiol 35 mcg	21, 28
Genora® 1/50 Nelova®1/50M Norethin® 1/50M Norinyl®1+50 Ortho-Novum®1/50	Combo	Norethindrone 1 mg	Mestranol 50 mcg	21, 28
Levlen® Levora® Nordette®	Combo	Levonorgestrel 0.15 mg	Ethinyl estradiol 20 mcg	21, 28
Micronor®	Progestin only	Norethindrone 0.35 mg	—	28
Norlestrin® 2.5/50	Combo	Norethindrone acetate 2.5 mg	Ethinyl estradiol 30 mcg	21
Nor-QD®	Progestin only	Norethindrone 0.35 mg	—	42
Ortho-Cept®	Combo	Desogestrel 0.15 mg	Ethinyl estradiol 30 mcg	21, 28
Ortho-Cyclen®	Combo	Norgestimate 0.25 mg	Ethinyl estradiol 35 mcg	21, 28
Nelova™ 10/11	Biphasic			
	1-10 d	Norethindrone 0.5 mg	Ethinyl estradiol 35 mcg	21, 28
	11-21 d	Norethindrone 1 mg	Ethinyl estradiol 35 mcg	
	22-28 d	Inert	—	
Ortho-Novum®10/11	Biphasic			
	1-10 d	Norethindrone 0.5 mg	Ethinyl estradiol 35 mcg	21, 28
	11-21 d	Norethindrone 1 mg	Ethinyl estradiol 35 mcg	
	22-28 d	Inert	—	
Ortho-Novum® 7/7/7	Triphasic			
	1-7 d	Norethindrone 0.5 mg	Ethinyl estradiol 35 mcg	21, 28
	8-14 d	Norethindrone 0.75 mg	Ethinyl estradiol 35 mcg	
	15-21 d	Norethindrone 1 mg	Ethinyl estradiol 35 mcg	
	22-28 d	Inert	—	

ORAL CONTRACEPTIVES *(Continued)*

Brand Name	Type	Progestin	Estrogen	Availability
Ortho Tri-Cyclen®	Triphasic			
	1-7 d	Norgestimate 0.18 mg	Ethinyl estradiol 35 mcg	21, 28
	8-14 d	Norgestimate 0.215 mg	Ethinyl estradiol 35 mcg	
	15-21 d	Norgestimate 0.25 mg	Ethinyl estradiol 35 mcg	
	22-28 d	Inert	—	
Ovcon® 35	Combo	Norethindrone 0.4 mg	Ethinyl estradiol 35 mcg	21, 28
Ovcon® 50	Combo	Norethindrone 1 mg	Ethinyl estradiol 50 mcg	21, 28
Ovral®	Combo	Norgestrel 0.5 mg	Ethinyl estradiol 50 mcg	21, 28
Ovrette®	Progestin only	Norgestrel 0.075 mg	—	28
Tri-Norinyl®	Triphasic			
	1-7 d	Norethindrone 0.5 mg	Ethinyl estradiol 35 mcg	21, 28
	8-16 d	Norethindrone 1 mg	Ethinyl estradiol 35 mcg	
	17-21 d	Norethindrone 0.5 mg	Ethinyl estradiol 35 mcg	
	22- 28 d	Inert	—	
Tri-Phasil® Tri-Levlen®	Triphasic			
	1-6 d	Levonorgestrel 0.05 mg	Ethinyl estradiol 30 mcg	21, 28
	7-11 d	Levonorgestrel 0.075 mg	Ethinyl estradiol 40 mcg	
	12-21 d	Levonorgestrel 0.125 mg	Ethinyl estradiol 30 mcg	
	22- 28 d	Inert	—	

Combo = monophasic combination.

Monophasic Oral Contraceptives
In Order of Decreasing Estrogen Content

Estrogen	Brand Name (Progestin Content)
Mestranol 50 mcg	Genora®1/50, Nelova®1/50M, Norethin®1/50M, Norinyl®1+50, Ortho-Novum®1/50 **(Norethindrone 1 mg)**
Ethinyl estradiol 50 mcg	Ovcon®-50 **(Norethindrone 1 mg)**
	Demulen ®1/50 **(Ethynodiol diacetate 1 mg)**
	Ovral® **(Norgestrel 0.5 mg)**
Ethinyl estradiol 35 mcg	Genora ®1/35, N.E.E ®1/35, Nelova®1/35E, Norethin®1/35E, Norinyl®1+35, Ortho-Novum®1/35 **(Norethindrone 1 mg)**
	Brevicon ®, Genora ®0.5/35, Modicon®, Nelova ®0.5/35E **(Norethindrone 0.5 mg)**
	Ovcon®-35 **(Norethindrone 0.4 mg)**
	Ortho-Cyclen® **(Norgestimate 0.25 mg)**
	Demulen® 1/35 **(Ethynodiol diacetate 1 mg)**
Ethinyl estradiol 30 mcg	Loestrin 21® 1.5/30, Loestrin®Fe 1.5/30 **(Norethindrone acetate 1.5 mg)**
	Lo/Ovral® **(Norgestrel 0.3 mg)**
	Desogen®, Ortho-Cept® **(Desogestrel 0.15 mg)**
Ethinyl estradiol 20 mcg	Levlen®, Levora®, Nordette® **(Levonorgestrel 0.15 mg)**
	Loestrin 21® 1/20, Loestrin®Fe 1/20 **(Norethindrone acetate 1 mg)**

Hormonal Effects of Progestins

	Progestin Effect	Estrogen Effect	Antiestrogen Effect	Androgen Effect
Norethynodrel	+1	+3	0	0
Norethindrone	+1	+1 (Low dose)	+1 (Higher doses)	+2
Norethindrone acetate	+1	+1	+3	+2
Ethynodiol diacetate	+2	+1 (Low dose)	+1 (Higher doses)	+2
Norgestimate	+3	0	+3	0
Desogestrel	+3	0/+1	+3	0/+1
Norgestrel/ levonorgestrel	+3	0	+2	+3

0 = no effect; +1 = slight effect; +2 = moderate effect; +3 = pronounced effect.

Adapted from *Facts and Comparisons*, St Louis, MO; Facts and Comparisons, Inc, 1996.

Signs/Symptoms of Hormonal Imbalance With Oral Contraceptives

Estrogen Excess	Fluid retention, edema, cyclic weight gain, "bloating," hypertension, breast fullness/tenderness, nausea, migraine headache, melasma, telangiectasia, cervical mucorrhea, and polyposis
Estrogen Deficiency	Increased spotting, early or midcycle breakthrough bleeding, hypomenorrhea
Progestin Excess	Fatigue, lethargy, depression, decreased libido, increased appetite, weight gain, breast regression, monilial vaginitis, hypomenorrhea, hair loss, hirsutism, acne, oily scalp. **Note:** Hair loss, hirsutism, acne, and oily scalp are effects of the androgenic activity of progestins.
Progestin Deficiency	Amenorrhea, late breakthrough bleeding, hypermenorrhea

FLUIDS, ELECTROLYTES, & NUTRITION

ENTERAL NUTRITIONAL PRODUCT FORMULARY, INFANTS

Milk Based Formulas[1]
(Indications: Feeding normal term infants or sick infants without special nutritional requirements)

	Human Milk	Enfamil® With Iron	Similac® With Iron
Calories /100 mL	67	68	68
Protein g/100 mL	1.0	1.45	1.40
Protein source	Mature Term human milk	Nonfat milk whey	Nonfat milk whey protein concentrate
Carbohydrate g/100 mL	6.8	7.3	7.3
Carbohydrate source	Lactose	Lactose	Lactose
Fat g/100 mL	4.0	3.6	3.65
Fat source	Human milk, fat	Palm olein, coconut, soy, and high oleic sunflower oils	High oleic safflower, soy and coconut oils
Osmolality mOsm/kg	300	300	300
Sodium mEq/L (mg/L)	7.8 (180)	8 (183)	6.8 (162)
Potassium mEq/L (mg/L)	13.5 (525)	18.7 (730)	18.2 (710)
Chloride mEq/L (mg/L)	11.9 (420)	12 (426)	12.2 (433)
Calcium mEq/L (mg/L)	14 (280)	26.4 (528)	26.4 (527)
Phosphorus mEq/L (mg/L)	9 (140)	20.5 (358)	18.8 (284)
Iron mg/L	0.3	12.2 (4.7)[2]	12.2 (4.7)[2]

[1]Information based on manufacturer's literature as of 2001 and is subject to change.

[2]Low iron formulation in parenthesis.

Hypercaloric Milk Based Formulas – 24[1,2]
(Indications: Fluid restriction, increased caloric demands)

	Enfamil® 24	Similac® 24
Calories /100 mL	81	80.6
Protein g/100 mL	1.74	2.2
Protein source	Nonfat milk and whey	Nonfat milk
Carbohydrate g/100 mL	8.8	8.5
Carbohydrate source	Lactose	Lactose
Fat g/100 mL	4.3	4.25
Fat source	Palm olein, coconut, soy, and high oleic sunflower oils	Soy and coconut oils
Osmolality mOsm/kg	360	380
Sodium mEq/L (mg/L)	9.6 (220)	12.1 (280)
Potassium mEq/L (mg/L)	22.3 (870)	27.4 (1070)
Chloride mEq/L (mg/L)	14.4 (510)	18.6 (660)
Calcium mEq/L (mg/L)	31.4 (628)	36.4 (730)
Phosphorus mEq/L (mg/L)	27.6 (427)	36.5 (565)
Iron mg/L	14.6 (5.7)[3]	14.5

[1]Information based on manufacturer's literature as of 2001 and is subject to change; 24 calories/oz

[2]To approximate values for the content of a 30 cal/oz formula (made by dilution of a powder formulation) multiply the value desired, found in a 20 cal/oz formula, by 1.5 (20 cal/oz formula contents for Enfamil® and Similac® are listed in preceding Milk Based Formula chart). For example, the fat in a 30 cal/oz Enfamil® formula = 1.5 x 3.6 = 5.4 g/100 mL.

[3]Low iron formulation in parentheses

FLUIDS, ELECTROLYTES, & NUTRITION *(Continued)*

Soy Formulas[1]
(Indications: Lactose deficiency, milk intolerance, or galactosemia)

	Prosobee®	Isomil®
Calories /100 mL	68	67.6
Protein g/100 mL	2	1.7
Protein source	Soy protein isolate L-methionine	Soy protein isolate L-methionine
Carbohydrate g/100 mL	6.8	6.9
Carbohydrate source	Corn syrup solids	Corn syrup and sucrose
Fat g/100 mL	3.6	3.69
Fat source	Palm olein, coconut, soy, and high oleic sunflower oils	High oleic safflower, soy and coconut oils
Osmolality mOsm/kg	200	200
Sodium mEq/L (mg/L)	10.6 (240)	12.8 (297)
Potassium mEq/L (mg/L)	20.6 (810)	18.9 (730)
Chloride mEq/L (mg/L)	14.7 (540)	11.5 (419)
Calcium mEq (mg/L)	35.5 (710)	35.1 (710)
Phosphorus mEq/L (mg/L)	36 (560)	32.9 (507)
Iron mg/L	12.2	12

[1]Information based on manufacturer's literature as of 2001 and is subject to change.

Hypercaloric Soy Formulas – 24[1,2]
(Indications: Fluid restriction, increased caloric demands)

	Prosobee® 24
Calories /100 mL	81.1
Protein g/100 mL	2.4
Protein source	Soy protein isolate
Carbohydrate g/100 mL	8.2
Carbohydrate source	Corn syrup solids
Fat g/100 mL	4.3
Fat source	Palm olein, coconut, soy, and high oleic sunflower oils
Osmolality mOsm/kg	240
Sodium mEq/L (mg/L)	12.7 (292)
Potassium mEq/L (mg/L)	25.2 (990)
Chloride mEq/L (mg/L)	19 (672)
Calcium mEq/L (mg/L)	38 (761)
Phosphorus mEq/L (mg/L)	38.9 (602)
Iron mg/L	15.2

[1]Information based on manufacturer's literature as of 2001 and is subject to change.

[2]To approximate values for the content of a 27 or 30 cal/oz formula (made by dilution of a powder based formulation), multiply the value desired, found in the 20 cal/oz formula (20 cal/oz formula contents for Prosobee® are listed in the preceding Soy Formulas chart), by the following factors: 1.35 (27 cal/oz) or 1.5 (30 cal/oz).

FLUIDS, ELECTROLYTES, & NUTRITION *(Continued)*

Casein Hydrolysate Formulas[1]
(Indication: For infants whose renal or cardiovascular functions
would benefit from lowered mineral levels)

	Similac® PM 60/40
Calories /100 mL	67.6
Protein g/100 mL	1.5
Protein source	Whey and caseinate
Carbohydrate g/100 mL	6.9
Carbohydrate source	Lactose
Fat g/100 mL	3.78
Fat source	Corn, soy and coconut oils
Osmolality mOsm/kg	280
Sodium mEq/L (mg/L)	6.8 (162)
Potassium mEq/L (mg/L)	14.9 (580)
Chloride mEq/L (mg/L)	11.5 (400)
Calcium mEq/L (mg/L)	19 (380)
Phosphorus mEq/L (mg/L)	12.3 (190)
Iron mg/L	4.7
Special uses	Renal and cardiovascular disease

[1]Information based on manufacturer's literature as of 2001 and is subject to change.

Casein Hydrolysate Formulas[1,2]

(Indication: For infants requiring low molecular weight peptides or amino acids)

	Nutramigen®	Pregestimil®	Alimentum®
Calories /100 mL	68	68	67.6
Protein g/100 mL	1.9	1.9	1.9
Protein source	Casein hydrolysate, L-cystine, L-tyrosine, and L-tryptophan	Casein hydrolysate, L-cystine, L-tyrosine, and L-tryptophan	Casein hydrolysate, L-cystine, L-tyrosine, and L-tryptophan
Carbohydrate g/100 mL	7.4	6.8	6.9
Carbohydrate source	Corn syrup solids and modified corn starch	Corn syrup solids, dextrose, and modified corn starch	Sucrose and modified tapioca starch
Fat g/100 mL	3.4	3.8	3.7
Fat source	Palm olein, soy, coconut, and high oleic sunflower oils	MCT oil, corn oil, and high oleic sunflower oil	Safflower, medium chain triglycerides, and soy oils
Osmolality mOsm/kg	320	320	370
Sodium mEq/L (mg/L)	13.8 (318)	11.5 (264)	12.8 (297)
Potassium mEq/L (mg/L)	19 (744)	18.9 (737)	20.3 (797)
Chloride mEq/L (mg/L)	16.4 (582)	16.4 (581)	15.5 (540)
Calcium mEq/L (mg/L)	31.8 (636)	31.8 (636)	35 (709)
Phosphorus mEq/L (mg/L)	27.3 (426)	28 (430)	32.7 (507)
Iron mg/L	12.2	12.8	12.2
Special uses	Sensitivity to intact proteins, galactosemia	Malabsorption, cystic fibrosis	Sensitivity to intact proteins, protein maldigest or fat malabsorption

[1]Information based on manufacturer's literature as of 2001 and is subject to change.

[2]To approximate values for the content of a 24, 27, or 30 cal/oz formula (made by dilution of a powder based formulation), multiply the value desired, found in the above 20 cal/oz formula, by the following factors: 1.2 (24 cal/oz), 1.35 (27 cal/oz), or 1.5 (30 cal/oz).

FLUIDS, ELECTROLYTES, & NUTRITION (Continued)

Other Infant and Pediatric Formulas[1] – Special Care
(Indication: Premature infant formulas designed for rapidly growing LBW infants)

	Preterm Human Milk	Preterm Human Milk + Similac® HMF[2] (1 pkt: 50 mL)	Special Care 20 With Fe	Special Care 24 With Fe	Neosure
Calories /100 mL	67	73	67.6	81	74.6
Protein g/100 mL	1.4	1.9	1.83	2.2	2
Protein source	Preterm human milk	Preterm human milk, nonfat milk and whey protein concentrate	Nonfat milk and whey protein concentrate	Nonfat milk and whey protein concentrate	Nonfat milk and whey protein concentrate
Carbohydrate g/100 mL	6.6	7.4	7.17	8.6	7.7
Carbohydrate source	Lactose	Corn syrup solids and lactose	Corn syrup solids and lactose	Corn syrup solids and lactose	Maltodextrin and lactose
Fat g/100 mL	3.9	4.0	3.67	4.4	4
Fat source	Preterm human milk	Preterm human milk, medium chain triglycerides	Medium chain triglycerides, soy, and coconut oils	Medium chain triglycerides, soy, and coconut oils	Medium chain triglycerides, soy, and coconut oils
Osmolality mOsm/kg	290	343	235	280	250
Sodium mEq/L (mg/L)	10.7 (248)	13.9 (321)	12.8 (290)	15.2 (350)	10.4 (246)
Potassium mEq/L (mg/L)	14.8 (570)	26.6 (1040)	22.3 (870)	26.6 (1045)	27 (1060)
Chloride mEq/L (mg/L)	15.4 (550)	20.4 (730)	15.5 (550)	18.6 (660)	15.7 (560)
Calcium mEq/L (mg/L)	15.4 (550)	40.9 (818)	60.8 (1220)	72.6 (1452)	39 (784)
Phosphorus mEq/L (mg/L)	8.2 (128)	29 (453)	43.7 (676)	47 (726)	29.6 (460)
Iron mg/L	1.2	2.9	12.2 (2.7)[3]	14.6 (3.2)[3]	13.4

[1]Information based on manufacturer's literature as of 2001 and is subject to change.

[2]HMF = human milk fortifier

[3]Low iron formulation in parentheses.

ENTERAL FORMULAS – PEDIATRIC

(A selection of the commonly used enteral feedings for children 1-10 years of age)

	Pediasure®	Peptamen Junior®	Vivonex® Pediatric	Boost®	Carnation Instant Breakfast®[1]	Ensure®	Kindercal®
Calories/oz	30	30	24	30	27	31	30
Calories/mL	1.0	1.06	0.8	1.0	0.93	1.04	1.0
Carbohydrate g/100 mL	11	13.8	13	17.4	14.4	16.7	13.5
Carbohydrate source	Maltodextrin, sucrose	Maltodextrin, corn starch	Maltodextrin, modified starch	Sucrose, corn syrup solids	Maltodextrin, sucrose, lactose	Maltodextrin, sucrose	Maltodextrin, sucrose
Protein g/100 mL	3.0	3.0	2.4	4.2	4.4	3.7	3.4
Protein source	Caseinate, whey protein conc	Hydrolyzed whey protein	L-amino acids	Milk protein conc	Nonfat milk	Caseinates, soy protein isolate	Caseinates
Fat g/100 mL	5.0	3.8	2.4	1.7	1.9	2.5	4.4
Fat source	High oleic safflower, soy, and MCT oils	MCT, soy, and canola oils	MCT and soy solids	Canola, sunflower, and corn oils	Butterfat	Corn oil	Canola, high oleic sunflower, corn, and MCT oils
Osmolality mOsm/kg	335	260 unflavored 360 vanilla	360	590-620	661-747	590	310
Sodium mg/100 mL (mEq/100 mL)	38 (1.7)	46 (2)	40 (1.7)	55 (2.4)	90 (3.9)	83 (3.6)	37 (1.6)
Potassium mg/100 mL (mEq/100 mL)	131 (3.4)	132 (3.4)	120 (3.1)	169 (4.3)	250 (6.4)	154 (3.9)	131 (3.3)
Iron (mg/100 mL)	1.4	1.4	1.0	1.5	—	1.9	1.1

[1]Mixed with 2% milk as directed.

FLUIDS, ELECTROLYTES, & NUTRITION *(Continued)*

ENTERAL FORMULAS – ADOLESCENTS, ADULTS

	Isocal®	Osmolite®	Osmolite HN®	Jevity®
Calories/mL	1.06	1.06	1.06	1.06
Carbohydrate g/100 mL	13.5	14.8	14.4	15.0
Carbohydrate source	Maltodextrin	Maltodextrin and corn syrup solids	Maltodextrin and corn syrup solids	Maltodextrin and corn syrup solids
Protein g/100 mL	3.4	3.7	4.4	4.4
Protein source	Caseinate, soy protein isolate	Caseinate, soy protein isolate	Caseinate, soy protein isolate	Caseinates
Fat g/100 mL	4.4	3.4	3.5	3.5
Fat source	Soy oil, MCT oil	High oleic safflower, canola, and MCT oils	High oleic safflower, canola, and MCT oils	High oleic safflower, canola, and MCT oils
Osmolality mOsm/kg	270	300	300	300
Sodium mg/100 mL (mEq/100 mL)	53 (2.3)	63 (2.7)	92 (4.0)	91.6 (4.0)
Potassium mg/100 mL (mEq/100 mL)	132 (3.4)	100 (2.6)	157 (4.0)	157 (4.0)

[1]Contains 13.6 g/L soy fiber.

ENTERAL FORMULAS WITH HIGH CALORIC DENSITY

	Ensure Plus®	Ensure Plus HN®	Comply®	TraumaCal®	Deliver®
Calories/mL	1.5	1.5	1.5	1.5	2
Carbohydrate g/100 mL	20.8	19.7	18	14.2	20
Carbohydrate source	Corn syrup solids, maltodextrin, sucrose	Maltodextrin, sucrose	Maltodextrin	Corn syrup solids, sucrose	Corn syrup
Protein g/100 mL	5.4	6.2	6.0	8.2	7.5
Protein source	Caseinate, soy protein isolate	Caseinate, soy protein isolate	Caseinates	Caseinates	Caseinates
Fat g/100 mL	4.8	4.9	6.1	6.8	10.2
Fat source	Canola, high oleic safflower and corn oils	Corn oil	Canola, high oleic sunflower, MCT and corn oils	Soy oil, MCT oil	Soy oil, MCT oil
Osmolality mOsm/kg	690	650	460	580	640
Sodium mg/100 mL (mEq/100 mL)	100 (4.3)	117 (5.1)	120 (5.2)	118 (5.1)	80 (3.5)
Potassium mg/100 mL (mEq/100 mL)	183 (4.7)	179 (4.6)	185 (4.7)	140 (3.6)	168 (4.3)

ENTERAL FORMULAS WITH MODIFIED PROTEIN – "ELEMENTAL"
Adolescents and Adults

	Criticare HN®	Peptamen®	Tolerex®	Vivonex Plus®
Calories/mL	1.06	1.0	1.0	1.0
Carbohydrate g/100 mL	22	12.7	23	19.0
Carbohydrate source	Maltodextrin, modified corn starch	Maltodextrin, corn starch	Maltodextrin	Maltodextrin, modified starch
Protein g/100 mL	3.8	4.0	2.1	4.5
Protein source	Hydrolyzed casein, L-amino acids	Hydrolyzed whey	L-amino acids	L-amino acids
Fat g/100 mL	0.53	3.9	0.15	0.67
Fat source	Safflower oil	Sunflower and MCT oils	Safflower oil	Soy oil
Osmolality mOsm/kg	650	270 unflavored 380 vanilla	550 unflavored 617-678 flavored	650
Sodium mg/100 mL (mEq/100 mL)	63 (2.7)	50 (2.2)	47 (2.0)	61 (2.7)
Potassium mg/100 mL (mEq/100 mL)	132 (3.4)	125 (3.2)	117 (3.0)	106 (2.7)

FLUIDS, ELECTROLYTES, & NUTRITION *(Continued)*

Nutritional Modules[1]

	Polycose® Liquid	Polycose® Powder	Promod® Powder[2]
Indication	Carbohydrate additive for use as a caloric supplement which is readily mixable in most foods, enteral formulas or beverages without appreciably altering their taste	Carbohydrate additive for use as a caloric supplement which is readily mixable in most foods, enteral formulas or beverages without appreciably altering their taste	Protein supplement which mixes readily in enteral formulas, most foods, or beverages without appreciably altering their taste
Calories	2/mL	3.8/g[3]	4.2/g
Protein (g)	—	—	0.76/g
Protein source	—	—	Whey protein concentrate
Carbohydrate (g)	0.5/mL	0.94/g	<0.1/g
Carbohydrate source	Glucose polymers	Glucose polymers	Lactose
Fat (g)	—	—	<0.09/g
Fat source	—	—	Soy lecithin
Osmolality mOsm/kg	900	900 in solution	—
Sodium mEq/L (mg/L)	<0.03/mL (<0.7/mL)	<0.05/g (<1.1/g)	<0.099/g (<2.3/g)
Potassium mEq/L (mg/L)	<0.002/mL (<0.06/mL)	<0.003/g (<0.1/g)	<0.25/g (<9.85/g)
Chloride mEq/L (mg/L)	<0.04/mL (<1.4/mL)	<0.06/g (<2.23/g)	—
Calcium mEq/L (mg/L)	<0.01/mL (<0.2/mL)	<0.02/g (<0.3/g)	<0.33/g (<6.67/g)
Phosphorus mEq/L (mg/L)	(<0.03/mL)	(<0.05/g)	(<5/g)
Iron mg/L	—	—	—

[1] These products are not complete formulations and should not be used as a sole source of nutrition.

[2] 1 scoop = 6.6 g, 1 tsp = 1.3 g, 1 tbsp = 4 g.

[3] 1 tsp (2 g) = 8 calories, 1 tbsp (6 g) = 23 calories, ¼ cup (24 g) = 95 calories.

Nutritional Modules[1]

	Vegetable Oil[2]	Microlipid®	MCT Oil®[3]	Whole Milk
Indications	Inexpensive fat source for calories and essential fatty acids	50% fat emulsion for use as a source of calories or essential fatty acids; it mixes easily and stays in emulsion	Fat supplement for use for patients who cannot efficiently digest and absorb long-chain fats	
Calories	8/mL	4.5/mL	7.67/mL	157/8 oz
Protein (g)	—	—	—	8/8 oz
Protein source	—	—	—	82% casein, 18% whey
Carbohydrate (g)	—	—	—	11/8 oz
Carbohydrate source	—	—	—	Lactose
Fat (g)	0.93/mL	0.5/mL[4]	0.93/mL	8.9/8 oz
Fat source	Corn, soybean, sunflower or safflower oils[5]	Safflower oil, polyglycerol esters, soy lecithin	Lipid fraction of coconut oil (consists primarily of C_8 and C_{10} saturated fatty acids)	Butter fat
Osmolality mOsm/kg	—	60	—	288
Sodium mEq/L (mg/L)	—	—	—	5.3/8 oz (122/8 oz)
Potassium mEq/L (mg/L)	—	—	—	9/8 oz (351/8 oz)
Chloride mEq/L (mg/L)	—	—	—	7/8 oz (247/8 oz)
Calcium mEq/L (mg/L)	—	—	—	14.4/8 oz (288/8 oz)
Phosphorus mEq/L (mg/L)	—	—	—	14.6/8 oz (227/8 oz)
Iron mg/L	—	—	—	0.12/8 oz

[1]These products are not complete formulations and should not be used as a sole source of nutrition.

[2]1 tbsp = 14 g.

[3]Does not contain essential fatty acids.

[4]1 tbsp = 5.9 g linoleic.

[5]% of linoleic from fat: soybean oil 51%, corn oil 58%, sunflower oil 65%, safflower oil 77%.

FLUID AND ELECTROLYTE REQUIREMENTS IN CHILDREN

Maintenance Fluids (Two methods)

Surface area method (most commonly used in children >10 kg): 1500-2000 mL/m^2/day

Body weight method

<10 kg	100 mL/kg/day
11-20 kg	1000 mL + 50 mL/kg (for each kg >10)
>20 kg	1500 mL + 20 mL/kg (for each kg >20)

Maintenance Electrolytes (See specific electrolyte in Alphabetical Listing of Drugs for more detailed information)

Sodium: 3-4 mEq/kg/day **or** 30-50 mEq/m^2/day
Potassium: 2-3 mEq/kg/day **or** 20-40 mEq/m^2/day

Dehydration Fluid Therapy

Goals of therapy:

- Restore circulatory volume to prevent shock (10% to 15% dehydration)
- Restore combined intracellular and extracellular deficits of water and electrolytes within 24 hours
- Maintain adequate water and electrolytes
- Resolve homeostatic distortions (eg, acidosis)
- Replace ongoing losses

Analysis of the Severity of Dehydration by Physical Signs

Clinical Sign	Mild*	Moderate*	Severe*
Pre-illness body weight	5% loss	10% loss	15% loss
Skin turgor	↓	Tenting	Tenting
Mucous membranes	Dry	Very dry	Parched
Skin color	Pale	Grey	Mottled
Urine output	↓	↓↓	Azotemic
Blood pressure	Normal	Normal, ↓	↓↓
Heart rate	Normal, ↑	↑	↑↑
Fontanelle (<7 mo)	Flat	Soft	Sunken
CNS	Consolable	Irritable	Lethargic/coma

*Postpubertal children and adults experience the same symptoms with mild, moderate, and severe dehydration associated with 3%, 6%, and 9% losses in body weight respectively.

Restoration of Circulatory Volume (10% to 15% dehydration estimate)

Fluid boluses of 20 mL/kg using crystalloid (eg, normal saline) or 10 mL/kg colloid (eg, 5% albumin) administered as rapidly as possible; repeat until improved circulation (eg, warm skin, decreased heart rate (towards normal), improved capillary refill time, urine output restored).

Classification of Dehydration (based upon the serum sodium concentration)

Isotonic	130-150 mEq/L
Hypotonic	<130 mEq/L
Hypertonic	>150 mEq/L

Estimated Water & Electrolyte Deficits in Dehydration
(moderate to severe)

Type of Dehydration	Water (mL/kg)	Na+ (mEq/kg)	K+ (mEq/kg)	Cl⁻ and HCO₃⁻ (mEq/kg)
Isotonic	100-150	8-10	8-10	16-20
Hypotonic	50-100	10-14	10-14	20-28
Hypertonic	120-180	2-5	2-5	4-10

Current Pediatric Diagnosis & Treatment, 10th ed, 1991.

Water deficit may also be calculated (in isotonic dehydration):

$$\text{Water deficit (mL)} \quad = \quad \frac{\%\ \text{dehydration x wt (kg) x 1000 g/kg}}{100}$$

Assessment of Water Loss in Relation to Serum Na⁺ Concentrations
Degree of Dehydration as % Body Weight

Serum Na⁺	Mild	Moderate	Severe
Isotonic	5%	10%	15%
Hypotonic (Na⁺< 130)	4%	6%	8%
Hypertonic (Na⁺ >150)	7%	12%	17%

Example of Fluid Replacement
(assume 10 kg infant with 10% isotonic dehydration)

	Water	Sodium (mEq)	Potassium (mEq)
Maintenance	1000 mL	40	20
Deficit*	1000 mL	80	80
Total	2000 mL	120	100

*Reduce this total by any fluid boluses given initially.

First 8 hours:

Replace ⅓ maintenance water	=	330 mL
Replace ½ deficit water	=	500 mL
Total		830 mL/8 h = 103 mL/h

Replace ½ of Na⁺ & K⁺ = 60 mEq sodium/803 mL; 50 mEq potassium/803 mL (It is suggested that the maximum potassium initially used is 40 mEq/L and is **not** started until urine output has been established.)

The actual order would appear as: D₅½NS at 103 mL/hour for 8 hours; add 40 mEq/L KCl after patient voids.

Second 16 hours:

Replace ⅔ maintenance water	=	670 mL
Replace ½ deficit water	=	500 mL
Total		1260 mL/16 h = 79 mL/h

Replace remainder of sodium and potassium.

The actual order would appear as: D₅⅓NS with KCl 40 mEq/L at 79 mL/hour for 16 hours. (Use of ¼NS may be more desirable for convenience.)

FLUID AND ELECTROLYTE REQUIREMENTS IN CHILDREN *(Continued)*

Analysis of Ongoing Losses

Electrolyte Composition of Biological Fluids (mEq/L)

Fluid Type	Sodium	Potassium	Chloride	Total HCO_3^-
Stomach	20-120	5-25	90-160	0-5
Duodenal drainage	20-140	3-30	30-120	10-50
Biliary tract	120-160	3-12	70-130	30-50
Small intestine Initial drainage	100-140	4-40	60-100	30-100
Small intestine Established drainage	4-20	4-10	10-100	40-120
Pancreatic	110-160	4-15	30-80	70-130
Diarrheal stool	10-25	10-30	30-120	10-50

Current Pediatric Diagnosis & Treatment, 9th ed, Appleton & Lange, 1987.

Because of the wide range of normal values, specific analyses are suggested in individual cases.

Alterations of Maintenance Fluid Requirements

Fever	Increase maintenance fluids by 5 mL/kg/day for each degree of temperature above 38°C
Hyperventilation	Increase maintenance fluids by 10-60 mL/100 kcal BEE (basal energy expenditure)
Sweating	Increase maintenance fluids by 10-25 mL/100 kcal BEE (basal energy expenditure)
Hyperthyroidism	Variable increase in maintenance fluids: 25%-50%
Renal disease	Monitor and analyze output; adjust therapy accordingly
Renal failure	Maintenance fluids are equal to insensible losses ($300 mL/m^3$) + urine replacement (mL for mL)
Diarrhea	Increase maintenance fluids on a mL/mL loss basis

Oral Rehydration

Due to the high worldwide incidence of dehydration from infantile diarrhea, effective, inexpensive oral rehydration solutions have been developed. In the U.S., a typical effective solution for rehydration contains 50-60 mEq/L sodium, 20-30 mEq/L potassium, 30 mEq/L bicarbonate or its equivalent, and sufficient chloride to provide electroneutrality. Two percent to 3% glucose facilitates electrolyte absorption and short-term calories. The following table describes the electrolyte/sugar content of commonly used oral rehydration solutions.

Composition of Frequently Used
Oral Electrolyte Replacement Solutions

Solutions	% CHO	Na⁺ (mEq/L)	K⁺ (mEq/L)	Cl⁻ (mEq/L)	HCO⁻ (mEq/L)
Normal saline		154		154	
Ringer's lactate		130	4	109	28
Dextrose 5% in 0.25% NaCl	5% glucose	38		38	
WHO solution	2% glucose or 4% sucrose	90	20	80	30 citrate
WHO solution, modified	2% glucose	55	25	30	50
Rehydralyte®	2.5% glucose	75	20	65	30 citrate
Ricelyte®	3% carbohydrate	50	25	45	34 citrate
Resol®	2% glucose	50	20	50	34 citrate
Rice water	2.5% carbohydrate	90	20	30	80
Pedialyte® (Ross)	2.5% glucose	45	20	35	30 citrate
Infalyte® (Penwalt)	3% glucose	50	25	45	34
Gatorade®	2.6% glucose, 2% fructose	23.5	<1	17	
Apple juice	3.2% glucose, 1.3% sucrose, 7.5% fructose	<1	25		
Orange juice 1:3 (dilution with water)	1% glucose, 1.2% fructose	<1	50		50 citrate
Grape juice	1.6% glucose, 2.1% fructose	0.2-0.7	8-11		8
One package cherry gelatin dissolved in 4 cups water		24	Needs added K⁺		
Coca-Cola®		1.6	<1		13.4 citrate
Pepsi-Coal®		6.5	0.8		
Beef broth		120	10		
Chicken broth		250	8		

Adapted from Aranda-Michel, J and Giannella RA, "Acute Diarrhea" A Practical Review," *Am J of Med,* 1999, 106:670-6.

PARENTERAL NUTRITION (PN)

The following information is intended as a brief overview of the use of PN in infants and children.

Goal: The therapeutic goal of PN in infants and children is both to maintain nutrition status and to achieve balanced somatic growth.

General Indications for Use

PN is the provision of required nutrients by the intravenous route to replenish, optimize, or maintain nutritional status.

Specific Indications

PN of **all** required nutrients (total parenteral nutrition) is indicated in patients for whom it is expected that it would be impossible or dangerous to enterally administer nutrition. PN in combination with enteral nutrition is indicated in patients who are expected to be unable to meet their nutritional needs by the enteral route alone within 5 days. Peripheral PN is indicated only for partial nutritional supplementation or as bridge therapy for patients awaiting central venous access.

1. Patients with an inability to absorb nutrients via the gastrointestinal tract which may include the following: severe diarrhea, short bowel syndrome, developmental anomalies of the GI tract, inflammatory bowel disease, cystic fibrosis, or anatomic or functional loss of GI integrity.

2. Severe malnutrition.

3. Severe catabolic states such as: burns, trauma, or sepsis.

4. Patients undergoing high dose chemotherapy, radiation, and bone marrow transplantation.

5. Patients whose clinical condition may necessitate complete bowel rest (eg, necrotizing enterocolitis, pancreatitis, GI fistulas, or recent GI surgery).

6. Intensive care low-birth-weight infants.

7. Neonatal asphyxia.

8. Meconium ileus.

9. Respiratory distress syndrome (RDS).

Nutritional Assessment

As many as 33% of hospitalized pediatric patients are malnourished and require nutritional therapy. The type of nutritional support indicated depends on the underlying disease, the degree of gastrointestinal function, and the severity of malnutrition. Acutely malnourished patients have an increased risk for serious infection, postoperative complications, and death. Indicators of acute protein-calorie malnutrition include low weight for height, low serum albumin, lymphopenia, decreased body fat folds, and decreased arm muscle area. Nutritional screening may be done by the dietitian. Those patients who are at nutritional risk should receive a complete nutritional assessment.

Nutritional Requirements

Approximate requirements for energy and protein at various ages for normal subjects are listed in the first table at the end of this section. Patients who are severely malnourished or markedly catabolic may require higher levels to achieve catch-up growth or meet increased requirements. Patients who are well-nourished and/or inactive may require less.

During parenteral nutrition, 10% to 16% of calories should be in the form of amino acids to achieve optimal benefit (approximately 2-3 g/kg/day in infants and 1.5-2.5 g/kg/day ideal body weight in older patients). Exceptions include patients with renal or hepatic failure (where less protein is indicated), or in the treatment of severe trauma, head injury, or sepsis (where more protein may be indicated).

PN ORDERING

Fluid Intake

The patient should be given a total volume of fluid reasonable for his/her age and cardiovascular status. It is generally safe to start with the fluid maintenance level of 1500 mL/m²/day in children (see Fluid and Electrolyte Requirements in Children). The fluid requirements in preterm infants are extremely variable due to much greater insensible water losses from radiant warmers and bili-lights. While the standard fluid maintenance of 100 mL/kg/day may be sufficient for term infants, intakes of up to 150 mL/kg/day may be necessary in the very low birth weight infants. Be sure to consider significant fluid intake from medications or other I.V. fluids and enteral diets in planning the fluids available for PN.

Dextrose

For central PN, dextrose is usually begun with a 10% to 12.5% solution or a solution providing dextrose at no more than 5 mg/kg/minute (in neonates and premature infants). The concentration is advanced, if tolerated, by 2.5% to 5% per day (2-2.5 mg/kg/minute increments in neonates and premature infants) to the desired caloric density, usually 20% to 25% dextrose. Fluid restricted patients often need 30% to 35% dextrose to meet their energy needs. For peripheral PN, 5% to 12.5% dextrose is utilized.

Dextrose calculations:

% Dextrose = dextrose (g)/100 mL
Dextrose calorie value = 3.4 kcal/g

$$\text{Dextrose infusion rate (mg/kg/minute)} = \frac{\text{rate (mL/h) x \% dextrose x 0.166}}{\text{weight (kg)}}$$

$$\text{\% Dextrose desired*} = \frac{\text{desired rate (mg/kg/min) x weight (kg)}}{0.166 \text{ x rate (mL/h)}}$$

*Do not use dextrose concentrations <5% due to hypotonicity.

Amino Acids

Amino acids may be described as either a "standard" mixture of essential and nonessential amino acids or "specialized" mixtures. Specialized mixtures are intended for use in patients whose physiologic or metabolic needs may not be met with the "standard" amino acid compositions. Examples of specialized solutions include:

TrophAmine®, Aminosyn® PF	Indicated for use in premature infants and young children due to addition of taurine, L-glutamic acid, L-aspartic acid, increased amounts of histidine, and reduction in amounts of methionine, alanine, phenylalanine, and glycine. Supplementation with a cysteine additive has been recommended.
HepatAmine®	Indicated for treatment in patients with hepatic encephalopathy due to cirrhosis or hepatitis or in patients with liver disease who are intolerant of standard amino acid solutions. Contains higher percentage of branched-chain amino acids and a lower percentage of aromatic amino acids than standard mixtures.
NephrAmine®, Aminosyn® RF	Indicated for use in patients with compromised renal function who are intolerant of standard amino acid solutions. Contains a mixture of essential amino acids and histidine.

PARENTERAL NUTRITION (PN) *(Continued)*

Amino acid calculations:

% amino acid	=	amino acid (g)/100mL
Grams of protein	=	grams of nitrogen x 6.25
% amino acid desired	=	(g amino acid/kg) x weight (kg) x 100
		total PN fluid volume (mL)

Fat Emulsion (FE)

There are three roles for intravenous fat in parenteral nutrition:

1. to provide nonprotein calories
2. to provide essential fatty acids and a "balanced" calorie source
3. to provide calories in catabolic patients with limited ability to excrete CO_2

The FE dosage is increased as tolerated daily (see General Guidelines for Initiation and Advancement for PN following). The maximum fat intake is 4 g/kg/day and no more than 60% of the total daily caloric intake. It is administered as a continuous infusion over 24 hours or at a rate no greater than 0.15-0.2 g/kg/hour via a Y-connector with the dextrose-amino acid I.V. line. In patients receiving cyclic PN, the FE should be administered over the duration of the PN infusion. The triglyceride concentration should be checked before the first infusion and daily as the dose is increased. Subsequently, it should be monitored at least weekly. Triglyceride concentrations should be maintained at <200 mg/dL in neonates, <350 mg/dL in renal patients, and <250 mg/dL in other patients. FE should be used cautiously in neonates with hyperbilirubinemia due to displacement of bilirubin from albumin by the free fatty acids. An increase in free bilirubin may increase the risk of kernicterus. Significant displacement occurs when the free fatty acid to serum albumin molar ratio (FFA/SA) >6. For example, infants with a total bilirubin >8-10 mg/dL (assuming an albumin concentration of 2.5-3 g/dL) should not receive more parenteral FE than required to meet the essential fatty acid requirement of 0.5-1 g/kg/day.

Note: Avoid use of 10% FE in preterm infants because a greater accumulation of plasma lipids occurs due to the greater phospholipid load of the 10% concentration.

Fat emulsion calculations:

20% FE = 20 g fat/100 mL = 2 kcal/mL

Desired 20% FE (mL)	=	(% total kcal as fat) x (total kcal)
		2 kcal/mL

or as an alternative

Desired 20% FE (mL)	=	FE (g/kg) x weight (kg) x 5 mL/g

General Guidelines for Initiation and Advancement of PN*

Age	Initiation and Advancement		Dextrose	Protein (g/kg/d)	Fat (g/kg/d)
Premature infant	Initial		4-6 mg/kg/min	0.5-1.5	0.5
	Daily increase		1-2.5 mg/kg/min	0.5-1	0.5
	Maximum		18 mg/kg/min	2.5-3	3
Term infant - 1 y	Initial		7-9 mg/kg/min	1-1.5	0.5-1
	Daily increase		1-2.5 mg/kg/min	1	0.5-1
	Maximum		21 mg/kg/min	2.5-3	4
Children 1-10 y	Initial dextrose concentration		10%-12.5%	1-1.5	1
	Daily increase		5% increments	1	1
	Maximum		15 mg/kg/min	2-2.5	3
>10 y	Initial dextrose concentration		10%-15%	1-1.5	1
	Daily increase		5% increments	1	1
	Maximum		8.5 mg/kg/min	1.5-2	3

*Rate of advancement may be limited by metabolic tolerance (eg, hyperglycemia, azotemia, hypertriglyceridemia)

MINERALS, TRACE ELEMENTS, AND VITAMINS

Guideline for Daily Electrolyte Requirements

	Neonates (mEq/kg)	Infants/Children (mEq/kg)	Adolescents
Sodium	2-5*	2-6	1-2 mEq/kg
Potassium	2-4	2-4	1-2 mEq/kg
Calcium gluconate†	3-4‡	1-2.5	10-20 mEq/d
Magnesium	0.3-0.5	0.3-0.5	10-30 mEq/d
Phosphate†	1-2 mmol/kg‡	0.5-1 mmol/kg	10-40 mmol/d

*Prematuare infants lose sodium in urine due to the immature resorptive function of kidney and diuretic use. Hyponatremia may lead to poor tissue growth and adverse developmental outcomes. Sodium content in PN may be adjusted to a maximum of 154 mEq/L (NS) to achieve normal sodium serum levels.

†Calcium-phosphate stability in parenteral nutrition solutions is dependent upon the pH of the solution, temperature, and relative concentration of each ion. The pH of the solution is primarily dependent upon the amino acid concentration. The higher the percentage amino acids the lower the pH, the more soluble the calcium and phosphate. Individual commercially available amino acid solutions vary significantly with respect to pH lowering potential and consequent calcium phosphate compatibility. See the pharmacist for specific calcium phosphate stability information.

‡A 1.7:1 calcium to phosphate ratio in PN allows for the highest absolute retention of both minerals and simulates the in utero accretion of calcium and phosphate.

Vitamins

A pediatric parenteral multivitamin product is indicated for children <11 years of age. Children >11 years of age may receive adult multivitamin formulations.

Dosage:

> Pediatric MVI:
> Neonates: 2 mL/kg/d; maximum 5 mL/d
> Infants and children ≤11 y: 5 mL
> Children >11 y and adults: Use adult formulation 10 mL/d

PARENTERAL NUTRITION (PN) *(Continued)*

Trace Mineral Daily Requirements*

	Infants	Children (≥3 mo to ≤5 y)	Older Children and Adolescents
Chromium†	0.2 mcg/kg	0.14-0.2 mcg/kg (max: 5 mcg)	10-15 mcg
Copper‡	20 mcg/kg	20 mcg/kg (max: 300 mcg)	0.3-0.5 mg
Iodide§	1 mcg/kg	1 mcg/kg	1 mcg/kg
Manganese‡	1 mcg/kg	2-10 mcg/kg (max: 50 mcg)	60-150 mcg
Selenium†¶	2-3 mcg/kg	2-3 mcg/kg (max: 30 mcg)	20-60 mcg
Zinc	400 mcg/kg (preterm) 300 mcg/kg (term <3 mo)	100 mcg/kg (max: 5 mg)	2.5-5 mg

*Recommended intakes of trace elements cannot be achieved through the use of a single pediatric trace element product. Only through the use of individualized trace element products can recommended intakes be achieved.

†Omit in patients with renal dysfunction.

‡Omit in patients with impaired biliary excretion or cholestatic liver disease.

§Percutaneous absorption from protein-bound iodine may be adequate.

¶Indicated for use in long-term parenteral nutrition patients.

These are recommended daily trace mineral requirements. Additional supplementation may be indicated in clinical conditions resulting in excessive losses. For example, additional zinc may be needed in situations of excessive gastrointestinal losses.

Developing the PN Goal Regimen

The purpose of this example is to illustrate the thought process in determining what dextrose and amino acid solution and fat emulsion intake would provide the desired daily fluid calorie and protein goals.

1. Calculate the fluid, protein, and caloric goals. Example:

    Weight = 10 kg
    Fluids = 100 mL/kg/day = 1000 mL
    Calories = 100 kcal/kg/day = 1000 kcal
    Protein = 2.5 g/kg/day = 25 g

2. If fat emulsion (FE) comprises 40% to 60% of the total daily calories, using the above example: 40% of 1000 kcal = 400 kcal.

    400 kcal ÷ 2 kcal/mL (20% FE) = 200 mL

3. To determine the goal dextrose concentration calculate the total daily calories remaining. Example:

    $$\begin{array}{ll} 1000 \text{ kcal} & \text{(total daily calories)} \\ -\ 400 \text{ kcal} & \text{(daily calories from fats)} \\ \hline 600 \text{ kcal} & \text{(total daily calories remaining)} \end{array}$$

4. Determine the concentration of dextrose to achieve the total daily calories remaining. Example:

    600 kcal ÷ 3.4 kcal/g x [100 ÷ 800 mL*] = 22%

    *Total daily fluids desired minus that from fats.

5. Calculate percent amino acid solution to achieve goal protein intake. Example:

    [25 g (total protein) ÷ 800 mL (total fluid)] x 100 = 3.1%

    This patient's goal regimen would be: dextrose 22%, amino acid 3.1%, 800 mL/day plus fat emulsion 20% 200 mL/day.

Suggested PN Monitoring Guidelines

Parameter	Suggested Frequency Initial/Hospitalized	Follow-up/Outpatient
Growth		
Weight	Daily	Daily to q visit
Height/length	Weekly	Weekly to q visit
Body composition (triceps skinfold, bone age)	Initially	Monthly to annually
Metabolic (Serum*)		
Electrolytes	Twice weekly	Weekly to q visit
BUN/creatinine	Weekly	Weekly to q visit
Acid-base status	Until stable	As indicated
Albumin/prealbumin	Weekly	Weekly to q visit
Glucose	Daily to weekly	Weekly to q visit
Triglyceride	Initially daily	Weekly to q visit
Liver function tests	Weekly	Weekly to q visit
Complete blood count/differential	Weekly	Weekly to q visit
Platelets, PT/PTT	Weekly	As indicated
Iron indices	As indicated	Biannually to annually
Trace elements	As indicated	Annually
Carnitine	As indicated	As indicated
Folate/vitamin B_{12}	As indicated	As indicated
Ammonia	As indicated	As indicated
Bilirubin, direct	Weekly	As indicated
Metabolic (Urine)		
Glucose	Twice daily	Daily to weekly
Ketone	Twice daily	Daily to weekly
Specific gravity	As indicated	As indicated
Urea nitrogen	As indicated	As indicated
Clinical Calculations		
Fluid balance	Daily	As indicated
Projected vs actual intake	Daily	Weekly to q visit
Calorie/protein intake	Daily	As indicated

Frequency depends on clinical condition.

*For metabolically unstable patients, need to check more frequently.

Adapted from "Guidelines for the Use of Parenteral and Enteral Nutrition in Adult and Pediatric Patients. ASPEN Board of Directors and The Clinical Guidelines Task Force," *JPEN J Parenter Enteral Nutr*, 2002, 26(1 Suppl):1-138SA.

Nutritional Guidelines for Pediatric Patients

Age	kcal/kg/d	Protein g/kg/d
Preterm neonate	120-140	3-4
Term infant - 1 y	90-120	2-3
1-7 y	75-90	1-1.2
12 y	60-75	1-1.2
12-18 y	30-60	0.8-0.9
>18 y	25-30	0.8

PARENTERAL NUTRITION (PN) *(Continued)*

PN kcal/mL*

Dextrose Concentration						
5%	10%	15%	20%	25%	30%	35%
0.17	0.34	0.51	0.68	0.85	1.02	1.19

Dextrose provides 3.4 kcal/g.

Intralipid 10% provides 1.1 kcal/mL.

Intralipid 20% provides 2 kcal/mL.

*Calories derived from amino acids are not included.

Reference

"Guidelines for the Use of Parenteral and Enteral Nutrition in Adult and Pediatric Patients. ASPEN Board of Directors and The Clinical Guidelines Task Force," *JPEN J Parenter Enteral Nutr*, 2002, 26(1 Suppl):1-138SA.

Y-Site Compatibility of Medications With TPN and Lipid*
(Administered in D_5W or NS via Y-connector into PN line)

Medication	PN	Lipid	Comments
Acetazolamide	I	—	Visual precipitate forms
Acyclovir	I	—	Visual precipitate forms
Albumin	C	I	May crack emulsion
Aldesleukin	C	C	
Alprostadil	—	—	
Amikacin	C	I	Causes oiling out of fat emulsion
Aminophylline	C	C	Incompatible with insulin
Amphotericin B	I	I	Visual precipitate forms
Ampicillin	I	I	Visual precipitate forms
Ampicillin/sulbactam	C	—	
Amrinone	—	—	
Atracurium	C	—	
Atropine	—	—	
Aztreonam	C	—	
Bicarbonate	I	I	Incompatible with many electrolytes; precipitate forms
Bumetanide	C	—	
Butorphanol	C	—	
Carboplatin	C	—	
Cefamandole	C	C	
Cefazolin	C	C	
Cefepime	—	—	
Cefonicid	—	—	
Cefoperazone	C	C	
Cefotaxime	C	C	
Cefotetan	C	C	
Cefoxitin	C	C	
Ceftazidime	C	C	
Ceftizoxime	C	C	
Ceftriaxone	C	C	
Cefuroxime	C	C	
Cephalothin	C	C	
Cephapirin	C	C	
Cephradine	I	—	Heavy precipitate of Ca/Phos due to increased pH

Y-Site Compatibility of Medications With TPN and Lipid*
(continued)

Medication	PN	Lipid	Comments
Chloramphenicol	C	C	
Chlorothiazide	I	—	Precipitate forms
Chlorpromazine	C	C	
Cimetidine	C	C	
Ciprofloxacin	C	C	
Cisatracurium	—	—	
Cisplatin	C	C	
Clindamycin	C	C	
Cyanocobalamin	C	C	
Cyclophosphamide	C	C	
Cyclosporine	C†	C	
Cytarabine	C†	—	
Dexamethasone (sodium phosphate)	C	C	
Digoxin	C	C	
Diphenhydramine	C	C	
Dobutamine	C	—	
Dopamine	C	C†	
Doxacurium	—	—	
Doxapram	—	—	
Doxorubicin	I	I	
Doxycycline	C	I	
Droperidol	C	I	
Epinephrine	C	—	
Epoetin alfa	C	—	
Erythromycin	C	C	
Etoposide	—	—	
Famotidine	C	C	
Fentanyl	C	C	
Filgrastim	I	C	Incompatible with salt solutions
Fluconazole	C	C	
Fluorouracil	C†	C	
Folic acid	C	C	
Foscarnet	C	—	
Fosphenytoin	C	—	
Furosemide	C	C	
Ganciclovir	I	—	Precipitate forms
Gentamicin	C	C	
Granisetron	C	—	
Haloperidol (lactate)	C	I	
Heparin	C	I	Free oil formation with 100 units/mL heparin
Hydralazine	C	—	
Hydrocortisone	C	C	
Hydromorphone	C	I†	Free oil formation
Hydroxyzine	C	C	
Idarubicin	C	—	
Ifosfamide	C	C	

PARENTERAL NUTRITION (PN) *(Continued)*

Y-Site Compatibility of Medications With TPN and Lipid*
(continued)

Medication	PN	Lipid	Comments
IL-2	C	—	
Imipenem/cilastatin	C	C	
Indomethacin	I	—	
Insulin, regular	C	C	
Iron dextran	C	I	Causes oiling out of fat emulsion
Isoproterenol	C	C	
Kanamycin	C	C	
Leucovorin	C	C	
Levofloxacin	—	—	
Levorphanol	C	I	Free oil formation
Lidocaine	C	C	
Lorazepam	C	I	
Mannitol (15%)	C	C	
Meperidine	C	C	
Meropenem	C	C	
Mesna	C	C	
Methotrexate	C†	C	Hazy subvisual precipitate
Methyldopa	C	I†	May crack emulsion
Methylprednisolone	C	C	
Metoclopramide	C†	C	
Metronidazole	C	C	
Midazolam	I	I	Precipitate forms
Milrinone	C	—	
Minocycline	I	I	
Mitoxantrone	C†	C	
Morphine	C	C†	
Nafcillin	C	C	
Netilmicin	C	C	
Nitroglycerin	C	C	
Norepinephrine	C	C	
Octreotide	I	C	
Ofloxacin	C	C	
Ondansetron	C	I	Free oil formation
Oxacillin	C	C	
Paclitaxel	C	C	
Penicillin G Na/K	C	C	
Pentobarbital	C	I	Free oil formation
Phenobarbital	C	I	Free oil formation
Phenytoin	I	I	Immediate precipitate
Phytonadione	C	C	
Piperacillin	C	C	
Piperacillin/tazobactam	C	C	
Propofol	C	—	
Ranitidine	C	C	
Sargramostim	C	—	
Sodium bicarbonate	I	I	Incompatible with many electrolytes; precipitate forms

Y-Site Compatibility of Medications With TPN and Lipid*
(continued)

Medication	PN	Lipid	Comments
Sodium nitroprusside	C	I	
Tacrolimus	C	C	
Thiamine	C	C	
Ticarcillin	C	C	
Ticarcillin/clavulanate	C	C	
Trimethoprim/ sulfamethoxazole	C	C	
Tobramycin	C	C	
Urokinase	C	—	
Vancomycin	C	—	
Vecuronium	C	—	
Verapamil	—	—	
Vitamin K	C	C	
Zidovudine	C	C	

C = compatible, may simultaneously infuse drug and TPN/lipid.

I = incompatible; drug should be given through a **separate** I.V. line or turn off the TPN/liquid during drug administration. Flush I.V. line with normal saline **before** and **after** drug administration.

— = information on compatibility not available. Give drug through a **separate** I.V. line or turn off TPN infusion during drug administration. Flush line with normal saline **before** and **after** drug administration.

*Compatibility does not reflect 3-in-one total nutrient admixture (including fat emulsion) solutions.

†Variable stability depending upon TPN composition (see Trissel, 2001).

Reference

Trissel LA, "Handbook on Injectable Drugs," 11th ed, Bethesda, MD: American Society of Health-System Pharmacists, Inc, 2001.

Pharmacologic considerations of mixing medications with PN solutions include:

- Adsorption — bag, bottle, tubing, filter
- Blood levels
- Site of injection/administration
- Flush
- Amino acid-dextrose concentrations
- pH factors
- Temperature
- Additives in solution
- Heparin dose

GROWTH CHARTS

CDC Growth Charts: United States

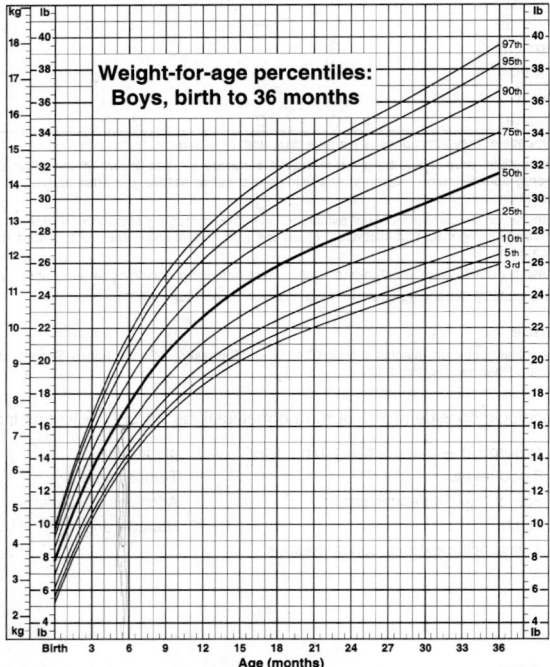

Weight-for-age percentiles:
Boys, birth to 36 months

SOURCE: Developed by the National Center for Health Statistics in collaboration with the
National Center for Chronic Disease Prevention and Health Promotion (2000).
Available at http://www.cdc.gov/growthcharts

CDC Growth Charts: United States

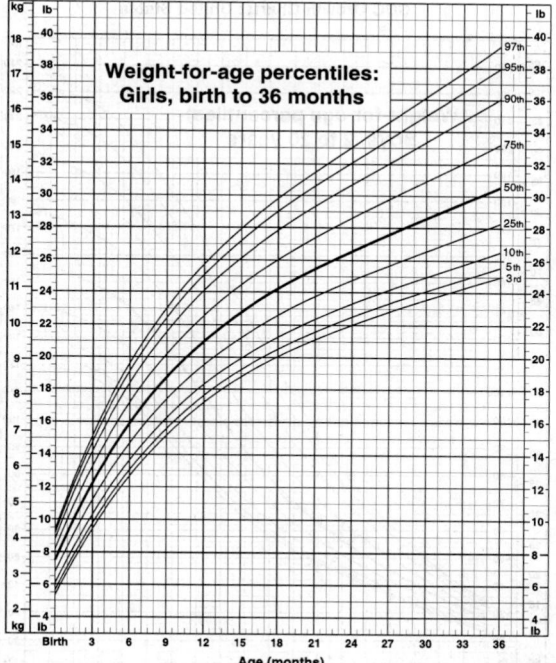

Weight-for-age percentiles:
Girls, birth to 36 months

SOURCE: Developed by the National Center for Health Statistics in collaboration with the
National Center for Chronic Disease Prevention and Health Promotion (2000).
Available at http://www.cdc.gov/growthcharts

CDC

GROWTH CHARTS *(Continued)*

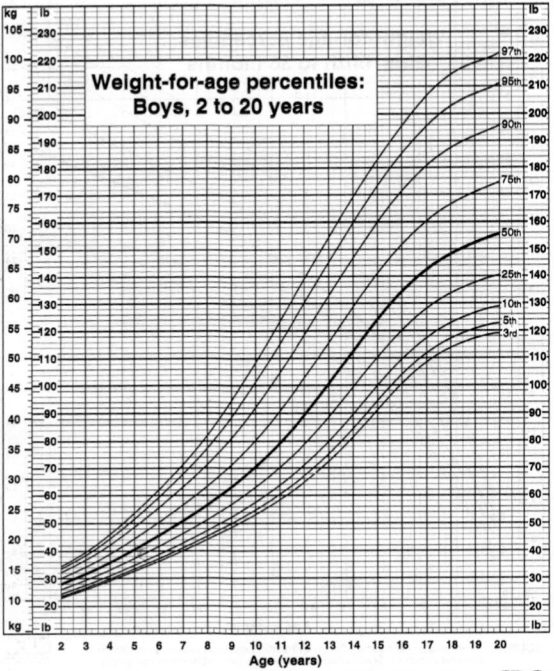

CDC Growth Charts: United States

**Weight-for-age percentiles:
Boys, 2 to 20 years**

SOURCE: Developed by the National Center for Health Statistics in collaboration with the
National Center for Chronic Disease Prevention and Health Promotion (2000).
Available at http://www.cdc.gov/growthcharts

CDC Growth Charts: United States

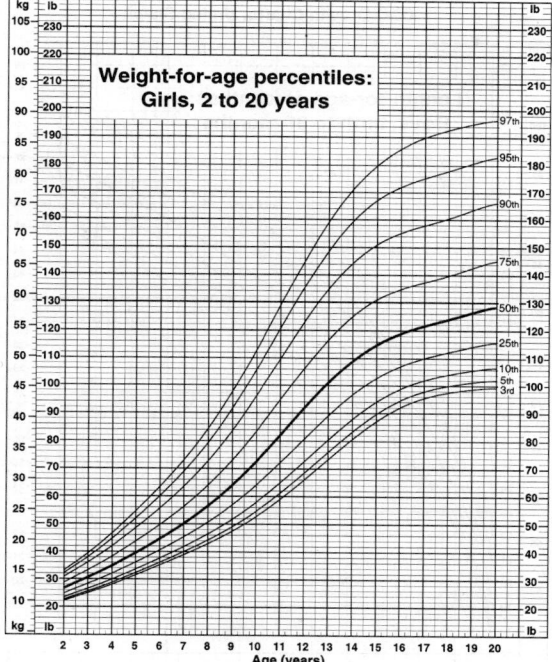

Weight-for-age percentiles: Girls, 2 to 20 years

SOURCE: Developed by the National Center for Health Statistics in collaboration with the National Center for Chronic Disease Prevention and Health Promotion (2000).
Available at http://www.cdc.gov/growthcharts

CDC Growth Charts: United States

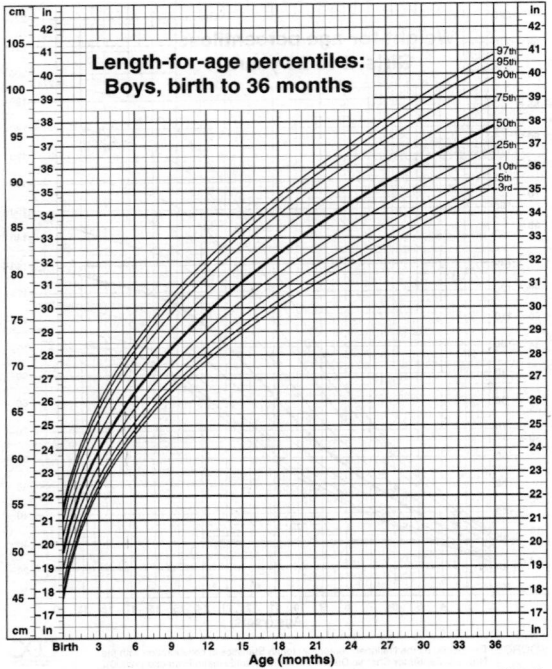

Length-for-age percentiles:
Boys, birth to 36 months

SOURCE: Developed by the National Center for Health Statistics in collaboration with the
National Center for Chronic Disease Prevention and Health Promotion (2000).
Available at http://www.cdc.gov/growthcharts

CDC Growth Charts: United States

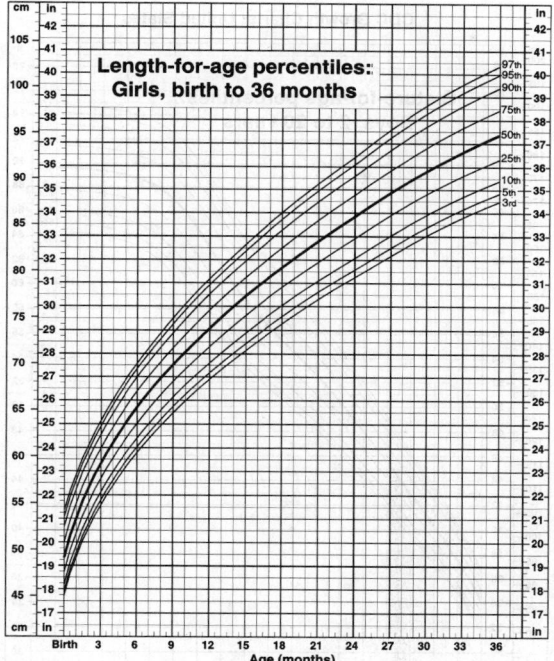

Length-for-age percentiles: Girls, birth to 36 months

SOURCE: Developed by the National Center for Health Statistics in collaboration with the National Center for Chronic Disease Prevention and Health Promotion (2000).
Available at http://www.cdc.gov/growthcharts

GROWTH CHARTS *(Continued)*

CDC Growth Charts: United States

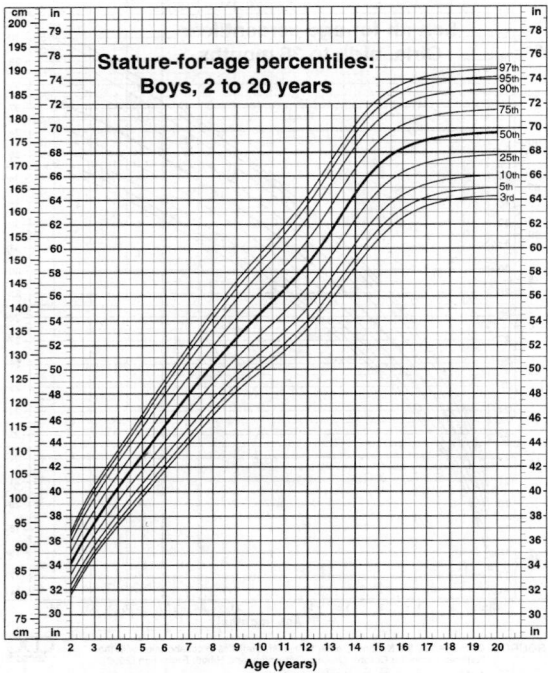

Stature-for-age percentiles:
Boys, 2 to 20 years

SOURCE: Developed by the National Center for Health Statistics in collaboration with the National Center for Chronic Disease Prevention and Health Promotion (2000).
Available at http://www.cdc.gov/growthcharts

CDC Growth Charts: United States

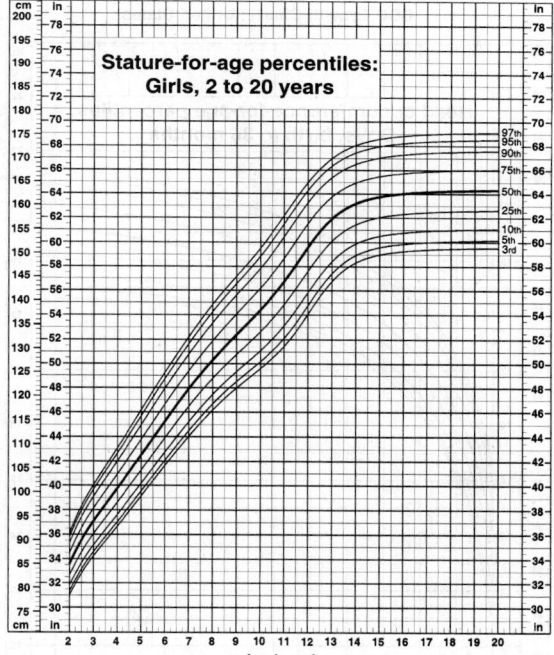

Stature-for-age percentiles: Girls, 2 to 20 years

SOURCE: Developed by the National Center for Health Statistics in collaboration with the National Center for Chronic Disease Prevention and Health Promotion (2000).
Available at http://www.cdc.gov/growthcharts

GROWTH CHARTS *(Continued)*

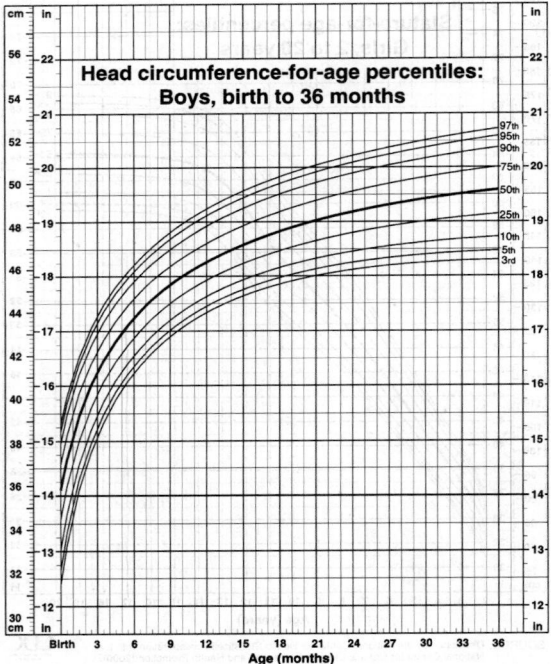

CDC Growth Charts: United States

Head circumference-for-age percentiles:
Boys, birth to 36 months

SOURCE: Developed by the National Center for Health Statistics in collaboration with the
National Center for Chronic Disease Prevention and Health Promotion (2000).
Available at http://www.cdc.gov/growthcharts

CDC

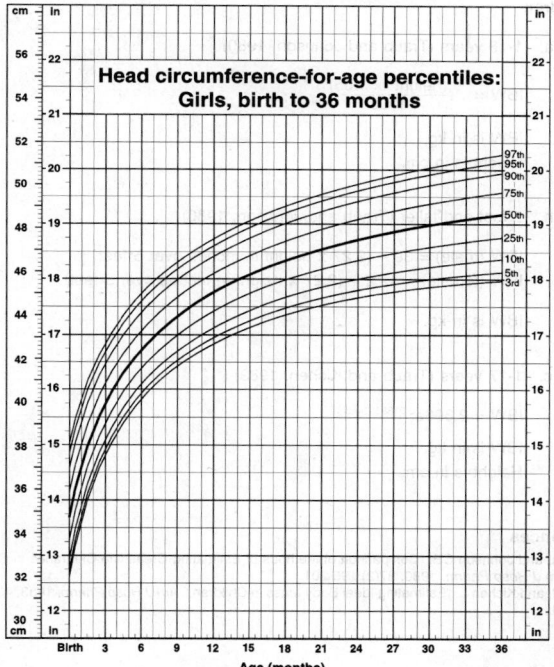

CDC Growth Charts: United States

Head circumference-for-age percentiles: Girls, birth to 36 months

SOURCE: Developed by the National Center for Health Statistics in collaboration with the National Center for Chronic Disease Prevention and Health Promotion (2000).
Available at http://www.cdc.gov/growthcharts

IDEAL BODY WEIGHT CALCULATION

Adults (18 years and older)

IBW (male) = 50 + (2.3 x height in inches over 5 feet)
IBW (female) = 45.5 + (2.3 x height in inches over 5 feet)

IBW is in kg.

Children

a. 1-18 years (Traub and Johnson, 1980)

$$IBW = \frac{(height^2 \times 1.65)}{1000}$$

IBW is in kg.
Height is in cm.

b. 5 feet and taller (Traub and Johnson, 1980)

IBW (male) = 39 + (2.27 x height in inches over 5 feet)
IBW (female) = 42.2 + (2.27 x height in inches over 5 feet)

IBW is in kg.

c. 1-17 years (Traub and Kichen, 1983)

$$IBW = 2.396e^{0.01883 \, (height)}$$

IBW is in kg.
Height is in cm.

References

Traub SL and Johnson CE, "Comparison of Methods of Estimating Creatinine Clearance in Children," *Am J Hosp Pharm*, 1980, 37(2):195-201.
Traub SL and Kichen L, "Estimating Ideal Body Mass in Children," *Am J Hosp Pharm*, 1983, 40(1):107-10.

BODY SURFACE AREA OF CHILDREN AND ADULTS

Calculating Body Surface Area in Children

In a child of average size, find weight and corresponding surface area on the boxed scale to the left; or, use the nomogram to the right. Lay a straightedge on the correct height and weight points for the child, then read the intersecting point on the surface area scale.

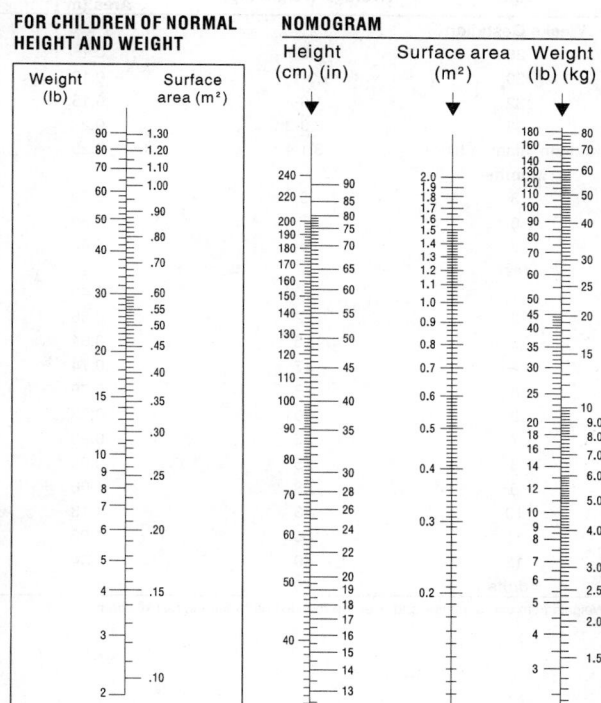

FOR CHILDREN OF NORMAL HEIGHT AND WEIGHT

NOMOGRAM

BODY SURFACE AREA FORMULA
(Adult and Pediatric)

$$\text{BSA (m}^2) = \sqrt{\frac{\text{Ht (in) x Wt (lb)}}{3131}} \quad \text{or, in metric: BSA (m}^2) = \sqrt{\frac{\text{Ht (cm) x Wt (kg)}}{3600}}$$

References

Lam TK and Leung DT, "More on Simplified Calculation of Body Surface Area," *N Engl J Med*, 1988, 318(17):1130 (Letter).

Mosteller RD, "Simplified Calculation of Body Surface Area", *N Engl J Med*, 1987, 317(17):1098 (Letter).

AVERAGE WEIGHTS AND SURFACE AREAS

Average Weight and Surface Area of Preterm Infants, Term Infants, and Children

Age	Average Weight (kg)*	Approximate Surface Area (m²)
Weeks Gestation		
26	0.9-1	0.1
30	1.3-1.5	0.12
32	1.6-2	0.15
38	2.9-3	0.2
40 (term infant at birth)	3.1-4	0.25
Months		
3	5	0.29
6	7	0.38
9	8	0.42
Year		
1	10	0.49
2	12	0.55
3	15	0.64
4	17	0.74
5	18	0.76
6	20	0.82
7	23	0.90
8	25	0.95
9	28	1.06
10	33	1.18
11	35	1.23
12	40	1.34
Adults	70	1.73

*Weights from age 3 months and over are rounded off to the nearest kilogram.

PHYSICAL DEVELOPMENT

Weight gain first 6 weeks

20 g/day

Birth weight

regained by day 14

doubles by age 4 mo

triples by age 12 mo

quadruples by age 2 y

Teeth

1st tooth 6-18 mo

teeth = age (mo) − 6
(until 30 mo)

Head circumference

35 cm at birth

44 cm by 6 mo

47 cm by 1 y

1 cm/mo for 1st y

3 cm/mo 2nd y

Length

increases 50% by age 1 y

doubles by age 4 y

triples by age 13 y

Tanner Stages of Sexual Development

Stage	Characteristics	Age at onset (mean ± SD)
Genital stages: Male		
1	Prepubertal	
2	Scrotum and testes enlarge; skin of scrotum reddens and rugations appear	11.4 ± 1.1 y
3	Penis lengthens; testes enlarge further	12.9 ± 1 y
4	Penis growth continues in length and width; glans develops adult form	13.8 ± 1 y
5	Development completed; adult appearance	14.9 ± 1.1 y
Breast development: Female		
1	Prepubertal	
2	Breast buds appear; areolae enlarge	11.2 ± 1.1 y
3	Elevation of breast contour; areolae enlarge	12.2 ± 1.1 y
4	Areolae and papilla form a secondary mound on breast	13.1 ± 1.2 y
5	Adult form	15.3 ± 1.7 y
Menarche		13.5 ± 1 y
Pubic hair: Both sexes		
1	Prepubertal, no coarse hair	
2	Longer, silky hair appears at base of penis or along labia	F: 11.7 ± 1.2 y M: 12 ± 1 y
3	Hair coarse, kinky, spreads over pubic bone	F: 12.4 ± 1.1 y M: 13.9 ± 1 y
4	Hair of adult quality but not spread to junction of medial thigh with perineum	F: 13 ± 1 y M: 14.4 ± 1.1 y
5	Spread to medial thigh	F: 14.4 ± 1.1 y M: 15.2 ± 1.1 y
6	"Male escutcheon"	Variable if occurs

Maximum growth rate

Male at 14.1±0.9 y

Female at 12.1±0.9 y

EMETOGENIC POTENTIAL OF SINGLE CHEMOTHERAPEUTIC AGENTS

Class I — Low (<10%)

Asparaginase/Pegaspargase
Bleomycin
Busulfan
Chlorambucil (oral)
Cladribine
Corticosteroids
Cyclophosphamide (oral)
Fludarabine

Hydroxyurea
Melphalan (oral)
Mercaptopurine
Methotrexate <50 mg/m^2
Thioguanine (oral)
Vinblastine
Vincristine

Class II — Moderately Low (10% to 30%)

Cytarabine <500 mg/m^2
Doxorubicin ≤20 mg/m^2
Etoposide
Fluorouracil <1000 mg/m^2
Gemcitabine
Interferon-beta

Lomustine
Methotrexate ≥50-250 mg/m^2
Mitomycin <8 mg/m^2
Paclitaxel
Raltitrexed
Thiotepa

Class III — Moderate (30% to 60%)

Amsacrine
Azacitidine
Cyclophosphamide <750 mg/m^2
Cytarabine 500-1000 mg/m^2
Daunorubicin
Docetaxel
Doxorubicin >20 mg to <60 mg/m^2
Epirubicin
Fluorouracil ≥1000 mg/m^2
Idarubicin

Ifosfamide
Irinotecan
Methotrexate >250 mg/m^2 to ≤1000 mg/m^2
Mitomycin ≥8 mg/m^2
Mitoxantrone
Teniposide
Topotecan
Tretinoin
Vinorelbine

Class IV — Moderately High (60% to 90%)

Actinomycin D
Aldesleukin
Carboplatin 200-400 mg/m^2
Carmustine <250 mg
Cisplatin <50 mg/m^2
Cyclophosphamide 750-1500 mg/m^2

Cytarabine >1000 mg/m^2
Dacarbazine <500 mg/m^2
Doxorubicin ≥60 mg/m^2
Melphalan 20-80 mg/m^2
Methotrexate >1000 mg/m^2
Procarbazine (oral)

Class V — High (>90%)

Busulfan (as part of BMT regimen)
Carboplatin >500 mg/m^2
Carmustine ≥250 mg/m^2
Cisplatin ≥50 mg/m^2
Cyclophosphamide ≥1500 mg/m^2

Dacarbazine ≥500 mg/m^2
Mechlorethamine
Melphalan >80 mg/m^2
Pentostatin

COMPATIBILITY OF CHEMOTHERAPY AND RELATED SUPPORTIVE CARE MEDICATIONS

Compatible: The drugs are physically compatible when mixed in the same container or infused through the same I.V. line simultaneously.

Y-site compatible: The drugs are physically compatible when infused through the same I.V. line simultaneously.

Incompatible: The drugs are physically incompatible when mixed in the same container, or infused through the same I.V. line simultaneously.

Variable compatibility: The compatibility of the drugs varies according to the concentration and/or diluent of the drugs. Please refer to the table at the end of this section for more information on variable compatibility.

Abbreviations

AA	Amino acid solution
BNS	Bacteriostatic normal saline
BWI	Bacteriostatic water for injection
D_5W	5% dextrose in water
D_5/NS	5% dextrose in 0.9% sodium chloride
$D_5/^1/_4NS$	5% dextrose in 0.225% sodium chloride
$D_5/^1/_2NS$	5% dextrose in 0.45% sodium chloride
D_5LR	5% dextrose in lactated Ringer's injection
$D_{10}W$	10% dextrose in water
$D_{10}W/0.01\%$ albumin	10% dextrose in water with 0.01% albumin
$D_{10}W/0.05\%$ albumin	10% dextrose in water with 0.05% albumin
$D_{10}W/0.1\%$ albumin	10% dextrose in water with 0.1% albumin
D_{10}/NS	10% dextrose in water in 0.9% sodium chloride
LR	Lactated Ringer's injection
NS	0.9% sodium chloride (normal saline)
SWI	Sterile water for injection
TPN	Total parenteral nutrition solution

COMPATIBILITY OF CHEMOTHERAPY AND RELATED SUPPORTIVE CARE MEDICATIONS *(Continued)*

Reported Compatibilities and Incompatibilities of Parenteral Dosage Forms

Aldesleukin

Compatible:

D_5W SWI

Y-Site Compatible:

Amikacin	Fluconazole	Ondansetron
Amphotericin	Foscarnet	Piperacillin
Calcium gluconate	Gentamicin	Potassium chloride
Cotrimoxazole	Heparin	Ranitidine
Diphenhydramine	Magnesium sulfate	Thiethylperazine
Dopamine	Metoclopramide	Ticarcillin
Fat emulsion	Morphine	Tobramycin

Incompatible:

Ganciclovir	Pentamidine	Promethazine
Heparin	Prochlorperazine	

Amifostine

Compatible:

NS

Y-Site Compatible:

Amikacin	Diphenhydramine	Mannitol
Aminophylline	Dobutamine	Mechlorethamine
Ampicillin	Dopamine	Meperidine
Ampicillin/sulbactam	Doxorubicin	Mesna
Aztreonam	Doxycycline	Methotrexate
Bleomycin	Droperidol	Methylprednisolone
Bumetanide	Enalaprilat	Metoclopramide
Buprenorphine	Etoposide	Metronidazole
Butorphanol	Famotidine	Mezlocillin
Calcium gluconate	Floxuridine	Mitomycin
Carboplatin	Fluconazole	Mitoxantrone
Carmustine	Fludarabine	Morphine
Cefamandole	Fluorouracil	Nalbuphine
Cefepime	Furosemide	Netilmicin
Cefotaxime	Gallium nitrate	Ondansetron
Cefotetan	Gemcitabine	Piperacillin
Cefoxitin	Gentamicin	Plicamycin
Ceftazidime	Granisetron	Potassium chloride
Ceftizoxime	Haloperidol	Promethazine
Ceftriaxone	Heparin	Ranitidine
Cefuroxime	Hydrocortisone sodium phosphate	Sodium bicarbonate
Cimetidine	Hydrocortisone sodium succinate	Streptozocin
Ciprofloxacin		Teniposide
Clindamycin	Hydromorphone	Thiotepa
Cotrimoxazole	Idarubicin	Ticarcillin
Cyclophosphamide	Ifosfamide	Ticarcillin/clavulanate
Cytarabine	Imipenem/cilastatin	Tobramycin
Dacarbazine	Leucovorin	Trimetrexate
Dactinomycin	Lorazepam	Vancomycin
Daunomycin	Magnesium sulfate	Vinblastine
Dexamethasone		Vincristine

Incompatible:

Acyclovir	Cisplatin	Minocycline
Amphotericin	Ganciclovir	Prochlorperazine
Chlorpromazine	Hydroxyzine	

Asparaginase

Compatible:

D$_5$W	NS	SWI

Y-Site Compatible:

Methotrexate	Sodium bicarbonate

Bleomycin

Compatible:

BNS	Dexamethasone	Leucovorin
BWI	Diphenhydramine	Metoclopramide
SWI	Droperidol	Phenytoin
Amikacin	Fluorouracil	Streptomycin
Amsacrine	Furosemide	Tobramycin
Ceftazidime	Gentamicin	Vinblastine
Cephapirin	Heparin	Vincristine
Cimetidine	Hydrocortisone sodium	
Dacarbazine	phosphate	

Y-Site Compatible:

Allopurinol	Doxorubicin, liposomal	Paclitaxel
Amifostine	Filgrastim	Piperacillin
Aztreonam	Fludarabine	Sargramostim
Cefepime	Gemcitabine	Teniposide
Cisplatin	Methotrexate	Thiotepa
Cyclophosphamide	Mitomycin	Vinorelbine
Doxorubicin	Ondansetron	

Incompatible:

Aminophylline	Diazepam	Nafcillin
Ascorbic acid	Doxapram	Penicillin G
Cefazolin	Hydrocortisone sodium	Terbutaline
Cephalothin	succinate	

Variable Compatibility:

D$_5$W	NS

Busulfan

Compatible:

D$_5$W	NS

Carboplatin

Compatible:

D$_5$W	Etoposide	Ifosfamide
SWI	Floxuridine	

Y-Site Compatible:

Allopurinol	Fludarabine	Propofol
Amifostine	Gemcitabine	Sargramostim
Aztreonam	Granisetron	Teniposide
Cefazolin	Ondansetron	Thiotepa
Doxorubicin, liposomal	Piperacillin	TPN
Filgrastim	Piperacillin/tazobactam	Vinorelbine

Incompatible:

Fluorouracil	Mesna	Sodium bicarbonate

Variable Compatibility:

D$_5$/NS	D$_5$/^{1}/$_2$NS	NS
D$_5$/^{1}/$_4$NS		

COMPATIBILITY OF CHEMOTHERAPY AND RELATED SUPPORTIVE CARE MEDICATIONS *(Continued)*

Carmustine

Compatible:
D_5W	SWI	Dacarbazine
NS		

Y-Site Compatible:
Amifostine	Gemcitabine	Sargramostim
Aztreonam	Ondansetron	Teniposide
Cefepime	Piperacillin	Thiotepa
Filgrastim	Piperacillin/tazobactam	Vinorelbine
Fludarabine		

Incompatible:
Allopurinol	Sodium bicarbonate	

Cisplatin

Compatible:
D_5/NS	Cephalothin	Ifosfamide
D_5/^{1}/$_4$NS	Cyclophosphamide	Leucovorin
D_5/^{1}/$_2$NS	Floxuridine	Mannitol
NS	Hydroxyzine	Mechlorethamine
Cefazolin	Hydroxyurea	Ondansetron

Y-Site Compatible:
Allopurinol	Filgrastim	Mitomycin
Aztreonam	Fludarabine	Morphine
Bleomycin	Fluorouracil	Paclitaxel
Bumetanide	Furosemide	Potassium chloride
Chlorpromazine	Ganciclovir	Prochlorperazine
Cimetidine	Gemcitabine	Promethazine
Dexamethasone	Granisetron	Propofol
Diphenhydramine	Heparin	Ranitidine
Doxapram	Hydromorphone	Sargramostim
Doxorubicin	Lorazepam	Teniposide
Doxorubicin, liposomal	Methotrexate	Thiotepa
Droperidol	Methylprednisolone	Vinorelbine
Famotidine	Metoclopramide	

Incompatible:
Amifostine	Gallium nitrate	Piperacillin
Amsacrine	Mesna	Piperacillin/tazobactam
Cefepime	Oxacillin	Sodium bicarbonate

Variable Compatibility:
D_5W	SWI	Etoposide

Cladribine

Compatible:
NS

Cyclophosphamide

Compatible:
D_5W	AA 4.25%/$D_{25}W$	Hydroxyzine
D_5/NS	Cisplatin	Mesna
D_5/LR	Dacarbazine	Methotrexate
NS	Etoposide	Mitoxantrone
LR	Fluorouracil	Ondansetron
SWI		

Y-Site Compatible:
Allopurinol	Cephalothin	Erythromycin
Amifostine	Cephapirin	Famotidine
Amikacin	Chloramphenicol	Filgrastim
Ampicillin	Chlorpromazine	Fludarabine
Azlocillin	Cimetidine	Furosemide
Aztreonam	Clindamycin	Gallium nitrate
Bleomycin	Cotrimoxazole	Ganciclovir
Cefamandole	Dexamethasone	Gemcitabine
Cefazolin	Diphenhydramine	Gentamicin
Cefepime	Doxapram	Granisetron
Cefoperazone	Doxorubicin	Heparin
Cefotaxime	Doxorubicin, liposomal	Hydromorphone
Cefoxitin	Doxycycline	Idarubicin
Ceftriaxone	Droperidol	Kanamycin

Leucovorin
Lorazepam
Methylprednisolone
Metoclopramide
Metronidazole
Mezlocillin
Minocycline
Mitomycin
Morphine
Moxalactam
Nafcillin

Oxacillin
Paclitaxel
Penicillin G
Piperacillin
Piperacillin/tazobactam
Prochlorperazine
Promethazine
Propofol
Ranitidine
Sargramostim
Sodium bicarbonate

Teniposide
Thiotepa
Ticarcillin
Ticarcillin/clavulanate
Tobramycin
TPN
Vancomycin
Vinblastine
Vincristine
Vinorelbine

Cytarabine

Compatible:

BNS
BWI
D₅W
D₅/NS
D₅/¼NS
D₅/½NS
D₅/LR
D₁₀/NS

NS
LR
AA 4.25%/D₂₅W
Corticotropin
Dacarbazine
Daunomycin
Etoposide
Hydroxyzine

Hydroxyurea
Lincomycin
Mitoxantrone
Ondansetron
Potassium chloride
Prednisolone
Sodium bicarbonate
Vincristine

Y-Site Compatible:

Amifostine
Amsacrine
Aztreonam
Cefepime
Chlorpromazine
Cimetidine
Dexamethasone
Diphenhydramine
Doxorubicin, liposomal
Droperidol
Famotidine

Filgrastim
Fludarabine
Furosemide
Gemcitabine
Granisetron
Heparin
Idarubicin
Lorazepam
Metoclopramide
Morphine
Paclitaxel

Piperacillin
Piperacillin/tazobactam
Prochlorperazine
Promethazine
Propofol
Ranitidine
Sargramostim
Teniposide
Thiotepa
TPN
Vinorelbine

Incompatible:

Allopurinol
Ceftazidime
Fluorouracil

Gallium nitrate
Ganciclovir
Insulin

Nafcillin
Oxacillin
Penicillin G

Variable Compatibility:

Cephalothin
Gentamicin

Hydrocortisone sodium
phosphate

Methylprednisolone

Dacarbazine

Compatible:

NS
SWI
Bleomycin
Carmustine
Cimetidine

Cyclophosphamide
Cytarabine
Dactinomycin
Doxorubicin
Fluorouracil

Mercaptopurine
Methotrexate
Ondansetron
Vinblastine

Y-Site Compatible:

Amifostine
Aztreonam
Doxorubicin, liposomal
Filgrastim
Fludarabine

Granisetron
Hydrocortisone sodium
phosphate
Lidocaine
Paclitaxel

Sargramostim
Teniposide
Thiotepa
Vinorelbine

Incompatible:

D₅W
Allopurinol
Cefepime

Hydrocortisone sodium
succinate

Piperacillin

Piperacillin/tazobactam

Variable Compatibility:

Heparin

Dactinomycin

Compatible:

D₅W
NS

SWI

Dacarbazine

Y-Site Compatible:

Allopurinol
Amifostine
Aztreonam
Cefepime

Fludarabine
Gemcitabine
Ondansetron
Sargramostim

Teniposide
Thiotepa
Vinorelbine

1291

COMPATIBILITY OF CHEMOTHERAPY AND RELATED SUPPORTIVE CARE MEDICATIONS (Continued)

Incompatible:

BNS   BWI   Filgrastim

Daunomycin

Compatible:

D$_5$W	SWI	Hydrocortisone sodium
NS	Cytarabine	succinate
LR	Etoposide	

Y-Site Compatible:

Amifostine	Methotrexate	Teniposide
Filgrastim	Ondansetron	Thiotepa
Gemcitabine	Sodium bicarbonate	Vinorelbine

Incompatible:

Allopurinol	Dexamethasone	Piperacillin
Aztreonam	Fludarabine	Piperacillin/tazobactam
Cefepime		

Dexrazoxane

Compatible:

D$_5$W

Y-Site Compatible:

Gemcitabine

Diphenhydramine

Compatible:

Amikacin	Glycopyrrolate	Penicillin G (sodium and
Aminophylline	Hydrocortisone sodium	potassium)
Ascorbic acid	succinate	Pentazocine
Atropine	Hydromorphone	Perphenazine
Bleomycin	Hydroxyzine	Prochlorperazine
Butorphanol	Lidocaine	Promazine
Cephapirin	Meperidine	Promethazine
Chlorpromazine	Methicillin	Ranitidine
Cimetidine	Methyldopa	Scopolamine
Colistimethate	Metoclopramide	Sufentanil
Dimenhydrinate	Midazolam	Thiothixene
Droperidol	Morphine	Polymyxin B
Erythromycin	Nalbuphine	Vitamin B complex
Fentanyl	Nafcillin	with C
Fluphenazine	Netilmicin	

Y-Site Compatible:

Acyclovir	Filgrastim	Methotrexate
Aldesleukin	Fluconazole	Ondansetron
Amifostine	Fludarabine	Paclitaxel
Amsacrine	Gallium nitrate	Piperacillin/tazobactam
Aztreonam	Gemcitabine	Potassium chloride
Ciprofloxacin	Granisetron	Sargramostim
Cisplatin	Heparin	Tacrolimus
Cyclophosphamide	Idarubicin	Teniposide
Cytarabine	Melphalan	Thiotepa
Doxorubicin	Meperidine	Vinorelbine

Incompatible:

Allopurinol	Cephalothin	Pentobarbital
Amobarbital	Dexamethasone	Secobarbital
Amphotericin	Foscarnet	Thiopental
Cefepime	Haloperidol	

Variable Compatibility:

Diatrizoate	Iodipamide

Docetaxel

Compatible:

D$_5$W	NS

Y-Site Compatible:

Gemcitabine

Incompatible:

Doxorubicin, liposomal

Doxorubicin

Compatible:

D$_5$W	LR	Ondansetron
NS	Dacarbazine	Vincristine

Y-Site Compatible:

Amifostine	Fludarabine	Paclitaxel
Aztreonam	Gemcitabine	Prochlorperazine
Bleomycin	Granisetron	Promethazine
Chlorpromazine	Hydromorphone	Propofol
Cimetidine	Leucovorin	Ranitidine
Cisplatin	Lorazepam	Sargramostim
Cyclophosphamide	Methotrexate	Sodium bicarbonate
Dexamethasone	Methylprednisolone	Teniposide
Diphenhydramine	Metoclopramide	Thiotepa
Famotidine	Mitomycin	Vinorelbine
Filgrastim	Morphine	

Incompatible:

Allopurinol	Gallium nitrate	Piperacillin/tazobactam
Aminophylline	Ganciclovir	TPN
Cefepime	Heparin	Paclitaxel
Cephalothin	Hydrocortisone sodium	
Diazepam	succinate	Tobramycin
Furosemide		

Variable Compatibility:

Fluorouracil	Vinblastine

Doxorubicin, Liposomal

Compatible:

D$_5$W

Y-Site Compatible:

Allopurinol	Dacarbazine	Leucovorin
Aldesleukin	Dexamethasone	Lorazepam
Aminophylline	Diphenhydramine	Magnesium sulfate
Ampicillin	Dobutamine	Mesna
Aztreonam	Dopamine	Methotrexate
Bleomycin	Droperidol	Methylprednisolone
Calcium chloride	Enalaprilat	Metronidazole
Calcium gluconate	Etoposide	Mezlocillin
Cefazolin	Famotidine	Netilmicin
Cefepime	Fluconazole	Ondansetron
Cefoperazone	Fluorouracil	Piperacillin
Cefoxitin	Furosemide	Potassium chloride
Ceftizoxime	Ganciclovir	Prochlorperazine
Ceftriaxone	Gentamicin	Ranitidine
Chlorpromazine	Granisetron	Ticarcillin
Cimetidine	Haloperidol	Ticarcillin/clavulanate
Ciprofloxacin	Heparin	Tobramycin
Cisplatin	Hydrocortisone sodium	Vancomycin
Clindamycin	succinate	Vinblastine
Cotrimoxazole	Hydromorphone	Vincristine
Cyclophosphamide	Ifosfamide	Vinorelbine
Cytarabine		

COMPATIBILITY OF CHEMOTHERAPY AND RELATED SUPPORTIVE CARE MEDICATIONS *(Continued)*

Incompatible:

Amphotericin	Mannitol	Morphine
Buprenorphine	Meperidine	Ofloxacin
Ceftazidime	Metoclopramide	Piperacillin/tazobactam
Docetaxel	Miconazole	Promethazine
Gallium nitrate	Mitoxantrone	Sodium bicarbonate
Hydroxyzine		

Droperidol

Compatible:

Atropine	Doxorubicin	Nalbuphine
Bleomycin	Fentanyl	Pentazocine
Butorphanol	Glycopyrrolate	Perphenazine
Chlorpromazine	Hydroxyzine	Prochlorperazine
Cimetidine	Meperidine	Promazine
Cisplatin	Metoclopramide	Promethazine
Cyclophosphamide	Midazolam	Scopolamine
Dimenhydrinate	Mitomycin	Vinblastine
Diphenhydramine	Morphine	Vincristine

Y-Site Compatible:

Amifostine	Idarubicin	Teniposide
Aztreonam	Melphalan	Thiotepa
Filgrastim	Ondansetron	Vinorelbine
Fluconazole	Paclitaxel	Vitamin B complex
Fludarabine		with C
Gemcitabine	Potassium chloride	
Hydrocortisone sodium	Sargramostim	
succinate		

Incompatible:

Allopurinol	Furosemide	Nafcillin
Cefepime	Heparin	Pentobarbital
Fluorouracil	Leucovorin	Piperacillin/tazobactam
Foscarnet	Methotrexate	

Erythropoietin

Compatible:

BNS	D_{10}/0.05% albumin	D_{10}/0.1% albumin

Incompatible:

D_{10}W	NS	SWI
D_{10}/0.01% albumin		

Etoposide

Compatible:

D_5W	Cyclophosphamide	Fluorouracil
NS	Cytarabine	Hydroxyzine
LR	Daunomycin	Ifosfamide
Carboplatin	Floxuridine	Ondansetron

Y-Site Compatible:

Allopurinol	Granisetron	Piperacillin/tazobactam
Amifostine	Haloperidol	Sargramostim
Aztreonam	Methotrexate	Sodium bicarbonate
Doxorubicin, liposomal	Paclitaxel	Teniposide
Fludarabine	Piperacillin	Vinorelbine
Gemcitabine		

Incompatible:

Cefoperazone	Cefepime	Gallium nitrate
Ceftazidime	Filgrastim	Idarubicin

Variable Compatibility:

Cisplatin	Mannitol	Potassium chloride

Filgrastim

Compatible:
  D₅W   SWI

Y-Site Compatible:

Acyclovir	Dexamethasone	Mechlorethamine
Allopurinol	Diphenhydramine	Meperidine
Amikacin	Doxorubicin	Mesna
Aminophylline	Doxycycline	Methotrexate
Ampicillin	Droperidol	Metoclopramide
Ampicillin/sulbactam	Enalaprilat	Miconazole
Aztreonam	Fat emulsion	Minocycline
Bleomycin	Floxuridine	Mitoxantrone
Bumetanide	Fluconazole	Morphine
Buprenorphine	Fludarabine	Nalbuphine
Butorphanol	Gallium nitrate	Netilmicin
Calcium gluconate	Ganciclovir	Ondansetron
Carboplatin	Gentamicin	Plicamycin
Carmustine	Haloperidol	Potassium chloride
Cefazolin	Hydrocortisone sodium	Promethazine
Cefotetan	phosphate	Ranitidine
Ceftazidime	Hydrocortisone sodium	Sodium bicarbonate
Chlorpromazine	succinate	Streptozocin
Cimetidine	Hydromorphone	Ticarcillin
Cisplatin	Hydroxyzine	Ticarcillin/clavulanate
Cotrimoxazole	Idarubicin	Tobramycin
Cyclophosphamide	Ifosfamide	Vancomycin
Cytarabine	Imipenem/cilastatin	Vinblastine
Dacarbazine	Leucovorin	Vincristine
Daunomycin	Lorazepam	Vinorelbine

Incompatible:

NS	Ceftizoxime	Mannitol
Amphotericin	Ceftriaxone	Methylprednisolone
Amsacrine	Cefuroxime	Metronidazole
Cefepime	Dactinomycin	Mezlocillin
Cefonicid	Etoposide	Mitomycin
Cefoperazone	Fluorouracil	Piperacillin
Cefotaxime	Furosemide	Prochlorperazine
Cefoxitin	Heparin	Thiotepa

Floxuridine

Compatible:

D₅W	Carboplatin	Fluorouracil
NS	Cisplatin	Heparin
SWI	Etoposide	Leucovorin

Y-Site Compatible:

Amifostine	Gemcitabine	Sargramostim
Aztreonam	Ondansetron	Teniposide
Filgrastim	Paclitaxel	Thiotepa
Fludarabine	Piperacillin/tazobactam	Vinorelbine

Incompatible:
  Allopurinol   Cefepime

Fludarabine

Compatible:
  D₅W   NS   SWI

Y-Site Compatible:

Allopurinol	Ceftriaxone	Fluorouracil
Amifostine	Cefuroxime	Furosemide
Amikacin	Cimetidine	Gemcitabine
Aminophylline	Cisplatin	Gentamicin
Ampicillin	Cotrimoxazole	Haloperidol
Ampicillin/sulbactam	Cyclophosphamide	Heparin
Amsacrine	Cytarabine	Hydrocortisone sodium
Aztreonam	Dacarbazine	phosphate
Bleomycin	Dactinomycin	Hydrocortisone sodium
Butorphanol	Dexamethasone	succinate
Carboplatin	Diphenhydramine	Hydromorphone
Carmustine	Doxorubicin	Ifosfamide
Cefazolin	Doxycycline	Imipenem/cilastatin
Cefepime	Droperidol	Lorazepam
Cefoperazone	Etoposide	Magnesium sulfate
Cefotaxime	Famotidine	Mannitol
Cefotetan	Filgrastim	Mechlorethamine
Ceftazidime	Floxuridine	Meperidine
Ceftizoxime	Fluconazole	Mesna

COMPATIBILITY OF CHEMOTHERAPY AND RELATED SUPPORTIVE CARE MEDICATIONS *(Continued)*

Methotrexate
Methylprednisolone
Metoclopramide
Mezlocillin
Minocycline
Mitoxantrone
Morphine
Multivitamins
Nalbuphine

Netilmicin
Ondansetron
Pentostatin
Piperacillin
Piperacillin/tazobactam
Potassium chloride
Promethazine
Ranitidine
Sodium bicarbonate

Teniposide
Tetracycline
Ticarcillin
Ticarcillin/clavulanate
Tobramycin
Vancomycin
Vinblastine
Vincristine
Vinorelbine

Incompatible:
Acyclovir
Amphotericin
Chlorpromazine

Daunomycin
Ganciclovir
Hydroxyzine

Miconazole

Prochlorperazine

Fluorouracil

Compatible:
D₅W
D₅/LR
NS
Bleomycin
Cephalothin

Cyclophosphamide
Dacarbazine
Etoposide
Floxuridine
Ifosfamide

Magnesium sulfate
Methotrexate
Mitoxantrone
Prednisolone
Vincristine

Y-Site Compatible:
Allopurinol
Amifostine
Aztreonam
Cefepime
Cisplatin
Doxorubicin, liposomal
Fludarabine
Furosemide
Gemcitabine

Granisetron
Heparin
Hydrocortisone sodium
    succinate
Mannitol
Metoclopramide
Mitomycin
Paclitaxel
Piperacillin

Piperacillin/tazobactam
Potassium chloride
Propofol
Sargramostim
Teniposide
Thiotepa
Vinblastine
Vitamin B complex

Incompatible:
Carboplatin
Cytarabine
Diazepam
Droperidol

Epirubicin
Filgrastim
Gallium nitrate

Ondansetron
TPN
Vinorelbine

Variable Compatibility:
Doxorubicin

Leucovorin

Gemcitabine

Compatible:
NS

Y-Site Compatible:
Amifostine
Amikacin
Aminophylline
Ampicillin
Ampicillin/sulbactam
Aztreonam
Bleomycin
Bumetanide
Buprenorphine
Butorphanol
Calcium gluconate
Carboplatin
Carmustine
Cefazolin
Cefonicid
Cefotetan
Cefoxitin
Ceftazidime
Ceftizoxime
Ceftriaxone
Cefuroxime
Chlorpromazine
Cimetidine
Ciprofloxacin
Cisplatin
Clindamycin
Cyclophosphamide
Cytarabine
Dactinomycin

Daunomycin
Dexamethasone
Dexrazoxane
Diphenhydramine
Dobutamine
Docetaxel
Dopamine
Doxorubicin
Doxycycline
Droperidol
Enalaprilat
Etoposide
Etoposide phosphate
Famotidine
Floxuridine
Fludarabine
Fluorouracil
Fluconazole
Gallium nitrate
Gentamicin
Granisetron
Haloperidol
Heparin
Hydrocortisone sodium
    phosphate
Hydrocortisone sodium
    succinate
Hydromorphone
Hydroxyzine

Idarubicin
Ifosfamide
Leucovorin
Lorazepam
Mannitol
Meperidine
Mesna
Metoclopramide
Metronidazole
Miconazole
Minocycline
Mitoxantrone
Morphine
Nalbuphine
Netilmicin
Ofloxacin
Ondansetron
Paclitaxel
Plicamycin
Potassium chloride
Promethazine
Ranitidine
Sodium bicarbonate
Streptozocin
Teniposide
Thiotepa
Ticarcillin
Ticarcillin/clavulanate
Tobramycin

Topotecan	Vinblastine	Vinorelbine
Trimethoprim	Vincristine	Zidovudine
Vancomycin		

Incompatible:

Acyclovir	Ganciclovir	Mezlocillin
Amphotericin	Imipenem/cilastatin	Mitomycin
Cefoperazone	Irinotecan	Piperacillin
Cefotaxime	Methotrexate	Piperacillin/tazobactam
Furosemide	Methylprednisolone	Prochlorperazine

Haloperidol

Compatible:

| Hydromorphone | Sufentanil | |

Y-Site Compatible:

Amifostine	Gemcitabine	Paclitaxel
Amsacrine	Lidocaine	Phenylephrine
Aztreonam	Lorazepam	Tacrolimus
Cimetidine	Melphalan	Teniposide
Dobutamine	Midazolam	Theophylline
Dopamine	Nitroglycerin	Thiotepa
Famotidine	Norepinephrine bitar-	TPN
Filgrastim	trate	Vinorelbine
Fludarabine	Ondansetron	

Incompatible:

Allopurinol	Foscarnet	Ketorolac
Cefepime	Gallium nitrate	Piperacillin/tazobactam
Diphenhydramine	Heparin	Sargramostim
Fluconazole	Hydroxyzine	

Variable Compatibility:

| Benztropine | Diamorphine | Sodium nitroprusside |
| Cyclizine | | |

Heparin

Compatible:

Aminophylline	Dopamine	Metronidazole
Amphotericin	Enalaprilat	Nafcillin
Ascorbic acid	Erythromycin	Norepinephrine
Bleomycin	Esmolol	Octreotide
Calcium gluconate	Floxacillin	Potassium chloride
Cefepime	Fluconazole	Prednisolone
Cephapirin	Flumazenil	Promazine
Chloramphenicol	Furosemide	Ranitidine
Cibenzoline	Isoproterenol	Sodium bicarbonate
Clindamycin	Lidocaine	Verapamil
Cloxacillin	Lincomycin	Vitamin B complex
Colistimethate	Methyldopate	with C
Dimenhydrinate	Methylprednisolone	

Y-Site Compatible:

Acyclovir	Esmolol	Minocycline
Aldesleukin	Estrogens, conjugated	Mitomycin
Allopurinol	Ethacrynate	Morphine
Amifostine	Famotidine	Neostigmine
Ampicillin	Fentanyl	Nitroglycerin
Ampicillin/sulbactam	Fludarabine	Ondansetron
Atracurium	Fluorouracil	Oxacillin
Atropine	Foscarnet	Oxytocin
Aztreonam	Gallium nitrate	Paclitaxel
Betamethasone sodium	Gemcitabine	Pancuronium
phosphate	Hydralazine	Penicillin G potassium
Cefazolin	Hydrocortisone sodium	Pentazocine
Cefotetan	succinate	Phytonadione
Ceftazidime	Insulin	Piperacillin
Ceftriaxone	Kanamycin	Piperacillin/tazobactam
Cephalothin	Leucovorin	Procainamide
Chlordiazepoxide	Lorazepam	Prochlorperazine
Chlorpromazine	Magnesium sulfate	Propranolol
Cimetidine	Melphalan	Pyridostigmine
Cisplatin	Menadiol sodium	Sargramostim
Cyanocobalamin	diphosphate	Scopolamine
Cyclophosphamide	Methicillin	Sodium nitroprusside
Cytarabine	Methotrexate	Streptokinase
Digoxin	Methoxamine	Succinylcholine
Diphenhydramine	Methyldopate	Tacrolimus
Edrophonium	Metoclopramide	Teniposide
Epinephrine	Metronidazole	Theophylline
Erythromycin	Midazolam	Thiotepa

COMPATIBILITY OF CHEMOTHERAPY AND RELATED SUPPORTIVE CARE MEDICATIONS *(Continued)*

Ticarcillin	Trimethaphan	Vincristine
Ticarcillin/clavulanate	Vercuronium	Vinorelbine
TPN	Vinblastine	ZIdovudine
Trimethobenzamide		

Incompatible:

Alteplase	Doxorubicin	Levorphanol
Amikacin	Doxycycline	Methadone
Amiodarone	Ergotamine	Methotrimeprazine
Amsacrine	Filgrastim	Phenytoin
Ciprofloxacin	Gentamicin	Polymyxin B
Codeine phosphate	Haloperidol	Streptomycin
Daunomycin	Hyaluronidase	Tobramycin
Diazepam	Idarubicin	Triflupromazine
Dobutamine	Labetatol	

Variable Compatibility:

Cephalothin	Hydrocortisone sodium	Promethazine
Dacarbazine	succinate	Quinidine gluconate
Diltiazem	Methylprednisolone	Vancomycin
Droperidol	Penicillin G sodium	

Hydroxyzine

Compatible:

Atropine	Etoposide	Pentazocine
Benzquinamide	Fentanyl	Mesna
Bupivacaine	Fluphenazine	Methotrexate
Butorphanol	Glycopyrrolate	Nafcillin
Chlorpromazine	Hydromorphone	Perphenazine
Cimetidine	Lidocaine	Procaine
Cisplatin	Meperidine	Prochlorperazine
Codeine	Methotrimeprazine	Promazine
Cyclophosphamide	Metoclopramide	Promethazine
Cytarabine	Midazolam	Scopolamine
Diphenhydramine	Morphine	Sufentanil
Doxapram	Nalbuphine	Thiothixene
Droperidol	Oxymorphone	

Y-Site Compatible:

Aztreonam	Gemcitabine	Teniposide
Ciprofloxacin	Melphalan	Thiotepa
Filgrastim	Ondansetron	Vinorelbine
Foscarnet	Sufentanil	

Incompatible:

Allopurinol	Fluconazole	Pentobarbital
Amifostine	Fludarabine	Phenobarbital
Aminophylline	Haloperidol	Piperacillin/tazobactam
Amobarbital	Ketorolac	Ranitidine
Cefepime	Paclitaxel	Sargramostim
Chloramphenicol	Penicillin G (sodium and	
Diphenhydramine	potassium)	

Idarubicin

Compatible:

D$_5$W	NS	LR
D$_5$/NS		

Y-Site Compatible:

Amifostine	Droperidol	Metoclopramide
Amikacin	Erythromycin	Potassium chloride
Aztreonam	Filgrastim	Ranitidine
Ciprofloxacin	Gemcitabine	Sargramostim
Cyclophosphamide	Imipenem/cilastatin	Thiotepa
Cytarabine	Magnesium sulfate	Vinorelbine
Diphenhydramine	Mannitol	

Incompatible:

Acyclovir	Furosemide	Methotrexate
Allopurinol	Gentamicin	Mezlocillin
Ampicillin/sulbactam	Heparin	Piperacillin/tazobactam
Cefazolin	Hydrocortisone sodium	Sodium bicarbonate
Cefepime	succinate	Teniposide
Ceftazidime	Lorazepam	Vancomycin
Dexamethasone	Meperidine	Vincristine
Etoposide		

Ifosfamide

Compatible:

D$_5$W	NS	Cisplatin
D$_5$/NS	LR	Etoposide
D$_5$/¼NS	SWI	Fluorouracil
D$_5$/LR	Carboplatin	

Y-Site Compatible:

Allopurinol	Gemcitabine	Sargramostim
Amifostine	Granisetron	Sodium bicarbonate
Aztreonam	Ondansetron	Teniposide
Doxorubicin, liposomal	Paclitaxel	Thiotepa
Filgrastim	Piperacillin	TPN
Fludarabine	Piperacillin/tazobactam	Vinorelbine
Gallium nitrate	Propofol	

Incompatible:

Cefepime	Methotrexate

Variable Compatibility:

Epirubicin	Mesna

Irinotecan

Compatible:
   D$_5$W

Incompatible:
   Gemcitabine

Leucovorin

Compatible:

BWI	NS	Bleomycin
D$_5$W	LR	Cisplatin
D$_{10}$/NS	SWI	Floxuridine

Y-Site Compatible:

Amifostine	Furosemide	Sodium bicarbonate
Aztreonam	Gemcitabine	Tacrolimus
Cefepime	Heparin	Teniposide
Cyclophosphamide	Methotrexate	Thiotepa
Doxorubicin	Metoclopramide	TPN
Doxorubicin, liposomal	Mitomycin	Vinblastine
Filgrastim	Piperacillin	Vincristine
Fluconazole	Piperacillin/tazobactam	

Incompatible:

Droperidol	Foscarnet	Trimetrexate

Variable Compatibility:
   Fluorouracil

Lorazepam

Compatible:

Cimetidine	Hydromorphone

Y-Site Compatible:

Acyclovir	Diltiazem	Melphalan
Albumin	Doxorubicin	Methotrexate
Amifostine	Erythromycin	Metronidazole
Amikacin	Etomidate	Morphine
Amoxicillin	Fentanyl	Paclitaxel
Amoxicillin/clavulanate	Filgrastim	Pancuronium
Amsacrine	Fluconazole	Piperacillin
Atracurium	Fludarabine	Piperacillin/tazobactam
Bumetanide	Furosemide	Potassium chloride
Cefepime	Gemcitabine	Ranitidine
Cefotaxime	Gentamicin	Tacrolimus
Ciprofloxacin	Granisetron	Teniposide
Cisplatin	Haloperidol	Thiotepa
Cotrimoxazole	Heparin	Vancomycin
Cyclophosphamide	Hydrocortisone sodium succinate	Vercuronium
Cytarabine		Vinorelbine
Dexamethasone	Kantaserin	Zidovudine

COMPATIBILITY OF CHEMOTHERAPY AND RELATED SUPPORTIVE CARE MEDICATIONS *(Continued)*

Incompatible:

Aldesleukin	Gallium nitrate	Sargramostim
Aztreonam	Idarubicin	Sufentanil
Buprenorphine	Imipenem/cilastatin	
Floxacillin	Ondansetron	Thiopental

Variable Compatibility:

Foscarnet

Mechlorethamine

Compatible:

NS   SWI

Y-Site Compatible:

Amifostine	Fludarabine	Sargramostim
Aztreonam	Granisetron	Teniposide
Filgrastim	Ondansetron	Vinorelbine

Incompatible:

D₅W	Cefepime	Methohexital
Allopurinol		

Melphalan

Compatible:

NS

Y-Site Compatible:

Acyclovir	Doxycycline	Methotrexate
Amikacin	Droperidol	Methylprednisolone
Aminophylline	Enalaprilat	Metoclopramide
Ampicillin	Etoposide	Metronidazole
Aztreonam	Famotidine	Miconazole
Bleomycin	Filgrastim	Minocycline
Bumetanide	Floxuridine	Mitomycin
Buprenorphine	Fluconazole	Mitoxantrone
Butorphanol	Fludarabine	Morphine
Calcium gluconate	Fluorouracil	Nalbuphine
Carboplatin	Furosemide	Netilmicin
Carmustine	Gallium nitrate	Ondansetron
Cefazolin	Ganciclovir	Pentostatin
Cefepime	Gentamicin	Piperacillin
Cefoperazone	Haloperidol	Plicamycin
Cefotaxime	Heparin	Potassium chloride
Cefotetan	Hydrocortisone sodium	Prochlorperazine
Ceftazidime	phosphate	Promethazine
Ceftriaxone	Hydrocortisone sodium	Ranitidine
Cefuroxime	succinate	Sodium bicarbonate
Cimetidine	Hydromorphone	Streptozocin
Cisplatin	Hydroxyzine	Teniposide
Cotrimoxazole	Idarubicin	Thiotepa
Cyclophosphamide	Ifosfamide	Ticarcillin
Cytarabine	Imipenem/cilastatin	Ticarcillin/clavulanate
Dacarbazine	Lorazepam	Tobramycin
Dactinomycin	Mannitol	Vancomycin
Daunomycin	Mechlorethamine	Vinblastine
Diazepam	Meperidine	Vincristine
Doxorubicin	Mesna	Vinorelbine

Incompatible:

D₅W	SWI	Chlorpromazine
LR	Amphotericin	

Mesna

Compatible:

BWI	LR	Hydroxyzine
D₅W	Cyclophosphamide	Ifosfamide
NS		

Y-Site Compatible:

Allopurinol	Gallium nitrate	Sargramostim
Amifostine	Gemcitabine	Sodium acetate
Aztreonam	Granisetron	Teniposide
Cefepime	Methotrexate	Thiotepa
Doxorubicin, liposomal	Ondansetron	TPN
Filgrastim	Paclitaxel	Vinorelbine
Fludarabine	Piperacillin/tazobactam	

Incompatible:

Carboplatin	Cisplatin	Chlorpromazine

Methadone

Incompatible:

Aminophylline	Phenytoin	Pentobarbital
Ammonium chloride	Heparin	Sodium bicarbonate
Amobarbital	Methicillin	
Chlorothiazide	Nitrofurantoin	Thiopental

Methotrexate

Compatible:

D₅W	Cyclophosphamide	Imipenem/cilastatin
NS	Cytarabine	Mercaptopurine
LR	Dacarbazine	Ondansetron
SWI	Fluorouracil	Sodium bicarbonate
Amino acid 4.25%/D₂₅W	Hydroxyzine	Vincristine
Cephalothin		

Y-Site Compatible:

Allopurinol	Doxorubicin, liposomal	Methylprednisolone
Amifostine	Etoposide	Mitomycin
Asparaginase	Famotidine	Morphine
Aztreonam	Filgrastim	Oxacillin
Bleomycin	Fludarabine	Paclitaxel
Cefepime	Furosemide	Piperacillin/tazobactam
Ceftriaxone	Gallium nitrate	Prochlorperazine
Cimetidine	Ganciclovir	Ranitidine
Cisplatin	Granisetron	Sargramostim
Daunomycin	Heparin	Teniposide
Dexchlorpheniramine	Hydromorphone	Thiotepa
Diphenhydramine	Leucovorin	Vinblastine
Doxapram	Lorazepam	Vindesine
Doxorubicin	Mesna	Vinorelbine

Incompatible:

Dexamethasone	Midazolam	Promethazine
Gemcitabine	Nalbuphine	Propofol
Idarubicin		
Ifosfamide	Prednisolone	TPN

Variable Compatibility:

Droperidol	Metoclopramide	Vancomycin

COMPATIBILITY OF CHEMOTHERAPY AND RELATED SUPPORTIVE CARE MEDICATIONS *(Continued)*

Metoclopramide

Compatible:

D₅W	Multivitamins	Potassium phosphate
NS	Potassium acetate	Verapamil
Clindamycin	Potassium chloride	TPN
Mannitol		

Y-Site Compatible:

Acyclovir	Fluconazole	Morphine
Aldesleukin	Fludarabine	Ondansetron
Amifostine	Fluorouracil	Paclitaxel
Aztreonam	Foscarnet	Piperacillin/tazobactam
Bleomycin	Gallium nitrate	Sargramostim
Ciprofloxacin	Gemcitabine	Sufentanil
Cisplatin	Heparin	Tacrolimus
Cyclophosphamide	Idarubicin	Teniposide
Cytarabine	Leucovorin	Thiotepa
Diltiazem	Melphalan	Vinblastine
Doxorubicin	Meperidine	Vincristine
Droperidol	Methotrexate	Vinorelbine
Famotidine	Mitomycin	Zidovudine
Filgrastim		

Incompatible:

Allopurinol	Cephalothin	Floxacillin
Ampicillin	Chloramphenicol	Furosemide
Calcium gluconate	Dexamethasone	Penicillin G potassium
Cefepime	Erythromycin	Sodium bicarbonate

Metronidazole

Compatible:

Amikacin	Cefuroxime	Heparin
Aminophylline	Cephalothin	Hydrocortisone
Cefazolin	Chloramphenicol	Moxalactam
Cefotaxime	Ciprofloxacin	Multielectrolyte concentrate
Cefotetan	Clindamycin	
Cefoxitin	Disopyramide	Multivitamins
Ceftazidime	Floxacillin	Netilmicin
Ceftizoxime	Fluconazole	Penicillin G potassium
Ceftriaxone	Gentamicin	Tobramycin

Y-Site Compatible:

Acyclovir	Gemcitabine	Perphenazine
Allopurinol	Heparin	Piperacillin/tazobactam
Amifostine	Hydromorphone	Sargramostim
Cefepime	Labetatol	Tacrolimus
Cyclophosphamide	Lorazepam	Teniposide
Diltiazem	Magnesium sulfate	Theophylline
Enalaprilat	Melphalan	Thiotepa
Esmolol	Meperidine	TPN
Fluconazole	Midazolam	Vinorelbine
Foscarnet	Morphine	

Incompatible:

Aztreonam	Dopamine	Filgrastim

Variable Compatibility:

Ampicillin	Cefamandole

Mitomycin

Compatible:
- NS
- LR
- Dexamethasone
- Hydrocortisone sodium succinate

Y-Site Compatible:
- Allopurinol
- Amifostine
- Bleomycin
- Cisplatin
- Cyclophosphamide
- Doxorubicin
- Droperidol
- Fluorouracil
- Furosemide
- Leucovorin
- Methotrexate
- Metoclopramide
- Ondansetron
- Teniposide
- Thiotepa
- Vinblastine
- Vincristine

Incompatible:
- Aztreonam
- Cefepime
- Filgrastim
- Gemcitabine
- Piperacillin/tazobactam
- Sargramostim
- Vinorelbine

Variable Compatibility:
- D_5W
- SWI
- Heparin

Mitoxantrone

Compatible:
- D_5W
- D_5/NS
- NS
- Cyclophosphamide
- Cytarabine
- Fluorouracil
- Potassium chloride

Y-Site Compatible:
- Allopurinol
- Amifostine
- Filgrastim
- Fludarabine
- Gemcitabine
- Ondansetron
- Sargramostim
- Teniposide
- Thiotepa
- Vinorelbine

Incompatible:
- Aztreonam
- Cefepime
- Doxorubicin, liposomal
- Heparin
- Paclitaxel
- Piperacillin
- Piperacillin/tazobactam
- Propofol

Variable Compatibility:
- Hydrocortisone sodium phosphate
- Hydrocortisone sodium succinate
- TPN

Ondansetron

Compatible:
- D_5W
- NS
- LR
- Cisplatin
- Cyclophosphamide
- Cytarabine
- Dacarbazine
- Dexamethasone
- Doxorubicin
- Etoposide
- Fluconazole
- Hydrocortisone sodium succinate
- Mannitol
- Meperidine
- Methotrexate
- Morphine
- Ranitidine

Y-Site Compatible:
- Aldesleukin
- Amifostine
- Amikacin
- Aztreonam
- Bleomycin
- Carboplatin
- Carmustine
- Cefazolin
- Cefotaxime
- Cefoxitin
- Ceftazidime
- Ceftizoxime
- Cefuroxime
- Chlorpromazine
- Cimetidine
- Dactinomycin
- Daunomycin
- Diphenhydramine
- Doxorubicin, liposomal
- Doxycycline
- Droperidol
- Famotidine
- Filgrastim
- Floxuridine
- Fludarabine
- Gallium nitrate
- Gemcitabine
- Gentamicin
- Haloperidol
- Heparin
- Hydrocortisone sodium phosphate
- Hydromorphone
- Hydroxyzine
- Ifosfamide
- Imipenem/cilastatin
- Magnesium sulfate
- Mechlorethamine
- Mesna
- Metoclopramide
- Miconazole
- Mitomycin
- Mitoxantrone
- Paclitaxel
- Pentostatin
- Piperacillin/tazobactam
- Potassium chloride
- Prochlorperazine
- Promethazine
- Sodium acetate
- Streptozocin
- Teniposide
- Thiotepa
- Ticarcillin
- Ticarcillin/clavulanate
- TPN
- Vancomycin
- Vinblastine
- Vincristine
- Vinorelbine

COMPATIBILITY OF CHEMOTHERAPY AND RELATED SUPPORTIVE CARE MEDICATIONS *(Continued)*

Incompatible:

Acyclovir	Amsacrine	Methylprednisolone
Allopurinol	Cefepime	Mezlocillin
Aminophylline	Cefoperazone	Piperacillin
Amphotericin	Furosemide	Sargramostim
Ampicillin	Ganciclovir	Sodium bicarbonate
Ampicillin/sulbactam	Lorazepam	

Variable Compatibility:

Fluorouracil

Paclitaxel

Compatible:

NS

Y-Site Compatible:

Acyclovir	Etoposide	Mannitol
Amikacin	Famotidine	Meperidine
Aminophylline	Floxuridine	Mesna
Ampicillin/sulbactam	Fluconazole	Methotrexate
Bleomycin	Fluorouracil	Metoclopramide
Butorphanol	Furosemide	Morphine
Calcium chloride	Ganciclovir	Nalbuphine
Carboplatin	Gemcitabine	Ondansetron
Cefepime	Gentamicin	Pentostatin
Cefotetan	Granisetron	Potassium chloride
Ceftazidime	Haloperidol	Prochlorperazine
Cefuroxime	Heparin	Propofol
Cimetidine	Hydrocortisone sodium phosphate	Ranitidine
Cyclophosphamide		Sodium bicarbonate
Cytarabine	Hydrocortisone sodium succinate	Thiotepa
Dacarbazine		TPN
Dexamethasone	Hydromorphone	Vancomycin
Diphenhydramine	Ifosfamide	Vinblastine
Doxorubicin	Lorazepam	Vincristine
Droperidol	Magnesium sulfate	

Incompatible:

Amphotericin	Doxorubicin, liposomal	Methylprednisolone
Chlorpromazine	Hydroxyzine	Mitoxantrone

Variable Compatibility:

D_5W	Cisplatin

Pentostatin

Compatible:

NS	LR

Y-Site Compatible:

Fludarabine	Paclitaxel	Sargramostim
Ondansetron		

Variable Compatibility:

D_5W

Phytonadione

Compatible:

Amikacin	Chloramphenicol	Doxapram
Calcium gluceptate	Cimetidine	Sodium bicarbonate
Cefapirin	Netilmicin	TPN

Y-Site Compatible:

Ampicillin	Hydrocortisone sodium	Tolazoline
Epinephrine	succinate	Vitamin B complex
Famotidine	Potassium chloride	with C
Heparin		

Incompatible:

Dobutamine	Ranitidine

Plicamycin

Compatible:

D$_5$W	SWI	Piperacillin
NS		

Y-Site Compatible:

Allopurinol	Filgrastim	Teniposide
Amifostine	Gemcitabine	Vinorelbine
Aztreonam	Piperacillin/tazobactam	

Incompatible:

Cefonicid

Prochlorperazine

Compatible:

Amikacin	Erythromycin	Sodium bicarbonate
Ascorbic acid	Ethacrinate	Vitamin B complex
Dexamethasone	Lidocaine	with C
Dimenhydrinate	Nafcillin	

Y-Site Compatible:

Amsacrine	Hydrocortisone sodium	Potassium chloride
Cisplatin	succinate	Sargramostim
Cyclophosphamide	Melphalan	Sufentanil
Cytarabine	Methotrexate	Teniposide
Doxorubicin	Ondansetron	Thiotepa
Fluconazole	Paclitaxel	Vinorelbine
Heparin		

Incompatible:

Aldesleukin	Cefepime	Gallium nitrate
Allopurinol	Cephalothin	Gemcitabine
Amifostine	Chloramphenicol	Methohexital
Aminophylline	Floxacillin	Penicillin G sodium
Amphotericin	Fludarabine	Piperacillin/tazobactam
Ampicillin	Foscarnet	Phenobarbital
Aztreonam	Filgrastim	Thiopental
Calcium gluceptate	Furosemide	

Variable Compatibility:

Calcium gluconate	Penicillin G potassium

COMPATIBILITY OF CHEMOTHERAPY AND RELATED SUPPORTIVE CARE MEDICATIONS *(Continued)*

Promethazine

Compatible:

Amikacin	Chloroquine	Vitamin B complex
Ascorbic acid	Netilmicin	with C

Y-Site Compatible:

Amifostine	Cytarabine	Melphalan
Amsacrine	Doxorubicin	Ondansetron
Aztreonam	Filgrastim	Sargramostim
Ciprofloxacin	Fluconazole	Teniposide
Cisplatin	Fludarabine	Thiotepa
Cyclophosphamide	Gemcitabine	Vinorelbine

Incompatible:

Aldesleukin	Chlorothiazide	Methohexital
Allopurinol	Floxacillin	Methotrexate
Aminophylline	Foscarnet	Penicillin G (sodium and
Cefepime	Furosemide	potassium)
Cefoperazone	Heparin	Pentobarbital
Cefotetan	Hydrocortisone sodium	Piperacillin/tazobactam
Ceftizoxime	succinate	Thiopental
Chloramphenicol	Methicillin	

Variable Compatibility:

Potassium chloride

Sargramostim

Compatible:

BWI	NS	SWI
D_5W		

Y-Site Compatible:

Allopurinol	Dacarbazine	Mechlorethamine
Amikacin	Dactinomycin	Meperidine
Aminophylline	Dexamethasone	Mesna
Aztreonam	Diphenhydramine	Methotrexate
Bleomycin	Dobutamine	Metoclopramide
Butorphanol	Doxorubicin	Metronidazole
Calcium gluconate	Doxycycline	Mezlocillin
Carboplatin	Droperidol	Miconazole
Carmustine	Etoposide	Minocycline
Cefazolin	Famotidine	Mitoxantrone
Cefepime	Fentanyl	Netilmicin
Cefotetan	Floxuridine	Pentostatin
Cefoxitin	Fluconazole	Piperacillin/tazobactam
Ceftizoxime	Fluorouracil	Potassium chloride
Ceftriaxone	Furosemide	Prochlorperazine
Cefuroxime	Gentamicin	Promethazine
Cimetidine	Heparin	Ranitidine
Cisplatin	Human immune globulin	Teniposide
Cotrimoxazole	Idarubicin	Ticarcillin
Cyclophosphamide	Ifosfamide	Ticarcillin/clavulanate
Cyclosporine	Magnesium sulfate	Vinblastine
Cytarabine	Mannitol	Vincristine

Incompatible:

Acyclovir	Hydrocortisone sodium	Mitomycin
Ampicillin	phosphate	Morphine
Ampicillin/sulbactam	Hydrocortisone sodium	Nalbuphine
Cefonicid	succinate	Ondansetron
Cefoperazone	Hydromorphone	Piperacillin
Chlorpromazine	Hydroxyzine	Sodium bicarbonate
Ganciclovir	Imipenem/cilastatin	Tobramycin
Haloperidol	Methylprednisolone	

Variable Compatibility:

Amphotericin	Ceftazidime	Vancomycin
Amsacrine		

Streptozocin

Compatible:

D₅W	NS	SWI

Y-Site Compatible:

Filgrastim	Ondansetron	Thiotepa
Gemcitabine	Teniposide	Vinorelbine
Granisetron		

Incompatible:

Allopurinol	Cefepime	Piperacillin/tazobactam
Aztreonam	Piperacillin	

Teniposide

Compatible:

D₅W	NS	LR

Y-Site Compatible:

Acyclovir	Dacarbazine	Mechlorethamine
Allopurinol	Dactinomycin	Meperidine
Amifostine	Daunomycin	Mesna
Amikacin	Dexamethasone	Methotrexate
Aminophylline	Diphenhydramine	Methylprednisolone
Amphotericin	Doxorubicin	Metoclopramide
Ampicillin	Doxycycline	Metronidazole
Ampicillin/sulbactam	Droperidol	Mezlocillin
Aztreonam	Enalaprilat	Miconazole
Bleomycin	Etoposide	Midazolam
Bumetanide	Famotidine	Mitomycin
Buprenorphine	Floxuridine	Mitoxantrone
Butorphanol	Fluconazole	Morphine
Calcium gluconate	Fludarabine	Nalbuphine
Carboplatin	Fluorouracil	Netilmicin
Carmustine	Furosemide	Ondansetron
Cefazolin	Gallium nitrate	Piperacillin
Cefonicid	Ganciclovir	Plicamycin
Cefoperazone	Gemcitabine	Potassium chloride
Cefotaxime	Gentamicin	Prochlorperazine
Cefotetan	Haloperidol	Promethazine
Cefoxitin	Heparin	Ranitidine
Ceftazidime	Hydrocortisone sodium phosphate	Sargramostim
Ceftizoxime		Sodium bicarbonate
Ceftriaxone	Hydrocortisone sodium succinate	Streptozocin
Cefuroxime		Thiotepa
Chlorpromazine	Hydromorphone	Ticarcillin
Cimetidine	Hydroxyzine	Ticarcillin/clavulanate
Cisplatin	Ifosfamide	Tobramycin
Corticotropin	Imipenem/cilastatin	Vancomycin
Cotrimoxazole	Leucovorin	Vinblastine
Cyclophosphamide	Lorazepam	Vincristine
Cytarabine	Mannitol	Vinorelbine

Incompatible:

Idarubicin

COMPATIBILITY OF CHEMOTHERAPY AND RELATED SUPPORTIVE CARE MEDICATIONS *(Continued)*

Thiethylperazine

Compatible:

NS	Hydromorphone	Ranitidine
Butorphanol	Midazolam	

Y-Site Compatible:

Aldesleukin

Incompatible:

Ketorolac	Perphenazine

Variable Compatibility:

Nalbuphine

Thiotepa

Compatible:

NS	SWI

Y-Site Compatible:

Acyclovir	Daunomycin	Mannitol
Allopurinol	Dexamethasone	Meperidine
Amifostine	Diphenhydramine	Mesna
Amikacin	Dobutamine	Methotrexate
Aminophylline	Dopamine	Methylprednisolone
Amphotericin	Doxorubicin	Metoclopramide
Ampicillin	Doxycycline	Metronidazole
Ampicillin/sulbactam	Droperidol	Mezlocillin
Aztreonam	Enalaprilat	Miconazole
Bleomycin	Etoposide	Mitomycin
Bumetanide	Famotidine	Mitoxantrone
Buprenorphine	Floxuridine	Morphine
Butorphanol	Fluconazole	Nalbuphine
Calcium gluconate	Fludarabine	Netilmicin
Carboplatin	Fluorouracil	Ofloxacin
Carmustine	Furosemide	Ondansetron
Cefazolin	Gallium nitrate	Paclitaxel
Cefepime	Ganciclovir	Piperacillin
Cefonicid	Gemcitabine	Piperacillin/tazobactam
Cefoperazone	Gentamicin	Plicamycin
Cefotaxime	Granisetron	Potassium chloride
Cefotetan	Haloperidol	Prochlorperazine
Cefoxitin	Heparin	Promethazine
Ceftazidime	Hydrocortisone sodium phosphate	Ranitidine
Ceftizoxime		Sodium bicarbonate
Ceftriaxone	Hydrocortisone sodium succinate	Streptozocin
Cefuroxime		Teniposide
Chlorpromazine	Hydromorphone	Ticarcillin
Cimetidine	Hydroxyzine	Ticarcillin/clavulanate
Ciprofloxacin	Idarubicin	Tobramycin
Cotrimoxazole	Ifosfamide	TPN
Cyclophosphamide	Imipenem/cilastatin	Vancomycin
Cytarabine	Leucovorin	Vinblastine
Dacarbazine	Lorazepam	Vincristine
Dactinomycin	Magnesium sulfate	

Incompatible:

Cisplatin	Filgrastim	Minocycline

Topotecan

Compatible:

D$_5$W	NS	LR

Y-Site Compatible:

Gemcitabine

Trimetrexate

Compatible:

D₅W

Y-Site Compatible:

Amifostine

Incompatible:

BNS	D₅/LR	Calcium chloride
D₅/NS	D₁₀/NS	Chloride ion
D₅/¼NS	NS	Leucovorin
D₅/½NS	LR	Potassium chloride

Vinblastine

Compatible:

BNS	NS	Bleomycin
D₅W	LR	Dacarbazine

Y-Site Compatible:

Allopurinol	Fludarabine	Paclitaxel
Amifostine	Fluorouracil	Piperacillin
Aztreonam	Gemcitabine	Piperacillin/tazobactam
Cisplatin	Leucovorin	Sargramostim
Cyclophosphamide	Methotrexate	Teniposide
Doxorubicin, liposomal	Metoclopramide	Vincristine
Droperidol	Mitomycin	Vinorelbine
Filgrastim	Ondansetron	

Incompatible:

Cefazolin   Furosemide

Variable Compatibility:

Doxorubicin   Heparin

Vincristine

Compatible:

D₅W	Bleomycin	Fluorouracil
NS	Cytarabine	Methotrexate
LR	Doxorubicin	

Y-Site Compatible:

Allopurinol	Filgrastim	Ondansetron
Amifostine	Fludarabine	Paclitaxel
Aztreonam	Gemcitabine	Piperacillin/tazobactam
Cisplatin	Granisetron	Sargramostim
Cyclophosphamide	Heparin	Teniposide
Doxapram	Leucovorin	Vinblastine
Doxorubicin, liposomal	Metoclopramide	Vinorelbine
Droperidol	Mitomycin	

Incompatible:

Cefepime	Idarubicin	Sodium bicarbonate
Furosemide		

COMPATIBILITY OF CHEMOTHERAPY AND RELATED SUPPORTIVE CARE MEDICATIONS *(Continued)*

Vinorelbine

Compatible:

D_5W	NS	LR
$D_5/^1/_2NS$		

Y-Site Compatible:

Amikacin	Doxycycline	Lorazepam
Aztreonam	Droperidol	Mannitol
Bleomycin	Enalaprilat	Mechlorethamine
Bumetanide	Etoposide	Meperidine
Buprenorphine	Famotidine	Mesna
Butorphanol	Filgrastim	Methotrexate
Calcium gluconate	Fluconazole	Metoclopramide
Carboplatin	Fludarabine	Metronidazole
Carmustine	Fluorouracil	Minocycline
Cefotaxime	Gallium nitrate	Mitoxantrone
Ceftazidime	Gemcitabine	Morphine
Ceftizoxime	Gentamicin	Nalbuphine
Chlorpromazine	Haloperidol	Netilmicin
Cimetidine	Heparin	Ondansetron
Cisplatin	Hydrocortisone sodium	Plicamycin
Cyclophosphamide	phosphate	Streptozocin
Cytarabine	Hydrocortisone sodium	Teniposide
Dacarbazine	succinate	Ticarcillin
Dactinomycin	Hydromorphone	Ticarcillin/clavulanate
Daunomycin	Hydroxyzine	Tobramycin
Dexamethasone	Idarubicin	Vinblastine
Diphenhydramine	Ifosfamide	Vincristine
Doxorubicin	Imipenem/cilastatin	Vindesine
Doxorubicin, liposomal		

Incompatible:

Acyclovir	Cefoperazone	Furosemide
Allopurinol	Cefotetan	Ganciclovir
Aminophylline	Ceftriaxone	Methylprednisolone
Amphotericin	Cefuroxime	Mitomycin
Ampicillin	Cotrimoxazole	Sodium bicarbonate
Cefazolin	Fluorouracil	Thiotepa

Drug	Variable Compatibility
Carboplatin	Solutions in saline are less stable than in dextrose.
Carmustine	Solutions should be dispensed in glass and protected from light. Solutions are stable for <8 hours under most circumstances.
Cisplatin	Must have a chloride concentration of at least 0.2% in the final solution. The commercial product has a NS concentration. Etoposide + mannitol + potassium chloride in normal saline precipitates within 24 hours; when in $D_5/^1/_2NS$, it is stable for 24 hours.
Dacarbazine	Heparin 100 units/mL with dacarbazine 25 mg/mL is **incompatible**. Heparin 100 units/mL with dacarbazine 10 mg/mL is **compatible**.
Filgrastim	Gentamicin is reported to be physically **compatible** for Y-site injection, but with a decrease in biologic activity. Imipenem/cilastatin with filgrastim 40 mcg/mL is reported to be physically **compatible** for Y-site injection, but with a decrease in biologic activity.
Fluorouracil	Doxorubicin 2 mg/mL with fluorouracil 50 mg/mL is **compatible** for 13 minutes. Doxorubicin 0.5-1 mg/mL with fluorouracil 50 mg/mL is **incompatible**. Fluorouracil with doxorubicin is **Y-site compatible**. Variable compatibility with leucovorin.
Mesna	**Compatible** with ifosfamide. **Incompatible** with ifosfamide and epinephrine.
Leucovorin	Variable compatibility with fluorouracil.
Mitomycin	Mitomycin 50 mg/L in NS has a color change and 10% loss of drug concentration in 12 hours. Mitomycin 1 g/L in SWI precipitates in 24 hours under refrigeration. Other temperatures and concentrations are reported to be stable. Mitomycin in D_5W is **incompatible** in 20 mg/L; **compatible** in 40 mg/L. Mitomycin 500 mg/L with heparin 33,300 units/L in NS is **compatible**. PVC containers of mitomycin 167 mg/L with heparin 33,300 units/L in NS is **compatible**. Glass containers of mitomycin 167 mg/L with heparin 33,300 units/L in NS are **incompatible**.
Pentostatin	Pentostatin 20 mg/mL in D_5W at room temperature: a 2% loss of drug in 24 hours; 8% to 10% loss in 48 hours; and a 10% loss in 54 hours. Under refrigeration, there is no loss in 96 hours. There is a 10% loss in 23 hours at room temperature of pentostatin 2 mg/mL in D_5W
Sargramostim	Amphotericin B 0.6 mg/mL in D_5W with sargramostim 10 mcg/mL in NS forms immediate precipitate. Amphotericin B 0.6 mg/mL in D_5W with sargramostim 10 mcg/mL in D_5W is **Y-site compatible**. Amsacrine with sargramostim in NS forms immediate precipitate. Amsacrine with sargramostim in D_5W is **Y-site compatible**. Ceftazidime 40 mg/mL in NS with sargramostim 10 mcg/mL in NS is **incompatible**, with particle formation within 4 hours. Ceftazidime 40 mg/mL with sargramostim 6 or 15 mcg/mL is **compatible** for 2 hours (Y-site **compatible**). Vancomycin 20 mg/mL and sargramostim 6 mcg/mL is **incompatible**. Vancomycin 10 mg/mL and sargramostim 10 mcg/mL is **Y-site compatible**. Vancomycin 20 mg/mL and sargramostim 15 mcg/mL is **Y-site compatible**.
Vancomycin	Vancomycin 5 mg/mL with methotrexate 30 mg/mL is **compatible** for 2 hours, precipitates within 4 hours. Other concentrations tested were **compatible** for 1 hour. Vancomycin with methotrexate is **Y-site compatible**.
Vinblastine	In various volumes, doxorubicin 2 mg/mL with vinblastine 1 mg/mL yields erratic assay results. Vinblastine with doxorubicin is **Y-site compatible**. Heparin 200 units/mL with vinblastine 1 mg/mL is **incompatible** in a syringe for 13 minutes. Heparin 500 units/mL with vinblastine 0.5 mg/mL is **compatible** in a syringe for 13 minutes.

COMPATIBILITY OF CHEMOTHERAPY AND RELATED SUPPORTIVE CARE MEDICATIONS *(Continued)*

Suggested Readings

Hall PD, Yui D, Lyons S, et al, "Compatibility of Filgrastim With Selected Antimicrobial Drugs During Simulated Y-Site Administration," *Am J Health-System Pharm*, 1997, 54:184-9.

McGuire TR, Narducci WA, and Fox JL, "Compatibility and Stability of Ondansetron Hydrochloride, Dexamethasone and Lorazepam in Injectable Solutions," *Am J Health-System Pharm*, 1993, 50:1410-4.

Najari Z and Rucho WJ, "Compatibility of Commonly Used Bone Marrow Drugs During Y-Site Delivery," *Am J Health-System Pharm*, 1997, 54:181-4.

Trissel LA, Chandler SW, and Folstad JT, "Visual Compatibility of Amsacrine With Selected Drugs During Simulated Y-Site Injection," *Am J Hospital Pharm*, 1990, 47:2525-8.

Trissel LA, Bready BB, Kwan JW, et al, "Visual Compatibility of Sargramostim With Selected Antineoplastic Agents, Anti-infectives, or Other Drugs During Simulated Y-Site Injection," *Am J Hospital Pharm*, 1992, 49:402-6.

Trissel LA and Martinez JF, "Physical Compatibility of Melphalan With Selected Drugs During Simulated Y-Site Administration," *Am J Hospital Pharm*, 1993, 50:2359-63.

Trissel LA and Martinez JF, Visual, "Turbidimetric and Particle-Content Assessment of Compatibility of Vinorelbine Tartrate With Selected Drugs During Simulated Y-Site Injection," *Am J Hospital Pharm*, 1994, 51:495-9.

Trissel LA and Martinez JF, "Physical Compatibility of Allopurinol Sodium With Selected Drugs During Simulated Y-Site Administration," *Am J Hospital Pharm*, 1994, 51:1792-9.

Trissel LA and Martinez JF, "Compatibility of Filgrastim With Selected Drugs During Simulated Y-Site Administration," *Am J Hospital Pharm*, 1994, 51:1907-13.

Trissel LA and Martinez JF, "Screening Teniposide For Y-Site Compatibility," *Hospital Pharm*, 1994, 29:1010, 1012-4, 1017.

Trissel LA, *Handbook on Injectable Drugs*, 9th Ed. Bethesda, MD: *Am Society Health-Systems Pharmacists*, 1996.

Trissel LA, *Supplement to Handbook on Injectable Drugs*, 9th Ed. Bethesda, MD: *Am Society of Health-Systems Pharmacists*, 1997.

Trissel LA, Gilbert DL, and Martinez JF, "Compatibility of Granisetron Hydrochloride With Selected Drugs During Simulated Y-Site Administration," *Am J Health-System Pharm*, 1997, 54:56-60.

Trissel LA, Gilbert DL, and Martinez JF, "Compatibility of Propofol With Selected Drugs During Simulated Y-Site Administration," *Am J Health-System Pharm*, 1997, 54:1287-92.

Trissel LA, Gilbert DL, Martinez JF, et al, "Compatibility of Parenteral Nutrient Solutions With Selected Drugs During Simulated Y-Site Administration," *Am J Health-System Pharm*, 1997, 54:1295-300.

Trissel LA, Gilbert DL, and Martinez JF, "Compatibility of Doxorubicin Hydrochloride Liposome With Selected Other Drugs During Simulated Y-Site Administration," *Am J Health-System Pharm*, 1997; 54:2708-13.

Trissel LA, Martinez JF, and Gilbert DL, "Compatibility of Gemcitabine Hydrochloride With 107 Selected Drugs During Simulated Y-Site Administration," *J Am Pharmaceutical Association*, 1999, 39 (4):514-18.

Zhang Y, Xu QA, Trissel LA, et al, "Compatibility and Stability of Paclitaxel Combined With Cisplatin and With Carboplatin in Infusion Solutions," *Ann Pharmacother*, 1997, 31 (12):1465-70.

HEMATOLOGIC ADVERSE EFFECTS OF DRUGS

Drug	Red Cell Aplasia	Thrombocy-topenia	Neutrope-nia	Pancytope-nia	Hemolysis
Acetazolamide		+	+	+	
Allopurinol			+		
Amiodarone	+				
Amphotericin B				+	
Amrinone		++			
Asparaginase		+++	+++	+++	++
Barbiturates		+		+	
Benzocaine					++
Captopril			++		+
Carbamazepine		++	+		
Cephalosporins			+		++
Chloramphenicol		+	++	+++	
Chlordiazepoxide			+	+	
Chloroquine		+			
Chlorothiazides		++			
Chlorpropamide	+	++	+	++	+
Chlortetracycline				+	
Chlorthalidone			+		
Cimetidine		+	++	+	
Codeine		+			
Colchicine				+	
Cyclophosphamide		+++	+++	+++	+
Dapsone					+++
Desipramine		++			
Digitalis		+			
Digitoxin		++			
Erythromycin		+			
Estrogen		+		+	
Ethacrynic acid			+		
Fluorouracil		+++	+++	+++	+
Furosemide		+	+		
Gold salts	+	+++	+++	+++	
Heparin		++		+	
Ibuprofen			+		+
Imipramine			++		
Indomethacin		+	++	+	
Isoniazid		+		+	
Isosorbide dinitrate					+
Levodopa					++
Meperidine		+			
Meprobamate		+	+	+	
Methimazole			++		
Methyldopa		++			+++
Methotrexate		+++	+++	+++	++
Methylene blue					+
Metronidazole			+		
Nalidixic acid					+
Naproxen				+	
Nitrofurantoin			++		+
Nitroglycerine		+			
Penicillamine		++	+		
Penicillins		+	++	+	+++
Phenazopyridine					+++
Phenothiazines		+	++	+++	+

HEMATOLOGIC ADVERSE EFFECTS OF DRUGS
(Continued)

Drug	Red Cell Aplasia	Thrombocytopenia	Neutropenia	Pancytopenia	Hemolysis
Phenylbutazone		+	++	+++	+
Phenytoin		++	++	++	+
Potassium iodide		+			
Prednisone		+			
Primaquine					+++
Procainamide			+		
Procarbazine		+	++	++	+
Propylthiouracil		+	++	+	+
Quinidine		+++	+		
Quinine		+++	+		
Reserpine		+			
Rifampicin		++	+		+++
Spironolactone			+		
Streptomycin		+		+	
Sulfamethoxazole with trimethoprim			+		
Sulfonamides	+	++	++	++	++
Sulindac	+	+	+	+	
Tetracyclines		+			+
Thioridazine			++		
Tolbutamide		++	+	++	
Triamterene					+
Valproate	+				
Vancomycin			+		

+ = rare or single reports.

++ = occasional reports.

+++ = substantial number of reports.

Adapted from D'Arcy PF and Griffin JP, eds, *Iatrogenic Diseases*, New York, NY: Oxford University Press, 1986, 128-30.

TUMOR LYSIS SYNDROME, MANAGEMENT

Tumor lysis syndrome (TLS) may be seen with any tumor that is undergoing rapid cell turnover as a result of high growth fraction or high cell death due to therapy. It occurs most often in Burkitt's lymphoma and T-cell ALL, both of which have large tumor burdens and high sensitivity to chemotherapy. Acute lysis of tumor cells results in the rapid release of potassium, phosphates, and nucleic acids into the circulation. Hypocalcemia, hyperuricemia, and renal failure may result. Secondary acute precipitation of calcium and urates in the kidney, tumor infiltration of the kidney, obstructive uropathy, and dehydration may increase the primary metabolic disturbances. The following chart reviews the management of TLS.

Therapy	Infants & Children	Adolescents & Adults
Hydration (patients typically present with dehydration; I.V. fluids should be started immediately)	3000-6000 mL/m²/day D_5W ¼ NS (+ sodium bicarbonate) Maintain urine output at ≥1 mL/kg/hour Maintain urine specific gravity at ≤1.010 Strict monitoring of I & O	3000-6000 mL/m²/day D_5W ¼ NS (+ sodium bicarbonate) Maintain urine output at 100-150 mL/hour Maintain urine specific gravity at ≤1.010 Strict monitoring of I & O
Alkalinization	50-100 mEq/L sodium bicarbonate in I.V. fluid Maintain urine pH at 7.0-7.5 Reduce bicarbonate if serum bicarbonate >30 mEq/L or urine pH >7.5	50-100 mEq/L sodium bicarbonate in I.V. fluid Maintain urine pH at 7.0-7.5 Reduce bicarbonate if serum bicarbonate >30 mEq/L or urine pH >7.5
Uric acid reduction	Allopurinol: I.V., oral: 200-400 mg/m²/day in 1-3 divided doses (maximum: 600 mg/day) Urate oxidase: I.V. (investigational, see protocol): 0.2 mg/kg/dose once or twice daily	Allopurinol: I.V.: 200-400 mg/m²/day in 1-3 divided doses (maximum: 600 mg/day) Oral: 600-800 mg/day in 1-2 doses
Diuretics (avoid if hypovolemic)	Furosemide: I.V.: 1 mg/kg/dose as needed Mannitol: I.V.: 0.25-0.5 g/kg/dose as needed	Furosemide: I.V.: 20-40 mg/dose as needed Mannitol: I.V.: 0.25-0.5 g/kg/dose as needed
Phosphate reduction	Aluminum hydroxide: Oral: 50 mg/kg/dose every 8 hours	Aluminum hydroxide: Oral: 30-40 mL/dose every 6-8 hours
Dialysis indications (peritoneal dialysis is much less efficient for reducing uric acid than other modalities, and is contraindicated in patients with abdominal tumors.)	Potassium level >6 mEq/L Uric acid level >10 mg/dL Creatinine >10 times normal Uremia Phosphorus >10 mg/dL or rapidly rising Symptomatic hypocalcemia Severe, unmanageable hypertension Volume overload	

Kelly KM and Lange B, "Oncologic Emergencies," *Pediatr Clin North Am*, 1997, 44(4):809-30.

ANTITHROMBOTIC THERAPY IN CHILDREN

Recommendations From the 6th American College of Chest Physicians (ACCP) Consensus Conference on Antithrombotic Therapy

Used with permission from Monagle P, Michelson AD, Bovill E, et al, "Antithrombotic Therapy in Children," *CHEST*, 2001, 119:344S-70S.

Abbreviations: APTT = activated partial thromboplastin time; BT = Blalock-Taussig; CVL = central venous line; DVT = deep venous thrombosis; FFP = fresh frozen plasma; INR = international normalized ratio; LMWH = low-molecular-weight heparin; OA = oral anticoagulant; PC = protein C; PE = pulmonary thromboembolism; PS = protein S; PT = prothrombin time; TE = thromboembolism

Venous Thromboembolic Disease in Children

First TE: ACCP recommends that children (>2 months of age) who have had an initial TE should be treated in the short term with doses of I.V. heparin that are sufficient to prolong the APTT to a range that corresponds to an anti-factor Xa level of 0.3-0.7 U/mL, or with doses of LMWH that are sufficient to achieve an anti-factor Xa level of 0.5-1 U/mL 4 hours after an injection (grade 1C+)*.

ACCP recommends that initial treatment with heparin or LMWH should be continued for 5-10 days. For patients in whom subsequent OA therapy will be used, it can be started as early as day 1 and heparin/LMWH therapy discontinued on day 6 if the INR is therapeutic on 2 consecutive days. For massive PEs or extensive DVTs, a longer period of heparin or LMWH therapy should be considered (grade 1C+).

ACCP recommends that anticoagulant therapy should be continued for at least 3 months using OAs to prolong the PT to a target INR of 2.5 (range, 2-3) or, alternatively, using LMWH to maintain an anti-factor Xa level of 0.5-1 U/mL (grade 2C).

For children who have experienced an idiopathic TE, ACCP recommends that treatment be continued for at least 6 months with either OAs or LMWH (grade 2C).

Following the initial 3 months of therapy, for children with a first CVL-related DVT, ACCP recommends prophylactic doses of OAs (INR, 1.5-1.8) or LMWH (anti-factor levels, 0.1-0.3) as an option until the CVL is removed (grade 2C).

Recurrent TE: For recurrent non-CVL-related TEs, following the initial 3 months of therapy (recommendation, 1-3 months), ACCP recommends that indefinite therapy with either therapeutic or prophylactic doses of OAs or LMWH be used (grade 2C).

For recurrent CVL-related TEs, following the initial 3 months of therapy, ACCP recommends that prophylactic doses of OAs (INR, 1.5-1.8) or LMWH (anti-factor Xa level, 0.1-0.3) be continued until removal of the CVL. If the recurrence occurs while that patient is receiving prophylactic therapy, ACCP recommends that therapeutic doses be continued until the CVL is removed or for a minimum of 3 months (all grade 2C).

Primary prophylaxis for Venous TE in Children: ACCP does *not* recommend primary prophylaxis for children with CVLs in general at this time, because there is no evidence for the efficacy or safety of this approach (grade 2C).

Remark: Short-term prophylactic anticoagulation therapy in high-risk situations such as immobility, significant surgery, or trauma is an option for children with known congenital prothrombotic disorders. However, to our knowledge, there are no published data on which to base a formal recommendation.

Venous Thromboembolic Disease in Newborns

Remark: There are insufficient data to make specific recommendations about anticoagulation therapy in the treatment of newborns with DVTs and PEs. Options include conventional anticoagulation therapy in age-appropriate doses, short-term anticoagulation therapy, or close monitoring of the thrombus with objective tests and use of anticoagulation therapy if thrombus extension occurs.

If anticoagulation therapy is used, ACCP recommends a short course (10-14 days) of I.V. heparin that is sufficient to prolong the APTT to the therapeutic range that corresponds to an anti-factor Xa level of 0.3-0.7 U/mL, or, alternatively, a short course of LMWH that is sufficient to achieve an anti-factor Xa level at the low end of the adult therapeutic range (0.5-1 U/mL) may be used (all grade 2C compared to no treatment). Longer courses of anticoagulant therapy, up to 3 months, may be required dependent on the location and extent of the thrombus. The thrombus should be closely monitored with objective tests for evidence of extension or recurrent disease. If the thrombus extends following discontinuation of heparin therapy, ACCP recommends oral anticoagulation therapy or extended LMWH therapy (grade 2C).

Thrombolytic Therapy for Venous Thromboembolic Disease

Remark: There are insufficient data to make specific recommendations about the use of thrombolytic agents in the treatment of venous TEs in neonates or children. Treatment needs to be individualized. If thrombolytic therapy is used, in the presence of physiologic or pathologic deficiencies of plasminogen, ACCP recommends supplementation with plasminogen (FFP) (grade 2C).

Congenital Prothrombotic Conditions

Homozygous PC-Deficient and PS-Deficient Patients: ACCP recommends that newborns with purpura fulminans due to a homozygous deficiency of PC or PS may be treated initially with replacement therapy (either FFP or PC concentrate) for approximately 6-8 weeks until the skin lesions have healed (grade 1C+).

Following resolution of the skin lesions, and under cover of replacement therapy, ACCP recommends that oral anticoagulation therapy be introduced with target INR values of approximately 3-4.5. Treatment duration with OAs is indefinite. ACCP recommends that replacement therapy with PC concentrate for PC-deficient patients may be used for long-term prophylaxis or as salvage therapy for recurrent skin lesions or thrombosis (grade 2C).

ACCP recommends that for patients with homozygous PC and PS deficiency but with measurable plasma concentrations, LMWH is a therapeutic option (grade 2C).

Treatment of Arterial Thromboembolism

Cardiac Catheterization: ACCP recommends that newborns and children requiring cardiac catheterization via an artery should undergo I.V. heparin prophylaxis (grade 1A).

ACCP recommends heparin doses of 100-150 U/kg as a bolus (grade 2A compared with 50 U/kg).

Remark: The initial dose and further administration of heparin therapy need further evaluation before definite recommendations can be given, in particular in small infants having procedural catheters.

ACCP recommends that clinicians *not* use aspirin alone (grade 1B).

Arterial TE: ACCP recommends that children or neonates with an arterial TE be treated with therapeutic doses of I.V. heparin (grade 1C).

Remark: There are insufficient data to make a recommendation about the optimal duration of therapy.

ACCP recommends that children or neonates with limb-threatening or organ-threatening arterial TEs who fail to respond to initial heparin therapy, and who have no known contraindications, be treated with thrombolytic therapy (grade 1C).

ANTITHROMBOTIC THERAPY IN CHILDREN *(Continued)*

Remark: The use of surgery to treat arterial thrombosis in children should be individualized. There are insufficient data to make specific recommendations in children.

Treatment of Kawasaki's Disease in Children

In addition to I.V. gamma globulin (2 g/kg as a single dose), children with Kawasaki's disease should receive aspirin, 80-100 mg/kg/day, during the acute phase (up to 14 days) as an anti-inflammatory agent, then aspirin, 3-5 mg/kg/day, for ≥7 weeks to prevent the formation of coronary aneurysm thrombosis (grade 1C).

Prosthetic Heart Valves in Children

Biological Prosthetic Heart Valves in Children: Children with biological prosthetic heart valves should be treated following adult recommendations and observed for evidence of valve dysfunction.

Mechanical Prosthetic Heart Valves in Children

ACCP recommends that children with mechanical prosthetic heart valves receive OA therapy (grade 1C+).

ACCP recommends levels of OA therapy that prolong the target INR to 3 (range, 2.5-3.5) (grade 1C+).

For children with mechanical prosthetic heart valves who suffer systemic embolisms despite adequate therapy with oral anticoagulation therapy, ACCP recommends the addition of aspirin, 6-20 mg/kg/day, to the regimen. Dipyridamole, 2-5 mg/kg/day, in addition to oral anticoagulation therapy is an alternative option (all grade 2C).

When full-dose oral anticoagulation therapy is contraindicated, ACCP recommends long-term therapy with OAs sufficient to increase the INR to 2.5 (range, 2-3) in combination with aspirin, 6-20 mg/kg/day, (grade 1C+) and dipyridamole, 2-5 mg/kg/day (grade 2C).

Other Cardiac Disorders

BT Shunts: ACCP recommends the initial treatment of patients with BT shunts with therapeutic amounts of heparin, followed by treatment with aspirin, at doses of 3-5 mg/kg/day, indefinitely (grade 2C).

Remark: Further clinical investigation is needed before definitive recommendations can be made.

Fontan Operations: ACCP recommends aspirin or therapeutic amounts of heparin followed by oral anticoagulation therapy to achieve a target INR of 2.5 (range, 2-3) as therapeutic options (grade 2C). The optimal duration of prophylaxis is unknown. Patients with fenestrations may benefit from treatment until closure.

Remark: Further clinical investigation is needed before definitive recommendations for primary postoperative prophylaxis can be made.

---

*The ACCP Consensus Conference on Antithrombotic Therapy uses grades of recommendations that are based on clarity of benefits versus risks of treatment (1 = clear risk/benefit, strong recommendation; 2 = unclear risk/benefit, weaker recommendation) and quality of the research methodology supporting the underlying evidence (A = randomized trials with consistent results; B = randomized trials with inconsistent results or with major weaknesses in methodology; C = observational studies and generalizations of randomized trials to another group of patients; C+ = observational studies with overwhelmingly compelling results or secure generalizations of randomized trials). The highest rating (1A) implies a strong recommendation; one that can be applied to most patients in most circumstances without reservations. The lowest rating (2C) implies a very weak recommendation; one in which other alternatives may be equally reasonable. For further information see Guyatt G, Schunemann H, Cook D, et al, "Grades of Recommendation for Antithrombotic Agents," *CHEST*, 2001, 119:3S-7S.

TOTAL BLOOD VOLUME

Age	Example Weight (kg) [age]	Approximate Total Blood Volume (mL/kg)*	Estimated Total Blood Volume (mL)
Premature infant	1.5	89-105	134-158
Term newborn	3.4	78-86	265-292
1-12 months	7.6 [6 months]	73-78	555-593
1-3 years	12.4 [2 years]	74-82	918-1017
4-6 years	18.2 [5 years]	80-86	1456-1565
7-18 years	45.5 [13 years]	83-90	3777-4095
Adults	70.0	68-88	4760-6160

*Approximate total blood volume information compiled from *Nathan and Oski's Hematology of Infancy and Childhood*, 5th ed, Nathan DG and Orkin SH, eds, Philadelphia, PA: WB Saunders, 1998.

HOTLINE PHONE NUMBERS

AIDS Hotline	800-590-2437
AMA Foreign Drug	312-464-4575
AMA Library Answer Center	312-464-4818
American Association of Poison Control Centers (AAPCC) Poison Prevention	202-625-3333
American College of Clinical Pharmacy (ACCP)	816-531-2177
American Dental Association (ADA)	800-621-8099
American Medical Association (AMA)	312-464-5000
American Pharmaceutical Association (APhA)	202-628-4410
American Association of Health-System Pharmacists	301-657-3000
Animal Poison Care Hotline (24-hours)	800-548-2423
Canadian Pharmaceutical Association	613-523-7877
Center for Disease Control	1-800-311-3435

Use this number for the following departments also:

- CDC Disease Information
- CDC Epidemiology Program
- CDC Immunity Division
- CDC Influenza Branch
- CDC International Travelers Information
- CDC Parasitic Division
- CDC STDs
- CDC Tuberculosis Section

FDA (Rare Diseases/Orphan Drugs)	800-300-7469
National Cancer Institute	301-496-1196
Asthma and Allergy Foundation of America	1-800-7-ASTHMA
Cancer Treatment (of NCI)	1-800-4-CANCER
Epilepsy Foundation of America	301-459-3700
National Council on Patient Information & Education	301-656-8565
National Institute of Health	301-496-4000
National Poison Center	202-362-3867
Emergency	800-222-1222
Parental Stress	800-632-8188
Pediatric Pharmacy Advocacy Group (PPAG) Membership and Drug Information	720-981-7356
Pesticides (Mon-Fri, 6:30 AM - 4:30 PM Pacific)	800-858-7378
Rocky Mountain Poison Control Information	800-525-6115

ENDOCARDITIS PROPHYLAXIS*

	Dosage for Adults	Dosage for Children†
DENTAL AND UPPER RESPIRATORY PROCEDURES		

Oral§

Amoxicillin¶	2 g 1 h before procedure	50 mg/kg 1 h before procedure

Penicillin allergy:

Clindamycin or	600 mg 1 h before procedure	20 mg/kg 1 h before procedure
Cephalexin or	2 g 1 h before procedure	50 mg/kg 1 h before procedure
Azithromycin or Clarithromycin	500 mg 1 h before procedure	15 mg/kg 1 h before procedure

Parenteral§

Ampicillin	2 g I.M. or I.V. 30 minutes before procedure	50 mg/kg I.M. or I.V. 30 minutes before procedure

Penicillin allergy:

Clindamycin or	600 mg I.V. 30 minutes before procedure	20 mg/kg I.V. 30 minutes before procedure
Cefazolin (not to be used in individuals with immediate-type hypersensitivity reaction to penicillins)	1 g I.M. or I.V. 30 minutes before procedure	25 mg/kg I.M. or I.V. 30 minutes before procedure

GASTROINTESTINAL AND GENITOURINARY PROCEDURES‡

Oral§

Amoxicillin for moderate risk patients	2 g 1 h before procedure	50 mg/kg 1 h before procedure

Parenteral§

Ampicillin for moderate risk patients	2 g I.M. or I.V. 30 minutes before procedure	50 mg/kg I.M. or I.V. 30 minutes before procedure
Ampicillin **plus**	2 g I.M. or I.V. 30 minutes before procedure; ampicillin 1 g I.M./I.V. or amoxicillin 1 g P.O. 6 h later	50 mg/kg I.M. or I.V. 30 minutes before procedure and 25 mg/kg I.M./I.V. or amoxicillin 25 mg/kg P.O. 6 h later
Gentamicin for high-risk patients	1.5 mg/kg (max: 120 mg) I.M. or I.V. 30 minutes before procedure	1.5 mg/kg I.M. or I.V. 30 minutes before procedure

ENDOCARDITIS PROPHYLAXIS* *(Continued)*

	Dosage for Adults	Dosage for Children†
Penicillin allergy:		
Vancomycin for moderate-risk patients	1 g I.V. infused **slowly over 1 h**; complete infusion within 30 minutes before procedure	20 mg/kg I.V. infused **slowly over 1 h**; complete infusion within 30 minutes before procedure
Vancomycin **plus**	1 g I.V. infused slowly over 1 h; complete infusion within 30 minutes before procedure	20 mg/kg I.V. infused slowly over 1 h; complete infusion within 30 minutes before procedure
Gentamicin for high-risk patients	1.5 mg/kg (max: 120 mg) I.M. or I.V. 30 minutes before procedure	1.5 mg/kg I.M. or I.V. 30 minutes before procedure

*Endocarditis prophylaxis recommended

High-risk category:

Prosthetic cardiac valves

Previous bacterial endocarditis

Complex cyanotic congenital heart disease (eg, single ventricle states, transposition of the great arteries, tetralogy of Fallot)

Surgically constructed systemic pulmonary shunts or conduits

Moderate-risk category:

Most other congenital cardiac malformations (other than high-risk category)

Acquired valvar dysfunction (eg, rheumatic heart disease)

Hypertrophic cardiomyopathy

Mitral valve prolapse with valvar regurgitation and/or thickened leaflets

†Children's dose should not exceed adult dosage.

‡For a review of the risk of bacteremia and endocarditis with various procedures, see Mandell GL, Bennett JE, Dolin R, eds, *Principles and Practice of Infectious Diseases*, 4th ed, New York, NY: Churchill Livingstone, 1995, 794.

§Oral regimens are more convenient and safer. Parenteral regimens are more likely to be effective; they are recommended especially for patients with prosthetic heart valves, those who have had endocarditis previously, or those taking continuous oral penicillin for rheumatic fever prophylaxis.

¶Amoxicillin is recommended because of its excellent bioavailability and good activity against streptococci and enterococci.

References
Dajani AS, Taubert KA, Wilson W, et al, "Prevention of Bacterial Endocarditis. Recommendations by the American Heart Association," *JAMA*, 1997, 277(22):1794-1801.

PEDIATRIC HIV

Selected tables from the Centers for Disease Control and Prevention, "Guidelines for the Use of Antiretroviral Agents in Pediatric HIV Infection," first published in *MMWR*, 1998:47(No.RR-4), April 17, 1998, updated as a "Living Document", December 14, 2001, located at (URL) http://www.aidsinfo.nih.gov.

Table 1. 1994 Revised Human Immunodeficiency Virus Pediatric Classification System: Immune Categories Based on Age-specific CD4+ T cell and Percentage*

Immune Category	<12 mo		1-5 y		6-12 y	
	No./mm^3	%	No./mm^3	%	No./mm^3	%
Category 1 no suppression	≥1500	≥25	≥1000	≥25	≥500	≥25
Category 2 moderate suppression	750-1499	15-24	500-999	15-24	200-499	15-24
Category 3 severe suppression	<750	<15	<500	<15	<200	<15

*Modified from: CDC,"1994 Revised Classification System for Human Immunodeficiency Virus Infection in Children Less Than 13 Years of Age," *MMWR*, 1994, 43(RR-12):1-10.

Table 2. 1994 Revised Human Immunodeficiency Virus Pediatric Classification System: Clinical Categories*

Category N: Not Symptomatic
Children who have no signs or symptoms considered to be the result of HIV infection or who have only **one** of the conditions listed in category A

Category A: Mildly Symptomatic
Children with **two** or more of the following conditions, but none of the conditions listed in categories B and C:

- Lymphadenopathy (≥0.5 cm at more than two sites; bilateral = one site)
- Hepatomegaly
- Splenomegaly
- Dermatitis
- Parotitis
- Recurrent or persistent upper respiratory infection, sinusitis, or otitis media

Category B: Moderately Symptomatic
Children who have symptomatic conditions, other than those listed for category A or category C, that are attributed to HIV infection. Examples of conditions in clinical category B include but are not limited to the following:

- Anemia (<8 g/dL), neutropenia (<1000/mm^3), or thrombocytopenia (<100,000/mm^3) persisting ≥30 days
- Bacterial meningitis, pneumonia, or sepsis (single episode)
- Candidiasis, oropharyngeal (ie, thrush) persisting for >2 months in children aged >6 months
- Cardiomyopathy
- Cytomegalovirus infection with onset before age 1 month
- Diarrhea, recurrent or chronic
- Hepatitis
- Herpes simplex virus (HSV) stomatitis, recurrent (ie, more than two episodes within 1 year)
- HSV bronchitis, pneumonitis, or esophagitis with onset before age 1 month
- Herpes zoster (ie, shingles) involving at least two distinct episodes or more than one dermatome
- Leiomyosarcoma

PEDIATRIC HIV *(Continued)*

- Lymphoid interstitial pneumonia (LIP) or pulmonary lymphoid hyperplasia complex
- Nephropathy
- Nocardiosis
- Fever lasting >1 month
- Toxoplasmosis with onset before age 1 month
- Varicella, disseminated (ie, complicated chickenpox)

Category C: Severely Symptomatic

Children who have any condition listed in the 1987 surveillance case definition for acquired immunodeficiency syndrome, with the exception of LIP (which is a category B condition).

*Centers for Disease Control and Prevention, "1994 Revised Classification System for Human Immunodeficiency Virus Infection in Children Less Than 13 Years of Age," *MMWR*, 1994, 43(RR-12):1-10.

Table 3. Indications for Initiation of Antiretroviral Therapy in Children With Human Immunodeficiency Virus (HIV) Infection*

- Clinical symptoms associated with HIV infection (ie, clinical categories A, B, or C [Table 2])
- Evidence of immune suppression, indicated by $CD4^+$ T cell absolute number or percentage (ie, immune category 2 or 3 [Table 1])
- Age <12 months - regardless of clinical, immunologic, or virologic status**
- For asymptomatic children ≥1 year of age with normal immune status, two options can be considered:

  Option 1: Initiate therapy – regardless of age or symptom status

  Option 2: Defer treatment in situations in which the risk for clinical disease progression is low and other factors (ie, concern for the durability of response, safety, and adherence) favor postponing treatment. In such cases, the healthcare provider should regularly monitor virologic, immunologic, and clinical status. Factors to be considered in deciding to initiate therapy include the following:

  - High or increasing HIV RNA copy number
  - Rapidly declining $CD4^+$ T cell number or percentage to values approaching those indicative of moderate immune suppression (ie, immune category 2 [Table 1])
  - Development of clinical symptoms

---

*Indications for initiation of antiretroviral therapy need to address issues of adherence. Postpubertal adolescents should follow the "Guidelines for the Use of Antiretroviral Agents in HIV-Infected Adults and Adolescents." (http://www.aidsinfo.nih.gov or see Adult and Adolescent HIV section in this Appendix).

**The Working Group recognizes that clinical trial data documenting therapeutic benefit from this approach are not currently available, and information on pharmacokinetics in infants under age 3-6 months is limited. This recommendation is based on expert opinion. Issues associated with adherence should be fully assessed, discussed, and addressed with the HIV-infected infant's caregivers before the decision to initiate therapy is made.

Table 4. Recommended Antiretroviral Regimens for Initial Therapy for Human Immunodeficiency Virus (HIV) Infection in Children

Strongly Recommended
Clinical trial evidence of clinical benefit and/or sustained suppression of HIV replication in adults and/or children.

- One highly active protease inhibitor (nelfinavir or ritonavir) plus two nucleoside analogue reverse transcriptase inhibitors (NRTIs)
    - Recommended dual NRTI combinations: the most data on use in children are available for the combinations of zidovudine (ZDV) and dideoxyinosine (ddI), ZDV and lamivudine (3TC), and stavudine (d4T) and ddI. More limited data are available for the combinations of d4T and 3TC, and ZDV and zalcitabine (ddC)*
- For children who can swallow capsules: the non-nucleoside reverse transcriptase inhibitor (NNRTI) efavirenz (Sustiva®)** plus two NRTIs, or efavirenz (Sustiva®) plus nelfinavir and one NRTI

Recommended as an Alternative
Clinical trial evidence of suppression of HIV replication, but 1) durability may be less in adults and/or children than with strongly recommended regimens or may not yet be defined; or 2) evidence of efficacy may not outweigh potential adverse consequences (ie, toxicity, drug interactions, cost, etc); 3) experience in infants and children is limited.

- Nevirapine and two NRTIs
- Abacavir in combination with ZDV and 3TC
- Lopinavir/ritonavir with two NRTIs or one NRTI and NNRTI†
- Indinavir (IDV) or saquinavir (SQV) soft gel capsule with two NRTIs for children who can swallow capsules.

Offer Only in Special Circumstances
Clinical trial evidence of either 1) virologic suppression that is less durable than for the Strongly Recommended or Alternative regimes; or 2) data are preliminary or inconclusive for use as initial therapy but may be reasonably offered in special circumstances.

- Two NRTIs
- Amprenavir in combination with two NRTIs or abacavir

Not Recommended
Evidence against use because 1) overlapping toxicity may occur, and/or 2) use may be virologically undesirable

- Any monotherapy§
- d4T and ZDV
- ddC* and ddI
- ddC* and d4T
- ddC* and 3TC

*ddC is not available commercially in a liquid preparation; although, a liquid formulation is available through a compassionate use program of the manufacturer (Hoffman-LaRoche Inc, (http://www.rocheusa.com), Nutley, New Jersey). ZDV and ddC is a less preferred choice for use in combination with a protease inhibitor.

**Efavirenz is currently available only in capsule form, although a liquid formulation is available through an expanded access program of the manufacturer, Bristol-Myers Squibb Company (http://www.bms.com). There are currently no data on appropriate dosage of efavirenz in children under age three years.

†The data presented to the Food and Drug Administration for review during the drug approval process provided significant data on the pharmacokinetics and safety in children receiving lopinavir/ritonavir (Kaletra™) for 24 weeks. The combination of lopinavir/ritonavir with either two NRTIs or one NRTI and an NNRTI may be moved up to the Strongly Recommended category as experience with this drug is gained by U.S. investigators.

§Except for ZDV chemoprophylaxis administered to HIV-exposed infants during the first 6 weeks of life to prevent perinatal HIV transmission; if an infant is confirmed as HIV-infected while receiving ZDV prophylaxis, therapy should be changed to a combination antiretroviral drug regimen.

PEDIATRIC HIV *(Continued)*

Table 5. Considerations for Changing Antiretroviral Therapy for Human Immunodeficiency Virus (HIV)-Infected Children

Virologic Considerations*

- Less than a minimally acceptable virologic response after 8-12 weeks of therapy. For children receiving antiretroviral therapy with two nucleoside analogue reverse transcriptase inhibitors (NRTIs) and a protease inhibitor, such a response is defined as a <10-fold (1.0 $\log_{10}$) decrease from baseline HIV RNA levels. For children who are receiving less potent antiretroviral therapy (ie, dual NRTI combinations), an insufficient response is defined as a <5-fold (0.7 $\log_{10}$) decrease in HIV RNA levels from baseline

- HIV RNA not suppressed to undetectable levels after 4-6 months of antiretroviral therapy†

- Repeated detection of HIV RNA in children who initially responded to antiretroviral therapy with undetectable levels‡

- A reproducible increase in HIV RNA copy number among children who have had a substantial HIV RNA response, but still have low levels of detectable HIV RNA. Such an increase would warrant change in therapy if, after initiation of the therapeutic regimen, a >3-fold (0.5 $\log_{10}$) increase in copy number for children aged ≥2 years and a >5-fold (0.7 $\log_{10}$) increase is observed for children aged <2 years

Immunologic Considerations*

- Change in immunologic classification (Table 1)§

- For children with CD4+ T cell percentages of <15% (ie, those in immune category 3), a persistent decline of five percentiles or more in CD4+ T cell percentage (eg, from 15% to 10%)

- A rapid and substantial decrease in absolute CD4+ T cell count (ie, a >30% decline in <6 months)

Clinical Considerations

- Progressive neurodevelopmental deterioration

- Growth failure defined as persistent decline in weight-growth velocity despite adequate nutritional support and without other explanation

- Disease progression defined as advancement from one pediatric clinical category to another (ie, from clinical category A to clinical category B)**

*At least two measurements (taken 1 week apart) should be performed before considering a change in therapy.

†The initial HIV RNA level of the child at the start of therapy and the level achieved with therapy should be considered when contemplating potential drug changes. For example, an immediate change in therapy may not be warranted if there is a sustained 1.5-2.0 $\log_{10}$ decrease in HIV RNA copy number, even if RNA remains detectable at low levels.

‡More frequent evaluation of HIV RNA levels should be considered if the HIV RNA increase is limited (ie, if when using an HIV RNA assay with a lower limit of detection of 1000 copies/mL, there is a ≤0.7 $\log_{10}$ increase from undetectable to approximately 5000 copies/mL in an infant <2 years of age).

§Minimal changes in CD4+ T cell percentile that may result in change in immunologic category (ie, from 26% to 24%, or 16% to 14%) may not be as concerning as a rapid substantial change in CD4+ percentile within the same immunologic category (ie, a drop from 35% to 25%).

**In patients with stable immunologic and virologic parameters, progression from one clinical category to another may not represent an indication to change therapy. Thus, in patients whose disease progression is not associated with neurologic deterioration or growth failure, virologic and immunologic considerations are important in deciding whether to change therapy.

ADULT AND ADOLESCENT HIV

Selected tables from the Centers for Disease Control and Prevention, "Report of the NIH Panel to Define Principles of Therapy of HIV Infection and Guidelines for the Use of Antiretroviral Agents in HIV-Infected Adults and Adolescents," first published in *MMWR*, 1998:47(No. RR-5), April 24, 1998, updated as a "Living Document," February 4, 2002, located at (URL) http://www.aidsinfo.nih.gov.

Indications for Plasma HIV RNA Testing*

Clinical Indication	Information	Use
Syndrome consistent with acute HIV infection	Establishes diagnosis when HIV antibody test is negative or indeterminate	Diagnosis†
Initial evaluation of newly diagnosed HIV infection	Baseline viral load "set point"	Decision to start or defer therapy
Every 3-4 months in patients not on therapy	Changes in viral load	Decision to start therapy
2-8 weeks after initiation of antiretroviral therapy	Initial assessment of drug efficacy	Decision to continue or change therapy
3-4 months after start of therapy	Maximal effect of therapy	Decision to continue or change therapy
Every 3-4 months in patients on therapy	Durability of antiretroviral effect	Decision to continue or change therapy
Clinical event or significant decline in CD4+ T cells	Association with changing or stable viral load	Decision to continue, initiate, or change therapy

*Acute illness (eg, bacterial pneumonia, tuberculosis, HSV, PCP, etc) and immunizations can cause increases in plasma HIV RNA for 2-4 weeks; viral load testing should not be performed during this time. Plasma HIV RNA results should usually be verified with a repeat determination before starting or making changes in therapy.

†Diagnosis of HIV infection determined by HIV RNA testing should be confirmed by standard methods (such as Western blot serology) performed 2-4 months after the initial indeterminate or negative test.

Recommendations for the Use of Drug Resistance Assays

Clinical Setting / Recommendation	Rationale
Recommended	
Virologic failure during HAART*	Determine the role of resistance in drug failure and maximize the number of active drugs in the new regimen, if indicated.
Suboptimal suppression of viral load after initiation of antiretroviral therapy	Determine the role of resistance and maximize the number of active drugs in the new regimen, if indicated.
Consider	
Acute HIV infection	Determine if drug-resistant virus was transmitted and change regimen accordingly.
Not Generally Recommended	
Chronic HIV infection prior to initiation of therapy	Uncertain prevalence of resistant virus. Current assays may not detect minor drug-resistant species.
After discontinuation of drugs	Drug-resistant mutations may become minor species in the absence of selective drug pressure. Current assays may not detect minor drug-resistant species.
Plasma viral load <1000 HIV RNA copies/mL	Resistance assays cannot be reliably performed because of low copy number of HIV RNA.

*HAART = highly active antiretroviral therapy.

ADULT AND ADOLESCENT HIV *(Continued)*

Risks and Benefits of Delayed Initiation of Therapy and of Early Therapy in the Asymptomatic HIV-Infected Patient

Risks and Benefits of Delayed Therapy *
Benefits of Delayed Therapy
- Avoid negative effects on quality of life (ie, inconvenience)
- Avoid drug-related adverse events
- Delay in development of drug resistance
- Preserve maximum number of available and future drug options when HIV disease risk is highest

Risks of Delayed Therapy
- Possible risk of irreversible immune system depletion
- Possible greater difficulty in suppressing viral replication
- Possible increased risk of HIV transmission

Risks and Benefits of Early Therapy *
Benefits of Early Therapy
- Control of viral replication easier to achieve and maintain
- Delay or prevention of immune system compromise
- Lower risk of resistance with complete viral suppression
- Possible decreased risk of HIV transmission†

Risks of Early Therapy
- Drug-related reduction in quality of life
- Greater cumulative drug-related adverse events
- Earlier development of drug resistance, if viral suppression is suboptimal
- Limitation of future antiretroviral treatment options

*See table, "Indications for the Initiation of Antiretroviral Therapy in the Chronically HIV-1 Infected Patient," for consensus recommendations regarding when to initiate therapy.

†The risk of viral transmission still exists; antiretroviral therapy cannot substitute for primary HIV prevention measures (eg, use of condoms and safer sex practices).

Goals of HIV Therapy and Tools to Achieve Them

Goals of Therapy
Maximal and durable suppression of viral load
Restoration and/or preservation of immunologic function
Improvement of quality of life
Reduction of HIV-related morbidity and mortality

Tools to Achieve Goals of Therapy
Maximize adherence to the antiretroviral regimen
Rational sequencing of drugs
Preservation of future treatment options
Use of resistance testing in selected clinical settings

Indications for the Initiation of Antiretroviral Therapy in the Chronically HIV-1 Infected Patient

Clinical Category	CD4⁺ T Cell Count	Plasma HIV RNA	Recommendation
Symptomatic (AIDS, severe symptoms)	Any value	Any value	Treat
Asymptomatic, AIDS	CD4⁺ T cells <200/mm³	Any value	Treat
Asymptomatic	CD4⁺ T cells >200/mm³ but <350/mm³	Any value	Treatment should generally be offered, though controversy exists.*
Asymptomatic	CD4⁺ T cells >350/mm³	>55,000 (by bDNA or RT-PCR)†	Some experts would recommend initiating therapy, recognizing that the 3-year risk of developing AIDS in untreated patients is >30% and some would defer therapy and monitor CD4⁺ T cell counts more frequently.
Asymptomatic	CD4⁺ T cells >350/mm³	<55,000 (by bDNA or RT-PCR)†	Many experts would defer therapy and observe, recognizing that the 3-year risk of developing AIDS in untreated patients is <15%.

*Clinical benefit has been demonstrated in controlled trials only for patients with CD4⁺ T cells <200/mm³. However, most experts would offer therapy at a CD4⁺ T cell threshold <350/mm³. A recent evaluation of data from the MACS cohort of 231 individuals with CD4⁺ T cell counts >200 and <350 cells/mm³ demonstrated that of 40 (17%) individuals with plasma HIV RNA <10,000 copies/mL, none progressed to AIDS by 3 years (Alvaro Munoz, personal communication). Of 28 individuals (29%) with plasma viremia of 10,000-20,000 copies/mL, 4% and 11% progressed to AIDS at 2 and 3 years, respectively. Plasma HIV RNA was calculated as RT-PCR values from measured bDNA values. For further information see "Considerations for Initiating Therapy in the Patient With Asymptomatic HIV Infection," found on page 7 of the "Guidelines for the Use of Antiretroviral Agents in HIV-Infected Adults and Adolescents" at http://www.aidsinfo.nih.gov.

†Although there was a 2- to 2.5-fold difference between RT-PCR and the first bDNA assay (version 2.0), with the current bDNA assay (version 3.0), values obtained by bDNA and RT-PCR are similar except at the lower end of the linear range (<1500 copies/mL).

ADULT AND ADOLESCENT HIV *(Continued)*

Recommended Antiretroviral Agents for Initial Treatment of Established HIV Infection

This table provides a guide to the use of available treatment regimens for individuals with no prior or limited experience on HIV therapy. In accordance with the established goals of HIV therapy, priority is given to regimens in which clinical trials data suggest the following: Sustained suppression of HIV plasma RNA (particularly in patients with high baseline viral load) and sustained increase in CD4+T cell count (in most cases over 48 weeks), and favorable clinical outcome (ie, delayed progression to AIDS and death). Particular emphasis is given to regimens that have been compared directly with other regimens that perform sufficiently well with regard to these parameters to be included in the "Strongly Recommended" category. Additional consideration is given to the regimen's pill burden, dosing frequency, food requirements, convenience, toxicity, and drug interaction profile compared with other regimens.

It is important to note that all antiretroviral agents, including those in the "Strongly Recommended" category, have potentially serious toxic and adverse events associated with their use (see individual drug monographs).

Antiretroviral drug regimens are comprised of one choice each from column A and column B. Drugs are listed in alphabetical, not priority order:

	Column A	Column B
Strongly Recommended	Efavirenz Indinavir Nelfinavir Ritonavir + Indinavir* Ritonavir/Lopinavir† Ritonavir + Saquinavir (SGC‡ or HGC‡)	Didanosine + Lamivudine Stavudine + Didanosine§ Stavudine + Lamivudine Zidovudine + Didanosine Zidovudine + Lamivudine
Recommended as Alternatives	Abacavir Amprenavir Delavirdine Nelfinavir + Saquinavir-SGC Nevirapine Ritonavir Saquinavir-SGC	Zidovudine + Zalcitabine
No Recommendation; Insufficient Data¶	Hydroxyurea in combination with antiretroviral drugs Ritonavir + Amprenavir Ritonavir + Nelfinavir Tenofovir♦	
Not Recommended; Should Not Be Offered (All monotherapies, whether from column A or B#)	Saquinavir-HGC•	Stavudine + Zidovudine Zalcitabine + Didanosine Zalcitabine + Lamivudine Zalcitabine + Stavudine

*Based on expert opinion.

†Co-formulated as Kaletra®.

‡Saquinavir-SGC, soft-gel capsule (Fortovase®); Saquinavir-HGC, hard-gel capsule (Invirase®).

§Pregnant women may be at increased risk for lactic acidosis and liver damage when treated with the combination of stavudine and didanosine. This combination should be used in pregnant women only when the potential benefit clearly outweighs the potential risk.

¶This category includes drugs or combinations for which information is too limited to allow a recommendation for or against use.

♦Data from clinical trials are limited to use in salvage. Data from trials of tenofovir as initial therapy may be available in the near future.

#Zidovudine monotherapy may be considered for prophylactic use in pregnant women with low viral load and high CD4+ T cell counts to prevent perinatal transmission.

•Use of saquinavir-HGC (Invirase®) is not recommended, except in combination with ritonavir.

Guidelines for Changing an Antiretroviral Regimen for Suspected Drug Failure

- Criteria for changing therapy include a suboptimal reduction in plasma viremia after initiation of therapy, reappearance of viremia after suppression to undetectable, significant increases in plasma viremia from the nadir of suppression, and declining $CD4^+$ T cell numbers.

- When the decision to change therapy is based on viral load determination, it is preferable to confirm with a second viral load test.

- Distinguish between the need to change a regimen due to drug intolerance or inability to comply with the regimen versus failure to achieve the goal of sustained viral suppression; single agents can be changed in the event of drug intolerance.

- In general, do not change a single drug or add a single drug to a failing regimen; it is important to use at least two new drugs and preferably to use an entirely new regimen with at least three new drugs. If susceptibility testing indicates resistance to only one agent in a combination regimen, it may be possible to replace only that drug; however, this approach requires clinical validation.

- Many patients have limited options for new regimens of desired potency; in some of these cases, it is rational to continue the prior regimen if partial viral suppression was achieved.

- In some cases, regimens identified as suboptimal for initial therapy are rational due to limitations imposed by toxicity, intolerance, or nonadherence. This especially applies in late-stage disease. For patients with no rational alternative options who have virologic failure with return of viral load to baseline (pretreatment levels) and a declining $CD4^+$ T cell count, there should be consideration for discontinuation of antiretroviral therapy.

- Experience is limited with regimens using combinations of two protease inhibitors or combinations of protease inhibitors with NNRTIs; for patients with limited options due to drug intolerance or suspected resistance, these regimens provide possible alternative treatment options.

- There is limited information about the value of restarting a drug that the patient has previously received. Susceptibility testing may be useful in this situation if clinical evidence suggestive of the emergence of resistance is observed. However, testing for phenotypic or genotypic resistance in peripheral blood virus may fail to detect minor resistant variants. Thus, the presence of resistance is more useful information in altering treatment strategies than the absence of detectable resistance.

- Avoid changing from ritonavir to indinavir, or vice versa, for drug failure, since high-level cross-resistance is likely.

- Avoid changing among NNRTIs for drug failure, since high-level cross-resistance is likely.

- The decision to change therapy and the choice of a new regimen requires that the clinician have considerable expertise in the care of people living with HIV. Physicians who are less experienced in the care of persons with HIV infection are strongly encouraged to obtain assistance through consultation with or referral to a clinician with considerable expertise in the care of HIV-infected patients.

ADULT AND ADOLESCENT HIV *(Continued)*

Acute Retroviral Syndrome: Associated Signs and Symptoms (Expected Frequency)

- Fever (96%)
- Lymphadenopathy (74%)
- Pharyngitis (70%)
- Rash (70%)
    - Erythematous maculopapular with lesions on face and trunk and sometimes extremities, including palms and soles
    - Mucocutaneous ulceration involving mouth, esophagus, or genitals
- Myalgia or arthralgia (54%)
- Diarrhea (32%)
- Headache (32%)
- Nausea and vomiting (27%)
- Hepatosplenomegaly (14%)
- Weight loss (13%)
- Thrush (12%)
- Neurologic symptoms (12%)
    - Meningoencephalitis or aseptic meningitis
    - Peripheral neuropathy or radiculopathy
    - Facial palsy
    - Guillain-Barré syndrome
    - Brachial neuritis
    - Cognitive impairment or psychosis

Zidovudine (ZDV) Perinatal Transmission Prophylaxis Regimen

Antepartum	Initiation at 14-34 weeks gestation and continued throughout pregnancy: A. PACTG 076 regimen: ZDV 100 mg 5 times daily B. Acceptable alternative regimen: ZDV 200 mg 3 times daily or ZDV 300 mg 2 times daily
Intrapartum	During labor, ZDV 2 mg/kg I.V. over 1 hour, followed by a continuous infusion of 1 mg/kg/hour I.V. until delivery
Postpartum	Oral administration of ZDV to the newborn (ZDV syrup, 2 mg/kg every 6 hours) for the first 6 weeks of life, beginning at 8-12 hours after birth

IMMUNIZATION GUIDELINES

Standards for Pediatric Immunization Practices

Standard 1.   Immunization services are readily available.

Standard 2.   There are no barriers or unnecessary prerequisites to the receipt of vaccines.

Standard 3.   Immunization services are available free or for a minimal fee.

Standard 4.   Providers utilize all clinical encounters to screen and, when indicated, immunize children.

Standard 5.   Providers educate parents and guardians about immunizations in general terms.

Standard 6.   Providers question parents or guardians about contraindications and, before immunizing a child, inform them in specific terms about the risks and benefits of the immunizations their child is to receive.

Standard 7.   Providers follow only true contraindications.

Standard 8.   Providers administer simultaneously all vaccine doses for which a child is eligible at the time of each visit.

Standard 9.   Providers use accurate and complete recording procedures.

Standard 10.   Providers co-schedule immunization appointments in conjunction with appointments for other child health services.

Standard 11.   Providers report adverse events following immunization promptly, accurately, and completely.

Standard 12.   Providers operate a tracking system.

Standard 13.   Providers adhere to appropriate procedures for vaccine management.

Standard 14.   Providers conduct semiannual audits to assess immunization coverage levels and to review immunization records in the patient populations they serve.

Standard 15.   Providers maintain up-to-date, easily retrievable medical protocols at all locations where vaccines are administered.

Standard 16.   Providers operate with patient-oriented and community-based approaches.

Standard 17.   Vaccines are administered by properly trained individuals.

Standard 18.   Providers receive ongoing education and training on current immunization recommendations.

Recommended by the National Vaccine Advisory Committee, April 1992.
Modified by the United States Public Health Service, 1993.
Endorsed by the American Academy of Pediatrics, May 1992.

The Standards represent the consensus of the National Vaccine Advisory Committee (NVAC) and of a broad group of medical and public health experts about what constitutes the most desirable immunization practices. It is recognized by the NVAC that not all of the current immunization practices of public and private providers are in compliance with the Standards. Nevertheless, the Standards are expected to be useful as a means of helping providers to identify needed changes, to obtain resources if necessary, and to actually implement the desirable immunization practices in the future.

IMMUNIZATION GUIDELINES *(Continued)*

Table 1. Dosage and Administration Guidelines for Vaccines Available in the United States

Vaccine	Dosage	Route of Administration	Type
DT[1]	0.5 mL	I.M.; do not give S.C.	Toxoids
Td[1]	0.5 mL	I.M.; do not give S.C.	Toxoids
DTaP (Acel-Imune®, Tripedia®, Infanrix®)[2]	0.5 mL	I.M.; do not give S.C.	Diphtheria and tetanus toxoids with inactivated acellular pertussis
DTaP-PRP-T (Tripedia®/ActHIB®, TriHIBit®)	0.5 mL	I.M.; do not give S.C.	Polysaccharide-protein conjugate with toxoids and inactivated bacteria
Haemophilus B conjugate vaccine	0.5 mL	I.M. PRP-D, HbOC, or PRP-T can be given S.C. in individuals at risk of hemorrhage	Polysaccharide protein conjugate
HibTITER® (HbOC),[3] manufactured by Lederle Laboratories	0.5 mL	I.M.	Oligosaccharide (diphtheria CRM_{197} protein conjugate)
PedvaxHIB® (PRP-OMP),[4] manufactured by MSD	0.5 mL	I.M.; do not give S.C.	Polysaccharide (meningococcal protein conjugate)
ActHIB®, OmniHIB® (PRP-T), manufactured by Pasteur Merieux Serums & Vaccines	0.5 mL	I.M.	Tetanus toxoid protein conjugate
Haemophilus B conjugate – PRP-OMP and hepatitis B (recombinant) (Comvax®)	0.5 mL	I.M.; do not give S.C.	Polysaccharide-protein conjugate with inactivated virus
Hepatitis A vaccine, inactivated		I.M.; do not give S.C.	Inactivated virus
Havrix®			
Children 2-18 y:	0.5 mL (720 ELISA units) with 2nd dose given 6-12 mo later		
Children >18 y and adults:	1 mL (1440 ELISA units) with 2nd dose given 6-12 mo later		
Vaqta®			
Children 2-17 y:	0.5 mL (25 units) with 2nd dose given 6-18 mo later		
Children >17 y and adults:	1 mL (50 units) with 2nd dose given 6 mo later		
Hepatitis B[5]		I.M. in the anterolateral thigh or in the deltoid muscle[7]	Yeast recombinant-derived inactivated viral antigen
Infants born to HB_sAg-negative mothers, children, and adolescents <20 y[6]			
Recombivax HB® (MSD)	5 mcg (0.5 mL)		
Engerix-B® (SKF)	10 mcg (0.5 mL)		

Infants born to HB_sAg-positive mothers (both immunization with hepatitis B and administration of 0.5 mL hepatitis B immune globulin is recommended for **infants** born to HB_sAg-positive mothers using different administration sites) within 12 hours of birth; administer vaccine at birth; repeat vaccine dose at 1 and 6 months following the initial dose

Recombivax HB® (MSD)	5 mcg (0.5 mL)		
Engerix-B® (SKF)	10 mcg (0.5 mL)		

Table 1. Dosage and Administration Guidelines for Vaccines Available in the United States *(continued)*

Vaccine	Dosage	Route of Administration	Type
Adolescents 11-15 y			
Recombivax HB® (MSD)	10 mcg (1 mL) 2nd dose given 4-6 mo after the first dose (alternate two-dose hepatitis B vaccination schedule)		
Adults ≥20 y			
Recombivax HB® (MSD)	10 mcg (1 mL)		
Engerix-B® (SKF)	20 mcg (1 mL)		
Dialysis patients and immunosuppressed patients			
Recombivax HB® (MSD)	<20 y: 20 mcg (0.5 mL); ≥20 y, 40 mcg (1 mL) using special dialysis formulation		
Engerix-B® (SKF)[8]	<20 y, 20 mcg (1 mL); ≥20 y, 40 mcg (2 mL), give as two 1 mL doses at different sites		
Influenza		I.M. (2 doses 4+ weeks apart in children <9 years of age not previously immunized; only 1 dose needed for annual updates)	Inactivated virus subvirion (split) (contraindicated in patients allergic to chicken eggs)
Split virus only in pediatric patients			
6-35 mo	0.25 mL (1 or 2 doses)		
3-8 y	0.5 mL (1 or 2 doses)		
≥9 y	0.5 mL (1 dose)		
Measles	0.5 mL	S.C.	Live virus (contraindicated in patients with anaphylactic allergy to neomycin)

Most areas: Two doses (1st dose at 15 months with MMR; 2nd dose at 4-6 years or 11-12 years, depending on local school entry requirements)

High-risk area: Two doses (1st dose at 12 months with MMR; 2nd dose as above)

Children 6-15 months in epidemic situations: Dose is given at the time of first contact with a health care provider; children <1 year of age should receive single antigen measles vaccine. If vaccinated before 1 year, revaccinate at 15 months with MMR. A 3rd dose is administered at 4-6 years or 11-12 years, depending on local school entry requirements.

Vaccine	Dosage	Route of Administration	Type
Meningococcal	0.5 mL[9]	S.C.	Polysaccharide
MMR[10]	0.5 mL	S.C.	Live virus
MR	0.5 mL	S.C.	Live virus
Mumps	0.5 mL	S.C.	Live virus
Pneumococcal heptavalent (Pnevnar®)[11]	0.5 mL	I.M.	Protein-conjugated polysaccharide
Pneumococcal polyvalent[12]	0.5 mL (≥2 y)	I.M. or S.C. (I.M. preferred)	Polysaccharide
Poliovirus (OPV) trivalent	0.5 mL	Oral	Live virus

IMMUNIZATION GUIDELINES *(Continued)*

Table 1. Dosage and Administration Guidelines for Vaccines Available in the United States *(continued)*

Vaccine	Dosage	Route of Administration	Type
Poliovirus (IPV)[13] trivalent	0.5 mL	S.C. or I.M.	Inactivated virus
Rabies			
Human diploid cell vaccine (Imovax®)	1 mL	I.M.[14] or	Inactivated virus
(HDCV)	0.1 mL	I.D.[15]	
Rabies vaccine adsorbed (RVA)	1 mL	I.M.[14]	Inactivated virus
Purified chick embryo cell (PCEC) (RabAvert™)	1 mL	I.M.[14]	Inactivated virus
Rubella	0.5 mL (≥12 mo)[16]	S.C.	Live virus
Tetanus (adsorbed)[17]	0.5 mL	I.M.	Toxoid
Tetanus (fluid)	0.5 mL	I.M., S.C.	Toxoid
Typhoid			
Injection, suspension (AKD and HP)		S.C.	Inactivated bacteria
Children 6 mo - 10 y: 0.25 mL; repeat dose in ≥4 weeks. Booster: 0.25 mL every 3 years.			
Children >10 y and adults: 0.5 mL; repeat dose in ≥4 weeks. Booster: 0.5 mL every 3 years.			
Oral (Vivotif® Berna)		P.O.	Live bacteria
Adults: Primary immunization: 1 capsule qod (days 1, 3, 5, and 7). Booster: Repeat primary immunization series every 5 years.			
Varicella (Varivax®)	0.5 mL	S.C.	Live virus
Children 12 mo - 12 y: Single 0.5 mL dose			
Adolescents ≥13 y and adults: 0.5 mL dose x 2 (second 0.5 mL dose is administered 4 to 8 weeks later)			
Yellow fever	0.5 mL[18]	S.C.	Live attenuated virus

[1]DT for use in children <7 years of age. Td contains same amount of tetanus toxoid as DT & DTP, but a reduced dose of diphtheria toxoid. Td for use in children ≥7 years of age.

[2]DTaP is the recommended vaccine for primary vaccination against diphtheria, tetanus, and pertussis; including completion of the series in children who have received 1 or more doses of whole-cell DTP. The occurrence of fever and local reactions is lower with acellular pertussis vaccine than with whole-cell DTP.

[3]The conjugate (HbCV) vaccine is preferred over the polysaccharide (HbPV) vaccine. In children with a high risk for *Haemophilus influenzae* type b disease and HbCV is unavailable, an acceptable alternate is to give HbPV at 18 months of age with a 2nd dose at 24 months of age. Children <5 years of age who were previously vaccinated with HbPV between 18-23 months of age should be revaccinated with a single dose of HbCV at least 2 months after the initial dose of HbPV. Either HbCV or HbPV can be administered up to the 5th birthday. However, they are generally not recommended for children >5 years of age.

[4]PRP-OMP (PedvaxHIB®) manufactured by Merck, Sharp & Dohme is initiated at 2 months of age for 3 doses (2 months, 4 months and 12 months). If initiated at 7-11 months of age, 3 doses are administered (initial 2 doses at 2-month intervals, 3rd dose at 15-18 months of age); if initiated at 12-14 months of age, 2 doses are administered at 2- to 3-month intervals between doses; if initiated at 15-59 months of age, 1 dose is administered.

[5]Hepatitis B vaccine can be given at the same time with DTP, HbOC, polio, and/or MMR; administer 3 doses at 0, 1, and 6 months).

[6]Administer to newborns at 0-2 days of age before hospital discharge; repeat at 1-2 months and 6-18 months following the initial dose. If not vaccinated at birth, administer at 2, 4, and 6-18 months of age.

[7]Aluminum-absorbed vaccines must be injected deep in the muscle mass and not S.C. because they can cause local irritation, inflammation, granuloma formation, and necrosis. Only patients (ie, hemophiliacs) who are at risk of hemorrhage following I.M. injections should receive hepatitis B vaccine S.C.

[8]Engerix-B® — an alternate schedule for postexposure prophylaxis or more rapid induction using 4 doses at 0, 1, 2, and 12 months of age is recommended.

[9]Indicated in children ≥2 years of age at risk (anatomic or functional asplenia, those with terminal complement component or properdin deficiencies, in epidemic or highly endemic areas. The American College Health Association recommends immunization of college students.

[10]See measles.

[11]Routine administration to all children ≤23 months at 2, 4, 6, and 12-15 months. Initial dose should be given no earlier than at 6 weeks of age. Recommended for children 24-59 months who are at high risk for invasive pneumococcal infection.

[12]Indicated for children with sickle cell disease; asplenia; nephrotic syndrome or chronic renal failure; conditions associated with immunosuppression; CSF leaks; HIV infection. Advisory Committee on Immunization Practices (ACIP) also recommends that patients ≥2 years of age with chronic cardiovascular disease, chronic pulmonary disease, diabetes mellitus, or chronic liver disease receive pneumococcal immunization. Patients ≥2 years of age living in special environments in which the risk of invasive pneumococcal disease is high (ie, Alaskan native and certain American Indian populations) should receive pneumococcal immunization.

[13]The primary series consists of 3 doses. The first 2 doses should be administered at an interval of 8 weeks beginning at 2 months of age (minimum age of 6 weeks). The 3rd dose should be given at 6-18 months of age. A booster dose of 0.5 mL should be given to all children who have completed the primary series, before entering school. However, if the 3rd dose of the primary series is given on or after the 4th birthday, a 4th dose is not required before entering school. When polio vaccine is given to persons >18 years of age, IPV should be given.

[14]In infants and small children, I.M. injection can be given into the midlateral aspect of the thigh; in older children and adults, I.M. injection can be given into the deltoid muscle. For postexposure prophylaxis, repeat doses are given on days 3, 7, 14, and 28 after the first dose. Initiate and complete immunization series with one vaccine product. Intradermal vaccine is not advised for postexposure prophylaxis.

[15]For pre-exposure prophylaxis against rabies for high-risk individuals, 1 mL I.M. or 0.1 mL intradermal is administered on days 0, 7, and 21 (or 28). Both I.M. and I.D. dosage forms are available. Preferred site for intradermal administration is the skin in the deltoid area. Patients taking chloroquine or mefloquine should only receive rabies vaccine by the I.M. route. Do **not** administer intradermally to minimize potential for vaccine failure.

[16]As MMR in a 2-dose schedule.

[17]Adsorbed preferred to fluid toxoid because of longer lasting immunity.

[18]≥9 months of age living in or traveling to endemic areas. Contraindicated in infants <4 months of age and in patients who have had an anaphylactic reaction to eggs. Increased risk of encephalitis associated with use of yellow fever vaccine in infants <9 months of age.

Note: For each vaccine, check the manufacturer's package insert for specific product information since preparations may change from time to time.

References

Advisory Committee on Immunization Practices, Measles Prevention, Recommendations of the Immunization Practices Advisory Committee, *MMWR Morb Mortal Wkly Rep*, 1989, 38(5-9):1-18.

Advisory Committee on Immunization Practices (ACIP) and the American Academy of Family Physicians (AAFP), "General Recommendations on Immunization," *MMWR Morb Mortal Wkly Rep*, 2002, 51(RR-2):1-36.

American Academy of Pediatrics, Report of the Committee on Infectious Diseases (Red Book), 25th ed, 2000.

American Academy of Pediatrics, Committee on Infectious Diseases, "Acellular Pertussis Vaccines: Recommendations for Use as the Fourth and Fifth Doses," *Pediatrics*, 1992, 90:121-3.

American Academy of Pediatrics, Committee on Infectious Diseases, "Universal Hepatitis B Immunization," *Pediatrics*, 1992, 89:795-800.

American Academy of Pediatrics, Committee on Infectious Diseases, "Recommendations for the Use of Live Attenuated Varicella Vaccine," *Pediatrics*, 1995, 95(5):791-6.

American Academy of Pediatrics, Committee on Infectious Diseases, "Policy Statement: Recommendations for the Prevention of Pneumococcal Infections, Including the Use of Pneumococcal Conjugate Vaccine (Prevnar®), Pneumococcal Polysaccharide Vaccine, and Antibiotic Prophylaxis," *Pediatrics*, 2000, 106(2 Pt 1): 362-6.

American Academy of Pediatrics, Committee on Infectious Diseases, "Recommended Childhood Immunization Schedule – United States, January-December 2002," *Pediatrics*, 2002, 109(1):162-4.

CDC, "Notice to Readers: Alternate Two-Dose Hepatitis B Vaccination Schedule for Adolescents Aged 11-15 Years," *MMWR Morb Mortal Wkly Rep*, 2000, 49(12):261.

IMMUNIZATION GUIDELINES (Continued)

Table 2. Currently Recommended Regimens for Routine *Haemophilus influenzae* Type b Conjugate Immunization for Children Immunized Beginning at 2-6 Months of Age[1]

Vaccine Product at Initiation	Total No. of Doses to Be Administered	Recommended Regimens
HbOC or PRP-T	4	3 doses at 2-month intervals initially; fourth dose at 12-15 months of age; any conjugate vaccine for dose 4[2]
PRP-OMP	3	2 doses at 2-month intervals initially; when feasible, same vaccine for doses 1 and 2; third dose at 12-15 months of age; any conjugate vaccine for dose 3[2]

[1]These vaccines may be given in combination products or as reconstituted products with DTaP or DTP, provided the combination or reconstituted vaccine is approved by the U.S. Food and Drug Administration for the child's age and the administration of the other vaccine component(s) also is justified.

[2]The safety and efficacy of PRP-OMP, PRP-T, HbOC, and PRP-D are likely to be equivalent for children ≥12 months of age. If a different product is given for dose 2, then the recommendations for that product (eg, HbOC or PRP-T) apply.

Adapted from "Report of the Committee on Infectious Diseases," *2000 Red Book*®, 25th ed, 268.

Table 3. Recommendations for Pneumococcal Conjugate Vaccine Use Among Healthy Children During Moderate and Severe Shortages

Age at First Vaccination (mo)	No Shortage[1]	Moderate Shortage	Severe Shortage
<6	2, 4, 6, and 12-15 months	2, 4, and 6 months (defer fourth dose)	2 doses at 2-month interval in first 6 months of life (defer third and fourth doses)
7-11	2 doses at 2-month interval; 12-15 month dose	2 doses at 2-month interval; 12-15-month dose	2 doses at 2-month interval (defer third dose)
12-23	2 doses at 2-month interval	2 doses at 2-month interval	1 dose (defer second dose)
>24	1 dose should be considered	No vaccination	No vaccination
Reduction in vaccine doses used[2]		21%	46%

[1]The vaccine schedule for no shortage is included as a reference. Providers should not use the no shortage schedule regardless of their vaccine supply until the national shortage is resolved.

[2]Assumes that approximately 85% of vaccine is administered to healthy infants beginning at age <7 months; approximately 5% is administered to high-risk infants beginning at age <7 months; and approximately 10% is administered to healthy children beginning at age 7-24 months. Actual vaccine savings will depend on a provider's vaccine use.

Adapted from the Advisory Committee on Immunization Practices, "Updated Recommendations on Use of Pneumococcal Conjugate Vaccine in a Setting of Vaccine Shortage," *MMWR Morb Mortal Wkly Rep*, 2001, 50(50):1140-2.

Table 4. Persons Who Should Receive Pre-exposure Hepatitis B Immunization

- All infants

- Children at high risk for early childhood HBV infection

- Adolescents: Hepatitis B vaccination should be given by or before 11-12 years of age. Special efforts should be made to vaccinate all adolescents, not only those at high risk

- Hemophiliac patients and other recipients of certain blood products

- Intravenous drug abusers

- Heterosexual persons who have had more than one sex partner in the previous 6 months and/or those with a recent episode of a sexually transmitted disease

- Sexually active men who have sex with men

- Household and sexual contacts of HB_sAg-positive persons

- Members of households with adoptees who are hepatitis B surface antigen-positive

- Children and other household contacts in populations of high HBV endemicity

- Staff and residents of institutions for the developmentally disabled

- Staff of nonresidential day care and school programs for developmentally disabled if attended by known HB_sAg-positive persons

- Hemodialysis patients

- Healthcare workers and others with occupational risk of exposure to blood or blood-contaminated body fluid

- International travelers to areas of high or intermediate HBV endemicity

- Inmates of long-term correctional facilities

Adapted from American Academy of Pediatrics, Report of the Committee on Infectious Diseases, *Red Book*, 25th ed, 2000, 296.

See **Table 5** for recommended Hepatitis B immunization schedule.

IMMUNIZATION GUIDELINES (Continued)

Table 5. Recommended Childhood and Adolescent Immunization Schedule - United States, 2003

Vaccine ▼ / Age ►	Birth	1 mo	2 mo	4 mo	6 mo	12 mo	15 mo	18 mo	24 mo	4-6 y	11-12 y	13-18 y
Hepatitis B[1]	HepB #1	only if mother HBsAg(-)									HepB series	
		HepB #2			HepB #3							
Diphtheria, tetanus, pertussis[2]			DTaP	DTaP	DTaP		DTaP			DTaP	Td	
H. influenzae type b[3]			Hib	Hib	Hib	Hib						
Inactivated polio			IPV	IPV		IPV				IPV		
Measles, mumps, rubella[4]						MMR #1				MMR #2	MMR #2	
Varicella[5]						Varicella					Varicella	
Pneumococcal[6]			PCV	PCV	PCV	PCV				PCV	PPV	
Hepatitis A[7]											Hepatitis A series	
Influenza[8]						Influenza (yearly)						

Vaccines below this line are for selected populations

This schedule indicates the recommended ages for routine administration of currently licensed childhood vaccines, as of December 1, 2002, for children through age 18 years. Any dose not given at the recommended age should be given at any subsequent visit when indicated and feasible. ▨ Indicates age groups that warrant special effort to administer those vaccines not previously given. Additional vaccines may be licensed and recommended during the year. Licensed combination vaccines may be used whenever any components of the combination are indicated and the vaccine's other components are not contraindicated. Providers should consult the manufacturers' package inserts for detailed recommendations.

[1] **Hepatitis B vaccine (HepB).** All infants should receive the first dose of hepatitis B vaccine soon after birth and before hospital discharge; the first dose may also be given by age 2 months if the infant's mother is HBsAg-negative. Only monovalent HepB can be used for the birth dose. Monovalent or combination vaccine containing HepB may be used to complete the series. Four doses of vaccine may be administered when a birth dose is given. The second dose should be given at least 4 weeks after the first dose, except for combination vaccines which cannot be administered before age 6 weeks. The third dose should be given at least 16 weeks after the first dose and at least 8 weeks after the second dose. The last dose in the vaccination series (third or fourth dose) should not be administered before age 6 months .

Infants born to HBsAg-positive mothers should receive HepB and 0.5 mL hepatitis B immune globulin (HBIG) within 12 hours of birth at separate sites. The second dose is recommended at age 1-2 months. The last dose in the vaccination series should not be administered before age 6 months. These infants should be tested for HBsAg and anti-HBs at 9-15 months of age.

Infants born to mothers whose HBsAg status is unknown should receive the first dose of the HepB series within 12 hours of birth. Maternal blood should be drawn as soon as possible to determine the mother's HBsAg status; if the HBsAg test is positive, the infant should receive HBIG as soon as possible (no later than age 1 week). The second dose is recommended at age 1-2 months. The last dose in the vaccination series should not be administered before age 6 months.

[2] **Diphtheria, tetanus toxoids, and acellular pertussis vaccine (DTaP).** The fourth dose of DTaP may be administered as early as age 12 months, provided 6 months have elapsed since the third dose and the child is unlikely to return at age 15-18 months. **Tetanus and diphtheria toxoids (Td)** is recommended at age 11-12 years if at least 5 years have elapsed since the last dose of tetanus and diphtheria toxoid-containing vaccine. Subsequent routine Td boosters are recommended every 10 years.

[3] *Haemophilus influenzae* **type b (Hib) conjugate vaccine.** Three Hib conjugate vaccines are licensed for infant use. If PRP-OMP (PedvaxHIB® or ComVax® [Merck]) is administered at ages 2 and 4 months, a dose at age 6 months is not required. DTaP/Hib combination products should not be used for primary immunization in infants at ages 2, 4, or 6 months, but can be used as boosters following any Hib vaccine.

[4] **Measles, mumps, and rubella vaccine (MMR).** The second dose of MMR is recommended routinely at age 4-6 years but may be administered during any visit, provided at least 4 weeks have elapsed since the first dose and that both doses are administered beginning at or after age 12 months. Those who have not previously received the second dose should complete the schedule by the 11- to 12-year old visit.

[5] **Varicella vaccine** is recommended at any visit at or after age 12 months for susceptible children (ie, those who lack a reliable history of chickenpox). Susceptible persons ≥13 years of age should receive 2 doses, given at least 4 weeks apart.

[6] The heptavalent **pneumococcal conjugate vaccine (PCV)** is recommended for all children ages 2-23 months. It is also recommended for certain children age 24-59 months. **Pneumococcal polysaccharide vaccine (PPV)** is recommended in addition to PCV for certain high-risk groups. See *MMWR Morb Mortal Wkly Rep*, 2000, 49(RR-9):1-38.

[7] **Hepatitis A vaccine** is recommended for children and adolescents in selected states and regions, and for certain high-risk groups; consult your local public health authority. Children and adolescents in these states, regions, and high-risk groups who have not been immunized against hepatitis A can begin the hepatitis A vaccination series during any visit. The two doses in the series should be administered at least 6 months apart. See *MMWR Morb Mortal Wkly Rep*, 1999, 48(RR-12): 1-37.

[8] **Influenza vaccine** is recommended annually for children age ≥6 months with certain risk factors (including but not limited to asthma, cardiac disease, sickle cell disease, HIV, diabetes, and household members of persons in groups at high risk; see *MMWR Morb Mortal Wkly Rep*, 2002, 51(RR-3):1-31), and can be administered to all others wishing to obtain immunity. In addition, healthy children age 6-23 months are encouraged to receive influenza vaccine if feasible because children in this age group are at substantially increased risk for influenza-related hospitalizations. Children ≤12 years of age should receive vaccine in a dosage appropriate for their age (0.25 mL if age 6-35 months or 0.5 mL if ≥3 years of age). Children ≤8 years of age who are receiving influenza vaccine for the first time should receive two doses separated by at least 4 weeks.

Approved by the Advisory Committee on Immunization Practices (www.cdc.gov/nip/acip), the American Academy of Pediatrics (www.aap.org), and the American Academy of Family Physicians (www.aafp.org).

FOR CHILDREN AND ADOLESCENTS WHO START LATE OR WHO ARE >1 MONTH BEHIND

Tables 6 and 7 give catch-up schedules and minimum intervals between doses for children who have delayed immunizations. There is no need to restart a vaccine series regardless of the time that has elapsed between doses. Use the chart appropriate for the child's age.

Table 6. Catch-up Schedule for Children Age 4 Months - 6 Years

Dose One (Minimum Age)	Minimum Interval Between Doses			
	Dose One to Dose Two	Dose Two to Dose Three	Dose Three to Dose Four	Dose Four to Dose Five
DTaP (6 wk)	4 wk	4 wk	6 mo	6 mo[1]
IPV (6 wk)	4 wk	4 wk	4 wk[2]	
HepB[3] (birth)	4 wk	8 wk (and 16 wk after first dose)		
MMR (12 mo)	4 wk[4]			
Varicella (12 mo)				
Hib[5] (6 wk)	**4 wk:** If 1st dose given at age <12 mo **8 wk (as final dose):** If 1st dose given at age 12-14 mo **No further doses needed:** If 1st dose given at age ≥15 mo	**4 wk[6]:** If current age <12 mo **8 wk (as final dose)[6]:** If current age ≥12 mo and 2nd dose given at age <15 mo **No further doses needed:** If previous dose given at age ≥15 mo	**8 wk (as final dose):** This dose only necessary for children age 12 mo - 5 y who received 3 doses before age 12 mo	
PCV[7] (6 wk)	**4 wk:** If 1st dose given at age <12 mo and current age <24 mo **8 wk (as final dose):** If 1st dose given at age ≥12 mo or current age 24-59 mo **No further doses needed:** For healthy children if 1st dose given at age ≥24 mo	**4 wk:** If current age <12 mo **8 wk (as final dose):** If current age ≥12 mo **No further doses needed:** For healthy children if previous dose given at age ≥24 mo	**8 wk (as final dose):** This dose only necessary for children age 12 mo - 5 y who received 3 doses before age 12 mo	

IMMUNIZATION GUIDELINES *(Continued)*

Table 7. Catch-up Schedule for Children Age 7-18 Years

Minimum Interval Between Doses		
Dose One to Dose Two	**Dose Two to Dose Three**	**Dose Three to Booster Dose**
Td: 4 wk	Td: 6 mo	Td[8]: **6 mo:** If 1st dose given at age <12 mo and current age <11 y **5 y:** If 1st dose given at age ≥12 mo and 3rd dose given at age <7 y and current age ≥11 y **10 y:** If 3rd dose given at age ≥7 y
IPV[9]: 4 wk	IPV[9]: 4 wk	IPV[9]
HepB: 4 wk	HepB: 8 wk (and 16 wk after first dose)	
MMR: 4 wk		
Varicella[10]: 4 wk		

Footnotes to Table 6 and Table 7

[1]**DTaP:** The fifth dose is not necessary if the fourth dose was given after the 4th birthday.

[2]**IPV:** For children who received an all-IPV or all-OPV series, a fourth dose is not necessary if third dose was given at age ≥4 years. If both OPV and IPV were given as part of a series, a total of four doses should be given, regardless of the child's current age.

[3]**HepB:** All children and adolescents who have not been immunized against hepatitis B should begin the hepatitis B vaccination series during any visit. Providers should make special efforts to immunize children who were born in, or whose parents were born in, areas of the world where hepatitis B virus infection is moderately or highly endemic.

[4]**MMR:** The second dose of MMR is recommended routinely at age 4-6 years, but may be given earlier if desired.

[5]**Hib:** Vaccine is not generally recommended for children age ≥5 years.

[6]**Hib:** If current age <12 months and the first 2 doses were PRP-OMP (PedvaxHIB® or ComVax®), the third (and final) dose should be given at age 12-15 months and at least 8 weeks after the second dose.

[7]**PCV:** Vaccine is not generally recommended for children age ≥5 years.

[8]**Td:** For children age 7-10 years, the interval between the third and booster dose is determined by the age when the first dose was given. For adolescents age 11-18 years, the interval is determined by the age when the third dose was given.

[9]**IPV:** Vaccine is not generally recommended for persons age ≥18 years.

[10]**Varicella:** Give 2-dose series to all susceptible adolescents age ≥13 years.

Table 8. Recommended Immunization Schedules for Children Not Immunized in the First Year of Life

Recommended Time/Age	Immunization(s)[1]	Comments
Younger Than 7 Years		
First visit	DTaP, Hib, HBV, MMR	If indicated, tuberculin testing may be done at same visit.
		If child is ≥5 y of age, Hib is not indicated in most circumstances.
Interval after first visit		
1 mo (4 wk)	DTaP, IPV, HBV, Var[2]	The second dose of IPV may be given if accelerated poliomyelitis immunization is necessary, such as for travelers to areas where polio is endemic.
2 mo	DTaP, Hib, IPV	Second dose of Hib is indicated only if the first dose was received when <15 mo.
≥8 mo	DTaP, HBV, IPV	IPV and HBV are not given if the third doses were given earlier.
Age 4-6 y (at or before school entry)	DTaP, IPV, MMR[3]	DTaP is not necessary if the fourth dose was given after the fourth birthday; IPV is not necessary if the third dose was given after the fourth birthday.
Age 11-12 y	See Table 5	
7-12 Years		
First visit	HBV, MMR, dT, IPV	
Interval after first visit		
2 mo (8 wk)	HBV, MMR,[3] Var,[4] dT, IPV	IPV also may be given 1 mo after the first visit if accelerated poliomyelitis immunization is necessary.
8-14 mo	HBV,[4] dT, IPV	IPV is not given if the third dose was given earlier.
Age 11-12 y	See Table 5	

[1] If all needed vaccines cannot be administered simultaneously, priority should be given to protecting the child against those diseases that pose the greatest immediate risk. In the United States, these diseases for children <2 years usually are measles and *Haemophilus influenzae* type b infection; for children >7 years, they are measles, mumps, and rubella. Before 13 years of age, immunity against hepatitis B and varicella should be ensured. DTaP, HBV, Hib, MMR, and Var can be given simultaneously at separate sites if failure of the patient to return for future immunizations is a concern.

[2] Varicella vaccine can be administered to susceptible children any time after 12 months of age. Unimmunized children who lack a reliable history of varicella should be immunized before their 13th birthday.

[3] Minimal interval between doses of MMR is 1 month (4 weeks).

[4] HBV may be given earlier in a 0-, 2-, and 4-month schedule.

Adapted from American Academy of Pediatrics, Report of the Committee on Infectious Diseases, *Red Book*, 25th ed, 2000.

IMMUNIZATION GUIDELINES *(Continued)*

Table 9. Spacing Live and Killed Antigen Administration Guidelines

Antigen Combinations	Recommended Minimum Interval Between Doses
≥2 killed antigens	None. May be given simultaneously or at any interval between doses. Vaccines associated with systemic reactions (cholera, plague, and parenteral typhoid) should be given on separate occasions.
Killed and live antigens	None. May be given simultaneously or at any interval between doses. (**Exception:** Concurrent administration of cholera and yellow fever vaccines should be avoided. Separate these vaccines by at least 3 weeks.)
≥2 live antigens parenteral	4-week minimum interval if not administered simultaneously. Live oral vaccines (eg, Ty21a typhoid vaccine, oral polio vaccine) can be administered simultaneously or at any interval before or after inactivated or live parenteral vaccines.

Table 10. Passive Immunization Agents — Immune Globulins

Immune Globulin	Dosage		Route
Hepatitis B (H-BIG®)			I.M.
percutaneous inoculation	0.06 mL/kg/dose (within 24 hours) (5 mL max)		
perinatal	0.5 mL/dose (within 12 hours of birth)		
sexual exposure	0.06 mL/kg/dose (within 14 days of contact) (5 mL max)		
Immune globulin (IG)			I.M.[1]
hepatitis A prophylaxis	0.02 mL/kg/dose (as soon as possible or within 2 weeks after exposure) (postexposure prophylaxis)		
<2 y:	0.06 mL/kg/dose (≥3 months or long-term exposure) repeat every 5 months with continuous exposure		
≥2 y:	0.02 mL/kg (3- to 5-month exposure) may be given to travelers whose departure is imminent with hepatitis A vaccine 0.06 mL/kg (long-term exposure) and hepatitis A vaccine		
hepatitis B	0.06 mL/kg/dose (H-BIG® should be used)		
hepatitis C	0.06 mL/kg/dose (percutaneous exposure)		
measles[2]	0.25 mL/kg/dose (max: 15 mL/dose) (within 6 days of exposure) 0.5 mL/kg/dose (max: 15 mL/dose) (immunocompromised children)		
Rabies[3]	20 IU/kg/dose (within 3 days)		
Tetanus (serious, contaminated, wounds; <3 previous tetanus vaccine doses)	250-500 units/dose		I.M.
Varicella-zoster[4] (VZIG)	Within 48 hours but not later than 96 hours after exposure		I.M.[5]
	0-10 kg	125 units = 1 vial	
	10.1-20 kg	250 units = 2 vials	
	20.1-30 kg	375 units = 3 vials	
	30.1-40 kg	500 units = 4 vials	
	>40 kg	625 units = 5 vials	

[1]Deep I.M. in the gluteal region for large doses only. Deltoid muscle or the anterolateral aspect of the thigh are preferred sites for injection. No greater than 5 mL/site in adults or large children; 1-3 mL/site in small children and infants. Max: 20 mL at one time. Pregnant women and infants should receive a thimerosol-free preparation.

[2]IG prophylaxis may not be indicated in a patient who has received IGIV within 3 weeks of exposure.

[3]1/2 of dose used to infiltrate the wound with the remaining 1/2 of dose given I.M. Rabies immune globulin is not recommended in previously HDCV immunized patients.

[4]Infants born to women who develop varicella within 5 days before or 48 hours after delivery should receive 125 units I.M. as a single dose.

[5]No greater than 2.5 mL of VZIG/one injection site. Doses >2.5 mL should be divided and administered at different sites.

Table 11. Suggested Intervals Between Administration of Immune Globulin Preparations for Various Indications and Measles Immunization[1]

Indication	Dose (including mg IgG/kg)	Time Interval (mo) Before Measles or Varicella Vaccination
Tetanus (TIG) prophylaxis	I.M.: 250 units (10 mg IgG/kg)	3
Hepatitis A (IG) prophylaxis		
Contact prophylaxis	I.M.: 0.02 mL/kg (3.3 mg IgG/kg)	3
International travel	I.M.: 0.06 mL/kg (10 mg IgG/kg)	3
Hepatitis B prophylaxis (HBIG)	I.M.: 0.06 mL/kg (10 mg IgG/kg)	3
Rabies immune globulin (RIG)	I.M.: 20 IU/kg (22 mg IgG/kg)	4
Varicella prophylaxis (VZIG)	I.M.: 125 units/10 kg (20-40 mg IgG/kg) (max: 625 units)	5
Measles prophylaxis (IG)		
Standard (ie, nonimmunocompromised contact)	I.M.: 0.25 mL/kg (40 mg IgG/kg)	5
Immunocompromised contact	I.M.: 0.50 mL/kg (80 mg IgG/kg)	6
Blood transfusion		
RBCs, washed	I.V.: 10 mL/kg (negligible IgG/kg)	0
RBCs, adenine-saline added	I.V.: 10 mL/kg (10 mg IgG/kg)	3
Packed RBCs	I.V.: 10 mL/kg (20-60 mg IgG/kg)	5
Whole blood cells	I.V.: 10 mL/kg (80-100 mg IgG/kg)	6
Plasma/platelet products	I.V.: 10 mL/kg (160 mg IgG/kg)	7
Replacement therapy for immune deficiencies	I.V.: 300-400 mg/kg (as IGIV)[2]	8
Immune thrombocytopenic purpura[3]	I.V.: 400 mg/kg (as IGIV)	8
	I.V.: 1000 mg/kg (as IGIV)	10
Kawasaki disease	I.V.: 2 g/kg (as IGIV)	11
RSV prophylaxis	I.V.: 750 mg/kg (as RSV-IVIG)	9
RSVIG monoclonal antibody (Syngis™)	I.M.: 15 mg/kg	None

[1]This table is not intended for determining the correct indications and dosage for the use of immune globulin preparations. Unvaccinated persons may not be fully protected against measles during the entire suggested time interval, and additional doses of immune globulin and/or measles vaccine may be indicated after measles exposure. The concentration of measles antibody in a particular immune globulin preparation can vary by lot. The rate of antibody clearance after receipt of an immune globulin preparation also can vary. The recommended time intervals are extrapolated from an estimated half-life of 30 days of passively acquired antibody and an observed interference with the immune response to measles vaccine for 5 months after a dose of 80 mg IgG/kg.

[2]Measles vaccination is recommended for most HIV-infected children who do not have evidence of severe immunosuppression, but it is contraindicated for patients who have congenital disorders of the immune system.

[3]Formerly referred to as idiopathic thrombocytopenic purpura.

Modified from *Red Book 2000: Report of the Committee on Infectious Diseases*, 25th ed, Elk Grove Village, IL: American Academy of Pediatrics, 390; Recommendations of the Advisory Committee on Immunization Practices (ACIP) and the American Academy of Family Physicians (AAFP), "General Recommendations on Immunization," *MMWR Morb Mortal Wkly Rep*, 2002, 51(RR-2), 1-36.

IMMUNIZATION GUIDELINES *(Continued)*

Table 12. Recommended for Routine Immunization of HIV-Infected Children — United States

Vaccine	Known HIV Infection	
	Asymptomatic	Symptomatic
DTaP	Yes	Yes
OPV	No	No
IPV	Yes	Yes
MMR	Yes	Yes*
Hib	Yes	Yes
Pneumococcal	Yes	Yes
Influenza†	Yes	Yes
Varicella	Consider	Consider
BCG	No	No
Hepatitis A	‡	‡
Hepatitis B	Yes	Yes

*Severely immunocompromised HIV-infected children should not receive MMR.

†Administer influenza vaccine each autumn and repeat annually for HIV-exposed infants ≥6 months of age, HIV-infected children and adolescents, and household contacts of HIV-infected persons.

‡The immune response in immunocompromised persons, including persons with HIV, may be suboptimal.

RECOMMENDATIONS FOR TRAVELERS

Table 13. Recommended Immunizations for Travelers to Developing Countries[1]

Immunizations	Length of Travel		
	Brief, <2 wk	Intermediate, 2 wk - 3 mo	Long-term Residential, >3 mo
Review and complete age-appropriate childhood schedule	+	+	+
• DTaP; poliovirus vaccine, and *H. influenzae* type b vaccine may be given at 4 wk intervals if necessary to complete the recommended schedule before departure			
• Measles: 2 additional doses given if younger than 12 mo of age at first dose			
• Varicella			
• Hepatitis B[2]			
Yellow fever[3]	+	+	+
Hepatitis A[4]	+	+	+
Typhoid fever[4]	±	+	+
Meningococcal disease[5]	±	±	±
Rabies[6]	±	+	+
Japanese encephalitis[3]	±	±	+

[1] + = recommended; ± = consider.

[2] If insufficient time to complete 6-month primary series, accelerated series can be given.

[3] For endemic regions, see *Health Information for International Travel* in *Red Book®*. For high-risk activities in areas experiencing outbreaks, vaccine is recommended even for brief travel.

[4] Indicated for travelers who will consume food and liquids in areas of poor sanitation.

[5] For endemic regions of Africa, during local epidemics, and travel to Saudi Arabia for the Hajj.

[6] Indicated for person with high risk of animal exposure, and for travelers to endemic countries.

Adapted from "Report of the Committee on Infectious Diseases," *2000 Red Book®*, 25th ed, 78.

Table 14. Recommendations for Pre-exposure Immunoprophylaxis of Hepatitis A Virus Infection for Travelers[1]

Age (y)	Likely Exposure (mo)	Recommended Prophylaxis
<2	<3	IG 0.02 mL/kg[2]
	3-5	IG 0.06 mL/kg[2]
	Long-term	IG 0.06 mL/kg at departure and every 5 mo if exposure to HAV continues[2]
≥2	<3[3]	HAV vaccine[4,5] **or**
	3-5[3]	HAV vaccine[4,5] **or** IG 0.06 mL/kg[2]
	Long-term	HAV vaccine[4,5]

[1] IG = immune globulin; HAV= hepatitis A virus.
[2] IG should be administered deep into a large muscle mass. Ordinarily, no more than 5 mL should be administered in one site in an adult or large child; lesser amounts (maximum 3 mL) should be given to small children and infants.
[3] Vaccine is preferable, but IG is an acceptable alternative.
[4] To ensure protection in travelers whose departure is imminent, IG also may be given.
[5] Dose and schedule of hepatitis A vaccine as recommended according to age.
Adapted from "Report of the Committee on Infectious Diseases," *2000 Red Book*®, 25th ed, 282.

CONTRAINDICATIONS AND PRECAUTIONS TO COMMONLY USED VACCINES

Vaccine	Contraindications	Precautions[1]	Vaccines Can Be Administered
General for all vaccines, including diphtheria and tetanus toxoids and acellular pertussis vaccine (DTaP); pediatric diphtheria-tetanus toxoid (DT); adult tetanus-diphtheria toxoid (Td); inactivated poliovirus vaccine (IPV); measles-mumps-rubella vaccine (MMR); *Haemophilus influenzae* type b vaccine (Hib); hepatitis A vaccine; hepatitis B vaccine; varicella vaccine; pneumococcal conjugate vaccine (PCV); influenza vaccine; and pneumococcal polysaccharide vaccine (PPV)	• Serious allergic reaction (eg, anaphylaxis) after a previous vaccine dose • Serious allergic reaction (eg, anaphylaxis) to a vaccine component	• Moderate or severe acute illnesses with or without a fever	• Mild acute illness with or without fever • Mild to moderate local reaction (ie, swelling, redness, soreness); low-grade or moderate fever after previous dose • Lack of previous physical examination in well-appearing person • Current antimicrobial therapy • Convalescent phase of illnesses • Premature birth (hepatitis B vaccine is an exception in certain circumstances)[2] • Recent exposure to an infectious disease • History of penicillin allergy, other nonvaccine allergies, receiving allergen extract immunotherapy • Temperature <40.5°C, fussiness or mild drowsiness after a previous dose of diphtheria toxoid-tetanus toxoid-pertussis vaccine (DTP)/DTaP • Family history of seizures[3] • Family history of sudden infant death syndrome • Family history of an adverse event after DTP or DTaP administration • Stable neurologic conditions (eg, cerebral palsy, well-controlled convulsions, developmental delay)
DTaP	• Severe allergic reaction after a previous dose or to a vaccine component • Encephalopathy (eg, coma, decreased level of consciousness, prolonged seizures) within 7 days of administration of previous dose of DTP or DTaP • Progressive neurologic disorder, including infantile spasms, uncontrolled epilepsy, progressive encephalopathy; defer DTaP until neurologic status clarified and stabilized	• Fever >40.5°C ≤48 hours after vaccination with a previous dose of DTP or DTaP • Collapse or shock-like state (ie, hypotonic hyporesponsive episode) ≤48 hours after receiving a previous dose of DTP/DTaP • Seizure ≤3 days of receiving a previous dose of DTP/DTaP[3] • Persistent, inconsolable crying lasting ≥3 hours, ≤48 hours after receiving a previous dose of DTP/DTaP • Moderate or severe acute illness with or without fever	Same as above

Vaccine	Contraindications	Precautions[1]	Vaccines Can Be Administered
DT, Td	• Severe allergic reaction after a previous dose or to a vaccine component	• Guillain-Barré syndrome ≤6 weeks after previous dose of tetanus toxoid-containing vaccine • Moderate or severe acute illness with or without fever	Same as above
IPV	• Severe allergic reaction to previous dose or vaccine component	• Pregnancy • Moderate or severe acute illness with or without fever	—
MMR[4]	• Severe allergic reaction after a previous dose or to a vaccine component • Pregnancy • Known severe immunodeficiency (eg, hematologic and solid tumors; congenital immunodeficiency; long-term immunosuppressive therapy,[5] or severely symptomatic human immunodeficiency virus [HIV] infection)	• Recent (≤11 months) receipt of antibody-containing blood product (specific interval depends on product) • History of thrombocytopenia or thrombocytopenic purpura • Moderate or severe acute illness with or without fever	• Positive tuberculin skin test • Simultaneous TB skin testing[6] • Breast-feeding • Pregnancy of recipient's mother or other close or household contact • Recipient is child-bearing-age female • Immunodeficient family member or household contact • Asymptomatic or mildly symptomatic HIV infection • Allergy to eggs
Hib	• Severe allergic reaction after a previous dose or to a vaccine component • Age <6 weeks	• Moderate or severe acute illness with or without fever	—
Hepatitis B	• Severe allergic reaction after a previous dose or to a vaccine component	• Infant weighing <2000 g[2] • Moderate or severe acute illness with or without fever	• Pregnancy • Autoimmune disease (eg, systemic lupus erythematosis or rheumatoid arthritis)
Hepatitis A	• Severe allergic reaction after a previous dose or to a vaccine component	• Pregnancy • Moderate or severe acute illness with or without fever	—
Varicella	• Severe allergic reaction after a previous dose or to a vaccine component • Substantial suppression of cellular immunity • Pregnancy	• Recent (≤11 months) receipt of antibody containing blood product (specific interval depends on product) • Moderate or severe acute illness with or without fever	• Pregnancy of recipient's mother or other close or household contact • Immunodeficient family member or household contact[7] • Asymptomatic or mildly symptomatic HIV infection • Humoral immunodeficiency (eg, agammaglobulinemia)
PCV	• Severe allergic reaction after a previous dose or to a vaccine component	• Moderate or severe acute illness with or without fever	—

CONTRAINDICATIONS AND PRECAUTIONS TO COMMONLY USED VACCINES *(Continued)*

Vaccine	Contraindications	Precautions[1]	Vaccines Can Be Administered
Influenza	• Severe allergic reaction to previous dose or vaccine component, including egg protein	• Moderate or severe acute illness with or without fever	• Nonsevere (eg, contact) allergy to latex or thimerosal • Concurrent administration of Coumadin® or aminophylline
PPV	• Severe allergic reaction after a previous dose or to a vaccine component	• Moderate or severe acute illness with or without fever	—

[1]Events or conditions listed as precautions should be reviewed carefully. Benefits and risks of administering a specific vaccine to a person under these circumstances should be considered. If the risk from the vaccine is believed to outweigh the benefit, the vaccine should not be administered. If the benefit of vaccination is believed to outweigh the risk, the vaccine should be administered. Whether and when to administer DTaP to children with proven or suspected underlying neurologic disorders should be decided on a case-by-case basis.

[2]Hepatitis B vaccination should be deferred for infants weighing <2000 g if the mother is documented to be hepatitis B surface antigen (Hb_sAg)-negative at the time of the infant's birth. Vaccination can commence at chronological age 1 month. For infants born to Hb_sAg-positive women, hepatitis B immunoglobulin and hepatitis B vaccine should be administered at or soon after birth regardless of weight.

[3]Acetaminophen or other appropriate antipyretic can be administered to children with a personal or family history of seizures at the time of DTaP vaccination and every 4-6 hours for 24 hours thereafter to reduce the possibility of postvaccination fever (source: American Academy of Pediatrics, Pickering LK, ed, "Active Immunization," *2000 Red Book®*, Report of the Committee on Infectious Diseases, 25th ed, Elk Grove Village, IL: American Academy of Pediatrics, 2000).

[4]MMR and varicella vaccines can be administered on the same day. If not administered on the same day, these vaccines should be separated by ≥28 days.

[5]Substantially immunosuppressive steroid dose is considered to be ≥2 weeks of daily receipt of 20 mg or 2 mg/kg body weight of prednisone or equivalent.

[6]Measles vaccination can suppress tuberculin reactivity temporarily. Measles-containing vaccine can be administered on the same day as tuberculin skin testing. If testing cannot be performed until after the day of MMR vaccination, the test should be postponed for ≥4 weeks after the vaccination. If an urgent need exists to skin test, do so with the understanding that reactivity might be reduced by the vaccine.

[7]If a vaccine experiences a presumed vaccine-related rash 7-25 days after vaccination, avoid direct contact with immunocompromised persons for the duration of the rash.

Adapted from "Recommendations and Reports," *MMWR Morb Mortal Wkly Rep,* 2002, 51(RR-2):9-10.

SKIN TESTS FOR DELAYED HYPERSENSITIVITY

Skin tests for delayed hypersensitivity are used diagnostically to assess previous infection (ie, PPD, histoplasmin, and coccidioidin) or used to evaluate cellular immune function by testing for anergy (ie, mumps, *Candida*, tetanus toxoid, trichophyton, PPD). Anergy, a defect in cell-mediated immunity, is characterized by a depressed response or lack of response to skin testing with injected antigens. Anergy has been associated with congenital and acquired immunodeficiencies, and malnutrition.

Candida 1:100

Dose = 0.1 mL intradermally (30% of children younger than 18 months of age and 50% older than 18 months of age respond)

Can be used as a control antigen

Coccidioidin 1:100

Dose = 0.1 mL intradermally (apply with PPD **and** a control antigen)
Mercury derivative used as a preservative for spherulin.

Histoplasmin 1:100

Dose = 0.1 mL intradermally (yeast derived)

Multitest CMI (*Candida*, diphtheria toxoid, tetanus toxoid, *Streptococcus*, old tuberculin, *Trichophyton*, *Proteus* antigen, and negative control)

Press loaded unit into the skin with sufficient pressure to puncture the skin and allow adequate penetration of all points.

Mumps 40 cfu per mL

Dose = 0.1 mL intradermally (contraindicated in patients allergic to eggs, egg products, or thimerosal)

Purified Protein Derivative 5 TU (PPD* Mantoux Tuberculin)

Screening for tuberculosis:

Children who have no risk factors but who reside in high-prevalence regions: skin test at 4-6 years and 11-16 years of age

Children exposed to HIV-infected individuals, homeless, residents of nursing homes, institutionalized adolescents, users of illicit drugs, incarcerated adolescents and migrant farm workers: skin test every 2-3 years

Children at high risk (children infected with HIV, incarcerated adolescents): annual skin testing

Dose = 0.1 mL intradermally

Definition of positive Mantoux skin test (regardless of previous BCG administration):

Reaction ≥5 mm for high-risk group (children in close contact with known or suspected infectious cases of tuberculosis; children suspected to have disease based on clinical and/or roentgenographic evidence; and children with underlying host factors (immunosuppressive conditions, receiving immunosuppressive therapy, and HIV infection).

Reaction ≥10 mm for children <4 years; those with medical diseases who are at increased risk for dissemination or for those at increased risk because of environmental exposure.

Reaction ≥15 mm for children ≥4 years of age including those with no risk factors.

*PPD 1 TU (first strength) is only used in individuals suspected of being highly sensitive. PPD 250 TU (second strength) is used only for individuals who fail to respond to a previous injection of 5 TU, or anergic patients in whom TB is suspected.

SKIN TESTS FOR DELAYED HYPERSENSITIVITY
(Continued)

Tetanus Toxoid 1:5

Dose = 0.1 mL intradermally (29% of children younger than 2 years of age and 78% older than 2 years of age respond if they have received 3 immunizing doses)

Can be used as a control antigen.

Tine Test

Indication: survey and screen for exposure to tuberculosis (grasp forearm firmly; stretch the skin of the volar surface tightly; apply the tines to the selected site; press for at least one second so that a circular halo impression is left on the skin)

General Information

1. Intradermal skin tests should be injected in the flexor surface of the forearm.

2. A pale wheal 6-10 mm in diameter should form over the needle tip as soon as the injection is administered. If no bleb forms, the injection must be repeated.

3. Space skin tests at least 2 inches apart to prevent reactions from overlapping.

4. Read skin tests for diameter of induration and presence of erythema at 24, 48, and 72 hours. Reactions occurring before 24 hours are indicative of an immediate rather than a delayed hypersensitivity reaction.

5. False-negative results may occur in patients with malnutrition, viral infections, febrile illnesses, immunodeficiency disorders, severe disseminated infections, uremia, patients who have received immunosuppressive therapy (steroids, antineoplastic agents), patients who have received a recent live attenuated virus vaccine (MMR, measles).

6. False-positive results may occur in patients sensitive to ingredients in the skin test solution such as thimerosal; cross-sensitivity between similar antigens; or with improper interpretation of skin test.

7. Side effects are pain, blisters, extensive erythema and necrosis at the injection site.

*Emergency equipment and epinephrine should be readily available to treat severe allergic reactions that may occur.

Recommended Interpretation of Skin Test Reactions

Reaction	Local Reaction	
	After Intradermal Injections of Antigens	After Dinitrochlorobenzene
1+	Erythema >10 mm and/or induration >1-5 mm	Erythema and/or induration covering <1/2 area of dosing site
2+	Induration 6-10 mm	Induration covering >1/2 area of dose site
3+	Induration 11-20 mm	Vesiculation and induration at dose site or spontaneous flare at days 7-14 at the site
4+	Induration >20 mm	Bulla or ulceration at dose site or spontaneous flare at days 7-14 at the site

References

American Academy of Pediatrics Committee on Infectious Diseases, "Screening for Tuberculosis in Infants and Children," *Pediatrics*, 1994, 93(1):131-4.
American Academy of Pediatrics Committee on Infectious Diseases, "Update on Tuberculosis Skin Testing of Children," *Pediatrics*, 1996, 97(2):282-4.

NORMAL LABORATORY VALUES FOR CHILDREN

Normal Values

CHEMISTRY

Albumin	0-1 y	2.0-4.0 g/dL
	1 y to adult	3.5-5.5 g/dL
Ammonia	Newborns	90-150 µg/dL
	Children	40-120 µg/dL
	Adults	18-54 µg/dL
Amylase	Newborns	0-60 units/L
	Adults	30-110 units/L
Bilirubin, conjugated, direct	Newborns	<1.5 mg/dL
	1 mo to adult	0-0.5 mg/dL
Bilirubin, total	0-3 d	2.0-10.0 mg/dL
	1 mo to adult	0-1.5 mg/dL
Bilirubin, unconjugated, indirect		0.6-10.5 mg/dL
Calcium	Newborns	7.0-12.0 mg/dL
	0-2 y	8.8-11.2 mg/dL
	2 y to adult	9.0-11.0 mg/dL
Calcium, ionized, whole blood		4.4-5.4 mg/dL
Carbon dioxide, total		23-33 mEq/L
Chloride		95-105 mEq/L
Cholesterol	Newborns	45-170 mg/dL
	0-1 y	65-175 mg/dL
	1-20 y	120-230 mg/dL
Creatinine	0-1 y	≤0.6 mg/dL
	1 y to adult	0.5-1.5 mg/dL
Glucose	Newborns	30-90 mg/dL
	0-2 y	60-105 mg/dL
	Children to Adults	70-110 mg/dL
Iron	Newborns	110-270 µg/dL
	Infants	30-70 µg/dL
	Children	55-120 µg/dL
	Adults	70-180 µg/dL
Iron binding	Newborns	59-175 µg/dL
	Infants	100-400 µg/dL
	Adults	250-400 µg/dL
Lactic acid, lactate		2-20 mg/dL
Lead, whole blood		<10 µg/dL
Lipase		
	Children	20-140 units/L
	Adults	0-190 units/L
Magnesium		1.5-2.5 mEq/L
Osmolality, serum		275-296 mOsm/kg
Osmolality, urine		50-1400 mOsm/kg
Phosphorus	Newborns	4.2-9.0 mg/dL
	6 wk to 19 mo	3.8-6.7 mg/dL
	19 mo to 3 y	2.9-5.9 mg/dL
	3-15 y	3.6-5.6 mg/dL
	>15 y	2.5-5.0 mg/dL

NORMAL LABORATORY VALUES FOR CHILDREN
(Continued)

Normal Values

CHEMISTRY

Potassium, plasma	Newborns	4.5-7.2 mEq/L
	2 d to 3 mo	4.0-6.2 mEq/L
	3 mo to 1 y	3.7-5.6 mEq/L
	1-16 y	3.5-5.0 mEq/L
Protein, total	0-2 y	4.2-7.4 g/dL
	>2 y	6.0-8.0 g/dL
Sodium		136-145 mEq/L
Triglycerides	Infants	0-171 mg/dL
	Children	20-130 mg/dL
	Adults	30-200 mg/dL
Urea nitrogen, blood	0-2 y	4-15 mg/dL
	2 y to Adult	5-20 mg/dL
Uric acid	Male	3.0-7.0 mg/dL
	Female	2.0-6.0 mg/dL

ENZYMES

Alanine aminotransferase (ALT) (SGPT)	0-2 mo	8-78 units/L
	>2 mo	8-36 units/L
Alkaline phosphatase (ALKP)	Newborns	60-130 units/L
	0-16 y	85-400 units/L
	>16 y	30-115 units/L
Aspartate aminotransferase (AST) (SGOT)	Infants	18-74 units/L
	Children	15-46 units/L
	Adults	5-35 units/L
Creatine kinase (CK)	Infants	20-200 units/L
	Children	10-90 units/L
	Adult male	0-206 units/L
	Adult female	0-175 units/L
Lactate dehydrogenase (LDH)	Newborns	290-501 units/L
	1 mo to 2 y	110-144 units/L
	>16 y	60-170 units/L

Blood Gases

	Arterial	Capillary	Venous
pH	7.35-7.45	7.35-7.45	7.32-7.42
pCO$_2$ (mm Hg)	35-45	35-45	38-52
pO$_2$ (mm Hg)	70-100	60-80	24-48
HCO$_3$ (mEq/L)	19-25	19-25	19-25
TCO$_2$ (mEq/L)	19-29	19-29	23-33
O$_2$ saturation (%)	90-95	90-95	40-70
Base excess (mEq/L)	-5 to +5	-5 to +5	-5 to +5

Thyroid Function Tests

T₄ (thyroxine)	1-7 d	10.1-20.9 µg/dL
	8-14 d	9.8-16.6 µg/dL
	1 mo to 1 y	5.5-16.0 µg/dL
	>1 y	4.0-12.0 µg/dL
FTI	1-3 d	9.3-26.6
	1-4 wk	7.6-20.8
	1-4 mo	7.4-17.9
	4-12 mo	5.1-14.5
	1-6 y	5.7-13.3
	>6 y	4.8-14.0
T₃	Newborns	100-470 ng/dL
	1-5 y	100-260 ng/dL
	5-10 y	90-240 ng/dL
	10 y to Adult	70-210 ng/dL
T₃ uptake		35%-45%
TSH	Cord	3-22 µIU/mL
	1-3 d	<40 µIU/mL
	3-7 d	<25 µIU/mL
	>7 d	0-10 µIU/mL

NORMAL LABORATORY VALUES FOR CHILDREN
(Continued)

Hematology Values

Age	Hgb (g/dL)	Hct (%)	RBC (mill/mm³)	RDW	MCV (fL)	MCH (pg)	MCHC (%)	PLTS (x 10³/mm³)
0-3 d	15.0-20.0	45-61	4.0-5.9	<18	95-115	31-37	29-37	250-450
1-2 wk	12.5-18.5	39-57	3.6-5.5	<17	86-110	28-36	28-38	250-450
1-6 mo	10.0-13.0	29-42	3.1-4.3	<16.5	74-96	25-35	30-36	300-700
7 mo to 2 y	10.5-13.0	33-38	3.7-4.9	<16	70-84	23-30	31-37	250-600
2-5 y	11.5-13.0	34-39	3.9-5.0	<15	75-87	24-30	31-37	250-550
5-8 y	11.5-14.5	35-42	4.0-4.9	<15	77-95	25-33	31-37	250-550
13-18 y	12.0-15.2	36-47	4.5-5.1	<14.5	78-96	25-35	31-37	150-450
Adult male	13.5-16.5	41-50	4.5-5.5	<14.5	80-100	26-34	31-37	150-450
Adult female	12.0-15.0	36-44	4.0-4.9	<14.5	80-100	26-34	31-37	150-450

WBC and Diff

Age	WBC (x 10³/mm³)	Segs	Bands	Lymphs	Monos	Eosinophils	Basophils	Atypical Lymphs	No. of NRBCs
0-3 d	9.0-35.0	32-62	10-18	19-29	5-7	0-2	0-1	0-8	0-2
1-2 wk	5.0-20.0	14-34	6-14	36-45	6-10	0-2	0-1	0-8	0
1-6 mo	6.0-17.5	13-33	4-12	41-71	4-7	0-3	0-1	0-8	0
7 mo to 2 y	6.0-17.0	15-35	5-11	45-76	3-6	0-3	0-1	0-8	0
2-5 y	5.5-15.5	23-45	5-11	35-65	3-6	0-3	0-1	0-8	0
5-8 y	5.0-14.5	32-54	5-11	28-48	3-6	0-3	0-1	0-8	0
13-18 y	4.5-13.0	34-64	5-11	25-45	3-6	0-3	0-1	0-8	0
Adults	4.5-11.0	35-66	5-11	24-44	3-6	0-3	0-1	0-8	0

Segs = segmented neutrophils.

Bands = band neutrophils.

Lymphs = lymphocytes.

Monos = monocytes.

NORMAL LABORATORY VALUES FOR CHILDREN
(Continued)

Erythrocyte Sedimentation Rates and Reticulocyte Counts

Sedimentation rate, Westergren	Children	0-20 mm/hour
	Adult male	0-15 mm/hour
	Adult female	0-20 mm/hour
Sedimentation rate, Wintrobe	Children	0-13 mm/hour
	Adult male	0-10 mm/hour
	Adult female	0-15 mm/hour
Reticulocyte count	Newborns	2%-6%
	1-6 mo	0%-2.8%
	Adults	0.5%-1.5%

Cerebrospinal Fluid Values, Normal

		% PMNs
Cell count		
Preterm mean	9 (0-25.4 WBC/mm^3)	57%
Term mean	8.2 (0-22.4 WBC/mm^3)	61%
>1 mo	0.7	0
Glucose		
Preterm	24-63 mg/dL	mean 50
Term	34-119 mg/dL	mean 52
Children	40-80 mg/dL	
CSF glucose/blood glucose		
Preterm	55-105%	
Term	44-128%	
Children	50%	
Lactic acid dehydrogenase	5-30 units/mL	mean 20 units/mL
Myelin basic protein	<4 ng/mL	
Pressure: Initial LP (mm H$_2$O)		
Newborns	80-110 (<110)	
Infants/children	<200 (lateral recumbent position)	
Respiratory movements	5-10	
Protein		
Preterm	65-150 mg/dL	mean 115
Term	20-170 mg/dL	mean 90
Children		
Ventricular	5-15 mg/dL	
Cisternal	5-25 mg/dL	
Lumbar	5-40 mg/dL	

APGAR SCORING SYSTEM

Sign	Score		
	0	1	2
Heart rate	Absent	Under 100 beats per minute	Over 100 beats per minute
Respiratory effort	Absent	Slow (irregular)	Good crying
Muscle tone	Limp	Some flexion of extremities	Active motion
Reflex irritability	No response	Grimace	Cough or sneeze
Color	Blue, pale	Pink body, blue extremities	All pink

From Apgar V, "A Proposal for a New Method of Evaluation of the Newborn Infant," *Anesth Analg*, 1953, 32:260.

FETAL HEART RATE MONITORING

Normal Heart Rates

Fetal heart rate (FHR) 120-160 bpm. Isolated accelerations are normal and considered reassuring. Mild (100-120 bpm) and transient bradycardias may be normal. Normal fetal heart rate tracings show beat-to-beat variability of 5-10 bpm (poor beat-to-beat variability suggests fetal hypoxia).

Abnormal Heart Rates

Bradycardia (FHR <120 bpm): Potential causes include fetal distress, drugs, congenital heart block (associated with maternal SLE, congenital cardiac defects).

Tachycardia (FHR >160 bpm): Potential causes include maternal fever, chorioamnionitis, drugs, fetal dysrhythmias, eg, SVT (with or without fetal CHF).

Decreased Beat-to-Beat Variability

Results from fetal CNS depression. Potential causes include fetal hypoxia, fetal sleep, fetal immaturity, and maternal narcotic/sedative administration.

Fetal Heart Rate Decelerations

Type 1 (early decelerations)

- Seen most commonly in late labor
- Mirror uterine contractions in time of onset, duration, and resolution
- Uniform shape
- Usually associated with good beat-to-beat variability
- Heart rate may dip to 60-80 bpm
- Associated with fetal head compression (increases vagal tone)
- Considered benign, and not representative of fetal hypoxia

APGAR SCORING SYSTEM *(Continued)*

Type 2 (late decelerations)

- Deceleration 10-30 seconds after onset of uterine contraction
- Heart rate fails to return to baseline after contraction is completed
- Asymmetrical shape (longer deceleration, shorter acceleration)
- Late decelerations of 10-20 bpm may be significant
- Probably associated with fetal CNS and myocardial depression

Type 3 (variable decelerations)

- Heart rate variations do not correlate with uterine contractions
- Variable shape and duration
- Occur occasionally in many normal labors
- Concerning if severe (HR <60 bpm), prolonged (duration >60 seconds), associated with poor beat-to-beat variability, or combined with late decelerations
- Associated with cord compression (including nuchal cord)

Reference
Manual of Neonatal Care, Joint Program in Neonatology, 1991.

CREATININE CLEARANCE ESTIMATING METHODS IN PATIENTS WITH STABLE RENAL FUNCTION

The following formulas provide an acceptable estimate of the patient's creatinine clearance except when:

a. The patient's serum creatinine is changing rapidly (either up or down).

b. Patients are markedly emaciated.

In these situations (a and b above), certain assumptions have to be made:

a. In patients with rapidly rising serum creatinines (ie, increasing by >0.5-0.7 mg/dL/day), it is best to assume that the patient's creatinine clearance is probably less than 10 mL/minute.

b. In emaciated patients, although their actual creatinine clearance is less than their calculated creatinine clearance (because of decreased creatinine production), it is not possible to predict easily how much less.

Estimation of creatinine clearance using serum creatinine and body length* (to be used when an adequate timed specimen cannot be obtained). **Note:** This formula may not provide an accurate estimation of creatinine clearance for infants <6 months of age or for patients with severe starvation or muscle wasting.

$$CL_{cr} = K \times L/S_{cr}$$

where:

Cl_{cr} = creatinine clearance in mL/minute/1.73 m^2

K = constant of proportionality that is age specific

Age	K
Low birth weight ≤1 y	0.33
Full-term ≤1 y	0.45
2-12 y	0.55
13-21 y female	0.55
13-21 y male	0.70

L = length in cm

S_{Cr} = serum creatinine concentration in mg/dL

Reference

Schwartz GJ, Brion LP, and Spitzer A, "The Use of Plasma Creatinine Concentration for Estimating Glomerular Filtration Rate in Infants, Children and Adolescents," *Ped Clin N Amer*, 1987, 34:571-90.

Children 1-18 years

Method 1: (Traub SL, Johnson CE, *Am J Hosp Pharm*, 1980, 37:195-201)

Equation:

$$Cl_{cr} = \frac{0.48 \times (height)}{S_{cr}}$$

where

Cl_{cr} = creatinine clearance in mL/min/1.73 m^2

S_{cr} = serum creatinine in mg/dL

Height = height in cm

Method 2: See nomogram.

CREATININE CLEARANCE ESTIMATING METHODS IN PATIENTS WITH STABLE RENAL FUNCTION *(Continued)*

Children 1-18 Years

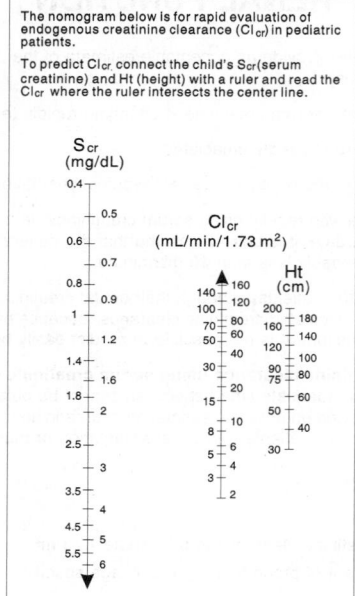

The nomogram below is for rapid evaluation of endogenous creatinine clearance (Cl_{cr}) in pediatric patients.

To predict Cl_{cr} connect the child's S_{cr} (serum creatinine) and Ht (height) with a ruler and read the Cl_{cr} where the ruler intersects the center line.

Adults 18 years and older

Method 1: (Cockroft DW and Gault MH, *Nephron*, 1976, 16:31-41)

Estimated creatinine clearance (Cl_{cr}) (mL/min):

$$\text{Male} = \frac{(140 - \text{age})\ \text{IBW (kg)}}{72 \times \text{serum creatinine}}$$

Female = Estimated Cl_{cr} male x 0.85

Note: The use of the patient's ideal body weight (IBW) is recommended for the above formula except when the patient's actual body weight is less than ideal. Use of the IBW is especially important in obese patients. See appendix Growth & Development section for Ideal Body Weight Calculation.

Method 2: (Jelliffe RW, *Ann Intern Med*, 1973, 79:604)

Estimated creatinine clearance (Cl_{cr}) (mL/min/1.73 m^2):

$$\text{Male} = \frac{98 - 0.8\ (\text{age} - 20)}{\text{serum creatinine}}$$

Female = Estimated Cl_{cr} male x 0.90

RENAL FUNCTION TESTS

Endogenous creatinine clearance vs age (timed collection)

Creatinine clearance (mL/min/1.73 m²) = $(Cr_uV/S_{Cr}T)$ (1.73/A)

where:

Cr_u	=	Urine creatinine concentration (mg/dL)
V	=	Total urine volume collected during sampling period (mL)
S_{Cr}	=	Serum creatinine concentration (mg/dL)
T	=	Duration of sampling period (min) (24 h = 1440 min)
A	=	Body surface area (m²)

Age-specific normal values

5-7 d	50.6±5.8 mL/min/1.73 m²
1-2 mo	64.6±5.8 mL/min/1.73 m²
5-8 mo	87.7±11.9 mL/min/1.73 m²
9-12 mo	86.9±8.4 mL/min/1.73 m²
≥18 mo	
male	124±26 mL/min/1.73 m²
female	109±13.5 mL/min/1.73 m²
Adults	
male	105±14 mL/min/1.73 m²
female	95±18 mL/min/1.73 m²

Note: In patients with renal failure (creatinine clearance <25 mL/min), creatinine clearance may be elevated over GFR because of tubular secretion of creatinine.

Serum BUN/Serum Creatinine Ratio

Serum BUN (mg/dL):serum creatinine (mg/dL)

Normal BUN:creatinine ratio is 10-15.

BUN:creatinine ratio >20 suggests prerenal azotemia (also seen with high urea-generation states such as GI bleeding).

BUN:creatinine ratio <5 may be seen with disorders affecting urea biosynthesis such as urea cycle enzyme deficiencies and with hepatitis.

Fractional Sodium Excretion

Fractional sodium secretion (FENa) = Na_uS_{Cr}/Na_sCr_u x 100%

where:

Na_u	=	Urine sodium (mEq/L)
Na_s	=	Serum sodium (mEq/L)
Cr_u	=	Urine creatinine (mg/dL)
S_{Cr}	=	Serum creatinine (mg/dL)

FENa <1% suggests prerenal failure
FENa >2% suggest intrinsic renal failure
(for newborns, normal FENa is approximately 2.5%)

Note: Disease states associated with a falsely elevated FENa include severe volume depletion (>10%), early acute tubular necrosis and volume depletion in chronic renal disease. Disorders associated with a lowered FENa include acute glomerulonephritis, hemoglobinuric or myoglobinuric renal failure, nonoliguric acute tubular necrosis, and acute urinary tract obstruction. In addition, FENa may be <1% in patients with acute renal failure **and** a second condition predisposing to sodium retention (eg, burns, congestive heart failure, nephrotic syndrome).

RENAL FUNCTION TESTS *(Continued)*

Urine Calcium/Urine Creatinine Ratio (spot sample)

Urine calcium (mg/dL): urine creatinine (mg/dL)

Normal values <0.21 (mean values 0.08 males, 0.06 females)

Premature infants show wide variability of calcium:creatinine ratio, and tend to have lower thresholds for calcium loss than older children. Prematures without nephrolithiasis had mean Ca:Cr ratio of 0.75±0.76. Infants with nephrolithiasis had mean Ca:Cr ratio of 1.32±1.03 (Jacinto, et al, *Pediatrics*, vol 81, p 31).

Urine Protein/Urine Creatinine Ratio (spot sample)

P_u/Cr_u	Total Protein Excretion (mg/m²/day)
0.1	80
1	800
10	8000

where:

$P_u =$	Urine protein concentration (mg/dL)
$Cr_u =$	Urine creatinine concentration (mg/dL)

Serum Osmolality

Predicted serum osmolality =

2 x Na (mEq/L) + BUN (mg/dL) / 2.8 + glucose (mg/dL) / 18

High Anion Gap (see Toxicology section)

ACID / BASE ASSESSMENT

Henderson-Hasselbalch Equation

$$pH = 6.1 + \log (HCO_3^- / (0.03) (pCO_2))$$

Alveolar Gas Equation

P_iO_2 = f_iO_2 x (total atmospheric pressure – vapor pressure of H_2O at 37°C)

= f_iO_2 x (760 mm Hg – 47 mm Hg)

PAO_2 = $P_iO_2 - PACO_2 / R$

Alveolar/arterial oxygen gradient = $PAO_2 - PaO_2$

Normal ranges:

Children	15-20 mm Hg
Adults	20-25 mm Hg

Where:

P_iO_2	=	Oxygen partial pressure of inspired gas (mm Hg) (150 mm Hg in room air at sea level)
f_iO_2	=	Fractional pressure of oxygen in inspired gas (0.21 in room air)
PAO_2	=	Alveolar oxygen partial pressure
$PACO_2$	=	Alveolar carbon dioxide partial pressure
PaO_2	=	Arterial oxygen partial pressure
R	=	Respiratory exchange quotient (typically 0.8, increases with high carbohydrate diet, decreases with high fat diet)

Acid/Base Disorders

Acute metabolic acidosis (<12 h duration)

$PaCO_2$ expected = 1.5 (HCO_3^-) + 8±2

or

expected change in pCO = (1-1.5) x change in HCO_3^-

Acute metabolic alkalosis (<12 h duration)

expected change in pCO_2 = (0.5-1) x change in HCO_3^-

Acute respiratory acidosis (<6 h duration)

expected change in HCO_3^- = 0.1 x pCO_2

Acute respiratory acidosis (>6 h duration)

expected change in HCO_3^- = 0.4 x change in pCO

Acute respiratory alkalosis (<6 h duration)

expected change in HCO_3^- = 0.2 x change in pCO

Acute respiratory alkalosis (>6 h duration)

expected change in HCO_3^- = 0.5 x change in pCO

ACUTE DYSTONIC REACTIONS, MANAGEMENT

1. **Confirm that patient has stable airway and adequate respiratory activity.**

2. Administer **one** of the following:

   Diphenhydramine 0.7-1 mg/kg/dose I.V./P.O. q4-6h prn **or**

   Hydroxyzine 0.5-1 mg/kg/dose I.M./P.O. q4-6h prn
   (adult dose: 25-100 mg I.M./P.O. q6h) **or**

   Children >3 years: Benztropine 0.02-0.05 mg/kg/dose or maximum of 1-2 mg I.V./P.O. (avoid use in children <3 years of age except in cases of extreme emergency)

Agents which predispose patients to acute dystonic reactions, such as phenothiazine neuroleptics or antiemetics, often have long therapeutic half-lives. Anticholinergic administration should therefore be continued for 6-24 hours after discontinuation of phenothiazine therapy.

PREPROCEDURE SEDATIVES IN CHILDREN

Purpose: The following table is a guide to aid the clinician in the selection of the most appropriate sedative to sedate a child for a procedure. One must also consider:

- Not all patients require sedation. It is dependent on the procedure and age of the child.

- When sedation is desired, one must consider the time of onset, the duration of action, and the route of administration.

- Each of the following drugs is well absorbed when given by the suggested routes and doses.

- Each drug was assigned an "intensity" based upon the class of drug, dose, and route.[1]

  - Conscious sedation: A medically controlled state of depressed consciousness that retains the patient's ability to independently and continuously maintain a patent airway, respond appropriately to physical stimulation and/or verbal commands. The protective reflexes are maintained.

  - Deep sedation: A medically controlled state of depressed consciousness associated with partial or complete loss of protective reflexes and inability to respond appropriately to physical stimulation and/or verbal commands.

- Those drugs classified as producing deep sedation require more frequent monitoring postprocedure.

- For painful procedures, an analgesic agent needs to be administered.

Sedatives Used to Produce Conscious Sedation

Drug	Route	Dose (mg/kg)	Onset (min)	Duration (h)	Comments
Chloral hydrate	P.O./P.R.	25-100	10-20	4-8	May cause hepatic neoplasms in rats; maximum single dose: infants: 1 g; children: 2 g
Diazepam[2,3] (Valium®)	P.O.	0.2-0.3 90 min prior	60-90	6-8	Maximum oral dose: 10 mg
	I.V.	0.1-0.2	1-3	6-8	Maximum dose I.V.: 5 mg; due to poor absorption and tissue irritation, I.M. route **not** recommended
	P.R.	0.2-0.4	2-10	6-8	May use I.V. solution rectally
"DPT" cocktail[4] (Demerol®, Phenergan®, Thorazine®)	I.M.	Demerol® 1-2, Phenergan® 0.5-1, Thorazine® 0.5-1	30	2-14	May be mixed in single syringe; I.M. only. This combination of agents may have a higher rate of adverse effects compared with alternative sedative/analgesics.
Fentanyl	Transmucosal	5-15 mcg/kg	5-15	1-2	Maximum transmucosal dose: 400 mcg
	I.M.	1-3 mcg/kg	7-15	1-2	
	I.V.	1-3 mcg/kg	Immediate	30-60 min	
Lorazepam[5] (Ativan®)	P.O.	0.05; 90-120 min prior	60	8-12	
	Deep I.M.	0.05; 90-120 min prior	30-60	8-12	
	I.V.	0.05; over 5-10 min	15-30	8-12	

PREPROCEDURE SEDATIVES IN CHILDREN *(Continued)*

Sedatives Used to Produce Conscious Sedation *(continued)*

Drug	Route	Dose (mg/kg)	Onset (min)	Duration (h)	Comments
Meperidine (Demerol®)	P.O.	2-4	10-15	2-4	Doses I.M./I.V. >2 mg/kg are considered deep sedation
	I.M.	0.5-2	10-15	2-4	
	I.V.	0.5-2	5	2-3	
Midazolam[6,7] (Versed®)	P.O.	0.2-0.4; 30-45 min prior	20-30	1-2	Maximum oral dose: 15 mg
	Deep I.M.	0.1-0.15; 30-60 min prior	15	1-2	Maximum total dose: 10 mg
	I.V.	**6 mo - 5 y:** 0.05-0.1; **6-12 y:** 0.025-0.05; **>12 y - Adult:** 2.5-5 mg (total dose); give over 10-20 min	1-5	1-2	Maximum concentration: 1 mg/mL; maximum I.M./I.V. dose: 6 mo - 5 y: 6 mg 6 y - Adult: 10 mg
	P.R.	0.3	20-30	1-2	Dilute injection in 5 mL NS; administer rectally
	Intranasal	0.2-0.3	5	30-60 min	Administer nasally: Use a 1 mL needleless syringe into the nares over 15 seconds; use 5 mg/mL concentration; ½ dose may be administered into each nare
Morphine	P.O.	0.2-0.5	20-30	3-5	
	I.M.	0.05-0.2	20-30	3-5	
	I.V.	0.05-0.2	10-15	2-5	

Note: See individual drug monographs for further information.

Sedatives Used to Produce Deep Sedation

Drug	Route	Dose (mg/kg)	Onset (min)	Duration (h)	Comments
Methohexital[8,9] (Brevital®)	I.M.	5-10	5	1-1.5	Maximum concentration for I.M./I.V.: 50 mg/mL; maximum I.M./I.V. dose: 200 mg. Greater incidence of adverse effects with I.V. use.
	I.V.	0.75-2	1	7-10 min	
	P.R.	20-35	5-10	1-1.5	Shorter duration of action than thiopental; rectal given as a 10% solution in sterile water; maximum dose rectal: 500 mg
Pentobarbital	P.O./ I.M./P.R.	2-6	10-25	1-4	Maximum I.M./I.V./P.O./P.R. dose: 100 mg
	I.V.	1-3	1	15 min	
Thiopental[10,4] (Pentothal)	I.V.	4-6	0.5-1	5-10 min	Variable rectal absorption; may use additional 12.5 mg/kg if necessary; maximum rectal dose: 1-1.5 g
	P.R.	25; immediately prior to procedure	10	1-5	

Note: See individual drug monographs for further information.

Sedatives Used to Produce Dissociative Anesthesia (Monitor as if deep sedation)

Drug	Route	Dose (mg/kg)	Onset (min)	Duration	Comments
Ketamine	P.O.	6-10; 30 min prior	30-45	10-30	Use only under direct supervision of physicians experienced in administering general anesthetics; has analgesic effects; may use injectable product orally diluted in a beverage of the patient's choice
	I.M.	3-7	7	12-25	
	I.V.	0.5-2	1	5-10	

Note: See individual drug monographs for further information.

Footnotes

1. Committee on Drugs, Section of Anesthesiology, American Academy of Pediatrics, "Guidelines for Monitoring and Management of Pediatric Patient During and After Sedation for Diagnostic and Therapeutic Procedures," *Pediatrics*, 1992, 89:1110-5.
2. Yager JY and Seshia SS, "Sublingual Lorazepam in Childhood Serial Seizures," *Am J Dis Child*, 1988, 142(9):931-2.
3. Fell D, Gough MB, Northan AA, et al, "Diazepam Premedication in Children," *Anaesthesia*, 1985, 40:12-7.
4. Burckart GJ, White III TJ, Siegle RL, et al, "Rectal Thiopental Versus an Intramuscular Cocktail for Sedating Children Before Computer Tomography," *Am J Hosp Pharm*, 1980, 37:222-4.
5. Burtles R and Astley B, "Lorazepam in Children," *Br J Anaesth*, 1983, 55:275-9.
6. Roelofse JA, van der Bijl P, Stegmann DH, et al, "Preanesthetic Medication With Rectal Midazolam in Children Undergoing Dental Extractions," *J Oral Maxillofac Surg*, 1990, 48(8):791-7.
7. Wilton NC, Leigh J, Rosen DR, et al, "Preanesthetic Sedation of Preschool Children Using Intranasal Midazolam," *Anesthesiology*, 1988, 60(6):972-5.
8. Elman DS and Denson JS, "Preanesthetic Sedation of Children With Intramuscular Methohexital Sodium," *Anesth Analg*, 1965, 44(5):494-8.
9. Miller JR, Grayson M, and Stoelting VK, "Sedation With Intramuscular Methohexital Sodium," *Am J Ophthalmol*, 1966, 62(1):38-43.
10. "Drug Evaluations," *AMA*, 1980.

FEBRILE SEIZURES

A febrile seizure is defined as a seizure occurring for no reason other than an elevated temperature. It does not have an infectious or metabolic origin within the CNS (ie, it is not caused by meningitis or encephalitis). Fever is usually >102°F rectally, but the more rapid the rise in temperature, the more likely a febrile seizure may occur. About 4% of children develop febrile seizures at one time of their life, usually occurring between 3 months and 5 years of age with the majority occurring at 6 months to 3 years of age. There are three types of febrile seizures:

1. **Simple** febrile seizures are nonfocal febrile seizures of less than 15 minutes duration. They do not occur in multiples.

2. **Complex** febrile seizures are febrile seizures that are either focal, have a focal component, are longer than 15 minutes in duration, or are multiple febrile seizures that occur within 30 minutes.

3. **Febrile status epilepticus** is a febrile seizure that is a generalized tonic clonic seizure lasting longer than 30 minutes.

Note: Febrile seizures should not be confused with true epileptic seizures associated with fever or "seizure with fever." "Seizure with fever" includes seizures associated with acute neurologic illnesses (ie, meningitis, encephalitis).

Long-term prophylaxis with phenobarbital may reduce the risk of subsequent febrile seizures. The 1980 NIH Consensus paper stated that after the first febrile seizure, long-term prophylaxis should be considered under any of the following:

1. Presence of abnormal neurological development or abnormal neurological exam

2. Febrile seizure was complex in nature:

    duration >15 minutes

    focal febrile seizure

    followed by transient or persistent neurological abnormalities

3. Positive family history of afebrile seizures (epilepsy)

Also consider long-term prophylaxis in certain cases if:

1. the child has multiple febrile seizures
2. the child is <12 months of age

Anticonvulsant prophylaxis is usually continued for 2 years or 1 year after the last seizure, whichever is longer. With the identification of phenobarbital's adverse effects on learning and cognitive function, many physicians will not start long-term phenobarbital prophylaxis after the first febrile seizure unless the patient has more than one of the above risk factors. Most physicians would start long-term prophylaxis if the patient has a second febrile seizure.

Daily administration of phenobarbital and therapeutic phenobarbital serum concentrations ≥15 mcg/mL decrease recurrence rates of febrile seizures. Valproic acid is also effective in preventing recurrences of febrile seizures, but is usually reserved for patients who have significant adverse effects to phenobarbital. The administration of rectal diazepam (as a solution or suppository) at the time of the febrile illness has been shown to be as effective as daily phenobarbital in preventing recurrences of febrile seizures. These rectal dosage forms are just now available in the United States. Some centers in the USA are still using the injectable form of diazepam rectally. The solution for injection is filtered prior to use if drawn from an ampul. A recent study suggests that oral diazepam, 0.33 mg/kg/dose given every 8 hours only when the child has a fever, may reduce the risk of recurrent febrile seizures (see Rosman, et al). (**Note:** A more recent study by Uhari (1995) showed that lower doses of diazepam, 0.2 mg/kg/dose, were not effective.) Carbamazepine and phenytoin are **not** effective in preventing febrile seizures.

References

Berg AT, Shinnar S, Hauser WA, et al, "Predictors of Recurrent Febrile Seizures: A Meta-Analytic Review," *J Pediatr*, 1990, 116(3):329-37.

Camfield PR, Camfield CS, Gordon K, et al, "Prevention of Recurrent Febrile Seizures," *J Pediatr*, 1995, 126(6):929-30.

NIH Consensus Statement, "Febrile Seizures: A Consensus of Their Significance, Evaluation and Treatment," *Pediatrics*, 1980, 66(6):1009-12.

Rosman NP, Colton T, Labazzo J, et al, "A Controlled Trial of Diazepam Administration During Febrile Illnesses to Prevent Recurrence of Febrile Seizures," *N Engl J Med*, 1993, 329(2):79-84.

Uhari M, Rantala H, Vainionpää L, et al, "Effect of Acetaminophen and of Low Intermittent Doses of Diazepam on Prevention of Recurrences of Febrile Seizures," *J Pediatr*, 1995, 126(6):991-5.

CAUSES OF NEONATAL SEIZURES

1. Trauma
   a. subdural hematoma
   b. intracortical hemorrhage
   c. cortical vein thrombosis

2. Asphyxia — subependymal hemorrhage

3. Congenital abnormalities (cerebral dysgenesis)
   a. lissencephaly
   b. schizencephaly

4. Hypertension

5. Metabolic
   a. hypocalcemia
      - hypomagnesemia
      - high phosphate load
      - IDM (infants of diabetic mothers)
      - hypoparathyroidism
      - maternal hyperparathyroidism
      - idiopathic
      - DiGeorge's syndrome
   b. hypoglycemia
      - galactosemia
      - IUGR (intrauterine growth retardation)
      - IDM (infants of diabetic mothers)
      - glycogen storage disease
      - idiopathic
      - methylmalonic acidemia
      - propionic acidemia
      - maple syrup urine disease
      - asphyxia
   c. electrolyte imbalance
      - hypernatremia
      - hypomagnesemia
      - hyponatremia

6. Infections
   a. bacterial meningitis
   b. cerebral abscess
   c. herpes encephalitis
   d. Coxsackie meningoencephalitis
   e. cytomegalovirus
   f. toxoplasmosis
   g. syphilis

7. Drug withdrawal
   a. methadone
   b. heroin
   c. barbiturate (short-acting, such as secobarbital and butalbital)
   d. propoxyphene
   e. benzodiazepines (chlordiazepoxide, diazepam)
   f. cocaine
   g. ethanol
   h. codeine

8. Pyridoxine dependency

9. Amino acid disturbances
   a. maple syrup urine disease
   b. urea cycle abnormalities
   c. nonketotic hyperglycinemia
   d. ketotic hyperglycinemia
   e. Leigh disease
   f. isovaleric acidemia

10. Toxins
    a. local anesthetics
    b. isoniazid
    c. lead
    d. indomethacin (from breast feeding)
    e. fentanyl

11. Familial seizures
    a. neurocutaneous syndromes
       • tuberous sclerosis
       • incontinentia pigmenti
    b. genetic syndromes
       • Zellweger's
       • Smith Lemli Opitz
       • neonatal adrenoleukodystrophy
    c. benign familial epilepsy

12. Cerebral hemorrhage
    a. intraventricular
    b. subarachnoid
    c. subdural

Adapted from Painter MJ, Bergman I, and Crumrie P, "Neonatal Seizures," *Pediatr Clin North Am*, 1986, 33:91-107.

ANTIEPILEPTIC DRUGS

Antiepileptic Drugs for Children and Adolescents by Seizure Type and Epilepsy Syndrome

Seizure Type or Epilepsy Syndrome	First Line Therapy	Alternatives
Partial seizures (with or without secondary generalization)	Carbamazepine	Valproate, phenytoin, gabapentin, lamotrigine, vigabatrin, phenobarbital, primidone; consider clonazepam, clorazepate, acetazolamide
Generalized tonic-clonic seizures	Valproate or carbamazepine	Phenytoin, phenobarbital, primidone; consider clonazepam
Childhood absence epilepsy		
Before 10 years of age	Ethosuximide or valproate	Methsuximide, acetazolamide, clonazepam, lamotrigine
After 10 years of age	Valproate	Ethosuximide, methsuximide, acetazolamide, clonazepam, lamotrigine; consider adding carbamazepine, phenytoin, or phenobarbital for generalized tonic-clonic seizures if valproate not tolerated
Juvenile myoclonic epilepsy	Valproate	Phenobarbital, primidone, clonazepam; consider carbamazepine, phenytoin, methsuximide, acetazolamide
Progressive myoclonic epilepsy	Valproate	Valproate plus clonazepam, phenobarbital
Lennox-Gastaut and related syndromes	Valproate	Clonazepam, phenobarbital, lamotrigine, ethosuximide, felbamate; consider methsuximide, ACTH or steroids, pyridoxine, ketogenic diet
Infantile spasms	ACTH or steroids	Valproate; consider clonazepam, vigabatrin (especially with tuberous sclerosis), pyridoxine
Benign epilepsy of childhood with centrotemporal spikes	Carbamazepine or valproate	Phenytoin; consider phenobarbital, primidone
Neonatal seizures	Phenobarbital	Phenytoin; consider clonazepam, primidone, valproate, pyridoxine

Adapted from Bourgeois BFD, "Antiepileptic Drugs in Pediatric Practice," *Epilepsia*, 1995, 36(Suppl 2):S34-S45.

COMA SCALES

Glasgow Coma Scale

Activity	Best Response	Score
Eye opening	Spontaneous	4
	Responds to voice	3
	Responds to pain	2
	No response	1
Verbal response	Oriented and appropriate	5
	Confused / disoriented conversation	4
	Inappropriate words	3
	Nonspecific sounds (incomprehensible)	2
	No response	1
Motor response	Follows commands	6
	Localizes pain	5
	Withdraws to pain	4
	Abnormal flexion (decorticate posturing)	3
	Abnormal extension (decerebrate posturing)	2
	No response	1

Modified Coma Scale for Infants

Activity	Best Response	Score
Eye opening	Spontaneous	4
	Responds to voice	3
	Responds to pain	2
	No response	1
Verbal response	Coos, babbles	5
	Irritable	4
	Cries to pain	3
	Moans to pain	2
	No response	1
Motor response	Normal spontaneous movements	6
	Withdraws to touch	5
	Withdraws to pain	4
	Abnormal flexion (decorticate posturing)	3
	Abnormal extension (decerebrate posturing)	2
	No response	1

Interpretation of Coma Scale Scores
Maximum Score: 15; Minimum Score: 3
(low score indicates greater severity of coma)

Range of Score	Interpretation
3- 8	Coma. Severe brain injury. Immediate action needed. Notify ICU staff STAT. Will require intubation regardless of respiratory status.
9-12	Lethargic. Needs close observation in special care unit. Frequent neuro checks. Notify ICU staff.
13-14	Needs observation
15	Normal

References

James HE, "Neurologic Evaluation and Support in the Child With an Acute Brain Insult," *Pediatr Ann*, 1986, 15(1):16-22.

Jennett B and Teasdale G, "Aspects of Coma After Severe Head Injury," *Lancet*, 1977, 1(8017): 878-81.

ASTHMA

Adapted from National Asthma Education and Prevention Program (NAEPP)
Expert Panel Report, "Guidelines for the Diagnosis and Management of Asthma
– Update on Selected Topics 2002," NIH Publication No. 02-5075
(www.nhlbi.nih.gov/guidelines/asthma/index.html)

MANAGEMENT OF ASTHMA IN INFANTS, CHILDREN, AND ADULTS

Goals of Asthma Treatment

- Minimal or no chronic symptoms day or night
- Minimal or no exacerbations
- No limitations on activities; no school/work missed
- Minimal use of inhaled short-acting beta$_2$-agonist (<1 time/day, <1 canister/month)
- Minimal or no adverse effects from medications
- Children >5 years of age and adults only: PEF >80% of personal best

Education

- Teach self-management.
- Teach about controlling environmental factors (avoidance of allergens or other factors that contribute to asthma severity).
- Review administration technique and compliance with patient.
- May use a written action plan to help educate.

Stepwise Approach for Managing Infants and Young Children (≤5 Years of Age) With Acute or Chronic Asthma[1]

Symptoms[2]	Long-Term Control (Daily Medications)
STEP 4: Severe Persistent	
Day: Continual Night: Frequent	• **Preferred treatment:** – **High dose inhaled corticosteroid** **AND** – **Long-acting inhaled beta$_2$-agonist** **AND**, if needed – Long-term oral corticosteroids (2 mg/kg/day, generally do not exceed 60 mg/day). (Make repeated attempts to reduce systemic corticosteroids and maintain control with high-dose inhaled corticosteroids.)
STEP 3: Moderate Persistent	
Day: Every day Night: >1 night/week	• **Preferred treatment:** – **Low-dose inhaled corticosteroid** **AND** **Long-acting inhaled beta$_2$-agonist** **OR** **Medium-dose inhaled corticosteroid** • Alternatives: – Low-dose inhaled corticosteroid and either leukotriene receptor antagonist or theophylline
	If needed (especially with recurring severe exacerbations): • **Preferred treatment:** – **Medium-dose inhaled corticosteroid and long-acting inhaled beta$_2$-agonist** • Alternatives: – Medium-dose inhaled corticosteroid and either leukotriene receptor antagonist or theophylline
STEP 2: Mild Persistent	
Day: >2 days/week but <1 time/day Night: >2 nights/month	• **Preferred treatment:** – **Low-dose inhaled corticosteroid (with nebulizer or MDI with holding chamber with or without face mask or DPI)** • Alternatives: Cromolyn (nebulizer is preferred or MDI with holding chamber) **OR** Leukotriene receptor antagonist

Stepwise Approach for Managing Infants and Young Children (≤5 Years of Age) With Acute or Chronic Asthma[1]

Symptoms[2]	Long-Term Control (Daily Medications)
STEP 1: Mild Intermittent	
Day: ≤2 days/week Night: ≤2 nights/month	No daily medication needed

[1]Classify severity. The presence of one of the features of severity is sufficient to place a patient in that category. An individual should be assigned to the most severe grade in which any feature occurs. The characteristics noted in this figure are general and may overlap because asthma is highly variable. Furthermore, an individual's classification may change over time.

[2]Patients at any level of severity can have mild, moderate, or severe exacerbations. Some patients with intermittent asthma experience severe and life-threatening exacerbations separated by long periods of normal lung function and no symptoms.

↓ **Step Down**
Review treatment every 1-6 month; a gradual stepwise reduction in treatment may be possible.

↑ **Step Up**
If control is not achieved, consider step up. But first: review patient medication technique, adherence, and environmental control (avoidance of allergens or other precipitant factors)

Quick Relief – All Patients

- Bronchodilator as needed for symptoms ≤2 times/week. Intensity of treatment will depend upon severity of exacerbation (see "Management of Asthma Exacerbations"). Either:
  - Preferred treatment: Inhaled short-acting beta$_2$-agonist by nebulizer or face mask and spacer/holding chamber
  - or
  - Alternative treatment: Oral beta$_2$-agonist
- With viral respiratory infection:
  - Bronchodilator q4-6h up to 24 hours (longer with physician consult) but, in general, repeat no more than once every 6 weeks.
  - Consider systemic corticosteroid if current exacerbation is severe or patient has history of severe exacerbations.
- Use of short-acting inhaled beta$_2$-agonist on a daily basis, or increasing use, indicates the need to initiate or titrate long-term control therapy.

Notes:

- **The stepwise approach presents guidelines to assist clinical decision making. Asthma is highly variable; clinicians should tailor specific medication plans to the needs and circumstances of individual patients.**
- Gain control as quickly as possible; then decrease treatment to the least medication necessary to maintain control.
- A rescue course of systemic corticosteroid may be needed at any time and step.
- In general, use of short-acting beta$_2$-agonist on a daily basis indicates the need for additional long-term control therapy.
- There are very few studies on asthma therapy for infants.
- Studies comparing medications in children <5 years of age are not available.
- Consultation with an asthma specialist is recommended for moderate or severe persistent asthma. Consider consultation for patient with mild persistent asthma.
- Initiation of long-term control therapy should be considered in infants and young children who have had >3 episodes of wheezing in the past year that lasted >1 day and affected sleep and who have risk factors for asthma.
- Inhaled corticosteroids improve health outcomes for children with mild-moderate persistent asthma. Monitor growth of children taking corticosteroids by any route. If growth appears slowed, weigh the benefits against the risks.
- Antibiotics are not recommended for treatment of acute asthma exacerbations except where there is evidence or suspicion of bacterial infection.

ASTHMA *(Continued)*

Stepwise Approach for Managing Asthma in Children >5 Years of Age, Adolescents, and Adults: Treatment[1]

Symptoms[2]	Lung Function[3]	Long-Term Control (Daily Medications)
STEP 4: Severe Persistent		
Day: Continual Night: Frequent	PEF/FEV_1 ≤60% PEF variability >30%	• **Preferred treatment:** – **High dose inhaled corticosteroid** **AND** – **Long-acting inhaled beta$_2$-agonist** **AND,** if needed – Long-term oral corticosteroids (2 mg/kg/day, generally do not exceed 60 mg/day). (Make repeated attempts to reduce systemic corticosteroids and maintain control with high-dose inhaled corticosteroids.)
STEP 3: Moderate Persistent		
Day: Every day Night: >1 night/week	PEF/FEV_1 >60% - <80% PEF variability >30%	• **Preferred treatment:** – **Low-medium dose inhaled corticosteroid** **AND** – **Long-acting inhaled beta$_2$-agonist** • Alternatives: – Increase inhaled corticosteroids within medium-dose range **OR** – Low-medium dose inhaled corticosteroids and either leukotriene receptor antagonist or theophylline
		If needed (especially with recurring severe exacerbations): • **Preferred treatment:** – Increase inhaled corticosteroids within medium-dose range, and add long-acting inhaled beta$_2$-agonist • Alternatives: – Increase inhaled corticosteroids in medium-dose range, and add either leukotriene receptor antagonist or theophylline
STEP 2: Mild Persistent		
Day: >2 days/week but <1 time/day Night: >2 nights/month	PEF/FEV_1 ≥80% PEF variability 20%-30%	• **Preferred treatment:** – **Low-dose inhaled corticosteroid** • Alternatives: Cromolyn, leukotriene receptor antagonist, nedocromil, or sustained release theophylline (serum concentration 5-15 mcg/mL)
STEP 1: Mild Intermittent		
Day: ≤2 days/week Night: ≤2 nights/month	PEF/FEV_1 ≥80% PEF variability <20%	No daily medication needed. A course of systemic corticosteroids is recommended for severe exacerbations.

[1]Classify severity. The presence of one of the features of severity is sufficient to place a patient in that category. An individual should be assigned to the most severe grade in which any feature occurs. The characteristics noted are general and may overlap because asthma is highly variable. Furthermore, an individual's classification may change over time.

[2]Patients at any level of severity can have mild, moderate, or severe exacerbations. Some patients with intermittent asthma experience severe and life-threatening exacerbations separated by long periods of normal lung function and no symptoms.

[3]PEF is % of personal best and FEV_1 is % predicted.

↓ **Step down**	↑**Step up**
Review treatment every 1-6 months; a gradual stepwise reduction in treatment may be possible.	If control is not maintained, consider step up. First, review patient medication technique, adherence, and environmental control.

Quick Relief – All Patients

- Short-acting bronchodilator: **Inhaled beta$_2$-agonists** as needed for symptoms.

- Intensity of treatment will depend on severity of exacerbation; see "Management of Asthma Exacerbations".

- Use of short-acting inhaled beta$_2$-agonists on a daily basis, or increasing use, indicates the need to initiate or titrate long-term control therapy.

Notes:

- **The stepwise approach presents general guidelines to assist clinical decision making; it is not intended to be a specific prescription. Asthma is highly variable; clinicians should tailor specific medication plans to the needs and circumstances of individual patients.**

- Gain control as quickly as possible; then decrease treatment to the least medication necessary to maintain control.

- A rescue course of systemic corticosteroids may be needed at any time and at any step.

- Some patients with intermittent asthma experience severe and life-threatening exacerbations separated by long periods of normal lung function and no symptoms. This may be especially common with exacerbations provoked by respiratory infections. A short course of systemic corticosteroids is recommended.

- At each step, patients should control their environment to avoid or control factors that make their asthma worse.

- Antibiotics are not recommended for treatment of acute asthma exacerbations except where there is evidence or suspicion of bacterial infection.

- Consultation with an asthma specialist is recommended for moderate or severe persistent asthma.

- Peak flow monitoring for patients with moderate-severe asthma should be considered.

ASTHMA (Continued)

Management of Asthma Exacerbations: Home Treatment[1]

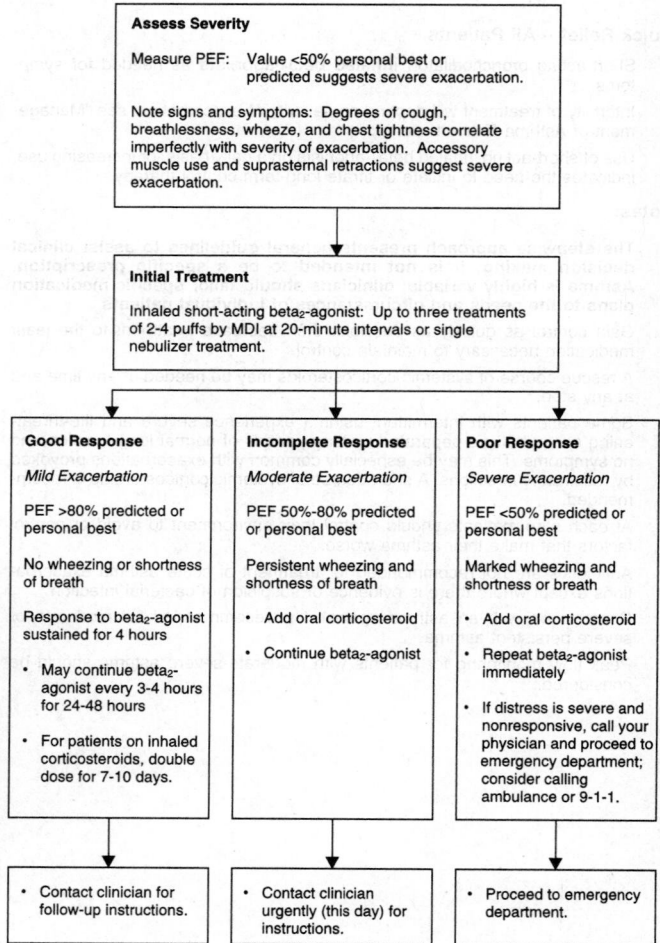

Assess Severity

Measure PEF: Value <50% personal best or predicted suggests severe exacerbation.

Note signs and symptoms: Degrees of cough, breathlessness, wheeze, and chest tightness correlate imperfectly with severity of exacerbation. Accessory muscle use and suprasternal retractions suggest severe exacerbation.

Initial Treatment

Inhaled short-acting beta2-agonist: Up to three treatments of 2-4 puffs by MDI at 20-minute intervals or single nebulizer treatment.

Good Response

Mild Exacerbation

PEF >80% predicted or personal best

No wheezing or shortness of breath

Response to beta2-agonist sustained for 4 hours

- May continue beta2-agonist every 3-4 hours for 24-48 hours

- For patients on inhaled corticosteroids, double dose for 7-10 days.

- Contact clinician for follow-up instructions.

Incomplete Response

Moderate Exacerbation

PEF 50%-80% predicted or personal best

Persistent wheezing and shortness of breath

- Add oral corticosteroid

- Continue beta2-agonist

- Contact clinician urgently (this day) for instructions.

Poor Response

Severe Exacerbation

PEF <50% predicted or personal best

Marked wheezing and shortness or breath

- Add oral corticosteroid

- Repeat beta2-agonist immediately

- If distress is severe and nonresponsive, call your physician and proceed to emergency department; consider calling ambulance or 9-1-1.

- Proceed to emergency department.

[1]Patients at high risk of asthma-related death should receive immediate clinical attention after initial treatment. Additional therapy may be required.

Management of Asthma Exacerbations: Emergency Department and Hospital-Based Care

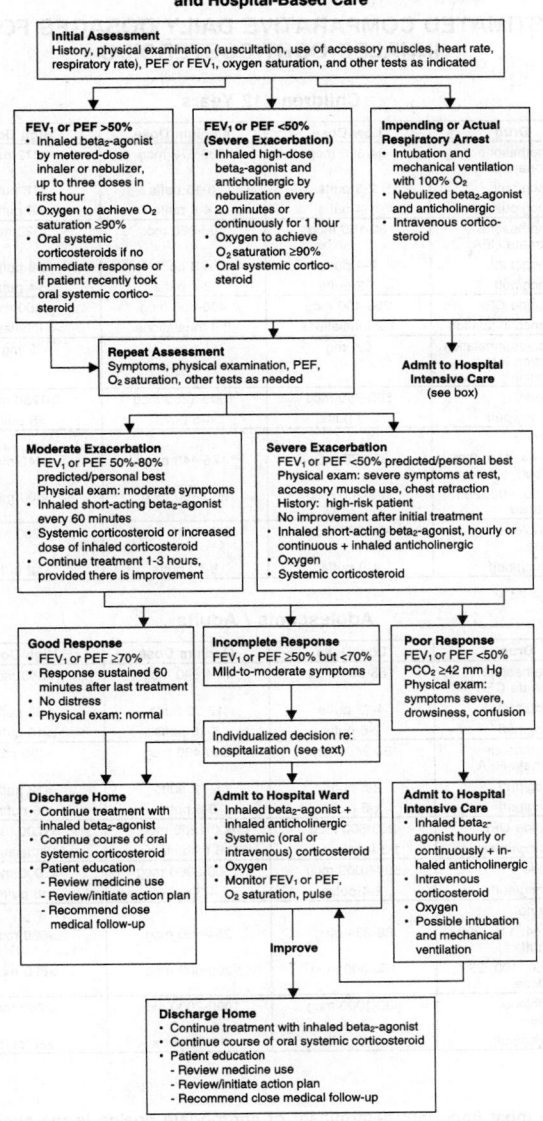

Initial Assessment
History, physical examination (auscultation, use of accessory muscles, heart rate, respiratory rate), PEF or FEV_1, oxygen saturation, and other tests as indicated

FEV_1 or PEF >50%
- Inhaled beta$_2$-agonist by metered-dose inhaler or nebulizer, up to three doses in first hour
- Oxygen to achieve O_2 saturation ≥90%
- Oral systemic corticosteroids if no immediate response or if patient recently took oral systemic corticosteroid

FEV_1 or PEF <50% (Severe Exacerbation)
- Inhaled high-dose beta$_2$-agonist and anticholinergic by nebulization every 20 minutes or continuously for 1 hour
- Oxygen to achieve O_2 saturation ≥90%
- Oral systemic corticosteroid

Impending or Actual Respiratory Arrest
- Intubation and mechanical ventilation with 100% O_2
- Nebulized beta$_2$-agonist and anticholinergic
- Intravenous corticosteroid

Repeat Assessment
Symptoms, physical examination, PEF, O_2 saturation, other tests as needed

Admit to Hospital Intensive Care
(see box)

Moderate Exacerbation
FEV_1 or PEF 50%-80% predicted/personal best
Physical exam: moderate symptoms
- Inhaled short-acting beta$_2$-agonist every 60 minutes
- Systemic corticosteroid or increased dose of inhaled corticosteroid
- Continue treatment 1-3 hours, provided there is improvement

Severe Exacerbation
FEV_1 or PEF <50% predicted/personal best
Physical exam: severe symptoms at rest, accessory muscle use, chest retraction
History: high-risk patient
No improvement after initial treatment
- Inhaled short-acting beta$_2$-agonist, hourly or continuous + inhaled anticholinergic
- Oxygen
- Systemic corticosteroid

Good Response
- FEV_1 or PEF ≥70%
- Response sustained 60 minutes after last treatment
- No distress
- Physical exam: normal

Incomplete Response
FEV_1 or PEF ≥50% but <70%
Mild-to-moderate symptoms

Poor Response
FEV_1 or PEF <50%
PCO_2 ≥42 mm Hg
Physical exam: symptoms severe, drowsiness, confusion

Individualized decision re: hospitalization (see text)

Discharge Home
- Continue treatment with inhaled beta$_2$-agonist
- Continue course of oral systemic corticosteroid
- Patient education
  - Review medicine use
  - Review/initiate action plan
  - Recommend close medical follow-up

Admit to Hospital Ward
- Inhaled beta$_2$-agonist + inhaled anticholinergic
- Systemic (oral or intravenous) corticosteroid
- Oxygen
- Monitor FEV_1 or PEF, O_2 saturation, pulse

Admit to Hospital Intensive Care
- Inhaled beta$_2$-agonist hourly or continuously + inhaled anticholinergic
- Intravenous corticosteroid
- Oxygen
- Possible intubation and mechanical ventilation

Improve

Discharge Home
- Continue treatment with inhaled beta$_2$-agonist
- Continue course of oral systemic corticosteroid
- Patient education
  - Review medicine use
  - Review/initiate action plan
  - Recommend close medical follow-up

ASTHMA *(Continued)*

ESTIMATED COMPARATIVE DAILY DOSAGES FOR INHALED CORTICOSTEROIDS

Children ≤12 Years

Drug	Low Dose	Medium Dose	High Dose
Beclomethasone dipropionate CFC	84-336 mcg	336-672 mcg	>672 mcg
42 mcg/puff	2-8 puffs	8-16 puffs	>16 puffs
84 mcg/puff	1-4 puffs	4-8 puffs	>8 puffs
Beclomethasone dipropionate HFA	80-160 mcg	160-320 mcg	>320 mcg
40 mcg/puff	2-4 puffs	4-8 puffs	>8 puffs
80 mcg/puff	1-2 puffs	2-4 puffs	>4 puffs
Budesonide DPI	200-400 mcg	400-800 mcg	>800 mcg
200 mcg/inhalation	1-2 inhalations	2-4 inhalations	>4 inhalations
Budesonide inhalation suspension for nebulization	0.5 mg	1 mg	2 mg
Flunisolide	500-750 mcg	1000-1250 mcg	>1250 mcg
250 mcg/puff	2-3 puffs	4-5 puffs	>5 puffs
Fluticasone			
MDI: 44, 110, 220 mcg/puff	88-176 mcg	176-440 mcg	>440 mcg
DPI: 50, 100, 250 mcg/dose	100-200 mcg	200-400 mcg	>400 mcg
Triamcinolone acetonide	400-800 mcg	800-1200 mcg	>1200 mcg
100 mcg/puff	4-8 puffs	8-12 puffs	>12 puffs

Adolescents / Adults

Drug	Low Dose	Medium Dose	High Dose
Beclomethasone dipropionate CFC	168-504 mcg	504-840 mcg	>840 mcg
42 mcg/puff	4-12 puffs	12-20 puffs	>20 puffs
84 mcg/puff	2-6 puffs	6-10 puffs	>10 puffs
Beclomethasone dipropionate HFA	80-240 mcg	240-480 mcg	>480 mcg
40 mcg/puff	2-6 puffs	6-12 puffs	>12 puffs
80 mcg/puff	1-3 puffs	3-6 puffs	>6 puffs
Budesonide DPI	200-600 mcg	600-1200 mcg	>1200 mcg
200 mcg/inhalation	1-3 inhalations	3-6 inhalations	>6 inhalations
Flunisolide	500-1000 mcg	1000-2000 mcg	>2000 mcg
250 mcg/puff	2-4 puffs	4-8 puffs	>8 puffs
Fluticasone			
MDI: 44, 110, 220 mcg/puff	88-264 mcg	264-660 mcg	>660 mcg
DPI: 50, 100, 250 mcg/dose	100-300 mcg	300-600 mcg	>600 mcg
Triamcinolone acetonide	400-1000 mcg	1000-2000 mcg	>2000 mcg
100 mcg/puff	4-10 puffs	10-20 puffs	>20 puffs

Notes:

- **The most important determinant of appropriate dosing is the clinician's judgment of the patient's response to therapy.** The clinician must monitor the patient's response on several clinical parameters and adjust the dose accordingly. The stepwise approach to therapy emphasizes that once control of asthma is achieved, the dose of mediation should be carefully titrated to the minimum dose required to maintain control, thus reducing the potential for adverse effect.
- The reference point for the range in the dosages for children is data on the safety on inhaled corticosteroids in children, which, in general, suggest that the dose

ranges are equivalent to beclomethasone dipropionate 200-400 mcg/day (low dose), 400-800 mcg/day (medium dose), and >800 mcg/day (high dose).

- Some dosages may be outside package labeling.

- Metered-dose inhaler (MDI) dosages are expressed as the actuator dose (the amount of drug leaving the actuator and delivered to the patient), which is the labeling required in the United States. This is different from the dosage expressed as the valve dose (the amount of drug leaving the valve, all of which is not available to the patient), which is used in many European countries and in some of the scientific literature. Dry powder inhaler (DPI) doses (eg, Turbuhaler) are expressed as the amount of drug in the inhaler following activation.

ESTIMATED CLINICAL COMPARABILITY OF DOSES FOR INHALED CORTICOSTEROIDS

Data from *in vitro* and in clinical trials suggest that the different inhaled corticosteroid preparations are not equivalent on a per puff or microgram basis. However, it is not entirely clear what implications these differences have for dosing recommendations in clinical practice because there are few data directly comparing the preparations. Relative dosing for clinical comparability is affected by differences in topical potency, clinical effects at different doses, delivery device, and bioavailability. The Expert Panel developed recommended dose ranges for different preparations based on available data and the following assumptions and cautions about estimating relative doses needed to achieve comparable clinical effect.

Relative Topical Potency Using Human Skin Blanching

- The standard test for determining relative topical anti-inflammatory potency is the topical vasoconstriction (MacKenzie skin blanching) test.

- The MacKenzie topical skin blanching test correlates with binding affinities and binding half-lives for human lung corticosteroid receptors (see following table) (Dahlberg, et al, 1984; Hogger and Rohdewald 1994).

- The relationship between relative topical anti-inflammatory effect and clinical comparability in asthma management is not certain. However, recent clinical trials suggest that different *in vitro* measures of anti-inflammatory effect is not certain. However, recent clinical trials suggest that different *in vitro* measures of anti-inflammatory effect correlate with clinical efficacy (Barnes and Pedersen 1993; Johnson 1996; Kamada, et al, 1996; Ebden, et al, 1986; Leblanc, et al, 1994; Gustaffson, et al, 1993; Lundback, et al, 1993; Barnes, et al, 1993; Fabbri, et al, 1993; Langdon and Capsey, 1994; Ayres, et al, 1995; Rafferty, et al, 1985; Bjorkander, et al, 1982, Stiksa, et al, 1982; Willey, et al, 1982.)

Medication	Topical Potency (Skin Blanching)[1]	Corticosteroid Receptor Binding Half-Life	Receptor Binding Affinity
Beclomethasone dipropionate (BDP)	600	7.5 hours	13.5
Budesonide (BUD)	980	5.1 hours	9.4
Flunisolide (FLU)	330	3.5 hours	1.8
Fluticasone propionate (FP)	1200	10.5 hours	18.0
Triamcinolone acetonide (TAA)	330	3.9 hours	3.6

[1]Numbers are assigned in reference to dexamethasone, which has a value of "1" in the MacKenzie test.

1383

ASTHMA *(Continued)*

Relative Doses to Achieve Similar Clinical Effects

- Clinical effects are evaluated by a number of outcome parameters (eg, changes in spirometry, peak flow rates, symptom scores, quick-relief beta$_2$-agonist use, frequency of exacerbations, airway responsiveness).

- The daily dose and duration of treatment may affect these outcome parameters differently (eg, symptoms and peak flow may improve at lower doses and over a shorter treatment time than bronchial reactivity) (van Essen-Zandvliet, et al, 1992; Haahtela, et al, 1991)

- Delivery systems influence comparability. For example, the delivery device for budesonide (Turbuhaler) delivers approximately twice the amount of drug to the airway as the MDI, thus enhancing the clinical effect (Thorsson, et al, 1994; Agertoft and Pedersen, 1993).

- Individual patients may respond differently to different preparations, as noted by clinical experience.

- Clinical trials comparing effects in reducing symptoms and improving peak expiratory flow demonstrate:

  - BDP and BUD achieved comparable effects at similar microgram doses by MDI (Bjorkander, et al, 1982; Ebden, et al, 1986; Rafferty, et al, 1985).

  - BDP achieved effects similar to twice the dose of TAA on a microgram basis.

Reference

National Asthma Education and Prevention Program (NAEPP), Clinical Practice Guidelines, Expert Panel Report 2, "Guidelines for the Diagnosis and Management of Asthma," NIH Publication No. 97-4051, July 1997.

NORMAL RESPIRATORY RATES

Hour After Birth	Average Respiratory Rate	Range
1st hour	60 breaths/minute	20-100
2-6 hours	50 breaths/minute	20-80
>6 hours	30-40 breaths/minute	20-60

Age (years)	Mean RR (breaths/minute)
0-2	25-30
3-9	20-25
10-18	16-20

BLOOD LEVEL SAMPLING TIME GUIDELINES

Drug	Infusion Time	Therapeutic Range	When to Draw Levels
Amikacin sulfate			
I.V.	30 min	Peak: 20-30 µg/mL	Peak: 30 min after end of 30 min infusion
		Trough: <10 µg/mL	Trough: Within 30 min before next dose
I.M.			Peak: 1 h after I.M. injection
			Trough: Within 30 min before next dose
Carbamazepine		4-12 µg/mL	Just before next dose
Chloramphenicol			
I.V.	30 min	Peak: 15-25 µg/mL	Peak: 90 min after end of 30 min infusion
			Trough: Just before next dose
P.O.			Peak: 2 h post-P.O. dose
Cyclosporine			
I.V./P.O.		BMT 100-200 ng/mL	Just before next dose
		Liver transplant 200-300 ng/mL	
		Renal transplant 100-200 ng/mL	
Digoxin			
I.V./P.O.		Age and disease related: 0.8-2 ng/mL	6 h postdose to just before next dose
Ethosuximide			
P.O.		40-100 µg/mL	Just before next dose
Flucytosine			
P.O.		25-100 µg/mL	Peak: 2 h postdose after at least 4 d of therapy
Fosphenytoin (measure phenytoin levels)			
I.V.		Phenytoin: 10-20 µg/mL	Peak: 2 h after end of an infusion
I.M.			Peak: 4 h after I.M. injection
Gentamicin			
I.V.	30 min	Peak: 4-10 µg/mL	Peak: 30 min after end of 30 min infusion
		Trough: 0.5-2 µg/mL	Trough: Within 30 min before next dose
I.M.			Peak: 1 h after I.M. injection
			Trough: Within 30 min before next dose
Phenobarbital		15-40 µg/mL	Trough: Just before next dose
Phenytoin			
P.O., I.V.		10-20 µg/mL	Trough: Just before next dose
I.V.			Post-load/Peak: 1 h after end of infusion
Theophylline			
I.V. bolus	30 min	10-20 µg/mL	Peak: 30 min after end of 30 min infusion
Continuous infusion			16-24 h after the start or change in a constant I.V. infusion
P.O. liquid, fast-release tablet (Somophyllin®, Slo-Phyllin® liquid & tablet)			Peak: 1 h postdose Trough: Just before next dose

Drug	Infusion Time	Therapeutic Range	When to Draw Levels
P.O. slow-release (Theo-Dur®, Slo-Phyllin® GC, Slo-bid®)			Peak: 4 h postdose Trough: Just before next dose
Tobramycin			
I.V.	30 min	Peak: 4-10 µg/mL	Peak: 30 min after end of 30 min infusion
		Trough: 0.5-2 µg/mL	Trough: Within 30 min before next dose
I.M.			Peak: 1 h post-I.M. injection
			Trough: Within 30 min before next dose
Trimethoprim			
I.V., dose 20 mg/kg	60 min	Peak: 5-10 µg/mL	Peak: 30 min after end of 60 min infusion
I.V., dose 8-10 mg/kg		Peak 1-3 µg/mL	
P.O.			Peak: 1 h postdose
Valproic acid			
P.O.		50-100 µg/mL	Trough: Just before next dose
Vancomycin	60 min	Peak: 25-40 µg/mL	Peak: 20-30 min after end of 60 min infusion*
		Trough: 5-15 µg/mL	Trough: Within 30 min before next dose

*Some institutions may draw vancomycin peak 1 hour after 1-hour infusion and accept the lower range of therapeutic.

OVERDOSE AND TOXICOLOGY*

Drug or Drug Class	Signs/Symptoms	Treatment/Comments
Acetaminophen	Nausea, vomiting, diaphoresis, delirium, fever, coma, vascular collapse, hepatic necrosis, transient azotemia, renal tubular necrosis	Assess severity of ingestion; doses ≥150 mg/kg for children and 7.5 g for adults are thought to be toxic. Obtain serum concentration ≥4 hours postingestion and use acetaminophen nomogram to evaluate need for acetylcysteine. Empty stomach with ipecac (if <1 hour postingestion) or gastric lavage. May administer activated charcoal for one dose, this may decrease absorption of acetylcysteine if given within 1 hour of acetylcysteine. For unknown ingested quantities and for significant ingestion, give acetylcysteine orally (diluted 1:4 with juice or carbonated beverage); initial: 140 mg/kg then give 70 mg/kg every 4 hours for 17 doses.
Alpha-adrenergic blocking agents	Hypotension, drowsiness	Induce emesis, give activated charcoal, additional treatment is symptomatic; use I.V. fluids, dopamine, or ephedrine to treat hypotension. Epinephrine may worsen hypotension due to beta effects.
Aminoglycosides	Ototoxicity, nephrotoxicity, neuromuscular toxicity	Hemodialysis or peritoneal dialysis may be useful in patients with decreased renal function.
Anticholinergics, antihistamines	Coma, hallucinations, delirium, tachycardia, dry skin, urinary retention, dilated pupils	For life-threatening arrhythmias or seizures physostigmine m ay be used.
Anticholinesterase agents	Nausea, vomiting, diarrhea, miosis, CNS depression, excessive salivation, excessive sweating, muscle weakness	Suction oral secretions, decontaminate skin, atropinize patient; atropine dose must be individualized. Infants and children: Initial dose: 0.01-0.02 mg/kg/dose; may need to increase as high as 0.05 mg/kg. Adults: Initial atropine dose: 1 mg; may need to increase to 2-5 mg/dose; pralidoxime (2-PAM) may need to be added for severe intoxications.
Barbiturates	Respiratory depression, circulatory collapse, bradycardia, hypotension, hypothermia, slurred speech, confusion	Repeated oral doses of activated charcoal given every 3-6 hours will increase clearance: Children: 1-2 g/kg/dose; adults: 30-60 g. Assure GI motility, adequate hydration, and renal function. Urinary alkalinization with I.V. sodium bicarbonate will increase renal elimination of longer-acting barbiturates (eg, phenobarbital).
Benzodiazepines	Respiratory depression, apnea, hypoactive reflexes, hypotension, slurred speech, unsteady gait, coma	For comatose patient, use gastric lavage with endotracheal tube in place to prevent aspiration; flumazenil, a benzodiazepine antagonist, can be used to reverse the effects of benzodiazepines. See Flumazenil monograph *on page 495* for dose. Action of flumazenil may be shorter than duration of benzodiazepine; repeat doses as needed. Norepinephrine, phenylephrine, or dopamine may be used to treat hypotension; dialysis is of limited value; support blood pressure and respiration.

Drug or Drug Class	Signs/Symptoms	Treatment/Comments
Beta-adrenergic blockers	Hypotension, bronchospasm, bradycardia, hyperglycemia, or hypoglycemia	Induce emesis, followed by activated charcoal; treat symptomatically; glucagon, atropine, isoproterenol, or cardiac pacing may be needed to treat bradycardia, conduction defects, or hypotension
Carbamazepine	Dizziness, drowsiness, ataxia, involuntary movements, opisthotonos, seizures, nausea, vomiting, agitation, nystagmus, coma, urinary retention, respiratory depression, tachycardia	Use supportive therapy, general poisoning management as needed; use repeated oral doses of activated charcoal given every 3-6 hours to decrease serum concentrations; children 1-2 g/kg/dose, adults: 30-60 g/dose; charcoal hemoperfusion may be needed; treat hypotension with I.V. fluids, dopamine, or norepinephrine; monitor EKG; diazepam may control convulsions but may exacerbate respiratory depression
Cardiac glycosides	Hyperkalemia may develop rapidly and result in life-threatening cardiac arrhythmias, progressive bradyarrhythmias, 2nd or 3rd degree heart block unresponsive to atropine, ventricular fibrillation, asystole	Obtain serum drug level, induce emesis or perform gastric lavage; give activated charcoal to reduce further absorption; atropine may reverse heart block, phenytoin will improve A-V conduction; digoxin immune Fab (digoxin specific antibody fragments) is used in life-threatening cases, each 38 mg of digoxin immune Fab binds with 0.5 mg of digoxin or digitoxin; see Digoxin Immune Fab monograph *on page 383* for dosing recommendations
Heparin	Severe hemorrhage	1 mg of protamine sulfate will neutralize approximately 90 units of heparin sodium (bovine) or 115 units of heparin sodium (porcine) or 100 units of heparin calcium (porcine)
Hydantoin derivatives	Nausea, vomiting, nystagmus, slurred speech, ataxia, coma	Gastric lavage or emesis; repeated oral doses of activated charcoal may increase clearance of phenytoin. Children: 1-2 g/kg/dose, adults: 30-60 g/dose activated charcoal every 3-6 hours until nontoxic serum concentration is obtained; assure adequate GI motility, supportive therapy; dialysis may be helpful.
Iron	Lethargy, nausea, vomiting, green or tarry stools, hypotension, weak rapid pulse, metabolic acidosis, shock, coma, hepatic necrosis, renal failure, local GI erosions	Induce emesis if awake or lavage with saline solution; give deferoxamine mesylate I.V. at 15 mg/kg/hour in cases of severe poisoning (serum Fe >350 mcg/mL) and continue chelation therapy for 24 hours after child is excreting normal color urine; urine output should be maintained at >2 mL/kg/hour to avoid hypovolemic shock
Isoniazid	Nausea, vomiting, blurred vision, CNS depression, intractable seizures, coma, metabolic acidosis	Control seizures with diazepam; if suspected ingestion of >80 mg/kg, give pyridoxine I.V. equal dose to the suspected overdose of isoniazid; lavage after seizure control is reached; force diuresis with I.V. fluids; hemo- or peritoneal dialysis may be beneficial in severe cases
Nonsteroidal anti-inflammatory drugs	Dizziness, abdominal pain, sweating, apnea, nystagmus, cyanosis, hypotension, coma	Induce emesis; give activated charcoal via NG tube; provide symptomatic and supportive care.

OVERDOSE AND TOXICOLOGY* *(Continued)*

Drug or Drug Class	Signs/Symptoms	Treatment/Comments
Opiates and morphine analogs	Respiratory depression, miosis, hypothermia, bradycardia, circulatory collapse, pulmonary edema, apnea	Establish airway and adequate ventilation; give naloxone 0.1 mg/kg for children up to 5 years of age or 20 kg; for those >5 years or 20 kg give 2 mg naloxone; repeat doses every 2-3 minutes if needed; additional doses may be needed every 20-60 minutes. May need to institute continuous infusion, as duration of action of opiates can be longer than duration of action of naloxone.
Phenothiazines	Deep, unarousable sleep, anticholinergic symptoms, extrapyramidal signs, diaphoresis, rigidity, tachycardia, cardiac dysrhythmias, hypotension, or hypertension	Emesis or gastric lavage; do **not** dialyze; use I.V. benztropine mesylate 0.02-0.05 mg/kg/dose or for adults 1-2 mg/dose slowly over 3-6 minutes for extrapyramidal signs; use loading dose of phenytoin 10-15 mg/kg slow I.V. push for ventricular dysrhythmias; use I.V. fluids and norepinephrine or phenylephrine to treat hypotension; avoid epinephrine which may cause hypotension due to phenothiazine-induced alpha-adrenergic blockade and unopposed epinephrine B_2 action; dantrolene orally 0.5 mg/kg/dose every 12 hours may help with the rigidity
Salicylates	Nausea, vomiting, respiratory alkalosis, hyperthermia, dehydration, hyperapnea, tinnitus, headache, dizziness, metabolic acidosis, coma	Induce emesis or gastric lavage immediately; give charcoal with cathartic via NG tube; correct fluid imbalance by giving D_5LR at 10-20 mL/kg/hour for 1-2 hours, more rapid fluid resuscitation may be needed for patients in shock; use sodium bicarbonate to correct metabolic acidosis and enhance renal elimination by alkalinizing the urine; give supplemental potassium after renal function has been determined to be adequate. Monitor electrolytes; obtain serum salicylate level ≥6 hours postingestion; use poisoning nomogram to assess the significance of the ingestion and the need for more aggressive measures.
Tricyclic antidepressants	Agitation, confusion, hallucinations, urinary retention, hypothermia, hypotension, tachycardia, arrhythmias, widened QRS complex, prolonged PR intervals	Maintain normal temperature; correct acidosis with sodium bicarbonate to increase protein binding and decrease free fraction; correction of acidosis may decrease cardiovascular toxicities; avoid disopyramide, procainamide, and quinidine; lidocaine, phenytoin or propranolol may be necessary; reserve physostigmine for refractory life-treating anticholinergic toxicities. For life-threatening arrhythmias or seizures: Children: I.V., slow: Physostigmine 0.01-0.03 mg/kg/dose up to 0.5 mg/dose over 2-3 minutes, repeat in 5 minutes (maximum total dose is 2 mg). Adolescents and adults: 2 mg/dose physostigmine, may repeat 1-2 mg in 20 minutes and give 1-4 mg slow I.V. over 5-10 minutes if signs and symptoms recur.
Warfarin	Internal or external hemorrhage, hematuria	For moderate overdoses, give oral or I.V. phytonadione; for severe hemorrhage, give fresh frozen plasma or whole blood

Drug or Drug Class	Signs/Symptoms	Treatment/Comments
Xanthine derivatives	Vomiting, abdominal pain, bloody diarrhea, tachycardia, extrasystoles, tachypnea, tonic/clonic seizures	Induce emesis, except in a convulsive patient; give activated charcoal orally; repeated oral doses of activated charcoal may increase clearance; children: 1-2 g/kg/dose, adults: 30-60 g/dose of activated charcoal every 3-6 hours until nontoxic serum concentrations are obtained. Assure adequate GI motility, supportive therapy; charcoal hemoperfusion can also be effective in decreasing serum concentrations.

*As for all overdoses and toxic ingestions, provide airway, breathing, and cardiac support; use appropriate general poisoning management and give general supportive therapy when needed (eg, I.V. fluids, blood pressure support, control seizures, etc). Consult more specific toxicology references (eg, Leikin JB and Paloucek FP, *Poisoning & Toxicology Handbook*, Hudson, OH: Lexi-Comp Inc, 1998, and Poisondex®) for further information.

COMMONLY USED ANTIDOTES FOR ACUTE OVERDOSES

While certain drugs may modify symptoms produced by a toxin, only a relatively few toxins have specific antidotes. The purpose of this chart is to identify those drugs, non-medicinal chemicals, plants, snakes, and spiders to which specific antidotes exist. Please refer to the specific monograph for dosing information. This information does not preclude the use of "conventional" therapeutic modalities for the treatment of intoxication (eg, emesis, lavage, charcoal, etc).

Poisoning Agent	Antidote(s)	Indications	Comments
Chemicals, Nonmedicinal			
Arsenic	Dimercaprol (BAL in Oil®)	• Symptomatic arsenic exposure	• Monitor for hypertension, tachycardia, hyperpyrexia, and urticaria • Pretreatment with diphenhydramine may diminish side effects
Calcium oxide	Edetate calcium disodium (EDTA) (Calcium Disodium Versenate®)	• Eye exposure from calcium oxide	• Immediate irrigation with saline followed by an irrigation with 0.01-0.05 M EDTA solution for at least 15 minutes
Carbon monoxide	Oxygen	• Any suspected carbon monoxide intoxication • Hyperbaric oxygen for any patient with signs and symptoms of severe intoxication regardless of the carboxyhemoglobin concentration • Patients with ischemic heart disease, acute ECG changes, anemia, seizure history, or pregnancy should receive hyperbaric oxygen if the carboxy hemoglobin (COHB) >20% or if any acute symptoms are present	
Carbamate insecticides	Atropine	• Symptomatic bradycardia • Myoclonic seizures, severe hallucinations, weakness, arrhythmias, excessive salivation, involuntary urination and defecation	• Caution should be used in patients with narrow-angle glaucoma, cardiovascular disease, or pregnancy • Plasma and/or erythrocyte cholinesterase levels will be depressed from normal
Copper	Penicillamine (Cuprimine®, Depen®)	• Symptomatic copper intoxication	• Little experience with chelation therapy in the setting of acute ingestion
Cyanide	Amyl nitrite, sodium nitrite, sodium thiosulfate (cyanide antidote kit)	• Begin treatment at the first sign of toxicity if exposure is known or strongly expected	• Do not use methylene blue to reduce elevated methemoglobin levels • Oxygen therapy may be useful when combined with sodium thiosulfate therapy

Poisoning Agent	Antidote(s)	Indications	Comments
Ethylene glycol	Ethanol **OR** Fomepizole (Antizol®)	• Ingestion of >0.25 mL/kg ethylene glycol • Ethylene glycol serum level >20 mg/dL • History or strong clinical suspicion of ingestion and at least two of the following criteria: Arterial pH <7.3 Serum bicarbonate <20 mEq/L Osmolality gap >10 mosm/L Urinary oxalate crystals present	• Goal: Blood ethanol concentration at least 100 mg/dL (22 mmol/L) • Indications for use of fomepizole over ethanol: Ingestion of multiple substances resulting in depressed level of consciousness, altered consciousness, lack of adequate intensive care staffing or laboratory support to monitor ethanol, critically-ill patient with anion gap metabolic acidosis of unknown origin and potential exposure to ethylene glycol, or patients with active hepatic disease • Continue therapy until ethylene glycol level <10 mg/dL • Monitor blood glucose especially in children as ethanol may cause hypoglycemia
Hydrazine	Pyridoxine (Vitamin B₆)	• Antidote for seizures and coma	
Hydrofluoric acid (HF)	Calcium gluconate	• Dermal burns (topical treatment with calcium gluconate gel for dermal exposures of HF <20% concentration) •S.C. injections of calcium gluconate for dermal exposures of HF >20% concentration or failure to respond to calcium gluconate gel	• Oral calcium also used as fluoride-binding agent following oral ingestion • Hypocalcemia occurs frequently following oral ingestion and dermal exposure • Topical calcium gels are not available commercially in U.S.; may be compounded; see Extemporaneous Preparations, Calcium Supplements *on page 200* •Injections of calcium gluconate should not be used in digital area
Hydrogen sulfide	Amyl nitrite **AND** Sodium nitrite	• Severe anoxia, if therapy can be started early – within one hour of exposure	• Do **NOT** use sodium thiosulfate
Lead	Edetate calcium disodium (EDTA) (Calcium Disodium Versenate®) **with or without** Dimercaprol (BAL in Oil®)	Use both calcium EDTA and BAL: • Symptoms of lead encephalopathy and/or blood lead level >70 mcg/dL • Symptomatic without encephalopathy or asymptomatic with blood lead level >70 µg/dL Use only EDTA for: • Asymptomatic with blood lead level 45-69 µg/dL	• Do not confuse or interchange therapy of **calcium** disodium edetate with disodium edetate (Chealamide®, Disotate®, Endrate®) – tetany and possibly fatal hypocalcemia may occur • Calcium EDTA should only be administered after adequate urine flow is established • If urine flow is not established, hemodialysis must accompany calcium EDTA dosing
	Succimer (Chemet®)	• Lead level >45 µg/dL in patients without encephalopathy or protracted vomiting	• Do not use with calcium disodium edetate or BAL

COMMONLY USED ANTIDOTES FOR ACUTE OVERDOSES
(Continued)

Poisoning Agent	Antidote(s)	Indications	Comments
Manganese	Edetate calcium disodium (EDTA) (Calcium Disodium Versenate®)		• Do not confuse or interchange therapy of **calcium** disodium edetate with disodium edetate (Chealamide®, Disotate®, Endrate®) – tetany and possibly fatal hypocalcemia may occur • Calcium EDTA should only be administered after adequate urine flow is established
Methanol	Ethanol **OR** Fomepizole (Antizol®)	• Anion gap metabolic acidosis associated with a history of methanol ingestion • Methanol blood level >20 mg/dL (6.2 mmoles/L) • Any symptomatic patient with a history of methanol ingestion	• Goal: Ethanol blood level 100-130 mg/dL (22-28 mmoles/L) • Continue therapy until methanol blood level <10 mg/dL • Fomepizole therapy is considered investigational
Organophosphate insecticides	Atropine Pralidoxime (2-PAM, Protopam®)	• Symptomatic bradycardia • Myoclonic seizures, severe hallucinations, weakness, arrhythmias, excessive salivation, involuntary urination and defecation	• Caution should be used in patients with narrow-angle glaucoma, cardiovascular disease, or pregnancy •Most effective when used in initial 24-36 hours after exposure • Plasma and/or erythrocyte cholinesterase levels will be depressed from normal
Drug / Drug Class			
Acetaminophen	Acetylcysteine (Mucomyst®)	• Serum acetaminophen level >150 µg/mL at 4 hours postingestion (see Acetaminophen *on page 36*) • Acute ingestion with dose ≥150 mg/kg (child) or 7.5 g (adolescent/adult) within 24 hours of presentation if results of plasma levels cannot be obtained within 8-10 hours of ingestion • Unknown quantity ingested and <24 hours have elapsed since the time of ingestion or unable to obtain serum acetaminophen levels within 12 hours of ingestion • Consider repeating an acetaminophen level 4-6 hours after an initial 4-hour level that is under the treatment range if extended release acetaminophen was ingested • Patients presenting >24 hours postacute ingestion who have measurable levels or biochemical evidence of hepatic injury	• Activated charcoal has been shown to adsorb acetylcysteine; therefore, administer activated charcoal before 4-hour acetaminophen level is drawn • If patient vomits within 1 hour of acetylcysteine dose, readminister the dose • I.V. N-acetylcysteine is available in the U.S. by investigational use only; contact a poison control center for further information

Poisoning Agent	Antidote(s)	Indications	Comments
Anticholinergics	Physostigmine (Antilirium®)	• Refractory seizures or arrhythmias unresponsive to conventional therapy • Symptoms should be life-threatening	• Due to potential for producing severe adverse effects, (eg, seizures, bradycardia) routine use of physostigmine is controversial • Atropine should be available to reverse life-threatening cholinergic effects of physostigmine
Baclofen	Physostigmine (Antilirium®)	• Distinguish anticholinergic delirium from other causes of altered mental status	• Long-lasting reversal of anticholinergic signs and symptoms is generally not achieved due to the relatively short duration of action of physostigmine • Atropine should be available to reverse life-threatening cholinergic effects of physostigmine
Benzodiazepines	Flumazenil (Romazicon®)	• Reverses sedative effects of benzodiazepines	• May precipitate benzodiazepine withdrawal in dependent patients • Not indicated for ethanol, barbiturate, general anesthetic, or narcotic overdose • Mixed drug overdose patients who have ingested drugs that increase the likelihood of seizures (eg, cocaine, lithium, cyclic antidepressants) are at extremely high risk for seizures when flumazenil is used • Action of flumazenil may be shorter than duration of benzodiazepines; repeat doses of flumazenil may be needed • Contraindicated in patients given benzodiazepines for potentially life-threatening conditions (eg, increased intracranial pressure, seizures) and patients with signs of serious cyclic-antidepressant overdosage
Beta-blockers	Isoproterenol (Isuprel®)	• Reversal of bradycardia and hypotension	
	Glucagon	• Reversal of bradycardia unresponsive to isoproterenol	• Glucagon activates adenyl cyclase system at a different site than isoproterenol • Requires liver glycogen stores for hyperglycemic response • I.V. glucose must also be given in treatment of hypoglycemia
Calcium channel blockers	Calcium chloride OR Calcium gluconate	• Reversal of cardiovascular effects of calcium channel blockers (calcium antagonists)	• Monitor serum calcium levels • Calcium is most effective in mild to moderate intoxications • May not be effective in correcting symptomatic bradyarrhythmias

COMMONLY USED ANTIDOTES FOR ACUTE OVERDOSES
(Continued)

Poisoning Agent	Antidote(s)	Indications	Comments
Digitalis glycosides	Digoxin immune Fab (Digibind®)	• Treatment of potentially life-threatening digoxin or digitoxin intoxication in carefully selected patients [serum digoxin level >10 ng/mL or ingestion of >4 mg (child) or >10 mg (adult)] • Life-threatening ventricular arrhythmias secondary to digoxin or digitoxin • Hyperkalemia (K⁺ >5 mEq/L) in the setting of digitalis toxicity • Life-threatening cardiac arrhythmias, progressive bradyarrhythmias, second or third degree heart block unresponsive to atropine	• Monitor potassium levels and continuous EKG • Digibind® interferes with the interpretation of serum digoxin/digitoxin levels
Heparin, Enoxaparin, Dalteparin	Protamine	• Severe hemorrhage	• Effect can be immediate and last for 2 hours • Protamine dosage related to anticoagulant dosage and time of anticoagulant administration • Monitor PTT • Monitor for hypotension
Insulin	Dextrose (25%-50%)	• Severe, symptomatic hypoglycemia	• Very hypertonic solutions; dilute with sterile water prior to I.V. administration
Iron	Deferoxamine (Desferal®)	• Serum iron level >350 µg/mL • Inability to obtain serum iron level within a reasonable time and patient is symptomatic	• Passing of vin rose colored urine indicates free iron was present • Discontinue therapy when urine returns to normal color • Monitor for hypotension during treatment
Isoniazid	Pyridoxine (Vitamin B₆)	• Ingestion of >80 mg/kg isoniazid	
Neuromuscular blocking agents, nondepolarizing (eg, pancuronium)	Edrophonium **OR** Neostigmine **OR** Pyridostigmine	• Reversal of neuromuscular blockade	• Atropine should be available to treat acute cholinergic crisis • Not effective for reversal of **depolarizing** neuromuscular blocking agents (eg, succinylcholine)

Poisoning Agent	Antidote(s)	Indications	Comments
Opiates	Naloxone (Narcan®)	• Reversal of symptoms associated with severe toxicity	• May precipitate withdrawal symptoms in patients with physical dependence to opiates • For prolonged intoxication, a continuous infusion may be used
Phenothiazines	Diphenhydramine (Benadryl®) **OR** Benztropine (Cogentin®)	• Reversal of phenothiazine-induced dystonic reactions	
	Sodium bicarbonate	• Reversal of "quinidine-like" cardiovascular effects (eg, prolonged QRS complex) – QRS duration >100 msec – Ventricular dysrhythmias and hypotension	• Goal is arterial pH of 7.45-7.55 and urine pH of 7.5-8 • Attempts at urine alkalinization may be dangerous in patients with renal dysfunction or where sodium and fluid overload may compromise respiratory or cardiac status
Tricyclic antidepressants	Sodium bicarbonate	• Reversal of "quinidine-like" cardiovascular effects (eg, prolonged QRS complex) – QRS duration >100 msec – Ventricular dysrhythmias and hypotension	• Goal is arterial pH of 7.45-7.55 and urine pH of 7.5-8 • Attempts at urine alkalinization may be dangerous in patients with renal dysfunction or where sodium and fluid overload may compromise respiratory or cardiac status
Warfarin	Phytonadione (Vitamin K_1)	• Large, acute ingestion • Prothrombin time greater than normal	• Vitamin K is relatively contraindicated in patients with prosthetic heart valves unless toxicity is life-threatening
Zinc	Edetate calcium disodium (EDTA) **and/or** Dimercaprol (BAL in Oil®)	• Symptomatic zinc ingestion	• Few case reports • Monitor zinc levels
Plants			
Foxglove Oleander	Digoxin immune Fab (Digibind®)	• Severely intoxicated patients who fail to respond to conventional therapy • Life-threatening ventricular arrhythmias, progressive bradyarrhythmias, or second- or third degree heart block not responsive to atropine • Hyperkalemia (K^+ >5 mEq/L) in the setting of digitalis toxicity	• Monitor potassium levels and continuous EKG
Mushroom (genus *Gyomitra*)	Pyridoxine (Vitamin B_6)		
Mushrooms containing muscarine (inocybe or clitocybe)	Atropine	•Myoclonic seizures, severe hallucinations, weakness, arrhythmias, excessive salivation, involuntary urination and defecation	•Atropine should only be used when indicated; otherwise use may result in anticholinergic poisoning

COMMONLY USED ANTIDOTES FOR ACUTE OVERDOSES
(Continued)

Poisoning Agent	Antidote(s)	Indications	Comments
Snake Bites			
Coral snakes (Eastern and Texas coral snakes only)	Antivenin *(Micrurus fulvius)*		• Not effective for Arizona or Sonoran coral snakes • Skin testing is recommended • Treatment for hypersensitivity reactions, including anaphylaxis, should be available
Pit vipers (Rattlesnakes, cottonmouths, copperheads)	Antivenin *(Crotalidae)* Polyvalent (equine origin)	• Administration within 4 hours of envenomation is ideal; however, administer within 30 hours in all severe cases of poisoning	• Skin testing is recommended • Treatment for hypersensitivity reactions, including anaphylaxis, should be available
Spiders, Scorpions			
Black widow spider	Antivenin *(Lactrodectus mactans)*	• Severe symptoms including respiratory failure, seizures, or pain and spasms not relieved by calcium, muscle relaxants, or analgesics • Symptomatic pregnant patients • Children <5 years or adults >60 years (at greatest risk for severe toxicity)	• Either dermal or conjunctival sensitivity testing should be done prior to administration of antivenin
Scorpion	Antivenin *(Centruroides)*		• No FDA-approved *Centruroides* antivenin in U.S.; only a *Centruroides exilicauda (sculpturatus)*-specific antivenin is available in Arizona (for intrastate use only)

Leikin JR and Paloucek FP, "Poisoning & Toxicology Compendium," Hudson, OH: Lexi-Comp, Inc, 1998.

Mowry JB, Furbee RB, and Chyka PA, "Poisoning," *Essentials of Critical Care Pharmacology*, 3rd ed, Baltimore, MD: Williams & Wilkens, 1994, 501-29.

Zed PJ and Krenzelok EP, "Treatment of Acetaminophen Overdose,"*Am J Health Syst Pharm*, 1999, 56(11):1081-91.

ANION GAP

Definition: The difference in concentration between unmeasured cation and anion equivalents in serum.

Anion gap = Na^+ - Cl^- - HCO_3^-
(The normal anion gap is 10-14 mEq/L.)

Differential diagnosis of increased anion gap

Organic anions
Lactate (sepsis, hypovolemia, large tumor burden)
Pyruvate
Uremia
Ketoacidosis (β-hydroxybutyrate and acetoacetate)
Amino acids and their metabolites
Other organic acids (eg, formate from methanol, glycolate from
ethylene glycol)

Inorganic anions
Hyperphosphatemia
Sulfates
Nitrates

Medications and toxins
Penicillins and cephalosporins
Salicylates (including aspirin)
Cyanide
Carbon monoxide

Differential diagnosis of decreased anion gap
Organic cations
Hypergammaglobulinemia

Inorganic cations
Hyperkalemia
Hypercalcemia
Hypermagnesemia

Medications and toxins
Lithium

Hypoalbuminemia

LABORATORY DETECTION OF DRUGS IN URINE

Agent	Time Detectable in Urine*
Alcohol	12-24 h
Amobarbital	2-4 d
Amphetamine	2-4 d
Butalbital	2-4 d
Cannabinoids	
Occasional use	2-7 d
Regular use	30 d
Cocaine (benzoylecgonine)	12-72 h
Codeine	2-4 d
Chlordiazepoxide	30 d
Diazepam	30 d
Ethanol	12-24 h
Heroin (morphine)	2-4 d
Hydromorphone	2-4 d
Marijuana	
Occasional use	2-7 d
Regular use	30 d
Methamphetamine	2-4 d
Methaqualone	2-4 d
Morphine	2-4 d
Pentobarbital	2-4 d
Phencyclidine (PCP)	
Occasional use	2-7 d
Regular use	30 d
Phenobarbital	30 d
Secobarbital	2-4 d

*The periods of detection for the various abused drugs listed above should be taken as estimates since the actual figures will vary due to metabolism, user, laboratory, and excretion.

Adapted from Chang JY, "Drug Testing and Interpretation of Results," *Pharmchem Newsletter*, 1989, 17:1.

OSMOLALITY

Definition: The summed concentrations of all osmotically active solute particles.

Predicted serum osmolality =

$2 \, Na^+$ (mEq/L) + glucose (mg/dL) / 18 + BUN (mg/dL) / 2.8

The normal range of serum osmolality is 285-295 mOsm/L.

Differential diagnosis of increased serum osmolal gap
(increased by >10 mOsm/L)

Medications and toxins
Alcohols (ethanol, methanol, isopropanol, glycerol, ethylene glycol)
Mannitol
Paraldehyde

SALICYLATE INTOXICATION

**Serum Salicylate Level and
Severity of Intoxication Single Dose
Acute Ingestion Nomogram**

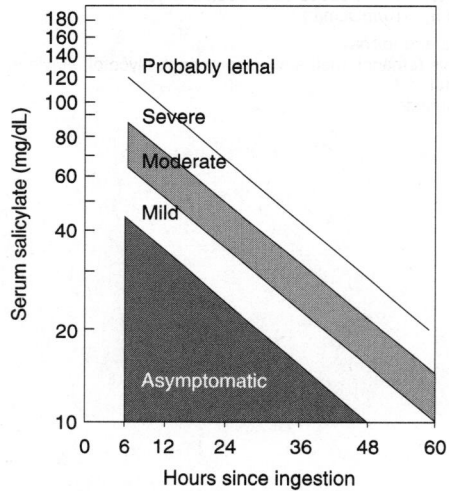

Nomogram relating serum salicylate concentration and expected severity of intoxication at varying intervals following the ingestion of a single dose of salicylate.
From Done AK, "Aspirin Overdosage: Incidence, Diagnosis, and Management," *Pediatrics*, 1978, 62:890-7 with permission.

ACETAMINOPHEN

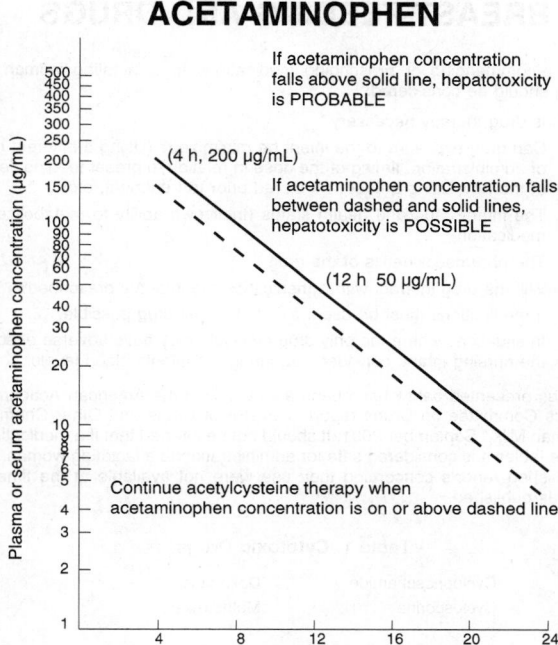

Nomogram relating plasma or serum acetaminophen concentration and probability of hepatotoxicity at varying intervals following ingestion of a single toxic dose of acetaminophen. Modified from Rumack BH, Matthew H, "Acetaminophen Poisoning and Toxicity", Pediatrics, 1975, 55:871-6,
© American Academy of Pediatrics, 1975, and from Rumack BH, et al, "Acetaminophen Overdose", Arch Intern Med, 1981, 141:380-5,
© American Medical Association.

BREAST-FEEDING AND DRUGS

Prior to recommending or prescribing medications to a lactating woman, the following should be considered:

- Is drug therapy necessary?
- Can drug exposure to the infant be minimized? (Using a different route of administration, timing of the dose in relation to breast-feeding, length of therapy, using breast milk stored prior to treatment, etc)
- The infants age and health status (their own ability to metabolize the medication)
- The pharmacokinetics of the drug
- Will the drug interact with a medication the infant is prescribed?
- If medications must be used, pick the safest drug possible.
- In situations where the only drug available may have adverse effects in the nursing infant, consider measuring the infants blood levels.

The tables presented below have been adapted from the American Academy of Pediatrics Committee on Drugs report "Transfer of Drugs and Other Chemicals Into Human Milk," September 2001. It should not be inferred that if a medication is not in the tables it is considered safe for administration to a lactating woman; only that published reports concerning their use were not available at the time the report was published.

Table 1. Cytotoxic Drugs

Cyclophosphamide	Doxorubicin
Cyclosporine	Methotrexate

These are medications thought to interfere with cellular metabolism in the nursing infant. Immune suppression may be possible; effects on growth or carcinogenesis are not known. In addition, doxorubicin is concentrated in human milk; methotrexate is associated with neutropenia in the nursing infant.

Table 2. Drugs of Abuse

Amphetamine	Marijuana
Cocaine	Phencyclidine
Heroin	

Drugs of abuse are not only dangerous to the nursing infant, but also to the mother. Women should be encouraged to avoid their use completely. Effects to the infant reported with amphetamine use in the mother include irritability and poor sleeping; it is also a substance that is concentrated in human milk. Cocaine may cause irritability, vomiting, diarrhea, tremors, or seizures in the infant. Heroin may also cause tremors as well as restlessness, vomiting, and poor feeding.

Nicotine, which was previously on this list, is associated with decreased milk production, decreased weight gain in the infant, and possible increased respiratory illness in the infant. Although there are still questions outstanding regarding smoking and breast-feeding, women should be counseled on the possible effects to their infants and offered aid to smoking cessation if appropriate.

Table 3. Radioactive Compounds That Require Temporary Cessation of Breast-Feeding

Drug	Recommended Time for Cessation of Breast-Feeding
Copper 64 (^{64}Cu)	Radioactivity in milk present at 50 h
Gallium 67 (^{67}Ga)	Radioactivity in milk present for 2 wk
Indium 111 (^{111}In)	Very small amount present at 20 h
Iodine 123 (^{123}I)	Radioactivity in milk present up to 36 h
Iodine 125 (^{125}I)	Radioactivity in milk present for 12 d
Iodine 131 (^{131}I)	Radioactivity in milk present 2-14 d, depending on study
Iodine[131]	If used for thyroid cancer, high radioactivity may prolong exposure to infant
Radioactive sodium	Radioactivity in milk present 96 h
Technetium-99m (^{99m}Tc), ^{99m}Tc macroaggregates, ^{99m}Tc O4	Radioactivity in milk present 15 h to 3 d

Consider pumping and storing milk prior to study for use during the radioactive period. Pumping should continue after the study to maintain milk production; however, this milk should be discarded until radioactivity is gone. Notify nuclear medicine physician prior to study that the mother is breast-feeding; a short-acting radionuclide may be appropriate. Contact Radiology Department after testing is complete to screen milk samples before resuming feeding.

Table 4a. Psychotropic Drugs Whose Effect on Nursing Infants Is Unknown But May Be of Concern

Antianxiety	Antidepressant	Antipsychotic
Alprazolam	Amitriptyline	Chlorpromazine
Diazepam	Amoxapine	Chlorprothixene
Lorazepam	Bupropion	Clozapine[1]
Midazolam	Clomipramine	Haloperidol
Perphenazine	Desipramine	Mesoridazine
Prazepam[1]	Dothiepin	Trifluoperazine
Quazepam	Doxepin	
Temazepam	Fluoxetine	
	Fluvoxamine	
	Imipramine	
	Nortriptyline	
	Paroxetine	
	Sertraline[1]	
	Trazodone	

[1]Drug is concentrated in human milk.

Psychotropic medications usually appear in the breast milk in low concentrations. Although adverse effects in the infant may be limited to a few case reports, the long half-life of these medications and their metabolites should be considered. In addition, measurable amounts may be found in the infants plasma and also brain tissue. Long-term effects are not known. Colic, irritability, feeding and sleep disorders, and slow weight gain are effects reported with fluoxetine. Chlorpromazine may cause galactorrhea in the mother, while drowsiness and lethargy have been reported in the nursing infant. A decline in developmental scores has been reported with chlorpromazine and haloperidol.

BREAST-FEEDING AND DRUGS *(Continued)*

Table 4b. Additional Drugs Whose Effect on Nursing Infants Is Unknown But May Be of Concern

Drug	Reported Effect in Nursing Infant
Amiodarone	Hypothyroidism
Chloramphenicol	Idiosyncratic bone marrow suppression
Clofazimine	Increase in skin pigmentation; high transfer of mothers dose to infant is possible
Lamotrigine	Therapeutic serum concentrations in infant
Metoclopramide[1]	
Metronidazole	
Tinidazole	

[1]Drug is concentrated in human milk.

No adverse effects to the infant have been reported for metoclopramide; however, it should be recognized that it is a dopaminergic agent. Metronidazole and tinidazole are *in vitro* mutagenic agents. In cases where single dose therapy is appropriate for the mother, breast-feeding may be discontinued for 12-24 hours to allow excretion of the medication.

Table 5. Drugs That Have Been Associated With Significant Effects on Some Nursing Infants and Should Be Given to Nursing Mothers With Caution[1]

Drug	Reported Effect
Acebutolol	Hypotension, bradycardia, tachypnea
5-Aminosalicylic acid	Diarrhea (one case)
Atenolol	Cyanosis, bradycardia
Bromocriptine	Suppresses lactation; may be hazardous to the mother
Aspirin (salicylates)	Metabolic acidosis (one case)
Clemastine	Drowsiness, irritability, refusal to feed, high-pitched cry, neck stiffness (one case)
Ergotamine	Vomiting, diarrhea, convulsions (doses used in migraine medications
Lithium	One-third to one-half therapeutic blood concentration in infants
Phenindone	Anticoagulant: increased prothrombin and partial thromboplastin time in one infant; not used in the United States
Phenobarbital	Sedation; infantile spasms after weaning from milk-containing phenobarbital, methemoglobinemia (one case)
Primidone	Sedation, feeding problems
Sulfasalazine (salicylazosulfapyridine)	Bloody diarrhea (one case)

[1]Blood concentration in the infant may be of clinical importance; measure when possible.

Table 6. Maternal Medication Usually Compatible With Breast-Feeding

Drug	Reported Effect
Acetaminophen	
Acetazolamide	
Acitretin	
Acyclovir[1]	
Alcohol (ethanol)	Large amounts may lead to drowsiness, diaphoresis, deep sleep, weakness, decreased linear growth, and/or abnormal weight gain. Ingestion of 1 g/kg/d decreases mothers milk ejection reflex.
Allopurinol	
Amoxicillin	
Antimony	
Atropine	
Azapropazone (apazone)	
Aztreonam	
B_1 (thiamine)	
B_6 (pyridoxine)	
B_{12}	
Baclofen	
Barbiturate	Refer to Table 5
Bendroflumethiazide	Lactation suppressed
Bishydroxycoumarin (Dicumarol®)	
Bromide	Rash, weakness, absence of cry with maternal intake of 5.4 g/d
Butorphanol	
Caffeine	Irritability and poor sleep may be seen with >2-3 cups/d; excreted slowly
Captopril	
Carbamazepine	
Carbetocin	
Carbimazole	Goiter
Cascara	
Cefadroxil	
Cefazolin	
Cefotaxime	
Cefoxitin	
Cefprozil	
Ceftazidime	
Ceftriaxone	
Chloral hydrate	Sleepiness
Chloroform	
Chloroquine	
Chlorothiazide	
Chlorthalidone	Slow excretion
Cimetidine[1]	
Ciprofloxacin	Theoretically, may affect cartilage in weight-bearing joints; pseudomembranous colitis reported in one infant
Cisapride	
Cisplatin	Not found in milk
Clindamycin	
Clogestone	

BREAST-FEEDING AND DRUGS *(Continued)*

Table 6. Maternal Medication Usually Compatible With Breast-Feeding *(continued)*

Drug	Reported Effect
Codeine	
Colchicine	
Contraceptive pill with estrogen and progesterone	Breast enlargement (rare), decreased milk production and protein count (unconfirmed)
Cycloserine	
D (vitamin)	Infant calcium levels should be monitored if mother receives pharmacologic doses
Danthron	Bowel activity increased
Dapsone	No effects reported, but sulfonamide detected in infants urine
Dexbrompheniramine maleate with d-isoephedrine	Crying, poor sleeping patterns, irritability
Diatrizoate	
Digoxin	
Diltiazem	
Dipyrone	
Disopyramide	
Domperidone	
Dyphylline[1]	
Enalapril	
Erythromycin[1]	
Estradiol	Withdrawal, vaginal bleeding
Ethambutol	
Ethanol	See alcohol
Ethosuximide	No effects reported, but detected in infants urine
Fentanyl	
Fexofenadine	
Flecainide	
Fleroxacin	In one report, a single 400 mg dose was administered to the mother and breast milk not given to infant for 48 hours
Fluconazole	
Flufenamic acid	
Fluorescein	
Folic acid	
Gadopentetic (Gadolinium)	
Gentamicin	
Gold salts	
Halothane	
Hydralazine	
Hydrochlorothiazide	
Hydroxychloroquine[1]	
Ibuprofen	
Indomethacin	Seizure (one case)
Iodides	May affect thyroid activity; see Iodine
Iodine	Goiter
Iodine (povidone-iodine/ vaginal douche)	Increased iodine levels in breast milk; iodine odor on infants skin
Iohexol	
Iopanoic acid	

Table 6. Maternal Medication Usually Compatible With Breast-Feeding *(continued)*

Drug	Reported Effect
Isoniazid	Metabolite secreted in breast milk; no hepatotoxicity reported in infant
Interferon alfa	
Ivermectin	
K₁ (vitamin)	
Kanamycin	
Ketoconazole	
Ketorolac	
Labetalol	
Levonorgestrel	
Levothyroxine	
Lidocaine	
Loperamide	
Loratadine	
Magnesium sulfate	
Medroxyprogesterone	
Mefenamic acid	
Meperidine	
Methadone	
Methimazole (active metabolite of carbimazole)	
Methyldopa	
Methprylon	Drowsiness
Metoprolol[1]	
Metrizamide	
Metrizoate	
Mexiletine	
Minoxidil	
Morphine	No effects reported but found in infants serum
Moxalactam	
Nadolol[1]	
Nalidixic acid	Hemolysis reported in infant with glucose-g-phosphate dehydrogenase deficiency
Naproxen	
Nefopam	
Nifedipine	
Nitrofurantoin	Hemolysis reported in infant with G6PD deficiency
Norethynodrel	
Norsteroids	
Noscapine	
Ofloxacin	Theoretically, may affect cartilage in weight-bearing joints
Oxprenolol	
Phenylbutazone	
Phenytoin	
Piroxicam	
Prednisolone	
Prednisone	
Procainamide	
Progesterone	
Propoxyphene	
Propranolol	

BREAST-FEEDING AND DRUGS *(Continued)*

Table 6. Maternal Medication Usually Compatible With Breast-Feeding *(continued)*

Drug	Reported Effect
Propylthiouracil	
Pseudoephedrine[1]	
Pyridostigmine	
Pyrimethamine	
Quinidine	
Quinine	
Riboflavin	
Rifampin	
Scopolamine	
Secobarbital	
Senna	
Sotalol	
Spironolactone	
Streptomycin	
Sulbactam	
Sulfapyridine	Use with caution in infants with G6PD deficiency and in ill, stressed, or premature infants
Sulfisoxazole	Use with caution in infants with G6PD deficiency and in ill, stressed, or premature infants
Sumatriptan	
Suprofen	
Terbutaline	
Terfenadine	
Tetracycline	Negligible absorption by infant; potential to stain infants unerupted teeth
Theophylline	Irritability
Thiopental	
Thiouracil	
Ticarcillin	
Timolol	
Tolbutamide	Jaundice is possible
Tolmetin	
Trimethoprim and sulfamethoxazole	
Triprolidine	
Valproic acid	
Verapamil	
Vitamin (see individual entries, eg, B_1, B_6, B_{12}, D, K)	
Warfarin	
Zolpidem	

[1]Drug is concentrated in human milk.

Table 7. Selected Food and Environmental Agents

Agent	Effect Related to Breast-Feeding
Aspartame	Use with caution if mother or infant has phenylketonuria
Chocolate	Irritability or increased bowel activity observed in infant when >16 oz/d consumed by mother
Fava beans	Hemolysis reported in infant with G6PD deficiency
Hexachlorobenzene	Skin rash, diarrhea, vomiting, dark urine, neurotoxicity, death
Hexachlorophene	No effects reported; however, possibility of milk contamination following nipple washing
Lead	Neurotoxicity possible
Mercury, methylmercury	Possible effects on neurodevelopment
Silicone breast implants	Breast-feeding not contraindicated
Vegetarian diet	B_{12} deficiency

References

American Academy of Pediatrics Committee on Drugs, "Transfer of Drugs and Other Chemicals Into Human Milk," *Pediatrics*, 2001, 108(3): 776-89.

2000 Red Book: Report of the Committee on Infectious Diseases, 25th ed, Elk Grove Village, IL: American Academy of Pediatrics, 2000, 98-104.

COMPATIBILITY OF MEDICATIONS MIXED IN A SYRINGE

	Atropine	Chlorpromazine	Codeine	Diphenhydramine	Droperidol	Fentanyl	Glycopyrrolate	Hydroxyzine	Meperidine	Metoclopramide	Midazolam	Morphine	Pentazocine	Pentobarbital†	Prochlorperazine	Promazine	Promethazine	Trimethobenzamide
Atropine		C	•	C	C	C	C	C	C	C	C	C	C	C	C	C	C	•
Chlorpromazine	C		•	C	C	C	C	C	C	C	C	C	C	X	C	C	C	•
Codeine	•	•		•	•	•	C	C	•	•	•	•	•	X	•	•	•	•
Diphenhydramine	C	C	•		C	C	C	C	C	C	C	C	C	X	C	C	C	•
Droperidol	C	C	•	C		C	C	C	C	C	C	C	C	X	C	C	C	•
Fentanyl	C	C	•	C	C		C	C	C	C	C	C	C	X	C	C	C	•
Glycopyrrolate	C	C	C	C	C	C		C	C	•	C	C	X	X	C	C	C	C
Hydroxyzine	C	C	C	C	C	C	C		C	C	C	C	C	X	C	C	C	•
Meperidine	C	C	•	C	C	C	C	C		C	C	X	C	X	C	C	C	•
Metoclopramide	C	C	•	C	C	C	•	C	C		C	C	•	•	C	C	C	•
Midazolam	C	C	•	C	C	C	C	C	C	C		C	C	X	X	C	C	C
Morphine	C	C	•	C	C	C	C	C	X	C	C		C	X	C*	C	C	C
Pentazocine	C	C	•	C	C	C	X	C	C	•	C	C		X	C	C	C	C
Pentobarbital†	C	X	X	X	X	X	X	X	X	•	X	X	X		X	X	X	•
Prochlorperazine	C	C	•	C	C	C	C	C	C	C	X	C*	C	X		C	C	•
Promazine	C	C	•	C	C	C	C	C	C	C	C	C	C	X	C		C	•
Promethazine	C	C	•	C	C	C	C	C	C	C	C	C	C	X	C	C		•
Trimethobenzamide	•	•	•	•	•	•	C	•	•	•	C	C	C	•	•	•	•	

C = physically compatible if used within 15 minutes after mixing in a syringe.
X = incompatible.
• = no documented information.
C* = potential incompatibility produced by certain manufacturers.
† = compatibility profile is characteristic of most barbiturate salts, such as phenobarbital and secobarbital.

The following combinations have been found to be compatible:
  atropine / meperidine / promethazine
  atropine / meperidine / hydroxyzine
  meperidine / promethazine / chlorpromazine

The following drugs should not be mixed with any other drugs in the same syringe:
  diazepam, chlordiazepoxide

References

Forman JK and Sourney PF, "Visual Compatibility of Midazolam Hydrochloride With Common Preoperative Injectable Medications," Am J Hosp Pharm, 1987, 44(10):2298-9.
King JC, "Guide to Parenteral Admixtures," St Louis, MO: Cutter Laboratories, 1986.
Parker WA, Hosp Pharm, 1984, 19:475-8.
Trissel LA, "Handbook on Injectable Drugs," 5th ed, Bethesda, MD: American Society of Health-System Pharmacists, Inc, 1988.
Stevenson JG and Patriarca C, "Incompatibility of Morphine Sulfate and Prochlorperazine Edisylate in Syringes," Am J Hosp Pharm, 1985, 42:2651.

CONTROLLED SUBSTANCES

Note: These are federal classifications. Your individual state may place a substance into a more restricted category. When this occurs, the more restricted category applies. Consult your state law.

Schedule I = C-I

The drugs and other substances in this schedule have no legal medical uses except research. They have a **high** potential for abuse. They include opiates, opium derivatives, and hallucinogens.

Schedule II = C-II

The drugs and other substances in this schedule have legal medical uses and a **high** abuse potential which may lead to severe dependence. They include former "Class A" narcotics, amphetamines, barbiturates, and other drugs.

Schedule III = C-III

The drugs and other substances in this schedule have legal medical uses and a **lesser** degree of abuse potential which may lead to **moderate** dependence. They include former "Class B" narcotics and other drugs.

Schedule IV = C-IV

The drugs and other substances in this schedule have legal medical uses and **low** abuse potential which may lead to **moderate** dependence. They include barbiturates, benzodiazepines, propoxyphenes and other drugs.

Schedule V = C-V

The drugs and other substances in this schedule have legal medical uses and **low** abuse potential which may lead to **moderate** dependence. They include narcotic cough preparations, diarrhea, preparations, and other drugs.

FEVER DUE TO DRUGS

Aminosalicylic acid
Antihistamines
Asparaginase
Barbiturates
Bleomycin
Cephalosporins
Iodides
Methyldopa
Penicillins
Phenolphthalein
Phenytoin
Procainamide
Quinidine
Sulfonamides
Thiouracil

Abstracted from Harrison's *Principles of Internal Medicine*, 12th ed, Wilson JD, ed, New York, NY: McGraw-Hill Book Co, 1991 and Tabor PA, "Drug-Induced Fever," *Drug Intell Clin Pharm*, 1986, 20:413-20.

DISCOLORATION OF FECES
DUE TO DRUGS

Black
Acetazolamide
Alcohols
Alkalies
Aluminum hydroxide
Aminophylline
Aminosalicylic acid
Amphetamine
Amphotericin
Antacids
Anticoagulants
Aspirin
Betamethasone
Bismuth
Charcoal
Chloramphenicol
Chlorpropamide
Clindamycin
Corticosteroids
Cortisone
Cyclophosphamide
Cytarabine
Dicumarol
Digitalis
Ethacrynic acid
Ferrous salts
Floxuridine
Fluorides
Fluorouracil
Halothane
Heparin
Hydralazine
Hydrocortisone
Ibuprofen
Indomethacin
Iodine drugs
Iron salts
Levarterenol
Levodopa
Manganese
Melphalan
Methylprednisolone

Methotrexate
Methylene blue
Oxyphenbutazone
Paraldehyde
Phenacetin
Phenolphthalein
Phenylbutazone
Phenylephrine
Phosphorous
Potassium salts
Prednisolone
Procarbazine
Pyrvinium
Reserpine
Salicylates
Sulfonamides
Tetracycline
Theophylline
Thiotepa
Triamcinolone
Warfarin

Blue
Chloramphenicol
Methylene blue

Dark Brown
Dexamethasone

Gray
Colchicine

Green
Indomethacin
Iron
Medroxyprogesterone

Greenish Gray
Oral antibiotics
Oxyphenbutazone
Phenylbutazone

Light Brown
Anticoagulants

Orange-Red
Phenazopyridine
Rifampin

Pink
Anticoagulants
Aspirin
Heparin
Oxyphenbutazone
Phenylbutazone
Salicylates

Red
Anticoagulants
Aspirin
Heparin
Oxyphenbutazone
Phenolphthalein
Phenylbutazone
Pyrvinium
Salicylates
Tetracycline syrup

Red-Brown
Oxyphenbutazone
Phenylbutazone
Rifampin

Tarry
Ergot preparations
Ibuprofen
Salicylates
Warfarin

White/Speckling
Aluminum hydroxide
Antibiotics (oral)
Indocyanine green

Yellow
Senna

Yellow-Green
Senna

Adapted from Drugdex® — Drug Consults, Micromedex, Vol 62, Denver, CO: Rocky Mountain Drug Consultation Center, 1998.

DISCOLORATION OF URINE DUE TO DRUGS

Black
Cascara
Cotrimoxazole
Ferrous salts
Iron dextran
Levodopa
Methocarbamol
Methyldopa
Naphthalene
Pamaquine
Phenacetin
Phenols
Quinine
Sulfonamides

Blue
Anthraquinone
DeWitt's pills
Indigo blue
Indigo carmine
Methocarbamol
Methylene blue
Mitoxantrone
Nitrofurans
Resorcinol
Triamterene

Blue-Green
Amitriptyline
Anthraquinone
DeWitt's pills
Doan's® pills
Indigo blue
Indigo carmine
Magnesium salicylate
Methylene blue
Resorcinol

Brown
Anthraquinone dyes
Cascara
Chloroquine
Hydroquinone
Levodopa
Methocarbamol
Methyldopa
Methocarbamol
Metronidazole
Nitrofurans
Nitrofurantoin
Pamaquine
Phenacetin
Phenols
Primaquine
Quinine
Rifabutin
Rifampin
Senna
Sodium diatrizoate
Sulfonamides

Brown-Black
Isosorbide mono- or
  dinitrate
Methyldopa
Metronidazole
Nitrates
Nitrofurans
Phenacetin
Povidone iodine
Quinine
Senna

Dark
p-Aminosalicylic acid
Cascara
Levodopa
Metronidazole
Nitrites
Phenacetin
Phenol
Primaquine
Quinine
Resorcinol
Riboflavin
Senna

Green
Amitriptyline
Anthraquinone
DeWitt's pills
Indigo blue
Indigo carmine
Indomethacin
Methocarbamol
Methylene blue
Nitrofurans
Phenols
Propofol
Resorcinol
Suprofen

Green-Yellow
DeWitt's pills
Methylene blue

Milky
Phosphates

Orange
Chlorzoxazone
Dihydroergotamine
  mesylate
Heparin sodium
Phenazopyridine
Phenindione
Rifabutin
Rifampin
Sulfasalazine
Warfarin

Orange-Red-Brown
Chlorzoxazone
Doxidan
Phenazopyridine
Rifampin
Warfarin

Orange-Yellow
Fluorescein sodium
Rifampin
Sulfasalazine

Pink
Aminopyrine
Anthraquinone dyes
Aspirin
Cascara
Danthron
Deferoxamine
Merbromin
Methyldopa
Phenazopyridone
Phenolphthalein
Phenothiazines
Phenytoin
Salicylates
Senna

Purple
Phenolphthalein

Red
Anthraquinone
Cascara
Chlorpromazine
Daunorubicin
Deferoxamine
Dihydroergotamine
  mesylate
Dimethyl sulfoxide
DMSO
Doxorubicin
Heparin
Ibuprofen
Methyldopa
Oxyphenbutazone
Phenacetin
Phenazopyridine
Phenolphthalein
Phenothiazines
Phensuximide
Phenylbutazone
Phenytoin
Rifampin
Senna

Red-Brown
Cascara
Deferoxamine
Methyldopa
Oxyphenbutazone
Pamaquine
Phenacetin
Phenazopyridine
Phenolphthalein
Phenothiazines
Phenylbutazone
Phenytoin
Quinine
Senna

Red-Purple
Chlorzoxazone
Ibuprofen
Phenacetin
Senna

Rust
Cascara
Chloroquine
Metronidazole
Nitrofurantoin
Pamaquine
Phenacetin
Quinacrine
Riboflavin
Senna
Sulfonamides

Yellow
Nitrofurantoin
Phenacetin
Quinacrine
Riboflavin
Sulfasalazine

Yellow-Brown
Aminosalicylate acid
Bismuth
Cascara
Chloroquine
DeWitt's pills
Methylene blue
Metronidazole
Nitrofurantoin
Pamaquine
Primaquine
Quinacrine
Senna
Sulfonamides

Yellow-Pink
Cascara
Senna

Adapted from Drugdex® — Drug Consults, Micromedex, Vol 62, Denver, CO: Rocky Mountain Drug Consultation Center, 1998.

DRUGS IN PREGNANCY

Medications Known to Be Teratogens

Alcohol	Isotretinoin
Androgens	Lithium
Anticonvulsants	Live vaccines
Antineoplastics	Methimazole
Cocaine	Penicillamine
Diethylstilbestrol	Tetracyclines
Etretinate	Warfarin
Iodides (including radioactive iodine)	

Medications Suspected to Be Teratogens

ACE inhibitors	Oral hypoglycemic drugs
Benzodiazepines	Progestogens
Estrogens	Quinolones

Medications With No Known Teratogenic Effects[1]

Acetaminophen	Narcotic analgesics
Cephalosporins	Penicillins
Corticosteroids	Phenothiazines
Docusate sodium	Thyroid hormones
Erythromycin	Tricyclic antidepressants
Multiple vitamins	

[1]No drug is absolutely without risk during pregnancy. These drugs appear to have a minimal risk when used judiciously in usual doses under the supervision of a medical professional.

Medications With Nonteratogenic Adverse Effects in Pregnancy

Antithyroid drugs	Diuretics
Aminoglycosides	Isoniazid
Aspirin	Narcotic analgesics (chronic use)
Barbiturates (chronic use)	Nicotine
Benzodiazepines	Nonsteroidal anti-inflammatory agents
Beta-blockers	Oral hypoglycemic agents
Caffeine	Propylthiouracil
Chloramphenicol	Sulfonamides
Cocaine	

Adapted from DiPiro JT, Talbert RL, Hayes PE, et al, "Therapeutic Considerations During Pregnancy and Lactation," *Pharmacotherapy: A Pathophysiologic Approach*, 4th ed, Stamford, CT: Appleton & Lange, 1999.

MILLIEQUIVALENT FOR SELECTED IONS

Approximate Milliequivalents — Weights of Selected Ions

Salt	mEq/g Salt	mg Salt/mEq
Calcium carbonate ($CaCO_3$)	20	50
Calcium chloride ($CaCl_2 \bullet 2H_2O$)	14	73
Calcium gluconate (Ca gluconate$_2 \bullet 1H_2O$)	4	224
Calcium lactate (Ca lactate$_2 \bullet 5H_2O$)	6	154
Magnesium sulfate ($MgSO_4$)	16	60
Magnesium sulfate ($MgSO_4 \bullet 7H_2O$)	8	123
Potassium acetate (K acetate)	10	98
Potassium chloride (KCl)	13	75
Potassium citrate (K_3 citrate$\bullet 1H_2O$)	9	108
Potassium iodide (KI)	6	166
Sodium bicarbonate ($NaHCO_3$)	12	84
Sodium chloride (NaCl)	17	58
Sodium citrate (Na_3 citrate$\bullet 2H_2O$)	10	98
Sodium iodide (NaI)	7	150
Sodium lactate (Na lactate)	9	112
Zinc sulfate ($ZnSO_4 \bullet 7H_2O$)	7	144

Valences and Approximate Weights of Selected Ions

Substance	Electrolyte	Valence	Ionic Wt
Calcium	Ca^{++}	2	40
Chloride	Cl^-	1	35.5
Magnesium	Mg^{++}	2	24
Phosphate	PO_4^{3-}	3	95*
	HPO_4^{2-}	2	96
	$H_2PO_4^-$	1	97
Potassium	K^+	1	39
Sodium	Na^+	1	23
Sulfate	SO_4^{2-}	2	96*

*The atomic weight of phosphorus is 31, and of sulfur is 32.

SEROTONIN SYNDROME

Diagnostic Criteria for Serotonin Syndrome

- Recent addition or dosage increase of any agent increasing serotonin activity or availability (usually within 1 day)
- Absence of abused substances, metabolic infectious etiology, or withdrawal
- No recent addition or dosage increase of a neuroleptic agent prior to onset of signs and symptoms
- Presence of three or more of the following: (% incidence)

Agitation (34%)
Abdominal pain (4%)
Ataxia/incoordination (40%)
Diaphoresis (45%)
Diarrhea (8%)
Hyperpyrexia (45%)
Hypertension/hypotension (35%)
Hyperthermia
Hyperreflexia (52%)
Mental status change – cognitive behavioral changes:
    Anxiety (15%)
    Euphoria/hypomania (21%)
    Confusion (51%)
    Agitation (34%)
    Disorientation
    Coma/unresponsiveness (29%)

Muscle rigidity (51%)
Mydriasis
Myoclonus (58%)
Nausea (23%)
Nystagmus (15%)
Restlessness/hyperactivity (48%)
Salivation (2%)
Seizures (12%)
Shivering (26%)
Sinus tachycardia (36%)
Tachypnea (26%)
Tremor (43%)
Unreactive pupils (20%)

Drugs (as Single Causative Agent) Which Can Induce Serotonin Syndrome

Specific serotonin reuptake inhibitors (SSRI)
MDMA (Ectasy)
Clomipramine

Drug Combinations Which Can Induce Serotonin Syndrome[1]

Alprazolam – Clomipramine
Amphetamines – MAO inhibitors
Amphetamines – SSRIs (Citalopram, Fluoxetine, Fluvoxamine, Paroxetine, Sertraline)
Amphetamines – Tricyclic antidepressants
Amitriptyline – Dihydroergotamine
Amitriptyline – Lithium – Trazodone
Amitriptyline – Sertraline
Anorexiants – MAO inhibitors
Bromocriptine – Levodopa/Carbidopa
Buspirone – Nefazodone
Buspirone – SSRIs (Citalopram, Fluoxetine, Fluvoxamine, Paroxetine, Sertraline)
Buspirone – Trazodone
Buspirone – Tricyclic antidepressants
Carbamazepine – Fluoxetine
Citalopram – Moclobemide
Clomipramine – Alprazolam
Clomipramine – Clorgiline
Clomipramine – Lithium
Clomipramine – MAO inhibitors
Clomipramine – Moclobemide

Clomipramine – S-adenosylmethionine
Clomipramine – Tranylcypromine
Clorgiline – Clomipramine
Dextromethorphan – MAO inhibitors
Dextromethorphan – SSRIs (Citalopram, Fluoxetine, Fluvoxamine, Paroxetine, Sertraline)
Dextropropoxyphene – Phenelzine – Trazodone
Dihydroergotamine – Amitriptyline
Dihydroergotamine – Paroxetine
Dihydroergotamine – SSRIs (Citalopram, Fluoxetine, Fluvoxamine, Paroxetine, Sertraline)
Dihydroergotamine – Tricyclic antidepressants
Fentanyl – SSRIs (Citalopram, Fluoxetine, Fluvoxamine, Paroxetine, Sertraline)
Fluoxetine – Carbamazepine
Fluoxetine – Remoxipride
Fluoxetine – Tryptophan
Levodopa/Carbidopa – Bromocriptine

Linezolid - SSRIs (Citalopram, Fluoxetine, Fluvoxamine, Paroxetine, Sertraline)
Linezolid – Tramadol
Linezolid – Tricyclic antidepressants
Lithium – Amitriptyline – Trazodone
Lithium – Clomipramine
Lithium – SSRIs (Citalopram, Fluoxetine, Fluvoxamine, Paroxetine, Sertraline)
Lithium – Tricyclic antidepressants
Lithium – Venlafaxine
Lysergic acid diethylamide (LSD) – SSRIs (Citalopram, Fluoxetine, Fluvoxamine, Paroxetine, Sertraline)
Metoclopramide – Sertraline
Metoclopramide – Venlafaxine
MAO inhibitors – Amphetamines
MAO inhibitors – Anorexiants
MAO inhibitors – Clomipramine
MAO inhibitors – Dextromethorphan
MAO inhibitors – Meperidine
MAO inhibitors – Nefazodone
MAO inhibitors – Serotonin agonists
MAO inhibitors – S-adenosylmethionine
MAO inhibitors – SSRIs (Citalopram, Fluoxetine, Fluvoxamine, Paroxetine, Sertraline)
MAO inhibitors – St John's Wort
MAO inhibitors – Tramadol
MAO inhibitors – Trazodone
MAO inhibitors – Tricyclic antidepressants
MAO inhibitors – Tryptophan
MAO inhibitors – Venlafaxine
Meperidine – MAO inhibitors
Meperidine – Moclobemide
Meperidine – Nefazodone
Meperidine – SSRIs (Citalopram, Fluoxetine, Fluvoxamine, Paroxetine, Sertraline)
Moclobemide – Citalopram
Moclobemide – Clomipramine
Moclobemide – Meperidine
Moclobemide – Pethidine
Moclobemide – SSRIs (Citalopram, Fluoxetine, Fluvoxamine, Paroxetine, Sertraline)
Moclobemide – Tricyclic antidepressants
Nefazodone – Buspirone
Nefazodone – MAO inhibitors
Nefazodone – Meperidine
Nefazodone – Serotonin agonists
Nefazodone – SSRIs (Citalopram, Fluoxetine, Fluvoxamine, Paroxetine, Sertraline)
Nefazodone – Trazodone
Nefazodone – Tramadol
Nefazodone – Valproic Acid
Nortriptyline – Trazodone

Paroxetine – Dihydroergotamine
Paroxetine – Trazodone
Pethidine – Moclobemide
Phenelzine – Trazodone – Dextropropoxyphene
Remoxipride – Fluoxetine
S-adenosylmethionine – Clomipramine
S-adenosylmethionine – MAO inhibitors
S-adenosylmethionine – SSRIs (Citalopram, Fluoxetine, Fluvoxamine, Paroxetine, Sertraline)
S-adenosylmethionine – Tricyclic antidepressants
Selegiline (high-dose) – SSRIs (Citalopram, Fluoxetine, Fluvoxamine, Paroxetine, Sertraline)
Selegiline (high-dose) – Tricyclic antidepressants
Selegiline (high-dose) – Venlafaxine
Serotonin agonists (Sumatriptan, others) – MAO inhibitors
Serotonin agonists (Sumatriptan, others) – Nefazodone
Serotonin agonists (Sumatriptan, others) – SSRIs (Citalopram, Fluoxetine, Fluvoxamine, Paroxetine, Sertraline)
Serotonin agonists (Sumatriptan, others) – TCAs
Serotonin agonists (Sumatriptan, others) – Tramadol
Sertraline – Amitriptyline
Sibutramine – SSRIs (Citalopram, Fluoxetine, Fluvoxamine, Paroxetine, Sertraline)
SSRIs – Amphetamines
SSRIs – Buspirone
SSRIs – Dextromethorphan
SSRIs – Dihydroergotamine
SSRIs – Fentanyl
SSRIs – Linezolid
SSRIs – Lithium
SSRIs – Lysergic acid diethylamide (LSD)
SSRIs – MAO inhibitors
SSRIs – Meperidine
SSRIs – Moclobemide
SSRIs – Nefazodone
SSRIs – S-adenosylmethionine
SSRIs – Selegiline (high-dose)
SSRIs – Serotonin agonists
SSRIs – Sibutramine
SSRIs – St John's Wort
SSRIs – Tramadol
SSRIs – Trazodone
SSRIs – Tricyclic antidepressants
SSRIs – Tryptophan
St John's Wort – MAO inhibitors

SEROTONIN SYNDROME *(Continued)*

St John's Wort – SSRIs (Citalopram, Fluoxetine, Fluvoxamine, Paroxetine, Sertraline)
St John's Wort – Tricyclic antidepressants
Sympathomimetics – Tricyclic antidepressants
Tramadol – Linezolid
Tramadol – MAO inhibitors
Tramadol – Nefazodone
Tramadol – Serotonin agonists
Tramadol – SSRIs (Citalopram, Fluoxetine, Fluvoxamine, Paroxetine, Sertraline)
Tramadol – TCAs
Tranylcypromine – Clomipramine
Trazodone – Buspirone
Trazodone – Lithium – Amitriptyline
Trazodone – MAO inhibitors
Trazodone – Nefazodone
Trazodone – Nortriptyline
Trazodone – Paroxetine
Trazodone – SSRIs (Citalopram, Fluoxetine, Fluvoxamine, Paroxetine, Sertraline) (theoretical)
Tricyclic antidepressants – Amphetamines
Tricyclic antidepressants – Buspirone
Tricyclic antidepressants – Dihydroergotamine

Tricyclic antidepressants – Linezolid
Tricyclic antidepressants – Lithium
Tricyclic antidepressants – MAO inhibitors
Tricyclic antidepressants – Moclobemide
Tricyclic antidepressants – S-adenosylmethionine
Tricyclic antidepressants – Serotonin agonists
Tricyclic antidepressants – SSRIs (Citalopram, Fluoxetine, Fluvoxamine, Paroxetine, Sertraline)
Tricyclic antidepressants – St John's Wort
Tricyclic antidepressants – Sympathomimetics
Tricyclic antidepressants – Tramadol
Tryptophan – Fluoxetine
Tryptophan – MAO inhibitors
Tryptophan – SSRIs (Citalopram, Fluoxetine, Fluvoxamine, Paroxetine, Sertraline)
Valproic acid – Nefazodone
Venlafaxine – Lithium
Venlafaxine – MAO inhibitors
Venlafaxine – Selegiline (high-dose)

[1]When administered within 2 weeks of each other.

Guidelines for Treatment of Serotonin Syndrome

Therapy is primarily supportive with intravenous crystalloid solutions utilized for hypotension and cooling blankets for mild hyperthermia. Norepinephrine is the preferred vasopressor. Chlorpromazine or dantrolene sodium may have a role in controlling fevers, although there is no proven benefit. Benzodiazepines are the first-line treatment in controlling rigors and thus, limiting fever and rhabdomyolysis, while clonazepam may be specifically useful in treating myoclonus. Endotracheal intubation and paralysis may be required to treat refractory muscular contractions. Tachycardia or tremor can be treated with beta-blocking agents; although due to its blockade of 5-HTIA receptors, the syndrome may worsen. Serotonin blockers such as diphenhydramine, cyproheptadine, or chlorpromazine have been used with variable efficacy. Methysergide and nitroglycerin (I.V. infusion with lorazepam) also has been utilized with variable efficacy in case reports. It appears that cyproheptadine is most consistently beneficial.

Recovery seen within 1 day in 70% of cases; mortality rate is about 11%.

References

Gardner DM and Lynd LD, "Sumatriptan Contraindications and the Serotonin Syndrome," *Ann Pharmacother*, 1998, 32(1):33-8

Gitlin MJ, "Venlafaxine, Monoamine Oxidase Inhibitors, and the Serotonin Syndrome," *J Clin Psychopharmacol*, 1997, 17:66-7.

Heisler MA, Guidery JR, and Arnecke B, "Serotonin Syndrome Induced by Administration of Venlafaxine and Phenelzine," *Ann Pharmacother*, 1996, 30:84.

Hodgman MJ, Martin TG, and Krenzelok EP, "Serotonin Syndrome Due to Venlafaxine and Maintenance Tranylcypromine Therapy," *Hum Exp Toxicol*, 1997, 16:14-7.

John L, Perreault MM, Tao T, et al, "Serotonin Syndrome Associated With Nefazodone and Paroxetine," *Ann Emerg Med*, 1997, 29:287-9.

LoCurto MJ, "The Serotonin Syndrome," *Emerg Clin North Am*, 1997, 15(3):665-75.

Martin TG, "Serotonin Syndrome," *Ann Emerg Med*, 1996, 28:520-6.

Mills K, "Serotonin Toxicity: A Comprehensive Review for Emergency Medicine," *Top Emerg Med*, 1993, 15:54-73.

Mills KC, "Serotonin Syndrome: A Clinical Update," *Crit Care Clin*, 1997, 13(4):763-83.

Nisijima K, Shimizu M, Abe T, et al, "A Case of Serotonin Syndrome Induced by Concomitant Treatment With Low-Dose Trazodone, and Amitriptyline and Lithium," *Int Clin Psychopharmacol*, 1996, 11:289-90.

Sobanski T, Bagli M, Laux G, et al, "Serotonin Syndrome After Lithium Add-On Medication to Paroxetine," *Pharmacopsychiatry*, 1997, 30:106-7.

Sporer, "The Serotonin Syndrome: Implicated Drugs, Pathophysiology and Management," *Drug Safety*, 1995, 13(2):94-104.

Sternbach H, "The Serotonin Syndrome," *Am J Psychiatry*, 1991, 146:705-7.

Van Berkum MM, Thiel J, Leikin JB, et al, "A Fatality Due to Serotonin Syndrome," *Medical Update for Psychiatrists*, 1997, 2:55-7.

SODIUM CONTENT OF SELECTED MEDICINALS

Name and Dosage Unit*	Sodium	
	mg	mEq
Antibiotics		
Amikacin sulfate, 1 g	29.9	1.3
Aminosalicylate sodium, 1 g	109	4.7
Ampicillin, suspension, 250 mg/5 mL, 5 mL	10	0.4
Ampicillin sodium, 1 g	66.7	3
Carbenicillin disodium, 382 mg (tablet)	23	1
Cefazolin sodium, 1 g	47	2
Cefotaxime sodium, 1 g	50.6	2.2
Cefoxitin sodium, 1 g	53	2.3
Ceftriaxone sodium, 1 g	60	2.6
Cefuroxime, 1 g	54.2	2.4
Chloramphenicol sodium succinate, 1 g	51.8	2.3
Dicloxacillin, 250 mg (capsule)	13	0.6
Erythromycin ethyl succinate, suspension 200 mg/5 mL	29	1.3
Erythromycin Base Filmtab®, 250 mg	70	3
Metronidazole, 500 mg I.V.	322	14
Nafcillin sodium, 1 g	66.7	2.9
Nitrofurantoin, suspension, 25 mg/5 mL	7	0.3
Penicillin G potassium, 1,000,000 units I.V.	7.6	0.3
Penicillin G sodium, 1,000,000 units I.V.	46	2
Penicillin V potassium, suspension, 250 mg/5 mL	38	1.7
Piperacillin sodium, 1 g	42.6	1.8
Ticarcillin disodium, 1 g	119.6	5.2
Antacids, Liquid (content per 5 mL)		
Amphojel®	<2.3	<0.1
ALternaGEL®	2	0.1
Basaljel®	2.4	0.1
Extra Strength Maalox®-Plus	0.65	≅0.05
Gaviscon®	13	0.57
Maalox®	1.3	0.06
Tums E-X™	<4.8	<0.2
Sodium Content of Miscellaneous Medicinals		
Acetazolamide sodium, 500 mg	47.2	2.05
Chlorothiazide sodium, 500 mg	57.5	2
Cisplatin, 10 mg	35.4	1.54
Edetate calcium disodium, 1 g	122	5.3
Fleet® Enema, 4.5 oz	5000†	218
Fleet® Phospho®-Soda, 20 mL	2217	96.4
Hydrocortisone sodium succinate, 1 g	47.5	2.07
Hypaque® M 75%, injection, 20 mL	200	8.7
Hypaque® M 90%, injection, 20 mL	220	9.6
Metamucil® Instant Mix (orange)	6	0.27
Methotrexate sodium, 100 mg vial	20	0.86
Methotrexate sodium, 100 mg vial (low sodium)	15	0.65
Naproxen sodium, 250 mg (tablet)	23	1

Name and Dosage Unit*	Sodium	
	mg	mEq
Neutra-Phos®, capsule and 75 mL reconstituted solution	164	7.13
Oragrafin® (capsule)	19	0.8
Pentobarbital sodium, 50 mg/mL	5	0.2
Phenobarbital sodium, 65 mg, 1 mL vial	6	0.3
Phenytoin sodium, 1 g	88	3.8
Promethazine expectorant, 5 mL	53	2.3
Shohl's solution modified, 1 mL	23	1
Sodium ascorbate, 500 mg acid equivalent	65.3	2.84
Sodium bicarbonate, 50 mL 8.4%	1150	50
Sodium nitroprusside, 50 mg	7.8	0.34
Sodium polystyrene sulfonate, 1 g	94.3‡	4.1
Thiopental sodium, 1 g	86.8	3.8
Valproate sodium, 250 mg/5 mL, 5 mL	23	1

*Product formulations and hence sodium content are subject to change by the manufacturer.

†Average systemic absorption 250-300 mg.

‡Total sodium content. Only about 33% is liberated in clinical use.

SUGAR-FREE LIQUID PHARMACEUTICALS

The following sugar-free liquid preparations are listed by therapeutic category and alphabetically within each category. Please note that product formulations are subject to change by the manufacturer. Some of these products may contain sorbitol, xylitol, or other sweeteners which may be partially metabolized to provide calories.

Analgesics
Acetaminophen Elixir (various)
APAP/APAP Plus
Aspirin/Buffered Aspirin (Medique®)
Bufferin® A/F Nite Time
Children's Anacin-3® Infants Drops
Children's Tylenol® Chewable Tablets
Extra Strength Tylenol® PM
Febrol® and Febrol® EX
Methadone Hydrochloride Intensol
MS-Ai®
Myapap® Drops
No Drowsiness Tylenol®
Pain-Off®
Paregoric USP (Abbott)
Sep-A-Soothe® II
St Joseph® Aspirin-Free Liquid and Drops
Tylenol® Drops

Antacids/Antiflatulents
Alcalak®
Aldroxicon®
Aluminum Hydroxide Suspension
Citrocarbonate® Granules
Di-Gel® Liquid (mint, lemon & orange flavored)
Gaviscon® Liquid
Maalox® Plus Suspension
Maalox® Suspension
Maalox® Therapeutic Concentrate
Magnesia and Alumina Oral Suspension USP (Abbott, Phillips Roxane)
Mallamint® Chewable Tablets
Medi-Seltzer®/Plus
Milk of Bismuth
Milk of Magnesia USP
Mylanta® Liquid
Mylanta®-II Liquid
Mylicon® Drops
Pepto-Bismol® Liquid and Tablets
Riopan Plus®
Riopan® Suspension
Titralac® Liquid
Titralac® Plus Liquid

Antiasthmatics
Alupent® Syrup
Elixophyllin® Elixir
Elixophyllin®-GG Liquid
Lufyllin® Elixir
Mucomyst®-10
Mucomyst®-20
Organidin® NR
Theolair™ 80 Syrup
Theophylline Elixir (Phillips Roxane)

Antidepressants
Sinequan® Oral Concentrate

Antidiarrheals

Corrective Mixture With Paregoric
Diasorb® Liquid and Tablets
Di-Gon® II
Diotame®
Donnagel®
Kalicon® Suspension
Kaolin Mixture With Pectin NF (Abbott)
Kaolin-Pectin Suspension (Phillips Roxane)
Konsyl® Powder
Lomanate®
Lomotil® Liquid
Paregoric USP (various)
Parepectolin® (various)
Pepto-Bismol®
St Joseph® Antidiarrheal

Antiepileptics

Mysoline® Suspension

Antihistamine-Decongestants

Actifed® With Codeine
Actifed® Syrup
Bromphen® Elixir
Dimetane® Decongestant Elixir
Dimetapp® Elixir
Hay-Febrol® Liquid
Isoclor® Liquid and Capsules
Naldecon® Pediatric Drops and Syrup
Naldecon® Syrup
Novahistine® Elixir
Phenergan® Fortis Syrup
Phenergan® Syrup
Rondec® DM Drops
Ryna® Liquid
S-T® Forte® Liquid
Tavist® Syrup
Vistaril® Oral Suspension

Anti-infectives

Augmentin® Suspension
Furadantin® Oral Suspension
Humatin®
Mandelamine® Suspension/Forte®
Minocin® Suspension
NegGram® Suspension
Sulfamethoxazole and Trimethoprim Suspension (Biocraft, Beecham, Burroughs Wellcome)
Vibramycin® Syrup

Corticosteroids

Decadron® Elixir
Dexamethasone Solution (Roxane)
Dexamethasone Intensol Solution
Pediapred® Oral Liquid

Cough Medicines

Anatuss® With Codeine Syrup
Anatuss® Syrup
Brown Mixture NF (Lannett)
Chlorgest-HD®
Codiclear® DH Syrup
Codimal® DM
Contac Jr® Liquid
Day-Night Comtrex®
Decoral® Forte®

SUGAR-FREE LIQUID PHARMACEUTICALS *(Continued)*

Dimetane®-DC Cough Syrup
Dimetane®-DX Cough Syrup
Entuss® Expectorant Liquid
Histafed® Pediatric Liquid
Hycomine® Syrup and Pediatric Syrup
Medicon® D
Medi-Synal®
Naldecon-DX® Pediatric Drops and Syrup
Naldecon-DX® Adult Liquid
Non-Drowsy Comtrex®
Organidin® NR
Potassium Iodide Solution (various)
Robitussin-CF® Liquid
Robitussin® Night Relief Liquid
Rondec®-DM Drops
Rondec®-DM Syrup
Ryna® Liquid
Ryna-C® Liquid
Ryna-CX® Liquid
Scot-Tussin® DM Syrup
Scot-Tussin® Expectorant
Scot-Tussin® DM Cough Chasers
Silexin® Cough Syrup
Sudodrin®/Sudodrin® Forte®
Terpin® Hydrate With Codeine Elixir (various)
Tolu-Sed® Cough Syrup
Tolu-Sed® DM
Tricodene® Liquid
Tussirex® Sugar-Free

Dental Preparations and Fluoride Preparations

Cepacol® Mouthwash
Cepastat® Mouthwash and Gargle
Chloraseptic® Mouthwash and Gargle
Fluorigard® Mouthrinse
Fluorinse®
Flura-Drops®
Flura-Loz®
Flura® Tablets
Gel-Kam®
Karigel®
Karigel® N
Luride® Drops
Luride® SF Lozi-Tabs
Luride® 0.25 and 0.5 Lozi-Tabs
Luride® Lozi-Tabs
Pediaflor® Drops
Phos-Flur® Rinse/Supplement
Point-Two® Mouthrinse
Prevident® Disclosing Drops
Thera-Flur® Gel and Drops

Diagnostic Agents

Gastrografin®

Dietary Substitutes

Co-Salt®

Iron Preparations/Blood Modifiers

Amicar® Syrup
Geritol® Complete Tablets
Geritonic™ Liquid
Hemo-Vite® Liquid
Iberet® Liquid

Iberet®-500 Liquid
Niferex®
Nu-Iron® Elixir
Vita-Plus H® Half Strength, Sugar-Free
Vita-Plus H®, Sugar-Free

Laxatives
Aromatic Cascara Fluidextract USP
Castor Oil
Castor Oil (flavored)
Castor Oil USP
Colace®, Liquid
Emulsoil®
Fiberall® Powder
Hydrocil® Instant Powder
Hypaque® Oral Powder
Kondremul®
Kondremul® With Cascara
Kondremul® With Phenolphthalein
Konsyl® Powder
Liqui-Doss®
Magnesium Citrate Solution NF
Metamucil® Instant Mix (lemon-lime or orange)
Metamucil® SF Powder
Milk of Magnesia
Milk of Magnesia/Cascara Suspension
Milk of Magnesia/Mineral Oil Emulsion (various)
Mineral Oil (various)
Neoloid® Liquid
NuLYTELY®
Sodium Phosphate & Biphosphate Oral Solution USP (Phillips Roxane)

Potassium Products
Cena-K® Solution
K-G® Elixir
Kaochlor-Eff® Tablets for Solution
Kaochlor® S-F Solution
Kaon® Elixir (grape and lemon-lime flavor)
Kaon-Cl® 20% Liquid
Kay Ciel® Elixir
Kay Ciel® Powder
Klor-Con®/25 Powder
Klor-Con® EF Tablets
Klor-Con® Liquid 20%
Klor-Con® Powder
Potassium Chloride Oral Solution USP 5%, 10%, and 20% (various)
Potassium Gluconate Elixir NF
Rum-K® Solution
Tri-K® Liquid

Sedatives-Tranquilizers-Antipsychotics
Butabarbital Sodium Elixir
Butisol Sodium® Elixir
Haldol® Concentrate
Loxitane® C Drops
Mellaril® Concentrate
Serentil® Concentrate
Thorazine® Concentrate

Vitamin Preparations-Nutritionals
Aquasol A® Drops
Bugs Bunny™ Chewable Tablets
Bugs Bunny™ Plus Iron Chewable Tablets
Bugs Bunny™ With Extra C Chewable Tablets
Bugs Bunny™ Plus Minerals Chewable Tablets
Calciferol™ Drops

SUGAR-FREE LIQUID PHARMACEUTICALS *(Continued)*

Caltrate® 600 Tablets
Cod Liver Oil (various)
DHT™ Intensol Solution (Roxane)
Drisdol® in Propylene Glycol
Flintstones™ Complete Chewable Tablets
Flintstones™ With Extra C Chewable Tablets
Flintstones™ Plus Iron Chewable Tablets
Oyst-Cal® 500 Tablets
Pediaflor®
PMS® Relief
Poly-Vi-Flor® Drops
Poly-Vi-Flor®/Iron Drops
Poly-Vi-Sol® Drops
Poly-Vi-Sol®/Iron Drops
Posture® Tablets
Spiderman™ Children's Chewable Vitamin Tablets
Spiderman™ Children's Plus Iron Tablets
Theragran® Jr Children's Chewable Tablets
Tri-Vi-Flor® Drops
Tri-Vi-Sol® Drops
Tri-Vi-Sol®/Iron Drops
Vi-Daylin® ADC Drops
Vi-Daylin® ADC/Fluoride Drops
Vi-Daylin® ADC Plus Iron Drops
Vi-Daylin® Drops
Vi-Daylin®/Fluoride Drops
Vi-Daylin® Plus Iron Drops
Vitalize®

Miscellaneous

Altace™ Capsules
Bicitra® Solution
Colestid® Granules
Digoxin® Elixir (Roxane)
Lipomul®
Lithium Citrate Syrup
Nicorette® Chewing Gum
Polycitra®-K Solution
Polycitra®-LC Solution
Tagamet® Liquid

References

Hill EM, Flaitz CM, and Frost GR, "Sweetener Content of Common Pediatric Oral Liquid Medications," *Am J Hosp Pharm*, 1988, 45:135-42.

Kumar A, Rawlings RD, and Beaman DC, "The Mystery Ingredients: Sweeteners, Flavorings, Dyes, and Preservatives in Analgesic/Antipyretic, Antihistamine/Decongestant, Cough and Cold, Antidiarrheal, and Liquid Theophylline Preparations," *Pediatrics*, 1993, 91:927-33.

"Sugar Free Products," *Drug Topics Red Book*, 1992, 17-8.

CARBOHYDRATE AND ALCOHOL CONTENT OF LIQUID MEDICATIONS FOR USE IN PATIENTS RECEIVING KETOGENIC DIETS

Generic Name	Carbohydrate g/5 mL				Ethyl Alcohol g/5 mL
	Sucrose	Sorbitol	Glycerin	Total	
Acetaminophen					
Tylenol® children's drops	0	0	0.43	0.43	0
Tylenol® children's elixir	1.6	1	0.43	3.03	0
Tylenol® children's suspension	3.7*	1	0.43	5.13	0
Tylenol® maximum strength liquid	5.49*	1	0	6.49	0
Acetaminophen/codeine					
Tylenol® elixir with codeine	3	0	0	3.0	0.35
Acyclovir					
Zovirax® suspension	0	0.3	0	0.3	0
Albuterol					
Ventolin® syrup	0	0	0	0	0
Proventil® syrup	0	0	0	0	0
AlOH/MgOH					
Maalox® Extra Strength Plus	0	0.5	0	0.5	0
Maalox® suspension	0	0.225	0	0.225	0
AlOH/MgOH/simethicone					
Mylanta® cherry cream liquid	0	0.6	0	0.6	0
Mylanta® double strength liquid	0	0.8	0	0.8	0
Mylanta® liquid	0	0.8	0	0.8	0
Mylanta® mint cream liquid	0	0.6	0	0.6	0
AlOH					
Alternagel®	0	0.6	0	0.6	0
Gaviscon® liquid	5.55§	0.36	0.51	6.42	0
AlOH gel (Roxane)					
Conc aluminum hydroxide gel	0	0.52	0	0.52	0
Alprazolam					
Alprazolam intensol®	0	0	0	0	0
Aminocaproic acid					
Amicar® syrup	0	0.7	0	0.7	0
Amoxicillin					
Amoxicillin 125 suspension (Biocraft)	2	0	0	2	0
Amoxicillin 250 suspension (Biocraft)	3	0	0	3	0
Trimox® suspension	3.3	0	0	3.3	0
Amoxicillin 125 suspension (Lederle)	2.08	0	0	2.08	0
Amoxicillin 250 suspension (Lederle)	1.923	0	0	1.923	
Amoxicillin/clavulanate					
Augmentin® 125 suspension	0	0	0	0	0
Augmentin® 250 suspension	0	0	0	0	0
Ampicillin					
Ampicillin 125 suspension (Lederle)	4.021	0	0	4.021	0
Ampicillin 250 suspension (Lederle)	4.024	0	0	4.024	0
Ampicillin 125 suspension (Biocraft)	2.6	0	0	2.6	0
Ampicillin 250 suspension (Biocraft)	2.6	0	0	2.6	0
Azithromycin					
Zithromax® 100 suspension	3.86	0	0	3.86	0
Zithromax® 200 suspension	3.87	0	0	3.87	0
Calcium carbonate (Roxane)					
CaCO$_3$ oral suspension	0	1.4	0	1.4	0
Calcium glubionate					
Neo-Calglucon®	0	0.45	0	0.45	0
Carbamazepine					
Tegretol® suspension	2	0.6	0	2.6	0

CARBOHYDRATE AND ALCOHOL CONTENT OF LIQUID MEDICATIONS FOR USE IN PATIENTS RECEIVING KETOGENIC DIETS *(Continued)*

Generic Name	Carbohydrate g/5 mL				Ethyl Alcohol g/5 mL
	Sucrose	Sorbitol	Glycerin	Total	
Cefaclor					
Ceclor® suspension	3	0	0	3	0
Cefadroxil					
Duricef® 125 suspension	2.55	0	0	2.55	0
Duricef® 250 suspension	2.43	0	0	2.43	0
Cefpodoxime					
Vantin® 50 suspension	2.94	0	0	2.94	0
Vantin® 100 suspension	2.94	0	0	2.94	0
Cefprozil					
Cefzil® suspension	2.03	0	0	2.03	0
Cefuroxime					
Ceftin® 125 suspension	3.214	0	0	3.214	0
Cephalexin					
Cephalexin 125 suspension (Lederle)	1.4	0	0	1.4	0
Cephalexin 250 suspension (Lederle)	1.2	0	0	1.2	0
Cephalexin 125 suspension (Biocraft)	2.6	0	0	2.6	0
Keflex® oral suspension	3	0	0	3	0
Cephradine					
Velosef® suspension	3.3	0	0	3.3	0
Chloral hydrate					
Chloral hydrate syrup (Geneva)	0	0	0.2	0.2	0
Chloral hydrate syrup (UDL Labs)	2.5	1.4	0	3.9	0
Chlorothiazide					
Diuril® oral suspension	2	0	0	2.0	0.025
Chlorpromazine					
Thorazine® concentrate	4.22	0	0	4.22	0
Cimetidine					
Tagamet® liquid	0	2.8	0	2.8	0.5
Cisapride					
Propulsid® suspension	0	3.85	0	3.85	0
Clarithromycin					
Biaxin® 125 suspension	3	0	0	3	0
Biaxin® 250 suspension	2.28	0	0	2.28	0
Clemastine					
Tavist® syrup	0	2.5	0	2.5	0
Clindamycin					
Cleocin® pediatric oral solution	1.825	0	0	1.825	0
Cloxacillin (Biocraft)					
Cloxacillin 250 suspension	2.4	0	0	2.4	0
Cyclosporine					
Sandimmune® oral solution	0	0	0	0	0.6
Dexamethasone (Roxane)					
Dexamethasone oral solution	0	1.2	0.5	1.7	0
Dexamethasone Intensol®	0	0	0	0	1.5
Diazepam					
Diazepam Intensol®	0	0	0	0	0.95
Diazepam solution	0	1	0	1	0
Dicyclomine					
Bentyl® liquid	0	0	0	4	0
Digoxin					
Lanoxin® elixir	1.5	0	0	1.5	0.5
Digoxin elixir (Roxane)	0	1	1	2.0	0.5
Diphenhydramine					
Benadryl® elixir cherry	0	0	0.3	0.3	0
Benadryl® elixir diet	0	2.25	0.6	2.85	0

Generic Name	Carbohydrate g/5 mL				Ethyl Alcohol g/5 mL
	Sucrose	Sorbitol	Glycerin	Total	
EES					
EES	3.5	0	0	3.5	0
EES/Sulfisoxazole					
EES/Sulfisoxazole (Lederle)	2	0	0	2	0
Pediazole®	1.95	0	0	1.95	0
Ethosuximide					
Zarontin® syrup	3	0	0.625	3.625	0
Famotidine					
Pepcid® oral suspension	1.186	0	0	1.186	0
Felbamate					
Felbatol® suspension	0	1.5	0	1.5	0
Ferrous gluconate					
Fergon®	2	0	0	2.0	0.436
Ferrous sulfate					
Fer-in-Sol® drops	1.9	1.55	0	3.45	0
Fer-in-Sol® syrup	3	0.325	0	3.325	0
Fer-Gen-Sol®	2	0	0	2.0	0.436
Fluconazole					
Diflucan® 50 suspension	2.88	0	0	2.88	0
Diflucan® 200 suspension	2.73	0	0	2.73	0
Fluoxetine					
Furazolidone					
Furoxone® oral solution	0	0	0.1893	0.1893	0
Furosemide					
Lasix® oral solution	1.75	0	0	1.75	0.25
Furosemide solution (10 mg/5 mL)	0	2.4	0	2.4	0
Furosemide solution (40 mg/5 mL)	0	2.4	0	2.4	0
Griseofulvin					
Grifulvin V® oral suspension	3.5	0	0	3.5	0
Haloperidol					
Haldol® concentrate	3.9¶	0	0	3.9	0
Haldoperidol Intensol®	0	0	0	0	0
Hydrochlorothiazide					
Hydrochlorothiazide solution	0	0	2	2	0
Hydrocortisone cypionate					
Cortef® oral suspension	0.4	0	0	0.4	0
Hydroxyzine					
Vistaril® suspension	0	5	0	5	0
Ibuprofen					
Pedia-Profen® suspension	0	1.55	0	1.55	0
Kaolin/pectin (Roxane)					
Kaolin Pectin suspension	0	0	0.1	0.1	0
Kaopectin					
Kaopectate® concentrated antidiarrheal regular	0.6	0	0	0.6	0
L-carnitine					
Carnitor® oral solution	0.2385	0	0	0.2385	0
Lactulose					
Cephulac® syrup	4.67¶	0	0	4.67	0
Chronulac® syrup	4.67¶	0	0	4.67	0
Lithium citrate					
Lithium citrate USP	0	2.7	0	2.7	0
Loperamide					
Imodium A-D®	3.7¶	0	0.43	4.13	0.26
Loperamide oral solution	0	0	3	3	0
Loracarbef					
Lorabid®	3	0	0	3	0
Lorazepam					
Lorazepam Intensol®	0	0	0	0	0
Metaproterenol (Biocraft)					
Metaproterenol syrup	0	1.7	0	1.7	0

CARBOHYDRATE AND ALCOHOL CONTENT OF LIQUID MEDICATIONS FOR USE IN PATIENTS RECEIVING KETOGENIC DIETS *(Continued)*

Generic Name	Carbohydrate g/5 mL				Ethyl Alcohol g/5 mL
	Sucrose	Sorbitol	Glycerin	Total	
Metaproterenol sulfate					
Alupent® syrup	0	1.4	0	1.4	0
Metaprel® syrup	0	1.4	0	1.4	0
Metoclopramide					
Metoclopramide syrup (Biocraft)	0	2.1	0	2.1	0
Metoclopramide Intensol®	0	1.4	0.5	1.9	0
Metoclopramide oral solution (Roxane)	0	1.4	0.5	1.9	0
Milk of Magnesia					
Concentrated Milk of Magnesia	0.4	1	0.2	1.6	0
Multivitamins					
Iberet® 250 liquid	0	3.61	0	3.61	0
Iberet® 500 liquid	0.62	2.1	0	2.72	0
Theragran® liquid	1.75	0	0	1.75	0
Poly-Vi-Sol® drops	0	0	4.25	4.25	0
Vi-Daylin® liquid	0.778	0	0.025	6.053	0
Vi-Daylin® multivitamin drops	0	0	4.8	4.8	0
Multivitamins with fluoride drops					
Poly-Vi-Flor® drops	0	0	4.25	4.25	0
Multivitamins with fluoride drops					
Tri-Vi-Flor® drops	0	0	4.25	4.25	0
Multivitamins with iron					
Poly-Vi-Flor® With Iron drops	0	0	3.9	3.9	0
Multivitamins with iron					
Tri-Vi-Flor® With Iron drops	0	0	3.9	3.9	0
Multivitamins with minerals					
Advanced Formula Centrum® liquid	1.67	0	0	1.67	0.335
Multivitamins/fluoride					
Vi-Daylin®/f	0	0	4.8	4.8	0
Naproxen					
Naprosyn® oral suspension	1.275	0.45	0	1.725	0
Nitrofurantoin					
Furadantin® suspension	0	0.7	0.7	1.4	0
Nystatin					
Nystatin oral suspension (Biocraft)	2.5	0	0.75	3.25	0.05
Nilstat® oral suspension	3	0	0	3	0
Oxybutynin					
Ditropan® syrup	4#	1.3	1.74	7.04	0
Paregoric					
Paregoric	0	0	0.25	0.25	2.25
PE/Triprolidine					
Children's Actifed® liquid	2.6	2.5	0	5.1	0
PE/PPA/chlorpheniramine/phenyltoloxamine					
Naldecon Ped® drops	0	1.14	0	1.14	0
Naldecon Ped® syrup	0	2	0	2	0
Naldecon syrup	0	2	0	2	0
Penicillin VK					
VeeTids®	3.5	0	0	3.5	0
Penicillin V Potassium (Biocraft)					
Penicillin VK 125® suspension	2.4	0	0	2.4	0
Phenobarbital (Lilly)					
Phenobarbital elixir	0.65	0	2.8	3.45	0.7125
Phenytoin					
Dilantin® suspension 125	1	0	0.385	1.385	0

Generic Name	Carbohydrate g/5 mL				Ethyl Alcohol g/5 mL
	Sucrose	Sorbitol	Glycerin	Total	
Potassium chloride					
Rum-K®	0	0.54	1.72	2.26	0
Kay Ciel® liquid	0	0	0	0	0.14
Potassium chloride oral solution 10% (Roxane)	0	0	0.25	0.25	0.25
Potassium chloride oral solution 20%	0	0	0.25	0.25	0.25
Kaochlor S-F®	0	0	0	0	0.25
Kaon® elixir (potassium gluconate)	0	0	0	0	0.25
Kaon-Cl® 20%	0	0	0	0	0.25
Klor-Con® powder	0	0	0	0	0
Klor-Con/25® powder	0	0	0	0	0
Potassium citrate					
Polycitra-K®	0	0	0	0	0
Potassium citrate/sodium citrate					
Polycitra®	0	0	0	0	0
Potassium iodide					
SSKI®	0	0	0	0	0
Prednisolone					
Pediapred®	0	1.53	0	1.53	0
Prelone® syrup	1.84	0	0	1.84	0.18
Prednisone					
Prednisone Intensol®	0	0	0	1.5	1.5
Prednisone solution (Roxane)	1.8•	0	0	1.8	0.25
Primadone					
Mysoline® suspension	0	0	0	0	0
Prochlorperazine					
Compazine® syrup	3.15	0	0	3.15	0
Propranolol (Roxane)					
Propranolol oral solution (20 mg/5 mL)	0	3.2	0	3.2	0
Propranolol oral solution (40 mg/5 mL)	0	3.2	0	3.2	0
Ranitidine					
Zantac® syrup	0	0.5	0	0.5	0.375
Senokot					
Senokot® syrup	3.3	0		3.3	0.35
Simethicone					
Mylicon® drops	0	0	0	0	0
Phazyme® liquid	0	0	0	0	0
Sodium citrate/citric acid					
Bicitra®	0	0	0	0	0
Sodium polystyrene sulfonate (Roxane)					
Sodium polystyrene sulfonate suspension	0	1.2	0	1.2	0.1
Sucralfate					
Carafate® suspension	0	0.7	0.77	1.47	0
Sulfisoxazole					
Gantrisin® pediatric suspension	2.77	0	0	2.77	0.14
Tetracycline					
Sumycin®	2.2	1.5	0	3.7	0
Theophylline					
Theolair® liquid	2.5	0.48	0	2.98	0
Theoclear-80® syrup	0	4	3.5	7.5	0
Elixophylline® elixir	0	0	0.312	0.312	0.86
Elixophylline GG® elixir	0	2.3	1.625	3.925	0
Slo-Phyllin® 80 syrup	0	2.87	0	2.87	0
Slo-Phyllin GG® syrup	0.93	0.6	0.83	2.36	0
Aminophylline oral solution (105 mg/5 mL)	0	0.7	1	1.7	0
Theophylline oral solution (Roxane)	0	2.3	0.5	2.8	0.4
Trimethoprim/Sulfamethoxazole					
Sulfamethoxazole/trimethoprim (Biocraft)	0	0.35	0.7	1.05	0
Septra® suspension	0	2.25	0	2.25	0
Bactrim® pediatric suspension	2.5	0.35	0.75	3.6	0

CARBOHYDRATE AND ALCOHOL CONTENT OF LIQUID MEDICATIONS FOR USE IN PATIENTS RECEIVING KETOGENIC DIETS *(Continued)*

Generic Name	Carbohydrate g/5 mL				Ethyl Alcohol g/5 mL
	Sucrose	Sorbitol	Glycerin	Total	
Valproic acid					
Depakene® syrup	3	0.75	0.75	4.5	0
Vancomycin					
Vancocin® oral solution	0	0	0	0	0
Vitamin A					
Aquasol A® drops	0	0	0	0	0
Vitamin D					
Drisdol®	0	0	0	0	0
Vitamin E					
Aquasol E® drops	0	1	0	1	0
Zidovudine					
Retrovir® syrup	3	0	0	3	0

Generic name abbreviations: DM: dextromethorphan; APAP: acetaminophen; PE: phenylephrine; Pyril: pyrilamine; PPA: phenylpropanolamine; EES: erythromycin ethylsuccinate

*Corn syrup

§Lactulose

•Fructose

¶Lactulose, galactose, lactose, and other sugars

#Glucose

Reference
Adapted from Feldstein TJ, "Carbohydrate and Alcohol Content of 200 Oral Liquid Medications for Use in Patients Receiving Ketogenic Diets," *Pediatrics*, 1996, 97:506-11.

ORAL MEDICATIONS THAT SHOULD NOT BE CRUSHED OR ALTERED

There are a variety of reasons for crushing tablets or capsule contents prior to administering to the patient. Patients may have nasogastric tubes which do not permit the administration of tablets or capsules; an oral solution for a particular medication may not be available from the manufacturer or readily prepared by pharmacy; patients may have difficulty swallowing capsules or tablets; or mixing of powdered medication with food or drink may make the drug more palatable.

Generally, medications which should not be crushed fall into one of the following categories.

- **Extended-Release Products**. The formulation of some tablets is specialized as to allow the medication within it to be slowly released into the body. This is sometimes accomplished by centering the drug within the core of the tablet, with a subsequent shedding of multiple layers around the core. Wax melts in the GI tract. Slow-K® is an example of this. Capsules may contain beads which have multiple layers which are slowly dissolved with time.

    Common Abbreviations for Extended-Release Products

CR	Controlled release
CRT	Controlled-release tablet
LA	Long-acting
SR	Sustained release
TR	Timed release
TD	Time delay
SA	Sustained action
XL	Extended length
XR	Extended release

- **Medications Which Are Irritating to the Stomach**. Tablets which are irritating to the stomach may be enteric-coated which delays release of the drug until the time when it reaches the small intestine. Enteric-coated aspirin is an example of this.

- **Foul-Tasting Medication**. Some drugs are quite unpleasant to taste so the manufacturer coats the tablet in a sugar coating to increase its palatability. By crushing the tablet, this sugar coating is lost and the patient tastes the unpleasant tasting medication.

- **Sublingual Medication**. Medication intended for use under the tongue should not be crushed. While it appears to be obvious, it is not always easy to determine if a medication is to be used sublingually. Sublingual medications should indicate on the package that they are intended for sublingual use.

- **Effervescent Tablets**. These are tablets which, when dropped into a liquid, quickly dissolve to yield a solution. Many effervescent tablets, when crushed, lose their ability to quickly dissolve.

Recommendations

1. It is not advisable to crush certain medications.

2. Consult individual monographs prior to crushing capsule or tablet.

3. If crushing a tablet or capsule is contraindicated, consult with your pharmacist to determine whether an oral solution exists or can be compounded.

ORAL MEDICATIONS THAT SHOULD
NOT BE CRUSHED OR ALTERED (Continued)

Drug Product	Dosage Form	Dosage Reasons/Comments
Accutane®	Capsule	Mucous membrane irritant
Aciphex™	Tablet	Slow release
Actifed 12® Hour	Capsule	Slow release[1]
Acutrim® (various)	Tablet	Slow release
Adalat® CC	Tablet	Slow release
Aerolate® SR, JR, III	Capsule	Slow release[1,2]
Allegra-D®	Tablet	Slow release
Allerest® 12-Hour	Capsule	Slow release
Artane® Sequels®	Capsule	Slow release[1,2]
Arthritis Bayer® Time Release	Capsule	Slow release
Arthrotec®	Tablet	Enteric-coated
A.S.A.® Enseals®	Tablet	Enteric-coated
Asacol®	Tablet	Slow release
Ascriptin® A/D	Tablet	Enteric-coated
Ascriptin® Extra Strength	Tablet	Enteric-coated
Atrohist® LA	Tablet	Slow release[1]
Atrohist® Plus	Tablet	Slow release[1]
Atrohist® Pediatric	Capsule	Slow release[1,2]
Azulfidine® EN-tabs®	Tablet	Enteric-coated
Baros	Tablet	Effervescent tablet[3]
Bayer® Aspirin EC	Caplet	Enteric-coated
Bayer® Aspirin, Low Adult 81 mg	Caplet	Enteric-coated
Bayer® Aspirin, Regular Strength 325 mg	Caplet	Enteric-coated
Betapen®-VK	Tablet	Taste[4]
Biaxin® XL	Tablet	Slow release
Bisacodyl	Tablet	Enteric-coated[5]
Bontril® Slow-Release	Capsule	Slow release
Breonesin®	Capsule	Slow release[1]
Brexin® L.A.	Capsule	Slow release
Calan® SR	Tablet	Slow release[6]
Cama® Arthritis Pain Reliever	Tablet	Multiple compressed tablet
Carbatrol®	Capsule	Slow release[2]
Carbiset-TR®	Tablet	Slow release
Cardene® SR	Capsule	Slow release
Cardizem®	Tablet	Slow release
Cardizem® CD	Capsule	Slow release[2]
Cardizem® SR	Capsule	Slow release[2]
Carter's Little Pills®	Tablet	Enteric-coated
Cartia® XT	Capsule	Slow release
Ceclor® CD	Tablet	Slow release
Ceftin®	Tablet	Taste[1] **Note:** Use suspension for children
CellCept®	Capsule, tablet	Teratogenic potential[7]
Charcoal Plus®	Tablet	Enteric-coated
Chloral Hydrate	Capsule	**Note:** Product is in liquid form within a special capsule[1]
Chlor-Trimeton® 12-Hour	Tablet	Slow release[1]
Choledyl® SA	Tablet	Slow release[1]
Cipro™	Tablet	Taste[4]
Claritin-D®	Tablet	Slow release
Claritin-D® 24-Hour	Tablet	Slow release
Codimal-L.A.®	Capsule	Slow release
Codimal-L.A.® Half	Capsule	Slow release
Colace®	Capsule	Taste[4]
Colestid®	Tablet	Slow release
Comhist® LA	Capsule	Slow release[2]
Compazine® Spansule®	Capsule	Slow release[1]
Congess SR, JR	Capsule	Slow release
Contac® 12-Hour	Capsule	Slow release[1,2]

Drug Product	Dosage Form	Dosage Reasons/Comments
Contac® Maximum Strength	Capsule	Slow release[1,2]
Cotazym-S®	Capsule	Enteric-coated[2]
Covera-HS™	Tablet	Slow release
Creon® 10, 20, 25	Capsule	Enteric-coated[2]
Cystospaz-M®	Capsule	Slow release
Cytovene®	Capsule	Skin irritant
Cytoxan®	Tablet	**Note:** Drug may be crushed, but maker recommends using injection
D.A.II™	Tablet	Slow release[6]
Dallergy®	Capsule	Slow release
Dallergy-D®	Capsule	Slow release
Dallergy-JR®	Capsule	Slow release
Deconamine® SR	Capsule	Slow release[1]
Defen L.A.®	Tablet	Slow release[6]
Demazin® Repetabs®	Tablet	Slow release[1]
Depakene®	Capsule	Slow-release-mucous membrane irritant[1]
Depakote®	Capsule	Enteric-coated
Desoxyn® Gradumets®	Tablet	Slow release
Desyrel®	Tablet	Taste[4]
Dexatrim®, Extended Duration	Tablet	Slow release
Dexedrine® Spansule®	Capsule	Slow release
Diamox® Sequels®	Capsule	Slow release
Dilacor® XR	Capsule	Slow release
Dilatrate-SR®	Capsule	Slow release
Dimetane® Extentab®	Tablet	Slow release[1]
Disobrom®	Tablet	Slow release
Disophrol® Chronotab®	Tablet	Slow release
Dital®	Capsule	Slow release
Ditropan® XL	Tablet	Slow release
Dolobid®	Tablet	Irritant
Donnatal® Extentab®	Tablet	Slow release[1]
Donnazyme®	Tablet	Enteric-coated
Drisdol®	Capsule	Liquid filled[8]
Drixoral®	Tablet	Slow release[1]
Drixoral® Plus	Tablet	Slow release
Drixoral®, various	Tablet	Slow release
Dulcolax®	Tablet	Enteric-coated[5]
Duratuss® GP	Tablet	Slow release[6]
Dura-Vent®/A	Tablet	Slow release[6]
Dura-Vent®/DA	Tablet	Slow release[6]
Dynabac®	Tablet	Enteric-coated
DynaCirc® CR	Tablet	Slow release
Easprin®	Tablet	Enteric-coated
EC-Naprosyn®	Tablet	Enteric-coated
Ecotrin® Adult Low Strength	Tablet	Enteric-coated
Ecotrin® Maximum Strength	Tablet	Enteric-coated
Ecotrin® Regular Strength	Tablet	Enteric-coated
E.E.S.® 400	Tablet	Enteric-coated[1]
Effexor® XR	Capsule	Slow release
Efidac/24®	Tablet	Slow release
Efidac® 24 Chlorpheniramine	Tablet	Slow release
E-Mycin®	Tablet	Enteric-coated
Endafed®	Capsule	Slow release
Entex® LA	Tablet	Slow release[1]
Entex® PSE	Tablet	Slow release
Equanil®	Tablet	Taste[4]
Ergomar®	Tablet	Sublingual form[9]
Eryc®	Capsule	Enteric-coated[2]
Ery-Tab®	Tablet	Enteric-coated
Erythrocin Stearate	Tablet	Enteric-coated
Erythromycin Base	Tablet	Enteric-coated
Eskalith CR®	Tablet	Slow release

ORAL MEDICATIONS THAT SHOULD
NOT BE CRUSHED OR ALTERED *(Continued)*

Drug Product	Dosage Form	Dosage Reasons/Comments
Exgest® LA	Tablet	Slow release
Extendryl JR	Capsule	Slow release
Extendryl SR	Capsule	Slow release[1]
Fe 50	Tablet	Slow release
Fedahist® Gyrocaps®	Capsule	Slow release[1]
Fedahist® Timecaps®	Capsule	Slow release[1]
Feldene®	Capsule	Mucous membrane irritant
Feocyte	Tablet	Slow release
Feosol®	Tablet	Enteric-coated[1]
Feosol®	Capsule	Slow release[1,2]
Feratab®	Tablet	Enteric-coated[1]
Fergon®	Capsule	Slow release[2]
Fero-Grad 500®	Tablet	Slow release
Ferro-Sequels®	Tablet	Slow release
FeverAll® Sprinkle	Capsule	Taste[2] **Note:** Capsule contents intended to be placed in a teaspoonful of water or soft food.
Flomax®	Capsule	Slow release
Fumatinic®	Capsule	Slow release
Gastrocrom®	Capsule	**Note:** Contents may be dissolved in water for administration.
Geocillin®	Tablet	Taste
Glucotrol® XL	Tablet	Slow release
Gris-PEG®	Tablet	**Note:** Crushing may result in precipitation of larger particles.
Guaifed®	Capsule	Slow release
Guaifed®-PD	Capsule	Slow release
Guaifenex® LA	Tablet	Slow release[6]
Guaifenex® PPA	Tablet	Slow release
Guaifenex® PSE	Tablet	Slow release[6]
GuaiMAX-D®	Tablet	Slow release
Humibid® DM	Tablet	Slow release
Humibid® DM Sprinkle	Capsule	Slow release[2]
Humibid® LA	Tablet	Slow release
Humibid® Sprinkle	Capsule	Slow release[2]
Hydergine® LC	Capsule	**Note:** Product is in liquid form within a special capsule[1]
Iberet®	Tablet	Slow release[1]
Iberet-500®	Tablet	Slow release[1]
ICAPS® Plus	Tablet	Slow release
ICAPS® Time Release	Tablet	Slow release
Ilotycin®	Tablet	Enteric-coated
Imdur™	Tablet	Slow release[6]
Inderal® LA	Capsule	Slow release
Inderide® LA	Capsule	Slow release
Indocin® SR	Capsule	Slow release[1,2]
Ionamin®	Capsule	Slow release
Isoptin® SR	Tablet	Slow release
Isordil® Sublingual	Tablet	Sublingual form[9]
Isordil® Tembid®	Tablet	Slow release
Isosorbide Dinitrate Sublingual	Tablet	Sublingual form[9]
Isosorbide SR	Tablet	Slow release
K+ 8®	Tablet	Slow release[1]
K+ 10®	Tablet	Slow release[1]
Kadian®	Capsule	Slow release[2]
Kaon-Cl®	Tablet	Slow release[1]
K-Dur®	Tablet	Slow release
K-Lease®	Capsule	Slow release[1,2]
Klor-Con®	Tablet	Slow release[1]
Klotrix®	Tablet	Slow release[1]

Drug Product	Dosage Form	Dosage Reasons/Comments
K-Lyte®	Tablet	Effervescent tablet[3]
K-Lyte/Cl®	Tablet	Effervescent tablet[3]
K-Lyte DS®	Tablet	Effervescent tablet[3]
K-Norm®	Capsule	Slow release
K-Tab®	Tablet	Slow release[1]
Levbid®	Tablet	Slow release[6]
Levsinex® Timecaps®	Capsule	Slow release
Lexxel®	Tablet	Slow release
Lithobid®	Tablet	Slow release
Lodine® XL	Tablet	Slow release
Lodrane LD®	Capsule	Slow release[2]
Mag-Tab® SR	Tablet	Slow release
Mestinon® Timespan®	Tablet	Slow release[1]
Mi-Cebrin®	Tablet	Enteric-coated
Mi-Cebrin® T	Tablet	Enteric-coated
Micro-K®	Capsule	Slow release[1,2]
Monafed®	Tablet	Slow release
Monafed® DM	Tablet	Slow release
Motrin®	Tablet	Taste[4]
MS Contin®	Tablet	Slow release[1]
Muco-Fen-DM®	Tablet	Slow release[6]
Muco-Fen-LA®	Tablet	Slow release[6]
Naldecon®	Tablet	Slow release[1]
Naprelan®	Tablet	Slow release
Nasatab LA®	Tablet	Slow release[6]
Nexium™	Capsule	Slow release[2]
Nicotinic Acid	Capsule, tablet	Slow release
Nitroglyn®	Capsule	Slow release[2]
Nitrong®	Tablet	Sublingual route[9]
Nitrostat®	Tablet	Sublingual route[9]
Nitro-Time®	Capsule	Slow release
Nolamine®	Tablet	Slow release
Nolex® LA	Tablet	Slow release
Norflex®	Tablet	Slow release
Norpace CR®	Capsule	Slow release form within a special capsule
Ondrox®	Tablet	Slow release
Optilets-500® Filmtab®	Tablet	Enteric-coated
Optilets-M-500® Filmtab®	Tablet	Enteric-coated
Oragrafin®	Capsule	**Note:** Product is in liquid form within a special capsule
Oramorph SR®	Tablet	Slow release[1]
Ornade® Spansule®	Capsule	Slow release
OxyContin®	Tablet	Slow release
Pancrease®	Capsule	Enteric-coated[2]
Pancrease® MT	Capsule	Enteric-coated[2]
PanMist® Jr, LA	Tablet	Slow release[6]
Panmycin®	Capsule	Taste
Pannaz®	Tablet	Slow release[6]
Papaverine Sustained Action	Capsule	Slow release
Pathilon® Sequels®	Capsule	Slow release[2]
Pavabid® Plateau®	Capsule	Slow release[2]
PBZ-SR®	Tablet	Slow release[1]
Pentasa®	Capsule	Slow release
Perdiem® Fiber Therapy	Granules	Wax coated
Peritrate® SA	Tablet	Slow release[6]
Permitil® Chronotab®	Tablet	Slow release[1]
Phazyme®	Tablet	Slow release
Phazyme® 95, 125	Tablet	Slow release
Phenergan®	Tablet	Taste[5]
Phyllocontin®	Tablet	Slow release
Plendil®	Tablet	Slow release
Pneumomist®	Tablet	Slow release[6]

ORAL MEDICATIONS THAT SHOULD
NOT BE CRUSHED OR ALTERED (Continued)

Drug Product	Dosage Form	Dosage Reasons/Comments
Polaramine® Repetabs®	Tablet	Slow release[1]
Prelu-2®	Capsule	Slow release
Prevacid®	Capsule	Slow release
Prilosec®	Capsule	Slow release
Pro-Banthine®	Tablet	Taste
Procainamide HCl SR	Tablet	Slow release
Procanbid®	Tablet	Slow release
Procardia®	Capsule	Delays absorption[1,4]
Procardia XL®	Tablet	Slow release **Note:** AUC is unaffected.
Profen® II	Tablet	Slow release[6]
Profen LA®	Tablet	Slow release[6]
Pronestyl-SR®	Tablet	Slow release
Propecia®	Tablet	**Note:** Women who are, or may become, pregnant, should not handle crushed or broken tablets
Proscar®	Tablet	**Note:** Women who are, or may become, pregnant, should not handle crushed or broken tablets
Protonix®	Tablet	Slow release
Proventil® Repetabs®	Tablet	Slow release[1]
Prozac®	Capsule	Slow release[2]
Quibron-T/SR®	Tablet	Slow release[1]
Quinaglute® Dura-Tabs®	Tablet	Slow release
Quinidex® Extentabs®	Tablet	Slow release
Quin-Release®	Tablet	Slow release
Respa-1st®	Tablet	Slow release[6]
Respa-DM®	Tablet	Slow release[6]
Respa-GF®	Tablet	Slow release[6]
Respahist®	Capsule	Slow release[2]
Respaire® SR	Capsule	Slow release
Respbid®	Tablet	Slow release
Ritalin-SR®	Tablet	Slow release
Robimycin®	Tablet	Enteric-coated
Rondec-TR®	Tablet	Slow release[1]
Ru-Tuss® DE	Tablet	Slow release
Sinemet CR®	Tablet	Slow release
Singlet for Adults®	Tablet	Slow release
Slo-bid™ Gyrocaps®	Capsule	Slow release[2]
Slo-Niacin®	Tablet	Slow release[6]
Slo-Phyllin GG®	Capsule	Slow release[1]
Slo-Phyllin® Gyrocaps®	Capsule	Slow release[1,2]
Slow FE®	Tablet	Slow release[1]
Slow FE® With Folic Acid	Tablet	Slow release
Slow-K®	Tablet	Slow release[1]
Slow-Mag®	Tablet	Slow release
Sorbitrate SA®	Tablet	Slow release
Sorbitrate® Sublingual	Tablet	Sublingual route
S-P-T	Capsule	**Note:** Liquid gelatin thyroid suspension.
Sudafed® 12-Hour	Capsule	Slow release[1]
Sudal® 60/500	Tablet	Slow release
Sudal® 120/600	Tablet	Slow release
Sudex®	Tablet	Slow release[6]
Sular®	Tablet	Slow release
Sustaire®	Tablet	Slow release[1]
Syn-RX	Tablet	Slow release
Syn-RX DM	Tablet	Slow release
Tavist-D®	Tablet	Multiple compressed tablet
Teczam®	Tablet	Slow release
Tedral® SA	Tablet	Slow release[1]

Drug Product	Dosage Form	Dosage Reasons/Comments
Tegretol®-XR	Tablet	Slow release
Teldrin® Maximum Strength	Capsule	Slow release[2]
Tepanil® Ten-Tab®	Tablet	Slow release
Tessalon® Perles	Capsule	Slow release
Theo-24®	Tablet	Slow release[1]
Theochron®	Tablet	Slow release
Theoclear® L.A	Capsule	Slow release[1]
Theo-Dur®	Tablet	Slow release[1]
Theo-Dur® Sprinkle	Capsule	Slow release[1,2]
Theolair SR®	Tablet	Slow release[1]
Theo-Sav®	Tablet	Slow release[6]
Theo-Time® SR	Tablet	Slow release
Theovent®	Capsule	Slow release[1]
Theo-X®	Tablet	Slow release
Thorazine® Spansule®	Capsule	Slow release
Tiamate®	Tablet	Slow release
Tiazac®	Capsule	Slow release
Toprol XL®	Tablet	Slow release[6]
Touro A&D™	Capsule	Slow release
Touro EX™	Tablet	Slow release
Touro LA™	Tablet	Slow release
T-Phyl®	Tablet	Slow release
Trental®	Tablet	Slow release
Triaminic®	Tablet	Enteric-coated[1]
Triaminic®-12	Tablet	Slow release[1]
Triaminic® TR	Tablet	Multiple compressed tablet[1]
Tri-Phen-Chlor® Time Release	Tablet	Slow release
Tri-Phen-Mine® SR	Tablet	Slow release
Triptone®	Tablet	Slow release
Tuss-LA®	Tablet	Slow release
Tuss-Ornade® Spansule®	Capsule	Slow release
Tylenol® Extended Relief	Capsule	Slow release
ULR-LA®	Tablet	Slow release
Ultrase®	Capsule	Enteric-coated[2]
Ultrase® MT	Capsule	Enteric-coated[2]
Uni-Dur®	Tablet	Slow release
Uniphyl®	Tablet	Slow release
Urocit®-K	Tablet	Wax-coated
Verelan®	Capsule	Slow release[2]
Volmax®	Tablet	Slow release
Wellbutrin® SR	Tablet	Anesthetize mucous membrane
Wygesic®	Tablet	Taste
ZORprin®	Tablet	Slow release
Zyban®	Tablet	Slow release
Zymase®	Capsule	Enteric-coated[2]

[1]Liquid dosage forms of the product are available; however, dose, frequency of administration, and manufacturers may differ from that of the solid dosage form.

[2]Capsule may be opened and the contents taken without crushing or chewing; soft food such as applesauce or pudding may facilitate administration; contents may generally be administered via nasogastric tube using an appropriate fluid, provided entire contents was washed down the tube.

[3]Effervescent tablets must be dissolved in the amount of diluent recommended by the manufacturer.

[4]The taste of this product in a liquid form would likely be unacceptable to the patient; administration via nasogastric tube should be acceptable.

[5]Antacids and/or milk may prematurely dissolve the coating of the tablet.

[6]Tablet is scored and may be broken in half without affecting release characteristics.

[7]Skin contact may enhance tumor production; avoid direct contact.

[8]Capsule may be opened and the liquid contents removed for administration.

[9]Tablets are made to disintegrate under the tongue.

Adapted from Mitchell JF, "Oral Dosage Forms That Should Not Be Crushed," *Hosp Pharm*, 2002, 37(2):213-4.

THERAPEUTIC CATEGORY & KEY WORD INDEX

NOTES

NOTES

NOTES

NOTES

NOTES

NOTES

NOTES

NOTES

NOTES

NOTES

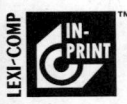

Other books offered by

LEXI-COMP

DRUG INFORMATION HANDBOOK (International edition available)
by Charles Lacy, RPh, PharmD, FCSHP; Lora L. Armstrong, RPh, PharmD, BCPS; Morton P. Goldman, PharmD, BCPS; and Leonard L. Lance, RPh, BSPharm

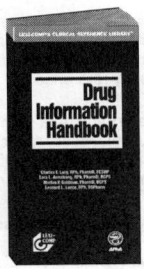

Specifically compiled and designed for the healthcare professional requiring quick access to concisely-stated comprehensive data concerning clinical use of medications.

The *Drug Information Handbook* is an ideal portable drug information resource, providing the reader with up to 29 key points of data concerning clinical use and dosing of the medication. Material provided in the Appendix section is recognized by many users to be, by itself, well worth the purchase of the handbook.

DRUG INFORMATION HANDBOOK P•O•C•K•E•T
by Charles Lacy, RPh, PharmD, FCSHP; Lora L. Armstrong, RPh, PharmD, BCPS; Morton P. Goldman, PharmD, BCPS; and Leonard L. Lance, RPh, BSPharm

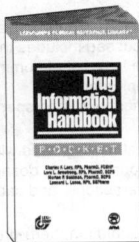

All medications found in the *Drug Information Handbook* are included in the abridged *Pocket* edition (select fields are extracted to maintain it's portability). It is specifically compiled and designed for the healthcare professional requiring quick access to concisely-stated comprehensive data concerning clinical use of medications.

The outstanding cross-referencing allows the user to quickly locate the brand name, generic name, synonym, and related information found in the Appendix making this a useful quick reference for medical professionals at any level of training or experience.

GERIATRIC DOSAGE HANDBOOK
by Todd P. Semla, PharmD, BCPS, FCCP; Judith L. Beizer, PharmD, FASCP; and Martin D. Higbee, PharmD, CGP

2000 "Book of the Year" — *American Journal of Nursing*

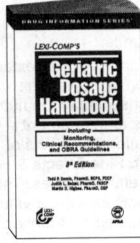

Many physiologic changes occur with aging, some of which affect the pharmacokinetics or pharmacodynamics of medications. Strong consideration should also be given to the effect of decreased renal or hepatic functions in the elderly, as well as the probability of the geriatric patient being on multiple drug regimens.

Healthcare professionals working with nursing homes and assisted living facilities will find the drug information contained in this handbook to be an invaluable source of helpful information.

An International Brand Name Index with names from 58 different countries is also included.

To order call toll free anywhere in the U.S.: 1-800-837-LEXI (5394)
Outside of the U.S. call: 330-650-6506 or online at www.lexi.com

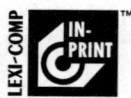

DRUG INFORMATION HANDBOOK FOR THE ALLIED HEALTH
PROFESSIONAL by Leonard L. Lance, RPh, BSPharm; Charles Lacy, RPh, PharmD, FCSHP; Lora L. Armstrong, RPh, PharmD, BCPS; and Morton P. Goldman, PharmD, BCPS

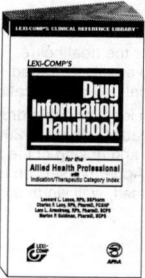

Working with clinical pharmacists, hospital pharmacy and therapeutics committees, and hospital drug information centers, the authors have assisted hundreds of hospitals in developing institution-specific formulary reference documentation.

The most current basic drug and medication data from those clinical settings have been reviewed, coalesced, and cross-referenced to create this unique handbook. The handbook offers quick access to abbreviated monographs for generic drugs.

This is a great tool for physician assistants, medical records personnel, medical transcriptionists and secretaries, pharmacy technicians, and other allied health professionals.

NATURAL THERAPEUTICS POCKET GUIDE
by Daniel L. Krinsky, RPh, MS; James B. LaValle, RPh, DHM, NMD, CCN; Ernest B. Hawkins, RPh, MS; Ross Pelton, RPh, PhD, CCN; Nancy Ashbrook Willis, BA, JD

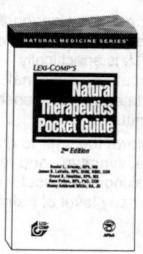

Provides condition-specific information on common uses of natural therapies. Each condition discussed includes the following: review of condition, decision tree, list of commonly recommended herbals, nutritional supplements, homeopathic remedies, lifestyle modifications, and special considerations.

Provides herbal/nutritional/nutraceutical monographs with over 10 fields including references, reported uses, dosage, pharmacology, toxicity, warnings & interactions, and cautions & contraindications.

The Appendix includes: drug-nutrient depletion, herb-drug interactions, drug-nutrient interaction, herbal medicine use in pediatrics, unsafe herbs, and reference of top herbals.

DRUG-INDUCED NUTRIENT DEPLETION HANDBOOK
by Ross Pelton, RPh, PhD, CCN; James B. LaValle, RPh, DHM, NMD, CCN; Ernest B. Hawkins, RPh, MS; Daniel L. Krinsky, RPh, MS

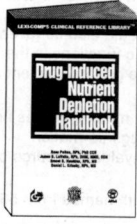

A complete and up-to-date listing of all drugs known to deplete the body of nutritional compounds.

This book is alphabetically organized and provides extensive cross-referencing to related information in the various sections of the book. Drug monographs identify the nutrients depleted and provide cross-references to the nutrient monographs for more detailed information on Effects of Depletion, Biological Function & Effect, Side Effects & Toxicity, RDA, Dosage Range, and Dietary Sources. This book also contains a Studies & Abstracts section, a valuable Appendix, and Alphabetical & Pharmacological Indexes.

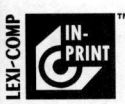

DRUG INFORMATION HANDBOOK FOR ADVANCED PRACTICE NURSING by Beatrice B. Turkoski, RN, PhD; Brenda R. Lance, RN, MSN; and Mark F. Bonfiglio, PharmD Foreword by: Margaret A. Fitzgerald, MS, RN, CS-FNP

1999 "Book of the Year" — *American Journal of Nursing*
Advanced Practice Nursing Category

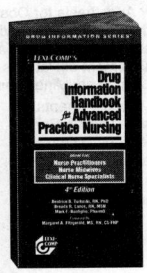

Designed specifically to meet the needs of nurse practitioners, clinical nurse specialists, nurse midwives, and graduate nursing students. The handbook is a unique resource for detailed, accurate information, which is vital to support the advanced practice nurse's role in patient drug therapy management. Over 4750 U.S., Canadian, and Mexican medications are covered in the 1000 monographs. Drug data is presented in an easy-to-use, alphabetically organized format covering up to 46 key points of information (including dosing for pediatrics, adults, and geriatrics). Cross-referenced to Appendix of over 230 pages of valuable comparison tables and additional information. Also included are two indexes, Pharmacologic Category and Controlled Substance, which facilitate comparison between agents.

DRUG INFORMATION HANDBOOK FOR NURSING
by Beatrice B. Turkoski, RN, PhD; Brenda R. Lance, RN, MSN; and Mark F. Bonfiglio, PharmD

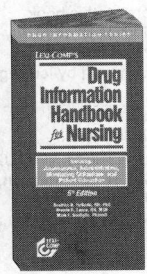

Registered Professional Nurses and upper-division nursing students involved with drug therapy will find this handbook provides quick access to drug data in a concise easy-to-use format.

Over 4000 U.S., Canadian, and Mexican medications are covered with up to 43 key points of information in each monograph. The handbook contains basic pharmacology concepts and nursing issues such as patient factors that influence drug therapy (ie, pregnancy, age, weight, etc) and general nursing issues (ie, assessment, administration, monitoring, and patient education). The Appendix contains over 230 pages of valuable information.

INFECTIOUS DISEASES HANDBOOK
by Carlos M. Isada, MD; Bernard L. Kasten Jr., MD; Morton P. Goldman, PharmD; Larry D. Gray, PhD; and Judith A. Aberg, MD

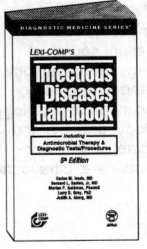

A four-in-one quick reference concerned with the identification and treatment of infectious diseases. Each of the four sections contain related information and cross-referencing to the other sections. The Disease Syndrome section provides the clinical presentation, differential diagnosis, diagnostic tests, and drug therapy recommended for treatment. The Organism section presents the microbiology, epidemiology, diagnosis, and treatment of each organism. The Laboratory Diagnosis section describes performance of specific tests and procedures. The Antimicrobial Therapy section presents important facts and considerations. Also contains an International Brand Name Index with names from 58 different countries.

To order call toll free anywhere in the U.S.: 1-800-837-LEXI (5394)
Outside of the U.S. call: 330-650-6506 or online at www.lexi.com

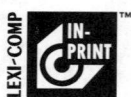

Other books offered by
LEXI-COMP

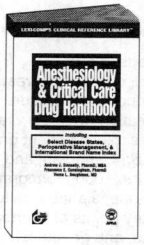
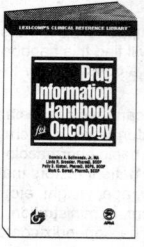
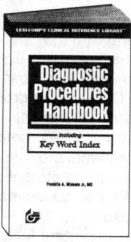

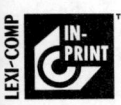

CLINICIAN'S GUIDE TO LABORATORY MEDICINE
—A Practical Approach by Samir P. Desai, MD and Sana Isa-Pratt, MD

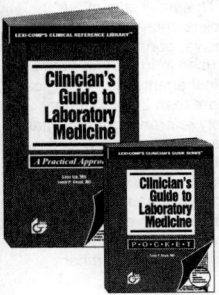

When faced with the patient presenting with abnormal laboratory tests, the clinician can now turn to the *Clinician's Guide to Laboratory Medicine: A Practical Approach*. This source is unique in its ability to lead the clinician from laboratory test abnormality to clinical diagnosis. Written for the busy clinician, this concise handbook will provide rapid answers to the questions that busy clinicians face in the care of their patients. No longer does the clinician have to struggle in an effort to find this information - *it's all here*.

Included is a **FREE** copy of *Clinician's Guide to Laboratory Medicine - Pocket*. Great to carry in your pocket! Perfect for use *"in the trenches"*.

CLINICIAN'S GUIDE TO INTERNAL MEDICINE
—A Practical Approach by Samir P. Desai, MD

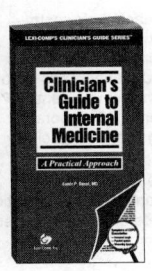

Provides quick access to essential information covering diagnosis, treatment, and management of commonly encountered patient problems in Internal Medicine.
- Up-to-date information in an easy-to-read format
- Clinically relevant information that is easily accessible
- Practical approaches that are not readily available in standard textbooks
- Algorithms to help you establish the diagnosis and select the appropriate therapy
- Numerous tables and boxes that summarize diagnostic and therapeutic strategies
- Ideal reference for use at the point-of-care

This is a reference companion that will provide you with the tools necessary to tackle even the most challenging problems in Internal Medicine.

CLINICIAN'S GUIDE TO DIAGNOSIS—A Practical Approach
by Samir Desai, MD

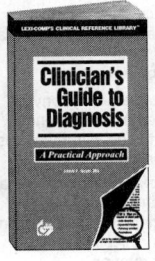

Symptoms are what prompt patients to seek medical care. In the evaluation of a patient's symptom, it is not unusual for healthcare professionals to ask "What do I do next?" This is precisely the question for which the *Clinician's Guide to Diagnosis: A Practical Approach* provides the answer. It will lead you from symptom to diagnosis through a series of steps designed to mimic the logical thought processes of seasoned clinicians. For the young clinician, this is an ideal book to help bridge the gap between the classroom and actual patient care. For the experienced clinician, this concise handbook offers rapid answers to the questions that are commonly encountered on a day-to-day basis. Let this guide become your companion, providing you with the tools necessary to tackle even the most challenging symptoms.

To order call toll free anywhere in the U.S.: 1-800-837-LEXI (5394)
Outside of the U.S. call: 330-650-6506 or online at www.lexi.com

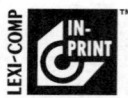
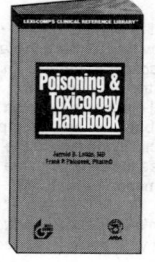
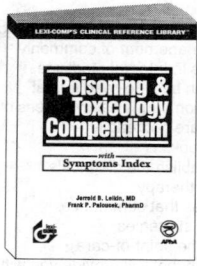
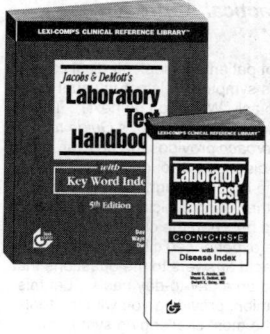

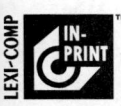
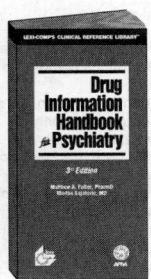
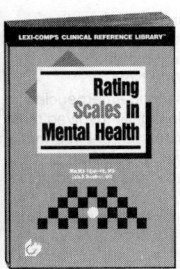
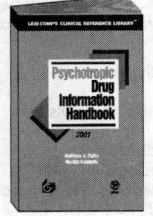

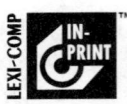

Other books offered by

LEXI-COMP

DRUG INFORMATION HANDBOOK FOR DENTISTRY
by Richard L. Wynn, BSPharm, PhD; Timothy F. Meiller, DDS, PhD; and
Harold L. Crossley, DDS, PhD

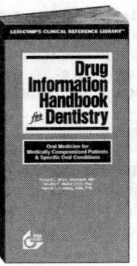

For all dental professionals requiring quick access to concisely-stated drug information pertaining to medications commonly prescribed by dentists and physicians.

Designed and written by dentists for all dental professionals as a portable, chair-side resource. Includes drugs commonly prescribed by dentists or being taken by dental patients and written in an easy-to-understand format. There are 24 key points of information for each drug including **Local Anesthetic/Vasoconstrictor, Precautions, Effects on Dental Treatment, and Drug Interactions.** Includes information on dental treatment for medically compromised patients and dental management of specific oral conditions.

Also contains Canadian & Mexican brand names.

CLINICIAN'S ENDODONTIC HANDBOOK
by Thom C. Dumsha, MS, DDS and James L. Gutmann, DDS, FACD, FICD

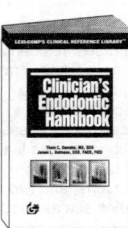

Designed for all general practice dentists.

- A quick reference addressing current endodontics
- Easy-to-use format and alphabetical index
- Latest techniques, procedures, and materials
- Root canal therapy: Why's and Why Nots
- Diagnosis and treatment of endodontic emergencies
- Facts/rationale of treating endodontically-involved teeth
- Straight-forward dental trauma management information
- Pulpal Histology, Access Openings, Bleaching, Resorption, Radiology, Restoration, and Periodontal / Endodontic Complications
- Frequently Asked Questions (FAQ) section and "Clinical Note" sections throughout.

DENTAL OFFICE MEDICAL EMERGENCIES
by Timothy F. Meiller, DDS, PhD; Richard L. Wynn, BSPharm, PhD; Ann Marie McMullin, MD; Cynthia Biron, RDH, EMT, MA; and Harold L. Crossley, DDS, PhD

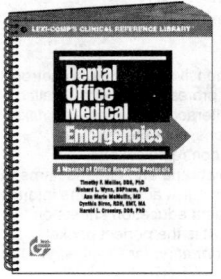

Designed specifically for general dentists during times of emergency. A tabbed paging system allows for quick access to specific crisis events. Created with urgency in mind, it is spiral bound and drilled with a hole for hanging purposes.

- Basic Action Plan for Stabilization
- Allergic / Drug Reactions
- Loss of Consciousness / Respiratory Distress / Chest Pain
- Altered Sensation / Changes in Affect
- Management of Acute Bleeding
- Office Preparedness / Procedures and Protocols
- Automated External Defibrillator (AED)
- Oxygen Delivery

To order call toll free anywhere in the U.S.: 1-800-837-LEXI (5394)
Outside of the U.S. call: 330-650-6506 or online at www.lexi.com

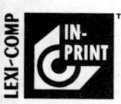

MANUAL OF CLINICAL PERIODONTICS
by Francis G. Serio, DMD, MS and Charles E. Hawley, DDS, PhD

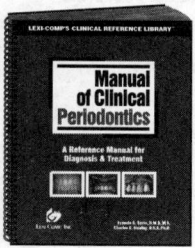

A reference manual for diagnosis and treatment including sample treatment plans. It is organized by basic principles and is visually-cued with over 220 high quality color photos. The presentation is in a "question & answer" format. There are 12 chapters tabbed for easy access: 1) Problem-based Periodontal Diagnosis; 2) Anatomy, Histology, and Physiology; 3) Etiology and Disease Classification; 4) Assessment, Diagnosis, and Treatment Planning; 5) Prevention and Maintenance; 6) Nonsurgical Treatment; 7) Surgical Treatment: Principles; 8) Repair, Resection, and Regeneration; 9) Periodontal Plastic Surgery; 10) Periodontal Emergencies; 11) Implant Considerations; 12) Appendix

ORAL SOFT TISSUE DISEASES
by J. Robert Newland, DDS, MS; Timothy F. Meiller, DDS, PhD; Richard L. Wynn, BSPharm, PhD; and Harold L.Crossley, DDS, PhD

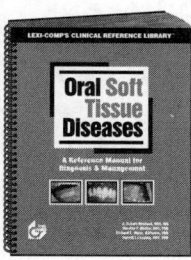

Designed for all dental professionals, a pictorial reference to assist in the diagnosis and management of oral soft tissue diseases, (over 160 photos).

Easy-to-use, sections include:

Diagnosis process: obtaining a history, examining the patient, establishing a differential diagnosis, selecting appropriate diagnostic tests, interpreting the results, etc.; White lesions; Red lesions; Blistering-sloughing lesions; Ulcerated lesions; Pigmented lesions; Papillary lesions; Soft tissue swelling (each lesion is illustrated with a color representative photograph); Specific medications to treat oral soft tissue diseases; Sample prescriptions; and Special topics.

ORAL HARD TISSUE DISEASES
by J. Robert Newland, DDS, MS

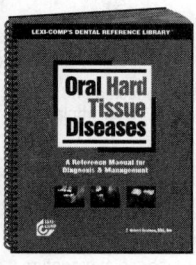

A reference manual for radiographic diagnosis, visually-cued with over 130 high quality radiographs and is designed to require little more than visual recognition to make an accurate diagnosis. Each lesion is illustrated by one or more photographs depicting the typical radiographic features and common variations. There are 12 chapters tabbed for easy access: 1) Periapical Radiolucent Lesions; 2) Pericoronal Radiolucent Lesions; 3) Inter-Radicular Radiolucent Lesions; 4) Periodontal Radiolucent Lesions; 5) Radiolucent Lesions Not Associated With Teeth; 6) Radiolucent Lesions With Irregular Margins; 7) Periapical Radiopaque Lesions; 8) Periocoronal Radiopaque Lesions; 9) Inter-Radicular Radiopaque Lesions; 10) Radiopaque Lesions Not Associated With Teeth; 11) Radiopaque Lesions With Irregular Margins; 12) Selected Readings / Alphabetical Index

To order call toll free anywhere in the U.S.: 1-800-837-LEXI (5394)
Outside of the U.S. call: 330-650-6506 or online at www.lexi.com

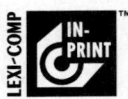
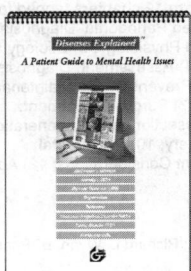
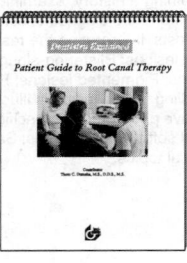
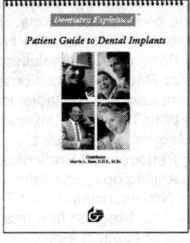

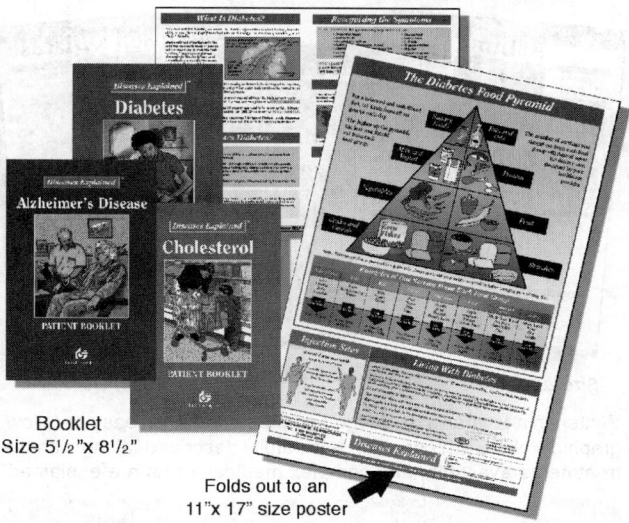

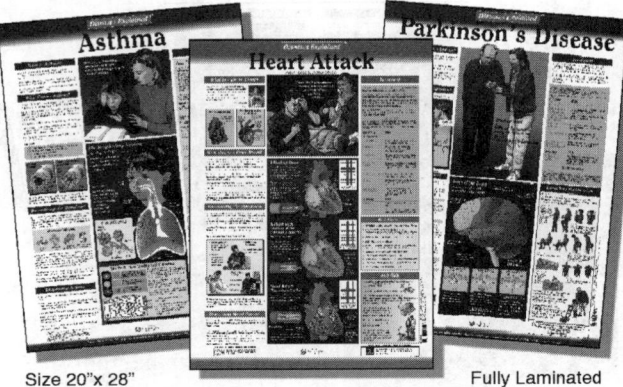

LEXI-COMP ON-HAND SOFTWARE LIBRARY
For Palm OS® and
Windows™ Powered Pocket PC Devices

 ™ Lexi-Comp's handheld software solutions provide quick, portable access to clinical information needed at the point-of-care. Whether you need laboratory test or diagnostic procedure information, to validate a dose, or to check multiple medications and natural products for drug interactions, Lexi-Comp has the information you need in the palm of your hand. Lexi-Comp also provides advanced linking technology to allow you to hyperlink to related information topics within a title or to the same topic in another title for more extensive information. No longer will you have to exit 5MCC to look up a dose in Lexi-Drugs or lab test information in Lexi-Diagnostic Medicine — seamlessly link between all databases to **save valuable time**.

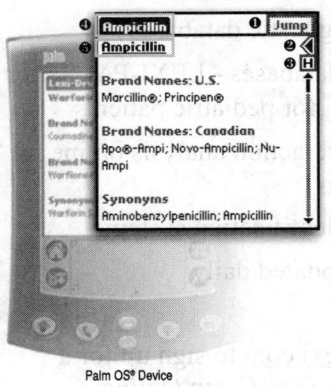

Palm OS® Device

New Navigational Tools:

❶ **"Jump"** provides a drop down list of available fields to easily navigate through information.

❷ **Back arrow** returns to the index from a monograph or to the "Installed Books" menu from the Index.

❸ **"H"** provides a linkable History to return to any of the last 12 Topics viewed during your session.

❹ **Title bar:** Tap the monograph or topic title bar to activate a menu to "Edit a Note" or return to the "Installed Books" menu.

❺ **Linking:** Link to another companion database by clicking the topic or monograph title link or within a database noted by various hyperlinked (colorized and underlined) text.

To order call toll free anywhere in the U.S.: 1-800-837-LEXI (5394
Outside of the U.S. call: 330-650-6506 or online at www.lexi.com